HOW TO FIND

THE BEST

NEW YORK METRO AREA

DOCTORS

HOW TO FIND
THE BEST
NEW YORK METRO AREA
DOCTORS

CASTLE CONNOLLY GUIDE

HOW TO FIND
THE BEST

NEW YORK METRO AREA

DOCTORS

For more information, please contact Castle Connolly Medical Ltd., 150 East 58th Street, New York, New York 10155, 212-980-8230. E-mail: CCMedical@aol.com. Web site: http://www.bestdocs.com

ISBN 1883769-08-6
ISBN 1883769-07-8 (pbk)

Printed in the United States of America

CASTLE CONNOLLY GUIDE

TABLE OF CONTENTS

SECTION TWO
Directory of Doctors

ABOUT THE PUBLISHERS

The mission of Castle Connolly Medical Ltd. is to help individuals and families find the best health care. The company was founded in 1992 by John K. Castle and John J. Connolly, Ed.D.

PUBLISHERS

John K. Castle is the Chairman of Castle Connolly Medical Ltd. He has spent much of the last two decades involved with health care institutions and issues. Mr. Castle served as Chairman of the Board of New York Medical College for eleven years, an institution where he has continued on the Board for more than twenty years.

Mr. Castle has been extensively involved in other health care and voluntary activities as well. He served for five years as a public commissioner on the Joint Commission on Accreditation of Healthcare Organizations (JCAHO), the body which accredits most public and private hospitals throughout the United States. Mr. Castle has also served as a trustee of five different hospitals in the metropolitan New York region and is a director emeritus of the United Hospital Fund as well as a trustee of the Whitehead Institute.

In addition to his health care activities, Mr. Castle has served on many voluntary boards including the Corporation of the Massachusetts Institute of Technology, as well as numerous corporate boards of directors, including the Equitable Life

ABOUT THE PUBLISHERS

Assurance Society of the United States. He is chairman of a leading merchant bank and has been chief executive of a major investment bank.

Mr. Castle holds a Bachelor of Science degree from MIT; an MBA with High Distinction from the Harvard Business School, where he was a Baker Scholar; and an honorary doctorate from New York Medical College.

John J. Connolly, Ed.D., is the President and CEO of Castle Connolly Medical Ltd. His experience in health care and education is extensive.

Dr. Connolly served as president of New York Medical College, the state's largest private medical college, for more than ten years. Dr. Connolly is a fellow of the New York Academy of Medicine, a member of the New York Academy of Sciences, a director of the New York Business Group on Health, a member of the President's Council of the United Hospital Fund, and a member of the Executive Committee of Funding First. Dr. Connolly has served as a trustee of two hospitals and as Chairman of the Board of one. He is extensively involved in health care and community activities, and serves on a number of voluntary and corporate boards, including the Board of the American Lyme Disease Foundation, of which he is a founder, the Friends of the National Library of Medicine, and the Board of Advisors of the Whitehead Institute. He has a Bachelor of Science degree from Worcester State College, a Master's degree from the University of Connecticut, and a Doctor of Education degree in College and University Administration from Teacher's College, Columbia University.

MEDICAL ADVISORY BOARD

We are pleased to have associated with Castle Connolly Medical Ltd. a distinguished group of medical leaders who offer invaluable advice and wisdom in our efforts to assist consumers in obtaining the best health care. While the Medical Advisory Board is not involved in the selection of doctors included in this edition of the Castle Connolly Guide, in addition to their valuable editorial comments many of them offered suggestions that helped us formulate appropriate selection criteria. We thank each member of the Medical Advisory Board for their valuable contributions.

CASTLE CONNOLLY MEDICAL ADVISORY BOARD

Charles Bechert, M.D.
Director
The Sight Foundation
Fort Lauderdale, FL

Roger Bulger, M.D.
President
Association of Academic Health Centers
Washington, DC

Harry J. Buncke, M.D.
Davies Medical Center
San Francisco, CA

Paul T. Calabresi, M.D.
Professor of Medicine and Medical Science
Chairman Emeritus
Department of Medicine
Brown University
Rhode Island Hospital
Providence, RI

Joseph Cimino, M.D.
Professor and Chairman
Community and Preventive Medicine
New York Medical College
Valhalla, NY

MEDICAL ADVISORY BOARD

FOREWORD

Dear Reader:

Choosing a doctor is one of the most important choices in your life. However, most of us put little effort into this selection. We simply pick a name from a list or get a recommendation from a friend.

Most of us have very little information about our doctors, and/or don't know where to get it. Now with the publication of the *Castle Connolly Guide—How To Find The Best Doctors*, you can learn about doctors' medical school education, residency training, fellowships, board certifications, hospital appointments and much more. The Guide also describes in simple terms what information about each doctor you should ascertain and how to evaluate it. This information gathering is essential for everyone who wants to find a good doctor to truly meet *his or her* health care needs.

FOREWORD

As an administrator and nurse who deals with the problems of health on a daily basis, I know well the importance of getting the best health care. Our center assists medical malpractice victims. The human tragedy we often encounter is heartbreaking.

In many cases, had the patient taken a few minutes to make a modest effort to learn more about their doctor's background, a serious incident may have been avoided.

That is why the *Castle Connolly Guide* is so important to consumers. In this new and rapidly changing health care environment, patients must be well informed. Many do not trust the health care system. They are not confident their HMO, their hospital, or even their doctor, is motivated to protect them and to ensure that they get excellent care.

The *Castle Connolly Guide* is a comprehensive guide chock full of valuable information. It is completely consumer-friendly, giving readers all they need to know to make intelligent, informed choices.

Use it well and in good health!

Sincerely,

Sandra Gainer RN
Associate Director
National Center for Patient Rights

INTRODUCTION

HOW THIS BOOK
CAN HELP
YOU IMPROVE
YOUR HEALTH

A savvy consumer, searching for a car, restaurant, house, or even a spouse, can easily find a guidebook to help. Yet, when it comes to choosing health care providers, the bookshelves are nearly bare.

How To Find The Best Doctors has been written to fill that void. It will guide you in making critical—even lifesaving—choices.

This book has two goals:

- *To provide you with a base of information and a framework of understanding so that you can participate in the important health care choices that will maximize your own health, your family's health, and the quality of your life.*

- *To provide detailed information on over 6,000 well-trained, highly competent physicians from which you may confidently choose your personal best doctors for your own health care needs and those of your family.*

INTRODUCTION

Medicine is often described as a combination of art and science. This description holds true for the process of selecting the best medical care. This book describes the "science" of making that selection. It is not magical or even difficult. It is simply a matter of knowing what information you should have and where to find it.

The "art" is what you will bring to the selection process. It is based upon your feelings, your needs, and the chemistry that develops between you and those who provide your health care. *How To Find The Best Doctors: New York Metro Area* will help you prepare for that interaction and guide you in getting the most from it.

Most important, *How To Find The Best Doctors: New York Metro Area* will tell you how to combine the art and science so that you can make the best choices.

HOW TO USE THIS BOOK

This book has been written as a basic, "how to" guide to selecting the best health care. The first section contains important information on how to choose the best doctors. Doctors are the most important providers of health care and whether you are part of an HMO or covered by traditional medical insurance, you want the very best doctor to attend to your health care needs. The second section contains the listings of doctors as well as information on the hospitals invited to participate in the Guide's Hospital Information Program. The third section includes information on Centers of Excellence – special programs and services – offered by a number of the hospitals participating in the Hospital Information Program. The fourth section offers 14 appendices presenting information that may be important and interesting.

There are two effective ways to use this book:

■ *Start at the beginning. This method will give you a broad understanding of the health care field and a clearer perspective of where you fit into it. This method will arm you with information necessary to make informed choices that will help you find the best doctors.*

■ *Study the doctor listings. While at least a brief reading of some or all of the introductory chapters is recommended so that, in the end, you will make well-informed choices, it is understandable that you may wish to go straight to the physician listings. The organization of these listings is outlined on pages 101 to 113. You will find guidelines for effectively using the listings on these pages.*

Each chapter begins with explanations of terms that may be new to you. Reviewing these terms will help you read the section easily.

In preparing this book, we've left little to chance or question. We hope to inspire you to assume that curious and insistent attitude as you make the health care choices that will take you and your family through life.

THE

DOCTOR

OF CHOICE

QUICK TIPS.

1. THE TIME TO ESTABLISH A RELATIONSHIP WITH A DOCTOR IS *WHILE YOU ARE HEALTHY*. THE BEST DOCTOR TO ESTABLISH YOUR RELATIONSHIP WITH IS THE ONE WHO IS MOST LIKELY TO KEEP YOU HEALTHY: A PRIMARY CARE DOCTOR.

2. PRIMARY MEANS FIRST, SO A PRIMARY CARE DOCTOR IS THE FIRST ONE YOU SEE FOR ANY HEALTH PROBLEM.

3. IT IS DIFFICULT FOR ANY DOCTOR, HOWEVER SKILLED, TO MAKE JUDGEMENTS BASED ON ONLY ONE VISIT OR A SINGLE TEST.

4. YOUR PRIMARY CARE DOCTOR CAN EDUCATE YOU ABOUT THE HOWS AND WHYS OF HEALTH MAINTENANCE AND DISEASE PREVENTION AND FOLLOW UP TO HELP YOU STAY FAITHFUL TO THE COURSE THE TWO OF YOU HAVE AGREED UPON.

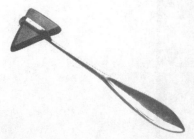

KEY TERMS
CHAPTER 1

LUPUS ERYTHEMATOSUS

An autoimmune disorder, also referred to as SLE, or simply lupus. It can cause inflammation and possible damage to a number of vital organs and is commonly marked by joint pain, facial and other rashes, abnormally high antibody levels, and diminished red blood cell levels.

LYME DISEASE

An infectious disease, transmitted through the bite of a deer tick, which may or may not produce a distinctive bull's-eye rash at the site of the tick bite. First identified in Lyme, Connecticut, the infection may also produce other symptoms, including flu-like aches, arthritic joint pain, and, in complicated cases, cardiac abnormalities.

MANAGED CARE

The process of integrating the finance and delivery of health care to control costs and improve quality. A managed care plan typically involves a group of practitioners who "manage" care for a specified population.

OSTEOPATH

A health care professional who has earned a degree in osteopathic medicine, a DO. Osteopathic Medicine emphasizes massage and bone manipulation while traditional western allopathic medicine emphasizes treatment with drugs and surgery.

PREVENTIVE MEDICINE/CARE

Health services that are aimed at maintaining good health and preventing illness. These services include routine physical examinations, immunizations, certain screening tests such as mammograms or Pap tests, as well as the practice of good health habits.

PRIMARY CARE PHYSICIAN

The first doctor consulted for any health problem, a Primary Care Physician is a specialist who offers basic, including preventive, medical care. It is important to maintain an ongoing relationship with your primary care physician.

SPECIALIST

A physician who practices one or more of the 25 specialties defined by the American Board of Medical Specialties (ABMS). The term is also used to denote a physician's area of practice, such as pediatrics, geriatrics, surgery, etc.

SUBSPECIALIST

A specialist who obtains further training and certification in one or more of the 70 subspecialties approved by the American Board of Medical Specialties.

QUICK TAKES

...Primary care physician. That's a hot term in health care today. Who is this physician? And how do you find one?...

CHAPTER 1

PRIMARY
CARE
PHYSICIANS

When it comes to choosing a doctor, too many people let the decision slide until they are sick or hurt and need medical attention fast. That's unfortunate if an illness that could have been managed successfully develops to a stage where it becomes difficult to control or cure. It's even more unfortunate if the illness could have been prevented in the first place.

The time to establish a relationship with a doctor is *while you are healthy,* and the best one to establish your relationship with is the one who is most likely to keep you healthy: a primary care doctor.

Primary means first, so a primary care doctor is the first one you see for any health problem. Primary also means basic, so a primary care doctor offers the kind of fundamental care that can keep you healthy.

YES, YOU DO NEED A DOCTOR WHEN YOU'RE HEALTHY.

Here are four good reasons why you should start your search for a primary care doctor now:

REASON ONE

A primary care doctor can put your medical condition in context. Context is important: this consists of your medical history, current condition as compared with past medical status, and changes in your body and environment over time. It is difficult for any doctor, however skilled, to make judgements based on only one visit or a single test. Conditions well out of normal range are easy to pick up, but extreme variations do not always occur, and a serious illness may develop slowly with only a gradual increase in symptoms. The operative word is continuity: ideally, your medical care should not be interrupted by changes in providers.

REASON TWO

A primary care doctor is better able to treat you as a whole person. Medicine has become very specialized and procedure-oriented, but the human body is not a loose collection of unrelated parts. It is a "whole," with strong interrelationships between all biological systems. Some of the poorest medical care results from people jumping from subspecialist to subspecialist. Despite talent, skill, and training, no specialist knows the patient well enough, or for long enough, to be able to take the whole person into consideration and track the normal patterns of evolution and change. We end up with a specialist for every organ and system instead of a doctor who will care for the whole person.

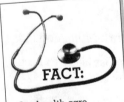

FACT:

Our health care system does not place enough emphasis on preventing illness; most health care dollars are spent on curative, rather than preventive, medicine.

REASON THREE

A primary care doctor can establish preventive programs. Our health care system does not place enough emphasis on preventing illness; most health care dollars are spent on curative, rather than preventive, medicine. But the status quo is slowly changing, and it is within primary care that the change is most evident. Your primary care doctor can educate you about the hows and whys of health maintenance and disease prevention and follow up to help you stay faithful to the course the two of you have agreed upon. Only an ongoing relationship makes this possible.

REASON FOUR

A primary care doctor can save you money. Managed care advocates, among others, have long deplored the waste inherent in a system in which patients can simply call any specialist any time they have an ache or pain or are not feeling well. Primary care doctors can monitor referrals to specialists, following the patient closely to put together a variety of observations, opinions, and test results in order to treat each person on an individual basis. This improves the quality of care and also controls costs.

A BUSINESSMAN IN HIS LATE FIFTIES, A LONG-TIME COMPETITIVE RUNNER, HAD SURGERY IN ONE OF NEW YORK'S TOP HOSPITALS TO REPAIR A BADLY TORN ACHILLES TENDON. AT HIS FIRST FOLLOW-UP VISIT TO THE ORTHOPEDIC SURGEON, HE WAS ASSURED THAT "EVERYTHING WAS HEALING PERFECTLY," THAT HE HAD NOTHING TO BE CONCERNED ABOUT, AND THAT HE WOULD SOON BE UP AND RUNNING AGAIN. SHORTLY

CHAPTER ONE

THEREAFTER, JUST BEFORE A SUMMER CAMPING TRIP, HE DECIDED TO HAVE HIS YEARLY PHYSICAL EXAMINATION. THE PRIMARY CARE DOCTOR EXAMINED THE SITE OF THE SURGERY, PROBING UP AND DOWN THE WHOLE LENGTH OF THE LEG. EXPLAINING THAT HE WAS CONCERNED ABOUT CERTAIN SWELLING AND DISCOLORATION, THE DOCTOR ARRANGED FOR A FURTHER EXAMINATION WITH ULTRASOUND IMAGING. THIS SOPHISTICATED TEST SHOWED THAT A BLOOD CLOT HAD FORMED IN THE UPPER PART OF THE LEG, WHICH COULD HAVE CAUSED SEVERE DISABILITY AND EVEN DEATH HAD IT GOTTEN INTO THE BLOODSTREAM AND TRAVELED TO THE HEART OR BRAIN. IT WAS THE PRIMARY CARE DOCTOR, CAREFULLY CONDUCTING A FULL PHYSICAL EXAM AND WHO KNEW THE PATIENT WELL, WHO DISCOVERED THE POTENTIALLY FATAL CONDITION.

Patients who visit specialists without some guidance from a primary care doctor may choose the wrong specialist based on a general observation and self-diagnosis about the problem or illness they're experiencing. While in some cases the problem may be obvious (for example, an eye injury), in others it may be more subtle. Diseases such as lupus erythematosus and Lyme disease, for example, often have myriad symptoms that are easily misinterpreted by laypersons; in fact, they are often difficult even for doctors to diagnose accurately. While certain problems may require the collaboration of several specialists, it is important to have a primary care doctor navigating the course.

Finally, it is estimated that almost half of all emergency room visits in some areas are for non-emergencies; it's the most expensive place to receive primary care. When people have primary care doctors, they tend to turn to them rather than to hospital emergency departments.

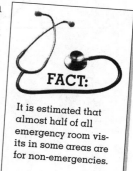

FACT:

It is estimated that almost half of all emergency room visits in some areas are for non-emergencies.

If you are enrolled in any kind of managed care program, health maintenance organization (HMO) or other, you will almost always be required to select a primary care doctor from its roster. Managed care executives recognize the necessity of a primary care doctor, not only for delivering quality health care, but also for controlling costs.

HOW TO FIND A DOCTOR

Unless you already have a primary care doctor you are satisfied with, you will have to find one. How? Here are five possible avenues to *begin* the process of finding the doctor that best suits your needs. Each has limits, however.

DOCTOR REFERRALS

If you are moving and are leaving a trusted doctor behind, get a recommendation or two before you go. Furthermore, ask in what context and how well your doctor knows the new doctor—they may not have met since medical school.

FRIENDS AND RELATIVES

Always keep in mind that such recommendations are based largely on what may be "simpatico," or a personal affinity. Ask why your friend likes the doctor. It might be because the fees are low or the doctor makes house calls or is warm and sociable—all valid considerations, but certainly not principal determinants. So be

QUICK TIPS.

5. ANY DOCTOR WITH A LICENSE CAN PRACTICE IN ANY SPECIALTY HE/SHE CHOOSES. BOARD CERTIFICATION IS YOUR ASSURANCE THAT THE DOCTOR HAS APPROPRIATE TRAINING FOR THE SPECIALTY.

6. WHEN CONSIDERING RECOMMENDATIONS, USE THE OLD NAVIGATIONAL TECHNIQUE OF TRIANGULATION: FOCUS ON DOCTORS WHOSE NAMES ARE MENTIONED BY THREE OR MORE PEOPLE.

7. HOSPITAL TELEPHONE REFERRAL LINES ARE NOT DESIGNED TO DISTINGUISH AMONG HUNDREDS OF DOCTORS WHO MAY BE MORE OR LESS WELL REGARDED BY OTHER DOCTORS, OR WHO MAY BE BETTER SUITED TO A PARTICULAR CALLER WHEN FACTORS OTHER THAN LOCATION, INSURANCE COVERAGE, AND OFFICE HOURS ARE TAKEN INTO CONSIDERATION.

8. MANY LOCAL MEDICAL SOCIETIES PUBLISH DIRECTORIES, SOME OF WHICH ARE INTENDED PRIMARILY FOR DOCTOR-TO-DOCTOR REFERRALS, WHILE OTHERS ARE DISTRIBUTED TO THE PUBLIC. THEY PROVIDE INFORMATION BUT DO NOT ADDRESS QUALITY.

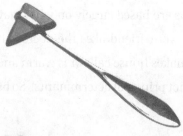

wary of the generalized recommendation that "Dr. Jones is just wonderful." When considering recommendations, use the old navigational technique of tri-angulation: focus on doctors whose names are mentioned by three or more people.

ONE WOMAN—A LONG-TIME CITY RESIDENT WHO MOVED TO THE SUBURBS TO BE NEAR HER CHILDREN—FOUND OUT THE HARD WAY ABOUT ADVICE WHEN SHE SELECTED A DOCTOR ON THE BASIS OF HER NEIGHBOR'S GLOWING PRAISE. DURING THE INITIAL VISIT, THE PATIENT'S NUMEROUS QUESTIONS ABOUT HER CHRONIC ARTHRITIS CONDITION WENT UNANSWERED WHILE THE DOCTOR MERELY PATTED HER ON THE SHOULDER AND ASSURED HER THAT HE WOULD "TAKE CARE OF EVERYTHING." WHILE THE PATERNALISTIC ATTITUDE MIGHT HAVE SUIT-ED THE NEIGHBOR'S NEEDS, IT FELL FAR SHORT FOR THIS SENIOR PATIENT, WHO WAS USED TO A GOOD GIVE-AND-TAKE WITH HER FORMER INTERNIST. SHE RESUMED HER SEARCH FOR A DOCTOR—THIS TIME WITH THE ADVICE OF HER FORMER DOCTOR, A MORE RELIABLE SOURCE THAN A FRIEND'S RECOMMENDATION.

HOSPITAL REFERRAL SERVICES

Hospital telephone referral lines are not designed to distinguish among hundreds of doctors who may be more or less well regarded by other doctors, or who may be better suited to a particular caller when factors other than location, insurance coverage, and office hours are taken into consideration. It would be impolitic for hospital referral services to rate their members. Their recommendations are based on specialty and geographic proximity, usually by way of a computer that rotates through the lists to "recommend" the next three names in line, and all members of the medical staff are eligible to participate.

MEDICAL SOCIETY DIRECTORIES

Many local medical societies publish directories, some of which are intended primarily for doctor-to-doctor referrals, while others are distributed to the public. These directories usually provide names, addresses, phone numbers, and specialties, and can be useful sources. However, they do not distinguish among doctors in any way. All members of the medical society, usually a countywide organization, are eligible for inclusion. This also applies to the referral lines offered by many medical societies.

ADVERTISING

Responding to advertising is the least effective way to find a doctor. While more and more health professionals now advertise, a practice which is no longer considered unethical, some stigma still remains. Advertising could lead you to a doctor who receives few or no referrals from colleagues and whose orientation to the profession is more entrepreneurial than medical. Most referral lines not sponsored by hospitals charge a fee to doctors who want to be listed. This is simply another form of advertising.

MANY WAYS TO SAY DOCTOR

In this book, the term "doctor" is used to describe only medical doctors who have received a doctor of medicine degree (MD) and osteopaths who have received a doctor of osteopathic medicine degree (DO). Doctors who have been trained in the British system may hold a degree of bachelor of medicine (MB), bachelor of surgery (BS), or bachelor of chirurgia (BCh), which is based on the ancient Greek term that refers to surgery.

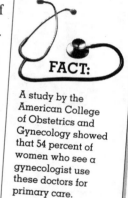

FACT:

A study by the American College of Obstetrics and Gynecology showed that 54 percent of women who see a gynecologist use these doctors for primary care.

The more formal term for any of these practitioners is "physician." However, most people use the more popular term "doctor," which is the one generally used in this book. Our discussions do not include other kinds of doctors such as dentists, podiatrists, psychologists, or chiropractors, who also deliver health care.

PRIMARY CARE: THE FUNDAMENTAL FOUR

There is not complete agreement in medicine on which specialties are practiced by the group of doctors known as primary care specialists. For the purposes of this book, we have included the following specialties: Internal Medicine; Pediatrics; Family Practice; and Obstetrics and Gynecology. Most adults choose general internists as their primary care doctors, and select pediatricians for their children. There is also a relatively new type of specialist, the family practitioner, who cares for both children and adults. In addition to such generalists, many women also select obstetrician/gynecologists as primary care providers.

- A GENERAL INTERNIST, specializing in internal medicine, is trained to treat all internal organs and systems of the body. Many internists are also board certified in a subspecialty, such as cardiology, gastroenterology, or geriatric medicine. Therefore, if you have a history of heart disease, you may wish to select an internist who has additional training in cardiology, but who primarily practices general internal medicine. On the other hand, your primary care doctor may refer you to a cardiologist when necessary, and both may treat you over a period of years. In fact, it is not unusual for a patient with a serious or complex illness to be followed by two or three doctors, with the primary care doctor "quarterbacking" the team.

- A FAMILY PRACTITIONER belongs to a relatively new specialty. Such doctors come closest to the general practitioner of the past. They are qualified to treat all family members, including children.

- A PEDIATRICIAN is the doctor you would choose for the care of your children. As with doctors in internal medicine, pediatricians often have a subspecialty such as cardiology, rheumatology, or endocrinology.

- OBSTETRICIANS and GYNECOLOGISTS are the subject of significant debate in terms of their appropriateness as primary care doctors. The American Board of Obstetrics and

Gynecology states that these doctors are specialists and are not generally trained for primary care. However, the reality is that many, particularly those who solely practice gynecology, often serve as a woman's primary care doctor. Gynecologists are divided on the issue. One recent study showed that 95 percent of visits to ob-gyns are self-referred and that about 60 percent of visits to these specialists are for diagnostic services and preventive services. Another study, by the American College of Obstetricians and Gynecologists, showed that 54 percent of women who see a gynecologist use these doctors for primary care. Reflecting the reality of current medical practice, we have included these specialists in the primary care category.

QUICK TIPS.

9. RESPONDING TO ADVERTISING IS THE LEAST EFFECTIVE WAY TO FIND A DOCTOR.

10. MANY WOMEN SELECT OBSTETRICIAN/GYNECOLOGISTS AS PRIMARY CARE PROVIDERS.

11. TO CHECK ON A DOCTOR'S (MD) BOARD CERTIFICATION CALL THE AMERICAN BOARD OF MEDICAL SPECIALTIES INFORMATION LINE ESTABLISHED FOR THAT PURPOSE (800) 776-2378.

12. SINCE MOST PEOPLE WILL OBTAIN ALL, OR CERTAINLY MOST, OF THEIR MEDICAL CARE NEAR WHERE THEY LIVE, IT IS IMPORTANT FOR YOU TO IDENTIFY WHICH DOCTORS ARE AMONG THE BEST IN YOUR OWN COMMUNITY.

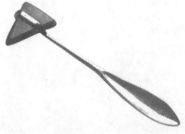

KEY TERMS
CHAPTER 2

ACADEMIC MEDICAL CENTER

A large medical complex that centers around a teaching hospital in which diversified residency programs are offered and where the medical school faculty practices full time with fellowship programs and major clinical research activities. Many hospitals call themselves medical centers to indicate a broader range of clinical services even if they do not have teaching programs.

BOARD CERTIFIED

Term signifying that a doctor is qualified for specialization by one of the American Board of Medical Specialties (ABMS) boards. Qualification includes completing an approved residency and passing a rigid exam.

BOARD ELIGIBLE

Term signifying that a doctor has completed an approved residency but has not yet taken the exam given by one of the ABMS recognized boards. The term conveys no official status in the eyes of the ABMS.

CLINICAL

Medical care that involves direct contact with patients.

CREDENTIALING

A process of screening conducted by hospitals by means of which they review the training and licenses of doctors applying to practice on their medical staffs.

INDEMNITY

A form of health insurance coverage that pays for health care but permits the patients to select their provider. Until 1990, indemnity insurance covered most insured people in the United States.

LICENSURE

Official credentials by individual states that permit a doctor to practice medicine in that state. In some states doctors may be licensed with no more than one year of post-graduate training.

RESIDENCY

A training period spent by a graduate of a medical school in a hospital before going into practice. Residents have earned a medical degree and, therefore, are doctors but must complete an approved residency and pass an exam to become board certified.

TERTIARY CARE

Medical services provided by a hospital or medical center that include complex treatments and procedures such as open heart surgery, organ transplants, and burn care.

QUICK TAKES

... You should consider four broad criteria in selecting a primary care doctor: professional preparation; professional reputation; office and practice arrangements; and professional or bedside manner...

CHAPTER 2

WHAT MAKES A DOCTOR "BEST"?

While the overwhelming majority of doctors are competent practitioners, some are less well trained or, for various other reasons, lack a desired level of professional skill or personal characteristics. They have met certain minimum standards, passed the necessary exams, and are licensed, but you would still be better off to avoid them. At the same time, among the many good doctors you could choose from, there will be some who are better for you and your family for a variety of reasons.

It is almost impossible to identify "the best" doctors in a particular specialty. There may be some who are generally acknowledged as leaders in a particular field, but that level of national reputation is typically built on appointments to important academic positions, innovative research, or the development of cutting-edge clinical techniques and treatments. Unless you are in need of those techniques and treatments, those doctors may not be the best for you. Since most people will obtain all, or certainly most, of their medical care near where they live, it is important for you to identify which doctors are among the best in your own community.

There are four basic criteria for selecting your own best doctor: Professional preparation; professional reputation; office and practice arrangements; and personal or bedside manner. The first three of these assessments can be made prior to your first visit, which is when you can make your fourth evaluation.

PROFESSIONAL PREPARATION

EDUCATION

Your review of your prospective doctor's education and training should begin with medical school. While you may feel that the institution where someone earned a bachelor's degree could be an indication of the quality of the doctor, most people in the medical field do not believe it plays a major role. A degree from a highly selective undergraduate college or university will help an aspiring doctor gain admission to a medical school, but once there, all students are peers. However, the information on undergraduate colleges, if important to you, is available in the American Board of Medical Specialties' (ABMS) *Compendium of Certified Medical Specialists* and other medical directories.

American medical schools are highly standardized, at least in terms of minimum quality. All US medical schools that grant medical degrees (MDs) and osteopathic degrees (DOs)

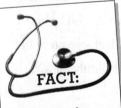

FACT:

All US medical schools that grant medical degrees (MDs) and osteopathic degrees (DOs) are accredited by a group known as the LCME (Liaison Committee for Medical Education).

are accredited by a group known as the LCME (Liaison Committee for Medical Education). Most are also accredited by the appropriate state agency, if one exists, and by regional accrediting agencies that accredit colleges and universities of all kinds.

Furthermore, US medical schools have universally high standards for admission, including success on the undergraduate level and on the Medical College Admissions Tests (MCATs). Although frequently criticized for being slow to change and for training too many specialists, the system of medical education in the United States has insured high quality in medical practice. One recent positive change is a strong effort in most medical schools to diversify the composition of the student body. While these schools have been less successful in enrolling racial minorities, the number of women in U.S. medical schools has increased to the point that they now make up about 40 percent of most classes. In certain specialties preferred by women medical graduates (pediatrics, for example), it is possible that in coming years the majority of specialists will be female.

FACT:

The number of women enrolled in medical school has increased to the point that they now make up about 40 percent of most classes.

Most doctors practicing in the United States are graduates of US medical schools. There are two other groups of doctors in practice who make up a relatively small proportion of the total doctor population. They are: (1) foreign nationals who graduated from foreign schools; and (2) US nationals who graduated from foreign schools. (Canadian medical schools are not considered foreign.)

FOREIGN MEDICAL GRADUATES

Foreign medical schools vary greatly in quality. Even some of the oldest and finest European schools have become virtually "open door," with huge numbers of unscreened students making teaching and learning difficult. Others are excellent and provided the model for our system of medical education.

The fact that someone graduated from a foreign school does not mean that he or she is a poor doctor. Foreign schools, like US schools, produce good doctors and poor doctors. Foreign medical graduates must pass the same exam taken by US graduates for licensure, but the failure rate for foreign graduates is significantly higher. In the first year of using the new United States Medical Licensing Exam (USMLE), 93 percent of US medical school graduates passed Step II, the clinical exam, as compared with 39 percent of the foreign graduates. It is clear that the quality of foreign schools, if not individual doctors, is not the same as US medical schools, at least as measured by our standards. Nonetheless, many communities and patients have been well served by foreign medical graduates practicing in this country—often in areas where it has been difficult to attract graduates of American schools.

RESIDENCY

Most doctors practicing today have at least three years of postgraduate (following the MD or DO) training in an approved residency program. This is not only an important step in the process of becoming a competent doctor, but it is also a requirement for board (specialty) certification. Most people assume that a prospective doctor needs to complete a three-year residency program to obtain a medical license. This is not true in some states. New York State, for example, requires only one postgraduate year. However, since all approved residencies last at least three years and some, such as those in neurosurgery, general surgery, orthopedic surgery, and urology, may extend for five or more years, it is important to know the details of a doctor's training. Licensure alone is not enough of a basis on which to make a good choice.

Without undertaking extensive and detailed research on every residency program, the best assessment you can make of a doctor's residency program is to see if it took place in a large medical center whose name you recognize. The more prestigious institutions tend to attract the best medical students, sometimes regardless of the quality of the individual residency program. If in doubt about a doctor's training, ask the doctor if the residency completed was in the specialty of the practice. If not, ask why.

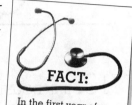

FACT:

In the first year of using the new United States Medical Licensing Exam (USMLE), 93 percent of US medical school graduates passed Step II, the clinical exam, as compared with 39 percent of the foreign graduates.

It is also important to be certain that a doctor completed a residency that has been approved by the appropriate governing board of the specialty, such as the American Board of Surgery, the American Board of Radiology, or the American Osteopathic Board of Pediatrics. These board groups are listed in Appendices A and B. If you are really concerned about a doctor's training, you should first call the hospital that offered the residency and ask if the residency was approved by the appropriate specialty group. If still in doubt, review the publication *Directory of Graduate Medical Education Programs,* often called the "green book," found in medical school or hospital libraries, which lists all approved residencies.

QUICK TIPS.

13. IF IN DOUBT ABOUT A DOCTOR'S TRAINING, ASK THE DOCTOR IF THE RESIDENCY COMPLETED WAS IN THE SPECIALTY OF THE PRACTICE. IF NOT, ASK WHY.

14. BOARD CERTIFICATION IS THE BEST WAY TO MEASURE COMPETENCE AND TRAINING.

15. THE EASIEST WAY YOU CAN ASSESS THE QUALITY OF A DOCTOR'S RESIDENCY PROGRAM IS TO SEE IF IT TOOK PLACE IN A LARGE MEDICAL CENTER WHOSE NAME YOU RECOGNIZE.

16. IF A DOCTOR DOES NOT HAVE ADMITTING PRIVILEGES OR IS NOT ON THE ATTENDING STAFF OF A HOSPITAL, YOU MAY WISH TO CONSIDER CHOOSING ANOTHER DOCTOR.

17. THERE ARE MANY EXCELLENT, WELL-TRAINED DOCTORS AT COMMUNITY HOSPITALS AND THEY SHOULD BE AS CAREFULLY EVALUATED AND CONSIDERED IN YOUR SEARCH AS A DOCTOR IN A LARGE INSTITUTION.

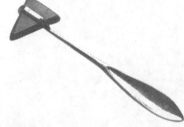

BOARD CERTIFICATION

With an MD or DO degree and a license, an individual may practice any kind of medicine—with or without additional special training. For example, doctors with a license but no special training may call themselves radiologists or pediatricians. This is why board certification is such an important factor. Twenty-five special-ties are recognized by the American Board of Medical Specialties (ABMS). Eighteen boards certify in 106 specialties under the aegis of the American Osteo-pathic Association (AOA). Doctors who have qualified for such specialization are called board certified; they have completed an approved residency and passed the board's exam. (See Appendix A for an approved ABMS list; see Appendix B for the AOA list; see Appendix C for a description of each specialty and subspecialty.) While many doctors who are not board certified do call themselves specialists, board certification is the best standard by which to measure competence and training.

You can be confident that doctors who are board certified have at a minimum the proper training in their specialty and have demonstrated their proficiency through supervision and testing. While there are many non-board certified doc-tors who are highly competent, it is more difficult to assess the level of their train-ing. Board certification alone does not guarantee competence, but it is a standard that reflects successful completion of an appropriate training program.

BOARD ELIGIBILITY

There are doctors without board certification who are highly competent, includ-ing many who have been more recently trained and are waiting to take the boards. They are sometimes described as "board eligible," a common term that is, however, frowned upon by the ABMS. Board eligible means that the doctor has completed an approved residency and is qualified to sit for the board exams, which may be given only infrequently. Most of the specialty boards permit unlimited attempts to pass the exam. Only the American Board of Internal Medicine (ABIM) continues to use and recognize the term board eligible. The other boards neither use the term, nor sanction its use. The description board eligible should not be viewed as a real qualification, especially if a doctor has been out of medical school long enough to have taken the certification exams. To the boards, a doctor is either board certified or not. In some cases, doctors who have failed the exams twice continue to call themselves board eligible. In osteopathic medicine, the board eligible status is recognized only for the first six years after completion of a residency.

In addition to the ABMS- and AOA-approved list of specialties and subspecialties, there is a wide variety of other doctors, and groups of doctors, who may call themselves specialists. There are, at present, at least 100 such groups called self-designated medical specialties. They range from doctors who are working to create a recognized body of knowledge and subspecialty training to less formal groups interested in a particular approach to the practice of medicine. These groups may or may not have standards for membership. There is no way of determining the true extent of their members' training, and they are not recognized by the ABMS or the AOA. While you should be cautious of doctors who claim they are specialists in these areas, many do have advanced training, and the groups at least offer a listing of people interested in a particular approach to medical care. Rely on board certification to assure yourself of basic competence, and use membership in one of these groups to indicate strong interest and possible additional training in a particular aspect of medicine. A list of these self-designated medical specialties may be found in Appendix D.

FELLOWSHIPS

The purpose of a fellowship is to provide advanced training in the clinical techniques and research of a particular subspecialty. In the US there are a variety of fellowship programs available to doctors, and they fall into two broad categories: approved and unapproved. Approved fellowships are those that are approved by the appropriate medical specialty board (e.g., the American Board of Radiology) and that lead to a subspecialty certificate. Fellowship programs that are not approved are often in the same areas of training as those that are, but they do not lead to a subspecialty certificate. Unfortunately, all too often, unapproved fellowships exist only to provide relatively inexpensive labor for the research and/or patient care activities of a clinical department in a medical school or hospital. In such cases, the learning that takes place is secondary and may be a good deal less than in an approved fellowship. On the other hand, any fellowship is better than none at all, and some unapproved fellowships have that status for a valid reason, which should not reflect negatively on the program. For example, the fellowship may have been recently created, with approval being sought. To check that a fellowship is an approved one, call the hospital where the training took place or the medical board for that specialty.

RECERTIFICATION

A relatively new focus of the specialty boards is the area of recertification. Until recently, board certification lasted for an unlimited time period. Now, almost all the boards have put time limits on the certification period. For example, in internal medicine, it is 10 years; in family practice, six, and under some circumstances, seven years; in anesthesiology there is no defined time period. In osteopathic medicine, most of the boards need to set a recertification period by 10 years. Many have done so already. These more stringent standards reflect an increasing emphasis, by both the

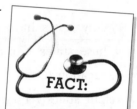

FACT:

Many states typically require a minimum number of continuing medical education (CME) credits for a doctor to maintain a medical license. Twenty-eight states require 150 CME credits over a three-year period. Osteopathic doctors are required to take 150 hours of CME credits within three years to maintain certification.

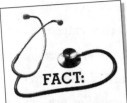

medical boards and state agencies responsible for licensing doctors, on recertification.

Since the policies of the boards vary widely, it is good procedure to ask a doctor if certification was awarded and when. If the date was seven to ten years ago, ask if he/she has been recertified. Unfortunately, many boards permit "grandfathering," whereby already certified doctors do not have to be recertified, and recertification demands apply only to newly certified doctors. Appendix A contains a list of the names and addresses of the boards and the certification period for each board specialty. Even if recertification is not required, it is good professional practice for doctors to undertake the process. It assures you, the patient, that they are attempting to stay current.

Many states have a continuing medical education requirement for doctors. These states typically require a minimum number of continuing medical education (CME) credits for a doctor to maintain a medical license. Twenty-eight states require 150 CME credits over a three-year period. Osteopathic doctors are required to take 150 hours of CME credits within three years to maintain certification.

PROFESSIONAL REPUTATION

There are doctors who meet every professional standard on paper, but who are simply not good doctors. In all probability the medical community has ascertained that and, while the individual may still practice medicine, his or her reputation will reflect that collective assessment. There are also doctors who are outstanding leaders in their fields because of research or professional activities, but who are not particularly strong or perhaps even active in patient care. It is important to distinguish that kind of professional reputation from a reputation as a competent, caring doctor in delivering patient care. In a consumer survey conducted by Towers Perrin, the management consulting firm, the chief criterion by which the respondents selected doctors was reputation. This was the most important factor for those enrolled in either managed care or indemnity plans.

HOSPITAL APPOINTMENT

Most doctors are on the medical staff of one or more hospitals and are known as attendings; some are not. If a doctor does not have admitting privileges or is not on the attending staff of a hospital, you may wish to consider choosing another doctor. It can be very difficult to ascertain whether the lack of hospital appointment is for a good reason or not. For example, it is understandable that some doctors who are raising families or heading toward retirement choose not to meet the demands (meetings, committees, etc.) of being an attending. However, if you need care in a hospital, the lack of such an appointment means that another doctor will have to oversee that care. In some specialties such as dermatology and psychiatry, doctors may conduct their entire practice in the office, and a hospital appointment is not as essential, or as good a criterion for assessment, as in other specialties.

While mistakes are made, most hospitals are quite careful about admissions to their medical staffs. The best hospitals are highly selective, so a degree of screening (or "credentialing") has been done for you. In other words, the best hospitals attract the best doctors. Since caring for a patient in the hospital is also often a team effort involving a number of specialists, the reputation of the hospital where the doctor admits patients carries special weight. Hospital medical staffs also review their colleagues to authorize them to perform specific procedures. In addition, they typically reappoint their medical staffs—and review them—every two or three years. In effect, this is an additional screening to protect patients. It is especially true of hospitals that have what are known as closed staffs, where it is impossible to obtain admitting privileges unless there is a vacancy that the administration and medical staff deem necessary to fill. Unfortunately, what a hospital appointment does not tell you is who on the medical staff is good, better, or best for you.

The reasons for a hospital's selectivity are easy to understand: no hospital, excellent or not, wishes to expose itself to liability, and every hospital wants to have the best reputation possible in order to attract patients. Obviously, the quality of the medical staff is immensely important in creating that reputation. Unfortunately, some hospitals are less diligent when a major group practice of doctors, all of whom have previously been affiliated with the institution, adds new members. In such cases, the hospital may almost automatically grant privileges without conducting the same intensive review given to individual doctors who are not members of a group practice. Also, some hospitals are less selective in granting privileges when beds are empty than when beds are full.

FACT:

Few hospitals permit doctors to practice in them unless they carry malpractice insurance. This not only protects the hospital, but the patient as well.

A last and very important reason why a hospital appointment is an essential requirement in your choice of a doctor is that many states permit doctors to practice *without* malpractice insurance. If you are injured as a result of the doctor's poor care, you could be without recourse. However, few hospitals permit doctors to practice in them unless they carry malpractice insurance. This not only protects the hospital, but the patient as well.

Many people believe that they should choose a doctor with an appointment at a major medical center as opposed to a community hospital. This assumption is incorrect on two counts. For one thing, there are many excellent, well-trained doctors at community hospitals and they should be as carefully evaluated and considered in your search as a doctor in a large institution. What's more, the term "medical center" has less significance today than it did years ago when the term was used to describe only the major university hospitals of medical schools. A true medical center is a teaching hospital which offers multiple residency programs and where the medical school faculty practices full-time with fellowship programs and major clinical research activities as an integral part of the teaching of medical students. These large centers are also involved in tertiary care, offering services such as organ transplants, burn care, and cardio-vascular surgery.

Today many community hospitals have added the term medical center to their name. They do this to indicate that they, too, offer advanced and sophisticated medical programs, as well as to compete with the academic medical centers for patients. With academic medical centers turning out many well-trained specialists and subspecialists who establish practices in nearby communities and then want to continue the highly specialized techniques they have learned, many community hospitals have initiated tertiary care programs of their own, further blurring the distinction between medical centers and hospitals.

In any case, most of our health care today is delivered *outside* of the hospital. Those who are hospitalized for acute illness (e.g., surgery, serious infection) will find that community hospitals and their staffs are well-suited to the task.

When extremely difficult and complex problems develop, or when tertiary care is needed, most communities have excellent academic medical centers. Of course, they offer primary care as well, especially to those who live nearby. This illustrates the point, once again, that medical care is a local issue.

QUICK TIPS.

18. DOCTORS WHO ARE FULL-TIME ACADEMICIANS MAY BE IN THE FOREFRONT OF NEW TECHNIQUES AND RESEARCH, BUT THEY ARE NOT NECESSARILY BETTER DOCTORS.

19. THE BEST CARE IS PROVIDED BY A COMBINATION OF PRIMARY CARE DOCTORS AND OTHER SPECIALISTS AND SUBSPECIALISTS.

20. DO NOT HESITATE TO ASK HOW FREQUENTLY YOUR DOCTOR HAS PERFORMED A PROCEDURE AND WITH WHAT DEGREE OF SUCCESS. PRACTICE MAY NOT LEAD TO PERFECTION, BUT IT IMPROVES SKILLS AND ENHANCES THE PROBABILITY OF SUCCESS.

21. CHECK THE DATE OF GRADUATION FROM MEDICAL SCHOOL OR COMPLETION OF RESIDENCY IF YOU WANT TO KNOW PRECISELY HOW LONG A DOCTOR HAS BEEN IN PRACTICE.

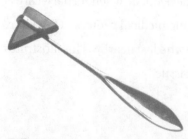

MEDICAL SCHOOL FACULTY APPOINTMENT

Many doctors have appointments on the faculties of medical schools. There is a range of categories from "straight" appointments—meaning full-time appointment as professor, associate professor, assistant professor, or instructor—to clinical ranks that may reflect lesser degrees of involvement in teaching or research. If someone carries what is known as a straight academic rank (i.e., professor of surgery, without clinical in the title), this usually means that the individual is engaged full-time in medical school research and/or teaching activities. The title professor of clinical surgery usually describes a doctor who has a full-time appointment in a medical school, but who puts a greater emphasis on clinical practice (patient care) than on research or teaching. The title clinical professor of surgery usually specifies a part-time or adjunct appointment and less direct involvement in medical school activities.

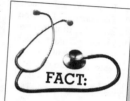

FACT:

The newest approaches and techniques in medicine, for the most part, are explored and developed by medical school faculties in their laboratories and clinical practice settings.

Doctors who are full-time academicians may be in the forefront of new techniques and research, but they are not necessarily better doctors. Nonetheless, you would be assured that they have the support of other faculty, residents, and medical students.

When you are seeking a subspecialist, a doctor's relationship to a medical school becomes more meaningful since medical school faculties tend to be made up of subspecialists. You are less likely to find large numbers of general or primary care practitioners engaged full-time on a medical school faculty. The newest approaches and techniques in medicine, for the most part, are explored and developed by medical school faculties in their laboratories and clinical practice settings. This is where they practice their subspecialties, as well as teach and perform research. Such leading specialists are not necessarily better doctors than com-

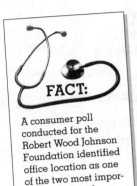

munity doctors—they are trained to provide a *different* kind of medical care. The best care is provided by a combination of primary care doctors and other specialists and subspecialists.

MEDICAL SOCIETY MEMBERSHIP

Most medical society memberships sound very prestigious and some are; however, there are many societies that are not selective and which virtually any doctor can join. In addition, membership in many of the more prestigious societies is based on research and publication, or on leadership in the field, and may have little to do with direct patient care. While it is clearly an honor to be invited to join these groups, membership may be less than helpful in discerning whether a doctor can meet your needs.

Board certified doctors are referred to as Diplomates of the Board. Some of the colleges of medical specialties (e.g., the American College of Radiology; the American College of Surgeons) have multiple levels of recognition. The first is basic membership and the second, more prestigious and difficult to obtain, is status as a Fellow. Fellowship status in the colleges is meaningful and is based on experience, professional achievement, and recognition by one's peers, including extensive experience in patient care. It should be viewed as a significant professional qualification.

EXPERIENCE

Experience is difficult to assess. Obviously, in most cases, an older doctor has more experience; on the other hand, a younger doctor has been more recently immersed in residency, the challenge of medical school, or even a fellowship, and may be the most up-to-date. If a doctor is board-certified, you may assume that assures at least a minimal amount of experience, but it could be as little as a year.

So check the date of graduation from medical school or completion of residency if you want to know precisely how long a doctor has been in practice.

The one type of experience you should specifically want to know about is that dealing with any special procedure, particularly a surgical one, that has recently been developed and introduced into practice. For example, many doctors using a new surgical technique for removing gallbladders—laparoscopic cholecystectomy—experienced a high percentage of problems because they were not properly trained. This prompted new standards to be issued by the American College of Surgeons to make sure doctors using this new approach would be adequately trained. Do not hesitate to ask how frequently your doctor has performed a procedure and with what degree of success. Practice may not lead to perfection, but it improves skills and enhances the probability of success.

OFFICE AND PRACTICE ARRANGEMENTS

Although clearly not as important as training or reputation, office and practice arrangements are usually of great significance to patients. Practice arrangements include office hours, office location, billing procedures, and office testing among the many factors that result in how well the office is run.

Many years ago most doctors practiced independently in private offices. They were called solo practitioners and usually had agreements with other doctors to respond to their patients' calls when they were unavailable. In recent decades, most doctors have entered group practices; indeed, this is becoming the most common way for young doctors to begin to practice. Two or more doctors in the same specialty, or in different specialties (a multi-specialty group), share offices and staff to lower their costs of operations. They also cover for each other on rotation for weekends, evenings, and vacations. As a patient you may prefer one of

QUICK TIPS.

22. IF YOU DON'T THINK YOU WILL BE SATISFIED HAVING YOUR OFFICE VISIT AND EXAMINATION CONDUCTED BY ANYONE BUT THE DOCTOR, YOU SHOULD DETERMINE UP FRONT HOW MANY MIDLEVEL PROVIDERS ARE ON STAFF AND HOW EXTENSIVE THEIR RESPONSIBILITIES ARE.

23. THE SITE OF THE OFFICE CAN BE VERY IMPORTANT IN CHOOSING A DOCTOR YOU MAY VISIT ON A REGULAR BASIS. IF THE LOCATION IS INCONVENIENT, YOU MAY BE DISCOURAGED FROM MAKING NEEDED VISITS.

24. YOU SHOULD DISCUSS ANY CHRONIC PROBLEMS WHEN FIRST ESTABLISHING A RELATIONSHIP WITH A DOCTOR. IN FACT, YOU MAY WANT TO FIND A DOCTOR WITH SPECIAL INTEREST OR TRAINING IN THAT PROBLEM.

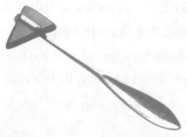

the following: a solo practitioner who is covered occasionally; a group where you usually, but not always, see the same doctor; or a multi-specialty group where, if a consultation or referral is necessary, the specialist is at the same location. The choice is really one of personal preference.

There are other factors relating to practice arrangements that may or may not be important to an individual choosing a doctor. One is the location of the office. A consumer poll conducted for the Robert Wood Johnson Foundation identified office location as one of the two most important factors in the selection of a doctor. (The other was a recommendation by a relative or friend.) Actually, the site of the office can be very important in choosing a doctor you may visit on a regular basis. If the location is inconvenient, you may be discouraged from making needed visits.

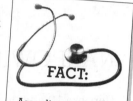

FACT:

According to an article in the professional journal *Family Practice Management*, these "midlevel providers," as they are called, "can handle 80 to 90 percent of the problems that occasion office visits."

Another important factor concerns the use of nurse practitioners and physician's assistants in the office. Licensed nurse practitioners are advanced practice nurses in primary care. They have additional training beyond the basic requirements for nursing licensure, usually a master's degree or special certificate. They perform a broad range of nursing functions as well as functions that, historically, have been performed by doctors, including assessing and diagnosing, conducting physical examinations, ordering diagnostic tests, implementing treatment plans and monitoring patient status. Physician's assistants are licensed to provide medical care in many states. Unlike nurses, they may practice only under a doctor's direction and supervision. According to an article in the professional journal *Family Practice Management*, these "midlevel providers," as they are called, "can handle 80 to 90 percent of the problems that occasion office visits." These providers have become more of a presence in health care in recent years, especially in medical groups and HMOs. If you don't think you will be satisfied having your office visit and examination conducted by anyone but the doctor, you should determine up front how many midlevel providers are on staff and how extensive their responsibilities are.

NARROWING THE CHOICE

Here are 10 additional questions that will guide you in assessing the practice patterns or arrangements of a doctor to see if they meet your needs. If there are other items not listed that are important to you, add them to the list before you make your initial appointment. You should try to obtain as much of the information as possible from the staff.

- *Are you currently accepting new patients and, if so, is a referral required?*

- *On average, how long does a patient have to wait for an appointment?*

- *Are you open on weekends? In the evening?*

- *If lab work and X-rays are performed in the office what are the qualifications of the people doing the test?*

- *Is full payment (or deductibles, co-payments) required at the time of the appointment?*

- *Do you accept my insurance plan? Medicare? Medicaid? Worker's Compensation? No-fault insurance?*

- *Do you accept credit cards and, if so, which do you accept?*

- *Do you accept patient phone calls?*

- *Will you care for a patient in the home?*

- *Is your office handicapped-accessible?*

If you have a chronic illness or disease, there may be certain additional aspects of a doctor's practice that could be particularly important to you. You should discuss any chronic problems when first establishing a relationship with a doctor. In fact, you may want to find a doctor with special interest or training in that problem.

FACT:

A recent *American Medical News* article suggested that 43 percent of internal medicine specialists and 65 percent of family practice specialists made one or more house calls a year.

House calls also continue to be important to some people. Yes, some doctors still do make house calls! In fact, a recent *American Medical News* article suggested that 43 percent of internal medicine specialists and 65 percent of family practice specialists made one or more house calls a year. However, it is important to point out that house calls have declined not because doctors are lazy or arrogant, but because of technology, liability risks, and time pressures. Important diagnostic equipment often cannot be carried around in a doctor's little black bag and is only available in the office or hospital. Also, the time required to visit one patient at home markedly reduces the time available to see other patients.

PERSONAL OR BEDSIDE MANNER

To many patients, once they have determined that a doctor is competent, the doctor's professional manner—also known as bedside manner—is the most important part of their choice. The Towers Perrin report cited earlier indicated that after reputation, communications skill was the most important factor sought in doctors. Patients want sensitive and caring doctors who listen carefully and demonstrate their concern. Studies show that these doctors are sued less often than others!

What characteristics make up a doctor's personal manner? The four described below may, when considered together, give you a clear idea of whether a particular doctor will be your personal "best."

■ **Listening.** Professional manner includes the doctor's willingness to listen to patients, be supportive and understanding, explain procedures, and exhibit concern and respect. These skills are expressed at the bedside, in the office, or in any setting where there is doctor/patient contact. Listening is also a valuable diagnostic tool. Unfortunately, these skills often have not been taught well in medical schools, and the lack of them forms the primary basis for complaints from patients. However, there is a growing emphasis on these vital interpersonal and communications skills in medical schools today, and with good reason. They are critically important to most patients.

■ **Cultural sensitivity.** Some patients may prefer doctors who speak their language or are familiar with their cultural background. The term "culturally competent physician" is a relatively new one describing doctors who have the skills and attitudes to deal with minority cultures.

■ **Ethical, religious, and philosophical views.** Religion, or at least views on issues such as abortion, utilization of life-sustaining measures, natural childbirth, breast-feeding, and other matters can also be important. It is perfectly appropriate to ask doctors questions about sensitive issues.

- ■ **Decision-making procedures.** Years ago patients took the words of the doctor as law, not to be questioned, or perhaps even discussed. That is not the case today. Consumers are better informed about health issues and may want to be actively involved in the decision-making affecting their health. Some patients do not feel this way and are comfortable accepting a doctor's diagnosis or course of treatment without question. Some doctors—in diminishing numbers, thankfully—feel uncomfortable with patients who want everything explained to them or want to be involved in decision-making. Consider how you feel about this issue and discuss it with your doctor to be certain you are on compatible wavelengths.

QUICK TIPS.

25. ALWAYS OBTAIN COPIES OF ALL MEDICAL RECORDS AND TESTS FOR YOUR FILES.

26. WHEN SELECTING A DOCTOR, ESPECIALLY A PRIMARY CARE DOCTOR, IT IS APPROPRIATE TO REQUEST AN EXPLORATORY INTERVIEW.

27. GOOD DOCTORS LISTEN, GOOD PATIENTS TALK.

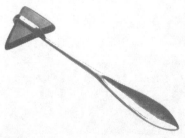

KEY TERMS
CHAPTER 3

AMERICAN MEDICAL ASSOCIATION

A partnership of physicians and their professional associations dedicated to promoting the art and science of medicine and the betterment of public health through establishing and promoting ethical, educational, and clinical standards for the medical profession. It represents the interests of physicians on the national level.

BASELINE TESTS

A series of basic, routine medical tests—such as electrocardiogram, complete blood count, blood pressure measurement, weight measurement, and chest X-ray—that are usually completed by a physician upon a patient s initial visit in order to provide a standard for comparison during subsequent health examinations.

GENERIC DRUGS

Prescription medications that have been marketed by one company under a proprietary or brand name and which may be sold, after the original exclusive 17-year patent expires, under a generic name or the name assigned to it during early stage of development. Most generic drugs are less expensive than proprietary versions and are just as effective except in cases when, because of different manufacturing processes, they are not bioequivalent or handled by the body in an identical manner.

THIRD PARTY PAYER

An organization such as indemnity insurance company or managed care organization that provides individual and group health insurance, or a governmental department which assumes responsibility for the payment of an individual's health care, either directly to the health care provider or by means of reimbursement to the individual (medicare and medicaid are such government programs).

QUICK TAKES

... The best doctor-patient relationship is based on a two-way dialogue. Be open and honest and seek a doctor who is the same...

CHAPTER 3

YOU AND YOUR DOCTOR: A TEAM

Trust and respect between doctors and patients have reached a low point in modern American society. A recent poll of consumers sponsored by the American Medical Association (AMA) concluded that approximately 70 percent of those who responded agreed with the statement that "people are beginning to lose faith in their doctors." (Despite concerns about doctors in general, much research has shown patients tend to rate their own doctors well.)

Trust between doctors and patients has declined for many reasons, including unrealistic expectations on the part of some patients and the patronizing attitudes of some doctors, which clash with the higher education level and medical sophistication of many patients. This has been further complicated by changing financial arrangements, particularly those involving the government and third-party payers, and the perception that some doctors seem to be motivated not by

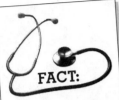

the values of the Hippocratic Oath (See Appendix E), but by those of the marketplace. The AMA poll cited earlier found that 69 percent of the respondents agreed that doctors "are too interested in making money." Perhaps a significant factor in creating this atmosphere is that in many cases the relationship between doctor and patient now has another dimension, the managed care organization. Another significant contributor is the huge amount of paperwork required from doctors. Generated by quality-assurance efforts, regulation, complex billing, and managed care procedures, this burden reduces the time doctors are able to spend with patients.

Given the formidable obstacles, it might seem impossible to find a primary care doctor who is well suited to your needs. If you have carefully read the preceding chapters, your work is half done. What remains is to find that special individual who fits the criteria.

THE INITIAL INTERVIEW

When selecting a doctor, especially a primary care doctor, it is appropriate to request an exploratory interview. Frequently, doctors will engage in such brief interviews at no charge or at a lower-than-standard fee. Others prefer to handle them by telephone. It is preferable to find out about a doctor's credentials, office hours, and billing procedures from the staff beforehand so you don't waste time asking about basic facts. This leaves time to ask the doctor questions that will allow you to determine what kind of relationship could develop.

ASK THE RIGHT QUESTIONS

The most important aspect of this session is to see if you can develop a positive doctor/patient relationship. Are you comfortable with the doctor's manner, style, and general personality? Do you feel a strong sense of trust in the doctor? Here are five questions to ask the doctor plus two questions to ask yourself that may lead you closer to a selection.

- *What is your experience in treating _____ (if you are seeking care for a particular illness or condition)?*

- *Are you open to treatments and therapies that do not rely heavily on medication?*

- *What preventive programs do you suggest for someone of my age, sex, and health status?*

- *How do you feel about involving patients in decision-making?*

- *What are your views on_____(ethical and moral issues of importance to you as a patient)?*

Even when the doctor is responding to your questions, you should ask yourself:

- *Is the doctor paying attention to me and really considering my questions or do the impersonal, "stock" answers indicate that the doctor's thoughts are elsewhere?*

- *Does this doctor speak about good health and prevention with the personal knowledge of someone who seems to practice it?*

If your prospective doctor seems to measure up to your standards, get the relationship off to a good start by making an appointment for a complete check-up. During this appointment, you will have an opportunity to share your medical and family history, and baseline tests will be performed to serve as a standard in the years ahead.

ONE WOMAN, IMBUED WITH HER NEW "TAKE CHARGE" ROLE IN HER HEALTH CARE, CARRIED THE INTERVIEWING PROCESS TO THE LIMIT WHEN SHE VISITED MORE THAN 20 DOCTORS FOR EXPLORATORY INTERVIEWS IN THE COURSE OF A SINGLE YEAR. EACH TIME THERE WAS SOME LITTLE PROBLEM: THE DOCTOR WAS BEHIND SCHEDULE, THE DOCTOR WAS VERY BRUSQUE, THE DOCTOR DISCUSSED EVERYTHING IN COMPLICATED MEDICAL LANGUAGE, EVEN ONE INSTANCE WHEN SHE CONCLUDED THAT THE DOCTOR WAS JUST TOO YOUNG. NOT ONLY WAS SHE IMPOSING ON THE PROFESSIONALISM OF THE DOCTORS WHO CONDUCTED THE INTERVIEWS WITH HER, BUT SHE WAS ACTUALLY NEGLECTING HER HEALTH CARE; DURING THAT YEAR, SHE NEVER HAD A SINGLE MEDICAL EXAMINATION. IF A SERIOUS HEALTH PROBLEM HAD BEEN IN THE DEVELOPING STAGES, A YEAR WOULD HAVE BEEN TOO LONG TO GO WITHOUT MEDICAL TREATMENT.

TALKING WITH YOUR DOCTOR

After you have selected your doctor, your first appointment should include an extensive medical history. Your doctor should spend time with you, ask questions, and listen to your responses carefully.

Medical students are often told, "Listen to your patients. They'll tell you what's wrong with them." This conveys an important lesson not only for doctors, but for patients: *Good doctors listen, good patients talk.*

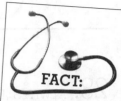

Analysis of doctor/patient conversations has revealed that many patients wait until the end of a conversation, even until they are saying goodbye, to tell their doctors what is really bothering them. This is just a small example of the dynamics of doctor/patient relationships. It is also a good example of a waste of valuable time—the doctor's and the patient's. One reason doctors need to be trained to be good listeners is that they frequently must ascertain what is troubling the patient not by what is said directly, but by what is said indirectly, not at all, or through body language and other signs. However, it is always easier, less time-consuming, and certainly more effective if a patient can describe problems completely and accurately.

FACT:

Analysis of doctor/patient conversations has revealed that many patients wait until the end of a conversation, even until they are saying goodbye, to tell their doctors what is really bothering them.

Before you even see a doctor, you should prepare thoroughly. You should have a complete record of your medical history, including a record of X-rays and any other diagnostic tests, as well as blood workups. You need information about childhood diseases, chronic conditions, hospitalizations, past and present medications, doses, and drug reactions, if any, and, if possible, something about the health history of your parents and even their siblings. Except for the last item, these are available to patients from their previous doctors or hospitals. That is why it is useful to obtain copies of all medical records and tests for your own files. Not only will this save you time and effort, but it may avoid additional testing and expense. Your doctor will also ask many seemingly personal questions about your work, education, sex life, and even drug and alcohol use. These are all part of a complete medical history and will help your doctor understand you better.

If you have a particular problem or concern, describe all your symptoms. Try not to minimize or exaggerate and, most of all, don't deny.

49

QUICK TIPS.

28. ALWAYS BRING A PAD AND PENCIL WITH YOU TO MEDICAL APPOINTMENTS. WHEN THE DOCTOR GIVES YOU INSTRUCTIONS, TAKE NOTES.

29. *THE PHYSICIAN'S DESK REFERENCE*, COMMONLY KNOWN AS THE PDR, IS AVAILABLE IN MOST LIBRARIES AND IS AN EXCELLENT RESOURCE FOR LEARNING MORE ABOUT MEDICATIONS. (THE PDR WEB PAGE IS AT http://www.medec.com)

30. DO NOT HESITATE TO ASK YOUR PHARMACIST ABOUT SIDE EFFECTS, GENERIC SUBSTITUTIONS, AND OTHER QUESTIONS RELATED TO YOUR MEDICATIONS.

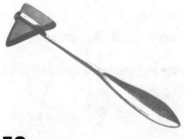

AN EXECUTIVE OF A LARGE COMPUTER SOFT-WARE FIRM ASSURED HIS DOCTOR THAT HE WAS "FEELING FIT," CHOOSING NOT TO MENTION THE SOMETIMES SEVERE PAIN IN HIS SCROTUM. SIX MONTHS LATER THE PAIN HAD WORSENED TO THE DEGREE THAT IT DEMANDED ATTENTION. UNFORTUNATELY, THE DIAGNOSIS WAS AD-VANCED TESTICULAR CANCER.

If you have questions to ask your doctor, make a list. Always bring a pad and pencil with you to medical appointments. When the doctor gives you instructions, take notes or ask the doctor to write them down for you. If a prescription is written, ask about doses, side effects, efficacy, and alternative medications, as well as generic substitutes. The *Physician's Desk Reference*, commonly known as the PDR, is available in most libraries and is an excellent resource for learning more about medications. There is also a PDR Web page on the Internet at http://www.medec.com. You can also get a great deal of information on medications from another health profession-al, your pharmacist. Do not hesitate to ask your pharmacist about side effects, generic substitutions, and other questions related to your medications. However, if the information you receive conflicts with that given by your doctor, consult with the doctor and follow his or her directions.

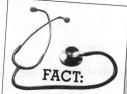

FACT:

Research has shown the average wait in a doctor's office is 20 minutes. However, the doctor who spends extra time with another patient probably is the doctor you want for yourself.

A MATTER OF TIME

Patients want and expect doctors who listen, express concern, explain conditions and procedures in a clear and understandable manner, discuss medications and their effects and side effects thoroughly, return calls, are available when needed and, perhaps most important, spend sufficient time with them. With increasing demands on their time, many doctors are left with an uneasy feeling of "running to stay in place." The end result may be a tendency, unintended for the most part, to rush through a patient visit. This situation contributes to the erosion of the doctor-patient relationship.

Also contributing to this problem is pervasive lateness on the part of doctors. Patients frequently complain that they spend hours in a doctor's waiting room, long past the appointed hour (research has shown the average wait is 20 minutes). Unfortunately, the duration of a patient visit is not always predictable. Unexpected delays may occur if the diagnosis is complicated or if a patient needs to discuss what is on his or her mind. The doctor who spends extra time with another patient is probably the doctor you want for yourself. If the lateness is excessive, persistent, and without apparent good reason, discuss it with your doctor and, if it is interfering with your relationship, consider changing doctors.

AFTER A DELAY OF TWO HOURS IN HIS DOCTOR'S OFFICE, ONE PATIENT, A SELF-EMPLOYED MARKETING CONSULTANT, MADE SURE THAT IT WOULD NEVER HAPPEN AGAIN. DID HE HAVE A SHOWDOWN WITH THE DOCTOR? DID HE DECIDE NEVER TO RETURN? NOT AT ALL. HE SIMPLY

MADE IT A POINT TO CALL THE DOCTOR'S OFFICE TWO HOURS BEFORE HIS SCHEDULED APPOINTMENT TO SEE HOW THE SCHEDULE WAS RUNNING. HE THEN ADJUSTED HIS OWN SCHEDULE TO COINCIDE WITH THE DOCTOR'S.

QUICK TIPS.

31. THE MORE COMPLEX AND DIFFICULT THE PROBLEM, THE MORE IMPORTANT REPUTATION IS. IN FACT, YOU MIGHT WELL NARROW YOUR FOCUS TO DOCTORS ON THE STAFFS OF CERTAIN MEDICAL CENTERS NOTED FOR EXCELLENCE WITH SPECIFIC PROBLEMS.

32. DOCTORS TYPICALLY REFER PATIENTS TO DOCTORS ON THE STAFFS OF THE SAME HOSPITALS WHERE THEY PRACTICE.

33. IN MANY CASES, INSURANCE COMPANIES WILL PAY FOR SECOND OPINIONS, BUT CHECK AHEAD OF TIME TO MAKE SURE YOUR INSURANCE PLAN DOES COVER THEM.

34. IF YOU ARE NOT COMFORTABLE WITH YOUR PRIMARY CARE DOCTOR'S REFERRAL, ASK FOR A NUMBER OF OPTIONS. IF NECESSARY, YOU MAY CONSIDER GOING "OUT OF NETWORK" EVEN IF YOU HAVE TO PAY SOME OR ALL OF THE FEE.

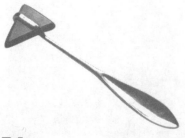

KEY TERMS CHAPTER 4

ALTERNATIVE THERAPY

Non-traditional forms of health care—including acupuncture, homeopathy, naturopathy, massage, reflexology, biofeedback, hypnotherapy, herbology, therapeutic touch, and prayer—that are often based on ancient healing methods and have not been tested in a conventional scientific manner.

CLINICAL TRIAL

An experimental trial of a new drug or therapy in a selected group of human volunteers who suffer from the condition for which the experimental drug or treatment is to be used.

DOUBLE BLIND STUDY

One form of a clinical trial in which two groups of volunteers—one group receiving the real drug or treatment and the other receiving a placebo or dummy—are followed for a specific period of time by researchers who do not know themselves who is receiving which therapy.

PROTOCOL

A rigid set of rules set up for a clinical trial by the Food and Drug Administration (FDA) which must be followed strictly by all researchers and volunteers participating in the trial.

QUICK TAKES

...The old adage, two heads are better than one often applies in health care, too. Expanded options include referrals, second opinions, alternative therapies, and clinical trials...

CHAPTER 4

STRENGTHENING
YOUR TEAM

WHEN YOU NEED A SPECIALIST

For the most part, selecting a specialist is similar to choosing a primary care doctor. There is one major difference, however; typically you will be referred to a specialist by your primary care doctor. Suggesting a consultation does not show a weakness on the part of the doctor. On the contrary, the real weakness lies in a reluctance to suggest consultations when advisable. Your primary care doctor will receive a written report from any consultation or referral. You should get a copy as well.

Ask your doctor why this particular specialist is being recommended. Find out about the specialist's training and experience. If your doctor has sent many patients to the same doctor for the same treatment, you should find out how successful the treatment was and if the patients were satisfied. You might also ask if the specialist would be the one selected for your doctor's personal care. You should feel comfortable about seeing the specialist and, if you are not, ask for another recommendation or you may want to find a different one on your own.

Frequently, patients do seek out specialists on their own. If you are attempting to find a specialist or subspecialist without the guidance of your primary care doctor, use the various kinds of selection procedures described in Chapters one, two and three. However, even greater emphasis should be placed on board certification in the relevant specialty. If you are trying to find someone to care for a very specific problem, make certain that the individual is well trained in that area. You may check to see if a doctor is board certified by calling the American Board of Medical Specialties at (800) 776-2378.

You will also want to know if the specialist you select is well respected. The more complex and difficult the problem, the more important reputation is. In fact, you might well narrow your focus to doctors on the staffs of certain medical centers noted for excellence with specific problems. There are a number of books and magazine articles listed in the annotated bibliography that offer views on the best medical centers for specific problems.

Last, make certain your doctor and the specialist communicate easily about your case. If you should have a problem with a specialist, or if you are not pleased with the care given, let your primary care doctor know about it right away.

EASY ACCESS TO SPECIALISTS AND SUBSPE-
CIALISTS, ESPECIALLY IN LARGE METROPOLITAN
AREAS, PRESENTS CERTAIN PROBLEMS IN COOR-
DINATION THAT A PATIENT SHOULD BE AWARE
OF. THIS DIFFICULTY IS PROBABLY EPITOMIZED
BY ONE WOMAN WHO WAS TREATED BY A

DERMATOLOGIST, AN OPHTHALMOLOGIST, A RHEUMATOLOGIST, A PSYCHIATRIST, AND AN ALLERGIST, —ALL OF WHOM HAD OFFICE SPACE IN HER VERY LARGE APARTMENT COMPLEX ON MANHATTAN'S UPPER WEST SIDE LEASED PRIMARILY TO DOCTORS, THUS ELIMINATING HER NEED TO TRAVEL ANYWHERE, OR, IN FACT, EVEN TO PUT ON HER COAT. FORTUNATELY, ALL WERE QUITE COMPETENT AND HAD ALL THE NECESSARY QUALIFICATIONS. UNFORTUNATELY, EACH WAS AFFILIATED WITH A DIFFERENT MEDICAL CENTER, WHICH MADE COORDINATING HER CARE WITH HER PRIMARY CARE DOCTOR VERY COMPLEX.

Doctors typically refer patients to doctors on the staffs of the same hospitals where they practice. There are good and poor reasons for this:

WHY DOCTORS USUALLY REFER TO DOCTORS IN THE SAME HOSPITALS

Good

■ They know the doctors better.

■ They continue to be involved in the case.

■ Coordination of multiple specialists may be easier.

Poor

■ It is easier.

■ They will get referrals back.

- **It reduces the chances of losing the patient.**

- **It may help build social or professional relationships.**

- **The hospital may pressure doctors to refer within the institution.**

In today's managed care environment doctor referrals are usually restricted to other doctors in the managed care organization's network. Sometimes the referring doctor may not even be familiar with the other doctor's qualifications. If you are not comfortable with your primary care doctor's referral, ask for a number of options. If necessary, you may consider going "out of network" even if you have to pay some or all of the fee.

SECOND OPINIONS

Second opinions are a valuable medical tool, too infrequently used in many instances, overused in others. Clearly, you do not want to get another doctor's opinion on every ailment or problem, but there are definitely times you should seek out a second opinion:

- **Before major surgery.**

- **When the diagnosis is serious or life-threatening.**

- **If a rare disease is diagnosed.**

- **If the diagnosis is uncertain.**

- **If you think the number of tests or procedures recommended is excessive.**

- ◼ If a test result has serious implications—a positive pap smear for example—have the test redone immediately before taking further action.

- ◼ If the treatment suggested is risky or expensive.

- ◼ If you are uncomfortable with the prescribed diagnosis and treatment.

- ◼ If a course of treatment is not working.

- ◼ If you question your doctor's competence.

- ◼ If your insurance company requires it.

Most doctors will be supportive if you request a second opinion, and many will recommend it. In many cases, insurance companies will pay for second opinions, but check ahead of time to make sure your insurance plan does cover them. In an HMO, you may have to be more assertive because one way HMOs control costs is by limiting second opinions. This is especially true if you want an opinion outside the plan's network.

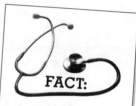

FACT:

A recent study conducted by the University of Florida estimated that 60 percent of all Americans use alternative therapies and total expenditures for alternative/complimentary treatments are between $18-22 billion.

Often, the opinion of a second doctor will affirm the opinion of the first, but the reassurance may be worth the time and extra cost. On the other hand, if the second opinion differs from the first, you have two remaining alternatives: seek the opinion of a third doctor, or educate yourself as much as possible by talking with both doctors and reading up on the problem, and trusting your instincts about which diagnosis is correct.

QUICK TIPS.

35. IN MANY CASES, INSURANCE COMPANIES WILL PAY FOR SECOND OPINIONS, BUT CHECK AHEAD OF TIME TO MAKE SURE YOUR INSURANCE PLAN DOES COVER THEM.

36. ONE WAY HMOS CONTROL COSTS IS BY LIMITING SECOND OPINIONS.

37. DOCTORS MAY HAVE DIFFERENT SOLUTIONS TO THE SAME PROBLEM—AND ANY ONE OR MORE COULD WORK.

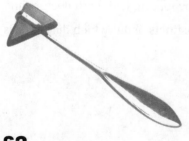

If the diagnosis is the same but the recommended treatments differ, remember that doctors may have different solutions to the same problem—and any one or more could work. For example, an orthopedic surgeon may recommend surgery to correct a knee injury while a physiatrist (a doctor certified in physical medicine and rehabilitation) may recommend rehabilitation. One might work better than the other or they could both work equally well. The choice may be based on your preference. Remember, however, that surgical solutions can rarely be reversed. It usually is best to try a medical solution first.

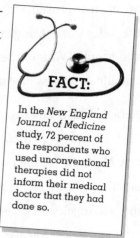

FACT:

In the *New England Journal of Medicine* study, 72 percent of the respondents who used unconventional therapies did not inform their medical doctor that they had done so.

ALTERNATIVE MEDICINE: EXPLORING YOUR OPTIONS

A recent study conducted by the University of Florida estimated that 60% of all Americans use alternative therapies and total expenditures for alternative/complementary treatments are between $18-$22 billion. The issue of alternative therapies is so important that the National Institutes of Health has created an Office of Alternative Medicine to examine their effectiveness.

One of the reasons conventional medical therapies are conventional is that most have been proven to be effective in a rigorous scientific manner. Most alternative therapies have not been tested under accepted scientific conditions—one, because they are relative newcomers in medicine and, two, because many of these alternative therapies don't fit into the exacting protocols set up in clinical testing.

You should always consider the possibility that alternative therapies, since they are often unproven, may do more harm than good. The alternative approaches in use today range from legitimate searches for new therapies to outright quackery and fraud. Without the guidance of the scientific and medical community, it is sometimes impossible for doctors, let alone consumers, to tell the difference.

Nonetheless, doctors are becoming more open to the use of alternative approaches. The term most often used to describe these therapies is "Alternative/Complementary Medicine," which suggests that such treatments work *with* Western medical practices. One study reported that about 30 percent of the doctors questioned in the Los Angeles area said that they were open to alternative practices in one form or another. Medical schools are also indicating a new interest in studying approaches to health that may complement the strengths of Western medicine. Some of the therapies being explored include mind-body medicine, hypnotherapy, biofeedback, chiropractic, vital energy, metabolic therapy, naturopathy, homeopathy, therapeutic touch, acupuncture, prayer, and the use of herbs.

In the *New England Journal of Medicine* study, 72 percent of the respondents who used unconventional therapies did not inform their medical doctor that they had done so. That is unfortunate, because such treatments could be greatly enhanced with the support and advice of a primary care doctor. More worrisome is the great danger that some people may seek alternative treatments in lieu of, rather than as a supplement to, more conventional and proven medical therapies. A classic and tragic example of this was the surge of patients who traveled to Mexico to seek a "magic bullet" cure for cancer promised by the drug Laetrile (made from apricot pits). There was no magic; indeed, patients lost money, hope, and, in some cases, the opportunity for timely use of proven treatment. If you do explore alternative therapies, be certain to let your doctor know about it. Some may be harmful, especially if you are undergoing another treatment under your doctor's direction.

To learn more about alternative medicine contact the Office of Alternative Medicine (See Appendix K). To locate a source of reliable information on the practice you are considering, see Appendix K.

HOW TO USE ALTERNATIVE/ COMPLEMENTARY MEDICINE WISELY AND WELL

■ Try to learn everything you can about the particular therapy you are interested in. Your local library may have materials on alternative medicine. Many consumer magazines feature articles on alternative medicine, and the librarian should be able to direct you to these publications.

■ Discuss your plans with your doctor. You might gain some insight into the therapy in terms of its possible risks. Furthermore, if you are currently under medical treatment, you should make certain that the two approaches will not conflict in some way.

■ If you start an alternative therapy and it does not appear to be providing relief, or worse, seems to be worsening the condition, contact your doctor immediately.

CLINICAL TRIALS: SHOULD YOU PARTICIPATE?

Each year, more than half a million Americans, some of them sick, but even more of them healthy, volunteer to take part in experimental trials of new drugs and therapies. Before drugs, vaccines, biological agents, and medical devices are made available for general use by doctors and their patients, they must go through extensive testing on animals and humans. The latter is called "clinical trials". There is probably at least one in process at some medical center for almost any serious disease.

On the plus side, a clinical trial offers the opportunity for prompt use of a drug or other treatment that seems promising, and comes with the bonus of regular and thorough medical examinations at no cost to you (some trials even make allowances for participants' travel and other expenses). Moreover, patients are encouraged to discuss all of their experiences regarding the trial. You will probably learn more about your condition and, therefore, feel more in control, which can have a very positive effect. On the downside, you may be giving up standard treatment for something that may or may not be better. There is even the possibility that you will not get a drug at all, because most trials are conducted by the double-blind method, in which half of the participants get the drug and half get a placebo, or "dummy" medicine. Even the doctors conducting the trials do not know who is getting which.

WHAT TO KNOW BEFORE YOU GET INVOLVED

If you are considering participating in a clinical trial, you will want to know:

■ **Who is the sponsor? Look for a federal government, major health organization, drug company, or university-sponsored trial.**

■ **Do any impartial authorities monitor the trial? Every hospital conducting research has an institutional review board (IRB) consisting of medical professionals and com-**

munity leaders to approve that hospital's participation. There are also data and safety monitoring boards that oversee trials.

■ Will there be pain or discomfort? Will diagnostic tests be involved? Get detailed answers to these concerns before you sign any form.

■ How often will I be examined? This depends on the guidelines of the trial (called the protocol). You should make every effort to keep your appointments.

■ Does my own doctor get a record) of my participation in the trial? Routine health information is sent to your doctor, but details relevant to a "blinded" trial are not disclosed until the trial is over.

■ Is the drug in this trial approved for treatment of any other disorder? If the answer is yes, you then know that the drug has a prior safety record.

■ After the study has ended, if I have responded well to the drug, will I be able to continue using it, even before it is approved?

■ Can I drop out?

If you are interested in participating in a clinical trial, make your desire known to your doctor, who can track down openings in trials being conducted by medical centers, private foundations, drug companies, and the federal government.

QUICK TIPS.

38. SURGICAL SOLUTIONS CAN RARELY BE REVERSED. IT USUALLY IS BEST TO TRY A MEDICAL SOLUTION FIRST.

39. YOU SHOULD ALWAYS CONSIDER THE POSSIBILITY THAT ALTERNATIVE THERAPIES, SIMPLY BECAUSE THEY ARE UNPROVEN, MAY DO MORE HARM THAN GOOD.

40. IF YOU DO EXPLORE ALTERNATIVE THERAPIES, BE CERTAIN TO LET YOUR DOCTOR KNOW ABOUT IT. SOME MAY BE HARMFUL, ESPECIALLY IF YOU ARE UNDERGOING ANOTHER TREATMENT UNDER YOUR DOCTOR'S DIRECTION.

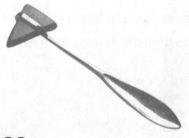

KEY TERMS
CHAPTER 5

NATIONAL PRACTITIONER DATA BANK

A computerized listing, created in 1986 by an Act of Congress, to track health professionals who are disciplined for unprofessional behavior and to deter them from simply moving their practices from one state to another.

PUBLIC CITIZEN'S HEALTH RESEARCH GROUP

A Washington, D.C. based consumer advocacy group that has been publicly critical of many medical practices that the group considers detrimental to public health care.

QUICK TAKES

... There's a big difference between doctor-hopping and changing doctors for a good reason. Most failed doctor-patient relationships can be attributed to some common complaints but sometimes it is a matter of self-defense...

CHAPTER 5

CHANGING
YOUR DOCTOR

Obviously, at times there are good reasons for changing doctors. Some are very simple and straightforward, such as a doctor's retirement, illness, or death, your own relocation, or a change in your health plan. About 40 percent of people enrolling in managed care plans have to change their doctor to one who is affiliated with the plan.

An onset of a chronic condition may also prompt a change to a different medical specialist, such as a rheumatologist or cardiologist, if a condition needs to be managed by a specialist other than a primary care doctor.

If you have continuing symptoms that your doctor has been unable to diagnose or if, after a diagnosis, your problems continue to linger without improvement, you should at least consider getting a second opinion and, depending on that opinion, possibly changing doctors. Doctors often have different approaches to the same problem. A different doctor may offer a different perspective and, perhaps, a solution.

You might also change doctors in order to find one who includes alternative medicine in the treatment or to find one who can help you enroll in a clinical trial.

People who have hostile feelings toward organized medicine tend to change doctors frequently; their complaints then become a self-fulfilling prophecy. They don't get continuous, quality care because it's impossible for anyone to deliver it. On the other hand, negative feelings may be prompted by unfortunate encounters with incompetent doctors or by the patronizing or otherwise inappropriate attitudes expressed by some doctors toward patients. Patients on the receiving end of such a relationship should continue their search for a doctor who better meets their needs.

EIGHT REASONS TO SAY GOODBYE

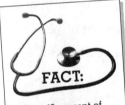

FACT:

About 40 percent of people enrolling in managed care plans have to change their doctor to one who is affiliated with the plan.

Here are the eight most common complaints about "doctors I don't go to anymore."

POOR BEDSIDE MANNER

Good medical care is more than diagnosis and treatment; it's also an attitude on the part of the doctor that sparks a sense of trust in the patient. Being under the care of a doctor who is impersonal, abrupt, bored, arrogant, condescending, or sarcastic, may in the end be counterproductive.

The doctor's aloofness could have a more serious explanation: substance abuse or psychological impairment, which according to a recent American Medical

Association report affects 30,000 to 40,000 physicians. Mood swings and detachment are signs to watch for.

TOO VAGUE AND EVASIVE

A doctor who dismisses problems with "it's nothing to worry about," or "let me take care of it," or who uses medical jargon isn't interested in having you as a partner in your health care. The effect of this evasiveness can be anger, fear, and confusion, leading to failure to follow directions and failure of treatment.

NEVER ON SCHEDULE

Medical emergencies can make appointment scheduling an inexact science, but when snafus become chronic, it's a sign of trouble. An explanation can ease the frustration, but make-up time should not be at your expense.

COULDN'T DIAGNOSE THE PROBLEM

Some conditions can't be diagnosed on-the-spot. Others aren't attributable to one specific cause. That doesn't excuse an incomplete workup, however, which may leave you with a condition that could have been treated earlier.

ORDERED TOO MANY TESTS

Sophisticated technology is available and doctors tend to use it, although some testing may not be necessary. The number of tests performed for diagnosis seems to be reduced in patient-doctor relationships where communication is strong.

DISCOURAGED SECOND OPINIONS

A doctor who dissuades you from talking to another doctor may perceive it as questioning his or her professional abilities.

DIDN'T PROTECT MY MEDICAL PRIVACY

No patient should have to discuss the reason for a visit, payment, or payment problems within earshot of other patients or staff.

Medical records can be requested by and turned over to insurance companies, lawyers, employers, and others without your consent, but you can certainly see them, too, to make sure they contain the proper information. In 27 states and the District of Columbia the law grants patients access to medical records from doctors and hospital records; in other states, a doctor may let you see them anyway.

UNPLEASANT OFFICE STAFF

Repeated incidents such as rudeness over the telephone, a brusque physician's assistant, or being kept waiting in an examining room for a long time before the doctor shows up are all annoying indications that a staff could do better.

The staff takes its cues from the chief. A doctor who doesn't demand the highest level of performance from a staff may be sending a message about his or her own laxity in diagnosis and treatment.

SHOULD YOU SWITCH?

If your doctor fits these important factors in a doctor-patient relationship, it may be time to consider finding a new doctor. But before you decide to part company with your doctor, ask yourself if you've been a responsible patient. Often problems arise when patients don't reveal their full medical history, or if they forget to alert their doctor about other drugs they are taking. A doctor-patient relationship is like a marriage—both sides have to work to make it successful.

If you're sure the problem isn't on your side, however, confront your doctor with your grievances. Or if it's easier for you, you may want to write them in a letter. Expressing your dissatisfaction may open the communication lines between you and your doctor. You might even end up in a better relationship with your present doctor. Sometimes doctors aren't aware that they are in the midst of a deteriorating relationship until a patient wants to leave.

But if you are still unhappy with your doctor and you've decided a change is necessary, you can make a clean break by simply going to another doctor. Keep in mind, however, that your most important concern should be continuity of care. So, unless the situation is intolerable or the doctor is impaired, stay with your current doctor until you have found another one that you like.

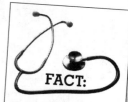

FACT:

In 23 states and the District of Columbia the law grants patients access to medical records held by physicians; in other states, a doctor may let you see them anyway.

Generally, medical records are kept by your doctor until you have found a new one. You will then have to sign a release with your new doctor approving the transfer of all your medical records to the new office. These records cannot be withheld for any reason, even if you have not yet paid your last bill.

Finally, don't feel embarrassed or guilty if you decide to change doctors. Remember, good quality medical care is your right!

IN ONE CASE INVOLVING A WOMAN IN HER MID-THIRTIES, THE DOCTOR-PATIENT RELATIONSHIP WAS SEVERED OVER WHAT WAS BASICALLY A CONFLICT IN PERSONALITIES: THE WOMAN WISHED TO HAVE MORE CONTROL OVER HER HEALTH CARE, AND THE DOCTOR WAS RELUCTANT TO GIVE IT. THE IMPASSE WAS REACHED

QUICK TIPS.

41. BEFORE YOU DECIDE TO PART COMPANY WITH YOUR DOCTOR, ASK YOURSELF IF YOU'VE BEEN A RESPONSIBLE PATIENT.

42. A DOCTOR-PATIENT RELATIONSHIP IS LIKE A MARRIAGE—BOTH SIDES HAVE TO WORK TO MAKE IT SUCCESSFUL.

43. EXPRESSING YOUR DISSATISFACTION MAY OPEN THE COMMUNICATION LINES BETWEEN YOU AND YOUR DOCTOR. YOU MIGHT EVEN END UP IN A BETTER RELATIONSHIP WITH YOUR PRESENT DOCTOR.

44. UNLESS THE SITUATION IS INTOLERABLE OR THE DOCTOR IS IMPAIRED, STAY WITH YOUR CURRENT DOCTOR UNTIL YOU HAVE FOUND ANOTHER ONE THAT YOU LIKE.

45. WHEN CHANGING DOCTORS YOU MAY HAVE TO SIGN A RELEASE WITH YOUR NEW DOCTOR APPROVING THE TRANSFER OF ALL YOUR MEDICAL RECORDS TO THE NEW OFFICE. THESE RECORDS CANNOT BE WITHHELD FOR ANY REASON, EVEN IF YOU HAVE NOT YET PAID YOUR LAST BILL.

BEFORE THE TWO COULD ATTEMPT ANY KIND OF A COMPROMISE, AND THE WOMAN WENT OFF IN SEARCH OF A DOCTOR WHO WOULD BETTER SUIT HER PERSONAL NEEDS. A YEAR LATER, AFTER A FRUITLESS SEARCH FOR A DOCTOR WHOSE MEDICAL EXPERTISE SHE RESPECTED, SHE RETURNED TO HER ORIGINAL DOCTOR.

SELF DEFENSE: AVOIDING QUESTIONABLE DOCTORS

In addition to finding good doctors, you also want to be able to identify and avoid doctors who have a history of professional problems. One way to do this is to make certain a doctor has not been disciplined by your state or, in fact, any state. You can call the appropriate state agency (listed in Appendix G) or check names in the book *16,638 Questionable Doctors,* published by the Public Citizens' Health Research Group. This book lists the names of doctors who have been disciplined by states or by the federal government. The disciplinary actions were taken for a variety of reasons, including overprescribing or misprescribing medications, criminal convictions, alcohol or drug abuse, and patient sexual abuse.

The Public Citizens' Health Research Group has been highly critical of state medical boards and their monitoring of the medical profession. The group's report compares state medical boards, ranks states by their disciplinary actions against doctors, and recommends actions for strengthening watchdog efforts.

The Public Citizens' Health Research Group believes that many states are not aggressive enough in monitoring doctors. They have been leading the call for public access to the National Practitioner Data Bank. The Data Bank was created in 1986 by an Act of Congress in order to track professionals who are disciplined for unprofessional behavior and to deter them from simply moving their practices from one state to another. The Data Bank became operational in 1990 and contains a record of adverse actions such as license removal, loss of clinical privileges, and professional society membership actions taken against doctors and other licensed health professionals, such as dentists. It contains the names of over 170,000 health practitioners who have either a licensing action or malpractice judgement or settlement against them. There is strong pressure from some medical groups either to do away with the Data Bank or to place even stricter controls on access. They support their position with examples of errors in the handling of sensitive information. It is unlikely that Congress would permit the elimination of the Data Bank, however. In fact, it is possible that at some time in the future, access may be made more available to the public. However, at the present time there is no public access to this information.

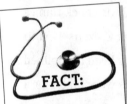

FACT:

The National Practitioner Data Bank contains the names of over 170,000 health practitioners who have either a licensing action or malpractice judgement or settlement against them. You can write directly to the National Practitioner Data Bank if you wish more information.

A data service used by lawyers to check on a doctor's or hospital's malpractice history is LEXIS/NEXIS, the computerized legal information service. Some libraries will do a LEXIS/NEXIS search for a fee, usually over $65.00. Public access to the listing of malpractice payments is one issue on which doctors are very sensitive, and rightfully so. Many malpractice payments are made by insurance companies over the objections of doctors because the insurers feel it's cheaper to settle than to fight. Yet doctors who feel they are blameless contend that these settlements reflect negatively on them. Also, since so many specialists, such as those in obstetrics and gynecology, are subject to more frequent lawsuits because of the nature of their practice, doctors are concerned about how patients will interpret a malpractice settlement.

People who believe they have a problem with a doctor, whether in regard to fees, treatment, or ethics, may contact the appropriate local medical society in the county in which the doctor practices, or the state medical society. State health departments are also places consumers may turn to for assistance or information on disciplinary actions taken against doctors. The health department, typically, will only divulge that an action has been taken but will not give you any specific information about it (See Appendix G for phone numbers and addresses).

Changing your doctor should not be considered a setback in your search for the best doctor to meet your needs. As you may have come to understand through-out preceding chapters in this book, the personal and treatment styles doctors bring to their practices vary greatly. What is important for you, as a patient, to realize is that these subtle and immeasurable characteristics can be as important as clinical skills. There is, in fact, substantial empirical and anecdotal evidence demonstrating that confidence in the healer and the healing process plays a major role in many cures. Your main objective is to find the therapy—in combination with the professional who is providing the therapy—that works best for you.

QUICK TIPS.

46. A DATA SERVICE USED BY LAWYERS TO CHECK ON A DOCTOR'S OR HOSPITAL'S MALPRACTICE HISTORY IS LEXIS/NEXIS, THE COMPUTERIZED LEGAL INFORMATION SERVICE. LEXIS WILL DO A SEARCH AND ISSUE A REPORT ON ANY MALPRACTICE AWARDS OR SETTLEMENTS ORDERED BY A COURT.

47. STATE HEALTH DEPARTMENTS ARE ALSO PLACES CONSUMERS MAY TURN TO FOR ASSISTANCE OR INFORMATION ON DISCIPLINARY ACTIONS TAKEN AGAINST DOCTORS.

48. THERE IS, IN FACT, SUBSTANTIAL EMPIRICAL AND ANECDOTAL EVIDENCE DEMONSTRATING THAT CONFIDENCE IN THE HEALER AND THE HEALING PROCESS PLAYS A MAJOR ROLE IN MANY CURES.

49. PEOPLE WHO BELIEVE THEY HAVE A PROBLEM WITH A DOCTOR, WHETHER IN REGARD TO FEES, TREATMENT, OR ETHICS, MAY CONTACT THE APPROPRIATE LOCAL MEDICAL SOCIETY IN THE COUNTY IN WHICH THE DOCTOR PRACTICES, OR THE STATE MEDICAL SOCIETY.

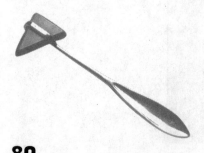

KEY TERMS
CHAPTER 6

CAPITATION

A method of payment to physicians and other health care providers whereby a fixed amount of money is allotted for each patient served.

EPO

An Exclusive Provider Organization is similar to a PPO except the patients must use only providers in the EPO.

GROUP MODEL HMO

A model of an HMO in which the HMO contracts with large multi-specialty groups of doctors to provide care, usually from a number of central locations.

HEALTH MAINTENANCE ORGANIZATION (HMO)

One type of managed care organization that provides for a wide range of comprehensive health care services for its members in return for a fixed, predetermined fee. The care is provided by a network or group of physicians affiliated with the organization and possibly other health care professionals.

IPA

An Independent Practice Association is one model of health maintenance organization (HMO) in which the organization contracts with individual doctors, or groups of doctors, to provide care for the enrolled patients in the doctors' own offices.

PHO

A Physician Hospital Organization is an organization of a hospital and its physicians that may contract with managed care organizations (MCO) or may become licensed as a MCO itself.

PPO

A Preferred Provider Organization is a managed care model that offers health care provided by a group of doctors and/or hospitals that have negotiated discounted rates, either capitated or fee-for-service, for enrollees while continuing to provide care for other patients. Patients typically pay less if they use the PPO provider.

PSO

A Provider Service Organization, sometimes called a provider service network (PSN), is a group of doctors that are organized to provide care to a large number of patients, typically under contract to managed care organizations.

STAFF MODEL HMO

A managed care model where the HMO employs the doctors, usually on salary. Care is provided out of a number of centralized locations.

QUICK TAKES

...The rules are different but they are not difficult to play by. The first step is to sort out the alphabet soup of models. The model of HMO usually determines how your care will be delivered and often your satisfaction with it...

CHAPTER 6

CHOOSING
A DOCTOR
IN AN HMO

Many people question the quality of doctors associated with HMOs. In some cases, especially when an HMO first enters a particular region, it may sign up virtually any licensed doctor who applies. At the same time, many HMO plans have rigorous selection standards and point out—correctly—that they screen their doctors carefully, while any doctor with a license can hang up a shingle and practice in the community.

At one time only doctors looking for new patients joined HMOs. Today, there is a new reality. Almost *all* doctors—over 80 percent—participate in some kind of managed care arrangement. So it is likely that you will find the best for your own care if you know how to work the system.

When managed care achieves a significant market penetration and begins to control the flow of large numbers of patients, more doctors sign on. Also, many hospitals encourage their doctors to sign on with as many different plans as possible in order to insure that the hospital does not lose any potential patients. Managed care now enrolls more than one out of every three people in the country, and over 75% of workers get health insurance through their employer. A doctor who has not joined an HMO could have few patients!

The main factor to focus on in assessing an HMO is its resources, primarily doctors and hospitals. First, is there an ample selection of primary care doctors near where you live and work? Second, are the doctors well qualified? This can be answered by following the approach outlined in this book for finding the best doctors. When choosing doctors, it is usually a good idea to call their offices to confirm they are still affiliated with the particular plan. Doctors frequently change affiliations with managed care plans. Also, it is a good idea to check on the procedure for using the doctor listed.

FACT:

Almost all doctors—over 80 percent—participate in some kind of managed care arrangement.

HMOs may list hundreds of doctors but not all of them are necessarily accessible to all members. A large HMO, for example, may restrict the number of specialists that primary care doctors can refer to for various reasons, including location, hospital capacity, and general resource allocation. So although you may see the name of an ophthalmologist, gynecologist, or other specialist you want to use, and indeed that doctor may be affiliated with the HMO, it does not necessarily follow that your primary care doctor is free to refer you to them. Those specialists may see HMO patients only on a certain basis—for specific procedures, for example, or in a certain geographic region—and then possibly only after a rigorous screening process. These possibilities illustrate the varying styles of operation you will find in managed care plans.

Doctors in HMOs are bound by the same professional ethics that guide all doctors. However, there is a major difference: In an HMO, the plan is responsible for providing you with care as well as with a doctor. If your doctor leaves the plan, you don't follow him or her. The plan provides a new doctor for you.

SELECTING DOCTORS IN AN HMO

Selecting a doctor in an HMO can be a greater challenge than selecting one when you have indemnity insurance that leaves you free to select a doctor without the restrictions of the plan. Obviously, in an HMO arrangement you need to select a doctor who belongs to that plan. Studies have shown that about 40 percent of enrollees in managed care plans have to choose a new doctor when they join. However, even in a plan of small size, you will usually have the option of choosing among a number of primary care doctors as well as other specialists and subspecialists. In doing so, utilize the same criteria you would apply to selecting a doctor in a fee-for-service practice.

The first doctor you select in an HMO plan is your primary care doctor. Typically, you will be sent a list with little information other than the doctor's name, specialty, and address. *Find out more about those doctors you may be considering.* Use the process described earlier in this book. If you make a selection and are not satisfied, request a change. Ask about the procedure for changing doctors before you join the plan.

When you need a specialist, it is your primary care doctor who will refer you, as in traditional indemnity plans. But, unlike indemnity plans in which you can find a specialist on your own if you choose, in managed care plans you must be referred to see a specialist. Again, your choices will be limited in selecting specialists, but be assertive. Ask for a choice of doctors and ask why your primary care doctor recommends a particular specialist. One disadvantage to the IPA model and the network referral process is that primary care doctors can end up making referrals to specialists and/or subspecialists they do not know. This may result in poor communication between the primary care doctor and the specialist, which is not in the patient's best interest. If you are not satisfied with the choices offered, ask to go outside the plan. Choice of providers outside a plan is built into certain managed care plans and is permitted in many others under certain conditions.

However, if you do not have a choice, or if the choices are not ones with which you agree, consider going outside the HMO. Although you are likely to have to pay more, it may be worth it if you get a correct diagnosis and appropriate treatment for your problem. In some cases, the HMO will agree to pay at least a consultation fee if you feel strongly that you need to discuss your problem with another doctor outside the HMO network. After the consultation, if you still feel the need for a different doctor, at least your choice will be based on more complete information.

One of the most popular plans offered by HMOs permits going outside of the network of doctors and hospitals—but at an added cost. The point of service or POS plan, one of the fastest growing offerings of many HMOs, permits the HMO member to use doctors, hospitals, and other services that are not part of the HMO network. Typically, the member will pay an additional fee for this choice—for example, 20 percent or 30 percent of the cost—whereas, if the member stays "in-network" the HMO will pay all or close to all of the cost.

When leaving the network of a POS, however, patients should find out exactly how much it will cost to do so. Some HMOs will pay a percentage of "appropriate and prevailing fees" while others will pay a percentage of their own fee schedule, which is usually lower.

HMO MODELS

Although a large alphabet soup of HMO models has appeared since the big move toward managed care began in the late 1980s, and we now have PPOs, PSOs, and EPOs, two models are most important to the health care consumer. One is the staff or group model where patients visit their doctors in a single, or perhaps in a few, locations and where all the doctors and most, if not all, diagnostic and treatment facilities are located. The second is the independent practice association or IPA model where doctors see patients in their private offices. Organizations such as PPOs, EPOs and PSOs tend to be organized on the IPA model.

Whether a group/staff model or an IPA, all HMOs require a primary care physician and all have certain protocols, usually involving referral by the primary care physician, to access a specialist.

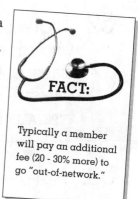

FACT:

Typically a member will pay an additional fee (20 - 30% more) to go "out-of-network."

DOCTOR COMPENSATION

There is virtually no difference in the types of doctors who practice in the two HMO models and each should be evaluated in terms of benefits to the individual patient. There is, however, a separate matter of how doctors in HMOs are compensated, and this issue has become a major concern to both patients and doctors.

HMOs compensate doctors in a number of ways. Doctors who are employed by staff model HMOs are usually on salary, perhaps with a quality bonus based on patient satisfaction. In group model HMOs the physician group has a contract with the HMO and the doctors are employed by the group, usually on salary and, again, often with a quality bonus.

87

QUICK TIPS.

50. THE MAIN FACTOR TO FOCUS ON IN ASSESSING AN HMO IS ITS RESOURCES, PRIMARILY DOCTORS AND HOSPITALS.

51. HMOS MAY LIST HUNDREDS OF DOCTORS BUT NOT ALL OF THEM ARE NECESSARILY ACCESSIBLE TO ALL MEMBERS.

52. WHEN YOU NEED A SPECIALIST, IT IS YOUR PRIMARY CARE DOCTOR WHO WILL REFER YOU, AS IN TRADITIONAL INDEMNITY PLANS. BUT, UNLIKE INDEMNITY PLANS IN WHICH YOU CAN FIND A SPECIALIST ON YOUR OWN IF YOU CHOOSE, IN MANAGED CARE PLANS YOU TYPICALLY MUST BE REFERRED TO SEE A SPECIALIST.

53. WHEN LEAVING THE NETWORK IN A POS PLAN PATIENTS SHOULD FIND OUT EXACTLY HOW MUCH IT WILL COST TO DO SO.

54. WHEN CHOOSING DOCTORS, IT IS USUALLY A GOOD IDEA TO CALL THEIR OFFICES TO CONFIRM THAT THEY ARE STILL AFFILIATED WITH THE PARTICULAR PLAN.

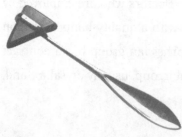

In the IPA model HMOs, or in PPOs, EPOs, PSOs and other types of managed care organizations the doctors are usually paid in one of two ways. In the past, the predominant payment method was a negotiated fee schedule, typically designed at some discount to the doctor's normal fee. Doctors simply traded the promise of higher volume for a reduced fee. Today, a major method of payment in an IPA is capitation. While this is fast becoming the most common method of payment in IPAs it is also the one generating the most controversy.

Under a capitated or capitation system doctors are paid a set amount per month or per year to provide care to a patient during that time period. So, for example, a primary care physician may be paid $15 per member per month.

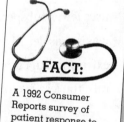

FACT:

A 1992 Consumer Reports survey of patient response to HMOs demonstrated that members were more satisfied with plans that paid their doctor on a fee basis than they were with those that paid on a capitated, or per person, basis.

HMOs have moved toward capitation as a method of payment because they found that discounted fee-for-service payment methods did not reduce costs as much as had been hoped, if at all. To make up for discounted fees of 20 percent, for instance, doctors simply scheduled 20 percent more patient visits so that their incomes would not decrease. Doctors openly comment that discounted fees translate to discounted time with patients!

Capitation has helped to control costs. However, it also has introduced a number of important ethical issues for doctors, other health care providers, and for patients. Many are troubled by the notion that a doctor could be placed in a situation that appears to promise rewards for *not* providing care. It is generally recognized that under a fee-for-service system doctors have an incentive to provide more care, even if it is not necessary, because they are paid by the amount of care they deliver. But the reverse is not accepted in such a benign fashion: the concept of a doctor being rewarded to provide *less* care is of major concern to many people, including many doctors.

Another technique involved in payment systems utilized by managed care companies is called "withholds" or "set-asides." This method is also used to motivate doctors to control costs and, as in capitation, raises similar ethical concerns. Under this method, for example, a group of pediatricians is contracted to care for 1,000 children. That contract is based on a budget of $15,000 a month. A certain amount of that budget, say 20 percent, is reserved for referrals to subspecialists and another 20 percent is set aside or withheld. If the group of doctors uses fewer subspecialist referrals than budgeted they receive the 20 percent that was set aside. If they use more subspecialist referrals than were budgeted the extra amount comes out of the set-aside. The more set-aside that is used for referrals, the less doctors will be able to receive from it.

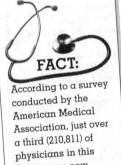

FACT:

According to a survey conducted by the American Medical Association, just over a third (210,811) of physicians in this country are now members of group practices, and, in 1995, those practices numbered 19,788, an increase of 361 percent since 1965.

A great deal of controversy has ensued over these payment mechanisms. Some states, in fact, are legislating to prohibit or restrict these practices. Individual "horror stories" of patients who have been denied appropriate care, such as not being referred to a subspecialist in a timely manner, have been used to demonstrate the issue in human terms.

Some studies demonstrate that when physician-run health plans are paid by capitation and are in control they reduce costs more substantially than other plans. Some doctors strongly support capitation. They believe it makes them, rather than managers, responsible for allocating resources and making medical decisions.

And, despite the outcry, most of the studies of HMO patients versus non-HMO patients demonstrate no differences in their health status.

In fact, there is a substantial body of research suggesting that HMO members receive more in the way of preventive services than do non-HMO populations.

If method of payment is an issue of concern to you, it may be wise to ask your doctor about the method of compensation in the HMO in which you are enrolled. If you believe the method would work against you as a patient you should discuss it with your doctor and ask if and how it influences the manner of care for patients. If you are not satisfied by the answer you may want to change doctors or, better yet, change HMOs, if possible.

While the wisest course of action is to ask about this issue before joining an HMO, rather than after you have become a member, most HMO members have not done this. If you believe you are not recieving appropriate care because of an HMO policy, you can contact your state health insurance department. (See Appendix G.)

In response to patient and physician concerns about payment policies, groups of doctors in various parts of the country have formed organizations to receive and investigate complaints against HMOs. You can contact them with any grievances you have about your HMO. (See Physicians Who Care, Appendix K.)

QUICK TIPS.

55. IF YOU BELIEVE YOU ARE NOT RECEIVING APPROPRIATE CARE BECAUSE OF AN HMO POLICY YOU CAN CONTACT YOUR STATE HEALTH OR INSURANCE DEPARTMENT.

56. TYPICALLY, YOU WILL BE SENT A LIST WITH LITTLE INFORMATION OTHER THAN THE DOCTOR'S NAME, SPECIALTY, AND ADDRESS. FIND OUT MORE ABOUT THOSE DOCTORS YOU MAY BE CONSIDERING.

57. IN SOME CASES, AN HMO WILL AGREE TO PAY AT LEAST A CONSULTATION FEE IF YOU FEEL STRONGLY THAT YOU NEED TO DISCUSS YOUR PROBLEM WITH ANOTHER DOCTOR OUTSIDE THE HMO NETWORK.

58. IF METHOD OF HMO PAYMENT TO PHYSICIANS IS AN ISSUE OF CONCERN TO YOU, IT MAY BE WISE TO ASK YOUR DOCTOR ABOUT THE METHOD OF COMPENSATION IN THE HMO IN WHICH YOU ARE ENROLLED.

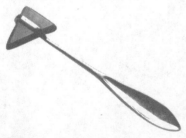

HOW DOCTORS AND PATIENTS FEEL ABOUT MANAGED CARE

People enrolled in HMOs tend to like them. However, most doctors do not like managed care—and understandably so! Managed care organizations negotiate deep discounts in fees for doctors. There is no reason doctors should prefer this process, but when managed care controls so many patients there is little choice but to join managed care and negotiate.

Managed care organizations also require doctors to do a substantial amount of paper work and to follow policies and procedures that control costs and monitor quality. All of this creates a level of business management most doctors resent.

At least a portion of these negative attitudes toward managed care can be ascribed to differences in the organization of medical practices in different parts of the country.

The northeast, south, and southwest regions have been the slowest to accept managed care. Doctors there generally resisted it more strongly than those in other parts of the country. Doctors in large group practices, which are more common in the far west and midwest than in the east, adapted to managed care more readily. In the northeast, where doctors practice solo or in small groups, the change has been greater and the adjustment more difficult.

However, most doctors have adapted and learned to practice successfully in this new medical environment. According to a survey conducted by the American Medical Association, just over a third (210,811) of physicians in this country are now members of group practices and in 1995 those practices numbered 19,788, an increase of 361 percent since 1965. From 1991 to 1995, the number of groups increased by 16.4 percent and the number of group physicians by 14.3 percent.

The survey shows that, in an environment that is organizationally complex, medical groups have changed how they are organized legally, with partnerships declining to 13.8 percent and professional corporations increasing to 77.9 percent. In the latter group, control of decision making remains largely in physician hands. This ability to retain decision making power has dramatically altered physicians' attitudes towards managed care.

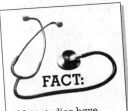

FACT:

Most studies have shown that enrollees in HMOs use about the same amount of health care resources at about the same rate as people not enrolled in HMOs, with the exception of hospital days, which HMOs reduce by about 30 percent.

The view of patients and the public, however, is decidedly more positive about managed care.

A study sponsored by the Medstat Group, J.D. Power and Associates and the New England Medical Center reported that in 20 markets across the United States, HMOs recieved more top scores than PPOs and fee-for-service plans.

The study asked plan members to assess their health plans on choice of providers, physician care, premiums and deductibles and access to care. HMOs topped fee-for-service and point-of-service plans in over half the markets.

One of the findings uncovered in a Louis Harris Associates poll of consumers was that the majority surveyed, 59 percent, believed the trend toward managed care was a good thing as compared to 28 percent who viewed it as a bad thing. Also, 48 percent as compared to 39 percent believed managed care would improve quality, and 59 percent versus 30 percent believed it would help contain the costs of care. Of note was that the response of those people in communities with a high penetration by managed care tended to be the most positive!

There are many studies that have examined the quality of care and the satisfaction of patients in managed care settings. Most show that members of HMOs and other managed care organizations are at least as satisfied or more satisfied with their care than people covered by indemnity insurance. Some studies have shown indemnity-covered people more satisfied, particularly when it relates to choice of doctors. In fact, the issue of greatest concern to HMO enrollees is usually access, particularly to specialists. Advocates of either view can point to studies to support managed care or to criticize it. The key may lay in the studies that have demonstrated that when individuals have a choice, and select a managed care plan, they tend to be more satisfied than those who have no choice.

In terms of quality the conclusion is similar. While critics may contend that the care delivered by managed care organizations is not adequate, and a study of Medicaid patients is frequently cited to support this view, the overwhelming majority of studies demonstrate no difference in the health status and quality of care of those people covered by managed care plans or by indemnity insurance.

The variability in the results of all of the studies on quality and satisfaction in managed care reinforces the important premise that as there are good doctors and poor doctors there are good HMOs and poor HMOs. It is important for consumers to know how to discern the difference and to put some effort, however modest, into finding the best.

POINTS TO REMEMBER

■ **To summarize, there is basically no difference in quality between doctors in HMOs and those in private practice. You can find excellent doctors if you're a member of an HMO and you can find poor ones, just as you can find excellent and poor doctors if you carry indemnity insurance. The key is making sure that you find the best available for your own needs and the needs of your family.**

Some simple guidelines to remember:

■ Review the credentials and training of any doctor who cares for you.

■ Make certain a doctor you select is taking new patients and the waiting period for an appointment is not unreasonable

■ Be sure the HMO has a sufficient number of specialists and subspecialists you may need to see and that they are of high quality. For example, if you have diabetes, you will want to make sure that the HMO has endocrinologists on staff or as part of its network. If you have coronary heart disease, you will want to make sure that the HMO has first rate cardiologists and an arrangement with an outstanding center where the doctors perform invasive and non-invasive diagnostic techniques and which has a good record for open heart surgery.

■ Determine beforehand the HMO's policy for patient referral to subspecialists, especially whether you will have a choice and how it may be exercised.

■ Inquire about the rules for changing doctors in the HMO if you are not satisfied with your initial choice. You will want to know not only the procedure but how often such change is allowed.

■ Ask about your options to go out of network and what your additional percentage of payment will be if you exercise this option. In determining what percentage the HMO pays, try to find out whether their payment is based on the HMO fee scale or "usual and customary" fees.

■ Ask your doctor about the HMO's compensation system. You want to be sure that the system for paying your doctor will not have a negative influence on your care.

QUICK TIPS.

59. IF YOU BELIEVE YOU ARE NOT RECEIVING APPROPRIATE CARE BECAUSE OF AN HMO POLICY YOU CAN CONTACT YOUR STATE HEALTH OR INSURANCE DEPARTMENT.

60. PEOPLE IN COMMUNITIES WITH A HIGH PENETRATION BY MANAGED CARE TENDED TO BE THE MOST POSITIVE ABOUT IT.

61. THE ISSUE OF GREATEST CONCERN TO HMO ENROLLEES IS USUALLY ACCESS, PARTICULARLY TO SPECIALISTS.

62. THE VARIABILITY IN THE RESULTS OF ALL OF THE STUDIES ON QUALITY AND SATISFACTION IN MANAGED CARE REINFORCES THE IMPORTANT PREMISE THAT AS THERE ARE GOOD DOCTORS AND POOR DOCTORS THERE ARE GOOD HMOS AND POOR HMOS.

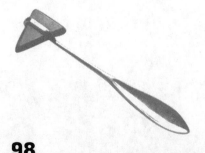

DIRECTORY

OF

DOCTORS

INCLUDES HOSPITAL

INFORMATION PROGRAM

DIRECTORY OF DOCTORS

SECTION TWO

HOW TO USE THE DIRECTORY OF DOCTORS

The third edition of the Castle Connolly Guide, *How to Find the Best Doctors: New York Metro Area*, contains vital information on more than 6,000 of the finest doctors in the region. Nominated by their peers, these doctors have met exacting criteria established by the Castle Connolly Medical Ltd. research staff. The result of the intensive screening process is a rigorously selected and outstanding group of doctors representing less than ten percent in the region, each one chosen for excellence in patient care.

WHY THIS BOOK IS YOUR BEST GUIDE

How to Find the Best Doctors is unique in a number of ways. The first edition of the Guide, published in 1994, was the first selective directory of doctors who practice in the New York metropolitan region. Our decision to publish a regional guide, rather than a countrywide directory of the best medical specialists was based on the simple and widely proven fact that most people, unless motivated by an extremely unusual health problem, will seek health care as close to home as possible. Health care consumers in the New York metropolitan region are very fortunate in the abundance of doctors—approximately 55,000—who practice in the area. On the other hand, making a selection of one out of such a multitude can be a daunting task; it's hard even to know where to start. With *How to Find the Best Doctors: New York Metro Area* in hand, you are already well on your way to finding the very best doctor for your individual needs and the needs of your family members.

With the profusion of outstanding academic medical centers, tertiary care teaching hospitals, and fine community hospitals in the region, virtually any medical procedure or treatment can be found close to home. By virtue of this fact, it would be a simple matter to compile a book identifying the outstanding leaders in medical research and academic medicine in the region. Although many of these doctors are included in the listings, their names are to be found among the many excellent and caring doctors who deliver outstanding patient care in every community in the New York metropolitan area. The goal—first and foremost—is to help you find the best doctors to meet your health care needs where you live and work. Again, a good reason why *How to Find the Best Doctors: New York Metro Area* is exceptional.

Further, the Castle Connolly Guide is different from most listings of doctors in its selection process. Our selection is predicated on an extensive nomination procedure and a set of exacting standards which each doctor nominated was required to meet. To you, this means that the basis for inclusion of every one of the 6,000-plus doctors in the listings was twofold: respect of their peers and medical excellence.

HOW CASTLE CONNOLLY SELECTED 6,000 OF THE BEST DOCTORS

How to Find the Best Doctors: New York Metro Area is the result of a meticulous search process that consumed the better part of six months. To begin the selection process, Castle Connolly Medical Ltd. randomly selected 20,000 board certified doctors from over 55,000 doctors who practice in the following counties:

New York State: Manhattan, Bronx, Kings, Queens, Richmond, Nassau, Suffolk, Rockland, Westchester

New Jersey: Bergen, Essex, Hudson, Mercer, Middlesex, Monmouth, Morris, Passaic, Somerset, Union

Connecticut: Fairfield (includes some Yale affiliated doctors in New Haven County)

A nomination form was mailed to each of the 20,000 doctors asking them to share with us the names of the best among their peers. We made it clear in this initial survey that we were not looking for the leaders in academic medicine and research, but rather *excellence in patient care*. Respondents were asked to nominate excellent, caring physicians "to whom you would send members of your own family." In addition, Castle Connolly Ltd. invited 6,000 nurses, who were also randomly selected from registered nurses in the region and more than 3,000 health care professionals in major medical centers and hospitals in the region to participate in the nomination process. These health care professionals included hospital executives, vice presidents of medical affairs, directors of clinical services, nursing vice presidents, and leading specialists and subspecialists. Following the extensive mail survey, follow-up telephone calls were made to the same group of health care leaders and to leading specialists to gather further nominations and validation of all nominations.

This process garnered nominations of over 17,500 different doctors. Using this pool of names, the Castle Connolly Medical Ltd. research staff set to work to validate and confirm the nominations. After thousands of personal telephone calls to trusted health care professionals in the region, as well as extensive review of the professional credentials of the nominated doctors, the research staff whittled down the initial list to a final selection of more than 6,000 doctors. These doctors were notified of their nomination and each was asked to complete a professional information form. These data forms became the basis for the information in the directory.

HOW *YOU* CAN SELECT
THE BEST DOCTORS

How can you begin to make a choice from such a compilation of names? There is, in fact, a basic, step-by-step process which varies somewhat depending on what your individual needs are as you approach the list. Here are the possibilities:

ONE: IF YOU ARE LOOKING FOR A DOCTOR IN A PARTICULAR COUNTY

The key: Physicians listed in the following pages are organized under the county where their office is located so that you can go directly to the section listing doctors in your county of residence (e.g., Fairfield, CT, Somerset, NJ, or Queens, NY).

Key fact: Like most health care consumers, you probably receive your health care locally. If you think about it, you usually have been treated by doctors close to where you live and in community hospitals. If necessary, you may be referred to regional specialists and nearby medical centers.

TWO: IF YOU ARE LOOKING FOR A PRIMARY CARE PHYSICIAN—A GENERALIST

The key: The doctors who practice predominantly primary care, in the specialties of internal medicine, family practice, pediatrics, and obstetrics/gynecology, are designated by the notation **PCP** in the listing.

Key fact: Every board certified physician is a specialist. The term "having boards" signifies that a physician has completed an approved residency in a given specialty and has passed a rigorous examination given by that particular board. Therefore, doctors who practice primary care—internists, family practitioners, pediatricians, and Ob/Gyns—are specialists in their respective fields, just as are urologists, otolaryngologists, and radiologists. They are also specialists in primary care.

THREE: IF YOU ARE LOOKING FOR A PHYSICIAN IN A PARTICULAR SPECIALTY

The Key: Each entry contains the specialty practiced by the doctor and, in most cases, the year of *initial* board certification.

Key Fact: Many physicians specialize in fields of medicine that are not primary care. These specialists have completed an approved residency in a given specialty and have passed a rigorous exam given by that specialty board. For example, some physicians are board certified in psychiatry, surgery, allergy and immunology, or dermatology.

Many doctors choose to specialize further. They choose an additional training program called a fellowship and upon completion of the program, they are required to take another exam in order to be certified as a subspecialist. An example of such subspecialization is an internist (initially board certified in internal medicine), who subspecializes in nephrology or cardiology. This doctor would be termed "double boarded" and would very likely practice nephrology or cardiology rather than internal medicine as a primary care physician.

FOUR: IF YOU ARE LOOKING FOR A DOCTOR WITH EXPERTISE IN A PARTICULAR DISEASE OR TECHNIQUE

The Key: Particular skills and interests of the doctors are found under the heading Special Practice Interest.

Key Fact: A physician may have a special practice interest in a particular field of medicine without actually being board certified in that area. Special practice interests should not be confused with a board certified medical specialty. For example, cosmetic surgery is not an American Board of Medical Specialties recognized specialty, but it may constitute a major practice activity for many plastic surgeons. Certain doctors may develop a reputation as "specialists" in AIDS, diabetes or arthroscopic surgery. None of these are recognized medical specialties, yet they are indications of a doctor's expertise in a disease or medical or surgical procedure which may be helpful if you have the disease or need the procedure.

Many doctors who have a strong interest in, or consider themselves "specializing in," a particular health problem or medical technique form special interest groups referred to as "self-designated medical specialties." These groups are often confused with recognized medical specialties, which they are not. Some of the groups would like to be recognized by the ABMS and may even work toward that goal. For example, adolescent medicine was a special interest and self-designated specialty that is now an ABMS recognized subspecialty.

Choosing a doctor with a special practice interest is an additional step to be considered after you have already narrowed your choices to particular specialists and/or subspecialists. An index of the special practice interests of the doctors in this book begins on pages 1212. Self-designated medical specialties are listed in Appendix D.

FIVE: IF YOU ARE LOOKING FOR A DOCTOR BY NAME

The Key: All doctors in this book are located in alphabetical order beginning on page 1276. This alphabetical listing will indicate the page on which information on the doctor's credentials can be found.

Key Fact: Most people start their search for a doctor through recommendation by family and friends. As a savvy health care consumer you realize that such recommendations are often based on personal "chemistry" and may be made by someone who actually knows very little about doctors or health care. Therefore, you will want to check the credentials of any recommended doctor and follow the additional recommendations we have outlined in Sections One and Two.

SIX: IF YOU ARE LOOKING FOR A DOCTOR AFFILIATED WITH YOUR HMO OR PPO

The Key: Each doctor's listing includes the first eight managed care organizations cited by the doctor and a (+) if the doctor belongs to more than five.

Key Fact: Most doctors have relationships with at least one managed care organization. Some doctors, in fact, listed 20 or more affiliations on their response form. In the listing, the HMO, PPO or other managed care organization is abbreviated; you will find the full names of the major HMOs and PPOs with which doctors in this book are affiliated on page 1203.

Since doctors' relationships with HMOs and PPOs change frequently and since we could not list all the managed care affiliations of the doctors, you should call the doctor's office to verify the information before you make an appointment.

SEVEN: IF YOU WANT DETAILED INFORMATION ON A PARTICULAR DOCTOR

The Key: Each doctor's listing includes a substantial amount of information about the doctor.

Key Fact: Wise choices in health care are made by consumers who have gathered as much information as possible about a particular doctor. If a professional information form was not returned by a doctor in time for inclusion in the book, our research staff verified certain major points of information (name address, telephone, hospital affiliation, and specialty) from public sources and we have included this limited information. Even if a doctor's full credentials are included in this book, it is possible that, since the time of publication, the doctor has moved his or her offices, changed telephone numbers, joined new medical groups, resigned from or joined hospital staffs, and, especially, changed relationships with HMOs and PPOs. Nonetheless, you can, in most cases, track down the doctor by using the following sources:

- Doctor's office—call the office number listed in the directory and ask for a new number.

- Hospitals—call the hospital listed in the directory and ask for help in locating a particular doctor.

- HMO or PPO—call the HMO or PPO listed and ask for further help.

- County Medical Societies—all county medical numbers are listed in Appendix H.

- State Medical Society—all state medical society numbers are listed in Appendix H.

- State Health Department—all state health

department numbers are listed in Appendix G. (In New York State, the State Education Department)

- American Board of Medical Specialties—a complete listing of ABMS Specialty Boards is found in Appendix A.

- American Osteopathic Association—a complete listing of AOA Specialty Boards is found in Appendix B.

CONCLUSION

You are now ready to work with our directory of more than 6,000 of the finest doctors in the New York Metropolitan area. Although you may be well-informed as a result of reading Sections One and Two of this book, it is possible that choosing the doctor will seem to be a complex endeavor. The tendency might be to try to get the job done as quickly as possible by picking a doctor based solely on the convenience of the office's location. To do so would be a big mistake. You want the best health care. You deserve it. A little effort will help you get the best.

There are many excellent doctors in the New York metropolitan region not listed in this book. You can identify them by using the process we have described in sections One and Two, or, if a doctor in this book is unable to meet your needs, ask about others whom that doctor regards highly.

We believe that this book will educate and enlighten you throughout its pages and that it will prove its value in the end—when you decide on the doctor with whom you plan to have a lasting relationship "in sickness and in health."

A. MEDICAL SPECIALTIES AND SUBSPECIALTIES

The following medical specialties and subspecialties are indicated by their abbreviations in the doctors' listings. Only those specialties and subspecialties for which we solicited nominations are included; therefore, certain specialties and subspecialties do not appear. For example, space medicine and anesthesia have been omitted. In the case of the former specialty, it is not one that most people would have an occasion to use. In the case of the latter specialty, it is one that is most often assigned rather than selected by patients. The exception here are anesthesiologists who specialize in pain management, who are included in the entries.

For a brief description of each specialty and subspecialty refer to Appendix C. Also, please note that specialties are indicated in bold and subspecialties in regular typeface. The four primary care specialties are in capital letters and bold italic. This list has been created for use in the *Castle Connolly Guide* to make it easy for you to find doctors in a given specialty or subspecialty. To review the official American Board of Medical Specialties (ABMS) organization of specialties, refer to Appendix A.

MEDICAL SPECIALTIES AND SUBSPECIALTIES

SPECIALTY & SUBSPECIALTY	ABBREVIATION	SPECIALTY & SUBSPECIALTY	ABBREVIATION
Addiction Psychiatry	AdP	**Emergency Medicine**	EM
Adolescent Medicine	AM	Endocrinology, Diabetes	
Allergy & Immunology	A&I	& Metabolism	EDM
Anesthesiology	Anes	*FAMILY PRACTICE*	FP
Cardiac Electrophysiology (Clinical)	CE	Forensic Psychiatry	FPsy
Cardiology (Cardiovascular Disease)	Cv	Gastroenterology	Ge
Child & Adolescent Psychiatry	ChAP	Geriatric Medicine	Ger
Child Neurology	ChiN	Geriatric Psychiatry	GerPsy
Colon & Rectal Surgery	CRS	Gynecologic Oncology*	GO
Critical Care Medicine	CCM	Hand Surgery	HS
Dermatology	D	Hematology	Hem
Diagnostic Radiology	DR	Infectious Disease	Inf

MEDICAL SPECIALTIES AND SUBSPECIALTIES

SPECIALTY & SUBSPECIALTY	ABBREVIATION
INTERNAL MEDICINE	IM
Maternal & Fetal Medicine	MF
Medical Genetics	MG
Medical Oncology*	Onc
Neonatal-Perinatal Medicine	NP
Nephrology	Nep
Neurological Surgery	NS
Neurology	N
Neurophysiology (Clinical)	C/NPh
Neuroradiology	NRad
Nuclear Medicine	NuM
Nuclear Radiology	NR
OBSTETRICS & GYNECOLOGY	ObG
Occupational Medicine	OM
Ophthalmology	Oph
Orthopaedic Surgery	OrS
Otolaryngology	Oto
Pain Management	PM
Pediatric Allergy & Immunology	PA&I
Pediatric Cardiology	PCd
Pediatric Critical Care Medicine	PCCM
Pediatric Emergency Medicine	PEM
Pediatric Endocrinology	PEn
Pediatric Gastroenterology	PGe
Pediatric Hematology–Oncology*	PHO
Pediatric Infectious Disease	PInf
Pediatric Nephrology	PNep

SPECIALTY & SUBSPECIALTY	ABBREVIATION
Pediatric Otolaryngology	POto
Pediatric Pulmonology	PPul
Pediatric Radiology	PR
Pediatric Rheumatology	PRhu
Pediatric Sports Medicine	PSpMed
Pediatric Surgery	PS
PEDIATRICS (GENERAL)	Ped
Physical Medicine & Rehabilitation	PMR
Plastic Surgery	PlS
Preventive Medicine	PrM
Psychiatry	Psyc
Public Health & General Preventive Medicine	PHGPM
Pulmonary Disease	Pul
Radiation Oncology*	RadRO
Radiology	Rad
Reproductive Endocrinology	RE
Rheumatology	Rhu
Sports Medicine	SM
Surgery	S
Surgical Critical Care	SCC
Thoracic Surgery (includes open heart surgery)	TS
Urology	U
Vascular & Interventional Radiology	VIR
Vascular Surgery (General)	GVS

Specialties in capital letters indicate Primary Care Specialties. However, many doctors will be certified in a subspecialty, but will practice predominantly primary care medicine. In our lists this will be indicated.

*Oncologists deal with Cancer

B. GUIDE TO SYMBOLS

♿	Handicapped accessible	🪙	Require payment of deductibles & co-payment at appointment
SA/SU	Open weekends	Mcr	Accept Medicare
☾	Evening office hours	Mcd	Accept Medicaid
☎	Calls by phone	WC	Accept Worker's Compensation
👤	Referral required	NFI	Accept no fault insurance
⊞	Accepting new patients	VISA	Accept Credit cards

Languages Spoken

Language	LangAbbr	Language	LangAbbr
		Italian	Itl
African	Afr	Japanese	Jpn
Afrikaans	Afk	Kannada	Kan
Albanian	Alb	Korean	Kor
Arabic	AR	Laotian	Lao
Armenian	Arm	Latvian	Lat
Ashanti	Ash	Lithuanian	Lth
Basque	Bsq	Malaysian	Mly
Bengali	Bng	Mandarin	Man
Bulgarian	Bul	Marathi	Mar
Burmese	Brm	Norwegian	Nwg
Cambodian	Cam	Pakistani	Pak
Cantonese	Can	Patois	Pat
Ceylonese	Cey	Persian	Per
Chinese	Chi	Polish	Pol
Creole	Cre	Portugese	Prt
Croatian	Crt	Punjabi	Pun
Czech	Czc	Romanian	Rom
Danish	Dan	Russian	Rus
Dutch	Dut	Serbian	Srb
East Indian	EIn	Serbo-Croatian	SCR
Estonian	Est	Signing	Sgn
Farsi	Frs	Sindhi	Sin
Filipino	Fil	Slovak	Slv
Finnish	Fin	Spanish	Sp
Flemish	Flm	Swahill	Swa
French	Fr	Tagalog	Tag
Gaelic	Gae	Taiwanese	Twn
German	Ger	Tamil	Tam
Greek	Grk	Telugy	Tel
Gujarati	Guj	Thai	Thai
Hebrew	Heb	Turkish	Trk
Hindi	Hin	Ukrainian	Ukr
Hungarian/Magyar	Hun	Urdu	Ur
Ilocano	Ilo	Uzbeki	Uzb
		Vietnamese	Vn
		Yiddish	Yd

C. SAMPLE LISTING

NAME

PRIMARY
ADMITTING HOSPITAL

OFFICE LOCATION
AND TELEPHONE NUMBER

MEDICAL SCHOOL
AND YEAR OF DEGREE

FACULTY APPOINTMENT(S)
AND MEDICAL SCHOOL

NETWORK
AFFILIATIONS

SPECIAL INTEREST(S)

Smith, John   IM   PCP
City Medical Center
150 E 58th, New York, NY 10155; **PH**: (212)
980-8230; **FAX**: (212) 980-1716; **BD CERT**:
IM 70, GE 74; **MS**: NY Med Coll 66; **RES**: IM,
Mt Sinai Med Ctr, NY 66-69; **FEL** :GE, St Vinct
Hosp, NY 70-72; **FAP**: Assoc Prof Clin Med,
SUNY Hlth Scie Ctr, Bklyn; *SI: Ulcers, Crohn's
Disease;* **HMO**: Aetna, Oxford, PHS, Metra
Health, Cigna, Preferred Care, PHCS, Premier+

🚹 🌙 📷 **LANG**: Sp, Heb, Rus 🏥 1️⃣ 🩸 1
Week Mcr WC **VISA** ●

DENOTES PRIMARY
CARE PHYSICIAN

SPECIALTY

BOARD
CERTIFICATION(S)
AND DATE(S)

RESIDENCY(IES)
AND LOCATIONS

INDICATES
DOCTOR
ACCEPTS MORE
THAN EIGHT
HEALTH
INSURANCE
PLANS

LENGTH OF
TIME BEFORE
APPOINTMENT

ALL SYMBOLS
ARE DEFINED ON
PAGE 112

FELLOWSHIP(S)
AND PROGRAM
LOCATION

In our listings of the professional information on doctors, we have abbreviated medical schools, hospitals and managed care affiliations. The abbreviations are designed to be self-explanatory, but if you need assistance, refer to the following appendices: Medical Schools, Appendix L; Hospitals, Appendix M; and HMOs, Appendix N.

HOSPITAL

INFORMATION

PROGRAM

THE HOSPITAL INFORMATION PROGRAM

Castle Connolly Medical Ltd. has received many requests from book buyers to provide information on hospitals in the New York Metro area. There are over 200 acute care and specialty hospitals in the region, many of which have extraordinary capabilities for superior patient care.

Therefore, in order to respond to these requests, we have invited a select group of outstanding hospitals to profile their services in the Castle Connolly Guide through the medium of paid advertorials. These selected hospitals were invited to sponsor the Hospital Information pages you will see in the Guide which are organized into three groupings: Major Medical Centers; Specialty Hospitals; Regional Medical Centers and Hospitals. This partnership with the participating hospitals is totally separate from the physician selection process which is based upon a totally independent review system.

The Major Medical Centers and Specialty Hospitals will be found on pages 118 to 137 prior to the listings of doctors. The Regional Medical Centers and Hospitals will be found at the beginning of each state or county section. The information presented will give you an overview of many of the programs and services offered by these hospitals, as well as such vital information as their accreditation and sponsorship. Also included in each hospital profile is the hospital's physican referral number, should you wish to ask the hospitals for recommendations of physicians not listed in the Castle Connolly Guide.

The "Centers of Excellence" section is also in response to requests by our readers. Not only are many people searching for the best doctor and hospital to meet their needs, but they want to know what hospitals have special programs or services focusing on a particular illness or health need. The "Centers of Excellence" section describes those special programs offered by the hospitals that are participating in the hospital information section of the Castle Connolly Guide. They reflect the depth of commitment to these special health care needs by the hospitals. Typically, the hospitals have recruited physicians, nurses and other staff with special interests and training and provided the attention and financial support necessary to develop these special programs. We believe you will find this information helpful in your search for the best health care — from both physicians and hospitals — for you and your family.

We are pleased to have these distinguished institutions as partners in our effort to provide you with useful information to help you meet your health care needs.

116

MAJOR MEDICAL CENTERS

The following pages contain vital information on six of the regions' Major Medical Centers. A Major Medical Center is an acute care hospital with tertiary care services, residency programs, a major affiliation with a medical school and clinical research programs. A major medical center draws its patients from a broad geographic region, even nationally and internationally and, in many instances, is the center of a network or consortium of hospitals.

The New York metropolitan region is nationally and internationally known for its major medical centers and their excellent programs and services. Many of the nation's leading academic centers are in this region and, in addition to superior patient care and cutting edge patient research, they produce thousands of talented, well trained physicians and other health professionals each year. Castle Connolly Medical Ltd. has invited a number of major medical centers in the region to sponsor the profiles and information that follows.

Major Medical Centers

CONTINUUM HEALTH PARTNERS, INC.

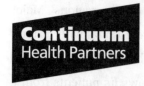

555 WEST 57TH STREET
NEW YORK, NY 10019
PHONE (800) 420-4004

Sponsorship	Voluntary Not-for-Profit
Beds	3,011 certified beds
Accreditation	Joint Commission on Accreditation of Healthcare Organizations (JCAHO), Accreditation Council for Graduate Medical Education, Medical Society of New York, in cooperation with the Accreditation Council for Continuing Medical Education

CONTINUUM HEALTH PARTNERS, INC.

In January of 1997, two prominent New York health care providers—Beth Israel Medical Center and St. Luke's-Roosevelt Hospital Center—united as Continuum Health Partners, Inc., bringing together their outstanding clinical resources and strong service traditions. In May of 1998, Long Island College Hospital, a major health care institution in Brooklyn, joined Continuum Health Partners, Inc., furthering the system's reputation as the premier provider of medical care in New York City. Together, the system has over 3,000 beds and represents more than 4,000 physicians and dentists. It also boasts a history of significant medical breakthroughs and some of the world's most modern facilities for medical diagnosis and treatment. The hospitals that make up Continuum Health Partners, Inc. feature major campuses all over Manhattan and in Brooklyn.

BETH ISRAEL MEDICAL CENTER

Beth Israel Medical Center has been serving the New York community for over a century. From its beginnings as a small dispensary serving the Lower East Side, Beth Israel has made it its mission "to provide the highest quality of patient care, with compassion and concern for each patient's well-being." While that mission still holds true today, Beth Israel Medical Center has grown into the largest provider of inpatient care in New York State, and one of the largest in the United States. It is the University Hospital and Manhattan Campus for the Albert Einstein College of Medicine and has one of the largest post-graduate teaching programs in the city.

Beth Israel is especially renowned for its many clinical areas of excellence, including:

Cardiology	Features The Heart Institute–a full range of diagnostic and treatment services. See sidebar.
Neurology	Features the Hyman-Newman Institute for Neurology and Neurosurgery (INN), a world-renowned center for the diagnosis and treatment of adults and children afflicted with neurological disorders. See sidebar.
Cancer	Features The Cancer Center–a comprehensive service for diagnosis, treatment and support of individuals with a wide range of cancers. See sidebar.
Orthopaedics	Offers diagnosis and treatment for all disorders of the musculoskeletal system. See sidebar.

Obstetrics	Combines the latest in high-tech delivery with alternative programs to provide the most comfortable birthing environment, with more than 5,700 births in 1996.
Pain Management	Features the first department for pain medicine and palliative care at a major teaching hospital in the country. See sidebar.
Spine Services	Features The Spine Institute, one of the first programs of its kind in New York to combine all the diagnostic and treatment services of spinal disorders of the back and neck under one roof. See sidebar.
HIV/AIDS Services	One of the largest providers of HIV/AIDS care in New York City with services such as The Peter Krueger Clinic for the Treatment of Immunological Disorders, and the Robert Mapplethorpe Residential Treatment Facility.
Chemical Dependency	The largest chemical dependency treatment program in the world, providing diagnosis, detoxification, treatment and aftercare.

ST. LUKE'S-ROOSEVELT HOSPITAL CENTER

Since their founding in 1846 and 1871, respectively, St. Luke's Hospital and Roosevelt Hospital has provided outstanding medical care to New Yorkers. Over the years, St. Luke's-Roosevelt pioneered many medical treatments and procedures, while remaining true to its mission to provide compassionate, state-of-the-art care to its patients. St. Luke's-Roosevelt is University Hospital for Columbia University College of Physicians and Surgeons and is one of the largest private teaching hospitals in the United States.

St. Luke's-Roosevelt Hospital Center is especially renowned for its many clinical areas of excellence, including:

Obstetrics	Special features include The Birthing Center, a home-like setting for labor, delivery and recovery; and services for high-risk pregnancies and births.
HIV/AIDS Services	Offers treatment and support of people living with HIV/AIDS through the Samuels Center for Comprehensive Care.
Cardiology	Features The Heart Center–comprehensive care for prevention, diagnosis and treatment of heart disease. See sidebar.
Hand Surgery	Features the C.V. Starr Hand Surgery Center, which uses the latest advances in the surgical treatment of injuries to the fingers, hand and wrist. See sidebar.
Diabetes	The Joslin Center for Diabetes offers patient-centered diabetes care and is the only New York City-based affiliate of the world-renowned center in Boston.
Emergency Services	Emergency medical services are available at both St. Luke's and Roosevelt, with a new level 1 trauma center at St. Luke's.
Sleep Disorders	New York's largest accredited sleep disorders center provides a full range of clinical services for sleep disorders.
Weight Management	The Theodore B. VanItallie Center for Nutrition and Weight Management is a program for the management of chronic obesity and related disorders, and one of only four centers in the country federally funded for obesity research.
Physical Rehabilitation	Independence Square is a unique rehabilitation service that incorporates elements of daily life in New York City into the clinical setting to help patients with disabling illnesses or injuries.
Chemical Dependency	The Smithers Alcoholism Treatment and Training Center has been an international leader in addiction treatment for over a quarter century, with a wide range of services to meet the needs of addiction problems.
Specialized Care	The Kathryn and Gilbert Miller Institute offers specialized health care–from occupational and physical therapy to primary care services–for actors, dancers, musicians and other performing artists.

THE LONG ISLAND COLLEGE HOSPITAL

The Long Island College Hospital has served the residents of Brooklyn and the wider metropolitan area since 1858. Today, LICH combines the best features of a major medical center, through teaching and research, with the personal approach of a community-centered hospital. Its mission–to provide the highest quality care in a caring environment–is emphasized every day throughout the hospital. As primary teaching affiliate of the SUNY Health Science Center at Brooklyn, The Long Island College Hospital offers training programs for resident physicians in more than 20 medical specialties.

The Long Island College Hospital is especially renowned for its many clinical areas of excellence, including:

Asthma / Allergies	Comprehensive services for asthma, allergies and immunology, and pulmonary medicine.
Bloodless Medicine	Features The New York Center for Bloodless Medicine and Surgery, with round-the-clock, on-site coordinators.
Cancer	Offers comprehensive cancer care, including extensive support services.
Dentistry	Offers high quality dental care with a wide range of leading edge services, including a Special Patient Care Center that provides dental care to physically and mentally challenged patients.
Nephrology	Established one of the largest renal dialysis programs in the country.
Neurology	Complete services for children and adults, including a comprehensive stroke center and the Stanley S. Lamm Institute for Child Neurology and Developmental Disabilities–one of the first centers in the nation for the treatment of neurological disabilities.
Ophthalmology	Features Brooklyn's only 24-hour ophthalmic trauma center with state-of-the-art equipment as well as the only facility in Brooklyn for the treatment of ocular cancer.
Otolaryngology	Comprehensive services include treatment for communicative disorders as well as head and neck surgery.
Pediatrics	Comprehensive, accessible pediatric medical and surgical services, including Brooklyn's only Cystic Fibrosis Center, treatment for digestive disorders and the borough's only Thalassemia treatment program.
Psychiatry	Full range of psychiatric services, including geriatric services and Brooklyn's only partial hospitalization program.
Urology	Features the New York Stone Center, the region's most comprehensive source for kidney stone treatment and prevention. Pioneered techniques for radical prostate surgery.
Women's Health	Provides a full range of women's health services, including a midwifery program and a hospital-based rape crisis intervention program.

Physician Referral	With more than 1,700 physicians in a wide range of specialties, The Referral Service can help you find a primary care physician or specialist affiliated with Beth Israel Medical Center, St. Luke's-Roosevelt Hospital Center or Long Island College Hospital. The Referral Staff is available Monday through Friday, from 8:30 a.m. to 6:00 p.m. Eastern Standard Time. A member of its multilingual staff can assist you in finding information about specialty care, convenient locations, insurance plans accepted and more. For a great doctor in your neighborhood, call **(800) 420-4004**.

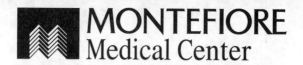

MONTEFIORE
Medical Center

**The University Hospital for the
Albert Einstein College of Medicine**

HENRY AND LUCY MOSES DIVISION	WEILER/EINSTEIN DIVISION
111 EAST 210TH STREET	1825 EASTCHESTER ROAD
BRONX, NY 10467-2490	BRONX, NY 10461-2373
PHONE (718) 920-4321	PHONE (718) 904-2000
FAX (718) 920-8543	FAX (718) 904-2189

Web Site www.montefiore.org

Sponsorship	Voluntary Not-for-Profit
Beds	1060
Accreditation	Joint Commission on Accreditation of Healthcare Organizations (JCAHO)

A PIONEER IN CLINICAL CARE, TEACHING, RESEARCH AND COMMUNITY OUTREACH

Montefiore Medical Center is internationally recognized as a leader in patient care, education, research and community service. Montefiore serves as a tertiary care referral center offering the most advanced care to patients from the entire New York City metropolitan area and across the nation. The medical center encompasses two acute care hospitals, two new ambulatory specialty care centers, a network of over 34 Montefiore Medical Group primary care offices in the Bronx and Westchester County, and one of the nation's largest home health agencies.

WESTCHESTER SPECIALTY PROGRAMS

Specialty centers in nearby Westchester County include the Fertility and Hormone Center in Dobbs Ferry, Women's Center in Larchmont, Laser & Eye Center in White Plains, and Multispecialty Center in Eastchester.

CENTERS OF EXCELLENCE

Heart Center
Comprehensive, state-of-the-art cardiac care for adults and children. (For more information, see Montefiore in the Centers of Excellence section.)

Cancer Care
Diagnosis and treatment of all major cancers. Montefiore, the clinical site for **The Albert Einstein Comprehensive Cancer Center, an NCI designated Cancer Center,** is finding and utilizing new treatments for colon, ovarian, cervical, breast, kidney and lung cancers, and acute leukemia...Active bone marrow transplant program; only center in NY to offer high-dose cytokine therapy for metastatic melanoma; first medical center in U.S. to treat melanoma and ovarian cancer with taxol; active radiation oncology service ...**The Albert Einstein Breast Center** enables women to obtain at one site, specialized breast cancer diagnoses and treatment....Only NY center in the **Women's Health Initiative**, a national study on heart disease, cancer and osteoporosis risk in post-menopausal women.

Neurosciences
Full range of subspecialty centers. **Epilepsy Center** has state-designated intensive care inpatient unit; physicians trained to administer ketogenic diet....**Stern Stroke Center** offers comprehensive treatment of all types of cerebrovascular disease; provides interventional stroke, tPA, other therapies.... **Sleep Disorders Center** treats patients with severe or long-standing problems associated with sleep and waking. Special **Narcolepsy Institute**.... **Headache Unit**, first facility of its kind in the world, treats rare forms of headache disorders; national studies on migraines, cluster and tension headaches.

Children's Health
Comprehensive pediatric care, with subspecialties in all areas. **Epilepsy Center** has intensive care unit; research focus on mechanisms of childhood seizures....**Center for Congenital Disorders** provides care to individuals with birth defects, including spina bifida, Down syndrome.... **Pediatric Otolaryngology** has special programs for communication disorders, audiology, speech, otitis media, adenotonsilar disorders.... **Pediatric Asthma Center** uses advanced pulmonary function tests and provides comprehensive treatment....**Adolescent AIDS/HIV Program** is the nation's oldest program of its kind for teens....New **Neonatal Intensive Care Unit**.

Women's Health
Full range of health and medical services for women of all ages. Unique subspecialties: a **Diabetes Pregnancy Program**....**Fertility and Hormone Center** in Dobbs Ferry, serves 900 couples annually for infertility problems with techniques such as IVF and ICSI or Intracytoplasmic Sperm Injection (for men with low sperm counts)....**Women's Health Laboratory**, a national leader in development of pregnancy screening tests for Tay-Sachs disease, Down syndrome and cystic fibrosis....**Perinatology Program** for high-risk pregnancies....Women's **Cancer** (see section on Cancer Care).... **Urinary Incontinence** specialists treat women over 65, one third of whom have this problem.

Other Specialties
Montefiore also has nationally recognized specialty programs in Ophthalmology (including laser surgery center), Diabetes, Thyroid Diseases, General Surgery, Vascular Surgery, Medicine, Urology, Rehabilitation Medicine, Radiology, Pathology, Orthopaedics, Plastic and Reconstructive Surgery, Kidney Transplantation and Psychiatry.

Physician Referral
Call 1-800-MD-MONTE (1-800-636-6683) to find a Montefiore physician.

THE MOUNT SINAI MEDICAL CENTER

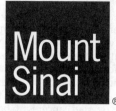

THE MOUNT SINAI
MEDICAL CENTER
ONE GUSTAVE L. LEVY PLACE
NEW YORK, NY 10029-6574
PHONE (212) 241-6500
1-800-MD-SINAI

Sponsorship	Voluntary Not-for-Profit
Beds	1,171
Accreditation	Joint Commission on Accreditation of Healthcare Organizations (JCAHO); Mount Sinai has nearly 25 clinical specialty departments recognized by their respective review organizations (e.g., American College, etc.)

GENERAL DESCRIPTION

The Mount Sinai Medical Center is home to one of the country's oldest and largest voluntary hospitals, and one of its premier medical schools. This partnership has enabled the merging of superb patient care, cutting-edge research and pioneering educational programs in a vibrant atmosphere. Here, in a preeminent academic health sciences institution, medical breakthroughs are swiftly and frequently ushered from the laboratory to the bedside. Indeed, since the Hospital's founding in 1852, Mount Sinai has been the source of some of the most important advances in medical history. Today, that legacy of innovation continues as we dedicate state-of-the-art resources to the most pressing medical issues of our time.

MEDICAL STAFF

The Mount Sinai Hospital has a medical staff of nearly 1,800 physicians in every medical and surgical specialty. More than 93% are board certified. Many of our physicians are nationally and internationally recognized for their expertise, and care for patients from around the globe. Listings of New York Magazine's 1998 "The Best Doctors in New York" included 114 Mount Sinai physicians; and 29 were named in American Health's 1996 listing of "The Best Doctors in America," making the staff one of the top five in the U.S.

TEACHING PROGRAMS

The Mount Sinai Hospital is a teaching facility with dozens of residency and fellowship programs in every specialty—from Anesthesiology to Urology. There are more than 800 residents and fellows, graduates of the finest medical schools, enrolled in our programs, all of which are approved by the Accreditation Council for Graduate Medical Education or the Council on Dental Education, and the appropriate medical specialty board.

SPECIAL PROGRAMS

Mount Sinai and its medical staff have been recognized for excellence in numerous specialties by unbiased sources, including outside physicians, and ranked among the best in our city and the country by such respected magazines as US News and World Report, American Health and New York.

Among those departments and services that are repeatedly singled out for excellence are the interdisciplinary Zena and Michael A. Wiener Cardiovascular Institute, which provides tertiary and quartenary care for those at risk for heart disease and those who suffer from acute cardiac illnesses. Our team of physicians and surgeons works with a full complement of rehabilitation experts and special services designed to help patients live life to the fullest.

Our Henry L. Schwartz Department of Geriatrics and Adult Development offers a full range of preventive care, inpatient and outpatient services for older adults. From outpatient care to a special inpatient unit designed to meet the special needs of the elderly, our services are guided by the principles of productive aging.

The Samuel Bronfman Department of Medicine's Division of Gastroenterology is consistently ranked among the best in the city. In addition to a full range of care and services, our staff works closely with members of our acclaimed Liver Transplant Team. These physicians performed the first liver transplantation surgery in New York State, and are recognized across the country as leaders in their field. Mount Sinai is also renowned for other transplantation surgery including combined organ transplantation. Our new Recanati/Miller Transplantation Institute integrates these diverse activities, to further clinical excellence, and facilitate research and the education and training of future leaders in transplantation.

At the Derald H. Ruttenberg Cancer Center, our pioneering scientists work tirelessly in the transformation of basic science findings into clinical applications. Through their efforts, Mount Sinai is developing exciting new ways to prevent and treat cancers of all kinds.

OTHER SERVICES

Mount Sinai's other special services include a Women's Health Center, a full range of inpatient and outpatient rehabilitation services, Home Care and a growing number of minimally invasive surgical procedures. We offer special services for individuals with Alzheimer's disease, for women with high-risk pregnancies and for children. Through The Mount Sinai Health System, our affiliated hospitals and long-term care facilities offer services throughout the New York/New Jersey metropolitan area.

PHYSICIAN REFERRAL

The Mount Sinai Hospital's free Physician Referral and Health Resource Service, 1-800-MD-SINAI (1-800-637-4624) is available to the general public weekdays from 8:30 am-6 pm. Staffed exclusively by registered nurses, the service provides: referrals to primary and specialty care physicians, as well as dentists, whose office hours, location and billing policies are right for individual callers; appointment scheduling assistance; and information on health promotion programs. All are on Mount Sinai's faculty and members of our leading medical staff.

THE NEW YORK AND PRESBYTERIAN HOSPITAL

THE NEW YORK HOSPITAL- CORNELL MEDICAL CENTER 525 EAST 68TH STREET NEW YORK, NY 10021 PHONE (212) 746-5454	COLUMBIA-PRESBYTERIAN MEDICAL CENTER 622 WEST 168TH STREET NEW YORK, NY 10032 PHONE (212) 305-2500

Sponsorship   Voluntary Not-for-Profit
Beds   2,170
Accreditation   Joint Commission on Accreditation of Healthcare Organizations (JCAHO), College of American Pathologists (CAP), Commission on Accreditation for Rehabilitation Facilities (CARF)

LOCATIONS

The New York and Presbyterian Hospital offers state-of-the-art inpatient and ambulatory services in two Manhattan locations — at New York Hospital-Cornell Medical Center (NYH) on the Upper East Side, and at Columbia-Presbyterian Medical Center (CPMC) in Washington Heights. The latest medical advances — some available nowhere else — are offered at both sites, assuring that patients receive only high-quality, efficient, and cost-effective health care.

MERGER

Patients throughout the tri-state area now have easy access to a broader range of traditional and innovative health care services as a result of an unprecedented merger between two major teaching hospitals — creating The New York and Presbyterian Hospital. The merger, which has brought together The New York Hospital and The Presbyterian Hospital, combines the best practices of these two world-renowned hospitals — in clinical care, teaching, research, and service to the communities of New York. With 2,170 beds, 87,000 discharges, and 841,000 outpatient visits annually, The New York and Presbyterian Hospital is the largest hospital in New York, and one of the largest and most comprehensive health care institutions in the world. Benefits to patients made possible by the merger include a new liver transplantation program, the Gamma Knife (a technology to treat brain tumors), and a center to treat spine disorders.

A SYSTEM OF QUALITY

To help meet the health care needs of residents throughout the metropolitan area, The New York and Presbyterian Hospital has developed a full-service network that includes acute-care and community hospitals, long-term-care facilities, home health agencies, ambulatory sites, physicians groups, and specialty institutions. With its members committed to providing high-quality, cost-effective, and conveniently accessible care, this network serves the residents of Manhattan, Brooklyn, Queens, and the Bronx, as well as Westchester, Long Island, New Jersey, Connecticut, and several upstate New York counties.

ACADEMIC AFFILIATIONS

The New York and Presbyterian Hospital is uniquely positioned as the primary teaching hospital for two of the nation's most prestigious medical schools: Cornell University Medical College and Columbia University College of Physicians and Surgeons. All faculty members hold appointments with both the hospital and at least one of the medical schools.

CENTERS OF EXCELLENCE OF
THE NEW YORK AND PRESBYTERIAN HOSPITAL (PARTIAL LISTING)

Pediatrics
The world-renowned Babies & Children's Hospital (which is found at the CPMC location) was the first hospital established for infants and children, and was the site of the first successful pediatric heart transplant surgery. The NYH location includes a renowned Perinatology Center (the first designated regional referral center for newborns), Pediatric Critical Care Center, and Pediatric Endocrinology Division.

Cardiac Care
At both locations, patients can access many of the nations leading cardio-thoracic surgeons. The heart transplant program (CPMC) is the country's largest, with surgeons known for their pioneering work in the development of partial artificial hearts and minimally invasive surgery. The cardiac catheterization program is the largest in New York State, and the bloodless cardiac surgery program is the first in the tri-state area (NYH). At both locations, cardiac patients receive world-class rehabilitative care designed to extend and improve their lives.

Burn Center
The largest and busiest burn center in the nation is located at the NYH site, where more than 1,300 inpatients and 4,000 outpatients are treated annually. Its research has led to significant improvements in the survival rate and quality of life for both adults and children.

Cancer Care
The Herbert Irving Comprehensive Cancer Center is only the second cancer center in the metropolitan area to have received the designation "comprehensive" from the National Institutes of Health (CPMC). Comprehensive cancer care is also provided at the NYH location.

Trauma Center
The New York and Presbyterian Hospital is one of only three hospitals in the country and the only one in New York to offer both a Level 1 Adult Trauma Unit (NYH) and a Level 1 Pediatric Trauma Unit (CPMC). (A "Level 1" designation indicates the highest standards of 24-hour preparedness and treatment.)

Aids Care
The Center for Special Studies provides continuous comprehensive care for men, women, and children with HIV/AIDS (NYH). Complete care is also available at the CPMC location. Both sites are New York State - and National Institutes of Health-designated AIDS centers.

Neurological Care
Both sites provide the latest in the research, diagnosis, and treatment of Alzheimer's and Parkinson's diseases, multiple sclerosis, movement disorders, aneurysms, epilepsy, brain tumors, and strokes. The CPMC location is widely recognized for treating the largest stroke caseload worldwide, having the lowest mortality rate for aneurysm surgery in the state, and being a pioneer in hypothermic arrest surgery.

Reproductive Medicine and Infertility
The hospital's two IVF programs are world-renowned: for treating more than 1,200 couples annually with a success rate that is double the national average (at NYH); and for being a national leader in treating women over the age of 40 (at CPMC).

Complementary Care Center
The New York and Presbyterian Hospital includes one of the first academic-based centers to investigate alternative methods of healing, including biofeedback and aromatherapy (CPMC).

Women's Health
Even before the merger, the two individual hospitals were among the nation's leaders in the field of women's health: The New York Hospital was the first to develop the PAP test, and a division of The Presbyterian Hospital, the Sloane Hospital for Women, was the first to perform amniocentesis and the first to perform surgery on a fetus *in utero*.

Gene Therapy
Innovative research programs at both locations have made recent advances in treating conditions such as cardiac ischemia and atherosclerosis, breast cancer, and cystic fibrosis.

Physician Referral
1-800-227-CPMC (for the Columbia-Presbyterian location)

1-800-822-2NYH (for the New York Hospital-Cornell location)

NYU MEDICAL CENTER

Tisch Hospital & Rusk Institute of Rehabilitation Medicine

550 FIRST AVENUE
NEW YORK, NY 10016
PHONE: (212) 263-7300 (GENERAL INFORMATION)
PHYSICIAN REFERRAL - 1- 888-7-MED-NYU

Sponsorship	**Private. Not-for-Profit**
Beds	**879 beds**
Accreditation	**Joint Commission on Accreditation of Healthcare Organizations,** Commission for Accreditation of Rehabilitation Facilities **(CARF)**

A LEADER IN PATIENT CARE

NYU Medical Center is one of the nation's leading biomedical resources, combining excellence in patient care, research and medical education. A not-for-profit institution, NYU Medical Center operates Tisch Hospital, a voluntary 705-bed tertiary care facility serving more than 29,402 inpatients annually, and the Rusk Institute of Rehabilitation Medicine, which has 174 beds and serves 1,000 inpatients and more than 77,000 outpatients annually. The Medical Center also includes the Hospital for Joint Diseases Orthopaedic Institute, which has 220 beds and is one of the nation's premier hospitals for treating orthopedic and rheumatological disorders, and NYU Downtown Hospital, a 330-bed facility

A DISTINGUISHED FACULTY

NYU School of Medicine has approximately 4,510 faculty members who are attending physicians at Tisch Hospital, Rusk Institute, the Hospital for Joint Diseases, NYU Downtown and Bellevue Hospital one of the largest and oldest municipal hospitals in North America, and an affiliate of NYU Medical Center. Many faculty members have distinguished national and international reputations.

A LEADER IN EDUCATION

NYU School of Medicine enrolls more than 650 students and has over 960 resident physicians who are graduates of the nation's finest medical schools. NYU School of Medicine offers a rich educational experience, providing residency programs in dermatology, gynecology, neurosurgery, medicine ophthalmology, orthopedics, pediatrics, psychiatry, radiology, surgery and urology.

CENTERS OF EXCELLENCE

Cancer	**The Rita J. & Stanley H. Kaplan Comprehensive Cancer Center** provides state-of-the-art cancer therapy and supportive care for patients with cancer, as well as diagnostic services for the early detection of cancer and educational programs on cancer prevention. Under the Kaplan's auspices are: **The Comprehensive Breast Cancer Center**, providing the latest treatments for breast cancer as well as genetic testing and counseling for patients and their families; **The Breast Imaging Center** offering diagnostic and screening services for the early diagnosis of breast cancer and **The Hassenfeld Children's Center for Cancer and Blood Disorders**, providing treatment for children with cancer and blood diseases in an exceptionally caring environment.
Cardiac Surgery	**NYU Medical Center's** cardiovascular surgeons were among the first nationwide to repair and replace diseased mitral heart valves without cracking open the chest. They are leaders in the development of minimally invasive techniques for heart valve and bypass surgery, which are less painful and require a much shorter recovery period.

Cardiology	NYU Medical Center has a longstanding commitment to provide excellent cardiac care. **The Pediatric Cardiology Program** provides comprehensive care to children who have congenital or acquired heart diseases. **The Joan and Joel Smilow Cardiac Prevention and Rehabilitation Center** provides an array of services for people at risk for heart disease and those recovering from cardiac surgery.
Child and Adolescent Mental Health	**The Child Study Center** is dedicated to advancing the understanding and treatment of child and adolescent mental health. It is the first and only program in New York to offer a comprehensive psychiatric program for children and their families.
Epilepsy	**The Comprehensive Epilepsy Center** is the largest facility of its kind on the East Coast. More than 2,000 adults and children receive help here each year. The Center's unique team approach includes evaluations with epileptologists, neuropsychologists and neurosurgeons, as well as diagnostic studies and therapies for seizure control. Special facilities are available for patients with an uncertain diagnosis, some of whom have been misdiagnosed with epilepsy.
Gamma Knife	**The Gamma Knife Unit** is the newest addition to one of the most technologically advanced neurosurgical departments in the country. The Gamma Knife offers many advantages over conventional surgery and is used to remove certain types of tumors, aneurysms, and arteriovenous malformations too deep within the brain to reach with a scalpel. Unlike conventional neurosurgery, the Gamma Knife is bloodless and patients usually return home the day after surgery.
Obstetrics & Gynecology	NYU Medical Center offers some of the most comprehensive services for women's health in the metropolitan area. Its medical staff is recognized nationally for pioneering many diagnostic techniques and for surgical innovations to treat a wide variety of diseases.
Organ Transplants	**The Mary Lea Richards Organ Transplantation Program** is one of the nation's leading centers for liver, kidney and pancreas transplants. The liver transplant program was ranked number one on the East Coast by the United Network for Organ Sharing and was among the top five nationally in a 1997 survey.
Pain Management	**The Pain Management Center** provides a comprehensive, holistic approach to managing acute and chronic pain. It offers extensive diagnostic and therapeutic services all in one location. The team consults with many specialists, creating an integrated approach individualized for each patient. Acute cancer and chronic pain management services are Center specialty services.
Plastic Surgery	**The Institute of Reconstructive Plastic Surgery** is internationally renowned. As the largest facility of its kind in the world, its staff performs 6,000 operations a year, treating problems ranging from facial reconstructive surgery to severe deformities stemming from congenital birth defects, injuries and burns. Its staff has pioneered techniques in craniofacial surgery, microsurgery, hand surgery, breast reconstruction and aesthetic surgery.
Pregnancy (High Risk)	NYU Medical Center provides a host of services for high-risk pregnancies. **The Program for IVF, Reproductive Surgery and Infertility** is at the leading edge of assisting couples who have trouble conceiving. **The Maternal-Fetal Medicine Program** helps women with risks, such as twins, triplets, hypertension, diabetes or heart problems. **The Recurrent Pregnancy Loss Program** enables women who have a history of miscarriage to bear healthy babies.
Skin Diseases	**The Charles C. Harris Skin and Cancer Unit** is an internationally acclaimed center for the treatment of serious and rare skin diseases, and also provides regular outpatient services in specialty clinics for a wide range of common skin problems.
Urology	NYU Medical Center's urologists are leaders in treating prostate disorders and prostate cancer as well as many other male and female urological problems. They also have helped pioneer the use of minimally invasive surgical techniques to preserve a man's sexual function after surgery for prostate cancer. They were also leaders in clinical trials for Viagra.
Physician Referral 1-888-7-MED-NYU	NYU Medical Center provides a free telephone referral service from 9 a.m. to 5 p.m. weekdays. The service is offered to the public and gives access to over 4,000 NYU physicians.

SAINT VINCENTS HOSPITAL AND MEDICAL CENTER

153 WEST 11TH STREET
NEW YORK, NY 10011
(212) 604-7000

CHARITY. SCIENCE. SERVICE.

With 783 inpatient beds, Saint Vincents Hospital is a major tertiary care and teaching hospital in the heart of Lower Manhattan. We're also the academic medical center of New York Medical College. Sponsored by the Sisters of Charity and the Archdiocese of New York, our resources and centers bring outstanding care to people in every stage of health, sickness and recovery – wherever they live or work in the city.

Serving an entire community means learning from and growing with the people we serve. Members of our staff take their cue from the Sisters of Charity who founded Saint Vincent's in 1849. Good medicine requires the best science. But its right hand is always compassion and understanding. Our caring nurses, doctors, social workers, counselors and volunteers are all people you can depend on in the worst of times. As well as for the best preventive medicine.

> *"I think the word that comes to mind is 'dignity.' They treat us as if our dignity were something very precious."*
>
> — *Carmen Velazquez, Daughter of a Patient*

Saint Vincent's is accredited by the Joint Commission for the Accreditation of Health Care Organizations. Ninety-three percent of our doctors are Board Certified, meaning they've met the highest standards in their chosen fields. Our experts bring the kind of insight and authority to their daily work that can turn a broken life into a renewed one. In settings like our Cystic Fibrosis Center, they're hastening future cures for chronic and terminal illnesses. They're leaders within the professional community. And as many patients testify, they're people you can trust with your life.

> *"To me his opinion is gold. I think that's the best thing you can say about a doctor."*
>
> — *Paul Weissman, Melanoma Patient*

CENTERS OF EXCELLENCE

Emergency Services

Our Emergency Room offers 24-hour access to a Level I Trauma Center where critical care experts handle the most complex emergencies. Their cardiac expertise has been recognized with a special heart care designation by the American Heart Association. Even patients with minor emergencies receive timely care through our Rapid Care Unit. There's also a separate adjoining area designed to soothe our youngest patients.

The Comprehensive Cardiovascular Center

Since we opened the nation's first coronary care unit in 1964, we've helped lengthen lives through free heart care screenings. Throughout our hospital – from the ER to the Intensive Care Unit – our cardiologists and cardiac surgeons are equally involved in every case, offering procedures that are minimally invasive whenever possible. We also offer internationally renowned experts in cardiac surgery. And some of the highest survival rate statistics of any hospital in the State of New York.

The Comprehensive Cancer Center

Helping our patients and their families meet the very special challenges they face is the central focus of The Saint Vincents Comprehensive Cancer Center. Largely because of this supportive philosophy that strengthens our excellent medical care, we've attracted some of the best cancer doctors in the world. In fact, our oncologists and other cancer experts have spearheaded leading research that has resulted in many of the newest breakthroughs in the diagnosis and treatment of cancer.

The Comprehensive HIV Center

Saint Vincent's is the city's premier one-stop source for HIV care and the latest-breaking therapies. From 1981 onward, our doctors and nurse practitioners have provided "leading edge" treatment and services. Newly expanded in 1997, our center addresses complex needs with more resources than ever. Testing, counseling, support groups, early intervention services and access to our innovative HIV-fighting drugs are all available in a compassionate setting. And, our patients and their families often describe our nursing care as second to none.

Women's Health

Each month, Saint Vincent's provides a wellspring of seminars and classes on women's health issues, including breast cancer, menopause, nutrition, healthy aging, childbirth, parenting and much more. Our Maternity Services offer the full range of birthing and gynecological options, with an open-minded regard for women's preferences and needs. Our affiliate, the Elizabeth Seton Childbearing Center is known throughout the city for its outstanding midwife care and intimate environment.

Choosing a Saint Vincent's Doctor.

Give our Doctor Directory a call at 1-888-4-SVH-DOC (1-888-478-4362) and we'll help you choose one of our outstanding doctors located throughout the city. Most participate in all major managed care plans.

SPECIALTY HOSPITALS

The New York metropolitan region is unique in its concentration of excellent specialty hospitals. Specialty Hospitals include those with a specific patient and disease focus such as cardiac care, psychiatric care and care of diseases and problems of eyes and ears. Many of these hospitals are nationally and internationally known for their outstanding care in these specialty areas and draw patients from the region and beyond who seek their excellent specialized care.

Castle Connolly Medical Ltd. has invited the following outstanding specialty hospitals to present important facts and information on their hospitals by sponsoring the profiles that follow.

Specialty Hospitals

CALVARY HOSPITAL

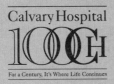

Calvary Hospital

For a Century, It's Where Life Continues

1740 EASTCHESTER ROAD
BRONX, NY 10461
PHONE (718) 518-2300
FAX (718) 518-2670

ds	200
creditation	Joint Commission on Accreditation of Healthcare Organizations (JCAHO) <u>with Commendation</u>; College of American Pathologists (CAP)

TRADITION OF CARING

ce its inception in 1899, this voluntary, not-for-profit, Archdiocesan hospital has specialized in wiading palliative care to adult patients in the advanced stages of cancer, addressing the symptoms of disease, not its cure. Calvary continues to embody this tradition of caring through the services and grams offered and through the dedication and concern shown by its staff members.

LLIATIVE CARE INSTITUTE

e Palliative Care Institute (PCI), Calvary's research and education arm, shares the hospital's expertise he care of advanced cancer patients with the community through its curriculum for medical students, gram for visiting physicians, distinguished lectures, palliative medicine conferences, palliative care inars, and the support of clinical investigation.

ROGRAMS OF CARE

ute Inpatient Specialty spital Services	Upon admission, patients are assigned a primary physician, registered nurse, social worker, registered dietitian, chaplin and case manager who work together with the patient and family to maximize physical, spiritual and emotional comfort.
tpatient Services	This Department works to control symptoms of advanced cancer for patients who do not require acute inpatient care. Personalized care plans are developed by an interdisciplinary team of clinicians in conjunction with the patient and family.
me Care	Calvary's Certified Home Health Agency provides a full range of home care services, (not limited to patients with advanced cancer), to support patients and their families.
spice	Please inquire about our new Hospice services.

JPPORT PROGRAMS

nily Support Group	These meetings give familes an opportunity to discuss the impact of the patient's illness on themselves.
ult Bereavement Group	Care for families does not end with the death of the patient. Bereavement groups are held throughout the year by Social Work and Pastoral Care.
l's Place	Structured activities help children ages 6 to 11 express their anticipatory grief.
cious Moments	This after school program teaches children ages 6 to 11 healthy ways of handling loss.
mmunity Cancer ient Support Group	Cancer patients in the community may join at any stage of illness from diagnosis to survivorship.
mmunity Cancer regivers Support Group	This weekly group teaches familes, friends, and caregivers of cancer patients new ways of coping with stressful situations related to cancer.
spite & Recreation gram	Allows adult patient visitors an opportunity to engage in activities designed to relieve stress.
ysician Referral	For further information about Calvary Hospital, please call (718) 518-2300, or visit our website at www.calvaryhospital.org.

FOUR WINDS HOSPITAL

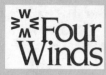

800 CROSS RIVER ROAD
KATONAH, NEW YORK 10536
PHONE (914) 763-8151
FAX (914) 763-9597

Sponsorship	Private
Beds	175 psychiatric
Accreditation	Joint Commission on Accreditation of Healthcare Organizations (JCAHO), New York State Office of Mental Health, NYS Office of Alcoholism and Substance Abuse Services (OASAS)

DESCRIPTION

Four Winds is an acute care psychiatric hospital. Inpatient and outpatient treatment services are prov ed for children, adolescents, adults, and older adults. Four Winds is the largest specialized provider child and adolescent mental health services in the Northeast.

ADMISSION INFORMATION

Quality treatment, delivered at the appropriate level, is not only clinically effective, but also cost-effecti Each individual is evaluated and placed into the appropriate program, either inpatient or outpatie depending on their needs at the time of their admission.

24 HOUR EVALUATION AND REFERRAL SERVICE

Four Winds accepts individuals 24 hours a day, 7 days a week. Consultations and evaluations can scheduled ahead of time, or done on a crisis basis. Individuals are triaged to the appropriate level of ca

INPATIENT TREATMENT PROGRAMS

Child	A multidisciplinary, experienced, caring, professional staff works with children age through 12 in homelike cottages. Intensive treatment incorporates play therapy a family therapy.
Adolescent	This service integrates individual, group and family therapy with a full compleme of educational, expressive, and recreational therapies. Special programs for dua diagnosed adolescents (psychiatric/substance abuse).
Adult	Acute treatment includes psychotherapy and pharmacological management, co bined with recreational and educational therapies. Special programs for dually dia nosed individuals and survivors of abuse and trauma.
Older Adult	This service focuses on individuals 60 years of age and older in need of treatment disorders specifically identified with the older generation.

OUTPATIENT TREATMENT SERVICES

CHOICES	A full service alcohol/chemical dependency outpatient center providing assessme interventions, early recovery group, ambulatory detox and acupuncture.
Partial Hospitalization	Adolescent and Adult alternative to inpatient treatment. Intensive, structured progra provides individual, group and family treatment. 1-800-528-6624, ext. 2200.
Adolescent Intensive	This after school group program provides intensive, structured outpatient treatme for individuals ages 13-17. 1-914-242-8888.
Consultation Services	Consultation and Evaluation Services including crisis evaluations are provided at fo locations: Westchester, New York City, Fishkill, NY, Fairfield, Ct. 1-800-528-6624.
Physician Referral	Four Winds provides triage services 24 hours a day, 7 days a week. For Admissions and Referrals call 1-800-546-1770.

HOSPITAL FOR JOINT DISEASES

301 East 17th Street (at Second Avenue)
New York, NY 10003
212-598-6000 FAX 212-260-1203
Website: www.hjd.com

Sponsorship	New York University Health System
Beds	220
Accreditation	Joint Commission on Accreditation of Healthcare Organizations (JCAHO)

PROFILE
The Hospital for Joint Diseases is one of the nation's leading orthopaedic, rheumatologic, neurologic, and rehabilitation specialty hospitals dedicated to the prevention and treatment of neuromusculoskeletal diseases. HJD is a voluntary, not-for-profit teaching hospital, and a member organization of the NYU Health System.

MEDICAL STAFF
The Hospital for Joint Diseases has 440 attending medical staff. Over 90% of the medical staff are Board certified.

TEACHING PROGRAMS
The Hospital for Joint Diseases offers a five-year residency program in Orthopaedic Surgery, and seven fellowships in Orthopaedic Surgery in the following areas: hand, spine, sports medicine, total joint replacement, shoulder, foot and ankle, and pediatrics.

SPECIAL PROGRAMS

Orthopaedic Surgery	Hip and Knee Replacement Center, Arthroscopic Surgery Bone Tumor Service, Foot and Ankle Surgery, Hand Surgery Limb Lengthening and Bone Growth, Occupational and Industrial Orthopaedic Care, Sports Medicine, Pediatric Orthopaedics Shoulder Institute, Center for Neuromuscular and Developmental Disorders, The Geriatric Hip Fracture Program, The Scoliosis Program The Spine Center, The Harkness Center for Dance Injuries 24-hour Urgent Orthopaedic Care
Center for Arthritis and Autoimmunity	Fibromyalgia, Lupus, Lyme Disease, Osteoarthritis, Osteoporosis Psoriatic Arthritis, Rheumatoid Arthritis, Scleroderma, Sjogren's Syndrome
Neurology	Orthopaedic Neurology, Initiative for Women with Disabilities Multiple Sclerosis, Epilepsy, Neuroimmunolgy, Neurohematology Cerebral Palsy, Attention Deficit Disorder, Pain Center
Rehabilitation Medicine	Physical and Occupational Therapy

OTHER SERVICES

Managed Care Plans	The Hospital for Joint Diseases participates in over 45 managed care plans covering 72 different products (i.e., HMO, POS, PPO, Medicare Medicaid, etc)
Physician Referral	The hospital offers a free telephone physician referral services, Monday — Friday, 8:00am — 4:00pm. The physician referral service can be reached at 1-888-HJD-DOCS (1-888-453-3627)

THE NEW YORK EYE & EAR INFIRMARY

SECOND AVENUE AT FOURTEENTH S
NEW YORK, NEW YORK 10003
PHONE (212) 979-4000
FAX (212) 228-0664

Sponsorship	Voluntary Not-for-Profit
Beds	103
Accreditation	Joint Commission on the Accreditation of Healthcare Organizations
	College of American Pathologists

ABOUT THE NEW YORK EYE AND EAR INFIRMARY

The New York Eye and Ear Infirmary is one of the world's leading facilities for the diagnosis and tre
ment of diseases of the eyes, ears, nose, throat and related conditions. A voluntary, not-for-profit insti
tion, the Infirmary is affiliated with New York Medical College and offers residency programs in op
thalmology and otolaryngology/head and neck surgery.

THE MEDICAL STAFF

The Medical Staff includes more than 500 attending physicians and surgeons throughout the metropc
tan area. Many are renowned for their breakthrough research introducing widely practiced technique:

RESEARCH AND EDUCATION

The New York Eye and Ear Infirmary is a national and international leader in research in its specialti
achieving many "firsts" in successful surgical procedures and medical treatments. Laboratories inclu
Cell Culture, Temporal Bone and the Aborn Center for Eye Research.

SPECIALTIES

Ophthalmology	Within this area are subspecialties of cataract, glaucoma, retina, cornea and refracti surgery, ocular plastic surgery, pediatric ophthalmology, and strabismus, neuro-op thalmology and ocular tumor. Laser, photography, fluorescein angiography and ele tro-physiological testing are among the most advanced services available anywhere
Otolaryngology	The department is in the forefront of treatment modalities using highly sophisticat endoscopic and laser equipment. Subspecialties include allergy, voice, rhinology, he & neck surgery, otology, neurotology, pediatric otolaryngology, audiology, speech the apy and hearing aid dispensing.
Plastic & Reconstructive Surgery	Microsurgical capabilities and premium patient accommodations provide an optimu environment for facial plasty, liposuction and repair of defects from disease or traum

RELATED SERVICES

New York Eye Trauma Center	An advanced program for emergency treatment of eye injuries, it handles a si nificant percentage of all cases reported to the National Eye Trauma Center.
Vision Correction Center	State-of-the art facility dedicated to all forms of laser refractive surgery performed an academic medical center which is in the forefront of teaching and research.
Ambulatory Surgery	A comprehensive Ambulatory Surgery Center is designed to expedite admission te: ing, pre-op preparation and post-op recovery in an efficient and comfortable setting
Pediatric Specialty Care	The city's only such center coordinating the services of eye and ear, nose and thrc specialists with other staff especially sensitive to the youngest patients.
Physician Referral	Call 1-800-449-HOPE (4673)

ST. FRANCIS HOSPITAL
THE HEART CENTER

100 PORT WASHINGTON BLVD.
ROSLYN, NY 11576
PHONE (516) 562-6000   FAX (516) 562-6909

onsorship	Voluntary Not-for-Profit
ds	279
creditation	Awarded *Accreditation With Commendation* from the Joint Commission on Accreditation of Healthcare Organizations for the third consecutive, three-year period
filiations	A member of Catholic Health Services of Long Island; a teaching affiliate of the Columbia University College of Physicians and Surgeons and The New York and Presbyterian Hospital

NATIONAL LEADER IN CARDIAC CARE

Francis Hospital, The Heart Center, New York's only specialty designated cardiac center, has the ghest cardiac caseload in the Northeast and the second largest in the United States.

ONSISTENT, OBJECTIVE EVIDENCE OF HIGH QUALITY

e Heart Center is committed to excellence in all aspects of cardiac care and to other medical and rgical services necessary to support the cardiovascular patient. The Hospital's nurse-to-patient tio is more than 2:1 and the patient satisfaction rate is a resounding 95%.

XPERIENCED IN CARDIAC CARE AND SURGERY

en Heart Surgery	Performed 2,574 open heart surgeries in 1997; the only New York hospital with a risk-adjusted mortality rate significantly below the statewide average for coronary bypass surgery, for all three-year periods analyzed by the New York State Department of Health (1989-1995).
rdiac Catheterization d Angioplasty	Site of 7,992 cardiac catheterizations and 2,357 coronary angioplasties in 1997 with the lowest mortality rate for coronary angioplasty in New York State.
rhythmia and cemaker Center	Largest pacemaker and arrhythmia program in the United States.
inimally Invasive eart Surgery	A leading center using the Port-Access™ device for bypass and valve surgery, with zero coronary mortality.

REVENTION, EDUCATION AND REHABILITATION PROGRAMS

e DeMatteis Center r Cardiac Research d Education	The only free-standing campus in the region dedicated to cardiac disease prevention, this facility is the site of more than 30 community education programs in fitness, safety, nutrition and cardiac health.
trafast CT scanner	A noninvasive and painless six-minute Ultrafast CT scan can detect calcification in the coronary arteries, an indication of atherosclerosis. The only one of its kind in the NY metro area, the scanner allows for early diagnosis of coronary artery disease, years before symptoms appear. Ideal for men ages 40-70; women ages 50-70.
rdiac Fitness Center	Four-phased medically supervised rehabilitation program for recovering heart patients and those at risk for heart disease.
pid Center	Offers coronary risk factor evaluation and modification, including lipid profiles, nutritional counseling and medical therapy.
ysician Referral	Physician listings are available by calling Medical Staff Affairs at (516) 562-6725 or through St. Francis Hospital's website at http://www. StFrancisHeartCenter.com.

REGIONAL MEDICAL CENTERS AND COMMUNITY HOSPITALS

The New York metropolitan region is fortunate to have a large number of truly excellent regional medical centers and community hospitals. Many of these institutions offer sophisticated services that in years past were offered only at academic medical centers. However, with advancements in medical technology, regional medical centers and community hospitals have access to the equipment, and by virtue of the medical schools and teaching hospitals in the region, the well-trained physicians and staff, to offer these programs.

Regional medical centers and community hospitals range in size from the small (100 beds) to the very large (800 beds) but they share a common theme: a primary focus on patient care.

We have invited a selected number of excellent community hospitals to provide readers of the Castle Connolly Guide with information on their institutions and services by sponsoring the following profiles.

THE STATE OF NEW YORK

PHYSICIAN'S LISTING

Information on hospitals in New York State may be found as follows:

NEW YORK (MANHATTAN) COUNTY

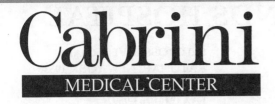

227 EAST 19TH STREET
NEW YORK, NY 10003
PHONE (212) 995-6000
PHYSICIAN REFERRAL
(212) CABRINI   (212) 222-7464
WEBSITE: www.cabrininy.org

onsorship	Voluntary, not-for-profit, sponsored by the Missionary Sisters of the Sacred Heart of Jesus
ds	444 acute, 30 psych, 45 hospice, 544 nursing home
ccreditation	Joint Commission on Accreditation of Healthcare Organizations (JCAHO), Accrediting Council for Graduate Medical Education, College of American Pathologists

ABRINI TRADITION

or over a century, Cabrini Medical Center has provided the New York metropolitan area with a strong adition of excellence in medical care. An acute care community-based teaching hospital, CMC is a member of The Mount Sinai Health System, an affiliate of Mount Sinai School of Medicine, and an associate ember of the Catholic Health Care Network. It is a Level II Trauma Center and 911 receiving hospital. ounded in 1892 by Mother Frances Xavier Cabrini, CMC continues to carry out her commitment to providing excellent health care in a caring, healing and compassionate environment.

PECIALTY SERVICES

abrini Medical Center has a dedicated, caring attending medical staff of 675. CMC's comprehensive specialty services are vast: ambulatory surgery, cancer care, eye care, ENT services, emergency cardiac care, ospice, pediatric hospice, laser and minimally invasive surgery (Indigo Laser Treatment for benign nlarged prostate and Advanced Breast Biopsy Instrumentation), oncology, osteoporosis screening, geriatric care, orthopedics, total joint replacement and other surgical specialties, rehabilitation medicine, urology, hyperbaric oxygen therapy, wound care, and certified home health care. Cabrini Center for Nursing nd Rehabilitation in Manhattan and St. Cabrini Nursing Home in Westchester County offer short/long-rm care.

OMPASSIONATE TOUCH

| ancer Center | CMC offers one of the most comprehensive and effective cancer care programs in New York, using the most sophisticated technology for screening and treatment, provided by a team of specialists in a patient-friendly, compassion-driven environment. |
| ospice Care | Renowned nationally as a model program, Cabrini Hospice is noted for its commitment to effectively and compassionately meet the needs of patients with advanced illness. |

QUALITY CARE

ound Care	Dramatized by its 82% healing rate, Cabrini Wound Care Center®, one of New York's most comprehensive, avoids amputation and heals chronic wounds by effectively combining aggressive medical treatment, after care, nutrition counseling and education. CMC has the only hyberbaric oxygen therapy center in Manhattan.
amily Medicine	CMC provides comprehensive primary care services that cater to families — from prenatal moms and children, to teens and grandparents — at Cabrini East Village, Cabrini Haven Plaza, Cabrini Madison Avenue and Cabrini Stuyvesant Polyclinic. These family practices provide internal medicine, preventive care, pediatrics and adolescent care, and women's health.
hysician Referral	Cabrini's referral services include information on 400 doctors, including education/training, insurances accepted, office hours and languages spoken. Information is also available on CMC primary care services and health education seminars/programs. For information, call 212-CABRINI (212-222-7464).

FOUR WINDS HOSPITAL

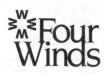

800 CROSS RIVER ROAD
KATONAH, NEW YORK 10536
PHONE (914) 763-8151
FAX (914) 763-9597

Sponsorship	Private
Beds	175 psychiatric
Accreditation	Joint Commission on Accreditation of Healthcare Organizations (JCAHO), New York State Office of Mental Health, NYS Office of Alcoholism and Substance Abuse Services (OASAS)

DESCRIPTION

Four Winds is an acute care psychiatric hospital. Inpatient and outpatient treatment services are provided for children, adolescents, adults, and older adults. Four Winds is the largest specialized provider child and adolescent mental health services in the Northeast.

ADMISSION INFORMATION

Quality treatment, delivered at the appropriate level, is not only clinically effective, but also cost-effectiv Each individual is evaluated and placed into the appropriate program, either inpatient or outpatien depending on their needs at the time of their admission.

24 HOUR EVALUATION AND REFERRAL SERVICE

Four Winds accepts individuals 24 hours a day, 7 days a week. Consultations and evaluations can l scheduled ahead of time, or done on a crisis basis. Individuals are triaged to the appropriate level of car

INPATIENT TREATMENT PROGRAMS

Child	A multidisciplinary, experienced, caring, professional staff works with children ages through 12 in homelike cottages. Intensive treatment incorporates play therapy ar family therapy.
Adolescent	This service integrates individual, group and family therapy with a full compleme of educational, expressive, and recreational therapies. Special programs for dual diagnosed adolescents (psychiatric/substance abuse).
Adult	Acute treatment includes psychotherapy and pharmacological management, con bined with recreational and educational therapies. Special programs for dually dia nosed individuals and survivors of abuse and trauma.
Older Adult	This service focuses on individuals 60 years of age and older in need of treatment f disorders specifically identified with the older generation.

OUTPATIENT TREATMENT SERVICES

CHOICES	A full service alcohol/chemical dependency outpatient center providing assessmen interventions, early recovery group, ambulatory detox and acupuncture.
Partial Hospitalization	Adolescent and Adult alternative to inpatient treatment. Intensive, structured progra provides individual, group and family treatment. 1-800-528-6624, ext. 2200.
Adolescent Intensive	This after school group program provides intensive, structured outpatient treatmer for individuals ages 13-17. 1-914-242-8888.
Consultation Services	Consultation and Evaluation Services including crisis evaluations are provided at fou locations: Westchester, New York City, Fishkill, NY, Fairfield, Ct. 1-800-528-6624.
Physician Referral	Four Winds provides triage services 24 hours a day, 7 days a week. For Admissions and Referrals call 1-800-546-1770.

LENOX HILL HOSPITAL

100 EAST 77TH STREET
NEW YORK, NY 10021
PHONE (212) 434-2000

Sponsorship	Voluntary Not-for-Profit
Beds	652 Beds
Accreditation	Joint Commission on Accreditation of Healthcare Organizations (JCAHO), College of American Pathologists, American Association of Blood Banks, Accreditation Council for Graduate Medical Education, Accreditation Council for Continuing Medical Education

GENERAL DESCRIPTION

Lenox Hill Hospital, which was founded in 1857, is an acute care, fully accredited teaching hospital with an outstanding reputation for providing the highest quality patient care and for pioneering innovative treatments. The hospital offers a wide range of medical, surgical, pediatric, obstetrical, gynecological and psychiatric services.

MEDICAL STAFF

Lenox Hill Hospital has over 1,200 physicians on staff—with outstanding national reputations in their fields. Over 90% are board certified.

TEACHING PROGRAMS

The hospital offers 13 residency programs and 8 fellowships and is a major teaching affiliate of NYU Medical Center.

SPECIAL PROGRAMS

Advanced Cardiovascular Services	The hospital is a pioneering leader in the treatment of coronary artery and vascular disease—performing the nation's first angioplasty and minimally invasive coronary bypass surgery. The medical and surgical cardiology and vascular staff work as a single coordinated, interdisciplinary team—focusing on each patient's cardiovascular needs.
Orthopedic Surgery	The hospital has earned an international reputation as a leader in orthopedic surgery and sports medicine. Its Center for Total Joint Replacement offers outstanding diagnostic and surgical services to patients requiring total hip and knee replacement. The hospital's orthopedic surgeons serve as team physicians to the NY Jets, Rangers and Islanders.
Maternal/Child Health	The hospital is renowned for its exceptional obstetrical services from prenatal to postpartum care, specializing in high-risk pregnancies and high-risk neonatal care. It offers a full range of services for all gynecological problems.
Primary Care and Internal Medicine	A large staff of outstanding primary care physicians and internists provides families with comprehensive medical care and coordinates their patients' total healthcare needs.
Otolaryngology—Head and Neck Surgery	This service is nationally recognized for its expertise in the medical, surgical and therapeutic treatment of ear, nose, throat and voice disorders in adults and children.
Lenox Hill Hospital Physician Referral Service	1-888-RIGHT-MD—(888-744-4683) helps callers find a Lenox Hill Hospital doctor or dentist who best suits their needs and accepts their insurance or managed care plans. Covering every medical specialty, Lenox Hill Hospital physicians provide the highest quality care. Its unique Appointment Scheduling Assistance Program (ASAP) arranges for same-day appointments. The right doctor is just a phone call away.

SPECIALTY & SUBSPECIALTY	ABBREVIATION	PAGE(S)
Addiction Psychiatry	AdP	149
Adolescent Medicine	AM	149
Allergy & Immunology	A&I	150-152
Anesthesiology	Anes	152
Cardiology (Cardiovascular Disease)	Cv	153-163
Child & Adolescent Psychiatry	ChAP	163-165
Child Neurology	ChiN	165-166
Colon & Rectal Surgery	CRS	166-167
Critical Care Medicine	CCM	167-168
Dermatology	D	169-177
Diagnostic Radiology	DR	177-179
Emergency Medicine	EM	179
Endocrinology, Diabetes & Metabolism	EDM	180-185
FAMILY PRACTICE	FP	186-187
Gastroenterology	Ge	187-196
Geriatric Medicine	Ger	196-198
Geriatric Psychiatry	GerPsy	198
Gynecologic Oncology*	GO	198-200
Hand Surgery	HS	200-201
Hematology	Hem	202-205
Infectious Disease	Inf	205-208
INTERNAL MEDICINE	IM	209-229
Maternal & Fetal Medicine	MF	229
Medical Genetics	MG	230
Medical Oncology*	Onc	230-237
Neonatal-Perinatal Medicine	NP	237-238
Nephrology	Nep	238-241
Neurological Surgery	NS	241-245
Neurology	N	245-254
Neuroradiology	NRad	254
Nuclear Medicine	NuM	255-256
OBSTETRICS & GYNECOLOGY	ObG	256-268
Ophthalmology	Oph	268-284
Orthopaedic Surgery	OrS	285-299
Otolaryngology	Oto	299-307
Pain Management	PM	308-309

SPECIALTY & SUBSPECIALTY	ABBREVIATION	PAGE(S)
Pediatric Allergy & Immunology	PA&I	309-310
Pediatric Cardiology	PCd	310-311
Pediatric Critical Care Medicine	PCCM	312
Pediatric Endocrinology	PEn	312-313
Pediatric Gastroenterology	PGe	314
Pediatric Hematology–Oncology*	PHO	315-316
Pediatric Infectious Disease	PInf	316
Pediatric Nephrology	PNep	317
Pediatric Pulmonology	PPul	317-318
Pediatric Radiology	PR	318
Pediatric Rheumatology	PRhu	318
Pediatric Surgery	PS	318-319
PEDIATRICS (GENERAL)	Ped	320-329
Physical Medicine & Rehabilitation	PMR	329-331
Plastic Surgery	PlS	332-340
Preventive Medicine	PrM	340
Psychiatry	Psyc	340-363
Pulmonary Disease	Pul	363-368
Radiation Oncology*	RadRO	368-370
Radiology	Rad	370-374
Reproductive Endocrinology	RE	374-375
Rheumatology	Rhu	376-381
Sports Medicine	SM	381-382
Surgery	S	382-395
Thoracic Surgery (includes open heart surgery)	TS	395-399
Urology	U	399-406
Vascular & Interventional Radiology	VIR	406-407
Vascular Surgery (General)	GVS	407-409

Specialties in capital letters indicate Primary Care Specialties. However, many doctors will be certified in subspecialty, but will practice predominantly primary care medicine. In our lists this will be indicated.

*Oncologists deal with Cancer

ADDICTION PSYCHIATRY

Paul, Edward (MD)   AdP
Bellevue Hosp Ctr
155 E 31st St 25J; New York, NY 10016; **BDCERT:**
Psyc 87; AdP 93; **MS:** Coll Physicians & Surgeons
82; **RES:** Psyc, NY Hosp-Cornell Med Ctr, New
York, NY; **FEL:** Psyc, NY Hosp-Cornell Med Ctr,
New York, NY; **SI:** *Addiction Psychiatry; Anxiety
Disorders;* **HMO:** CIGNA Oxford PHS MCC
♿ 🔋 📷 📻 💻 **S** A Few Days

Weiss, Carol J (MD)   AdP
NY Hosp-Cornell Med Ctr
55 E 72nd St; New York, NY 10021; (212) 988-
1209; **BDCERT:** Psyc 89; AdP 93; **MS:** Johns
Hopkins U 83; **RES:** NY Hosp-Cornell Med Ctr, New
York, NY 87; **FEL:** Substance Abuse, NY Hosp-
Cornell Med Ctr, New York, NY 87-89; **FAP:** Asst
Clin Prof Cornell U; **SI:** *Drug & Alcohol Abuse*
LANG: Heb; 📷 📻 💻 A Few Days

ADOLESCENT MEDICINE

Cohall, Alwyn (MD)   AM
St Luke's Roosevelt Hosp Ctr
126 W 60th St; New York, NY 10023; (212) 523-
6900; **BDCERT:** Ped 86; **MS:** UMDNJ-NJ Med Sch,
Newark 80; **RES:** Montefiore Med Ctr, Bronx, NY
80-83; **FEL:** AM, Mount Sinai Med Ctr, New York,
NY 83-84; **HOSP:** Columbia-Presbyterian Med Ctr;
HMO: Oxford Sanus Chubb US Hlthcre
♿ 📷 💻 **S** Immediately 💳 *VISA* 💳 💳

Lopez, Ralph (MD)   AM   **PCP**
Lenox Hill Hosp
418 E 71st St; New York, NY 10021; (212) 772-
8989; **BDCERT:** Ped 72; **MS:** NYU Sch Med 67;
RES: Bellevue Hosp Ctr, New York, NY; Children's
Hosp, Boston, MA; **FEL:** Children's Hosp, Boston,
MA; **HOSP:** NY Hosp-Cornell Med Ctr; **SI:** *School
Problems; Eating Disorders;* **HMO:** Metlife
LANG: Sp; ♿ 🔋 📷 📻 💻 Immediately 💳

Marks, Andrea (MD)   AM   **PCP**
Mount Sinai Med Ctr
AdolescentYoung Adult Medicine, 14 E 90th St;
New York, NY 10128; (212) 987-1414; **BDCERT:**
Ped 77; AM 94; **MS:** Univ Penn 72; **RES:** Ped,
Children's Hosp, Boston, MA 72-74; **FEL:** AM,
Children's Hosp, Boston, MA 74-75; **FAP:** Assoc
Clin Prof Mt Sinai Sch Med; **SI:** *Eating Disorders;
Adolescent Gynecology*
♿ 📷 📻 💻 **S** 1 Week *VISA* 💳

Pegler, Cynthia (MD)   AM   **PCP**
Lenox Hill Hosp
418 E 71st St; New York, NY 10021; (212) 772-
8989; **BDCERT:** Ped 88; AM 94; **MS:** Albany Med
Coll 84; **RES:** Ped, N Shore Univ Hosp-Manhasset,
Manhasset, NY 87; **FEL:** AM, N Shore Univ Hosp-
Manhasset, Manhasset, NY 87-90; **FAP:** Clin Instr
Ped Cornell U; **HMO:** Aetna Hlth Plan Metlife
♿ 🔋 📷 📻 💻 A Few Days 💳 *VISA* 💳

Guide to symbols and abbreviations can be found on pages 110-113.

149

ALLERGY & IMMUNOLOGY

Buchbinder, Ellen (MD)   A&I
Mount Sinai Med Ctr
111 E 88th St Apt B; New York, NY 10128; (212) 410-3246; **BDCERT:** A&I 83; IM 81; **MS:** Tulane U 78; **RES:** IM, New England Deaconess Hosp, Boston, MA 78-81; **FEL:** A&I, Mass Gen Hosp, Boston, MA 81-83; **FAP:** Asst Clin Prof Mt Sinai Sch Med; **SI:** *Asthma; Allergies;* **HMO:** Oxford PHCS Beech Street Prudential CIGNA +

LANG: Sp; 🚹 📞 🚹 🏧 💲   A Few Days

Chandler, Michael (MD)   A&I
Mount Sinai Med Ctr
115 E 61st St Fl 12; New York, NY 10021; (212) 486-6715; **BDCERT:** IM 84; A&I 87; **MS:** Wayne State U Sch Med 81; **RES:** IM, Northwestern Mem Hosp, Chicago, IL 81-84; **FEL:** A&I, Northwestern Mem Hosp, Chicago, IL 84-86; **FAP:** Clin Instr Mt Sinai Sch Med; **HOSP:** Lenox Hill Hosp; **SI:** *Sinusitis; Asthma;* **HMO:** Oxford PHCS United Healthcare CIGNA PHS +

🚹 📷 🚹 🏧 💲 📇   Immediately **VISA** 💳

Cunningham-Rundles, Charlotte (MD & PhD)   A&I
Mount Sinai Med Ctr
5 E 98th St; New York, NY 10029; (212) 241-4014; **BDCERT:** IM 72; **MS:** Columbia P&S 69; **RES:** Bellevue Hosp Ctr, New York, NY 69-72; New York University Med Ctr, New York, NY 69-74; **FEL:** A&I, New York University Med Ctr, New York, NY 72-74; **FAP:** Prof Mt Sinai Sch Med; **HOSP:** Beth Israel Med Ctr; **SI:** *Immunodeficiency; Clinical Immunology;* **HMO:** Oxford

🚹 🚹 🏧 💲   2-4 Weeks 🏧 **VISA** 💳 🏧

Davis, William J (MD)   A&I
Columbia-Presbyterian Med Ctr
3959 Broadway 107N; New York, NY 10032; (212) 305-2300; **BDCERT:** A&I 74; **MS:** Columbia P&S 65; **RES:** Bellevue Hosp Ctr, New York, NY; Ped, Columbia-Presbyterian Med Ctr, New York, NY; **FEL:** Nat Inst Health, Bethesda, MD; A&I, Columbia-Presbyterian Med Ctr, New York, NY

🚹 📷 🚹 🏧 💲   Immediately

Dworetzky, Murray (MD)   A&I
NY Hosp-Cornell Med Ctr
115 E 61st St Fl 12; New York, NY 10021; (212) 838-3421; **BDCERT:** A&I 72; IM 51; **MS:** SUNY Hlth Sci Ctr 42; **RES:** Path, City Hosp, New York, NY 42-46; U Chicago Hosp, Chicago, IL 47; **FEL:** IM, Mayo Clinic, Rochester, MN 47-50; **FAP:** Clin Prof Med Cornell U; **SI:** *Allergic Rhinitis; Urticaria;* **HMO:** None

🚹 📷 🚹 🏧 📇   1 Week

Feldman, B Robert (MD)   A&I
Columbia-Presbyterian Med Ctr
Allergy Division, The NYPresbyterian Hosp, 3959 Broadway; New York, NY 10032; (212) 305-2300; **BDCERT:** Ped 68; A&I 72; **MS:** U Hlth Sci/Chicago Med Sch 59; **RES:** Ped, Michael Reese Hosp Med Ctr, Chicago, IL 60-62; **FEL:** A&I, Michael Reese Hosp Med Ctr, Chicago, IL 62-63; A&I, Columbia-Presbyterian Med Ctr, New York, NY 63-64; **FAP:** Clin Prof Ped Columbia P&S; **SI:** *Asthma; Allergic Rhinitis;* **HMO:** Oxford ABC Health Blue Choice PHS Empire Blue Cross & Shield +

🚹 📷 🚹 🏧 💲 📇   A Few Days

Frenkel, Renata (MD)   A&I
St Luke's Roosevelt Hosp Ctr
30 W 60th St 1U; New York, NY 10023; (212) 265-1990; **BDCERT:** A&I 79; **MS:** Austria 68; **RES:** St Luke's Roosevelt Hosp Ctr, New York, NY 71-73; **FEL:** St Luke's Roosevelt Hosp Ctr, New York, NY 73-75; **FAP:** Assoc Columbia P&S; **HOSP:** Lenox Hill Hosp; **SI:** *Asthma; Allergies;* **HMO:** Oxford US Hlthcre CIGNA Aetna Hlth Plan Prucare +

LANG: Ger, Rus; 🚹 📞 📷 🚹 🏧 💲 📇   Immediately

Grieco, Michael (MD) A&I
St Luke's Roosevelt Hosp Ctr

University Medical Practice Assoc, 425 W 59th St; New York, NY 10019; (212) 523-7090; **BDCERT:** A&I 66; Inf 72; **MS:** SUNY Downstate 57; **RES:** IM, St Luke's Roosevelt Hosp Ctr, New York, NY 57-58; **FEL:** A&I, St Luke's Roosevelt Hosp Ctr, New York, NY 62-63; Inf, Bellevue Hosp Ctr, New York, NY 62-64; **FAP:** Prof of Clin Med Columbia P&S; *SI: Asthma; Immunological Disorders*; **HMO:** Oxford Aetna Hlth Plan Anthem Health CIGNA PHCS +

🚻 📷 🔧 🛏 💲 🏧 2-4 Weeks 💳 **VISA** 💳

Grubman, Samuel (MD) A&I
St Vincents Hosp & Med Ctr NY

32 W 18th St 5th FL; New York, NY 10011; (212) 647-6466; **BDCERT:** Ped 89; A&I 89; **MS:** Mt Sinai Sch Med 83; **RES:** Ped, New York University Med Ctr, New York, NY 83-86; **FEL:** A&I, Albert Einstein Med Ctr, Bronx, NY 86-88; **FAP:** Asst Prof Path NY Med Coll; *SI: Food and Environmental Allergies; Asthma*; **HMO:** Oxford Blue Cross & Blue Choice Prucare PHS Aetna-US Healthcare +

LANG: Sp, Heb; 🚻 📞 📷 🔧 🛏 💲 🏧 🏧 🏧
A Few Days 💳 **VISA** 💳

Kadar, Avraham (MD) A&I
Beth Israel Med Ctr

Diagnostic Ctr for Immunology, Allergy & Asthma, 530 Park Ave; New York, NY 10021; (212) 755-3456; **BDCERT:** A&I 88; **MS:** Israel 83; **RES:** Tel Hashomer Hosp, Tel Aviv, Israel 83; Montefiore Med Ctr, Bronx, NY 83-86; **FEL:** A&I, Nat Inst Health, Bethesda, MD; **FAP:** Asst Clin Prof A&I Albert Einstein Coll Med; **HOSP:** Northern Westchester Hosp Ctr; *SI: Diagnostic Laboratory Immunology*; **HMO:** Oxford

LANG: Heb; 🚻 🏧 📞 📷 🔧 🛏 💲 2-4 Weeks 💳
VISA 💳 💳

Macris, Nicholas T (MD) A&I
Lenox Hill Hosp

1430 2nd Ave Ste 102; New York, NY 10021; (212) 249-2940; **BDCERT:** A&I 74; **MS:** SUNY Hlth Sci Ctr 58; **RES:** IM, Lenox Hill Hosp, New York, NY 58-59; IM, Lenox Hill Hosp, New York, NY 61-63; **FEL:** A&I, Rockefeller Univ Hosp, New York, NY 63-65; A&I, NY Hosp-Cornell Med Ctr, New York, NY; **FAP:** Clin Prof Med Cornell U; **HOSP:** NY Hosp-Cornell Med Ctr; *SI: Allergy and Asthma; Lupus*; **HMO:** None

LANG: Grk, Sp, Fr; 🚻 📷 🛏 💲 🏧 2-4 Weeks

Mazza, David Stephen (MD) A&I
St Luke's Roosevelt Hosp Ctr

7 Lexington Ave 3; New York, NY 10010; (212) 677-7170; **BDCERT:** A&I 89; Ped 83; **MS:** Univ Vt Coll Med 77; **RES:** Ped, New York University Med Ctr, New York, NY 77-80; **FEL:** Ped, Bellevue Hosp Ctr, New York, NY 80-82; A&I, St Luke's Roosevelt Hosp Ctr, New York, NY 87-89; **FAP:** Asst Prof Columbia P&S; **HOSP:** St Vincents Hosp & Med Ctr NY; *SI: Asthma; Allergy—Hayfever*; **HMO:** Aetna Hlth Plan CIGNA Oxford Prucare United Healthcare +

🚻 📞 📷 🔧 🛏 💲 🏧 2-4 Weeks 💳 **VISA** 💳

Rubin, James (MD) A&I
Beth Israel Med Ctr

35 E 35th St 202; New York, NY 10016; (212) 685-4225; **BDCERT:** IM 68; A&I 71; **MS:** NY Med Coll 60; **RES:** Beth Israel Med Ctr, New York, NY 60-61; Beth Israel Med Ctr, New York, NY 62-64; **FEL:** A&I, Jewish Hosp Med Ctr, Brooklyn, NY 64-65; **FAP:** Assoc Clin Prof Med Albert Einstein Coll Med; *SI: Asthma; Sinusitis*; **HMO:** Oxford Aetna Hlth Plan United Healthcare Prucare Empire +

LANG: Sp; 🚻 📞 📷 🔧 🛏 💲 🏧 🏧 A Few Days
VISA 💳

Shepherd, Gillian M (MD)   A&I
NY Hosp-Cornell Med Ctr
235 E 67th St Ste 203; New York, NY 10021;
(212) 288-9300; **BDCERT:** IM 79; A&I 81; **MS:** NY
Med Coll 76; **RES:** IM, Lenox Hill Hosp, New York,
NY 76-79; **FEL:** A&I, NY Hosp-Cornell Med Ctr,
New York, NY 79-81; **FAP:** Assoc Clin Prof Med
Cornell U; **HOSP:** Mem Sloan Kettering Cancer Ctr;
SI: Allergic Reactions, Hives; Asthma; **HMO:** Oxford
21st Century Empire Blue Cross & Shield United
Healthcare CIGNA +

LANG: Sp; ⬛ 🔲 🔲 🔲 💲 🔲 1 Week 🔲 *VISA*
🔲

Slankard, Marjorie (MD)   A&I
Columbia-Presbyterian Med Ctr
16 E 60th St; New York, NY 10022; (212) 326-
8410; **BDCERT:** IM 74; A&I 77; **MS:** Univ Mo-
Columbia Sch Med 71; **RES:** Med, NY Hosp-Cornell
Med Ctr, New York, NY 72-74; IM, Rockefeller Univ
Hosp, New York, NY 72-73; **FEL:** A&I, NY Hosp-
Cornell Med Ctr, New York, NY 74-76; Tumor
Immunology, Mount Sinai Med Ctr, New York, NY
76-80; **FAP:** Assoc Clin Prof Med Columbia P&S;
HOSP: Valley Hosp; *SI: Asthma; Sinus Disease*; **HMO:**
Oxford Aetna Hlth Plan Chubb Merrill Lynch
Prucare +

LANG: Sp; ⬛ 🔲 🔲 🔲 🔲 💲 2-4 Weeks 🔲 *VISA*
🔲

Young, Stuart (MD)   A&I
Mount Sinai Med Ctr
121 E 60th St; New York, NY 10022; (212) 826-
0815; **BDCERT:** Ped 70; A&I 72; **MS:** SUNY Hlth
Sci Ctr 63; **RES:** Ped, Kings County Hosp Ctr,
Brooklyn, NY 63-65; Ped, Univ Hosp SUNY Bklyn,
Brooklyn, NY 65-66; **FEL:** A&I, Nat Jewish Med Ctr,
Denver, CO 68-70; **FAP:** Assoc Clin Prof Med Mt
Sinai Sch Med; *SI: Asthma; Nasal and Sinus Allergy*;
HMO: Aetna Hlth Plan Oxford CIGNA United
Healthcare PHS +

LANG: Sp; ⬛ 🔲 🔲 🔲 🔲 🔲 🔲 Immediately
VISA 🔲

ANESTHESIOLOGY

Leff, Alan (MD)   Anes
New York University Med Ctr
Pain Mgmt & Rehab Med Svcs, 247 3rd Ave Ste
302; New York, NY 10010; (212) 228-4141;
BDCERT: Anes 73; PM 96; **MS:** NYU Sch Med 65;
RES: Anes, Columbia-Presbyterian Med Ctr, New
York, NY 66-68; **FEL:** PM, Mem Sloan Kettering
Cancer Ctr, New York, NY 93; **FAP:** Asst Clin Prof
Anes NYU Sch Med; **HOSP:** Cabrini Med Ctr; *SI:
Back Pain; Neck Pain*; **HMO:** Oxford Blue Cross

⬛ 🔲 🔲 🔲 🔲 🔲 🔲 🔲 Immediately

Statile, Lorna (MD)   Anes
Cabrini Med Ctr
148 W 23rd St 9H; New York, NY 10011; (212)
995-6163; **BDCERT:** Anes 86; **MS:** Belgium 78;
RES: IM, St Vincent's Med Ctr-Bridgeport,
Bridgeport, CT 79-81; Anes, New York University
Med Ctr, New York, NY 81-83; **FEL:** N Anes, New
York University Med Ctr, New York, NY 83; **FAP:**
Clin Instr NYU Sch Med

Wilson, Roger (MD)   Anes
Mem Sloan Kettering Cancer Ctr
450 E 63rd St 3J; New York, NY 10021; (212)
639-6848; **BDCERT:** Anes 71; CCM 86; **MS:**
UMDNJ-NJ Med Sch, Newark 66; **RES:** Columbia-
Presbyterian Med Ctr, New York, NY 67-69; **FEL:**
Columbia-Presbyterian Med Ctr, New York, NY;
HMO: None

⬛ 🔲 🔲 🔲 🔲 🔲 💲 🔲 🔲 🔲 🔲 Immediately

CARDIOLOGY (CARDIOVASCULAR DISEASE)

Ambrose, John (MD)　　　Cv
Mount Sinai Med Ctr

Mt Sinai Hosp, 5 E 98th St; New York, NY 10029; (212) 241-3263; **BDCERT:** IM 75; Cv 77; **MS:** NY Med Coll 72; **RES:** IM, Mount Sinai Med Ctr, New York, NY 72-75; **FEL:** Cv, Mount Sinai Med Ctr, New York, NY 75-77; **FAP:** Prof Med Mt Sinai Sch Med; *SI: Cardiac Catheterization; Coronary Angioplasty*

LANG: Sp; 🖮 🖮 🆔 📠 2-4 Weeks

Askanas, Alexander (MD)　　　Cv
Beth Israel Med Ctr

1085 Park Ave; New York, NY 10128; (212) 369-3080; **BDCERT:** IM 72; Cv 74; **MS:** Poland 60; **RES:** VA Med Ctr-Manh, New York, NY 69-71; **FEL:** Cv, VA Med Ctr-Manh, New York, NY 71-72; *SI: Irregular Heart Beat; Chest Pains*; **HMO:** US Hlthcre Prucare CIGNA

LANG: Rus; 🖮 🖮 🆔 💲 📠 2-4 Weeks

Berdoff, Russell (MD)　　　Cv
Beth Israel Med Ctr

67 Irving Pl 7th Fl; New York, NY 10003; (212) 979-9224; **BDCERT:** IM 78; Cv 81; **MS:** NY Med Coll 75; **RES:** IM, Georgetown U Hosp, Washington, DC 75-78; **FEL:** Cv, Johns Hopkins Hosp, Baltimore, MD 78-80; **FAP:** Asst Prof of Clin Med Albert Einstein Coll Med; *SI: Consulting Cardiology; Cardiovascular MRI*; **HMO:** Oxford US Hlthcre Empire Blue Cross Multiplan United Healthcare +

LANG: Pol, Sp; 🖮 🖮 🆔 📠 Immediately 🖮 **VISA** 🔴

Berger, Marvin (MD)　　　Cv
Beth Israel Med Ctr

Beth Israel Medical Center, 1st Ave & 16th St Fl 11; New York, NY 10003; (212) 420-2068; **BDCERT:** IM 69; Cv 77; **MS:** U Hlth Sci/Chicago Med Sch 61; **RES:** IM, Beth Israel Med Ctr, New York, NY 61-64; **FEL:** Cv, Mount Sinai Med Ctr, New York, NY 64-65; **FAP:** Assoc Prof Albert Einstein Coll Med; *SI: Echocardiography*; **HMO:** Aetna-US Healthcare Oxford Empire Blue Choice NYLCare CIGNA +

🖮 1 Week 🖮 **VISA** 🔴

Bernaski, Edward (MD)　　　Cv
St Vincents Hosp & Med Ctr NY

Gramercy Park Medical Assoc, 60 Gramercy Park N; New York, NY 10010; (212) 254-1220; **BDCERT:** IM 90; Cv 95; **MS:** St Louis U 85; **RES:** IM, Cabrini Med Ctr, New York, NY 85-88; Cv, Univ Hosp SUNY Buffalo, Buffalo, NY 88-91; **FAP:** Clin Instr IM NY Med Coll; **HOSP:** Cabrini Med Ctr; *SI: Echocardiography; Stress Testing*; **HMO:** Oxford PHS CIGNA GHI United Healthcare +

LANG: Sp; 🖮 🖮 🖮 🆔 💲 📠 A Few Days

Blake, James (MD)　　　Cv
NY Hosp-Cornell Med Ctr

340 E 64th St; New York, NY 10021; (212) 755-8700; **BDCERT:** IM 84; Cv 87; **MS:** Albert Einstein Coll Med 81; **RES:** NY Hosp-Cornell Med Ctr, New York, NY 81-82; NY Hosp-Cornell Med Ctr, New York, NY 82-84; **FEL:** Cv, NY Hosp-Cornell Med Ctr, New York, NY 84-87; **FAP:** Clin Prof Cornell U; *SI: Thallium Stress Testing; Echocardiography*; **HMO:** Oxford Blue Cross PHCS 32BJ

LANG: Sp, Rus; 🖮 🆔 💲 📠 1 Week **VISA** 🔴

Blumenthal, David S (MD)　　　Cv
NY Hosp-Cornell Med Ctr

407 E 70th St; New York, NY 10021; (212) 861-3222; **BDCERT:** IM 78; Cv 81; **MS:** Cornell U 75; **RES:** NY Hosp-Cornell Med Ctr, New York, NY 75-78; **FEL:** Cv, Johns Hopkins Hosp, Baltimore, MD 78-80; *SI: Valvular Heart Disease; Arteriosclerosis*; **HMO:** None

🖮 🖮 🆔 📠 1 Week

Borer, Jeffrey (MD) Cv
NY Hosp-Cornell Med Ctr

Chief, Division of Cardiovascular Pathophysiology, 525 E 68th St; New York, NY 10021; (212) 746-4646; **BDCERT:** IM 73; Cv 75; **MS:** Cornell U 69; **RES:** Mass Gen Hosp, Boston, MA 69-70; Mass Gen Hosp, Boston, MA 70-71; **FEL:** Nat Inst Health, Bethesda, MD 71-74; Guy's Hosp Univ of London, London, England 74; **FAP:** Prof Cv; **SI:** *Heart Valve Disease; Coronary Artery Disease*; **HMO:** Metlife

LANG: Sp; ♿ ☎ ⌚ Mcr 🅰🅼🅴🆇 *VISA* ⬤

Braff, Robert (MD) Cv
St Vincents Hosp & Med Ctr NY

36 7th Ave 420; New York, NY 10011; (212) 242-3337; **BDCERT:** IM 76; Cv 81; **MS:** SUNY Hlth Sci Ctr 73; **RES:** St Vincents Hosp & Med Ctr NY, New York, NY 73-76; **FEL:** Cv, Georgetown U Hosp, Washington, DC 76-78; **SI:** *Coronary Intervention; Echocardiography*; **HMO:** GHI Magnacare Aetna Hlth Plan Oxford Empire Blue Cross & Shield +

LANG: Sp; ♿ ☎ ♿ ⌚ 🆂 Mcr 1 Week

Burack, Bernard (MD) Cv
Lenox Hill Hosp

2A E 77th St; New York, NY 10021; (212) 988-6655; **BDCERT:** IM 58; **MS:** Creighton U 49; **RES:** Montefiore Med Ctr, Bronx, NY; **FEL:** NY Hosp-Cornell Med Ctr, New York, NY; **FAP:** Asst Clin Prof Med Albert Einstein Coll Med; **HOSP:** Montefiore Med Ctr; **SI:** *Sleep Medicine*

LANG: Yd, Ger, Heb; ♿ ☎ ♿ Mcr Mod Immediately

Cemaletin, Nevber (MD) Cv
Lenox Hill Hosp

184 E 70th St 1B; New York, NY 10021; (212) 744-6296; **BDCERT:** IM 88; Cv 89; **MS:** NY Med Coll 84; **RES:** Lenox Hill Hosp, New York, NY 84-87; **FEL:** Cv, Lenox Hill Hosp, New York, NY 87-89; **HOSP:** Manhattan Eye, Ear & Throat Hosp

♿ ☎ ♿ ⌚ 🆂 Mcr A Few Days

Cole, William Joseph (MD) Cv
NYU Downtown Hosp

170 William St 8th Fl; New York, NY 10038; (212) 732-5499; **BDCERT:** IM 83; Cv 87; **MS:** NYU Sch Med 80; **RES:** Cv, NYU Med Ctr/Bellevue Hospital, New York, NY 80-84; **FAP:** Asst Prof of Clin Med NYU Sch Med; **HOSP:** New York University Med Ctr; **HMO:** Multiplan

♿ ☎ ⌚ 🆂 Mcr A Few Days

Colombo, Antonio (MD) Cv
Lenox Hill Hosp

Cardiology—Interventional Cardiology, 100 E 77th St; New York, NY 10021; (212) 434-2606; **BDCERT:** IM 82; Cv 86; **MS:** Italy 75; **RES:** IM, Cabrini Med Ctr, New York, NY 77-78; IM, Cabrini Med Ctr, New York, NY 78-81; **FEL:** Cv, VA Med Ctr, Long Beach, CA 81-83; Cv, St Joseph's Hosp-Queens, Flushing, NY 83-84; **FAP:** Clin Prof Med NYU Sch Med; **SI:** *Coronary Angioplasty; Vascular Stents*; **HMO:** US Hlthcre CIGNA Blue Cross & Blue Shield Oxford Aetna Hlth Plan +

LANG: Sp; ♿ ☎ ♿ ⌚ 🆂 Mcr Mod WC NFI Immediately

Colvin, Stephen (MD) Cv
New York University Med Ctr

530 1st Ave Ste 9V; New York, NY 10016; (212) 263-6384; **BDCERT:** Cv 73; **MS:** Albert Einstein Coll Med 69; **RES:** New York University Med Ctr, New York, NY 69-76; **FEL:** Cv, New York University Med Ctr, New York, NY 76-78; **FAP:** Assoc Clin Prof S NYU Sch Med; **SI:** *Minimally Invasive Cardiac Surgery; Congenital Heart Disease*; **HMO:** Health Source

LANG: Sp; ♿ ◖ ☎ ♿ ⌚ Mcr Mod WC NFI Immediately

Coppola, John (MD) Cv
St Vincents Hosp & Med Ctr NY

32 W 18th St FL4; New York, NY 10011; (212) 647-6420; **BDCERT:** IM 81; Cv 83; **MS:** NY Med Coll 78; **RES:** St Vincents Hosp & Med Ctr NY, New York, NY; **FEL:** Cv, St Vincents Hosp & Med Ctr NY, New York, NY; **HMO:** US Hlthcre Oxford Aetna Hlth Plan Prucare Blue Choice +

♿ ☎ ⌚ 🆂 Mcr Mod 2-4 Weeks 🅰🅼🅴🆇 *VISA* ⬤ ▦

Drusin, Ronald (MD) Cv
Columbia-Presbyterian Med Ctr
161 Fort Washington Ave; New York, NY 10032;
(212) 305-5371; **BDCERT:** IM 73; Cv 75; **MS:**
Columbia P&S 66; **RES:** IM, Bellevue Hosp Ctr, New
York, NY 66-67; IM, Columbia-Presbyterian Med
Ctr, New York, NY 67-69; **FEL:** Cv, Columbia-
Presbyterian Med Ctr, New York, NY 71-73; **FAP:**
Prof of Clin Med Columbia P&S; **SI:** *Cardiovascular
Disease;* **HMO:** Oxford Empire Blue Cross & Shield
Health Source Aetna Hlth Plan Prudential +
🔲 🔲 🔲 🔲 1 Week

Fox, Arthur Charles (MD) Cv
New York University Med Ctr
NYU Med Ctr, 530 1st Ave 4G; New York, NY
10016; (212) 263-7229; **BDCERT:** IM 75; Cv 75;
MS: NYU Sch Med 48; **RES:** Bellevue Hosp Ctr, New
York, NY 48-52; **FEL:** Cv, Bellevue Hosp Ctr, New
York, NY 55-57; **FAP:** Prof Med; **HOSP:** Bellevue
Hosp Ctr; **SI:** *Cardiology, Difficult Diagnoses*
🔲 🔲 🔲 🔲 A Few Days

Friedman, Sanford (MD) Cv `PCP`
Mount Sinai Med Ctr
941 Park Ave; New York, NY 10028; (212) 988-
3772; **BDCERT:** IM 73; Cv 76; **MS:** Tufts U 71; **RES:**
Med, Mt Sinai Med Ctr, New York, NY 71-74; **FEL:**
Cv, Mt Sinai Med Ctr, New York, NY 74-76; **FAP:** Sr
Clin Instr Mt Sinai Sch Med; **HOSP:** Beth Israel Med
Ctr; **SI:** *Preventive Cardiology; Diagnostic Cardiology;*
HMO: Oxford United Healthcare Empire First
Health
LANG: Sp; 🔲 🔲 🔲 🔲 🔲 1 Week

Fuchs, Richard (MD) Cv
NY Hosp-Cornell Med Ctr
310 E 72nd St; New York, NY 10021; (212) 717-
2254; **BDCERT:** IM 79; Cv 81; **MS:** Harvard Med
Sch 76; **RES:** NY Hosp-Cornell Med Ctr, New York,
NY 76-79; **FEL:** Cv, Johns Hopkins Hosp, Baltimore,
MD 79-82; **FAP:** Assoc Clin Prof Med Cornell U; **SI:**
Coronary Artery Disease; Valvular Heart Disease
🔲 🔲 🔲 🔲 🔲 1 Week *VISA* 🔲

Fuster, Valentin (MD & PhD) Cv
Mount Sinai Med Ctr
1 Gustave Levy Plaza Box 1030; New York, NY
10029; (212) 241-7911; **BDCERT:** IM 76; Cv 77;
MS: Spain 67; **RES:** IM, Mayo Clinic, Rochester, MN
72; **FEL:** Mayo Clinic, Rochester, MN 74; **FAP:** Prof
Cv Mt Sinai Sch Med; **SI:** *Arteriosclerosis;
Cardiovascular Diseases;* **HMO:** Oxford US Hlthcre
Aetna-US Healthcare Premier

LANG: Sp; 🔲 🔲 🔲 🔲 1 Week 🔲 *VISA* 🔲 🔲

Garfein, Oscar (MD) Cv
St Luke's Roosevelt Hosp Ctr
425 W 59th St 8B; New York, NY 10019; (212)
586-0435; **BDCERT:** IM 71; Cv 75; **MS:** Columbia
P&S 65; **RES:** IM, Columbia-Presbyterian Med Ctr,
New York, NY 65-67; IM, Mass Gen Hosp, Boston,
MA 69-70; **FEL:** Cv, Beth Israel Med Ctr, Boston,
MA 70-71; Cv, St Luke's Roosevelt Hosp Ctr, New
York, NY 71-72; **FAP:** Assoc Clin Prof Columbia
P&S; **SI:** *Coronary Artery Disease; Pacemaker
Implantation;* **HMO:** Oxford Aetna Hlth Plan
LANG: Sp; 🔲 🔲 🔲 🔲 🔲 🔲 1 Week

Gertler, Menard (MD) Cv
New York University Med Ctr
317 E 34th St Fl 9; New York, NY 10016; (212)
689-5621; **BDCERT:** IM 52; Cv 54; **MS:** Canada
43; **RES:** IM, McGill Teaching Hosp, Montreal,
Canada 44; **FEL:** Mass Gen Hosp, Boston, MA 47-
50; **FAP:** Clin Prof Med Cornell U; **HOSP:** Lenox Hill
Hosp; **SI:** *Preventive & Early Intervention; Coronary
Heart Disease;* **HMO:** Aetna Hlth Plan GHI US
Hlthcre Oxford
LANG: Fr; 🔲 🔲 🔲 🔲 🔲 🔲 A Few Days

Giardina, Elsa-Grace (MD) Cv
Columbia-Presbyterian Med Ctr
16 E 60th St; New York, NY 10016; (212) 326-
8540; **BDCERT:** IM 71; Cv 83; **MS:** NY Med Coll 68;
RES: St Luke's Roosevelt Hosp Ctr, New York, NY
65-69; Columbia-Presbyterian Med Ctr, New York,
NY 69-72; **FEL:** Cv, Columbia-Presbyterian Med
Ctr, New York, NY 69-72; **FAP:** Prof Columbia P&S;
SI: *Heart Disease; Arrhythmias*
LANG: Sp; 🔲 🔲 🔲 🔲 🔲 🔲 A Few Days 🔲
VISA 🔲

Guide to symbols and abbreviations can be found on pages 110-113.

155

Gliklich, Jerry (MD)   Cv
Columbia-Presbyterian Med Ctr
161 Ft Washington Ave Ste 645; New York, NY 10032; (212) 305-5588; **BDCERT:** IM 78; Cv 81; **MS:** Columbia P&S 75; **RES:** IM, NY Hosp-Cornell Med Ctr, New York, NY 75-78; **FEL:** Columbia-Presbyterian Med Ctr, New York, NY 78-81; **HMO:** None

♿ ▣ ▣ **$** 2-4 Weeks

Goldberg, Harvey (MD)   Cv
NY Hosp-Cornell Med Ctr
New York Cardiology Associates, 425 E 61st St Fl 6; New York, NY 10021; (212) 752-2000; **BDCERT:** IM 79; Cv 81; **MS:** Cornell U 72; **RES:** IM, NY Hosp-Cornell Med Ctr, New York, NY 76-79; **FEL:** PCd, NY Hosp-Cornell Med Ctr, New York, NY; **FAP:** Assoc Clin Prof Cornell U

LANG: Sp, Rus, Crt; ♿ ▣ ▣ ▣ **$** A Few Days **VISA** ●

Goldman, Martin (MD)   Cv
Mount Sinai Med Ctr
1 Gustave Levy Pl; New York, NY 10029; (212) 241-3078; **BDCERT:** Cv 79; **MS:** Albert Einstein Coll Med 76; **RES:** Med, Harvard Med Sch, Cambridge, MA 76-78; **FEL:** Cv, Mount Sinai Med Ctr, New York, NY 79-81; **FAP:** Prof NYU Sch Med; *SI: Echocardiography; Valvular Heart Disease*

♿ ▣ ▣ ▣ **$** Mc A Few Days **VISA** ●

Grossman, Will (MD)   Cv
Beth Israel Med Ctr
30 E 72nd St FL1; New York, NY 10021; (212) 535-5110; **BDCERT:** IM 72; Cv 77; **MS:** NYU Sch Med 57; **RES:** Cincinnati Gen Hosp, Cincinnati, OH 58-59; Med, Henry Ford Hosp, Detroit, MI 61-63; **FEL:** Cv, NJ Coll Med, Newark, NJ 63-64; **FAP:** Instr Med Mt Sinai Sch Med

Halperin, Jonathan (MD)   Cv
Mount Sinai Med Ctr
Mount Sinai Hospital, 5 E 98th St Fl 10; New York, NY 10029; (212) 427-1540; **BDCERT:** IM 80; Cv 81; **MS:** Boston U 75; **RES:** Boston U Med Ctr, Boston, MA 75-77; **FEL:** Cv, Boston U Med Ctr, Boston, MA 78-80; **FAP:** Prof Mt Sinai Sch Med; *SI: Peripheral Vascular Disease*

♿ ▣ ▣ **$** Mc Mc 4+ Weeks **VISA** ●

Hecht, Alan (MD)   Cv
Mount Sinai Med Ctr
994 5th Ave; New York, NY 10028; (212) 535-6690; **BDCERT:** IM 84; Cv 86; **MS:** Northwestern U 81; **RES:** IM, Mount Sinai Med Ctr, New York, NY 82-84; **FEL:** IM, Mount Sinai Med Ctr, New York, NY 84-86; **FAP:** Clin Instr Mt Sinai Sch Med; **HOSP:** Beth Israel Med Ctr; *SI: Preventive Cardiology; Stress Echocardiography;* **HMO:** Blue Cross & Blue Shield Oxford GHI Prucare United Healthcare +

♿ ▣ ▣ ▣ Mc A Few Days

Horowitz, Steven (MD)   Cv
Beth Israel Med Ctr
1st Ave & 16th St; New York, NY 10003; (212) 420-4560; **BDCERT:** IM 75; Cv 79; **MS:** NY Med Coll 72; **RES:** IM, Beth Israel Med Ctr, New York, NY 72-75; **FEL:** Cv, Mount Sinai Med Ctr, New York, NY 76-78; **HMO:** Oxford

♿ ▣ ▣ Mc 1 Week **VISA** ●

Infantino, Michael (MD)   Cv
St Vincents Hosp & Med Ctr NY
32 W 18th St; New York, NY 10011; (212) 647-6420; **BDCERT:** IM 84; Cv 87; **MS:** SUNY Hlth Sci Ctr 81; **RES:** IM, Staten Island Univ Hosp, Staten Island, NY 81-84; **FEL:** Cv, St Vincents Hosp & Med Ctr NY, New York, NY; **FAP:** Asst Prof NY Med Coll; **HOSP:** St Vincent's Med Ctr-Richmond; **HMO:** Oxford US Hlthcre Magnacare Aetna Hlth Plan

LANG: Sp; ♿ ▣ ▣ **$** Mc 2-4 Weeks **VISA** ● ●

Inra, Lawrence A (MD)   Cv   `PCP`
NY Hosp-Cornell Med Ctr

407 E 70th St; New York, NY 10011; (212) 249-1011; **BDCERT:** IM 79; Cv 81; **MS:** Johns Hopkins U 76; **RES:** IM, NY Hosp-Cornell Med Ctr, New York, NY 76-79; **FEL:** Cv, Mount Sinai Med Ctr, New York, NY 79-81; **FAP:** Asst Clin Prof Med Cornell U; **SI:** *Coronary Artery Disease; Hypercholesterolemia;* **HMO:** None

🦽 🔂 🏧 💲   1 Week

Kamen, Mazen (MD)   Cv
NY Hosp-Cornell Med Ctr

520 E 72nd St; New York, NY 10021; (212) 879-6600; **BDCERT:** IM 90; Cv 95; **MS:** NYU Sch Med 83; **RES:** New York University Med Ctr, New York, NY 83-86; **FEL:** NY Hosp-Cornell Med Ctr, New York, NY; **FAP:** Asst Prof Med Cornell U; **SI:** *Valvular Heart Diseases; Hypercholesterolemia;* **HMO:** Aetna Hlth Plan Oxford CIGNA

LANG: Fr, Sp; 🦽 🌙 🔂 🔩 🏧   A Few Days

Killip, Thomas (MD)   Cv
Beth Israel Med Ctr

1st Ave & 16th St administration; New York, NY 10003; (212) 420-4010; **BDCERT:** IM 60; Cv 68; **MS:** Cornell U 52; **RES:** Strong Mem Hosp, Rochester, NY 52-53; NY Hosp-Cornell Med Ctr, New York, NY 53-55; **FEL:** Cv, NY Hosp-Cornell Med Ctr, New York, NY 55-57; **HMO:** Aetna Hlth Plan HealthNet US Hlthcre Oxford Sanus +

🦽 🔂 🔩 🏧 Mcr WC NFI   Immediately

Kligfield, Paul (MD)   Cv
NY Hosp-Cornell Med Ctr

525 E 68th St; New York, NY 10021; (212) 746-4686; **BDCERT:** IM 73; Cv 75; **MS:** Harvard Med Sch 70; **RES:** Beth Israel Med Ctr, Boston, MA 70-72; **FEL:** Cv, St Georges Hosp, London, England 72-73; NY Hosp-Cornell Med Ctr, New York, NY 73-75; **FAP:** Prof Med Cornell U; **SI:** *Exercise Testing; Cardiac Rehabilitation;* **HMO:** Aetna Hlth Plan Metlife Oxford

🦽 🔂 🏧 Mcr   2-4 Weeks ▨ **VISA** 💳

Kloth, Howard (MD)   Cv
New York University Med Ctr

650 1st Ave Fl 6; New York, NY 10016; (212) 889-5800; **BDCERT:** IM 64; Cv 75; **MS:** Albany Med Coll 57; **RES:** Boston Med Ctr, Boston, MA 57; Bellevue Hosp Ctr, New York, NY 60-63; **FAP:** Asst Clin Prof NYU Sch Med

🔂 🔩 🏧 💲 Mcr   1 Week ▨ **VISA** 💳

Kronzon, Itzhak (MD)   Cv
New York University Med Ctr

560 1st Ave HW228; New York, NY 10016; (212) 263-5665; **BDCERT:** IM 79; Cv 81; **MS:** Israel 64; **RES:** Med, Jerusalem Hosp, Israel 68-69; **FEL:** Cv, Albert Einstein Med Ctr, Bronx, NY 71-73; Cv, New York University Med Ctr, New York, NY 73-74; **FAP:** Prof Med NYU Sch Med; **SI:** *Echocardiography; Valve Disease;* **HMO:** Oxford Prucare US Hlthcre

LANG: Heb; 🦽 🔂 🏧 💲 Mcr   Immediately ▨ **VISA** 💳

Kuhn, Leslie (MD)   Cv
Mount Sinai Med Ctr

1050 5th Ave; New York, NY 10028; (212) 876-9009; **BDCERT:** IM 57; Cv 60; **MS:** SUNY Hlth Sci Ctr 48; **RES:** Mount Sinai Med Ctr, New York, NY 48-49; Boston Med Ctr, Boston, MA 49-51; **FEL:** Cv, Mount Sinai Med Ctr, New York, NY; **FAP:** Clin Prof Med Mt Sinai Sch Med

🦽 🔂 🔩 🏧

Kutnick, Richard (MD)   Cv
Lenox Hill Hosp

898 Park Ave; New York, NY 10021; (212) 879-2628; **BDCERT:** IM 79; Cv 81; **MS:** Tufts U 76; **RES:** Lenox Hill Hosp, New York, NY 76-77; Lenox Hill Hosp, New York, NY 77-79; **FEL:** Cv, Lenox Hill Hosp, New York, NY 79-81; **HOSP:** Beth Israel Med Ctr; **SI:** *Echocardiography;* **HMO:** Oxford

🦽 🌙 🔂 🔩 🏧 💲   Immediately

Laragh, John (MD)   Cv
NY Hosp-Cornell Med Ctr

520 E 70th St 4th Fl; New York, NY 10021; (212) 746-2210; **BDCERT:** IM 55; **MS:** Cornell U 48; **RES:** Med, Columbia-Presbyterian Med Ctr, New York, NY 49-51; **FEL:** Cv, Columbia-Presbyterian Med Ctr, New York, NY 50-52; **FAP:** Chief & Prof Cv Cornell U; **SI:** *High Blood Pressure; Heart Attack;* **HMO:** None

♿ 🍽 M̄cr 1 Week ▨ **VISA** ●

Lewis, Benjamin (MD)   Cv
Lenox Hill Hosp

16 E 60th St; New York, NY 10022; (212) 326-8425; **BDCERT:** IM 810; Cv 83; **MS:** UC San Francisco 77; **RES:** IM, Hosp of U Penn, Philadelphia, PA 77-78; IM, Columbia-Presbyterian Med Ctr, New York, NY 78-80; **FEL:** Cv, Brigham & Women's Hosp, Boston, MA 80-82; **FAP:** Asst Prof Columbia P&S; **HOSP:** Columbia-Presbyterian Med Ctr; **SI:** *Women's Health; Mitral Valve Prolapse;* **HMO:** Oxford

LANG: Sp, Rus, Fr; ♿ 🍽 Ⓢ 1 Week ▨ **VISA** ●

Matos, Jeffrey (MD)   Cv
Lenox Hill Hosp

920 Park Ave; New York, NY 10028; (212) 772-6389; **BDCERT:** IM 80; CE 94; **MS:** Harvard Med Sch 75; **RES:** Beth Israel Med Ctr, Boston, MA 75-76; Harvard Med Sch, Cambridge, MA 77; **FEL:** Peter Bent Brigham Hosp, Boston, MA 78-80; **SI:** *Heart Beat Abnormalities;* **HMO:** United Healthcare Aetna Hlth Plan CIGNA

♿ 📷 🍽 Ⓢ M̄cr 2-4 Weeks

Mattes, Leonard (MD)   Cv
Mount Sinai Med Ctr

1199 Park Ave 1F; New York, NY 10128; (212) 876-7045; **BDCERT:** IM 72; Cv 75; **MS:** Tulane U 62; **RES:** IM, Mount Sinai Med Ctr, New York, NY 65-67; Cv, Mount Sinai Med Ctr, New York, NY 68-69; **FEL:** Cv, Mount Sinai Med Ctr, New York, NY 67-68; **FAP:** Assoc Prof Mt Sinai Sch Med

LANG: Sp; ♿ 📷 🍽 M̄cr 1 Week ▨ **VISA** ●

Mazzara, James (MD)   Cv
St Vincents Hosp & Med Ctr NY

153 W 11th St; New York, NY 10011; (212) 604-2224; **BDCERT:** IM 69; Cv 73; **MS:** NY Med Coll 63; **RES:** IM, St Vincents Hosp & Med Ctr NY, New York, NY 66-69; **FEL:** Cv, St Vincents Hosp & Med Ctr NY, New York, NY 69-70; **FAP:** Prof of Clin Med NY Med Coll

♿ 🍽 M̄cr M̄cd 2-4 Weeks

Moses, Jeffrey W (MD)   Cv
Lenox Hill Hosp

Advanced Heart Physicians & Surgeons Network, 130 E 77th St; New York, NY 10021; (212) 434-2606; **BDCERT:** IM 77; Cv 81; **MS:** Univ Penn 74; **RES:** IM, Presbyterian Med Ctr, Philadelphia, PA 74; IM, Presbyterian Med Ctr, Philadelphia, PA 75; **FEL:** Cv, Presbyterian Med Ctr, Philadelphia, PA 78; **FAP:** Clin Prof Med NYU Sch Med; **SI:** *Coronary Angioplasty; Vascular Stents*

📷 🚗 🍽 M̄cr NFI

Mueller, Richard (MD)   Cv
NY Hosp-Cornell Med Ctr

133 E 58th St; New York, NY 10022; (212) 593-9800; **BDCERT:** Cv 90; IM 90; **MS:** UC San Francisco 87; **RES:** IM, N Shore Univ Hosp-Manhasset, Manhasset, NY 87-88; Mem Sloan Kettering Cancer Ctr, New York, NY 88-89; **FEL:** Cv, NY Hosp-Cornell Med Ctr, New York, NY; **FAP:** Instr Med Cornell U; **HOSP:** St Luke's Roosevelt Hosp Ctr; **SI:** *Bone Density Tests;* **HMO:** Aetna Hlth Plan United Healthcare Oxford Sanus-NYLCare GHI +

LANG: Sp; ♿ SA 📞 📷 🚗 🍽 M̄cr A Few Days ▨ **VISA** ● ▣

Oz, Mehmet (MD)   Cv
Columbia-Presbyterian Med Ctr

Milstein 7435, 177 Ft Washington Ave; New York, NY 10032; (212) 305-4434; **BDCERT:** S 92; Cv 94; **MS:** Univ Penn 86; **RES:** Columbia-Presbyterian Med Ctr, New York, NY 87-91; **FAP:** Asst Prof Columbia P&S; **HOSP:** St Michael's Med Ctr; **SI:** *Coronary Bypass; Heart Failure;* **HMO:** Oxford Blue Cross

LANG: Sp, Fr, Trk; ♿ 📞 📷 🚗 🍽 M̄cr M̄cd WC Immediately

Packer, Milton (MD)   Cv
Columbia-Presbyterian Med Ctr

177 Fort Washington Ave Fl 5; New York, NY
10032; (212) 305-7500; **BDCERT:** IM 76; Cv 79;
MS: Jefferson Med Coll 73; **RES:** IM, Albert Einstein
Med Ctr, Bronx, NY 73-76; **FEL:** Cv, Mount Sinai
Med Ctr, New York, NY 76-78; **SI:** *Heart Failure*

Pinkernell, Bruce (MD)   Cv
St Luke's Roosevelt Hosp Ctr

425 W 59th St 8B; New York, NY 10019; (212)
376-3180; **BDCERT:** IM 71; Cv 73; **MS:** NY Med
Coll 64; **RES:** IM, St Vincents Hosp & Med Ctr NY,
New York, NY 64-67; **FEL:** Cv, St Vincents Hosp,
New York, NY 67-69; **FAP:** Assoc Clin Prof Med
Columbia P&S; **SI:** *Cardiology*

LANG: Sp; 🦽 👱 🎬 💲 Mcr 1 Week

Porder, Joseph (MD)   Cv
Mount Sinai Med Ctr

1160 5th Ave 102; New York, NY 10029; (212)
860-5500; **BDCERT:** IM 85; Cv 87; **MS:** Columbia
P&S 82; **RES:** IM, Mount Sinai Med Ctr, New York,
NY 82-85; **FEL:** Cv, Mount Sinai Med Ctr, New
York, NY 85-87; **FAP:** Clin Instr Mt Sinai Sch Med;
SI: *Preventive Cardiology; Nutritional Medicine;* **HMO:**
Oxford Metlife Blue Choice Aetna Hlth Plan

📞 👱 🎬 Mcr WC A Few Days

Post, Martin (MD)   Cv
NY Hosp-Cornell Med Ctr

425 E 61st St; New York, NY 10021; (212) 752-
2000; **BDCERT:** IM 74; **MS:** SUNY Syracuse 67;
RES: Ohio State U Hosp, Columbus, OH; **FEL:** Cv, NY
Hosp-Cornell Med Ctr, New York, NY; **FAP:** Asst
Prof Cornell U; **HOSP:** Lenox Hill Hosp; **SI:**
Arteriosclerosis; Hyperlipidemia; **HMO:** None

🦽 SA 👱 🎬 💲 Mcr A Few Days 🔳 **VISA** 💳

Reichstein, Robert (MD)   Cv
Mount Sinai Med Ctr

1185 Park Ave 1L; New York, NY 10128; (212)
996-2900; **BDCERT:** IM 80; Cv 83; **MS:** U Hlth
Sci/Chicago Med Sch 77; **RES:** IM, Mount Sinai Med
Ctr, New York, NY 78-81; **FEL:** Cv, Mount Sinai
Med Ctr, New York, NY 81-84; **FAP:** Asst Prof Med
Mt Sinai Sch Med; **SI:** *Diseases of the Aorta;*
Preventive Cardiology

LANG: Sp; 🦽 👱 🎬 🛏️

Reiffel, James (MD)   Cv
Columbia-Presbyterian Med Ctr

161 Fort Washington Ave; New York, NY 10032;
(212) 305-5206; **BDCERT:** Cv 74; CE 92; **MS:**
Columbia P&S 69; **RES:** Med, Columbia-
Presbyterian Med Ctr, New York, NY 69-72; **FEL:**
CE, Columbia-Presbyterian Med Ctr, New York, NY
72-74; **FAP:** Prof Columbia P&S; **SI:** *Arrhythmias;*
Electrophysiology

🦽 👱 💲 Mcr 2-4 Weeks

Rentrop, K Peter (MD)   Cv
St Vincents Hosp & Med Ctr NY

Gramercy Cardiac Diagnostic Services, 38 E 22nd
St; New York, NY 10010; (212) 475-8066;
BDCERT: IM 73; **MS:** Germany 66; **RES:** IM, Detroit
Med Ctr, Detroit, MI 69-70; IM, Cleveland Clinic
Hosp, Cleveland, OH 70-71; **FEL:** Cv, Cleveland
Clinic Hosp, Cleveland, OH 71-73; **FAP:** Lecturer
Med NY Med Coll; **HOSP:** St Luke's Roosevelt Hosp
Ctr; **SI:** *Early Diagnosis & Treatment; Coronary Artery*
Disease; **HMO:** GHI Oxford Aetna-US Healthcare
United Healthcare Empire Blue Cross & Shield +

LANG: Ger, Grk, Cam, Rus; 🦽 📞 👱 🎬 💲 Mcr
Mcr WC NFl A Few Days

Riegelhaupt, Elliot (MD)   Cv   **PCP**
Mount Sinai Med Ctr

64 E 94th St 1E; New York, NY 10128; (212) 439-
6690; **BDCERT:** IM 79; Cv 83; **MS:** Albert Einstein
Coll Med 76; **RES:** Montefiore Med Ctr, Bronx, NY
76-79; **FEL:** Cv, Mount Sinai Med Ctr, New York,
NY 80-82; **HOSP:** Beth Israel Med Ctr

Romanello, Paul (MD)   Cv
Lenox Hill Hosp

Park East Cardiology, 1421 3rd Ave; New York, NY 10028; (212) 535-6340; **BDCERT:** IM 87; Cv 89; **MS:** SUNY Hlth Sci Ctr 83; **RES:** IM, Lenox Hill Hosp, New York, NY 83-87; **FEL:** Cv, Lenox Hill Hosp, New York, NY 87-89; *SI: Cholesterol Problems; Coronary Artery Disease;* **HMO:** Oxford CIGNA PHCS Blue Choice Aetna-US Healthcare +

LANG: Sp, Rus; 🦽 🔲 🖼 🏥 💲 Mcr   A Few Days
VISA ●●

Rose, Eric A (MD)   Cv
Columbia-Presbyterian Med Ctr

ColumbiaPresbyterian Med Ctr, 177 Ft Washington Ave; New York, NY 10032; (212) 305-6380; **BDCERT:** TS 83; **MS:** Columbia P&S 75; **RES:** TS, Columbia-Presbyterian Med Ctr, New York, NY 80-81; **HMO:** Aetna Hlth Plan Chubb Sanus Oxford

Rosenfeld, Isadore (MD)   Cv
NY Hosp-Cornell Med Ctr

Cornell Cardiology Consultants, 125 E 72nd St; New York, NY 10021; (212) 628-6100; **MS:** McGill U 51; **RES:** Royal Victoria Hosp, Montreal, Canada 52-53; Johns Hopkins Hosp, Baltimore, MD 53-54; **FEL:** Cv, Jewish Gen Hosp, Montreal, Canada; Mount Sinai Med Ctr, New York, NY; **FAP:** Prof Med Cornell U; **HOSP:** Mem Sloan Kettering Cancer Ctr; *SI: Cardiology*

LANG: Sp, Ger, Fr, Rom, Chi; 🔲 🖼 🏥 💲 Mcr
1 Week 🖩 **VISA** ●● 🖼

Rozanski, Alan (MD)   Cv
St Luke's Roosevelt Hosp Ctr

421 W 114th St; New York, NY 10025; (212) 523-4011; **BDCERT:** IM 78; Cv 83; **MS:** Tufts U 75; **RES:** IM, Mount Sinai Med Ctr, New York, NY 75-77; **FEL:** Cv, Mount Sinai Med Ctr, New York, NY 78-80; NuM, Cedars-Sinai Med Ctr, Los Angeles, CA 80-82; **FAP:** Assoc Prof Columbia P&S; *SI: Nuclear Cardiology; Preventive Cardiology;* **HMO:** Oxford Aetna Hlth Plan 1199 GHI Amerihealth +

🦽 🔲 🏥 Mcr Mcd Immediately

Scheidt, Stephen (MD)   Cv
NY Hosp-Cornell Med Ctr

520 E 70th St; New York, NY 10021; (212) 746-2150; **BDCERT:** IM 74; Cv 74; **MS:** Columbia P&S 65; **RES:** Montefiore Med Ctr, Bronx, NY 65-66; Med, Bellevue Hosp Ctr, New York, NY 66-68; **FEL:** Cv, NY Hosp-Cornell Med Ctr, New York, NY 68-70; **FAP:** Prof Cornell U; **HMO:** Aetna-US Healthcare CIGNA Magnacare Empire Blue Cross & Shield Multiplan +

LANG: Ger; 🦽 🔲 🏥 💲 Mcr Mcd

Schiffer, Mark (MD)   Cv
Lenox Hill Hosp

1421 3rd Ave; New York, NY 10028; (212) 535-6340; **BDCERT:** IM 80; Cv 83; **MS:** Northwestern U 77; **RES:** Med, Lenox Hill Hosp, New York, NY 78-81; **FEL:** Cv, Lenox Hill Hosp, New York, NY 81-83; **FAP:** Assoc Clin Prof IM NYU Sch Med; **HMO:** Oxford US Hlthcre Blue Choice CIGNA PHCS +

Schiller, Myles (MD)   Cv
NY Hosp-Cornell Med Ctr

NY Hosp/Cornell Med Ctr, 525 E 68th St PedCAR; New York, NY 10021; (212) 746-3250; **BDCERT:** Ped 78; PCd 79; **MS:** U Hlth Sci/Chicago Med Sch 73; **RES:** Ped, NY Hosp-Cornell Med Ctr, New York, NY 74-75; **FEL:** PCd, NY Hosp-Cornell Med Ctr, New York, NY 76-77; **FAP:** Assoc Clin Prof Ped Cornell U; *SI: Congenital Heart Disease; Interventional Cardiology*

🦽 🔲 🖼 🏥 💲 Mcr Mcd Immediately **VISA** ●●

Schulman, Ira (MD)   Cv
NYU Downtown Hosp

170 William St 818; New York, NY 10038; (212) 233-5308; **BDCERT:** IM 77; Cv 79; **MS:** NYU Sch Med 74; **RES:** IM, Bellevue Hosp Ctr, New York, NY 74-77; **FEL:** Cv, Montefiore Med Ctr, Bronx, NY 77-79; **FAP:** Asst Prof Med Cornell U; **HOSP:** New York University Med Ctr; *SI: Angina; Heart Failure;* **HMO:** Aetna Hlth Plan Oxford United Healthcare PHCS

LANG: Chi, Sp; 🦽 🅲 🔲 🖼 🏥 💲 Immediately

Schwartz, Miles (MD) Cv
St Luke's Roosevelt Hosp Ctr
102 E 81st St; New York, NY 10028; (212) 288-
1850; **BDCERT:** IM 58; Cv 67; **MS:** NY Med Coll 51;
RES: IM, VA Med Ctr-Bronx, Bronx, NY 52-53; IM,
VA Med Ctr-Bronx, Bronx, NY 53-54; **FEL:** Cv,
Bronx VA Hosp, Bronx, NY 54-55
⚕ 📷 🛏 💲 Mcr Immediately

Schwartz, William (MD) Cv
Lenox Hill Hosp
302 W 86th St 12 A; New York, NY 10024; (718)
721-1500; **BDCERT:** IM 78; Cv 81; **MS:** Albert
Einstein Coll Med 75; **RES:** Med, Bronx Municipal
Hosp Center, Bronx, NY 75-76; Med, Bronx
Municipal Hosp Center, Bronx, NY 76-78; **FEL:** Cv,
Bronx Municipal/Albert Einstein Med Ctr, Bronx,
NY 78-79; **HOSP:** Mount Sinai Med Ctr; **HMO:**
Aetna Hlth Plan Oxford PHS
LANG: Sp; ⚕ 📞 📷 🛉 🛏 💲 Mcr Mcd Immediately
▨▨ *VISA* ⬤

Seinfeld, David (MD) Cv **PCP**
Lenox Hill Hosp
MidManhattan Medical Associates, 35 E 75th St
Ground Fl; New York, NY 10021; (212) 288-1538;
BDCERT: IM 76; Cv 79; **MS:** Albert Einstein Coll
Med 73; **RES:** Montefiore Med Ctr, Bronx, NY 73-
76; **FEL:** Cv, Montefiore Med Ctr, Bronx, NY 76-78;
HOSP: Montefiore Med Ctr; **HMO:** Oxford 32BJ
LANG: Heb, Yd; ⚕ 📷 🛉 🛏 💲 Mcr A Few Days
VISA ⬤

Sherman, Warren (MD) Cv
Beth Israel Med Ctr
305 1st Ave; New York, NY 10003; (212) 420-
2806; **BDCERT:** IM 80; Cv 83; **MS:** SUNY Syracuse
77; **RES:** Rochester Gen Hosp, Rochester, NY 77-
80; **FEL:** Cv, Oregon Health Sci U Hosp, Portland,
OR; *SI: Cardiac Catheterization; Angioplasty;* **HMO:**
CIGNA HIP Network Oxford GHI Aetna Hlth Plan +
LANG: Sp, Rus, Chi; ⚕ 📷 🛉 🛏 💲 Mcr Mcd WC
A Few Days ▨▨ *VISA* ⬤

Siegal, Michael S (MD) Cv
St Luke's Roosevelt Hosp Ctr
18 E 53rd St 12th Fl; New York, NY 10022; (212)
319-1700; **BDCERT:** IM 80; **MS:** Harvard Med Sch
70; **RES:** New York University Med Ctr, New York,
NY 78-80; **FEL:** Cv, Mount Sinai Med Ctr, New
York, NY 80-82; **HOSP:** Lenox Hill Hosp; **HMO:**
None
LANG: Sp, Fr, Yd, Ger, Itl; ⚕ 📞 📷 🛉 🛏 💲
Immediately *VISA* ⬤

Squire, Anthony (MD) Cv
Mount Sinai Med Ctr
1120 Park Ave 1C; New York, NY 10128; (212)
410-4800; **BDCERT:** IM 81; Cv 83; **MS:** Mt Sinai
Sch Med 78; **RES:** Mount Sinai Med Ctr, New York,
NY 78-81; **FEL:** Cv, Mount Sinai Med Ctr, New
York, NY; *SI: Angina; Echocardiology;* **HMO:** Oxford
US Hlthcre Prucare United Healthcare Blue Cross &
Blue Shield +
LANG: Sp; ⚕ 📷 🛏 💲 Mcr Immediately ⬤

Stein, Richard A (MD) Cv
Lenox Hill Hosp
178 E 85th St; New York, NY 10028; (212) 434-
2600; **BDCERT:** IM 73; Cv 75; **MS:** NYU Sch Med
67; **RES:** IM, Univ Hosp SUNY Bklyn, Brooklyn, NY
68-69; **FEL:** Cv, Univ Hosp SUNY Bklyn, Brooklyn,
NY 72-74; **FAP:** Prof SUNY Hlth Sci Ctr; *SI: Cardiac
Prevention and Rehabilitation; Cardiac Exercise;* **HMO:**
Oxford Empire Blue Cross & Shield GHI
LANG: Fr, Sp; ⚕ 📞 📷 🛉 🛏 Mcr WC Immediately
▨▨

Steinberg, Gregory (MD) Cv
St Luke's Roosevelt Hosp Ctr
St LukesRoosevelt HospitalCenter, 428 W 59th St
8A; New York, NY 10019; (212) 841-0987;
BDCERT: IM 85; Cv 87; **MS:** England 78; **RES:** IM,
Midway Hosp-Gillingham, Kent, England 79-80;
IM, St Luke's Roosevelt Hosp Ctr, New York, NY 80-
81; **FEL:** IM, St Luke's Roosevelt Hosp Ctr, New
York, NY 82-85; Cv, St Luke's Roosevelt Hosp Ctr,
New York, NY 85-87; **FAP:** Assoc Prof of Clin Med
Columbia P&S; *SI: General Cardiology; General
Internal Medicine;* **HMO:** Oxford Chubb Aetna-US
Healthcare Prudential PHS +
LANG: Fr; ⚕ 📞 📷 🛏 💲 Mcr 1 Week

Tenenbaum, Joseph (MD)   Cv
Columbia-Presbyterian Med Ctr

161 Ft Washington Ave; New York, NY 10032;
(212) 305-5288; **BDCERT:** IM 77; Cv 79; **MS:**
Harvard Med Sch 74; **RES:** Columbia-Presbyterian
Med Ctr, New York, NY 74-77; **FEL:** Cv, Mount
Sinai Med Ctr, New York, NY 77-79; **FAP:** Clin Prof
Columbia P&S; **SI:** *Valvular Heart Disease; Coronary
Heart Disease;* **HMO:** Oxford

🛆 🔂 💲 Mcr 4+ Weeks

Tyberg, Theodore (MD)   Cv   PCP
NY Hosp-Cornell Med Ctr

New York Cardiology Associates, 425 E 61st St 6th
Fl; New York, NY 10021; (212) 752-2000;
BDCERT: Cv 81; **MS:** Rush Med Coll 75; **RES:** IM,
NY Hosp-Cornell Med Ctr, New York, NY 75-78;
FEL: Cv, Yale-New Haven Hosp, New Haven, CT
78-80; **FAP:** Assoc Clin Prof Med Cornell U; **HOSP:**
Lenox Hill Hosp; **SI:** *Hyperlipidemia*

LANG: Fr, Sp, Rus, Heb; 🛆 🔂 🐍 🛏 💲 Mcr
A Few Days ▨ *VISA* 💳

Unger, Allen (MD)   Cv
Mount Sinai Med Ctr

12 E 86th St; New York, NY 10028; (212) 734-
6000; **BDCERT:** Cv 78; IM 67; **MS:** SUNY Syracuse
60; **RES:** Mount Sinai Med Ctr, New York, NY 61-
67; **FEL:** Cv, Mount Sinai Med Ctr, New York, NY
65-66; **FAP:** Asst Clin Prof Mt Sinai Sch Med; **SI:**
Hypercholesterolemia; Hypertension

🛆 🔂 🐍 🛏 Mcr A Few Days ▨ *VISA* 💳

Varriale, Philip (MD)   Cv
Cabrini Med Ctr

222 E 19th St 2D; New York, NY 10003; (212)
777-3219; **BDCERT:** IM 66; Cv 70; **MS:** SUNY Hlth
Sci Ctr 59; **RES:** VA Med Ctr-Brooklyn, Brooklyn,
NY 60-62; St Vincents Hosp & Med Ctr NY, New
York, NY 62-63; **FEL:** St Vincents Hosp & Med Ctr
NY, New York, NY 63-64; **FAP:** Assoc Clin Prof
Med NY Med Coll; **HOSP:** St Vincents Hosp & Med
Ctr NY; **SI:** *Pacemaker Therapy; Coronary Care;* **HMO:**
GHI Blue Cross 32BJ 1199

🛆 🅲 🔂 🐍 🛏 💲 Mcr Mcd 1 Week

Weisenseel, Arthur (MD)   Cv
Mount Sinai Med Ctr

12 E 86th St; New York, NY 10028; (212) 734-
6000; **BDCERT:** IM 69; Cv 73; **MS:** Georgetown U
63; **RES:** IM, Mount Sinai Med Ctr, New York, NY
64-66; **FEL:** Mount Sinai Med Ctr, New York, NY
66-67; **FAP:** Asst Clin Prof Mt Sinai Sch Med; **SI:**
Vascular Disease; Hyperlipidemia; **HMO:** None

LANG: Sp, Slv, Rom; 🔂 🐍 🛏 💲 Mcr A Few Days
▨ *VISA* 💳 💳

Weisfeldt, Myron L (MD)   Cv
Columbia-Presbyterian Med Ctr

630 W 168th St; New York, NY 10032; (212)
305-5838; **MS:** Johns Hopkins U 65; **RES:**
Columbia-Presbyterian Med Ctr, New York, NY 65-
67; Mass Gen Hosp, Boston, MA 69-70; **FEL:** Cv,
Mass Gen Hosp, Boston, MA; **FAP:** Prof Columbia
P&S; **HMO:** Oxford Prudential

🔂 Mcr Mcd 2-4 Weeks

Wilentz, James (MD)   Cv
Beth Israel Med Ctr

1st Ave & 16th St FL11; New York, NY 10003;
(212) 420-2806; **BDCERT:** IM 79; **MS:** NYU Sch
Med 76; **RES:** IM, Peter Bent Brigham Hosp, Boston,
MA 77-79; **FEL:** Grace Hosp, Detroit, MI 85-86;
Med, Boston U Med Ctr, Boston, MA 82-84; **FAP:**
Asst Clin Prof Med Cornell U

Wolk, Michael (MD)   Cv
NY Hosp-Cornell Med Ctr

520 E 72nd St LC1; New York, NY 10021; (212)
988-2881; **BDCERT:** IM 71; Cv 73; **MS:** Columbia
P&S 64; **RES:** Univ Hosp SUNY Bklyn, Brooklyn, NY
64-67; **FEL:** New England Med Ctr, Boston, MA 67-
69; NY Hosp-Cornell Med Ctr, New York, NY 69-
70; **FAP:** Clin Prof Med Cornell U; **SI:** *Angina;
Myocardial Infarction;* **HMO:** PHCS PHS American
Health Plan Anthem Health

🛆 🔂 🛏 💲 Mcr A Few Days

Zaremski, Benjamin (MD)   Cv
Beth Israel Med Ctr

510 E 80th St; New York, NY 10021; (212) 517-0022; **BDCERT:** IM 86; **MS:** Dominican Republic 81; **RES:** NY Med Coll, New York, NY 82-84; **FEL:** NY Med Coll, New York, NY 84-86; **HOSP:** Lenox Hill Hosp; **SI:** *Heart Disease*; **HMO:** Oxford Aetna Hlth Plan Magnacare PHCS PHS +

LANG: Sp, Heb, Fr; 🚻 🈯 🔲 🕮 🕮 💲 Mcr Immediately

CHILD & ADOLESCENT PSYCHIATRY

Abright, Arthur Reese (MD)ChAP
St Vincents Hosp & Med Ctr NY

203 W 12th St; New York, NY 10011; (212) 604-8213; **BDCERT:** Psyc 78; ChAP 81; **MS:** Univ Texas, Houston 73; **RES:** Med/Psyc, St Vincents Hosp & Med Ctr NY, New York, NY 73-74; Psyc, NY Hosp-Cornell Med Ctr, New York, NY 74-77; **FEL:** ChAP, NY Hosp-Cornell Med Ctr, New York, NY 77-79; **FAP:** Assoc Prof NY Med Coll; **SI:** *Depression and Bipolar Disorder; Attention Deficit Disorder*

🚻 🈯 🔲 🕮 💲 1 Week

Bird, Hector (MD)   ChAP
Columbia-Presbyterian Med Ctr

New York State Psychiatric Institute/ Columbia Presbyterian, 145 Central Park West 1CC; New York, NY 10023; (212) 874-5311; **BDCERT:** Psyc 75; ChAP 77; **MS:** Yale U Sch Med 65; **RES:** Psyc, Columbia-Presbyterian Med Ctr, New York, NY 68-71; ChAP, Columbia-Presbyterian Med Ctr, New York, NY 70-72; **FEL:** Psyc, William A White Inst, New York, NY 72-77; **FAP:** Clin Prof Psyc Columbia P&S; **SI:** *Depression; Personality Disorders*

LANG: Sp; 🚻 🔲 🕮 💲 wc

Fox, Sarah J (MD)   ChAP
Columbia-Presbyterian Med Ctr

210 W 89th St 1E; New York, NY 10024; (212) 874-4558; **BDCERT:** Psyc 91; ChAP 94; **MS:** Tufts U 82; **RES:** Ped, Jacobi Med Ctr, Bronx, NY 82-83; Psyc, Albert Einstein Med Ctr, Bronx, NY 83-85; **FEL:** ChAP, Columbia-Presbyterian Med Ctr, New York, NY 85-87; NYS Psychiatric Institute, New York, NY 86-95; **FAP:** Instr Columbia P&S; **SI:** *Child and Adolescent Psychiatry; Psychoanalysis*

🚻 🔲 🕮 💲 1 Week

Green, Arthur (MD)   ChAP
Columbia-Presbyterian Med Ctr

350 Central Park West Apt 13I; New York, NY 10025; (212) 678-4338; **BDCERT:** ChAP 69; Psyc 64; **MS:** Holland 57; **RES:** Univ Hosp SUNY Bklyn, Brooklyn, NY 58-60; St Luke's Roosevelt Hosp Ctr, New York, NY 60-61; **FEL:** Psychoanalysis, NYS Psychiatric Institute, New York, NY 60-67; ChAP, NYS Psychiatric Institute, New York, NY 75-79; **FAP:** Clin Prof Psyc Columbia P&S; **SI:** *Traumatic Stress; Psychotherapy/Psychoanalysis*

LANG: Dut, Fr; 🚻 🔲 🕮 wc NfI A Few Days

Green, Wayne Hugo (MD)   ChAP
Bellevue Hosp Ctr

Bellevue Children & Adolescent Psychiatric Clinic, 1st Ave & 27th St Admin A259; New York, NY 10016; (212) 562-4991; **BDCERT:** ChAP 78; Psyc 75; **MS:** NYU Sch Med 67; **RES:** Psyc, Bellevue Hosp Ctr, New York, NY 70-72; **FEL:** ChAP, Bellevue Hosp Ctr, New York, NY 72-74; **FAP:** Assoc Prof of Clin Psyc NYU Sch Med; **HOSP:** New York University Med Ctr; **SI:** *Psychopharmacology; Outpatient Treatment*; **HMO:** Centercare Metroplus

🚻 🔲 🕮 Mcr Mol A Few Days

Harrison-Ross, Phyllis (MD)ChAP
Metropolitan Hosp Ctr

41 Central Park West 10 C; New York, NY 10023; (212) 799-8055; **MS:** Wayne State U Sch Med 59; **RES:** Ped, NY Hosp-Cornell Med Ctr, New York, NY 60-62; Psyc, Jacobi Med Ctr, Bronx, NY 62-64; **FEL:** ChAP, Jacobi Med Ctr, Bronx, NY 64-66; **FAP:** Prof NY Med Coll; **SI:** *Multicultural Competency*; **HMO:** Metroplus Centercare Fidelis

🚻 🈯 🔲 🕮 💲 2-4 Weeks

Hertzig, Margaret (MD)   ChAP
NY Hosp-Cornell Med Ctr

525 E 68th St Box 147; New York, NY 10021; (212) 821-0726; **BDCERT:** ChAP 68; ChAP 75; **MS:** NYU Sch Med 60; **RES:** Bellevue Hosp Ctr, New York, NY 61-65; **FAP:** Prof Cornell U; *SI: Developmental Disabilities; Attention Deficit Disorders*

⬛ ⬛ ⬛ ⬛ ⬛ 1 Week

Hirsch, Glenn S (MD)   ChAP
New York University Med Ctr

182 E 79th St; New York, NY 10021; (212) 263-8704; **BDCERT:** Psyc 84; ChAP 85; **MS:** Albert Einstein Coll Med 79; **RES:** Psyc, NY Hosp-Cornell-Westchester, White Plains, NY 79-82; **FEL:** ChAP, Columbia-Presbyterian Med Ctr, New York, NY 82-84; **FAP:** Asst Prof of Clin Psyc NYU Sch Med; *SI: Tourette's; Anxiety*

⬛ ⬛ ⬛ ⬛ ⬛ 1 Week

Kestenbaum, Clarice (MD) ChAP
Columbia-Presbyterian Med Ctr

NYSPI, 722 W 168th St 9th Fl Unit 60; New York, NY 10032; (212) 873-1020; **BDCERT:** Psyc 71; ChAP 75; **MS:** USC Sch Med 60; **RES:** Psyc, Columbia-Presbyterian Med Ctr, New York, NY 61-64; ChAP, Columbia-Presbyterian Med Ctr, New York, NY 64-65; **FEL:** Columbia-Presbyterian Med Ctr, New York, NY; **FAP:** Prof of Clin Columbia P&S; *SI: Child and Adolescent Psychiatry; Psychoanalysis;* **HMO:** None

⬛

Koplewicz, Harold (MD)   ChAP
New York University Med Ctr

550 1st Ave; New York, NY 10021; (212) 263-6205; **BDCERT:** ChAP 83; **MS:** Albert Einstein Coll Med 78; **RES:** Jacobi Med Ctr, Bronx, NY; NY Hosp-Cornell-Westchester, White Plains, NY; **FEL:** Columbia-Presbyterian Med Ctr, New York, NY; **FAP:** Prof NYU Sch Med; **HOSP:** Bellevue Hosp Ctr; *SI: Pediatric Psychopharmacology*

⬛ ⬛ ⬛ ⬛ ⬛ ⬛ 4+ Weeks

Kron, Leo (MD)   ChAP
St Luke's Roosevelt Hosp Ctr

30 E 76th St; New York, NY 10021; (212) 861-7001; **BDCERT:** Psyc 76; ChAP 86; **MS:** U British Columbia Fac Med 61; **RES:** Psyc, Montefiore Med Ctr, Bronx, NY 73-76; **FEL:** ChAP, St Luke's Roosevelt Hosp Ctr, New York, NY; **FAP:** Asst Prof Psyc Columbia P&S; *SI: Psychopharmacology; Psychoanalytic Therapy*

⬛ ⬛ ⬛ ⬛ ⬛ 2-4 Weeks

Lewis, Dorothy Otnow (MD)ChAP
Bellevue Hosp Ctr

550 1st Ave; New York, NY 10016; (212) 263-6208; **BDCERT:** Psyc 72; **MS:** Yale U Sch Med 63; **RES:** Psyc, Yale-New Haven Hosp, New Haven, CT 65-67; **FEL:** ChAP, Yale-New Haven Hosp, New Haven, CT 68-69; **FAP:** Prof NYU Sch Med; **HOSP:** Yale-New Haven Hosp

LANG: Fr; ⬛

Lewis, Owen (MD)   ChAP
Columbia-Presbyterian Med Ctr

11 E 87th St; New York, NY 10128; (212) 996-8196; **BDCERT:** Psyc 82; **MS:** Mt Sinai Sch Med 76; **RES:** Psyc, NY Hosp-Cornell Med Ctr, New York, NY 76-80; ChAP, NY Hosp-Cornell Med Ctr, New York, NY 80-82; **FAP:** Assoc Clin Prof Psyc Columbia P&S; *SI: Psychotherapy; Psychopharmacology*

⬛ ⬛ ⬛ ⬛ ⬛ 2-4 Weeks

Moreau, Donna (MD)   ChAP
Columbia-Presbyterian Med Ctr

110 East End Ave; New York, NY 10028; (212) 772-9205; **BDCERT:** Psyc 85; ChAP 91; **MS:** SUNY Hlth Sci Ctr 76; **RES:** Psyc, NY Hosp-Cornell Med Ctr, New York, NY 80-84; **FEL:** ChAP, NY Hosp-Cornell Med Ctr, New York, NY 84-86; **FAP:** Assoc Clin Prof Psyc Columbia P&S; *SI: Psychopharmacology & Depression; Anxiety*

⬛ ⬛ ⬛ ⬛ 1 Week

Shaffer, David (MD)   ChAP
Columbia-Presbyterian Med Ctr
722 W 168th St; New York, NY 10032; (212)
543-5947; **MS:** England 61; **RES:** Hosp For Sick
Children, London, England 63-66; U Coll Hosp,
London, England 62; **FEL:** Yale-New Haven Hosp,
New Haven, CT 66-67; U of London, London,
England 65-69; **FAP:** Prof Columbia P&S; *SI:*
Suicidal Adolescents; Anxiety Disorders

♿ 📷 ▤ 📅 2-4 Weeks

Spencer, Elizabeth (MD)   ChAP
Bellevue Hosp Ctr
22 E 36th St Ste 2D; New York, NY 10016; (212)
684-3810; **BDCERT:** Psyc 90; ChAP 92; **MS:** Geo
Wash U Sch Med 79; **RES:** Ped, U MD Hosp,
Baltimore, MD 79-82; Psyc, New York University
Med Ctr, New York, NY 84-86; **FEL:** Behavorial
Ped, U MD Hosp, Baltimore, MD 82-84; ChAP, New
York University Med Ctr, New York, NY 86-88;
FAP: Asst Prof Psyc NYU Sch Med; **HOSP:** New
York University Med Ctr; **HMO:** None

1 Week

Youngerman, Joseph (MD) ChAP
Bronx Children's Psych Ctr
122 E 82nd St; New York, NY 10021; (212) 249-
1449; **BDCERT:** Psyc 76; **MS:** Harvard Med Sch 68;
RES: Psyc, Albert Einstein Med Ctr, Bronx, NY 71-
73; **FEL:** ChAP, Albert Einstein Med Ctr, Bronx, NY
73-75; **FAP:** Asst Clin Prof Psyc Albert Einstein Coll
Med

CHILD NEUROLOGY

Aron, Alan (MD)   ChiN
Mount Sinai Med Ctr
5 E 98th St; New York, NY 10029; (212) 831-
4393; **BDCERT:** Ped 63; N 67; **MS:** Columbia P&S
58; **RES:** Columbia-Presbyterian Med Ctr, New
York, NY 59-61; **FEL:** Ped N, Columbia-
Presbyterian Med Ctr, New York, NY 61-64; *SI:*
Neurofibromatosis; Seizure Disorders; **HMO:** US
Hlthcre Oxford

LANG: Sp; ♿ 📷 ▤ 📅 S M N 2-4 Weeks 👄
VISA 💳 💳

Chutorian, Abe (MD)   ChiN
NY Hosp-Cornell Med Ctr
525 E 68th St Box 91; New York, NY 10021; (212)
746-3278; **BDCERT:** Ped 62; N 65; **MS:** U
Manitoba 57; **RES:** Ped, Children's Hosp of Los
Angeles, Los Angeles, CA 58-60; **FEL:** N, Columbia-
Presbyterian Med Ctr, New York, NY 60-63; **HOSP:**
Hosp For Special Surgery; *SI: Brain Tumors; Seizures*;
HMO: Blue Choice Oxford NYLCare 32BJ United
Healthcare +

♿ 📷 📅 S M N 1 Week 👄 **VISA** 💳

DeVivo, Darryl C (MD)   ChiN
Columbia-Presbyterian Med Ctr
710 W 168th St; New York, NY 10032; (212)
305-5244; **BDCERT:** N 72; **MS:** U Va Sch Med 78;
RES: Ped, Mass Gen Hosp, Boston, MA 65-66; Mass
Gen Hosp, Boston, MA 66-67; **FAP:** Prof Columbia
P&S; *SI: Neuromuscular Diseases*; **HMO:** Oxford

♿ 📷 ▤ 📅 S **VISA** 💳 💳

Fish, Irving (MD)   ChiN
New York University Med Ctr
University Neurology Assoc, 650 1st Ave Fl 4; New
York, NY 10016; (212) 213-8469; **MS:** Canada
64; **RES:** ChiN, Children's Hosp, Halifax, Canada
64-65; NY Hosp-Cornell Med Ctr, New York, NY
65-68; **FEL:** NY Hosp-Cornell Med Ctr, New York,
NY 68-69; **FAP:** Dir ChiN NYU Sch Med; **HOSP:**
Bellevue Hosp Ctr; *SI: Headaches—Pediatric*; **HMO:**
Oxford US Hlthcre

♿ 📷 ▤ 📅 S 1 Week

Gold, Arnold (MD)   ChiN
Columbia-Presbyterian Med Ctr
Pediatric Neurology, 720 W 168th St; New York,
NY 10032; (212) 305-5483; **BDCERT:** N 62; Ped
60; **MS:** Switzerland 54; **RES:** Charity Hosp, New
Orleans, LA 54-55; Ped, Children's Hosp Med Ctr,
Cincinnati, OH 55-58; **FEL:** ChiN, Columbia-
Presbyterian Med Ctr, New York, NY 58-61; **FAP:**
Clin Prof N Columbia P&S; *SI: Learning Disabilities;*
Developmental Disabilities

LANG: Fr; ♿ 🔍 📷 ▤ 📅 S 2-4 Weeks

Guide to symbols and abbreviations can be found on pages 110-113.

165

Lell, Mary-Elizabeth (MD)   ChiN
St Vincents Hosp & Med Ctr NY

153 W 11th St Rm 457; New York, NY 10011;
(212) 604-7494; **BDCERT:** Ped 80; ChiN 76; **MS:**
Univ Penn 68; **RES:** N, Med Ctr Hosp of VT,
Burlington, VT 69-71; Ped, St Louis Children's
Hosp, St Louis, MO 71-72; **FEL:** ChiN, Columbia-
Presbyterian Med Ctr, New York, NY 72-74; **FAP:**
Assoc Prof of Clin N NY Med Coll; *SI: Neonatal
Neurology; Learning Difficulties;* **HMO:** Blue Cross &
Blue Shield Prucare US Hlthcre Aetna Hlth Plan
PHS +

LANG: Sp; 🔲 🔲 🔲 🔲 🔲   1 Week

Molofsky, Walter (MD)   ChiN
Beth Israel Med Ctr

Beth Israel Medical CtrNorth Divison, 170 E End
Ave; New York, NY 10128; (212) 870-9407;
BDCERT: ChiN 86; Ped 82; **MS:** NYU Sch Med 76;
RES: Ped, Columbia-Presbyterian Med Ctr, New
York, NY 76-78; **FEL:** ChiN, Columbia-Presbyterian
Med Ctr, New York, NY 78-81; **FAP:** Assoc Prof
Albert Einstein Coll Med; **HOSP:** Roosevelt Hosp; *SI:
Headaches; Muscle Disease;* **HMO:** Oxford Prudential
Aetna Hlth Plan CIGNA Blue Cross & Blue Shield +

LANG: Sp; 🔲 🔲 🔲 🔲 🔲 🔲 🔲 🔲   1 Week 🔲
VISA 🔲 🔲

Nordli, Douglas (MD)   ChiN
Columbia-Presbyterian Med Ctr

BH-11N, 3959 Broadway Ste 8; New York, NY
10032; (212) 305-7549; **BDCERT:** N 89; Ped 89;
MS: Columbia P&S 84; **RES:** Ped, Babies Hosp, New
York, NY 84-86; ChiN, Columbia-Presbyterian Med
Ctr, New York, NY 86-89; **FEL:** C/NPh, Columbia-
Presbyterian Med Ctr, New York, NY 89-90; **FAP:**
Dir Ped Columbia P&S; *SI: Epilepsy Pediatric*

🔲 🔲 🔲 🔲 🔲 🔲 🔲   4+ Weeks 🔲 **VISA** 🔲 🔲

COLON & RECTAL SURGERY

Brandeis, Steven (MD)   CRS
NYU Downtown Hosp

251 E 33rd St Fl 2; New York, NY 10016; (212)
696-5411; **BDCERT:** S 81; CRS 82; **MS:** NYU Sch
Med 75; **RES:** S, Bellevue Hosp Ctr-NYU, New York,
NY 75-80; **FEL:** CRS, RWJ Univ Hosp-New
Brunswick, New Brunswick, NJ 80-81; **HOSP:** New
York University Med Ctr; *SI: Hemorrhoids;* **HMO:**
Aetna Hlth Plan US Hlthcre CIGNA Blue Cross
Oxford +

LANG: Sp, Rus, Czc; 🔲 🔲 🔲 🔲 🔲 🔲 🔲
A Few Days

Cohen, Alfred M (MD)   CRS
Mem Sloan Kettering Cancer Ctr

1275 York Ave; New York, NY 10021; (212) 639-
6698; **BDCERT:** S 76; **MS:** Johns Hopkins U 67;
RES: Mass Gen Hosp, Boston, MA; **FEL:** Nat Cancer
Inst, Bethesda, MD

🔲 🔲 🔲 🔲 🔲 🔲   Immediately 🔲 **VISA** 🔲

Freed, Jeffrey (MD)   CRS
VA Med Ctr-Bronx

969 Park Ave; New York, NY 10028; (212) 396-
0050; **BDCERT:** S 89; **MS:** SUNY Downstate 70;
RES: Montefiore Med Ctr, Bronx, NY 85-89; **HOSP:**
Lenox Hill Hosp

Gingold, Bruce (MD)   CRS
St Vincents Hosp & Med Ctr NY

36 7th Ave 507; New York, NY 10011; (212) 675-
2997; **BDCERT:** S 77; CRS 76; **MS:** Jefferson Med
Coll 70; **RES:** S, St Vincents Hosp & Med Ctr NY,
New York, NY 70-75; **FEL:** CRS, Cleveland Clinic
Hosp, Cleveland, OH 75-76; **FAP:** Assoc Clin Prof S
NY Med Coll; **HOSP:** Beth Israel Med Ctr; *SI: Rectal
Cancer; Colonoscopy;* **HMO:** Aetna Hlth Plan CIGNA
Oxford Prucare Blue Choice +

LANG: Rus, Fr, Ger; 🔲 🔲 🔲 🔲 🔲   2-4 Weeks

Gorfine, Stephen (MD)　　**CRS**
Mount Sinai Med Ctr

25 E 69th St; New York, NY 10021; (212) 517-
8600; **BDCERT:** CRS 88; **MS:** Univ Mass Sch Med
78; **RES:** IM, Mount Sinai Med Ctr, New York, NY
78-81; SM, Mount Sinai Med Ctr, New York, NY
81-85; **FEL:** CRS, Ferguson Clinic, Grand Rapids,
MI; **FAP:** Assoc Clin Prof Mt Sinai Sch Med; *SI: Anal
Diseases;* **HMO:** Oxford

LANG: Sp, Fr; 🔒 📷 👤 🛏 $ Mcr NFI A Few Days 📧
VISA 💳 💳

Gottesman, Lester (MD)　　**CRS**
St Luke's Roosevelt Hosp Ctr

Madison Surgical Assoc, 425 W 59th St 9A; New
York, NY 10019; (212) 523-8417; **BDCERT:** CRS
88; **MS:** Univ Pittsburgh 78; **RES:** St Luke's
Roosevelt Hosp Ctr, New York, NY 78-83; **FEL:** S
Onc, Mem Sloan Kettering Cancer Ctr, New York,
NY 84-85; Ferguson Clinic, Grand Rapids, MI 86-
87; **FAP:** Asst Prof Columbia P&S; *SI: Functional
Colon Problems; Inflammatory Bowel Disease;* **HMO:**
Magnacare Oxford Aetna Hlth Plan Chubb
Prudential +

LANG: Fr, Sp, Ger; 🔒 📷 👤 🛏 $ Mcr A Few Days
📧 *VISA* 💳

Sohn, Norman (MD)　　**CRS**
Lenox Hill Hosp

Somerset Surgical Assoc, 475 E 72nd St 102; New
York, NY 10021; (212) 249-9010; **BDCERT:** CRS
71; **MS:** NYU Sch Med 63; **RES:** S, New York
University Med Ctr, New York, NY 66-70; **FEL:**
Colorectal S, Lahey Clinic, Burlington, MA 70-71;
FAP: Asst Clin Prof Cornell U; *SI: Benign Rectal
Disorders; Crohn's Disease;* **HMO:** Oxford

🔒 📷 👤 🛏 $ Mcr WC NFI Immediately 📧 *VISA*
💳

Steinhagen, Randolph (MD) CRS
Mount Sinai Med Ctr

5 E 98th St 11th Fl; New York, NY 10029; (212)
241-3336; **BDCERT:** S 83; CRS 85; **MS:** Wayne
State U Sch Med 77; **RES:** S, Mount Sinai Med Ctr,
New York, NY 77-82; **FEL:** CRS, Cleveland Clinic
Hosp, Cleveland, OH 82-83; **FAP:** Assoc Prof Mt
Sinai Sch Med; *SI: Colon and Rectal Cancer; Colitis &
Ileitis;* **HMO:** Aetna Hlth Plan Oxford Metlife

🔒 📷 👤 🛏 $ Mcr A Few Days 📧 *VISA* 💳 💳

Weinstein, Michael (MD)　　**CRS**
Lenox Hill Hosp

475 E 72nd St 102; New York, NY 10021; (212)
249-9010; **BDCERT:** CRS 76; S 74; **MS:** SUNY Hlth
Sci Ctr 68; **RES:** Albert Einstein Med Ctr, Bronx, NY
69-70; Beth Israel Med Ctr, New York, NY 70-73;
FEL: CRS, Muhlenberg Regional Med Ctr, Plainfield,
NJ 75-76; **HMO:** Oxford Prucare PHCS PHS First
Option +

🔒 📷 👤 🛏 $ Mcr A Few Days 📧 *VISA* 💳

Whelan, Richard (MD)　　**CRS**
Columbia-Presbyterian Med Ctr

161 Ft Washington Ave Rm 522; New York, NY
10032; (212) 305-6136; **BDCERT:** S 89; **MS:**
Columbia P&S 82; **RES:** Columbia-Presbyterian
Med Ctr, New York, NY 82-87; **FEL:** CRS, U MN
Med Ctr, Minneapolis, MN; **HMO:** Chubb Travelers
GHI Oxford

🔒 📞 📷 👤 🛏 Mcr Mod Immediately

CRITICAL CARE ANESTHESIOLOGY

Kaufman, Brian (MD)CCM (Anes)
New York University Med Ctr

New York Critical Care Associates, 550 1st Ave;
New York, NY 10016; (212) 263-5078; **BDCERT:**
Anes 88; CCM 87; **MS:** SUNY Buffalo 77; **RES:** IM,
Albany Med Ctr, Albany, NY 78-80; Anes, New
York University Med Ctr, New York, NY 84-87;
FEL: CCM, Ellis Hosp, Schenectady, NY 80-82; **FAP:**
Assoc Clin Prof NYU Sch Med; *SI: Respiratory
Failure; Shock*

Mcr Mod

Guide to symbols and abbreviations can be found on pages 110-113.

167

CRITICAL CARE MEDICINE

Benjamin, Ernest (MD)   CCM
Mount Sinai Med Ctr
Mt Sinai Medical Center - Surgical ICU Box 1264, 1 Gustave Levy Pl; New York, NY 10029; (212) 241-8867; **BDCERT:** CCM 89; Anes 88; **MS:** France 71; **RES:** Anes, Univ of Claude Bernard, France 71-78; IM, North General Hosp, New York, NY 80-82; **FEL:** Anes, Mount Sinai Med Ctr, New York, NY 79-80; Anes, Mount Sinai Med Ctr, New York, NY 82-83; **FAP:** Assoc Prof Anes Mt Sinai Sch Med; *SI: Acute Respiratory Distress Syndrome;* **HMO:** Most

LANG: Fr, Cre, Sp, Chi; 🧑 ☖ ☎ 🧍 🛏 Mcr Mcd WC NFI Immediately ▦ **VISA** ● ▦

Brusco, Louis (MD)   CCM
St Luke's Roosevelt Hosp Ctr
St Lukes, 1111 Amsterdam Ave; New York, NY 10025; (212) 523-2500; **BDCERT:** IM 88; CCM 93; **MS:** Columbia P&S 85; **RES:** Anes, Columbia-Presbyterian Med Ctr, New York, NY 88-90; Med, St Lukes-Roosevelt Hosp, New York, NY 86-88; **FEL:** CCM (Anes), Columbia-Presbyterian Med Ctr, New York, NY 91; **FAP:** Asst Clin Prof Anes Columbia P&S; *SI: Critical Care Medicine; Anesthesiology;* **HMO:** 1199 32BJ Chubb HIP Network US Hlthcre +

LANG: Fr, Sp, Itl, Rus, Chi; 🧑 ☖ 🛏 Mcr Mcd WC NFI Immediately **VISA** ●

Carlon, Graziano (MD)   CCM
Mem Sloan Kettering Cancer Ctr
1275 York Ave; New York, NY 10021; (212) 639-6673; **BDCERT:** Anes 79; CCM 86; **MS:** Italy 69; **RES:** PM, NY Hosp-Cornell Med Ctr, New York 76-78

Greenbaum, Dennis (MD)   CCM
St Vincents Hosp & Med Ctr NY
St Vincent's Hospital Medical Center, 153 W 11th St; New York, NY 10011; (212) 604-8061; **BDCERT:** IM 74; **MS:** Georgetown U 68; **RES:** IM, St Vincents Hosp & Med Ctr NY, New York, NY 69-70; Med, St Vincents Hosp & Med Ctr NY, New York, NY 72-74; **FEL:** CCM, Presbyterian U Hosp, Pittsburgh, PA 74-75; *SI: Respiratory Failure; Shock;* **HMO:** Aetna-US Healthcare Oxford Empire Blue Cross & Shield

LANG: Itl; 🧑 ☖ 🧍 🛏 Mcr Mcd WC NFI

Steiger, David (MD)   CCM
Hosp For Joint Diseases
301 E 17th St; New York, NY 10003; (212) 598-6091; **BDCERT:** IM 87; CCM 95; **MS:** England 81; **RES:** Med, St Luke's Roosevelt Hosp Ctr, New York, NY 84-87; Med, St Luke's Roosevelt Hosp Ctr, New York, NY 88-89; **FEL:** Pul, UC San Francisco Med Ctr, San Francisco, CA 89-94; **FAP:** Asst Prof Med NYU Sch Med; *SI: Asthma; Pulmonary Embolism;* **HMO:** Blue Cross & Blue Choice Oxford Magnacare

🧑 🕿 ☎ 🧍 🛏 ⓢ Mcr WC NFI A Few Days ▦ **VISA** ● ▦

Wagner, Ira (MD)   CCM
St Vincents Hosp & Med Ctr NY
St Vincent's Hospital of New York, 153 W 11th St Ste 1050E; New York, NY 10011; (212) 604-8336; **BDCERT:** IM 80; CCM 89; **MS:** SUNY Downstate 76; **RES:** Med, St Vincents Hosp & Med Ctr NY, New York, NY 77-79; **FEL:** CCM, U of Pittsburgh Med Ctr, Pittsburgh, PA 79-80; **FAP:** Assoc Prof Med NYU Sch Med; **HMO:** Oxford Blue Choice Aetna-US Healthcare

🧑 🕿 ⓢ Mcr Mcd WC 4+ Weeks

DERMATOLOGY

Abrahams, Irving (MD)   **D**
Columbia-Presbyterian Med Ctr
Dept of Dermatology, Columbia Presbyterian
Medical Center, 161 Fort Washington Ave Ste 750;
New York, NY 10032; (212) 305-5301; **BDCERT:**
D 60; **MS:** SUNY Downstate 54; **RES:** D, Columbia-
Presbyterian Med Ctr, New York, NY 55-58; **IM:**
Kings County Hosp Ctr, Brooklyn, NY 54-55; **FAP:**
Assoc Clin Prof D Columbia P&S; *SI: Dermatologic
Surgery; Geriatric Dermatology;* **HMO:** Oxford Empire
Blue Choice PHS Chubb

LANG: Sp; 🔲 🔲 🔲 🔲 🔲 🔲 🔲 2-4 Weeks **VISA**
🔲

Albom, Michael (MD)   **D**
New York University Med Ctr
33 E 70th St; New York, NY 10021; (212) 517-
2121; **BDCERT:** S 76; D 77; **MS:** Boston U 70; **RES:**
Boston U Med Ctr, Boston, MA 71-74; **FEL:**
Microsurgery, New York University Med Ctr, New
York, NY 74-75; **FAP:** Clin Prof D NYU Sch Med;
HOSP: Manhattan Eye, Ear & Throat Hosp; *SI:
Moh's Micrographic Surgery; Liposuction; Lasers;
Botox;* **HMO:** Oxford CIGNA Prucare Independent
Health Plan Aetna-US Healthcare +

🔲 🔲 🔲 🔲 A Few Days 🔲 **VISA** 🔲 🔲

Ashinoff, Robin (MD)   **D**
New York University Med Ctr
NYU Medical Center, 530 1st Ave 7R; New York,
NY 10016; (212) 263-7019; **BDCERT:** D 89; **MS:**
NYU Sch Med 85; **RES:** NY Hosp-Cornell Med Ctr,
New York, NY 85-86; D, New York University Med
Ctr, New York, NY 86-89; **FEL:** Dermatologic S,
New York University Med Ctr, New York, NY 89-
91; **FAP:** Asst Prof NYU Sch Med; **HOSP:** Bellevue
Hosp Ctr; *SI: Skin Cancer; Botox;* **HMO:** Oxford Blue
Cross & Blue Shield Aetna Hlth Plan CIGNA Blue
Choice +

🔲 🔲 🔲 🔲 🔲 🔲 🔲 Immediately 🔲 **VISA** 🔲

Auerbach, Robert (MD)   **D**
New York University Med Ctr
Dermatology Associates, 440 E 57th St; New York,
NY 10022; (212) 935-9610; **BDCERT:** D 64; **MS:**
NYU Sch Med 58; **RES:** U Chicago Hosp, Chicago, IL
59-61; Nat Cancer Inst, Bethesda, MD 61-63;
HOSP: Bellevue Hosp Ctr; *SI: Skin Tumors Benign &
Malignant; Psoriasis;* **HMO:** Oxford Aetna Hlth Plan
US Hlthcre NYLCare Blue Choice +

LANG: Sp, Yd; 🔲 🔲 🔲 🔲 🔲 🔲 🔲 Immediately
🔲 **VISA** 🔲

Avram, Marc R (MD)   **D**
Long Island Coll Hosp
927 5th Ave; New York, NY 10021; (212) 734-
4007; **BDCERT:** D 94; **MS:** SUNY Downstate 89;
RES: D, Harvard Med Sch, Cambridge, MA 90-94;
FAP: Asst Prof D NYU Sch Med; *SI: Surgical Hair
Transplant;* **HMO:** None

🔲 🔲 🔲 🔲 🔲 🔲 🔲 2-4 Weeks 🔲 **VISA** 🔲

Bickers, David (MD)   **D**
Columbia-Presbyterian Med Ctr
Columbia University Dermatology Associates, 16 E
60th St 300; New York, NY 10032; (212) 326-
8465; **BDCERT:** D 74; **MS:** U Va Sch Med 67; **RES:**
New York University Med Ctr, New York, NY 70-
73; **FEL:** Pharmacology, Rockefeller Univ Hosp,
New York, NY 71-74; **FAP:** Prof D Columbia P&S;
SI: Photosensitivity; **HMO:** Oxford Empire Blue
Choice Multiplan PHS

🔲 🔲 🔲 🔲 🔲 🔲 1 Week **VISA** 🔲

Brademas, Mary Ellen (MD)   **D**
New York University Med Ctr
11 5th Ave; New York, NY 10003; (212) 477-
1515; **BDCERT:** D 83; **MS:** Georgetown U 79; **RES:**
D, Johns Hopkins Hosp, Baltimore, MD 80-81; New
York University Med Ctr, New York, NY 81-83;
FAP: Asst Clin Instr NYU Sch Med; *SI: Nails;
Cosmetic Dermatology*

🔲 🔲 🔲 🔲 🔲 🔲 Immediately 🔲 **VISA** 🔲

Guide to symbols and abbreviations can be found on pages 110-113.

169

Brodey, Marvin (MD)   D
Lenox Hill Hosp

876 Park Ave; New York, NY 10021; (212) 734-4365; **BDCERT:** D 56; **MS:** Columbia P&S 49; **RES:** Columbia-Presbyterian Med Ctr, New York, NY 51-53; *SI: Skin Cancers; X-Ray Therapy*; **HMO:** Most

LANG: Fr, Ger, Sp, Itl, Chi; ⬚ ⬚ ⬚ ⬚ ⬚ ⬚ ⬚ ⬚ ⬚ ⬚ Immediately

Bystryn, Jean Claude (MD)   D
New York University Med Ctr

530 1st Ave 7F; New York, NY 10016; (212) 263-7333; **BDCERT:** D 70; **MS:** NYU Sch Med 62; **RES:** Med, Montefiore Med Ctr, Bronx, NY 63-64; D, New York University Med Ctr, New York, NY 66-69; **FEL:** VIR, USC Med Ctr, Los Angeles, CA 68-69; A&I, New York University Med Ctr, New York, NY 69-72; **FAP:** Prof NYU Sch Med; *SI: Skin Cancer Melanoma; Bullous Diseases*; **HMO:** Oxford United Healthcare CIGNA PHS

LANG: Fr; ⬚ ⬚ ⬚ ⬚ ⬚ 1 Week

Cipollaro, Vincent (MD)   D
NY Hosp-Cornell Med Ctr

1016 5th Ave; New York, NY 10028; (212) 879-1670; **BDCERT:** D 65; **MS:** Italy 58; **RES:** D, VA Med Ctr-Bronx, Bronx, NY 60-62; **FEL:** D, NY Hosp-Cornell Med Ctr, New York, NY 63; **FAP:** Sr Prof Cornell U; *SI: Skin Cancer*; **HMO:** None

LANG: Sp, Itl; ⬚ ⬚ ⬚ ⬚ ⬚ A Few Days

Clark, Sheryl (MD)   D
NY Hosp-Cornell Med Ctr

109 E 61st St; New York, NY 10021; (212) 750-2905; **BDCERT:** D 88; **MS:** Case West Res U 82; **RES:** Mount Sinai Hosp, Cleveland, OH 82-83; Barnes Hosp, St Louis, MO 85-88; **FEL:** Barnes Hosp, St Louis, MO 84-85; **FAP:** Asst Clin Prof Cornell U; *SI: Melanoma; Atypical Moles*; **HMO:** United Healthcare Multiplan Oxford 32BJ Blue Cross & Blue Shield +

⬚ ⬚ ⬚ ⬚ ⬚ Immediately ⬚ **VISA** ⬚

Cohen, Steven (DO)   D
Beth Israel Med Ctr

10 Union Square East; New York, NY 10003; (212) 420-3000; **BDCERT:** D 78; **MS:** Penn State U-Hershey Med Ctr 71; **RES:** D, Yale-New Haven Hosp, New Haven, CT 74-77; **HOSP:** Beth Israel North; *SI: Psoriasis, Environmental and Occupational Skin Disease*; **HMO:** Oxford US Hlthcre Prucare Blue Choice

Davis, Joyce (MD)   D
Beth Israel Med Ctr

69 5th Ave 1A; New York, NY 10003; (212) 242-3066; **BDCERT:** D 83; **MS:** Albert Einstein Coll Med 79; **RES:** IM, Beth Israel Med Ctr, New York, NY 79-80; D, Mount Sinai Med Ctr, New York, NY 80-83; **FAP:** Clin Instr Mt Sinai Sch Med; **HOSP:** Mount Sinai Med Ctr; *SI: Acne; Collagen, Liposuction*

LANG: Fr; ⬚ ⬚ ⬚ ⬚ ⬚ ⬚ ⬚ Immediately ⬚ **VISA** ⬚ ⬚

de Leo, Vincent A (MD)   D
St Luke's Roosevelt Hosp Ctr

425 W 59th St; New York, NY 10019; (212) 246-3967; **BDCERT:** D 76; **MS:** LSU Sch Med, New Orleans 69; **RES:** Columbia-Presbyterian Med Ctr, New York, NY 73-77; **FEL:** Columbia-Presbyterian Med Ctr, New York, NY; *SI: Contact Allergic Dermatitis; Photosensitivity*; **HMO:** Aetna Hlth Plan Oxford Blue Cross & Blue Shield US Hlthcre 1199 +

⬚ ⬚ ⬚ ⬚ ⬚ ⬚ ⬚ 4+ Weeks **VISA** ⬚

Demar, Leon (MD)   D
St Luke's Roosevelt Hosp Ctr

985 5th Ave; New York, NY 10021; (212) 988-9010; **BDCERT:** D 77; **MS:** NYU Sch Med 73; **RES:** Stanford Med Ctr, Stanford, CA 74-75; Columbia-Presbyterian Med Ctr, New York, NY 75-77; **HOSP:** Columbia-Presbyterian Med Ctr; *SI: Skin Cancer; Pediatric Dermatology*; **HMO:** Oxford Travelers Chubb PHCS Aetna Hlth Plan +

⬚ ⬚ ⬚ ⬚ ⬚ ⬚ Immediately **VISA** ⬚

Franks Jr, Andrew G (MD)   D
New York University Med Ctr

Gramercy Park Dermatology, 60 Gramercy Park N
1N; New York, NY 10010; (212) 475-2312;
BDCERT: D 77; IM 75; MS: NY Med Coll 71; RES:
IM, Beth Israel Med Ctr, Boston, MA 73-74; D,
Columbia-Presbyterian Med Ctr, New York, NY 74-
75; FEL: Rhu, Columbia-Presbyterian Med Ctr, New
York, NY 75-77; FAP: Assoc Clin Prof D NYU Sch
Med; HOSP: Lenox Hill Hosp; HMO: Oxford Chubb
Magnacare

⬛ 🔲 🔲 $ Mcr Immediately **VISA** ⬛

Freedberg, Irwin M (MD)   D
New York University Med Ctr

530 1st Ave; New York, NY 10016; (212) 263-
5889; BDCERT: D 63; MS: Harvard Med Sch 56;
RES: D, Harvard Med Sch, Cambridge, MA 62;
HOSP: Bellevue Hosp Ctr; *SI: Psoriasis; Severe Skin
Disease*; HMO: Oxford Blue Cross & Blue Shield
Aetna Hlth Plan United Healthcare Prucare +

LANG: Sp; 🔲 🔲 🔲 🔲 $ Mcr 1 Week ⬛ **VISA**
⬛

Friedman-Kien, Alvin (MD)   D
New York University Med Ctr

Nyu Medical Ctr, 530 1st Ave 7C; New York, NY
10016; (212) 263-7380; BDCERT: D 65; MS: Yale
U Sch Med 60; RES: D, Mass Gen Hosp, Boston, MA
61-62; D, Nat Inst Health, Bethesda, MD 62-64;
FEL: D, New York University Med Ctr, New York,
NY 64-65; FAP: Prof D NY Med Coll; HMO:
Prudential CIGNA

LANG: Fr, Nwg, Swd; 🔲 🔲 🔲 🔲 $ Mcr
A Few Days ⬛ **VISA** ⬛

Gendler, Ellen (MD)   D
New York University Med Ctr

40 E 72nd St; New York, NY 10021; (212) 288-
8222; BDCERT: D 85; MS: Columbia P&S 81; RES:
D, New York University Med Ctr, New York, NY 81-
82; FAP: Assoc Clin Prof NYU Sch Med; *SI: Cosmetic
Dermatology*

LANG: Sp; 🔲 🔲 🔲 🔲 $ 1 Week ⬛ **VISA** ⬛

Geronemus, Roy (MD)   D
New York Eye & Ear Infirmary

317 E 34th St Ste 11N; New York, NY 10016;
(212) 686-7306; BDCERT: D 83; MS: U Miami Sch
Med 79; RES: New York University Med Ctr, New
York, NY 79-80; HOSP: Mount Sinai Med Ctr;
HMO: Blue Choice Oxford PHS Metlife US Hlthcre +
🔲 🔲 🔲 🔲 $ Mcr 1 Week ⬛

Gordon, Marsha (MD)   D
Mount Sinai Med Ctr

5 E 98th St; New York, NY 10029; (212) 831-
4119; BDCERT: D 88; MS: Univ Penn 84; RES: D,
Mount Sinai Med Ctr, New York, NY 85-88; Cooper
Hosp, Camden, NJ 84-85; FAP: Assoc Clin Prof Mt
Sinai Sch Med; *SI: General Dermatology; Aging Skin*
🔲 🔲 🔲 🔲 $ Mcr 2-4 Weeks ⬛ **VISA** ⬛

Granstein, Richard (MD)   D
NY Hosp-Cornell Med Ctr

Cornell Dermatology Consultants, 525 E 68th St
Rm 1340; New York, NY 10021; (212) 746-7274;
BDCERT: D 83; MS: UCLA 78; RES: D, Mass Gen
Hosp, Boston, MA 79-81; FEL: Harvard Med Sch,
Cambridge, MA 82-84; Nat Cancer Inst, Bethesda,
MD 81-82; FAP: Chrmn Cornell U; *SI: Skin Cancer;
Psoriasis*; HMO: Empire Blue Cross & Shield Oxford
Aetna-US Healthcare Prudential CIGNA +
🔲 🔲 🔲 $ Mcr 2-4 Weeks ⬛ **VISA** ⬛

Greenberg, Robert (MD)   D
New York University Med Ctr

117 E 72nd St; New York, NY 10021; (212) 861-
2580; BDCERT: D 77; MS: U Mich Med Sch 70;
RES: U Miami Hosp, Miami, FL 73-74; U Miami
Hosp, Miami, FL 74-75; FEL: New York University
Med Ctr, New York, NY 75-77; FAP: Asst Clin Prof
NYU Sch Med; HOSP: Lenox Hill Hosp; *SI: Cosmetic
Dermatology; Laser Skin Surgery*; HMO: Blue Choice
PHCS Oxford CIGNA PHS +
🔲 🔲 🔲 🔲 🔲 $ Mcr A Few Days ⬛ **VISA** ⬛

Greenspan, Alan (MD)   D
New York University Med Ctr

39 Broadway 1911; New York, NY 10006; (212) 509-5200; **BDCERT:** D 84; **MS:** Northwestern U 79; **RES:** Northwestern Mem Hosp, Chicago, IL 79-81; D, New York University Med Ctr, New York, NY 81-84; **FAP:** Asst Clin Prof NYU Sch Med; **HOSP:** NYU Downtown Hosp; **SI:** *General Dermatology; Skin Cancer;* **HMO:** Oxford United Healthcare Aetna Hlth Plan GHI Blue Cross +

LANG: Heb, Fr; 🦽 📞 🔒 👤 🏥 🅂 Mcr WC
A Few Days 🔲 **VISA** 💳

Hatcher, Virgil (MD)   D
New York University Med Ctr

161 Madison Ave; New York, NY 10016; (212) 686-2888; **BDCERT:** D 82; **MS:** UC San Francisco 78; **RES:** D, New York University Med Ctr, New York, NY 79-82; **SI:** *Psoriasis; Viral Skin Infections;* **HMO:** Oxford US Hlthcre Blue Choice CIGNA Prudential +

🦽 📞 👤 🏥 🅂 Mcr   2-4 Weeks 🔲 **VISA** 💳

Hochman, Herbert (MD)   D
Lenox Hill Hosp

1020 Park Ave; New York, NY 10028; (212) 861-1656; **BDCERT:** D 77; **MS:** Tulane U 70; **RES:** D, Albert Einstein Med Ctr, Bronx, NY 73-75; **SI:** *General Dermatology; Skin Cancer*

👤 🏥 🅂   A Few Days 🔲 **VISA** 💳 💳

Jacobs, Michael (MD)   D
NY Hosp-Cornell Med Ctr

407 E 70th St Fl 2; New York, NY 10021; (212) 772-7190; **BDCERT:** D 81; **MS:** Cornell U 77; **RES:** Baylor Med Ctr, Dallas, TX 77-78; NY Hosp-Cornell Med Ctr, New York, NY 78-81; **FAP:** Asst Clin Prof Cornell U; **HOSP:** Hosp For Special Surgery; **SI:** *Skin Cancer; Lupus*

🦽 🔒 👤 🏥 🅂   A Few Days

Kantor, Irwin (MD)   D
Mount Sinai Med Ctr

Mt Sinai Dermatology Assocs, 5 E 98th St Bx1048; New York, NY 10029; (212) 369-4548; **BDCERT:** D 60; **MS:** England 50; **RES:** D, Mt Sinai Hospital, New York, NY 53-54; D, Grad Sch Med U Penn, Philadelphia, PA 55-56; **FAP:** Prof D Mt Sinai Sch Med; **HMO:** Blue Shield Oxford Aetna-US Healthcare PHS Chubb +

LANG: Sp, Fr, Ger, Yd; 🦽 🔒 👤 🏥 🅂 Mcr WC NFI
A Few Days 🔲 **VISA** 💳

Katz, Bruce (MD)   D
Columbia-Presbyterian Med Ctr

The Skin & Laser Asthetics Ctr, 14 E 82nd St; New York, NY 10028; (212) 734-5599; **BDCERT:** D 83; 83; **MS:** McGill U 77; **RES:** D, Columbia-Presbyterian Med Ctr, New York, NY 79-82; **FAP:** Assoc Clin Prof Columbia P&S; **HOSP:** St Luke's Roosevelt Hosp Ctr; **SI:** *Laser Surgery; Cosmetic Surgery;* **HMO:** Oxford Aetna-US Healthcare United Healthcare NYLCare Blue Choice +

LANG: Sp, Fr, Rus; 🦽 🅂🅄 📞 🔒 👤 🏥 🅂   1 Week
🔲 **VISA** 💳

Kenet, Barney (MD)   D
NY Hosp-Cornell Med Ctr

160 E 72nd St; New York, NY 10021; (212) 535-9753; **BDCERT:** D 92; **MS:** Brown U 88; **RES:** D, NY Hosp-Cornell Med Ctr, New York, NY 89-92; **SI:** *Cosmetic Dermatology; Liposuction Botox*

📞 🔒 🏥 🅂   A Few Days 🔲

Kline, Mitchell (MD)   D
NY Hosp-Cornell Med Ctr

53 E 67th St 117; New York, NY 10021; (212) 517-6555; **BDCERT:** D 85; **MS:** Univ Penn 85; **RES:** Hosp of U Penn, Philadelphia, PA 87; NY Hosp-Cornell Med Ctr, New York, NY 90; **FAP:** Clin Instr Cornell U; **SI:** *Skin Cancer Surgery;* **HMO:** Oxford Blue Cross & Blue Shield PHCS

🅂🅄 📞 👤 🏥 🅂 WC   1 Week 🔲 **VISA** 💳

Konecky, Elizabeth (MD)   **D**
St Luke's Roosevelt Hosp Ctr

133 E 73rd St; New York, NY 10021; (212) 861-9000; **BDCERT:** D 82; **MS:** Mt Sinai Sch Med 78; **RES:** Beth Israel Med Ctr, New York, NY 78-79; Univ Hosp SUNY Bklyn, Brooklyn, NY 79-82; **HOSP:** Columbia-Presbyterian Med Ctr

LANG: Fr, Yd, Heb, Tag; 🔊 🎦 ▦ **VISA** 💳 💳

Kopf, Alfred (MD)   **D**
New York University Med Ctr

Dermatology Medical Assoc, 350 5th Ave 7805; New York, NY 10118; (212) 689-5050; **BDCERT:** D 57; **MS:** Cornell U 51; **RES:** D, New York University Med Ctr, New York, NY; **FAP:** Assoc Prof NYU Sch Med; *SI: Malignant Melanoma; Dysplastic Moles*

🔊 🎦 🎭 ▦ ▦ **VISA** 💳 💳

Kurtin, Stephen (MD)   **D**
Mount Sinai Med Ctr

111 E 71st St; New York, NY 10021; (212) 772-1717; **BDCERT:** D 70; **MS:** Columbia P&S 65; **RES:** Med, Mount Sinai Med Ctr, New York, NY 65-66; D, New York University Med Ctr, New York, NY 66-69; **FAP:** Asst Clin Prof Mt Sinai Sch Med; *SI: Skin Aging; Collagen Injections*

🎦 🎭 ▦ 💲 Mcr A Few Days **VISA** 💳

Lebwohl, Mark (MD)   **D**
Mount Sinai Med Ctr

Mount Sinai Hospital, 5 E 98th St; New York, NY 10029; (212) 876-7199; **BDCERT:** D 83; **MS:** Harvard Med Sch 78; **RES:** IM, Mount Sinai Med Ctr, New York, NY 78-81; D, Mount Sinai Med Ctr, New York, NY 81-83; **FAP:** Chrmn D Mt Sinai Sch Med; *SI: Skin Cancer; Psoriasis*

LANG: Sp, Heb; 🔊 🎦 🎭 ▦ 💲 Mcr Immediately

Lefkovits, Albert M (MD)   **D**
Mount Sinai Med Ctr

1040 Park Ave; New York, NY 10028; (212) 861-9600; **MS:** NY Med Coll 62; **RES:** D, Univ Hosp SUNY Bklyn, Brooklyn, NY 63-65; D, Mount Sinai Med Ctr, New York, NY 65-66; **FEL:** Mount Sinai Med Ctr, New York, NY 66-67; **FAP:** Asst Clin Prof D Mt Sinai Sch Med; *SI: Facial Rejuvenation; Cancer of the Skin*

LANG: Fr; 🔊 🎦 🎭 ▦ 💲 A Few Days ▦ **VISA** 💳 💳

Lombardo, Peter C (MD)   **D**
St Luke's Roosevelt Hosp Ctr

Sutton Place Dermatology, 445 E 58th St; New York, NY 10022; (212) 838-0270; **BDCERT:** D 67; **MS:** Albany Med Coll 59; **RES:** D, Columbia-Presbyterian Med Ctr, New York, NY 62-65; IM, St Luke's Roosevelt Hosp Ctr, New York, NY 65; **FAP:** Assoc Prof Columbia P&S; **HOSP:** Columbia-Presbyterian Med Ctr; *SI: Skin, Hair & Nail Problems; Skin Rejuvenation—Laser;* **HMO:** Oxford Blue Cross Aetna Hlth Plan Prudential

LANG: Sp, Itl; 🔊 🎦 🎭 ▦ 💲 Mcr 2-4 Weeks ▦ **VISA** 💳 💳

Orbuch, Philip (MD)   **D**
New York University Med Ctr

200 E 36th St; New York, NY 10016; (212) 532-5355; **BDCERT:** D 86; **MS:** Israel 81; **RES:** D, New York University Med Ctr, New York, NY 82-85; **FEL:** D, New York University Med Ctr, New York, NY 85-86; **HOSP:** Bellevue Hosp Ctr; *SI: Pediatric Dermatology; Skin Cancers;* **HMO:** Oxford Aetna Hlth Plan GHI United Healthcare Blue Cross +

LANG: Sp, Heb, Yd; 🔊 🎭 🔊 🎦 🎭 ▦ 💲 Mcr A Few Days ▦ **VISA** 💳 💳

Orentreich, David (MD)   **D**
Mount Sinai Med Ctr

909 5th Ave; New York, NY 10021; (212) 794-0800; **BDCERT:** D 84; **MS:** Columbia P&S 80; **RES:** St Luke's Roosevelt Hosp Ctr, New York, NY 80-81; D, Mount Sinai Med Ctr, New York, NY 81-84; *SI: Dermatologic Surgery; Liposuction;* **HMO:** None

LANG: Jpn, Sp, Itl, Chi; 🔊 🎦 🎭 ▦ Mcr ▦ **VISA** 💳 💳

Orentreich, Norman (MD)   D
NY Hosp-Cornell Med Ctr

909 5th Ave; New York, NY 10021; (212) 794-0800; **BDCERT:** D 53; **MS:** NYU Sch Med 48; **RES:** Queens Hosp Ctr, Jamaica, NY 48-50; D, Mem Sloan Kettering Cancer Ctr, New York, NY 50-53; **FAP:** Clin Prof NYU Sch Med; **SI:** *Endocrinology; Hair Loss*

LANG: Itl, Chi, Sp, Jpn, Sgn; ⬛ ⬛ ⬛ ⬛ ⬛ ⬛ 1 Week ⬛ **VISA** ⬛ ⬛

Orlow, Seth (MD)   D
New York University Med Ctr

Dermatologic Associates, 530 1st Ave Ste 7R; New York, NY 10016; (212) 263-5889; **BDCERT:** D 90; **MS:** Albert Einstein Coll Med 86; **RES:** Ped A&I, Mount Sinai Med Ctr, New York, NY 86-87; D, Yale-New Haven Hosp, New Haven, CT 87-89; **FEL:** Ped D, Yale-New Haven Hosp, New Haven, CT 89-90; **FAP:** Assoc Prof D NYU Sch Med; **HOSP:** Lenox Hill Hosp; **SI:** *Pediatric & Teenage Dermatology; Hemangiomas Moles, Eczema;* **HMO:** Oxford Chubb CIGNA United Healthcare +

⬛ ⬛ ⬛ ⬛ **VISA** ⬛

Perez, Maritza (MD)   D
St Luke's Roosevelt Hosp Ctr

425 W 59th St; New York, NY 10019; **BDCERT:** D 89; **MS:** U Puerto Rico 80; **RES:** D, U of Puerto Rico School of Med, , PR 81-84; **FEL:** Immunodermatology, Columbia-Presbyterian Med Ctr, New York, NY 85-87; Dermatologic S, New York University Med Ctr, New York, NY 93-94; **FAP:** Assoc Prof Columbia P&S; **SI:** *Melanoma/Skin Cancer; Hair Transplant;* **HMO:** Oxford

LANG: Sp; ⬛ ⬛ ⬛ ⬛ ⬛ ⬛ ⬛ ⬛ A Few Days ⬛ **VISA** ⬛

Petratos, Marinos (MD)   D
Cabrini Med Ctr

35 E 35th St; New York, NY 10016; (212) 532-7020; **MS:** UMDNJ-NJ Med Sch, Newark 60; **RES:** Bellevue Hosp Ctr, New York, NY 66; **SI:** *Cosmetic Dermatology; Peels & Collagen Injections;* **HMO:** Blue Shield GHI

LANG: Grk, Sp; ⬛ ⬛

Podwal, Mark (MD)   D
Bellevue Hosp Ctr

55 E 73rd St; New York, NY 10021; (212) 288-7488; **BDCERT:** D 75; **MS:** NYU Sch Med 70; **RES:** Bellevue Hosp Ctr, New York, NY 72-74; **HOSP:** New York University Med Ctr; **HMO:** Oxford Chubb HealthNet 1199

LANG: Sp; ⬛ ⬛ ⬛ ⬛ Immediately

Poh, Maureen (MD)   D
St Luke's Roosevelt Hosp Ctr

425 W 59th St # 5C; New York, NY 10019; (212) 246-3865; **BDCERT:** D 73; **MS:** U Tenn Ctr Hlth Sci, Memphis 67; **RES:** Barnes Hosp, St Louis, MO 69-72; **HOSP:** Columbia-Presbyterian Med Ctr

Prioleau, Philip G (MD)   D
NY Hosp-Cornell Med Ctr

1035 5th Ave C; New York, NY 10028; (212) 794-3548; **BDCERT:** D 83; S 73; **MS:** Med U SC, Charleston 67; **RES:** S, U of VA Health Sci Ctr, Charlottesville, VA 72; PlS, Duke U Med Ctr, Durham, NC 75; **FEL:** Path, Barnes Hosp, St Louis, MO 79; DP, New York University Med Ctr, New York, NY 81; **FAP:** Assoc Clin Prof D Cornell U; **SI:** *Melanoma; Mohs Micrographic Surgery;* **HMO:** None

⬛ ⬛ ⬛ A Few Days **VISA** ⬛

Prystowsky, Janet (MD)   D
Columbia-Presbyterian Med Ctr

161 Fort Washington Ave Ste 638; New York, NY 10032; (212) 305-5293; **BDCERT:** D 87; **MS:** U Chicago-Pritzker Sch Med 83; **RES:** U Chicago Hosp, Chicago, IL 84; D, Hosp of U Penn, Philadelphia, PA 87; **FAP:** Asst Prof Columbia P&S; **HOSP:** St Luke's Roosevelt Hosp Ctr; **SI:** *Skin Cancer Laser; Leg Ulcers; Spider Veins*

⬛ ⬛ ⬛ ⬛ ⬛ ⬛ A Few Days **VISA** ⬛

Rabhan, Nathan B (MD) D
Beth Israel Med Ctr

136 E 36th St 1A; New York, NY 10016; (212) 685-1337; **BDCERT:** D 70; IM 68; **MS:** Med Coll Ga 61; **RES:** IM, Sinai Hosp of Baltimore, Baltimore, MD 61-65; D, New York University Med Ctr, New York, NY 67-69; *SI: Connective Tissue and Bullous Diseases; Phototherapy Psoriasis;* **HMO:** None

LANG: Rus, Pol, Yd; 🅰 🅰 🅰 🆂 A Few Days

Ramsay, David L (MD) D
New York University Med Ctr

New York Univ Med Ctr, 530 1st Ave; New York, NY 10016; (212) 683-6283; **BDCERT:** D 74; **MS:** Ind U Sch Med 69; **RES:** D, New York University Med Ctr, New York, NY 70-73; **FEL:** Nat Inst Health, Bethesda, MD 72-73; *SI: Lymphomas of Skin; Oncology;* **HMO:** None

🅰 🅰 🅲 🅰 🅰 🅰 A Few Days

Reisch, Milton (MD) D
Montefiore Med Ctr

30 E 40th St; New York, NY 10016; (212) 697-4290; **BDCERT:** D 53; **MS:** U Md Sch Med 46; **RES:** Brooke Army Med Ctr, San Antonio, TX 46-47; VA Med Ctr-Bronx, Bronx, NY 50-52; **FAP:** Clin Prof Albert Einstein Coll Med; **HOSP:** New York University Med Ctr; *SI: Skin Cancer*

🅰 🅰 🅰 Immediately

Rigel, Darrell (MD) D
New York University Med Ctr

35 E 35th St; New York, NY 10016; (212) 684-6140; **BDCERT:** D 83; **MS:** Geo Wash U Sch Med 78; **RES:** IM, NY Hosp-Cornell Med Ctr, New York, NY 78-79; D, New York University Med Ctr, New York, NY 79-82; **FEL:** Skin S, New York University Med Ctr, New York, NY 82-83; **FAP:** Clin Prof D NYU Sch Med; *SI: Skin Cancer; Skin Surgery;* **HMO:** Aetna Hlth Plan Oxford US Hlthcre GHI +

LANG: Sp; 🅰 🅲 🅰 🅰 🅰 🅰 A Few Days 🖼 🕋

Robins, Perry (MD) D
New York University Med Ctr

530 First Ave; New York, NY 10016; (212) 263-7222; **BDCERT:** D 91; **MS:** Germany 60; **RES:** D, VA Med Ctr, Bronx, NY 61-62; D, NYU Med Ctr, New York, NY 63; **FAP:** Prof D NYU Sch Med; **HOSP:** Bellevue Hosp Ctr; *SI: Dermatological Surgery; Melanoma/Skin Cancer;* **HMO:** Oxford

🅰 🅰 🅰 🅰 2-4 Weeks 🖼 **VISA** 🕋

Romano, John (MD) D
St Vincents Hosp & Med Ctr NY

36 7th Ave 423; New York, NY 10011; (212) 242-5815; **BDCERT:** D 80; **MS:** Cornell U 73; **RES:** S, Jacobi Med Ctr, Bronx, NY 73-74; IM, St Vincents Hosp & Med Ctr NY, New York, NY 74-76; **FEL:** D, NY Hosp-Cornell Med Ctr, New York, NY 76-78; **FAP:** Asst Clin Prof D Cornell U; **HOSP:** NY Hosp-Cornell Med Ctr; *SI: Treatment of Aging Skin; Skin Cancer Screening;* **HMO:** Oxford Aetna Hlth Plan Prucare CIGNA PHS +

🅰 🅲 🅰 🅰 🅰 🅰 🅰 A Few Days 🖼 **VISA** 🕋 🅰

Sadick, Neil (MD) D
New York University Med Ctr

772 Park Ave; New York, NY 10021; (212) 772-7242; **BDCERT:** IM 80; D 83; **MS:** SUNY Hlth Sci Ctr 77; **RES:** IM, N Shore Univ Hosp-Manhasset, Manhasset, NY 78-80; Mem Sloan Kettering Cancer Ctr, New York, NY 78-80; **FEL:** D, NY Hosp-Cornell Med Ctr, New York, NY; **FAP:** Assoc Clin Prof Cornell U; **HOSP:** NY Hosp-Cornell Med Ctr; *SI: Laser Surgery; Varicose Veins;* **HMO:** MDNY NYLCare Blue Cross & Blue Shield Sel Pro Independent Health Plan +

LANG: Sp, Ger, Heb; 🅰 🅰 🅲 🅰 🅰 🅰 🅰 Immediately 🖼 **VISA** 🕋

Scher, Richard K (MD) D
Columbia-Presbyterian Med Ctr

16 E 60th St; New York, NY 10022; (212) 326-8465; **BDCERT:** D 60; **MS:** Howard U 55; **RES:** D, New York University Med Ctr, New York, NY 56-59; **FAP:** Prof Columbia P&S; *SI: Nail Disorders; Nail Surgery*

🅰 🅰 🅰 🅰 🅰 🅰 1 Week **VISA** 🕋

Guide to symbols and abbreviations can be found on pages 110-113.

175

Schultz, Neal (MD) D
Mount Sinai Med Ctr

1040 Parl Ave; New York, NY 10028; (212) 861-9600; **BDCERT:** D 78; **MS:** Columbia P&S 73; **RES:** IM, Mount Sinai Med Ctr, New York, NY 74-75; D, Mount Sinai Med Ctr, New York, NY 75-78; **FAP:** Clin Instr Mt Sinai Sch Med; **HOSP:** Lenox Hill Hosp; **SI:** Cosmetic Dermatology; Aesthetic Laser Surgery

♿ ⬛ 🔧 🏠 Immediately ▨ **VISA** 💳 ▨

Scott, Rachelle (MD) D
NY Hosp-Cornell Med Ctr

525 E 68th St Ste 318; New York, NY 10021; (212) 472-8025; **BDCERT:** D 85; Ped 82; **MS:** NY Med Coll 79; **RES:** U Chicago Hosp, Chicago, IL 79; NY Hosp-Cornell Med Ctr, New York, NY 85; **FEL:** Ambulatory Ped, Columbia-Presbyterian Med Ctr, New York, NY 81; **FAP:** Assoc Prof D Cornell U; **SI:** Pediatric Dermatology; Inflammatory Skin Disease; **HMO:** Oxford Blue Choice Aetna-US Healthcare US Hlthcre GHI +

LANG: Sp; ♿ ⬛ 🔧 🏠 💲 Mcr NFI ▨ **VISA** 💳 ▨

Shelton, Ronald M (MD) D
Mount Sinai Med Ctr

625 Park Ave; New York, NY 10021; (212) 517-6767; **BDCERT:** D 90; **MS:** SUNY Hlth Sci Ctr 84; **RES:** S, Long Island Jewish Med Ctr, New Hyde Park, NY 84-85; D, Brooke Army Med Ctr, San Antonio, TX 87-90; **FEL:** Dermatologic S, UC San Francisco Med Ctr, San Francisco, CA 92-93; **FAP:** Asst Prof Mt Sinai Sch Med; **SI:** Liposuction,; Laser Resurfacing; **HMO:** Aetna Hlth Plan Beech Street Prucare Oxford PHCS +

♿ ⬛ 🏠 💲 Mcr 2-4 Weeks **VISA** 💳 ▨

Shupack, Jerome (MD) D
Bellevue Hosp Ctr

530 1st Ave 7F; New York, NY 10016; (212) 263-7344; **BDCERT:** D 70; **MS:** Columbia P&S 63; **RES:** Med, Mount Sinai Med Ctr, New York, NY 64; D, New York University Med Ctr, New York, NY 67-70; **FEL:** New York University Med Ctr, New York, NY 71; **FAP:** Clin Prof D NYU Sch Med; **SI:** Rare Skin Diseases; Psoriasis; **HMO:** Oxford

♿ ⬛ 🔧 🏠 💲 2-4 Weeks ▨ **VISA** 💳

Sibulkin, David (MD) D
St Luke's Roosevelt Hosp Ctr

30 E 60th St Rm 206; New York, NY 10022; (212) 753-1470; **BDCERT:** D 73; **MS:** NYU Sch Med 66; **RES:** Bellevue Hosp Ctr, New York, NY 69-72; **HOSP:** Columbia-Presbyterian Med Ctr; **HMO:** Oxford Guardian CIGNA Health Source Blue Cross PPO +

♿ ⬛ 🏠 💲 Mcr Immediately

Silvers, David (MD) D
Columbia-Presbyterian Med Ctr

630 W 168th St; New York, NY 10032; (212) 305-2155; **BDCERT:** D 73; DP 74; **MS:** Duke U 68; **RES:** D, New York University Med Ctr, New York, NY 69-71; **FEL:** DP, Armed Forces Inst Path, Washington, DC 71-73; **FAP:** Clin Prof Columbia P&S; **SI:** Melanoma; Other Skin Tumors

Mcr

Sobel, Howard (MD) D
Lenox Hill Hosp

132 E 76th St 2G; New York, NY 10021; (212) 288-0060; **MS:** Albert Einstein Coll Med 75; **RES:** Emory U Hosp, Atlanta, GA 79; **HOSP:** Beth Israel Med Ctr; **HMO:** Oxford Aetna Hlth Plan PHCS PHS

♿ 🅂🅂 🌙 🔧 ⬛ 🏠 💲 Mcr Immediately ▨ **VISA** 💳

Soter, Nicholas A (MD) D
New York University Med Ctr

560 1st Ave Suite 7R; New York, NY 10016; (212) 263-7680; **BDCERT:** D 70; A&I 85; **MS:** U Tex SW, Dallas 65; **RES:** Baylor Med Ctr, Dallas, TX 66-68; Mass Gen Hosp, Boston, MA 68-69; **FEL:** Harvard Med Sch, Cambridge, MA 71-73; **FAP:** Prof D NYU Sch Med; **SI:** Urticaria (hives); Pruritus (itching); **HMO:** Oxford Chubb Blue Cross & Blue Shield CIGNA Aetna Hlth Plan +

LANG: Sp; ♿ 🅂🅂 🌙 🔧 🏠 💲 Mcr A Few Days ▨ **VISA** 💳

Tesser, Mark (MD)   D
Mount Sinai Med Ctr

1107 Park Ave; New York, NY 10128; (212) 996-9600; **BDCERT:** IM 77; D 80; **MS:** Albert Einstein Coll Med 74; **RES:** IM, Mount Sinai Med Ctr, New York, NY 74-77; D, Mount Sinai Med Ctr, New York, NY 77-79; **FAP:** Clin Instr Mt Sinai Sch Med; **HOSP:** Beth Israel Med Ctr; **SI:** *General Dermatology*; **HMO:** Oxford PHCS Blue Choice United Healthcare Multiplan +

♿ 📷 🚹 🏥 **S** **Mcr**   A Few Days ▤

Toback, Arnold C (MD)   D
Columbia-Presbyterian Med Ctr

2 E 69th St; New York, NY 10021; (212) 737-1440; **BDCERT:** IM 83; D 86; **MS:** Boston U 80; **RES:** IM, Med Ctr Hosp of VT, Burlington, VT 80-83; D, Columbia-Presbyterian Med Ctr, New York, NY 83-86; **SI:** *Cosmetic Dermatology; Skin Cancer*

♿ **C** 📷 🚹 🏥 **S** **Mcr**   A Few Days

Vogel, Louis (MD)   D
New York University Med Ctr

16 Park Ave 1D; New York, NY 10016; (212) 447-5443; **BDCERT:** D 83; IM 80; **MS:** Boston U 77; **RES:** IM, New York University Med Ctr, New York, NY 78-80; D, New York University Med Ctr, New York, NY 80-82; **FAP:** Asst Clin Prof NYU Sch Med; **SI:** *Warts*; **HMO:** Empire Blue Choice Aetna Hlth Plan

LANG: Sp, Fr; ♿ **C** 🚹 🏥 **S** **Mcr**   2-4 Weeks ▤

Walther, Robert (MD)   D
Columbia-Presbyterian Med Ctr

16 E 60th St 300; New York, NY 10022; (212) 326-8465; **BDCERT:** D 78; IM 77; **MS:** U NC Sch Med 73; **RES:** Med, U Miami Hosp, Miami, FL 73-75; D, Columbia-Presbyterian Med Ctr, New York, NY 75-78; **FAP:** Clin Prof Columbia P&S; **SI:** *Psoriasis; Skin Cancer*; **HMO:** Oxford Aetna Hlth Plan

♿ 📷 🚹 🏥 **Mcr**   1 Week ▤ **VISA** ●

Warner, Robert (MD)   D
Mount Sinai Med Ctr

580 Park Ave; New York, NY 10021; (212) 752-3692; **BDCERT:** D 81; **MS:** SUNY Hlth Sci Ctr 77; **RES:** Kings County Hosp Ctr, Brooklyn, NY 77-78; Mount Sinai Med Ctr, New York, NY 78-81; **FAP:** Clin Instr Mt Sinai Sch Med; **SI:** *Cosmetic Dermatology; Dermatologic Surgery*; **HMO:** Oxford Blue Choice CIGNA PHS PHCS +

LANG: Sp; **C** 📷 🚹 🏥 **S** **Mcr**   A Few Days **VISA** ●

DIAGNOSTIC RADIOLOGY

Abiri, Michael (MD)   DR
St Luke's Roosevelt Hosp Ctr

West Side Radiology, 425 W 59th St; New York, NY 10019; (212) 523-4247; **BDCERT:** DR 78; **MS:** Iran 72; **RES:** Rad, St Luke's Roosevelt Hosp Ctr, New York, NY 75-78; **SI:** *Ultrasound*; **HMO:** Oxford US Hlthcre Prudential Aetna Hlth Plan CIGNA +

♿ 🇸🇩 **C** 🏥 **S** **Mcr** **Mcd** **WC** **NFI** ▤ **VISA** ●

Atlas, Scott (MD)   DR
Mount Sinai Med Ctr

1 Gustave Levy Pl Box 1234; New York, NY 10029; (212) 241-3423; **BDCERT:** DR 85; **MS:** U Chicago-Pritzker Sch Med 81; **RES:** Northwestern Mem Hosp, Chicago, IL 82-85; **FEL:** NR, Hosp of U Penn, Philadelphia, PA 85-87; **FAP:** Prof NR Mt Sinai Sch Med

♿ 🇸🇩 📷 🏥 **Mcr** **Mcd**   Immediately

Austin, John (MD)   DR
Columbia-Presbyterian Med Ctr

622 W 168th St; New York, NY 10032; (212) 305-9024; **BDCERT:** Rad 70; **MS:** Yale U Sch Med 65; **RES:** Rad, UC San Francisco Med Ctr, San Francisco, CA 66-70; **FEL:** Rad, UC San Francisco Med Ctr, San Francisco, CA; **FAP:** Lecturer Rad Columbia P&S; **SI:** *Chest Radiology; Lung Cancer*; **HMO:** Oxford

♿ **Mcr** **Mcd**

Guide to symbols and abbreviations can be found on pages 110-113.

177

Barone, Clement (MD) DR

1440 York Ave P1; New York, NY 10021; (212) 988-1303; **BDCERT:** Rad 74; **MS:** NY Med Coll 68; **RES:** Mount Sinai Med Ctr, New York, NY 72-74; **SI:** *Women's Imaging*; **HMO:** US Hlthcre Aetna Hlth Plan Oxford United Healthcare Blue Choice +

LANG: Sp, Ar, Vn, Fr; ♿ 🏥 💲 Mcr WC NFI Immediately **VISA** 💳

Chang, James (MD) DR
St Vincents Hosp & Med Ctr NY

36 7th Ave; New York, NY 10011; (212) 604-8742; **BDCERT:** DR 73; **MS:** Tufts U 68; **RES:** St Vincents Hosp & Med Ctr NY, New York, NY 72; **FEL:** St Vincents Hosp & Med Ctr NY, New York, NY 73; **HMO:** Aetna Hlth Plan Empire Blue Choice Oxford

Cohen, Burton A (MD) DR
Mount Sinai Med Ctr

Doctors' Offices, MD, PC, 1 E 82nd St; New York, NY 10028; (212) 535-9770; **BDCERT:** DR 79; **MS:** NY Med Coll 75; **RES:** Rad, Mount Sinai Med Ctr, New York, NY 76-79; **HMO:** Oxford Unicare Primary Plus Blue Cross Multiplan Prucare +

LANG: Sp, Fr, Rus, Yd, Heb; ♿ 🎥 🏥 💲 Mcr WC NFI Immediately ▦ **VISA** 💳

Dershaw, D David (MD) DR
Mem Sloan Kettering Cancer Ctr

1275 York Ave; New York, NY 10021; (212) 639-7295; **BDCERT:** DR 78; **MS:** Jefferson Med Coll 74; **RES:** DR, NY Hosp-Cornell Med Ctr, New York, NY 75-78; **FEL:** Diagnostic Ultrasound, Thomas Jefferson U Hosp, Philadelphia, PA 78-79; **FAP:** Prof Rad Cornell U; **SI:** *Diagnostic Ultrasound; Mammography—Breast Cancer*; **HMO:** None

♿ 🏥 💲 1 Week ▦ **VISA** 💳 💳

Drayer, Burton P (MD) DR
Mount Sinai Med Ctr

Gustave Levy Pl; New York, NY 10029; (212) 241-6403; **BDCERT:** N 76; DR 78; **MS:** U Chicago-Pritzker Sch Med 71; **RES:** N, Med Ctr Hosp of VT, Burlington, VT 72-75; Rad, U of Pittsburgh Med Ctr, Pittsburgh, PA 75-78; **FEL:** NR, U of Pittsburgh Med Ctr, Pittsburgh, PA 75-78; **FAP:** Prof Mt Sinai Sch Med; **SI:** *Aging Brain; Stroke*; **HMO:** Oxford United Healthcare GHI PHS US Hlthcre +

LANG: Sp, Rus, Chi, Ar, Fr; ♿ 🏥 📞 🎥 🏥 💲 Mcr Mol WC NFI Immediately ▦ **VISA** 💳

Lipset, Richard (MD) DR
St Luke's Roosevelt Hosp Ctr

1000 10th Ave; New York, NY 10019; (212) 523-7035; **BDCERT:** DR 94; **MS:** SUNY Downstate 87; **RES:** DR, St Luke's Roosevelt Hosp, New York, NY 88-92; **FEL:** Body Imaging, Yale-New Haven Hosp, New Haven, CT 92-93; **FAP:** Asst Prof of Clin Rad Columbia P&S; **SI:** *Ultrasound*; **HMO:** Most

LANG: Sp; ♿ 🏥 📞 🎥 🏥 💲 Mcr Mol WC NFI A Few Days ▦ **VISA** 💳

Maklansky, Daniel (MD) DR
Mount Sinai Med Ctr

1075 Park Ave Apt 1D; New York, NY 10128; (212) 289-5611; **BDCERT:** Rad 62; **MS:** SUNY Downstate 56; **RES:** Rad, Mount Sinai Med Ctr, New York, NY 59-62; **FAP:** Assoc Clin Prof Mt Sinai Sch Med; **SI:** *Gastrointestinal Radiology*; **HMO:** Oxford Aetna Hlth Plan Empire Sanus

LANG: Sp; 🎥 🏥 💲 Mcr WC NFI Immediately ▦ **VISA** 💳 💳

Megibow, Alec Jeffrey (MD) DR
New York University Med Ctr

550 1st Ave; New York, NY 10016; (212) 263-5222; **MS:** SUNY Syracuse 74; **RES:** DR, Bellevue Hosp Ctr, New York, NY 74-77; **FEL:** Abdominal Imaging, New York University Med Ctr, New York, NY 77-78; **FAP:** Prof NYU Sch Med; **SI:** *Abdominal Imaging*; **HMO:** Oxford United Healthcare Prucare US Hlthcre CIGNA +

LANG: Sp; ♿ 🎥 🏥 💲 Mcr Mol Immediately ▦ **VISA** 💳 💳

Mitnick, Julie (MD) DR
New York University Med Ctr

Murray Hill Radiology, 650 1st Ave; New York, NY 10018; (212) 686-4440; **BDCERT:** DR 77; **MS:** NYU Sch Med 77; **RES:** Lenox Hill Hosp, New York, NY 72-73; **FAP:** Asst Prof DR NYU Sch Med; **HMO:** Oxford Aetna Hlth Plan PHCS

LANG: Sp, Grk, Rus; ⌨ 🔲 🔲 🔲 🔲 2-4 Weeks ▨
VISA 🔴

Nelson, Peter (MD) DR
New York University Med Ctr

Rad Dept, 550 1st Ave; New York, NY 10016; (212) 263-6325; **BDCERT:** Rad 93; **MS:** LSU Sch Med, New Orleans 86; **RES:** Rad, Barnes Hosp, St Louis, MO 4; **FEL:** NR, Barnes Hosp, St Louis, MO 2; **FAP:** Asst Prof NY Med Coll; **SI:** *Interventional Neuroradiology; Cerebrovascular Radiology;* **HMO:** Oxford US Hlthcre Prudential Aetna Hlth Plan

LANG: Sp, Prt, Can, Bng, Jpn; ⌨ 🔲 🔲 🔲 🔲 🔲 🔲
🔲

Norton, Karen (MD) DR
Mount Sinai Med Ctr

Radiology Associates, 1 Gustave Levy Pl; New York, NY 10029; (212) 241-7418; **BDCERT:** Rad 84; **MS:** Mt Sinai Sch Med 80; **RES:** Ped, New York University Med Ctr, New York, NY 80-81; Rad, Mount Sinai Med Ctr, New York, NY 81-84; **FEL:** Ped Imaging, Mount Sinai Med Ctr, New York, NY 84-85; **FAP:** Assoc Prof PR Mt Sinai Sch Med; **HMO:** Oxford Aetna Hlth Plan Guardian PHS CIGNA +

⌨ 🔲 🔲 🔲 🔲 🔲 🔲 🔲 🔲 A Few Days

Som, Peter (MD) DR
Mount Sinai Med Ctr

1 Gustave Levy Pl; New York, NY 10029; (212) 241-7420; **BDCERT:** Rad 72; **MS:** NYU Sch Med 67; **RES:** Rad, Mount Sinai Med Ctr, New York, NY 71; **FAP:** Prof Rad Mt Sinai Sch Med; **SI:** *Head and Neck Imaging;* **HMO:** Aetna Hlth Plan Blue Choice Blue Cross & Blue Shield CIGNA Metlife +

LANG: Sp; ⌨ 🔲 🔲 🔲 🔲 🔲 🔲 A Few Days ▨
VISA 🔴

EMERGENCY MEDICINE

Almond, Gregory (MD) EM
Metropolitan Hosp Ctr

1901 1st Ave; New York, NY 10029; (212) 423-7175; **BDCERT:** EM 91; **MS:** Med U SC, Charleston 86; **RES:** Metropolitan Hosp Ctr, New York, NY 86-89; **FAP:** Assoc Clin Prof EM NY Med Coll; **SI:** *Stroke; Trauma*

LANG: Ar, Sp; ⌨ 🔲 🔲 🔲 🔲 🔲 🔲 🔲 🔲
Immediately ▨ **VISA** 🔴 🔲

Goldfrank, Lewis (MD) EM
Bellevue Hosp Ctr

462 1st Ave; New York, NY 10016; (212) 561-3346; **BDCERT:** IM 73; EM 80; **MS:** Belgium 70; **RES:** IM, Montefiore Med Ctr, Bronx, NY 71-73; **FAP:** Assoc Prof NYU Sch Med; **SI:** *Medical Toxicology*

LANG: Fr, Sp, Chi; ⌨ 🔲 🔲 🔲 🔲 🔲 🔲 🔲 🔲 🔲

Husk, Gregg (MD) EM
Beth Israel Med Ctr

Beth Israel Medical Center, 1st Ave & 16th St; New York, NY 10003; (212) 420-2847; **BDCERT:** EM 96; **MS:** U Chicago-Pritzker Sch Med 75; **RES:** IM, Bronx Municipal Hosp, Bronx, NY 75-78

Lynn, Stephan (MD) EM
St Luke's Roosevelt Hosp Ctr

1000 10th Ave; New York, NY 10019; (212) 523-3330; **BDCERT:** EM 83; S 79; **MS:** Columbia P&S 73; **RES:** St Luke's Roosevelt Hosp Ctr, New York, NY 73-78; **FAP:** Assoc Prof Columbia P&S

⌨ 🔲 🔲 🔲 🔲 🔲 🔲 🔲 🔲 🔲 Immediately

ENDOCRINOLOGY, DIABETES & METABOLISM

Barandes, Martin (MD)   EDM
Manhattan Eye, Ear & Throat Hosp

155 E 76th St; New York, NY 10021; (212) 249-0622; **BDCERT:** EDM 75; NuM 72; **MS:** Albany Med Coll 63; **RES:** IM, St Luke's Roosevelt Hosp Ctr, New York, NY 65-66; IM, Mem Sloan Kettering Cancer Ctr, New York, NY 66-67; **FEL:** Mathematical Biology, Nat Inst Health, Bethesda, MD 64-65; EDM/NuM, NY Hosp-Cornell Med Ctr, New York, NY 67-71; **HOSP:** St Vincents Hosp & Med Ctr NY; **SI:** *Thyroid Disease; Cardiology-Nuclear Medicine;* **HMO:** Aetna Hlth Plan GHI Aetna-US Healthcare 32BJ United Healthcare +

LANG: Sp; ⯑ ⯑ ⯑ ⯑ ⯑ Mcr Mcd Immediately ▦
VISA ⬤

Bergman, Donald (MD)   EDM
Mount Sinai Med Ctr

1199 Park Ave Suite 1F; New York, NY 10128; (212) 876-7333; **BDCERT:** IM 75; EDM 77; **MS:** Jefferson Med Coll 71; **RES:** ObG, Mount Sinai Med Ctr, New York, NY 71-72; Med, Mount Sinai Med Ctr, New York, NY 72-75; **FEL:** EDM, Mount Sinai Med Ctr, New York, NY 75-77; **FAP:** Assoc Clin Prof Med Mt Sinai Sch Med; **HOSP:** Beth Israel North; **SI:** *Osteoporosis; Thyroid Disorders;* **HMO:** Oxford

⯑ ⯑ ⯑ ⯑ ⯑ A Few Days ▦ **VISA** ⬤

Bernstein, Gerald (MD)   EDM
Lenox Hill Hosp

35 E 75th St; New York, NY 10021; (212) 288-1538; **BDCERT:** IM 66; **MS:** Tufts U 59; **RES:** VA Med Ctr-Bronx, Bronx, NY 60; Montefiore Med Ctr, Bronx, NY 63; **FEL:** EDM, Montefiore Med Ctr, Bronx, NY; **HOSP:** Montefiore Med Ctr; **SI:** *Thyroid;* **HMO:** Oxford

⯑ ⯑ ⯑ ⯑ ⯑ Immediately **VISA** ⬤

Bilezikian, John Paul (MD)   EDM
Columbia-Presbyterian Med Ctr

630 W 168th St PH8W864; New York, NY 10032; (212) 305-6238; **BDCERT:** IM 75; EDM 77; **MS:** Columbia P&S 69; **RES:** IM, Columbia-Presbyterian Med Ctr, New York, NY 73-75; **FEL:** EDM, Nat Inst Health, Bethesda, MD 71-73; **FAP:** Prof Med Columbia P&S; **SI:** *Hyperparathyroidism; Osteoporosis;* **HMO:** PHS Blue Choice Oxford Health First Prudential +

LANG: Sp; ⯑ ⯑ ⯑ ⯑ ⯑ Mcr WC NFI 4+ Weeks ▦
VISA ⬤

Bloomgarden, Zachary (MD)   EDM
Mount Sinai Med Ctr

35 E 85th St; New York, NY 10028; (212) 879-5933; **BDCERT:** IM 77; EDM 79; **MS:** Albert Einstein Coll Med 74; **RES:** Montefiore Med Ctr, Bronx, NY 74-77; **FEL:** EDM, Vanderbilt U Med Ctr, Nashville, TN 77-79; **FAP:** Assoc Clin Prof Med Mt Sinai Sch Med; **SI:** *Diabetes; Obesity;* **HMO:** Blue Choice PHCS 32BJ 1199

LANG: Sp, Fr; ⯑ ⯑ ⯑ ⯑ Mcr 2-4 Weeks

Blum, Conrad (MD)   EDM   ▣PCP
Columbia-Presbyterian Med Ctr

16 E 60th St Ste 320; New York, NY 10022; (212) 326-8421; **BDCERT:** IM 76; EDM 77; **MS:** Northwestern U 71; **RES:** IM, Columbia-Presbyterian Med Ctr, New York, NY 71-72; IM, Peter Bent Brigham Hosp, Boston, MA 75-76; **FEL:** EDM, Northwestern Mem Hosp, Chicago, IL 76; **FAP:** Prof of Clin Med Columbia P&S; **SI:** *Cholesterol and Triglycerides; Thyroid Diseases;* **HMO:** None

⯑ ⯑ ⯑ ⯑ ⯑ A Few Days

Blum, Manfred (MD)   EDM
New York University Med Ctr

530 1st Ave 4E; New York, NY 10016; (212) 263-7444; **BDCERT:** IM 64; **MS:** NYU Sch Med 57; **RES:** IM, Montefiore Med Ctr, Bronx, NY 58-59; **SI:** *Thyroid;* **HMO:** None

Bockman, Richard (MD & PhD) EDM
Hosp For Special Surgery
535 E 70th St; New York, NY 10021; (212) 606-1458; **BDCERT:** IM 75; **MS:** Yale U Sch Med 68; **RES:** Bellevue Hosp Ctr, New York, NY 73-75; **FEL:** EDM, NY Hosp-Cornell Med Ctr, New York, NY 73; **HOSP:** NY Hosp-Cornell Med Ctr; **SI:** *Osteoporosis; Metabolic Bone Disorders*; **HMO:** Oxford PHS NY Hosp Hlth GHI

♿ 📷 📅 **S** Mcr 2-4 Weeks

Bukberg, Phillip (MD) EDM
St Vincents Hosp & Med Ctr NY
36 7th Ave Ste 517; New York, NY 10011; (212) 807-8129; **BDCERT:** EDM 79; IM 77; **MS:** SUNY Downstate 73; **RES:** IM, St Vincents Hosp & Med Ctr NY, New York, NY 75-77; **FEL:** EDM, Mem Sloan Kettering Cancer Ctr, New York, NY 77-79; Metabolism, Mount Sinai Med Ctr, New York, NY 79-81; **SI:** *Cholesterol Disorders; Diabetes Mellitus*; **HMO:** Oxford Prucare Aetna-US Healthcare

♿ 📷 📅 **S** Mcr 2-4 Weeks

Davies, Terry (MD) EDM
Mount Sinai Med Ctr
Box 1055 Mt Sinai Hospital, 1 Gustave Levy Pl; New York, NY 10029; (212) 241-6627; **MS:** England 71; **RES:** U of Newcastle-Upon-Tyne, Newcastle-Upon-Tyne, England; **FEL:** U of Newcastle-Upon-Tyne, Newcastle-Upon-Tyne, England; Nat Inst Health, Bethesda, MD; **FAP:** Prof Mt Sinai Sch Med; **HMO:** Most

♿ 🌙 📷 📅 **S** Mcr 2-4 Weeks **VISA** 💳

Drexler, Andrew (MD) EDM
New York University Med Ctr
1200 5th Ave; New York, NY 10029; (212) 684-6116; **BDCERT:** IM 77; EDM 81; **MS:** NYU Sch Med 72; **RES:** IM, Barnes Hosp, St Louis, MO 75-76; **FEL:** EDM, Washignton U Med, Washignton, DC 76-78; **HOSP:** Mount Sinai Med Ctr; **SI:** *Diabetes—Type 1; Diabetes and Pregnancy*

♿ 📷 📅 **S** Mcr 2-4 Weeks

Felig, Philip (MD) EDM
Lenox Hill Hosp
1056 5th Ave; New York, NY 10028; (212) 534-5900; **BDCERT:** IM 68; **MS:** Yale U Sch Med 61; **RES:** IM, Yale-New Haven Hosp, New Haven, CT 61-67; **FEL:** EDM, Peter Bent Brigham Hosp, Boston, MA 67-69; **HOSP:** Beth Israel North; **SI:** *Diabetes; Thyroid Disorders*

LANG: Sp, Heb; ♿ 📷 📷 📅 **S** A Few Days

Futterweit, Walter (MD) EDM
Mount Sinai Med Ctr
1172 Park Ave; New York, NY 10128; (212) 876-6400; **BDCERT:** IM 65; EDM 72; **MS:** NYU Sch Med 57; **RES:** Montefiore Med Ctr, Bronx, NY 58-60; **FEL:** EDM, Mount Sinai Med Ctr, New York, NY 60-61; **FAP:** Clin Prof Med Mt Sinai Sch Med; **SI:** *Polycystic Ovary Syndrome; Acne Hair Growth Excess Loss*; **HMO:** Oxford Premier

LANG: Ger; 📅 **S** Mcr 1 Week **AMERICAN** **VISA** 💳

Gabrilove, J Lester (MD) EDM
Mount Sinai Med Ctr
Mt Sinai Hospital, 5 E 98th St FL11; New York, NY 10029; (212) 241-7975; **BDCERT:** IM 48; **MS:** NYU Sch Med 40; **RES:** Mount Sinai Med Ctr, New York, NY; **FEL:** EDM, Yale-New Haven Hosp, New Haven, CT 45; Mount Sinai Med Ctr, New York, NY 46-48; **FAP:** Prof Med Mt Sinai Sch Med; **SI:** *General Endocrinology; Adrenal Diseases*

♿ 📷 📅 Mcr A Few Days 💳 **VISA** 💳 💳

Gershberg, Herbert (MD) EDM
New York University Med Ctr
614 2nd Ave 2; New York, NY 10016; (212) 686-0240; **BDCERT:** IM 52; **MS:** Med Coll Va 41; **RES:** Yale-New Haven Hosp, New Haven, CT 45-48; New York University Med Ctr, New York, NY 48; **FEL:** New York University Med Ctr, New York, NY; **HOSP:** Beth Israel North; **SI:** *Diabetes; Thyroid*

Guide to symbols and abbreviations can be found on pages 110-113.

181

Gershengorn, Marvin (MD) EDM
NY Hosp-Cornell Med Ctr

1300 York Ave; New York, NY 10021; (212) 746-6275; **BDCERT:** IM 74; **MS:** NYU Sch Med 71; **RES:** IM, Strong Mem Hosp, Rochester, NY 71-73; **FEL:** EDM, Nat Inst Health, Bethesda, MD; **FAP:** Prof Cornell U

🖬 🛇 Mcr Mcd

Gittler, Robert (MD)   EDM
Lenox Hill Hosp

116 E 66th St; New York, NY 10021; (212) 288-0478; **BDCERT:** IM 56; **MS:** Univ Vt Coll Med 49; **RES:** Beth Israel Med Ctr, New York, NY 52; **FEL:** EDM, U Mich Med Ctr, Ann Arbor, MI 52-54; **FAP:** Assoc Clin Prof Albert Einstein Coll Med; **HOSP:** Beth Israel Med Ctr

LANG: Fr; 🖬 🛗 🛇 Mcr   A Few Days

Goland, Robin (MD)   EDM
Columbia-Presbyterian Med Ctr

Department of Medicine, 622 W 168th St; New York, NY 10032; (212) 305-3788; **BDCERT:** IM 83; **MS:** Columbia P&S 80; **RES:** Med, Columbia-Presbyterian Med Ctr, New York, NY 80-84; **FEL:** EDM, Columbia-Presbyterian Med Ctr, New York, NY 84-87; **FAP:** Assoc Prof Med Columbia P&S; **HMO:** Oxford Prudential Blue Cross & Blue Choice Chubb PHS +

🖬 🖬 🖬 🛗 🛇 Mcr 🎟 *VISA* 💳

Greene, Loren (MD)   EDM
New York University Med Ctr

NYU Medical Ctr, 530 1st Ave 4B; New York, NY 10016; (212) 263-7449; **BDCERT:** IM 78; EDM 81; **MS:** NYU Sch Med 75; **RES:** New York University Med Ctr, New York, NY 75-78; **FEL:** New York University Med Ctr, New York, NY 78-80; **FAP:** Assoc Clin Prof Med NYU Sch Med; **HOSP:** Cabrini Med Ctr; *SI: Thyroid, Pituitary; Osteoporosis, Menopause*

LANG: Sp; 🖬 🖬 🖬 🛗 🛇 Mcr   2-4 Weeks

Hurley, James (MD)   EDM
NY Hosp-Cornell Med Ctr

525 E 68th St ST221; New York, NY 10021; (212) 746-6290; **BDCERT:** IM 68; NuM 72; **MS:** Cornell U 61; **RES:** NY Hosp-Cornell Med Ctr, New York, NY 61-64; **FEL:** EDM, NY Hosp-Cornell Med Ctr, New York, NY 64-65; **FAP:** Assoc Prof Med; *SI: Hyperthyroidism; Thyroid Cancer*

🖬 🖬 🛗 Mcr Mcd   2-4 Weeks 🎟 *VISA* 💳

Imperato-Mcginley, Julianne (MD)   EDM
PCP
NY Hosp-Cornell Med Ctr

525 E 68th St; New York, NY 10021; (212) 746-6276; **MS:** SUNY Downstate 65; **RES:** Lenox Hill Hosp, New York, NY 68-69; **HOSP:** New York Methodist Hosp

Jacobs, David R (MD)   EDM
Lenox Hill Hosp

311 E 79th St; New York, NY 10021; (212) 628-0300; **BDCERT:** IM 63; EDM 72; **MS:** Case West Res U 56; **RES:** Lenox Hill Hosp, New York, NY 56-57; Mount Sinai Med Ctr, New York, NY 57-59; **FEL:** EDM, Mount Sinai Med Ctr, New York, NY 59-60; **FAP:** Clin Prof Med NYU Sch Med; **HOSP:** Mount Sinai Med Ctr; *SI: Thyroid Diseases; Osteoporosis*

LANG: Fr; 🖬 🛗   1 Week

Jacobs, Thomas (MD)   EDM
Columbia-Presbyterian Med Ctr

161 Fort Washington Ave; New York, NY 10032; (212) 305-5578; **BDCERT:** IM 73; **MS:** Johns Hopkins U 68; **RES:** Columbia-Presbyterian Med Ctr, New York, NY 68-73; **FEL:** EDM, U WA Med Ctr, Seattle, WA; **FAP:** Clin Prof Med Columbia P&S; *SI: Pituitary Disorders; Calcium-Skeletal Metabolism*

🖬 🖬 🛗 🛇   1 Week

Kalin, Marcia (MD) EDM
Beth Israel Med Ctr
Beth Israel Med Ctr Dept of Medicine, 1st Ave & 16th St 10th Fl; New York, NY 10003; (212) 420-3917; **BDCERT:** IM 88; EDM 89; **MS:** Mt Sinai Sch Med 80; **RES:** IM, Overlook Hosp, Summit, NJ 80-81; IM, Beth Israel Med Ctr, New York, NY 83-85; **FEL:** EDM, Beth Israel Med Ctr, New York, NY 85-88; **FAP:** Asst Prof Albert Einstein Coll Med; **SI:** *Diabetes*

LANG: Sp; ⬧ ⬧ ⬧ ⬧ ⬧ 1 Week ▦ **VISA** ⬧ ⬧

Kleinberg, David (MD) EDM
New York University Med Ctr
530 1st Ave Ste 4G; New York, NY 10016; (212) 263-6772; **BDCERT:** IM 72; EDM 75; **MS:** U Miami Sch Med 66; **RES:** IM, Maimonides Med Ctr, Brooklyn, NY 67-68; IM, Columbia-Presbyterian Med Ctr, New York, NY 70-71; **FEL:** EDM, Columbia-Presbyterian Med Ctr, New York, NY 68-70; **FAP:** Prof NYU Sch Med; **SI:** *Pituitary Disease; Neuro Endocrinology*; **HMO:** Chubb Health Source CIGNA

⬧ ⬧ ⬧ ⬧ ⬧ ⬧ 1 Week

Klyde, Barry J (MD) EDM PCP
NY Hosp-Cornell Med Ctr
520 E 72nd St LO; New York, NY 10021; (212) 772-3333; **BDCERT:** IM 77; EDM 81; **MS:** Stanford U 74; **RES:** IM, NY Hosp-Cornell Med Ctr, New York, NY 74-77; **FEL:** EDM, NY Hosp-Cornell Med Ctr, New York, NY 77-79; **FAP:** Assoc Clin Prof IM Cornell U; **SI:** *Thyroid; Sexual Dysfunction*; **HMO:** None

LANG: Sp; ⬧ ⬧ ⬧ ⬧ ⬧ ⬧ 1 Week ▦ **VISA** ⬧

Laufer, Ira (MD) EDM
New York University Med Ctr
247 3rd Ave L1; New York, NY 10010; (212) 475-2535; **BDCERT:** IM 62; **MS:** NYU Sch Med 53; **RES:** Bellevue Hosp Ctr, New York, NY 56-58; New York University Med Ctr, New York, NY 58-59; **FEL:** EDM, New York University Med Ctr, New York, NY 57-58; **FAP:** Assoc Clin Prof Med NYU Sch Med; **HOSP:** Cabrini Med Ctr; **SI:** *Diabetic Neuropathy; Adult Diabetes*

⬧ ⬧ ⬧ ⬧ ⬧ ⬧ 1 Week

Levy, Brian (MD) EDM
New York University Med Ctr
Murray Hill Medical Group, PC, 317 E 34th St 7th Fl; New York, NY 10016; (212) 726-7426; **BDCERT:** IM 83; EDM 85; **MS:** Johns Hopkins U 79; **RES:** IM, VA Med Ctr-Manh, New York, NY 80-83; **FEL:** EDM, NYU Medical Center, New York, NY 83-85; **FAP:** Asst Lecturer Med NYU Sch Med; **SI:** *Thyroid Diseases; Diabetes*

⬧ ⬧ ⬧ ⬧ ⬧ ⬧ ▦ **VISA** ⬧

Mahler, Richard J (MD) EDM
NY Hosp-Cornell Med Ctr
220 E 69th St; New York, NY 10021; (212) 879-4073; **BDCERT:** IM 87; **MS:** NY Med Coll 59; **RES:** IM, NY Med Coll, New York, NY 60-63; **FEL:** EDM,; EDM, NY Academy of Med, New York, NY 63-64; **FAP:** Assoc Clin Prof Cornell U; **HOSP:** Lenox Hill Hosp; **HMO:** None

⬧ ⬧ ⬧ 2-4 Weeks

McConnell, Robert (MD) EDM
Columbia-Presbyterian Med Ctr
161 Ft Washington Ave Rm210; New York, NY 10032; (212) 305-5579; **BDCERT:** EDM 81; IM 79; **MS:** Columbia P&S 73; **RES:** IM, Barnes Hosp, St Louis, MO 73-75; **FEL:** EDM, Columbia-Presbyterian Med Ctr, New York, NY 75-78; **FAP:** Assoc Clin Prof Med Columbia P&S; **SI:** *Thyroid Diseases*; **HMO:** Oxford Blue Cross Cambridge Net Prudential Multiplan +

⬧ ⬧ ⬧ ⬧ ⬧ 2-4 Weeks

McEvoy, Robert (MD) EDM
Mount Sinai Med Ctr
Mt Sinai Med Ctr, 1176 5th Ave Box 1659; New York, NY 10029; (212) 241-6936; **BDCERT:** Ped 90; PEn 91; **MS:** U Minn 73; **RES:** Pen, Mount Sinai Med Ctr, New York, NY 81-84; **FAP:** Prof Mt Sinai Sch Med; **HOSP:** Englewood Hosp & Med Ctr; **SI:** *Diabetes; Low Blood Sugar*; **HMO:** Oxford US Hlthcre

⬧ ⬧ ⬧ ⬧ ⬧ ⬧ ⬧ Immediately

Mechanick, Jeffrey (MD)   EDM
Mount Sinai Med Ctr
1192 Park Ave; New York, NY 10128; (212) 831-
2100; **BDCERT:** EDM 93; **MS:** Mt Sinai Sch Med 85;
RES: IM, Baylor Coll Med, Houston, TX 85-88; **FEL:**
EDM, Mount Sinai Med Ctr, New York, NY 88-90;
FAP: Assoc Clin Prof Med Mt Sinai Sch Med; *SI:*
Nutrition Support—TPN; **HMO:** Oxford Premier PHS
Affordable Hlth Plan

🚫 🖼 🏧 💲 Mcr   2-4 Weeks▦ **VISA** ⬤

Merker, Edward (MD)   EDM
Cabrini Med Ctr
35 E 85th St; New York, NY 10028; (212) 288-
1110; **BDCERT:** EDM 77; Ger 94; **MS:** NYU Sch
Med 65; **RES:** IM, Mount Sinai Med Ctr, New York,
NY 68-70; **FEL:** EDM, Mount Sinai Med Ctr, New
York, NY 70-72; **FAP:** Asst Clin Prof Mt Sinai Sch
Med; **HOSP:** Lenox Hill Hosp; *SI: Diabetes Mellitus;*
Metabolic Bone Disease; **HMO:** Most

LANG: Fr, Rom, Sp, Rus, Ukr; 🚫 🌙 🖼 🏧 💲 Mcr Mol
A Few Days **VISA** ⬤

Park, Constance (MD & PhD)EDM
Columbia-Presbyterian Med Ctr
635 Madison Ave 8th Fl; New York, NY 10022;
(212) 317-4567; **BDCERT:** IM 80; EDM 97; **MS:**
Albert Einstein Coll Med 74; **RES:** Bellevue Hosp Ctr,
New York, NY 74-75; Bellevue Hosp Ctr, New
York, NY 75-76; **FEL:** EDM, Albert Einstein Med
Ctr, Bronx, NY 76-78; **FAP:** Assoc Clin Prof Med
Columbia P&S; **HMO:** None

LANG: Sp, Fr; 🚫 🖼 🚹 🏧 💲 Mcr NFl 2-4 Weeks▦
VISA ⬤ ▭

Poretsky, Leonid (MD)   EDM
NY Hosp-Cornell Med Ctr
525 E 68th St; New York, NY 10028; (212) 746-
6290; **BDCERT:** IM 83; EDM 95; **MS:** Russia 77;
RES: Coney Island Hosp, Brooklyn, NY 80-83; **FEL:**
Beth Israel Med Ctr, Boston, MA 83-85; **FAP:** Assoc
Prof Cornell U; *SI: Diabetes; Thyroid*
LANG: Rus; 🚫 🖼 🚹 🏧 💲 Mcr 4+ Weeks

Quagliarello, John (MD)   EDM
New York University Med Ctr
530 1st Ave 10Q; New York, NY 10016; (212)
263-6358; **BDCERT:** 79; RE 81; **MS:** McGill U 70;
RES: ObG, New York University Med Ctr, New York,
NY 70-77; **FEL:** RE, New York University Med Ctr,
New York, NY 77-79; **FAP:** Assoc Prof NYU Sch
Med; *SI: Laparoscopic Hysterioscopic Surgery; Clinical*
Infertility; **HMO:** Oxford

🚫 🌙 🖼 🏧 💲 A Few Days **VISA** ⬤

Richard, Jack (MD)   EDM
NY Hosp-Cornell Med Ctr
407 E 70th St 4th FL; New York, NY 10021; (212)
861-6677; **BDCERT:** IM 74; EDM 75; **MS:** Cornell U
53; **RES:** IM, NY Hosp-Cornell Med Ctr, New York,
NY 53-54; IM, NY Hosp-Cornell Med Ctr, New
York, NY 56-60; **FEL:** EDM, NY Hosp-Cornell Med
Ctr, New York, NY 58-59; **FAP:** Clin Prof Cornell U;
SI: General Endocrinology; Thyroid Disease; **HMO:**
None

LANG: Sp, Grk; 🚫 🖼 🏧 Mcr 1 Week

Seplowitz, Alan (MD)   EDM
Columbia-Presbyterian Med Ctr
161 Fort Washington Ave; New York, NY 10032;
(212) 305-5503; **BDCERT:** IM 75; EDM 77; **MS:**
Columbia P&S 72; **RES:** Columbia-Presbyterian
Med Ctr, New York, NY 72-74; **FEL:** EDM,
Columbia-Presbyterian Med Ctr, New York, NY 76-
78; **FAP:** Assoc Clin Prof Med Columbia P&S; *SI:*
Thyroid Diseases; Diabetes Mellitus; **HMO:** Oxford
CIGNA PHS Guardian Blue Choice +

🚫 🖼 🏧 💲 2-4 Weeks

Shane, Elizabeth (MD)   EDM
Columbia-Presbyterian Med Ctr
Metabolic Bone Disease Program, 180 Ft
Washington Ave; New York, NY 10032; (212)
305-2663; **BDCERT:** IM 78; EDM 81; **MS:** U
Toronto 75; **RES:** IM, Toronto Gen Hosp, Toronto,
Canada 75-76; IM, Columbia-Presbyterian Med
Ctr, New York, NY 76-78; **FEL:** EDM, Columbia-
Presbyterian Med Ctr, New York, NY 78-81; **FAP:**
Prof of Clin Med Columbia P&S; *SI:*
Osteoporosis/Hyperparathyroid; Transplantation Bone
Disease; **HMO:** Oxford Prudential Empire Blue Cross
& Shield Multiplan PHS +

🚫 🖼 🚹 🏧 💲 Mcr Mol 2-4 Weeks▦ **VISA** ⬤

Silverberg, Shonni J (MD)   EDM
Columbia-Presbyterian Med Ctr
622 W 168th St; New York, NY 10032; (212)
305-2663; **BDCERT:** EDM 85; IM 83; **MS:** Cornell U
80; **RES:** IM, NY Hosp-Cornell Med Ctr, New York,
NY 81-83; **FEL:** EDM, Columbia-Presbyterian Med
Ctr, New York, NY 83-86; **FAP:** Assoc Prof Med
Columbia P&S; *SI: Osteoporosis; Primary
Hyperparathyroid;* **HMO:** Oxford
⌖ ⌂ ⚥ ⊞ Mcr 4+ Weeks 💳 **VISA** ●

Siris, Ethel (MD)   EDM
Columbia-Presbyterian Med Ctr
Harkness Pavillion-Toni Spabile Ctr for the
Prevention and Treatment of Osteoporosis-Columb
Presb Med Ctr, 180 W Ft Washington Ave; New
York, NY 10032; (212) 305-2663; **BDCERT:** IM
74; EDM 77; **MS:** Columbia P&S 71; **RES:**
Columbia-Presbyterian Med Ctr, New York, NY 71-
74; **FEL:** Nat Inst Health, Bethesda, MD; EDM,
Columbia-Presbyterian Med Ctr, New York, NY 76-
77; **FAP:** Prof Columbia P&S; *SI: Osteoporosis;
Paget's Disease of Bone;* **HMO:** Oxford Blue Choice
⌖ ⌂ ⚥ ⊞ $ Mcr 2-4 Weeks 💳 **VISA** ●

Szabo, Andrew John (MD)   EDM
Lenox Hill Hosp
220 E 69th St 3; New York, NY 10021; (212) 628-
5626; **BDCERT:** IM 87; EDM 89; **MS:** McGill U 59;
RES: IM, Montreal Children's Hosp, Montreal,
Canada 60-64; IM, Queen Mary Veteran's Hosp,
Montreal, Canada 61-62; **FEL:** EDM, Montreal Gen
Hosp, Montreal, Canada 62-63; Diabetes, New
England Deaconess Hosp, Boston, MA 64-65; **FAP:**
Assoc Clin Prof Med Cornell U; **HOSP:** NY Hosp-
Cornell Med Ctr; *SI: Diabetes; Hyperthyroidism;*
HMO: Chubb PHCS PHS Oxford Metlife +
LANG: Hun; ⌖ ⌂ ⊞ $ Mcr Immediately

Wallach, Stanley (MD)   EDM
Hosp For Joint Diseases
305 2nd Ave Ste 16; New York, NY 10003; (212)
598-6093; **BDCERT:** IM 60; EDM 72; **MS:** SUNY
Hlth Sci Ctr 53; **RES:** Kings County Hosp Ctr,
Brooklyn, NY 53-54; U UT Hosp, Salt Lake City, UT
54-56; **FEL:** EDM, Mass Gen Hosp, Boston, MA 56-
57; **HOSP:** New York University Med Ctr; *SI:
Osteoporosis; Paget's Disease;* **HMO:** Oxford Blue
Cross & Blue Shield Aetna Hlth Plan US Hlthcre
LANG: Sp; ⌖ ⌂ ⚥ ⊞ Mcr 2-4 Weeks

Wardlaw, Sharon (MD)   EDM
Columbia-Presbyterian Med Ctr
630 W 168th St; New York, NY 10032; (212)
305-3725; **BDCERT:** IM 78; EDM 79; **MS:** Cornell U
75; **RES:** IM, Case Western Reserve U Hosp,
Cleveland, OH; **FEL:** EDM, Columbia-Presbyterian
Med Ctr, New York, NY; **FAP:** Assoc Prof Columbia
P&S; *SI: Neuroendocrinology; Pituitary Disease;* **HMO:**
Oxford Empire Blue Cross & Shield Prucare
⌖ ⌂ ⚥ ⊞ $ Mcr 1 Week **VISA** ●

Zumoff, Barnett (MD)   EDM
Beth Israel Med Ctr
Beth Israel Med Ctr Div of Endocrinology, 1st Ave at
16th St 5BH20; New York, NY 10003; (212) 420-
4008; **BDCERT:** IM 58; EDM 73; **MS:** SUNY
Downstate 49; **RES:** Med, Jewish Hosp Med Ctr,
Brooklyn, NY 51-52; Med, Kings County Hosp Ctr,
Brooklyn, NY 54-55; **FEL:** EDM, Mem Sloan
Kettering Cancer Ctr, New York, NY 55-57; **FAP:**
Prof Med Albert Einstein Coll Med; *SI: Hormones
Male Female Adrenology; Diabetes;* **HMO:** Oxford
1199
LANG: Yd; ⌖ ⌂ ⚥ ⊞ $ Mcr NFl 1 Week 💳 **VISA**
● ▦

FAMILY PRACTICE

Calman, Neil (MD) FP PCP
Beth Israel Med Ctr

Institute Urban Family Health, 16 E 16th St 4th Fl;
New York, NY 10003; (212) 924-7744; **BDCERT:**
FP 97; Ger 88; **MS:** Rush Med Coll 75; **RES:** FP,
Montefiore Med Ctr, Bronx, NY 75-78; **FAP:** Prof
Albert Einstein Coll Med; **HOSP:** Bronx Lebanon
Hosp Ctr; **SI:** *Family Health Care;* **HMO:** Oxford
Aetna-US Healthcare ABC Health NYLCare

LANG: Sp; ⬚ ⬚ ⬚ ⬚ ⬚ ⬚ ⬚ 1 Week **VISA** ⬚

Clements, Jerry (MD) FP PCP
Beth Israel Med Ctr

25 5th Ave 1A; New York, NY 10003; (212) 477-
1750; **BDCERT:** FP 87; **MS:** West Indies 83; **RES:** St
Joseph's Med Ctr-Stamford, Stamford, CT 83-86;
HOSP: St Vincents Hosp & Med Ctr NY; **SI:** *Office
Gynecology; Office Pediatrics*

⬚ ⬚ ⬚ ⬚ ⬚ ⬚ A Few Days ⬚

Falencki, John J (MD) FP PCP
Beth Israel Med Ctr

Village Family Practice, 25 5th Ave 1A; New York,
NY 10003; (212) 477-1750; **BDCERT:** FP 76; FP
82; **MS:** Wayne State U Sch Med 72; **RES:** FP,
Group Health Co-Op Puget Sound, Seattle, WA 74-
76; FP, Hosp of St Raphael, New Haven, CT 73-74;
FAP: Clin Instr Ped Mt Sinai Sch Med; **HOSP:** St
Vincents Hosp & Med Ctr NY

LANG: Sp; ⬚ ⬚ ⬚ ⬚ ⬚ ⬚ ⬚ ⬚ A Few Days
⬚ **VISA** ⬚ ⬚

Leeds, Gary (MD) FP PCP
Beth Israel Med Ctr

Family Medical Group, 77 W 15th St; New York,
NY 10011; (212) 206-7717; **BDCERT:** FP 96; **MS:**
Brown U 78; **RES:** FP, Georgetown U Hosp,
Washington, DC 78-81; **FAP:** Clin Instr Albert
Einstein Coll Med; **HOSP:** Cabrini Med Ctr; **HMO:**
US Hlthcre Oxford CIGNA United Healthcare

LANG: Prt, Sp; ⬚ ⬚ ⬚ ⬚ ⬚ ⬚ A Few Days

Levy, Albert (MD) FP PCP
Beth Israel Med Ctr

911 Park Ave; New York, NY 10021; (212) 288-
7193; **BDCERT:** FP 94; Ger 96; **MS:** Brazil 73; **RES:**
FP, Kings County Hosp Ctr, Brooklyn, NY 78-80;
FAP: Asst Prof Albert Einstein Coll Med; **HOSP:**
Montefiore Med Ctr; **SI:** *Hypertension; Diabetes;*
HMO: Aetna Hlth Plan NYLCare US Hlthcre
Prucare Oxford +

LANG: Prt, Sp, Fr; ⬚ ⬚ ⬚ ⬚ ⬚ ⬚ ⬚ ⬚
Immediately ⬚ **VISA** ⬚

Ravetz, Valerie (MD) FP PCP
St Vincents Hosp & Med Ctr NY

51 E 25th St 7FL; New York, NY 10010; (212)
684-7455; **BDCERT:** FP 90; **MS:** Temple U 86; **RES:**
Community Hosp, Glen Cove, NY 89; **SI:** *Young
Women and Office Gynecology; Preventive Care;* **HMO:**
First Health Oxford PHS United Healthcare
Multiplan +

⬚ ⬚ ⬚ ⬚ ⬚ 1 Week ⬚ **VISA** ⬚ ⬚

Schiller, Robert (MD) FP PCP
Beth Israel Med Ctr

16 E 16th St; New York, NY 10003; (212) 206-
5252; **BDCERT:** FP 85; **MS:** NYU Sch Med 82; **RES:**
Montefiore Med Ctr, Bronx, NY 83-85; **FEL:**
Montefiore Med Ctr, Bronx, NY; **HOSP:** Bronx
Lebanon Hosp Ctr

⬚ ⬚ ⬚ ⬚ ⬚ ⬚ ⬚ ⬚ ⬚ ⬚ ⬚ 2-4 Weeks ⬚
VISA ⬚

Tamarin, Steven (MD) FP PCP
St Luke's Roosevelt Hosp Ctr

441 West End Ave; New York, NY 10024; (212)
496-2133; **BDCERT:** FP 80; **MS:** Mexico 75; **RES:**
FP, Univ Hosp SUNY Bklyn, Brooklyn, NY 77-80;
FAP: Asst Clin Prof FP Columbia P&S; **HOSP:** Beth
Israel Med Ctr; **SI:** *Family Care;* **HMO:** PHS Oxford
Aetna Hlth Plan CIGNA NYLCare +

LANG: Sp; ⬚ ⬚ ⬚ ⬚ ⬚ ⬚ ⬚ A Few Days ⬚
VISA ⬚

Tesher, Martin (MD) FP `PCP`
Beth Israel North
1112 Park Ave; New York, NY 10128; (212) 534-1500; **BDCERT:** FP 91; **MS:** Queens U 62; **RES:** Toronto East Gen, Toronto, Canada 62-63; Herrick Mem Hosp, Berkeley, CA 63-64; **SI:** *Pain Management/Headaches; Obesity/Back Pain*

LANG: Itl, Sp; 🔊 🅲 🔾 👹 🛏 💲 ᴹᶜʳ Immediately ▨ *VISA* ●

Wang, Christopher (MD) FP `PCP`
Columbia-Presbyterian Med Ctr
64 Nagle Ave; New York, NY 10040; (212) 567-2291; **BDCERT:** FP 97; Ger 94; **MS:** Boston U 80; **RES:** FP, Montefiore Med Ctr, Bronx, NY 81-83; **HMO:** Oxford Prucare Aetna-US Healthcare GHI 1199 +

🔾 👹 🛏 💲 ᴹᶜʳ ᴹᵒᵈ 2-4 Weeks ▨ *VISA* ●

GASTROENTEROLOGY

Ackert, John (MD) Ge
New York University Med Ctr
Concord Medical Group, 232 E 30th St; New York, NY 10016; (212) 889-5544; **BDCERT:** IM 75; Ge 77; **MS:** NYU Sch Med 72; **RES:** Bellevue Hosp Ctr, New York, NY 72-75; **FEL:** Ge, Bellevue Hosp Ctr, New York, NY; **HMO:** Aetna Hlth Plan Blue Choice Blue Cross & Blue Shield CIGNA HIP Network +

LANG: Sp, Hin; 🔾 🛏 💲 ᴹᶜʳ Immediately ▨ *VISA* ●

Aisenberg, James (MD) Ge
Mount Sinai Med Ctr
21 E 87th St; New York, NY 10128; (212) 996-6633; **BDCERT:** IM 90; Ge 93; **MS:** Harvard Med Sch 87; **RES:** IM, Columbia-Presbyterian Med Ctr, New York, NY 87-90; **FEL:** Ge, Mount Sinai Med Ctr, New York, NY 90-93; **FAP:** Asst Clin Prof Mt Sinai Sch Med; **SI:** *Colonoscopy; Diarrhea Diseases*; **HMO:** Oxford PHS Aetna Hlth Plan United Healthcare Empire Blue Choice +

LANG: Sp, Fr; 🔾 🔾 👹 🛏 💲 ᴹᶜʳ 1 Week ▨ *VISA* ●

Attia, Albert (MD) Ge `PCP`
St Luke's Roosevelt Hosp Ctr
350 W 58th St; New York, NY 10019; (212) 307-7210; **BDCERT:** IM 70; **MS:** Cornell U 58; **RES:** St Luke's Roosevelt Hosp Ctr, New York, NY 59-61; **FEL:** Ge, Seton Hall, Jersey City, NJ 61-63; **FAP:** Assoc Clin Prof Med Columbia P&S; **SI:** *Inflammatory Bowel Disease; Colon Cancer and Colitis*; **HMO:** Oxford PHCS CIGNA Blue Choice United Healthcare +

LANG: Sp; 🔾 👹 🛏 💲 A Few Days

Basuk, Paul M (MD) Ge
NY Hosp-Cornell Med Ctr
520 E 70th St; New York, NY 10021; (212) 746-4901; **BDCERT:** IM 83; Ge 87; **MS:** Northwestern U 80; **RES:** IM, UC San Francisco Med Ctr, San Francisco, CA 81-83; **FEL:** Ge, UC San Francisco Med Ctr, San Francisco, CA 85-87; **FAP:** Asst Prof Med Cornell U; **SI:** *Bile Duct Disorders; Colon Polyps and Cancer*; **HMO:** Aetna Hlth Plan Sanus Oxford Blue Choice NYLCare +

LANG: Sp; 🔾 🔾 🛏 ᴹᶜʳ ᴹᵒᵈ A Few Days ▨ *VISA* ●

Bearnot, H Robert (MD) Ge
New York University Med Ctr
245 E 35th St; New York, NY 10016; (212) 684-3601; **BDCERT:** IM 78; Ge 81; **MS:** NYU Sch Med 73; **RES:** IM, Bellevue Hosp Ctr, New York, NY; **FEL:** Ge, Columbia Presbyterian Med Ctr, New York, NY

Bednarek, Karl (MD) Ge `PCP`
Beth Israel Med Ctr
305 1st Ave; New York, NY 10003; (212) 420-4434; **BDCERT:** Ge 93; **MS:** Mt Sinai Sch Med 82; **RES:** Beth Israel Med Ctr, New York, NY 83-86; **FEL:** Ge, Beth Israel Med Ctr, New York, NY 86-88; **HOSP:** Hosp For Joint Diseases; **HMO:** Oxford Blue Choice Blue Cross & Blue Shield Metlife Sanus +

🔾 🔾 👹 🛏 💲 ᴹᶜʳ ᵂᶜ ᴺᶠ¹ Immediately

Ben-Zvi, Jeffrey (MD)   Ge
Beth Israel Med Ctr

Jeffrey S BenZvi, MD, FACP, FACG, 911 Park Ave;
New York, NY 10021; (212) 772-8730; **BDCERT:**
IM 86; Ge 91; **MS:** Columbia P&S 83; **RES:** IM, St
Luke's Roosevelt Hosp Ctr, New York, NY 83-86;
FEL: Ge, St Luke's Roosevelt Hosp Ctr, New York,
NY 86-88; **FAP:** Asst Prof of Clin Med Columbia
P&S; **HOSP:** Beth Israel Med Ctr-Kings Hwy; *SI:
Hepatitis; Inflammatory Bowel Disease*; **HMO:** Oxford
Guardian Blue Choice Magnacare

LANG: Heb, Sp, Rus, Yd, Hun; 🅰 💳 🔲 🔲 🔲 🔲
🔲 🔲 2-4 Weeks 🔲 *VISA* 💳 🔲

Berenson, Murray (MD)   Ge   PCP
St Vincents Hosp & Med Ctr NY

Internal Medical Gastroecterology, 115 E 61st St Fl
14; New York, NY 10021; (212) 421-8340;
BDCERT: IM 69; **MS:** NYU Sch Med 61; **RES:** St
Vincents Hosp & Med Ctr NY, New York, NY 61-63;
FEL: Ge, Hosp of U Penn, Philadelphia, PA; **HMO:**
None

🔲 🔲 🔲 🔲 🔲 Immediately

Bodenheimer Jr, Henry (MD)   Ge
Mount Sinai Med Ctr

5 E 98th St; New York, NY 10029; (212) 241-
1424; **BDCERT:** IM 78; Ge 81; **MS:** Tufts U 75; **RES:**
Mount Sinai Med Ctr, New York, NY 75-78; **FEL:**
Liver Disease, Mount Sinai Med Ctr, New York, NY
78-79; Ge, Rhode Island Hosp, Providence, RI 79-
81; **FAP:** Prof Mt Sinai Sch Med; *SI: Hepatitis;
Transplantation*; **HMO:** Oxford Health Source PHS
Blue Cross & Blue Shield Blue Choice +

🔲 🔲 🔲 🔲 🔲 🔲 🔲 *VISA* 💳

Cantor, Michael C (MD)   Ge
NY Hosp-Cornell Med Ctr

310 E 72nd St GrFl; New York, NY 10021; (212)
472-3333; **BDCERT:** IM 85; Ge 89; **MS:** Columbia
P&S 82; **RES:** IM, NY Hosp-Cornell Med Ctr, New
York, NY 82-85; **FEL:** Ge, NY Hosp-Cornell Med Ctr,
New York, NY 86-88; **FAP:** Asst Clin Prof Med
Cornell U; *SI: Colon Cancer Detection; Hepatitis and
Liver Disease*; **HMO:** Metlife Oxford

🔲 🔲 🔲 🔲 A Few Days 🔲 *VISA* 💳

Chapman, Mark (MD)   Ge
Mount Sinai Med Ctr

12 E 86th St; New York, NY 10028; (212) 861-
2000; **BDCERT:** IM 68; Ge 70; **MS:** SUNY
Downstate 61; **RES:** IM, Mount Sinai Med Ctr, New
York, NY 61-62; Ge, Montefiore Med Ctr, Bronx,
NY 62-63; **FEL:** Mount Sinai Med Ctr, New York,
NY 63-64; **FAP:** Assoc Clin Prof Med Mt Sinai Sch
Med; *SI: Inflammatory Bowel Disease*

LANG: Sp, Yd; 🔲 🔲 🔲 2-4 Weeks 💳

Cohen, Larry (MD)   Ge
Mount Sinai Med Ctr

21 E 87th St; New York, NY 10128; (212) 996-
6633; **BDCERT:** IM 81; Ge 83; **MS:** Hahnemann U
78; **RES:** IM, Mount Sinai Med Ctr, New York, NY
78-79; **FEL:** Ge, Mount Sinai Med Ctr, New York,
NY 81-83; **FAP:** Asst Prof Mt Sinai Sch Med; *SI:
Swallowing Disorders; Gastroesophageal Reflux*; **HMO:**
Oxford

🔲 🔲 🔲 🔲 🔲 🔲 A Few Days 🔲 *VISA* 💳

Cohen, Seth (MD)   Ge
Beth Israel Med Ctr

60 East End Ave; New York, NY 10028; (212) 734-
8874; **BDCERT:** IM 89; Ge 91; **MS:** Columbia P&S
86; **RES:** IM, Mount Sinai Med Ctr, New York, NY
86-89; Ge, St Luke's Roosevelt Hosp Ctr, New York,
NY 89-91; **FEL:** Beth Israel Med Ctr, New York, NY
91-92; **FAP:** Asst Clin Prof Columbia P&S; **HMO:**
US Hlthcre Oxford CIGNA Magnacare Prudential +

Connor, Bradley A (MD)   Ge   PCP
NY Hosp-Cornell Med Ctr

Travel Health Svc, 50 E 69th St; New York, NY
10021; (212) 570-4000; **BDCERT:** IM 82; Ge 85;
MS: U Tex SW, Dallas 78; **RES:** IM, U Hosp-S TX
Med Ctr, San Antonio, TX 78-81; **FEL:** Ge, NY
Hosp-Cornell Med Ctr, New York, NY; **FAP:** Asst
Clin Prof Med Cornell U; **HOSP:** Beth Israel Med Ctr;
SI: Travel Medicine; Parasitology; **HMO:** Oxford
Guardian PHCS United Healthcare Empire Blue
Cross & Shield +

LANG: Sp, Rus; 🔲 🔲 🔲 🔲 🔲 Immediately 💳

188

Cooper, Robert (MD)　　　Ge
NY Hosp-Cornell Med Ctr
50 E 70th St; New York, NY 10021; (212) 717-4967; **BDCERT:** IM 83; Ge 85; **MS:** Cornell U 81; **RES:** IM, NY Hosp-Cornell Med Ctr, New York, NY 81-82; IM, NY Hosp-Cornell Med Ctr, New York, NY 82-84

♿ 📷 📺 **S** **Mcr** 4+ Weeks ▨

Dieterich, Douglas (MD)　　Ge　　PCP
New York University Med Ctr
Liberty Medical LLP, 345 E 37th St 300; New York, NY 10016; (212) 986-3330; **BDCERT:** Ge 87; **MS:** Yale U Sch Med 74; **RES:** New York University Med Ctr, New York, NY 78; Bellevue Hosp Ctr, New York, NY 81; **HOSP:** Bellevue Hosp Ctr; **SI:** *Hepatitis; AIDS;* **HMO:** Oxford Aetna Hlth Plan United Healthcare Independent Health Plan Blue Cross +

LANG: Sp; ♿ 📷 🚑 📺 **S** **Mcr** A Few Days ▨
VISA ●

Field, Steven (MD)　　　Ge
New York University Med Ctr
245 E 35th St; New York, NY 10016; (212) 686-9477; **BDCERT:** IM 80; Ge 83; **MS:** NYU Sch Med 77; **RES:** IM, Bellevue Hosp Ctr, New York, NY 77-81; **FEL:** Ge, Mount Sinai Med Ctr, New York, NY 81-83; **FAP:** Asst Prof of Clin NYU Sch Med; **SI:** *Inflammatory Bowel Disease;* **HMO:** Oxford CIGNA United Healthcare

♿ 📷 🚑 📺 **S** **Mcr** 1 Week

Foong, Anthony (MD)　　Ge
St Vincents Hosp & Med Ctr NY
210 Canal St 601; New York, NY 10013; (212) 693-2100; **BDCERT:** IM 84; Ge 87; **MS:** Tufts U 81; **RES:** U, U MD Hosp, Baltimore, MD 82-84; **FEL:** Ge, St Luke's Roosevelt Hosp Ctr, New York, NY 84-86; **SI:** *Gastrointestinal Endoscopy; Hemorrhoid Treatment;* **HMO:** Oxford GHI Blue Shield Aetna Hlth Plan Guardian +

♿ Ⓢ 📷 🚑 📺 **S** **Mcr** Immediately

Freiman, Hal (MD)　　　Ge
St Vincents Hosp & Med Ctr NY
59 W 12th St 1D; New York, NY 10011; (212) 206-0074; **BDCERT:** IM 81; Ge 83; **MS:** Albany Med Coll 78; **RES:** IM, St Vincents Hosp & Med Ctr NY, New York, NY 78-81; **FEL:** Ge, NY Med Coll, Valhalla, NY 81-83; **FAP:** Asst Clin Prof Med NY Med Coll; **SI:** *Ulcer disease; Colon Cancer Screening;* **HMO:** Oxford Blue Choice Prucare US Hlthcre Prucare +

♿ 📷 🚑 📺 **S** **Mcr** **Mcd** 2-4 Weeks

Friedlander, Charles (MD)　　Ge
New York University Med Ctr
Concorde Medical Group, 232 E 30th St; New York, NY 10016; (212) 889-5544; **BDCERT:** IM 74; Ge 77; **MS:** SUNY Downstate 68; **RES:** Bellevue Hosp Ctr, New York, NY 68-71; **FEL:** Ge, New York University Med Ctr, New York, NY 74-76; **SI:** *Colonoscopy;* **HMO:** Oxford

♿ 📷 🚑 📺 **S** **Mcr** A Few Days ▨ **VISA** ●

Friedman, Gerald (MD)　　　Ge
Mount Sinai Med Ctr
1751 York Ave; New York, NY 10128; (212) 860-6660; **BDCERT:** IM 65; Ge 71; **MS:** SUNY Buffalo 57; **RES:** Montefiore Med Ctr, Bronx, NY 58-59; Mount Sinai Med Ctr, New York, NY 59-60; **FEL:** Ge, Mount Sinai Med Ctr, New York, NY; **FAP:** Clin Prof Med Mt Sinai Sch Med; **HOSP:** Beth Israel North; **SI:** *Irritable Bowel Syndrome; Inflammatory Bowel Disease;* **HMO:** Oxford

LANG: Sp, Chi, Yd; ♿ 📷 🚑 📺 **S** **Mcr** 2-4 Weeks

Gerson, Charles (MD)　　　Ge
Mount Sinai Med Ctr
80 Central Park West; New York, NY 10023; (212) 496-6161; **BDCERT:** IM 70; Ge 72; **MS:** SUNY Downstate 62; **RES:** IM, Bellevue Hosp Ctr, New York, NY 62-64; IM, Mount Sinai Med Ctr, New York, NY 64-65; **FEL:** Ge, Bellevue Hosp Ctr, New York, NY 67-68; Ge, Mount Sinai Med Ctr, New York, NY 68-69; **FAP:** Assoc Clin Prof Mt Sinai Sch Med; **SI:** *Irritable Bowel Syndrome; Diarrheal Diseases;* **HMO:** Oxford Sel Pro PHCS Blue Choice Premier +

♿ 📷 🚑 📺 **S** **Mcr** A Few Days **VISA** ●

Goldberg, Myron (MD)   Ge
Lenox Hill Hosp

110 E 59th St Ste 10B; New York, NY 10022;
(212) 583-2900; **BDCERT:** IM 77; Ge 79; **MS:**
Albert Einstein Coll Med 71; **RES:** Montefiore Med
Ctr, Bronx, NY 72-73; Lenox Hill Hosp, New York,
NY 73-74; **FEL:** Ge, Columbia-Presbyterian Med
Ctr, New York, NY 76-77; Ge, Lenox Hill Hosp,
New York, NY 77-78; **FAP:** Assoc Clin Prof Med
NYU Sch Med; **SI:** *Inflammatory Bowel Disease;*
Endoscopy—Colonoscopy; **HMO:** Chubb Blue Choice
Blue Cross & Blue Shield CIGNA HealthNet +

LANG: Sp; 🔒 📷 👤 🏥 Mcr A Few Days *VISA* 💳

Goldin, Howard (MD)   Ge
NY Hosp-Cornell Med Ctr

646 Park Ave; New York, NY 10021; (212) 249-
0404; **BDCERT:** IM 68; Ge 73; **MS:** Cornell U 61;
RES: IM, NY Hosp-Cornell Med Ctr, New York, NY
62-64; **FEL:** Ge, NY Hosp-Cornell Med Ctr, New
York, NY 64-66; **FAP:** Clin Prof Cornell U; **HOSP:**
Rockefeller Univ Hosp; **SI:** *Inflammatory Bowel*
Disease; GI Endoscopy

🔒 📷 👤 🏥 💲 Immediately *VISA* 💳

Green, Peter (MD)   Ge
Columbia-Presbyterian Med Ctr

161 Fort Washington Ave; New York, NY 10032;
(212) 305-5590; **MS:** Australia 70; **RES:** North
Shore Hosp, Sidney, Australia 71-74; **FEL:** Ge,
North Shore Hosp, Sidney, Australia; Beth Israel
Med Ctr, Boston, MA; **FAP:** Assoc Prof of Clin Med
Columbia P&S; **SI:** *Celiac Disease; Endoscopy;* **HMO:**
Oxford PHS Blue Cross & Blue Shield

🔒 📷 👤 🏥 💲 Mcd 2-4 Weeks

Grendell, James H (MD)   Ge
NY Hosp-Cornell Med Ctr

525 E 68th St; New York, NY 10021; (212) 746-
4400; **BDCERT:** IM 78; Ger 81; **MS:** Ohio State U
75; **RES:** IM, Beth Israel Med Ctr, Boston, MA 75-
78; **FEL:** Ge, UC San Francisco Med Ctr, San
Francisco, CA 78-81; **FAP:** Prof Med Ohio U, Coll
Osteo Med; **SI:** *Diseases of the Pancreas; Liver Diseases;*
HMO: Oxford Empire Blue Cross & Shield Aetna
Hlth Plan Prudential PHS +

LANG: Sp, Rus; 🔒 📷 👤 🏥 💲 Mcr Mcd 2-4 Weeks
🔳 *VISA* 💳 💳

Hammerman, Hillel (MD)   Ge   PCP
Beth Israel North

178 East End Ave; New York, NY 10128; (212)
288-1030; **BDCERT:** IM 81; Ge 83; **MS:** Cornell U
78; **RES:** Baltimore City Hosp, Baltimore, MD; **FEL:**
Lahey Clinic, Burlington, MA 81-83; **SI:**
Inflammatory Bowel Disorder; **HMO:** Oxford PHCS
CIGNA United Healthcare Prucare +

🔒 📷 👤 🏥 💲 Mcr Immediately

Harary, Albert (MD)   Ge
Lenox Hill Hosp

654 Madison Ave 6th Fl; New York, NY 10021;
(212) 355-5222; **BDCERT:** IM 82; Ge 85; **MS:**
Columbia P&S 79; **RES:** U Miami Hosp, Miami, FL
79-82; **FEL:** U Miami Hosp, Miami, FL 82-84; **FAP:**
Asst Clin Prof NYU Sch Med; **HOSP:** St Luke's
Roosevelt Hosp Ctr; **HMO:** Oxford CIGNA

LANG: Sp, Fr; 🔒 👤 🏥 💲 Mcr A Few Days 💳
VISA 💳 💳

Holt, Peter (MD)   Ge
St Luke's Roosevelt Hosp Ctr

15 W 81st St Ste 15D; New York, NY 10024; (212)
523-3680; **BDCERT:** IM 66; **MS:** England 54; **RES:**
London Hosp, London, England 54-55; St Luke's
Roosevelt Hosp Ctr, New York, NY 57-59; **FEL:** Ge,
Mass Gen Hosp, Boston, MA 59-61; **FAP:** Prof Med
Columbia P&S; **SI:** *Chronic Diarrhea; Inflammatory*
Bowel Disease; **HMO:** Oxford PHS PHCS CIGNA
Chubb +

LANG: Ger, Fr; 📞 👤 🏥 💲 Mcr 1 Week

Horowitz, Lawrence (MD)   Ge
New York University Med Ctr

Tisch Hosp, 530 1st Ave; New York, NY 10016;
(212) 263-7236; **BDCERT:** IM 62; Ge 66; **MS:**
SUNY Downstate 55; **RES:** IM, Albert Einstein Med
Ctr, Bronx, NY 66-68; Ge, VA Med Ctr-Manh, New
York, NY 68-69; **FAP:** Clin Prof Med NYU Sch Med;
SI: *Esophageal Disorders; Irritable Bowel Syndrome*

🔒 SU 📷 👤 🏥 💲 Mcr A Few Days

Jacobson, Ira (MD)   Ge
NY Hosp-Cornell Med Ctr

50 E 69th St; New York, NY 10021; (212) 734-5200; **BDCERT:** IM 82; Ge 85; **MS:** Columbia P&S 79; **RES:** UC San Francisco Med Ctr, San Francisco, CA 79-82; **FEL:** Ge, Mass Gen Hosp, Boston, MA 82-84; Harvard Med Sch, Cambridge, MA; **FAP:** Assoc Clin Prof Med Cornell U; *SI: Hepatitis & Liver Diseases; Gastrointestinal Endoscopy*

♿ 🅿 🛏 💲 Ⓜ 2-4 Weeks

Janowitz, Henry (MD)   Ge
Mount Sinai Med Ctr

1075 Park Ave; New York, NY 10128; (212) 289-4962; **BDCERT:** IM 55; Ge 54; **MS:** Columbia P&S 39; **RES:** IM, Mount Sinai Med Ctr, New York, NY 46; Path, Mount Sinai Med Ctr, New York, NY 47; **FAP:** Clin Prof Mt Sinai Sch Med; *SI: Inflammatory Bowel Disease; Crohn's Disease*; **HMO:** Oxford Aetna Hlth Plan

LANG: Ger, Yd; ♿ 🅾 🅿 🛏 💲 Ⓜ A Few Days

Klion, Franklin (MD)   Ge
Mount Sinai Med Ctr

1060 5th Ave; New York, NY 10128; (212) 369-1515; **BDCERT:** IM 65; **MS:** NY Med Coll 58; **RES:** Med, Mount Sinai Med Ctr, New York, NY 62-64; **FEL:** Ge,; Hem,; **FAP:** Clin Prof Mt Sinai Sch Med; *SI: Hepatitis; Chronic Liver Disease*; **HMO:** Oxford

LANG: Itl; ♿ 🅾 🛏 💲 Ⓜ Immediately *VISA* ●

Knapp, Albert B (MD)   Ge
Lenox Hill Hosp

21 E 79th St; New York, NY 10021; (212) 737-3446; **BDCERT:** IM 82; Ge 87; **MS:** Columbia P&S 79; **RES:** IM, Albert Einstein Med Ctr, Bronx, NY 79-82; **FEL:** Ge, Brigham & Women's Hosp, Boston, MA 82-85; **FAP:** Asst Prof NYU Sch Med; **HOSP:** St Vincents Hosp & Med Ctr NY; *SI: Colonoscopy and Gastroscopy; Liver Disease*

LANG: Fr; ♿ 🅾 🅿 🛏 💲 A Few Days ▦

Korelitz, Burton I (MD)   Ge
Lenox Hill Hosp

45 E 85th St; New York, NY 10028; (212) 988-3800; **BDCERT:** IM 58; Ge 61; **MS:** Boston U 51; **RES:** Mount Sinai Med Ctr, New York, NY 51-52; Boston VA Med Ctr, Boston, MA 52-53; **FEL:** Beth Israel Med Ctr, Boston, MA 53-54; Mount Sinai Med Ctr, New York, NY 54-56; **FAP:** Clin Prof NYU Sch Med; *SI: Inflammatory Bowel Disease; Crohn's Disease*; **HMO:** None

LANG: Sp; ♿ 🅾 🛏 💲 Ⓜ A Few Days ▦ *VISA*

Kornbluth, Arthur Asher (MD) Ge
Mount Sinai Med Ctr

1751 York Ave; New York, NY 10128; (212) 369-2490; **BDCERT:** IM 89; Ge 91; **MS:** SUNY Hlth Sci Ctr 84; **RES:** IM, Albert Einstein Med Ctr, Bronx, NY 84-88; **FEL:** Ge, Mount Sinai Med Ctr, New York, NY; **FAP:** Assoc Clin Prof Mt Sinai Sch Med; *SI: Inflammatory Bowel Disease; Endoscopy*; **HMO:** Oxford Blue Cross United Healthcare PHCS Guardian +

LANG: Yd, Rus, Sp, Chi; ♿ 🅾 🅿 🛏 💲 Ⓜ Immediately *VISA* ●

Kotler, Donald P (MD)   Ge
St Luke's Roosevelt Hosp Ctr

G I Immunology, 421 W 113th St SR1301; New York, NY 10025; (212) 523-3670; **BDCERT:** IM 76; Ge 79; **MS:** Albert Einstein Coll Med 73; **RES:** IM, Jacobi Med Ctr, Bronx, NY 73-76; **FEL:** Ge, Hosp of U Penn, Philadelphia, PA 76-78; **FAP:** Prof Med Columbia P&S; *SI: HIV Infection; Malnutrition*; **HMO:** Oxford Blue Choice Multiplan GHI Chubb +

LANG: Sp; ♿ Ⓒ 🅾 🛏 Ⓜ Ⓜ 2-4 Weeks

Krumholz, Michael (MD)   Ge
Lenox Hill Hosp

111 E 80th St 1C; New York, NY 10021; (212) 734-5533; **BDCERT:** IM 83; **MS:** Mt Sinai Sch Med 80; **RES:** IM, Beth Israel, New York, NY 81-84; **FEL:** Ge, Lenox Hill, New York, NY 84-86

Guide to symbols and abbreviations can be found on pages 110-113.

191

Kummer, Bart (MD) Ge
NYU Downtown Hosp
19 Beekman St Fl 6; New York, NY 10038; (212) 406-7050; **BDCERT:** IM 82; Ge 85; **MS:** Cornell U 79; **RES:** IM, Harlem Hosp Ctr, New York, NY 79-82; **FEL:** Ge, St Luke's Roosevelt Hosp Ctr, New York, NY 83-85; **FAP:** Instr NYU Sch Med; **HOSP:** New York University Med Ctr; **SI:** *Cancer Prevention and Screening; Abdominal Pain Syndromes*; **HMO:** Empire Oxford Chubb Magnacare +

LANG: Fr, Sp; ⛊ ⛁ ⛫ ⛻ ⛿ Mcr WC NFI A Few Days 🎫 **VISA** 💳 🖋

Lambroza, Arnon (MD) Ge
NY Hosp-Cornell Med Ctr
950 Park Ave; New York, NY 10028; (212) 517-7570; **BDCERT:** IM 87; Ge 91; **MS:** Albert Einstein Coll Med 84; **RES:** IM, Hosp of U Penn, Philadelphia, PA 84-87; **FEL:** Ge, NY Hosp-Cornell Med Ctr, New York, NY 88-90; **FAP:** Asst Clin Prof Cornell U; **SI:** *Swallowing Disorders; Gastroesophageal Reflux*; **HMO:** Oxford United Healthcare

LANG: Sp; ⛊ ⛁ ⛫ ⛻ ⛿ Mcr A Few Days 🎫 **VISA** 💳

Lebwohl, Oscar (MD) Ge
Columbia-Presbyterian Med Ctr
161 Fort Washington Ave; New York, NY 10032; (212) 305-4037; **BDCERT:** IM 75; Ge 77; **MS:** Harvard Med Sch 72; **RES:** Mount Sinai Med Ctr, New York, NY 72-75; **FEL:** Columbia-Presbyterian Med Ctr, New York, NY 75-76; Mount Sinai Med Ctr, New York, NY 76-77; **FAP:** Assoc Clin Prof Med Columbia P&S; **SI:** *Colonoscopy and Gastroscopy; Inflammatory Bowel Disease*; **HMO:** Oxford Empire Blue Choice Physician's Health Plan Prudential

⛊ ⛁ ⛫ ⛻ ⛿ Mcr A Few Days

Lewis, Blair (MD) Ge
Mount Sinai Med Ctr
1067 5th Ave; New York, NY 10128; (212) 369-6600; **BDCERT:** IM 85; **MS:** Albert Einstein Coll Med 82; **RES:** IM, Montefiore Med Ctr, Bronx, NY 82-85; **FEL:** Ge, Mount Sinai Med Ctr, New York, NY 85-87; **FAP:** Assoc Clin Prof Mt Sinai Sch Med; **HOSP:** Beth Israel North; **SI:** *Colonoscopy and Endoscopy; Internal Bleeding*; **HMO:** US Hlthcre Oxford PHCS PHS

LANG: Sp; ⛊ ⛁ ⛫ ⛻ Mcr Immediately **VISA** 💳

Lichtiger, Simon (MD) Ge
Mount Sinai Med Ctr
1185 Park Ave; New York, NY 10128; (212) 831-4900; **BDCERT:** IM 83; **MS:** NYU Sch Med 79; **RES:** Albert Einstein Med Ctr, Bronx, NY 79-83; **FEL:** Ge, Mount Sinai Med Ctr, New York, NY 83-85; **FAP:** Assoc Prof Med Mt Sinai Sch Med; **SI:** *Inflammatory Bowel Disease*; **HMO:** Oxford PHCS

⛊ ⛁ ⛫ ⛻ ⛿ A Few Days

Lightdale, Charles (MD) Ge
Columbia-Presbyterian Med Ctr
161 Fort Washington Ave; New York, NY 10032; (212) 305-3423; **BDCERT:** IM 72; Ge 73; **MS:** Columbia P&S 66; **RES:** Yale-New Haven Hosp, New Haven, CT 66-68; NY Hosp-Cornell Med Ctr, New York, NY 68-69; **FEL:** Ge, NY Hosp-Cornell Med Ctr, New York, NY 71-73; Mem Sloan Kettering Cancer Ctr, New York, NY 71-73; **FAP:** Prof Columbia P&S; **SI:** *Endoscopic Ultrasonography; Barrett's Esophagus*; **HMO:** Oxford PHS Blue Choice Prudential 1199 +

LANG: Sp; ⛊ ⛁ ⛫ ⛻ ⛿ Mcr Immediately

Lindner, Arthur (MD) Ge
New York University Med Ctr
Nyu Medical Ctr, 530 1st Ave 4K; New York, NY 10016; (212) 263-7270; **BDCERT:** IM 77; **MS:** U Rochester 54; **RES:** IM, U Mich Med Ctr, Ann Arbor, MI 55-58; **FEL:** Ge, Mount Sinai Med Ctr, New York, NY 60-62; **FAP:** Assoc Lecturer Med NYU Sch Med; **HMO:** PHS Oxford Chubb Independent Health Plan United Healthcare +

Lombardo, Robert (MD) Ge PCP
Lenox Hill Hosp
70 E 77th St 1B; New York, NY 10021; (212) 861-0132; **BDCERT:** IM 74; Ge 75; **MS:** NY Med Coll 70; **RES:** IM, St Luke's Roosevelt Hosp Ctr, New York, NY 71-73; **FEL:** Ge, St Luke's Roosevelt Hosp Ctr, New York, NY 73-74; Ge, Mem Sloan Kettering Cancer Ctr, New York, NY; **FAP:** Adjct Clin Prof Columbia P&S; **HOSP:** St Luke's Roosevelt Hosp Ctr; **SI:** *Irritable Bowel Syndrome; Inflammatory Bowel Disease*; **HMO:** Oxford CIGNA Chubb Aetna Hlth Plan PHS +

⛊ ⛁ ⛫ ⛻ ⛿ Mcr A Few Days 🎫 **VISA** 💳

Lucak, Basil K (MD)   Ge
New York University Med Ctr
345 E 37th St 308; New York, NY 10016; (212) 867-2851; **BDCERT:** IM 77; Ge 81; **MS:** NYU Sch Med 74; **RES:** IM, NY Hosp-Cornell Med Ctr, New York, NY 74-76; IM, VA Med Ctr-Northport, Northport, NY 76-77; **FEL:** Ge, Bellevue Hosp Ctr, New York, NY 77-79; **FAP:** Asst Clin Prof NYU Sch Med; **HOSP:** VA Med Ctr-Manh; *SI: Nutritional Health; Stress & Intestinal Health;* **HMO:** Oxford

LANG: Czc; ♿ 🔲 💊 🛏 💲 Mcr 1 Week 🟦 **VISA** ⬤

Lustbader, Ian (MD)   Ge   **PCP**
New York University Med Ctr
245 E 35th St; New York, NY 10016; (212) 685-5252; **BDCERT:** IM 85; Ge 87; **MS:** Columbia P&S 82; **RES:** IM, St Luke's Roosevelt Hosp Ctr, New York, NY 82-85; **FEL:** Ge, Bellevue Hosp Ctr, New York, NY 85-87; **FAP:** Asst Clin Prof NYU Sch Med; *SI: Hepatitis and Hepatitis "C"; Inflammatory Bowel Disease;* **HMO:** Oxford GHI Blue Cross Aetna Hlth Plan United Healthcare +

LANG: Sp; 📞 🔲 💊 🛏 💲 Mcr A Few Days 🟦

Magun, Arthur (MD)   Ge
Columbia-Presbyterian Med Ctr
161 Fort Washington Ave; New York, NY 10032; (212) 305-5287; **BDCERT:** IM 81; Ge 83; **MS:** Mt Sinai Sch Med 77; **RES:** IM, Columbia-Presbyterian Med Ctr, New York, NY 77-80; **FEL:** Ge, Columbia-Presbyterian Med Ctr, New York, NY 80-83; **FAP:** Assoc Prof Columbia P&S; *SI: Hepatitis; Ulcerative Colitis;* **HMO:** Oxford

♿ 📞 💊 🛏 💲 Mcr A Few Days

Markowitz, David (MD)   Ge
Columbia-Presbyterian Med Ctr
161 Ft Washington Ave; New York, NY 10032; (212) 305-1024; **BDCERT:** IM 88; Ge 91; **MS:** Columbia P&S 85; **RES:** Columbia-Presbyterian Med Ctr, New York, NY 85-88; **FEL:** Ge, Columbia-Presbyterian Med Ctr, New York, NY 88-91; **FAP:** Asst Prof of Clin Med Columbia P&S; *SI: Esophageal Diseases; Endoscopy*

♿ 🔲 💊 🛏 💲

Meyers, Samuel (MD)   Ge
Mount Sinai Med Ctr
120 E 90th St; New York, NY 10128; (212) 534-7002; **BDCERT:** IM 74; Ge 75; **MS:** SUNY Hlth Sci Ctr 71; **RES:** Albert Einstein Med Ctr, Bronx, NY 71-73; **FEL:** Ge, Mount Sinai Med Ctr, New York, NY 73-75; **FAP:** Clin Prof Mt Sinai Sch Med; *SI: Inflammatory Bowel Disease*

♿ 🔲 💊 🛏 1 Week

Miskovitz, Paul (MD)   Ge
NY Hosp-Cornell Med Ctr
50 E 70th St; New York, NY 10021; (212) 717-4966; **BDCERT:** IM 78; Ge 81; **MS:** Cornell U 75; **RES:** NY Hosp-Cornell Med Ctr, New York, NY 75-78; **FEL:** Ge, NY Hosp-Cornell Med Ctr, New York, NY; **FAP:** Assoc Clin Prof Med Cornell U; *SI: Gastrointestinal/Endoscopy; Digestive & Liver Diseases;* **HMO:** Oxford

LANG: Sp; ♿ 🔲 🛏 💲 Mcr A Few Days 🟦

Nagler, Jerry (MD)   Ge
NY Hosp-Cornell Med Ctr
407 E 70th St Fl 5; New York, NY 10021; (212) 628-7777; **BDCERT:** IM 76; Ge 83; **MS:** Yale U Sch Med 73; **RES:** IM, Columbia-Presbyterian Med Ctr, New York, NY 73-76; **FEL:** Ge, NY Hosp-Cornell Med Ctr, New York, NY 76-78; **FAP:** Asst Clin Prof Med Cornell U; *SI: Inflammatory Bowel Disease; Colitis*

♿ 🔲 💊 🛏 💲 Mcr 2-4 Weeks

Ottaviano, Lawrence (MD)   Ge
Cabrini Med Ctr
Lower Manhattam Gastroenterology Grp, PC, 60 Gramercy Park North 1B; New York, NY 10010; (212) 242-2412; **BDCERT:** IM 88; Ge 93; **MS:** West Indies 84; **RES:** IM, Cabrini Med Ctr, New York, NY 84-87; **FEL:** Ge, Cabrini Med Ctr, New York, NY 87-89; **HOSP:** St Vincents Hosp & Med Ctr NY; *SI: Peptic Ulcer; Colitis;* **HMO:** Oxford Blue Cross & Blue Shield Anthem Health Centercare Aetna Hlth Plan +

LANG: Sp; ♿ 📞 🔲 💊 🛏 Mcr 1 Week

Guide to symbols and abbreviations can be found on pages 110-113.

193

Pochapin, Mark (MD)　　　Ge
NY Hosp-Cornell Med Ctr

435 E 70th St J314; New York, NY 10021; (212) 746-4014; **BDCERT:** IM 91; Ge 93; **MS:** Cornell U 88; **RES:** IM, NY Hospital, New York, NY 89-91; **FEL:** Ge, Montefiore/Albert Einstein Med Ctr, Bronx, NY 91-93; **HMO:** Blue Choice Aetna Hlth Plan Oxford Prudential

LANG: Sp; ♿ 🅿 👥 💲 Mcr Mcd WC NFI 🅰 **VISA** 💳 💳

Present, Daniel (MD)　　　Ge
Mount Sinai Med Ctr

12 E 86th St; New York, NY 10028; (212) 861-2000; **BDCERT:** IM 66; **MS:** SUNY Downstate 59; **RES:** IM, Mount Sinai Med Ctr, New York, NY 62-64; **FEL:** Ge, Mount Sinai Med Ctr, New York, NY 64-66; **FAP:** Clin Prof Med Mt Sinai Sch Med; *SI: Crohn's Disease; Ulcerative Colitis*

LANG: Sp; 📷 👥 💲　4+ Weeks 🅰 **VISA** 💳

Robilotti, James (MD)　　　Ge
St Vincents Hosp & Med Ctr NY

29 Washington Sq West 111; New York, NY 10011; (212) 475-4030; **BDCERT:** IM 72; **MS:** UMDNJ-NJ Med Sch, Newark 65; **RES:** St Vincents Hosp & Med Ctr NY, New York, NY 66-67; **FEL:** Ge, St Vincents Hosp & Med Ctr NY, New York, NY 68-69; Ge, St Vincents Hosp & Med Ctr NY, New York, NY 69-70; **FAP:** Asst Clin Prof NY Med Coll; *SI: Irritable Bowel; Peptic Ulcer*; **HMO:** CIGNA Oxford Blue Shield 1199 +

♿ 📞 👥 💲 Mcr Mcd

Romeu, Jose (MD)　　　Ge
Mount Sinai Med Ctr

1107 5th Ave; New York, NY 10128; (212) 534-6747; **BDCERT:** IM 73; Ge 75; **MS:** NYU Sch Med 70; **RES:** IM, Mount Sinai Med Ctr, New York, NY 70-73; **FEL:** Ge, Mount Sinai Med Ctr, New York, NY 73-75; **FAP:** Asst Prof Mt Sinai Sch Med; **HOSP:** Lenox Hill Hosp; *SI: Therapeutic Endoscopy ERCP; Colon-Liver-Pancreas Cancer*; **HMO:** Guardian Independent Health Plan Oxford 32BJ +

LANG: Sp, Prt, Fr, Itl, Crt; ♿ 📷 🅿 👥 Mcr Immediately 🅰 **VISA** 💳 💳

Rubin, Moshe (MD)　　　Ge
Columbia-Presbyterian Med Ctr

16 E 60th St; New York, NY 10022; (212) 326-5538; **BDCERT:** IM 86; Ge 88; **MS:** Yale U Sch Med 83; **RES:** NY Hosp-Cornell Med Ctr, New York, NY 83-86; **FEL:** Columbia-Presbyterian Med Ctr, New York, NY 86-88; **FAP:** Assoc Clin Prof Columbia P&S; *SI: Endoscopy; Colonoscopy*; **HMO:** Oxford Blue Cross & Blue Shield PHCS

♿ 🅿 👥 💲 Mcr

Rubin, Peter (MD)　　　Ge
Mount Sinai Med Ctr

12 E 86th St; New York, NY 10028; (212) 861-1829; **BDCERT:** IM 73; **MS:** U Rochester 70; **RES:** Mount Sinai Med Ctr, New York, NY 70-73; **FEL:** Mount Sinai Med Ctr, New York, NY 73-75; *SI: GI Endoscopy; Colitis and Crohn's*; **HMO:** Oxford

LANG: Sp, Rus; ♿ 📷 🅿 👥 💲 Mcr　A Few Days 🅰 **VISA** 💳

Ruoff, Michael (MD)　　　Ge
New York University Med Ctr

NYU Medical Ctr, 530 1st Ave 7F; New York, NY 10016; (212) 263-7275; **BDCERT:** IM 69; Ge 72; **MS:** NYU Sch Med 63; **RES:** Ge, New York University Med Ctr, New York, NY 66-67; Med, Bellevue Hosp Ctr, New York, NY 64-66; **FAP:** Clin Prof Med NYU Sch Med; **HMO:** Independent Health Plan

Sachar, David (MD)　　　Ge
Mount Sinai Med Ctr

Gastroenterology Consultants, 5 E 98th St Fl11; New York, NY 10029; (212) 241-4299; **BDCERT:** Ge 72; IM 69; **MS:** Harvard Med Sch 63; **RES:** Beth Israel Med Ctr, Boston, MA 63-65; **FEL:** Ge, Mount Sinai Med Ctr, New York, NY 68-70; **FAP:** Prof Med Mt Sinai Sch Med; *SI: Crohn's Disease; Ulcerative Colitis*

LANG: Sp; ♿ 📷 👥 💲 Mcr Mcd　4+ Weeks 🅰 **VISA** 💳

Salik, James (MD)   Ge
New York University Med Ctr

232 E 30th St; New York, NY 10016; (212) 889-5544; **BDCERT:** IM 83; Ge 85; **MS:** NYU Sch Med 80; **RES:** IM, Bellevue Hosp Ctr, New York, NY 80-83; **FEL:** Ge, Bellevue Hosp Ctr, New York, NY 83-85; **FAP:** Asst Prof NYU Sch Med; **HOSP:** Beth Israel North; *SI: Diseases of the Esophagus,; Stomach, Liver, and Colon;* **HMO:** Aetna Hlth Plan United Healthcare Oxford

LANG: Sp, Chi, Rom, Grk; ♿ 📞 📷 🧑 🏧 💲 Mcr A Few Days ▦ *VISA* ⬤

Schmerin, Michael (MD)   Ge
NY Hosp-Cornell Med Ctr

1060 Park Ave 1G; New York, NY 10128; (212) 348-3166; **BDCERT:** IM 76; Ge 77; **MS:** Jefferson Med Coll 73; **RES:** NY Hosp-Cornell Med Ctr, New York, NY 73-75; **FEL:** Ge, NY Hosp-Cornell Med Ctr, New York, NY 75-77; **HOSP:** Lenox Hill Hosp; *SI: Colonoscopy; Gastroscopy*

📷 🧑 🏧 💲 1 Week

Schneider, Lewis (MD)   Ge
Columbia-Presbyterian Med Ctr

16 E 60th St 322; New York, NY 10022; (212) 326-8426; **BDCERT:** IM 81; **MS:** SUNY Downstate 78; **RES:** IM, Columbia-Presbyterian Med Ctr, New York, NY 78-81; **FEL:** Ge, Columbia-Presbyterian Med Ctr, New York, NY 81-83; **FAP:** Asst Prof Med Columbia P&S; *SI: Colon Cancer Screening; Colon Polyps Colitis;* **HMO:** Oxford Blue Cross & Blue Shield

♿ 📷 🧑 🏧 Mcr A Few Days

Shike, Moshe (MD)   Ge
Mem Sloan Kettering Cancer Ctr

1275 York Ave; New York, NY 10021; (212) 639-7230; **BDCERT:** IM 77; Ge 81; **MS:** Israel 75; **RES:** IM, Mt Auburn Hosp, Cambridge, MA 75-76
LANG: Heb, Fr;

Shinya, Hiromi (MD)   Ge
Beth Israel Med Ctr

305 E 55th St 102; New York, NY 10022; (212) 751-9714; **MS:** Japan 61; **RES:** S, Beth Israel Med Ctr, New York, NY 63-68; **FEL:** S, Beth Israel Med Ctr, New York, NY 68-70; **FAP:** Clin Prof S Albert Einstein Coll Med; *SI: GI Endoscopy; Nutritional Counseling;* **HMO:** 1199 Oxford

LANG: Jpn, Chi, Sp; 📷 🧑 🏧 💲 Mcr Immediately *VISA* ⬤

Siegel, Jerome H (MD)   Ge
Beth Israel Med Ctr

60 E End Ave; New York, NY 10028; (212) 734-8874; **BDCERT:** Ge 78; **MS:** Med Coll Ga 60; **RES:** VA Med Ctr-Bronx, Bronx, NY 63-65; Ge, VA Med Ctr-Bronx, Bronx, NY 65-66; **FEL:** Ge & Liver Disease, Royal Free Hosp, London, England 74-75; **HOSP:** Beth Israel North; **HMO:** Oxford Metlife CIGNA Aetna Hlth Plan Metlife +

LANG: Sp, Fr; ♿ 📷 🧑 🏧 💲 Mcr NFl Immediately ▦ *VISA* ⬤

Stein, Jeffrey Alan (MD)   Ge   PCP
Columbia-Presbyterian Med Ctr

161 Ft Washington Ave; New York, NY 10032; (212) 305-5444; **BDCERT:** IM 71; Ge 73; **MS:** Harvard Med Sch 65; **RES:** Columbia-Presbyterian Med Ctr, New York, NY 66-67; **FEL:** Ge, Columbia-Presbyterian Med Ctr, New York, NY 70-71; **FAP:** Clin Prof Columbia P&S; *SI: Gallbladder Disease; Ulcer Disease;* **HMO:** Oxford CIGNA Aetna Hlth Plan

♿ 📷 🏧 💲 Mcr A Few Days

Steinberg, Herman (MD)   Ge
NY Hosp-Cornell Med Ctr

646 Park Ave; New York, NY 10021; (212) 249-0404; **BDCERT:** IM 54; **MS:** Albany Med Coll 45; **RES:** Med, Queens Hosp Ctr, Jamaica, NY 48-51; Ge, Lenox Hill Hosp, New York, NY 51-52; **FEL:** Ge, NY Hosp-Cornell Med Ctr, New York, NY 52-53; Ge, Bellevue Hosp Ctr, New York, NY 53-55; **FAP:** Med Cornell U; *SI: Inflammatory Bowel Disease; Abdominal Pain*

📷 🧑 🏧 💲 Mcr A Few Days

Guide to symbols and abbreviations can be found on pages 110-113.

195

Tobias, Hillel (MD)   Ge
New York University Med Ctr

Concorde Medical Group, 232 E 30th St; New York,
NY 10016; (212) 889-5544; **BDCERT:** IM 67; Ge
79; **MS:** Washington U, St Louis 60; **RES:** IM,
Bellevue Hosp Ctr, New York, NY 60-63; **FEL:** Ge,
Royal Free Hosp, London, England 63-65; Mount
Sinai Med Ctr, New York, NY 65-67; **FAP:** Assoc
Prof NYU Sch Med; **HOSP:** Beth Israel North; *SI:*
Liver Diseases; Hepatitis; **HMO:** Oxford Guardian
Aetna Hlth Plan Blue Choice Chubb +

⬧ 🅰 🆀 🎬 🆂 🔢 A Few Days 💳 **VISA** ⬤

Warner, Richard (MD)   Ge
Mount Sinai Med Ctr

1751 York Ave; New York, NY 10128; (212) 722-
2100; **BDCERT:** IM 59; Ge 69; **MS:** U Cincinnati
51; **RES:** Med, Mount Sinai Med Ctr, New York, NY
51-54; Med, VA Med Ctr-Bronx, Bronx, NY 52-53;
FEL: Ge, Mount Sinai Med Ctr, New York, NY 57-
58; **FAP:** Assoc Clin Prof Mt Sinai Sch Med; **HOSP:**
Beth Israel North; *SI: Neuroendocrine Carcinoids;*
Tumors; **HMO:** None

LANG: Swd; ⬧ 🅰 🎬 🆂 🔢 2-4 Weeks **VISA** ⬤

Waye, Jerome (MD)   Ge
Mount Sinai Med Ctr

650 Park Ave Fl 1; New York, NY 10021; (212)
439-7779; **BDCERT:** IM 65; Ge 70; **MS:** Boston U
58; **RES:** IM, Mount Sinai Med Ctr, New York, NY
58-62; **FEL:** Ge, Mount Sinai Med Ctr, New York,
NY 58-62; **FAP:** Clin Prof Mt Sinai Sch Med;
HOSP: Lenox Hill Hosp; *SI: Colon Cancer;*
Colonoscopy; **HMO:** None

🅰 🎬 🆂 🔢 2-4 Weeks **VISA** ⬤

Weiss, Robert (MD)   Ge
Beth Israel Med Ctr

2 W 86th St 4; New York, NY 10024; (212) 769-
1700; **BDCERT:** IM 87; Ge 89; **MS:** Mt Sinai Sch
Med 83; **RES:** IM, Beth Israel Med Ctr, New York,
NY 83-86; **FEL:** Ge, Mount Sinai Med Ctr, New
York, NY 86-88; Ge, City Hosp, New York, NY;
FAP: Clin Instr Albert Einstein Coll Med; *SI: Peptic*
Ulcer Disease; Colon Cancer Prevention; **HMO:** CIGNA
PHS Oxford GHI

LANG: Heb, Sp; ⬧ 🅰 🆀 🎬 🆂 🔢 A Few Days

Werther, J Lawrence (MD)   Ge
Mount Sinai Med Ctr

1060 5th Ave Str Lvl; New York, NY 10128; (212)
369-1515; **BDCERT:** IM 60; Ge 66; **MS:** Columbia
P&S 51; **RES:** IM, Mount Sinai Med Ctr, New York,
NY 51-52; Path, Mount Sinai Med Ctr, New York,
NY 52-53; **FEL:** Ge, Mount Sinai Med Ctr, New
York, NY 56-57; **HMO:** Oxford

⬧ 🅰 🆀 🎬 🆂 🔢 A Few Days 💳 **VISA** ⬤

Winawer, Sidney G (MD)   Ge
Mem Sloan Kettering Cancer Ctr

1275 York Ave; New York, NY 10021; (212) 639-
7675; **BDCERT:** IM 65; **MS:** SUNY Hlth Sci Ctr 56;
RES: VA Med Ctr-Manh, New York, NY 59-61;
Maimonides Med Ctr, Brooklyn, NY 61-62; **FEL:** Ge,
Boston Med Ctr, Boston, MA 62-64; **FAP:** Prof Med
Cornell U

⬧ 🆀 🎬 🔢 4+ Weeks 💳 **VISA** ⬤ 💳

Zakim, David (MD)   Ge
NY Hosp-Cornell Med Ctr

525 E 68th St; New York, NY 10021; (212) 746-
4419; **BDCERT:** IM 68; **MS:** SUNY Hlth Sci Ctr 61;
RES: NY Hosp-Cornell Med Ctr, New York, NY 62-
63; **FEL:** NY Hosp-Cornell Med Ctr, New York, NY
64-65; **FAP:** Prof Med Cornell U; *SI: Liver Disease*

⬧ 🅰 🎬 🆂 🔢 🆆🅲 🅽🅵🅸 A Few Days 💳 **VISA** ⬤

GERIATRIC MEDICINE

Adelman, Ronald (MD)   Ger
NY Hosp-Cornell Med Ctr

NY Hosp-Cornell Med Ctr, 525 E 68th St Bx 46;
New York, NY 10021; (212) 746-1677; **BDCERT:**
Ger 82; **MS:** Albert Einstein Coll Med 78; **RES:**
Montefiore Med Ctr, Bronx, NY 78-81; **FAP:** Dir Ger
Cornell U; *SI: Communications between Doctors and*
Patients; **HMO:** Aetna Hlth Plan Cost Care Blue
Choice Oxford

⬧ 🆂 🔢 🔢 2-4 Weeks 💳 **VISA** ⬤ 💳

Ahronheim, Judith (MD) Ger PCP
St Vincents Hosp & Med Ctr NY

Medical Associates of St Vincents, 32 W 18th St 3rd
Fl; New York, NY 10011; (212) 647-6400;
BDCERT: IM 79; Ger 88; **MS:** Univ IL Coll Med 76;
RES: IM, Univ Hosp SUNY Bklyn, Brooklyn, NY 76-
79; **FEL:** Ger, Long Island Jewish Med Ctr, New
Hyde Park, NY 79-80; **SI:** *Alzheimer's Disease;*
Geriatric Medication

⬧ ⬧ ⬧ ⬧ ⬧ 2-4 Weeks

Bloom, Patricia (MD) Ger PCP
St Luke's Roosevelt Hosp Ctr

University Medical Practice Associates, 1090
Amsterdam Ave; New York, NY 10025; (212) 523-
5727; **BDCERT:** IM 78; Ger 88; **MS:** U Minn 75;
RES: IM, Montefiore Med Ctr, Bronx, NY 75-78;
FAP: Assoc Clin Prof Med Columbia P&S; **SI:**
Dementia; Geriatric Assessment; **HMO:** Oxford
Empire Blue Cross & Shield CIGNA Aetna-US
Healthcare PHS +

LANG: Sp; ⬧ ⬧ ⬧ ⬧ ⬧ ⬧ 2-4 Weeks *VISA*
⬧ ⬧

Cassel, Christine (MD) Ger
Mount Sinai Med Ctr

Dept of Geriatrics & Adult Develop/ Mt Sinai Med
Ctr, 1 Gustave Levy Pl; New York, NY 10029;
(212) 241-4840; **BDCERT:** IM 79; **MS:** U Md Sch
Med 76; **RES:** IM, Children's Hosp Med Ctr, San
Francisco, CA 77-79; UC San Francisco Med Ctr,
San Francisco, CA 78-79; **FEL:** Ger, Portland VA
Hospital, Portland, OR 79-81

Finkelstein, Martin Samuel (MD) Ger
PCP
New York University Med Ctr

NYU Medical Ctr, 530 1st Ave 4J; New York, NY
10016; (212) 263-7043; **BDCERT:** IM 70; Ge 88;
MS: NYU Sch Med 64; **RES:** IM, Bellevue Hosp Ctr,
New York, NY 64-66; Stamford U Med Ctr,
Stamford, CT 66-67; **FEL:** Inf, Stamford U Med Ctr,
Stamford, CT 67-68; **HMO:** Oxford United
Healthcare Prucare

⬧ ⬧ ⬧ ⬧ ⬧ ⬧ 1 Week

Freedman, Michael L (MD) Ger
New York University Med Ctr

550 1st Ave 4J; New York, NY 10016; (212) 263-
7043; **BDCERT:** IM 71; Ger 88; **MS:** Tufts U 63;
RES: IM, Bellevue Hosp Ctr, New York, NY 64-65;
Bellevue Hosp Ctr, New York, NY 68-69; **FEL:** Nat
Inst Health, Bethesda, MD 65-68; **FAP:** Prof NYU
Sch Med; **SI:** *Geriatrics; Alzheimer's Disease*

Kellogg, F Russell (MD) Ger PCP
St Vincents Hosp & Med Ctr NY

36 7th Ave Ste 414; New York, NY 10011; (212)
691-6633; **BDCERT:** IM 78; Ger 97; **MS:** NY Med
Coll 74; **RES:** St Vincents Hosp & Med Ctr NY, New
York, NY 74-77; **SI:** *Preventive Health Care; Diabetes;*
HMO: Oxford Blue Choice

⬧ ⬧ ⬧ ⬧ ⬧ ⬧ A Few Days

Lachs, Mark (MD) Ger
NY Hosp-Cornell Med Ctr

NY Hosp Cornell Med Ctr, 525 E 68th St Box 46;
New York, NY 10021; (212) 746-1677; **BDCERT:**
IM 88; Ger 92; **MS:** NYU Sch Med 85; **RES:** Hosp of
U Penn, Philadelphia, PA 85-88; **FEL:** Ger, RWJ
Univ Hosp-New Brunswick, New Brunswick, NJ;
Yale-New Haven Hosp, New Haven, CT; **FAP:** Assoc
Prof Med Cornell U

⬧ ⬧ ⬧ ⬧ 2-4 Weeks

Leipzig, Rosanne (MD) Ger
Mount Sinai Med Ctr

Mt Sinai Medical Hospital, 1 Gustave Levy Pl; New
York, NY 10029; (212) 241-4274; **BDCERT:** IM
82; Ger 88; **MS:** U Mich Med Sch 78; **RES:** IM,
Strong Mem Hosp, Rochester, NY 79-82; **FEL:**
Pharmacology, NY Hosp-Cornell Med Ctr, New
York, NY 83-85; **FAP:** Assoc Prof Mt Sinai Sch Med

⬧ ⬧ ⬧ ⬧ ⬧ ⬧ 4+ Weeks

Libow, Leslie (MD) Ger **PCP**
Mount Sinai Med Ctr

Mt Sinai Hosp, PO Box 1070; New York, NY
10029; (212) 824-7646; **BDCERT:** IM 65; Ger 88;
MS: U Hlth Sci/Chicago Med Sch 58; **RES:** Mount
Sinai Med Ctr, New York, NY 58-59; Bronx VA
Hospital, Bronx, NY 59-60; **FEL:** Mount Sinai Med
Ctr, New York, NY 63-64; **FAP:** Prof Ger Mt Sinai
Sch Med; **SI:** *Diagnostic & Management Problems;
Quality of Life Problems*

🚹 🔒 🐍 🛏 Mcr Mcd 2-4 Weeks

Meier, Diane (MD) Ger
Mount Sinai Med Ctr

5 E 98th St 5th Flr; New York, NY 10029; (212)
241-8258; **BDCERT:** IM 81; Ger 88; **MS:**
Northwestern U 77; **RES:** IM, Oregon Health Sci U
Hosp, Portland, OR 81; **FEL:** Ger, VA Med Ctr,
Portland, OR 83; **HMO:** Premier Blue Cross & Blue
Shield CIGNA US Hlthcre

🔒 🐍 🛏 💲 Mcr Mcd A Few Days

Paris Cammer, Barbara (MD) Ger **PCP**
Mount Sinai Med Ctr

Mount Sinai Hospital, One Gustave Levy Pl Box
1070; New York, NY 10029; (212) 824-7646;
BDCERT: IM 82; Ger 88; **MS:** SUNY Downstate 77;
RES: IM, St Vincents Hosp & Med Ctr NY, New
York, NY 78-80; **FEL:** Ger, Mount Sinai Med Ctr,
New York, NY 83-86; **FAP:** Asst Clin Prof Ger Mt
Sinai Sch Med; **HMO:** US Hlthcre Oxford Prudential
LANG: Heb; 🚹 🔒 🐍 🛏 Mcr Mcd 2-4 Weeks

Sherman, Fredrick (MD) Ger **PCP**
Mount Sinai Med Ctr

1470 Madison Ave; New York, NY 10029; (212)
824-7646; **BDCERT:** IM 75; Ger 88; **MS:** Temple U
72; **RES:** Hosp Med College of PA, Philadelphia, PA
75; **FAP:** Assoc Clin Prof Ger Mt Sinai Sch Med; **SI:**
Alzheimer's Disease; Falls in the elderly; **HMO:** Oxford
Prudential US Hlthcre Multiplan

🚹 🔒 🐍 🛏 Mcr Mcd A Few Days

GERIATRIC
PSYCHIATRY

Butler, Robert (MD) GerPsy
Mount Sinai Med Ctr

12165 5th Ave Suite 552; New York, NY 10029;
(212) 241-4633; **BDCERT:** Psyc 61; **MS:** Columbia
P&S 53; **RES:** Psyc, Nat Inst Mental Health,
Bethesda, MD 59-60; **FEL:** Psyc, Chestnut Lodge
Hosp, Rockville, ME 58-59

🚹 🔒 Mcr Immediately

Reisberg, Barry (MD) GerPsy
New York University Med Ctr

550 1st Ave THN314; New York, NY 10016; (212)
889-7579; **BDCERT:** Psyc 76; 91; **MS:** NY Med Coll
72; **RES:** Psyc, Metropolitan Hosp Ctr, New York,
NY 72-75; **FEL:** Behavior Therapy, U London,
London, England 75; **HOSP:** Bellevue Hosp Ctr; **SI:**
Alzheimer's Disease; Memory Problems

🚹 🅂🅄 🌙 🔒 🐍 🛏 💲 Mcr 2-4 Weeks

Serby, Michael J (MD) GerPsy
Mount Sinai Med Ctr

1 Gustave Levy Pl Bx 1230; New York, NY 10029;
(212) 241-3737; **BDCERT:** Psyc 79; Ger 91; **MS:**
Emory U Sch Med 69; **RES:** Psyc, Bellevue Hosp Ctr,
New York, NY 73-76; **SI:** *Alzheimer's Disease;
Psychopharmacology*

🚹 🌙 🔒 🐍 🛏 💲 1 Week

GYNECOLOGIC
ONCOLOGY

Barakat, Richard (MD) GO
Mem Sloan Kettering Cancer Ctr

1275 York Ave Rm C1091; New York, NY 10021;
(212) 639-2453; **BDCERT:** ObG 92; **MS:** SUNY
Hlth Sci Ctr 85; **RES:** Bellevue Hosp Ctr, New York,
NY 85-89; **FEL:** GO, Mem Sloan Kettering Cancer
Ctr, New York, NY 89; **HOSP:** NY Hosp-Cornell
Med Ctr; **SI:** *Uterine Cancer; Ovarian Cancer*

🚹 🔒 🐍 🛏 💲 Mcr Mcd Immediately **VISA** 💳
💳

Barber, Hugh (MD)　　　GO
Lenox Hill Hosp

122 E 76th St 1C; New York, NY 10021; (212)
734-6555; **BDCERT:** ObG 56; **MS:** Columbia P&S
44; **RES:** Lenox Hill Hosp, New York, NY 48-51; S,
Mem Sloan Kettering Cancer Ctr, New York, NY
52-54; **FAP:** Clin Prof ObG Cornell U; **SI:**
Mastectomy; Tumors; **HMO:** None

⬥ 🔲 🏠 💲 Ⓜ　Immediately

Birnbaum, Stanley (MD)　　　GO
NY Hosp-Cornell Med Ctr

449 E E 68th St 8; New York, NY 10021; (212)
628-1500; **BDCERT:** ObG 60; **MS:** Cornell U 51;
RES: NY Hosp-Cornell Med Ctr, New York, NY 52-
56; **FAP:** Prof ObG Cornell U; **SI:** *Vaginal Repair
Surgery; Minimally Invasive Surgery*

LANG: Fr; ⬥ 🔲 🏠 🏠 💲 Ⓜ　A Few Days ▦
VISA ⬤

Caputo, Thomas A (MD)　　　GO
NY Hosp-Cornell Med Ctr

525 E 68th St; New York, NY 10021; (212) 746-
3179; **BDCERT:** ObG 71; **MS:** UMDNJ-NJ Med Sch,
Newark 65; **RES:** Martland Hosp, Newark, NJ 65-
69; **FEL:** GO, Emory U Hosp, Atlanta, GA 72-74;
HMO: Oxford Blue Cross & Blue Shield CIGNA PHS
United Healthcare +

⬥ 🔲 🏠 Ⓜ Ⓜ　A Few Days ▦ ***VISA*** ⬤

Cohen, Carmel (MD)　　　GO
Mount Sinai Med Ctr

1 Gustave Levy Pl; New York, NY 10029; (212)
427-9898; **BDCERT:** ObG 67; **MS:** Tulane U 58;
RES: ObG, Mount Sinai Med Ctr, New York, NY 59-
65; **FEL:** GO, Mount Sinai Med Ctr, New York, NY;
HMO: Aetna Hlth Plan Oxford

⬥ 🔲 🏠 🏠 💲 Ⓜ Ⓜ　A Few Days ▦ ***VISA*** ⬤

Curtin, John P (MD)　　　GO
Mem Sloan Kettering Cancer Ctr

1275 York Ave; New York, NY 10021; (212) 639-
2493; **BDCERT:** 96; **MS:** Creighton U 79; **RES:** ObG,
U MN Med Ctr, Minneapolis, MN 79-84; **FEL:** GO,
Mem Sloan Kettering Cancer Ctr, New York, NY;
FAP: Assoc Prof Cornell U; **SI:** *Ovarian Cancer;
Cervical Cancer*

⬥ 🔲 🏠 🏠 Ⓜ Ⓜ　1 Week ▦ ***VISA*** ⬤

Dottino, Peter (MD)　　　GO　🄿🄲🄿
Mount Sinai Med Ctr

Group for Women, 800A 5th Ave Ste 405; New
York, NY 10021; (212) 888-8439; **BDCERT:** ObG
86; GO 87; **MS:** Georgetown U 79; **RES:** SUNY
Downstate, Brooklyn, NY; **FEL:** GO, Mount Sinai
Med Ctr, New York, NY; **HOSP:** Hackensack Univ
Med Ctr; **SI:** *Laparoscopic Gynecologic Surgery*

⬥ 🌙 🏠 🏠 Ⓜ　2-4 Weeks ▦ ***VISA*** ⬤ 🖅

Economos, Katherine (MD)　GO
NY Hosp-Cornell Med Ctr

Cornell Medical College Division of Gynecologic
Oncology, 525 E 68th St J130; New York, NY
10021; (212) 746-3198; **BDCERT:** GO 98; ObG 96;
MS: SUNY Downstate 86; **RES:** ObG, Maimonides
Med Ctr, Brooklyn, NY 86-90; **FEL:** GO, U Texas SW
Med Ctr, Dallas, TX 90-93; **FAP:** Asst Prof Cornell
U; **HOSP:** New York Methodist Hosp; **SI:** *Gynecologic
Cancer*; **HMO:** Oxford US Hlthcre Magnacare Blue
Choice +

LANG: Grk, Heb; ⬥ 🔲 🏠 💲 Ⓜ　1 Week ▦ ***VISA***
⬤ 🖅

Hirsch, Lissa (MD)　　　GO　🄿🄲🄿
Lenox Hill Hosp

755 Park Ave; New York, NY 10021; (212) 570-
2222; **BDCERT:** ObG 86; **MS:** UMDNJ-NJ Med Sch,
Newark 79; **RES:** New York University Med Ctr,
New York, NY 79-83

🔲 🏠 🏠 💲 Ⓜ　Immediately ***VISA*** ⬤

Hoskins, William (MD)　　GO
Mem Sloan Kettering Cancer Ctr

PO Box 226, 1275 York Ave; New York, NY
10021; (212) 639-7766; **BDCERT:** ObG 73; GO 79;
MS: U Tenn Ctr Hlth Sci, Memphis 65; **RES:** Naval
Med Ctr, Oakland, CA 71; **FEL:** GO, U Miami Hosp,
Miami, FL 76; **FAP:** Prof ObG Cornell U; **SI:** *Ovarian
Cancer; Gynecological Cancers*; **HMO:** Blue Cross &
Blue Shield

⬥ 🔲 🏠 Ⓜ Ⓜ　1 Week ▦ ***VISA*** ⬤ 🖅

Guide to symbols and abbreviations can be found on pages 110-113.

199

Killackey, Maureen (MD)   GO
St Luke's Roosevelt Hosp Ctr

425 W 59th St; New York, NY 10019; (212) 582-3723; **BDCERT:** ObG 85; GO 87; **MS:** Cornell U 78; **RES:** ObG, NY Hosp-Cornell Med Ctr, New York, NY 79-82; **FEL:** GO, Mem Sloan Kettering Cancer Ctr, New York, NY 82-84; **FAP:** Assoc Lecturer Columbia P&S; **SI:** *Gynecologic Cancers; Colposcopy;* **HMO:** Aetna Hlth Plan Oxford CIGNA PHS Prucare +

LANG: Sp; 🔲 🔲 🔲 🔲 🔲 A Few Days ▨ **VISA**

Liu, Paul (MD)   GO
Beth Israel Med Ctr

Dept of OB/GYN, 1st Ave & 16th St 8 Baird; New York, NY 10003; (212) 420-4236; **BDCERT:** ObG 97; **MS:** U Chicago-Pritzker Sch Med 90; **RES:** ObG, Columbia-Presbyterian Med Ctr, New York, NY 90-91; ObG, Columbia-Presbyterian Med Ctr, New York, NY 91-94; **FEL:** GO, Hosp of U Penn, Philadelphia, PA 94-96; **FAP:** Asst Clin Prof; **HOSP:** Englewood Hosp & Med Ctr; **SI:** *Genetic Based Cancer; Ovarian—Endometrial;* **HMO:** PHS HIP Network Empire Oxford Prudential +

LANG: Prt, Chi, Sp; 🔲 🔲 🔲 🔲 🔲 🔲 🔲 A Few Days

Smith, Daniel (MD)   GO
Columbia-Presbyterian Med Ctr

161 Fort Washington Ave; New York, NY 10032; (212) 305-3410; **BDCERT:** ObG 82; GO 83; **MS:** Harvard Med Sch 72; **RES:** S, Mass Gen Hosp, Boston, MA 78-79; ObG, Los Angeles Cty Hosp, Los Angeles CA 75-78; **FEL:** ObG, Mem Sloan Kettering Cancer Ctr, New York, NY 79-81; **HMO:** Oxford Blue Cross & Blue Shield

LANG: Sp; 🔲 🔲 🔲 🔲 🔲 🔲 Immediately

HAND SURGERY

Athanasian, Edward (MD)   HS
Hosp For Special Surgery

535 E 70th St; New York, NY 10021; (212) 606-1962; **BDCERT:** OrS 97; **MS:** Columbia P&S 88; **RES:** S, Beth Israel Med Ctr, Boston, MA 88-89; OrS, Hosp For Special Surgery, New York, NY 89-93; **FEL:** HS, Mayo Clinic, Rochester, MN 93-94; OrS, Mem Sloan Kettering Cancer Ctr, New York, NY 94-95; **FAP:** Asst Instr Cornell U; **HOSP:** Mem Sloan Kettering Cancer Ctr; **SI:** *Tumors of Soft Tissue & Bone; Fractures;* **HMO:** Blue Cross & Blue Shield PHCS Amerihealth Multiplan Sel Pro +

🔲 🔲 🔲 🔲 🔲 🔲 🔲 🔲 A Few Days ▨ **VISA** 🔲

Beasley, Robert (MD)   HS
New York University Med Ctr

Hand Surgery Associates, 310 E 30th St; New York, NY 10016; (212) 685-3834; **BDCERT:** PlS 68; **MS:** U Tenn Ctr Hlth Sci, Memphis 55; **RES:** St Luke's Roosevelt Hosp Ctr, New York, NY 57; US Army Hosp, Fort Irvin 59; **HOSP:** Bellevue Hosp Ctr; **HMO:** Blue Choice Chubb HealthNet Metlife

Botwinick, Nelson (MD)   HS
NYU Downtown Hosp

19 Beekman St; New York, NY 10038; (212) 513-7711; **BDCERT:** OrS 88; HS 98; **MS:** NYU Sch Med 80; **RES:** OrS, New York University Med Ctr, New York, NY 81-85; **FEL:** OrS, New York University Med Ctr, New York, NY 85-86; **HOSP:** New York University Med Ctr; **SI:** *Carpal Tunnel/Repetitive Stress Disorders; Upper Extremity Surgery;* **HMO:** Oxford United Healthcare Aetna-US Healthcare Blue Choice Prucare +

LANG: Chi, Sp, Rus, Fr, Itl; 🔲 🔲 🔲 🔲 🔲 🔲 🔲 A Few Days ▨ **VISA**

Grad, Joel (MD) **HS**
St Vincents Hosp & Med Ctr NY
Hand Surgery Associates, 310 E 30th St; New York, NY 10016; (212) 685-3834; **BDCERT:** OrS 84; HS 94; **MS:** SUNY Downstate 76; **RES:** S, St Vincents Hosp & Med Ctr NY, New York, NY 76-78; OrS, New York University Med Ctr, New York, NY 78-81; **FEL:** HS, Hand Surg Assoc, New York, NY 81-82; **FAP:** Asst Prof NYU Sch Med; **HOSP:** NY Hosp-Cornell Med Ctr; ***SI:** Upper Extremity Surgery*; **HMO:** Oxford Magnacare Metlife Blue Choice PHCS +
LANG: Sp; ☎ 🧍 📅 $ [WC] Immediately AMEX VISA MasterCard Discover

King, William (MD) **HS**
Hosp For Joint Diseases
159 E 74th St; New York, NY 10021; (212) 744-1620; **BDCERT:** OrS 88; **MS:** Columbia P&S 74; **RES:** S, St Luke's Roosevelt Hosp Ctr, New York, NY 74-76; OrS, Columbia-Presbyterian Med Ctr, New York, NY 76-79; **FEL:** HS Microsurgery, U CO Hosp, Denver, CO 79-80; **FAP:** Mt Sinai Sch Med; **HOSP:** Beth Israel Med Ctr; ***SI:** Compression Neuropathy; Repetitive Stress Injury*
LANG: Sp, Fr, Itl; ♿ ☎ 🧍 📅 $ [Mcr] [WC] [NFI]
A Few Days

Malone, Charlie (MD) **HS**
Beth Israel Med Ctr
317 E 34th St; New York, NY 10016; (212) 683-4263; **BDCERT:** OrS 76; HS 93; **MS:** Georgetown U 69; **RES:** OrS, Nassau County Med Ctr, East Meadow, NY 69-74; **FEL:** HS, New York University Med Ctr, New York, NY 74-75; **FAP:** Prof OrS NYU Sch Med; ***SI:** Sports Injuries; Arthritic Conditions of Hand*; **HMO:** Most
LANG: Sp; ♿ 🧍 📅 $ [Mcr] [WC] [NFI] 4+ Weeks AMEX VISA MasterCard Discover

McCormack Jr, Richard R (MD) **HS**
Hosp For Special Surgery
523 E 72nd St 2nd Fl; New York, NY 10021; (212) 606-1230; **BDCERT:** OrS 83; HS 92; **MS:** Cornell U 75; **RES:** S, St Luke's Roosevelt Hosp Ctr, New York, NY 75-77; OrS, Hosp For Special Surgery, New York, NY 77-80; **FEL:** HS, St Luke's Roosevelt Hosp Ctr, New York, NY 80-81; **FAP:** Assoc OrS Cornell U; **HOSP:** NY Hosp-Cornell Med Ctr; ***SI:** Dupuytren's Contracture; Wrist Problems*
♿ ☎ 🧍 📅 $ [Mcr] [NFI] 1 Week VISA MasterCard

Posner, Martin (MD) **HS**
Hosp For Joint Diseases
2 E 88th St; New York, NY 10128; (212) 348-6644; **BDCERT:** OrS 70; HS 89; **MS:** U Hlth Sci/Chicago Med Sch 62; **RES:** OrS, Hosp For Joint Diseases, New York, NY 62-67; **FEL:** HS, Orthopaedic Hosp, Los Angeles, CA 67-68; HS, Derbyshire Royal Infirmary, Derbyshire Royal Infirmary; **FAP:** Assoc Clin Prof OrS Mt Sinai Sch Med; **HOSP:** Lenox Hill Hosp; ***SI:** Arthritis Deformity; Nerve, Tendon Problems*; **HMO:** Oxford
LANG: Sp; ☎ 🧍 📅 $ [WC] [NFI] 2-4 Weeks VISA MasterCard

Weiland, Andrew J (MD) **HS**
Hosp For Special Surgery
535 E 70th St; New York, NY 10021; (212) 606-1575; **BDCERT:** OrS 77; HS 89; **MS:** Bowman Gray 68; **RES:** S, U Mich Med Ctr, Ann Arbor, MI 68-69; Johns Hopkins Hosp, Baltimore, MD 72-75; **FEL:** U Mich Med Ctr, Ann Arbor, MI 69-70; **FAP:** Prof OrS Cornell U; **HOSP:** NY Hosp-Cornell Med Ctr; ***SI:** Microvascular Surgery*; **HMO:** Oxford
♿ 📅 $ [Mcr] [WC] [NFI] 1 Week AMEX VISA MasterCard Discover

HEMATOLOGY

Aledort, Louis (MD) Hem
Mount Sinai Med Ctr
19 E 98th St; New York, NY 10029; (212) 860-0205; **BDCERT:** IM 66; **MS:** Albert Einstein Coll Med 59; **RES:** U of VA Health Sci Ctr, Charlottesville, VA 59-61; Nat Inst Health, Bethesda, MD 61-63; **FEL:** Hem, Strong Mem Hosp, Rochester, NY; **HMO:** Aetna Hlth Plan
[icons] Immediately [icons] **VISA** [icon]

Amorosi, Edward (MD) Hem
New York University Med Ctr
530 1st Ave Ste 9N; New York, NY 10016; (212) 263-7300; **BDCERT:** IM 66; Hem 72; **MS:** NYU Sch Med 59; **RES:** Francis Delafield Hosp, New York, NY 62-63
[icons] Immediately [icons] **VISA** [icon]

Astrow, Alan (MD) Hem
St Vincents Hosp & Med Ctr NY
170 W 12th St; New York, NY 10011; (212) 604-2427; **BDCERT:** IM 83; Hem 86; **MS:** Yale U Sch Med 80; **RES:** IM, Boston Med Ctr, Boston, MA 81-83; **FEL:** Hem Onc, New York University Med Ctr, New York, NY 83-86; **FAP:** Asst Clin Prof Med NY Med Coll; **HMO:** Aetna Hlth Plan Oxford CIGNA PHS US Hlthcre +
[icons] Immediately

Cho, John (MD) Hem
St Vincents Hosp & Med Ctr NY
170 W 12th St; New York, NY 10011; (212) 604-7221; **MS:** Univ Pittsburgh 87; **RES:** Med, St Vincents Hosp & Med Ctr NY, New York, NY 87-90; **FEL:** Hem, St Vincents Hosp & Med Ctr NY, New York, NY 90-91; Onc, New York University Med Ctr, New York, NY 91-92; **FAP:** Asst Prof Med NY Med Coll; **SI:** Head & Neck Cancer; Lymphoma; **HMO:** Oxford Blue Cross Aetna Hlth Plan Multiplan
LANG: Sp; [icons] 1 Week [icons] **VISA** [icon]

Cuttner, Janet (MD) Hem
Mount Sinai Med Ctr
5 E 98th St; New York, NY 10029; (212) 860-9055; **BDCERT:** IM 84; Hem 86; **MS:** Med Coll PA 57; **RES:** Kings County Hosp Ctr, Brooklyn, NY 58-60; Med, Kings County Hosp, Brooklyn, NY 60-61; **FEL:** Hem, Mount Sinai Med Ctr, New York, NY 61-63; **FAP:** Prof Med Mt Sinai Sch Med; **SI:** Leukemia; Lymphoma
[icons] **VISA**

Diaz, Michael (MD) Hem
Mount Sinai Med Ctr
112 Park Ave; New York, NY 10128; (212) 876-4500; **BDCERT:** IM 79; Hem 86; **MS:** St Louis U 71; **RES:** MF, Lenox Hill Hosp, New York, NY 72-74; **FEL:** Hem, Mount Sinai Med Ctr, New York, NY 74-76; **FAP:** Asst Clin Prof Med Mt Sinai Sch Med; **HOSP:** NY Hosp Med Ctr of Queens; **SI:** Coagulation Anemia; Lymphoma Oncology; **HMO:** Oxford
LANG: Sp; [icons] A Few Days

Diuguid, David L (MD) Hem
Columbia-Presbyterian Med Ctr
161 Ft Washington Ave; New York, NY 10032; (212) 305-8039; **BDCERT:** Hem 86; Onc 85; **MS:** Cornell U 79; **RES:** IM, Boston U Med Ctr, Boston, MA 79-83; **FEL:** Hem Onc, New England Med Ctr, Boston, MA 83-87; **FAP:** Asst Prof Columbia P&S; **SI:** Blood Clotting Disorders; **HMO:** Oxford Aetna Hlth Plan Chubb PHS
[icons] A Few Days

Fruchtman, Steven (MD) Hem
Mount Sinai Med Ctr
5 E 98th St 1275; New York, NY 10029; (212) 241-6021; **BDCERT:** IM 81; **MS:** NY Med Coll 77; **RES:** Univ Hosp SUNY Bklyn, Brooklyn, NY 77-81; **FEL:** Mount Sinai Med Ctr, New York, NY; Fred Hutchinson Cancer Research Ctr, Seattle, WA; **SI:** Bone Marrow Transplantation; Polycylthemia Vera; **HMO:** Aetna Hlth Plan Blue Cross & Blue Shield CIGNA HIP Network Metlife +
[icons] A Few Days [icons] **VISA** [icon]

Greenberg, Michael L (MD) Hem
Mount Sinai Med Ctr

5 E 98th St 10th Fl; New York, NY 10029; (212) 876-8220; **BDCERT:** Hem 74; Onc 75; **MS:** Univ Nebr Coll Med 58; **RES:** IM, Mount Sinai Med Ctr, New York, NY 61-62; IM, VA Med Ctr-Manh, New York, NY 59-60; **FEL:** Hem, Mount Sinai Med Ctr, New York, NY 60-61; **FAP:** Prof Mt Sinai Sch Med; **HMO:** Aetna-US Healthcare Oxford GHI CIGNA Blue Choice +

LANG: Sp, Chi; 🗄 🕿 🕎 🏧 💲 Mcr A Few Days 🗎
VISA 💳

Gulati, Subhash C (MD & PhD)Hem
NY Hosp-Cornell Med Ctr

449 E 68th St 10; New York, NY 10021; (212) 535-1514; **BDCERT:** IM 80; Onc 83; **MS:** U Miami Sch Med 76; **RES:** Buffalo Gen Hosp, Buffalo, NY 76-78; **FEL:** Mem Sloan Kettering Cancer Ctr, New York, NY 78-80; **HOSP:** Wyckoff Heights Med Ctr; **SI:** *Bone Marrow Transplantation; Lymphoma;* **HMO:** Blue Choice GHI Oxford United Healthcare Aetna Hlth Plan +

LANG: Hin, Sp, Chi; 🗄 🌙 🕿 🕎 🏧 💲 Mcr WC NFI Immediately

Herzig, Geoffrey P (MD) Hem
St Vincents Hosp & Med Ctr NY

170 W 12th St; New York, NY 10011; (212) 604-6021; **MS:** Case West Res U 67; **RES:** Bronx Muncipal Hosp Ctr, Bronx, NY 68-69; **FEL:** Hem, Barnes Hosp, St Louis, MO 72-73

Hirschman, Richard J (MD) Hem
Cabrini Med Ctr

247 3rd Ave 401; New York, NY 10010; (212) 228-0471; **BDCERT:** Hem 72; Onc 73; **MS:** Johns Hopkins U 65; **RES:** NY Hosp-Cornell Med Ctr, New York, NY; Columbia-Presbyterian Med Ctr, New York, NY; **FEL:** Columbia-Presbyterian Med Ctr, New York, NY; **FAP:** Asst Clin Prof Mt Sinai Sch Med; **HOSP:** Beth Israel Med Ctr; **HMO:** Oxford Aetna Hlth Plan Prucare CIGNA

LANG: Sp, Fr; 🗄 🕿 🕎 🏧 Mcr Immediately 🗎
VISA 💳

Hymes, Kenneth (MD) Hem
New York University Med Ctr

NYU Medical Ctr, 530 1st Ave 9N; New York, NY 10016; (212) 263-7226; **BDCERT:** IM 78; Hem 80; **MS:** SUNY Syracuse 75; **RES:** IM, Barnes Hosp, St Louis, MO 75-78; **FEL:** Hem, New York University Med Ctr, New York, NY 78-80; Onc, New York University Med Ctr, New York, NY 80-81; **FAP:** Assoc Prof NYU Sch Med; **SI:** *Coagulation Disorder; Cutaneous Lymphoma;* **HMO:** Oxford Blue Cross & Blue Shield CIGNA Prudential

LANG: Ger, Sp; 🗄 🕿 🏧 💲 Mcr 1 Week

Lerner, Robert (MD) Hem
Univ Hosp SUNY Bklyn

Lymphedema Services, PC, 245 E 63rd St Ste 106; New York, NY 10021; (212) 688-6107; **BDCERT:** S 62; **MS:** NYU Sch Med 55; **RES:** S, Jewish Hosp Med Ctr, Brooklyn, NY 55-60; **FEL:** S, Mem Sloan Kettering Cancer Ctr, New York, NY 60-61; **FAP:** Clin Prof S SUNY Downstate; **SI:** *Lymphedema-Lymphology; Head & Neck Surgery*

LANG: Fr, Ger; 🗄 🕿 🕎 🏧 💲 NFI A Few Days
VISA 💳

Mears, John Gregory (MD) Hem
Columbia-Presbyterian Med Ctr

161 Ft Washington Ave; New York, NY 10032; (212) 305-3506; **BDCERT:** IM 76; Hem 78; **MS:** Columbia P&S 73; **RES:** Boston U Med Ctr, Boston, MA 73-75; **FEL:** Hem Onc, Columbia-Presbyterian Med Ctr, New York, NY; **HMO:** Blue Cross & Blue Shield Chubb Oxford Anthem Health Prudential +

Moskovits, Tibor (MD) Hem
New York University Med Ctr

NYU Medical Ctr, 530 1st Ave 9N; New York, NY 10016; (212) 263-7082; **BDCERT:** Med 89; Hem 92; **MS:** SUNY Downstate 85; **RES:** Med, Beth Israel Med Ctr, New York, NY 85-86; Med, Beth Israel Med Ctr, New York, NY 86-89; **FEL:** Hem, New York University Med Ctr, New York, NY; **FAP:** Instr NYU Sch Med; **HOSP:** NYU Downtown Hosp; **SI:** *Lymphoma Breast Cancer;* **HMO:** Oxford Blue Choice US Hlthcre United Healthcare

LANG: Rus, Sp; 🗄 🌙 🕿 🕎 🏧 💲 Mcr 1 Week

Guide to symbols and abbreviations can be found on pages 110-113.

203

Ossias, A Lawrence (MD)   Hem
Mount Sinai Med Ctr

1112 Park Ave; New York, NY 10128; (212) 427-9333; **BDCERT:** Hem 72; Onc 79; **MS:** Yale U Sch Med 65; **RES:** Strong Mem Hosp, Rochester, NY 65-66; Albert Einstein Med Ctr, Bronx, NY 68-70; **FEL:** Mount Sinai Med Ctr, New York, NY 70-72; **FAP:** Asst Clin Prof Med Mt Sinai Sch Med; **HOSP:** Beth Israel North; **SI:** *Hematological Oncology*; **HMO:** None

LANG: Fr; 🚻 🗂 👤 🛏 💲   A Few Days ▦ **VISA** ⬤

Rand, Jacob (MD)   Hem
Mount Sinai Med Ctr

Mt Sinai Hospital, 5 E 98th St; New York, NY 10029; (212) 289-6400; **BDCERT:** IM 77; Hem 78; **MS:** Albert Einstein Coll Med 73; **RES:** Montefiore Med Ctr, Bronx, NY 73-74; Mount Sinai Med Ctr, New York, NY 74-76; **FEL:** Hem, Montefiore Med Ctr, Bronx, NY; **FAP:** Prof Mt Sinai Sch Med; **SI:** *Bleeding and Clotting Disorders; Hematology*; **HMO:** Oxford US Hlthcre Blue Cross & Blue Shield Aetna Hlth Plan +

🚻 🗂 👤 🛏 💲 🅼   Immediately

Raphael, Bruce (MD)   Hem
New York University Med Ctr

530 1st Ave Ste 9N; New York, NY 10016; (212) 263-7085; **BDCERT:** IM 78; Hem 80; **MS:** McGill U 75; **RES:** IM, Jewish Gnrl Hosp, Montreal, Canada 75-77; **FEL:** Onc, Mem Sloan Kettering Cancer Ctr, New York, NY 77-78; Onc, New York University Med Ctr, New York, NY 78-80; **FAP:** Assoc Prof NYU Sch Med; **HOSP:** NYU Downtown Hosp; **SI:** *Lymphoma; Leukemia*; **HMO:** Oxford Aetna Hlth Plan United Healthcare CIGNA

LANG: Fr, Sp, Rus; 🚻 🗂 🛏 💲 🅼   1 Week ▦ **VISA** ⬤

Ruggiero, Joseph (MD)   Hem
NY Hosp-Cornell Med Ctr

428 E 72nd St Ste 300; New York, NY 10021; (212) 746-2083; **BDCERT:** IM 80; Hem 82; **MS:** NYU Sch Med 77; **RES:** NY Hosp-Cornell Med Ctr, New York, NY 77-80; **FEL:** Hem, NY Hosp-Cornell Med Ctr, New York, NY 80-83; Onc, NY Hosp-Cornell Med Ctr, New York, NY 80-83; **FAP:** Assoc Prof Cornell U; **SI:** *Breast Cancer; Colon Cancer*

🚻 🗂 👤 🛏 💲 🅼   2-4 Weeks ▦ **VISA** ⬤

Scigliano, Eileen (MD)   Hem   PCP
Mount Sinai Med Ctr

5 E 98th St; New York, NY 10029; (212) 241-6021; **BDCERT:** IM 84; Hem 88; **MS:** Israel 81; **RES:** Kings County Hosp, Brooklyn, NY 81-84; **FEL:** Hem, VA Med Ctr-B'klyn, Brooklyn, NY 84-85; Mount Sinai, New York, NY 85-88; **HMO:** US Hlthcre Oxford GHI Aetna Hlth Plan CIGNA +

🚻 🗂 🛏 💲 🅼 🅼   Immediately ▦ **VISA** ⬤ ▦

Straus, David (MD)   Hem
Mem Sloan Kettering Cancer Ctr

1275 York Ave; New York, NY 10021; (212) 639-8365; **BDCERT:** Hem 76; Onc 77; **MS:** Med Coll Wisc 69; **RES:** IM, Montefiore Med Ctr, Bronx, NY 69-72; **FEL:** Hem, Beth Israel Med Ctr, Boston, MA 72-73; Hem Onc, Mem Sloan Kettering Cancer Ctr, New York, NY 75-77; **FAP:** Prof Cornell U; **SI:** *Lymphoma; Multiple Myeloma*; **HMO:** Empire Blue Cross & Shield

🚻 🗂 👤 🛏 🅼 🅼   1 Week ▦ **VISA** ⬤ ▦

Waxman, Samuel (MD)   Hem
Mount Sinai Med Ctr

1150 5th Ave 1A; New York, NY 10128; (212) 289-2828; **BDCERT:** IM 71; Hem 72; **MS:** SUNY Downstate 63; **RES:** IM, Mount Sinai Med Ctr, New York, NY 64-66; **FEL:** Hem, Mount Sinai Med Ctr, New York, NY 66-70; **FAP:** Clin Prof Med Mt Sinai Sch Med; **HMO:** Oxford

🗂 🛏 🅼 ▦ **VISA** ⬤

Weiss, Harvey (MD)   Hem
St Luke's Roosevelt Hosp Ctr

1000 10th Ave LLA35; New York, NY 10019; (212) 523-7281; **BDCERT:** IM 62; Hem 76; **MS:** Harvard Med Sch 55; **RES:** Bellevue Hosp Ctr, New York, NY 55-56; VA Med Ctr-Manh, New York, NY 56-58; **FEL:** Hem, Mount Sinai Med Ctr, New York, NY 59-60; **FAP:** Prof Med Columbia P&S

🗂 🅼   A Few Days

Wisch, Nathaniel (MD)   Hem
Lenox Hill Hosp

12 E 86th St; New York, NY 10028; (212) 861-6660; **BDCERT:** Onc 77; Hem 72; **MS:** Northwestern U 58; **RES:** Mount Sinai Med Ctr, New York, NY 60-61; Montefiore Med Ctr, Bronx, NY 61-62; **FEL:** Onc, Mount Sinai Med Ctr, New York, NY; **FAP:** Assoc Prof Med Mt Sinai Sch Med; **HOSP:** Mount Sinai Med Ctr; **SI:** *Lymphoma; Breast Cancer*

🔲 🔲 🔲 🔲 🔲 🔲 1 Week **VISA** 💳

Zaharia, Veronica (MD)   Hem
Cabrini Med Ctr

237 E 20th St Ste 1H; New York, NY 10003; (212) 995-0422; **MS:** Hungary 75; **RES:** IM, Long Island Coll Hosp, Brooklyn, NY 83-84; IM, Brookdale Univ Hosp Med Ctr, Brooklyn, NY 84-86; **FEL:** Hem Onc, Brookdale Univ Hosp Med Ctr, Brooklyn, NY 86-88; Hem Onc, Cabrini Med Ctr, New York, NY 88-89; **FAP:** Clin Instr NY Med Coll; **HOSP:** NYU Downtown Hosp; **SI:** *Leukemia; Lymphoma; Multiple Myeloma; Anemia;* **HMO:** Empire Blue Cross & Shield GHI 32BJ 1199 +

LANG: Rom, Sp, Hun, Ger, Fr; 🔲 🔲 🔲 🔲 🔲 🔲 🔲 Immediately

Zalusky, Ralph (MD)   Hem
Beth Israel Med Ctr

1st Ave & 16th St; New York, NY 10003; (212) 420-4185; **BDCERT:** IM 64; Hem 72; **MS:** Boston U 57; **RES:** Duke U Med Ctr, Durham, NC 57-59; Duke U Med Ctr, Durham, NC 61-62; **FEL:** Hem, Boston Med Ctr, Boston, MA 59-61; **FAP:** Prof Med Albert Einstein Coll Med; **SI:** *Leukemias - Lymphoma; Coagulation Defects;* **HMO:** 1199 Blue Choice Blue Cross & Blue Shield Choicecare HealthNet +

🔲 🔲 🔲 🔲 🔲 Immediately 💳 **VISA**

INFECTIOUS DISEASE

Armstrong, Donald (MD)   Inf
Mem Sloan Kettering Cancer Ctr

Infectious Disease, 1275 York Ave; New York, NY 10021; (212) 639-7809; **BDCERT:** IM 67; **MS:** Columbia P&S 57; **RES:** Med, Bellevue Hosp Ctr, New York, NY 58-59; Med, Mem Sloan Kettering Cancer Ctr, New York, NY 59-61; **FEL:** Inf, Nat Inst Health, Bethesda, MD 61-63; Inf, Children's Hosp of Philadelphia, Philadelphia, PA 63-66; **FAP:** Prof Cornell U; **HOSP:** NY Hosp-Cornell Med Ctr; **SI:** *Immune Compromised Host; AIDS Fungal Infections*

🔲 🔲 🔲 🔲 🔲 🔲 🔲 A Few Days

Baum, Stephen (MD)   Inf
Beth Israel Med Ctr

305 1st Ave; New York, NY 10003; (212) 420-4050; **BDCERT:** IM 72; Inf 72; **MS:** NYU Sch Med 62; **RES:** Boston Med Ctr, Boston, MA 66-67; **FEL:** Inf, Nat Inst Health, Bethesda, MD 64-67

🔲 🔲 🔲 🔲 1 Week

Brause, Barry (MD)   Inf   PCP
Hosp For Special Surgery

215 E 68th St; New York, NY 10021; (212) 570-6122; **BDCERT:** IM 73; Inf 76; **MS:** Univ Pittsburgh 70; **RES:** NY Hosp-Cornell Med Ctr, New York, NY 71-73; **FEL:** Inf, NY Hosp-Cornell Med Ctr, New York, NY 73-75; **FAP:** Clin Prof Med Cornell U; **HOSP:** NY Hosp-Cornell Med Ctr; **SI:** *Infectious Diseases of Bones/Joints; Lyme Disease;* **HMO:** Most

🔲 🔲 🔲 🔲 A Few Days 💳

Brown, Arthur E (MD)   Inf
Mem Sloan Kettering Cancer Ctr

1275 York Ave; New York, NY 10021; (212) 639-8475; **MS:** Jefferson Med Coll 71; **RES:** Med, St Luke's Roosevelt Hosp Ctr, New York, NY 74-76; Med, USPHS Hosp, Baltimore, MD 73-74; **FEL:** Inf, Mem Sloan Kettering Cancer Ctr, New York, NY 76-78; **FAP:** Prof Cornell U; **HOSP:** NY Hosp-Cornell Med Ctr; **SI:** *AIDS*

🔲 🔲 🔲 🔲 🔲 🔲 🔲 A Few Days 💳 **VISA** 💳 💳

Busillo, Christopher (MD)   Inf
NYU Downtown Hosp

N Y Downtown Medical Assoc, 170 William St FL7; New York, NY 10038; (212) 238-0102; **BDCERT:** IM 91; Inf 92; **MS:** Italy 86; **RES:** IM, Cabrini Med Ctr, New York, NY 86-89; **FEL:** Inf, Cabrini Med Ctr, New York, NY 89-91; **HOSP:** Cabrini Med Ctr; **SI:** *AIDS; Travel Medicine;* **HMO:** Oxford United Healthcare Empire Prudential Health Source +

LANG: Itl, Sp, Chi, Pol; 🔲 🔲 🔲 🔲 🔲 A Few Days 💳 **VISA** 💳 💳

Guide to symbols and abbreviations can be found on pages 110-113.

205

Garvey, Glenda Josephine (MD)Inf
Columbia-Presbyterian Med Ctr
Presby Hosp, 622 W 168th St; New York, NY
10032; (212) 305-3272; **BDCERT:** IM 93; CCM
89; **MS:** Albany Med Coll 90; **RES:** IM, Columbia-
Presbyterian Med Ctr, New York, NY 69-72; **FEL:**
Inf, Columbia-Presbyterian Med Ctr, New York, NY
72-74; **FAP:** Prof Columbia P&S; *SI: Infections;*
Endocarditis

Giordano, Michael F (MD)   Inf   PCP
NY Hosp-Cornell Med Ctr
525 E 68 St; New York, NY 10021; (212) 746-
2397; **BDCERT:** IM 87; Inf 90; **MS:** Cornell U 84;
RES: IM, NY Hosp-Cornell Med Ctr, New York, NY
85-87; **FEL:** Inf, NY Hosp-Cornell Med Ctr, New
York, NY 87-88; **FAP:** Asst Prof Cornell U; *SI:*
HIV/AIDS; Tropical Medicine

🦽 🆘 📠 👤 🛏 💲   A Few Days 📧 **VISA** 💳

Gumprecht, Jeffrey Paul (MD) Inf
Mount Sinai Med Ctr
Glenn Hammer PC, 1100 Park Ave; New York, NY
10128; (212) 427-9550; **BDCERT:** IM 87; Inf 90;
MS: Albany Med Coll 83; **RES:** Med, Mount Sinai
Hosp, Cleveland, OH 84-87; Med, Mount Sinai
Hosp, Cleveland, OH 88; **FEL:** Albert Einstein Med
Ctr, Bronx, NY 90; **FAP:** Asst Instr; *SI: HIV;*
Medicine for travel, tropics; **HMO:** Oxford PHS PHCS

📠 👤 🛏 💲 📧   2-4 Weeks 📧 **VISA** 💳

Hammer, Glenn (MD)   Inf   PCP
Mount Sinai Med Ctr
1100 Park Ave; New York, NY 10128; (212) 427-
9550; **BDCERT:** IM 73; Inf 74; **MS:** NYU Sch Med
69; **RES:** IM, Mount Sinai Med Ctr, New York, NY
69-72; **FEL:** Inf, Mount Sinai Med Ctr, New York,
NY 72-74; **HOSP:** Beth Israel North; *SI: Lyme*
Disease; Chronic Fatigue Syndrome; **HMO:** Oxford
Aetna Hlth Plan

👤 🛏 💲 📧   Immediately 📧 **VISA** 💳

Hartman, Barry Jay (MD)   Inf
NY Hosp-Cornell Med Ctr
407 E 70th St; New York, NY 10021; (212) 744-
4882; **BDCERT:** IM 76; Inf 80; **MS:** Penn State U-
Hershey Med Ctr 73; **RES:** NY Hosp-Cornell Med
Ctr, New York, NY 73-76; **FEL:** Inf, NY Hosp-
Cornell Med Ctr, New York, NY 78-81; **FAP:** Clin
Prof Med Cornell U; *SI: Surgical Infection;*
Endocarditis; **HMO:** None

🦽 📠 👤 🛏 💲 📧   2-4 Weeks

Helfgott, David (MD)   Inf   PCP
NY Hosp-Cornell Med Ctr
311 E 79th St; New York, NY 10021; (212) 879-
6004; **BDCERT:** IM 86; Inf 88; **MS:** Yale U Sch Med
83; **RES:** IM, NY Hosp-Cornell Med Ctr, New York,
NY 83-86; **FEL:** Inf, NY Hosp-Cornell Med Ctr, New
York, NY 86-89; **FAP:** Asst Clin Prof Cornell U;
HOSP: Beth Israel North; *SI: Infectious Diseases;*
Travel Medicine; **HMO:** Oxford PHCS Blue Choice
NYLCare

🦽 📠 👤 🛏 💲   Immediately 📧 **VISA** 💳

Jacobs, Jonathan (MD)   Inf   PCP
NY Hosp-Cornell Med Ctr
449 E 68th St 1A; New York, NY 10021; (212)
734-1365; **BDCERT:** IM 83; Inf 86; **MS:** Yale U Sch
Med 80; **RES:** NY Hosp-Cornell Med Ctr, New York,
NY 80-83; **FEL:** Inf, NY Hosp-Cornell Med Ctr, New
York, NY 83-86; **FAP:** Assoc Clin Prof Med Cornell
U; **HMO:** None

🦽 📠 👤 🛏 💲   Immediately 📧 **VISA** 💳

Kislak, Jay Ward (MD)   Inf
St Vincents Hosp & Med Ctr NY
Travelers Medical Ctr, 31 Washington Sq West FL4;
New York, NY 10011; (212) 475-8833; **BDCERT:**
IM 65; **MS:** Yale U Sch Med 58; **RES:** Inf, Bellevue-
NYU, New York, NY 62-63; IM, Bellevue-NYU,
New York, NY 61-62; **FEL:** Inf, Thorndike Meml-
Harvard, Boston, MA 63-65

Lerner, Chester (MD)   Inf
New York University Med Ctr
170 William St; New York, NY 10038; (212) 238-0106; **BDCERT:** IM 81; Inf 84; **MS:** Univ Pittsburgh 78; **RES:** IM, Lenox Hill Hosp, New York, NY 78-81; **FEL:** Inf, Lenox Hill Hosp, New York, NY 81-83; *SI: HIV Infection/AIDS; Travel Medicine*; **HMO:** Oxford United Healthcare Aetna-US Healthcare Blue Cross & Blue Shield Prudential +

⬧ ⬧ ⬧ ⬧ ⬧ ⬧ 1 Week ▓▓ *VISA* ⬤ ▭

Louie, Eddie (MD)   Inf   PCP
NY Hosp-Cornell Med Ctr
345 E 37th St; New York, NY 10016; (212) 682-9202; **BDCERT:** IM 82; Inf 86; **MS:** NYU Sch Med 79; **RES:** IM, Kings County Hosp Ctr, Brooklyn, NY 79-83; **FEL:** Inf, New York University Med Ctr, New York, NY 83-85; **FAP:** Asst Clin Prof NYU Sch Med; *SI: Lyme Disease; AIDS*; **HMO:** Oxford United Healthcare CIGNA PHS

⬧ ⬧ ⬧ ⬧ ⬧ ⬧ 1 Week

Mildvan, Donna (MD)   Inf
Beth Israel Med Ctr
Chief Division of Infectious Diseases Beth Israel Med Ctr, 1st Ave at 16th St; New York, NY 10003; (212) 420-4005; **BDCERT:** IM 72; Inf 72; **MS:** Johns Hopkins U 67; **RES:** IM, Mount Sinai Med Ctr, New York, NY 67-70; **FEL:** Inf, Mount Sinai Med Ctr, New York, NY 70-72; **FAP:** Prof Med Albert Einstein Coll Med; *SI: AIDS Antiviral Therapy; HIV Infection*; **HMO:** 1199 Aetna Hlth Plan Beech Street Oxford US Hlthcre +

⬧ ⬧ ⬧ ⬧ ⬧ ⬧ 4+ Weeks

Miller, Dennis (MD)   Inf
Lenox Hill Hosp
4 E 76th St; New York, NY 10021; (212) 472-1237; **BDCERT:** IM 85; **MS:** Rush Med Coll 82; **RES:** IM, Lenox Hill Hosp, New York, NY 83-85; **FEL:** Inf, Lenox Hill Hosp, New York, NY 85-87; *SI: Lyme Disease; AIDS*; **HMO:** Oxford Blue Choice United Healthcare PHS PHCS +

⬧ ⬧ ⬧ ⬧ ⬧ ⬧ 1 Week *VISA* ⬤

Neibart, Eric (MD)   Inf
Mount Sinai Med Ctr
1100 Park Ave; New York, NY 10128; (212) 427-9550; **BDCERT:** IM 83; Inf 86; **MS:** UMDNJ-NJ Med Sch, Newark 80; **RES:** Mount Sinai Med Ctr, New York, NY 80-83; **FEL:** Inf, Mount Sinai Med Ctr, New York, NY 84-86; **FAP:** Asst Prof Mt Sinai Sch Med; *SI: Travel Medicine; AIDS*; **HMO:** Oxford PHS PHCS

⬧ ⬧ ⬧ ⬧ ⬧ A Few Days ▓▓ *VISA* ⬤

Perlman, David (MD)   Inf
Beth Israel Med Ctr
1st Ave at 16th St; New York, NY 10003; (212) 420-4470; **BDCERT:** Inf 88; IM 86; **MS:** Albert Einstein Coll Med 83; **RES:** IM, NY Hosp-Cornell Med Ctr, New York, NY 83-86; **FEL:** Inf, Montefiore Med Ctr, Bronx, NY 86-8; **FAP:** Assoc Med; **HOSP:** Beth Israel North; **HMO:** Most

⬧ ⬧ ⬧ ⬧ ⬧ ⬧ ⬧ A Few Days ▓▓ *VISA* ⬤ ▭

Polsky, Bruce (MD)   Inf
Mem Sloan Kettering Cancer Ctr
1275 York Ave; New York, NY 10021; (212) 639-8361; **BDCERT:** IM 83; Inf 86; **MS:** Wayne State U Sch Med 80; **RES:** IM, Montefiore Med Ctr, Bronx, NY 81-83; **FEL:** Inf, Mem Sloan Kettering Cancer Ctr, New York, NY 83-86; **FAP:** Assoc Prof Med Cornell U; *SI: Viral Infections; AIDS & HIV Disease*

LANG: Fr; ⬧ ⬧ ⬧ ⬧ 1 Week ▓▓ *VISA* ⬤

Press, Robert (MD)   Inf
New York University Med Ctr
530 1st Ave Ste 4G; New York, NY 10016; (212) 263-7229; **BDCERT:** IM 76; **MS:** NYU Sch Med 73; **RES:** IM, Beth Israel Med Ctr, Boston, MA 73-75; IM, New York University Med Ctr, New York, NY 75-76; **FEL:** Montefiore Med Ctr, Bronx, NY 76-78; **FAP:** Assoc Clin Prof Med NYU Sch Med; **HOSP:** Manhattan Eye, Ear & Throat Hosp; *SI: Surgical Infections; Infections in Hospitals*

⬧ ⬧ ⬧ ⬧ ⬧ 2-4 Weeks

Romagnoli, Mario (MD)   Inf
Columbia-Presbyterian Med Ctr

16 E 60th St; New York, NY 10022; (212) 326-8420; **BDCERT:** IM 79; **MS:** Columbia P&S 76; **RES:** Med, Columbia-Presbyterian Med Ctr, New York, NY 76-79; **FEL:** Inf, Beth Israel Med Ctr, Boston, MA 79-81; **FAP:** Assoc Prof Columbia P&S; *SI: AIDS/HIV Infection; Chronic Bone & Joint Infection;* **HMO:** Oxford

LANG: Sp, Itl, Fr; ⬛ ⬛ ⬛ ⬛ ⬛ ⬛   A Few Days

Rosenberg, Amy (MD)   Inf   PCP
St Luke's Roosevelt Hosp Ctr

St Lukes Roosevelt Hosp Ctr, 1111 Amsterdam Ave; New York, NY 10025; (212) 523-1758; **BDCERT:** IM 90; Inf 92; **MS:** Israel 87; **RES:** IM, St Luke's Roosevelt Hosp Ctr, New York, NY 87-90; **FEL:** Inf, Mem Sloan Kettering Cancer Ctr, New York, NY 90-93; **FAP:** Asst Clin Prof Med Columbia P&S

⬛ ⬛ ⬛ ⬛ ⬛ ⬛   A Few Days

Sanjana, Veeraf (MD & PhD)   Inf   PCP
Cabrini Med Ctr

310 E 14th St; New York, NY 10003; (212) 473-8088; **BDCERT:** IM 81; Inf 90; **MS:** U Miami Sch Med 77; **RES:** Albert Einstein Med Ctr, Bronx, NY 77-78; Cabrini Med Ctr, New York, NY 78-79; **FEL:** Cabrini Med Ctr, New York, NY 87-89; *SI: AIDS; HIV;* **HMO:** Oxford CIGNA Magnacare Blue Cross PHS +

LANG: Slv, Prt; ⬛ ⬛ ⬛ ⬛ ⬛ ⬛ ⬛

Simberkoff, Michael S (MD)   Inf
VA Med Ctr-Manh

423 E 23rd St; New York, NY 10010; (212) 951-3417; **BDCERT:** IM 69; Inf 72; **MS:** NYU Sch Med 62; **RES:** IM, Bellevue Hosp Ctr, New York, NY 62-67; **FEL:** Inf, New York University Med Ctr, New York, NY 67-69; **FAP:** Assoc Med NYU Sch Med; **HOSP:** New York University Med Ctr; *SI: HIV/AIDS; Pneumonia;* **HMO:** None

⬛ ⬛ ⬛ ⬛   1 Week

Soave, Rosemary (MD)   Inf
NY Hosp-Cornell Med Ctr

1300 York Ave; New York, NY 10021; (212) 746-6320; **BDCERT:** IM 79; **MS:** Cornell U 76; **RES:** NY Hosp-Cornell Med Ctr, New York, NY 76-79; **FEL:** Mem Sloan Kettering Cancer Ctr, New York, NY 79-80; Inf, NY Hosp-Cornell Med Ctr, New York, NY 80-82; *SI: Cryptosporidioses; Transplant Infections*

LANG: Itl; ⬛ ⬛ ⬛ ⬛ ⬛ ⬛

Tapper, Michael (MD)   Inf
Lenox Hill Hosp

100 E 77th St; New York, NY 10021; (212) 434-3440; **BDCERT:** IM 73; Inf 76; **MS:** Columbia P&S 70; **RES:** IM, Harlem Hosp Ctr, New York, NY 70-73; **FEL:** Inf, Mem Sloan Kettering Cancer Ctr, New York, NY 73-75; **FAP:** Clin Prof Med NYU Sch Med; *SI: AIDS/HIV Disease; Infection Hospital Acquired*

⬛ ⬛ ⬛

Wetherbee, Roger (MD)   Inf   PCP
New York University Med Ctr

530 1st Ave 4C; New York, NY 10016; (212) 263-7300; **BDCERT:** IM 74; Inf 97; **MS:** NYU Sch Med 69; **RES:** Bellevue Hosp Ctr, New York, NY 69-70; VA Med Ctr-Manh, New York, NY 73-74; **FEL:** Nat Inst Health, Bethesda, MD 70-72; VA Med Ctr-Manh, New York, NY 74-75; **FAP:** Assoc Clin Prof Med NYU Sch Med; *SI: Hepatitis, Fever of Unk Origin; HIV Primary Care;* **HMO:** Aetna Hlth Plan Oxford US Hlthcre Prucare Blue Cross & Blue Shield +

⬛ ⬛ ⬛ ⬛ ⬛ ⬛ ⬛   A Few Days

Yancovitz, Stanley (MD)   Inf
Beth Israel Med Ctr

317 E 17th St; New York, NY 10003; (212) 420-2600; **BDCERT:** IM 73; Inf 76; **MS:** SUNY Hlth Sci Ctr 67; **RES:** Metropolitan Hosp Ctr, New York, NY; Beth Israel Med Ctr, New York, NY; **FEL:** Inf, Mount Sinai Med Ctr, New York, NY; **FAP:** Assoc Prof Med Albert Einstein Coll Med; **HMO:** Oxford CIGNA US Hlthcre Aetna-US Healthcare Empire Blue Cross & Shield +

⬛ ⬛ ⬛ ⬛ ⬛ ⬛ ⬛   A Few Days ⬛ **VISA** ⬛ ⬛

INTERNAL MEDICINE

Adler, Mitchell (MD)   IM   PCP
New York University Med Ctr
Murray Hill Medical Group, 317 E 34th St; New
York, NY 10016; (212) 726-7499; **BDCERT:** IM
83; **MS:** NYU Sch Med 80; **RES:** IM, Bellevue Hosp
Ctr, New York, NY 80-83; Bellevue Hosp Ctr, New
York, NY 83-84; **FAP:** Asst Prof of Clin Med NYU
Sch Med; **SI:** *Sports Medicine; Geriatrics;* **HMO:**
CIGNA Health Source Oxford PHS

⬧ ⬧ ⬧ ⬧ ⬧ ⬧ ⬧ A Few Days ▦ *VISA* ⬤

Akhavan, Iraj (MD)   IM   PCP
St Clare's Hosp & Health Ctr
300 W 49th St; New York, NY 10019; (212) 331-
7661; **BDCERT:** IM 79; **MS:** Iran 71; **RES:** IM,
Westchester County Med Ctr, Valhalla, NY 74-75;
IM, New Rochelle Hosp Med Ctr, New Rochelle, NY
75-78; **FEL:** Pul, Harlem Hosp Ctr, New York, NY
78-80; **HOSP:** St Luke's Roosevelt Hosp Ctr; **SI:**
Chronic Lung Diseases; Asthma; **HMO:** Oxford Blue
Cross & Blue Shield Senior Plan GHI Aetna-US
Healthcare +

LANG: Slv, Fil, Frs; ⬧ ⬧ ⬧ ⬧ ⬧ ⬧ ⬧ ⬧
A Few Days

Altman, Kenneth (MD)   IM   PCP
St Luke's Roosevelt Hosp Ctr
425 W 59th St 4G; New York, NY 10019; (212)
246-1264; **BDCERT:** IM 65; **MS:** Columbia P&S 54;
RES: Lenox Hill Hosp, New York, NY 57-60; St
Luke's Roosevelt Hosp Ctr, New York, NY 60-61;
FEL: NuM, Mount Sinai Med Ctr, New York, NY;
FAP: Asst Clin Prof Med Columbia P&S; **SI:**
Gastroenterology; **HMO:** Oxford CIGNA Prucare US
Hlthcre Blue Cross & Blue Shield +

LANG: Fr, Sp, Ger, Yd, Heb; ⬧ ⬧ ⬧ ⬧ ⬧
A Few Days

Ascheim, Robert (MD)   IM
NY Hosp-Cornell Med Ctr
435 E 57th St #1A; New York, NY 10022; (212)
421-4333; **BDCERT:** IM 69; **MS:** Tufts U 62; **RES:**
IM, Bellevue Hosp Ctr, New York, NY 65-68; Cv,
Mem Sloan Kettering Cancer Ctr, New York, NY
65-67; **FEL:** Cv, NY Hosp-Cornell Med Ctr, New
York, NY 68-70

Baldwin, David (MD)   IM   PCP
Bellevue Hosp Ctr
20 E 68th St 1A; New York, NY 10021; (212) 737-
8989; **BDCERT:** IM 52; **MS:** U Rochester 45; **RES:**
Med, Barnes Hosp, St Louis, MO 45-46; Med,
Bellevue Hosp Ctr, New York, NY 46-48; **FEL:** Nep,
New York University Med Ctr, New York, NY 48-
50; **FAP:** Prof Med NYU Sch Med; **HOSP:** New York
University Med Ctr; **SI:** *Kidney Diseases;
Hypertension;* **HMO:** Oxford Chubb United
Healthcare Health Source CIGNA +

⬧ ⬧ ⬧ ⬧ ⬧ ⬧ 1 Week

Bardes, Charles L (MD)   IM
NY Hosp-Cornell Med Ctr
525 E 68th St; New York, NY 10021; (212) 746-
1333; **BDCERT:** IM 89; **MS:** Univ Penn 86; **RES:** NY
Hosp-Cornell Med Ctr, New York, NY 86-89; **FAP:**
Assoc Prof Cornell U; **SI:** *Preventive Medicine;* **HMO:**
Oxford Blue Choice Aetna Hlth Plan

⬧ ⬧ ⬧ ⬧ ⬧ 4+ Weeks

Barnes, Edward (MD)   IM
Bellevue Hosp Ctr

317 E 34th St; New York, NY 10016; (212) 726-7434; **BDCERT:** IM 87; **MS:** Mt Sinai Sch Med 84; **RES:** Bellevue Med Ctr, New York, NY 84-87

Baskin, David (MD)   IM   **PCP**
St Luke's Roosevelt Hosp Ctr

185 W End Ave 1M; New York, NY 10023; (212) 595-7701; **BDCERT:** IM 85; **MS:** Boston U 82; **RES:** St Luke's Roosevelt Hosp Ctr, New York, NY 82-85; *SI: Preventive Care; Cholesterol*

LANG: Sp; ♿ 🄲 🄰 🄼 🄳 🄢 Mcr   A Few Days

Beer, Maurice (MD)   IM   **PCP**
Lenox Hill Hosp

270 West End Ave 1N; New York, NY 10024; (212) 496-0880; **BDCERT:** IM 76; **MS:** NY Med Coll 73; **RES:** IM, Flower Fifth Ave Hosp, New York, NY 73-76; IM, Metropolitan Hosp Ctr, New York, NY 73-76; **HOSP:** St Luke's Roosevelt Hosp Ctr; *SI: Functional & Alternative Medicine; Nutritional Medicine*; **HMO:** Oxford Chubb Aetna Hlth Plan CIGNA PHS +

LANG: Rus, Sp, Yd, Heb; ♿ 🄰 🄼 🄳 🄢 Mcr   2-4 Weeks 🔲 *VISA* ⬤

Benjamin, Bry (MD)   IM   **PCP**
NY Hosp-Cornell Med Ctr

14 E 63rd St; New York, NY 10021; (212) 207-3780; **BDCERT:** IM 56; Ger 88; **MS:** Harvard Med Sch 47; **RES:** Cincinnati Gen Hosp, Cincinnati, OH 50-51; NY Hosp-Cornell Med Ctr, New York, NY 54-55; **HOSP:** Beth Israel Med Ctr; *SI: Geriatrics*; **HMO:** US Hlthcre Well Care Oxford Independent Health Plan

LANG: Sp; ♿ 🄰 🄼 🄳 Mcr Med   1 Week *VISA* ⬤

Benovitz, Harvey (MD)   IM   **PCP**
St Luke's Roosevelt Hosp Ctr

265 Central Park West; New York, NY 10024; (212) 877-2100; **BDCERT:** IM 72; **MS:** Albert Einstein Coll Med 62; **RES:** U of Pittsburgh Med Ctr, Pittsburgh, PA 62-64; U of Pittsburgh Med Ctr, Pittsburgh, PA 64-67; **FEL:** EDM, St Luke's Roosevelt Hosp Ctr, New York, NY 67-70; **FAP:** Asst Clin Prof Columbia P&S; *SI: Thyroid; Diabetes Mellitus*; **HMO:** Aetna Hlth Plan Oxford CIGNA NYLCare PHS +

🄲 🄰 🄼 🄳 🄢 Mcr   A Few Days 🔲

Bernot, Robert (MD)   IM   **PCP**
St Luke's Roosevelt Hosp Ctr

30 W 60th St 1D; New York, NY 10023; (212) 581-3553; **BDCERT:** IM 70; **MS:** SUNY Buffalo 60; **RES:** IM, VA Med Ctr-Manh, New York, NY 60-63; IM, St Luke's Roosevelt Hosp Ctr, New York, NY 64-65; **FEL:** Ge, Lahey Clinic, Burlington, MA 63-64; **FAP:** Asst Clin Prof Med Columbia P&S; **HMO:** Oxford Health Source PHS +

♿ 🄰 🄼 🄳 NFI   A Few Days

Bevelaqua, Frederick (MD)   IM
New York University Med Ctr

650 1st Ave; New York, NY 10016; (212) 213-6796; **BDCERT:** IM 78; Pul 80; **MS:** NYU Sch Med 74; **RES:** Hosp of U Penn, Philadelphia, PA 74-75; New York University Med Ctr, New York, NY 75-78; **FEL:** Pul/CCM, New York University Med Ctr, New York, NY 78-80; **FAP:** Asst Prof NYU Sch Med; *SI: Asthma; Chronic Respiratory Disease*

♿ 🄲 🄰 🄼 🄳 🄢 Mcr   A Few Days 🔲 *VISA* ⬤ 🔲

Bruno, Michael (MD)   IM   PCP
Lenox Hill Hosp

110 E 59th St Fl 9A; New York, NY 10022; (212) 583-2820; **BDCERT:** IM 53; **MS:** Columbia P&S 45; **RES:** IM, Bellevue Hosp Ctr, New York, NY 48-51

🔲 🔲 🔲 1 Week ▦ **VISA**

Bruno, Peter (MD)   IM   PCP
Beth Israel Med Ctr

110 E 59th St 9A; New York, NY 10022; (212) 583-2820; **BDCERT:** IM 79; **MS:** Hahnemann U 75; **RES:** IM, Lenox Hill, New York, NY 75-78; **FEL:** IM, Lenox Hill, New York, NY 78-79; **FAP:** Assoc Clin Prof Med NYU Sch Med; **HOSP:** Lenox Hill Hosp; **SI:** *Pre-Operative Evaluation; Sports Medicine*; **HMO:** Oxford United Healthcare

LANG: Sp; 🔲 🔲 🔲 🔲 🔲 🔲 🔲 🔲 🔲
A Few Days ▦ **VISA** ● ●

Burke, Gary R (MD)   IM   PCP
St Luke's Roosevelt Hosp Ctr

University Medical Practice Associates, 1090 Amsterdam Ave 4TH; New York, NY 10025; (212) 523-5727; **BDCERT:** IM 76; **MS:** U Minn 73; **RES:** Med, UC Davis Med Ctr, Sacramento, CA 74-76; Med, Med Coll WI, Milwaukee, WI 74-76; **FAP:** Asst Clin Prof Columbia P&S; **HMO:** Aetna-US Healthcare CIGNA Oxford NYLCare PHS +

LANG: Sp, Fr; 🔲 🔲 🔲 🔲 🔲 🔲 🔲 A Few Days ▦ **VISA** ● ●

Burroughs, Valentine (MD)   IM   PCP
North General Hosp

Mid Manhattan Medical Associates, 654 Madison Ave Fl 6; New York, NY 10021; (212) 355-5222; **BDCERT:** IM 78; EDM 81; **MS:** U Mich Med Sch 75; **RES:** Columbia-Presbyterian Med Ctr, New York, NY 76-78; Columbia-Presbyterian Med Ctr, New York, NY 78-79; **FEL:** EDM, New York University Med Ctr, New York, NY 79-81; **FAP:** Asst Prof Columbia P&S; **HOSP:** St Luke's Roosevelt Hosp Ctr; **SI:** *Diabetes; Thyroid Diseases*; **HMO:** Oxford PHS Aetna Hlth Plan CIGNA Blue Cross & Blue Shield +

🔲 🔲 🔲 🔲 🔲 🔲 🔲 A Few Days ▦ **VISA** ●
🔲

Bush, Michael (MD)   IM   PCP
Lenox Hill Hosp

48 E 75th St; New York, NY 10021; (212) 583-2820; **BDCERT:** IM 81; **MS:** SUNY Hlth Sci Ctr 78; **RES:** IM, Lenox Hill Hosp, New York, NY 79-82; Lenox Hill Hosp, New York, NY 78-79; **FAP:** Asst Clin Prof Med NYU Sch Med; **HMO:** Oxford Chubb

🔲 🔲 🔲 🔲 🔲 🔲 Immediately ▦ **VISA** ●

Carmichael, David (MD)   IM   PCP
Columbia-Presbyterian Med Ctr

New York Physicians, PC, 635 Madison Ave 8thFL; New York, NY 10022; (212) 317-4566; **BDCERT:** IM 79; Ger 94; **MS:** Albert Einstein Coll Med 76; **RES:** IM, Jacobi Med Ctr, Bronx, NY 76-77; IM, Bronx Lebanon Hosp Ctr, Bronx, NY 77-79; **FEL:** Ger, Columbia-Presbyterian Med Ctr, New York, NY 79-80; **FAP:** Assoc Clin Prof Columbia P&S; **SI:** *Health Maintenance; Travel Medicine*; **HMO:** Oxford

LANG: Fr, Sp; 🔲 🔲 🔲 🔲 🔲 🔲 A Few Days ▦
VISA ● 🔲

Case, David B (MD)   IM   PCP
NY Hosp-Cornell Med Ctr

New York Physicians, PC, 635 Madison Ave Fl 7; New York, NY 10022; (212) 857-4660; **BDCERT:** IM 74; **MS:** Columbia P&S 68; **RES:** Johns Hopkins Hosp, Baltimore, MD 68-70; **FEL:** Columbia-Presbyterian Med Ctr, New York, NY 70-72; **FAP:** Assoc Clin Prof Cornell U; **HOSP:** Columbia-Presbyterian Med Ctr; **SI:** *High Blood Pressure; Cardiovascular Risk Reduction*; **HMO:** None

LANG: Sp; 🔲 🔲 🔲 🔲 🔲 2-4 Weeks **VISA** ●

Cervia, Joseph (MD)   IM   PCP
NY Hosp-Cornell Med Ctr

505 E 70th St 524; New York, NY 10021; (212) 946-6320; **BDCERT:** IM 89; Inf 90; **MS:** NY Med Coll 84; **RES:** IM, Brookdale Univ Hosp Med Ctr, Brooklyn, NY 85-88; **FEL:** Inf, NY Hosp-Cornell Med Ctr, New York, NY 88-90; **FAP:** Assoc Prof Med Cornell U; **SI:** *HIV/AIDS; Infectious Disease*; **HMO:** Blue Choice Magnacare US Hlthcre Aetna Hlth Plan

🔲 🔲 🔲 🔲 🔲 🔲 🔲 A Few Days

Guide to symbols and abbreviations can be found on pages 110-113.

211

Charap, Peter (MD) IM PCP
Mount Sinai Med Ctr

234 Central Park West 1; New York, NY 10024;
(212) 579-2200; **BDCERT:** IM 87; **MS:** Mt Sinai
Sch Med 84; **RES:** IM, Mount Sinai Med Ctr, New
York, NY 84-87; **FAP:** Asst Clin Prof Mt Sinai Sch
Med; **HOSP:** Beth Israel Med Ctr; *SI: Preventive
Medicine*; **HMO:** Oxford Aetna Hlth Plan CIGNA
PHS NYLCare +

LANG: Sp; ♿ 🄲 🔲 🔳 🄼 💲 Ⓜ A Few Days ▦
VISA 💳

Cimino, James (MD) IM PCP
Columbia-Presbyterian Med Ctr

622 W 168th St; New York, NY 10032; (212)
305-6262; **BDCERT:** IM 84; **MS:** NY Med Coll 81;
RES: St Vincents Hosp & Med Ctr NY, New York, NY
81-84; **FEL:** Med Informatics, Mass Gen Hosp,
Boston, MA; **FAP:** Assoc Prof Columbia P&S; **HMO:**
Blue Choice

♿ 🔲 🄼 💲 Ⓜ Ⓜ 4+ Weeks

Clain, David (MD) IM
St Luke's Roosevelt Hosp Ctr

305 1st Ave; New York, NY 10003; (212) 420-
4521; **BDCERT:** IM 80; **MS:** South Africa 59; **RES:**
Charing Cross Hosp, London, England 64-65;
Birmingham Gen Hosp, Birmingham, AL 63-64;
FEL: Royal Free Hosp, London, England 64-65;
FAP: Prof Albert Einstein Coll Med; **HOSP:** Beth
Israel Med Ctr; *SI: Viral Hepatitis Chronic*; **HMO:**
Aetna Hlth Plan Oxford Prudential CIGNA +

LANG: Sp; ♿ 🔲 🔳 💲 Ⓜ ▦ *VISA* 💳

Cohen, Michael (MD) IM
Columbia-Presbyterian Med Ctr

161 Fort Washington Ave; New York, NY 10032;
(212) 305-5440; **BDCERT:** IM 71; **MS:** Johns
Hopkins U 65; **RES:** Columbia-Presbyterian Med
Ctr, New York, NY 66-71; **FEL:** Cv, Columbia-
Presbyterian Med Ctr, New York, NY 69-70; *SI:
Angina; Hypertension*

🔲 🔳 💲 2-4 Weeks

Cohen, Richard P (MD) IM PCP
NY Hosp-Cornell Med Ctr

235 E 67th St; New York, NY 10021; (212) 734-
6464; **BDCERT:** IM 78; **MS:** Cornell U 75; **RES:** IM,
NY Hosp-Cornell Med Ctr, New York, NY 75-78;
FEL: Inf, NY Hosp-Cornell Med Ctr, New York, NY
78-79; **FAP:** Assoc Prof Cornell U; *SI: Diagnostic
Problems Complex*

LANG: Sp; ♿ 🔲 🄼 🔳 4+ Weeks

Collens, Richard (MD) IM PCP
St Luke's Roosevelt Hosp Ctr

MidManhattan Med Assocs PC, 697 West End Ave;
New York, NY 10025; (212) 222-7071; **BDCERT:**
IM 73; Cv 73; **MS:** NY Med Coll 66; **RES:** Jacobi Med
Ctr, Bronx, NY 66-70; **FEL:** Mount Sinai Med Ctr,
New York, NY 70-71; Bronx Muncipal Hosp Ctr,
Bronx, NY 71-72; **FAP:** Assoc Clin Prof Med; **HOSP:**
Lenox Hill Hosp; **HMO:** Aetna-US Healthcare
Oxford CIGNA Metlife PHS +

♿ 🄲 🔲 🄼 🔳 💲 Ⓜ Immediately ▦ *VISA* 💳

Coller, Barry (MD) IM
Mount Sinai Med Ctr

1 Gustave Levy Pl; New York, NY 10029; (212)
241-4200; **BDCERT:** IM 73; Hem 74; **MS:** NYU Sch
Med 70; **RES:** IM, Bellevue Hosp Ctr, New York, NY
70-71; **FEL:** Hem, Nat Inst Health, Bethesda, MD;
SI: Coagulation Disorder; Platelets; **HMO:** Aetna Hlth
Plan Blue Cross & Blue Shield Oxford

LANG: Sp; ♿ 🔳 Ⓜ Ⓜ 🅆 🄽 2-4 Weeks *VISA* 💳

Constantiner, Arturo (MD) IM PCP
NYU Downtown Hosp

19 Beekman St FL6; New York, NY 10038; (212)
349-8455; **BDCERT:** IM 79; Nep 95; **MS:** Mexico
75; **RES:** IM, Elmhurst Hosp Ctr, Elmhurst, NY 76-
79; **FEL:** Nep, Mount Sinai Med Ctr, New York, NY
79-81; **FAP:** Asst Clin Prof NYU Sch Med; *SI: High
Blood Pressure; Renal Diseases*; **HMO:** Oxford
Unicare Primary Plus Aetna-US Healthcare Blue
Choice Magnacare +

LANG: Sp, Heb, Fr, Chi; ♿ 🄲 🔲 🄼 🔳 Ⓜ 🅆 🄽
A Few Days ▦ *VISA* 💳

Cox, D Sayer (MD)   IM   PCP
NY Hosp-Cornell Med Ctr
530 E 72nd St; New York, NY 10021; (212) 879-4003; **BDCERT:** IM 60; **MS:** Columbia P&S 52; **RES:** Pul, NY Hosp-Cornell Med Ctr, New York, NY 54-56; **FEL:** EDM, NY Hosp-Cornell Med Ctr, New York, NY 55-56; **FAP:** Assoc Clin Prof Med Cornell U; **SI:** *Anti-Aging Medicine; Preventive Medicine;* **HMO:** None

LANG: Fr, Sp, Ger, Itl; 🦽 🔁 🎦 A Few Days **VISA** 💳

Cunningham, Ward (MD)   IM   PCP
Mount Sinai Med Ctr
240 E 68th St; New York, NY 10021; (212) 737-8973; **BDCERT:** IM 76; **MS:** NYU Sch Med 71; **RES:** IM, Bellevue Hosp Ctr, New York, NY 71-72; IM, Bellevue Hosp Ctr, New York, NY 72-73; **FEL:** Immunology, Mem Sloan Kettering Cancer Ctr, New York, NY 72-76; Onc, Mem Sloan Kettering Cancer Ctr, New York, NY 72-76; **FAP:** Asst Clin Prof Mt Sinai Sch Med; **HOSP:** Beth Israel Med Ctr; **SI:** *Immunology; Allergy*

🆑 🔁 🎦 💲 A Few Days 💳 **VISA** 💳

Davidson, Morton (MD)   IM   PCP
Beth Israel Med Ctr
227 E 19th St Fl 5; New York, NY 10016; (212) 995-6896; **BDCERT:** IM 68; **MS:** U Chicago-Pritzker Sch Med 59; **RES:** IM, Bellevue Hosp Ctr, New York, NY 60-64; **FEL:** Inf, Bellevue Hosp Ctr, New York, NY 64-67; **FAP:** Assoc Prof Med NYU Sch Med; **HOSP:** Cabrini Med Ctr; **SI:** *HIV Infection & AIDS; Hepatitis;* **HMO:** Oxford Blue Cross & Blue Shield

LANG: Sp, Fr, Rus; 🦽 🈁 🆑 🔁 🈲 🎦 💲 ⓜ

Davis, Anne (MD)   IM
Bellevue Hosp Ctr
550 1st Ave; New York, NY 10016; (212) 263-6479; **BDCERT:** IM 58; Pul 66; **MS:** Columbia P&S 49; **RES:** IM, Bellevue Hosp Ctr, New York, NY 49-50; **FEL:** Pul, Columbia-Presbyterian Med Ctr, New York, NY 55-58; EDM, Bellevue Hosp Ctr, New York, NY 54-55; **FAP:** Assoc Prof of Clin Med NYU Sch Med; **HOSP:** New York University Med Ctr; **SI:** *Chronic Obstructive Lung Disease; Tuberculosis*

🔁 ⓜ ⓜ 1 Week

DeBellis, Robert H (MD)   IM   PCP
Columbia-Presbyterian Med Ctr
161 Ft Washington Ave; New York, NY 00032; (212) 305-5325; **MS:** Columbia P&S 58; **RES:** Jacobi Med Ctr, Bronx, NY 58-61; **FEL:** Columbia-Presbyterian Med Ctr, New York, NY 61-64; **SI:** *Breast Cancer; Lymphoma;* **HMO:** Aetna Hlth Plan

🦽 🔁 🈲 🎦 💲 ⓜ A Few Days

Dermksian, George (MD)   IM   PCP
St Luke's Roosevelt Hosp Ctr
925 Park Ave; New York, NY 10028; (212) 535-2620; **BDCERT:** IM 61; **MS:** Cornell U 54; **RES:** St Luke's Roosevelt Hosp Ctr, New York, NY 54-56; St Luke's Roosevelt Hosp Ctr, New York, NY 58-60; **FAP:** Clin Prof Med Columbia P&S; **SI:** *Cardiovascular Diseases;* **HMO:** None

LANG: Arm; 🔁 🎦 💲 ⓜ A Few Days

Devereux, Richard (MD)   IM
NY Hosp-Cornell Med Ctr
NY Hosp/Cornell Med Ctr—Int Med Dep't, 525 E 68th St; New York, NY 10021; (212) 746-4655; **BDCERT:** IM 74; **MS:** Univ Penn 71; **RES:** IM, NY Hosp-Cornell Med Ctr, New York, NY 71-74; **FEL:** Cv, Hosp of U Penn, Philadelphia, PA 74-76; **HMO:** Aetna Hlth Plan Blue Choice CIGNA Magnacare

🦽 🈲 💲 ⓜ 2-4 Weeks

Distenfeld, Ariel (MD)   IM
Cabrini Med Ctr
227 E 19th St Rm 238; New York, NY 10003; (212) 945-6082; **BDCERT:** IM 64; Hem 74; **MS:** NYU Sch Med 57; **RES:** IM, Bellevue Hosp Ctr, New York, NY 57-60; **FEL:** Hem, New York University Med Ctr, New York, NY 60-61; **FAP:** Assoc Clin Prof NYU Sch Med; **HOSP:** New York University Med Ctr; **SI:** *General Hematology;* **HMO:** Blue Choice Oxford Aetna-US Healthcare CIGNA GHI +

LANG: Heb; 🦽 🔁 🎦 💲 ⓜ ⓜ 1 Week

Drapkin, Arnold (MD)   IM **PCP**
Mount Sinai Med Ctr

1050 5th Ave; New York, NY 10028; (212) 289-0101; **BDCERT:** IM 62; **MS:** SUNY Syracuse 55; **RES:** IM, Jacobi Med Ctr, Bronx, NY 56-58; IM, Jacobi Med Ctr, Bronx, NY 59-60; **FEL:** Cv, Jacobi Med Ctr, Bronx, NY 58-59; **FAP:** Asst Clin Prof Med Mt Sinai Sch Med; **SI:** *Preventive Medicine; Diagnostic Problems*; **HMO:** None

LANG: Sp; 🦽 📷 🛏 A Few Days 💳 **VISA** 💳

Edelson, Henry (MD)   IM **PCP**
Lenox Hill Hosp

133 E 58th St 909; New York, NY 10022; (212) 593-9800; **BDCERT:** IM 89; **MS:** NYU Sch Med 84; **RES:** IM, Bellevue Hosp Ctr, New York, NY 87; **HMO:** Prucare Aetna Hlth Plan CIGNA Chubb GHI +

🦽 📷 🛏 💲 Mcr A Few Days **VISA** 💳 💳

Edsall, John (MD)   IM
Columbia-Presbyterian Med Ctr

161 Fort Washington Ave Rm311; New York, NY 10032; (212) 305-5261; **BDCERT:** IM 63; **MS:** England 48; **RES:** Kings College, Cambridge, England 48-52; Harefield Hosp, Middlesex, England; **FEL:** Chest, Bellevue Hosp Ctr, New York, NY 56-57; **FAP:** Clin Prof Med Columbia P&S; **SI:** *Asthma; Emphysema*

🦽 📷 📷 🛏 💲 A Few Days

El-Sadr, Wafaa (MD)   IM
Harlem Hosp Ctr

Harlem Hospital—Int Med, 506 Lenox Ave Rm 310; New York, NY 10037; (212) 939-2936; **BDCERT:** IM 86; **MS:** Egypt 74; **RES:** Columbia-Presbyterian Med Ctr, New York, NY; Inf, VA Med Ctr-Manh, New York, NY 79-80

Engel, Milton (MD)   IM
Mount Sinai Med Ctr

1036 Park Ave; New York, NY 10028; (212) 879-3200; **MS:** Switzerland 61; **RES:** Mount Sinai Med Ctr, New York, NY; **FEL:** Long Island Coll Hosp, Brooklyn, NY

Etingin, Orli (MD)   IM **PCP**
NY Hosp-Cornell Med Ctr

1315 York Ave; New York, NY 10021; (212) 746-2066; **BDCERT:** IM 84; **MS:** Albert Einstein Coll Med 80; **RES:** NY Hosp-Cornell Med Ctr, New York, NY 80-83; **FEL:** NY Hosp-Cornell Med Ctr, New York, NY 83-86; **HMO:** PHCS PHS

🦽 📷 📷 🛏 💲 Mcr 1 Week 💳 **VISA** 💳 💳

Faust, Michael (MD)   IM **PCP**
New York University Med Ctr

345 E 37th St; New York, NY 10016; (212) 986-3330; **BDCERT:** IM 81; Ge 83; **MS:** NYU Sch Med 78; **RES:** New York University Med Ctr, New York, NY 78-81; Bellevue Hosp Ctr, New York, NY 78-81; **FEL:** Ge, New York University Med Ctr, New York, NY 81-83; Bellevue Hosp Ctr, New York, NY 81-83

🦽 📷 📷 🛏 💲 Mcr A Few Days

Feltheimer, Seth (MD)   IM **PCP**
Columbia-Presbyterian Med Ctr

161 Ft Washington Ave Ste 535; New York, NY 10032; (212) 305-8669; **BDCERT:** IM 84; **MS:** Spain 81; **RES:** Med, Interfaith Med Ctr, Brooklyn, NY 81-84; **FEL:** Med, Columbia-Presbyterian Med Ctr, New York, NY; **FAP:** Assoc Clin Prof Columbia P&S; **SI:** *Preventive Medicine; Medical Problems in Surgery*; **HMO:** Oxford Aetna Hlth Plan CIGNA NYLCare Blue Choice +

LANG: Swa; 🦽 📷 📷 🛏 Mcr A Few Days 💳 **VISA** 💳

Feuer, Martin (MD)   IM **PCP**
Beth Israel Med Ctr

889 Lexington Ave; New York, NY 10021; (212) 744-5433; **BDCERT:** IM 66; **MS:** NYU Sch Med 59; **RES:** Mount Sinai Med Ctr, New York, NY 60-62; **FEL:** Pul, Montefiore Med Ctr, Bronx, NY 62-63; **SI:** *Bronchitis*; **HMO:** Blue Choice Oxford PHS United Healthcare

🦽 📷 📷 🛏 Mcr WC NFI Immediately **VISA**

Fiedler, Robert (MD)   IM
Mount Sinai Med Ctr
1175 Park Ave; New York, NY 10128; (212) 289-6500; **BDCERT:** IM 70; **MS:** Albert Einstein Coll Med 64; **RES:** IM, DC Gen Hosp, Washington, DC 65-66; IM, VA Med Ctr-Bronx, Bronx, NY 66-67; **FEL:** EDM, Mount Sinai Med Ctr, New York, NY 67-69; **FAP:** Assoc Clin Prof Mt Sinai Sch Med

Fisch, Morton (MD)   IM
Lenox Hill Hosp
800A 5th Ave 301; New York, NY 10021; (212) 755-7711; **BDCERT:** IM 67; **MS:** SUNY Hlth Sci Ctr 57; **RES:** Lenox Hill Hosp, New York, NY 60-63
[⌷] [▣] [✦] [▦] [⑊] 1 Week [▦] **VISA** ●

Fisher, Laura (MD)   IM   PCP
NY Hosp-Cornell Med Ctr
449 E 68th St 8; New York, NY 10021; (212) 717-5920; **BDCERT:** IM 87; **MS:** Brown U 84; **RES:** Inf, NY Hosp-Cornell Med Ctr, New York, NY 84-87; **FEL:** Inf, Mass Gen Hosp, Boston, MA 87-89; **SI:** Travel medicine; Lyme disease; **HMO:** United Healthcare CIGNA PHS Guardian
[⌷] [▣] [✦] [▦] [⑊] Immediately **VISA** ●

Fishman, Donald (MD)   IM   PCP
St Luke's Roosevelt Hosp Ctr
74 E 90th St; New York, NY 10128; (212) 369-8144; **BDCERT:** IM 76; Pul 78; **MS:** Univ Penn 73; **RES:** IM, U Mich Med Ctr, Ann Arbor, MI 73-76; **FEL:** Pul, New York University Med Ctr, New York, NY 76-78; Bellevue Hosp Ctr, New York, NY 76-78; **FAP:** Asst Clin Prof Columbia P&S; **HOSP:** Lenox Hill Hosp; **SI:** Asthma; Bronchoscopy; **HMO:** Oxford PHS Blue Choice Health Source PHCS +
[▣] [✦] [▦] [⑊] 1 Week **VISA** ●

Fried, Richard (MD)   IM   PCP
St Luke's Roosevelt Hosp Ctr
15 W 72nd St 1N; New York, NY 10023; (212) 580-4840; **BDCERT:** IM 72; Inf 74; **MS:** Columbia P&S 68; **RES:** St Luke's Roosevelt Hosp Ctr, New York, NY 68-72; **FEL:** Inf, Stanford Med Ctr, Stanford, CA 73-74; **FAP:** Assoc Clin Prof Med Columbia P&S; **SI:** Infections; Lyme Disease; **HMO:** Oxford CIGNA Blue Cross PHS +
[⌷] [▣] [✦] [▦] [⑊] [Mcr] A Few Days

Friedman, Jeffrey (MD)   IM   PCP
New York University Med Ctr
Murray Hill Medical Group PC, 317 E 34th St 1001; New York, NY 10016; (212) 726-7440; **BDCERT:** IM 86; **MS:** NYU Sch Med 83; **RES:** Bellevue Hosp Ctr, New York, NY 83-87; **FAP:** Asst Clin Prof IM NYU Sch Med; **HOSP:** Hosp For Joint Diseases; **SI:** Preventive Med; **HMO:** Oxford Aetna Hlth Plan CIGNA Metlife PHS +
LANG: Sp; [⌷] [●] [▣] [✦] [▦] [⑊] [Mcr] Immediately [▦] **VISA** ●

Gabriel, James (MD)   IM
St Luke's Roosevelt Hosp Ctr
425 W 59th St; New York, NY 10019; (212) 977-9600; **BDCERT:** IM 56; **MS:** Harvard Med Sch 49; **RES:** IM, VA Med Ctr-Brooklyn, Brooklyn, NY 50-53; **FEL:** Ge, VA Med Ctr-Brooklyn, Brooklyn, NY 53-55; **FAP:** Assoc Clin Prof Columbia P&S; **SI:** Endoscopy; **HMO:** Blue Choice Health Source CIGNA Independent Health Plan
LANG: Grk; [⌷] [▣] [✦] [▦] [⑊] [Mcr] 1 Week [▦] **VISA** ●

Gilbert, Richard (MD)   IM
Columbia-Presbyterian Med Ctr
NYU Medical Ctr, 530 1st Ave 3A; New York, NY 10016; (212) 263-7300; **BDCERT:** IM 72; Nep 76; **MS:** NYU Sch Med 58; **RES:** IM, New York University Med Ctr, New York, NY 69-72; Nep, Albert Einstein Med Ctr, Bronx, NY 74-76; **FEL:** Nep, Montefiore Med Ctr, Bronx, NY 76-77

Gitlow, Stanley (MD)   IM
Mount Sinai Med Ctr
1107 5th Ave; New York, NY 10128; (212) 722-5731; **BDCERT:** IM 57; **MS:** SUNY Hlth Sci Ctr 48; **RES:** Mount Sinai Med Ctr, New York, NY 48-49; Mount Sinai Med Ctr, New York, NY 51-52; **FEL:** Univ Hosp SUNY Bklyn, Brooklyn, NY 50-51; VA Med Ctr-Bronx, Bronx, NY 49-50; **FAP:** Clin Prof Med Mt Sinai Sch Med; **SI:** Addiction Medicine
[⌷] [▣] [▦] [⑊] A Few Days

Globus, David (MD)   IM   PCP
NY Hosp-Cornell Med Ctr

340 E 72nd St; New York, NY 10021; (212) 988-3838; **BDCERT:** IM 65; **MS:** Washington U, St Louis 54; **RES:** U of Alabama Hosp, Birmingham, AL 57-58; NY Hosp-Cornell Med Ctr, New York, NY 60-62; **FEL:** Nep, NY Hosp-Cornell Med Ctr, New York, NY 58-60; **FAP:** Assoc Clin Prof Med Cornell U

🔲 👥 🏥 💲   A Few Days

Goldstein, Marvin (MD)   IM   PCP
Mount Sinai Med Ctr

1225 Park Ave 1E; New York, NY 10128; (212) 410-7100; **BDCERT:** IM 64; Nep 76; **MS:** Med Coll Va 57; **RES:** IM, Mount Sinai Med Ctr, New York, NY 58-59; **FEL:** Nep, Mount Sinai Med Ctr, New York, NY 60-61; **FAP:** Clin Prof Med Mt Sinai Sch Med; **HOSP:** Beth Israel North; **SI:** *Hypertension;* **HMO:** Aetna-US Healthcare Blue Choice Oxford United Healthcare

LANG: Sp; ♿ 🔲 👥 🏥 💲 Mcr Mcd   Immediately

Goldstein, Paul (MD)   IM
St Vincents Hosp & Med Ctr NY

80 5th Ave Suite 1601; New York, NY 10011; (212) 645-8500; **BDCERT:** IM 85; **MS:** NY Med Coll 82; **RES:** St Vincents Hosp & Med Ctr NY, New York, NY

Goldstone, Jonas (MD)   IM   PCP
Lenox Hill Hosp

125 E 74th St; New York, NY 10021; (212) 879-3725; **BDCERT:** IM 62; Onc 75; **MS:** Harvard Med Sch 55; **RES:** Boston Med Ctr, Boston, MA 55-57; **FEL:** Hem, Cleveland Metro Gen Hosp, Cleveland, OH 59-61; **FAP:** Clin Prof Columbia P&S; **HOSP:** St Luke's Roosevelt Hosp Ctr; **SI:** *Breast Tumors; Hematologic Tumors;* **HMO:** Oxford CIGNA US Hlthcre

♿ 🔲 👥 🏥 💲 Mcr   1 Week

Goodrich, Charles (MD)   IM   PCP
NY Hosp-Cornell Med Ctr

51 E 73rd St Ste 2B; New York, NY 10021; (212) 628-0804; **BDCERT:** IM 59; PrM 59; **MS:** Harvard Med Sch 51; **RES:** Seattle VA Hosp, Seattle, WA 52-53; Bellevue Hosp Ctr, New York, NY 55-56; **FEL:** NY-Cornell, New York, NY 57-58; **SI:** *Preventive Medicine; Nutrition; Stress Management*

LANG: Fr, Sp; 🌙 🔲 👥 🏥 Mcr   2-4 Weeks *VISA* ⬤

Grayson, Martha (MD)   IM   PCP
St Vincents Hosp & Med Ctr NY

Medical Associates of Saints Vincents Hospital, 32 W 18th St; New York, NY 10011; (212) 647-6464; **BDCERT:** IM 82; **MS:** Albert Einstein Coll Med 79; **RES:** Montefiore Med Ctr, Bronx, NY 79-82; **FAP:** Assoc NY Med Coll; **SI:** *Preventive Medicine;* **HMO:** Oxford Aetna-US Healthcare PHS Prudential

♿ 🔲 🏥 💲 Mcr Mcd   2-4 Weeks 🟦 *VISA* ⬤

Greene, Jeffrey (MD)   IM   PCP
Bellevue Hosp Ctr

345 E 37th St 208; New York, NY 10016; (212) 682-2844; **BDCERT:** IM 79; Inf 82; **MS:** NYU Sch Med 76; **RES:** Bellevue Hosp Ctr, New York, NY 77-79; **FEL:** Inf, Bellevue Hosp Ctr, New York, NY 80-82; **FAP:** Assoc Clin Prof Med NYU Sch Med; **HOSP:** Univ Hosp SUNY Stony Brook; **SI:** *Infectious Disease; AIDS Medicine;* **HMO:** Empire Blue Cross & Shield Oxford CIGNA United Healthcare

♿ 🌙 🔲 👥 🏥 💲 Mcr   A Few Days

Grieco, Anthony (MD)   IM
New York University Med Ctr

530 1st Ave 4h; New York, NY 10016; (212) 263-7272; **BDCERT:** IM 68; Rad 44; **MS:** NYU Sch Med 63; **RES:** New York University Med Ctr, New York, NY 63-68; Bellevue Hosp Ctr, New York, NY 63-68; **HMO:** Oxford

♿

Halperin, Ira (MD)   **IM**
St Vincents Hosp & Med Ctr NY

2 5th Ave 9; New York, NY 10011; (212) 254-
5940; **BDCERT:** IM 70; **MS:** NYU Sch Med 62; **RES:**
St Vincents Hosp & Med Ctr NY, New York, NY 62-
66; **FEL:** Hem, Mount Sinai Med Ctr, New York, NY
68-69; **SI:** *Leukemia; Myeloproliferative Disorder*;
HMO: Oxford PHS PHCS Multiplan Cost Care +

LANG: Sp; 🔲 🔲 🔲 🔲 A Few Days

Hart, Catherine (MD)   **IM**   **PCP**
NY Hosp-Cornell Med Ctr

310 E 72th St 2; New York, NY 10021; (212) 396-
3272; **BDCERT:** IM 84; **MS:** Univ Penn 80; **RES:** NY
Hosp-Cornell Med Ctr, New York, NY 80-83; **FEL:**
Inf, NY Hosp-Cornell Med Ctr, New York, NY 83-85

🔲 🔲 🔲 🔲 🔲 A Few Days 🔲 **VISA**

Hembree, Wylie (MD)   **IM**
Columbia-Presbyterian Med Ctr

161 Fort Washington Ave; New York, NY 10032;
(212) 305-5549; **BDCERT:** IM 72; EDM 73; **MS:**
Washington U, St Louis 64; **RES:** Med, Beth Israel
Med Ctr, Boston, MA 64-66; Med, Columbia-
Presbyterian Med Ctr, New York, NY 70-71; **FEL:**
Nat Cancer Inst, Bethesda, MD 66-68; Nat Cancer
Inst, Bethesda, MD 68-70; **FAP:** Assoc Clin Prof
Med Columbia P&S; **SI:** *Andrology*; **HMO:** Empire
Blue Cross & Shield Prudential

🔲 🔲 🔲 🔲 🔲 2-4 Weeks

Hoffman, Ira (MD)   **IM**   **PCP**
Lenox Hill Hosp

800 5th Ave A301; New York, NY 10021; (212)
755-7711; **BDCERT:** IM 69; **MS:** SUNY Downstate
56; **RES:** Long Island Coll Hosp, Brooklyn, NY 56-
60; Lenox Hill Hosp, New York, NY 56; **FAP:** Clin
Prof NYU Sch Med

🔲 🔲 🔲 🔲 🔲 🔲 Immediately **VISA** 🔲

Horbar, Gary (MD)   **IM**   **PCP**
Lenox Hill Hosp

6 E 85th St; New York, NY 10028; (212) 570-
9119; **BDCERT:** IM 79; **MS:** NY Med Coll 76; **RES:**
IM, Lenox Hill Hosp, New York, NY 76-80; **FAP:**
Asst Clin Prof NYU Sch Med; **HMO:** Oxford Health
Source

🔲 🔲 🔲 🔲 A Few Days

Houghton, Alan (MD)   **IM**   **PCP**
Mem Sloan Kettering Cancer Ctr

1275 York Ave; New York, NY 10021; (212) 639-
7595; **BDCERT:** IM 77; **MS:** U Conn Sch Med 74;
RES: Thomas Jefferson U Hosp, Philadelphia, PA
75; U Conn Hlth Ctr, Farmington, CT 76; **FEL:** Onc,
Mem Sloan Kettering Cancer Ctr, New York, NY;
FAP: Prof Cornell U; **SI:** *Melanoma*

🔲 🔲 🔲 🔲 A Few Days 🔲 **VISA** 🔲 🔲

Januzzi, James (MD)   **IM**   **PCP**
St Vincents Hosp & Med Ctr NY

29 Washington Sq West; New York, NY 10011;
(212) 982-5551; **BDCERT:** IM 72; Ge 77; **MS:** NY
Med Coll 66; **RES:** St Vincents Hosp & Med Ctr NY,
New York, NY 70-72; **FAP:** Asst Prof of Clin Med
NY Med Coll; **SI:** *Gastroenterology*

LANG: Itl; 🔲 🔲 🔲 🔲 🔲 🔲 2-4 Weeks

Johnson, Warren (MD)   **IM**
NY Hosp-Cornell Med Ctr

Division of International Medicine & Infectious
Disease, 1300 York Ave A431; New York, NY
10021; (212) 746-3620; **BDCERT:** IM 71; Inf 74;
MS: Columbia P&S 62; **RES:** NY Hosp-Cornell Med
Ctr, New York, NY 62-64; NY Hosp-Cornell Med
Ctr, New York, NY 68-69; **FEL:** Inf, NY Hosp-
Cornell Med Ctr, New York, NY 66-68; **FAP:** Prof
Cornell U

🔲 🔲 🔲 🔲 🔲 1 Week 🔲 **VISA**

Kahn, Martin (MD)   **IM**
NY Hosp-Cornell Med Ctr

530 1st Ave Ste 4H; New York, NY 10016; (212)
263-7228; **BDCERT:** IM 70; Cv 75; **MS:** NYU Sch
Med 63; **RES:** IM, Bellevue Hosp Ctr, New York, NY
64-65; IM, Bellevue Hosp Ctr, New York, NY 67-
70; **FEL:** Cv, Bellevue Hosp Ctr, New York, NY 70-
72; **FAP:** Prof of Clin Med NYU Sch Med; **HOSP:**
United Hosp Med Ctr

Kairam, Indira (MD)   IM
St Clare's Hosp & Health Ctr
945 W End Ave 1 D; New York, NY 10023; (212) 865-7355; **BDCERT:** IM 78; **MS:** India 73; **RES:** IM, St Clare's Hosp & Health Ctr, New York, NY; **FEL:** Ge, St Clare's Hosp & Health Ctr, New York, NY 78-80; **HOSP:** Roosevelt Hosp; **SI:** *Colon Cancer; Hepatitis*

LANG: Srb, Hin; 🔲 🔲 🔲 🔲 🔲 🔲 1 Week

Kaminsky, Donald (MD)   IM
Beth Israel Med Ctr
67 Irving Pl; New York, NY 10003; (212) 353-8787; **BDCERT:** IM 82; **MS:** Geo Wash U Sch Med 79; **RES:** IM, Beth Israel Med Ctr, New York, NY; **FEL:** Inf, Beth Israel Med Ctr, New York, NY; **SI:** *AIDS; Tropical Medicine*

🔲 🔲 🔲 🔲 🔲 🔲 🔲 🔲 A Few Days 🔲 **VISA** 🔲 🔲

Karp, Adam (MD)   IM   PCP
Hosp For Joint Diseases
301 E 17th St; New York, NY 10003; (212) 598-6738; **BDCERT:** IM 90; **MS:** Albert Einstein Coll Med 87; **RES:** IM, Maimonides Med Ctr, Brooklyn, NY 87-90; **FEL:** Ger, New York University Med Ctr, New York, NY 90-92; **HOSP:** New York University Med Ctr; **HMO:** Oxford Chubb Empire Blue Cross & Shield

🔲 🔲 🔲 🔲 🔲 Immediately 🔲 **VISA** 🔲 🔲

Kaufman, Cindy (MD)   IM
Englewood Hosp & Med Ctr
227 Madison St 427; New York, NY 10002; (212) 238-7448; **BDCERT:** IM 90; **MS:** NYU Sch Med 87; **RES:** IM, Mt Sinai Med Ctr, New York, NY 87-90; **FEL:** EDM, NYU Med Ctr, New York, NY 90; **HMO:** Blue Cross & Blue Shield

Kaufman, David Lyons (MD) IM   PCP
St Vincents Hosp & Med Ctr NY
314 W 14th St Fl 5; New York, NY 10014; (212) 620-0144; **BDCERT:** IM 80; **MS:** NY Med Coll 77; **RES:** St Vincents Hosp & Med Ctr NY, New York, NY 77-80; **FAP:** Asst Prof Med NY Med Coll; **SI:** *HIV Medicine; Infectious Diseases*; **HMO:** Oxford Prucare United Healthcare Empire Blue Cross & Shield PHCS +

LANG: Sp, Fr; 🔲 🔲 🔲 🔲 🔲 🔲 🔲 A Few Days

Kennedy, James (MD)   IM   PCP
New York University Med Ctr
650 1st Ave; New York, NY 10016; (212) 689-7768; **BDCERT:** IM 78; **MS:** NYU Sch Med 72; **RES:** Bellevue Hosp Ctr, New York, NY 73-77; **HMO:** United Healthcare Oxford PHS Prucare Health Source +

🔲 🔲 🔲 🔲 1 Week 🔲 **VISA** 🔲

Kennish, Arthur (MD)   IM   PCP
Mount Sinai Med Ctr
108 E 96th St; New York, NY 10128; (212) 410-6610; **BDCERT:** IM 80; Cv 83; **MS:** Albert Einstein Coll Med 77; **RES:** Mount Sinai Med Ctr, New York, NY 77-80; **FEL:** Cv, Mount Sinai Med Ctr, New York, NY 80-82; **HOSP:** Beth Israel North; **SI:** *Mitral Valve Prolapse*; **HMO:** Oxford United Healthcare Blue Choice Aetna Hlth Plan PHS +

LANG: Sp; 🔲 🔲 🔲 🔲 🔲 🔲 2-4 Weeks 🔲 **VISA** 🔲 🔲

Kimball, Annetta (MD)   IM
St Luke's Roosevelt Hosp Ctr
30 E 60th St 508; New York, NY 10022; (212) 371-8900; **BDCERT:** IM 72; Ge 73; **MS:** Boston U 68; **RES:** St Luke's Roosevelt Hosp Ctr, New York, NY 68-70; Mount Sinai Med Ctr, New York, NY 70-71; **FEL:** Ge, Mount Sinai Med Ctr, New York, NY 71-73; **SI:** *Liver Diseases; Inflammatory Bowel Disease*

🔲 🔲 🔲 🔲 🔲 2-4 Weeks

Kinn, Mark (MD)   IM   PCP
St Luke's Roosevelt Hosp Ctr

240 Central Park South 2P; New York, NY 10019; (212) 245-8910; **BDCERT:** IM 80; **MS:** NYU Sch Med 77; **RES:** IM, St Luke's Roosevelt Hosp Ctr, New York, NY 77-80; **FAP:** Asst Clin Prof Med Columbia P&S; **HMO:** Aetna Hlth Plan United Healthcare Oxford PHCS Prucare +

LANG: Fr; ⟨symbols⟩ Immediately ⟨symbol⟩

Kurtz, Robert C (MD)   IM
Mem Sloan Kettering Cancer Ctr

1275 York Ave; New York, NY 10021; (212) 639-7620; **BDCERT:** IM 71; Ge 77; **MS:** Jefferson Med Coll 68; **RES:** NY Hosp-Cornell Med Ctr, New York, NY 71; **FEL:** NY Hosp-Cornell Med Ctr, New York, NY 73; **FAP:** Prof Cornell U; **SI:** *Hepatobiliary Diseases; GI Oncology*

LANG: Sp; ⟨symbols⟩ A Few Days

Lamm, Steven (MD)   IM   PCP
New York University Med Ctr

12 E 86th St; New York, NY 10028; (212) 988-1146; **BDCERT:** IM 77; **MS:** NYU Sch Med 74; **RES:** IM, New York University Med Ctr, New York, NY 74-78; **FEL:** New York University Med Ctr, New York, NY 78; **FAP:** Asst Clin Prof Med NYU Sch Med; **HOSP:** Lenox Hill Hosp; **SI:** *Sexual Dysfunction; Obesity;* **HMO:** Oxford Multiplan United Healthcare

LANG: Sp, Itl, Pol; ⟨symbols⟩ A Few Days
VISA ⟨symbol⟩

Langelier, Carolyn (MD)   IM   PCP
New York University Med Ctr

317 E 34th St 1001; New York, NY 10016; (212) 726-7424; **BDCERT:** IM 93; **MS:** Cornell U 89; **RES:** New York University Med Ctr, New York, NY 89-92; **SI:** *Preventive Health Care; Travel Medicine;* **HMO:** Oxford Aetna Hlth Plan CIGNA Health Source PHS +

LANG: Sp, Prt; ⟨symbols⟩ Immediately
⟨symbol⟩ *VISA* ⟨symbol⟩

Lax, James (MD)   IM   PCP
St Luke's Roosevelt Hosp Ctr

160 E 72nd St; New York, NY 10021; (212) 988-5740; **BDCERT:** IM 84; Ge 87; **MS:** NYU Sch Med 81; **RES:** St Luke's Roosevelt Hosp Ctr, New York, NY; **FEL:** St Luke's Roosevelt Hosp Ctr, New York, NY; **FAP:** Assoc Columbia P&S; **HOSP:** Beth Israel Med Ctr; **SI:** *Liver Disease; Colitis;* **HMO:** Aetna Hlth Plan Chubb Blue Choice United Healthcare Oxford +

LANG: Sp, Fr; ⟨symbols⟩ 1 Week

Lebowitz, Arthur (MD)   IM   PCP
New York University Med Ctr

Concorde Medical Group, 650 1st Ave Fl 3S; New York, NY 10016; (212) 725-1474; **BDCERT:** IM 70; **MS:** NYU Sch Med 65; **RES:** NC Mem Hosp, Chapel Hill, NC 65-67; Bellevue Hosp Ctr, New York, NY 67-68; **FEL:** Inf, Bellevue Hosp Ctr, New York, NY 68-70; **FAP:** Asst Clin Prof Med NYU Sch Med; **HOSP:** Bellevue Hosp Ctr; **SI:** *Women's Health Issues*

LANG: Sp; ⟨symbols⟩ 2-4 Weeks ⟨symbol⟩ *VISA* ⟨symbol⟩

Lee, Marjorie (MD)   IM   PCP
Cabrini Med Ctr

222 E 19th St 1E; New York, NY 10003; (212) 533-1185; **BDCERT:** IM 76; Pul 78; **MS:** SUNY Hlth Sci Ctr 73; **RES:** Kaiser Hosp, San Francisco, CA 73-74; Kaiser Hosp, Oakland, CA 74-76; **FEL:** Cabrini Med Ctr, New York, NY 76-77; Yale-New Haven Hosp, New Haven, CT 77-79; **SI:** *Asthma;* **HMO:** Oxford United Healthcare Empire Blue Choice Magnacare PHS +

LANG: Can, Man, Sp; ⟨symbols⟩ A Few Days

Guide to symbols and abbreviations can be found on pages 110-113.

219

Legato, Marianne J (MD)   **IM**   `PCP`
Columbia-Presbyterian Med Ctr

962 Park Ave; New York, NY 10028; (212) 737-5663; **BDCERT:** IM 93; **MS:** NYU Sch Med 62; **RES:** ObG, Bellevue Hosp Ctr, New York, NY 62-64; ObG, Columbia-Presbyterian Med Ctr, New York, NY 64-65; **FEL:** Cv, Columbia-Presbyterian Med Ctr, New York, NY 65-68; St Luke's Roosevelt Hosp Ctr, New York, NY 65-68; **FAP:** Clin Instr NYU Sch Med; **HOSP:** St Luke's Roosevelt Hosp Ctr; **SI:** *Menopause & Osteoporosis; Fibroids, OB Care & Genetics;* **HMO:** None

LANG: Fr; 🚻 🈳 🔲 🔲 🎬 🅢 🔲 A Few Days **VISA** 🔲

Leifer, Edgar (MD & PhD)   **IM**   `PCP`
Columbia-Presbyterian Med Ctr

161 Ft Washington Ave; New York, NY 10032; (212) 305-5307; **BDCERT:** IM 53; **MS:** Columbia P&S 46; **RES:** Columbia-Presbyterian Med Ctr, New York, NY 46-47; Columbia-Presbyterian Med Ctr, New York, NY 49-51; **FAP:** Prof of Clin Med Columbia P&S

🚻 🔲 🎬 🔲 2-4 Weeks

Levere, Richard (MD)   **IM**
Rockefeller Univ Hosp

Rockefeller University Hospital, 1230 York Ave; New York, NY 10021; (212) 327-8762; **BDCERT:** IM 63; **MS:** SUNY Hlth Sci Ctr 56; **RES:** Bellevue Hosp Ctr, New York, NY 56-58; Kings County Hosp Ctr, Brooklyn, NY 60-61; **FEL:** SUNY Hlth Sci Ctr, Brooklyn, NY 61-63; Rockefeller Univ Hosp, New York, NY 63-65; **FAP:** Prof Med NYU Sch Med; **HOSP:** New York University Med Ctr; **SI:** *Porphyria;* **HMO:** Oxford Aetna Hlth Plan US Hlthcre HIP Network CIGNA

🚻 🔲 🎬 🔲 🔲 2-4 Weeks

Levine, Randy (MD)   **IM**
St Luke's Roosevelt Hosp Ctr

University Med Practice Assoc, 25 Central Park West 1Z; New York, NY 10019; (212) 397-7266; **BDCERT:** IM 82; **MS:** SUNY Buffalo 79; **RES:** Montefiore Med Ctr, Bronx, NY 79-82; **FEL:** Hem, Montefiore Med Ctr, Bronx, NY; **HOSP:** Lenox Hill Hosp; **SI:** *Hematological Malignancies; AIDS Related Malignancies;* **HMO:** Oxford Blue Choice Aetna Hlth Plan PHS PHCS +

🔲 🔲 🎬 🅢 🔲 1 Week

Lewin, Margaret (MD)   **IM**   `PCP`
Lenox Hill Hosp

114 E 72nd St 1E; New York, NY 10021; (212) 737-7910; **BDCERT:** IM 80; Onc 84; **MS:** Case West Res U 77; **RES:** IM, NY Hosp-Cornell Med Ctr, New York, NY 77-80; **FEL:** Hem, NY Hosp-Cornell Med Ctr, New York, NY 80-83; Onc, NY Hosp-Cornell Med Ctr, New York, NY 80-83; **FAP:** Asst Clin Prof Cornell U; **HOSP:** NY Hosp-Cornell Med Ctr; **SI:** *Preventive Health Care; Breast Cancer;* **HMO:** Oxford Chubb Aetna Hlth Plan

🚻 🔲 🔲 🎬 🅢 🔲 Immediately 🔲 **VISA** 🔲

Lewin, Sharon (MD)   **IM**   `PCP`
St Luke's Roosevelt Hosp Ctr

139 W 82nd St 1C; New York, NY 10024; (212) 496-7200; **BDCERT:** IM 78; Inf 80; **MS:** Canada 75; **RES:** Wadsworth VA Hosp, Los Angeles, CA 75-78; **FEL:** Bellevue Hosp Ctr, New York, NY 78-80; **SI:** *Travel Medicine; HIV;* **HMO:** Oxford Blue Choice

🔲 🔲 🎬 🅢 🔲 2-4 Weeks 🔲

Liguori, Michael (MD)   **IM**   `PCP`
St Vincents Hosp & Med Ctr NY

80 5th Ave 1601; New York, NY 10011; (212) 645-8500; **BDCERT:** IM 85; **MS:** Mt Sinai Sch Med 81; **RES:** St Vincents Hosp & Med Ctr NY, New York, NY 81-84; **SI:** *HIV Medicine; Geriatrics;* **HMO:** Oxford Blue Choice PHS

🚻 🔲 🔲 🅢 2-4 Weeks 🔲 **VISA** 🔲

Lipton, Mark (MD)　　　　**IM**　**PCP**
New York University Med Ctr
New York Medical Associates, 907 5th Ave; New
York, NY 10021; (212) 570-2077; **BDCERT:** IM
81; Cv 85; **MS:** NYU Sch Med 78; **RES:** Bellevue
Hosp Ctr, New York, NY 78-81; **FEL:** Cv, New York
University Med Ctr, New York, NY 83-85; **HOSP:**
Beth Israel Med Ctr; **SI:** *Preventive Cardiology;*
Coronary Heart Disease; **HMO:** Oxford CIGNA PHS
United Healthcare Prudential +
🄲 🄰 🅈 🎟 🅂 🄼𝒸𝓇　A Few Days

Logan, Bruce (MD)　　　　**IM**　**PCP**
NYU Downtown Hosp
19 Beekman St Fl 6; New York, NY 10038; (212)
608-6634; **BDCERT:** IM 78; **MS:** Columbia P&S 71;
RES: Harlem Hosp Ctr, New York, NY 72-73; **FAP:**
Assoc Clin Prof NYU Sch Med; **SI:** *Cholesterol;*
Preventative Medicine; **HMO:** Oxford
🅰 🄲 🄰 🅈 🎟 🅂 🄼𝒸𝓇　1 Week 💳 **VISA** 💳

Lupiano, John (MD)　　　　**IM**　**PCP**
St Clare's Hosp & Health Ctr
57 W 57th St; New York, NY 10019; (212) 330-
0609; **BDCERT:** IM 87; **MS:** SUNY Buffalo 84; **RES:**
IM, NY Hosp-Cornell-Med Ctr, New York, NY 85-
87; **HOSP:** St Luke's Roosevelt Hosp Ctr; **HMO:** Blue
Cross & Blue Shield Oxford
🄲 🄰 🅈 🎟 🅂 🄼𝒸𝓇　Immediately

Mackenzie, C Ronald (MD)　**IM**　**PCP**
Hosp For Special Surgery
535 E 70th St; New York, NY 10021; (212) 606-
1669; **BDCERT:** IM 81; Rhu 81; **MS:** U Calgary 77;
RES: FP, Calgary Gen Hosp, Calgary,Canada 78;
IM, U Manitoba, Winnipeg, Canada; **FEL:** Rhu, NY
Hosp-Cornell Med Ctr, New York, NY 81-83; Hosp
For Special Surgery, New York, NY 88-92; **FAP:**
Assoc Prof of Clin Med Cornell U; **HOSP:** NY Hosp-
Cornell Med Ctr
LANG: Sp; 🅰 🄰 🅈 🎟 🅂 🄼𝒸𝓇　4+ Weeks

Manson, Aaron (MD)　　　　**IM**
Columbia-Presbyterian Med Ctr
ColumbiaPresbyterian Hospital, 161 Ft
Washington Ave Rm 540; New York, NY 10032;
(212) 305-3804; **BDCERT:** AM 79; **MS:** Univ Penn
76; **RES:** Syracuse,; **FAP:** Assoc Clin Prof Med
Columbia P&S
🅰 🅈 🎟 🅂

Markenson, Joseph (MD)　　**IM**
NY Hosp-Cornell Med Ctr
535 E 70th St 303; New York, NY 10021; (212)
606-1261; **BDCERT:** IM 76; Rhu 78; **MS:** SUNY
Downstate 70; **RES:** NY Hosp-Cornell Med Ctr, New
York, NY 73-75; **FEL:** Rhu, Hosp For Special
Surgery, New York, NY 75-76; **FAP:** Clin Prof Med
Cornell U; **HOSP:** Hosp For Special Surgery; **HMO:**
Aetna Hlth Plan Blue Cross & Blue Shield CIGNA
🅰 🄰 🎟 🅂 🄼𝒸𝓇 🅆𝒸 🄽𝒻𝒾

Marsh Jr, Franklin (MD)　**IM**　**PCP**
NY Hosp-Cornell Med Ctr
342 E 67th St; New York, NY 10021; (212) 288-
8820; **BDCERT:** IM 81; Ge 85; **MS:** SUNY Buffalo
78; **RES:** IM, Harlem Hosp Ctr, New York, NY 78-
82; **FEL:** Ge, NY Hosp-Cornell Med Ctr, New York,
NY 92-95; **FAP:** Asst Clin Instr Cornell U; **HOSP:**
Beth Israel Med Ctr; **SI:** *Colon Cancer Screening;*
Digestive Disorders; **HMO:** NYLCare United
Healthcare PHCS Oxford CIGNA +
🅰 🆂🅄 🄲 🄰 🅈 🎟 🅂 🄼𝒸𝓇 🄼𝒸𝒹　1 Week

Matta, Raymond (MD)　　　**IM**
Mount Sinai Med Ctr
1120 Park Ave; New York, NY 10128; (212) 410-
5800; **BDCERT:** IM 73; Cv 75; **MS:** Univ Pittsburgh
69; **RES:** IM, Mass Gen Hosp, Boston, MA 69-71;
Cv, Peter Bent Brigham Hosp, Boston, MA 73-75;
FAP: Assoc Prof Mt Sinai Sch Med

Mayer, Lloyd (MD)　　　　**IM**
Mount Sinai Med Ctr
1 Gustave Levy Pl; New York, NY 10029; (212)
241-0764; **BDCERT:** IM 79; Ge 81; **MS:** Mt Sinai
Sch Med 76; **RES:** Bellevue Hosp Ctr, New York, NY
76-79; **FEL:** Mount Sinai Med Ctr, New York, NY
🅰 🄰 🎟 🅂 🄼𝒸𝓇　1 Week 💳 **VISA** 💳 💳

Mernick, Mitchel (MD)   IM   PCP
Beth Israel Med Ctr

Park Ave Medical & Nutrition, PC, 10 E 38th St Fl 4; New York, NY 10016; (212) 686-0901; **BDCERT:** IM 85; **MS:** Mt Sinai Sch Med 82; **RES:** IM, Beth Israel Med Ctr, New York, NY 82-85; **FEL:** Onc, Beth Israel Med Ctr, New York, NY 85-87; **FAP:** Clin Instr Albert Einstein Coll Med; **HOSP:** Cabrini Med Ctr; *SI: Wellness-Nutrition Cancer; Complementary Medicine;* **HMO:** Oxford United Healthcare Aetna-US Healthcare Empire Blue Choice +

LANG: Heb, Sp, Rus, Can, Yd; ⛄ 🅂🅄 🌙 📷 🔆 🎞 💲 🄼🄲 🅆🄲 🅽🄵🄵 Immediately ▦ *VISA* ⬤

Meyer, Richard (MD)   IM   PCP
Mount Sinai Med Ctr

1111 Park Ave; New York, NY 10128; (212) 427-7700; **BDCERT:** IM 75; Hem 77; **MS:** Mt Sinai Sch Med 72; **RES:** IM, Mount Sinai Med Ctr, New York, NY 72-75; **FEL:** Onc, Mount Sinai Med Ctr, New York, NY 78; Hem, Mount Sinai Med Ctr, New York, NY 75-77; **FAP:** Assoc Clin Prof Mt Sinai Sch Med; *SI: Leukemia; Head and Neck Malignancy;* **HMO:** Oxford Blue Choice Aetna Hlth Plan PHS Vytra +

⛄ 📷 🔆 🎞 💲 🄼🄲 A Few Days *VISA* ⬤

Midoneck, Shari (MD)   IM
NY Hosp-Cornell Med Ctr

1315 York Ave; New York, NY 10021; (212) 746-2088; **BDCERT:** IM 92; Inf 94; **MS:** Cornell U 89; **RES:** NY Hosp-Cornell Med Ctr, New York, NY 90-92; *SI: Infectious Diseases;* **HMO:** Oxford Blue Cross & Blue Shield Blue Choice Multiplan PHS

⛄ 🎞 🄼🄲 2-4 Weeks *VISA* ⬤

Milano, Andrew (MD)   IM
New York University Med Ctr

NYU Medical Center, 530 1st Ave 4K; New York, NY 10016; (212) 263-7483; **BDCERT:** IM 70; Ge 72; **MS:** NYU Sch Med 64; **RES:** IM, Bellevue Hosp Ctr, New York, NY 64-67; **FEL:** Ge, Bellevue Hosp Ctr, New York, NY 67-68; **FAP:** Clin Prof Med NYU Sch Med; *SI: GI Diseases; Endoscopy;* **HMO:** Oxford Metlife Chubb

⛄ 📷 🎞 💲 Immediately

Minkowitz, Susan (MD)   IM   PCP
St Vincents Hosp & Med Ctr NY

260 E Broadway; New York, NY 10028; (212) 475-4093; **BDCERT:** IM 88; Pul 90; **MS:** NY Med Coll 84; **RES:** IM, Metropolitan Hosp Ctr, New York, NY 84-87; **FEL:** Pul, Montefiore Med Ctr, Bronx, NY 87-89; **FAP:** Asst. Prof Med NYU Sch Med; *SI: Asthma; Emphysema;* **HMO:** Oxford CIGNA Blue Choice US Hlthcre

LANG: Sp; ⛄ 🅂🅄 🌙 📷 🔆 🎞 💲 🄼🄲 🄼🄳 🅽🄵🄵 A Few Days

Mirsky, Stanley (MD)   IM   PCP
Lenox Hill Hosp

4 E 70th St 1A; New York, NY 10021; (212) 861-4224; **BDCERT:** IM 65; **MS:** Northwestern U 55; **RES:** Joslin Cilinic, Boston, MA 57-58; Mount Sinai Med Ctr, New York, NY 58-59; **HOSP:** Mount Sinai Med Ctr; *SI: Diabetes;* **HMO:** Blue Cross & Blue Shield Metlife

LANG: Sp, Ger; ⛄ 📷 🔆 🎞 🄼🄲 A Few Days

Mullen, Michael (MD)   IM   PCP
Cabrini Med Ctr

232 E 20th St; New York, NY 10003; (212) 995-6904; **BDCERT:** IM 85; Inf 86; **MS:** Spain 81; **RES:** Jewish Hosp Med Ctr, Brooklyn, NY 81-84; **FEL:** Inf, Cabrini Med Ctr, New York, NY 84-86; **HOSP:** Beth Israel Med Ctr; **HMO:** Blue Choice Oxford PHS

⛄ 🌙 📷 🔆 🎞 🄼🄲 🄼🄳 A Few Days

Nash, Thomas (MD)   IM   PCP
NY Hosp-Cornell Med Ctr

310 E 72nd St; New York, NY 10021; (212) 734-6612; **BDCERT:** Pul 85; Inf 84; **MS:** NYU Sch Med 78; **RES:** NY Hosp-Cornell Med Ctr, New York, NY; **FEL:** Inf, NY Hosp-Cornell Med Ctr, New York, NY; Pul, Mem Sloan Kettering Cancer Ctr, New York, NY; *SI: Asthma; Lung Infections*

⛄ 📷 🔆 🎞 💲 A Few Days ▦ *VISA* ⬤

Nelson, Deena (MD) IM **PCP**
Mem Sloan Kettering Cancer Ctr

635 Madison Ave; New York, NY 10022; (212) 857-4670; **BDCERT:** IM 80; **MS:** Albert Einstein Coll Med 77; **RES:** NY Hosp-Cornell Med Ctr, New York, NY 77-79; Barnes Hosp, St Louis, MO 79-80; **HOSP:** NY Hosp-Cornell Med Ctr

LANG: Sp; 🔲 🔲 🔲 🔲 1 Week ▦ **VISA** ●

Nydick, Martin (MD) IM **PCP**
NY Hosp-Cornell Med Ctr

475 E 72nd St L2; New York, NY 10021; (212) 249-1260; **BDCERT:** IM 65; **MS:** Columbia P&S 57; **RES:** IM, Bellevue Hosp Ctr, New York, NY 64-65; **FEL:** EDM, Nat Inst Health, Bethesda, MD 60-62; U WA Med Ctr, Seattle, WA 62-64; **HOSP:** Hosp For Special Surgery

🔲 🔲 🔲 🔲 🔲 🔲 🔲 Immediately ▦

Orsher, Stuart (MD) IM **PCP**
Lenox Hill Hosp

9 E 79th St; New York, NY 10021; (212) 535-7763; **BDCERT:** IM 83; **MS:** Hahnemann U 75; **RES:** Lenox Hill Hosp, New York, NY 75-78; **HOSP:** Beth Israel North

🔲 🔲 🔲 🔲 **VISA** ●

Padilla, Maria (MD) IM
Mount Sinai Med Ctr

PO Box 1232; New York, NY 10029; (212) 241-5656; **BDCERT:** IM 78; **MS:** Mt Sinai Sch Med 75; **RES:** IM, Mount Sinai Med Ctr, New York, NY 83-86; **FEL:** Pul, Mount Sinai Med Ctr, New York, NY 86-88; Pul, Mount Sinai Med Ctr, New York, NY 88-90; *SI: Chronic and End-Stage Disease; Lung Transplantation;* **HMO:** Aetna Hlth Plan PHS Beech Street Oxford PHCS +

LANG: Sp, Fr; 🔲 🔲 🔲 🔲 🔲 🔲 2-4 Weeks ▦ **VISA** ●

Perla, Elliott (MD) IM **PCP**
Metropolitan Hosp Ctr

Metropolitan Hosp CtrDept of Med, 1901 1st Ave; New York, NY 10029; (212) 423-6771; **BDCERT:** IM 77; Pul 80; **MS:** NY Med Coll 74; **RES:** IM, Mount Sinai Med Ctr, New York, NY 74-77; **FEL:** Pul, Metropolitan Hosp Ctr, New York, NY 77-79; **FAP:** Assoc Prof of Clin Med NY Med Coll; *SI: Asthma*

🔲 🔲 🔲 🔲 A Few Days

Perskin, Michael (MD) IM **PCP**
New York University Med Ctr

135 E 37th St; New York, NY 10016; (212) 679-1410; **BDCERT:** IM 89; **MS:** Brown U 86; **RES:** St Luke's Roosevelt Hosp Ctr, New York, NY 86-89; **FEL:** Ger, New York University Med Ctr, New York, NY; **HOSP:** Hosp For Joint Diseases; *SI: Geriatrics;* **HMO:** Oxford Aetna Hlth Plan Chubb

🔲 🔲 🔲 🔲 🔲 🔲 A Few Days ▦ **VISA** ● ●

Postley, John E (MD) IM **PCP**
Columbia-Presbyterian Med Ctr

635 Madison Ave; New York, NY 10022; (212) 317-4646; **BDCERT:** IM 73; **MS:** Columbia P&S 68; **RES:** Columbia-Presbyterian Med Ctr, New York, NY 68-69; Columbia-Presbyterian Med Ctr, New York, NY 71-73; **FAP:** Asst Clin Prof Columbia P&S; **HMO:** None

🔲 🔲 🔲 🔲 🔲 2-4 Weeks **VISA**

Primack, Marshall (MD) IM
Columbia-Presbyterian Med Ctr

101 Central Park West; New York, NY 10023; (212) 769-2570; **BDCERT:** EDM 72; IM 72; **MS:** Johns Hopkins U 65; **RES:** Med, Bellevue Hosp Ctr, New York, NY 66-68; **FEL:** EDM, Columbia-Presbyterian Med Ctr, New York, NY 68-71; **FAP:** Asst Prof of Clin Med Columbia P&S; **HOSP:** St Luke's Roosevelt Hosp Ctr

LANG: Sp; 🔲 🔲 🔲 🔲 🔲 🔲 1 Week

Racanelli, Joseph (MD)   IM   PCP
Beth Israel Med Ctr

1107 Park Ave; New York, NY 10128; (212) 876-4070; **MS:** Mexico 75; **RES:** Med, Winthrop Univ Hosp, Mineola, NY 77-81; **HOSP:** Cabrini Med Ctr; **HMO:** Independent Health Plan Oxford Blue Choice United Healthcare 1199 +

LANG: Sp; 🔳 🔳 🔳 🔳 🔳 🔳 A Few Days

Rackow, Eric (MD)   IM
St Vincents Hosp & Med Ctr NY

32 W 18th St; New York, NY 10011; (212) 647-6400; **BDCERT:** IM 75; Cv 77; **MS:** SUNY Hlth Sci Ctr 71; **RES:** IM, Univ Hosp SUNY Bklyn, Brooklyn, NY 71-72; Kings County Hosp Ctr, Brooklyn, NY 72-73; **FEL:** Cv, Univ Hosp SUNY Bklyn, Brooklyn, NY 73-75; **FAP:** Prof Med NY Med Coll; **HMO:** Oxford Blue Cross & Blue Shield US Hlthcre US Hlthcre PHS +

🔳 🔳 🔳 🔳 🔳 🔳 🔳 Immediately 🔳 *VISA* 🔳

Reape, Donald (MD)   IM   PCP
NYU Downtown Hosp

New York Downtown Med Assoc, 170 William St; New York, NY 10038; (212) 238-0110; **BDCERT:** IM 85; **MS:** Italy 82; **RES:** IM, Univ Hosp SUNY Bklyn, Brooklyn, NY 82-85; **SI:** *High Blood Pressure; Cholesterol;* **HMO:** Oxford Aetna Hlth Plan CIGNA Prucare United Healthcare +

LANG: Itl, Sp, Chi, Prt, Yd; 🔳 🔳 🔳 🔳 🔳 🔳 🔳 🔳 Immediately 🔳 *VISA* 🔳 🔳

Reidenberg, Marcus (MD)   IM
NY Hosp-Cornell Med Ctr

1300 York Ave 70; New York, NY 10021; (212) 746-6227; **BDCERT:** IM 67; **MS:** Temple U 58; **RES:** Temple U Hosp, Philadelphia, PA 62-65; **FEL:** Temple U Hosp, Philadelphia, PA 59-60; **FAP:** Prof Cornell U; **SI:** *Clinical Pharmacology;* **HMO:** Blue Cross & Blue Shield

🔳 🔳 🔳 🔳 Immediately

Rivlin, Richard (MD)   IM
Mem Sloan Kettering Cancer Ctr

Memorial Sloan Kettering Cancer Ctr, 1275 York Ave; New York, NY 10021; (212) 639-8352; **BDCERT:** IM 69; **MS:** Harvard Med Sch 59; **RES:** Med, Bellevue Hosp Ctr, New York, NY 59-60; Med, Johns Hopkins Hosp, Baltimore, MD 60-61; **FEL:** EDM, Nat Inst Health, Bethesda, MD 61-64; Med, Johns Hopkins Hosp, Baltimore, MD 64-66; **FAP:** Prof Med Cornell U; **HOSP:** NY Hosp-Cornell Med Ctr; **SI:** *Cancer Prevention; Nutrition;* **HMO:** Blue Cross & Blue Shield

LANG: Sp; 🔳 🔳 🔳 🔳 🔳 2-4 Weeks 🔳 *VISA* 🔳 🔳

Rodman, John (MD)   IM
Lenox Hill Hosp

435 E 57th St 1A; New York, NY 10022; (212) 752-3043; **BDCERT:** IM 75; **MS:** Columbia P&S 70; **RES:** NY Hosp-Cornell Med Ctr, New York, NY; **FEL:** Nep, NY Hosp-Cornell Med Ctr, New York, NY; **HOSP:** NY Hosp-Cornell Med Ctr; **SI:** *Nephrology; Hypertension*

LANG: Sp; 🔳 🔳 🔳 🔳 🔳 🔳 🔳 A Few Days

Rogers, Murray (MD)   IM
Lenox Hill Hosp

800A 5th Ave; New York, NY 10021; (212) 755-7711; **BDCERT:** IM 68 Pul 71; **MS:** Univ Penn 55; **RES:** IM, VA Med Ctr-Bronx, Bronx, NY 56-58; IM, Lenox Hill Hosp, New York, NY 58-59; **FAP:** Assoc Prof Clin Med NYU Sch Med; **SI:** *Pulmonary Diseases; Bronchoscopy & Laser Surgery;* **HMO:** None

LANG: Sp, Ger, Dut, Yd; 🔳 🔳 🔳 🔳 🔳 1 Week 🔳 *VISA* 🔳 🔳

Rosenbluth, Michael (MD)   IM
Lenox Hill Hosp

912 5th Ave; New York, NY 10021; (212) 737-2274; **MS:** NYU Sch Med 56; **RES:** Bellevue Hosp Ctr, New York, NY 56-59; **FEL:** NY Hosp-Cornell Med Ctr, New York, NY 59-60; London Sch of Tropical Med, London, England 60-61; **FAP:** Asst Clin Prof Med Cornell U; **HOSP:** NY Hosp-Cornell Med Ctr; **SI:** *Parasitology*

LANG: Fr; 🔳 🔳 🔳 🔳

Sayad, Karim (MD)   IM
Cabrini Med Ctr
60 Gramercy Park N; New York, NY 10010; (212) 254-1220; **BDCERT:** IM 86; **MS:** Mexico 79; **RES:** IM, Cabrini Med Ctr, New York, NY 81-85; **FEL:** Ge, Cabrini Med Ctr, New York, NY 85-87; **HOSP:** St Vincents Hosp & Med Ctr NY; **SI:** *Peptic Ulcer; Colitis*; **HMO:** Aetna-US Healthcare Blue Cross & Blue Shield CIGNA Magnacare Oxford +

LANG: Sp, Ar, Fr; ♿ ☎ 👥 🏨 💲 Mcr Mcd   2-4 Weeks

Schneebaum, Cary (MD)   IM
Beth Israel Med Ctr
240 1st Ave Mh; New York, NY 10009; (212) 529-4020; **BDCERT:** IM 81; **MS:** SUNY Hlth Sci Ctr 81; **RES:** Beth Israel Med Ctr, New York, NY 81-84; **FEL:** Beth Israel Med Ctr, New York, NY 84-86; **SI:** *Gastroenterology*; **HMO:** Aetna Hlth Plan Prucare Oxford Metlife Blue Choice +

LANG: Pol; ☎ 👥 🏨 💲 Mcr Mcd   A Few Days

Schneider, Steven (MD)   IM   `PCP`
Lenox Hill Hosp
Madison Medical, 110 E 59th St Ste 10A; New York, NY 10022; (212) 583-2880; **BDCERT:** IM 79; **MS:** Johns Hopkins U 76; **RES:** Presbyterian Med Ctr, Philadelphia, PA 77-79; **FAP:** Asst Clin Prof Cornell U; **HOSP:** Mount Sinai Med Ctr; **SI:** *Occupational Medicine*; **HMO:** Oxford CIGNA Prucare United Healthcare Blue Choice +

LANG: Sp, Fr, Ger; ♿ ☎ 👥 🏨 💲 Mcr Mcd WC A Few Days 💳 **VISA** 💳 💳

Seitzman, Peter (MD)   IM   `PCP`
Lenox Hill Hosp
18 E 77th St 1B; New York, NY 10021; (212) 288-8382; **BDCERT:** IM 77; **MS:** NYU Sch Med 74; **RES:** Lenox Hill Hosp, New York, NY 74-77; Lenox Hill Hosp, New York, NY 77-78; **HOSP:** NY Hosp-Cornell Med Ctr

LANG: Sp; ♿ ☎ 👥 🏨 💲 Mcr Mcd   Immediately 💳 **VISA** 💳 💳

Seltzer, Terry (MD)   IM
New York University Med Ctr
530 1st Ave 4G; New York, NY 10016; (212) 263-8717; **BDCERT:** IM 80; **MS:** Harvard Med Sch 77; **RES:** Bellevue Hosp Ctr, New York, NY 77-80; **FEL:** Bellevue Hosp Ctr, New York, NY 80-82; **FAP:** Asst Clin Prof NYU Sch Med; **SI:** *Diabetes; Thyroid Disorders*; **HMO:** Oxford Chubb United Healthcare Health Source +

♿ ☎ 👥 🏨 💲   Immediately

Seremetis, Stephanie (MD)   IM
Mount Sinai Med Ctr
Women's Health Program, 5 E 98th St; New York, NY 10029; (212) 241-8818; **BDCERT:** IM 82; **MS:** SUNY Hlth Sci Ctr 78; **RES:** IM, Mount Sinai Med Ctr, New York, NY 78-81; **FEL:** Hem, Mount Sinai Med Ctr, New York, NY 81-83; **FAP:** Assoc Prof Mt Sinai Sch Med; **SI:** *Bleeding Disorders; Women's Health*; **HMO:** Oxford Aetna-US Healthcare PHS Beech Street PHCS +

♿ ☎ 👥 🏨 💲 Mcr   4+ Weeks 💳 **VISA** 💳 💳

Seriff, Nathan (MD)   IM
Lenox Hill Hosp
130 E 77th St Fl 9; New York, NY 10021; (212) 988-0005; **BDCERT:** IM 62; Pul 68; **MS:** U Tex Med Br, Galveston 54; **RES:** Mount Sinai Med Ctr, New York, NY 54-56; VA Med Ctr-Brooklyn, Brooklyn, NY 56-58; **FEL:** Pul, VA Med Ctr-Bronx, Bronx, NY 59; Mount Sinai Med Ctr, New York, NY 58; **SI:** *Pulmonary Function Testing*

LANG: Yd, Sp; ♿ ☎ 🏨 💲 Mcr   A Few Days 💳 **VISA**

Shimony, Rony (MD)   IM
Lenox Hill Hosp
800A 5th Ave 301; New York, NY 10021; (212) 750-0506; **BDCERT:** IM 87; Cv 87; **MS:** SUNY Buffalo 84; **RES:** IM, Lenox Hill Hosp, New York, NY 84-85; IM, Lenox Hill Hosp, New York, NY 85-87; **FEL:** Cv, Lenox Hill Hosp, New York, NY 87-89; CE, Lenox Hill Hosp, New York, NY 89-92; **SI:** *Coronary Artery Disease; Syncope, Atrial Fibrillation*; **HMO:** Multiplan Oxford Blue Choice 1199

LANG: Man, Heb, Sp, Rus; ♿ 📞 ☎ 👥 🏨 💲 Mcr   2-4 Weeks 💳 **VISA** 💳

Shorofsky, Morris (MD)   IM   PCP
NY Hosp-Cornell Med Ctr
Morris Shorosky MD,PC, 166 E 61st St Suite 1C;
New York, NY 10021; (212) 751-0777; **BDCERT:**
IM 78; Ger 88; **MS:** Switzerland 59; **RES:** IM, Mount
Sinai Med Ctr, New York, NY 63-64; IM, Beth Israel
Med Ctr, New York, NY 64-65; **FAP:** Asst Clin Prof
Cornell U; **HOSP:** Beth Israel Med Ctr; **SI:** *Primary
Care*; **HMO:** Aetna-US Healthcare Oxford Prucare
United Healthcare NYLCare +

LANG: Ger; 🗀 🎟 Mcr WC NFI 1 Week

Siegel, George (MD)   IM
Beth Israel Med Ctr
240 E 82nd St; New York, NY 10028; (212) 517-
4770; **BDCERT:** IM 68; EDM 72; **MS:** Albany Med
Coll 59; **RES:** Montefiore Med Ctr, Bronx, NY 61-
63; Flower Fifth Ave Hosp, New York, NY 60-61;
FEL: EDM, Mount Sinai Med Ctr, New York, NY 63-
64; **FAP:** Asst Clin Prof Mt Sinai Sch Med; **HOSP:**
Beth Israel North; **SI:** *Thyroid Disease; Diabetes*;
HMO: Oxford Blue Choice Metlife

🗀 🎎 🎟 $ Mcr 2-4 Weeks **VISA** 💮

Silverman, David (MD)   IM   PCP
New York University Med Ctr
239 Central Park West; New York, NY 10024;
(212) 496-1929; **BDCERT:** IM 79; **MS:** Columbia
P&S 76; **RES:** IM, Bellevue Hosp Ctr, New York, NY
77-80; Bellevue Hosp Ctr, New York, NY 80-81;
FEL: Inf, Bellevue Hosp Ctr, New York, NY 81-82;
FAP: Assoc Clin Prof NYU Sch Med; **HOSP:** Bellevue
Hosp Ctr; **SI:** *Preventive Health Care; Diagnostics*

LANG: Sp; 🗒 🗀 🎟 **VISA** 💮

Sirota, David King (MD)   IM
Mount Sinai Med Ctr
1175 Park Ave; New York, NY 10128; (212) 427-
5600; **BDCERT:** IM 72; EDM 77; **MS:** Washington
U, St Louis 60; **RES:** Jacobi Med Ctr, Bronx, NY 60-
65; **FEL:** EDM, Mount Sinai Med Ctr, New York, NY
65-67; **FAP:** Assoc Clin Prof Med Mt Sinai Sch Med;
SI: *Thyroid Diseases; Geriatric Care*

LANG: Sp; 🗒 🗀 🎎 🎟 Mcr 2-4 Weeks

Sivak, Steven L (MD)   IM   PCP
St Vincents Hosp & Med Ctr NY
Medical Practice Center, 32 W 18th St 3rd FL; New
York, NY 10011; (212) 647-6464; **BDCERT:** IM
79; **MS:** NY Med Coll 76; **RES:** Metropolitan Hosp,
Philadelphia, PA 76-77; **FEL:** Metropolitan Hosp,
Philadelphia, PA 77-79; **HMO:** Oxford PHS Prucare

LANG: Sp; 🗒 🗀 $ Mcr Mcd 4+ Weeks 📇 **VISA** 💮
💳

Sklaroff, Herschel (MD)   IM   PCP
Mount Sinai Med Ctr
1175 Park Ave; New York, NY 10128; (212) 289-
6500; **BDCERT:** IM 69; **MS:** Univ Penn 61; **RES:**
Cv/Med, Mt Sinai, New York, NY 62-66; **FAP:**
Assoc Prof Mt Sinai Sch Med; **SI:** *Cardiology*

🗀 🎎 🎟 Mcr NFI 2-4 Weeks

Snyder, Arthur (MD)   IM   PCP
Columbia-Presbyterian Med Ctr
New York Physicians, PC, 635 Madison Ave Fl 8;
New York, NY 10022; (212) 857-4590; **BDCERT:**
IM 59; Rhu 74; **MS:** Columbia P&S 50; **RES:** IM,
Columbia-Presbyterian Med Ctr, New York, NY 51-
53; IM, Boston VA Med Ctr, Boston, MA 53-54;
FEL: Rhu, Columbia-Presbyterian Med Ctr, New
York, NY 54-56; **FAP:** Asst Clin Prof Columbia P&S;
SI: *Rheumatoid Arthritis; Osteoarthritis*; **HMO:**
Oxford PHS CIGNA Blue Choice Multiplan +

🗒 🗀 🎎 🎟 $ Mcr A Few Days 📇 **VISA** 💮 💳

Sperber, Kirk (MD)   IM
Mount Sinai Med Ctr
5 E 98th St; New York, NY 10029; (212) 241-
0764; **BDCERT:** IM 85; A&I 87; **MS:** UMDNJ-NJ
Med Sch, Newark 83; **RES:** St Michael's Med Ctr,
Newark, NJ 82-85; **FEL:** Mount Sinai Med Ctr, New
York, NY 85-88; Mount Sinai Med Ctr, New York,
NY 88-90; **FAP:** Assoc Prof Mt Sinai Sch Med; **SI:**
HIV Infection; Immunodeficiency; **HMO:** None

LANG: Sp; 🗒 🗀 🎎 🎟 $ Mcr Immediately 📇
VISA 💮 💳

Spero, Marc (MD)   IM   **PCP**
Lenox Hill Hosp

MidManhattan Medical Associates, 654 Madison Ave 6th Fl; New York, NY 10021; (212) 355-5222; **BDCERT:** IM 77; Pul 79; **MS:** Albert Einstein Coll Med 73; **RES:** IM, Jacobi Med Ctr, Bronx, NY 73-74; IM, St Luke's Roosevelt Hosp Ctr, New York, NY 75-77; **FEL:** St Luke's Roosevelt Hosp Ctr, New York, NY 77-79; **FAP:** Instr Med NYU Sch Med; **HOSP:** St Luke's Roosevelt Hosp Ctr; **SI:** Asthma; Diving Medicine; **HMO:** Oxford US Hlthcre Aetna Hlth Plan CIGNA Chubb +

LANG: Heb, Sp, Yd; ♿ ⓐ 🅗 ⏱ 💲 Ⓜ A Few Days
▦ **VISA** ●

Stein, Richard (MD)   IM
Mount Sinai Med Ctr

Renal Internists Assoc, PO Box 1121; New York, NY 10029; (212) 241-4060; **BDCERT:** IM 66; Nep 72; **MS:** SUNY Hlth Sci Ctr 58; **RES:** IM, Kings County Hosp Ctr, Brooklyn, NY 58-59; IM, Maimonides Med Ctr, Brooklyn, NY 59-61; **FEL:** Nep, Mount Sinai Med Ctr, New York, NY 61-63; **FAP:** Prof Mt Sinai Sch Med; **SI:** Renal Failure—Dialysis; Kidney Stones; **HMO:** Oxford Aetna Hlth Plan

♿ ⓐ 🅗 ⏱ Ⓜ 1 Week ▦ **VISA** ● 💳

Stein, Sidney (MD)   IM   **PCP**
Beth Israel Med Ctr

2 E 76th St; New York, NY 10021; (212) 879-7776; **BDCERT:** IM 82; Pul 88; **MS:** SUNY Hlth Sci Ctr 79; **RES:** IM, Beth Israel Med Ctr, New York, NY 80-82; **FEL:** Pul, Beth Israel Med Ctr, New York, NY 82-84; **FAP:** Asst Clin Prof Albert Einstein Coll Med; **HOSP:** Beth Israel North; **SI:** Asthma; Chronic Bronchitis; **HMO:** Oxford PHS Blue Choice Independent Health Plan PHCS +

♿ ⓐ 🅗 ⏱ Ⓜ A Few Days

Stein, William (MD)   IM   **PCP**
Mount Sinai Med Ctr

853 5th Ave; New York, NY 10021; (212) 744-8000; **BDCERT:** IM 67; Cv 76; **MS:** McGill U 58; **RES:** Mount Sinai Med Ctr, New York, NY 58-61; **FEL:** Cv, Mount Sinai Med Ctr, New York, NY 61-63; **FAP:** Asst Prof IM Mt Sinai Sch Med

ⓐ 🅗 Ⓜ Immediately

Steinberg, Charles (MD)   IM
NY Hosp-Cornell Med Ctr

525 E 68th St; New York, NY 10021; (212) 746-4100; **BDCERT:** IM 71; Inf 74; **MS:** Cornell U 64

Strauss, Michael (MD)   IM   **PCP**
Beth Israel Med Ctr

310 E 14th St North Bldg FL 3; New York, NY 10003; (212) 777-3077; **BDCERT:** IM 83; **MS:** Belgium 80; **RES:** Cabrini Med Ctr, New York, NY 80-83; **HOSP:** New York Eye & Ear Infirmary; **SI:** Acupuncture; **HMO:** Oxford Blue Cross 1199 GHI PHS +

LANG: Fr; ♿ 🅢 ⓐ 🅗 ⏱ 💲 Ⓜ Immediately

Sweeting, Joseph (MD)   IM
Columbia-Presbyterian Med Ctr

161 Fort Washington Ave 4; New York, NY 10032; (212) 305-5424; **BDCERT:** IM 64; Ge 72; **MS:** Columbia P&S 56; **RES:** Columbia-Presbyterian Med Ctr, New York, NY 56-58; Columbia-Presbyterian Med Ctr, New York, NY 61-62; **FEL:** Ge, Columbia-Presbyterian Med Ctr, New York, NY 62-63; **FAP:** Prof of Clin Med Columbia P&S; **SI:** Inflammatory Bowel Disease; Irritable Bowel Syndrome; **HMO:** Oxford Empire Blue Cross & Shield
♿ ⓐ 🅗 ⏱ Ⓜ 1 Week

Swerdlow, Frederick H (MD)   IM
Mount Sinai Med Ctr

1088 Park Ave; New York, NY 10128; (212) 860-4000; **BDCERT:** IM 74; Rhu 78; **MS:** SUNY Hlth Sci Ctr 70; **RES:** Mount Sinai Med Ctr, New York, NY; **FEL:** IM, Mount Sinai Med Ctr, New York, NY; Rhu, Mount Sinai Med Ctr, New York, NY 74-75; **FAP:** Assoc Prof Med Mt Sinai Sch Med; **HMO:** Oxford Aetna Hlth Plan

LANG: Sp, Rus, Yd; ♿ ⓐ 🅗 ⏱ 💲 Ⓜ 1 Week

Taylor, William (MD)   IM   **PCP**
New York University Med Ctr

530 1st Ave; New York, NY 10016; (212) 263-7413; **BDCERT:** IM 76; **MS:** NYU Sch Med 57; **RES:** Bellevue Hosp Ctr, New York, NY 57-64; **HMO:** Oxford
♿ ⓐ 🅗 ⏱ Ⓜ 1 Week

Troy, Kevin (MD)   **IM**
Mount Sinai Med Ctr

5 E 98th St; New York, NY 10029; (212) 860-
9055; **BDCERT:** IM 82; Hem 84; **MS:** U Conn Sch
Med 79; **RES:** IM, Lenox Hill Hosp, New York, NY
79-82; **FEL:** HS, Mount Sinai Med Ctr, New York,
NY 82-84; **FAP:** Assoc Clin Prof Mt Sinai Sch Med;
SI: Leukemia Lymphoma; Hodgkin's Disease; **HMO:**
Oxford Vytra Aetna-US Healthcare Blue Choice
PHCS +

♿ 📷 💉 📅 **S** **Mcr** A Few Days

Turino, Gerard M (MD)   **IM**
St Luke's Roosevelt Hosp Ctr

1000 10th Ave; New York, NY 10019; (212) 523-
5919; **BDCERT:** IM 56; **MS:** Columbia P&S 48; **RES:**
IM, Bellevue Hosp Ctr, New York, NY 49-50; IM,
Bellevue Hosp Ctr, New York, NY 53-54; **FEL:** Pul,
Columbia-Presbyterian Med Ctr, New York, NY 54-
56; Pul, Columbia-Presbyterian Med Ctr, New
York, NY 56-60; **FAP:** Lecturer Med Columbia P&S;
HOSP: Columbia-Presbyterian Med Ctr; *SI: Chronic
Obstructive Lung Disease; Asthma—Emphysema;*
HMO: Oxford Blue Cross & Blue Shield PHS
Prudential

♿ 📷 💉 📅 **Mcr** **Mcd** **WC** **NFI** A Few Days

Underberg, James (MD)   **IM**   PCP
New York University Med Ctr

Murray Hill Medical Group, 317 E 34th St 1001;
New York, NY 10016; (212) 725-5556; **BDCERT:**
IM 89; **MS:** Univ Penn 86; **RES:** Bellevue Hosp Ctr,
New York, NY 89; **HOSP:** Hosp For Joint Diseases;
HMO: Oxford Health Source PHS United Healthcare
CIGNA +

♿ 📞 📷 💉 📅 **S** **Mcr** A Few Days 📰 **VISA** 💳

Villamena, Patricia (MD)   **IM**
Beth Israel Med Ctr

1st Ave & 16th St; New York, NY 10003; (212)
420-2377; **BDCERT:** IM 89; **MS:** NY Med Coll 77;
RES: Metropolitan Hosp Ctr, New York, NY 77-80;
FEL: Beth Israel Med Ctr, New York, NY 84-86

♿ 📷 📅 **S** Immediately

Walfish, Jacob (MD)   **IM**   PCP
Mount Sinai Med Ctr

1150 Park Ave; New York, NY 10128; (212) 831-
5000; **BDCERT:** IM 77; Ge 79; **MS:** Harvard Med
Sch 74; **RES:** IM, Mount Sinai Med Ctr, New York,
NY 74-77; **FEL:** Ge, Mount Sinai Med Ctr, New
York, NY 77-79; **FAP:** Asst Clin Prof Med Mt Sinai
Sch Med; **HMO:** Oxford Aetna Hlth Plan CIGNA
Blue Choice

LANG: Yd, Heb; 📶 📞 📷 💉 📅 **S** **Mcr** Immediately

Weinstein, Jay (MD)   **IM**   PCP
St Vincents Hosp & Med Ctr NY

32 W 18th St Fl 3; New York, NY 10011; (212)
647-6464; **BDCERT:** IM 91; **MS:** Hahnemann U
87; **HMO:** US Hlthcre Oxford PHS

♿ 📷 💉 📅 **S** **Mcr** 1 Week 📰 **VISA** 💳

Weintraub, Gerald (MD)   **IM**   PCP
St Luke's Roosevelt Hosp Ctr

74 E 90th St; New York, NY 10128; (212) 348-
4741; **BDCERT:** IM 61; Ge 67; **MS:** NYU Sch Med
54; **RES:** St Luke's Roosevelt Hosp Ctr, New York,
NY 57-58; Bellevue Hosp Ctr, New York, NY 58-
59; **FEL:** Mount Sinai Med Ctr, New York, NY 59-
60; **FAP:** Assoc Clin Prof Columbia P&S; **HMO:**
Prucare Multiplan Oxford PHS PHCS +

LANG: Yd; ♿ 📷 💉 📅 **S** **Mcr** A Few Days **VISA**

Whiteside, Timothy (MD)   **IM**
Cabrini Med Ctr

227 E 19th St; New York, NY 10003; (212) 995-
6093; **BDCERT:** IM 83; **MS:** 80; **RES:** IM, Univ Hosp
SUNY Bklyn, Brooklyn, NY 80-83; **FEL:** Hem Onc,
VA Med Ctr-Brooklyn, Brooklyn, NY 83-86; *SI:
Emergency Medicine; Hyperbaric Medicine;* **HMO:**
Blue Cross Mt Sinai Hlth

Wiseman, Paul (MD)   **IM**   PCP
St Luke's Roosevelt Hosp Ctr

101 Central Park West Fl 1; New York, NY 10023;
(212) 496-5800; **BDCERT:** IM 87; **MS:** Albert
Einstein Coll Med 81; **RES:** Montefiore Med Ctr,
Bronx, NY 81-84; **FAP:** Clin Instr Med Columbia
P&S; **HOSP:** Beth Israel Med Ctr; *SI: Preventive
Medicine;* **HMO:** None

LANG: Sp; ♿ 📷 📅 **S** 1 Week

Wolf, David J (MD)   IM
NY Hosp-Cornell Med Ctr

115 E 61st St; New York, NY 10021; (212) 688-
7100; **BDCERT:** IM 76; Hem 79; **MS:** SUNY Hlth
Sci Ctr 73; **RES:** NY Hosp-Cornell Med Ctr, New
York, NY; Mem Sloan Kettering Cancer Ctr, New
York, NY; **FEL:** Onc, NY Hosp-Cornell Med Ctr, New
York, NY; NY Hosp-Cornell Med Ctr, New York,
NY; **HOSP:** Beth Israel North

Yaffe, Bruce (MD)   IM
Lenox Hill Hosp

121 E 84th St; New York, NY 10028; (212) 879-
4700; **BDCERT:** IM 79; Ge 80; **MS:** Geo Wash U
Sch Med 76; **RES:** IM, Mount Sinai Med Ctr, New
York, NY 77-79; **FEL:** Hem, Mount Sinai Med Ctr,
New York, NY 79-80; Ge, Lenox Hill Hosp, New
York, NY 80-82; **HMO:** Aetna Hlth Plan Oxford
United Healthcare Multiplan PHCS +

🔲 🔲 🔲 🔲 🔲 🔲 Immediately ▥ **VISA**

Yanoff, Allen (MD)   IM   PCP
Lenox Hill Hosp

9 E 63rd St; New York, NY 10021; (212) 593-
7170; **BDCERT:** IM 71; **MS:** Albert Einstein Coll
Med 66; **RES:** Lincoln Med & Mental Hlth Ctr,
Bronx, NY 66-70; **HOSP:** Montefiore Med Ctr;
HMO: None

🔲 🔲 🔲 🔲 🔲 A Few Days ▥ **VISA** ⬤

Young, Iven (MD)   IM
St Vincents Hosp & Med Ctr NY

130 W 12th St 7D; New York, NY 10011; (212)
675-9332; **BDCERT:** IM 66; **MS:** NYU Sch Med 59;
RES: VA Med Ctr-Manh, New York, NY 60-63; **FEL:**
New York University Med Ctr, New York, NY 63-
66; **FAP:** Assoc Clin Prof Med NY Med Coll; **HOSP:**
New York University Med Ctr; **SI:** *Thyroid;*
Osteoporosis; **HMO:** Oxford Blue Cross & Blue Choice
PHS

🔲 🔲 🔲 🔲 🔲 1 Week

Zeale, Peter (MD)   IM
St Vincents Hosp & Med Ctr NY

32 W 18th St; New York, NY 10011; (212) 647-
6430; **BDCERT:** IM 82; **MS:** Georgetown U 79; **RES:**
IM, St Vincents Hosp & Med Ctr NY, New York, NY
80-83

🔲 🔲 🔲 🔲 🔲 🔲 2-4 Weeks

MATERNAL & FETAL MEDICINE

Gugliucci, Camillo (MD)   MF
Lenox Hill Hosp

950 Park Ave; New York, NY 10028; (212) 988-
1833; **BDCERT:** ObG 70; **MS:** Italy 57; **RES:** ObG,
Metropolitan Hosp Ctr, New York, NY 58-62; **FEL:**
ObG, Metropolitan Hosp Ctr, New York, NY 62-63;
FAP: Assoc Clin Prof ObG NY Med Coll; **SI:** *Diabetes
in Pregnancy; Multiple Births;* **HMO:** None

LANG: Itl; 🔲 🔲 🔲 A Few Days

Lockwood, Charles (MD)   MF
New York University Med Ctr

NYU Medical Ctr, 530 1st Ave Ste 7V; New York,
NY 10016; (212) 263-7021; **BDCERT:** ObG 88; MF
89; **MS:** Univ Penn 81; **RES:** ObG, Hosp of U Penn,
Philadelphia, PA 81-85; **FEL:** MF, Yale-New Haven
Hosp, New Haven, CT 85-87; **HMO:** Oxford Empire
Blue Cross CIGNA Prucare Multiplan

🔲 🔲 🔲 🔲 🔲 1 Week

MEDICAL GENETICS

Davis, Jessica (MD)   MG
NY Hosp-Cornell Med Ctr

525 E 68th St; New York, NY 10021; (212) 746-1496; **BDCERT:** MG 84; **MS:** Columbia P&S 59; **RES:** Ped, St Luke's Roosevelt Hosp Ctr, New York, NY 61-62; **FEL:** MG, Albert Einstein Med Ctr, Bronx, NY; Cytogenetics, Albert Einstein Med Ctr, Bronx, NY; **FAP:** Assoc Prof of Clin Ped Cornell U; **HOSP:** Hosp For Special Surgery; **SI:** *Marfan's Syndrome; Mental Retardation;* **HMO:** Blue Shield United Healthcare Oxford Prudential US Hlthcre +

LANG: Fr, Sp; 🔲 🔲 🔲 🔲 🔲 🔲 🔲 Immediately 🔲 **VISA** 🔲 🔲

Desnick, Robert (MD)   MG
Mount Sinai Med Ctr

Box 1498, 5th Avenue at 100th St St; New York, NY 10029; (212) 241-6944; **BDCERT:** MG 82; **MS:** U Minn 71; **RES:** Ped, U MN Med Ctr, Minneapolis, MN 71-72; **FAP:** Chrmn MG Mt Sinai Sch Med; **SI:** *Inherited Diseases; Metabolic Diseases;* **HMO:** Aetna Hlth Plan Blue Cross & Blue Shield

🔲 🔲 🔲 🔲 🔲 🔲 A Few Days 🔲 **VISA** 🔲

Gilbert, Fred (MD)   MG
NY Hosp-Cornell Med Ctr

1300 York Ave; New York, NY 10021; (212) 746-3475; **BDCERT:** MG 82; **MS:** Albert Einstein Coll Med 66; **RES:** Med, Barnes Hosp, St Louis, MO 66-68; Med, Nat Inst Health, Bethesda, MD 68-71; **FEL:** MG, Yale-New Haven Hosp, New Haven, CT 71-74; **FAP:** Assoc Prof Cornell U; **SI:** *Cancer Genetic Testing*

LANG: Sp, Chi; 🔲 🔲 🔲 🔲 🔲 🔲 🔲 🔲 🔲 **VISA** 🔲 🔲

Penchaszadeh, Victor (MD)   MG
Beth Israel Med Ctr

1st Ave & 16th St 6BH10; New York, NY 10003; (212) 420-4179; **BDCERT:** MG 89; **MS:** Argentina 64; **RES:** Ped, Childrens Hosp, Buenos Aires, Argentina 65-68; **FEL:** MG, Johns Hopkins Hosp, Baltimore, MD 68-70; **FAP:** Prof Ped Albert Einstein Coll Med; **SI:** *Prenatal Diagnosis; Birth Defects;* **HMO:** Aetna Hlth Plan Oxford CIGNA HIP Network US Hlthcre +

LANG: Sp, Fr, Rus, Chi, Grk; 🔲 🔲 🔲 🔲 🔲 🔲 A Few Days 🔲 **VISA** 🔲

Willner, Judith P (MD)   MG
Mount Sinai Med Ctr

1 Gustave Levy Pl; New York, NY 10029; (212) 241-6947; **BDCERT:** Ped 78; MG 82; **MS:** NYU Sch Med 71; **RES:** Ped, Children's Hosp Nat Med Ctr, Washington, DC 71-72; Ped, Children's Hosp Nat Med Ctr, Washington, DC 72-73; **FEL:** MG, Mount Sinai Med Ctr, New York, NY 74-77; **FAP:** Assoc Prof Mt Sinai Sch Med; **HOSP:** Englewood Hosp & Med Ctr; **SI:** *Genetic Disorders; Genetic Prenatal Diagnosis;* **HMO:** Oxford Aetna Hlth Plan US Hlthcre

LANG: Sp, Chi, Fr, Prt; 🔲 🔲 🔲 🔲 🔲 🔲 🔲 A Few Days 🔲 **VISA** 🔲

MEDICAL ONCOLOGY

Antman, Karen (MD)   Onc
Columbia-Presbyterian Med Ctr

177 Fort Washington Ave; New York, NY 10032; (212) 305-8602; **BDCERT:** IM 77; **MS:** Columbia P&S 74; **RES:** Columbia-Presbyterian Med Ctr, New York, NY 74-77; **FEL:** Onc, Dana-Farber Cancer Inst, Boston, MA; **HMO:** Blue Choice Chubb Oxford PHS Prucare +

🔲 🔲 🔲 🔲 🔲 A Few Days 🔲 **VISA** 🔲

Bajorin, Dean (MD)   Onc
Mem Sloan Kettering Cancer Ctr

1275 York Ave; New York, NY 10021; (212) 639-6708; **BDCERT:** Onc 81; **MS:** NY Med Coll 78; **RES:** Hartford Hosp, Hartford, CT 79-81; **SI:** *Genitourinary Malignancies; Bladder Cancer*

🔲 🔲 🔲 🔲 🔲 🔲 2-4 Weeks

Bander, Neil (MD)   Onc
NY Hosp-Cornell Med Ctr

Cornell University Med College, 525 E 68th St; New York, NY 10021; (212) 746-5460; **BDCERT:** U 83; **MS:** U Conn Sch Med 74; **RES:** New York University Med Ctr, New York, NY 74-77; U, U Conn Hlth Ctr, Farmington, CT 77-81; **FEL:** U Onc, Mem Sloan Kettering Cancer Ctr, New York, NY 83; **FAP:** Assoc Prof Cornell U; **SI:** *Urologic Oncology*

♿ 📷 🚹 🗓 $ Mcr   4+ Weeks

Barbasch, Avi (MD)   Onc
Mount Sinai Med Ctr

1050 Park Ave; New York, NY 10028; (212) 860-3292; **BDCERT:** IM 97; **MS:** Mexico 75; **RES:** IM, Elmhurst Hosp Ctr, Elmhurst, NY 77-80; **FEL:** Onc, Roswell Park Cancer Inst, Buffalo, NY 80-82; **FAP:** Asst Clin Prof Med Mt Sinai Sch Med; **SI:** *Breast Cancer; Colon Cancer*

LANG: Sp; 📷 🚹 🗓 Mcr   1 Week [AMEX] **VISA** ●

Berman, Ellin (MD)   Onc
Mem Sloan Kettering Cancer Ctr

1275 York Ave; New York, NY 10021; (212) 639-7762; **BDCERT:** IM 80; Onc 85; **MS:** Harvard Med Sch 77; **RES:** Boston U Med Ctr, Boston, MA 77-78; **FEL:** Hem Onc, Mem Sloan Kettering Cancer Ctr, New York, NY; **SI:** *Leukemia; Lymphoma*

♿ 📷 🚹 🗓 Mcr Mcd WC NFl   Immediately

Blum, Ronald (MD)   Onc
St Vincents Hosp & Med Ctr NY

153 W 11th St; New York, NY 10011; (212) 604-6011; **BDCERT:** IM 75; **MS:** SUNY Buffalo 70; **RES:** Johns Hopkins Hosp, Baltimore, MD 70; Harvard Med Sch, Cambridge, MA; **FEL:** Harvard Med Sch, Cambridge, MA 74; **HMO:** Oxford Aetna Hlth Plan Chubb

♿ 📷 🚹 🗓 $ Mcr WC   Immediately

Bosl, George (MD)   Onc
Mem Sloan Kettering Cancer Ctr

1275 York Ave; New York, NY 10021; (212) 639-8473; **BDCERT:** IM 76; **MS:** Creighton U 73; **RES:** NY Hosp-Cornell Med Ctr, New York, NY 73-76; **FEL:** Onc, U MN Med Ctr, Minneapolis, MN 77-79; **SI:** *Testicular Cancer*

LANG: Sp; ♿ 📷 🗓 Mcr Mcd   A Few Days

Brower, Mark (MD)   Onc
NY Hosp-Cornell Med Ctr

310 E 72nd St; New York, NY 10021; (212) 717-2995; **BDCERT:** Hem 82; Onc 79; **MS:** Johns Hopkins U 74; **RES:** IM, NY Hosp-Cornell Med Ctr, New York, NY 74-77; **FEL:** Onc, NY Hosp-Cornell Med Ctr, New York, NY 77-79; Hem Onc, NY Hosp-Cornell Med Ctr, New York, NY 79-80; **FAP:** Assoc Clin Prof Med Cornell U; **HOSP:** Beth Israel North; **SI:** *Breast Cancer; Bleeding Disorders*

LANG: Sp; ♿ 📷 🚹 🗓   1 Week

Brown, John C (MD)   Onc
Beth Israel Med Ctr

54 Gramercy Park N; New York, NY 10010; (212) 529-9100; **BDCERT:** IM 76; Onc 78; **MS:** Bowman Gray 73; **RES:** NY Hosp-Cornell Med Ctr, New York, NY 73-74; NY Hosp-Cornell Med Ctr, New York, NY 74-75; **FEL:** Hem, Mem Sloan Kettering Cancer Ctr, New York, NY 76-78; Univ Hosp SUNY Syracuse, Syracuse, NY 75; **HOSP:** Hosp For Joint Diseases; **HMO:** Oxford PHS Prucare Aetna-US Healthcare

♿ 📷 🚹 🗓 Mcr   2-4 Weeks [AMEX]

Cohen, Seymour (MD)   Onc
Mount Sinai Med Ctr

Oncology Consultants Inc, 1045 5th Ave; New York, NY 10028; (212) 249-9141; **BDCERT:** Onc 73; **MS:** Univ Pittsburgh 62; **RES:** IM, Montefiore Med Ctr, Bronx, NY 63-64; IM, Mount Sinai Med Ctr, New York, NY 64-65; **FEL:** Hem, Mount Sinai Med Ctr, New York, NY 65-67; Hem, Long Island Jewish Med Ctr, New Hyde Park, NY 68-69; **FAP:** Assoc Clin Prof Med Mt Sinai Sch Med; **HOSP:** NY Hosp Med Ctr of Queens; **SI:** *Breast Cancer; Melanoma*; **HMO:** Oxford

LANG: Fr, Yd; ♿ 📷 🚹 🗓 Mcr   A Few Days **VISA** ●

Guide to symbols and abbreviations can be found on pages 110-113.

231

Coleman, Morton (MD) Onc
NY Hosp-Cornell Med Ctr

407 E 70th St 3rd Fl; New York, NY 10021; (212) 861-1383; **BDCERT:** IM 71; Hem 72; **MS:** Med Coll Va 63; **RES:** NY Hosp-Cornell Med Ctr, New York, NY 67-68; Grady Mem Hosp, Atlanta, GA 63-65; **FEL:** Hem Onc, NY Hosp-Cornell Med Ctr, New York, NY 68-70; **FAP:** Clin Prof Med Cornell U; *SI: Lymphoma-Hodgkin's Disease; Myeloma—Leukemia*; **HMO:** None

LANG: Itl, Yd, Ger; ♿ ⊡ ⧄ ⊞ Ⓜ A Few Days
VISA ⊜

Gaynor, Mitchell (MD) Onc
NY Hosp-Cornell Med Ctr

Strang Cancer Prevention Center, 428 E 72nd St Suite 200; New York, NY 10021; (212) 410-3820; **BDCERT:** IM 85; Onc 87; **MS:** Univ Texas, Houston 82; **RES:** NY Hosp-Cornell Med Ctr, New York, NY 82-85; **FEL:** Hem Onc, NY Hosp-Cornell Med Ctr, New York, NY 85-88; **FAP:** Asst Clin Prof Cornell U; *SI: Breast Cancer; Nutrition*

LANG: Sp; ♿ ⧄ ⊞ Ⓢ A Few Days

Gee, Timothy S (MD) Onc
St Vincents Hosp & Med Ctr NY

St Vincent Comprehensive Cancer Center, 170 W 12th St; New York, NY 10011; (212) 604-6010; **BDCERT:** IM 67; **MS:** UC San Francisco 60; **RES:** Med, UC San Francisco Med Ctr, San Francisco, CA 63-65; Med, UC San Francisco Med Ctr, San Francisco, CA 65-66; **FEL:** Hem, San Francisco Gen Hosp, San Francisco, CA 66-67; Onc, Mem Sloan Kettering Cancer Ctr, New York, NY 67-69; *SI: Leukemia; Lymphoma*; **HMO:** Oxford Blue Cross & Blue Shield

LANG: Sp, Chi; ♿ ⊡ ⊞ Ⓜ Ⓜ

Gold, Ellen (MD) Onc
Beth Israel Med Ctr

Beth Israel Medical Center, 10 Union Square East; New York, NY 10003; (212) 420-4642; **BDCERT:** Hem 90; Onc 89; **MS:** NY Med Coll 83; **RES:** Med, Beth Israel Med Ctr, New York, NY 83-86; **FEL:** Hem Onc, Beth Israel Med Ctr, New York, NY 86-87; Hem Onc, Columbia-Presbyterian Med Ctr, New York, NY 87-89; **FAP:** Asst Prof Albert Einstein Coll Med; *SI: Breast Cancer; Lymphoma & Blood Disorders*; **HMO:** Oxford PHS Health First US Hlthcre Chubb +

LANG: Sp; ♿ ⊡ ⊞ Ⓢ Ⓜ 1 Week

Goldberg, Arthur (MD) Onc
Lenox Hill Hosp

121 E 79th St; New York, NY 10021; (212) 249-0030; **BDCERT:** IM 74; Onc 75; **MS:** SUNY Hlth Sci Ctr 65; **RES:** NY Hosp-Cornell Med Ctr, New York, NY 69; Bellevue Hosp Ctr, New York, NY 72; **FEL:** IM, Mem Sloan Kettering Cancer Ctr, New York, NY; **HOSP:** Mount Sinai Med Ctr; *SI: Breast Cancer; Prostate Cancer*; **HMO:** Oxford

♿ ⊡ ⧄ ⊞ Ⓢ Ⓜ Immediately ▓ *VISA* ⊜

Golde, David (MD) Onc
Mem Sloan Kettering Cancer Ctr

1275 York Ave; New York, NY 10021; (212) 639-2000; **BDCERT:** IM 72; Onc 73; **MS:** McGill U 66; **RES:** Nat Inst Health, Bethesda, MD 68-70; UC San Francisco Med Ctr, San Francisco, CA 70-71; **FEL:** Hem, Nat Inst Health, Bethesda, MD 69-70; Cancer Research Inst, Los Angeles, CA; **FAP:** Prof Med Cornell U; *SI: Leukemia; Lymphoma*

LANG: Sp; ♿ ⊡ ⊞ Ⓜ Ⓜ 1 Week ▓ *VISA* ⊜ ◪

Goldsmith, Michael (MD) Onc
Mount Sinai Med Ctr

1045 5th Ave; New York, NY 10028; (212) 628-6800; **BDCERT:** IM 76; Onc 77; **MS:** Albert Einstein Coll Med 71; **RES:** Mount Sinai Med Ctr, New York, NY 74-75; **FEL:** Neoplastic Disease, Mount Sinai Med Ctr, New York, NY 75; **FAP:** Asst Clin Prof Med Mt Sinai Sch Med; **HOSP:** NY Hosp Med Ctr of Queens; *SI: Breast Cancer; Gastrointestinal Cancers*; **HMO:** Oxford CIGNA Aetna Hlth Plan NYLCare

♿ ⊡ ⧄ ⊞ Ⓢ Ⓜ A Few Days ▓ *VISA* ⊜

Grace, William (MD)   Onc
St Vincents Hosp & Med Ctr NY

36 7th Ave Ste 511; New York, NY 10011; (212)
675-6826; **BDCERT:** IM 76; Onc 77; **MS:** Boston U
69; **RES:** IM, St Vincents Hosp & Med Ctr NY, New
York, NY 70-71; **FEL:** Hem Onc, Dartmouth
Hitchcock Med Ctr, Lebanon, NH 74-76; **FAP:**
Assoc Clin Prof Med NY Med Coll; **SI:** *Breast Cancer;*
Liver Cancer; **HMO:** Oxford US Hlthcre PHS Blue
Cross & Blue Shield

LANG: Sp, Itl; ☒ ☒ ☒ ☒ ☒ ☒ Immediately
☒ **VISA** ☒

Grossbard, Lionel (MD)   Onc
Columbia-Presbyterian Med Ctr

161 Fort Washington Ave; New York, NY 10032;
(212) 305-8399; **BDCERT:** Hem 74; Onc 75; **MS:**
Columbia P&S 61; **RES:** Columbia-Presbyterian
Med Ctr, New York, NY 61-64; **FEL:** Hem Onc,
Columbia-Presbyterian Med Ctr, New York, NY 66-
68; **FAP:** Clin Prof Columbia P&S; **SI:** *Breast Cancer;*
Lymphoma; **HMO:** Oxford Blue Shield PHS
Independent Health Plan Multiplan +

☒ ☒ ☒ ☒ ☒ A Few Days

Gruenstein, Steven (MD)   Onc
Beth Israel Med Ctr

12 E 86th St; New York, NY 10028; (212) 861-
6660; **BDCERT:** Onc 91; Hem 94; **MS:** Italy 84;
RES: Metropolitan Hosp Ctr, New York, NY 84-87;
FEL: Beth Israel Med Ctr, New York, NY 87-90;
FAP: Clin Instr Mt Sinai Sch Med; **HOSP:** Lenox Hill
Hosp; **SI:** *Hematological/Malignancies; Breast Cancer;*
HMO: Oxford Blue Choice CapCare Chubb Empire +

LANG: Sp, Itl, Fr; ☒ ☒ ☒ ☒ ☒ ☒ ☒ 1 Week **VISA**
☒

Hirshaut, Yashar (MD)   Onc
New York Comm Hosp of Bklyn

860 5th Ave; New York, NY 10021; (212) 861-
1799; **BDCERT:** IM 72; Onc 75; **MS:** Albert Einstein
Coll Med 63; **RES:** IM, Montefiore Med Ctr, Bronx,
NY 63-65; **FEL:** Onc, Nat Cancer Inst, Bethesda, MD
65-68; Mem Sloan Kettering Cancer Ctr, New York,
NY 68-70; **FAP:** Assoc Clin Prof Cornell U; **HOSP:**
Mount Sinai Med Ctr

LANG: Ger, Heb, Sp; ☒ ☒ ☒ ☒ ☒ ☒ ☒ ☒
A Few Days

Hochster, Howard (MD)   Onc
New York University Med Ctr

530 1st Ave 9R; New York, NY 10016; (212) 263-
7249; **BDCERT:** IM 83; Onc 85; **MS:** Yale U Sch
Med 80; **RES:** New York University Med Ctr, New
York, NY 80-83; **FEL:** New York University Med
Ctr, New York, NY 83-85; Jules Bordet Inst,
Brussels, Belgium 85-86; **FAP:** Assoc Prof NYU Sch
Med; **SI:** *Gastrointestinal Cancers; Gynecologic*
Cancers; **HMO:** Oxford Chubb Aetna Hlth Plan

LANG: Sp, Fr, Ger, Heb; ☒ ☒ ☒ ☒ ☒ ☒ 1 Week

Holland, James F (MD)   Onc
Mount Sinai Med Ctr

5 E 98th St; New York, NY 10029; (212) 241-
6361; **BDCERT:** IM 55; **MS:** Columbia P&S 47; **RES:**
Columbia-Presbyterian Med Ctr, New York, NY 47-
49; **FEL:** Onc, Francis Delafield Hosp, New York, NY
51-53; **SI:** *Breast Cancer* ☒

☒ ☒ ☒ Immediately ☒ **VISA** ☒

Jagannath, Sundar (MD)   Onc
St Vincents Hosp & Med Ctr NY

170 W 12th St NR 1421; New York, NY 10011;
(212) 604-6068; **BDCERT:** IM 80; Onc 85; **MS:**
India 89; **RES:** Bronx Lebanon Hosp Ctr, Bronx, NY
77-79; Harper Hosp, Detroit, MI 79-80; **FEL:** Onc,
MD Anderson Cancer Ctr, Houston, TX 80-82;
FAP: Prof Onc NY Med Coll; **SI:** *Multiple Myeloma;*
HMO: Most

☒ ☒ ☒ ☒ ☒ ☒ ☒ ☒ ☒ A Few Days ☒ **VISA**
☒ ☒

Jarowski, Charles (MD)   Onc
NY Hosp-Cornell Med Ctr

400 E 77th St 1A; New York, NY 10021; (212)
794-9500; **BDCERT:** Onc 77; Hem 78; **MS:** Cornell
U 72; **RES:** NY Hosp-Cornell Med Ctr, New York,
NY 73-75; **FEL:** Hem Onc, NY Hosp-Cornell Med
Ctr, New York, NY 75-78; **SI:** *Breast Cancer; Lung*
Cancer; **HMO:** Oxford PHS PHCS 32BJ Multiplan +

LANG: Pol, Hin; ☒ ☒ ☒ ☒ ☒ 1 Week

Kabakow, Bernard (MD) Onc
Beth Israel Med Ctr

70 E 10th St; New York, NY 10003; (212) 674-4455; **BDCERT:** Onc 73; Rad 80; **MS:** Univ Vt Coll Med 53; **RES:** Kings County Hosp Ctr, Brooklyn, NY 54-55; Mount Sinai Med Ctr, New York, NY 55-57; **FEL:** Montefiore Med Ctr, Bronx, NY 56-58; **HOSP:** Cabrini Med Ctr; **HMO:** Aetna Hlth Plan Blue Choice HealthNet CIGNA

🦽 📞 📷 🚺 🛏 Mcr Mcd WC NFI Immediately

Kelsen, David (MD) Onc
Mem Sloan Kettering Cancer Ctr

1275 York Ave; New York, NY 10021; (212) 639-8470; **BDCERT:** GO 76; Onc 79; **MS:** Hahnemann U 72; **RES:** Temple U Hosp, Philadelphia, PA 72-76; **FEL:** Onc, Mem Sloan Kettering Cancer Ctr, New York, NY 76-78; **SI:** *Colon Cancer*

LANG: Heb; 🦽 📷 🚺 🛏 Mcr Mcd 2-4 Weeks

Kemeny, Nancy (MD) Onc
Mem Sloan Kettering Cancer Ctr

1275 York Ave; New York, NY 10021; (212) 639-8068; **BDCERT:** IM 74; Onc 82; **MS:** UMDNJ-NJ Med Sch, Newark 71; **RES:** Med, St Luke's Roosevelt Hosp Ctr, New York, NY 72-74; **FEL:** Onc, Mem Sloan Kettering Cancer Ctr, New York, NY 74-76; **FAP:** Prof Med Cornell U; **SI:** *Colon Cancer; Rectal Cancer*

LANG: Hun, Sp, Jpn, Kor; 🦽 🚺 🛏 Mcr Mcd 2-4 Weeks 💳 **VISA**

Kris, Mark (MD) Onc PCP
Mem Sloan Kettering Cancer Ctr

1275 York Ave; New York, NY 10021; (212) 639-7590; **BDCERT:** IM 80; Onc 83; **MS:** Cornell U 77; **RES:** IM, NY Hosp-Cornell Med Ctr, New York, NY 77-80; Mem Sloan Kettering Cancer Ctr, New York, NY 81-82; **FEL:** Onc, Mem Sloan Kettering Cancer Ctr, New York, NY; **SI:** *Thoracic Oncology*

🦽 📷 🚺 🛏 Mcr Mcd WC Immediately 💳 **VISA** 💳

Krown, Susan (MD) Onc
Mem Sloan Kettering Cancer Ctr

1275 York Ave; New York, NY 10021; (212) 639-7426; **BDCERT:** Onc 77; **MS:** SUNY Hlth Sci Ctr 71; **RES:** Mount Sinai Med Ctr, New York, NY 71-74; **FEL:** Onc, Mem Sloan Kettering Cancer Ctr, New York, NY 75-77; Clinical Immunology, Mem Sloan Kettering Cancer Ctr, New York, NY 74-75; **FAP:** Prof Med Cornell U; **SI:** *AIDS Associated Cancers*; **HMO:** None

LANG: Sp; 🦽 📷 🛏 Mcr Mcd 1 Week

Malamud, Stephen (MD) Onc
Beth Israel Med Ctr

305 1st Ave; New York, NY 10003; (212) 420-4512; **BDCERT:** IM 81; Onc 83; **MS:** Albert Einstein Coll Med 78; **RES:** Beth Israel Med Ctr, New York, NY 79-81; **FEL:** Onc, Mount Sinai Med Ctr, New York, NY 81-83; **FAP:** Asst Prof Albert Einstein Coll Med; **HOSP:** Hosp For Joint Diseases; **SI:** *Lung Cancer; Gastrointestinal Cancers*; **HMO:** US Hlthcre Prudential Aetna Hlth Plan Oxford Blue Choice +

LANG: Sp, Fr, Dut; 🦽 📷 🛏 💲 Mcr Mcd A Few Days 💳 **VISA** 💳

Moore, Anne (MD) Onc
NY Hosp-Cornell Med Ctr

New York Hosp, 428 E 72nd St Ste 300; New York, NY 10021; (212) 746-2085; **BDCERT:** IM 73; Onc 77; **MS:** Columbia P&S 69; **RES:** Med, NY Hosp-Cornell Med Ctr, New York, NY 70-73; Ge, Rockefeller Univ Hosp, New York, NY 72-73; **SI:** *Breast Cancer*

LANG: Sp, Fr, Rus, Ar; 🦽 📷 🚺 💲 Mcr 4+ Weeks 💳 **VISA** 💳

Nachman, Ralph L (MD) Onc
NY Hosp-Cornell Med Ctr

NY Hospital Cornell Medical Center, 520 E 70th St Ste 341; New York, NY 10021; (212) 746-2075; **BDCERT:** IM 63; Onc 79; **MS:** Vanderbilt U Sch Med 56; **RES:** Path CP, NY Hosp-Cornell Med Ctr, New York, NY 57-58; IM, Montefiore Med Ctr, Bronx, NY 60-62; **FEL:** IM, NY Hosp-Cornell Med Ctr, New York, NY 62-63; **FAP:** Chrmn Med Cornell U; **SI:** *Blood Coagulation Problem; Thrombocytopenia*; **HMO:** Oxford Empire CIGNA Blue Choice Multiplan +

🦽 📷 Mcr Mcd 2-4 Weeks 💳 **VISA** 💳

Norton, Larry (MD) Onc
Mem Sloan Kettering Cancer Ctr
205 E 64th St; New York, NY 10021; (212) 639-5438; **BDCERT:** IM 72; Onc 77; **MS:** Columbia P&S 72; **RES:** Albert Einstein Med Ctr, Bronx, NY 72-74; **HMO:** Blue Cross & Blue Shield

Offit, Kenneth (MD) Onc
Mem Sloan Kettering Cancer Ctr
1275 York Ave; New York, NY 10021; (212) 639-6760; **BDCERT:** IM 85; Onc 87; **MS:** Harvard Med Sch 82; **RES:** Mem Sloan Kettering Cancer Ctr, New York, NY 86-87; **FEL:** Mem Sloan Kettering Cancer Ctr, New York, NY 87-88; Mem Sloan Kettering Cancer Ctr, New York, NY 85-88; **FAP:** Assoc Prof Cornell U; **SI:** *Cancer Genetic Testing*

 ♿ 🏠 🏥 Mcr Mcl 2-4 Weeks 🟦 **VISA** 💳 💳

Oratz, Ruth (MD) Onc
New York University Med Ctr
530 1st Ave 9R; New York, NY 10016; (212) 263-7218; **BDCERT:** IM 85; Onc 89; **MS:** Albert Einstein Coll Med 82; **RES:** IM, Bellevue Hosp Ctr, New York, NY 82-85; **FEL:** Onc, Bellevue Hosp Ctr, New York, NY 85-88; **SI:** *Breast Cancer; Melanoma*; **HMO:** Chubb Oxford

 ♿ 🏠 🏥 🏥 💲 Mcr 2-4 Weeks

Oster, Martin (MD) Onc
Columbia-Presbyterian Med Ctr
161 Fort Washington Ave; New York, NY 10032; (212) 305-8231; **BDCERT:** IM 74; Onc 75; **MS:** Columbia P&S 71; **RES:** Mass Gen Hosp, Boston, MA 71-73; **FEL:** Onc, Nat Cancer Inst, Bethesda, MD 73-76; **FAP:** Assoc Prof Columbia P&S; **SI:** *Breast Cancer Chemotherapy; Gastrointestinal Cancer*; **HMO:** Oxford Prucare

 ♿ 🏠 🏥 🏥 Mcr A Few Days

Pasmantier, Mark (MD) Onc
NY Hosp-Cornell Med Ctr
407 E 70th St; New York, NY 10021; (212) 517-5900; **BDCERT:** Hem 74; Onc 75; **MS:** NYU Sch Med 66; **RES:** IM, Harlem Hosp Ctr, New York, NY 69-70; **FEL:** Hem, Montefiore Med Ctr, Bronx, NY 70-71; Onc, NY Hosp-Cornell Med Ctr, New York, NY 71-72; **FAP:** Assoc Prof Cornell U; **SI:** *Lung Cancer; Ovarian Cancer*; **HMO:** Empire Blue Cross & Shield Sanus

 ♿ 🏠 🏥 🏥 💲 Mcr A Few Days **VISA** 💳

Portlock, Carol S (MD) Onc
Mem Sloan Kettering Cancer Ctr
Lymphoma Service, MSKCC, 1275 York Ave; New York, NY 10021; (212) 639-8109; **BDCERT:** IM 76; Onc 77; **MS:** Stanford U 71; **RES:** Stanford Med Ctr, Stanford, CA 71-74; **FEL:** Stanford Med Ctr, Stanford, CA 74-76; **SI:** *Non Hodgkin's Lymphomas; Hodgkin's Disease*

 ♿ 🏥 1 Week

Ratner, Lynn (MD) Onc
Mount Sinai Med Ctr
12 E 86th St; New York, NY 10028; (212) 861-6660; **BDCERT:** IM 71; Onc 73; **MS:** Albert Einstein Coll Med 64; **RES:** Bellevue Hosp Ctr, New York, NY 64-65; Bellevue Hosp Ctr, New York, NY &; **FEL:** Mem Sloan Kettering Cancer Ctr, New York, NY 70; **HOSP:** Lenox Hill Hosp; **SI:** *Medical Oncology; Breast Cancer*; **HMO:** Oxford Blue Cross & Blue Shield

LANG: Sp, Itl, Yd; ♿ Mcr 🟦 **VISA** 💳

Sara, Gabriel (MD) Onc
St Luke's Roosevelt Hosp Ctr
30 W 60th St A; New York, NY 10023; (212) 977-9292; **BDCERT:** Onc 87; Hem 86; **MS:** Lebanon 80; **RES:** IM, Univ Hosp SUNY Bklyn, Brooklyn, NY 82-84; IM, Brooklyn Hosp Ctr, Brooklyn, NY 81-82; **FEL:** Hem Onc, Columbia-Presbyterian Med Ctr, New York, NY 86-87; Hem Onc, St Luke's Roosevelt Hosp Ctr, New York, NY 84-86; **FAP:** Asst Clin Prof Med Columbia P&S; **SI:** *Breast, Gastrointestinal, and Lung Cancers; Lymphoma*; **HMO:** Oxford Select Chubb Cost Care Magnacare +

LANG: Fr, Sp; ♿ 🏠 🏥 💲 2-4 Weeks

Scher, Howard (MD)   Onc
Mem Sloan Kettering Cancer Ctr

1275 York Ave; New York, NY 10021; (212) 639-7585; **BDCERT:** IM 79; **MS:** NYU Sch Med 76; **RES:** Med, Bellevue Hosp Ctr, New York, NY 77-80; **FEL:** Onc, Mem Sloan Kettering Cancer Ctr, New York, NY 80-83; **HMO:** Blue Cross & Blue Shield

♿ 🅟 🅟 🈺 🆂 ⓂⒸⓇ   A Few Days

Sherman, William H (MD)   Onc
Columbia-Presbyterian Med Ctr

161 Fort Washington Ave AP9-922; New York, NY 10032; (212) 305-3856; **BDCERT:** IM 75; Onc 78; **MS:** Jefferson Med Coll 69; **RES:** IM, U IL Med Ctr, Chicago, IL 69-71; **FEL:** Onc, Columbia-Presbyterian Med Ctr, New York, NY 74-77; **FAP:** Assoc Prof Columbia P&S; **SI:** *Pancreatic Cancer; Myeloma;* **HMO:** Oxford Empire Blue Cross & Blue Choice Bronx Health Multiplan +

LANG: Sp; ♿ ⓒ 🅟 🅟 🈺 🆂 ⓂⒸⓇ   A Few Days

Silver, Richard (MD)   Onc
NY Hosp-Cornell Med Ctr

1440 York Ave P4; New York, NY 10021; (212) 288-5040; **BDCERT:** IM 62; Onc 73; **MS:** Cornell U 53; **RES:** IM, NY Hosp-Cornell Med Ctr, New York, NY 54-56; Hem, NY Hosp, New York, NY 56-57; **FEL:** Nat Cancer Inst, Bethesda, MD 57-58; **FAP:** Clin Prof Med Cornell U; **SI:** *Leukemia-Lymphoma; Myeloproliferative Disease*

♿ 🅟 🈺 🆂 ⓂⒸⓇ   A Few Days 🔲 *VISA* ⬤

Speyer, James (MD)   Onc
New York University Med Ctr

530 1st Ave Ste 9R; New York, NY 10016; (212) 263-6304; **BDCERT:** Onc 79; Hem 78; **MS:** Johns Hopkins U 74; **RES:** Columbia-Presbyterian Med Ctr, New York, NY 75-76; **FEL:** Onc, Columbia-Presbyterian Med Ctr, New York, NY 76-77; Onc, Nat Cancer Inst, Bethesda, MD 77-79

♿ 🅟 🅟 🈺 🆂 ⓂⒸⓇ   1 Week

Spriggs, David (MD)   Onc
Mem Sloan Kettering Cancer Ctr

1275 York Ave; New York, NY 10021; (212) 639-2203; **BDCERT:** Onc 85; **MS:** U Wisc Med Sch 77; **RES:** Columbia-Presbyterian Med Ctr, New York, NY; **FEL:** Onc, Dana-Farber Cancer Inst, Boston, MA; **FAP:** Assoc Prof Cornell U; **SI:** *Gynecologic Cancer; New Drug Development;* **HMO:** None

♿ 🅟 🈺 ⓂⒸⓇ Ⓜⓞⓓ

Stoopler, Mark (MD)   Onc
Columbia-Presbyterian Med Ctr

161 Fort Washington Ave; New York, NY 10032; (212) 305-8230; **BDCERT:** Onc 81; IM 78; **MS:** Cornell U 75; **RES:** IM, N Shore Univ Hosp-Glen Cove, Glen Cove, NY 75-78; IM, Mem Sloan Kettering Cancer Ctr, New York, NY 75-78; **FEL:** Onc, Mem Sloan Kettering Cancer Ctr, New York, NY 78-80; **FAP:** Assoc Clin Prof Med Columbia P&S; **SI:** *Lung Cancer; Esophagus Cancer;* **HMO:** Blue Choice Oxford Independent Health Plan PHS Multiplan +

♿ 🅟 🅟 🈺 🆂 ⓂⒸⓇ   1 Week

Taub, Robert (MD & PhD)   Onc
Columbia-Presbyterian Med Ctr

161 Fort Washington Ave 731; New York, NY 10032; (212) 305-4076; **BDCERT:** Onc 87; Hem 74; **MS:** Yale U Sch Med 61; **RES:** IM, New England Med Ctr, Boston, MA 65-66; **FEL:** Hem, New England Med Ctr, Boston, MA 68; **FAP:** Prof Columbia P&S; **SI:** *Sarcoma-Mesothelioma; Melanoma;* **HMO:** Oxford

LANG: Yd; ♿ 🅟 🈺 🆂 ⓂⒸⓇ Ⓦⓒ   1 Week

Tepler, Jeffrey (MD)   Onc
NY Hosp-Cornell Med Ctr

310 E 72nd St; New York, NY 10021; (212) 650-1780; **BDCERT:** Onc 87; Hem 88; **MS:** Yale U Sch Med 82; **RES:** IM, NY Hosp-Cornell Med Ctr, New York, NY 82-85; **FEL:** Hem Onc, NY Hosp-Cornell Med Ctr, New York, NY 85-88; **FAP:** Asst Clin Prof Med Cornell U; **SI:** *Breast Cancer; Lymphoma—Leukemia;* **HMO:** Oxford United Healthcare

LANG: Sp; ♿

Vogel, James M (MD) Onc
Mount Sinai Med Ctr

1125 Park Ave; New York, NY 10128; (212) 369-4250; **BDCERT:** Hem 72; Onc 73; **MS:** Columbia P&S 62; **RES:** IM, Mount Sinai Med Ctr, New York, NY 63-64; IM, Mount Sinai Med Ctr, New York, NY 66-67; **FEL:** Onc, Nat Cancer Inst, Bethesda, MD 64-66; Hem, Mount Sinai Med Ctr, New York, NY 67-68; **FAP:** Assoc Prof Med Mt Sinai Sch Med; **HOSP:** Beth Israel Med Ctr; *SI: Breast Cancer; Lymphoma;* **HMO:** Aetna Hlth Plan Blue Choice GHI CIGNA

LANG: Sp; 🔲 🔲 🔲 🔲 A Few Days **VISA** 🔲

Wernz, James (MD) Onc
New York University Med Ctr

530 1st Ave 9R; New York, NY 10016; (212) 263-7257; **BDCERT:** IM 76; Onc 81; **MS:** U Wash, Seattle 73; **RES:** St Luke's Roosevelt Hosp Ctr, New York, NY 73-76; **FEL:** Hem Onc, New York University Med Ctr, New York, NY 76-79; *SI: Breast Cancer; Lung Cancer;* **HMO:** Oxford Health Source CIGNA PHS United Healthcare +

🔲 🔲 🔲 🔲 🔲 🔲 A Few Days

NEONATAL-PERINATAL MEDICINE

Cohen-Addad, Nicole (MD) NP
St Vincents Hosp & Med Ctr NY

153 W 11th St Ste 839; New York, NY 10011; (212) 604-7884; **BDCERT:** Ped 81; NP 83; **MS:** France 74; **RES:** ped, Bretonneau Hosp, Paris, France 75-76; Ped, Children's Hosp of MI, Detroit, MI 76-77; **FEL:** Ped, Children's Hosp of MI, Detroit, MI 77-78; **HMO:** Prudential US Hlthcre Blue Choice Oxford PHS +

🔲 🔲 🔲 🔲

Driscoll, John (MD) NP
Columbia-Presbyterian Med Ctr

3959 Broadway 114S; New York, NY 10032; (212) 305-2934; **BDCERT:** Ped 70; **MS:** Bowman Gray 62; **RES:** Ped, Children's Hosp of Pittsburgh, Pittsburgh, PA 62-63; Columbia-Presbyterian Med Ctr, New York, NY 67-69; **FEL:** NP, Columbia-Presbyterian Med Ctr, New York, NY 69-71

🔲 🔲 🔲 🔲 🔲 🔲 Immediately 🔲 **VISA** 🔲 🔲

Fischer, Rita (MD) NP
St Vincents Hosp & Med Ctr NY

St Vincent's Hospital, 153 W 11th St Rm 841; New York, NY 10011; (212) 604-7883; **BDCERT:** Ped 79; **MS:** SUNY Downstate 70; **RES:** Ped, Columbia-Presbyterian Med Ctr, New York, NY 70-72; Ped, St Luke's Roosevelt Hosp Ctr, New York, NY 72-74; **FAP:** Asst Prof NY Med Coll; *SI: Care of Premature Infants;* **HMO:** Oxford Empire Blue Cross & Shield GHI Aetna-US Healthcare

🔲 🔲 🔲 🔲

Holzman, Ian (MD) NP
Mount Sinai Med Ctr

NewBorn Associates, 1 Gustave Levy Pl 1513; New York, NY 10029; (212) 241-5446; **BDCERT:** Ped 75; **MS:** Univ Pittsburgh 71; **RES:** Children's Hosp of Pittsburgh, Pittsburgh, PA 71-75; **FEL:** NP, U CO Hosp, Denver, CO; **FAP:** Prof Mt Sinai Sch Med; *SI: Nutrition; Enterocolitis;* **HMO:** Aetna Hlth Plan CIGNA Chubb Oxford PHCS +

LANG: Sp; 🔲 🔲 🔲 🔲 🔲 Immediately 🔲 **VISA** 🔲

Kandall, Stephen (MD) NP
Beth Israel Med Ctr

1st Ave & 16th St; New York, NY 10003; (212) 420-4170; **BDCERT:** Ped 70; NP 75; **MS:** NYU Sch Med 65; **RES:** Ped, Albert Einstein Med Ctr, Bronx, NY 65-69; **FEL:** NP, UC San Francisco Med Ctr, San Francisco, CA 71-72; **HMO:** Oxford US Hlthcre Sanus Blue Choice

🔲 🔲 🔲 🔲 🔲 🔲 🔲

Guide to symbols and abbreviations can be found on pages 110-113.

237

Krauss, Alfred N (MD) NP
NY Hosp-Cornell Med Ctr

525 E 68th St N 506; New York, NY 10021; (212) 746-3530; **BDCERT:** Ped 68; NP 75; **MS:** Cornell U 63; **RES:** Ped, NY Hosp-Cornell Med, New York, NY 64-67; **FEL:** Ped, Cornell-NY Hosp, New York, NY 64-69; **FAP:** Assoc Prof Ped Cornell U; **SI:** *Neonatology*
🔶

Mercado, Myra (MD) NP
St Luke's Roosevelt Hosp Ctr

129 Wadsworth Ave 4; New York, NY 10033; (212) 781-5889; **BDCERT:** Ped 95; **MS:** Dominica 82; **RES:** Ped, Lincoln Med & Mental Hlth Ctr, Bronx, NY 85-88; **FEL:** NP, Bellevue Hosp Ctr, New York, NY 93-96; **HMO:** US Hlthcre

LANG: Sp; 🔶 🔶 🔶 🔶 🔶 🔶 🔶 🔶 Immediately

Shahrivar, Farrokh (MD) NP
St Luke's Roosevelt Hosp Ctr

501 E 79th St; New York, NY 10021; (212) 523-3760; **BDCERT:** Ped 74; NP 75; **MS:** Iran 66; **RES:** Ped, St Luke's Roosevelt Hosp Ctr, New York, NY 70-71; Ped, St Luke's Roosevelt Hosp Ctr, New York, NY 71-72; **FEL:** NP, St Christopher's Hosp for Children, Philadelphia, PA 72-73; NP, Albert Einstein Med Ctr, Bronx, NY; **FAP:** Assoc Clin Prof Ped Columbia P&S; **HOSP:** Beth Israel Med Ctr

Yellin, Paul (MD) NP
NYU Downtown Hosp

170 William St; New York, NY 10038; (212) 312-5052; **BDCERT:** NP 84; Ped 84; **MS:** NYU Sch Med 79; **RES:** Ped, Bellevue Hosp Ctr, New York, NY 79-82; **FEL:** NP, Columbia-Presbyterian Med Ctr, New York, NY 82-84; **HOSP:** Bellevue Hosp Ctr

🔶 🔶 🔶 🔶 🔶 🔶 🔶 🔶 *VISA* 🔶 🔶

NEPHROLOGY

Ames, Richard (MD) Nep
St Luke's Roosevelt Hosp Ctr

16 E 90th St 2CA; New York, NY 10128; (212) 410-1245; **BDCERT:** IM 67; **MS:** Columbia P&S 58; **RES:** Boston Med Ctr, Boston, MA 58-61; **FEL:** HyprT, Columbia-Presbyterian Med Ctr, New York, NY 61-63; **FAP:** Clin Prof Med Columbia P&S; **HOSP:** St Clare's Hosp & Health Ctr; **SI:** *High Blood Pressure; Renal Dialysis*; **HMO:** Oxford Independent Health Plan Blue Choice Multiplan CIGNA +

LANG: Fr, Grk; 🔶 🔶 🔶 🔶 🔶 🔶 A Few Days

Appel, Gerald (MD) Nep
Columbia-Presbyterian Med Ctr

622 W 168th St 4124; New York, NY 10032; (212) 305-3273; **BDCERT:** IM 75; Nep 78; **MS:** Albert Einstein Coll Med 72; **RES:** Columbia-Presbyterian Med Ctr, New York, NY 72-75; **FEL:** Nep, Columbia-Presbyterian Med Ctr, New York, NY 75-76; Yale-New Haven Hosp, New Haven, CT 76-78; **SI:** *Glomerulonephritis; Lupus, Kidney Disease*; **HMO:** Oxford Empire Blue Choice Chubb Prucare

🔶 🔶 🔶 🔶 🔶 2-4 Weeks 🔶 *VISA* 🔶

August, Phyllis (MD) Nep
NY Hosp-Cornell Med Ctr

Cornell Medical Ctr, 525 E 68th St 463; New York, NY 10021; (212) 746-2189; **BDCERT:** IM 80; Nep 82; **MS:** Yale U Sch Med 77; **RES:** IM, NY Hosp-Cornell Med Ctr, New York, NY 78-80; **FEL:** Hypertension, NY Hosp-Cornell Med Ctr, New York, NY 80-83; **FAP:** Prof Med Cornell U; **SI:** *Hypertension; Kidney Disease*; **HMO:** Aetna-US Healthcare United Healthcare Prudential Oxford USA +

LANG: Sp; 🔶 🔶 🔶 🔶 🔶 🔶 1 Week 🔶 *VISA* 🔶

Burns, Godfrey (MD) Nep
St Vincents Hosp & Med Ctr NY

130 W 12th St; New York, NY 10011; (212) 790-8322; **BDCERT:** IM 72; Nep 76; **MS:** Howard U 67; **RES:** Med, St Vincents Hosp & Med Ctr NY, New York, NY 68-70; **FEL:** Renal Disease, St Vincents Hosp & Med Ctr NY, New York, NY 70-71

Cheigh, Jhoong (MD)   Nep
NY Hosp-Cornell Med Ctr

Rogosin Kidney Center, 525 E 68th St; New York, NY 10021; (212) 746-3096; **BDCERT:** IM 71; Nep 72; **MS:** South Korea 60; **RES:** Med, Mount Sinai Med Ctr, New York, NY 66-70; **FEL:** Nep, NY Hosp-Cornell Med Ctr, New York, NY 70-72; **FAP:** Clin Prof Med Cornell U; **SI:** *Chronic Renal Failure; Dialysis;* **HMO:** Oxford Aetna Hlth Plan Blue Choice Prudential US Hlthcre +

LANG: Kor; 🚹 📠 🏥 💲 Mcr Mcd 1 Week **VISA** ⬤ 💳

Cohen, David (MD)   Nep
Columbia-Presbyterian Med Ctr

622 W 168th St PH4124; New York, NY 10032; (212) 305-3273; **BDCERT:** Nep 84; **MS:** Albert Einstein Coll Med 77; **RES:** Mount Sinai Med Ctr, New York, NY 77-80; **FEL:** Columbia-Presbyterian Med Ctr, New York, NY 80-81; Immunology & Transplant, Harvard Med Sch, Cambridge, MA 81-83; **FAP:** Assoc Prof Columbia P&S; **SI:** *Kidney Transplantation; Glomerulonephritis;* **HMO:** Oxford Aetna Hlth Plan CIGNA Blue Cross & Blue Shield

LANG: Sp, Fr; 🚹 📠 📠 🏥 💲 Mcr Mcd WC NFI 1 Week ▓ **VISA**

De Fabritus, Albert (MD)   Nep
St Vincents Hosp & Med Ctr NY

36 7th Ave 517; New York, NY 10011; (212) 807-8817; **BDCERT:** IM 76; Nep 78; **MS:** NY Med Coll 73; **RES:** IM, St Vincents Hosp & Med Ctr NY, New York, NY 73-76; **FEL:** Nep, NY Hosp-Cornell Med Ctr, New York, NY 76-78; **FAP:** Asst Prof Med NY Med Coll; **SI:** *Hypertension; Urinary Tract Infection;* **HMO:** Aetna-US Healthcare Oxford United Healthcare PHS Guardian +

LANG: Sp; 🚹 📠 📠 🏥 💲 Mcr 1 Week

Glabman, Sheldon (MD)   Nep
Mount Sinai Med Ctr

1175 Park Ave; New York, NY 10128; (212) 534-3968; **BDCERT:** IM 64; **MS:** U Hlth Sci/Chicago Med Sch 57; **RES:** Mount Sinai Med Ctr, New York, NY 58-63; **FEL:** NY Hosp-Cornell Med Ctr, New York, NY 60-62; **HOSP:** Beth Israel Med Ctr; **HMO:** Oxford

📠 🏥 💲 Mcr A Few Days

Kaufman, Allen M (MD)   Nep
Beth Israel North

Chief Division of Nephrology and Hypertension, 170 East End Ave Ste 400; New York, NY 10128; (212) 870-9400; **BDCERT:** IM 78; Nep 80; **MS:** U Rochester 75; **RES:** Mount Sinai Med Ctr, New York, NY; **FEL:** Nep, Mount Sinai Med Ctr, New York, NY; **FAP:** Assoc Clin Prof Med Albert Einstein Coll Med; **HOSP:** Mount Sinai Med Ctr; **SI:** *Kidney Dialysis; Diabetic Kidney Disease*

LANG: Sp, Jpn; 🚹 SA SU 🅲 📠 📠 🏥 💲 Mcr Mcd WC NFI Immediately ▓ **VISA** ⬤ 💳 🔲

Lowenstein, Jerome (MD)   Nep
New York University Med Ctr

530 1st Ave Ste 4D; New York, NY 10016; (212) 263-7439; **BDCERT:** IM 64; Nep 76; **MS:** NYU Sch Med 57; **RES:** IM, Bellevue Hosp Ctr, New York, NY 60-63; **FEL:** Nep, Bellevue Hosp Ctr, New York, NY 63-67; **FAP:** Prof Med NYU Sch Med; **SI:** *Hypertension; Renal Disease;* **HMO:** Oxford

🚹 📠 💲 Mcr 2-4 Weeks

Matalon, Robert (MD)   Nep
New York University Med Ctr

NYU Medical Ctr, 530 1st Ave 4A; New York, NY 10016; (212) 263-7239; **BDCERT:** IM 70; Nep 70; **MS:** NYU Sch Med 64; **RES:** IM, Bellevue Hosp Ctr, New York, NY 64-67; **FEL:** Nep, New York University Med Ctr, New York, NY 67-69; **FAP:** Assoc Clin Prof Med NYU Sch Med; **HOSP:** NYU Downtown Hosp; **SI:** *Dialysis; Kidney Failure;* **HMO:** Oxford CIGNA PHS United Healthcare Consumer Hlth Network +

🚹 📠 🏥 💲 Mcr

Meltzer, Jay I (MD)   Nep   PCP
Columbia-Presbyterian Med Ctr

903 Park Ave; New York, NY 10021; (212) 988-4488; **BDCERT:** IM 61; **MS:** Columbia P&S 53; **RES:** Columbia-Presbyterian Med Ctr, New York, NY 55-58; Med, Bellevue Hosp Ctr, New York, NY 58-59; **HOSP:** NY Hosp-Cornell Med Ctr; **SI:** *Hypertension; Kidney Disease;* **HMO:** None

LANG: Sp, Ger; 🚹 📠 🏥 Mcr A Few Days

Guide to symbols and abbreviations can be found on pages 110-113.

239

Michelis, Michael (MD)   Nep
Lenox Hill Hosp

130 E 77th St Fl 5; New York, NY 10021; (212) 988-3506; **BDCERT:** IM 69; **MS:** Geo Wash U Sch Med 63; **RES:** Lenox Hill Hosp, New York, NY 63-65; Hosp Med College of PA, Philadelphia, PA 65-67; **FEL:** Renal Disease, U of Pittsburgh Med Ctr, Pittsburgh, PA 69-70; **FAP:** Clin Prof Med NYU Sch Med; **SI:** *Hypertension; Salt & Fluid Problems;* **HMO:** Aetna Hlth Plan GHI CIGNA Oxford Prucare +

LANG: Sp; 🚹 🅰 🚼 🏥 🅂 Mcr Mod Immediately

Saal, Stuart (MD)   Nep
NY Hosp-Cornell Med Ctr

505 E 70th St HT230; New York, NY 10021; (212) 746-1553; **BDCERT:** IM 74; **MS:** NY Med Coll 71; **RES:** St Luke's Roosevelt Hosp Ctr, New York, NY 74; **FEL:** NY Hosp-Cornell Med Ctr, New York, NY 76

🚹 🅰 🏥 Mcr 1 Week

Sherman, Raymond (MD)   Nep
NY Hosp-Cornell Med Ctr

407 E 70th St Fl 4; New York, NY 10021; (212) 879-8245; **BDCERT:** IM 69; Nep 74; **MS:** SUNY Hlth Sci Ctr 61; **RES:** St Luke's Roosevelt Hosp Ctr, New York, NY 61-64; Strong Mem Hosp, Rochester, NY 64-65; **FEL:** Nep, NY Hosp-Cornell Med Ctr, New York, NY 67-69; **FAP:** Clin Prof Med Cornell U; **SI:** *Abnormal Kidney Function; Hypertension;* **HMO:** Blue Choice

🚹 🅰 🏥 🅂 A Few Days

Stenzel, Kurt H (MD)   Nep
NY Hosp-Cornell Med Ctr

505 E 70th St; New York, NY 10021; (212) 746-6117; **BDCERT:** IM 88; Nep 92; **MS:** Cornell U 58; **RES:** Bellevue Hosp Ctr, New York, NY 58-60; Bellevue Hosp Ctr, New York, NY 62-63; **FEL:** Nep, NY Hosp-Cornell Med Ctr, New York, NY 63-66; **FAP:** Prof Cornell U; **SI:** *Dialysis; Transplantation;* **HMO:** Oxford United Healthcare Blue Choice Magnacare US Hlthcre +

LANG: Sp, Chi, Kor; 🚹 🅰 🚼 🏥 Mcr Mod 1 Week

Stern, Leonard (MD)   Nep
Columbia-Presbyterian Med Ctr

622 W 168th St; New York, NY 10032; (212) 305-3273; **BDCERT:** IM 78; Nep 80; **MS:** NY Med Coll 75; **RES:** Jacobi Med Ctr, Bronx, NY 75-78; **FEL:** Montefiore Med Ctr, Bronx, NY 78-79; Yale-New Haven Hosp, New Haven, CT 79-81; **FAP:** Asst Prof of Clin Med Columbia P&S; **SI:** *Dialysis; Kidney Transplantation*

LANG: Sp; 🚹 🅰 🏥 🅂 Mcr Mod 2-4 Weeks

Wang, John (MD)   Nep
NY Hosp-Cornell Med Ctr

505 E 70th St 213; New York, NY 10021; (212) 746-3097; **BDCERT:** IM 85; Nep 86; **MS:** Cornell U 79; **RES:** Long Island Jewish Med Ctr, New Hyde Park, NY 79; Laguardia Hosp, Forest Hills, NY 82; **FEL:** Nep, NY Hosp-Cornell Med Ctr, New York, NY; **HMO:** Sanus-NYLCare

🚹 🅰 🚼 🏥 Mcr Mod Immediately 🔲 **VISA** 🔴

Wasser, Walter (MD)   Nep
Cabrini Med Ctr

Lifecare Dialysis Ctr, 211 W 61st St; New York, NY 10023; (212) 977-3100; **BDCERT:** IM 79; Nep 84; **MS:** Albert Einstein Coll Med 76; **RES:** IM, Maimonides Med Ctr, Brooklyn, NY 77-78; IM, Mount Sinai Med Ctr, New York, NY 78-79; **FEL:** Nep, Mount Sinai Med Ctr, New York, NY 79-81; Bacteriology & Immunology, Rockefeller Univ Hosp, New York, NY 81-83; **FAP:** Asst Clin Prof Med Cornell U; **HOSP:** Beth Israel Med Ctr; **SI:** *Hemodialysis; Glomerulonephritis;* **HMO:** Oxford US Hlthcre PHS United Healthcare Prucare +

LANG: Sp, Rus, Chi; 🚹 🅰 🚼 🏥 Mcr Mod A Few Days

Weiss, Stanley (MD)   Nep
Beth Israel Med Ctr

1085 Park Ave; New York, NY 10028; (212) 369-2844; **BDCERT:** IM 72; Nep 76; **MS:** NYU Sch Med 65; **RES:** IM, Montefiore Med Ctr, Bronx, NY 66-67; IM, Montefiore Med Ctr, Bronx, NY 67-68; **FEL:** Renal Disease, Montefiore Med Ctr, Bronx, NY 68-69; **HOSP:** St Clare's Hosp & Health Ctr; **SI:** *Hypertension; Kidney Failure*

🚹 🅰 🚼 🏥 Mcr Immediately

Weisstuch, Joseph (DO)   Nep
New York University Med Ctr
NYU Medical Ctr, 530 1st Ave 7F; New York, NY
10016; (212) 263-0705; **BDCERT:** IM 88; Nep 92;
MS: NYU Sch Med 85; **RES:** IM, New York
University Med Ctr, New York, NY 85-89; **FEL:** Nep,
Bellevue Hosp Ctr, New York, NY 89-91; **FAP:** Asst
Clin Prof NYU Sch Med; **HOSP:** Hosp For Joint
Diseases; **HMO:** Oxford CIGNA Aetna Hlth Plan
Blue Cross & Blue Shield Health Source +

LANG: Sp, Heb, Yd; ♿ ⌂ ⅲ 💲 Mcr Mcd
Immediately

Williams, Gail S (MD)   Nep
Columbia-Presbyterian Med Ctr
161 Ft Washington Ave APb51; New York, NY
10032; (212) 305-5376; **BDCERT:** IM 72; Nep 74;
MS: Columbia P&S 68; **RES:** IM, Columbia-
Presbyterian Med Ctr, New York, NY 72-73; **FEL:**
Ped, Columbia-Presbyterian Med Ctr, New York,
NY 70-72; **FAP:** Assoc Clin Prof Med Columbia
P&S; **SI:** *Dialysis; Transplantation;* **HMO:** Oxford
Crespo Prudential

♿ ⅲ 💲 2-4 Weeks

Winston, Jonathan (MD)   Nep
Mount Sinai Med Ctr
Mount Sinai Medical Center, 5 E 98th St Bx1121;
New York, NY 10029; (212) 241-4060; **BDCERT:**
IM 80; Nep 84; **MS:** Geo Wash U Sch Med 77; **RES:**
Long Island Jewish Med Ctr, New Hyde Park, NY
77-80; **FEL:** Nep, Mount Sinai Med Ctr, New York,
NY 80-82; **SI:** *Kidney Disease; Kidney Transplantation*

♿ ⌂ ⅳ ⅲ Mcr Mcd A Few Days

Zabetakis, Paul (MD)   Nep
Lenox Hill Hosp
130 E 77th St Fl 5; New York, NY 10021; (212)
861-3534; **BDCERT:** Nep 75; **MS:** U Tenn Ctr Hlth
Sci, Memphis 72; **RES:** U of Pittsburgh Med Ctr,
Pittsburgh, PA 72-75; **FEL:** Yale-New Haven Hosp,
New Haven, CT 75-77; **FAP:** Assoc Clin Prof Med
NYU Sch Med; **SI:** *Hypertension; Kidney Failure;*
HMO: Oxford Blue Cross CIGNA PHS Multiplan +

LANG: Sp; ♿ ⌂ ⅲ 💲 Mcr Mcd Immediately

Zackson, David A (MD)   Nep
NY Hosp-Cornell Med Ctr
525 E 68th St Rm F2020; New York, NY 10021;
(212) 746-6290; **BDCERT:** IM 64; **MS:** NYU Sch
Med 57; **RES:** IM, Kingsbridge VA Med Ctr, Bronx,
NY 58-60; **FEL:** Nep, Montefiore Med Ctr, Bronx,
NY 60-61; **SI:** *Osteoporis; Calcium Deficiency;* **HMO:**
None

♿ ⌂ 💲 Mcr 1 Week ▓ *VISA* 💳 📇

NEUROLOGICAL SURGERY

Bederson, Joshua (MD)   NS
Mount Sinai Med Ctr
Box 1136; New York, NY 10029; (212) 241-2377;
BDCERT: NS 93; **MS:** UC San Francisco 84; **RES:** N,
UC San Francisco Med Ctr, San Francisco, CA 84-
90; **FEL:** Cerebrovascular S, Barrow Neurological
Inst, Phoenix, AZ; Microneurosurgery, U Hosp
Zurich, Zurich, Switzerland; **FAP:** Assoc Prof Mt
Sinai Sch Med; **HOSP:** Elmhurst Hosp Ctr; **SI:**
Cerebrovascular Surgery; Aneurysm; **HMO:** Oxford
Empire Blue Cross & Shield Aetna Hlth Plan PHCS
Health Source +

LANG: Sp, Itl, Chi, Jpn, Fr; ♿ ⌂ ⅳ ⅲ Mcr Mcd
A Few Days ▓ *VISA* 💳 📇

Benjamin, Vallo (MD)   NS
New York University Med Ctr
530 1st Ave 7W; New York, NY 10016; (212)
263-5013; **BDCERT:** NS 67; **MS:** Iran 58; **RES:**
Bellevue Hosp Ctr, New York, NY 60-64; **FEL:** NS,
New York University Med Ctr, New York, NY 65-
66; **FAP:** Prof N NYU Sch Med; **HOSP:** Beth Israel
North; **SI:** *Skull Base Tumors—Meningiomas;
Complex Spinal Surgery*

LANG: Sp, Frs; ♿ ⌂ ⅳ ⅲ 💲 NFl Immediately
VISA 💳

Guide to symbols and abbreviations can be found on pages 110-113.

241

Camins, Martin B (MD)   NS
Mount Sinai Med Ctr

205 E 68th St T 1C; New York, NY 10021; (212) 570-0100; **BDCERT:** NS 80; **MS:** U Hlth Sci/Chicago Med Sch 69; **RES:** NS, Columbia-Presbyterian Med Ctr, New York, NY 71-75; N, Columbia-Presbyterian Med Ctr, New York, NY 70-71; **FEL:** NS, Nat Hosp for Nervous Disease, London, England 73; New York University Med Ctr, New York, NY 76-77; **FAP:** Assoc Clin Prof NS Mt Sinai Sch Med; **HOSP:** Lenox Hill Hosp; *SI: Brain Tumor Microsurgery; Spine-Cervical-Lumbar*

LANG: Sp; ⓵ ⓸ ⓹ ⓺ ⓼ Mcr WC NFI   Immediately

Cooper, Paul (MD)   NS
New York University Med Ctr

550 1st Ave; New York, NY 10016; (212) 263-6514; **BDCERT:** NS 77; **MS:** U Va Sch Med 66; **RES:** S, U Hosp of Cleveland, Cleveland, OH 67-68; NS, New York University Med Ctr, New York, NY 70-75; **FAP:** Prof NS NYU Sch Med; *SI: Spinal Surgery; Pituitary Surgery;* **HMO:** Oxford Aetna-US Healthcare United Healthcare CIGNA Blue Cross PPO +

LANG: Fr; ⓵ ⓸ ⓺ ⓼ Mcr WC NFI   1 Week

De Los Reyes, Raul (MD)   NS
Beth Israel North

Beth Israel Med Ctr - North, 170 East End Ave 523; New York, NY 10128; (212) 870-9260; **BDCERT:** NS 86; **MS:** U Tex Med Br, Galveston 77; **RES:** NS, Henry Ford Hosp, Detroit, MI 78-83; **FEL:** Microneurosurgery, Henry Ford Hosp, Detroit, MI 83; **FAP:** Assoc Prof NS Albert Einstein Coll Med; **HOSP:** Beth Israel Med Ctr; *SI: Brain Aneurysms-Vascular; Lower Back;* **HMO:** Oxford Aetna-US Healthcare NYLCare Prucare CIGNA +

LANG: Sp, Grk; ⓵ ⓸ ⓺ ⓼ Mcr WC NFI   A Few Days
▩ *VISA* ⬤

Digiacinto, George (MD)   NS
St Luke's Roosevelt Hosp Ctr

425 W 59th St; New York, NY 10019; (212) 523-8500; **BDCERT:** N 81; **MS:** Harvard Med Sch 70; **RES:** S, St Luke's Roosevelt Hosp Ctr, New York, NY 70-72; Columbia-Presbyterian Med Ctr, New York, NY 74-78; **FEL:** NS, Columbia-Presbyterian Med Ctr, New York, NY 74-78; **FAP:** Instr N Columbia P&S; **HOSP:** Beth Israel North; *SI: Spine Surgery; Brain Tumors;* **HMO:** CIGNA Blue Cross & Blue Shield Oxford Chubb Aetna-US Healthcare +

LANG: Sp; ⓵ ⓸ ⓹ ⓺ ⓼ Mcr Mcd WC NFI   Immediately

Fodstad, Harald (MD)   NS
New York Methodist Hosp

130 E 18th St 17 H; New York, NY 10003; (718) 780-5328; **MS:** Switzerland 67; **RES:** NS, Umea Univ Hosp, Sweden 71-7; **FEL:** N Phys, Neurological Clinic, Tokyo, Japan 76; **FAP:** Assoc Prof Cornell U; *SI: Parkinson's Disease; Brain & Spine Surgery;* **HMO:** Oxford Fidelis Health First First Option Empire Blue Choice +

LANG: Fr, Ger, Sp, Man; ⓵ ⓸ ⓹ ⓺ Mcr Mcd
A Few Days ▩ *VISA* ⬤

Fraser, Richard (MD)   NS
NY Hosp-Cornell Med Ctr

525 E 68th St; New York, NY 10021; (212) 746-2385; **BDCERT:** NS 71; **MS:** U British Columbia Fac Med 61; **RES:** NS, Stanford Med Ctr, Stanford, CA 65; NS, Columbia-Presbyterian Med Ctr, New York, NY 66-70; **FEL:** NS, Columbia-Presbyterian Med Ctr, New York, NY 67; NS, Nat Inst Health, Bethesda, MD 71; **FAP:** Chf NS Cornell U; **HOSP:** Hosp For Special Surgery; *SI: Brain Surgery; Epilepsy;* **HMO:** Aetna Hlth Plan Magnacare Oxford Sanus

⓵ ⓺ ⓸ ⓹ ⓺ Mcr   Immediately

Gamache, Francis (MD) NS
NY Hosp-Cornell Med Ctr
Cornell University Med College, 523 E 72nd St 7th
FL; New York, NY 10021; (212) 746-2388;
BDCERT: NS 82; **MS:** Cornell U 71; **RES:** NS, NY
Hosp-Cornell Med Ctr, New York, NY 78-79; **FEL:**
Neurotrauma, Md Inst Emer Med Svcs, Baltimore,
MD 78; Univ of Western Ontario, London, Canada
78-79; **FAP:** Assoc Prof NS Cornell U; **HOSP:** Hosp
For Special Surgery; **SI:** *Brain and Vascular Tumors;*
Spine & Syringomyelia; **HMO:** Empire PHCS Oxford
NYLCare PHS +

LANG: Sp, Ger, Itl; 🦽 📷 🛏 💲 Mcr wc NFI
Immediately 📧 *VISA* 💳 📧

Ghajar, Jamshid (MD) NS
New York University Med Ctr
1300 York Ave 650; New York, NY 10021; (212)
746-2396; **BDCERT:** NS 93; **MS:** Cornell U 81; **RES:**
NYU Med Ctr, New York, NY 81-85; **FAP:** Asst Clin
Prof NYU Sch Med; **HOSP:** Jamaica Med Ctr

🦽 🛏 Mcr Mcd

Golfinos, John (MD) NS
New York University Med Ctr
530 1st Ave Ste 8R; New York, NY 10016; (212)
263-8002; **MS:** Columbia P&S 88; **RES:** NS, Barrow
Neurological Inst, Phoenix, AZ 89-95; **FAP:** Asst
Prof NYU Sch Med; **SI:** *Brain Tumors; Minimally*
Invasive Surgery; **HMO:** Oxford United Healthcare
Blue Cross & Blue Shield

LANG: Slv, Grk, Fr; 🦽 SA/SU 📷 🛏 🛏 Mcr Mcd wc NFI
A Few Days 📧 *VISA* 💳

Goodman, Robert R (MD) NS
Columbia-Presbyterian Med Ctr
710 W 168th St Rm 428; New York, NY 10032;
(212) 305-3774; **BDCERT:** NS 93; **MS:** Johns
Hopkins U 82; **RES:** NS, Columbia-Presbyterian
Med Ctr, New York, NY 82-89; **HOSP:** Holy Name
Hosp; **SI:** *Epilepsy; Parkinson's Disease;* **HMO:** Oxford
Empire Blue Choice Prudential PHS Medichoice +

LANG: Sp, Heb; 🦽 📷 🛏 🛏 💲 Mcr Mcd wc NFI
1 Week 📧 *VISA* 💳

Gutin, Philip (MD) NS
Mem Sloan Kettering Cancer Ctr
Dept of Neurological SurgeryMem Sloan Kettering,
1275 York Ave; New York, NY 10021; (212) 639-
8556; **BDCERT:** NS 81; **MS:** Univ Penn 71; **RES:**
NS, UC San Francisco Med Ctr, San Francisco, CA
72-79; **FAP:** Prof Cornell U; **HOSP:** NY Hosp-
Cornell Med Ctr; **SI:** *Brain Tumors; Stereotactic*
Surgery; **HMO:** Empire Blue Cross

🦽 📷 🛏 🛏 Mcr Mcd AMERICAN *VISA* 💳 📧

Jafar, Jafar (MD) NS
New York University Med Ctr
560 1st Ave Suite 8R; New York, NY 10016; (212)
263-6312; **BDCERT:** NS 84; **MS:** Iran 76; **RES:** U
Chicago Hosp, Chicago, IL 76-82; **FAP:** Assoc Prof
NYU Sch Med; **SI:** *Brain Aneurysms; Skull Base*
Tumors; **HMO:** CIGNA Aetna Hlth Plan Prucare

LANG: Fr, Sp, Ar, Per; 🦽 📞 📷 🛏 🛏 💲 Mcr
Immediately

Kelly, Patrick (MD) NS
New York University Med Ctr
NYU Med Ctr Dept NeurSurg, 530 1st Ave Ste 8R;
New York, NY 10016; (212) 263-8002; **BDCERT:**
NS 78; **MS:** SUNY Buffalo 66; **RES:** NS,
Northwestern Mem Hosp, Chicago, IL 70-72; NS, U
TX Med Branch Hosp, Galveston, TX 72-74; **FEL:**
SM, St Anne Hosp, Paris, France 77; **FAP:** Chrmn
NS NYU Sch Med; **HOSP:** Lenox Hill Hosp; **SI:** *Brain*
Tumor Removal; Movement Disorder Surgery

LANG: Slv, Flm, Grk; 🦽 📷 🛏 🛏 💲 A Few Days
📧 *VISA* 💳

Lavyne, Michael H (MD) NS
NY Hosp-Cornell Med Ctr
523 E 72nd St; New York, NY 10021; (212) 717-
0200; **BDCERT:** NS 82; **MS:** Cornell U 72; **RES:**
Mass Gen Hosp, Boston, MA 73-79; **FEL:** N, Beth
Israel Med Ctr, Boston, MA 73-74; **FAP:** Assoc Prof
of Clin S Cornell U; **HOSP:** Hosp For Special Surgery;
SI: *Spinal Surgery; Acoustic/Skull Base Surgery*

🦽 📷 🛏 💲 Mcr 1 Week 📧 *VISA* 💳

McCormick, Paul C (MD)   NS
Columbia-Presbyterian Med Ctr
710 W 168th St 406; New York, NY 10032; (212) 305-7976; **BDCERT:** NS 93; **MS:** Columbia P&S 82; **RES:** NS, Columbia-Presbyterian Med Ctr, New York, NY 84-89; **FAP:** Assoc Prof NS Columbia P&S; **HOSP:** Valley Hosp; **SI:** *Spinal Disorders/Back Pain; Herniated Disk/Stenosis;* **HMO:** Oxford

♿ 🅿 🏨 $ WC 2-4 Weeks 💳 **VISA** 💳

McMurtry, James (MD)   NS
Columbia-Presbyterian Med Ctr
The Neurological Institute, 710 W 168th St 212; New York, NY 10032; (212) 305-5595; **BDCERT:** NS 65; **MS:** Baylor 57; **RES:** S, Baylor Coll Med, Houston, TX 58-59; NS, Columbia-Presbyterian Med Ctr, New York, NY 60-63; **FEL:** NS, Columbia-Presbyterian Med Ctr, New York, NY 63-65; **FAP:** Prof of Clin NS Columbia P&S; **SI:** *Brain Tumors; Spinal Surgery;* **HMO:** Blue Choice Oxford Prucare

LANG: Sp; ♿ SA 🅿 🚻 🏨 Mcr WC NFI A Few Days

Moore, Frank (MD)   NS
Mount Sinai Med Ctr
1158 5th Ave; New York, NY 10029; (212) 410-6990; **BDCERT:** NS 92; **MS:** France 83; **RES:** NS, Mount Sinai Med Ctr, New York, NY 84-89; NS, Mount Sinai Med Ctr, New York, NY; **HOSP:** Englewood Hosp & Med Ctr; **SI:** *Brain Tumors/Aneurysms; Spinal Cord Tumors/Discs;* **HMO:** PHCS Oxford PHS Medichoice United Healthcare +

LANG: Fr, Sp, Ger; ♿ 🅿 🚻 🏨 $ Mcr WC NFI A Few Days

Murali, Raj (MD)   NS
St Vincents Hosp & Med Ctr NY
Manhattan Neurosurgical Associates PC, 153 W 11th St NR 8; New York, NY 10011; (212) 604-7767; **BDCERT:** NS 82; **MS:** India 68; **RES:** New York University Med Ctr, New York, NY; **FAP:** Assoc Prof NY Med Coll; **HOSP:** Bellevue Hosp Ctr; **SI:** *Spine Surgery; Skull Base Surgery;* **HMO:** Oxford Magnacare Aetna Hlth Plan Anthem Health PHCS +

♿ 🅿 🚻 🏨 $ Mcr Mcd WC NFI 1 Week

Post, Kalmon (MD)   NS
Mount Sinai Med Ctr
Mount Sinai Hospital, 5 E 98th St FL7; New York, NY 10029; (212) 241-0933; **BDCERT:** NS 78; **MS:** NYU Sch Med 67; **RES:** S, Bellevue Hosp Ctr, New York, NY 68-69; NS, Bellevue Hosp Ctr, New York, NY 71-75; **FAP:** Dir NS Mt Sinai Sch Med

Raynor, Richard B (MD)   NS
Cabrini Med Ctr
112 E 74th St; New York, NY 10021; (212) 535-1255; **BDCERT:** NS 66; **MS:** Univ Vt Coll Med 55; **RES:** NS, Columbia-Presbyterian Med Ctr, New York, NY 58-61; **FAP:** Clin Prof NYU Sch Med; **HOSP:** St Vincents Hosp & Med Ctr NY; **SI:** *Spine Surgery; Brain Tumors*

♿ 🅿 🚻 🏨 $ Mcr WC NFI A Few Days

Sachdev, Ved (MD)   NS
Mount Sinai Med Ctr
1148 5th Ave 1B; New York, NY 10128; (212) 289-5490; **BDCERT:** NS 76; **MS:** India 55; **RES:** St Joseph's Hosp, Lorain, OH 69; Mount Sinai Med Ctr, New York, NY 70-73; **FEL:** Royal Coll of Surgeons, England 62-63; **SI:** *Microneurosurgery Brain; Microneurosurgery Spine;* **HMO:** Oxford

LANG: Ur, Hin; ♿ 🅿 🏨 $ Mcr WC NFI A Few Days 💳

Sisti, Michael (MD)   NS
Columbia-Presbyterian Med Ctr
Neurosurgical Associates Of New York, 710 W 168th St A; New York, NY 10032; (212) 305-1728; **BDCERT:** NS 91; **MS:** Columbia P&S 81; **RES:** NS, Columbia-Presbyterian Med Ctr, New York, NY 83-88; **FEL:** NS, Nat Inst Health, Bethesda, MD 82-83; **FAP:** Asst Prof NS Columbia P&S; **SI:** *Brain Tumors; AVMS;* **HMO:** Oxford Prucare PHS Empire Independent Health Plan +

♿ 🅿 🚻 🏨 $ Mcr NFI A Few Days 💳 **VISA** 💳

Snow, Robert (MD) NS
NY Hosp-Cornell Med Ctr

523 E 72nd St; New York, NY 10021; (212) 717-0256; **BDCERT:** NS 89; **MS:** Stanford U 81; **RES:** NS, NY Hosp-Cornell Med Ctr, New York, NY 82-86; **FAP:** Assoc Clin Prof NS Cornell U; **SI:** *Spinal Surgery; Pituitary Tumors;* **HMO:** Oxford United Healthcare US Hlthcre CIGNA PHS +

LANG: Sp, Itl; ♿ ☎ 🏥 💲 Mcr WC   A Few Days **VISA** ⬤

Solomon, Robert (MD) NS
Columbia-Presbyterian Med Ctr

710 W 168th St; New York, NY 10032; (212) 305-4118; **BDCERT:** NS 88; **MS:** Johns Hopkins U 80; **RES:** Columbia-Presbyterian Med Ctr, New York, NY 80-86; **SI:** *Cerebral Aneurysms; Arteriovenous Malformations;* **HMO:** Oxford

LANG: Sp; ♿ ☎ 🏥 🏥 💲 Mcr Mcd   Immediately 🔲 **VISA** ⬤ 🔲

Steinberger, Alfred A (MD) NS
Mount Sinai Med Ctr

1158 5th Ave; New York, NY 10029; (212) 410-6990; **BDCERT:** NS 85; **MS:** Columbia P&S 76; **RES:** NS, Columbia-Presbyterian Med Ctr, New York, NY 77-81; Columbia-Presbyterian Med Ctr, New York, NY 81-82; **FAP:** Asst Clin Prof Mt Sinai Sch Med; **HOSP:** Englewood Hosp & Med Ctr; **SI:** *Brain Tumors/Aneurysms; Spinal Cord Tumors;* **HMO:** Oxford PHCS PHS Multiplan

♿ ☎ 🏥 💲 Mcr WC NFI   1 Week

Sundaresan, Narayan (MD) NS
Mount Sinai Med Ctr

1148 5th Ave; New York, NY 10128; (212) 876-7575; **BDCERT:** NS 80; **MS:** India 69; **RES:** NS, Northwestern Mem Hosp, Chicago, IL 71-77; **FEL:** N Onc, Mem Sloan Kettering Cancer Ctr, New York, NY 74; **FAP:** Clin Prof Mt Sinai Sch Med; **HOSP:** Lenox Hill Hosp; **SI:** *Spine Tumors & Discs; Brain Tumors;* **HMO:** Oxford Sel Pro Premier

♿ ☎ 🏥 🏥 💲 Mcr WC NFI   A Few Days **VISA** ⬤ 🔲

Wisoff, Jeffrey H (MD) NS
New York University Med Ctr

550 1st Ave; New York, NY 10016; (212) 263-6419; **BDCERT:** NS 90; 96; **MS:** Geo Wash U Sch Med 78; **RES:** Mount Sinai Med Ctr, New York, NY 78-79; NS, New York University Med Ctr, New York, NY 79-84; **FEL:** Ped NS, New York University Med Ctr, New York, NY 84-85; **FAP:** Assoc Prof Ped NYU Sch Med; **HOSP:** Bellevue Hosp Ctr; **SI:** *Brain Tumors Pediatric; Hydrocephalus;* **HMO:** Oxford Chubb US Hlthcre Empire Blue Cross & Shield United Healthcare +

LANG: Sp; ♿ ☎ 🏥 🏥 💲 Mcr Mcd WC   Immediately **VISA** ⬤

NEUROLOGY

Allen, Jeffrey (MD) N
Beth Israel Med Ctr

Beth Israel Medical Center NorthPed Neurology/NeuroOncology, 170 E End Ave; New York, NY 10128; (212) 870-9407; **BDCERT:** N 77; **MS:** Harvard Med Sch 69; **RES:** Ped A&I, Montreal Children's Hosp, Montreal, Canada 90-92; Montreal Neur Inst, Montreal, Canada 92-95; **FAP:** Prof NYU Sch Med; **SI:** *Brain Tumors; Cerebral Palsy;* **HMO:** Oxford Blue Cross Aetna Hlth Plan US Hlthcre

LANG: Sp, Prt, Fr; ♿ ☎ 🏥 🏥 💲 Mcr Mcd   A Few Days 🔲 **VISA** ⬤ 🔲

Apatoff, Brian R (MD & PhD) N
NY Hosp-Cornell Med Ctr

New York Hospital Cornell Med Ctr Dept of Neurology, 520 E 70th St; New York, NY 10021; (212) 746-4504; **BDCERT:** N 91; **MS:** U Chicago-Pritzker Sch Med 84; **RES:** N, Columbia-Presbyterian Med Ctr, New York, NY 87-90; **FEL:** Multiple Sclerosis, Columbia-Presbyterian Med Ctr, New York, NY 90-92; **FAP:** Asst Prof N Cornell U; **SI:** *Multiple Sclerosis;* **HMO:** +

♿ ☾ ☎ 🏥 🏥 Mcr 🔲 **VISA** ⬤

Balmaceda, Casilda (MD)   N
Columbia-Presbyterian Med Ctr

710 W 168th St Ste 202; New York, NY 10032;
(212) 305-4572; **BDCERT:** N 93; **MS:** Columbia
P&S 87; **RES:** IM, Montefiore Med Ctr, Bronx, NY
89-90; N, Columbia-Presbyterian Med Ctr, New
York, NY 88-91; **FEL:** N Onc, Mem Sloan Kettering
Cancer Ctr, New York, NY 91-93; **FAP:** Columbia
P&S; *SI: Brain Tumors-Astrocytoma; Meningioma;*
HMO: Oxford Aetna Hlth Plan Prudential GHI Blue
Cross & Blue Shield +

LANG: Sp, Fr, Itl; 🖐 🕮 🕐 🖬 🖬 🎬 Mcr
Immediately ▦ *VISA* 💳 💳

Belok, Lennart (MD)   N
Beth Israel Med Ctr

410 E 20th St MG; New York, NY 10009; (212)
254-9716; **BDCERT:** N 83; IM 77; **MS:** NY Med
Coll 73; **RES:** IM, Beth Israel Med Ctr, New York,
NY 73-76; Nep, New York University Med Ctr, New
York, NY 76-79; **HOSP:** Cabrini Med Ctr; **HMO:**
Oxford Prucare United Healthcare Blue Cross &
Blue Shield GHI +

LANG: Sp; 🎬 🅂 Mcr WC NFI   A Few Days

Braun, Carl (MD)   N
St Luke's Roosevelt Hosp Ctr

1090 Amsterdam Ave; New York, NY 10025;
(212) 523-3650; **BDCERT:** N 72; **MS:** Univ Penn
62; **RES:** Med, St Luke's Roosevelt Hosp Ctr, New
York, NY 62-63; N, Columbia-Presbyterian Med
Ctr, New York, NY 64-67; **FAP:** Clin Prof N
Columbia P&S; *SI: Nerve and Muscle Diseases;*
Headache; **HMO:** Oxford PHS CIGNA United
Healthcare NYLCare +

LANG: Jpn; 🖐 🕐 🎬 🅂 Mcr WC NFI   4+ Weeks

Bressman, Susan (MD)   N
Beth Israel Med Ctr

Beth Israel Medical Center, Dept of Neurology, 10
Union Square East 2R; New York, NY 10032; (212)
844-8379; **BDCERT:** N 83; **MS:** Columbia P&S 77;
RES: Med, NY Hosp-Cornell Med Ctr, New York, NY
77-78; N, Columbia-Presbyterian Med Ctr, New
York, NY 78-81; **FEL:** Movement Disorder,
Columbia-Presbyterian Med Ctr, New York, NY 81-
83; **FAP:** Prof Albert Einstein Coll Med; *SI:*
Parkinson's Disease; Dystonia; **HMO:** Oxford Bronx
Health PHS

LANG: Sp, Heb, Itl, Rus; 🖐 🕐 🎬 🅂 Mcr Mcl   1 Week
▦ *VISA* 💳 💳

Bronster, David (MD)   N
Mount Sinai Med Ctr

3 E 83rd St; New York, NY 10028; (212) 772-
0008; **BDCERT:** N 84; **MS:** Mt Sinai Sch Med 79;
RES: Cabrini Med Ctr, New York, NY 79-80; Mount
Sinai Med Ctr, New York, NY 80-83; **FAP:** Assoc
Clin Prof Mt Sinai Sch Med; *SI: Dizziness; Headache;*
HMO: Oxford Aetna Hlth Plan CIGNA PHCS United
Healthcare +

LANG: Sp; 🕐 🎬 🅂 Mcr   Immediately ▦ *VISA* 💳

Brust, John (MD)   N
Harlem Hosp Ctr

506 Lenox Ave 16101; New York, NY 10037;
(212) 939-4244; **BDCERT:** N 71; **MS:** Columbia
P&S 62; **RES:** N, Columbia-Presbyterian Med Ctr,
New York, NY 66-69; IM, Columbia-Presbyterian
Med Ctr, New York, NY 63-65; **HOSP:** Columbia-
Presbyterian Med Ctr

🖐 🕐 🖬 🎬 Mcr Mcl NFI   A Few Days

Cafferty, Maureen (MD)   N
St Luke's Roosevelt Hosp Ctr

1090 Amsterdam Ave 8B; New York, NY 10025;
(212) 636-4994; **BDCERT:** N 87; IM 82; **MS:**
Columbia P&S 79; **RES:** St Luke's Roosevelt Hosp
Ctr, New York, NY; N, Columbia-Presbyterian Med
Ctr, New York, NY; **FAP:** Asst Lecturer N Columbia
P&S; *SI: Multiple Sclerosis;* **HMO:** Oxford Blue Cross
Prucare CIGNA HealthNet +

🖐 🕐 🖬 🎬 🅂 Mcr   A Few Days

Caronna, John J (MD) N
NY Hosp-Cornell Med Ctr
Department of Neurology Cornell Univ Med Coll, 520 E 70th St Ste 607; New York, NY 10021; (212) 746-2304; **BDCERT:** N 74; **MS:** Cornell U 65; **RES:** IM, NY Hosp-Cornell Med Ctr, New York, NY 65-67; N, NY Hosp-Cornell Med Ctr, New York, NY 69-71; **FEL:** Neuroscience, NY Hosp-Cornell Med Ctr, New York, NY 72-73; **FAP:** Prof of Clin N Cornell U; ***SI:*** *Stroke; Coma*; **HMO:** Oxford Empire Blue Cross & Shield Prestige NYLCare MCI +
♿ ☎ 📅 $ [Mcr] 1 Week [AMEX] VISA [MasterCard]

Charney, Jonathan (MD) N
Mount Sinai Med Ctr
1111 Park Ave 1A; New York, NY 10128; (212) 831-2886; **BDCERT:** N 77; **MS:** NY Med Coll 69; **RES:** N, Columbia-Presbyterian Med Ctr, New York, NY 71-73; N, Baylor Med Ctr, Dallas, TX 70-71; **FAP:** Asst Clin Prof Mt Sinai Sch Med; **HOSP:** Beth Israel Med Ctr; ***SI:*** *Headaches; Stroke*
♿ Immediately

Chokroverty, Sudhans (MD) N
St Vincents Hosp & Med Ctr NY
153 W 11th St Cronin 466; New York, NY 10011; (212) 604-2401; **BDCERT:** N 71; **MS:** India 56; **RES:** VA Hosp, Hines, IL 66-67; **FEL:** C/NPh, Northwestern Mem Hosp, Chicago, IL 68-69; **FAP:** Prof N NY Med Coll; **HOSP:** VA Med Ctr-Manh; ***SI:*** *Sleep Medicine; Movements Disorders*; **HMO:** Oxford Cost Care Multiplan Prudential GHI +
LANG: Sp, Hin, Bng; ♿ ☎ 👤 📅 $ [Mcr] [WC] [NFI]
1 Week

Coddon, David R (MD) N
Mount Sinai Med Ctr
Neurology Faculty Associates, 5 E 98th St Faculty Practice As; New York, NY 10029; (212) 369-5888; **MS:** NYU Sch Med 53; **RES:** Mount Sinai Med Ctr, New York, NY 54-57; **FEL:** Nat Inst Health, Bethesda, MD 55; **FAP:** Assoc Clin Prof N Mt Sinai Sch Med; **HOSP:** Englewood Hosp & Med Ctr; ***SI:*** *Headaches, Head Injuries; Epilepsy*; **HMO:** Aetna-US Healthcare Affordable Hlth Plan Beech Street PHCS PHS +
♿ ☎ 👤 📅 $ [WC] [NFI] A Few Days [AMEX] VISA [MasterCard]

Coll, Raymond (MD) N
NY Hosp-Cornell Med Ctr
1365 York Ave; New York, NY 10021; (212) 249-0840; **BDCERT:** N 74; **MS:** South Africa 61; **RES:** N, NY Hosp-Cornell Med Ctr, New York, NY 68-71; **FAP:** Assoc Clin Prof N Cornell U
LANG: Heb; ☎ 👤 📅 $ [Mcr] [NFI] A Few Days

Daras, Michael (MD) N
Metropolitan Hosp Ctr
Metropoitan Hospital Faculty Practice, 1901 1st Ave; New York, NY 10029; (212) 423-6676; **BDCERT:** N 80; **MS:** Greece 69; **RES:** Psyc, Elmhurst Mem Hosp, Elmhurst, IL 73-76; N, NY Med Coll, New York, NY 76-79; **FEL:** Albert Einstein Med Ctr, Bronx, NY 79-80; **FAP:** Prof of Clin N NY Med Coll; **HOSP:** St Vincents Hosp & Med Ctr NY; ***SI:*** *Neural. Complications of Drugs*
LANG: Grk; ♿ [Mcr] [Mcd] [WC] [NFI] A Few Days

De Angelis, Lisa (MD) N
Mem Sloan Kettering Cancer Ctr
1275 York Ave; New York, NY 10021; (212) 639-7123; **BDCERT:** N 86; **MS:** Columbia P&S 80; **RES:** N, Columbia-Presbyterian Med Ctr, New York, NY; **FEL:** N Onc, Mem Sloan Kettering Cancer Ctr, New York, NY
♿ ☎ 👤 📅 [Mcr] A Few Days [AMEX] VISA [MasterCard]

Devinsky, Orrin (MD) N
Hosp For Joint Diseases
301 E 17th St 1101; New York, NY 10003; (212) 598-6412; **BDCERT:** N 90; **MS:** Harvard Med Sch 83; **RES:** NY Hosp-Cornell Med Ctr, New York, NY 83-86; **FEL:** Epilepsy, Nat Inst Health, Bethesda, MD 86-88; C/NPh, Nat Inst Health, Bethesda, MD; **HOSP:** New York University Med Ctr; ***SI:*** *Epilepsy*; **HMO:** CIGNA Oxford US Hlthcre United Healthcare
LANG: Sp; ♿ [SA SU] ☾ ☎ 👤 📅 [Mcr] [Mcd] [WC] [NFI]
A Few Days

Effron, Charles (MD)   N
Mount Sinai Med Ctr

5 E 94th St; New York, NY 10128; (212) 987-6110; **BDCERT:** N 89; **MS:** Brown U 83; **RES:** IM, Beth Israel Med Ctr, New York, NY 83-84; N, Mount Sinai Med Ctr, New York, NY 84-87; **FAP:** Instr Mt Sinai Sch Med; **HMO:** Guardian Travelers PHS

🔲 🏨 💲 ⓦ A Few Days

Fahn, Stanley (MD)   N
Columbia-Presbyterian Med Ctr

The Center for Parkinson's Diseases & Other Movement Disorders, 710 W 168th St 3rdfl, rm350; New York, NY 10032; (212) 305-5277; **BDCERT:** N 58; **MS:** UC San Francisco 58; **RES:** N, Woods Hole, MA 57; N, Columbia-Presbyterian Med Ctr, New York, NY 59-62; **FAP:** Prof N Columbia P&S; **SI:** *Movement Disorders; Parkinson's Disease;* **HMO:** None

LANG: Sp; 🔲 🏨 💲 ⓜ 4+ Weeks 🔲 **VISA** 🔲 🔲

Fetell, Michael R (MD)   N
Columbia-Presbyterian Med Ctr

710 W 168th St 425; New York, NY 10032; (212) 305-5571; **BDCERT:** N 78; **MS:** Albert Einstein Coll Med 72; **RES:** Albert Einstein Med Ctr, Bronx, NY 73-76; **FEL:** Columbia-Presbyterian Med Ctr, New York, NY 76-77; **FAP:** Prof Columbia P&S; **SI:** *Neuro-Oncology; Brain Tumor;* **HMO:** Oxford Prudential

LANG: Fr, Itl; 🔲 🏨 ⓜ A Few Days 🔲 **VISA** 🔲

Fink, Matthew Earl (MD)   N
Beth Israel Med Ctr

Beth Israel Hosp NeuroFierman Hall, 317 E 17th St; New York, NY 10003; (212) 420-5621; **BDCERT:** IM 80; N 83; **MS:** Univ Pittsburgh 78; **RES:** IM, Boston Med Ctr, Boston, MA 77-80; N, Columbia-Presby, New York, NY 78-79; **FAP:** Assoc Prof NR Columbia P&S; **HMO:** Blue Choice GHI Oxford PHS

ⓜ

Foo, Sun-hoo (MD)   N
New York University Med Ctr

650 1st Ave Fl 4; New York, NY 10016; (212) 213-0270; **BDCERT:** N 80; IM 76; **MS:** Taiwan 72; **RES:** IM, St Vincent's Med Ctr-Bridgeport, Bridgeport, CT 74-76; N, New York University Med Ctr, New York, NY 76-77; **FAP:** Assoc Prof NYU Sch Med; **HOSP:** NYU Downtown Hosp; **HMO:** Aetna Hlth Plan Chubb Oxford Metlife PHS +

LANG: Can, Man; 🔲 🔲 🔲 🏨 💲 ⓜ A Few Days

Forster, George (MD)   N
Mount Sinai Med Ctr

1160 5th Ave Ste 107; New York, NY 10029; (212) 410-6400; **BDCERT:** N 80; **MS:** Italy 71; **RES:** IM, Maimonides Med Ctr, Brooklyn, NY 71-74; N, Mount Sinai Med Ctr, New York, NY 74-77; **FAP:** Asst Clin Prof Mt Sinai Sch Med; **SI:** *Multiple Sclerosis; Clinical Neurology;* **HMO:** Oxford PHS Guardian +

LANG: Itl, Sp; 🔲 🔲 🏨 ⓜ A Few Days 🔲 **VISA** 🔲

Gendelman, Seymour (MD)   N
Mount Sinai Med Ctr

5 E 98th Street Fl 7; New York, NY 10029; (212) 241-8172; **BDCERT:** N 71; Psyc 71; **MS:** Geo Wash U Sch Med 64; **RES:** Mount Sinai Med Ctr, New York, NY 65-68; **HMO:** Oxford PHCS

🔲 🔲 🔲 🏨 💲 ⓜ ⓦ Ⓝ 1 Week 🔲 **VISA** 🔲

Goodgold, Albert (MD)   N
New York University Med Ctr

530 1st Ave Ste 5A; New York, NY 10016; (212) 263-7205; **MS:** Switzerland 55; **RES:** N, Bellevue Hosp Ctr, New York, NY 57-60; **FAP:** Prof of Clin N NYU Sch Med; **SI:** *Spinal Cord Root Disorders; Multiple Sclerosis;* **HMO:** None

LANG: Ger, Itl; 🔲 🔲 🏨 💲 ⓜ 1 Week

Gopinathan, Govindan (MD)   N
New York University Med Ctr

650 1st Ave Fl 4; New York, NY 10016; (212) 213-9559; **BDCERT:** N 80; **MS:** India 73; **RES:** Coney Island Hosp, Brooklyn, NY 73-75; New York University Med Ctr, New York, NY 75-78; **FEL:** Movement Disorder, Nat Inst Health, Bethesda, MD 78-80; **FAP:** Clin Prof NYU Sch Med; **SI:** *Parkinson's Disease; Headache;* **HMO:** Oxford Aetna Hlth Plan CIGNA

⬛ ⬛ ⬛ ⬛ ⬛ A Few Days

Herbstein, Diego (MD)   N
NY Hosp-Cornell Med Ctr

11 E 68th St; New York, NY 10021; (212) 794-2281; **BDCERT:** N 76; **MS:** Argentina 68; **RES:** IM, Fernandez Hosp, Buenos Aires, Argentina 69-70; N, Albert Einstein Med Ctr, Bronx, NY 70-73; **FEL:** N, Jacobi Med Ctr, Bronx, NY 73-74; **FAP:** Asst Clin Prof N Cornell U; **HOSP:** Lenox Hill Hosp; **SI:** *Cerebrovascular Disease; Parkinson's Disease*

LANG: Sp, Fr; ⬛ ⬛ ⬛ ⬛ ⬛ ⬛ ⬛ ⬛
A Few Days

Herman, Peter (MD)   N
Mount Sinai Med Ctr

226 E 79th St; New York, NY 10021; (212) 737-9720; **BDCERT:** N 80; **MS:** France 64; **RES:** New York University Med Ctr, New York, NY 68; Flower Fifth Ave Hosp, New York, NY 66-67; **FEL:** N, Mount Sinai Med Ctr, New York, NY 66; **FAP:** Assoc Clin Prof Mt Sinai Sch Med; **HOSP:** Beth Israel Med Ctr; **SI:** *Strokes; Headaches;* **HMO:** US Hlthcre PHS Well Care

LANG: Fr, Sp, Fil; ⬛ ⬛ ⬛ ⬛ ⬛ ⬛ ⬛
Immediately ⬛

Hiesiger, Emile (MD)   N
New York University Med Ctr

530 1st Ave 5A; New York, NY 10016; (212) 263-6123; **BDCERT:** N 83; **MS:** NY Med Coll 78; **RES:** N, New York University Med Ctr, New York, NY 79-82; **FEL:** N, Mem Sloan Kettering Cancer Ctr, New York, NY 82-84; N, NY Hosp-Cornell Med Ctr, New York, NY 82-84; **FAP:** Assoc Clin Prof NRad NYU Sch Med; **HOSP:** Beth Israel North; **SI:** *Interventional Pain Management; Oncology Pain;* **HMO:** None

LANG: Sp, Fr; ⬛ ⬛ ⬛ ⬛ ⬛ 2-4 Weeks ⬛ *VISA* ⬛

Horwich, Mark (MD)   N
NY Hosp-Cornell Med Ctr

523 E 72nd St 7th Floor; New York, NY 10021; (212) 717-0212; **BDCERT:** N 74; **MS:** Harvard Med Sch 67; **RES:** Med, Duke U Med Ctr, Durham, NC 67-69; N, NY Hosp-Cornell Med Ctr, New York, NY 69-72; **FAP:** Prof N Cornell U; **SI:** *Headache;* **HMO:** Metlife NYLCare HealthNet Oxford United Healthcare +

⬛ ⬛ ⬛ ⬛ ⬛ ⬛ Immediately ⬛ *VISA* ⬛

Jonas, Saran (MD)   N
New York University Med Ctr

530 1st Ave 5A; New York, NY 10016; (212) 263-7202; **BDCERT:** N 67; **MS:** Columbia P&S 56; **RES:** IM, New York University Med Ctr, New York, NY 56-62; N, Bellevue Hosp Ctr, New York, NY 62-64; **HOSP:** Bellevue Hosp Ctr

⬛ ⬛ ⬛ ⬛ ⬛ ⬛ ⬛ Immediately

Kolodny, Edwin H (MD)   N
New York University Med Ctr

NYU Medical Ctr Dept of Neurology, 550 1st Ave; New York, NY 10016; (212) 263-6347; **BDCERT:** MG 87; N 71; **MS:** NYU Sch Med 62; **RES:** IM, Bellevue Hosp Ctr, New York, NY 62-64; N, Mass Gen Hosp, Boston, MA 64-67; **FEL:** Neurochemistry, Nat Inst of Neur Dis & Stroke, Bethesda, MD 67-70; **FAP:** Chrmn N NYU Sch Med; **SI:** *Neurogenetics; Developmental Disabilities;* **HMO:** Blue Cross Oxford Chubb Prudential

⬛ ⬛ ⬛ ⬛ ⬛ ⬛ 2-4 Weeks

Kupersmith, Mark J (MD)   N
Beth Israel North

INN, BI North, 170 E End Ave 3B; New York, NY 10128; (212) 870-9418; **BDCERT:** Oph 81; N 81; **MS:** Northwestern U 76; **RES:** N, New York University Med Ctr, New York, NY; Oph, New York University Med Ctr, New York, NY; **FAP:** Prof NYU Sch Med; **HOSP:** New York Eye & Ear Infirmary; **SI:** *Neuro-Ophthalmology*

⬛ ⬛ ⬛ ⬛ ⬛ ⬛ 2-4 Weeks

Lange, Dale J (MD) N
Columbia-Presbyterian Med Ctr

710 W 168th St; New York, NY 10032; (212)
305-5706; BDCERT: N 85; MS: NY Med Coll 78;
RES: IM, Albany Med Ctr, Albany, NY 78-79; N,
New England Med Ctr, Boston, MA 79-82; FEL:
Neuromuscular Diseases, Columbia-Presbyterian
Med Ctr, New York, NY 82-83; FAP: Assoc Prof N
Columbia P&S; SI: *Neuromuscular Disease*; HMO:
Oxford Aetna Hlth Plan PHS

🔲 🌙 🔲 🔲 🔲 Mcr WC NFI Immediately ▓▓ **VISA**
🔲

Latov, Norman (MD) N
Columbia-Presbyterian Med Ctr

710 W 168th St Rm 237; New York, NY 10032;
(212) 305-5704; BDCERT: N 89; MS: Univ Penn
75; RES: Boston Med Ctr, Boston, MA 75-76;
Columbia-Presbyterian Med Ctr, New York, NY 76-
79; FEL: Immunology, Columbia-Presbyterian Med
Ctr, New York, NY; FAP: Prof Columbia P&S; SI:
Peripheral Neuropathy; Neuropathy; HMO: Oxford
Prucare Blue Choice Multiplan Chubb +

🔲 🌙 🔲 🔲 🔲 🔲 Mcr 1 Week ▓▓ **VISA** 🔲

Levine, David (MD) N
New York University Med Ctr

400 E 34th St; New York, NY 10016; (212) 263-
7744; BDCERT: N 76; MS: Harvard Med Sch 68;
RES: Mass Gen Hosp, Boston, MA 71-74; FEL: N,
Mass Gen Hosp, Boston, MA; SI: *Memory Disorders;
Stroke*; HMO: CIGNA Oxford Aetna-US Healthcare
Prucare Chubb +

🔲 🔲 🔲 🔲 🔲 Mcr NFI A Few Days

Lovelace, Robert Edward (MD) N
Columbia-Presbyterian Med Ctr

710 W 168th St 157; New York, NY 10032; (212)
305-1326; MS: England 53; RES: Middlesex Hosp,
London,England 57-60; Queen Elizabeth Hosp,
Birmingham,England 60-62; FEL: Mayo Clinic,
Rochester, MN 62-63; FAP: Prof N Columbia P&S;
HOSP: Harlem Hosp Ctr; SI: *Lou Gehrig's Disease;
Myasthenia Gravis*; HMO: Oxford Blue Choice

🔲 🔲 Mcr 4+ Weeks ▓▓ **VISA** 🔲 🔲

Mauskop, Alexander (MD) N
Long Island Coll Hosp

New York Headache Center, 30 E 76 St; New York,
NY 10027; (212) 794-3550; BDCERT: N 87; PM
95; MS: Russia 79; RES: IM, Brookdale Univ Hosp
Med Ctr, Brooklyn, NY 80-81; N, Univ Hosp SUNY
Bklyn, Brooklyn, NY 81-84; FEL: PMR, Mem Sloan
Kettering Cancer Ctr, New York, NY 84-86; FAP:
Assoc Clin Prof N SUNY Downstate; HOSP: Beth
Israel Med Ctr; SI: *Headaches; Pain*; HMO: Aetna
Hlth Plan Oxford US Hlthcre GHI

LANG: Rus, Hun; 🌙 🔲 🔲 🔲 🔲 Mcr 2-4 Weeks

Miller, James R (MD) N
Columbia-Presbyterian Med Ctr

710 W 168th St; New York, NY 10032; (212)
305-5508; BDCERT: N 74; MS: NYU Sch Med 64;
RES: IM, Bellevue Hosp Ctr, New York, NY 64-66;
N, Columbia-Presbyterian Med Ctr, New York, NY
68-71; FEL: Neurovirology, Rockefeller Univ Hosp,
New York, NY 71-74

🔲 🔲 🔲 🔲 🔲 Mcr A Few Days ▓▓ **VISA** 🔲

Mohr, Jay Preston (MD) N
Columbia-Presbyterian Med Ctr

710 W 168th St 514; New York, NY 10032; (212)
305-8033; BDCERT: N 71; MS: U Va Sch Med 63;
RES: Columbia-Presbyterian Med Ctr, New York,
NY 65-66; Mass Gen Hosp, Boston, MA 66-69; FEL:
N, Mass Gen Hosp, Boston, MA 67-69; FAP: Prof N
Columbia P&S; SI: *Stroke; TIA*; HMO: Oxford CIGNA
Empire Blue Cross & Shield Blue Choice PHCS +

LANG: Sp, Fr, Ger; 🔲 🔲 🔲 🔲 Mcr 2-4 Weeks

Nass, Ruth (MD) N
New York University Med Ctr

400 E 34th St Ste RR311; New York, NY 10016;
(212) 263-7753; BDCERT: ChiN 81; Ped 80; MS:
Albert Einstein Coll Med 75; RES: Ped, NY Hosp-
Cornell Med Ctr, New York, NY 75-77; ChiN,
Columbia-Presbyterian Med Ctr, New York, NY 77-
78; FEL: ChiN, NY Hosp-Cornell Med Ctr, New
York, NY 81-82; FAP: Prof of Clin N NYU Sch Med;
SI: *Learning Disabilities; Attention Deficit Disorders*;
HMO: Oxford US Hlthcre

🔲 🔲 🔲 🔲 1 Week

Nealon, Nancy (MD) N
NY Hosp-Cornell Med Ctr

815 Park Ave; New York, NY 10021; (212) 288-8600; **BDCERT:** IM 78; N 84; **MS:** Penn State U-Hershey Med Ctr 75; **RES:** N, NY Hosp-Cornell Med Ctr, New York, NY 75-81; **FEL:** Nerve & Muscle, Columbia-Presbyterian Med Ctr, New York, NY 81-82; N Onc, Mem Sloan Kettering Cancer Ctr, New York, NY 82-83; **FAP:** Asst N Cornell U; *SI: Migraine; Back Pain;* **HMO:** Oxford PHS Blue Cross PPO

⬤ ⬤ ⬤ ⬤ ⬤ ⬤ Immediately

Nelson, Jeffrey (MD) N
New York University Med Ctr

650 1st Ave FL 4; New York, NY 10016; (212) 213-9570; **BDCERT:** N 83; **MS:** Cornell U 78; **RES:** Bellevue Hosp Ctr, New York, NY 79-82; *SI: Spinal Cord Nerve Muscle*

⬤ Immediately

Neophytices, Andreas (MD) N
New York University Med Ctr

285 Riverside Dr 6A; New York, NY 10025; (718) 278-7700; **BDCERT:** Psyc 78; N 78; **MS:** Greece 70; **RES:** S, Long Island Jewish Med Ctr, New Hyde Park, NY 72-73; N, New York University Med Ctr, New York, NY 73-76; **FEL:** Nat Inst Health, Bethesda, MD 76-78; **FAP:** Assoc Clin Prof N NYU Sch Med; *SI: Spinal Disorders;* **HMO:** Oxford Aetna-US Healthcare United Healthcare US Hlthcre

LANG: Grk; ⬤ ⬤ ⬤ ⬤ ⬤ ⬤ ⬤ ⬤ 1 Week

Olanow, C Warren (MD) N
Mount Sinai Med Ctr

Mt Sinai Med Ctr, 1 Gustave Levy Pl Box 1137; New York, NY 10029; (212) 241-6500; **BDCERT:** N 70; **MS:** U Toronto 65; **RES:** N, Toronto Gen Hosp, Toronto, Canada 67-68; N, Columbia-Presbyterian Med Ctr, New York, NY 68-70; **FEL:** Neuroanatomy, Columbia-Presbyterian Med Ctr, New York, NY 70-71; **FAP:** Chrmn Mt Sinai Sch Med; *SI: Parkinson's Disease; Movement Disorders;* **HMO:** Oxford

LANG: Sp, Fr; ⬤ ⬤ ⬤ ⬤ ⬤ 4+ Weeks ▦ **VISA** ⬤

Olarte, Marcelo (MD) N
Columbia-Presbyterian Med Ctr

710 W 168th St; New York, NY 10032; (212) 305-1832; **BDCERT:** N 76; **MS:** Argentina 70; **RES:** N, St Vincents Hosp & Med Ctr NY, New York, NY 71-74; **FEL:** Neuromuscular Disease, Columbia-Presbyterian Med Ctr, New York, NY 74-75; **FAP:** Assoc Prof Columbia P&S; **HOSP:** Harlem Hosp Ctr; *SI: Muscle Diseases-Headaches; Electrodiagnostic Medicine;* **HMO:** Oxford

LANG: Sp, Itl; ⬤ ⬤ ⬤ ⬤ ⬤ ⬤ ⬤ 2-4 Weeks ▦ **VISA** ⬤ ⬤

Pedley, Timothy (MD) N
Columbia-Presbyterian Med Ctr

710 W 168th St 1401; New York, NY 10032; (212) 305-1742; **BDCERT:** N 75; **MS:** Yale U Sch Med 69; **RES:** IM, Stanford Med Ctr, Stanford, CA 69-70; N, Stanford Med Ctr, Stanford, CA 70-73; **FEL:** Epilepsy, Stanford Med Ctr, Stanford, CA 73-75; *SI: Epilepsy; Seizure Disorders;* **HMO:** Oxford Chubb PHS

⬤ ⬤ ⬤ ⬤ 2-4 Weeks ▦ **VISA** ⬤ ⬤

Petito, Frank (MD) N
NY Hosp-Cornell Med Ctr

New York Cornell Medical Ctr, 520 E 70th St; New York, NY 10021; (212) 746-2309; **BDCERT:** N 72; **MS:** Columbia P&S 67; **RES:** NY Hosp-Cornell Med Ctr, New York, NY 67-70; **FAP:** Prof of Clin N Cornell U; *SI: Multiple Sclerosis; Headache*

⬤ ⬤ ⬤ ⬤ 4+ Weeks ▦ **VISA**

Plum, Fred (MD) N
NY Hosp-Cornell Med Ctr

525 E 68th St Ste 607; New York, NY 10021; (212) 746-6141; **BDCERT:** N 56; **MS:** Cornell U 47; **RES:** NY Hosp-Cornell Med Ctr, New York, NY 48-49; **FAP:** Sr Prof Cornell U; *SI: Stroke;* **HMO:** Empire Magnacare Multiplan NYLCare United Healthcare +

⬤ ⬤ ⬤ ⬤ ⬤ 2-4 Weeks ▦ **VISA** ⬤ ⬤

Guide to symbols and abbreviations can be found on pages 110-113.

251

Posner, Jerome (MD)   **N**
Mem Sloan Kettering Cancer Ctr

1275 York Ave; New York, NY 10021; (212) 639-7047; **BDCERT:** N 62; **MS:** U Wash, Seattle 55; **RES:** U WA Med Ctr, Seattle, WA 55-59; **FEL:** U WA Med Ctr, Seattle, WA 61-63; **FAP:** Prof N Cornell U; *SI: Brain Tumors; Paraneoplastic Syndromes*

🔲 🔲 🔲 🔲 Mcr Mcd NFI 1 Week

Rapoport, Samuel (MD)   **N**
NY Hosp-Cornell Med Ctr

515 E 72nd St; New York, NY 10021; (212) 570-0642; **BDCERT:** N 86; **MS:** Cornell U 76; **RES:** NY Hosp-Cornell Med Ctr, New York, NY 78-82; **FEL:** Rockefeller Univ Hosp, New York, NY 78; **HOSP:** Lenox Hill Hosp; *SI: Neck, Back Pain— Radiculopathies; Peripheral Neuropathy*

LANG: Sp, Fr, Yd, Heb, Rus; 🔲 🔲 🔲 💲 1 Week
💳 **VISA** 💳

Raps, Mitchell S (MD)   **N**
Mount Sinai Med Ctr

1045 Park Ave; New York, NY 10028; (212) 860-1900; **BDCERT:** N 86; **MS:** Mt Sinai Sch Med 80; **RES:** Psyc, Mount Sinai Med Ctr, New York, NY 80-82; N, Mount Sinai Med Ctr, New York, NY 82-85; **FAP:** Asst Clin Prof Mt Sinai Sch Med; **HOSP:** NYU Downtown Hosp; **HMO:** Oxford

LANG: Sp; 🔲 🔲 🔲 💲 Mcr 1 Week

Reich, Edward (MD)   **N**
Lenox Hill Hosp

55 E 72nd St; New York, NY 10021; (212) 794-2777; **BDCERT:** N 80; **MS:** SUNY Buffalo 66; **RES:** Mount Sinai Med Ctr, New York, NY 70; **HOSP:** Mount Sinai Med Ctr

🔲 🔲 🔲 💲 Mcr WC NFI Immediately 💳 **VISA** 💳

Rizzo, Frank (MD)   **N**
Beth Israel North

1155 Park Ave; New York, NY 10128; (212) 369-3430; **BDCERT:** N 72; **MS:** U Mich Med Sch 60; **RES:** Henry Ford Hosp, Detroit, MI 63-65; Mount Sinai Med Ctr, New York, NY 65-68; **FEL:** Neuroendocrinology, Mount Sinai Med Ctr, New York, NY 68-70; **FAP:** Asst Prof Mt Sinai Sch Med; **HOSP:** Mount Sinai Med Ctr; *SI: Dizziness; Headache*; **HMO:** Oxford PHS Aetna Hlth Plan CIGNA Beech Street +

LANG: Sp, Itl; 🔲 🔲 🔲 Mcr NFI

Rowan, A James (MD)   **N**
Mount Sinai Med Ctr

5 E 98th St; New York, NY 10029; (212) 831-1473; **BDCERT:** N 71; **MS:** Stanford U 61; **RES:** IM, Boston VA Med Ctr, Boston, MA 62-63; N, Columbia-Presbyterian Med Ctr, New York, NY 63-66; **FEL:** EEG, London Hosp, London, England; **FAP:** Prof N Mt Sinai Sch Med; **HOSP:** VA Med Ctr-Bronx; *SI: Epilepsy; Seizure Disorders*; **HMO:** Oxford Aetna Hlth Plan US Hlthcre

🔲 🔲 🔲 Mcr 1 Week

Rowland, Lewis P (MD)   **N**
Columbia-Presbyterian Med Ctr

710 W 168th St; New York, NY 10032; (212) 305-4119; **BDCERT:** Psyc 55; N 55; **MS:** Yale U Sch Med 48; **RES:** IM, Yale-New Haven Hosp, New Haven, CT 49-50; N, Columbia-Presbyterian Med Ctr, New York, NY 50-53; *SI: Neuromuscular; Motor Neuron; Myasthenia*; **HMO:** Oxford Blue Choice Prucare PHS

🔲 🔲 🔲 💲 Mcr 2-4 Weeks 💳 **VISA** 💳 💳

Rudolph, Steven (MD)   **N**
Mount Sinai Med Ctr

1175 Park Ave; New York, NY 10128; (212) 423-0610; **BDCERT:** N 81; **MS:** SUNY Hlth Sci Ctr 76; **RES:** Med, Brookdale Univ Hosp Med Ctr, Brooklyn, NY 76-77; N, Mount Sinai Med Ctr, New York, NY 77-80; **FEL:** Oph, Mount Sinai Med Ctr, New York, NY 80-82; **FAP:** Asst Prof Mt Sinai Sch Med; **HOSP:** Beth Israel Med Ctr; *SI: Stroke; Neuro-Ophthalmology*; **HMO:** Oxford Aetna Hlth Plan

🔲 🔲 🔲 💲 Mcr 1 Week

Sacco, Ralph L (MD) N
Columbia-Presbyterian Med Ctr
710 W 168th St Rm 547; New York, NY 10032; (212) 305-1710; **BDCERT:** N 89; **MS:** Boston U 83; **RES:** IM, St Luke's Roosevelt Hosp Ctr, New York, NY 83-84; N, Columbia-Presbyterian Med Ctr, New York, NY 84-87; **FEL:** Cv, Columbia-Presbyterian Med Ctr, New York, NY 87-89; PHGPM, Columbia-Presbyterian Med Ctr, New York, NY 87-89; **FAP:** Assoc Prof Columbia P&S; **SI:** *Stroke*; **HMO:** Oxford PHS Blue Choice Prudential CIGNA +

LANG: Sp; ♿ 📷 🏥 💲 Mcr 2-4 Weeks ▨ *VISA* 🔵 ▨

Sadiq, Saud (MD) N
St Luke's Roosevelt Hosp Ctr
The Multiple Sclerosis Research & Treatment Center, 425 W 59th St Ste 7C; New York, NY 10032; (212) 305-5508; **MS:** Africa 79; **RES:** IM, England 85; N, U of Texas Med Sch, Houston, TX 88; **FEL:** Neuroimmunology, Columbia-Presbyterian Med Ctr, New York, NY 91; **FAP:** Assoc Prof Albert Einstein Coll Med; **SI:** *Multiple Sclerosis; Neuroimmunology*

LANG: Swa, Trk, Hin, Ur, Rom; ♿ 🚑 📞 📷 📹 🏥 💲 Mcr A Few Days ▨ *VISA* 🔵

Schaefer, John A (MD) N
NY Hosp-Cornell Med Ctr
523 E 72nd St; New York, NY 10021; (212) 717-0231; **BDCERT:** N 79; **MS:** Australia 68; **RES:** St Vincent Hosp, Victoria, Australia 69-73; **FEL:** NY Hosp-Cornell Med Ctr, New York, NY 79-75

♿ 📷 📹 🏥 💲 Mcr Immediately ▨ *VISA* 🔵 ▨

Sciarra, Daniel (MD) N
Columbia-Presbyterian Med Ctr
710 W 168th St 214; New York, NY 10032; (212) 305-5248; **BDCERT:** N 49; **MS:** Harvard Med Sch 43; **RES:** Boston Med Ctr, Boston, MA 43-44; Boston Med Ctr, Boston, MA 44-45; **FEL:** N, Montefiore Med Ctr, Bronx, NY 47-48; **FAP:** Prof of Clin N Columbia P&S; **SI:** *Dementia; Brain Tumor Spinal Problem*; **HMO:** None

LANG: Itl; ♿ 📷 🏥 Mcr Immediately

Sivak, Mark (MD) N
Mount Sinai Med Ctr
Mount Sinai Hospital, 5 E 98th St FL7; New York, NY 10029; (212) 241-6719; **BDCERT:** N 78; **MS:** KY Med Sch, Louisville 72; **RES:** NR, Mount Sinai Med Ctr, New York, NY; **FEL:** Mount Sinai Med Ctr, New York, NY; **SI:** *Myasthenia-Gravis; Lou Gehrig's Disease*; **HMO:** Oxford Aetna Hlth Plan Vytra Beech Street +

♿ 📷 📹 Mcr Mod NFI Immediately ▨ *VISA*

Smallberg, Gerald (MD) N
Lenox Hill Hosp
1010 5th Ave; New York, NY 10028; (212) 535-5348; **BDCERT:** N 77; **MS:** Yale U Sch Med 69; **RES:** U Mich Med Ctr, Ann Arbor, MI 69-71; Hosp of U Penn, Philadelphia, PA 73-75; **FEL:** Columbia-Presbyterian Med Ctr, New York, NY 75-76; **FAP:** Asst Clin Prof NYU Sch Med; **HMO:** CIGNA PHCS United Healthcare PHS

♿ 📷 📹 🏥 💲 Mcr WC NFI A Few Days

Snyder, David (MD) N
NY Hosp Med Ctr of Queens
NY Neurological Assoc, 11 E 68th St 6D; New York, NY 10021; (212) 794-2281; **BDCERT:** N 75; **MS:** U Md Sch Med 69; **RES:** N, U MD Hosp, Baltimore, MD 70-73; **FEL:** N Path, Albert Einstein Med Ctr, Bronx, NY; **HOSP:** Lenox Hill Hosp; **SI:** *Multiple Sclerosis*

♿ 🚑 📷 📹 🏥 💲 Mcr Mod WC A Few Days

Stacy, Charles B (MD) N
Mount Sinai Med Ctr
1107 5th Ave; New York, NY 10128; (212) 876-8614; **BDCERT:** N 83; **MS:** Cornell U 77; **RES:** Med, Mount Sinai Med Ctr, New York, NY 77-79; N, Mount Sinai Med Ctr, New York, NY 79-82; **FEL:** Pain, Mem Sloan Kettering Cancer Ctr, New York, NY 82-83; **HOSP:** Beth Israel North; **HMO:** Oxford Aetna Hlth Plan

♿ 📷 🏥 💲 Mcr 1 Week ▨ *VISA* 🔵

Tuchman, Alan (MD)   N
St Vincents Hosp & Med Ctr NY

48 E 81st St; New York, NY 10028; (212) 772-9305; **BDCERT:** N 79; **MS:** U Cincinnati 72; **RES:** N, Mount Sinai Med Ctr, New York, NY 73-76; **FEL:** Multiple Sclerosis, Albert Einstein Med Ctr, Bronx, NY 78-79; **FAP:** Prof N NY Med Coll; **HOSP:** Our Lady of Mercy Med Ctr; **SI:** *Seizures; Multiple Sclerosis;* **HMO:** Oxford Blue Choice

♿ 🅲 🔄 🎯 🏨 💲 Mcr WC 1 Week

Tuhrim, Stanley (MD)   N
Mount Sinai Med Ctr

5 E 98th St 7Fl.; New York, NY 10029; (212) 831-1473; **BDCERT:** N 83; **MS:** Mt Sinai Sch Med 79; **RES:** Mount Sinai Med Ctr, New York, NY 80-83; **FEL:** Cerebrovascular Disease, U MD Hosp, Baltimore, MD 83-84; **FAP:** Assoc Prof Mt Sinai Sch Med; **SI:** *Stroke; Cerebrovascular Disease;* **HMO:** Oxford Aetna Hlth Plan Vytra PHCS CIGNA +

LANG: Sp; ♿ 🔄 🏨 💲 Mcr A Few Days ▦ *VISA* ⬤

Weinberg, Harold (MD)   N
New York University Med Ctr

650 1st Ave FL4; New York, NY 10016; (212) 213-9339; **BDCERT:** N 79; **MS:** Albert Einstein Coll Med 78; **RES:** N, Columbia-Presbyterian Med Ctr, New York, NY 79-82; **FEL:** Neuromuscular Disease, Columbia-Presbyterian Med Ctr, New York, NY 82; **FAP:** Assoc Clin Prof N NYU Sch Med; **SI:** *Neuromuscular Disease*

♿ 🔄 🏨 💲 2-4 Weeks

Weinberger, Jessie (MD)   N
Mount Sinai Med Ctr

5 E 98th St; New York, NY 10029; (212) 831-1473; **BDCERT:** N 76; **MS:** Johns Hopkins U 71; **RES:** IM, Bellevue Hosp Ctr, New York, NY 71-72; N, Mount Sinai Med Ctr, New York, NY 72-75; **FEL:** Cv, Hosp of U Penn, Philadelphia, PA 77-78; **FAP:** Prof Mt Sinai Sch Med; **HOSP:** North General Hosp; **SI:** *Transient Ischemic Attacks; Stroke;* **HMO:** Oxford Blue Choice Aetna Hlth Plan Premier American Health Plan +

LANG: Sp, Fr, Ger; ♿ 🅲 🔄 🏨 Mcr Mcd NFI A Few Days ▦ *VISA*

Weiss, Arthur H (MD)   N
Mount Sinai Med Ctr

1056 5th Ave; New York, NY 10128; (212) 831-1055; **BDCERT:** N 64; **MS:** SUNY Hlth Sci Ctr 57; **RES:** Mount Sinai Med Ctr, New York, NY 58-63; **FEL:** Columbia-Presbyterian Med Ctr, New York, NY 64; **FAP:** Asst Clin Prof Mt Sinai Sch Med; **HOSP:** Lenox Hill Hosp; **SI:** *Parkinson's Disease; Epilepsy;* **HMO:** Aetna Hlth Plan Chubb PHS CIGNA Oxford +

♿ 🔄 🏨 💲 Mcr WC NFI 1 Week

NEURORADIOLOGY

Berenstein, Alejando (MD) NRad
Beth Israel Med Ctr

Center of Endovascular Surgery, 170 E End Ave 3F; New York, NY 10128; (212) 870-9660; **BDCERT:** Rad 76; NR 95; **MS:** Mexico 69; **RES:** Rad, Mount Sinai Med Ctr, New York, NY 73-76; **FEL:** NR, New York University Med Ctr, New York, NY 76-78; **FAP:** Prof Rad NYU Sch Med; **SI:** *Brain Artery/Vein Malformation; Cerebral Aneurysm;* **HMO:** Oxford

LANG: Heb, Sp; ♿ 🔄 🏨 💲 Mcr Mcd NFI 1 Week

Chase, Norman (MD)   NRad
New York University Med Ctr

Faculty Practice Radiology, 550 1st Ave; New York, NY 10016; (212) 263-6246; **BDCERT:** Rad 59; N 95; **MS:** U Cincinnati 53; **RES:** Rad, Columbia-Presbyterian Med Ctr, New York, NY 56-58; **FAP:** Prof Rad NYU Sch Med; **SI:** *Stroke; Brain Tumors;* **HMO:** Oxford Aetna Hlth Plan United Healthcare Prucare PHS +

♿ 🔄 🏨 Mcr WC NFI A Few Days ▦ *VISA* ⬤

NUCLEAR MEDICINE

Abdel-Dayem, Hussein M (MD)NuM
St Vincents Hosp & Med Ctr NY

153 W 11th St; New York, NY 10011; (212) 604-8783; **BDCERT:** Rad 72; NuM 72; **MS:** Egypt 59; **RES:** Cairo Univ Hosp, Cairo, Egypt 60-63; NuM, Roswell Park Cancer Inst, Buffalo, NY 70-71; **FEL:** RadRO, Roswell Park Cancer Inst, Buffalo, NY; **FAP:** Prof NY Med Coll; *SI: Nuclear Medicine-Neurology; Cardiology;* **HMO:** GHI Oxford Blue Cross & Blue Shield

LANG: Chi, Sp, Ar; 🦽 ☎ 🏨 M̄c̄r̄ M̄c̄d̄ W̄C̄ N̄F̄Ī Immediately

Becker, David V (MD)   NuM
NY Hosp-Cornell Med Ctr

525 E 68th St ST221; New York, NY 10021; (212) 746-4583; **BDCERT:** NuM 72; **MS:** NYU Sch Med 48; **RES:** Maimonides Med Ctr, Brooklyn, NY 49-50; NY Hosp-Cornell Med Ctr, New York, NY 52-54; **FEL:** Biophysics, Mem Sloan Kettering Cancer Ctr, New York, NY 50-52; **FAP:** Prof Rad Cornell U; *SI: Hyperthyroidism & Thyroid Cancer;* **HMO:** None

🦽 ☎ 🏨 M̄c̄r̄ 2-4 Weeks

De Puey, Ernest (MD)   NuM
St Luke's Roosevelt Hosp Ctr

Amsterdam Ave & 114th St; New York, NY 10025; (212) 523-3398; **BDCERT:** IM 76; NuM 78; **MS:** Baylor 73; **RES:** IM, Baylor Med Ctr, Dallas, TX 73-75; NuM, Baylor Med Ctr, Dallas, TX 75-77; **FEL:** NuM, Baylor Med Ctr, Dallas, TX 78; *SI: Nuclear Cardiology*

🦽 🏨 M̄c̄r̄ M̄c̄d̄ W̄C̄ N̄F̄Ī Immediately

Goldfarb, Richard (MD)   NuM
Beth Israel Med Ctr

55 E 34th St; New York, NY 10016; (212) 252-6070; **BDCERT:** Rad 75; DR 75; **MS:** NY Med Coll 70; **RES:** DR, St Luke's Roosevelt Hosp Ctr, New York, NY 71-74; **FEL:** NuM, St Luke's Roosevelt Hosp Ctr, New York, NY 74-75; **FAP:** Assoc Prof Rad Albert Einstein Coll Med; **HOSP:** St Luke's Roosevelt Hosp Ctr; *SI: Thyroid*

🦽 S̄Ā C̄ ☎ 🏨 S̄ M̄c̄r̄ M̄c̄d̄ W̄C̄ N̄F̄Ī Immediately
VISA 💳 💳 💳

Goldsmith, Stanley J (MD)   NuM
NY Hosp-Cornell Med Ctr

NY HospCornell Medical Center, 525 E 68th St Starr221; New York, NY 10021; (212) 746-4588; **BDCERT:** NuM 72; IM 69; **MS:** SUNY Downstate 62; **RES:** IM, Kings County Hosp Ctr, Brooklyn, NY 65-67; **FEL:** EDM, Mount Sinai Med Ctr, New York, NY 67-68; **FAP:** Prof Rad Cornell U; *SI: Cancer Radionuclide Therapy; Thyroid Disease*

LANG: Sp, Rus, Can, Itl, Fr; 🦽 ☎ 🦽 🏨 M̄c̄r̄ M̄c̄d̄ W̄C̄ N̄F̄Ī A Few Days

Kramer, Elissa (MD)   NuM
New York University Med Ctr

Tisch Hospital, 560 1st Ave 2nd Fl; New York, NY 10016; (212) 263-7410; **BDCERT:** NuM 82; DR 82; **MS:** NYU Sch Med 77; **RES:** Rad, Bellevue Hosp Ctr, New York, NY 78-80; **FEL:** NuM, Bellevue Hosp Ctr, New York, NY 80-82; **FAP:** Prof NYU Sch Med; **HOSP:** NYU Downtown Hosp; *SI: Tumor Imaging;* **HMO:** Aetna-US Healthcare Oxford Blue Choice PPO United Healthcare +

LANG: Sp; 🦽 S̄Ā C̄ ☎ 🏨 S̄ M̄c̄r̄ M̄c̄d̄ W̄C̄ A Few Days 🖼 **VISA** 💳

Larson, Steven (MD)   NuM
Mem Sloan Kettering Cancer Ctr

1275 York Ave F 212; New York, NY 10021; (212) 639-7373; **BDCERT:** NuM 72; IM 73; **MS:** U Wash, Seattle 65; **RES:** IM, Virginia Mason Hosp, Seattle, WA 68-70; NuM, Natl Inst Health, Bethesda, MD 70-72; **FAP:** Chf NuM Columbia P&S; *SI: Nuclear Oncology; Proton Emission Tomography;* **HMO:** Blue Cross & Blue Shield Oxford

☎ 🏨 M̄c̄r̄ W̄C̄ 1 Week

Liebeskind, Arie (MD)   NuM
Montefiore Med Ctr-Weiler/Einstein Div

Park Avenue Radiologists, PC, 525 Park Ave; New York, NY 10021; (212) 888-1000; **BDCERT:** NuM 72; RadRO 70; **MS:** Albert Einstein Coll Med 65; **RES:** Rad, Albert Einstein Med Ctr, Bronx, NY 70-74; Rad, Jacobi Med Ctr, Bronx, NY 66-69; **FEL:** NR, Albert Einstein Med Ctr, Bronx, NY 70-72; **FAP:** Instr Rad Albert Einstein Coll Med; *SI: Fine Needle Aspiration;* **HMO:** Blue Cross & Blue Shield CIGNA GHI Oxford Aetna Hlth Plan +

LANG: Sp, Chi, Hin, Fr, Heb; 🦽 S̄Ā C̄ ☎ 🏨 S̄ M̄c̄r̄ M̄c̄d̄ W̄C̄ N̄F̄Ī Immediately 🖼 **VISA** 💳 💳

Pierson, Richard (MD)   NuM
St Luke's Roosevelt Hosp Ctr

1111 Amsterdam Ave; New York, NY 10025; (212) 523-3385; **BDCERT:** NuM 72; **MS:** Columbia P&S 55; **RES:** St Luke's Roosevelt Hosp Ctr, New York, NY 55-56; St Luke's Roosevelt Hosp Ctr, New York, NY 58-60; **FEL:** St Luke's Roosevelt Hosp Ctr, New York, NY 60-61; **FAP:** Prof Columbia P&S

LANG: Fr, Chi; 🚹 📷 🏥 📅 💲 Mcr A Few Days

Sanger, Joseph J (MD)   NuM
New York University Med Ctr

560 1st Ave 2nd Fl; New York, NY 10016; (212) 263-7410; **BDCERT:** NuM 80; **MS:** NYU Sch Med 77; **RES:** Rad, New York University Med Ctr, New York, NY 77-79; **FEL:** NuM, New York University Med Ctr, New York, NY 79-81; **HOSP:** NYU Downtown Hosp; **HMO:** Oxford Chubb Metlife Aetna Hlth Plan

🚹 SA/SO 🌙 📷 📅 💲 Mcr Immediately ▨ **VISA** ⬤

Scharf, Stephen (MD)   NuM
Lenox Hill Hosp

Lenox Hill Hosp, 100 E 77th St; New York, NY 10021; (212) 434-2630; **BDCERT:** IM 77; NuM 79; **MS:** Albert Einstein Coll Med 74; **RES:** IM, Bronx Muncipal Hosp Ctr, Bronx, NY 75-76; NuM, Albert Einstein Med Ctr, Bronx, NY 76-78; **FEL:** Nep, Albert Einstein Med Ctr, Bronx, NY 77-79; **FAP:** Asst Clin Prof Albert Einstein Coll Med; **HMO:** Vytra Oxford Blue Choice Prucare Aetna Hlth Plan +

LANG: Sp; 🚹 📷 📅 Mcr Mod WC Immediately ▨ **VISA** ⬤ ▥

OBSTETRICS & GYNECOLOGY

Allen, Machelle (MD)   ObG
Bellevue Hosp Ctr

110 Bleecker St 26 B; New York, NY 10016; (212) 263-6337; **BDCERT:** ObG 91; **MS:** UC San Francisco 75; **RES:** Rad, UC San Francisco Med Ctr, San Francisco, CA 76-77; ObG, Albert Einstein Med Ctr, Bronx, NY 78-81; **FEL:** ObG/MF, Columbia-Presbyterian Med Ctr, New York, NY 82-84; **FAP:** Asst Prof NYU Sch Med; **SI:** *HIV Infection; Substance Abuse;* **HMO:** Metroplus

🚹 📷 🏥 📅 Mcr Mod WC NFI A Few Days

Antoine, Clarel (MD)   ObG   `PCP`
New York University Med Ctr

Obstetrics and Gynecology, 530 1st Ave Ste 10Q; New York, NY 10016; (212) 263-6541; **BDCERT:** ObG 82; **MS:** Columbia P&S 75; **RES:** ObG, Columbia-Presbyterian Med Ctr, New York, NY 75-79; **FEL:** MF, Bellevue Hosp Ctr, New York, NY 79-81; **FAP:** Dir ObG NYU Sch Med; **HOSP:** Bellevue Hosp Ctr; **SI:** *High Risk Pregnancy*

LANG: Sp, Fr; 🚹 📷 🏥 📅 💲 Mcr Immediately

Baxi, Laxmi (MD)   ObG   `PCP`
Columbia-Presbyterian Med Ctr

161 Ft Washington Ave; New York, NY 10032; (212) 305-5899; **BDCERT:** ObG 80; MF 87; **MS:** India 62; **RES:** ObG, King Edward M Hosp, Bombay, India 64-69; St Peter's Med Ctr, New Brunswick, NJ 76-77; **FEL:** MF, Columbia-Presbyterian Med Ctr, New York, NY 77-79; **FAP:** Prof Columbia P&S; **SI:** *Preteen Delivery; Pregnancy Loss;* **HMO:** Oxford Empire PHCS

LANG: Hin, Guj, Mar, Sin; 🚹 📷 🏥 📅 💲 Mcr 1 Week

Beatty, Edward (MD)   ObG   `PCP`
Beth Israel Med Ctr

279 E 3rd St; New York, NY 10009; (212) 477-8849; **BDCERT:** ObG 74; **MS:** SUNY Hlth Sci Ctr 60; **RES:** ObG, Beth Israel Med Ctr, New York, NY 67-69

LANG: Sp; 🚹 SA/SO 📷 🏥 📅 💲 Mcr Mod Immediately ▨ **VISA** ⬤ ▥

Berkowitz, Richard (MD)   ObG
Mount Sinai Med Ctr

5 E 98th St; New York, NY 10029; (212) 241-5681; **BDCERT:** ObG 74; MF 79; **MS:** NYU Sch Med 65; **RES:** Kings County Hosp Ctr, Brooklyn, NY 65-66; NY Hosp-Cornell Med Ctr, New York, NY 68-71; **FEL:** Johns Hopkins Hosp, Baltimore, MD 72; **FAP:** Chrmn ObG Mt Sinai Sch Med; *SI: Obstetrical Ultrasound; Invasive Fetal Procedures;* **HMO:** Oxford Aetna Hlth Plan Empire Blue Cross & Shield Premier Mt Sinai Hlth +

LANG: Fr; 🔊 📷 🅿 🛏 💲 A Few Days 💳 **VISA** 🏧

Berman, Alvin (MD)   ObG
Mount Sinai Med Ctr

111 E 88th St B; New York, NY 10128; (212) 722-5757; **BDCERT:** ObG 78; **MS:** South Africa 69; **RES:** ObG, Mount Sinai Med Ctr, New York, NY 72-75; ObG, Mount Sinai Med Ctr, New York, NY 75-76; **FEL:** NP, Mount Sinai Med Ctr, New York, NY 76-77; *SI: Perimenopausal; General Gynecology;* **HMO:** Oxford Aetna Hlth Plan PHCS Premier

LANG: Afr; 🔊 🌙 📷 🅿 🛏 💲 A Few Days **VISA** 🏧

Blanco, Jody (MD)   ObG   PCP
Columbia-Presbyterian Med Ctr

161 Fort Washington Ave; New York, NY 10032; (212) 305-1107; **BDCERT:** ObG 88; **MS:** SUNY Hlth Sci Ctr 81; **RES:** Columbia-Presbyterian Med Ctr, New York, NY 81-85; **FEL:** Pelvic S & Urogynecology, UC Irvine Med Ctr, Orange, CA 85; *SI: Pelvic Reconstruction; Abnormal Pap Smears;* **HMO:** Oxford Aetna Hlth Plan GHI Prudential US Hlthcre +

🔊 📷 🅿 🛏 💲 Mcr 1 Week

Bowe, Edward (MD)   ObG
Columbia-Presbyterian Med Ctr

161 Fort Washington Ave; New York, NY 10032; (212) 305-4037; **BDCERT:** ObG 69; **MS:** Columbia P&S 61; **RES:** Columbia-Presbyterian Med Ctr, New York, NY 62-67; **FAP:** Clin Prof ObG Columbia P&S; *SI: Maternal-Fetal Medicine;* **HMO:** Oxford Aetna Hlth Plan Blue Cross & Blue Shield

🔊 📷 🅿 🛏 💲 Mcr Mcr 2-4 Weeks 💳 **VISA**

Breitstein, Robert (MD)   ObG
St Luke's Roosevelt Hosp Ctr

425 W 59th St; New York, NY 10019; (212) 523-3473; **BDCERT:** ObG 69; **MS:** SUNY Downstate 60; **RES:** Kings County Hosp Ctr, Brooklyn, NY 61-65; **FAP:** Asst Clin Prof NYU Sch Med; *SI: Endometriosis; Laser Surgery;* **HMO:** Oxford United Healthcare Multiplan Prucare CIGNA +

LANG: Sp, Fr; 🔊 🌙 📷 🅿 🛏 💲 Mcr Mcl 2-4 Weeks

Brodman, Michael (MD)   ObG
Mount Sinai Med Ctr

Klingenstein Pavillion-Mount Sinai Medical Center, One Gustave Levy Pl; New York, NY 10029; (212) 241-8762; **BDCERT:** ObG 88; **MS:** Mt Sinai Sch Med 82; **RES:** ObG, Mount Sinai Med Ctr, New York, NY 82-86; **FEL:** Mount Sinai Med Ctr, New York, NY 86-87; **FAP:** Assoc Prof Mt Sinai Sch Med; *SI: Incontinence Female; Laparoscopic Surgery;* **HMO:** Oxford Aetna Hlth Plan

🔊 📷 🅿 🛏 💲 Mcr WC 2-4 Weeks 💳 **VISA** 🏧

Caplan, Ronald (MD)   ObG   PCP
NY Hosp-Cornell Med Ctr

12 E 69th St; New York, NY 10021; (212) 517-8333; **BDCERT:** ObG 69; **MS:** Canada 62; **RES:** S, Royal Victoria Hosp, Montreal, Canada 63; ObG, Royal Victoria Hosp, Montreal, Canada 64-67; **FAP:** Assoc Clin Prof Cornell U; *SI: Laparoscopic Surgery; Hysteroscopic Surgery;* **HMO:** Oxford Aetna Hlth Plan GHI

LANG: Chi, Sp; 📷 🅿 🛏 💲 Immediately 💳 **VISA** 🏧

Cherry, Sheldon (MD)   ObG   PCP
Mount Sinai Med Ctr

1160 Park Ave; New York, NY 10128; (212) 860-2600; **BDCERT:** ObG 67; **MS:** Columbia P&S 58; **RES:** Columbia-Presbyterian Med Ctr, New York, NY 59-62; *SI: High Risk Pregnancies; Infertility;* **HMO:** Aetna Hlth Plan

🌙 📷 🅿 🛏 💲 Mcr Immediately 💳 **VISA** 🏧

Guide to symbols and abbreviations can be found on pages 110-113.

257

Chervenak, Frank (MD)   ObG
NY Hosp-Cornell Med Ctr

525 E 68th St J130; New York, NY 10021; (212) 746-3046; **BDCERT:** ObG 84; **MF** 84; **MS:** Jefferson Med Coll 76; **RES:** NY Med Coll, New York, NY 77-79; St Luke's Roosevelt Hosp Ctr, New York, NY 79-81; **FEL:** MF, Yale-New Haven Hosp, New Haven, CT 81-83; **HMO:** Oxford Empire Blue Cross & Shield United Healthcare US Hlthcre PHCS +

🦽 📷 🛗 🅿️ 💲 Immediately ▨ **VISA** 💳

Chin, Jean (MD)   ObG
Mount Sinai Med Ctr

1130 Park Ave; New York, NY 10128; (212) 348-2525; **BDCERT:** ObG 82; **MS:** Columbia P&S 76; **RES:** ObG, Mount Sinai Med Ctr, New York, NY; **HOSP:** Beth Israel North

📞 📷 🅿️ 🛗 💲 A Few Days **VISA** 💳

Corio, Laura (MD)   ObG   `PCP`
Mount Sinai Med Ctr

62 E 88th St 201; New York, NY 10128; (212) 860-6700; **BDCERT:** ObG 84; **MS:** UMDNJ-NJ Med Sch, Newark 78; **RES:** Mount Sinai Med Ctr, New York, NY 79-82; **SI:** *Perimenopause/Menopause; High Risk Obstetrics*; **HMO:** None

LANG: Sp; 🦽 📞 📷 🅿️ 🛗 💲 Mcr A Few Days ▨
VISA 💳

Cox, Kathryn (MD)   ObG
NY Hosp-Cornell Med Ctr

124 E 72nd St; New York, NY 10021; (212) 535-2600; **BDCERT:** ObG 81; **MS:** U Mich Med Sch 75; **RES:** NY Hosp-Cornell Med Ctr, New York, NY 75-79; **SI:** *Pregnancy after Age 35; Conservative GYN Surgery*; **HMO:** None

SA/SO 📷 🛗 💲 Mcr 4+ Weeks ▨ **VISA** 💳

Cutler, Lawrence (MD)   ObG   `PCP`
NY Hosp-Cornell Med Ctr

42 E 75th St; New York, NY 10021; (212) 535-2700; **BDCERT:** ObG 86; **MS:** U Chicago-Pritzker Sch Med 80; **RES:** ObG, NY Hosp-Cornell Med Ctr, New York, NY 81-84; **FAP:** Instr Cornell U; **SI:** *High Risk Pregnancy; Recurrent Miscarriages*; **HMO:** None

📷 🅿️ 🛗 💲 A Few Days

Dantuono, Louise (MD)   ObG
New York University Med Ctr

35 E 35th St 1C; New York, NY 10016; (212) 679-7970; **BDCERT:** ObG 51; **MS:** Med Coll PA 42; **RES:** Bellevue Hosp Ctr, New York, NY 43-46; Queens Hosp Ctr, Jamaica, NY 42; **FAP:** Clin Prof NYU Sch Med; **HOSP:** Bellevue Hosp Ctr; **SI:** *Menopausal Syndrome; Gynecology Checkups*

🦽 📷 🅿️ 🛗 Mcr WC NFI 1 Week

Debrovner, Charles (MD)   ObG
New York University Med Ctr

338 E 30th St; New York, NY 10016; (212) 683-0090; **BDCERT:** ObG 67; **MS:** NYU Sch Med 60; **RES:** Bellevue Hosp Ctr, New York, NY 61-65; **HOSP:** St Luke's Roosevelt Hosp Ctr; **SI:** *Infertility; Menopause*; **HMO:** Oxford Aetna Hlth Plan Chubb PHCS

🦽 SA/SO 📷 🅿️ 🛗 💲 Mcr NFI A Few Days **VISA** 💳

Degann, Sona (MD)   ObG   `PCP`
NY Hosp-Cornell Med Ctr

211 E 70th St; New York, NY 10021; (212) 249-0900; **BDCERT:** ObG 90; **MS:** Johns Hopkins U 83; **RES:** NY Hosp-Cornell Med Ctr, New York, NY 83-87; **HMO:** None

LANG: Fr, Sp, Arm, Ar; 🦽 📷 🅿️ 🛗 💲 Mcr
4+ Weeks **VISA** 💳

Diamond, Sharon (MD)   ObG   `PCP`
Mount Sinai Med Ctr

61 E 86th St 1; New York, NY 10028; (212) 876-2200; **BDCERT:** ObG 85; **MS:** Mt Sinai Sch Med 79; **RES:** Mount Sinai Med Ctr, New York, NY 79-82; **SI:** *Abnormal Pap Smears; Menopause*

🦽 📷 🅿️ 🛗 💲 2-4 Weeks **VISA** 💳

Edersheim, Terri (MD)   ObG   `PCP`
NY Hosp-Cornell Med Ctr

523 E 72nd St Fl 9; New York, NY 10021; (212) 472-5340; **BDCERT:** ObG 87; **MS:** Albert Einstein Coll Med 80; **RES:** NY Hosp-Cornell Med Ctr, New York, NY 80-84; **FEL:** NP, NY Hosp-Cornell Med Ctr, New York, NY 84-86; **SI:** *High Risk Obstetrics; Multiple Pregnancies*; **HMO:** HMO

🦽 📷 🅿️ 🛗 💲 A Few Days ▨ **VISA**

Essig, Mitchell (MD) ObG
Beth Israel Med Ctr

88 Univ Pl Fl 9; New York, NY 10003; (212) 243-4050; **BDCERT:** ObG 82; **MS:** NY Med Coll 75; **RES:** Beth Israel Med Ctr, New York, NY 75-79; **FEL:** EDM, Bellevue Hosp Ctr, New York, NY 79-81; **HOSP:** New York University Med Ctr; **SI:** IVF

🚫 🏥 📞 📷 🧑 🏧 $ Mcr Immediately ▒ **VISA** 💳 💳

Freuman, Henry (MD) ObG **PCP**
Lenox Hill Hosp

1430 2nd Ave Ste 101; New York, NY 10021; (212) 517-3322; **BDCERT:** ObG 73; **MS:** Israel 63; **RES:** ObG, Brooklyn Jewish Hosp, Brooklyn, NY 68-72; **HOSP:** Beth Israel North; **SI:** Fibroids; Treatment without Hysterectomy; Infertility. Cysts.; **HMO:** Most

🏧 📞 📷 🧑 🏧 Immediately **VISA**

Friedman, Frederick (MD) ObG **PCP**
Mount Sinai Med Ctr

5 E 98th St 1174; New York, NY 10029; (212) 241-8762; **BDCERT:** ObG 91; **MS:** SUNY Hlth Sci Ctr 85; **RES:** ObG, Mount Sinai Med Ctr, New York, NY 85-89; **FAP:** Asst Prof ObG Mt Sinai Sch Med; **SI:** Well Woman Care; Contraception; **HMO:** Oxford Blue Cross Blue Choice Aetna Hlth Plan

LANG: Sp; 🚫 📷 🧑 🏧 $ Mcr 2-4 Weeks ▒ **VISA** 💳 💳

Friedman, Lynn (MD) ObG **PCP**
Mount Sinai Med Ctr

229 E 79th St; New York, NY 10021; (212) 737-3282; **BDCERT:** ObG 98; **MS:** NYU Sch Med 84; **RES:** ObG, Mount Sinai Med Ctr, New York, NY 84-88; **FAP:** Asst Clin Instr Mt Sinai Sch Med; **SI:** Recurrent Miscarriage; Infertility Issues; **HMO:** Oxford

LANG: Sp; 🚫 📞 📷 🧑 🏧 $ Mcr 4+ Weeks **VISA** 💳

Gershowitz, Judith (MD) ObG
Beth Israel Med Ctr

New York Gynecological & Obstetrical Assoc, 145 E 32nd St; New York, NY 10016; (212) 684-5522; **BDCERT:** ObG 83; **MS:** NY Med Coll 75; **RES:** ObG, Beth Israel Med Ctr, New York, NY 75-79; **FAP:** Asst Albert Einstein Coll Med; **HMO:** Oxford US Hlthcre Aetna Hlth Plan GHI 1199 +

🚫 📷 🧑 🏧 $ Mcr 4+ Weeks ▒ **VISA** 💳

Goldman, Gary (MD) ObG **PCP**
NY Hosp-Cornell Med Ctr

519 E 72nd St Ste 202; New York, NY 10021; (212) 535-6100; **BDCERT:** ObG 92; **MS:** SUNY Hlth Sci Ctr 86; **RES:** ObG, NY Hosp-Cornell Med Ctr, New York, NY 86-90; **FAP:** Clin Instr Cornell U; **SI:** Endometriosis; Laparoscopy; **HMO:** Oxford

🚫 📷 🧑 🏧 $ 1 Week **VISA** 💳

Goldstein, Dov (MD) ObG
St Luke's Roosevelt Hosp Ctr

Central Park West Fertility Center, 55 Central Park West; New York, NY 10023; (212) 721-4545; **BDCERT:** ObG 89; **MS:** Israel 75; **RES:** ObG, Rothschild U, Israel 75-80; ObG, Maimonides Med Ctr, Brooklyn, NY 83-86; **FEL:** RE, Columbia-Presbyterian Med Ctr, New York, NY 81; RE, Univ Hosp SUNY Bklyn, Brooklyn, NY 81-83; **FAP:** Assoc Instr ObG Columbia P&S; **HOSP:** Beth Israel Med Ctr; **SI:** In Vitro Fertilization; Ovulation; **HMO:** Oxford NYLCare Aetna Hlth Plan PHCS

LANG: Chi, Fr, Heb, Rus, Itl; 🚫 🏧 📞 📷 🧑 🏧 $ Mcr A Few Days ▒ **VISA** 💳 💳

Goldstein, Martin (MD) ObG
Mount Sinai Med Ctr

1192 Park Ave; New York, NY 10128; (212) 996-0400; **BDCERT:** ObG 73; **MS:** SUNY Hlth Sci Ctr 66; **RES:** ObG, Mount Sinai Med Ctr, New York, NY 67-71; **SI:** Laparoscopic & Laser Surgery; Urinary Incontinence

🚫 📷 🧑 🏧 $ Mcr 1 Week **VISA** 💳

Guide to symbols and abbreviations can be found on pages 110-113.

259

Grant, Susan (MD) ObG `PCP`
Lenox Hill Hosp
242 W 76th St; New York, NY 10023; (212) 769-0755; **BDCERT:** ObG 85; **MS:** Med Coll PA 79; **RES:** St Luke's Roosevelt Hosp Ctr, New York, NY 79-83; **HOSP:** St Luke's Roosevelt Hosp Ctr
LANG: Sp; ⚕ 🅲 🔲 🔳 🔳 🆂 A Few Days

Grunebaum, Amos (MD) ObG `PCP`
St Luke's Roosevelt Hosp Ctr
425 W 59th St 5A; New York, NY 10019; (212) 333-5533; **BDCERT:** ObG 88; MF 96; **MS:** Germany 74; **RES:** ObG, Univ Hosp SUNY Bklyn, Brooklyn, NY 78-82; **FEL:** MF, Univ Hosp SUNY Bklyn, Brooklyn, NY 82-84; **FAP:** Asst Prof Columbia P&S; **SI:** *Preconception Counseling; High Risk Pregnancy;* **HMO:** Aetna Hlth Plan Blue Cross & Blue Shield CIGNA Oxford
LANG: Gae, Sp, Fr, Yd; ⚕ 🔳 🅲 🔲 🔳 🔳 🆂 🔳
1 Week 🔳 *VISA* 💳 💳

Grunfeld, Lawrence (MD) ObG
Mount Sinai Med Ctr
Reproductive Medicine Associates, LLP, 58 E 79th St; New York, NY 10021; (212) 744-1855; **BDCERT:** RE 89; ObG 87; **MS:** Mt Sinai Sch Med 79; **RES:** ObG, Albert Einstein, Bronx, NY 80-84; **FEL:** RE, Albert Einstein/Yale U, Bronx, NY 84-87; **FAP:** Asst Prof Mt Sinai Sch Med; **SI:** *Infertility;* **HMO:** Oxford PHS PHCS Aetna Hlth Plan
🔳 🔲 🔳 🔳 🆂 A Few Days 🔳 *VISA* 💳

Gruss, Leslie (MD) ObG `PCP`
Beth Israel Med Ctr
568 Broadway 304; New York, NY 10012; (212) 966-7600; **BDCERT:** ObG 89; **MS:** Med Coll PA 83; **RES:** Montefiore Med Ctr, Bronx, NY 83-87; **SI:** *Laparoscopy & Hysteroscopy; General Gynecology;* **HMO:** Oxford United Healthcare PHCS Prucare
⚕ 🅲 🔲 🔳 🔳 🆂 🔳 Immediately *VISA* 💳

Handszer, Bernardo (MD) ObG
Lenox Hill Hosp
120 Central Park South 1C; New York, NY 10019; (212) 246-1119; **BDCERT:** ObG 72; **MS:** Colombia 59; **RES:** ObG, Hosp San Juan Dedios, Bogota, Columbia 61-65; St Luke's Roosevelt Hosp Ctr, New York, NY 68-70; **HOSP:** St Luke's Roosevelt Hosp Ctr; **SI:** *Colposcopy;* **HMO:** American Health Plan Multiplan PHCS Health Source Oxford +
LANG: Sp; 🔲 🔳 🔳 🆂 Immediately 🔳 *VISA* 💳

Ho, Alison G (MD) ObG
New York University Med Ctr
145 E 32nd St; New York, NY 10016; (212) 679-2213; **BDCERT:** ObG 89; **MS:** Univ Penn 82; **RES:** ObG, New York University Med Ctr, New York, NY 82-86; **FAP:** Asst Prof NYU Sch Med
⚕ 🔲 🔳 🔳 🆂 A Few Days

Holland, Claudia (MD) ObG `PCP`
Columbia-Presbyterian Med Ctr
161 Ft Washington Ave 409; New York, NY 10032; (212) 305-5572; **BDCERT:** ObG 87; **MS:** Mt Sinai Sch Med 81; **RES:** ObG, New York University Med Ctr, New York, NY 81-85; **FAP:** Asst Prof NYU Sch Med; **SI:** *Obstetrics; Prenatal Evaluation;* **HMO:** CIGNA Oxford NYLCare United Healthcare GHI +
LANG: Sp, Fr, Itl; ⚕ 🔲 🔳 🔳 🆂 🔳 A Few Days

Hoskins, Iffath (MD) ObG
New York University Med Ctr
NYU Downtown OBGYN Associates, 170 William St; New York, NY 10038; (212) 312-5840; **BDCERT:** ObG 86; **MS:** Pakistan 75; **RES:** Psyc, St Elizabeth's Hosp, Washington, DC 77-79; ObG, Nat Naval Med Ctr, Bethesda, MD 79-82; **FEL:** MF, Walter Reed Army Med Ctr, Washington, DC 83-85; **FAP:** Assoc Prof; **SI:** *High Risk Pregnancy; Infections in Pregnancy;* **HMO:** Oxford Aetna Hlth Plan Prudential Blue Cross & Blue Shield CIGNA +
LANG: Chi, Sp; ⚕ 🅲 🔲 🔳 🔳 🆂 🔳 🔳
Immediately 🔳 *VISA* 💳 💳

Husami, Nabil (MD)   **ObG**
Columbia-Presbyterian Med Ctr

12 W 72nd St; New York, NY 10032; (212) 650-0355; **BDCERT:** ObG 79; **MS:** Lebanon 72; **RES:** American U Med Ctr, Beirut, Lebanon 72-75; Columbia-Presbyterian Med Ctr, New York; NY 75-76; **FEL:** RE, Columbia-Presbyterian Med Ctr, New York, NY 76-78; **SI:** *Endometriosis; Laparoscopic*

🔲

Hutson, J Milton (MD)   **ObG** **PCP**
NY Hosp-Cornell Med Ctr

523 E 72nd St Flr 9; New York, NY 10021; (212) 472-5340; **BDCERT:** ObG 83; MF 85; **MS:** U Ala Sch Med 75; **RES:** U Hosp, Cincinnati, OH 75-79; **FEL:** MF, Columbia-Presbyterian Med Ctr, New York, NY 80-82; **SI:** *Multiple Pregnancies*

♿ 🔲 👤 🏥 💲 A Few Days 🔲 **VISA** 💳

Jacobs, Allan J (MD)   **ObG**
Beth Israel Med Ctr

10 Union Square East; New York, NY 10003; (212) 844-8570; **BDCERT:** ObG 79; GO 83; **MS:** USC Sch Med 72; **RES:** Parkland Mem Hosp, Dallas, TX 73-76; **FEL:** GO, Mount Sinai Med Ctr, New York, NY 78-80; **HOSP:** Victory Memorial Hosp; **SI:** *Gynecologic Oncology;* **HMO:** First Health GHI HIP Network Oxford NYLCare +

LANG: Sp; ♿ 🔲 🏥 🔲 🔲 🔲 1 Week

James, David F (MD)   **ObG** **PCP**
Lenox Hill Hosp

Ob Gyn Assoc, 45 E 85th St; New York, NY 10028; (212) 535-4611; **BDCERT:** ObG 71; **MS:** England 64; **RES:** ObG, Lenox Hill Hosp, New York, NY 64-69; **FAP:** Asst Clin Prof ObG Cornell U; **HOSP:** NY Hosp-Cornell Med Ctr; **SI:** *Menopause;* **HMO:** Oxford Sel Pro Magnacare Oxford United Healthcare +

LANG: Fr; ♿ 🔲 🔲 👤 🏥 💲 🔲 A Few Days 🔲 **VISA** 💳 🔲

Jones, James (MD)   **ObG**
St Vincents Hosp & Med Ctr NY

Saint Vincent's Hospital, 153 W 11th St Rm 903; New York, NY 10011; (212) 604-2512; **BDCERT:** ObG 72; RE 74; **MS:** SUNY Hlth Sci Ctr 60; **RES:** Long Island Coll Hosp, Brooklyn, NY 60-64; **FEL:** RE, UC San Francisco Med Ctr, San Francisco, CA 64-67; **SI:** *Infertility/Amenorrhea; Hirsutism;* **HMO:** Prucare US Hlthcre Empire Blue Cross & Shield Oxford Blue Shield +

LANG: Sp; ♿ 🔲 🔲 👤 🏥 🔲 🔲 A Few Days

Juan, Paul L (MD)   **ObG**
St Vincents Hosp & Med Ctr NY

130 W 12th St; New York, NY 10011; (212) 604-7838; **BDCERT:** ObG 80; **MS:** Canada 61; **RES:** ObG, St Vincents Hosp & Med Ctr NY, New York, NY 62-66; **FAP:** Asst Clin Prof NY Med Coll

Kaminsky, Sari J (MD)   **ObG** **PCP**
Metropolitan Hosp Ctr

Metropolitan Hospital, 1901 1st Ave Flr3 Rm3A; New York, NY 10029; (212) 423-6796; **BDCERT:** ObG 77; **MS:** SUNY Hlth Sci Ctr 71; **RES:** ObG, Univ Hosp SUNY Bklyn, Brooklyn, NY 71-75; **FAP:** Assoc Prof ObG NY Med Coll; **HOSP:** Westchester Med Ctr

♿ 🔲 👤 🔲 🔲

Kent, Joan (MD)   **ObG**
NY Hosp-Cornell Med Ctr

235 E 67th St; New York, NY 10021; (212) 772-2900; **BDCERT:** ObG 90; **MS:** Cornell U 84; **RES:** ObG, NY Hosp-Cornell Med Ctr, New York, NY 84-88; **FAP:** Clin Instr ObG Cornell U

♿ 💲 🔲 2-4 Weeks **VISA** 💳

Kerenyi, Thomas (MD)   **ObG**
Mount Sinai Med Ctr

1126 Park Ave; New York, NY 10128; (212) 427-7400; **BDCERT:** ObG 69; **MS:** Cornell U 60; **RES:** ObG, Mount Sinai Med Ctr, New York, NY 60-65; **FEL:** NP, Barnes Hosp, St Louis, MO 65-67; **FAP:** Assoc Clin Prof Mt Sinai Sch Med

LANG: Hun, Sp; 🔲 👤 🏥 💲 A Few Days **VISA** 💳

Kessler, Alan (MD)   ObG   `PCP`
NY Hosp-Cornell Med Ctr

Cornell University Medical College, 525 E 68th St;
New York, NY 10021; (212) 746-1036; **BDCERT:**
ObG 85; **MS:** Mexico 78; **RES:** NY Hosp-Cornell Med
Ctr, New York, NY 79-83; **FAP:** Assoc Prof ObG
Cornell U; **HOSP:** New York Eye & Ear Infirmary; *SI:*
Multiple Gestations; Benign Gynecologic Surgery

LANG: Sp; 🦽 🎥 👥 🏥 💲 ▥ Immediately ▨
VISA

Kim, Joyce M (MD)   ObG   `PCP`
Mount Sinai Med Ctr

1130 Park Ave; New York, NY 10128; (212) 348-
2525; **BDCERT:** ObG 92; **MS:** Mt Sinai Sch Med 86;
RES: Mount Sinai Med Ctr, New York, NY 86-90;
SI: Laser Surgery; General Obstetrics

📞 🎥 👥 🏥 💲 ▥ Immediately **VISA** 💳

Krause, Cynthia (MD)   ObG
Mount Sinai Med Ctr

5 E 98th St Box 1521; New York, NY 10029; (212)
241-8216; **BDCERT:** ObG 88; **MS:** Duke U 80; **RES:**
IM, Baltimore City Hosp, Baltimore, MD 80-82;
ObG, Mount Sinai Med Ctr, New York, NY 82-86;
FAP: Asst Prof Mt Sinai Sch Med; *SI: Menopause;*
Ultrasound; **HMO:** PHCS Beech Street Oxford

🦽 🎥 👥 🏥 💲 ▥ 4+ Weeks ▨ **VISA** 💳

Lafontant, Jennifer (MD)   ObG   `PCP`
St Barnabas Hosp-Bronx

Also ofc on Brxdale Av, Brx NY, 121 E 60th St 8NE;
New York, NY 10022; (212) 308-9101; **BDCERT:**
ObG 85; **MS:** West Indies 76; **RES:** ObG, St Luke's
Roosevelt Hosp Ctr, New York, NY 78-80; ObG,
Metropolitan Hosp Ctr, New York, NY 80-81; **FAP:**
Asst Clin Prof Columbia P&S; **HOSP:** Columbia-
Presbyterian Med Ctr; *SI: Colposcopy; Laparoscopy;*
HMO: US Hlthcre GHI 1199 Prudential Oxford +

LANG: Sp, Fr, Cre; 🦽 🆘 📞 🎥 👥 🏥 💲 ▥ ▥
Immediately ▨ **VISA** 💳

Ledger, William (MD)   ObG
NY Hosp-Cornell Med Ctr

525 E 68th St Ste J130; New York, NY 10021;
(212) 746-3009; **BDCERT:** ObG 67; **MS:** Univ Penn
58; **RES:** ObG, Temple U Hosp, Philadelphia, PA 61-
64; **HMO:** Oxford United Healthcare Blue Choice US
Hlthcre Physician's Health Plan +

LANG: Hun; 🦽 🎥 👥 💲 ▥ 2-4 Weeks

Levine, Richard U (MD)   ObG
Columbia-Presbyterian Med Ctr

161 Ft Washington Ave 436; New York, NY
10032; (212) 305-5300; **BDCERT:** ObG 74; **MS:**
Cornell U 66; **RES:** Columbia-Presbyterian Med Ctr,
New York, NY 75; Bellevue Hosp Ctr, New York,
NY 66-67; **FEL:** ObG, Sweden; **FAP:** Prof ObG
Columbia P&S; *SI: Abnormal Pap Smears;*
Gynecologic Surgery; **HMO:** Oxford Blue Cross & Blue
Shield Aetna Hlth Plan CIGNA Prucare +

LANG: Sp, Fr; 🦽 🎥 👥 🏥 💲 ▥ 1 Week

Lieberman, Beth (MD)   ObG   `PCP`
New York University Med Ctr

333 E 30th St; New York, NY 10016; (212) 689-
4468; **BDCERT:** ObG 80; **MS:** NYU Sch Med 73;
RES: ObG, Bellevue Hosp Ctr, New York, NY 73-77;
FAP: Asst Clin Prof ObG NYU Sch Med; **HOSP:**
Bellevue Hosp Ctr; *SI: Menopause; Weight Reduction*

LANG: Rus, Fr; 🦽 📞 🎥 👥 🏥 💲 Immediately ▨
VISA 💳

Lissak, Louis (MD)   ObG
NY Hosp-Cornell Med Ctr

328 E 75th St; New York, NY 10021; (212) 535-
6737; **BDCERT:** ObG 77; **MS:** U Hlth Sci/Chicago
Med Sch 69; **RES:** ObG, NY Hosp-Cornell Med Ctr,
New York, NY 70-74; **FAP:** Clin Instr Cornell U; *SI:*
Laparoscopic Surgery; Obstetrics; **HMO:** Aetna Hlth
Plan Oxford Blue Cross & Blue Shield PHS

LANG: Sp; 🦽 🎥 👥 🏥 💲 ▥ ▥ Immediately ▨
VISA 💳

Lustig, Ilana (MD) ObG
New York University Med Ctr

233 E 31st St; New York, NY 10016; (212) 696-9536; **BDCERT:** ObG 84; **MS:** Geo Wash U Sch Med 77; **RES:** Yale-New Haven Hosp, New Haven, CT 77-81; **FEL:** Bellevue Hosp Ctr, New York, NY 81-83; **FAP:** NYU Sch Med; *SI: High Risk Pregnancy*; **HMO:** Oxford

🔲 📧 🎚 💲 4+ Weeks

Maggio, John (DO) ObG
St Vincents Hosp & Med Ctr NY

205 E 69th St; New York, NY 10021; (212) 628-1212; **BDCERT:** ObG 78; **MS:** Chicago Coll Osteo Med 68; **RES:** St Clare's Hosp & Health Ctr, New York, NY 70-74; **FAP:** Asst Clin Prof NY Med Coll; **HOSP:** St Clare's Hosp & Health Ctr; *SI: Urinary Incontinence-Fem; Laparoscopy*; **HMO:** Aetna Hlth Plan Blue Choice Magnacare PHS Oxford +

♿ 🌙 🔲 📧 🎚 💲 Immediately

Maidman, Jack (MD) ObG
Columbia-Presbyterian Med Ctr

21 W 86th St; New York, NY 10024; (212) 799-2818; **BDCERT:** ObG 82; **MS:** UC San Francisco 62; **RES:** Kings Cty Hosp Ctr, Brooklyn, NY 63-68; **FEL:** GO, Kings County Hosp, Brooklyn, NY 67-69; Hosp U Penn, Philadelphia, PA 69-70

Manning, Frank (MD) ObG
Columbia-Presbyterian Med Ctr

Dept of Obstetrics & Gynecology, 622 W 168th St; New York, NY 10032; **BDCERT:** ObG 80; MF 83; **MS:** U Manitoba 70; **RES:** ObG, U Manitoba, Winnipeg,Canada 71-75; **FEL:** Med, University of Oxford, Oxford, England 75-77; Med, U South California, Los Angeles, CA 77-79; **FAP:** Prof Columbia P&S; *SI: Fetal Assessment; Prenatal Diagnosis Treatment*

LANG: Fr, Itl, Sp, Ger; ♿ 🔲 🌙 🔲 🎚 💲 📧 📧 📧 🔲

Martens Jr, Frederick W (MD)ObG
NY Hosp-Cornell Med Ctr

449 E 68th St; New York, NY 10021; (212) 628-1500; **BDCERT:** ObG 67; **MS:** Cornell U 57; **RES:** ObG, NY Hosp-Cornell Med Ctr, New York, NY 58-63; **FAP:** Prof Cornell U; *SI: GYN Surgery; Post Menopausal Hormones*; **HMO:** None

🔲 📧 🎚 📧 A Few Days 📧 **VISA** 📧

Matera-Abouzahr, Cristina (MD)ObG
Columbia-Presbyterian Med Ctr

860 5th Ave; New York, NY 10021; (212) 639-9122; **BDCERT:** ObG 94; RE 96; **MS:** NYU Sch Med 86; **RES:** ObG, Columbia-Presbyterian Med Ctr, New York, NY 86-90; **FEL:** Columbia-Presbyterian Med Ctr, New York, NY 90-92; **FAP:** Assoc Prof Columbia P&S; *SI: Infertility; Laparoscopy & Hysteroscopy*

LANG: Sp; ♿ 🔲 📧 🎚 💲 📧 2-4 Weeks **VISA** 📧

McCaffrey, Raymond (MD) ObG [PCP]
Columbia-Presbyterian Med Ctr

16 E 60th St; New York, NY 10128; (212) 722-8888; **BDCERT:** ObG 68; **MS:** Cornell U 58; **RES:** NY Hosp-Cornell Med Ctr, New York, NY 58-59; Columbia-Presbyterian Med Ctr, New York, NY 59-64; **HMO:** Oxford Blue Cross & Blue Shield HealthNet PHS 1199 +

♿ 📧 🔲 📧 🎚 💲 1 Week

McGill, Frances (MD) ObG
St Vincents Hosp & Med Ctr NY

32 W 18th St 5th FL; New York, NY 10011; (212) 647-6490; **BDCERT:** ObG 97; **MS:** Grenada 81; **RES:** ObG, Women & Infants Hosp, Providence, RI 82-85; **FAP:** Assoc Prof of Clin ObG NY Med Coll; *SI: Menopause; GYN Care for Breast Cancer*; **HMO:** Blue Cross & Blue Shield United Healthcare Oxford Prucare CIGNA +

♿ 🔲 📧 🎚 💲 📧 2-4 Weeks **VISA** 📧

Guide to symbols and abbreviations can be found on pages 110-113.

263

Meiland, Hanne (MD) ObG
NY Hosp-Cornell Med Ctr

211 E 70th St; New York, NY 10021; (212) 249-0900; **BDCERT:** ObG 90; **MS:** Denmark 81; **RES:** ObG, Copenhagen Univ Hosp, Copenhagen, Denmark 82-86; ObG, NY Hosp-Cornell Med Ctr, New York, NY 87-90; *SI: Menopause*

LANG: Dan, Sp, Ger, Fr; ⬅ 🔲 🔲 🔲 🔲 2-4 Weeks

Melnick, Hugh (MD) ObG
Lenox Hill Hosp

Advanced Family Services, PC, 1625 3rd Ave ; New York, NY 10128; (212) 369-8700; **BDCERT:** ObG 76; **MS:** Temple U 72; **RES:** ObG, Lenox Hill Hosp, New York, NY 72-76; **FEL:** Immunology, U Birmingham, Birmingham, England 69; **HOSP:** Beth Israel Med Ctr; *SI: In Vitro Fertilization*

LANG: Sp, Rus, Fr, Pol; ⬅ 🔲 🔲 🔲 🔲 🔲
Immediately 🔲 *VISA* 🔲

Moreno, Fernando (MD) ObG
Beth Israel Med Ctr

151 E 83rd St 1D; New York, NY 10028; (216) 535-5022; **BDCERT:** ObG 88; **MS:** NY Med Coll 90; **RES:** St Vincents Hosp & Med Ctr NY, New York, NY; **HOSP:** St Vincents Hosp & Med Ctr NY

Moss, Richard (MD) ObG
Mount Sinai Med Ctr

1160 Park Ave; New York, NY 10128; (212) 860-2600; **BDCERT:** ObG 65; ObG 79; **MS:** SUNY Hlth Sci Ctr 57; **RES:** Mount Sinai Med Ctr, New York, NY 57-62; **FAP:** Asst Clin Prof Mt Sinai Sch Med; *SI: Menopause; Colposcopy*; **HMO:** Aetna Hlth Plan US Hlthcre

LANG: Fr, Yd, Sp; 🔲 🔲 🔲 🔲 Immediately 🔲
VISA 🔲

Nash, Warner (MD) ObG
Lenox Hill Hosp

799 Park Ave; New York, NY 10021; (212) 288-3290; **BDCERT:** ObG 62; **MS:** Columbia P&S 53; **RES:** Columbia-Presbyterian Med Ctr, New York, NY 53-57; **FEL:** MF, Francis Delafield Hosp, New York, NY 57-58

🔲 🔲 🔲 🔲 Immediately

Ordorica, Steven (MD) ObG
New York University Med Ctr

530 1st Ave Ste 10Q; New York, NY 10016; (212) 263-5982; **BDCERT:** ObG 90; MF 92; **MS:** SUNY Hlth Sci Ctr 83; **RES:** ObG, New York University Med Ctr, New York, NY 83-87; **FEL:** MF, New York University Med Ctr, New York, NY 87-89; **FAP:** Asst Prof NYU Sch Med

LANG: Sp; ⬅ 🔲 🔲 🔲 🔲 🔲 🔲 Immediately

Panter, Gideon (MD) ObG
NY Hosp-Cornell Med Ctr

653 Park Ave; New York, NY 10021; (212) 737-7727; **BDCERT:** ObG 67; **MS:** Cornell U 60; **RES:** Columbia Presbyterian Med Ctr, New York, NY 61-65; **FEL:** NY Hosp-Cornell Med Ctr, New York, NY 60

Pascario, Ben (MD) ObG `PCP`
Lenox Hill Hosp

8 E 83rd St; New York, NY 10028; (212) 628-2400; **BDCERT:** ObG 77; **MS:** Romania 61; **RES:** ObG, St Luke's Roosevelt Hosp Ctr, New York, NY 71-75; **HOSP:** Beth Israel North

LANG: Itl, Fr, Sp; ⬅ 🔲 🔲 🔲 🔲 🔲 A Few Days

Porges, Robert (MD) ObG
New York University Med Ctr

530 1st Ave Ste 5H; New York, NY 10016; (212) 263-6362; **BDCERT:** ObG 63; **MS:** SUNY Downstate 55; **RES:** ObG, Mount Sinai Med Ctr, New York, NY 56-57; ObG, Bronx Muncipal Hosp Ctr, Bronx, NY 57-60; **FAP:** Prof NYU Sch Med; *SI: Pelvic Organ Prolapse*

LANG: Ger, Sp; 🔲 🔲 🔲 🔲 🔲

Randolph, Paula (MD) ObG `PCP`
Columbia-Presbyterian Med Ctr

635 Madison Ave; New York, NY 10022; (212) 317-4544; **BDCERT:** ObG 89; **MS:** Columbia P&S 83; **RES:** Columbia-Presbyterian Med Ctr, New York, NY 87; *SI: Surgery-Laparoscopy; Vulvar Cutaneous Disease*; **HMO:** Oxford Aetna Hlth Plan Empire Sanus Metlife +

LANG: Fr, Sp; ⬅ 🔲 🔲 🔲 🔲 🔲 🔲 Immediately
🔲 *VISA*

Rehnstrom, Jaana (MD) ObG
St Luke's Roosevelt Hosp Ctr

103 5th Ave; New York, NY 10003; (212) 366-4765; **BDCERT:** ObG 88; **MS:** Finland 79; **RES:** St Luke's Roosevelt Hosp Ctr, New York, NY 83-86; **HOSP:** Lenox Hill Hosp; *SI: Abnormal Pap Smears; Bleeding,Contraception*; **HMO:** PHCS Multiplan Oxford Blue Choice

LANG: Fin, Swd, Sp; ♿ 🅲 🔄 🔧 🏨 🅂 Mcr
A Few Days *VISA* 💳

Rehrer, Lisa (MD) ObG
St Vincents Hosp & Med Ctr NY

103 5th Ave FL8; New York, NY 10003; (212) 691-8833; **BDCERT:** ObG 94; **MS:** Ind U Sch Med 84; **RES:** New York University Med Ctr, New York, NY 85-89; **FAP:** Assoc Prof NYU Sch Med; **HMO:** Oxford Aetna Hlth Plan US Hlthcre PHS

Reiss, Ronald (MD) ObG **PCP**
United Hosp Med Ctr

124 E 84th St; New York, NY 10028; (212) 749-3113; **BDCERT:** ObG 83; **MS:** Belgium 76; **RES:** ObG, St Luke's Roosevelt Hosp Ctr, New York, NY 76-80; **HOSP:** Lenox Hill Hosp; *SI: Infertility*; **HMO:** Aetna Hlth Plan Oxford GHI United Healthcare Health Source +

LANG: Fr, Tag; 🅲 🔄 🔧 🏨 🅂 Mcr A Few Days 💳
VISA 💳 💳

Rodke, Gae (MD) ObG
St Luke's Roosevelt Hosp Ctr

146 Central Park West 1G; New York, NY 10023; (212) 496-9800; **BDCERT:** ObG 88; **MS:** Albert Einstein Coll Med 81; **RES:** Univ Hosp SUNY Stony Brook, Stony Brook, NY 81-82; ObG, Univ Hosp SUNY Stony Brook, Stony Brook, NY 82-86; **FAP:** Asst Clin Prof Columbia P&S; *SI: Vulvovaginal Disease; Gynecological Surgery*

🅲 🔧 🏨 🅂 💳 💳 💳

Rothbard, Malcolm (MD) ObG
Lenox Hill Hosp

108 E 66th St 1B; New York, NY 10021; (212) 861-2629; **BDCERT:** ObG 72; **MS:** SUNY Downstate 65; **RES:** ObG, Kingsbrook Jewish Med Ctr, Brooklyn, NY 69-70; **FEL:** Metropolitan Hosp Ctr, New York, NY 69-70

LANG: Sp; 🏨 🅂 Immediately

Rothe, Desider (MD) ObG
NY Hosp-Cornell Med Ctr

653 Park Ave; New York, NY 10021; (212) 535-2175; **BDCERT:** ObG 74; **MS:** Hungary 61; **RES:** ObG, NY Hosp-Cornell Med Ctr, New York, NY 71-72; **FAP:** Assoc Prof ObG Cornell U

LANG: Fr, Hun; 🅲 🔄 🔧 🏨 🅂 Mcr Mcr 2-4 Weeks
💳

Rubell, Donald (MD) ObG **PCP**
Cabrini Med Ctr

46 E 73rd St; New York, NY 10021; (212) 772-3535; **BDCERT:** ObG 75; **MS:** NYU Sch Med 68; **RES:** New York University Med Ctr, New York, NY 73; **HOSP:** Beth Israel Med Ctr; **HMO:** Centercare Blue Choice PHS NYLCare

🅲 🔄 🔧 🏨 🅂 Mcr A Few Days 💳 *VISA* 💳

Ryan, Samuel (MD) ObG
NY Hosp-Cornell Med Ctr

449 E 68th St 8; New York, NY 10021; (212) 628-1500; **BDCERT:** ObG 63; **MS:** Ireland 54; **RES:** NY Hosp-Cornell Med Ctr, New York, NY 56-61; **FEL:** Christie Hosp, Manchester,England 61-63; **FAP:** Clin Prof Cornell U

🔄 🔧 🏨 🅂 A Few Days *VISA* 💳

Sailon, Peter (MD) ObG
Lenox Hill Hosp

955 Park Ave; New York, NY 10028; (212) 879-9191; **BDCERT:** ObG 82; **MS:** Italy 76; **RES:** S, Univ Hosp SUNY Bklyn, Brooklyn, NY 76-77; ObG, St Luke's Roosevelt Hosp Ctr, New York, NY 77-80; **FEL:** Infertility, St Luke's Roosevelt Hosp Ctr, New York, NY 80-81; **FAP:** Instr Columbia P&S; **HOSP:** St Luke's Roosevelt Hosp Ctr; *SI: Hysteroscopic Surgery; Laparoscopic Surgery*

LANG: Itl; ♿ 🅲 🔄 🔧 🏨 🅂 1 Week

Guide to symbols and abbreviations can be found on pages 110-113.

265

Sandler, Benjamin (MD)   ObG
Mount Sinai Med Ctr

Reproductive Medicine Associates, 58 E 79th St;
New York, NY 10021; (212) 744-1855; **BDCERT:**
ObG 90; **MS:** Mexico 82; **RES:** ObG, Michael Reese
Hosp Med Ctr, Chicago, IL 83-87; **FEL:** RE, Mount
Sinai Med Ctr, New York, NY 87-89; **FAP:** Asst Clin
Prof ObG Mt Sinai Sch Med; **SI:** *Infertility;*
Reproductive Surgery; **HMO:** Oxford PHCS

LANG: Sp; 🆂🗂 🔟 👤 🏨 💲 A Few Days 💳 **VISA**
😊

Sarosi, Peter (MD)   ObG
Beth Israel Med Ctr

88 University Pl FL9; New York, NY 10003; (212)
243-4050; **BDCERT:** ObG 84; ObG 95; **MS:**
Hungary 76; **RES:** ObG, Beth Israel Med Ctr, New
York, NY 76-80; **FEL:** Inf, New York University Med
Ctr, New York, NY 80-82; **HOSP:** St Clare's Hosp &
Health Ctr; **SI:** *Menopause;* **HMO:** Oxford CIGNA
Aetna-US Healthcare Independent Health Plan
PHCS +

LANG: Rus, Sp, Heb; ♿ 🔟 👤 🏨 💲 Mcr 2-4 Weeks
💳 **VISA** 😊

Sassoon, Robert (MD)   ObG   PCP
NY Hosp-Cornell Med Ctr

12 E 69th St; New York, NY 10021; (212) 517-
8333; **BDCERT:** ObG 87; **MS:** Cornell U 81; **RES:**
ObG, NY Hosp-Cornell Med Ctr, New York, NY 81-
85; **FAP:** Asst Clin Prof Cornell U; **SI:** *Laparoscopic &*
Gynecologic Surgery; High Risk Obesity.; **HMO:** None

LANG: Fr, Ar, Sp, Heb; 🌙 🔟 👤 🏨 Mcr 2-4 Weeks
VISA 😊

Scher, Jonathan (MD)   ObG
Mount Sinai Med Ctr

1126 Park Ave; New York, NY 10128; (212) 427-
7400; **BDCERT:** ObG 81; **MS:** South Africa 64; **RES:**
ObG, Kings College Hosp, London, England 70-72;
FEL: Gynecology, Mt Sinai, New York, NY 80-80;
SI: *Recurrent Miscarriages*

Schoen, Roy M (MD)   ObG
Lenox Hill Hosp

17 E 82nd St; New York, NY 10028; (212) 861-
4422; **BDCERT:** Psyc 78; ObG 85; **MS:** Israel 71;
RES: Psyc, NY Hosp-Cornell Med Ctr, New York, NY
71-72; ObG, Lenox Hill Hosp, New York, NY 78-82;
FEL: ChAP, Babies Hosp, New York, NY 72-73; **SI:**
PMS; Cervical Abnormalities; **HMO:** Oxford Chubb
Guardian

LANG: Sp; 🔟 👤 🏨 💲 Mcr Immediately

Schwartz, Judith (MD)   ObG
Mount Sinai Med Ctr

Eastside Womens ObGyn Assoc, 134 E 93rd St Fl 2;
New York, NY 10128; (212) 348-7800; **BDCERT:**
ObG 88; **MS:** Mt Sinai Sch Med 82; **RES:** ObG,
Mount Sinai Med Ctr, New York, NY 82-86; **FAP:**
Asst Clin Prof Mt Sinai Sch Med

LANG: Sp; ♿ 🌙 🔟 👤 🏨 💲 Mcr 2-4 Weeks

Sloan, Don (MD)   ObG   PCP
Lenox Hill Hosp

1435 2nd Ave Ste 2R; New York, NY 10019; (212)
439-0781; **BDCERT:** ObG 70; **MS:** SUNY Hlth Sci
Ctr 63; **RES:** ObG, Temple U Hosp, Philadelphia, PA
63-67; **FEL:** Human Sexuality, Masters & Johnson
Inst, St Louis, MO 70-73; **FAP:** Assoc Prof ObG NY
Med Coll; **HOSP:** Beth Israel Med Ctr; **SI:** *Marital*
Counseling; **HMO:** None

LANG: Fr; ♿ 🌙 🔟 🏨 💲 2-4 Weeks

Snyder, Jon (MD)   ObG
New York University Med Ctr

530 1st Ave Ste 10N; New York, NY 10016; (212)
263-6356; **BDCERT:** ObG 78; **MS:** NYU Sch Med
72; **RES:** Bellevue Hosp Ctr, New York, NY 72-76;
HOSP: Bellevue Hosp Ctr; **SI:** *Ultrasound;* **HMO:**
Oxford Health Source Blue Choice PPO

♿ 🔟 👤 🏨 💲 Mcr 1 Week **VISA** 😊

Steadman, E Thomas (MD) ObG
NY Hosp-Cornell Med Ctr

449 E 68th St 8; New York, NY 10021; (212) 628-
1500; **BDCERT:** ObG 66; **MS:** Cornell U 57; **RES:**
NY Hosp-Cornell Med Ctr, New York, NY 58-63

♿ 🔟 👤 🏨 Mcr **VISA** 😊

Strider, William (MD)   ObG
NYU Downtown Hosp

170 William St Flr 8; New York, NY 10038; (212)
406-1471; **BDCERT:** ObG 84; **MS:** NYU Sch Med
78; **RES:** Bellevue Hosp Ctr, New York, NY 78-82;
FAP: Asst Clin Prof NYU Sch Med; **HOSP:** St
Vincents Hosp & Med Ctr NY; **SI:** *Pap Smear
Abnormalities; Pelvic Surgery*; **HMO:** Aetna Hlth
Plan Blue Cross & Blue Shield Oxford GHI

LANG: Sp; 🔲 🔲 🔲 🔲 🔲 🔲 1 Week

Strongin, Michael J (MD)   ObG
Lenox Hill Hosp

45 E 85th St; New York, NY 10028; (212) 535-
4611; **BDCERT:** ObG 79; **MS:** Boston U 73; **RES:**
ObG, NY Hosp-Cornell Med Ctr, New York, NY 73-
77; **FAP:** Asst Clin Prof ObG Cornell U; **HOSP:** NY
Hosp-Cornell Med Ctr

Sullum, Stanford (MD)   ObG   PCP
Mount Sinai Med Ctr

1136 5th Ave; New York, NY 10128; (212) 876-
4630; **BDCERT:** ObG 79; **MS:** Jefferson Med Coll 73;
RES: Mount Sinai Med Ctr, New York, NY 73-77;
FAP: Asst Clin Prof Mt Sinai Sch Med

🔲 🔲 🔲 🔲 🔲 Immediately

Tanz, Alfred (MD)   ObG
Lenox Hill Hosp

266 E 78th St; New York, NY 10021; (212) 861-
2277; **BDCERT:** ObG 57; ObG 81; **MS:** NY Med Coll
48; **RES:** Flower Fifth Ave Hosp, New York, NY 48-
52; **FEL:** GO, NY Med Coll, New York, NY 48-49;
FAP: Clin Prof ObG NY Med Coll; **HOSP:** Beth Israel
North; **HMO:** Chubb

LANG: Sp; 🔲 🔲 🔲 🔲 🔲 🔲 Immediately

Tretter, Wolfgang (MD)   ObG   PCP
Columbia-Presbyterian Med Ctr

899 Park Ave; New York, NY 10021; (212) 305-
5360; **BDCERT:** ObG 66; **MS:** Germany 52; **RES:** St
Vincent Med Ctr, Los Angeles, CA 56-57; ObG,
Columbia-Presbyterian Med Ctr, New York, NY 58-
63

LANG: Ger; 🔲 🔲 🔲 🔲 A Few Days

Van Praagh, Ian (MD)   ObG   PCP
Lenox Hill Hosp

103 E 86th St; New York, NY 10028; (212) 427-
5774; **BDCERT:** ObG 66; **MS:** Canada 55; **RES:**
ObG, Toronto Gen Hosp, Toronto, Canada 55-61;
FEL: Reproductive Physiology, Case Western
Reserve U Hosp, Cleveland, OH 62-63; Middlesex
Hosp, Middletown, NJ 63-?; **HOSP:** St Luke's
Roosevelt Hosp Ctr; **SI:** *Colposcopy; Family Planning*;
HMO: Oxford Aetna Hlth Plan Chubb Blue Choice
CIGNA +

LANG: Fr, Sp; 🔲 🔲 🔲 🔲 🔲 🔲 A Few Days

Wallach, Robert C (MD)   ObG
New York University Med Ctr

700 Park Ave; New York, NY 10021; (212) 666-
5566; **BDCERT:** ObG 67; GO 74; **MS:** Yale U Sch
Med 69; **RES:** Beth Israel Med Ctr, New York, NY
60-61; ObG, Beth Israel Med Ctr, New York, NY 61-
65; **FEL:** GO, Univ Hosp SUNY Bklyn, Brooklyn, NY

🔲 🔲 🔲 🔲 🔲 A Few Days

Wan, Livia (MD)   ObG
New York University Med Ctr

320 E 30th St; New York, NY 10016; (212) 683-
8111; **BDCERT:** ObG 71; **MS:** Taiwan 58; **RES:**
Maimonides Med Ctr, Brooklyn, NY 59-60;
Philadelphia Gen Hosp, Philadelphia, PA 60-63;
FEL: Pennsylvania Hosp, Philadelphia, PA 63-68;
HOSP: Bellevue Hosp Ctr; **SI:** *Laparoscopic Surgery;
Vaginal Surgery*; **HMO:** Chubb Oxford Aetna Hlth
Plan

🔲 🔲 🔲 🔲 1 Week

Wolf, Leonard (MD)   ObG   PCP
New York University Med Ctr

905 5th Ave Fl 1; New York, NY 10021; (212)
535-8833; **BDCERT:** ObG 65; **MS:** Ireland 49; **RES:**
Jessop Hosp, Sheffield, England 52-55; **FEL:** Mount
Sinai Med Ctr, New York, NY 58-60; **FAP:** Assoc
Prof NYU Sch Med; **HOSP:** Beth Israel North; **SI:**
Liver & Vaginal Diseases; **HMO:** Oxford Chubb
CIGNA

LANG: Fr, Sp; 🔲 🔲 🔲 🔲 🔲 Immediately

Guide to symbols and abbreviations can be found on pages 110-113.

267

Yale, Suzanne (MD) ObG
Lenox Hill Hosp

768 Park Ave; New York, NY 10021; (212) 744-9300; **BDCERT:** ObG 84; **MS:** UMDNJ-RW Johnson Med Sch 77; **RES:** ObG, Lenox Hill Hosp, New York, NY 81

  ♿ 📷 ⚕ 🏥 💲 Mcr 2-4 Weeks

Yeh, Ming-neng (MD) ObG
Columbia-Presbyterian Med Ctr

161 Fort Washington Ave; New York, NY 10032; (212) 305-5239; **BDCERT:** ObG 74; **MS:** Taiwan 64; **RES:** Brooklyn Hosp Ctr, Brooklyn, NY 67-68; St Luke's Roosevelt Hosp Ctr, New York, NY 68-71; **FEL:** Columbia-Presbyterian Med Ctr, New York, NY; **FAP:** Clin Prof ObG Columbia P&S; **SI:** *High Risk Pregnancy; Ultrasound;* **HMO:** Aetna Hlth Plan Oxford Health Source CIGNA Blue Cross & Blue Shield +

  ♿ 📷 ⚕ 🏥 💲 Mcr NFI A Few Days ▨ VISA ⬤

Young, Bruce (MD) ObG **PCP**
New York University Med Ctr

NYU Medical Center, 530 1st Ave Ste 5G; New York, NY 10016; (212) 263-6359; **BDCERT:** ObG 70; MF 75; **MS:** NYU Sch Med 63; **RES:** ObG, New York University Med Ctr, New York, NY 64-68; Bellevue Hosp Ctr, New York, NY 64-68; **FEL:** RE, New York University Med Ctr, New York, NY 68; **FAP:** Prof NYU Sch Med; **HOSP:** VA Med Ctr-Manh; **SI:** *Infertility & Miscarriage; Gynecological Surgery*

LANG: Fr, Sp; ♿ 📷 🏥 💲 Mcr 2-4 Weeks

OPHTHALMOLOGY

Abell, Penny (MD) Oph
Mount Sinai Med Ctr

5 E 98th St; New York, NY 10029; (212) 241-0939; **BDCERT:** Oph 80; **MS:** SUNY Buffalo 75; **RES:** Yale-New Haven Hosp, New Haven, CT 76; New York University Med Ctr, New York, NY 77-80; **FEL:** Eye, Ear, Nose & Throat Hosp, New Orleans, LA 80-82; **FAP:** Prof Oph Mt Sinai Sch Med; **SI:** *Cornea;* **HMO:** Oxford United Healthcare CIGNA Aetna Hlth Plan Chubb +

  ♿ ⚕ 🏥 💲 Mcr Mcd WC Immediately ▨ VISA ⬤

Accardi, Frank (MD) Oph
New York Eye & Ear Infirmary

4 Lexington Ave Fl 1; New York, NY 10010; (212) 228-5300; **BDCERT:** Oph 87; **MS:** Italy 79; **RES:** Cabrini Med Ctr, New York, NY 79-82; Univ Hosp SUNY Bklyn, Brooklyn, NY 82-85; **FEL:** Cornea, Univ Hosp SUNY Bklyn, Brooklyn, NY; **HOSP:** Cabrini Med Ctr; **SI:** *Cornea—Contact Lens; Cataracts;* **HMO:** United Healthcare Guardian US Hlthcre Oxford HIP Network +

LANG: Itl, Sp; ♿ 🌙 📷 ⚕ 🏥 💲 Mcr Mcd 1 Week ▨ VISA ⬤

Angioletti, Louis (MD) Oph
New York Eye & Ear Infirmary

7 Gramercy Park W; New York, NY 10003; (212) 505-8510; **BDCERT:** Oph 75; **MS:** NY Med Coll 66; **RES:** New York Eye & Ear Infirmary, New York, NY 70-73; **FEL:** New York Eye & Ear Infirmary, New York, NY 73-74; **SI:** *Retina;* **HMO:** Oxford CIGNA Metlife US Hlthcre

  ♿ 📷 ⚕ 🏥 💲 Mcr Mcd WC NFI Immediately

Barasch, Kenneth (MD) Oph
Manhattan Eye, Ear & Throat Hosp

115 E 39th St; New York, NY 10016; (212) 687-4106; **BDCERT:** Oph 68; **MS:** Cornell U 60; **RES:** NY Hosp-Cornell Med Ctr, New York, NY 63-66; **FAP:** Assoc Clin Prof NYU Sch Med; **HOSP:** Lenox Hill Hosp; **SI:** *Diagnosis and Treatment of Corneal Disease and Cataracts;* **HMO:** Blue Choice PHS Health Source Blue Choice

LANG: Fr, Sp; ♿ 📷 ⚕ 🏥 💲 Mcr Mcd WC NFI Immediately ▨ VISA ⬤

Barker, Barbara (MD) Oph
New York Eye & Ear Infirmary

11 E 86th St; New York, NY 10028; (212) 289-2244; **BDCERT:** Oph 81; **MS:** Mt Sinai Sch Med 76; **RES:** Mt Sinai-Beth Israel Hosp, New York, NY 77-80; **FEL:** Glaucoma, Beth Israel Med Ctr, New York, NY 80-81; Cornea & Retina S, Beth Israel Med Ctr, New York, NY 81-82; **FAP:** Assoc Clin Prof Mt Sinai Sch Med; **SI:** *Glaucoma; Cornea-Anterior Segment;* **HMO:** Aetna Hlth Plan Blue Choice Oxford HealthNet 32BJ +

  ♿ 🌙 📷 🏥 💲 Mcr Mcd WC 1 Week VISA ⬤

Behrens, Myles (MD)   Oph
Columbia-Presbyterian Med Ctr
635 W 165th St; New York, NY 10032; (212)
305-5415; **BDCERT:** Oph 71; **MS:** Columbia P&S
62; **RES:** Columbia-Presbyterian Med Ctr, New
York, NY 62-64; Oph, Columbia-Presbyterian Med
Ctr, New York, NY 67-70; **FEL:** N, UC San Francisco
Med Ctr, San Francisco, CA; **FAP:** Prof Oph
Columbia P&S; **SI:** *Neuro-Ophthalmology*; **HMO:**
Oxford Prudential Blue Choice
♿ 📷 👤 🏥 💲   1 Week

Best, Milton (MD)   Oph
Lenox Hill Hosp
1165 Park Ave 1A; New York, NY 10128; (212)
427-5183; **BDCERT:** Oph 68; **MS:** NY Med Coll 62;
RES: Metropolitan Hosp Ctr, New York, NY 63-66;
SI: *Cataract Surgery; Laser Surgery*; **HMO:** Oxford
CIGNA Empire PHCS PHS +
♿ 📷 🏥 💲 Mcr   A Few Days

Brown, Alan (MD)   Oph
St Luke's Roosevelt Hosp Ctr
127 W 79th St; New York, NY 10024; (212) 724-
4430; **BDCERT:** Oph 82; **MS:** Cornell U 77; **RES:** St
Luke's Roosevelt Hosp Ctr, New York, NY 78-81;
FEL: Cornea & External Disease, Park Ridge Hosp,
Rochester, NY 81-82; **FAP:** Asst Instr Columbia
P&S; **HMO:** Blue Cross & Blue Shield HealthNet
Prucare Oxford Aetna Hlth Plan +

Buxton, Douglas (MD)   Oph
Manhattan Eye, Ear & Throat Hosp
310 E 14th St 403; New York, NY 10003; (212)
777-7290; **BDCERT:** Oph 87; **MS:** Cornell U 82;
RES: Oph, New York Eye & Ear Infirmary, New
York, NY 93; **FEL:** New York Eye & Ear Infirmary,
New York, NY 86-88; **SI:** *Corneal Diseases; Myopia*;
HMO: CIGNA Prudential Aetna Hlth Plan United
Healthcare PHCS +
LANG: Sp, Fr; ♿ 🏥 🔌 📷 🏥 💲 Mcr Mcd
Immediately 🔲 **VISA** ⬤

Buxton, Jorge (MD)   Oph
New York Eye & Ear Infirmary
310 E 14th St 403; New York, NY 10003; (212)
777-7290; **BDCERT:** Oph 51; **MS:** Argentina 47;
RES: New York Eye & Ear Infirmary, New York, NY
48-52
👤 🏥 💲 Mcr   A Few Days

Carr, Ronald (MD)   Oph
New York University Med Ctr
NYU Medical Ctr, 530 1st Ave 3B; New York, NY
10016; (212) 263-7360; **BDCERT:** Oph 64; **MS:**
Johns Hopkins U 58; **RES:** New York University
Med Ctr, New York, NY 59-63; **FEL:** New York
University Med Ctr, New York, NY 62-63; Nat Inst
Health, Bethesda, MD 63-65; **FAP:** Prof NY Med
Coll; **HOSP:** Bellevue Hosp Ctr; **SI:** *Macular
Degeneration; Retinal Disease*; **HMO:** Oxford Prucare
CIGNA United Healthcare Health Source +
♿ 📷 👤 🏥 Mcr   A Few Days

Chaiken, Barry (MD)   Oph
Manhattan Eye, Ear & Throat Hosp
625 Park Ave; New York, NY 10021; (212) 249-
1976; **BDCERT:** Oph 81; **MS:** Columbia P&S 76;
RES: Oph, Mount Sinai Med Ctr, New York, NY 77-
80; **FAP:** Clin Instr Med Columbia P&S; **HOSP:** St
Luke's Roosevelt Hosp Ctr; **SI:** *Cataract Surgery;
Refractive Surgery*
♿ 📷 👤 🏥 💲 Mcr   Immediately **VISA** ⬤

Chang, Stanley (MD)   Oph
Columbia-Presbyterian Med Ctr
Vitreoretinal Specialists PC, 425 W 59th St Ste 3B;
New York, NY 10019; (212) 307-0777; **BDCERT:**
Oph 79; **MS:** Columbia P&S 74; **RES:** Retina, Mass
Eye & Ear Infirmary, Boston, MA 76-78; **FEL:**
Bascom Palmer Eye Inst, Miami, FL 78-79; **FAP:**
Chrmn Columbia P&S; **HOSP:** St Luke's Roosevelt
Hosp Ctr; **SI:** *Vitreous—Retina—Macula*
LANG: Chi, Ger, Sp; ♿ 🏥 💲 Mcr **VISA** ⬤

Charles, Norman (MD) Oph
New York Eye & Ear Infirmary
620 Park Ave; New York, NY 10021; (212) 772-6920; BDCERT: Oph 71; MS: NYU Sch Med 63; RES: Oph, New York University Med Ctr, New York, NY 66-70; FAP: Clin Prof Oph NYU Sch Med; HOSP: New York University Med Ctr; SI: Cataracts; Eyelid Tumors

LANG: Fr, Ger; 🔲 🔲 🔲 🔲 Immediately

Chern, Relly (MD) Oph
Manhattan Eye, Ear & Throat Hosp
923 5th Ave; New York, NY 10021; (212) 628-0160; BDCERT: Oph 83; MS: Albert Einstein Coll Med 76; RES: IM, Bronx Lebanon Hosp Ctr, Bronx, NY 76-77; Oph, Montefiore Med Ctr, Bronx, NY 77-80; HOSP: Montefiore Med Ctr; HMO: Oxford Aetna-US Healthcare Blue Cross & Blue Shield

LANG: Fr, Sp, Rom, Rus; 🔲 🔲 🔲 🔲 🔲 🔲 🔲 🔲 🔲 A Few Days

Chu, Wing (MD) Oph
Manhattan Eye, Ear & Throat Hosp
17 E 72nd St; New York, NY 10021; (212) 288-3301; BDCERT: Oph 78; MS: SUNY Hlth Sci Ctr 72; RES: N Shore Univ Hosp, Manhasset, NY 72-74; New York Eye & Ear Infirmary, New York, NY 74-77; FEL: Mass Eye & Ear Infirmary, Boston, MA 77-79; FAP: Assoc Clin Prof Oph Columbia P&S; HOSP: St Luke's Roosevelt Hosp Ctr; SI: Corneal Transplants; Cataract Surgery; HMO: None

LANG: Sp, Chi; 🔲 🔲 🔲 🔲 A Few Days 🔲 VISA 🔲

Cohen, Ben (MD) Oph
Manhattan Eye, Ear & Throat Hosp
140 E 80th St Fl 1; New York, NY 10021; (212) 772-0600; BDCERT: Oph 83; MS: NY Med Coll 76; RES: U Chicago Hosp, Chicago, IL 77-80; FEL: Retina, Manhattan Eye, Ear & Throat Hosp, New York, NY 80-81; Retina, Mass Eye & Ear Infirmary, Boston, MA; HOSP: Mount Sinai Med Ctr; HMO: Aetna Hlth Plan Prucare Metlife

🔲 🔲 🔲 🔲 🔲 🔲 🔲 🔲 🔲 Immediately

Cohen, Leeber (MD) Oph
New York Eye & Ear Infirmary
11 5th Ave B; New York, NY 10003; (212) 777-1644; BDCERT: Oph 89; MS: SUNY Hlth Sci Ctr 83; RES: Onc, Univ Hosp SUNY Bklyn, Brooklyn, NY 83-84; Oph, Univ Hosp SUNY Bklyn, Brooklyn, NY 84-87; HOSP: St Vincents Hosp & Med Ctr NY; SI: Retinitis; Refractive Surgery; HMO: Aetna Hlth Plan Oxford Magnacare Blue Choice

LANG: Heb, Sp; 🔲 🔲 🔲 🔲 🔲 🔲 🔲 🔲 A Few Days 🔲 VISA 🔲

Coleman, D J (MD) Oph
NY Hosp-Cornell Med Ctr
Cornell Ophthalmology Associates, 520 E 70th St; New York, NY 10021; (212) 746-5588; BDCERT: Oph 69; MS: SUNY Buffalo 60; RES: Oph, Columbia-Presbyterian Med Ctr, New York, NY 64-67; FEL: Retina, Columbia-Presbyterian Med Ctr, New York, NY 67-68; FAP: Prof Oph Cornell U; SI: Retina Diseases; Ocular Tumors; HMO: Oxford Blue Choice Magnacare Multiplan CIGNA +

LANG: Grk, Sp; 🔲 🔲 🔲 🔲 🔲 🔲 🔲 2-4 Weeks 🔲 VISA 🔲 🔲

Copland, Richard (MD) Oph
New York Eye & Ear Infirmary
310 E 14th St; New York, NY 10003; (212) 979-4428; BDCERT: Oph 75; MS: NY Med Coll 69; RES: New York Eye & Ear Infirmary, New York, NY; HOSP: Beth Israel Med Ctr; SI: Complicated Cataracts; Laser Refractive Surgery; HMO: Oxford Centercare Blue Cross Prudential +

LANG: Chi, Sp; 🔲 🔲 🔲 🔲 🔲 🔲 🔲 2-4 Weeks 🔲 VISA

Cykiert, Robert (MD) Oph
New York University Med Ctr
345 E 37th St 210; New York, NY 10016; (212) 922-1430; BDCERT: Oph 81; MS: NY Med Coll 76; RES: Montefiore Med Ctr, Bronx, NY 77-80; FEL: Cornea, Wills Eye Hosp, Philadelphia, PA 80-81; FAP: Asst Clin Prof NYU Sch Med; HMO: Oxford Aetna Hlth Plan Blue Choice CIGNA US Hlthcre +

D'Amico, Robert (MD)   Oph
St Vincent's Med Ctr-Richmond

36 7th Ave 506; New York, NY 10011; (212) 807-8866; **BDCERT:** Oph 64; **MS:** Geo Wash U Sch Med 55; **RES:** Temple U Hosp, Philadelphia, PA 56-57; **FEL:** Castroviejo Hosp, New York, NY 61-62; **HOSP:** Bayley Seton Hosp; **HMO:** Empire Blue Choice Magnacare Oxford Prucare HIP Network +

♿ 🌙 📷 🚼 🏥 Mcr Immediately

Della Rocca, Robert (MD)   Oph
New York Eye & Ear Infirmary

310 E 14th St Rm 319; New York, NY 10003; (212) 421-4505; **BDCERT:** Oph 75; **MS:** Creighton U 67; **RES:** New York Eye & Ear Infirmary, New York, NY; **FEL:** Oculoplastic S, Manhattan Eye, Ear & Throat Hosp, New York, NY; Oculoplastic S, Albany Med Ctr, Albany, NY; **HMO:** Sanus Oxford Metlife US Hlthcre

Dinnerstein, Stephen (MD) Oph
New York Eye & Ear Infirmary

36 E 36th St 1J; New York, NY 10016; (212) 889-4944; **BDCERT:** Oph 76; **MS:** NY Med Coll 70; **RES:** Oph, Univ Hosp SUNY Bklyn, Brooklyn, NY 71-74; **FAP:** Instr Mt Sinai Sch Med; **SI:** *Cataract; Glaucoma;* **HMO:** Oxford Aetna-US Healthcare United Healthcare Blue Shield GHI +

LANG: Sp, Ger, Fr; ♿ 🌙 📷 🚼 🏥 💲 Mcr WC A Few Days

Dodick, Jack M (MD)   Oph
Manhattan Eye, Ear & Throat Hosp

535 Park Ave; New York, NY 10023; (212) 288-7638; **BDCERT:** Oph 69; **MS:** U Toronto 63; **RES:** Oph, Manhattan Eye, Ear & Throat Hosp, New York, NY 64-67; **FEL:** S, NY Med Coll, New York, NY 67-68; **SI:** *Cataract Surgery; Laser Surgery;* **HMO:** None

📷 🚼 🏥 💲 Mcr 1 Week 💳 *VISA* 💳

Eggers, Howard M (MD)   Oph
Columbia-Presbyterian Med Ctr

635 W 165th St; New York, NY 10032; (212) 305-5409; **BDCERT:** Oph 78; **MS:** Columbia P&S 71; **RES:** Oph, Columbia-Presbyterian Med Ctr, New York, NY 72-75; **FEL:** Ped Oph, Indiana U Med Ctr, Indianapolis, IN 75; Ped Oph, U IA Hosp, Iowa City, IA 76; **FAP:** Prof Columbia P&S; **SI:** *Strabismus; Pediatric Ophthalmology;* **HMO:** Oxford CIGNA Health Source Empire Blue Choice Prudential +

♿ 📷 🚼 🏥 💲 Mcr NFI 2-4 Weeks

Eichenbaum, Joseph (MD)   Oph
Mount Sinai Med Ctr

1050 Park Ave; New York, NY 10028; (212) 289-7200; **BDCERT:** Oph 80; **MS:** Yale U Sch Med 73; **RES:** Oph, New York University Med Ctr, New York, NY 74-77; **FAP:** Assoc Clin Prof Mt Sinai Sch Med; **HOSP:** Manhattan Eye, Ear & Throat Hosp

LANG: Sp, Heb; ♿ 🌙 📷 🚼 🏥 💲 Mcr Immediately

Farris, R Linsy (MD)   Oph
Columbia-Presbyterian Med Ctr

635 W 165th St 202; New York, NY 10032; (212) 305-5418; **BDCERT:** Oph 68; **MS:** Duke U 61; **RES:** Columbia-Presbyterian Med Ctr, New York, NY 64-67; **FAP:** Prof Columbia P&S; **HOSP:** Harlem Hosp Ctr; **SI:** *Cornea; Cataract;* **HMO:** Aetna Hlth Plan Oxford Chubb Prudential Empire Blue Cross & Shield +

LANG: Sp; ♿ 🌆 🌙 📷 🚼 🏥 💲 Mcr A Few Days
VISA 💳 💳

Finger, Paul (MD)   Oph
New York Eye & Ear Infirmary

The New York Eye & Ear Infirmary, 310 E 14th St Ste 319; New York, NY 10003; (212) 979-4293; **BDCERT:** Oph 90; **MS:** Tulane U 82; **RES:** St Vincents Hosp & Med Ctr NY, New York, NY 82-83; Manhattan Eye, Ear & Throat Hosp, New York, NY 83-86; **FEL:** NY Hosp-Cornell Med Ctr, New York, NY 86-87; **FAP:** Assoc Prof Oph NYU Sch Med; **HOSP:** N Shore Univ Hosp-Forest Hills; **SI:** *Eye, Eyelid, Orbital Tumors;* **HMO:** Blue Choice HealthNet Chubb PHCS

LANG: Sp, Rus; ♿ 📷 🏥 💲 Mcr Mcd A Few Days

Fisher, Yale (MD)　　　　Oph
NY Hosp-Cornell Med Ctr
519 E 72nd St Ste 203; New York, NY 10021; (212) 861-9797; **BDCERT:** Oph 73; **MS:** Cornell U 67; **RES:** Manhattan Eye, Ear & Throat Hosp, New York, NY 68-71; **FAP:** Clin Prof Oph Cornell U; **HOSP:** Manhattan Eye, Ear & Throat Hosp; *SI: Vitreoretinal Surgery;* **HMO:** Blue Choice Blue Cross & Blue Shield Travelers Prucare

LANG: Sp; 🔲 📷 🔲 🛏 $ Mcr WC　A Few Days 📧 **VISA**

Fong, Raymond (MD)　　　　Oph
Manhattan Eye, Ear & Throat Hosp
109 Lafayette St Fl 4; New York, NY 10013; (212) 274-1900; **BDCERT:** Oph 87; **MS:** Cornell U 81; **RES:** Manhattan Eye, Ear & Throat Hosp, New York, NY 82-85; **HOSP:** NYU Downtown Hosp; *SI: Cataract Surgery; Laser Surgery;* **HMO:** Oxford US Hlthcre GHI Blue Cross & Blue Shield

🔲 SA SU 📷 🛏 $ Mcr Mcd　A Few Days

Forbes, Max (MD)　　　　Oph
Columbia-Presbyterian Med Ctr
635 W 165th St Ste 308; New York, NY 10032; (212) 927-1854; **BDCERT:** Oph 65; **MS:** U Chicago-Pritzker Sch Med 57; **RES:** Oph, Barnes Hosp, St Louis, MO 58-60; Oph, Barnes Hosp, St Louis, MO 61-62; **FEL:** Oph, Columbia-Presbyterian Med Ctr, New York, NY 60-61; Glaucoma, Barnes Hosp, St Louis, MO 62-63; **FAP:** Prof of Clin Oph Columbia P&S; *SI: Glaucoma; Cataracts;* **HMO:** Oxford Empire Prudential Multiplan

🔲 📷 🔲 🛏 $ Mcr　2-4 Weeks

Fox, Martin (MD)　　　　Oph
New York Eye & Ear Infirmary
Cornea & Refractive Surgery Practice of NY & NJ, 16 E 52nd St 503; New York, NY 10022; (212) 838-1053; **BDCERT:** Oph 81; **MS:** Hahnemann U 76; **RES:** Boston U Med Ctr, Boston, MA 77-80; **FEL:** Corneal S, New York Eye & Ear Infirmary, New York, NY 80-81; **HOSP:** Beth Israel Med Ctr; *SI: Refractive Surgery; Diseases of the Cornea;* **HMO:** Magnacare Sel Pro United Healthcare Aetna Hlth Plan Anthem Health +

LANG: Tag, Sp; 🔲 📷 🔲 🛏 $ Mcr WC　A Few Days

Friedberg, Dorothy (MD)　　　　Oph
New York University Med Ctr
310 Lexington Ave; New York, NY 10016; (212) 687-0265; **BDCERT:** Oph 79; **MS:** NYU Sch Med 74; **RES:** Oph, Montefiore Med Ctr, Bronx, NY 75-78; **HOSP:** New York Eye & Ear Infirmary; *SI: Eye Problems in AIDS;* **HMO:** NYLCare CIGNA Oxford Aetna Hlth Plan US Hlthcre +

🔲 🔲 🛏 $ Mcr WC NFI　1 Week

Friedman, Alan (MD)　　　　Oph
New York Eye & Ear Infirmary
120 E 36th St 1C; New York, NY 10016; (212) 683-5180; **BDCERT:** Oph 65; **MS:** Harvard Med Sch 59; **RES:** Bellevue Hosp Ctr, New York, NY 60-63; **FEL:** Glaucoma, Bellevue Hosp Ctr, New York, NY 63-64; **FAP:** Assoc Clin Prof NYU Sch Med; **HOSP:** New York University Med Ctr; *SI: Cataract Implant Surgery; Laser Surgery;* **HMO:** Oxford Chubb

LANG: Sp; 🔲 📷 🔲 🛏 $　A Few Days

Friedman, Robert (MD)　　　　Oph
Lenox Hill Hosp
67 E 78th St; New York, NY 10021; (212) 772-6202; **BDCERT:** Oph 88; **MS:** Albert Einstein Coll Med 83; **RES:** Lenox Hill Hosp, New York, NY 84-87; Columbia-Presbyterian Med Ctr, New York, NY 84; **FEL:** Vitreoretinal S, Manhattan Eye, Ear & Throat Hosp, New York, NY; **HOSP:** New York Eye & Ear Infirmary; *SI: Cataracts; Vitreoretinal Surgery*

LANG: Heb; 🔲 📷 🛏 $ Mcr Mcd　Immediately 📧 **VISA** 💳

Fuchs, Wayne (MD)　　　　Oph
Mount Sinai Med Ctr
121 E 60th St Fl 5; New York, NY 10022; (212) 319-8205; **BDCERT:** Oph 85; **MS:** Mt Sinai Sch Med 79; **RES:** U Miami Hosp, Miami, FL 79-80; Mount Sinai Med Ctr, New York, NY 80-83; **FEL:** Vitreoretinal S, NY Hosp-Cornell Med Ctr, New York, NY; **FAP:** Assoc Clin Prof Mt Sinai Sch Med; **HOSP:** Manhattan Eye, Ear & Throat Hosp; *SI: Diabetic Retinopathy; Macular Degeneration;* **HMO:** Oxford Empire Blue Cross & Shield

🔲 📷 🔲 🛏 $ Mcr Mcd　2-4 Weeks

Gallin, Pamela (MD) Oph
Columbia-Presbyterian Med Ctr
635 W 165th St Ste 224; New York, NY 10032;
(212) 305-5407; **BDCERT:** Oph 83; **MS:**
Washington U, St Louis 78; **RES:** Oph, Mount Sinai
Med Ctr, New York, NY 79-82; **FEL:** Ped Oph,
Children's Hosp Nat Med Ctr, Washington, DC;
Strabismus, Columbia-Presbyterian Med Ctr, New
York, NY; *SI: Pediatric Ophthalmology; Adult
Strabismus;* **HMO:** Oxford
♿ 📷 🚹 🏦 **$** A Few Days ▩ **VISA** ●

Guillory, Samuel (MD) Oph
Mount Sinai Med Ctr
1103 Park Ave; New York, NY 10128; (212) 860-
5400; **BDCERT:** Oph 80; **MS:** Mt Sinai Sch Med 75;
RES: Mount Sinai Med Ctr, New York, NY; **FEL:** NY
Hosp-Cornell Med Ctr, New York, NY; *SI: Cataracts;
Refractive Surgery;* **HMO:** None
♿ 📷 🚹 **$** A Few Days ▩ **VISA** ●

Haddad, Heskel (MD) Oph
Beth Israel Med Ctr
1125 Park Ave; New York, NY 10128; (212) 427-
1246; **BDCERT:** Oph 65; **MS:** Israel 53; **RES:** Barnes
Hosp, St Louis, MO 60-64; **FEL:** Ped Oph, Univ
Pacific, 62-63; **FAP:** Clin Prof NY Med Coll; **HOSP:**
St Luke's Roosevelt Hosp Ctr; *SI: Pediatric
Strabismus; Metabolic Diabetes;* **HMO:** US Hlthcre
Blue Cross PPO Blue Choice Aetna Hlth Plan
LANG: Heb, Ar, Fr, Rus, Ger; ♿ 📷 🚹 🏦 **$** Mcr Mcd
WC NFI Immediately

Haight, David (MD) Oph
Manhattan Eye, Ear & Throat Hosp
799 Park Ave; New York, NY 10021; (212) 772-
9474; **BDCERT:** Oph 85; **MS:** Johns Hopkins U 80;
RES: Oph, Manhattan Eye, Ear & Throat Hosp, New
York, NY 81-84; **FEL:** Cornea & Refractive S,
Manhattan Eye, Ear & Throat Hosp, New York, NY
84-85; **FAP:** Lecturer Columbia P&S; **HOSP:** Beth
Israel North; *SI: Refractive Laser Surgery; Corneal
Transplants;* **HMO:** GHI Aetna-US Healthcare
Oxford Blue Cross PPO CIGNA +
♿ 💳 📷 🚹 🏦 **$** Mcr 1 Week ▩ **VISA** ●

Harmon, Gregory K (MD) Oph
NY Hosp-Cornell Med Ctr
520 E 70th St 823; New York, NY 10021; (212)
746-2475; **BDCERT:** Oph 91; **MS:** Mt Sinai Sch
Med 82; **RES:** Oph, NY Hosp-Cornell Med Ctr, New
York, NY 83-86; **FEL:** Glaucoma, NY Hosp-Cornell
Med Ctr, New York, NY 86-87; **FAP:** Assoc Dir Oph;
HOSP: Columbia-Presbyterian Med Ctr; *SI:
Glaucoma; Cataracts;* **HMO:** Blue Choice Oxford
Multiplan CIGNA Magnacare +
LANG: Sp; ♿ 📷 🏦 **$** Mcr Mcd WC NFI A Few Days
▩ **VISA** ●

Harrison, Raymond (MD) Oph
Manhattan Eye, Ear & Throat Hosp
121 E 60th St; New York, NY 10022; (212) 755-
3838; **BDCERT:** Oph 65; **MS:** England 48; **RES:**
Boston Med Ctr, Boston, MA 57-59; **FEL:** Mass Eye
& Ear Infirmary, Boston, MA; *SI: Glaucoma*
♿ 📷 Mcr A Few Days

Heinemann, Murk-Hein (MD)Oph
Mem Sloan Kettering Cancer Ctr
520 E 70th St STARR 811; New York, NY 10021;
(212) 746-2483; **BDCERT:** Oph 82; **MS:** Cornell U
76; **RES:** Yale-New Haven Hosp, New Haven, CT
77-80; **FEL:** New York Hospital, New York, NY 81-
82; **HMO:** Blue Cross Blue Shield Oxford PHCS
United Healthcare +

Hornblass, Albert (MD) Oph
Manhattan Eye, Ear & Throat Hosp
Oculoplastic Surgery, 130 E 67th St; New York, NY
10021; (212) 879-6824; **BDCERT:** Oph 70; PlS 72;
MS: U Cincinnati 64; **RES:** Univ Hosp SUNY Bklyn,
Brooklyn, NY 65-69; **FEL:** Oph, Manhattan Eye, Ear
& Throat Hosp, New York, NY 71-72; **FAP:** Prof
Oph SUNY Downstate; **HOSP:** Hackensack Univ
Med Ctr; *SI: Cosmetic eyelid surgery; Eye Cancer;*
HMO: Blue Cross & Blue Shield Anthem Health
Health Source HealthNet Oxford +
LANG: Sp, Fr, Heb, Yd, Ger; ♿ 📷 🚹 🏦 **$** WC NFI
VISA

Howard, George (MD) Oph
Columbia-Presbyterian Med Ctr
635 W 165th St; New York, NY 10032; (212) 305-5400; **BDCERT:** Oph 65; **MS:** Albany Med Coll 59; **RES:** Mass Eye & Ear Infirmary, Boston, MA 61-64; **FEL:** Onc, Columbia-Presbyterian Med Ctr, New York, NY; **SI:** *Cataract*; **HMO:** Aetna Hlth Plan Blue Choice Oxford Aetna Hlth Plan Prudential +

🔥 📷 🛏 💲 1 Week ▦

Kazim, Michael (MD) Oph
Columbia-Presbyterian Med Ctr
Pvt Office, 635 W 165th St; New York, NY 10032; (212) 305-5477; **BDCERT:** Oph 89; **MS:** Columbia P&S 84; **RES:** Oph, Columbia-Presbyterian Med Ctr, New York, NY 85-88; **FEL:** Orbital S, Allegheny Gen Hosp, Pittsburgh, PA 89-90; PlS, Children's Hosp of Philadelphia, Philadelphia, PA 88-89; **FAP:** Asst Clin Prof Oph Columbia P&S; **SI:** *Oculoplastic, Orbital Surgery; Orbital Surgery*

📷 📷 🛏 💲 �Mcr A Few Days **VISA** 💳

Kelly, Stephen E (MD) Oph
Manhattan Eye, Ear & Throat Hosp
Cataract & Corneal Associates, PC, 154 E 71st St; New York, NY 10021; (212) 628-2202; **BDCERT:** Oph 76; **MS:** Washington U, St Louis 70; **RES:** New York Eye & Ear Infirmary, New York, NY 72-75; **FEL:** Manhattan Eye, Ear & Throat Hosp, New York, NY 75-76; **FAP:** Lecturer Columbia P&S; **HOSP:** Lenox Hill Hosp; **SI:** *Laser Vision Correction; Cataract Surgery*; **HMO:** Oxford Empire Blue Shield Aetna-US Healthcare PHCS CIGNA +

LANG: Sp; 📷 📷 🛏 💲 Mcr WC A Few Days **VISA** 💳

Kelman, Charles D (MD) Oph
New York Eye & Ear Infirmary
220 Madison Ave; New York, NY 10016; (212) 736-9696; **BDCERT:** Oph 63; **MS:** Switzerland 56; **RES:** Wills Eye Hosp, Philadelphia, PA 58-60; **SI:** *Cataract Extraction; Lens Implantation*; **HMO:** Oxford US Hlthcre

LANG: Fr, Rus, Pol, Heb, Yd; 🔥 📷 📷 🛏 Mcr WC Immediately **VISA** 💳

Klapper, Daniel (MD) Oph
Manhattan Eye, Ear & Throat Hosp
7 W 81st St 1A; New York, NY 10024; (212) 874-2726; **BDCERT:** Oph 91; **MS:** Albert Einstein Coll Med 84; **RES:** Brookdale Univ Hosp Med Ctr, Brooklyn, NY 84-88; **FAP:** Assoc Albert Einstein Coll Med; **HOSP:** Beth Israel Med Ctr; **SI:** *Glaucoma; Cataract*; **HMO:** Oxford Aetna Hlth Plan Blue Choice GHI PHS +

LANG: Ger, Yd, Heb, Sp; 🔥 📞 📷 📷 🛏 💲 Mcr Immediately ▦ **VISA** 💳

Klein, Noah (MD) Oph
Beth Israel Med Ctr
51 E 25th St Fl 3; New York, NY 10010; (212) 696-9013; **BDCERT:** Oph 85; **MS:** Albert Einstein Coll Med 80; **RES:** IM, New York University Med Ctr, New York, NY 80-81; Oph, Long Island Jewish Med Ctr, New Hyde Park, NY 81-84; **HOSP:** New York Eye & Ear Infirmary; **SI:** *Diabetic Eye Disease; Glaucoma*; **HMO:** Oxford Blue Choice United Healthcare US Hlthcre

LANG: Heb, Yd, Sp; 🔥 📞 📷 📷 🛏 💲 Mcr 1 Week ▦

Koplin, Richard (MD) Oph
New York Eye & Ear Infirmary
Ophthalmic Consultants, 310 E 14th St; New York, NY 10003; (212) 505-6550; **BDCERT:** Oph 75; **MS:** NY Med Coll 69; **RES:** Oph, New York Eye & Ear Infirmary, New York, NY 70-73; **FAP:** Assoc Prof NY Med Coll; **HOSP:** Beth Israel Med Ctr; **SI:** *High Risk Cataract Surgery; Refractive Surgery*; **HMO:** Oxford CIGNA Prudential Blue Cross

LANG: Sp, Chi; 🔥 📷 📷 🛏 💲 Mcr WC 2-4 Weeks ▦ **VISA** 💳

Leib, Martin L (MD)   Oph
Columbia-Presbyterian Med Ctr

Edward Harkness Eye Institute, 635 W 165th St Ste 230; New York, NY 10032; (212) 305-2303; **BDCERT:** Oph 82; PlS 91; **MS:** NY Med Coll 74; **RES:** S, Mount Sinai Med Ctr, New York, NY 75-76; Oph, McGill Teaching Hosp, Montreal, Canada 76-79; **FEL:** Orbital PlS, Columbia-Presbyterian Med Ctr, New York, NY 79-80; **FAP:** Assoc Clin Prof Oph Columbia P&S; **HOSP:** St Luke's Roosevelt Hosp Ctr; **SI:** *Orbital Tumors—Cosmetic Surgery; Cataract Implants;* **HMO:** Oxford Blue Choice Blue Cross

LANG: Fr, Heb, Grk, Itl; ♿ 🌙 🅿 👥 🏥 💲 Mcr Immediately *VISA* 💳

L'Esperance, Francis A (MD) Oph
Columbia-Presbyterian Med Ctr

1 E 71 St; New York, NY 10021; (212) 249-1140; **BDCERT:** Oph 62; **MS:** Harvard Med Sch 56; **RES:** Oph, Mass Eye & Ear Infirmary, Boston, MA 57-60; **FAP:** Prof of Clin Oph Columbia P&S; **HOSP:** Manhattan Eye, Ear & Throat Hosp; **SI:** *Vitreoretinal; Laser Surgery;* **HMO:** Blue Cross & Blue Shield Oxford

🅿 👥 🏥 💲 2-4 Weeks 💳 *VISA* 💳

Lester, Richard (MD)   Oph
St Luke's Roosevelt Hosp Ctr

132 E 76th St 2D; New York, NY 10021; (212) 861-4455; **BDCERT:** Oph 81; **MS:** Univ Texas, Houston 75; **RES:** USC Med Ctr, Los Angeles, CA 75-76; St Luke's Roosevelt Hosp Ctr, New York, NY 77-80; **FEL:** Retina, Northwestern Mem Hosp, Chicago, IL; **FAP:** Clin Instr Columbia P&S; **HOSP:** Lenox Hill Hosp; **SI:** *Diabetic Eye Disease; Contact Lens Problems;* **HMO:** Oxford PHS United Healthcare Blue Cross & Blue Shield US Hlthcre +

LANG: Dut, Fr; ♿ 🅿 👥 🏥 💲 Mcr A Few Days

Levitzky, Munro (MD)   Oph
New York University Med Ctr

161 Madison Ave Fl 6; New York, NY 10016; (212) 725-5225; **BDCERT:** Oph 70; **MS:** Columbia P&S 61; **RES:** IM, Bellevue Hosp Ctr, New York, NY 62-63; Oph, Bellevue Hosp Ctr, New York, NY 65-69; **HOSP:** New York Eye & Ear Infirmary; **HMO:** Metlife Oxford Chubb US Hlthcre

♿ 🌙 🅿 👥 🏥 💲 Mcr A Few Days

Lieberman, Theodore (MD) Oph
Mount Sinai Med Ctr

70 E 96th St; New York, NY 10128; (212) 722-5477; **BDCERT:** Oph 67; **MS:** Yale U Sch Med 58; **RES:** Barnes Hosp, St Louis, MO 62-65; **FEL:** N, Mount Sinai Med Ctr, New York, NY 59-60; **SI:** *Glaucoma; Neuro-Ophthalmology;* **HMO:** Oxford Beech Street PHCS PHS

LANG: Sp; ♿ 🅿 🏥 💲 Mcr NFI 1 Week

Liebowitz, Solomon (MD)   Oph
New York Eye & Ear Infirmary

36 E 36th St; New York, NY 10016; (212) 686-1313; **BDCERT:** Oph 66; **MS:** NYU Sch Med 57; **RES:** New York Eye & Ear Infirmary, New York, NY 62-64; **HOSP:** Beth Israel Med Ctr; **HMO:** Blue Cross & Blue Shield Sanus-NYLCare Oxford US Hlthcre GHI +

♿ 🅿 👥 🏥 💲 Mcr WC 1 Week 💳 *VISA* 💳 💳

Lisman, Richard (MD)   Oph
Manhattan Eye, Ear & Throat Hosp

635 Park Ave; New York, NY 10021; (212) 585-1405; **BDCERT:** Oph 81; **MS:** NYU Sch Med 76; **RES:** Oph, Manhattan Eye, Ear & Throat Hosp, New York, NY 80; **FEL:** PIS, NY Hosp-Cornell Med Ctr, New York, NY 81-82; PIS, New York Eye & Ear Infirmary, New York, NY 82; **FAP:** Clin Prof Oph NYU Sch Med; **HOSP:** New York University Med Ctr; **SI:** *Eyelid Reconstruction; Cosmetic Eyelid Surgery;* **HMO:** Prudential CIGNA Oxford PHS Aetna Hlth Plan +

LANG: Sp; ♿ 🅿 👥 🏥 💲 Mcr NFI 1 Week 💳 *VISA* 💳

Luntz, Maurice (MD)   Oph
Manhattan Eye, Ear & Throat Hosp

121 E 60th St; New York, NY 10022; (212) 751-3301; **BDCERT:** Oph 79; **MS:** South Africa 52; **RES:** Groote Schuur Hosp, Cape Town, South Africa 53-55; St Mary's Hosp, London, England 57; **FEL:** Glaucoma & Cataract, Oxford Eye Hosp, Oxford, England; **HOSP:** Beth Israel Med Ctr; **SI:** *Glaucoma Surgery; Cataract Surgery;* **HMO:** HIP Network Aetna Hlth Plan Travelers Oxford PHS +

♿ 🅿 👥 🏥 💲 Mcr Immediately 💳 *VISA* 💳

Mackay, Cynthia J (MD)   Oph
Columbia-Presbyterian Med Ctr
69 E 71st St; New York, NY 10021; (212) 772-
6050; **BDCERT:** Oph 82; **MS:** SUNY Hlth Sci Ctr 77;
RES: Columbia-Presbyterian Med Ctr, New York,
NY 78-81; **FEL:** Retina, New York University Med
Ctr, New York, NY 81-82; Retina, Bellevue Hosp
Ctr, New York, NY 81-82; **HOSP:** Manhattan Eye,
Ear & Throat Hosp; *SI: Diabetic Retinopathy; Macular
Degeneration*; **HMO:** Oxford HealthNet Blue Choice
Aetna Hlth Plan Prucare +

LANG: Sp, Fr, Ger; ⬚ ⬚ ⬚ ⬚ ⬚ Immediately
VISA ⬤

Mamelok, Alfred E (MD)   Oph
Manhattan Eye, Ear & Throat Hosp
115 E 61st St; New York, NY 10021; (212) 832-
9228; **BDCERT:** Oph 54; **MS:** NY Med Coll 46; **RES:**
Coney Island Hosp, Brooklyn, NY 47-48;
Manhattan Eye, Ear & Throat Hosp, New York, NY
51-53; **FAP:** Assoc Clin Prof Oph Cornell U; **HOSP:**
NY Hosp-Cornell Med Ctr; *SI: Uveitis; Medical
Problems*; **HMO:** None

LANG: Fr, Ger; ⬚ ⬚ ⬚ ⬚ ⬚ ⬚ ⬚ A Few Days

Mandelbaum, Sid (MD)   Oph
Manhattan Eye, Ear & Throat Hosp
178 E 71st St; New York, NY 10021; (212) 650-
0400; **BDCERT:** Oph 82; **MS:** Yale U Sch Med 76;
RES: Oph, Los Angeles Cty Hosp, Los Angeles, CA
78-81; **FEL:** Corneal Disease, Bascom Palmer Eye
Inst, Miami, FL 81-82; **FAP:** Assoc Clin Instr Oph
Albert Einstein Coll Med; **HOSP:** Long Island Jewish
Med Ctr; *SI: Corneal Diseases; Refractive Surgery*;
HMO: Oxford US Hlthcre PHS Independent Health
Plan Aetna Hlth Plan +

⬚ ⬚ ⬚ ⬚ ⬚ ⬚ 2-4 Weeks

McVeigh, Anne Marie (MD) Oph
St Vincents Hosp & Med Ctr NY
36 7th Ave 519; New York, NY 10011; (212) 929-
3747; **BDCERT:** Oph 89; **MS:** NY Med Coll 82; **RES:**
St Vincents Hosp & Med Ctr NY, New York, NY 82;
Oph, St Vincents Hosp & Med Ctr NY, New York,
NY 83-86; **HOSP:** Cabrini Med Ctr; **HMO:** Oxford
Blue Choice Chubb

⬚ ⬚ ⬚ ⬚ ⬚ ⬚ Immediately

Medow, Norman (MD)   Oph
NY Hosp-Cornell Med Ctr
225 E 64th St; New York, NY 10021; (212) 628-
0032; **BDCERT:** Oph 75; **MS:** SUNY Hlth Sci Ctr 66;
RES: Manhattan Eye, Ear & Throat Hosp, New
York, NY 69-72; **FAP:** Assoc Clin Prof Cornell U;
HOSP: Manhattan Eye, Ear & Throat Hosp; *SI:
Pediatric Cataracts Cornea; Pediatric Glaucoma*

LANG: Sp, Ger, Itl; ⬚ ⬚ ⬚ ⬚ 1 Week

Melton, R Christine (MD)   Oph
Cabrini Med Ctr
222 E 19th St 1C; New York, NY 10003; (212)
475-3791; **BDCERT:** Oph 82; **MS:** Canada 77; **RES:**
Oph, St Vincents Hosp & Med Ctr NY, New York,
NY 78-81; **FAP:** Asst Clin Prof NY Med Coll; **HOSP:**
New York Eye & Ear Infirmary; **HMO:** Aetna-US
Healthcare Oxford GHI 1199

LANG: Sp, Fr; ⬚ ⬚ ⬚ ⬚ ⬚ ⬚ ⬚ A Few Days

Merhige, Kenneth (MD)   Oph
St Luke's Roosevelt Hosp Ctr
114th St & Amsterdam Ave; New York, NY 10025;
(212) 523-2562; **BDCERT:** Oph 85; **MS:** Cornell U
80; **RES:** Oph, St Luke's Roosevelt Hosp Ctr, New
York, NY; **FEL:** Vitreoretinal, NY Hosp-Cornell Med
Ctr, New York, NY; **HMO:** Oxford GHI US Hlthcre
Aetna Hlth Plan CIGNA +

⬚ ⬚ ⬚ Immediately **VISA** ⬤

Merriam, John C (MD)   Oph
Columbia-Presbyterian Med Ctr
Edward Sl Harkness Eye Institute, 635 W 165th St;
New York, NY 10032; (212) 305-5402; **BDCERT:**
Oph 83; **MS:** Harvard Med Sch 77; **RES:** PIS,
Brigham & Women's Hosp, Boston, MA 78; Oph,
Mass Eye & Ear Infirmary, Boston, MA 79-82; **FEL:**
UC San Francisco Med Ctr, San Francisco, CA 82-
83; Moorefields Eye Hosp, London, England; **FAP:**
Assoc Prof Columbia P&S; **HOSP:** Harlem Hosp Ctr;
SI: Cataract; Opthalmic Plastic Surgery; **HMO:** Aetna
Hlth Plan Blue Choice Oxford Chubb Independent
Health Plan +

⬚ ⬚ ⬚ ⬚ A Few Days

Millman, Arthur (MD) Oph
New York Eye & Ear Infirmary
Manhattan Ctr for Facial Plastic Surgery, 345 E 37th St 212; New York, NY 10016; (212) 697-9797; **BDCERT:** Oph 87; PlS 88; **MS:** Northwestern U 81; **RES:** Oph, New York Eye & Ear Infirmary, New York, NY 85-87; **FEL:** PlS, IL Eye & Ear Infirmary, Chicago, IL 86-87; PlS, New York Eye & Ear Infirmary, New York, NY 86-87; **FAP:** Asst Prof NY Med Coll; **HOSP:** Lenox Hill Hosp; **HMO:** Most
LANG: Sp, Grk, Heb; ♿ ☾ ☎ 👤 📅 $ [Mcr] 1 Week American Express VISA MasterCard

Mindel, Joel (MD) Oph
Mount Sinai Med Ctr
Mt Sinai Hospital, 5 E 98th St; New York, NY 10029; (212) 241-8800; **BDCERT:** Oph 70; **MS:** U Md Sch Med 64; **RES:** U Mich Med Ctr, Ann Arbor, MI 66-69; **FEL:** N Oph, Columbia-Presbyterian Med Ctr, New York, NY 65-66; **FAP:** Assoc Prof Oph; **HOSP:** VA Med Ctr-Bronx; ***SI:*** *Neuro-Ophthalmology; Ocular Pharmacology*; **HMO:** Oxford
♿ 📅 $ [Mcr] A Few Days American Express VISA MasterCard

Mitchell, John P (MD) Oph
St Luke's Roosevelt Hosp Ctr
1901 Madison Ave; New York, NY 10027; (212) 662-8300; **BDCERT:** Oph 78; **MS:** Cornell U 73; **RES:** Oph, Harlem Hosp Ctr, New York, NY 74-77; **FEL:** Oph, Columbia-Presbyterian Med Ctr, New York, NY 77-78; **FAP:** Asst Prof Columbia P&S; ***SI:*** *Neurologic Diseases of Eye; Cataracts and Glaucoma*; **HMO:** Oxford Blue Cross & Blue Shield US Hlthcre GHI Aetna Hlth Plan +
LANG: Sp, Cre; ♿ [SA SU] ☾ ☎ 👤 📅 $ [Mcr] [Mcd] A Few Days American Express VISA MasterCard

Muchnick, Richard (MD) Oph
NY Hosp-Cornell Med Ctr
69 E 71st St; New York, NY 10021; (212) 744-1726; **BDCERT:** Oph 75; **MS:** Cornell U 67; **RES:** NY Hosp-Cornell Med Ctr, New York, NY; **FEL:** Oph Plastic & Reconstruct S, UC San Francisco Med Ctr, San Francisco, CA; Strabismus, Manhattan Eye, Ear & Throat Hosp, New York, NY; **FAP:** Assoc Clin Prof Oph Cornell U; **HOSP:** Manhattan Eye, Ear & Throat Hosp; ***SI:*** *Pediatric Ophthalmology*; **HMO:** Blue Choice Aetna Hlth Plan HealthNet Oxford HIP Network +
LANG: Sp, Yd; ♿ ☎ 👤 📅 $ [Mcr] [NFI] 1 Week VISA MasterCard

Muldoon, Thomas (MD) Oph
New York Eye & Ear Infirmary
310 E 14th St; New York, NY 10003; (212) 979-4595; **BDCERT:** Oph 71; **MS:** U Rochester 62; **RES:** S, St Luke's Roosevelt Hosp Ctr, New York, NY 65-66; Oph, New York Eye & Ear Infirmary, New York, NY 66-69; **FEL:** New York Eye & Ear Infirmary, New York, NY 69-70; **FAP:** Assoc Clin Prof NY Med Coll; **HOSP:** Beth Israel Med Ctr; ***SI:*** *Retinal Detachments; Diabetic Retinopathy*; **HMO:** Oxford CIGNA Prucare US Hlthcre Aetna Hlth Plan +
♿ ☎ 👤 📅 $ [Mcr] [WC] [NFI] Immediately

Nadel, Alfred (MD) Oph
Lenox Hill Hosp
515 E 79th St; New York, NY 10021; (212) 288-9841; **BDCERT:** Oph 69; **MS:** Columbia P&S 60; **RES:** IL Eye & Ear Infirmary, Chicago, IL 63-66; **FEL:** NY Hosp-Cornell Med Ctr, New York, NY 66-67; **HOSP:** Brookdale Univ Hosp Med Ctr; ***SI:*** *Retina; Vitreous Disease*; **HMO:** Aetna Hlth Plan Blue Cross & Blue Shield CIGNA HIP Network
LANG: Fr, Sp, Grk; ♿ ☾ ☎ 👤 📅 $ [Mcr] [Mcd]
Immediately

Newhouse, Robert P (MD)　Oph
Manhattan Eye, Ear & Throat Hosp

30 W 60th St 1 Y; New York, NY 10022; (212) 265-7733; **BDCERT:** Oph 67; **MS:** Albany Med Coll 56; **RES:** Ped, Mount Sinai Med Ctr, New York, NY 61-62; Oph, NY Polyclinic Hosp, New York, NY 62-64; **FEL:** Glaucoma, Manhattan Eye, Ear & Throat Hosp, New York, NY 64-65; **FAP:** Asst Instr Columbia P&S; **HOSP:** St Luke's Roosevelt Hosp Ctr; *SI: Glaucoma;* **HMO:** Aetna Hlth Plan United Healthcare Blue Choice US Hlthcre HealthNet +

LANG: Ger, Sp; 🦽 📷 🚗 🏥 Mcr Mcd WC NFI 2-4 Weeks

Newton, Michael (MD)　Oph
Manhattan Eye, Ear & Throat Hosp

64 E 86th St; New York, NY 10028; (212) 861-0146; **BDCERT:** Oph 78; **MS:** Tufts U 71; **RES:** Oph, Mount Sinai Med Ctr, New York, NY 74-77; **FEL:** Corneal S, AB Nesburn MD, Los Angeles, CA 77-78; **FAP:** Assoc Clin Prof Mt Sinai Sch Med; **HOSP:** Mount Sinai Med Ctr; *SI: Cataract and Corneal Surgery; Laser Refractive Surgery;* **HMO:** Oxford

🦽 ♿ 📷 🚗 🏥 💲 Mcr 1 Week ▨ **VISA** ⬤

Nightingale, Jeffrey (MD)　Oph
New York Eye & Ear Infirmary

211 Central Park West; New York, NY 10024; (212) 877-7188; **BDCERT:** Oph 77; **MS:** SUNY Hlth Sci Ctr 73; **RES:** Bronx Lebanon Hosp, Bronx, NY 73-76; **FEL:** NY Eye & Ear Infirmary, New York, NY 76-77; **HOSP:** Our Lady of Mercy Med Ctr

Noble, Kenneth (MD)　Oph
New York University Med Ctr

161 Madison Ave FL5; New York, NY 10016; (212) 683-2533; **BDCERT:** Oph 75; **MS:** NYU Sch Med 68; **RES:** Oph, New York University Med Ctr, New York, NY 70-74; **FEL:** Retina, New York University Med Ctr, New York, NY 73-74; **FAP:** Assoc Prof NYU Sch Med; *SI: Medical Retina; Uvetis;* **HMO:** Oxford Blue Cross CIGNA GHI Aetna Hlth Plan +

🦽 📷 🚗 🏥 Mcr Immediately **VISA** ⬤

Obstbaum, Stephen (MD)　Oph
Lenox Hill Hosp

115 E 39th St; New York, NY 10016; (212) 687-4106; **BDCERT:** Oph 74; **MS:** NY Med Coll 67; **RES:** Oph, Flower Fifth Ave - NY Med Coll, New York, NY 68-72; **FEL:** Glaucoma, Washington U Hosp, St Louis, MO 72-73; **FAP:** Clin Prof Oph NYU Sch Med; *SI: Cataract; Glaucoma;* **HMO:** Blue Choice PHS PHCS Oxford CIGNA +

LANG: Sp; 📷 🏥 💲 Mcr A Few Days ▨ **VISA** ⬤

Odell, Peter (MD)　Oph
NY Hosp-Cornell Med Ctr

116 E 63rd St; New York, NY 10021; (212) 421-8025; **BDCERT:** Oph 76; **MS:** Tufts U 68; **RES:** Oph, NY Hosp-Cornell Med Ctr, New York, NY 71-74; **FEL:** Oph PlS, Manhattan Eye, Ear & Throat Hosp, New York, NY 75; **FAP:** Assoc Clin Prof Oph Cornell U; *SI: Cataracts; Ophthalmic Plastic Surgery*

🦽 📷 🚗 🏥 2-4 Weeks

Podell, David (MD)　Oph
Lenox Hill Hosp

67 E 78th St; New York, NY 10021; (212) 628-2323; **BDCERT:** Oph 66; **MS:** Queens U 57; **RES:** Lenox Hill Hosp, New York, NY 58-61; NY Med Coll, New York, NY 58-59; **HOSP:** Beth Israel Med Ctr

Podos, Steven (MD)　Oph
Mount Sinai Med Ctr

5 E 98th St; New York, NY 10029; (212) 241-6752; **BDCERT:** Oph 68; **MS:** Harvard Med Sch 62; **RES:** Barnes Hosp, St Louis, MO 64-67; **FEL:** Glaucoma, Nat Inst Health, Bethesda, MD 67-69; **FAP:** Chrmn Mt Sinai Sch Med; *SI: Glaucoma;* **HMO:** PHS Aetna Hlth Plan CIGNA Chubb Oxford +

LANG: Sp; 🦽 🏥 Mcr Mcd WC 2-4 Weeks ▨ **VISA** ⬤ ▨

Poole, Thomas (MD) Oph
Manhattan Eye, Ear & Throat Hosp
4 E 77th St; New York, NY 10021; (212) 288-1200; **BDCERT:** Oph 74; **MS:** Harvard Med Sch 66; **RES:** NY Hosp-Cornell Med Ctr, New York, NY 69-72; **FEL:** Retina, NY Hosp-Cornell Med Ctr, New York, NY 72-73; **HOSP:** Lenox Hill Hosp; *SI: Retinal Disorders; Macular Degeneration;* **HMO:** Oxford Blue Cross & Blue Shield GHI Aetna-US Healthcare Magnacare +

🗐 🛏 💲 Mcr Mcd WC NFI 1 Week

Prince, Andrew (MD) Oph
New York Eye & Ear Infirmary
178 E 71st St; New York, NY 10021; (212) 717-2200; **BDCERT:** Oph 87; **MS:** SUNY Downstate 81; **RES:** Univ Hosp SUNY Bklyn, Brooklyn, NY; **FEL:** Glaucoma, New York Eye & Ear Infirmary, New York, NY; **FAP:** Assoc Prof NYU Sch Med; **HOSP:** Catholic Med Ctr Bklyn & Qns; *SI: Glaucoma; Cataract;* **HMO:** Aetna-US Healthcare Oxford Blue Cross & Blue Shield PHS

LANG: Sp, Rus; 🚫 🗐 🚹 🛏 💲 Mcr 1 Week **VISA** 💳

Raab, Edward (MD) Oph
Mount Sinai Med Ctr
5 E 98th St 7th Fl; New York, NY 10029; (212) 369-0988; **BDCERT:** Oph 66; **MS:** NYU Sch Med 58; **RES:** Mount Sinai Med Ctr, New York, NY 64; **FEL:** Ped Oph, Children's Hosp Nat Med Ctr, Washington, DC 66-67; **FAP:** Prof Oph Mt Sinai Sch Med; *SI: Pediatric Cataracts; Ocular Plastic Surgery;* **HMO:** Oxford Aetna Hlth Plan HIP Network

LANG: Fr, Sp; 🚫 🗐 🚹 🛏 💲 Mcr Mcd WC NFI A Few Days 📷 **VISA** 💳

Relland, Maureen (MD) Oph
St Vincents Hosp & Med Ctr NY
36 7th Ave; New York, NY 10011; (212) 645-7771; **BDCERT:** Oph 71; **MS:** NY Med Coll 64; **RES:** Oph, St Vincents Hosp & Med Ctr NY, New York, NY 65-68; **FEL:** Mount Sinai Med Ctr, New York, NY 68-70; Oph, St Vincents Hosp & Med Ctr NY, New York, NY 75-78; **HOSP:** Bayley Seton Hosp; *SI: Cataracts; Plastic Eye Surgery*

LANG: Fr, Sp; 🚫 🗐 🚹 🛏 💲 WC NFI 1 Week 📷 **VISA** 💳

Reppucci, Vincent (MD) Oph
Columbia-Presbyterian Med Ctr
Vitreoretinal Specialists, 425 W 59th St Ste 3B; New York, NY 10019; (212) 307-0777; **BDCERT:** Oph 89; **MS:** Albert Einstein Coll Med 83; **RES:** Columbia-Presbyterian Med Ctr, New York, NY 84-87; **FEL:** NY Hosp-Cornell Med Ctr, New York, NY 87-88; **FAP:** Asst Prof Columbia P&S; **HOSP:** Danbury Hosp; *SI: Vitreoretinal Surgery; Complicated Retina Detach*

LANG: Sp, Itl; 🚫 🛏 💲 Mcr A Few Days 📷 **VISA** 💳

Richards, Renee (MD) Oph
Manhattan Eye, Ear & Throat Hosp
40 Park Ave; New York, NY 10016; (212) 532-1168; **BDCERT:** Oph 65; **MS:** U Rochester 59; **RES:** Manhattan Eye, Ear & Throat Hosp, New York, NY 61-63; **FEL:** Columbia-Presbyterian Med Ctr, New York, NY; Oregon Health Sci U Hosp, Portland, OR; *SI: Pediatric Ophthalmology; Eye Muscles—Double Vision*

🚫 🛏 💲 Mcr NFI 4+ Weeks 📷 **VISA** 💳

Ritch, Robert (MD) Oph
New York Eye & Ear Infirmary
310 E 14th St Fl 3; New York, NY 10003; (212) 477-7540; **BDCERT:** Oph 77; **MS:** Albert Einstein Coll Med 72; **RES:** Oph, Mount Sinai Med Ctr, New York, NY 73-76; **FEL:** Mount Sinai Med Ctr, New York, NY 76-77; Mount Sinai Med Ctr, New York, NY 77-88; **FAP:** Prof NY Med Coll; *SI: Glaucoma; Cataract;* **HMO:** Aetna Hlth Plan CIGNA Blue Cross & Blue Shield

LANG: Fr, Ger, Sp, Jpn, Chi; 🚫 🗐 🚹 🛏 💲 Mcr Immediately 📷 **VISA** 💳 💳

Guide to symbols and abbreviations can be found on pages 110-113.

279

Roberts, Calvin (MD)   Oph
NY Hosp-Cornell Med Ctr

520 E 70th St; New York, NY 10021; (212) 746-3937; **BDCERT:** Oph 82; **MS:** Columbia P&S 78; **RES:** Oph, Columbia-Presbyterian Med Ctr, New York, NY 78-81; **FEL:** Cornea, Mass Gen Hosp, Boston, MA 81-82; Cornea, Harvard Med Sch, Cambridge, MA 81-82; **FAP:** Prof Cornell U; *SI: Cataract Surgery; Laser Vision Correction;* **HMO:** Oxford Aetna-US Healthcare NYLCare United Healthcare Blue Cross & Blue Shield +

LANG: Sp; 🚻 🔲 🔲 🔲 🔲 🔲 2-4 Weeks 🔲 🔲 🔲

Rodriguez-Sains, Rene (MD) Oph
Manhattan Eye, Ear & Throat Hosp

178 E 71st St; New York, NY 10021; (212) 535-0315; **BDCERT:** Oph 82; **MS:** NYU Sch Med 77; **RES:** New York University Med Ctr, New York, NY 77-78; Manhattan Eye, Ear & Throat Hosp, New York, NY 78-81; **FEL:** Oph Onc & PlS, Manhattan Eye, Ear & Throat Hosp, New York, NY 81-82; **HOSP:** Lenox Hill Hosp; *SI: Eyelid Tumors; Cosmetic Eyelid Surgery;* **HMO:** Blue Cross & Blue Shield Metlife Chubb Oxford

LANG: Sp, Fr; 🚻 🔲 🔲 🔲 🔲 🔲 🔲 Immediately 🔲 *VISA* 🔲

Rosen, Richard (MD)   Oph
New York Eye & Ear Infirmary

NY Eye and Ear Infirmary Faculty Practice, 310 E 14th St 319SB; New York, NY 10003; (212) 979-4288; **BDCERT:** Oph 91; **MS:** U Miami Sch Med 85; **RES:** Oph, New York Eye & Ear Infirmary, New York, NY 86-89; **FEL:** Retina Vitreous, New York Eye & Ear Infirmary, New York, NY 89-91; **FAP:** Asst Prof NY Med Coll; **HOSP:** Beth Israel Med Ctr; *SI: Retinal Detachment, Tears; Diabetes—Macular Degeneration;* **HMO:** Oxford GHI CIGNA Blue Cross NYLCare +

🚻 🔲 🔲 🔲 🔲 🔲 🔲 🔲 Immediately

Rosenbaum, Jacob (MD)   Oph
Mount Sinai Med Ctr

115 E 39th St; New York, NY 10016; (212) 681-0883; **BDCERT:** Oph 91; **MS:** Germany 72; **RES:** Kings County Hosp Ctr, Brooklyn, NY 74-77; **FEL:** Kings County Hosp Ctr, Brooklyn, NY 77-78; **FAP:** Asst Clin Prof Mt Sinai Sch Med; *SI: Diabetes of Aged; Macular Degeneration;* **HMO:** Oxford Blue Cross Magnacare US Hlthcre

LANG: Ger, Hun, Yd; 🚻 🔲 🔲 🔲 🔲 🔲 🔲 A Few Days

Rosenthal, Jeanne L (MD)   Oph
New York Eye & Ear Infirmary

20 E 9th St; New York, NY 10003; (212) 674-2970; **BDCERT:** Oph 85; **MS:** SUNY Downstate 79; **RES:** Oph, New York Eye & Ear Infirmary, New York, NY 80-83; **FEL:** Retina Vitreous, New York Eye & Ear Infirmary, New York, NY 83-85; **FAP:** Asst Clin Prof Oph NY Med Coll; **HMO:** Oxford Blue Choice GHI Anthem Health Amerihealth +

Rudick, A Joseph (MD)   Oph
Manhattan Eye, Ear & Throat Hosp

150 Broadway 1110; New York, NY 10038; (212) 233-2344; **BDCERT:** Oph 90; **MS:** Univ Penn 83; **RES:** Manhattan Eye, Ear & Throat Hosp, New York, NY 88; **HOSP:** NYU Downtown Hosp; *SI: Cataract Surgery; Refractive Surgery;* **HMO:** Oxford Metlife Aetna-US Healthcare Blue Cross & Blue Choice GHI +

LANG: Sp; 🚻 🔲 🔲 🔲 🔲 🔲 🔲 🔲 🔲 🔲 Immediately 🔲 *VISA* 🔲

Schneider, Howard (MD)   Oph
Mount Sinai Med Ctr

Fifth Ave Eye Associates, 1034 5th Ave; New York, NY 10028; (212) 628-2300; **BDCERT:** Oph 70; **MS:** U Rochester 64; **RES:** Northwestern Mem Hosp, Chicago, IL 64-67; *SI: Glaucoma;* **HMO:** 1199 Aetna Hlth Plan Magnacare Blue Cross PPO Blue Choice +

LANG: Sp, Fr, Yd, Rus, Itl; 🚻 🔲 🔲 🔲 🔲 🔲 Immediately 🔲 *VISA* 🔲 🔲

Schubert, Herman N (MD)   Oph
Columbia-Presbyterian Med Ctr
635 W 165th St Rm206; New York, NY 10032;
(212) 305-6534; **BDCERT:** Oph 87; Path 79; **MS:**
Germany 74; **RES:** Path, Columbia-Presbyterian
Med Ctr, New York, NY 79; Oph, Columbia-
Presbyterian Med Ctr, New York, NY 85; **FEL:**
Retina, Wills Eye Hosp, Philadelphia, PA 85-87;
FAP: Prof Columbia P&S; **HOSP:** Southampton
Hosp; *SI: Vitreoretinal; Diabetic Retinopathy;* **HMO:**
Oxford Blue Choice PHS Aetna Hlth Plan Blue Cross
+

LANG: Sp, Ger, Fr; 🦽 🔒 👥 🏠 $ Mcr NFI
Immediately

Schutz, James (MD)   Oph
Manhattan Eye, Ear & Throat Hosp
Eye Surgeons PC, 485 Park Ave; New York, NY
10022; (212) 753-6464; **BDCERT:** Oph 75; **MS:**
Harvard Med Sch 69; **RES:** S, Mass Gen Hosp,
Boston, MA 69-70; Oph, Manhattan Eye, Ear &
Throat Hosp, New York, NY 70-73; **FAP:** Assoc
Clin Prof Cornell U; **HOSP:** NY Hosp-Cornell Med
Ctr; *SI: Cataract; Retina;* **HMO:** Oxford CIGNA
United Healthcare PHS

LANG: Flm, Itl; 🔒 👥 🏠 $ Mcr WC   A Few Days

Seedor, John (MD)   Oph
New York Eye & Ear Infirmary
Ophthalmic Consultants, 310 E 14th St; New York,
NY 10003; (212) 979-4428; **BDCERT:** Oph 87;
MS: Hahnemann U 81; **RES:** Bryn Mawr Hosp,
Bryn Mawr, PA 82; New York Eye & Ear Infirmary,
New York, NY 85; **FEL:** Cornea & Refractive S,
Emory U Hosp, Atlanta, GA; **HOSP:** Beth Israel Med
Ctr; *SI: Refractive Surgery; Corneal Transplantation;*
HMO: US Hlthcre CIGNA Oxford GHI

LANG: Sp, Chi; 🦽 🔒 👥 🏠 $ Mcr WC NFI
A Few Days 🏧 **VISA** 💳

Serle, Janet (MD)   Oph
Mount Sinai Med Ctr
Mt Sinai Medical Ctr, 5 E 98th St 7th Fl; New York,
NY 10029; (212) 241-0939; **BDCERT:** Oph 87;
MS: Harvard Med Sch 80; **RES:** Oph, Mount Sinai
Med Ctr, New York, NY 82-85; **FEL:** Glaucoma,
Mount Sinai Med Ctr, New York, NY 81-82;
Glaucoma, Mount Sinai Med Ctr, New York, NY
85-86; **FAP:** Assoc Prof Mt Sinai Sch Med; *SI:*
Glaucoma; Cataracts; **HMO:** Oxford PHS PHCS

LANG: Sp, Fr, Rus; 🦽 👥 🏠 $ Mcr Mcd WC   1 Week
🏧 **VISA** 💳

Shabto, Uri (MD)   Oph
New York Eye & Ear Infirmary
310 E 14th St; New York, NY 10003; (212) 677-
2000; **BDCERT:** Oph 91; **MS:** Harvard Med Sch 86;
RES: Oph, New York Eye & Ear Infirmary, New
York, NY 88-90; **FEL:** Retina Vitreous, Montefiore
Med Ctr, Bronx, NY 90-91; **HOSP:** Beth Israel Med
Ctr; *SI: Diabetic Eye Disease; Macular Diseases;* **HMO:**
Blue Cross Guardian PHS Unicare Primary Plus
Aetna-US Healthcare +

LANG: Sp; 🦽 🔒 👥 🏠 $ Mcr Mcd WC NFI
Immediately

Sherman, Spencer (MD)   Oph
Manhattan Eye, Ear & Throat Hosp
Manhattan Ophthalmology Assoc, 166 E 63rd St;
New York, NY 10021; (212) 753-8300; **BDCERT:**
Oph 70; **MS:** Columbia P&S 62; **RES:** Oph, Mount
Sinai Med Ctr, New York, NY 65-68; **FAP:** Assoc
Clin Prof Mt Sinai Sch Med; **HOSP:** Mount Sinai
Med Ctr; *SI: Refractive Eye Surgery; Cataract Surgery;*
HMO: Aetna Hlth Plan Blue Choice Oxford Prucare
Chubb +

LANG: Sp, Fr, Fil; 🦽 🔒 👥 🏠 $ Mcr WC
A Few Days 🏧 **VISA** 💳 💳

Shulman, Julius (MD)   Oph
Mount Sinai Med Ctr
229 E 79th St 1L; New York, NY 10021; (212)
861-6200; **BDCERT:** Oph 76; **MS:** SUNY Hlth Sci
Ctr 69; **RES:** Oph, Mount Sinai Med Ctr, New York,
NY 72-75; **HMO:** Metlife Aetna Hlth Plan Blue
Choice Oxford US Hlthcre +

LANG: Sp; 🦽 🌙 🔒 👥 🏠 $ Mcr   1 Week 🏧 **VISA**
💳 💳

Solomon, Joel (MD) Oph
New York University Med Ctr

530 1st Ave 3B; New York, NY 10016; (212) 263-7537; **BDCERT:** Oph 87; **MS:** Cornell U 81; **RES:** IM, Albany Med Ctr, Albany, NY 81-83; Oph, New York University Med Ctr, New York, NY 83-86; **FEL:** Cornea, Med Coll WI, Milwaukee, WI 86-87; *SI: Laser Surgery for Myopia; Cataract & Corneal Surgery;* **HMO:** Blue Cross & Blue Shield Oxford CIGNA Aetna Hlth Plan

♿ 📷 📺 📺 **S** **Mcr** 2-4 Weeks

Soloway, Barrie D (MD) Oph
New York Eye & Ear Infirmary

160 E 56th St Ste 300; New York, NY 10022; (212) 758-3838; **BDCERT:** Oph 87; **MS:** Penn State U-Hershey Med Ctr 80; **RES:** New York Eye & Ear Infirmary, New York, NY 82-85; **FEL:** New York Eye & Ear Infirmary, New York, NY; **HOSP:** Lenox Hill Hosp; *SI: Glaucoma;* **HMO:** Aetna Hlth Plan Oxford Blue Cross & Blue Shield CIGNA GHI +

LANG: Sp, Hun, Yd, Itl; ♿ ☎ 📷 📺 **S** **Mcr** **Mcd** **WC** **NFI** A Few Days ▨ **VISA** ● □

Spaide, Richard (MD) Oph
St Vincents Hosp & Med Ctr NY

Vitreous Retina Macula Consint, 519 72nd St 203; New York, NY 10011; (212) 861-9797; **BDCERT:** Oph 87; **MS:** Jefferson Med Coll 81; **RES:** St Vincents Hosp & Med Ctr NY, New York, NY 82-85; **FEL:** Manhattan Eye, Ear & Throat Hosp, New York, NY 89-90; **FAP:** Asst Clin Prof Oph NY Med Coll; **HOSP:** Manhattan Eye, Ear & Throat Hosp; *SI: Retinal Diseases; Macular Degeneration;* **HMO:** Oxford GHI US Hlthcre Blue Choice

LANG: Sp; ♿ 📷 📺 📺 **Mcr** **NFI** A Few Days **VISA** ●

Speaker, Mark (MD) Oph
New York Eye & Ear Infirmary

310 E 14th St 401; New York, NY 10003; (212) 260-0600; **BDCERT:** Oph 87; **MS:** Albert Einstein Coll Med 82; **RES:** New York Eye & Ear Infirmary, New York, NY 83-86; **FEL:** Wills Eye Hosp, Philadelphia, PA 86-87; **FAP:** Assoc Clin Prof Oph NY Med Coll; **HOSP:** Beth Israel Med Ctr; *SI: Cornea-External Diseases; Refractive Surgery;* **HMO:** Blue Choice Blue Cross & Blue Shield HIP Network US Hlthcre

LANG: Sp, Fr, Itl; ♿ ☎ 📷 📺 **S** **Mcr** **Mcd** **WC** **NFI** A Few Days **VISA** ●

Starr, Michael (MD) Oph
Lenox Hill Hosp

515 E 79th St; New York, NY 10128; (212) 717-0222; **BDCERT:** Oph 78; **MS:** Mt Sinai Sch Med 72; **RES:** N, Mount Sinai Med Ctr, New York, NY 73; Oph, Lenox Hill Hosp, New York, NY 74-77; **FEL:** Cornea, UC San Francisco Med Ctr, San Francisco, CA; **FAP:** Assoc Mt Sinai Sch Med; **HOSP:** Manhattan Eye, Ear & Throat Hosp; *SI: Refractive Surgery; Corneal-Cataract-Surgery*

LANG: Fr; ♿ 📷 📺 **S** Immediately **VISA** ●

Steele, Mark (MD) Oph
Lenox Hill Hosp

317 E 34th St FL11; New York, NY 10016; (212) 532-0058; **BDCERT:** Oph 91; **MS:** NYU Sch Med 86; **RES:** Oph, New York University Med Ctr, New York, NY 87-90; **FEL:** Ped Oph, Wills Eye Hosp, Philadelphia, PA 90-91; **FAP:** Asst Clin Prof NYU Sch Med; **HOSP:** NYU Downtown Hosp; *SI: Pediatric Ophthalmology;* **HMO:** Oxford Prudential Aetna-US Healthcare Empire Blue Cross & Blue Shield +

Sudarsky, R David (MD)   Oph
Manhattan Eye, Ear & Throat Hosp
4 E 77th St; New York, NY 10021; (212) 288-
1200; **BDCERT:** Oph 58; **MS:** Yale U Sch Med 49;
RES: Med, Grace New Haven Hosp, New Haven, CT
49-51; OrS, Mass Eye & Ear Infirmary, Boston, MA;
FEL: US Naval Med Research Lab, 51-54; Retina,
Mass Eye & Ear Infirmary, Boston, MA 54-56; **FAP:**
Assoc Clin Prof Oph Columbia P&S; **HOSP:** Lenox
Hill Hosp; **SI:** *Macular Degeneration; Retina*; **HMO:**
Blue Choice US Hlthcre Magnacare Physician's
Health Plan Sel Pro +

LANG: Fr; 🔲 🛏 🏧 A Few Days

Teich, Steven (MD)   Oph
Mount Sinai Med Ctr
111 E 80th St 1A; New York, NY 10021; (212)
734-9170; **BDCERT:** Oph 80; **MS:** Boston U 75;
RES: Mount Sinai Med Ctr, New York, NY 79; **FEL:**
Med Retina, Montefiore Med Ctr, Bronx, NY 80-81;
FAP: Assoc Clin Prof Mt Sinai Sch Med; **HOSP:** Beth
Israel Med Ctr; **HMO:** Oxford PHCS Blue Choice

LANG: Prt, Sp; 🦽 🔲 🚗 💲 🏧 Immediately 📠
VISA 💳

Topilow, Harvey (MD)   Oph
New York Eye & Ear Infirmary
1016 5th Ave; New York, NY 10028; (212) 288-
3860; **BDCERT:** Oph 80; **MS:** Columbia P&S 75;
RES: Albert Einstein Med Ctr, Bronx, NY 76-79;
FEL: Mass Eye & Ear Infirmary, Boston, MA 79-81;
FAP: Assoc Clin Prof Oph Albert Einstein Coll Med;
HOSP: Montefiore Med Ctr; **SI:** *Retinal Detachment
Diabetes; Macular Degeneration*; **HMO:** Oxford
Empire Blue Cross & Blue Shield

🦽 🔲 🚗 🛏 💲 🏧 ♿ 🏧 Immediately

Toueg, Elia (MD)   Oph
New York Eye & Ear Infirmary
New York Health Care, 55 E 34th St Fl 2; New
York, NY 10016; (212) 252-6020; **BDCERT:** Oph
73; **MS:** Egypt 50; **RES:** Egypt 51-53; Beth Israel
Med Ctr, New York, NY 69-71; **FEL:** Cairo Univ
Hosp, Cairo, Egypt 56; **FAP:** Asst Prof Mt Sinai Sch
Med; **HOSP:** Mount Sinai Med Ctr; **SI:** *Cataract
Surgery; Glaucoma*; **HMO:** US Hlthcre CIGNA Oxford
Aetna-US Healthcare

LANG: Fr, Ar, Sp; 🦽 🏧 🔲 🚗 🛏 💲 🏧 ♿
A Few Days 📠 **VISA** 💳

Trokel, Stephen (MD)   Oph
Columbia-Presbyterian Med Ctr
16 E 60th St; New York, NY 10021; (212) 305-
5477; **BDCERT:** Oph 67; **MS:** Columbia P&S 65;
RES: Columbia-Presbyterian Med Ctr, New York,
NY 64-66; **HOSP:** Manhattan Eye, Ear & Throat
Hosp; **HMO:** Aetna Hlth Plan Blue Choice Oxford
🦽 🔲 🛏 💲 🏧 🏧 A Few Days **VISA** 💳

Walsh, Joseph (MD)   Oph
New York Eye & Ear Infirmary
310 E 14th St Fl 3, Bldg S; New York, NY 10003;
(212) 979-4447; **BDCERT:** Oph 76; **MS:**
Georgetown U 66; **RES:** Boston U Med Ctr, Boston,
MA 67-68; New York Eye & Ear Infirmary, New
York, NY 70-73; **FEL:** Retina, Montefiore Med Ctr,
Bronx, NY 73-74; **FAP:** Chrmn NY Med Coll;
HOSP: Beth Israel Med Ctr; **SI:** *Retina; Diabetic
Retinopathy*; **HMO:** Blue Choice CIGNA Oxford
LANG: Sp, Itl; 🦽 🔲 🛏 💲 🏧 1 Week

Wang, Frederick (MD)   Oph
New York Eye & Ear Infirmary
30 E 40th St; New York, NY 10016; (718) 548-
7100; **BDCERT:** Oph 80; **MS:** Albert Einstein Coll
Med 72; **RES:** Ped, Jacobi Med Ctr, Bronx, NY 74;
Oph, Albert Einstein Med Ctr, Bronx, NY 79; **FEL:**
Children's Hosp Nat Med Ctr, Washington, DC 80;
FAP: Clin Prof Albert Einstein Coll Med; **HOSP:**
Montefiore Med Ctr; **SI:** *Eye Muscle & Alignment;
Pediatric Eye Disorders*; **HMO:** United Healthcare
Magnacare Aetna-US Healthcare US Hlthcre
Oxford +

LANG: Sp, Ger; 🦽 🔲 🚗 🛏 💲 🏧 2-4 Weeks

Weiss, Michael (MD & PhD) Oph
Columbia-Presbyterian Med Ctr
635 W 165th St; New York, NY 10032; (212)
305-9925; **BDCERT:** Oph 87; **MS:** Columbia P&S
81; **RES:** Columbia-Presbyterian Med Ctr, New
York, NY; **FAP:** Assoc Prof Columbia P&S; **HOSP:**
Manhattan Eye, Ear & Throat Hosp; **HMO:** Oxford
Aetna Hlth Plan Chubb Blue Choice Multiplan +
LANG: Heb; 🦽 🔲 🚗 🛏 🏧

Guide to symbols and abbreviations can be found on pages 110-113.

283

Whitmore, Wayne (MD)   Oph
NY Hosp-Cornell Med Ctr

116 E 68th St; New York, NY 10021; (212) 249-3030; **BDCERT:** Oph 82; **MS:** Dartmouth Med Sch 77; **RES:** Oph, NY Hosp-Cornell Med Ctr, New York, NY 78-81; **FEL:** Oph Onc, NY Hosp-Cornell Med Ctr, New York, NY 81-82; **FAP:** Asst Clin Prof Cornell U; **HOSP:** Manhattan Eye, Ear & Throat Hosp; *SI: Cataract; Glaucoma;* **HMO:** +

LANG: Sp; ♿ ⚅ 🅿 🏥 $ Immediately ▨ **VISA** ⬤

Wisnicki, H Jay (MD)   Oph
Beth Israel Med Ctr

10 Union Square East 4th Ave Ste 3B; New York, NY 10003; (212) 844-8080; **BDCERT:** Oph 87; **MS:** SUNY Hlth Sci Ctr 81; **RES:** Oph, Mount Sinai Med Ctr, New York, NY; **FEL:** Ped Oph, Johns Hopkins Hosp, Baltimore, MD; **HOSP:** Mount Sinai Med Ctr; **HMO:** US Hlthcre Metlife Sanus HIP Network

♿ ⚅ 🅿 🏥 $ Mcr   A Few Days

Wong, Raymond (MD)   Oph
New York Eye & Ear Infirmary

210 Canal St 409; New York, NY 10013; (212) 227-5451; **BDCERT:** Oph 90; **MS:** SUNY Hlth Sci Ctr 84; **RES:** Oph, Yale-New Haven Hosp, New Haven, CT 85-88; **FEL:** Retina Vitreous, UCLA Med Ctr, Los Angeles, CA 88-90; **FAP:** Asst Clin Prof Oph NY Med Coll; **HOSP:** Cabrini Med Ctr; *SI: Diabetic Retinopathy; Retinal Detachment Surgery;* **HMO:** Oxford Blue Cross & Blue Shield Prudential Aetna-US Healthcare PHCS +

♿ 🏧 ☎ ⚅ 🅿 🏥 $ Mcr Mcd   Immediately

Yagoda, Arnold (MD)   Oph
Lenox Hill Hosp

67 E 78th St; New York, NY 10021; (212) 744-2513; **BDCERT:** Oph 80; **MS:** Cornell U 75; **RES:** Med, VA Med Ctr-Manh, New York, NY 75-76; Oph, Lenox Hill Hosp, New York, NY 76-79; **FEL:** Retina, Montefiore Med Ctr, Bronx, NY 79-80; **FAP:** Asst Clin Prof Albert Einstein Coll Med; **HOSP:** Montefiore Med Ctr; *SI: Diabetic Retinopathy; Macular Degeneration;* **HMO:** Oxford GHI Aetna Hlth Plan Blue Cross Guardian +

LANG: Sp, Fr, Heb, Yd; ☎ ⚅ 🅿 🏥 $ Mcr Mcd   1 Week

Yannuzzi, Lawrence (MD)   Oph
Manhattan Eye, Ear & Throat Hosp

VitreousRetina Macula Consultants of NY, 519 E 72nd St 203; New York, NY 10021; (212) 861-9797; **BDCERT:** Oph 70; **MS:** Boston U 63; **RES:** Oph, Manhattan Eye, Ear & Throat Hosp, New York, NY 65-68; **FAP:** Clin Prof Oph Columbia P&S; *SI: Macular Degeneration; Diabetic Retinopathy*

LANG: Sp; ♿ ⚅ 🅿 🏥 $ Mcr   1 Week ▨ **VISA** ⬤

Young, Charles (MD)   Oph
NYU Downtown Hosp

Associate Ophthalmologists, 150 Broadway 1110; New York, NY 10038; (212) 232-2344; **BDCERT:** Oph 87; **MS:** LSU Med Ctr, Shreveport 80; **RES:** Ochsner Fdn Hosp, New Orleans, LA 84; **FAP:** Asst Clin Prof NYU Sch Med; **HMO:** Oxford Affordable Hlth Plan Magnacare Prucare Blue Choice +

♿ ⚅ 🅿 🏥 $ Mcr WC   A Few Days ▨ **VISA** ⬤

Zinn, Keith (MD)   Oph
Manhattan Eye, Ear & Throat Hosp

Manhattan Eye Surgeons, 1044 5th Ave; New York, NY 10028; (212) 535-5030; **BDCERT:** Oph 72; **MS:** SUNY Hlth Sci Ctr 65; **RES:** Oph, Mount Sinai Med Ctr, New York, NY 69-71; **FEL:** Corneal S, Mass Eye & Ear Infirmary, Boston, MA 68-69; Retinal S, Mass Eye & Ear Infirmary, Boston, MA 71-73; **FAP:** Clin Prof Oph Mt Sinai Sch Med; **HOSP:** Mount Sinai Med Ctr; *SI: Diabetic Eye Disease; Cataract and Laser Surgery;* **HMO:** Oxford GHI Aetna-US Healthcare Blue Cross & Blue Shield

LANG: Sp, Grk, Pol, Itl, Fr; ⚅ 🅿 🏥 $ Mcr   Immediately ▨ **VISA** ⬤

Zweifach, Philip (MD)   Oph
Manhattan Eye, Ear & Throat Hosp

131 E 69th St; New York, NY 10021; (212) 535-1508; **BDCERT:** Oph 68; **MS:** Cornell U 61; **RES:** Oph, NY Hosp-Cornell Med Ctr, New York, NY 63-66; N, Boston Med Ctr, Boston, MA 62-63; **FEL:** N/Oph, Mass Eye & Ear Infirmary, Boston, MA 66-67; **FAP:** Assoc Clin Prof Oph Cornell U

ORTHOPAEDIC SURGERY

Adler, Edward (MD)   OrS
Hosp For Joint Diseases
1245 Madison Ave; New York, NY 10128; (212) 427-3986; **BDCERT:** OrS 92; **MS:** UMDNJ-NJ Med Sch, Newark 84; **RES:** UMDNJ-NJ Med Schl, Newark, NJ 85-89; **SI:** *Joint Replacement*
🔲 🔳 ▦ 🆂 Mcr WC NFI A Few Days 🔲 **VISA** 💳

Alexiades, Michael (MD)   OrS
Lenox Hill Hosp
159 E 74th St 2nd FL; New York, NY 10021; (212) 734-1288; **BDCERT:** OrS 91; **MS:** Cornell U 83; **RES:** OrS, Lenox Hill Hosp, New York, NY 84-88; S, Children's Hosp, Boston, MA 86; **FEL:** Arthritis S, Hosp For Special Surgery, New York, NY 88; **FAP:** Asst Prof Cornell U; **HOSP:** Hosp For Special Surgery; **SI:** *Joint Replacement Surgery; Sports Medicine;* **HMO:** Sanus Oxford United Healthcare CIGNA Blue Cross & Blue Shield +
LANG: Grk, Sp; 🔲 🔳 ▦ ▦ 🆂 Mcr WC NFI
A Few Days 🔲 **VISA** 💳

Altchek, David (MD)   OrS
Hosp For Special Surgery
525 E 71st St; New York, NY 10021; (212) 606-1909; **BDCERT:** OrS 90; **MS:** Cornell U 82; **RES:** OrS, Hosp For Special Surgery, New York, NY 83-87; **FEL:** SM, Hosp For Special Surgery, New York, NY 87-88; **FAP:** Asst Prof S Cornell U; **HOSP:** NY Hosp-Cornell Med Ctr; **SI:** *Arthroscopic Surgery; Shoulder, Knee, Elbow*
🔲 🔳 ▦ ▦ 🆂 1 Week 🔲 💳 💳

Andrews, David (MD)   OrS
Columbia-Presbyterian Med Ctr
161 Fort Washington Ave; New York, NY 10032; (212) 305-5226; **BDCERT:** OrS 65; **MS:** Columbia P&S 56; **RES:** Bellevue Hosp Ctr, New York, NY 57-58; Columbia-Presbyterian Med Ctr, New York, NY 58-61; **HOSP:** Hosp For Special Surgery
🔲 🔳 ▦ ▦ 🆂 Mcr WC NFI Immediately

Bauman, Phillip (MD)   OrS
St Luke's Roosevelt Hosp Ctr
Orthopaedic Associates of New York, 343 W 58th St; New York, NY 10019; (212) 765-2260; **BDCERT:** OrS 90; **MS:** Columbia P&S 81; **RES:** St Luke's Roosevelt Hosp Ctr, New York, NY 81-83; OrS, Columbia-Presbyterian Med Ctr, New York, NY 84-87; **HOSP:** Columbia-Presbyterian Med Ctr; **SI:** *Sports Medicine; Reconstructive Surgery;* **HMO:** Aetna Hlth Plan Oxford Blue Choice PHS PHCS +
LANG: Fr, Sp; 🔲 🔳 ▦ ▦ 🆂 Mcr WC A Few Days 🔲 **VISA** 💳

Besser, Walter (MD)   OrS
Hosp For Joint Diseases
300 E 57th St; New York, NY 10022; (212) 486-4308; **BDCERT:** OrS 77; **MS:** Spain 68; **RES:** LI/Brooklyn Jewish Hosp, Brooklyn, NY 71-74; Hosp for Special Surg, New York, NY; **HOSP:** Western Queens Comm Hosp; **SI:** *Total Joint Replacement;* **HMO:** Oxford Aetna-US Healthcare Blue Choice United Healthcare
LANG: Sp, Itl, Fr; 🔲 🅲 🔳 ▦ ▦ Mcr Mod WC
A Few Days

Bigliani, Louis (MD)   OrS
Columbia-Presbyterian Med Ctr
161 Fort Washington Ave; New York, NY 10032; (212) 305-4037; **BDCERT:** OrS 79; **MS:** Loyola U-Stritch Sch Med, Maywood 73; **RES:** S, St Luke's Roosevelt Hosp Ctr, New York, NY 72-74; OrS, Columbia-Presbyterian Med Ctr, New York, NY 74-77; **FEL:** Columbia-Presbyterian Med Ctr, New York, NY 78; **FAP:** Prof OrS Columbia P&S; **SI:** *Shoulder Surgery*
🔲 ▦ 🆂 Mcr 2-4 Weeks

Bonamo, John (MD)   OrS
New York University Med Ctr
530 1st Ave Ste 8U; New York, NY 10016; (212) 263-7352; **BDCERT:** OrS 74; **MS:** NY Med Coll 68; **RES:** S, Staten Island Univ Hosp, Staten Island, NY 68-70; OrS, New York University Med Ctr, New York, NY 70-73; **FEL:** Basel, Switerland; **FAP:** Assoc Prof NYU Sch Med; **SI:** *Knee Arthroscopy; Knee Ligament Reconstruction;* **HMO:** Oxford United Healthcare Prudential Aetna Hlth Plan Health Source +
LANG: Sp; 🔲 ▦ 🔳 ▦ 🆂 Mcr A Few Days

Brisson, Paul (MD)   OrS
Cabrini Med Ctr

942 5th Ave; New York, NY 10021; (212) 734-4504; **BDCERT:** OrS 93; **MS:** U Montreal 79; **RES:** McGill Teaching Hosp, Montreal, Canada 83-87; **FEL:** Hosp For Joint Diseases, New York, NY 88; Spinal S, Buffalo Gen Hosp, Buffalo, NY 89; **HOSP:** New York Methodist Hosp; **HMO:** Oxford CIGNA US Hlthcre Blue Cross HealthNet +

LANG: Fr, Sp; 🔲 🔲 🔲 🔲 **S** 🔲 🔲 🔲 🔲 2-4 Weeks **VISA** ⬤

Bronson, Michael (MD)   OrS
Lenox Hill Hosp

Saga Sports Medical Ctr, 159 E 74th St Fl 2; New York, NY 10021; (212) 734-2646; **BDCERT:** OrS 84; **MS:** NY Med Coll 76; **RES:** OrS, Lenox Hill Hosp, New York, NY 76-80; **FEL:** Hip & Knee S, Columbia-Presbyterian Med Ctr, New York, NY; **SI:** *Joint Replacement; Sports Medicine;* **HMO:** Oxford US Hlthcre CIGNA Aetna Hlth Plan United Healthcare +

LANG: Sp; 🔲 🔲 🔲 🔲 **S** 🔲 🔲 🔲 Immediately

Bryk, Eli (MD)   OrS
Beth Israel Med Ctr

10 Union Square East; New York, NY 10003; (212) 844-8548; **BDCERT:** OrS 90; **MS:** Columbia P&S 82; **RES:** Columbia-Presbyterian Med Ctr, New York, NY 81-84; Columbia-Presbyterian Med Ctr, New York, NY 84-87; **FAP:** Assoc Clin Prof OrS Albert Einstein Coll Med; **HOSP:** Kingsbrook Jewish Med Ctr; **SI:** *Hip & Knee Joint Replacement; Arthroscopic Surgery of Knee;* **HMO:** Aetna-US Healthcare Oxford Blue Cross & Blue Shield Blue Choice United Healthcare +

LANG: Sp, Sgn; 🔲 🔲 🔲 🔲 **S** 🔲 🔲 🔲 Immediately **VISA** ⬤

Burke, Stephen W (MD)   OrS
Hosp For Special Surgery

535 E 70th St; New York, NY 10021; (212) 606-1180; **BDCERT:** OrS 77; **MS:** Cornell U 71; **RES:** OrS, U UT Hosp, Salt Lake City, UT 72-76; **FEL:** LSU Med Ctr, Shreveport, LA 78-79; Children's Hosp, New Orleans, LA 78-80; **FAP:** Assoc Prof OrS Cornell U; **HOSP:** New York University Med Ctr; **SI:** *Pediatric/Adolescent; Clubfoot;* **HMO:** Oxford Blue Cross & Blue Shield United Healthcare Multiplan

🔲 🔲 🔲 🔲 **S** 🔲 A Few Days ⬛ **VISA** ⬤

Capozzi, James (MD)   OrS
Mount Sinai Med Ctr

200 E 62nd St; New York, NY 10021; (212) 758-7444; **BDCERT:** OrS 89; **MS:** Mt Sinai Sch Med 81; **RES:** Mount Sinai Med Ctr, New York, NY 81-86; **FEL:** New England Baptist Hosp, Boston, MA; **HOSP:** St Francis Hosp-Roslyn; **SI:** *Reconstructive Surgery—;* **HMO:** Oxford Aetna Hlth Plan GHI PHCS

🔲 🔲 🔲 🔲 **S** 🔲 🔲 🔲 A Few Days **VISA** ⬤

Casden, Andrew (MD)   OrS
Beth Israel Med Ctr

Spine Institute, 10 Union Square East 5P; New York, NY 10003; (212) 844-8674; **BDCERT:** OrS 91; **MS:** Cornell U 83; **RES:** Hosp For Joint Diseases, New York, NY 84-88; **FEL:** Spine S, Rush Presbyterian-St Lukes Med Ctr, Chicago, IL 88-89; **FAP:** Asst Prof OrS Mt Sinai Sch Med; **SI:** *Scoliosis; Spinal Disorders;* **HMO:** Aetna Hlth Plan Oxford CIGNA

🔲 🔲 🔲 **S** 🔲 🔲 🔲 1 Week ⬛ **VISA** ⬤

Chorney, Gail (MD)   OrS
Hosp For Joint Diseases

301 E 17th St; New York, NY 10003; (212) 598-6211; **BDCERT:** OrS 89; **MS:** Boston U 78; **RES:** OrS, Tufts Univ Hosp, Boston, MA 80-84; S, Baylor Coll Med, Houston, TX 78-80; **FAP:** Asst Prof NYU Sch Med; **HOSP:** New York University Med Ctr; **SI:** *Congenital Anomalies; Pediatric Sports Medicine;* **HMO:** Travelers Oxford Blue Choice Aetna-US Healthcare Magnacare +

LANG: Sp; 🔲 🔲 🔲 🔲 **S** 🔲 Immediately ⬛ **VISA** ⬤ ▦

Cornell, Charles (MD) OrS
Hosp For Special Surgery
535 E 70th St; New York, NY 10021; (212) 606-1414; **BDCERT:** OrS 88; **MS:** Cornell U 80; **RES:** Hosp For Special Surgery, New York, NY 82-85; **FEL:** Trauma, U WA Med Ctr, Seattle, WA 85-86; **HOSP:** NY Hosp Med Ctr of Queens

Craig, Edward V (MD) OrS
Hosp For Special Surgery
The Hosp for Special Surg, 535 E 70th St; New York, NY 10021; (212) 606-1966; **BDCERT:** OrS 84; **MS:** Columbia P&S 73; **RES:** IM, Columbia-Presbyterian Med Ctr, New York, NY 73-76; OrS, Columbia-Presbyterian Med Ctr, New York, NY 77-80; **FEL:** S, Columbia-Presbyterian Med Ctr, New York, NY 80-81; HS, Columbia-Presbyterian Med Ctr, New York, NY 81-82; **FAP:** Prof of Clin S Cornell U; *SI: Shoulder & Sports Med; Arthroscopy & Arthritis;* **HMO:** Empire Blue Cross & Shield United Healthcare Multiplan Health Source PHS +

🔲 🔲 🔲 🔲 🔲 🔲 🔲 🔲 1 Week ▦ **VISA** 🔴

Cuomo, Frances (MD) OrS
Hosp For Joint Diseases
Hospital for Joint Diseases, 301 E 17th St; New York, NY 10003; (212) 598-6183; **BDCERT:** OrS 91; **MS:** NYU Sch Med 83; **RES:** S, Beth Israel Med Ctr, New York, NY; OrS, Lenox Hill Hosp, New York, NY 84-88; **FEL:** OrS, Columbia-Presbyterian Med Ctr, New York, NY 88-89; **FAP:** Asst Prof OrS NYU Sch Med; **HOSP:** New York University Med Ctr; *SI: Shoulder Problems; Elbow Problems;* **HMO:** Empire Blue Cross & Blue Shield Blue Choice GHI Oxford +

LANG: Sp, Rus; 🔲 🔲 🔲 🔲 🔲 🔲 🔲 🔲 Immediately ▦ **VISA** 🔴

Di Cesare, Paul (MD) OrS
Hosp For Joint Diseases
301 E 17th St; New York, NY 10003; (212) 598-6521; **BDCERT:** OrS 94; **MS:** USC Sch Med 86; **RES:** LA Cnty-USC Med Ctr, Los Angeles, CA 86-91; **HOSP:** New York University Med Ctr; *SI: Reconstructive Surgery; Joint Replacement Surgery;* **HMO:** Blue Cross & Blue Shield Magnacare Multiplan 1199 GHI +

Dick, Harold (MD) OrS
Columbia-Presbyterian Med Ctr
161 Fort Washington Ave; New York, NY 10032; (212) 305-5561; **BDCERT:** OrS 68; **MS:** NYU Sch Med 60; **RES:** Columbia-Presbyterian Med Ctr, New York, NY 62-66; Mem Sloan Kettering Cancer Ctr, New York, NY; **FEL:** NY Hosp-Cornell Med Ctr, New York, NY; Microsurgery, Montreal, Canada 77

🔲 🔲 🔲 🔲 🔲 🔲 🔲 Immediately ▦ **VISA** 🔴

Eaton, Richard (MD) OrS
St Luke's Roosevelt Hosp Ctr
1000 10th Ave; New York, NY 10019; (212) 523-7590; **BDCERT:** OrS 66; HS 89; **MS:** Univ Penn 55; **RES:** OrS, Harvard Med Sch, Cambridge, MA 59-62; **FEL:** HS, St Luke's Roosevelt Hosp Ctr, New York, NY; *SI: Joint Reconstruction(Hand); Sports Medicine(Hand);* **HMO:** PHCS

🔲 🔲 🔲 🔲 🔲 Immediately ▦ **VISA** 🔴

Eftekhar, Nas (MD) OrS
Columbia-Presbyterian Med Ctr
Colum-Presby Hosp—Orth Surg, 161 Fort Washington Ave; New York, NY 10032; (212) 305-5368; **BDCERT:** OrS 71; **MS:** Iran 60; **RES:** Johns Hopkins Hosp, Baltimore, MD 63; U, IL Research & Ed Hosp, Chicago, IL; **FEL:** Wrightington Hosp Ctr For Hip Surg, Wrightington, England 67-68; New York Orthopaedic Hosp, New York, NY 69-70

🔲 🔲 🔲 🔲 🔲 🔲 1 Week

El-Dakkak, Mohammed (MD)OrS
Cabrini Med Ctr
Orthopedic Surgery & Sports Medicine, 247 3rd Ave 402; New York, NY 10010; (212) 475-2335; **BDCERT:** OrS 89; **MS:** Egypt 70; **RES:** S, Cabrini Med Ctr, New York, NY 76-79; OrS, Bellevue Hosp Ctr, New York, NY 79-82; **FEL:** SM, New York University Med Ctr, New York, NY; **HOSP:** Hosp For Joint Diseases; *SI: Sports Medicine; Total Joint Re Hip Knee;* **HMO:** Blue Cross & Blue Shield 1199 Well Care

LANG: Sp; 🔲 🔲 🔲 🔲 🔲 🔲 🔲 🔲 1 Week ▦ **VISA** 🔴

Guide to symbols and abbreviations can be found on pages 110-113.

287

Errico, Thomas (MD)　　　OrS
New York University Med Ctr
NYU Medical Ctr, 530 1st Ave 8U; New York, NY 10016; (212) 263-7182; **BDCERT:** OrS 86; **MS:** UMDNJ-NJ Med Sch, Newark 78; **RES:** New York University Med Ctr, New York, NY 79-83; **FEL:** Spinal S, U Toronto Gen Hosp, Toronto, Canada 83-84; **FAP:** Assoc Clin Prof NYU Sch Med; **HOSP:** Overlook Hosp; *SI: Spinal Reconstructive Surgery; Scoliosis;* **HMO:** Oxford Aetna Hlth Plan Blue Cross & Blue Shield CIGNA Prucare +

🦽 📷 🔧 🏥 💲 Mcr WC NFI 2-4 Weeks 🃏 **VISA** 💳

Fabian, Dennis (DO)　　　OrS
St Vincents Hosp & Med Ctr NY
95 University Pl; New York, NY 10003; (212) 604-1350; **BDCERT:** OrS 80; **MS:** Philadelphia Coll Osteo Med 72; **RES:** OS, Metropolitan Hosp Ctr, New York, NY 74-77; S, St Vincents Hosp & Med Ctr NY, New York, NY 72-74; **FEL:** S, Hosp For Special Surgery, New York, NY 77-78; **HMO:** Oxford Blue Choice Prucare Guardian

Feldman, Robert (MD)　　　OrS
Hosp For Joint Diseases
1317 3rd Ave Fl 7; New York, NY 10021; (212) 570-6600; **BDCERT:** OrS 88; **MS:** SUNY Hlth Sci Ctr 78; **RES:** S, Lenox Hill Hosp, New York, NY 78-79; OrS, Hosp For Joint Diseases, New York, NY 79-83; **FEL:** Foot & Ankle, Hosp For Special Surgery, New York, NY 83; **FAP:** Asst Clin Prof NYU Sch Med; **HOSP:** Cabrini Med Ctr; *SI: Foot & Ankle; Arthroscopy & Sports Med;* **HMO:** Prucare NYLCare CIGNA US Hlthcre Oxford +

LANG: Fr, Man, Jpn, Can; 🦽 📞 📷 🔧 🏥 💲 Mcr WC NFI Immediately 🃏 **VISA** 💳

Ferriter, Pierce (MD)　　　OrS
Lenox Hill Hosp
1160 Park Ave; New York, NY 10128; (212) 249-8144; **BDCERT:** OrS 88; **MS:** UMDNJ-RW Johnson Med Sch 79; **RES:** Lenox Hill Hosp, New York, NY 80; OrS, Lenox Hill Hosp, New York, NY 79-85; **FEL:** Spine, Buffalo Gen Hosp, Buffalo, NY 85-86; **HMO:** Oxford Blue Choice

🦽 📞 📷 🔧 🏥 💲 Mcr WC NFI Immediately 🃏 **VISA** 💳

Figgie, Mark (MD)　　　OrS
Hosp For Special Surgery
535 E 70th St 337; New York, NY 10021; (212) 606-1932; **BDCERT:** OrS 90; **MS:** Case West Res U 81; **RES:** OrS, U Hosp of Cleveland, Cleveland, OH 81-86; **FEL:** Biomechanics, Hosp For Special Surgery, New York, NY 86; OrS, Hosp For Special Surgery, New York, NY 87-88; **FAP:** Instr Cornell U; **HOSP:** NY Hosp-Cornell Med Ctr; *SI: Total Joint Replacement; Shoulder and Elbow Surgery;* **HMO:** Oxford PHCS PHS United Healthcare Health Source +

LANG: Sp; 🦽 📷 🔧 🏥 💲 Mcr WC NFI 1 Week

Flatow, Evan (MD)　　　OrS
Columbia-Presbyterian Med Ctr
161 Fort Washington Ave; New York, NY 10032; (212) 305-5599; **BDCERT:** OrS 89; **MS:** Columbia P&S 81; **RES:** S, St Luke's Roosevelt Hosp Ctr, New York, NY 82-83; OrS, Columbia-Presbyterian Med Ctr, New York, NY 83-85; **FEL:** Shoulder, Columbia-Presbyterian Med Ctr, New York, NY 86-87; **FAP:** Prof Columbia P&S; *SI: Shoulder Surgery;* **HMO:** Oxford CIGNA Blue Choice

🦽 📷 🔧 🏥 💲 Mcr WC NFI 2-4 Weeks

Frankel, Victor H (MD)　　　OrS
Hosp For Joint Diseases
301 E 17th St; New York, NY 10003; (212) 598-6523; **BDCERT:** OrS 61; **MS:** Univ Penn 51; **RES:** S, Charlotte Mem Hosp, Charlotte, NC 55; Hosp For Joint Diseases, New York, NY 58; **FEL:** Biomechanics, U of Uppsala, Uppsala, Sweden 60; *SI: Total Hip & Knee Joint Replacement*

LANG: Sp, Swd; 🦽 📷 🔧 🏥 Mcr WC NFI A Few Days **VISA**

Giannaris, Theodore (MD)　　　OrS
St Clare's Hosp & Health Ctr
901 5th Ave; New York, NY 10021; (212) 879-0307; **BDCERT:** OrS 77; **MS:** Greece 65; **RES:** OrS, St Vincents Hosp & Med Ctr NY, New York, NY 73-74; NY Polyclinic Hosp, New York, NY 72-75; **FEL:** St Giles Hosp For Crippled Children, Brooklyn, NY 74; **FAP:** Clin Instr NY Med Coll; **HOSP:** Western Queens Comm Hosp; *SI: Fractures Joint Replacement; Arthroscopy;* **HMO:** Oxford Blue Cross & Blue Choice Aetna Hlth Plan

🦽 📷 🏥 💲 Mcr Mod WC NFI 2-4 Weeks

Gilbert, Marvin (MD)   OrS
Mount Sinai Med Ctr
1100 Park Ave; New York, NY 10128; (212) 289-0700; **BDCERT:** OrS 72; **MS:** Columbia P&S 64; **RES:** OrS, Mount Sinai Med Ctr, New York, NY 65-69; **FAP:** Assoc Clin Prof Med Mt Sinai Sch Med; **HOSP:** Beth Israel North; **SI:** *Joint Replacement; Reconstructive Surgery*

LANG: Sp, Fr; 🦽 📷 🛏 Mcr WC NFI   1 Week **VISA** 💳

Glickel, Steven (MD)   OrS
St Luke's Roosevelt Hosp Ctr
1000 10th Ave; New York, NY 10019; (212) 523-7590; **BDCERT:** OrS 85; HS 89; **MS:** Harvard Med Sch 76; **RES:** S, Columbia-Presbyterian Med Ctr, New York, NY 76-78; OrS, Harvard Comb Ortho Prgm, Boston, MA 78-81; **FEL:** HS, Columbia-Presbyterian Med Ctr, New York, NY 81-82; St Luke's Roosevelt Hosp Ctr, New York, NY 82-83; **FAP:** Asst Clin Prof Columbia P&S; **HOSP:** Beth Israel North; **SI:** *Hand/Wrist; Elbow;* **HMO:** Aetna Hlth Plan Chubb Oxford Prucare Magnacare +

LANG: Sp, Chi; 🦽 📷 🛏 🛏 S Mcr Mod WC   A Few Days 💳 **VISA** 💳

Goodwin, Charles (MD)   OrS
Hosp For Special Surgery
New York Physcians P C, 635 Madison Ave; New York, NY 10022; (212) 317-4600; **BDCERT:** OrS 85; **MS:** U Cincinnati 76; **RES:** S, St Luke's Roosevelt Hosp Ctr, New York, NY 76-79; OrS, Columbia-Presbyterian Med Ctr, New York, NY 79-82; **FEL:** Spine S, Univ of Toronto, Toronto, Canada 82-83; **FAP:** Asst Prof OrS Cornell U; **HOSP:** St Luke's Roosevelt Hosp Ctr; **SI:** *Sports Medicine; Spine Surgery;* **HMO:** Oxford

🦽 📷 🛏 🛏 S Mcr   A Few Days 💳 **VISA** 💳

Grant, Alfred (MD)   OrS
Hosp For Joint Diseases
301 E 17th St 310; New York, NY 10003; (212) 598-6605; **BDCERT:** OrS 66; **MS:** U Hlth Sci/Chicago Med Sch 57; **RES:** Hosp For Joint Diseases, New York, NY 62; Montefiore Med Ctr, Bronx, NY 59; **FAP:** Clin Prof OrS NYU Sch Med; **HOSP:** New York University Med Ctr; **SI:** *Pediatric Orthopaedics; Neuromuscular Diseases;* **HMO:** HIP Network Oxford United Healthcare Chubb Multiplan +

LANG: Hin, Sp, Yd; 🦽 📷 🛏 🛏 S WC NFI   1 Week 💳 **VISA** 💳 💳

Green, Steven (MD)   OrS
Mount Sinai Med Ctr
2 E 88th St; New York, NY 10128; (212) 348-6644; **BDCERT:** OrS 77; HS 89; **MS:** Albert Einstein Coll Med 70; **RES:** OrS, Mount Sinai Med Ctr, New York, NY 72-75; **FEL:** HS, Thomas Jefferson U Hosp, Philadelphia, PA 77-78; **HOSP:** Hosp For Joint Diseases; **SI:** *Hand Surgery;* **HMO:** Oxford PHCS HIP Network

📷 🛏 🛏 S WC NFI   Immediately

Haher, Thomas R (MD)   OrS
St Vincents Hosp & Med Ctr NY
36 7th Ave 502; New York, NY 10028; (212) 604-3990; **BDCERT:** OrS 86; **MS:** NY Med Coll 75; **RES:** OrS, NY Med Coll, New York, NY 75-80; **FEL:** Ped OrS, Shriners Hosp, Chicago, IL 80-81; Scoliosis, Rush Presbyterian-St Lukes Med Ctr, Chicago, IL 81-82; **FAP:** Prof NY Med Coll; **HOSP:** Long Island Coll Hosp; **SI:** *Scoliosis; Low Back Pain;* **HMO:** Oxford Empire GHI US Hlthcre Blue Choice +

LANG: Sp; 🦽 📞 📷 🛏 🛏 S Mcr Mod WC NFI   A Few Days

Hamilton, William (MD) OrS
St Luke's Roosevelt Hosp Ctr

Orthopaedic Associates of NY, 343 W 58th St; New York, NY 10019; (212) 765-2260; **BDCERT:** OrS 71; **MS:** Columbia P&S 64; **RES:** St Luke's Roosevelt Hosp Ctr, New York, NY 65-66; OrS, Columbia-Presbyterian Med Ctr, New York, NY 66-69; **FEL:** Newington Children's Hosp, Newington, CT 69-70; Newington Children's Hosp, Newington, CT; **FAP:** Clin Prof OrS Columbia P&S; **HOSP:** Beth Israel North; **SI:** *Sports Medicine Foot/Ankle; Ballet Dancers-Surgery*

LANG: Sp, Fr; 🚹 🔒 👥 🛏 $ WC 2-4 Weeks 📧 **VISA** 💳

Hannafin, Jo (MD & PhD) OrS
Hosp For Special Surgery

523 E 72nd St 3rd Floor; New York, NY 10021; (212) 606-1469; **BDCERT:** OrS 94; **MS:** Albert Einstein Coll Med 85; **RES:** S, Montefiore Med Ctr, Bronx, NY 86-90; OrS, Montefiore Med Ctr, Bronx, NY 90-91; **FEL:** SM, Hosp For Special Surgery, New York, NY; **FAP:** Asst Prof Cornell U; **HOSP:** NY Hosp-Cornell Med Ctr; **SI:** *Female Athlete; Sports Medicine;* **HMO:** Aetna Hlth Plan Oxford PHCS Blue Choice PHS +

LANG: Sp; 🚹 🔒 👥 🛏 $ Mcr WC NFi Immediately 📧 **VISA** 💳

Harwin, Steven F (MD) OrS
Beth Israel North

Park Avenue Center for Reconstructive Joint Surgery, 910 Park Ave; New York, NY 10021; (212) 861-9800; **BDCERT:** OrS 76; **MS:** SUNY Hlth Sci Ctr 71; **RES:** Albert Einstein Med Ctr, Bronx, NY 75; **FAP:** Asst Prof Albert Einstein Coll Med; **SI:** *Total Joint Replacement; Sports Surgery Arthroscopy;* **HMO:** Aetna Hlth Plan Oxford PHS GHI CIGNA +

LANG: Sp; 🚹 🔒 👥 🛏 $ Mcr WC NFi 1 Week

Hausman, Michael (MD) OrS
Mount Sinai Med Ctr

5 E 98th St; New York, NY 10029; (212) 241-1658; **BDCERT:** OrS 89; HS 90; **MS:** Yale U Sch Med 79; **RES:** Yale-New Haven Hosp, New Haven, CT 82-85; **FEL:** HS, St Luke's Roosevelt Hosp Ctr, New York, NY; **HOSP:** Manhattan Eye, Ear & Throat Hosp; **SI:** *Microvascular Reconstruction; Elbow Problems*

LANG: Sp, Heb, Itl; 🚹 🛏 $ Mcr WC 📧

Healey, John (MD) OrS
Mem Sloan Kettering Cancer Ctr

1275 York Ave 61; New York, NY 10021; (212) 639-7610; **BDCERT:** OrS 86; **MS:** Univ Vt Coll Med 78; **RES:** OrS, Hosp for Special Surgery, New York, NY 79-83; **FEL:** OrS Onc, Mem Sloan Kettering Cancer Ctr, New York, NY 83-84; OrS, Hosp For Special Surgery, New York, NY 83-84; **FAP:** Assoc Prof OrS Cornell U; **HOSP:** Hosp For Special Surgery; **SI:** *Bone and Soft Tissue Tumor Sarcoma*

🚹 🌙 🔒 👥 🛏 Mcr 2-4 Weeks **VISA** 💳

Helfet, David L (MD) OrS
Hosp For Special Surgery

535 E 70th St; New York, NY 10021; (212) 606-1888; **BDCERT:** OrS 84; **MS:** Africa 75; **RES:** S, Edendale Hospital, Pietermaritzburg, South Africa 75-77; OrS, Johns Hopkins Hosp, Baltimore, MD 77-81; **FEL:** Trauma Arthroplasty, Inselspital, Bern, Switzerland 81; SM, UCLA Med Ctr, Los Angeles, CA 81-82; **FAP:** Assoc Prof Cornell U; **HOSP:** NY Hosp-Cornell Med Ctr; **SI:** *Complex Fractures; Unhealed Fractures;* **HMO:** Oxford

LANG: Fr, Sp, Grk, Rus, Itl; 🚹 🔒 🛏 $ Mcr WC NFi Immediately

Hershman, Elliott (MD) OrS
Lenox Hill Hosp

Manhattan Orthopaedics, 130 E 77th St Fl 8; New York, NY 10021; (212) 744-8114; **BDCERT:** OrS 87; OrS 97; **MS:** U Rochester 79; **RES:** OrS, Lenox Hill Hosp, New York, NY 79-84; **FEL:** SM, Cleveland Clinic Hosp, Cleveland, OH; **SI:** *Arthroscopic Knee Surgery; Knee Ligament Injuries;* **HMO:** Oxford United Healthcare Chubb

🚹 🔒 🛏 $ Mcr WC Immediately 📧 **VISA** 💳

Hotchkiss, Robert (MD)   OrS
Hosp For Special Surgery

535 E 70th St; New York, NY 10021; (212) 606-1964; **BDCERT:** OrS 89; **MS:** Johns Hopkins U 80; **RES:** S, Johns Hopkins Hosp, Baltimore, MD 82; OrS, Johns Hopkins Hosp, Baltimore, MD 82-85; **FEL:** OrS, Johns Hopkins Hosp, Baltimore, MD 81; Hand/Microvascular S, Union Mem Hosp, Baltimore, MD 86-87; **FAP:** Asst Lecturer S Cornell U; **HOSP:** NY Hosp-Cornell Med Ctr; *SI: Hand/Wrist/Elbow; Microvascular Surgery*

LANG: Rus; ♿ 🅿 👤 🛏 $ Mcr WC NFI 2-4 Weeks
AMEX VISA ●

Inglis, Allan (MD)   OrS
Beth Israel North

1725 York Ave; New York, NY 10128; (212) 410-2379; **BDCERT:** OrS 63; **MS:** U Rochester 54; **RES:** Hosp For Special Surgery, New York, NY 56-60; **FEL:** Mem Sloan Kettering Cancer Ctr, New York, NY; HS, Hosp For Special Surgery, New York, NY 61-62; **FAP:** Prof Cornell U; **HOSP:** Hosp For Special Surgery; *SI: Joint Replacement; Arthritis Surgery*; **HMO:** Blue Choice Independent Health Plan

LANG: Sp; ♿ 🅿 👤 🛏 Mcr WC NFI Immediately

Insall, John (MD)   OrS
Beth Israel North

170 East End Ave; New York, NY 10128; (212) 870-9760; **BDCERT:** OrS 68; **MS:** England 56; **RES:** Shriners Hosp For Crippled Children, Montreal, Canada; Royal Victoria Hosp, Montreal, Canada; **FEL:** Hosp For Special Surgery, New York, NY; Royal National Orthopaedic Hosp, London, England

♿ 🅿 🛏 Mcr NFI Immediately

Jaffe, Fredrick (MD)   OrS
Beth Israel Med Ctr

401 E 55th St; New York, NY 10022; (212) 759-5500; **BDCERT:** OrS 74; **MS:** Tufts U 68; **RES:** S, NY Hosp-Cornell Med Ctr, New York, NY 68-70; OrS, Hosp For Joint Diseases, New York, NY 70-73; **FEL:** Hosp For Joint Diseases, New York, NY 74; **FAP:** Asst Prof of Clin OrS Mt Sinai Sch Med; *SI: Hip Replacement; Knee Replacement*; **HMO:** Aetna Hlth Plan Oxford US Hlthcre Prucare Blue Cross & Blue Shield +

LANG: Sp; ♿ 🅿 👤 🛏 $ Mcr WC NFI A Few Days
AMEX VISA ● 🅿

Jaffe, William (MD)   OrS
Hosp For Joint Diseases

JNR Sports Medcine, 1095 Park Ave; New York, NY 10128; (212) 427-7750; **BDCERT:** OrS 72; **MS:** Temple U 63; **RES:** OrS, Hosp For Joint Diseases, New York, NY 65-69; **FEL:** S, Centre for HIP Surg, Wigan, Eng 69-70; S, Harvard Med Sch, Cambridge, MA 69-70; **FAP:** Clin Prof NYU Sch Med; *SI: Total Hip Surgery; Knee Surgery*; **HMO:** United Healthcare Aetna-US Healthcare Oxford Empire Blue Choice PHCS +

♿ 🅿 👤 🛏 $ Mcr WC NFI 1 Week **VISA** ●

Kelly, Michael (MD)   OrS
Beth Israel North

170 East End Ave Fl 4; New York, NY 10128; (212) 870-9747; **BDCERT:** OrS 88; **MS:** Georgetown U 79; **RES:** S, St Vincents Hosp & Med Ctr NY, New York, NY 79-81; OrS, Columbia-Presbyterian Med Ctr, New York, NY 81-84; **FEL:** Hosp For Special Surgery, New York, NY 84-85; **FAP:** Asst Prof Albert Einstein Coll Med; **HOSP:** Beth Israel Med Ctr; *SI: Knee Sports Injuries; Total Knee Replacement*; **HMO:** Oxford Aetna Hlth Plan United Healthcare CIGNA PHS +

♿ 🅿 👤 🛏 $ Mcr WC NFI A Few Days

Kenan, Samuel (MD)   OrS
Hosp For Joint Diseases

301 E 17th St; New York, NY 10003; (212) 598-6350; **MS:** Israel 76; **RES:** Hadassah Hosp, Jerusalem, Israel 78-84; **FEL:** OrS, Hosp For Joint Diseases, New York, NY 85-87; **HOSP:** New York University Med Ctr

♿ SA/SU 🅿 🛏 $ Mcr Mcd

Kiernan, Howard (MD)   OrS
Columbia-Presbyterian Med Ctr

161 Fort Washington Ave Rm211; New York, NY 10032; (212) 305-5241; **BDCERT:** OrS 75; **MS:** NYU Sch Med 66; **RES:** Columbia-Presbyterian Med Ctr, New York, NY 70-73; **HMO:** Blue Cross & Blue Shield PHS PHS Prudential

Guide to symbols and abbreviations can be found on pages 110-113.

291

Koval, Kenneth (MD)   OrS
Hosp For Joint Diseases

301 E 17th St; New York, NY 10003; (212) 598-6137; **BDCERT:** OrS 92; **MS:** NYU Sch Med 84; **RES:** Hosp For Joint Diseases, NY, NY 85-89; **FEL:** OrS, Tampa Gen Hosp, Tampa, FL; **FAP:** Asst Prof NYU Sch Med; **SI:** *Orthopaedic Traumatology; Reconstructive Surgery;* **HMO:** HIP Network US Hlthcre Oxford

LANG: Sp; 🖥 🏠 🛏 💲 Mcr Mcd WC NFI   Immediately
VISA 💳

Krinick, Ronald M (MD)   OrS
NYU Downtown Hosp

Seaport Orthopaedic Associates, 19 Beekman St; New York, NY 10038; (212) 513-7711; **BDCERT:** OrS 97; **MS:** NYU Sch Med 79; **RES:** OrS, New York University Med Ctr, New York, NY 80-84; Southwestern Orth Med Group, Inglewood, CA; **FEL:** SM, New York University Med Ctr, New York, NY 84; **FAP:** Assoc Clin Prof OrS NYU Sch Med; **HOSP:** Hosp For Joint Diseases; **SI:** *Sports Medicine; Orthopaedic Surgery;* **HMO:** Aetna-US Healthcare Oxford Prudential CIGNA United Healthcare +

LANG: Sp, Chi, Rus, Ger; 🖥 🏠 🛏 💲 Mcr WC NFI
A Few Days

Kuflik, Paul (MD)   OrS
Beth Israel Med Ctr

10 Union Square East 4E; New York, NY 10003; (212) 598-6796; **BDCERT:** OrS 89; **MS:** SUNY Hlth Sci Ctr 81; **RES:** OrS, Hosp For Joint Diseases, New York, NY 82-86; **FEL:** Spine S, Toronto Gen Hosp, Toronto, Canada 86; **HMO:** Oxford US Hlthcre Choicecare Aetna Hlth Plan +

LANG: Heb, Sp, Rus; 🖥 🏠 🛏 💲 Mcr WC NFI   2-4 Weeks **VISA** 💳

Laskin, Richard (MD)   OrS
Hosp For Special Surgery

535 E 70th St; New York, NY 10021; (212) 606-1041; **BDCERT:** OrS 72; **MS:** NYU Sch Med 64; **RES:** S, Bronx Muncipal Hosp Ctr, Bronx, NY 64-66; OrS, Albert Einstein Med Ctr, Bronx, NY 68-71; **FAP:** Prof Cornell U; **SI:** *Total Knee Replacement; Total Hip Replacement;* **HMO:** Oxford Aetna Hlth Plan United Healthcare Blue Choice PHS +

LANG: Can, Sp; 🖥 🏠 🛏 🛏 💲 Mcr   A Few Days

Lehman, Wallace B (MD)   OrS
Hosp For Joint Diseases

Hosp for Joint DiseasesChief, Ped Orth Surgery, 301 E 17th St Rm 835; New York, NY 10003; (212) 598-6403; **BDCERT:** OrS 66; **MS:** SUNY Hlth Sci Ctr 58; **RES:** Hosp For Joint Diseases, New York, NY 58-63; **FAP:** Clin Prof OrS NYU Sch Med; **HOSP:** Beth Israel Med Ctr; **SI:** *Pediatric Orthopedic Surgery*

LANG: Heb, Yd; 🖥 🏠 🛏 💲   Immediately 💳
VISA 💳

Lenzo, Salvatore (MD)   OrS
Hosp For Joint Diseases

207 E 16th St 21; New York, NY 10003; (212) 529-2052; **BDCERT:** OrS 88; **MS:** NYU Sch Med 81; **RES:** OrS, Bellevue Hosp Ctr, New York, NY 82-86; **FEL:** S, Bellevue Hosp Ctr, New York, NY 86-87; **FAP:** Assoc Prof OrS NYU Sch Med; **HOSP:** New York University Med Ctr; **SI:** *Carpal Tunnel Syndrome; Arthritis;* **HMO:** Oxford United Healthcare Prucare United Healthcare

LANG: Sp, Itl; 🖥 🏠 🛏 🛏 💲 Mcr Mcd WC NFI
Immediately 💳 **VISA** 💳

Levy, Howard (MD)   OrS
Beth Israel Med Ctr

401 E 55th St; New York, NY 10022; (212) 759-5500; **BDCERT:** OrS 93; HS 94; **MS:** SUNY Hlth Sci Ctr 83; **RES:** OrS, U Miami Hosp, Miami, FL 84-89; **FEL:** SM, U of Alabama Hosp, Birmington, AL 89; HS, St Luke's Roosevelt Hosp Ctr, New York, NY 90; **FAP:** Clin Instr OrS Albert Einstein Coll Med; **SI:** *Arthroscopy; Sports Injuries;* **HMO:** Oxford CIGNA Metlife Aetna Hlth Plan Guardian +

LANG: Sp; 🖥 📞 🏠 🛏 🛏 💲 WC NFI   Immediately 💳

Levy, Roger (MD)   OrS
Mount Sinai Med Ctr

Dept of Orthopaedics, Mount Sinai Med Ctr, 58 98th St 9th Fl; New York, NY 10029; (212) 241-7080; **BDCERT:** OrS 67; **MS:** SUNY Downstate 59; **RES:** OrS, Mount Sinai Med Ctr, New York, NY 59-64; **FEL:** S, Mount Sinai Med Ctr, New York, NY 65; **SI:** *Joint Replacement; Arthroscopic Surgery;* **HMO:** Aetna Hlth Plan US Hlthcre Oxford Premier PHCS +

🖥 🏠 🛏 🛏 💲 Mcr Mcd WC NFI   A Few Days **VISA** 💳

Lichtblau, Sheldon (MD)   OrS
Mount Sinai Med Ctr

5 E 98th St 9th Fl; New York, NY 10029; (212) 241-4049; **BDCERT:** OrS 62; **MS:** U Hlth Sci/Chicago Med Sch 53; **RES:** S, VA Med Ctr-Bronx, Bronx, NY 55-56; OrS, Hosp For Special Surgery, New York, NY 56-59; *SI: Geriatric Orthopedics; Hip Fractures;* **HMO:** Aetna Hlth Plan Blue Cross PPO Oxford US Hlthcre Affordable Hlth Plan +

🚳 ☎ ♿ 🏧 S Mcr Mcd WC NFI Immediately ▦
VISA 💳

Lubliner, Jerry (MD)   OrS
Hosp For Joint Diseases

215 E 73rd St # 1C; New York, NY 10021; (212) 249-8200; **BDCERT:** N 88; OrS 88; **MS:** SUNY Hlth Sci Ctr 81; **RES:** Beth Israel Med Ctr, NY, NY 81; Hosp For Joint Diseases, New York, NY 81-85; **FEL:** SM, U West Ontario, Ottawa, Canada 85; **HOSP:** Beth Israel North; *SI: Knee & Shoulder Surgery; Sports Medicine;* **HMO:** Oxford Aetna Hlth Plan Prucare Blue Choice CIGNA +

🚳 ☎ ♿ 🏧 Mcr WC NFI Immediately ▦ **VISA** 💳
💳

McCann, Peter (MD)   OrS
Beth Israel North

170 East End Ave Fl 4; New York, NY 10128; (212) 870-9764; **BDCERT:** OrS 88; **MS:** Columbia P&S 80; **RES:** S, St Vincents Hosp & Med Ctr NY, New York, NY 80-82; OrS, Columbia-Presbyterian Med Ctr, New York, NY 82-85; **FEL:** Shoulder & Elbow S, Columbia-Presbyterian Med Ctr, New York, NY; **FAP:** Asst Clin Prof OrS Albert Einstein Coll Med; *SI: Rotator Cuff Injury; Shoulder Dislocations;* **HMO:** CIGNA HIP Network Prucare Oxford Guardian +

📞 ☎ 🏧 Mcr NFI A Few Days ▦ **VISA**

Melone Jr, Charles P (MD)   OrS
Beth Israel Med Ctr

317 E 34th St 3rd Fl; New York, NY 10016; (212) 683-4263; **BDCERT:** OrS 93; **MS:** Georgetown U 69; **RES:** S, Nassau County Med Ctr, East Meadow, NY 70-71; OrS, Nassau County Med Ctr, East Meadow, NY 71-74; **FEL:** HS, New York University Med Ctr, New York, NY 74-75; **FAP:** Prof OrS NYU Sch Med; **HOSP:** New York University Med Ctr; *SI: Reconstruction of Arthritic Hand; Fractures of Hand & Wrist;* **HMO:** Chubb Oxford CIGNA PHS +

LANG: Sp; 🚳 ☎ ♿ 🏧 S Mcr WC NFI 1 Week ▦
VISA 💳

Menche, David (MD)   OrS
Hosp For Joint Diseases

Hosp Joint Dis Orth Inst,Sport Ctr, 303 2nd Ave 3; New York, NY 10003; (212) 598-6484; **BDCERT:** OrS 97; **MS:** NYU Sch Med 79; **RES:** OrS, Hosp For Joint Diseases, New York, NY 80-84; **FEL:** SM, Gothenburg, Sweden 84-85; **FAP:** Asst Prof of Clin OrS NYU Sch Med; **HOSP:** New York Methodist Hosp; *SI: Knee Surgery; Orthopaedic Reconstruction;* **HMO:** Guardian Blue Choice CIGNA Oxford +

LANG: Sp; 🚳 📞 ☎ ♿ 🏧 S Mcr WC NFI 1 Week ▦
VISA 💳 💳

Mendoza, Francis (MD)   OrS
Lenox Hill Hosp

159 E 74th St; New York, NY 10021; (212) 628-9600; **BDCERT:** OrS 84; **MS:** Columbia P&S 76; **RES:** OrS, Columbia-Presbyterian Med Ctr, New York, NY 78-81; S, St Luke's Roosevelt Hosp Ctr, New York, NY 76-78; **FEL:** Columbia-Presbyterian Med Ctr, New York, NY 81-86; *SI: Shoulder/Elbow/Surgery; Sports Medicine;* **HMO:** None

🚳 ☎ 🏧 S Mcr WC NFI 2-4 Weeks

Minkoff, Jeffrey (MD)   OrS
Beth Israel Med Ctr

333 E 56th St; New York, NY 10022; (212) 319-6500; **BDCERT:** OrS 73; **MS:** SUNY Downstate 67; **RES:** S, Bronx Muni Hosp, Bronx, NY 68-69; OrS, Lenox Hill Hosp, New York, NY 69-71; **FAP:** Assoc Clin Prof Med NYU Sch Med; **HOSP:** Lenox Hill Hosp; **HMO:** Oxford Chubb

LANG: Sp; 🚳 ☎ ♿ 🏧 S Mcr NFI A Few Days ▦
VISA 💳

Guide to symbols and abbreviations can be found on pages 110-113.

293

Moskovich, Ronald (MD)   OrS
Hosp For Joint Diseases

301 E 17th St; New York, NY 10003; (212) 598-6622; **BDCERT:** OrS 91; **MS:** South Africa 78; **RES:** St George's Hosp, London, England 80-84; Hosp For Joint Diseases, New York, NY 84-88; **FEL:** UC Davis Med Ctr, Sacramento, CA 88; Natl Hosp For Neurology, London, England 89; **FAP:** Asst Prof NYU Sch Med; **HOSP:** New York University Med Ctr; **SI:** *Spinal Deformity; Spinal Injury;* **HMO:** Oxford Independent Health Plan

♿ 📷 🚗 🛏 **S** Mcr WC NFI 2-4 Weeks ▤ **VISA** ◉

Neuwirth, Michael (MD)   OrS
Beth Israel Med Ctr

Beth Israel Med Ctr - Spine Institute,; New York, NY 10003; (212) 844-8680; **BDCERT:** OrS 80; **MS:** SUNY Hlth Sci Ctr 74; **RES:** OrS, Hosp For Joint Diseases, New York, NY 77-78; **FEL:** Rush Presbyterian-St Lukes Med Ctr, Chicago, IL; **HOSP:** New York University Med Ctr; **HMO:** US Hlthcre HIP Network Oxford

♿ 📷 🚗 🛏 **S** WC NFI A Few Days ▤ **VISA** ◉ ▤

Nicholas, James (MD)   OrS
Lenox Hill Hosp

130 E 77th St; New York, NY 10021; (212) 737-3301; **BDCERT:** OrS 55; **MS:** SUNY Downstate 45; **RES:** Lenox Hill, New York, NY 45-46; Staten Island Hospital, Staten Island, NY 49-50; **FEL:** Shriners Hospital, Chicago, IL 48-50; **FAP:** Prof of Clin Med Cornell U; **HOSP:** Hosp For Special Surgery; **SI:** *Sports Medicine; Knee Surgery;* **HMO:** None

LANG: Grk, Sp; ♿ 📷 🚗 🛏 Mcr Mcd A Few Days

Nicholas, Stephen (MD)   OrS
Lenox Hill Hosp

130 E 77th St; New York, NY 10021; (212) 737-3301; **BDCERT:** OrS 94; **MS:** NY Med Coll 86; **RES:** OrS, Hosp For Special Surgery, New York, NY 87-91; **FEL:** SM, Lenox Hill Hosp, New York, NY 91-92; **SI:** *Knee Surgery; Shoulder Surgery;* **HMO:** Oxford United Healthcare Magnacare US Hlthcre Blue Choice +

LANG: Grk, Sp; ♿ 📷 🚗 🛏 **S** Mcr WC NFI 2-4 Weeks ▤ **VISA** ◉

Nisonson, Barton (MD)   OrS
Lenox Hill Hosp

130 E 77th St; New York, NY 10021; (212) 570-9120; **BDCERT:** OrS 74; **MS:** Columbia P&S 66; **RES:** Columbia-Presbyterian Med Ctr, New York, NY 70-73; **FEL:** Columbia-Presbyterian Med Ctr, New York, NY 72-73; **SI:** *Knee Surgery; Shoulder Surgery;* **HMO:** PHCS Sel Pro

♿ 📷 🚗 🛏 **S** 1 Week

O'Brien, Stephen J (MD)   OrS
Hosp For Special Surgery

Hosp For Special Surgery—Orth Surgery, 535 E 70th St; New York, NY 10021; (212) 606-1011; **BDCERT:** OrS 89; **MS:** U Va Sch Med 81; **RES:** OrS, Hosp For Special Surgery, New York, NY 82-86; **FEL:** SM, Hosp For Special Surgery, New York, NY 86-87; **FAP:** Assoc Prof OrS Cornell U; **HMO:** PHCS Chubb

LANG: Sp; ♿ 🅐 📷 🚗 🛏 **S** Mcr WC NFI 2-4 Weeks **VISA** ◉

O'Leary, Patrick (MD)   OrS
Lenox Hill Hosp

1160 Park Ave; New York, NY 10128; (212) 249-8100; **BDCERT:** OrS 76; **MS:** Ireland 68; **RES:** St Luke's Roosevelt Hosp Ctr, New York, NY 69-72; Hosp For Special Surgery, New York, NY 72-75; **FEL:** Spine, U Toronto Gen Hosp, Toronto, Canada 75-76; **HOSP:** Hosp For Special Surgery

SA SU 🅐 📷 🚗 🛏 **S** Mcr WC NFI 1 Week

Parisien, J Serge (MD)   OrS
Hosp For Joint Diseases

1070 Park Ave # 1; New York, NY 10128; (212) 534-1212; **BDCERT:** OrS 73; **MS:** Haiti 63; **RES:** S, Mercy Hosp, Philadelphia, PA 68-69; OrS, Hosp For Joint Diseases, New York, NY 69-72; **FAP:** Clin Prof NYU Sch Med; **HOSP:** New York University Med Ctr; **SI:** *Sports Medicine/Arthroscopy;* **HMO:** Oxford GHI 1199 US Hlthcre United Healthcare +

LANG: Fr, Cre, Sp; ♿ 📷 🚗 🛏 **S** WC NFI A Few Days

Patterson, Andrew (MD)　　OrS
St Luke's Roosevelt Hosp Ctr

Orthopaedic Associates Of NY, 343 W 58th St; New York, NY 10019; (212) 765-2260; **BDCERT:** OrS 66; **MS:** Columbia P&S 58; **RES:** S, St Luke's Roosevelt Hosp Ctr, New York, NY 59-60; OrS, Columbia-Presbyterian Med Ctr, New York, NY 60-63; **FAP:** Clin Prof Columbia P&S; **HMO:** Aetna Hlth Plan PHCS Oxford US Hlthcre

LANG: Sp; ⓔ ⓐ 🎗 ⛨ 🄢 Mcr wc Nfi 1 Week ▥ **VISA** ⬤

Pearl, Richard (MD)　　OrS
Cabrini Med Ctr

942 5th Ave; New York, NY 10021; (212) 734-4504; **MS:** Mexico 74; **RES:** Mount Sinai Med Ctr, New York, NY 76-77; New York University Med Ctr, New York, NY 77-80; **FEL:** New England Baptist Hosp, Boston, MA; **HOSP:** New York Methodist Hosp; **SI:** *Total Hip Replacements; Total Knee Replacements;* **HMO:** US Hlthcre Oxford PHS Independent Health Plan Blue Choice +

LANG: Fr, Sp; ⓔ ⓐ 🎗 ⛨ 🄢 Mcr wc Nfi A Few Days **VISA** ⬤

Pellicci, Paul (MD)　　OrS
Hosp For Special Surgery

535 E 70th St; New York, NY 10021; (212) 606-1010; **BDCERT:** OrS 82; **MS:** Cornell U 75; **RES:** S, NY Hosp-Cornell Med Ctr, New York, NY 75-76; OrS, Hosp For Special Surgery, New York, NY 77-80; **FEL:** Brigham & Women's Hosp, Boston, MA 80-81; NY Hosp-Cornell Med Ctr, New York, NY; **FAP:** Assoc Prof S Cornell U; **HOSP:** NY Hosp-Cornell Med Ctr; **SI:** *Total Hip Replacement; Total Knee Replacement;* **HMO:** Metlife Oxford United Healthcare PHS PHCS +

LANG: Sp, Itl, Fr; ⓔ ⓐ 🎗 ⛨ Mcr wc 2-4 Weeks

Phillips, Donna (MD)　　OrS
New York University Med Ctr

24 E 12th St 603; New York, NY 10003; (212) 645-1111; **BDCERT:** OrS 80; **MS:** Baylor 81; **RES:** Baylor Med Ctr, Dallas, TX 83; Indiana U Med Ctr, Indianapolis, IN 87; **FEL:** Ped OrS, TX Scottish Rite Hosp, Dallas, TX; **HOSP:** St Vincents Hosp & Med Ctr NY; **SI:** *Foot Deformity; Scoliosis;* **HMO:** Oxford CIGNA Chubb Magnacare Prucare +

LANG: Sp; ⓔ ⓐ 🎗 ⛨ 🄢 Immediately

Pitman, Mark (MD)　　OrS
Hosp For Joint Diseases

305 2nd Ave 3; New York, NY 10003; (212) 598-6025; **BDCERT:** OrS 65; **MS:** Univ Vt Coll Med 56; **RES:** Hosp For Joint Diseases, New York, NY 57-61; **FEL:** SM, Stockholm, Sweden; **FAP:** Assoc Clin Prof OrS NYU Sch Med; **SI:** *Chondrocyte Implantation; Arthroscopy;* **HMO:** CIGNA Prucare Blue Shield Magnacare

ⓔ ⓐ 🎗 ⛨ 🄢 Mcr wc Nfi A Few Days ▥ **VISA** ⬤

Price, Andrew (MD)　　OrS
New York University Med Ctr

530 1st Ave 8U; New York, NY 10016; (212) 263-8247; **BDCERT:** OrS 90; **MS:** NYU Sch Med 80; **RES:** New York University Med Ctr, New York, NY 81-85; **FEL:** Ped OrS, Newington Children's Hosp, Newington, CT 85-86; **FAP:** Assoc Lecturer NYU Sch Med; **HOSP:** Bellevue Hosp Ctr; **SI:** *Erb's Palsy; Pediatric Orthopedics;* **HMO:** Oxford United Healthcare CIGNA Health Source

LANG: Sp; ⓔ ⓐ 🎗 ⛨ 🄢 Nfi A Few Days **VISA** ⬤

Pruzansky, Mark E (MD)　　OrS
Mount Sinai Med Ctr

975 Park Ave; New York, NY 10028; (212) 249-8700; **BDCERT:** OrS 80; HS 92; **MS:** Mt Sinai Sch Med 74; **RES:** OrS, Mount Sinai Med Ctr, New York, NY 75-78; **FEL:** HS, So Baptist, New Orleans, LA 78; HS, Pacific Presbyterian, San Francisco, CA 79; **FAP:** Asst Prof OrS Mt Sinai Sch Med; **HOSP:** Beth Israel North; **SI:** *Hand/Microsurgery/Sports Medicine; Knees/Shoulders;* **HMO:** Blue Cross & Blue Shield CIGNA Oxford PHS PHCS +

LANG: Ger, Sp; ⓔ ⓐ 🎗 ⛨ 🄢 Mcr wc Nfi Immediately ▥ **VISA** ⬤

Ranawat, Chitranjan (MD)   OrS
Lenox Hill Hosp

Center for Total Joint Replacement Lenox Hill Hosp, 130 E 77th St 11th Flr; New York, NY 10021; (212) 434-4700; **BDCERT:** OrS 69; **MS:** India 62; **RES:** India 62; S, MY Hosp, India 59-63; **FEL:** Hosp For Special Surgery, New York, NY 66-67; PlS, Hosp For Special Surgery, New York, NY; **HOSP:** Hosp For Special Surgery; **HMO:** Oxford US Hlthcre Blue Choice Multiplan United Healthcare +

♿ 🔲 🔲 🔲 **$**   2-4 Weeks **VISA** 💳

Raskin, Keith (MD)   OrS
New York University Med Ctr

317 E 34th St 3rd Fl; New York, NY 10016; (212) 683-4263; **BDCERT:** OrS 91; **MS:** Geo Wash U Sch Med 83; **RES:** OrS, New York University Med Ctr, New York, NY 84-88; **FEL:** HS, Union Mem Hosp, Baltimore, MD; **FAP:** Chf HS NYU Sch Med; **HOSP:** Bellevue Hosp Ctr

Root, Leon (MD)   OrS
Hosp For Special Surgery

535 E 70th St; New York, NY 10021; (212) 606-1330; **BDCERT:** OrS 64; **MS:** NY Med Coll 55; **RES:** OrS, St Joseph's Hosp-Paterson, Paterson, NJ; **FEL:** OrS, Hosp For Special Surgery, New York, NY; **HOSP:** NY Hosp-Cornell Med Ctr; **HMO:** Aetna Hlth Plan Blue Choice Chubb

🔲 🔲 **$** 🔲   2-4 Weeks ▨ **VISA** 💳

Rose, Donald J (MD)   OrS
Hosp For Joint Diseases

JNR Sports Medicine, PC, 1095 Park Ave; New York, NY 10128; (212) 427-7750; **BDCERT:** OrS 89; **MS:** Rutgers U 80; **RES:** S, Beth Israel Med Ctr, New York, NY 80-81; OrS, Hosp For Joint Diseases, New York, NY 81-85; **FEL:** SM, Temple U Hosp, Philadelphia, PA 85-86; **FAP:** Asst Clin Prof NYU Sch Med; **HOSP:** New York University Med Ctr; *SI: Arthroscopy; Sports/Dance Injuries;* **HMO:** AARP Aetna-US Healthcare GHI PHS United Healthcare +

LANG: Sp; ♿ 🔲 🔲 🔲 **$** 🔲 🔲   A Few Days **VISA** 💳

Rose, Howard Anthony (MD)OrS
Hosp For Special Surgery

535 E 70th St Ste 373; New York, NY 10021; (212) 606-1278; **BDCERT:** OrS 85; **MS:** Geo Wash U Sch Med 77; **RES:** OrS, Hosp For Special Surgery, New York, NY 78-82; **FEL:** SM, Brigham & Women's Hosp, Boston, MA 82-83; SM, Brigham & Women's Hosp, Boston, MA 82-83; **FAP:** Clin Instr Cornell U; *SI: Arthroscopy; Joint Replacement;* **HMO:** Oxford Aetna-US Healthcare PHCS PHS GHI +

LANG: Fr, Ger, Sp, Itl; ♿ 🔲 🔲 🔲 🔲 **$** 🔲 🔲 🔲   Immediately ▨ **VISA** 💳

Rosenwasser, Melvin (MD)   OrS
Columbia-Presbyterian Med Ctr

161 Fort Washington Ave Rm 251; New York, NY 10032; (212) 305-4037; **BDCERT:** OrS 85; **MS:** Columbia P&S 76; **RES:** St Luke's Roosevelt Hosp Ctr, New York, NY 76-79; Columbia-Presbyterian Med Ctr, New York, NY 79-82; **FEL:** HS, Columbia-Presbyterian Med Ctr, New York, NY; **HMO:** Aetna Hlth Plan Blue Choice Oxford 1199 Multiplan +

♿ 🔲 🔲 🔲 🔲 **$** 🔲 🔲 🔲   A Few Days ▨ **VISA** 💳 💳

Roye, David (MD)   OrS
Columbia-Presbyterian Med Ctr

3959 Broadway; New York, NY 10032; (212) 305-5475; **BDCERT:** OrS 76; **MS:** Columbia P&S 75; **RES:** S, St Luke's Roosevelt Hosp Ctr, New York, NY 75-76; Columbia-Presbyterian Med Ctr, New York, NY 75-79; **FEL:** Ped OrS, Hosp For Sick Children, Toronto, Canada; *SI: Pediatric Orthopaedic Surgery;* **HMO:** Aetna Hlth Plan Blue Choice HealthNet Travelers Oxford +

LANG: Sp; ♿ 🔲 🔲 🔲 **$**   4+ Weeks ▨ **VISA** 💳 💳

Rozbruch, Jacob (MD)   OrS
Beth Israel Med Ctr

East 72nd St Orthopaedic Surgery Specialists, 420 E 72nd St 1J; New York, NY 10021; (212) 744-9857; **BDCERT:** OrS 80; Ped 79; **MS:** SUNY Buffalo 73; **RES:** OrS, Hosp For Special Surgery, New York, NY 76-79; S, NY Hosp-Cornell Med Ctr, New York, NY 75-76; **FEL:** NY Hosp-Cornell Med Ctr, New York, NY 74-75; OrS, Beth Israel North, New York, NY 87-94; *SI: Joint Replacement; Spine Surgery; Shoulder/Reconstruction;* **HMO:** Oxford PHS Beech Street Health Source Blue Choice +

LANG: Sp, Itl, Rus, Ger, Heb; ♿ 🔲 🔲 🔲 💲 Mcr WC NFI 1 Week ▨ **VISA** 💳 💳

Salvati, Eduardo (MD)   OrS
Hosp For Special Surgery

535 E 70th St; New York, NY 10021; (212) 606-1472; **BDCERT:** OrS 72; **MS:** Argentina 63; **RES:** OrS, University of Florence, Florence, Italy 63-65; OrS, University of Buenos Aires, Buenos Aires, Argentina 66-69; **FEL:** Hip S, Hosp For Special Surgery, New York, NY 69-72; **FAP:** Clin Prof OrS Cornell U; *SI: Hip Replacement; Knee Replacement;* **HMO:** United Healthcare PHS Multiplan Oxford

LANG: Sp, Itl; ♿ 🔲 🔲 🔲 💲 Mcr WC NFI 2-4 Weeks

Sands, Andrew (MD)   OrS
Beth Israel Med Ctr

10 Union Square East Ste 3M; New York, NY 10003; (212) 844-8550; **BDCERT:** OrS 92; **MS:** NY Med Coll 85; **RES:** OrS, Lenox Hill Hosp, New York, NY 86-90; **FEL:** Foot S, Harborview Medical Ctr, Seattle, WA 93-94; **HOSP:** Kingsbrook Jewish Med Ctr; **HMO:** Aetna Hlth Plan Blue Choice Blue Cross & Blue Shield CIGNA

Scott, W Norman (MD)   OrS
Beth Israel North

170 East End Ave Fl 4; New York, NY 10128; (212) 870-9740; **BDCERT:** OrS 78; **MS:** Cornell U 72; **RES:** OrS, Hosp For Special Surgery, New York, NY 74-77; S, St Luke's Roosevelt Hosp Ctr, New York, NY 73-74; **FAP:** Cornell U; **HOSP:** Lenox Hill Hosp; *SI: Knee Cartilage & Ligament; Total Knee Replacements;* **HMO:** Oxford CIGNA Aetna-US Healthcare Blue Choice +

♿ 🔲 🔲 🔲 💲 Mcr Mcd WC NFI Immediately ▨ **VISA** 💳

Sculco, Thomas (MD)   OrS
Hosp For Special Surgery

535 E 70th St; New York, NY 10021; (212) 606-1475; **BDCERT:** OrS 76; **MS:** Columbia P&S 69; **RES:** S, St Luke's Roosevelt Hosp Ctr, New York, NY 69-71; OrS, Hosp For Special Surgery, New York, NY 71-74; **FEL:** OrS, London Hosp, London, England 74-75; **FAP:** Prof S Cornell U; **HOSP:** NY Hosp-Cornell Med Ctr; *SI: Total Hip Replacement; Total Knee Replacement;* **HMO:** Oxford Blue Cross & Blue Shield NYLCare Aetna Hlth Plan IPA +

LANG: Sp; ♿ 🔲 💲 Mcr NFI 4+ Weeks ▨ **VISA** 💳

Siffert, Robert (MD)   OrS
Mount Sinai Med Ctr

955 5th Ave; New York, NY 10021; (212) 288-7900; **BDCERT:** OrS 52; **MS:** NYU Sch Med 43; **RES:** Mount Sinai Med Ctr, New York, NY 46-49; **FAP:** Prof Mt Sinai Sch Med; *SI: General Orthopedics; Pediatric Orthopedics;* **HMO:** Oxford Aetna Hlth Plan Blue Choice

LANG: Sp, Rus; ♿ 🔲 🔲 🔲 💲 Mcr WC NFI Immediately **VISA** 💳

Guide to symbols and abbreviations can be found on pages 110-113.

297

Springfield, Dempsey (MD)   OrS
Mount Sinai Med Ctr

Leni and Peter W May Dept of Orthopaedics, 5 E
98th St; New York, NY 10029; (212) 241-8311;
BDCERT: OrS 92; **MS:** U Fla Coll Med 71; **RES:** S, U
of Alabama Hosp, Birmingham, AL 71-72; OrS, U
FL Shands Hosp, Gainesville, FL 72-76; **FEL:**
Musculoskeletal Pathology, U FL Shands Hosp,
Gainesville, FL 74; U FL Shands Hosp, Gainesville,
FL 78-79; **FAP:** Chrmn & Prof Mt Sinai Sch Med; *SI:*
Musculoskeletal Tumors; Bone Transplants; **HMO:**
Oxford Aetna-US Healthcare Blue Choice CIGNA
PPO Blue Cross & Blue Shield +

🔲 🔲 🔲 🔲 🔲 🔲 🔲   A Few Days 🔲 **VISA** 🔲

Stuchin, Steven (MD)   OrS
Hosp For Joint Diseases

301 E 17th St 1402; New York, NY 10003; (212)
598-6708; **BDCERT:** OrS 84; **MS:** Columbia P&S
76; **RES:** S, St Luke's Roosevelt Hosp Ctr, New York,
NY 76-78; OrS, Hosp For Special Surgery, New
York, NY 78-81; **FEL:** HS, Thomas Jefferson U Hosp,
Philadelphia, PA 81-82; **FAP:** Assoc Prof OrS NYU
Sch Med; **HOSP:** New York University Med Ctr; *SI:*
Hip & Knee Replacement; Hand Surgery-Arthritis
Surgery; **HMO:** Oxford CIGNA US Hlthcre GHI
United Healthcare +

🔲 🔲 🔲 🔲 🔲 🔲 🔲 🔲   1 Week 🔲 **VISA** 🔲

Testa, Noel (MD)   OrS
New York University Med Ctr

NYU Medical Ctr, 530 1st Ave 7F; New York, NY
10016; (212) 263-7284; **BDCERT:** OrS 74; **MS:**
NY Med Coll 66; **RES:** S, St Vincents Hosp & Med Ctr
NY, New York, NY 67-68; OrS, New York
University Med Ctr, New York, NY 70-73; **FEL:** New
England Baptist Hosp, Boston, MA 73-74

Truchly, George (MD)   OrS
Cabrini Med Ctr

227 E 19th St Ste 316D; New York, NY 10003;
(212) 979-0773; **BDCERT:** OrS 61; **MS:** Austria
46; **RES:** S, Mercy Hosp, Canton, OH 51-52; OrS,
Bellevue Hosp Ctr, New York, NY 53-56; **FAP:** Prof
of Clin OrS NYU Sch Med; *SI: Shoulder Surgery; Spine*
Surgery; **HMO:** Aetna Hlth Plan CIGNA Empire
Blue Choice GHI +

LANG: Ger, Hun, Slv, Rus, Ukr; 🔲 🔲 🔲 🔲 🔲 🔲
🔲 🔲   A Few Days

Ulin, Richard (MD)   OrS
Mount Sinai Med Ctr

1095 Park Ave; New York, NY 10128; (212) 860-
0905; **BDCERT:** OrS 92; **MS:** Columbia P&S 62;
RES: Hosp For Joint Diseases, New York, NY 63-67;
FEL: Rancho Los Amigos Med Ctr, Downey, CA;
FAP: Clin Prof Mt Sinai Sch Med; *SI: Pediatric*
Orthopedics; Scoliosis; **HMO:** Oxford Aetna Hlth Plan
US Hlthcre Guardian Blue Choice +

LANG: Sp, Itl; 🔲 🔲 🔲 🔲 🔲 🔲 🔲 🔲 🔲   2-
4 Weeks

Waller, John F (MD)   OrS
Lenox Hill Hosp

110 E 59th St Ste 10B; New York, NY 10022;
(212) 583-2920; **BDCERT:** OrS 79; **MS:** NY Med
Coll 71; **RES:** OrS, Lenox Hill Hosp, New York, NY
74-77; **FEL:** Foot & Ankle, Hosp For Special
Surgery, New York, NY 78; *SI: Foot & Ankle*
Problems; **HMO:** Oxford United Healthcare Select
Premier Magnacare +

🔲 🔲 🔲 🔲 🔲 🔲 🔲 🔲   A Few Days 🔲 **VISA**
🔲

Warren, Russell (MD)   OrS
Hosp For Special Surgery

535 E 70th St; New York, NY 10021; (212) 606-
1178; **BDCERT:** OrS 74; **MS:** SUNY Hlth Sci Ctr 66;
RES: St Luke's Roosevelt Hosp Ctr, New York, NY
66-68; Hosp For Special Surgery, New York, NY
70-73; **FEL:** Shoulder S, Columbia-Presbyterian
Med Ctr, New York, NY 76; **FAP:** Prof OrS Cornell
U; **HOSP:** NY Hosp-Cornell Med Ctr; *SI: Shoulder*
Surgery; Knee Instability

LANG: Sp; 🔲 🔲 🔲 🔲 🔲 🔲   2-4 Weeks

Weiner, Lon S (MD)   OrS
Lenox Hill Hosp
130 E 77th St; New York, NY 10021; (212) 434-4880; **BDCERT:** OrS 90; **MS:** Mt Sinai Sch Med 82; **RES:** Mount Sinai Med Ctr, New York, NY 82-87; **FEL:** Ped OrS, Hosp For Special Surgery, New York, NY 87-88; **HOSP:** Mount Sinai Med Ctr; *SI: Trauma; Fractures Adult/Pediatric;* **HMO:** Oxford PHCS Empire Blue Choice US Hlthcre

LANG: Sp; ♿ ⏰ 👪 🏥 $ Mcr Mcd WC NFI
Immediately 💳 **VISA** 💳

Wickiewicz, Thomas (MD)   OrS
Hosp For Special Surgery
525 E 71st St; New York, NY 10021; (212) 606-1450; **BDCERT:** OrS 84; **MS:** UMDNJ-NJ Med Sch, Newark 76; **RES:** Hosp For Special Surgery, New York, NY 78-81; **FEL:** SM, Hosp For Special Surgery, New York, NY 77-78; SM, UCLA Med Ctr, Los Angeles, CA 81; **HMO:** Aetna Hlth Plan Blue Choice Metlife PHCS

♿ 📞 ⏰ 👪 🏥 $ Mcr   A Few Days

Windsor, Russell (MD)   OrS
Hosp For Special Surgery
535 E 70th St; New York, NY 10021; (212) 606-1166; **BDCERT:** OrS 86; **MS:** Georgetown U 78; **RES:** Thomas Jefferson U Hosp, Philadelphia, PA 79; Hosp of U Penn, Philadelphia, PA 79-83; **FEL:** Knee Reconstruction, Hosp For Special Surgery, New York, NY 83-84; **HOSP:** NY Hosp-Cornell Med Ctr

♿ ⏰ 👪 🏥 $ Mcr   Immediately **VISA** 💳

Zambetti, George (MD)   OrS
St Luke's Roosevelt Hosp Ctr
343 W 58th St; New York, NY 10019; (212) 765-2260; **BDCERT:** OrS 83; **MS:** Albany Med Coll 76; **RES:** St Luke's Roosevelt Hosp Ctr, New York, NY 76-78; Columbia-Presbyterian Med Ctr, New York, NY 78-81; **HOSP:** Columbia-Presbyterian Med Ctr; *SI: Sports Medicine; Knee Reconstruction;* **HMO:** Aetna Hlth Plan Oxford Prucare US Hlthcre

LANG: Sp; ♿ ⏰ 👪 🏥 $ Mcr WC NFI   Immediately
💳 **VISA** 💳

Zuckerman, Joseph (MD)   OrS
Hosp For Joint Diseases
Hospital for Joint Diseases, 301 E 17th St 14th Fl; New York, NY 10003; (212) 598-6674; **BDCERT:** OrS 86; OrS 92; **MS:** Med Coll Wisc 78; **RES:** OrS, U WA Med Ctr, Seattle, WA 79-83; **FEL:** S, Brigham & Women's Hosp, Boston, MA 83-84; S, Mayo Clinic, Rochester, MN 84; **FAP:** Assoc Prof NYU Sch Med; **HOSP:** New York University Med Ctr; *SI: Hip & Knee Replacement; Shoulder Surgery;* **HMO:** Oxford Aetna-US Healthcare GHI Chubb

LANG: Sp; ♿ ⏰ 👪 🏥 $ Mcr Mcd WC NFI
Immediately 💳 **VISA** 💳

OTOLARYNGOLOGY

Anand, Vijay (MD)   Oto
Manhattan Eye, Ear & Throat Hosp
205 E 64th St 101; New York, NY 10021; (212) 832-3222; **BDCERT:** Oto 82; **MS:** India 75; **RES:** Our Lady of Mercy Med Ctr, Bronx, NY 76-78; Manhattan Eye, Ear & Throat Hosp, New York, NY 79-82; **FEL:** Head & Neck S, Mercy Hosp, Pittsburgh, PA; **HOSP:** Lenox Hill Hosp; *SI: Endoscopic Sinus Surgery; Head and Neck Surgery;* **HMO:** Prucare CIGNA United Healthcare Magnacare Multiplan +

LANG: Sp; ♿ 📞 ⏰ 👪 🏥 $ Immediately 💳
VISA 💳

April, Max (MD)   Oto
Lenox Hill Hosp
New York Otolaryngology Institute, 186 E 76th St; New York, NY 10021; (212) 327-3000; **BDCERT:** Oto 90; **MS:** Boston U 85; **RES:** Boston U Med Ctr, Boston, MA 90; **FEL:** Johns Hopkins Hosp, Baltimore, MD 91; *SI: Pediatric Sinus Disease; Neck Masses*

♿ 📞 ⏰ 🏥 $ A Few Days **VISA** 💳

Guide to symbols and abbreviations can be found on pages 110-113.

299

Aviv, Jonathan (MD)   Oto
Columbia-Presbyterian Med Ctr

Columbia Presbyterian Assoc, 16 E 60th St 360; New York, NY 10022; (212) 326-8475; **BDCERT:** Oto 90; **MS:** Columbia P&S 85; **RES:** Mount Sinai Med Ctr, New York, NY 85-87; Oto, Mount Sinai Med Ctr, New York, NY 87-90; **FEL:** GVS, Mount Sinai Med Ctr, New York, NY 90-91; **FAP:** Assoc Prof Oto Columbia P&S; **SI:** *Sinus Surgery; Swallowing & Voice Disorder;* **HMO:** Oxford Aetna Hlth Plan CIGNA Chubb Prucare +

LANG: Sp, Heb; 🔲 🔲 🔲 🔲 🔲 🔲 Immediately ▓
VISA 💳 💳

Bernard, Peter (MD)   Oto
Mount Sinai Med Ctr

55 E 87th St; New York, NY 10128; (212) 289-1731; **BDCERT:** Oto 87; **MS:** Mt Sinai Sch Med 82; **RES:** S, Lenox Hill Hosp, New York, NY; **FEL:** Oto, Mount Sinai Med Ctr, New York, NY 84-87; **FAP:** Asst Prof Mt Sinai Sch Med; **HMO:** None

LANG: Sp; 🔲 🔲 🔲 🔲 🔲 Immediately ▓ **VISA** 💳

Biller, Hugh (MD)   Oto
Mount Sinai Med Ctr

Faculty Practice, 5 E 98th St; New York, NY 10029; (212) 241-9410; **BDCERT:** Oto 68; **MS:** Med Coll Wisc 60; **RES:** Johns Hopkins Hosp, Baltimore, MD 64-67; **FAP:** Prof Oto Mt Sinai Sch Med; **SI:** *Head & Neck Surgery;* **HMO:** None

🔲 🔲 🔲 🔲 🔲 A Few Days ▓ **VISA** 💳 💳

Blaugrund, Stanley (MD)   Oto
Lenox Hill Hosp

115 E 61st St Fl 12; New York, NY 10021; (212) 758-6330; **BDCERT:** Oto 64; **MS:** Univ Texas, Houston 55; **RES:** Oto, Mount Sinai Medical Center, New York, NY 52-62; S, Mount Sinai Med Ctr, New York, NY 58; **FEL:** Head & Neck S, St Vincents Hosp & Med Ctr NY, New York, NY 62-65; **SI:** *Sinonasal Surgery; Laryngeal Surgery;* **HMO:** None

LANG: Sp; 🔲 🔲 🔲 🔲 🔲 🔲 Immediately

Blitzer, Andrew (MD)   Oto
St Luke's Roosevelt Hosp Ctr

Head & Neck Surgical Group, 425 W 59th St 10th Fl; New York, NY 10019; (212) 262-9500; **BDCERT:** Oto 77; **MS:** Mt Sinai Sch Med 73; **RES:** S, Beth Israel Med Ctr, New York, NY 73-74; Oto, Mount Sinai Med Ctr, New York, NY 74-77; **FAP:** Prof Columbia P&S; **HOSP:** Columbia-Presbyterian Med Ctr; **SI:** *Voice & Swallowing; Nasal & Sinus Diseases*

LANG: Rus, Sp, Fr; 🔲 🔲 🔲 🔲 🔲 🔲 1 Week ▓
VISA 💳

Brookler, Kenneth (MD)   Oto
Lenox Hill Hosp

Neurotologic Associates, PC, 111 E 77th St; New York, NY 10021; (212) 861-6900; **BDCERT:** Oto 68; **MS:** Canada 62; **RES:** Winnipeg Gen Hosp, Winnipeg, Canada 63; Mayo Clinic, Rochester, MN 64-67; **FEL:** Oto, Mayo Clinic, Rochester, MN 68; **HOSP:** Manhattan Eye, Ear & Throat Hosp; **SI:** *Dizziness; Hearing Loss/Tinnitus*

🔲 🔲 🔲 🔲 🔲 1 Week **VISA** 💳

Catalano, Peter (MD)   Oto
Mount Sinai Med Ctr

Otolaryngology Assoc, 5 E 98th St FL 8; New York, NY 10029; (212) 241-9410; **BDCERT:** Oto 90; **MS:** Mt Sinai Sch Med 85; **RES:** S, Cedars-Sinai Med Ctr, Los Angeles, CA 85-87; Oto, Mount Sinai Med Ctr, New York, NY 87-90; **FAP:** Assoc Prof Mt Sinai Sch Med; **SI:** *Skull Base Surgery; Ear-Nose-Throat*

LANG: Sp, Itl, Chi, Heb, Kor; 🔲 🔲 🔲 🔲 🔲 🔲 🔲 A Few Days ▓ **VISA** 💳 💳

Cho, Hyun (MD)   Oto
Beth Israel Med Ctr

114 E 61st St; New York, NY 10021; (212) 888-3784; **BDCERT:** Oto 82; **MS:** South Korea 64; **RES:** S, Beth Israel Med Ctr, New York, NY 68-72; Oto, Columbia-Presbyterian Med Ctr, New York, NY 79-82; **FEL:** Head & Neck S, Beth Israel Med Ctr, New York, NY 72-74; **FAP:** Assoc Prof Albert Einstein Coll Med; **HOSP:** N Shore Univ Hosp-Forest Hills; **SI:** *Head & Neck Oncology; Laryngology*

LANG: Kor, Chi, Sp, Czc; 🔲 🔲 🔲 🔲 🔲 🔲 🔲 A Few Days

Close, Lanny Garth (MD)   Oto
Columbia-Presbyterian Med Ctr

Columbia Presbyterian Assoc, 16 E 60th St 360;
New York, NY 10022; (212) 326-8475; **BDCERT:**
Oto 77; **MS:** Baylor 72; **RES:** Johns Hopkins Hosp,
Baltimore, MD 72-74; Baylor Coll Med, Houston,
TX 74-77; **FEL:** Head & Neck S, MD Anderson
Cancer Ctr, Houston, TX 78-79; **FAP:** Prof
Columbia P&S; **SI:** *Sinus Disease; Head & Neck
Cancer;* **HMO:** Oxford Aetna-US Healthcare Blue
Choice Anthem Health Empire +

LANG: Sp, Kor; 🔊 📷 💊 🏥 💲 Mcr NFI A Few Days
🏦 **VISA** 💳

Cohen, Noel (MD)   Oto
New York University Med Ctr

530 1st Ave; New York, NY 10016; (212) 263-
7373; **BDCERT:** Oto 63; **MS:** Germany 57; **RES:**
Oto, New York University Med Ctr, New York, NY
59-62

Dolitsky, Jay (MD)   Oto
New York Eye & Ear Infirmary

310 E 14th St; New York, NY 10003; (212) 979-
4200; **BDCERT:** Oto 90; **MS:** SUNY Hlth Sci Ctr 81;
RES: New York University Med Ctr, New York, NY
84-86; Manhattan Eye, Ear & Throat Hosp, New
York, NY 87-90; **FEL:** Ped Oto, Children's Hosp of
Pittsburgh, Pittsburgh, PA; **HOSP:** Beth Israel Med
Ctr; **SI:** *Pediatric Sinusitis;* **HMO:** GHI Oxford Aetna
Hlth Plan PHCS Multiplan +

🔊 📷 💊 🏥 💲 Mcr Mcd Immediately 🏦 **VISA** 💳

Dropkin, Lloyd (MD)   Oto
NY Hosp-Cornell Med Ctr

449 E 68th St 11; New York, NY 10021; (212)
535-9191; **BDCERT:** Oto 76; **MS:** Cornell U 70;
RES: NY Hosp-Cornell Med Ctr, New York, NY 70-
76; **HMO:** Aetna Hlth Plan Blue Choice Magnacare
Metlife

🔊 📷 💊 🏥 Immediately

Eberle, Robert (MD)   Oto
St Vincents Hosp & Med Ctr NY

130 W 12th St; New York, NY 10011; (212) 807-
7720; **BDCERT:** S 63; Oto 66; **MS:** Northwestern U
54; **RES:** S, Cook Cty Hosp, Chicago, IL 58-62; Oto,
U Chicago Hosp, Chicago, IL 63-66; **FEL:** Path, U
Hosp Zurich, Zurich, Switzerland 55-56; Head &
Neck S, , NY; **HOSP:** Lawrence Hosp; **SI:** *Head &
Neck Cancer; Thyroid & Parathyroid;* **HMO:** Blue
Cross Oxford Aetna-US Healthcare Magnacare

LANG: Sp, Ger; 🔊 📷 💊 🏥 💲 Mcr WC NFI
A Few Days

Edelstein, David (MD)   Oto
Manhattan Eye, Ear & Throat Hosp

210 E 64th St Fl 3; New York, NY 10021; (212)
605-3789; **BDCERT:** Oto 85; **MS:** Boston U 80;
RES: S, Mount Sinai Med Ctr, New York, NY 80-81;
Oto, Mount Sinai Med Ctr, New York, NY 81-84;
FAP: Clin Prof Cornell U; **HOSP:** Lenox Hill Hosp; **SI:**
Nasal and Sinus Disease; Endoscopic & Laser Surgery;
HMO: Oxford Magnacare PHS Multiplan Premier +

LANG: Sp, Grk; 🔊 💳 📷 💊 🏥 💲 Mcr Immediately
🏦 **VISA** 💳

Eden, Avrim (MD)   Oto
Mount Sinai Med Ctr

Mt Sinai Otolaryngology Associates, 5 E 98th St FL
8; New York, NY 10029; (212) 241-9410;
BDCERT: Oto 74; **MS:** South Africa 68; **RES:** Oto, U
Toronto Gen Hosp, Toronto, Canada 70-74; **FEL:**
Oto, U Hosp Zurich, Zurich, Switzerland 74-75;
FAP: Prof Oto Mt Sinai Sch Med; **SI:** *Middle & Inner
Ear Disease; Meniere's Disease;* **HMO:** Aetna-US
Healthcare Oxford PHCS Blue Choice CIGNA +

LANG: Sp; 🔊 📷 💊 🏥 💲 Mcr 2-4 Weeks 🏦 **VISA**
💳

Gold, Scott (MD)   Oto
Beth Israel Med Ctr

New York Otolaryngology Group, 36 E 36th St
200; New York, NY 10016; (212) 889-8575;
BDCERT: Oto 83; **MS:** Mt Sinai Sch Med 79; **RES:**
Oto, Mount Sinai Med Ctr, New York, NY 80-83;
HOSP: Mount Sinai Med Ctr; **SI:** *Sinus Disease;
Endoscopic Sinus Surgery;* **HMO:** CIGNA PHCS
Oxford Cost Care PHS +

LANG: Sp; 🔊 📷 💊 🏥 💲 Mcr A Few Days 🏦
VISA 💳

Guide to symbols and abbreviations can be found on pages 110-113.

301

Green, Robert (MD) Oto
Mount Sinai Med Ctr

1035 5th Ave B; New York, NY 10028; (212) 288-6262; **BDCERT:** Oto 81; **MS:** Harvard Med Sch 77; **RES:** S, Mount Sinai Med Ctr, New York, NY 77-78; Oto, Mount Sinai Med Ctr, New York, NY 78-81; **FAP:** Assoc Clin Prof Mt Sinai Sch Med; **SI:** *Endoscopic Sinus Surgery;* **HMO:** Oxford Blue Choice Aetna Hlth Plan CIGNA PHCS +

LANG: Sp; 🔲 🔳 🔳 🔳 Immediately **VISA**

Guida, Robert (MD) Oto
NY Hosp-Cornell Med Ctr

520 E 70th St 541; New York, NY 10021; (212) 746-2212; **BDCERT:** Oto 89; **MS:** Hahnemann U 83; **RES:** Hosp of U Penn, Philadelphia, PA; New York Eye & Ear Infirmary, New York, NY; **FEL:** Oregon Health Sci U Hosp, Portland, OR; **HOSP:** Manhattan Eye, Ear & Throat Hosp; **HMO:** Aetna Hlth Plan Blue Choice Magnacare Metlife Multiplan +

🔲 🔳 🔳 🔳 🔳 🔳 A Few Days 🔳 **VISA** 🔳

Haddad, Joseph (MD) Oto
Columbia-Presbyterian Med Ctr

3959 Broadway BHN501; New York, NY 10032; (212) 305-8933; **BDCERT:** Oto 88; **MS:** NYU Sch Med 83; **RES:** S, Columbia-Presbyterian Med Ctr, New York, NY 83-85; Oto, Columbia-Presbyterian Med Ctr, New York, NY 85-88; **FEL:** Ped Oto, U of Pittsburgh Med Ctr, Pittsburgh, PA; **HMO:** Oxford Aetna Hlth Plan Chubb

🔲 🔳 🔳 🔳 🔳 Immediately 🔳 **VISA** 🔳

Hammerschlag, Paul E (MD) Oto
New York University Med Ctr

650 1st Ave; New York, NY 10016; (212) 889-2600; **BDCERT:** Oto 78; **MS:** Albert Einstein Coll Med 72; **RES:** Virginia Mason Hosp, Seattle, WA 73-74; Mass Eye & Ear Infirmary, Boston, MA 74-77; **FEL:** Oto, Harvard Med Sch, Cambridge, MA 76-77; **HOSP:** Beth Israel Med Ctr; **SI:** *Vertigo;* **HMO:** Magnacare CIGNA Oxford US Hlthcre

LANG: Sp; 🔲 🔳 🔳 🔳 🔳 🔳 Immediately **VISA** 🔳

Harrison, Theodore J (MD) Oto
Beth Israel Med Ctr

2 5th Ave Ste 1; New York, NY 10011; (212) 254-2020; **BDCERT:** Oto 82; **MS:** Jefferson Med Coll 76; **RES:** S, Hahnemann U Hosp, Philadelphia, PA 77-78; EM, Sacred Heart Hosp, Norristown, PA 78-79; **FEL:** Thomas Jefferson U Hosp, Philadelphia, PA 79-80; Univ of Med & Dent NJ Hosp, Newark, NJ 80-82; **FAP:** Clin Instr Mt Sinai Sch Med; **HOSP:** Cabrini Med Ctr; **SI:** *Nasal-Sinus Disorders-Head/Neck Surgery; Facial Plastic Surgery;* **HMO:** 1199 Unicare Primary Plus HIP Network Blue Cross PHS +

LANG: Yd; A Few Days

Hoffman, Ronald (MD) Oto
New York University Med Ctr

1430 2nd Ave; New York, NY 10021; (212) 535-2298; **BDCERT:** Oto 76; **MS:** Jefferson Med Coll 71; **RES:** New York University Med Ctr, New York, NY 73-76; **FEL:** Ont N, Lenox Hill Hosp, New York, NY; **FAP:** Prof Oto NYU Sch Med; **HOSP:** Lenox Hill Hosp; **SI:** *Skull Base Surgery;* **HMO:** PHS Oxford

🔲 🔳 🔳 🔳 🔳 🔳 1 Week **VISA** 🔳

Jacobs, Joseph (MD) Oto
New York University Med Ctr

530 1st Ave 3; New York, NY 10016; (212) 263-7398; **BDCERT:** Oto 78; **MS:** Albert Einstein Coll Med 74; **RES:** Oto, New York University Med Ctr, New York, NY 78; **FEL:** PIS, UCLA Med Ctr, Los Angeles, CA 78-79; **FAP:** Prof NYU Sch Med; **SI:** *Nasal & Sinus Disorders;* **HMO:** Blue Choice

🔲 🔳 🔳 🔳 🔳 🔳 🔳 Immediately 🔳 **VISA** 🔳

Jones, Jacqueline (MD) Oto
NY Hosp-Cornell Med Ctr

520 E 70th St Ste 541; New York, NY 10021; (212) 746-2236; **BDCERT:** Oto 89; **MS:** Cornell U 84; **RES:** Oto, Hosp of U Penn, Philadelphia, PA 84-89; **FEL:** Ped Oto, Children's Hosp, Boston, MA 89-90; **FAP:** Assoc Prof Cornell U; **HOSP:** Lenox Hill Hosp; **SI:** *Pediatric Sinus Disease; Airway Problems In Children;* **HMO:** Oxford United Healthcare Blue Cross & Blue Shield CIGNA Aetna Hlth Plan +

LANG: Sp, Chi; 🔲 🔳 🔳 🔳 🔳 🔳 🔳 2-4 Weeks 🔳 **VISA** 🔳 🔳

Josephson, Jordan S (MD)   Oto
Manhattan Eye, Ear & Throat Hosp
111 E 77th St; New York, NY 10021; (212) 717-
1773; **BDCERT:** Oto 88; **MS:** SUNY Hlth Sci Ctr 83;
RES: Long Island Jewish Med Ctr, New Hyde Park,
NY 84-88; **FEL:** Johns Hopkins Hosp, Baltimore,
MD; *SI: Chronic Sinusitis; Rhinoplasty*

LANG: Fr, Fil, Sp; 🔲 🔲 🔲 🔲 🔲 🔲 🔲 🔲 🔲
Immediately 🔲 **VISA** 🔲

Kimmelman, Charles P (MD) Oto
Manhattan Eye, Ear & Throat Hosp
210 E 64th St; New York, NY 10021; (212) 605-
3789; **BDCERT:** Oto 79; **MS:** Temple U 75; **RES:**
Lankenau Hosp, Philadelphia, PA 76; Hosp of U
Penn, Philadelphia, PA 79; **HOSP:** Lenox Hill Hosp;
SI: Sinus & Ear Surgery; Disorders of Taste and Smell;
HMO: Oxford Magnacare Premier Sel Pro Cost Care
+

🔲 🔲 🔲 🔲 🔲 🔲 🔲 1 Week 🔲 **VISA** 🔲

Kohan, Darius (MD)   Oto
New York University Med Ctr
800 5th Ave 502A; New York, NY 10021; (212)
319-2400; **BDCERT:** Oto 90; **MS:** NYU Sch Med
84; **RES:** S, Beth Israel Med Ctr, New York, NY 84-
86; Oto, New York University Med Ctr, New York,
NY 86-90; **FEL:** Ont N, New York University Med
Ctr, New York, NY 90-91; **FAP:** Asst Prof NYU Sch
Med; **HOSP:** Beth Israel Med Ctr; *SI: Hearing Loss &*
Tinnitus; Surgery for Ear Disease; **HMO:** Oxford
CIGNA Aetna Hlth Plan US Hlthcre NYLCare +

LANG: Sp, Fr, Itl, Rom; 🔲 🔲 🔲 🔲 🔲 🔲 🔲
A Few Days 🔲 **VISA** 🔲

Komisar, Arnold (MD)   Oto
Lenox Hill Hosp
1317 3rd Ave Fl 10; New York, NY 10021; (212)
861-8888; **BDCERT:** Oto 79; **MS:** Hahnemann U
75; **RES:** S, Beth Israel Med Ctr, New York, NY 75-
76; Oto, Mount Sinai Med Ctr, New York, NY 76-
79; **HOSP:** Manhattan Eye, Ear & Throat Hosp; *SI:*
Head and Neck Tumors; Sinus Disease; **HMO:** Oxford
Aetna Hlth Plan PHCS United Healthcare Blue
Cross & Blue Shield +

🔲 🔲 🔲 🔲 🔲 🔲 Immediately 🔲 **VISA** 🔲

Krauss, Denis (MD)   Oto
Mem Sloan Kettering Cancer Ctr
MSKCC, 1275 York Ave Box 285; New York, NY
10021; (212) 639-5621; **BDCERT:** Oto 90; **MS:** U
Rochester 85; **RES:** S, Cleveland Clinic Hosp,
Cleveland, OH 85-87; Oto, Cleveland Clinic Hosp,
Cleveland, OH 87-90; **FEL:** Head & Neck S, Mem
Sloan Kettering Cancer Ctr, New York, NY 90-91;
FAP: Asst Prof Cornell U; *SI: Sinus and Skull Base*
Cancer; Larynx Cancer

🔲 🔲 🔲 🔲 🔲 A Few Days 🔲 **VISA**

Krespi, Yosef (MD)   Oto
St Luke's Roosevelt Hosp Ctr
Head & Neck Surgical Group, 425 W 59th St 4E;
New York, NY 10019; (212) 262-4444; **BDCERT:**
Oto 81; **MS:** Israel 73; **RES:** S, Mount Sinai Med Ctr,
New York, NY 74-76; Oto, Mount Sinai Med Ctr,
New York, NY 76-80; **FEL:** S, Northwestern Mem
Hosp, Chicago, IL 80-81; **FAP:** Clin Prof Columbia
P&S; *SI: Laser Surgery; Sleep Disorders*; **HMO:** Blue
Choice US Hlthcre Oxford Prudential

LANG: Fr, Sp, Heb, Rus, Trk; 🔲 🔲 🔲 🔲 🔲 🔲 🔲
A Few Days 🔲 **VISA** 🔲 🔲

Kuhel, William (MD)   Oto
NY Hosp-Cornell Med Ctr
520 E 70th St 541; New York, NY 10021; (212)
746-2220; **BDCERT:** Oto 88; **MS:** U Mich Med Sch
83; **RES:** S, St Vincents Hosp & Med Ctr NY, New
York, NY 83-85; Oto, Indiana U Med Ctr,
Indianapolis, IN 85-88; **FEL:** S, MD Anderson
Cancer Ctr, Houston, TX 88-89; **FAP:** Assoc Clin
Prof Oto Cornell U; *SI: Head & Neck Surgery; Thyroid-*
Parathyroid Surgery

🔲 🔲 🔲 🔲 🔲 🔲 🔲 A Few Days

Kuriloff, Daniel (MD)　　Oto
St Luke's Roosevelt Hosp Ctr

Head & Neck Surgical Group, 425 W 59th St 10th
Fl; New York, NY 10019; (212) 262-5555;
BDCERT: Oto 88; **MS:** Mt Sinai Sch Med 82; **RES:**
Oto, New York Eye & Ear Infirmary, New York, NY
84-88; S, Albany Med Ctr, Albany, NY 88-89; **FEL:**
Head & Neck Onc, U Mich Med Ctr, Ann Arbor, MI
89-90; **FAP:** Assoc Prof Columbia P&S; **HOSP:**
Columbia-Presbyterian Med Ctr; **SI:** *Thyroid Tumors;*
Sinusitis; **HMO:** Oxford CIGNA Guardian Blue
Choice Empire +

⬛⬛ ⬛ ⬛ ⬛ ⬛ ⬛ ⬛ A Few Days ▦ *VISA*
⬛

Lawson, William (MD)　　Oto
Mount Sinai Med Ctr

Otolaryngology Assoc, 5 E 98th St Fl 8; New York,
NY 10029; (212) 241-9410; **BDCERT:** Oto 74; **MS:**
NYU Sch Med 65; **RES:** S, Bronx VA Hosp, Bronx,
NY 66-67; Oto, Mt Sinai Hosp, New York, NY 69-
70; **FEL:** Oto, Mount Sinai Med Ctr, New York, NY
70-73; **FAP:** Prof Oto Mt Sinai Sch Med; **SI:** *Facial*
Plastic Reconstruction; Sinus Surgery

⬛ ⬛ ⬛ ⬛ ⬛ ⬛ ⬛ 2-4 Weeks ▦ *VISA* ⬛

Lee, Norris K (MD)　　Oto
NY Hosp-Cornell Med Ctr

Cornell University Med Ctr, 520 E 70th St Starr
541; New York, NY 10021; (212) 746-2216;
BDCERT: Oto 90; **MS:** NYU Sch Med 82; **RES:** S,
Cedars-Sinai Med Ctr, Los Angeles, CA 82-84; Oto,
Montefiore Med Ctr, Bronx, NY 84-88; **FEL:** Head &
Neck S, MD Anderson Cancer Ctr, Houston, TX 88-
90; **FAP:** Asst Prof Cornell U; **HOSP:** Manhattan
Eye, Ear & Throat Hosp; **SI:** *Endoscopic Sinus*
Surgery; Tumors of Head Neck Region; **HMO:** Oxford
32BJ Aetna Hlth Plan CIGNA Blue Cross +

⬛ ⬛ ⬛ ⬛ ⬛ ⬛ ⬛ Immediately

Levenson, Mark (MD)　　Oto
Manhattan Eye, Ear & Throat Hosp

3 E 71st St; New York, NY 10021; (212) 535-
5392; **BDCERT:** Oto 83; **MS:** NY Med Coll 72; **RES:**
Manhattan Eye, Ear & Throat Hosp, New York, NY
80-83; **FEL:** Ont N, Manhattan Eye, Ear & Throat
Hosp, New York, NY 83-84; **FAP:** Asst Clin Prof
Cornell U; **HOSP:** Lenox Hill Hosp; **SI:** *Otosclerosis*
Surgery; Cholesteatoma Surgery; **HMO:** Oxford
Chubb CIGNA Blue Cross & Blue Shield HIP
Network +

LANG: Sp, Prt, Can; ⬛ ⬛ ⬛ ⬛ ⬛ A Few Days
▦ *VISA* ⬛

Linstrom, Christopher (MD) Oto
New York Eye & Ear Infirmary

Department of Otolaryngology, 310 E 14th St; New
York, NY 10003; (212) 979-4200; **BDCERT:** Oto
87; **MS:** Canada 82; **RES:** NY Hosp-Cornell Med Ctr,
New York, NY 84-87; **FEL:** Michigan Ear Inst,
Farmington Hills, MI 87-89; **HOSP:** St Vincents
Hosp & Med Ctr NY; **SI:** *Hearing Loss;* **HMO:** Aetna
Hlth Plan Blue Cross & Blue Shield GHI US Hlthcre
Oxford

LANG: Srb, Fr, Ger; ⬛ ⬛ ⬛ ⬛ ⬛ ⬛ A Few Days
▦ *VISA* ⬛

Markowitz, Arlene (MD)　　Oto
Columbia-Presbyterian Med Ctr

133 E 73rd St; New York, NY 10021; (212) 861-
9000; **BDCERT:** Oto 90; **MS:** Columbia P&S 84;
RES: Columbia-Presbyterian Med Ctr, New York,
NY 90; **HOSP:** Beth Israel Med Ctr; **HMO:** Oxford
PHCS

⬛ ⬛ ⬛ ⬛ ⬛ 1 Week ▦ *VISA* ⬛

Parisier, Simon (MD)　　Oto
Manhattan Eye, Ear & Throat Hosp

186 E 76th St; New York, NY 10021; (212) 535-
6400; **BDCERT:** Oto 67; **MS:** Boston U 61; **RES:**
Mount Sinai Med Ctr, New York, NY 62-66; **HOSP:**
Mount Sinai Med Ctr; **SI:** *Otology; Cochlear Implants*
LANG: Sp; ⬛ ⬛ ⬛ ⬛ ⬛ ⬛ 2-4 Weeks *VISA* ⬛

Pastorek, Norman (MD)　Oto
NY Hosp-Cornell Med Ctr

12 E 88th St; New York, NY 10128; (212) 987-4700; **BDCERT:** Oto 70; **MS:** Univ IL Coll Med 64; **RES:** S, Hines VA Hosp, Chicago, IL 66; Oto, U IL Med Ctr, Chicago, IL 66-69; **FAP:** Clin Prof Cornell U; **HOSP:** Manhattan Eye, Ear & Throat Hosp; *SI: Aesthetic Facial Surgery*

⬛ ⬛ ⬛ ⬛ ⬛ ⬛ 4+ Weeks *VISA*

Persky, Mark (MD)　Oto
New York University Med Ctr

NYU Medical Ctr, 530 1st Ave 3C; New York, NY 10016; (212) 263-7277; **BDCERT:** Oto 76; **MS:** SUNY Syracuse 72; **RES:** S, Montefiore Med Ctr, Bronx, NY 72-73; Oto, New York University Med Ctr, New York, NY 73-76; **FEL:** Head & Neck S, Beth Israel Med Ctr, New York, NY 76-77; *SI: Head & Neck Tumors*

⬛ ⬛ ⬛ ⬛ ⬛ ⬛ A Few Days ⬛ *VISA* ⬛

Pincus, Robert (MD)　Oto
Beth Israel Med Ctr

36A E 36th St Ste 200; New York, NY 10016; (212) 889-8575; **BDCERT:** Oto 83; **MS:** U Mich Med Sch 78; **RES:** Lenox Hill Hosp, New York, NY 78-79; Mount Sinai Med Ctr, New York, NY 80-83; **HOSP:** St Vincents Hosp & Med Ctr NY; *SI: Sinus-Head-Neck Surgery; Rhinoplasty-Reconstructive;* **HMO:** Aetna Hlth Plan CIGNA PHCS Oxford GHI +

LANG: Sp; ⬛ ⬛ ⬛ ⬛ ⬛ ⬛ ⬛ 1 Week ⬛ *VISA* ⬛ ⬛

Pollack, Geoffrey (MD)　Oto
St Luke's Roosevelt Hosp Ctr

211 Central Park West; New York, NY 10024; (212) 873-6175; **BDCERT:** Oto 84; **MS:** Columbia P&S 79; **RES:** Mount Sinai Med Ctr, New York, NY 79-81; Columbia-Presbyterian Med Ctr, New York, NY 81-84; **FAP:** Clin Instr Oto Columbia P&S; *SI: Head & Neck Surgery; Pediatric & Adult ENT*

LANG: Sp; ⬛ ⬛ ⬛ ⬛ 2-4 Weeks *VISA* ⬛

Sacks, Steven (MD)　Oto
Mount Sinai Med Ctr

1035 5th Ave B; New York, NY 10028; (212) 288-6262; **BDCERT:** Oto 81; **MS:** Washington U, St Louis 77; **RES:** Oto, Mount Sinai Med Ctr, New York, NY 77-81; *SI: Sinus Surgery; Thyroid & Parathyroid;* **HMO:** Oxford Blue Cross & Blue Shield GHI Aetna Hlth Plan PHS +

⬛ ⬛ ⬛ ⬛ ⬛ ⬛ A Few Days ⬛ *VISA* ⬛

Savetsky, Lawrence (MD)　Oto
Columbia-Presbyterian Med Ctr

161 Ft Washington Ave; New York, NY 10032; (212) 305-5335; **BDCERT:** Oto 62; **MS:** SUNY Hlth Sci Ctr 55; **RES:** Columbia-Presbyterian Med Ctr, New York, NY 58-61; **FAP:** Clin Prof Oto Columbia P&S; *SI: Otology; Nasal & Sinus Diseases;* **HMO:** Oxford Empire

LANG: Ger, Fr; ⬛ ⬛ ⬛ ⬛ ⬛ A Few Days

Schaefer, Steven (MD)　Oto
New York Eye & Ear Infirmary

310 E 14th St; New York, NY 10003; (212) 979-4200; **BDCERT:** Oto 78; **MS:** UC Irvine 72; **RES:** S, UCLA Med Ctr, Los Angeles, CA 72-74; Oto, Stanford Med Ctr, Stanford, CA 73-74; **HOSP:** St Vincents Hosp & Med Ctr NY; *SI: Sinus Surgery; Head & Neck Oncologic Surgery;* **HMO:** Oxford Aetna Hlth Plan Blue Cross & Blue Shield Prudential CIGNA +

LANG: Fr, Sp, Rus; ⬛ ⬛ ⬛ ⬛ ⬛ ⬛ Immediately ⬛ *VISA* ⬛

Schley, W Shain (MD)　Oto
NY Hosp-Cornell Med Ctr

525 E 68th St; New York, NY 10021; (212) 746-2223; **BDCERT:** Oto 73; **MS:** Emory U Sch Med 66; **RES:** S, St Luke's Roosevelt Hosp Ctr, New York, NY 66-68; Oto, NY Hosp-Cornell Med Ctr, New York, NY 70-73; **FAP:** Chrmn Oto Cornell U; **HMO:** None

⬛ ⬛ ⬛ ⬛ ⬛ ⬛ ⬛ ⬛ ⬛ Immediately ⬛ *VISA* ⬛ ⬛

Guide to symbols and abbreviations can be found on pages 110-113.

305

Schneider, Kenneth L (MD) Oto
New York University Med Ctr

530 1st Ave Ste 3C; New York, NY 10016; (212) 263-7165; **BDCERT:** Oto 82; **MS:** SUNY Hlth Sci Ctr 78; **RES:** S, Mount Sinai Med Ctr, New York, NY 78-79; Oto, New York University Med Ctr, New York, NY 79-82; **FEL:** Head & Neck S, Montefiore Med Ctr, Bronx, NY 82-83; **FAP:** Assoc Prof of Clin Oto NYU Sch Med; **SI:** *Sleep Apnea; Sinus Disease*; **HMO:** Oxford Aetna Hlth Plan US Hlthcre

♿ ⚀ ⚁ ⚂ $ Mcr A Few Days [AMEX] *VISA* ♣

Schvey, Malcolm H (MD) Oto
Columbia-Presbyterian Med Ctr

903 Park Ave; New York, NY 10021; (212) 744-4644; **BDCERT:** Oto 61; **MS:** Holland 56; **RES:** Columbia-Presbyterian Med Ctr, New York, NY 58-61; **HOSP:** Lenox Hill Hosp; **HMO:** Most

♿ ⚀ ⚁ ⚂ Mcr Immediately

Sculerati, Nancy (MD) Oto
New York University Med Ctr

NYU Medical Ctr, 530 1st Ave 3C; New York, NY 10016; (212) 263-7300; **BDCERT:** Oto 86; **MS:** NYU Sch Med 81; **RES:** S, New York University Med Ctr, New York, NY 81-83; Oto, New York University Med Ctr, New York, NY 83-86; **FEL:** Ped, Children's Hosp of Pittsburgh, Pittsburgh, PA 86-88; **FAP:** Assoc Prof NYU Sch Med; **SI:** *Ear Problems; Snoring*; **HMO:** CIGNA Oxford United Healthcare GHI PHS +

♿ ⚀ ⚁ ⚂ $ 1 Week

Selesnick, Samuel H (MD) Oto
NY Hosp-Cornell Med Ctr

520 E 70th St Ste 541; New York, NY 10021; (212) 746-2282; **BDCERT:** Oto 90; **MS:** NYU Sch Med 85; **RES:** Oto, Manhattan Eye, Ear & Throat Hosp, New York, NY 87-90; SM, St Vincents Hosp & Med Ctr NY, New York, NY 86-87; **FEL:** Skull Base S, UC San Francisco Med Ctr, San Francisco, CA 90-91; **FAP:** Assoc Prof Cornell U; **HOSP:** Mem Sloan Kettering Cancer Ctr; **SI:** *Acoustic Neuromas; Cholesteatoma*; **HMO:** Aetna-US Healthcare Oxford Blue Choice United Healthcare PHS +

♿ ⚀ ⚂ $ WC NFI 1 Week [AMEX] *VISA* ♣ ▣

Shemen, Larry (MD) Oto
Jamaica Med Ctr

233 E 69th St Ste 1D; New York, NY 10021; (212) 472-8882; **BDCERT:** Oto 83; **MS:** Canada 78; **RES:** Oto, St Michaels-Weilesley, 82-83; S, Cedar-Sinai Med Ctr, Los Angeles, CA 81-82; **FEL:** HS, Meml Sloan Kettering, New York, NY 83-84; **HOSP:** Catholic Med Ctr Bklyn & Qns; **SI:** *Head and Neck Surgery*; **HMO:** Oxford Aetna Hlth Plan

Shugar, Joel (MD) Oto
Mount Sinai Med Ctr

55 E 87th St; New York, NY 10128; (212) 289-1731; **BDCERT:** Oto 78; **MS:** McGill U 72; **RES:** S, Jewish Gen Hosp, Montreal, Canada 72-74; Oto, Mount Sinai Med Ctr, New York, NY 75-78; **FEL:** Oto, Mount Sinai Med Ctr, New York, NY 74-75; **FAP:** Assoc Clin Prof Oto Mt Sinai Sch Med; **HOSP:** Lenox Hill Hosp; **HMO:** None

♿ ⚀ ⚁ ⚂ $ Mcr A Few Days [AMEX] *VISA* ♣

Slavit, David H (MD) Oto
Lenox Hill Hosp

105 E 73rd St; New York, NY 10021; (212) 517-9177; **BDCERT:** Oto 92; **MS:** Mt Sinai Sch Med 86; **RES:** Oto, Mayo Clinic, Rochester, MN 86-91; **FAP:** Asst Prof SUNY Hlth Sci Ctr; **HOSP:** Univ Hosp SUNY Bklyn; **SI:** *Voice Disorders; Sinus Disease*; **HMO:** PHS CIGNA Oxford Aetna Hlth Plan Chubb +

LANG: Lat, Sp; ⚀ ⚁ ⚂ Mcr WC NFI Immediately [AMEX] *VISA* ♣

Stern, Jordan (MD) Oto
New York Eye & Ear Infirmary

Department of Otolaryngology, 310 E 14th St; New York, NY 10003; (212) 979-4200; **BDCERT:** Oto 90; **MS:** Geo Wash U Sch Med 85; **RES:** S, Mount Sinai Med Ctr, New York, NY 85; Oto, New York Eye & Ear Infirmary, New York, NY 86-90; **FAP:** Asst Prof NY Med Coll; **HOSP:** Beth Israel Med Ctr; **SI:** *Head & Neck Tumor Surgery; Voice Disorders*; **HMO:** Oxford Aetna Hlth Plan Blue Cross

LANG: Sp, Fr, Rus; ♿ ♤ ⚂ $ Mcr Immediately [AMEX] *VISA* ♣ ▣

Stingle, Walter (MD)   Oto
Lenox Hill Hosp

755 Park Ave; New York, NY 10021; (212) 879-3445; **BDCERT:** Oto 76; **MS:** Columbia P&S 69; **RES:** Oto, St Luke's Roosevelt Hosp Ctr, New York, NY 73-76; **FAP:** Asst Clin Prof Columbia P&S; **HOSP:** St Luke's Roosevelt Hosp Ctr; *SI: Sleep Apnea and Snoring; Nasal and Sinus Problems*; **HMO:** Oxford Aetna-US Healthcare Prucare Blue Cross Blue Choice +

LANG: Sp; 🔾 🔾 🔾 🔾 🔾 🔾 🔾 A Few Days

Storper, Ian (MD)   Oto
Columbia-Presbyterian Med Ctr

161 Fort Washington Ave; New York, NY 10032; (212) 305-5820; **BDCERT:** Oto 95; **MS:** Univ Penn 88; **RES:** Oto, UCLA, Los Angeles, CA 88-94; **FEL:** Oto/N Oto, Ear Rsrch Foundation, , TN 94-95; **FAP:** Asst Prof Columbia P&S

🔾 🔾 🔾 🔾 🔾 1 Week **VISA** 🔾

Tobias, Geoffrey (MD)   Oto
Mount Sinai Med Ctr

815 Park Ave; New York, NY 10021; (212) 245-0202; **BDCERT:** Oto 78; **MS:** Tufts U 73; **RES:** Oto, Mount Sinai Med Ctr, New York, NY 75-78; **HOSP:** Englewood Hosp & Med Ctr; *SI: Rhinoplasty; Repair Failed Rhinoplasty*; **HMO:** Oxford US Hlthcre HMO Blue CIGNA Chubb +

🔾 🔾 🔾 🔾 🔾 🔾 🔾 🔾 🔾 A Few Days

Urken, Mark (MD)   Oto
Mount Sinai Med Ctr

Otolaryngology Assoc, 5 E 98th St Fl 8; New York, NY 10029; (212) 241-9410; **BDCERT:** Oto 86; **MS:** U Va Sch Med 81; **RES:** St Elizabeth's Med Ctr, Boston, MA 81-83; Mount Sinai Med Ctr, New York, NY 83-86; **FEL:** Microvascular S, Mercy Hosp, Pittsburgh, PA 86-87; **FAP:** Assoc Prof Mt Sinai Sch Med; **HOSP:** Elmhurst Hosp Ctr

LANG: Sp; 🔾 🔾 🔾 🔾 🔾 🔾 🔾 🔾 🔾

Volpi, David (MD)   Oto
Lenox Hill Hosp

262 Central Park West; New York, NY 10024; (212) 873-6036; **BDCERT:** Oto 88; **MS:** Hahnemann U 82; **RES:** Hosp Med College of PA, Philadelphia, PA; New York Eye & Ear Infirmary, New York, NY; **FAP:** Clin Instr NY Med Coll; **HOSP:** New York Eye & Ear Infirmary; *SI: Sinus Disease; Sleep Related Disorder*; **HMO:** Aetna Hlth Plan Oxford CIGNA

LANG: Sp; 🔾 🔾 🔾 🔾 🔾 Immediately 🔾 **VISA** 🔾

Ward, Robert (MD)   Oto
NY Hosp-Cornell Med Ctr

186 E 76th St Flr2; New York, NY 10021; (212) 327-3000; **BDCERT:** Oto 86; **MS:** Cornell U 81; **RES:** Oto, NY Hosp-Cornell Med Ctr, New York, NY 81; **FEL:** Ped Oto, Children's Hosp, Boston, MA 86-87; **HOSP:** Lenox Hill Hosp; **HMO:** PHCS PHS Oxford United Healthcare

LANG: Sp; 🔾 🔾 🔾 🔾 🔾 🔾 A Few Days **VISA** 🔾

Wazen, Jack (MD)   Oto
Columbia-Presbyterian Med Ctr

161 Fort Washington Ave 512; New York, NY 10032; (212) 305-1618; **BDCERT:** Oto 83; **MS:** Lebanon 78; **RES:** Columbia-Presbyterian Med Ctr, New York, NY 83; **FEL:** Ont N, Ear Research Foundation, Sarasota, FL 83-84; **FAP:** Assoc Prof Columbia P&S; *SI: Meniere's Disease; Acoustic Neuroma*; **HMO:** Oxford Empire Chubb Aetna Hlth Plan

LANG: Fr, Ar, Sp, Kor; 🔾 🔾 🔾 🔾 🔾 🔾 🔾 🔾 🔾 Immediately 🔾 **VISA** 🔾

PAIN MANAGEMENT

Dubois, Michel (MD)   PM
New York University Med Ctr

Pain Management Ctr, 530 1st Ave Ste 9T; New York, NY 10016; (212) 263-7316; **BDCERT:** Anes 85; PM 93; **MS:** France 74; **RES:** Anes, Georgetown U Hosp, Washington, DC 78-80; **FEL:** N Anes, Georgetown U Hosp, Washington, DC 83; **FAP:** Prof NYU Sch Med; **HOSP:** Bellevue Hosp Ctr; **SI:** *Chronic Neck and Lower Back Pain; Neuropathic Pain;* **HMO:** Oxford Aetna-US Healthcare Health Plus

LANG: Sp, Fr, Chi, Grk; A Few Days

Foley, Kathleen M (MD)   PM
Mem Sloan Kettering Cancer Ctr

1275 York Ave; New York, NY 10021; (212) 639-7050; **BDCERT:** N 77; **MS:** Cornell U 69; **RES:** N, NY Hosp-Cornell Med Ctr, New York, NY 69-70; **FEL:** MG, NY Hosp-Cornell Med Ctr, New York, NY 70-71; **FAP:** Prof N Cornell U

Gevirtz, Clifford (MD & PhD) PM
Metropolitan Hosp Ctr

1901 1st Ave Rm 1215A; New York, NY 10029; (212) 423-6803; **BDCERT:** Anes 97; PM 93; **MS:** Tulane U 81; **RES:** S, Montefiore Med Ctr, Bronx, NY 81-82; Anes, Jacobi Med Ctr, Bronx, NY 82-85; **FEL:** Anes, Mass Gen Hosp, Boston, MA 85-86; **FAP:** Assoc Prof NY Med Coll; **SI:** *Heroin Detox; Palliative Medicine;* **HMO:** Centercare GHI

LANG: Sp, Fr; **VISA**

Jain, Subhash (MD)   PM
Mem Sloan Kettering Cancer Ctr

Memorial Sloan Kettering Hospital, 1275 York Ave; New York, NY 10021; (212) 639-6851; **BDCERT:** Anes 94; **MS:** India 68; **RES:** S, St Vincent's Med Ctr-Richmond, Staten Island, NY; Anes, NY Hosp-Cornell Med Ctr, New York, NY; **FAP:** Assoc Prof Cornell U; **HOSP:** NY Hosp-Cornell Med Ctr; **SI:** *Cancer and Pelvic Pain; Neuropathic Pain*

LANG: Sp, Hin, Fr; A Few Days **VISA**

Kestenbaum, Alan (MD)   PM
NY Hosp-Cornell Med Ctr

525 E 68th St M0026; New York, NY 10021; (212) 746-2960; **BDCERT:** Anes 90; PM 96; **MS:** Boston U 85; **RES:** Anes, Long Island Jewish Med Ctr, New Hyde Park, NY 85-88; **FEL:** PM, Mem Sloan Kettering Cancer Ctr, New York, NY 88-89; **FAP:** Asst Prof Cornell U; **SI:** *Low Back Pain; Cancer Pain;* **HMO:** Oxford GHI Blue Cross & Blue Shield +

LANG: Sp; 2-4 Weeks **VISA**

Kreitzer, Joel (MD)   PM
Mount Sinai Med Ctr

Pain Management Service, 5 E 98th St 6th Fl.; New York, NY 10280; (212) 241-6372; **BDCERT:** Anes 90; PM 93; **MS:** Albert Einstein Coll Med 85; **RES:** Anes, Mount Sinai Med Ctr, New York, NY 86-89; **FEL:** Pain Management, Mount Sinai Med Ctr, New York, NY 88-89; **FAP:** Asst Prof Mt Sinai Sch Med; **SI:** *Back Pain; Cancer Pain;* **HMO:** Oxford PHCS Aetna-US Healthcare 32BJ Beech Street +

A Few Days **VISA**

Lewis-Mantell, Laura (MD)   PM
Beth Israel Med Ctr

110 East End Ave 1K; New York, NY 10028; (212) 472-5756; **MS:** NY Med Coll 83; **RES:** Anes, St Vincents Hosp Med Ctr, New York, NY 84-85; **FEL:** Anes, St Vincents Hosp Med Ctr, New York, NY 85-87; **SI:** *Back Pain;* **HMO:** None

Marcus, Norman (MD)   PM
Lenox Hill Hosp

NY Pain Treatment Program, 130 E 77th St Fl 7; New York, NY 10021; (212) 249-2200; **BDCERT:** PM 93; **MS:** SUNY Syracuse 67; **RES:** Psyc, Albert Einstein Med Ctr, Bronx, NY 68-71; **FEL:** Psychosomatic Medicine, Montefiore Med Ctr, Bronx, NY 72-74; Muscle Pain Evaluation & Treatment, Lenox Hill Hosp, New York, NY 91-96; **SI:** *Back Pain and Neck Pain; Cancer Pain & Headaches;* **HMO:** US Hlthcre

VISA

Moqtaderi, Farideh (MD)   **PM**
Mount Sinai Med Ctr
1060 5th Ave; New York, NY 10128; (212) 426-
9200; **BDCERT:** Anes 73; **MS:** Iran 66; **RES:** Anes,
Mount Sinai Med Ctr, New York, NY 67-69; Anes,
Mem Sloan Kettering Cancer Ctr, New York, NY
69-71; **FEL:** Anes, NY Med Coll, New York, NY 71-
73; **FAP:** Asst Clin Prof Anes Mt Sinai Sch Med; *SI:*
Muscle and Joint Pain, Stress Headache; Acupuncture
LANG: Frs; 🚫 🌓 📷 🏥 🛏 $ �︎ 🚫 1 Week 📠
VISA ⬤

Ngeow, Jeffrey (MD)   **PM**
Hosp For Special Surgery
535 E 70th St; New York, NY 10021; (212) 606-
1059; **BDCERT:** Anes 80; PM 94; **MS:** England 71;
RES: S, Boston U Med Ctr, Boston, MA 74; PM,
Peter Bent Brigham Hosp, Boston, MA 75-77; **FEL:**
PM, New England Med Ctr, Boston, MA 77-78;
FAP: Assoc Clin Prof Cornell U; *SI: Musculoskeletal*
Pain; Acupuncture
LANG: Can, Per; 🚫 📷 🏥 🛏 $ 🚫 A Few Days

Portenoy, Russell (MD)   **PM**
Beth Israel Med Ctr
Beth Israel Med Ctr, Dept of Pain Medicine &
Palliative Care, 1st Ave & 16th St; New York, NY
10003; (212) 844-1505; **BDCERT:** N 85; **MS:** U
Md Sch Med 80; **RES:** N, Albert Einstein Med Ctr,
Bronx, NY 81-84; Mem Sloan Kettering Cancer Ctr,
New York, NY 84-85; **FAP:** Chrmn PM Albert
Einstein Coll Med; *SI: Pain Management; Palliative*
Care; **HMO:** Oxford Fidelis US Hlthcre
🚫 📷 🏥 🛏 $ 🚫 🔲 2-4 Weeks

Rosner, Howard (MD)   **PM**
NY Hosp-Cornell Med Ctr
NY Hospital Cornell Med CtrDept of Anes, Pain Mgt
Service, 525 E 68th St; New York, NY 10021;
(212) 746-2960; **BDCERT:** Anes 89; PM 93; **MS:** U
Miami Sch Med 80

Stamatos, John (MD)   **PM**
St Vincents Hosp & Med Ctr NY
95 University Pl Fl 8; New York, NY 10003; (212)
604-1300; **BDCERT:** Anes 92; PM 93; **MS:**
Uniformed Srvs U 87; **RES:** Anes, Walter Reed
Army Med Ctr, Washington, DC 88-91; **FEL:** PM,
Walter Reed Army Med Ctr, Washington, DC 90-
91; **FAP:** Asst Prof NY Med Coll; *SI: Cancer Pain*
Management; Lower Back Pain; **HMO:** Oxford Blue
Cross & Blue Choice
LANG: Grk, Sp, Itl; 🚫 📷 🏥 🛏 $ 🚫 🚫 🚫
A Few Days **VISA**

PEDIATRIC ALLERGY & IMMUNOLOGY

Ehrlich, Paul (MD)   **PA&I**
New York University Med Ctr
35 E 35th St 202; New York, NY 10016; (212)
685-4225; **BDCERT:** PA&I 77; **MS:** NYU Sch Med
70; **RES:** New York University Med Ctr, New York,
NY 70-73; Bellevue Hosp Ctr, New York, NY 70-
73; **FEL:** Walter Reed Army Med Ctr, Washington,
DC 75-77; **HOSP:** Beth Israel Med Ctr; *SI: Asthma;*
Childhood Asthma; **HMO:** Oxford Aetna-US
Healthcare Prudential NYLCare
LANG: Fr, Sp; 🚫 📷 🏥 🛏 $ 🚫 🔲 🚫
Immediately **VISA** ⬤

Haines, Kathleen (MD)   **PA&I**
Hosp For Joint Diseases
305 2nd Ave Ste 16; New York, NY 10003; (212)
598-6516; **BDCERT:** A&I 92; **MS:** Albert Einstein
Coll Med 75; **RES:** Ped, NY Hosp-Cornell Med Ctr,
New York, NY 75-77; **FEL:** A&I, NY Hosp-Cornell
Med Ctr, New York, NY 77-80; **HOSP:** New York
University Med Ctr; *SI: Chronic Arthritis; Rhinitis—*
Urticaria; **HMO:** Oxford Aetna-US Healthcare US
Hlthcre Oxford Prucare +
🚫 🏥 🛏 $ 🚫 A Few Days

Rappaport, Irwin (MD) PA&I
NY Hosp-Cornell Med Ctr

530 E 20th St 20MG; New York, NY 10009; (212) 777-8407; **BDCERT:** A&I 72; Ped 67; **MS:** Med Coll Va 62; **RES:** Bellevue Hosp Ctr, New York, NY 62-63; Ped, NY Hosp-Cornell Med Ctr, New York, NY 63-65; **FEL:** A&I, St Vincents Hosp & Med Ctr NY, New York, NY 65-66; **HMO:** Oxford PHCS PHS Independent Health Plan +

🔲 👪 🏥 Immediately

PEDIATRIC CARDIOLOGY

Arnon, Rica (MD) PCd
Mount Sinai Med Ctr

The Mount Sinai Ped Cardiology Group, 1 Gustave Levy Pl 1201; New York, NY 10029; (212) 241-7578; **BDCERT:** Ped 72; PCd 73; **MS:** SUNY Hlth Sci Ctr 67; **RES:** Ped, Univ Hosp SUNY Bklyn, Brooklyn, NY 67-70; **FEL:** PCd, Univ Hosp SUNY Bklyn, Brooklyn, NY 70-73; **FAP:** Assoc Clin Prof Mt Sinai Sch Med; **HOSP:** Elmhurst Hosp Ctr; **SI:** *Heart Disease Pediatric; Exercise In Children;* **HMO:** Aetna Hlth Plan Oxford US Hlthcre Blue Cross & Blue Shield HIP Network +

LANG: Sp, Fr, Heb; 👪 🔲 👪 🏥 $ Mcd A Few Days 💳 *VISA* 💳 💳

Artman, Michael (MD) PCd
New York University Med Ctr

New York University Med Ctr, 530 1st Ave 9U; New York, NY 10016; (212) 263-5940; **BDCERT:** Ped 83; PCd 85; **MS:** Tulane U 78; **RES:** Ped, Vanderbilt U Med Ctr, Nashville, TN 79-81; **FEL:** PCd, Vanderbilt U Med Ctr, Nashville, TN 81-83; **FAP:** Prof PCd NYU Sch Med

LANG: Sp; 👪 🔲 🏥 $ Mcd 1 Week 💳 *VISA* 💳 💳

Barst, Robyn (MD) PCd
Columbia-Presbyterian Med Ctr

3959 Broadway BH262N; New York, NY 10032; (212) 305-8509; **BDCERT:** Ped 80; PCd 81; **MS:** U NC Sch Med 76; **RES:** Ped A&I, Columbia-Presbyterian Med Ctr, New York, NY 76-79; **FEL:** PCd, Columbia-Presbyterian Med Ctr, New York, NY 79-81; PPul, Columbia-Presbyterian Med Ctr, New York, NY 81-83; **FAP:** Assoc Prof Ped Columbia P&S; **SI:** *Pulmonary Hypertension;* **HMO:** Empire CIGNA Multiplan PHS Prucare +

👪 🔲 👪 🏥 $ Mcr Mcd NFI A Few Days 💳 *VISA* 💳

Borg, Morton (MD) PCd
Beth Israel Med Ctr

1st Ave & 16th St; New York, NY 10003; (212) 420-4542; **BDCERT:** PCd 88; **MS:** Albert Einstein Coll Med 81; **RES:** Ped, Brookdale Univ Hosp Med Ctr, Brooklyn, NY 82-84; **FEL:** PCd, NY Hosp-Cornell Med Ctr, New York, NY 84-86; **FAP:** Asst Prof Albert Einstein Coll Med; **SI:** *Fetal Echocardiology;* **HMO:** Oxford US Hlthcre CIGNA Prucare NYLCare +

👪 SA/SD 🔲 🏥 $ Mcd 1 Week

Danilowicz, Delores (MD) PCd
New York University Med Ctr

560 1st Ave; New York, NY 10016; (212) 263-5656; **BDCERT:** Ped 86; PCd 86; **MS:** NYU Sch Med 60; **RES:** Ped, Jacobi Med Ctr, Bronx, NY 60-63; **FEL:** PCd, Jacobi Med Ctr, Bronx, NY 63-65; Johns Hopkins Hosp, Baltimore, MD 65-66; **FAP:** Prof NYU Sch Med; **HOSP:** Lenox Hill Hosp; **SI:** *Heart Diseases Pediatric; Congenital Heart In Adults*

LANG: Sp, Ger; 👪 🔲 $ Mcr Mcd

Friedman, Deborah (MD) PCd PCP
NY Hosp-Cornell Med Ctr

525 E 68th St; New York, NY 10021; (212) 746-3566; **BDCERT:** PCd 83; PCCM 92; **MS:** U Chicago-Pritzker Sch Med 77; **RES:** Albert Einstein Med Ctr, Bronx, NY 77-80; **FEL:** PCd, New York University Med Ctr, New York, NY; **HMO:** Sanus US Hlthcre Aetna Hlth Plan Metlife PHS +

👪 ☕ 🔲 👪 🏥 $ Mcr Mcd NFI A Few Days 💳 *VISA* 💳 💳

Gersony, Welton (MD)   **PCd**
Columbia-Presbyterian Med Ctr

Babies and Children Hosp of New York, 3959 Broadway 2nd Fl North; New York, NY 10032; (212) 305-8509; **BDCERT:** Ped 63; **MS:** SUNY Hlth Sci Ctr 58; **RES:** Ped, Rainbow Babies & Children's Hosp, Cleveland, OH 58-61; **HMO:** Prudential Oxford Chubb NYLCare

Golinko, Richard J (MD)   **PCd**
Mount Sinai Med Ctr

1 Gustave Levy Pl; New York, NY 10029; (212) 241-8662; **BDCERT:** Ped 61; PCd 62; **MS:** NY Med Coll 56; **RES:** Children's Hosp of Philadelphia, Philadelphia, PA 56-57; **FEL:** Med, Children's Hosp, Boston, MA 59-60; Albert Einstein Med Ctr, Bronx, NY; **HMO:** Most

♿ Immediately ▨ **VISA** ▧

Hordof, Allan (MD)   **PCd**
Columbia-Presbyterian Med Ctr

3959 Broadway Rm 255; New York, NY 10032; (212) 305-4432; **BDCERT:** Ped 71; PCd 73; **MS:** NYU Sch Med 66; **RES:** Ped, Children's Hosp of Buffalo, Buffalo, NY 67-68; Ped, Babies Hosp, New York, NY 68-69; **FEL:** Ped, Babies Hosp, New York, NY 71-72; Ped, Babies Hosp, New York, NY 72-73; **FAP:** Prof Ped Columbia P&S; **SI:** *Cardiac Arrhythmias; Congenital Heart Disease*

♿ ▨ ▨ ▨ Immediately

Krongrad, Ehud (MD)   **PCd**
Columbia-Presbyterian Med Ctr

3959 Broadway; New York, NY 10032; (212) 305-8509; **BDCERT:** Ped 70; PCd 74; **MS:** Israel 66; **RES:** Maimonides Med Ctr, Brooklyn, NY 67-69; **FEL:** Mayo Clinic, Rochester, MN 69-71; **SI:** *Pediatric Cardiology; Syncope;* **HMO:** Aetna Hlth Plan PHS Oxford Chubb Blue Choice +

LANG: Yd, Heb; ♿ ▨ ▨ ▨ ▨ A Few Days

Liu, Lena (MD)   **PCd**
St Vincents Hosp & Med Ctr NY

130 W 12th St; New York, NY 10011; (212) 604-7880; **BDCERT:** Ped 63; PCd 68; **MS:** Taiwan 57; **RES:** Kings County Hosp Ctr, Brooklyn, NY 60-63; **FEL:** Babies Hosp, New York, NY 64-67; **HMO:** Oxford Prucare HealthNet Champus Blue Choice +

♿ ▨ ▨ ▨ ▨ A Few Days

Parness, Ira (MD)   **PCd**
Mount Sinai Med Ctr

Mount Sinai Med Ctr, 1 Gustave Levy Pl #1201; New York, NY 10029; (212) 241-8662; **BDCERT:** Ped 82; PCd 85; **MS:** SUNY Hlth Sci Ctr 79; **RES:** Ped, Brookdale Univ Hosp Med Ctr, Brooklyn, NY 79-82; **FEL:** PCd, Children's Hosp, Boston, MA 82-85; **FAP:** Assoc Prof Mt Sinai Sch Med; **SI:** *Pediatric Echocardiography; Fetal Echocardiography;* **HMO:** Oxford Blue Cross & Blue Shield US Hlthcre Premier Affordable Hlth Plan +

LANG: Sp, Kor, Heb; ♿ ▨ ▨ ▨ ▨ ▨ Immediately

Steinfeld, Leonard (MD)   **PCd**
Mount Sinai Med Ctr

Mount Sinai Hospital, 1 Gustave Levy Pl; New York, NY 10029; (212) 241-7210; **BDCERT:** Ped 60; PCd 61; **MS:** SUNY Downstate 53; **RES:** Ped, Mount Sinai Med Ctr, New York, NY 54-56; **FEL:** PCd, Mount Sinai Med Ctr, New York, NY 56-59; **FAP:** Prof Mt Sinai Sch Med; **SI:** *Pediatric Cardiology; Echocardiography;* **HMO:** Blue Cross Aetna Hlth Plan HIP Network GHI Oxford +

LANG: Sp; ♿ ▨ ▨ ▨ ▨ ▨ ▨ ▨ Immediately ▨ **VISA** ▨ ▨

Steinherz, Laurel (MD)   **PCd**
Mem Sloan Kettering Cancer Ctr

1275 York Ave; New York, NY 10021; (212) 639-8103; **BDCERT:** Ped 76; PCd 78; **MS:** Albert Einstein Coll Med 70; **RES:** Ped, NY Hosp-Cornell Med Ctr, New York, NY 70-71; Ped, St Louis Children's Hosp, St Louis, MO 71-72; **FEL:** PCd, NY Hosp-Cornell Med Ctr, New York, NY 73-75; **FAP:** Assoc Prof Cornell U; **HOSP:** NY Hosp-Cornell Med Ctr; **SI:** *Cardiac Compl Bone Mr Trans*

LANG: Sp, Heb, Rus; ♿ ▨ ▨ ▨ ▨ A Few Days

Guide to symbols and abbreviations can be found on pages 110-113.

311

PEDIATRIC CRITICAL CARE MEDICINE

Greenwald, Bruce M (MD) PCCM
NY Hosp-Cornell Med Ctr

525 E 68th St G6329; New York, NY 10021; (212) 746-3056; **BDCERT:** Ped 87; PCCM 90; **MS:** NYU Sch Med 82; **RES:** Ped, Bellevue Hosp Ctr, New York, NY 82-86; **FEL:** PCCM, NY Hosp-Cornell Med Ctr, New York, NY 86-88; **FAP:** Assoc Prof of Clin Ped Cornell U; *SI: Respiratory Failure; Circulatory Shock*

🔲 🆂🆄 🌙 🔳 🔳 Mcr Mcd WC NFI Immediately ▦ **VISA** 💳 💳

Notterman, Daniel A (MD)PCCM
NY Hosp-Cornell Med Ctr

Box 437, 525 E 68th St ,N; New York, NY 10021; (212) 746-3056; **BDCERT:** Ped 83; PCCM 87; **MS:** NYU Sch Med 78; **RES:** Bellevue Hosp Ctr, New York, NY 78-81; **FEL:** NY Hosp-Cornell Med Ctr, New York, NY 83; **FAP:** Assoc Prof Cornell U

LANG: Sp, Chi; 🔲 🆂🆄 🌙 🔳 🔳 Mcd WC NFI ▦ **VISA** 💳 💳

Weingarten, Jacqueline (MD)PCCM
Montefiore Med Ctr

GPGP/VC4, 622 W 168th St; New York, NY 10032; (212) 342-3200; **BDCERT:** Ped 89; **MS:** Cornell U 86; **RES:** Ped, Columbia-Presbyterian Med Ctr, New York, NY 86-89; Ped, Columbia-Presbyterian Med Ctr, New York, NY 89-90; **FAP:** Assoc Clin Prof Ped Columbia P&S; *SI: Respiratory Failure; Nutrition;* **HMO:** Health First US Hlthcre PHS

LANG: Sp; 🔲 🆂🆄 🌙 🔳 🔳 🔳 Mcr Mcd WC NFI Immediately

Zucker, Howard A (MD) PCCM
Columbia-Presbyterian Med Ctr

Columbia Presbyterain, 3959 Broadway 2n259; New York, NY 10032; (212) 305-4432; **BDCERT:** PCCM 92; PCd 94; **MS:** Geo Wash U Sch Med 82; **RES:** Ped, Johns Hopkins Hosp, Baltimore, MD 82-85; PrM, Hosp of U Penn, Philadelphia, PA 85-87; **FEL:** PCd, Children's Hosp of Philadelphia, Philadelphia, PA; Children's Hosp, Boston, MA; **FAP:** Asst Prof Columbia P&S; *SI: Pediatric Cardiology; Pediatric Intensive Care;* **HMO:** Oxford Aetna Hlth Plan Prudential Blue Choice Chubb +

🔲 🔳 🔳 🔳 1 Week ▦▦ **VISA** 💳

PEDIATRIC ENDOCRINOLOGY

Aranoff, Gaya S (MD) PEn
Columbia-Presbyterian Med Ctr

3959 Broadway 50; New York, NY 10032; (212) 305-6559; **BDCERT:** Ped 80; PEn 86; **MS:** Albert Einstein Coll Med 75; **RES:** Ped, St Luke's Roosevelt Hosp Ctr, New York, NY 79-80; **FEL:** PEn, Columbia-Presbyterian Med Ctr, New York, NY 79-80; PEn, Columbia-Presbyterian Med Ctr, New York, NY 84-85; **FAP:** Assoc ClinP Columbia P&S; *SI: Pediatric Endo Testing; Pediatric Endo Except Diabetes;* **HMO:** Oxford Chubb CIGNA Blue Choice Aetna Hlth Plan +

LANG: Sp, Heb; 🔲 🔳 🔳 🔳 Mcd 4+ Weeks ▦▦ **VISA** 💳

David, Raphael (MD) PEn
New York University Med Ctr

530 1st Ave; New York, NY 10016; (212) 263-6462; **BDCERT:** Ped 65; PEn 78; **MS:** Switzerland 54; **RES:** Ped, Sinai Hosp of Baltimore, Baltimore, MD; Ped, Johns Hopkins Hosp, Baltimore, MD; **FEL:** EDM, Johns Hopkins Hosp, Baltimore, MD; **FAP:** Prof NYU Sch Med; **HOSP:** Bellevue Hosp Ctr; *SI: Growth Disorders; Puberty Disorders*

LANG: Fr; 🔲 🔳 🔳 🔳 $ 1 Week

Greig, Fenella (MD)   PEn
Mount Sinai Med Ctr
1 Gustave Levy Pl Bx1659; New York, NY 10029;
(212) 241-6936; **BDCERT:** Ped 83; PEn 83; **MS:** Mt
Sinai Sch Med 76; **RES:** Ped, Beth Israel Med Ctr,
New York, NY 77-79; Ped, NY Hosp-Cornell Med
Ctr, New York, NY 79-80; **FEL:** PEn, NY Hosp-
Cornell Med Ctr, New York, NY 79-80; **FAP:** Assoc
Prof Mt Sinai Sch Med; **SI:** *Diabetes in Young
Children; Thyroid Disease;* **HMO:** Aetna Hlth Plan
Oxford CIGNA US Hlthcre

LANG: Sp; ⬛ ⬛ ⬛ ⬛ ⬛ ⬛   A Few Days ⬛
VISA ⬛

Kohn, Brenda (MD)   PEn
Long Island Coll Hosp
Endocrinology, Diabetes & Metabolism, 475 E 72nd
St Ste 101; New York, NY 10021; (212) 249-
4408; **BDCERT:** Ped 81; EDM 83; **MS:** Albert
Einstein Coll Med 76; **RES:** Ped, New York
University Med Ctr, New York, NY 76-77; Ped, New
York University Med Ctr, New York, NY 77-79;
FEL: NY Hosp-Cornell Med Ctr, New York, NY 80-
83; Adolescent RE, Nat Inst Health, Bethesda, MD
80-83; **FAP:** Assoc Prof of Clin Ped SUNY Hlth Sci
Ctr; **HOSP:** Lenox Hill Hosp; **SI:** *Hypothalamic
Pituitary Disorders; Disorders of Growth;* **HMO:**
Oxford Empire Blue Cross & Shield PHCS Guardian
Blue Choice +

LANG: Fr, Heb, Yd, Itl; ⬛ ⬛ ⬛   A Few Days

Levine, Lenore (MD)   PEn
Columbia-Presbyterian Med Ctr
Director of Pediatric Endocrinology, 622 W 168th
St; New York, NY 10032; (212) 305-6559;
BDCERT: Ped 64; PEn 78; **MS:** NYU Sch Med 58;
RES: Ped, Bellevue Hosp Ctr, New York, NY 58-60;
FEL: Ped, NY Hosp-Cornell Med Ctr, New York, NY
60-61; PEn, NY Hosp-Cornell Med Ctr, New York,
NY 67-69; **FAP:** Prof Columbia P&S; **HOSP:** St
Luke's Roosevelt Hosp Ctr; **SI:** *Growth Disorders;
Adrenal Disorders;* **HMO:** Oxford Blue Choice PHS
CIGNA

LANG: Sp; ⬛ ⬛ ⬛ ⬛ ⬛   2-4 Weeks ⬛ **VISA**
⬛

New, Maria (MD)   PEn
NY Hosp-Cornell Med Ctr
525 E 68th St; New York, NY 10021; (212) 746-
3450; **BDCERT:** Ped 60; **MS:** Univ Penn 54; **RES:**
NY Hosp-Cornell Med Ctr, New York, NY 55-57;
FEL: NY Hosp-Cornell Med Ctr, New York, NY 61-
64; **FAP:** Chrmn Ped Cornell U; **SI:** *Disorders of
Puberty; Genetic Disorders of Hormones*

⬛ ⬛ ⬛ ⬛ ⬛ ⬛ ⬛   2-4 Weeks ⬛ **VISA** ⬛ ⬛

Oberfield, Sharon (MD)   PEn
Columbia-Presbyterian Med Ctr
Division of Pediatric Endocrinology, 622 W 168th
St; New York, NY 10032; (212) 305-6559;
BDCERT: Ped 79; **MS:** Cornell U 74; **RES:** Ped, NY
Hosp-Cornell Med Ctr, New York, NY 74-76; **FEL:**
PEn, NY Hosp-Cornell Med Ctr, New York, NY 76-
79; **FAP:** Prof Columbia P&S; **SI:** *Growth Disorders;
Adrenal Disorders;* **HMO:** Oxford

LANG: Sp; ⬛ ⬛ ⬛ ⬛ ⬛   2-4 Weeks ⬛ **VISA**
⬛

Sklar, Charles A (MD)   PEn
Mem Sloan Kettering Cancer Ctr
1275 York Ave; New York, NY 10021; (212) 639-
8138; **BDCERT:** Ped 79; PEn 80; **MS:** USC Sch Med
74; **RES:** Children's Hosp of Los Angeles, Los
Angeles, CA 74-76; **FEL:** PEn, UC San Francisco
Med Ctr, San Francisco, CA 76-79; **HOSP:** NY
Hosp-Cornell Med Ctr; **SI:** *Late Complications of
Cancer; Pituitary Disease;* **HMO:** None

⬛ ⬛ ⬛ ⬛ ⬛   2-4 Weeks

PEDIATRIC GASTROENTEROLOGY

Bangaru, Babu (MD) PGe
New York University Med Ctr
530 1st Ave Ste 3A; New York, NY 10016; (212) 263-7868; **BDCERT:** Ped 78; PGe 90; **MS:** India 70; **RES:** St Luke's Roosevelt Hosp Ctr, New York, NY; **FEL:** Liver Disease, Albert Einstein Med Ctr, Bronx, NY 76-78; Ge & Nutrition, Emory U Hosp, Atlanta, GA 78-79; **FAP:** Assoc Clin Prof Ped NYU Sch Med; **HOSP:** NY Hosp Med Ctr of Queens; ***SI:*** *Nutritional Problems Pediatric*; **HMO:** Aetna Hlth Plan Prucare CIGNA Oxford +

LANG: Hin; ♿ ☎ 📅 $ 1 Week

Illueca, Marta (MD) PGe
NY Hosp-Cornell Med Ctr
525 E 68th St M436; New York, NY 10021; (212) 746-3520; **BDCERT:** Ped 90; **MS:** Panama 84; **RES:** Ped, NY Hosp-Cornell Med Ctr, New York, NY 85-88; **FEL:** NY Hosp-Cornell Med Ctr, New York, NY 88-90; **FAP:** Asst Prof Cornell U; ***SI:*** *Pediatric Endoscopy; Acid-Peptic Diseases*; **HMO:** Aetna Hlth Plan US Hlthcre CIGNA Blue Choice Magnacare +

LANG: Sp; ♿ ☎ 📅 $ [Mcd] [NFI] 1 Week

Le Leiko, Neal S (MD) PGe
Mount Sinai Med Ctr
Pediatric Gastroenterology, 1 Gustave Levy Place Bx1656; New York, NY 10029; (212) 241-5415; **BDCERT:** Ped 76; PGe 90; **MS:** NY Med Coll 71; **RES:** Mount Sinai Med Ctr, New York, NY 71-74; **FEL:** PGe, Children's Hosp, Boston, MA 76-79; **FAP:** Prof Mt Sinai Sch Med; ***SI:*** *Short Gut Syndrome; Inflammatory Bowel Disease*; **HMO:** Oxford US Hlthcre Aetna-US Healthcare Blue Cross

♿ ☎ 👤 📅 $ [Mcr] A Few Days American Express VISA MasterCard

Levy, Joseph (MD) PGe
Columbia-Presbyterian Med Ctr
Childrens Digestive Health Ctr, 3959 Broadway BHN726; New York, NY 10032; (212) 305-5693; **BDCERT:** Ped 79; PGe 90; **MS:** Israel 73; **RES:** Hebrew U, Jerusalem, Israel 72; Ped, Beth Israel Med Ctr, New York, NY 75-77; **FEL:** PGe, Columbia-Presbyterian Med Ctr, New York, NY 77-79; **FAP:** Prof of Clin Ped Columbia P&S; ***SI:*** *Crohn's Colitis and Short Bowel; Reflux Abdominal Pain*; **HMO:** Empire Blue Cross & Shield Blue Choice Guardian Merrill Lynch Select +

LANG: Sp, Heb, Fr; ♿ ☎ 📅 $ [Mcd] 2-4 Weeks American Express VISA MasterCard

Mones, Richard (MD) PGe [PCP]
Columbia-Presbyterian Med Ctr
401 W 118th St 2; New York, NY 10027; (212) 666-4610; **BDCERT:** Ped 77; PGe 97; **MS:** NY Med Coll 71; **RES:** Ped, Columbia-Presbyterian Med Ctr, New York, NY 71-73; Ped, Columbia-Presbyterian Med Ctr, New York, NY 75-77; **FEL:** Ped, Columbia-Presbyterian Med Ctr, New York, NY; **FAP:** Assoc Clin Prof Columbia P&S; **HOSP:** St Luke's Roosevelt Hosp Ctr; ***SI:*** *Inflammatory Bowel Disease*; **HMO:** Oxford Aetna Hlth Plan Empire Blue Choice Healthease +

LANG: Sp, Fr, Cre; ♿ [SA SU] ☎ 👤 📅 $ Immediately VISA MasterCard

Spivak, William (MD) PGe
Montefiore Med Ctr
475 E 72nd St 101; New York, NY 10021; (212) 249-3300; **BDCERT:** Ped 81; PGe 90; **MS:** Albert Einstein Coll Med 76; **RES:** Ped, Jacobi Med Ctr, Bronx, NY; **FEL:** Ge, Children's Hosp, Boston, MA; **FAP:** Assoc Prof PGe Albert Einstein Coll Med; **HOSP:** Lenox Hill Hosp; ***SI:*** *Colitis; Crohn's Disease*; **HMO:** Oxford CIGNA PHCS Multiplan Blue Cross & Blue Shield +

♿ ☎ 👤 📅 $ A Few Days VISA MasterCard

Guide to symbols and abbreviations can be found on pages 110-113.

PEDIATRIC HEMATOLOGY-ONCOLOGY

Aledo, Alexander (MD) PHO
NY Hosp-Cornell Med Ctr
525 E 68th St P 695; New York, NY 10021; (212) 746-3447; **BDCERT:** Ped 89; PHO 96; **MS:** NYU Sch Med 84; **RES:** Ped, NY Hosp-Cornell Med Ctr, New York, NY 84-87; **FEL:** PHO, Mem Sloan Kettering Cancer Ctr, New York, NY 87-90; **FAP:** Asst Prof Cornell U; **HOSP:** NY Hosp Med Ctr of Queens; *SI: Sarcomas of Adolescents; Pediatric Oncology*; **HMO:** Oxford Blue Cross Health Plus United Healthcare

LANG: Sp; 🔲 🔲 🔲 🔲 🔲 🔲 🔲 Immediately 🔲 *VISA* 🔲 🔲

Finlay, Jonathan (MD) PHO
New York University Med Ctr
Stephen Hassenfeld Center For Childhood Cancer and Blood Disorders, 317 E 34th St 8th Floor; New York, NY 10021; (212) 263-6725; **BDCERT:** Ped 84; PHO 87; **MS:** England 73; **RES:** Ped, Birmingham, England 73-75; Manchester, England 76; **FEL:** U Wisconsin Hosp ; **FAP:** Prof Ped NYU Sch Med; **HOSP:** Bellevue Hosp Ctr; *SI: Brain Tumors; Childhood Lymphoma*

LANG: Sp; 🔲 🔲 🔲 🔲 🔲 🔲 🔲

Garvin, James (MD) PHO
Columbia-Presbyterian Med Ctr
3959 Broadway; New York, NY 10032; (212) 305-9770; **BDCERT:** Ped 82; PHO 84; **MS:** Jefferson Med Coll 76; **RES:** Children's Hosp of Philadelphia, Philadelphia, PA 76-78; Middlesex Hosp, London, England 78-79; **FEL:** Hem Onc, Children's Hosp, Boston, MA 79-82; *SI: Bone Marrow Transplantation; Brain Tumor*; **HMO:** Aetna Hlth Plan Empire Blue Cross PHS Prudential Oxford +

LANG: Sp; 🔲 🔲 🔲 🔲 🔲 🔲 🔲 Immediately 🔲 *VISA* 🔲

Giardina, Patricia (MD) PHO
NY Hosp-Cornell Med Ctr
525 E 68th St Rm P695; New York, NY 10021; (212) 746-3405; **BDCERT:** Ped 74; **MS:** NY Med Coll 68; **RES:** NY Hosp-Cornell Med Ctr, New York, NY 69-70; **FEL:** NY Hosp-Cornell Med Ctr, New York, NY 71-72; **HMO:** Aetna Hlth Plan Blue Cross & Blue Shield CIGNA Metlife Prucare +

Karpatkin, Margaret (MD) PHO
New York University Med Ctr
550 1st Ave; New York, NY 10016; (212) 263-6428; **BDCERT:** Ped 80; PHO 80; **MS:** England 57; **RES:** St George's Hosp, London, England 57-61; **FEL:** Hem, St George's Hosp, London, England 61-64; **FAP:** Prof Ped NYU Sch Med; **HOSP:** Bellevue Hosp Ctr; *SI: Blood Clotting Disorders; Platelet Disorders*; **HMO:** Oxford CIGNA Aetna Hlth Plan United Healthcare Prucare +

LANG: Sp, Fr; 🔲 🔲 🔲 🔲 🔲 1 Week

Kernan, Nancy A (MD) PHO
Mem Sloan Kettering Cancer Ctr
1275 York Ave; New York, NY 10021; (212) 639-7250; **BDCERT:** PHO 84; **MS:** Cornell U 78; **RES:** Children's Hosp Nat Med Ctr, Washington, DC 78-81; **FEL:** PHO, Mem Sloan Kettering Cancer Ctr, New York, NY 81-84; *SI: Bone Marrow Transplantation*

🔲 🔲 🔲 🔲 🔲 🔲 Immediately 🔲 *VISA* 🔲

Lipton, Jeffrey F (MD) PHO
Mount Sinai Med Ctr
Mt Sinai Med Ctr, 1184 5th Ave Rm 720; New York, NY 10029; (212) 241-6031; **BDCERT:** Ped 81; **MS:** Jefferson Med Coll 87; **RES:** Path, New England Med Ctr, Boston, MA 88-89; Path, Beth Israel Med Ctr, New York, NY 90-94; **FEL:** Med Infomatics, New England Med Ctr, Boston, MA 89-90; **HOSP:** Englewood Hosp & Med Ctr; *SI: Pediatric Hematology-Oncology Only*; **HMO:** Most

LANG: Sp; 🔲 🔲 🔲 🔲 🔲 🔲 🔲 2-4 Weeks 🔲 *VISA* 🔲 🔲

Guide to symbols and abbreviations can be found on pages 110-113.

315

O'Reilly, Richard (MD)   PHO
Mem Sloan Kettering Cancer Ctr

1275 York Ave; New York, NY 10021; (212) 639-5957; **BDCERT:** PHO 73; Ped 74; **MS:** U Rochester 68; **RES:** Children's Hosp, Boston, MA 71-72

Piomelli, Sergio (MD)   PHO
Columbia-Presbyterian Med Ctr

3959 Broadway; New York, NY 10032; (212) 305-6531; **MS:** Italy 54; **RES:** Med, Univ of Naples Med Sch, Naples, Italy 55-57; **FEL:** Med, New England Med Ctr, Boston, MA 57-58; **FAP:** Prof Ped Columbia P&S; **SI:** *Sickle Cell Anemia; Thalassemia;* **HMO:** Bronx Health Oxford 1199 Empire Blue Cross & Shield Multiplan +

LANG: Sp, Itl, Fr; 🗲 🖸 🏧 🅂 🏧 Immediately 🖼
VISA 💳

Rausen, Aaron (MD)   PHO
New York University Med Ctr

317 E 34th St 8th Fl; New York, NY 10016; (212) 263-7144; **BDCERT:** Ped 60; PHO 74; **MS:** SUNY Downstate 54; **RES:** Bellevue Hosp Ctr, New York, NY 54-56; Mount Sinai Med Ctr, New York, NY 58-59; **FEL:** Hem Onc, Children's Hosp, Boston, MA; **HOSP:** Lenox Hill Hosp

🗲 🖸 🖩 🏧 🏧 Immediately

Sitarz, Anneliese (MD)   PHO
Columbia-Presbyterian Med Ctr

Babies & Childrens Hosp, Harkness Pavilion, 180 Fort Washington Ave; New York, NY 10032; (212) 305-9770; **BDCERT:** Ped 59; PHO 74; **MS:** Columbia P&S 54; **RES:** Children's Hosp, Boston, MA 54-55; Columbia-Presbyterian Med Ctr, New York, NY 55-57; **FEL:** Hem Onc, Columbia-Presbyterian Med Ctr, New York, NY 57-65; **FAP:** Prof of Clin Ped Columbia P&S; **SI:** *Acute Lymphoblastic Leukemia; Neuroblastoma;* **HMO:** Aetna-US Healthcare Oxford Prudential CIGNA United Healthcare +

LANG: Sp, Ger; 🗲 🖸 🖩 🏧 🏧 A Few Days 🖼
VISA 💳 🖼

Truman, John (MD)   PHO
Columbia-Presbyterian Med Ctr

630 W 168th St; New York, NY 10032; **BDCERT:** PHO 74; **MS:** Canada 60; **RES:** Mass Gen Hosp, Boston, MA 61-63; **FEL:** Mass Gen Hosp, Boston, MA 63-65; **FAP:** Clin Prof Ped Columbia P&S

Weiner, Michael (MD)   PHO
Columbia-Presbyterian Med Ctr

Columbia Presbyterian Medical Center, 180 Fort Washington Ave; New York, NY 10032; (212) 305-5808; **BDCERT:** Ped 80; **MS:** SUNY Syracuse 72; **RES:** Ped, Montefiore Med Ctr, Bronx, NY 72-74; **FEL:** PHO, New York University Med Ctr, New York, NY 74-76; Ped Onc, Johns Hopkins Hosp, Baltimore, MD 77; **FAP:** Prof of Clin Ped Columbia P&S; **SI:** *Hodgkin's Disease; Leukemia;* **HMO:** Oxford Prudential CIGNA Anthem Health PHS +

LANG: Sp; 🗲 🖩 🕿 🖸 🖩 🏧 🅂 🏧 Immediately
🖼 **VISA** 💳 🖼

PEDIATRIC INFECTIOUS DISEASE

Krasinski, Keith M (MD)   Ped Inf
Bellevue Hosp Ctr

Pediatric Infectious Diseases & Immunology, 550 1st Ave; New York, NY 10016; (212) 263-6427; **BDCERT:** Ped 80; Ped Inf 94; **MS:** Univ IL Coll Med 76; **RES:** Ped, Children's Med Ctr, Dallas, TX 77-79; **FEL:** Ped Inf, U Texas SW Med Ctr, Dallas, TX 79-81; **FAP:** Prof Ped NYU Sch Med; **SI:** *HIV/AIDS; Bacterial Infections*

LANG: Sp, Fr, Cre, Rus; 🗲 🖩 🏧 A Few Days

Noel, Gary (MD)   Ped Inf
NY Hosp-Cornell Med Ctr

NY Hosp-Cornell Med Ctr—Ped Inf Dis Dept, 525 E 68th St; New York, NY 10021; (212) 746-3326; **BDCERT:** Ped 85; Ped Inf 94; **MS:** Cornell U 80; **RES:** NY Hosp-Cornell Med Ctr, New York, NY 81-83; **FEL:** Boston Med Ctr, Boston, MA 83-85; **SI:** *Lyme Disease; HIV;* **HMO:** Aetna Hlth Plan Blue Choice Magnacare

🗲 🖸 🖩 🏧 🅂 🏧 🏧 🔲 🔲 1 Week 🖼 **VISA** 💳

PEDIATRIC NEPHROLOGY

Johnson, Valerie (MD)   PNep
NY Hosp-Cornell Med Ctr

525 E 68th St N0008; New York, NY 10021; (212) 746-3260; **BDCERT:** Ped 84; **MS:** Cornell U 77; **RES:** Ped, Mount Sinai Med Ctr, New York, NY 77-79; **FEL:** Nep, Albert Einstein Med Ctr, Bronx, NY 79-82; **FAP:** Assoc Clin Prof Ped Cornell U; *SI: Nephritic Syndrome; Glomerulonephritis;* **HMO:** Oxford US Hlthcre Blue Choice Aetna Hlth Plan Prucare +

LANG: Pol, Sp, Fr, Itl, Ar; 🅰 🔟 🖼 🎚 🅂 Mcr Mcd NFI Immediately ▨ **VISA** ●

Lieberman, Kenneth (MD) PNep
Mount Sinai Med Ctr

Pediatric Nephrology, 1 Gustave Levy Pl; New York, NY 10029; (212) 241-6187; **BDCERT:** Ped 81; PNep 83; **MS:** Albert Einstein Coll Med 77; **RES:** Ped, Mount Sinai Med Ctr, New York, NY 77-79; **FEL:** Nep, NY Hosp-Cornell Med Ctr, New York, NY 79-81; **FAP:** Assoc Prof Mt Sinai Sch Med; **HOSP:** Maimonides Med Ctr; *SI: Kidney Disease; Hypertension;* **HMO:** Oxford US Hlthcre Aetna Hlth Plan Travelers Premier +

LANG: Sp, Fr; 🅰 🔟 🖼 🎚 Mcr Mcd Immediately ▨ **VISA** ●

Seigle, Robert (MD)   PNep
Columbia-Presbyterian Med Ctr

3959 Broadway 701; New York, NY 10032; (212) 305-5825; **BDCERT:** Ped 80; PNep 82; **MS:** Columbia P&S 74; **RES:** Ped, Columbia-Presby, New York, NY 75-78; **FEL:** PNep, Albert Einstein, New York, NY 78-81; **FAP:** Asst Prof Columbia P&S; **HMO:** Aetna Hlth Plan Blue Choice Blue Cross & Blue Shield Oxford US Hlthcre +

PEDIATRIC PULMONOLOGY

Dimaio, Mary (MD)   PPul
NY Hosp-Cornell Med Ctr

525 E 68th St Rm J114; New York, NY 10021; (212) 427-4703; **BDCERT:** Ped 87; PPul 92; **MS:** SUNY Hlth Sci Ctr 81; **RES:** N Shore Univ Hosp-Manhasset, Manhasset, NY 85; **FEL:** Mount Sinai Med Ctr, New York, NY 85-88

Kattan, Meyer (MD)   PPul
Mount Sinai Med Ctr

5 E 98th St; New York, NY 10029; (212) 241-7788; **BDCERT:** Ped 80; PPul 86; **MS:** McGill U 73; **RES:** Children's Hosp Med Ctr, Cincinnati, OH 73-75; **FEL:** Ped Pul, Hosp For Sick Children, Toronto, Canada 75-78; **FAP:** Prof Mt Sinai Sch Med; *SI: Asthma; Cystic Fibrosis*

🅰 🎚 🅂 Mcr

Lamm, Carin (MD)   PPul
Mount Sinai Med Ctr

One Gustave Levy Pl Box 1202B; New York, NY 10029; (212) 241-9787; **BDCERT:** Ped 87; PPul 86; **MS:** NYU Sch Med 75; **RES:** Ped, Mount Sinai Med Ctr, New York, NY 76-79; **FEL:** PPul, Mount Sinai Med Ctr, New York, NY 79-81; **FAP:** Asst Prof Mt Sinai Sch Med; *SI: Sleep Disorders; Asthma;* **HMO:** Oxford Blue Choice US Hlthcre Guardian PHCS +

🅰 🔟 🖼 🎚 🅂 1 Week ▨ ●

Mellins, Robert (MD)   PPul
Columbia-Presbyterian Med Ctr

Pediatric Pulmonary Division, 3959 Broadway; New York, NY 10032; (212) 305-5122; **BDCERT:** Ped 58; PPul 95; **MS:** Johns Hopkins U 52; **RES:** Ped, NY Hosp-Cornell Med Ctr, New York, NY 55-56; Columbia-Presbyterian Med Ctr, New York, NY 56-57; **FEL:** Pul, Columbia-Presbyterian Med Ctr, New York, NY 61-64; **FAP:** Prof Columbia P&S; *SI: Asthma/Chronic Cough; Pneumonia;* **HMO:** Oxford PHS Prudential CIGNA Blue Choice +

LANG: Fr, Grk; 🅰 🔟 🖼 🎚 🅂 1 Week ▨ **VISA** ● ▨

Guide to symbols and abbreviations can be found on pages 110-113.

317

Valacer, David J (MD)   **PPul**
NY Hosp-Cornell Med Ctr

525 E 68th St J116; New York, NY 10021; (212) 746-3313; **BDCERT:** PPul 94; Ped 84; **MS:** Univ Vt Coll Med 79; **RES:** Columbia-Presbyterian Med Ctr, New York, NY 79-82; **FEL:** A&I, UC San Francisco Med Ctr, San Francisco, CA 82-84; **HOSP:** New York Methodist Hosp; **SI:** *Lung Disease—Allergic; Asthma;* **HMO:** Aetna Hlth Plan Blue Choice Blue Cross & Blue Shield HealthNet Metlife +

♿ 🔶 🔳 ⊞ 🅂   Immediately ▨ *VISA* 💳 ▨

PEDIATRIC RADIOLOGY

Berdon, Walter (MD)   **PR**
Columbia-Presbyterian Med Ctr

3959 Broadway; New York, NY 10032; (212) 305-9864; **BDCERT:** Rad 62; PR 95; **MS:** SUNY Syracuse 55; **RES:** PR, Montefiore Med Ctr, Bronx, NY 59-62; **SI:** *Newborn Radiology; Childhood Tumors*

PEDIATRIC RHEUMATOLOGY

Eichenfield, Andrew (MD)Ped Rhu
Mount Sinai Med Ctr

Box 1198, Div of Pediatric Rheumatology, Mt Sinai Med Ctr; New York, NY 10029; (212) 241-1865; **BDCERT:** Ped 83; Rhu 92; **MS:** U Hlth Sci/Chicago Med Sch 78; **RES:** Ped, Mount Sinai Med Ctr, New York, NY 78-81; **FEL:** Rhu, Children's Hosp of Philadelphia, Philadelphia, PA 82-84; **FAP:** Asst Prof Ped Mt Sinai Sch Med; **SI:** *Juvenile Arthritis; Lyme Disease;* **HMO:** Aetna Hlth Plan Prucare Oxford Affordable Hlth Plan US Hlthcre +

♿ 🔶 🔳 ⊞ 🅂 ▨ ▨   1 Week ▨ *VISA* 💳

Lehman, Thomas (MD)   **Ped Rhu**
Hosp For Special Surgery

535 E 70th St; New York, NY 10021; (212) 606-1151; **BDCERT:** Ped 79; PR 92; **MS:** Jefferson Med Coll 74; **RES:** Ped, Children's Hosp of Los Angeles, Los Angeles, CA 74-76; Ped, UC San Francisco Med Ctr, San Francisco, CA 76-77; **FEL:** PR, Children's Hosp of Los Angeles, Los Angeles, CA 77-79; Rhu, Nat Inst Health, Bethesda, MD 81-83; **FAP:** Prof Ped Cornell U; **HOSP:** NY Hosp-Cornell Med Ctr; **SI:** *Lupus; Juvenile Rheumatoid Arthritis*

LANG: Sp, Itl, Prt; ♿ 🔶 🔳 ⊞ 🅂   A Few Days ▨ *VISA* 💳

PEDIATRIC SURGERY

Altman, R Peter (MD)   **PS**
Columbia-Presbyterian Med Ctr

15 W 81st St 16E; New York, NY 10024; (212) 305-5804; **BDCERT:** TS 71; PS 75; **MS:** NY Med Coll 61; **RES:** Mount Sinai Med Ctr, New York, NY 61-62; New England Med Ctr, Boston, MA 62-67; **FEL:** TS, Children's Hosp Nat Med Ctr, Washington, DC 67-69; Geo Wash U Med Ctr, Washington, DC 68; **FAP:** Prof S Columbia P&S; **SI:** *Liver & Biliary Disease; Chest Wall Surgery;* **HMO:** Oxford Blue Choice PHS GHI US Hlthcre +

♿ 🔶 ⊞ 🅂 ▨   Immediately

Beck, A Robert (MD)   **PS**
Beth Israel Med Ctr

112 E 83rd St; New York, NY 10028; (212) 861-0260; **BDCERT:** S 65; PS 75; **MS:** Albany Med Coll 58; **RES:** S, Mount Sinai Med Ctr, New York, NY 59-64; **FEL:** PS, Children's Hosp of Buffalo, Buffalo, NY 64-66; **FAP:** Clin Prof PS Mt Sinai Sch Med; **HOSP:** Mount Sinai Med Ctr; **SI:** *Newborn Surgery; Hernias;* **HMO:** HIP Network Aetna Hlth Plan Blue Shield CIGNA US Hlthcre +

🔶 ⊞   A Few Days

Dolgin, Stephen (MD)   PS
Mount Sinai Med Ctr

Mt Sinai Hospital, 5 E 98th St 12th; New York, NY 10029; (212) 241-3699; **BDCERT:** S 83; PS 93; **MS:** NYU Sch Med 77; **RES:** S, Harvard Med Sch, Cambridge, MA 77-82; **FEL:** PS, Childrens Mem Med Ctr, Chicago, IL; **FAP:** Chf PS Mt Sinai Sch Med; **SI:** *Newborn Operations; Inflammatory Bowel Disease;* **HMO:** GHI Oxford Aetna Hlth Plan Blue Cross & Blue Shield Blue Choice +

LANG: Sp, Rus; 🚻 🔂 👾 🎴 Med NFI   A Few Days

Epstein, Fred (MD)   PS
Beth Israel Med Ctr

317 E 34th St 1012; New York, NY 10016; (212) 870-9600; **BDCERT:** NS 72; **MS:** NY Med Coll 63; **RES:** New York University Med Ctr, New York, NY 65-70; **HOSP:** NYU Downtown Hosp; **SI:** *Pediatric Neurosurgery*

Ginsburg, Howard (MD)   PS
New York University Med Ctr

530 1st Ave 10 W; New York, NY 10016; (212) 263-7391; **BDCERT:** S 78; PS 84; **MS:** U Cincinnati 72; **RES:** New York University Med Ctr, New York, NY 72-77; **FEL:** PS, Columbia-Presbyterian Med Ctr, New York, NY 77-79; Ped U, Mass Gen Hosp, Boston, MA 79-80; **FAP:** Assoc Prof S NYU Sch Med; **HOSP:** Beth Israel Med Ctr; **SI:** *Neonatal Surgery; Pediatric Urology;* **HMO:** Oxford Aetna-US Healthcare GHI Guardian US Hlthcre +

🚻 🔂 👾 🎴 S Mcr Med   A Few Days 📷 **VISA** 💳 📠

La Quaglia, Michael (MD)   PS
Mem Sloan Kettering Cancer Ctr

1275 York Ave 1106; New York, NY 10021; (212) 639-7002; **BDCERT:** PS 85; **MS:** UMDNJ-NJ Med Sch, Newark 76; **RES:** S, Mass Gen Hosp, Boston, MA 76-83; **FEL:** PdS, Children's Hosp, Boston, MA 85-86; Mass Gen Hosp, Boston, MA 84-85; **FAP:** Assoc Prof Cornell U; **HOSP:** NY Hosp-Cornell Med Ctr

🚻 🔂 👾 🎴 Mcr Med NFI   Immediately

Schullinger, John (MD)   PS
Columbia-Presbyterian Med Ctr

3959 Broadway; New York, NY 10032; (212) 305-5871; **BDCERT:** S 64; PS 75; **MS:** Columbia P&S 55; **RES:** Columbia-Presbyterian Med Ctr, New York, NY 58-64; **FEL:** Babies Hosp, New York, NY 64

🚻 🔂 👾 🎴 Med   Immediately

Stolar, Charles (MD)   PS
Columbia-Presbyterian Med Ctr

Division of Pediatric Surgery, 3959 Broadway; New York, NY 10032; (212) 305-2305; **BDCERT:** S 81; PS 85; **MS:** Georgetown U 74; **RES:** U IL Med Ctr, Chicago, IL 74-80; **FEL:** Children's Hosp Nat Med Ctr, Washington, DC 80-82; **FAP:** Prof Columbia P&S; **SI:** *Neonatal Surgery; Pediatric Surgical Oncology*

LANG: Sp; 🚻 🔂 👾 🎴 S Med

Stylianos, Steven (MD)   PS
Columbia-Presbyterian Med Ctr

3959 Broadway; New York, NY 10032; (212) 305-8861; **BDCERT:** S 89; PS 94; **MS:** NYU Sch Med 83; **RES:** S, Columbia-Presbyterian Med Ctr, New York, NY 83-88; Children's Hosp, Boston, MA 90-92; **FEL:** Ped Trauma, New England Med Ctr, Boston, MA 88-90; **FAP:** Assoc Prof PS Columbia P&S; **SI:** *Laparoscopy in Infants;* **HMO:** Aetna Hlth Plan Oxford US Hlthcre GHI

LANG: Sp, Grk; 🚻 🔂 🎴 S Med   A Few Days

Velcek, Francisca (MD)   PS
Lenox Hill Hosp

Ped Surgery and Urology Associates, 965 5th Ave; New York, NY 10021; (212) 744-9396; **BDCERT:** S 74; PS 97; **MS:** Philippines 66; **RES:** S, St Clare's Hosp & Health Ctr, New York, NY 66-71; **FEL:** PdS, Univ Hosp SUNY Bklyn, Brooklyn, NY 73-75; PdS, Univ Hosp SUNY Bklyn, Brooklyn, NY 72-73; **FAP:** Prof S SUNY Hlth Sci Ctr; **HOSP:** Long Island Coll Hosp; **SI:** *Pediatric Adolescent Gynecology; Anorectal Malformations;* **HMO:** Oxford CIGNA Prucare GHI US Hlthcre +

LANG: Sp, Fil, Crt, Czc, Ilo; 🚻 SA 🔂 🔂 👾 🎴 S Med NFI   A Few Days

PEDIATRICS

Agre, Fred (MD)   Ped
St Luke's Roosevelt Hosp Ctr
1000 10th Ave; New York, NY 10019; (212) 523-3359; **BDCERT:** Ped 67; **MS:** Duke U 61; **RES:** Duke U Med Ctr, Durham, NC; Jacobi Med Ctr, Bronx, NY 63-64

Allendorf, Dennis (MD)   Ped   **PCP**
Columbia-Presbyterian Med Ctr
ColuPresby Westside Pediatrics also 21 W 86 St Ofc, 401 W 118th St 2; New York, NY 10027; (212) 666-4610; **BDCERT:** Ped 87; **MS:** NY Med Coll 70; **RES:** St Luke's Roosevelt Hosp Ctr, New York, NY 71-72; Columbia-Presbyterian Med Ctr, New York, NY 73; **FAP:** Asst Clin Prof Ped Columbia P&S; **HOSP:** St Luke's Roosevelt Hosp Ctr; **SI:** *Congenital Malformations; Congenital Deformations;* **HMO:** Magnacare HealthNet Guardian Blue Cross & Blue Shield Healthease +
LANG: Sp, Fr; ♿ 🏧 📷 👤 🏥 $ A Few Days **VISA** 💳

Arpadi, Stephen M (MD)   Ped   **PCP**
St Luke's Roosevelt Hosp Ctr
1111 Amsterdam Ave; New York, NY 10025; (212) 523-5818; **BDCERT:** Ped 87; **MS:** Geo Wash U Sch Med 82; **RES:** Ped, Children's Hosp Nat Med Ctr, Washington, DC 82-85; **FAP:** Asst Prof Ped Columbia P&S; **SI:** *AIDS/HIV*
LANG: Sp; ♿ 📷 👤 🏥 Mcr Mcd A Few Days

Bizzoco, Sabina (MD)   Ped
NY Hosp-Cornell Med Ctr
NY Hospital / Cornell Medical Center, 525 E 68th St; New York, NY 10021; (212) 821-0560; **BDCERT:** Ped 89; **MS:** Mexico 82; **RES:** New York University Med Ctr, New York, NY; Bellevue Hosp Ctr, New York, NY; **FEL:** NY Hosp-Cornell Med Ctr, New York, NY; **FAP:** Asst Prof Ped Cornell U; **SI:** *Pediatric Emergency Medicine*
LANG: Sp; ♿ 🏧 📷 👤 🏥 Mcr Mcd WC Immediately

Bonforte, Richard (MD)   Ped   **PCP**
Beth Israel Med Ctr
350 E 17th St; New York, NY 10003; (212) 420-4098; **BDCERT:** Ped 70; **MS:** Georgetown U 65; **RES:** Ped, Mount Sinai Med Ctr, New York, NY 65-68; **FEL:** Ped, Mount Sinai Med Ctr, New York, NY 70-72; **FAP:** Prof Albert Einstein Coll Med; **SI:** *Cystic Fibrosis; Asthma;* **HMO:** Oxford Prudential Aetna-US Healthcare Blue Choice Health First +
♿ 📷 👤 🏥 $ Mcr Mcd WC NFI A Few Days 💳 **VISA** 💳

Borkowsky, William (MD)   Ped
New York University Med Ctr
550 1st Ave; New York, NY 10016; (212) 561-3612; **BDCERT:** Ped 79; Inf 79; **MS:** NYU Sch Med 79; **RES:** Bellevue Hosp Ctr, New York, NY 72-75; **FEL:** Inf, New York University Med Ctr, New York, NY 75-78; **FAP:** Prof NYU Sch Med; **HOSP:** Bellevue Hosp Ctr
♿ 📷 👤 Mcd Immediately

Bowen, Shawn (MD)   Ped   **PCP**
Montefiore Med Ctr
New York Children's Health Project, 317 E 64th St; New York, NY 10021; (212) 535-9779; **BDCERT:** Ped 96; **MS:** Columbia P&S 93; **RES:** Montefiore Med Ctr, Bronx, NY 94-96; **FAP:** Instr Ped Albert Einstein Coll Med; **SI:** *Homeless Families; Mobile Medical Offices;* **HMO:** +
LANG: Sp; 📷 👤 🏥 Mcd Immediately

Burstin, Harris E (MD)   Ped   **PCP**
New York University Med Ctr
Pediatric AssociatesNew York, 317 E 34th St FL3; New York, NY 10016; (212) 725-6300; **BDCERT:** Ped 82; CCM 90; **MS:** Mexico 77; **RES:** Ped, New York University Med Ctr, New York, NY 78-82; **HOSP:** Beth Israel Med Ctr; **SI:** *Asthma and Allergies; Hospitalized Sick Children;* **HMO:** Aetna Hlth Plan Health Source Oxford United Healthcare PHS +
LANG: Sp, Yd, Itl; ♿ 🏧 📷 👤 🏥 $ A Few Days **VISA** 💳

Bussel, James (MD) Ped
NY Hosp-Cornell Med Ctr
525 E 68th St; New York, NY 10021; (212) 746-3416; **BDCERT:** Ped 79; Hem 81; **MS:** Columbia P&S 75; **RES:** Ped, Children's Hosp Med Ctr, Cincinnati, OH 76; **FEL:** PHO, NY Hosp-Cornell Med Ctr, New York, NY 78-81; Mem Sloan Kettering Cancer Ctr, New York, NY 78-81; **HOSP:** Lenox Hill Hosp; **HMO:** Aetna Hlth Plan Blue Choice Blue Cross & Blue Shield CIGNA HealthNet +

🔲 🔲 🔲 🔲 🔲 🔲 Mcr Mcd NFl A Few Days 🔲 **VISA** 🔲
🔲

Bye, Michael R (MD) Ped
Valley Hosp
Columbia Presbyterian - Babies and Children's Hospital, 3959 Broadway; New York, NY 10032; (212) 305-5122; **BDCERT:** Ped 80; Pul 86; **MS:** SUNY Buffalo 76; **RES:** Ped, Children's Hosp of Buffalo, Buffalo, NY 79; Ped, Children's Hosp of Buffalo, Buffalo, NY 79-82; **FAP:** Prof Ped Columbia P&S; **HOSP:** Columbia-Presbyterian Med Ctr; *SI: Asthma; Cough;* **HMO:** Oxford CIGNA Blue Cross & Blue Shield PHS Chubb +

🔲 🔲 🔲 🔲 🔲 Mcr Mcd 🔲 **VISA** 🔲

Coffey, Robert (MD) Ped **PCP**
St Vincents Hosp & Med Ctr NY
Soho Pediatric Group, 568 Broadway 205; New York, NY 10012; (212) 334-3366; **BDCERT:** Ped 80; **MS:** U Okla Coll Med 74; **RES:** Jacobi Med Ctr, Bronx, NY 74-77; **FEL:** Bronx Muncipal Hosp Ctr, Bronx, NY 77-78; **HOSP:** Beth Israel Med Ctr; **HMO:** Oxford Aetna Hlth Plan PHCS PHS Empire +

🔲 🔲 🔲 🔲 🔲 🔲 🔲 Immediately **VISA** 🔲

Cohen, Michel (MD) Ped **PCP**
St Vincents Hosp & Med Ctr NY
13 Harrison St; New York, NY 10013; (212) 226-7666; **BDCERT:** Ped 93; **MS:** France 89; **RES:** New York University Med Ctr, New York, NY 90-91; Long Island Jewish Med Ctr, New Hyde Park, NY; **HOSP:** NYU Downtown Hosp; **HMO:** Oxford PHS Aetna Hlth Plan

🔲 🔲 🔲 🔲 🔲 🔲 NFl Immediately

Cooper, Louis Z (MD) Ped
St Luke's Roosevelt Hosp Ctr
1000 10th Ave; New York, NY 10019; (212) 523-3365; **MS:** Yale U Sch Med 57; **RES:** Mass Gen Hosp, Boston, MA 57-58; Boston VA Med Ctr, Boston, MA 58-59; **FEL:** New England Med Ctr, Boston, MA 61-64; **FAP:** Prof Ped Columbia P&S; **HOSP:** Columbia-Presbyterian Med Ctr; *SI: Rubella Virus Infections During Pregnancy; Immunizations*

🔲 🔲 🔲 Mcr Mcd Immediately 🔲 **VISA** 🔲 🔲

Davies, Edward (MD) Ped **PCP**
Lenox Hill Hosp
50 E 77th St; New York, NY 10021; (212) 744-8530; **BDCERT:** Ped 63; **MS:** NYU Sch Med 57; **RES:** Bellevue Hosp Ctr, New York, NY 59; NY Hosp-Cornell Med Ctr, New York, NY 60; **HOSP:** NY Hosp-Cornell Med Ctr

🔲 🔲 🔲 🔲 🔲 🔲 Immediately 🔲 **VISA** 🔲

Elbirt-Bender, Paula (MD) Ped **PCP**
Mount Sinai Med Ctr
983 Park Ave; New York, NY 10028; (212) 737-1190; **BDCERT:** Ped 88; **MS:** Hahnemann U 79; **RES:** Mount Sinai Med Ctr, New York, NY 79-82; **FEL:** PPul, Mount Sinai Med Ctr, New York, NY; **HOSP:** Lenox Hill Hosp; *SI: Early Child Development; Adolescent Issues;* **HMO:** Oxford

🔲 🔲 🔲 🔲 🔲 🔲 Immediately 🔲 **VISA** 🔲

Ferrier, Genevieve (MD) Ped **PCP**
St Vincents Hosp & Med Ctr NY
West 11th Street, 46 W 11th St; New York, NY 10011; (212) 529-4330; **BDCERT:** Ped 91; **MS:** Mt Sinai Sch Med 88; **RES:** Ped, Children's Hosp of Los Angeles, Los Angeles, CA 88-91; **HOSP:** New York University Med Ctr; *SI: Child Development;* **HMO:** Oxford US Hlthcre Blue Cross Blue Choice

LANG: Fr, Sp; 🔲 🔲 🔲 🔲 🔲 Immediately **VISA** 🔲 🔲

Franklin, Bonita (MD)   Ped
Beth Israel Med Ctr
327 Rector Pl; New York, NY 10280; **BDCERT:** Ped
82; **MS:** SUNY Hlth Sci Ctr 76; **RES:** Ped, Mount
Sinai Med Ctr, New York, NY 78-79; Bronx
Municipal Hospital, Bronx, NY 77-78; **FEL:** Mt
Sinai, New York, NY 79-81; **HOSP:** Parkway Hosp;
HMO: Aetna Hlth Plan

⬤ ⬤ ⬤ ⬤ ⬤ Immediately

Gaerlan, Pureza (MD)   Ped
St Vincents Hosp & Med Ctr NY
36 7th Ave 509; New York, NY 10011; (212) 604-
8895; **BDCERT:** Ped 64; **MS:** Philippines 57; **RES:**
Albert Einstein Med Ctr, Bronx, NY 58-61; **FEL:**
Babies Hosp, New York, NY; Hem Onc, MD
Anderson Cancer Ctr, Houston, TX; **HMO:** Oxford
US Hlthcre Blue Cross & Blue Shield Prucare
Champus +

⬤ ⬤ ⬤ ⬤ ⬤ ⬤ Immediately

Gershon, Anne (MD)   Ped
Columbia-Presbyterian Med Ctr
650 W 168th St 4427; New York, NY 10032;
(212) 305-1556; **BDCERT:** Ped 69; Inf 94; **MS:**
Cornell U 64; **RES:** Ped, NY Hosp-Cornell Med Ctr,
New York, NY 66-68; **FEL:** Inf, New York
University Med Ctr, New York, NY; Inf, Oxford
Univ, Oxford, England

A Few Days

Gidwani, Sonia (MD)   Ped
St Luke's Roosevelt Hosp Ctr
Dep't of Pediatrics, 1090 Amsterdam Ave 3rd Flr;
New York, NY 10025; (212) 523-6900; **BDCERT:**
Ped 93; **MS:** India 90; **RES:** Sucheta Kripalani Hosp,
New Delhi, India 89-90; Ped, Univ of Med & Dent
NJ Hosp, Newark, NJ 90-93; **FEL:** PEn, Cornell U
Med Coll, Ithaca, NY 93-94

⬤ ⬤ 1 Week

Glaser, Stephen (MD)   Ped   PCP
Columbia-Presbyterian Med Ctr
3959 Broadway; New York, NY 10032; (212)
305-8585; **BDCERT:** Ped 69; **MS:** NYU Sch Med
64; **RES:** Ped, Case Western Reserve U Hosp,
Cleveland, OH 64-66; Ped, Babies Hosp, New York,
NY 66-67; **FEL:** PHO, Columbia-Presbyterian Med
Ctr, New York, NY 69-70; **FAP:** Asst Prof Columbia
P&S; **HMO:** Empire Oxford CIGNA Prucare PHS +

⬤ ⬤ ⬤ ⬤ ⬤ ⬤ ⬤ Immediately

Goldstein, Judith (MD)   Ped   PCP
Lenox Hill Hosp
1111 Park Ave; New York, NY 10128; (212) 369-
4670; **BDCERT:** Ped 77; **MS:** SUNY Hlth Sci Ctr 71;
RES: Lenox Hill Hosp, New York, NY 72-75; **HOSP:**
NY Hosp-Cornell Med Ctr; **SI:** *Newborns & Infants;*
Infectious Disease; **HMO:** Oxford Chubb Empire Blue
Cross & Shield Metlife

LANG: Ger, Hun, Itl, Sp, Fr; ⬤ ⬤ ⬤ ⬤ ⬤ ⬤
A Few Days ▦ **VISA** ⬤

Gribetz, Donald (MD)   Ped   PCP
Mount Sinai Med Ctr
1176 5th Ave 7; New York, NY 10029; (212) 289-
1401; **BDCERT:** Ped 53; **MS:** NYU Sch Med 47;
RES: Kingsbrook Jewish Med Ctr, Brooklyn, NY 48-
50; **FEL:** EDM, Mass Gen Hosp, Boston, MA 50-53;
HMO: None

⬤ ⬤ ⬤ ⬤ Immediately ▦ **VISA**

Gribetz, Irwin (MD)   Ped   PCP
Mount Sinai Med Ctr
1176 5th Ave 7; New York, NY 10029; (212) 876-
1855; **BDCERT:** Ped 61; **MS:** NY Med Coll 54; **RES:**
Mount Sinai Med Ctr, New York, NY 54-58; Ped,
Mount Sinai Med Ctr, New York, NY 55-57; **FEL:**
Pul, Harvard Med Sch, Cambridge, MA 57-58;
FAP: Prof Ped Mt Sinai Sch Med; **SI:** *Asthma*

LANG: Heb; ⬤ ⬤ ⬤ ⬤ ⬤ Immediately ▦ **VISA**
⬤

Grunfeld, Paul (MD)　　Ped　**PCP**
Lenox Hill Hosp
1111 Park Ave; New York, NY 10128; (212) 534-3000; **BDCERT:** Ped 80; **MS:** Romania 60; **RES:** Ped, Lenox Hill Hosp, New York, NY 71-73; **FEL:** PCd, Lenox Hill Hosp, New York, NY 73-75; *SI: Asthma/ Allergic Illnesses; Speech & Hearing Problems*; **HMO:** Oxford CIGNA Aetna Hlth Plan Guardian +

LANG: Rom, Ger, Hun, Sp, Pol; ⬆ 🅂 🄲 🄰 🄷 🄷
🅂 ▒ **VISA** ● ▬ ▬

Heagarty, Margaret (MD)　　Ped　**PCP**
Harlem Hosp Ctr
506 Lenox Ave; New York, NY 10037; (212) 939-4013; **BDCERT:** Ped 66; **MS:** Univ Penn 61; **RES:** Ped, St Christopher's Hosp for Children, Philadelphia, PA 61-62; Ped, St Christopher's Hosp for Children, Philadelphia, PA 62-64; **FEL:** Ped, Harvard Med Sch, Cambridge, MA 64-66; **FAP:** Prof Ped Columbia P&S; *SI: Pediatric AIDS; Low Income Children*

⬆ 🅂 🄷 Mcd WC Immediately

Inamdar, Sarla (MD)　　Ped　**PCP**
Metropolitan Hosp Ctr
68 Greenacres Ave; New York, NY 10029; (212) 423-6628; **BDCERT:** Ped 74; **MS:** India 69; **RES:** Flower Fifth Ave Hosp, New York, NY; Metropolitan Hosp Ctr, New York, NY 70-72; **FAP:** Prof of Clin Ped NY Med Coll; **HOSP:** Hosp Ctr at Orange

⬆ 🄰 🄷 🄷 Mcd Mcd A Few Days

Kahn, Max (MD)　　Ped　**PCP**
New York University Med Ctr
390 West End Ave; New York, NY 10024; (212) 787-1444; **BDCERT:** Ped 80; **MS:** Columbia P&S 75; **RES:** Jacobi Med Ctr, Bronx, NY 75-78; **FAP:** Assoc Clin Prof NYU Sch Med; **HOSP:** White Plains Hosp Ctr; **HMO:** Oxford CIGNA PHS United Healthcare

LANG: Fr, Sp, Alb; ⬆ 🅂 🄲 🄰 🄷 🄷 🅂
A Few Days **VISA** ●

Kaufman, David M (MD)　　Ped
Mount Sinai Med Ctr
3 E 83rd St; New York, NY 10028; (212) 737-4911; **BDCERT:** Ped 80; **MS:** Boston U 75; **RES:** Ped, NY Hosp-Cornell Med Ctr, New York, NY 75-77; N, Mount Sinai Med Ctr, New York, NY 77-78; **FEL:** ChiN, Mount Sinai Med Ctr, New York, NY 78-80; **FAP:** Asst Clin Prof Mt Sinai Sch Med; **HOSP:** Lenox Hill Hosp; *SI: Epilepsy; Headaches*; **HMO:** Oxford

LANG: Sp; ⬆ 🄰 🄷 🅂 2-4 Weeks ▒ **VISA** ●

Kotin, Neal (MD)　　Ped　**PCP**
Mount Sinai Med Ctr
1125 Park Ave; New York, NY 10128; (212) 289-1400; **BDCERT:** Ped 89; PPul 89; **MS:** Albany Med Coll 82; **RES:** Ped, Johns Hopkins Hosp, Baltimore, MD 83-85; **FEL:** PPul, Mount Sinai Med Ctr, New York, NY 85-88; **FAP:** Asst Prof Ped Mt Sinai Sch Med; **HMO:** Oxford CIGNA

LANG: Sp, Heb; ⬆ 🄲 🄰 🄷 🄷 🅂 Immediately
VISA ●

Landreth, Barbara (MD)　　Ped　**PCP**
NY Hosp-Cornell Med Ctr
115 E 67th St 1 C; New York, NY 10021; (212) 980-8230; **BDCERT:** Ped 92; **MS:** NYU Sch Med 87; **RES:** Ped, NY Hosp-Cornell Med Ctr, New York, NY 87-88; Ped, NY Hosp-Cornell Med Ctr, New York, NY 88-90; **FAP:** Instr Cornell U; **HOSP:** Lenox Hill Hosp; **HMO:** None

LANG: Sp; ⬆ 🅂 🄲 🄰 🄷 🄷 🅂 Immediately
VISA ●

Larsen, John (MD)　　Ped　**PCP**
Mount Sinai Med Ctr
1175 Park Ave; New York, NY 10128; (212) 427-0540; **BDCERT:** Ped 79; **MS:** SUNY Hlth Sci Ctr 74; **RES:** Ped, Mount Sinai Med Ctr, New York, NY 74-77; **FEL:** Ped Inf, Mount Sinai Med Ctr, New York, NY 77-78; **FAP:** Assoc Clin Prof Mt Sinai Sch Med; *SI: Pediatric Infectious Diseases*; **HMO:** Oxford Health Source

⬆ 🄰 🄷 🄷 🅂 Mcd A Few Days ▒ ●

Larson, Signe S (MD)   Ped   PCP
Mount Sinai Med Ctr
1175 Park Ave; New York, NY 10128; (212) 427-0540; **BDCERT:** Ped 84; PEn 89; **MS:** SUNY Hlth Sci Ctr 78; **RES:** FP, Vancouver Gen Hosp, Vancouver, Canada 78-79; Ped, St Luke's Roosevelt Hosp Ctr, New York, NY 79-82; **FEL:** PEn, Mount Sinai Med Ctr, New York, NY 82-84; **FAP:** Asst Prof Mt Sinai Sch Med; **HMO:** Oxford

A Few Days **VISA**

Lazarus, George (MD)   Ped   PCP
Columbia-Presbyterian Med Ctr
106 E 78th; New York, NY 10021; (212) 744-0840; **BDCERT:** Ped 76; **MS:** Columbia P&S 71; **RES:** Babies Hosp, New York, NY 71-72; Babies Hosp, New York, NY 72-74; **FAP:** Assoc Clin Prof Ped Columbia P&S; **HOSP:** Lenox Hill Hosp; **SI:** General Pediatrics; Adolescent Health

A Few Days

Lazarus, Herbert (MD)   Ped   PCP
New York University Med Ctr
Pediatric and Adolescent Medicine, LLP, 390 West End Ave; New York, NY 10024; (212) 787-1444; **BDCERT:** Ped 87; PR 92; **MS:** UMDNJ-NJ Med Sch, Newark 83; **RES:** New York University Med Ctr, New York, NY; **FEL:** Ped Rhu, Hosp For Joint Diseases, New York, NY; **HOSP:** Lenox Hill Hosp; **SI:** Juvenile Arthritis; Systemic Lupus; **HMO:** Oxford United Healthcare CIGNA PHS

LANG: Sp; A Few Days **VISA**

Levin, Linda (MD)   Ped   PCP
Mount Sinai Med Ctr
312 E 94th St; New York, NY 10128; (212) 423-2887; **BDCERT:** Ped 87; AM 94; **MS:** NYU Sch Med 82; **RES:** Montefiore Med Ctr, Bronx, NY 83-85; **FEL:** AM, Montefiore Med Ctr, Bronx, NY 85-86; **FAP:** Assoc Clin Prof Ped Mt Sinai Sch Med; **SI:** Adolescent AIDS Program; **HMO:** Most

LANG: Sp, Fr; 4+ Weeks

Levitzky, Susan (MD)   Ped   PCP
Beth Israel Med Ctr
161 Madison Ave Fl 6; New York, NY 10016; (212) 213-1960; **BDCERT:** Ped 72; **MS:** Univ IL Coll Med 67; **RES:** Bellevue Hosp Ctr, New York, NY 67-68; Beth Israel Med Ctr, New York, NY 68-70; **FAP:** Asst Prof Albert Einstein Coll Med; **SI:** Asthma; **HMO:** Oxford

LANG: Sp; A Few Days

Lipper, Evelyn (MD)   Ped
NYU Downtown Hosp
New York Hospital-Division of Child Development, 525 E 68th St; New York, NY 10021; (212) 746-3392; **BDCERT:** Ped 76; **MS:** Albert Einstein Coll Med 71; **RES:** Ped, Babies Hosp, New York, NY 72-73; Ped, Bronx Muncipal Hosp Ctr, Bronx, NY 74-75; **FAP:** Assoc Prof of Clin Ped Cornell U; **SI:** Learning Disabilities; Behavioral Problems; **HMO:** Empire Blue Cross Oxford PHS United Healthcare Empire +

LANG: Sp; 4+ Weeks **VISA**

McCarton, Cecelia (MD)   Ped
Montefiore Med Ctr-Weiler/Einstein Div
The McCarton Ctr for Developmental Pediatrics, 108 E 96th St; New York, NY 10128; (212) 996-9019; **BDCERT:** Ped 87; **MS:** Albert Einstein Coll Med 73; **RES:** Albert Einstein Med Ctr, Bronx, NY 70-74; **FEL:** Human Dev Bio, Albert Einstein Med Ctr, Bronx, NY; **FAP:** Prof Albert Einstein Coll Med; **HOSP:** Montefiore Med Ctr; **SI:** Developmental Pediatrics; **HMO:** None

4+ Weeks **VISA**

McHugh, Margaret (MD)   Ped
Bellevue Hosp Ctr
1st Ave & 27th St; New York, NY 10016; (212) 562-6321; **BDCERT:** Ped 75; **MS:** Georgetown U 70; **RES:** NY Med Coll, New York, NY 70-73; **FEL:** Ped, Columbia-Presbyterian Med Ctr, New York, NY 73-75; **HOSP:** New York University Med Ctr; **SI:** Adolescent Health Care; Child Protection; **HMO:** Centercare

Immediately

Meislin, Aaron G (MD)   Ped   `PCP`
New York University Med Ctr
530 1st Ave; New York, NY 10016; (212) 263-7219; **BDCERT:** Ped 59; **MS:** NYU Sch Med 54; **RES:** Ped, Bellevue Hosp Ctr, New York, NY 54-56; Ped, Mount Sinai Hosp, Cleveland, OH 56-57; **FEL:** Hem, Mount Sinai Med Ctr, New York, NY 57-78; **FAP:** Prof of Clin Ped NYU Sch Med; **HOSP:** Bellevue Hosp Ctr; **SI:** *Pediatric Rheumatology;* **HMO:** Oxford Well Care Metlife Aetna Hlth Plan

⟐ ▣ ▨ ⬚ $ Immediately

Meyers, Paul (MD)   Ped
Mem Sloan Kettering Cancer Ctr
1275 York Ave; New York, NY 10021; (212) 639-5952; **BDCERT:** Ped 78; **MS:** Mt Sinai Sch Med 73; **RES:** Mount Sinai Med Ctr, New York, NY 73-76; **FEL:** Hem Onc, NY Hosp-Cornell Med Ctr, New York, NY 76-79; Hem Onc, Mem Sloan Kettering Cancer Ctr, New York, NY 77-79; **FAP:** Assoc Clin Prof Ped Cornell U; **HOSP:** NY Hosp-Cornell Med Ctr; **SI:** *Bone Cancer; Childhood Cancer*

LANG: Sp, Fr; ⟐ ▣ ▨ ⬚ Mcr Mcd   Immediately

Mitchell, Michael (MD)   Ped   `PCP`
Beth Israel Med Ctr
Greenwich Village Pediatrics, 24 E 12th St; New York, NY 10003; (212) 929-3313; **BDCERT:** Ped 85; **MS:** Dominican Republic 81; **RES:** Ped, Beth Israel Med Ctr, New York, NY 82-85; **FAP:** Albert Einstein Coll Med; **SI:** *Natural Remedies;* **HMO:** Oxford Aetna Hlth Plan Blue Cross & Blue Shield Multiplan Anthem Health +

LANG: Sp; ⟐ ▣ ▨ ⬚ $ Immediately ▦ *VISA* ⬤

Monti, Louis G (MD)   Ped   `PCP`
Mount Sinai Med Ctr
BSM Pediatrics, PC, 55 E 87th St IG; New York, NY 10128; (212) 722-0707; **BDCERT:** Ped 85; **MS:** Mt Sinai Sch Med 80; **RES:** Mount Sinai Med Ctr, New York, NY 80-83; **FEL:** Ped Inf, Children's Hosp of Los Angeles, Los Angeles, CA 83-84; **FAP:** Asst Clin Prof Mt Sinai Sch Med; **SI:** *Pediatric Infectious Disease*

LANG: Itl, Sp; ▥ ◖ ▣ ▨ ⬚ $ A Few Days ▦ *VISA* ⬤ ▨

Murphy, Ramon J C (MD)   Ped   `PCP`
Mount Sinai Med Ctr
1175 Park Ave, 1175 Park Ave; New York, NY 10128; (212) 427-0540; **BDCERT:** Ped 74; **MS:** Northwestern U 69; **RES:** Med, Cook Cty Hosp, Chicago, IL 69-70; Ped, Childrens Mem Med Ctr, Chicago, IL 70-71; **FEL:** Ped, Babies Hosp, New York, NY 71-73; Mount Sinai Med Ctr, New York, NY 73-74; **FAP:** Assoc Clin Prof Ped Mt Sinai Sch Med; **SI:** *Adolescent Medicine*

LANG: Sp; ⟐ ▣ ▨ ⬚ $ Mcd   1 Week ▦ *VISA* ⬤

Nash, Martin (MD)   Ped
Columbia-Presbyterian Med Ctr
Babies & Childrens Hosp of New York, 3959 Broadway 701; New York, NY 10032; (212) 305-5825; **BDCERT:** Ped 69; **MS:** Duke U 64; **RES:** Georgetown U Hosp, Washington, DC 65; Columbia-Presbyterian Med Ctr, New York, NY 65-67; **FEL:** Albert Einstein Med Ctr, Bronx, NY 67-69; **FAP:** Prof Columbia P&S; **SI:** *Nephritic Syndrome; Renal Failure;* **HMO:** Oxford Empire Blue Cross & Shield US Hlthcre Health Source

⟐ ▣ ⬚ Mcr Mcd   1 Week ▦ *VISA* ⬤

Newman-Cedar, Meryl (MD) Ped
NY Hosp-Cornell Med Ctr
215 E 79th St 1C; New York, NY 10021; (212) 737-7800; **BDCERT:** Ped 87; **MS:** SUNY Downstate 81; **RES:** Ped, NY Hospital, New York, NY; **FEL:** NY Hospital, New York, NY; **FAP:** Clin Instr Cornell U; **HOSP:** Lenox Hill Hosp; **SI:** *Child Development*

LANG: Sp; ⟐ ▧ ◖ ▣ ▨ ⬚   Immediately *VISA* ⬤ ▨

Pitt, Jane (MD)   Ped
Columbia-Presbyterian Med Ctr
622 W 168th St; New York, NY 10032; (212) 305-2790; **BDCERT:** Ped 69; Ped Inf 98; **MS:** Harvard Med Sch 64; **RES:** Children's Hosp, Boston, MA 64-66; **FEL:** New England Med Ctr, Boston, MA 66-67; Children's Hosp, Boston, MA 67-70; **FAP:** Assoc Prof Columbia P&S; **SI:** *Immune Deficiency;* **HMO:** Empire Blue Cross & Shield Aetna Hlth Plan Chubb Oxford Prudential +

LANG: Fr, Ger; ⟐ ◖ ▣ ▨ $ Mcr Mcd   2-4 Weeks ▦ *VISA* ⬤ ▨

Poon, Eric (MD) Ped `PCP`
NYU Downtown Hosp
170 William St FL3; New York, NY 10038; (212)
312-5350; **BDCERT:** Ped 88; **MS:** Mexico 82;
HMO: Oxford Blue Cross & Blue Shield

Popper, Laura (MD) Ped `PCP`
Mount Sinai Med Ctr
8 E 77th St 1B; New York, NY 10021; (212) 794-
2136; **BDCERT:** Ped 81; **MS:** Columbia P&S 74;
RES: Babies Hosp, New York, NY 74-76; **FEL:**
Ambulatory Ped, Babies Hosp, New York, NY 76-
77; **SI:** *Adolescent Care;* **HMO:** Oxford
🔲 🔲 🔲 🔲 Immediately 🔲 *VISA* 🔲 🔲

Prezioso, Paula (MD) Ped `PCP`
New York University Med Ctr
Pediatric AssociatesNew York, 317 E 34th St FL3;
New York, NY 10016; (212) 725-6300; **BDCERT:**
Ped 91; **MS:** SUNY Downstate 87; **RES:** Bellevue
Hosp Ctr, New York, NY 87-90; Bellevue Hosp Ctr,
New York, NY 90-91; **FAP:** Asst Clin Prof NYU Sch
Med; **SI:** *Behavioral Pediatrics; Adolescent Medicine;*
HMO: Aetna Hlth Plan US Hlthcre Aetna Hlth Plan
CIGNA +
🔲 🔲 🔲 🔲 🔲 🔲 Immediately *VISA* 🔲

Quittell, Lynne (MD) Ped
Columbia-Presbyterian Med Ctr
3959 Broadway; New York, NY 10032; (212)
305-5122; **BDCERT:** Ped 86; **MS:** Israel 81; **RES:**
Schneider Children's Hosp, New Hyde Park, NY 81-
84; **FEL:** St Christopher's Hosp for Children,
Philadelphia, PA; **HMO:** Aetna Hlth Plan Chubb
Oxford PHS
🔲 🔲 🔲 🔲 A Few Days 🔲 *VISA* 🔲

Raucher, Harold (MD) Ped `PCP`
Mount Sinai Med Ctr
1125 Park Ave; New York, NY 10128; (212) 289-
1400; **BDCERT:** Ped 83; Ped Inf 94; **MS:** Mt Sinai
Sch Med 78; **RES:** Ped, Mount Sinai Hosp,
Cleveland, OH 78-80; **FEL:** Inf, Mount Sinai Med
Ctr, New York, NY 80-82; **FAP:** Assoc Prof Mt Sinai
Sch Med; **HOSP:** Lenox Hill Hosp; **SI:** *Behavioral
Pediatrics; Infectious Diseases*
🔲 🔲 🔲 🔲 🔲 🔲 🔲 Immediately *VISA* 🔲 🔲

Rocchio, Joseph (MD) Ped `PCP`
St Vincents Hosp & Med Ctr NY
59 W 12th St 1C; New York, NY 10011; (212)
255-7733; **MS:** Italy 77; **RES:** Ped, St Vincents
Hosp & Med Ctr NY, New York, NY 77-78; Ped, St
Vincents Hosp & Med Ctr NY, New York, NY 78-80;
FEL: Ped Pul, St Vincents Hosp & Med Ctr NY, New
York, NY 80-81; **SI:** *Infant Child; Adolescent;* **HMO:**
1199 Aetna Hlth Plan US Hlthcre
🔲 🔲 🔲 🔲 🔲 Immediately 🔲 *VISA* 🔲

Rosello, Lori (MD) Ped `PCP`
St Vincents Hosp & Med Ctr NY
46 W 11th St; New York, NY 10011; (212) 529-
4330; **BDCERT:** Ped 90; **MS:** Albert Einstein Coll
Med 87; **RES:** Columbia-Presbyterian Med Ctr, New
York, NY 87-90; **FAP:** Asst Clin Prof NYU Sch Med;
HOSP: New York University Med Ctr; **SI:** *General
Pediatrics;* **HMO:** Oxford Blue Choice US Hlthcre
Magnacare United Healthcare +
🔲 🔲 🔲 🔲 🔲 🔲 Immediately *VISA* 🔲

Rosen, Tove S (MD) Ped
Columbia-Presbyterian Med Ctr
Dept of Pediatrics, 3959 Broadway; New York, NY
10032; (212) 305-8500; **BDCERT:** Ped 71; **NP:** 75;
MS: SUNY Hlth Sci Ctr 65; **RES:** Ped, St Luke's
Roosevelt Hosp Ctr, New York, NY 68-70; **FEL:** NP,
Columbia-Presbyterian Med Ctr, New York, NY 72-
75; **FAP:** Prof of Clin Ped Columbia P&S; **SI:**
Neonatology; Drug Abuse
🔲

Rosenbaum, Michael (MD) Ped `PCP`
NY Hosp-Cornell Med Ctr
West End Pediatrics, 450 W End Ave; New York,
NY 10024; (212) 769-3070; **BDCERT:** Ped 88;
PEn 91; **MS:** Cornell U 82; **RES:** Columbia-
Presbyterian Med Ctr, New York, NY 82-85; **FEL:**
EDM, NY Hosp-Cornell Med Ctr, New York, NY 85-
88; **HOSP:** Lenox Hill Hosp; **SI:** *Nutrition; Growth;*
HMO: Oxford
LANG: Sp; 🔲 🔲 🔲 🔲 🔲 🔲 🔲 Immediately 🔲
VISA 🔲 🔲

Rosenfeld, Suzanne (MD)   Ped   PCP
NY Hosp-Cornell Med Ctr

West End Pediatrics, 450 West End Ave; New York, NY 10024; (212) 769-3070; **BDCERT:** Ped 86; **MS:** Columbia P&S 80; **RES:** Mount Sinai Med Ctr, New York, NY 81; Columbia-Presbyterian Med Ctr, New York, NY 83; **FEL:** Ped, NY Hosp-Cornell Med Ctr, New York, NY 84; **HOSP:** St Luke's Roosevelt Hosp Ctr

LANG: Sp; 🚹 📠 🅲 📷 👪 🛏 💲 Immediately ▦ **VISA** 💳

Rubinstein, Beatriz (MD)   Ped   PCP
Lenox Hill Hosp

50 E 77th St; New York, NY 10021; (212) 249-2447; **MS:** Argentina 62; **RES:** Lenox Hill Hosp, New York, NY; **FEL:** University of Vienna, Vienna, Austria; Rockefeller Univ Hosp, New York, NY; *SI: Acne*

LANG: Sp, Prt, Fr, Ger; 📠 🅲 📷 👪 🛏 Immediately ▦ **VISA** 💳 📷

Sanford, Marie (MD)   Ped   PCP
St Vincents Hosp & Med Ctr NY

59 W 12th St; New York, NY 10011; (212) 255-7733; **BDCERT:** Ped 94; **MS:** Mt Sinai Sch Med 91; **RES:** Ped, Mount Sinai Med Ctr, New York, NY 91-95; **FAP:** Asst Prof Ped NY Med Coll; **HMO:** Blue Cross & Blue Shield CIGNA Oxford Aetna-US Healthcare GHI +

🚹 🅲 📷 👪 🛏 💲 A Few Days

Saphir, Richard L (MD)   Ped   PCP
Mount Sinai Med Ctr

BSM Pediatrics PC, 55 E 87th St 1G; New York, NY 10128; (212) 722-4950; **BDCERT:** Ped 63; **MS:** SUNY Hlth Sci Ctr 58; **RES:** Mount Sinai Med Ctr, New York, NY 58-61; **FAP:** Clin Prof Ped Mt Sinai Sch Med; *SI: Newborns; Adolescents*; **HMO:** None

📠 🅲 📷 👪 🛏 💲 1 Week ▦ **VISA** 💳 📷

Schwartz, Stephen (MD)   Ped   PCP
New York University Med Ctr

530 1st Ave 3A; New York, NY 10016; (212) 263-7220; **BDCERT:** Ped 73; **MS:** NYU Sch Med 68; **RES:** Bellevue Hosp Ctr, New York, NY 68-71; **HOSP:** Long Island Coll Hosp; **HMO:** US Hlthcre Blue Choice Chubb

🚹 📷 👪 🛏 💲 Immediately

Seed, William T (MD)   Ped   PCP
NY Hosp-Cornell Med Ctr

56 E 76th St; New York, NY 10021; (212) 249-5544; **BDCERT:** Ped 68; **MS:** Cornell U 62; **RES:** Ped, NY Hosp-Cornell Med Ctr, New York, NY 63-65; **FEL:** NY Hosp-Cornell Med Ctr, New York, NY 65-66; **FAP:** Assoc Prof Cornell U; **HOSP:** Lenox Hill Hosp; **HMO:** None

LANG: Sp; 📷 👪 🛏 💲 Immediately **VISA** 💳

Silverman, Joseph (MD)   Ped   PCP
Columbia-Presbyterian Med Ctr

3 E 85th St; New York, NY 10028; (212) 535-7774; **BDCERT:** Ped 62; **MS:** Columbia P&S 56; **RES:** Babies Hosp, New York, NY 59-61; *SI: Anorexia Nervosa; Bulimia*

🚹 📷 👪 🛏 A Few Days

Skog, Donald (MD)   Ped   PCP
NY Hosp-Cornell Med Ctr

215 E 79th St 1C; New York, NY 10021; (212) 737-7800; **BDCERT:** Ped 77; **MS:** UMDNJ-NJ Med Sch, Newark 71; **RES:** Ped, NY Hosp-Cornell Med Ctr, New York, NY 72-74; **FAP:** Asst Prof Cornell U; **HOSP:** Lenox Hill Hosp

📷 👪 🛏 💲 Immediately **VISA** 💳

Smith, David (MD)   Ped   PCP
NY Hosp-Cornell Med Ctr

450 E 69th St; New York, NY 10021; (212) 988-0600; **BDCERT:** Ped 63; **MS:** NYU Sch Med 56; **RES:** Kings County Hosp Ctr, Brooklyn, NY 56-57; NY Hosp-Cornell Med Ctr, New York, NY 59-61; **HOSP:** Lenox Hill Hosp

🚹 📷 🛏 Immediately **VISA** 💳

Guide to symbols and abbreviations can be found on pages 110-113.

327

Softness, Barney (MD)   Ped   PCP
Columbia-Presbyterian Med Ctr

West End Pediatrics, 450 W End Ave; New York, NY 10024; (212) 769-3070; **BDCERT:** Ped 86; **PEn** 86; **MS:** Columbia P&S 80; **RES:** Ped, Babies Hosp, New York, NY; **FEL:** EDM, NY Hosp-Cornell Med Ctr, New York, NY; **FAP:** Asst Prof Columbia P&S; **HOSP:** NY Hosp-Cornell Med Ctr; *SI: Growth and Development*

🔧 🏧 💳 📷 🔧 🛏 💲 Immediately 🔲 **VISA** 💳

Spielman, Gerald (MD)   Ped   PCP
NY Hosp-Cornell Med Ctr

44 E 65th St 1B; New York, NY 10021; (212) 734-5655; **BDCERT:** Ped 71; **MS:** Albert Einstein Coll Med 66; **RES:** NY Hosp-Cornell Med Ctr, New York, NY 66-70; **HOSP:** New York Methodist Hosp; **HMO:** Oxford

📷 🔧 🛏 💲 A Few Days 🔲 💳

Stein, Barry B (MD)   Ped   PCP
Mount Sinai Med Ctr

1125 Park Ave; New York, NY 10128; (212) 289-1400; **BDCERT:** Ped 87; **MS:** South Africa 80; **RES:** Ped, Mount Sinai Med Ctr, New York, NY 83-86; **FAP:** Asst Clin Prof Mt Sinai Sch Med; **HMO:** None

LANG: Sp, Heb; 🔧 💳 📷 🔧 🛏 💲 A Few Days **VISA** 💳 💳

Stone, Richard K (MD)   Ped   PCP
Metropolitan Hosp Ctr

1901 1st Ave 1B2; New York, NY 10029; (212) 423-8131; **BDCERT:** Ped 73; **MS:** NY Med Coll 68; **RES:** Ped, NY Med Coll, New York, NY 68-71; **FAP:** Assoc Prof NY Med Coll; *SI: Primary Care; Behavioral Pediatrics;* **HMO:** Metroplus Centercare Fidelis

LANG: Sp; 🔧 📷 🔧 🛏 Ⓜ 1 Week 🔲 **VISA** 💳

Traister, Michael (MD)   Ped   PCP
Bellevue Hosp Ctr

390 West End Ave; New York, NY 10024; (212) 787-1444; **BDCERT:** Ped 80; **MS:** NY Med Coll 75; **RES:** Ped, Bronx Muncipal Hosp Ctr, Bronx, NY 76-78; **FEL:** Bellevue Hosp Ctr, New York, NY 78-79; **FAP:** Asst Prof of Clin Ped NYU Sch Med; **HMO:** CIGNA PHS United Healthcare

🔧 🏧 💳 📷 🔧 🛏 💲 4+ Weeks **VISA** 💳

van Gilder, Max (MD)   Ped   PCP
Columbia-Presbyterian Med Ctr

241 Central Park West 16; New York, NY 10024; (212) 787-1788; **BDCERT:** Ped 76; **MS:** Tulane U 71; **RES:** Montefiore Med Ctr, Bronx, NY 71-74; **FAP:** Asst Clin Prof Ped Columbia P&S; **HOSP:** St Luke's Roosevelt Hosp Ctr; **HMO:** Oxford Blue Choice Aetna-US Healthcare PHS Prucare +

LANG: Sp; 🏧 💳 📷 🔧 🛏 💲 A Few Days 🔲 **VISA** 💳 💳

Wallace, Claudina (MD)   Ped
Harlem Hosp Ctr

Dept of Pediatrics, Harlem Hosp; New York, NY 10037; (212) 939-2352; **BDCERT:** Ped 77; **MS:** Howard U 67; **RES:** Harlem Hosp Ctr, New York, NY 62-70; **FEL:** St Luke's Roosevelt Hosp Ctr, New York, NY

Weinberger, Sylvain M (MD) Ped   PCP
Beth Israel Med Ctr

326 E 18 St; New York, NY 10003; (212) 598-0331; **BDCERT:** Ped 82; **NP** 83; **MS:** Belgium 77; **RES:** Ped, Long Island Jewish Med Ctr, New Hyde Park, NY 79; **FEL:** NP, Long Island Jewish Med Ctr, New Hyde Park, NY 79-81; **HMO:** Oxford Chubb United Healthcare CIGNA Blue Choice +

LANG: Fr, Itl, Heb, Hun; 💳 📷 🔧 🛏 💲 Immediately 🔲 **VISA** 💳

Wishnick, Marcia M (MD & PhD)   Ped
PCP
New York University Med Ctr

157 E 81st St 1A; New York, NY 10028; (212) 879-7014; **BDCERT:** Ped 79; **MS:** NYU Sch Med 74; **RES:** Ped, New York University Med Ctr, New York, NY 74-77; **FAP:** Clin Prof Ped NYU Sch Med; **HOSP:** Mount Sinai Med Ctr; *SI: Developmental Pediatrics; Genetics—Adolescents;* **HMO:** US Hlthcre Oxford Aetna Hlth Plan Prucare CIGNA +

LANG: Sp, Rus, Grk, Itl, Fr; 🔧 🏧 💳 📷 🔧 🛏 💲 Immediately **VISA** 💳

Yapalater, Greg (MD)   Ped   `PCP`
Lenox Hill Hosp
1020 Park Ave; New York, NY 10028; (212) 289-8683; **BDCERT:** Ped 92; **MS:** France 81; **RES:** Lenox Hill Hosp, New York, NY 84; *SI: Infant Nutrition*; **HMO:** None

LANG: Fr; 🚹 ⛑ 🄲 📷 🛏 💲   Immediately ▦
VISA 💳

Zimmerman, Sol (MD)   Ped   `PCP`
New York University Med Ctr
Pediatric Associates of NYC, PC, 317 E 34th St; New York, NY 10016; (212) 725-6300; **BDCERT:** Ped 77; **MS:** NYU Sch Med 72; **RES:** Bellevue Hosp Ctr, New York, NY 72-75; Bellevue Hosp Ctr, New York, NY 77-78; **FAP:** Assoc Clin Prof Ped NYU Sch Med; **HOSP:** Beth Israel Med Ctr; *SI: Development and Behavior; Psychogenic Illness*; **HMO:** Oxford United Healthcare Aetna Hlth Plan CIGNA PHS +

🚹 ⛑ 📷 🄿 🛏 💲   2-4 Weeks *VISA* 💳

PHYSICAL MEDICINE & REHABILITATION

Ahn, Jung (MD)   PMR
New York University Med Ctr
400 E 34th St 421; New York, NY 10016; (212) 263-6122; **BDCERT:** PMR 80; **MS:** South Korea 70; **RES:** New York University Med Ctr, New York, NY; **FEL:** Spinal Cord Injuries, New York University Med Ctr, New York, NY; **FAP:** Assoc Clin Prof NYU Sch Med; *SI: Spinal Disorders; Stroke*; **HMO:** Oxford Aetna Hlth Plan Chubb United Healthcare

🚹 📷 🄿 🛏 💲 Mcr WC NFI   1 Week

Bodack, Mark (MD)   PMR
NY Hosp-Cornell Med Ctr
NY Hosp, 525 E 68th St; New York, NY 10021; (212) 746-1500; **BDCERT:** PMR 95; **MS:** Ireland 90; **RES:** PMR, NY Hosp-Cornell Med Ctr, New York, NY 91-94; **FAP:** Asst Prof Cornell U; *SI: Low Back Pain; Electrodiagnostic Studies*; **HMO:** Oxford CIGNA NYLCare Blue Choice Multiplan +

LANG: Sp, Bul; 🚹 🄲 📷 🄿 🛏 💲 Mcr WC NFI
A Few Days ▦ *VISA* 💳

Brown, Andrew (MD)   PMR
NYU Downtown Hosp
Downtown Physical Medicine Rehabilitation, 19 Beekman St; New York, NY 10038; (212) 513-7711; **BDCERT:** PMR 88; **MS:** West Indies 82; **RES:** PMR, Mount Sinai Med Ctr, New York, NY 84-87; **FAP:** Clin Instr Cornell U; *SI: Disability Evaluations; Electromyography*; **HMO:** Aetna Hlth Plan Blue Choice CIGNA GHI Oxford +

LANG: Sp, Chi, Rus, Ger, Itl; 🚹 📷 🛏 💲 Mcr WC NFI
A Few Days ▦ *VISA* 💳 🖼

Downey, John (MD)   PMR
Columbia-Presbyterian Med Ctr
622 W 168th St; New York, NY 10032; (212) 305-5954; **BDCERT:** PMR 64; **MS:** Canada 54; **RES:** PMR, Columbia-Presbyterian Med Ctr, New York, NY 54-58; IM, Peter Bent Brigham Hosp, Boston, MA 56-57; **FEL:** Oxford Univ, Oxford, England

🚹 📷 🛏 💲   A Few Days ▦ *VISA* 💳

Fazzari, Patrick (MD)   PMR
St Luke's Roosevelt Hosp Ctr
425 W 59th Street 8B; New York, NY 10019; (212) 376-3184; **BDCERT:** Ped 72; PMR 75; **MS:** Albany Med Coll 67; **RES:** Ped, Montefiore Med Ctr, Bronx, NY 68-70; PMR, Albert Einstein Med Ctr, Bronx, NY 70-72; **FAP:** Assoc Clin Prof Columbia P&S; *SI: Back Pain and Neck Pain; Performing Artists*; **HMO:** Oxford CIGNA Prucare Chubb Anthem Health +

LANG: Sp; 🚹 📷 🄿 🛏 💲 Mcr WC NFI   1 Week ▦
VISA 💳 🖼

Focseneanu, Marius (MD)   PMR
Beth Israel Med Ctr
1st Ave & 16th St Fl 3; New York, NY 10003; (212) 420-2757; **BDCERT:** PMR 79; **MS:** Romania 59; **RES:** PMR, Elmhurst Hosp Ctr, Elmhurst, NY 74-77; **FAP:** Asst Prof PMR Albert Einstein Coll Med; *SI: Rehabilitation, Acute In-Patient*; **HMO:** Blue Choice Blue Cross & Blue Shield Metlife Sanus-NYLCare

LANG: Rom; 🚹 📷 🄿 🛏 Mcr Mcd WC NFI   1 Week
VISA 💳

Goldberg, Robert (DO) PMR
St Vincents Hosp & Med Ctr NY

314 W 14th St Fl 1; New York, NY 10014; (212) 929-9009; **BDCERT:** PMR 82; **MS:** Philadelphia Coll Osteo Med 77; **RES:** St Vincents Hosp & Med Ctr NY, New York, NY 78-80; **FEL:** St Vincents Hosp & Med Ctr NY, New York, NY 80-81; **SI:** *Sports Medicine; Manipulation;* **HMO:** Health Source

LANG: Sp, Hin; 🔲 🔲 🔲 🔲 🔲 Mcr WC NFI Immediately
VISA 💳

Gotlin, Robert S (DO) PMR
Beth Israel Med Ctr

170 E End Ave; New York, NY 10128; (212) 870-9028; **BDCERT:** PMR 92; **MS:** Nova SE Univ, Coll Osteo Med 87; **RES:** PMR, Mount Sinai Med Ctr, New York, NY 88-91; **FAP:** Asst Prof Albert Einstein Coll Med; **SI:** *Sports Medicine; Orthopaedic Rehabilitation;* **HMO:** Aetna Hlth Plan Oxford CIGNA GHI Metlife +

LANG: Sp; 🔲 🔲 🔲 🔲 🔲 🔲 Mcr WC NFI
A Few Days 💳 **VISA** 💳 💳

Grynbaum, Bruce (MD) PMR
Rusk Institute

400 E 34th St RR119; New York, NY 10016; (212) 263-6477; **BDCERT:** PMR 52; **MS:** Columbia P&S 43; **RES:** Mount Sinai Hosp, Cleveland, OH 46-47; New York University Med Ctr, New York, NY 47-50; **FAP:** Clin Prof NYU Sch Med; **HOSP:** St Vincents Hosp & Med Ctr NY; **SI:** *Low Back Pain; Stroke*

LANG: Sp, Czc, Ger, Rus, Itl; 🔲 🔲 🔲 🔲 🔲 WC NFI
A Few Days

Hryhorowych, Arthur N (MD)PMR
Cabrini Med Ctr

67 Irving Place South 6th Fl; New York, NY 10003; (212) 673-7500; **BDCERT:** PMR 86; **MS:** Mexico 80; **RES:** Bronx Lebanon Hosp Ctr, Bronx, NY 82-84; **HOSP:** Beth Israel Med Ctr; **SI:** *Sports Medicine*

Inwald, Gary (DO) PMR
St Vincents Hosp & Med Ctr NY

24 E 12th St 302; New York, NY 10003; (212) 807-6599; **BDCERT:** PMR 83; **MS:** Mich St U 76; **RES:** PMR, St Vincents Hosp & Med Ctr NY, New York, NY 79-82; **HMO:** Blue Choice Blue Cross & Blue Shield HealthNet Oxford Prucare +

LANG: Sp; 🔲 🔲 🔲 🔲 🔲 🔲 Mcr WC NFI

Lachmann, Elisabeth A (MD)PMR
NY Hosp-Cornell Med Ctr

Dept of Rehabilitation Medicine, Box 142, 525 E 68th 18th Flr; New York, NY 10021; (212) 746-1500; **BDCERT:** PMR 92; **MS:** Med Coll PA 87; **RES:** PMR, NY Hosp-Cornell Med Ctr, New York, NY 88-91; **IM,** N Shore Univ Hosp-Manhasset, Manhasset, NY 87-88; **FAP:** Asst Prof Cornell U; **SI:** *Musculoskeletal Medicine; Low Back Pain;* **HMO:** Blue Choice Oxford Aetna Hlth Plan United Healthcare CIGNA +

LANG: Sp; 🔲 🔲 🔲 🔲 🔲 🔲 Mcr Mcd WC NFI
Immediately 💳 **VISA** 💳

Lanyi, Valery (MD) PMR
Rusk Institute

400 E 34th St Rm 314; New York, NY 10016; (212) 263-6197; **BDCERT:** PMR 68; **MS:** Hungary 54; **RES:** New York University Med Ctr, New York, NY 58-61; **FAP:** Prof PMR NYU Sch Med; **SI:** *Arthritis; Stroke;* **HMO:** CIGNA 1199 Health Source Aetna-US Healthcare Oxford +

🔲 🔲 🔲 🔲 Mcr Mcd WC NFI 1 Week

Lee, Mathew H (MD) PMR
New York University Med Ctr

400 E 34th St Rm 600; New York, NY 10016; (212) 263-6105; **BDCERT:** PMR 66; **MS:** U Md Sch Med 56; **RES:** New York University Med Ctr, New York, NY 62-64; **FAP:** Lecturer PMR NYU Sch Med; **SI:** *Acupuncture; Chronic Pain;* **HMO:** None

🔲 🔲 🔲 WC A Few Days

Lieberman, James (MD) PMR
Columbia-Presbyterian Med Ctr
Rehabilitation Medicine Assoc, 630 W 168th St 38;
New York, NY 10032; (212) 305-4818; **BDCERT:**
PMR 81; N 71; **MS:** UC San Francisco 63; **RES:** N, U
Mich Med Ctr, Ann Arbor, MI 64-65; N, Yale-New
Haven Hosp, New Haven, CT 65-67; **FEL:** PMR, UC
Davis Med Ctr, Sacramento, CA 78-80; **FAP:**
Chrmn Columbia P&S; **HMO:** Oxford Empire
Prucare Multiplan

 🔵 📷 🛏 💲 Mcr WC 4+ Weeks▓ **VISA** 💳

Ma, Dong M (MD) PMR
New York University Med Ctr
400 E 34th St; New York, NY 10016; (212) 263-
6338; **BDCERT:** PMR 79; **MS:** South Korea 68;
RES: New York University Med Ctr, New York, NY;
FEL: New York University Med Ctr, New York, NY;
FAP: Assoc Clin Prof NYU Sch Med; **SI:**
Electromyography; Musculoskeletal Disorders; **HMO:**
Oxford United Healthcare Health Source Aetna-US
Healthcare PHS +

LANG: Kor; 🔵 📷 🚹 🛏 💲 Mcr WC NFI Immediately

Moldover, Jonathan (MD) PMR
Beth Israel Med Ctr
Beth Israel Spine Institute, 10 Union Square East 5
P; New York, NY 10003; (212) 844-8689;
BDCERT: PMR 79; **MS:** Columbia P&S 74; **RES:** IM,
Strong Mem Hosp, Rochester, NY 74-76; PMR,
Columbia-Presbyterian Med Ctr, New York, NY 76-
78; **FAP:** Assoc Prof Albert Einstein Coll Med; **SI:**
Spine Rehabilitation; Chronic Pain; **HMO:** Oxford

LANG: Sp; 🔵 📷 🚹 🛏 💲 Mcr Mod WC NFI 2-4 Weeks
VISA 💳

Myers, Stanley (MD) PMR
Columbia-Presbyterian Med Ctr
Columbia Presbyterian Rehabilitation Associates,
180 Fort Washington Ave HP1171; New York, NY
10032; (212) 305-3344; **BDCERT:** PMR 71; **MS:**
SUNY Hlth Sci Ctr 61; **RES:** IM, Maimonides Med
Ctr, Brooklyn, NY 62-64; PMR, Columbia-
Presbyterian Med Ctr, New York, NY 67-69; **FEL:**
Neuromuscular Disease, Maimonides Med Ctr,
Brooklyn, NY 64-65; **FAP:** Prof Columbia P&S; **SI:**
Neuromuscular Diseases; Stroke; **HMO:** CIGNA
Oxford Chubb Empire Blue Cross & Shield Multiplan
+

 🔵 📷 🛏 💲 Mcr 1 Week▓ **VISA** 💳

Nagler, Willibald (MD) PMR
NY Hosp-Cornell Med Ctr
New York Hospital Box 142, 525 E 68th St Rm
F1809; New York, NY 10021; (212) 746-1503;
BDCERT: PMR 67; **MS:** 58; **RES:** Med, Roswell Park
Cancer Inst, Buffalo, NY 60-63; **FEL:** Med, NY
Hosp-Cornell Med Ctr, New York, NY 63-66; PMR,
NY Hosp-Cornell Med Ctr, New York, NY 66-67;
FAP: Prof &Chrmn Cornell U; **HOSP:** Columbia-
Presbyterian Med Ctr; **SI:** *Cervical and Lumbar Spine;
Problems Rehab of Cancer*; **HMO:** Aetna-US
Healthcare Prestige Anthem Health Pomco 32BJ +

LANG: Sp, Ger; 🔵 📷 🚹 🛏 💲 Mcr 2-4 Weeks▓
VISA 💳

Ragnarsson, Kristjan (MD) PMR
Mount Sinai Med Ctr
5 E 98th St; New York, NY 10029; (212) 241-
5736; **BDCERT:** PMR 76; **MS:** Iceland 69; **RES:**
PMR, New York University Med Ctr, New York, NY
71-74; **FEL:** Spinal Cord Injuries, New York
University Med Ctr, New York, NY 74-75; **FAP:**
Prof Mt Sinai Sch Med; **HMO:** Oxford Blue Choice

 🔵 📷 🚹 🛏 💲 Mcr 2-4 Weeks▓ **VISA** 💳

Thornhill, Herbert (MD) PMR
Harlem Hosp Ctr
506 Lenox Ave; New York, NY 10037; (212) 939-
4401; **BDCERT:** PMR 64; **MS:** Howard U 55; **RES:**
IM, Freedman's Hosp, Washington, DC 56-57; **FEL:**
Pul, Montefiore Med Ctr, Bronx, NY 65; **SI:**
Rehabilitation of Adults

LANG: Sp, Fr; 🔵 📷 🚹 🛏 Mod WC NFI Immediately

PLASTIC SURGERY

Abouzahr, Kamel (MD)   PlS
Columbia-Presbyterian Med Ctr
860 5th Ave; New York, NY 10021; (212) 585-3100; **BDCERT:** PlS 90; **MS:** Lebanon 79; **RES:** New York University Med Ctr, New York, NY 82-85; St Louis U Hosp, St Louis, MO 85-87; **FEL:** HS, New York University Med Ctr, New York, NY 87-88; **HOSP:** New York Eye & Ear Infirmary; **HMO:** Oxford PHS

🖬 🖬 🖬 🖬 🖬   A Few Days

Almeyda, Elizabeth (MD)   PlS
St Luke's Roosevelt Hosp Ctr
75 Central Park West; New York, NY 10023; (212) 501-0600; **BDCERT:** PlS 88; **MS:** U Rochester 78; **RES:** S, St Luke's Roosevelt Hosp Ctr, New York, NY 78-83; **FEL:** PlS, NY Hosp-Cornell Med Ctr, New York, NY 83-85; **FAP:** Clin Instr Columbia P&S; *SI: Breast Reconstruction; Liposuction;* **HMO:** Oxford Blue Cross & Blue Shield Prucare PHS GHI +

LANG: Sp; 🖬 🖬 🖬 🖬 🖬 🖬 🖬 🖬   1 Week **VISA** 💳

Altchek, Edgar (MD)   PlS
Beth Israel Med Ctr
102 E 78th St; New York, NY 10021; (212) 734-9266; **BDCERT:** PlS 74; **MS:** NY Med Coll 65; **RES:** Beth Israel Med Ctr, New York, NY 66-69; **FEL:** PlS, Mount Sinai Med Ctr, New York, NY 69-72; **FAP:** Assoc Clin Prof Mt Sinai Sch Med; **HOSP:** Mount Sinai Med Ctr

Antell, Darrick (MD)   PlS
St Luke's Roosevelt Hosp Ctr
Center for Specialty Care Inc, 850 Park Ave; New York, NY 10021; (212) 988-4040; **BDCERT:** PlS 90; **MS:** MC Ohio, Toledo 82; **RES:** Stanford Med Ctr, Stanford, CA 82-85; PlS, NY Hosp-Cornell Med Ctr, New York, NY 85-87; **FAP:** Asst Clin Prof S Columbia P&S; **HOSP:** Beth Israel Med Ctr; *SI: Facial Cosmetic Surgery; Liposuction*

🖬 🖬 🖬 🖬 🖬 🖬   2-4 Weeks 🖬 **VISA** 💳

Ascherman, Jeffrey (MD)   PlS
Columbia-Presbyterian Med Ctr
161 Ft Washington Ave; New York, NY 10032; (212) 305-9612; **BDCERT:** PlS 97; **MS:** Columbia P&S 88; **RES:** S, Columbia-Presbyterian Med Ctr, New York, NY 88-91; PlS, Columbia-Presbyterian Med Ctr, New York, NY 91-94; **FAP:** Asst Prof S Columbia P&S; **HOSP:** New York Eye & Ear Infirmary; *SI: Breast Surgery; Cosmetic Surgery;* **HMO:** Oxford Aetna-US Healthcare Prudential

LANG: Fr, Sp; 🖬 🖬 🖬 🖬 🖬 🖬 🖬 🖬
A Few Days 🖬 **VISA** 💳

Aston, Sherrell (MD)   PlS
Manhattan Eye, Ear & Throat Hosp
50 E 71st; New York, NY 10021; (212) 249-6000; **BDCERT:** PlS 76; **MS:** U Va Sch Med 68; **RES:** UCLA Med Ctr, Los Angeles, CA 68-73; New York University Med Ctr, New York, NY 73-75; **FEL:** S, Johns Hopkins Hosp, Baltimore, MD 70; **FAP:** Prof S NYU Sch Med; **HOSP:** New York University Med Ctr; *SI: Face Lifting; Body Contouring;* **HMO:** None

🖬 🖬 🖬 🖬 🖬 🖬   4+ Weeks

Baker, Daniel (MD)   PlS
Manhattan Eye, Ear & Throat Hosp
630 Park Ave; New York, NY 10021; (212) 734-9695; **BDCERT:** PlS 78; **MS:** Columbia P&S 68; **RES:** New York University Med Ctr, New York, NY 75-77; *SI: Cosmetic Surgery;* **HMO:** None

🖬 🖬 🖬 🖬   4+ Weeks

Birnbaum, Jay (MD)   PlS
Mount Sinai Med Ctr
74 E 79th St 1A; New York, NY 10021; (212) 472-3040; **BDCERT:** PlS 89; **MS:** Med U SC, Charleston 80; **RES:** S, Mount Sinai Med Ctr, New York, NY; PlS, Mount Sinai Med Ctr, New York, NY 86; **FEL:** France; **FAP:** Assoc Prof Mt Sinai Sch Med; **HOSP:** Beth Israel Med Ctr; *SI: Aesthetic Surgery; Breast Reconstruction;* **HMO:** Blue Cross & Blue Shield

LANG: Fr, Sp; 🖬 🖬 🖬   2-4 Weeks 🖬 **VISA** 💳

Casson, Phillip (MD)　　　PlS
New York University Med Ctr

800 5th Ave 203; New York, NY 10021; (212)
758-6609; **BDCERT:** PlS 71; S 68; **MS:** Australia
49; **RES:** PlS, New York University Med Ctr, New
York, NY 63-65; S, Mem Sloan Kettering Cancer
Ctr, New York, NY 61-63; **FEL:** S, New York
University Med Ctr, New York, NY 65-67; **FAP:**
Prof PlS NYU Sch Med; **HOSP:** New York Eye & Ear
Infirmary; **HMO:** Blue Choice United Healthcare
Metlife

⬚ ⬚ ⬚ ⬚ ⬚ ⬚　A Few Days▩ *VISA* ● ▩

Cenedese, Luis (MD)　　　PlS
Beth Israel Med Ctr

715 Park Ave; New York, NY 10021; (718) 836-
0325; **BDCERT:** PlS 92; **MS:** SUNY Downstate 81;
RES: S, Beth Israel Med Ctr, New York, NY 81-85;
PlS, Mount Sinai Med Ctr, New York, NY 85-88;
FEL: HS, Thomas Jefferson U Hosp, Philadelphia, PA
88-89; **FAP:** Clin Instr Albert Einstein Coll Med;
HOSP: Cabrini Med Ctr; **HMO:** Oxford Blue Choice
Guardian GHI NYLCare +

LANG: Sp, Itl, Fr; ⬚ ⬚ ⬚ ⬚ ⬚ ⬚ ⬚ ⬚
Immediately▩ *VISA* ●

Chiu, David T W (MD)　　　PlS
Columbia-Presbyterian Med Ctr

161 Ft Washington Ave 601; New York, NY
10032; (212) 305-8252; **BDCERT:** PlS 82; HS 90;
MS: Columbia P&S 73; **RES:** Barnes Hosp, St Louis,
MO 74-77; Columbia-Presbyterian Med Ctr, New
York, NY 77-79; **FEL:** HS, New York University
Med Ctr, New York, NY 80; **FAP:** Prof Columbia
P&S; **HOSP:** New York Eye & Ear Infirmary; *SI:*
Hand Surgery-Microsurgery; Cosmetic surgery

LANG: Chi; ⬚ ⬚ ⬚ ⬚ ⬚ ⬚ ⬚ ⬚ ⬚　2-4 Weeks
VISA ●

Chun, Jin (MD)　　　PlS
Mount Sinai Med Ctr

Mt Sinai Hospital, 5 E 98th St; New York, NY
10029; (212) 241-3699; **BDCERT:** PlS 93; **MS:** U
Va Sch Med 83; **RES:** S, Eastern VA Med Sch,
Norfolk, VA 83-86; PlS, Albany Med Ctr, Albany,
NY 88-90; **FEL:** S, MicroSurgery Research Ctr,
Virginia, VA 86-87; HS, Westchester County Med
Ctr, Valhalla, NY 87-88; *SI: Cancer Reconstruction;*
Cosmetic Surgery; **HMO:** Blue Cross Aetna-US
Healthcare Oxford GHI

LANG: Sp, Rus, Grk, Kor; ⬚ ⬚ ⬚ ⬚ ⬚ ⬚ ⬚ ⬚
▩ *VISA* ●

Colen, Helen S (MD)　　　PlS
Manhattan Eye, Ear & Throat Hosp

784 Park Ave; New York, NY 10021; (212) 772-
1300; **BDCERT:** PlS 83; **MS:** NYU Sch Med 72; **RES:**
S, U Colorado, Denver, CO 79; PlS, St Luke's
Roosevelt Hosp Ctr, New York, NY 81; **FEL:**
Microsurg, Bellevue Hosp Ctr, New York, NY; **FAP:**
Clin Instr S SUNY Hlth Sci Ctr; **HOSP:** NYU
Downtown Hosp; *SI: Cosmetic Surgery—*
Rhinoplasty; Breast & Facial Reconstruction; **HMO:**
None

LANG: Sp; ⬚ ⬚ ⬚ ⬚ ⬚ ⬚　2-4 Weeks▩ *VISA*
●

Colen, Stephen (MD)　　　PlS
New York University Med Ctr

784 Park Ave 7F; New York, NY 10021; (212)
988-8900; **BDCERT:** PlS 83; S 79; **MS:**
Hahnemann U 74; **RES:** S, U CO Hosp, Denver, CO
74-79; **FEL:** PlS, New York University Med Ctr, New
York, NY; **FAP:** Assoc Prof NYU Sch Med; **HOSP:**
Manhattan Eye, Ear & Throat Hosp; *SI: Cosmetic*
Facial Surgery; Cosmetic Breast & Body

⬚ ⬚ ⬚ ⬚　2-4 Weeks▩ *VISA* ●

Craig-Scott, Susan (MD)　　PlS
Beth Israel North

150 E 77th St; New York, NY 10021; (212) 737-
8860; **BDCERT:** PlS 87; **MS:** Columbia P&S 74;
RES: St Luke's Roosevelt Hosp Ctr, New York, NY
75-79; New York University Med Ctr, New York,
NY 79-81; **FEL:** PlS, New York University Med Ctr,
New York, NY 79-81; SHd, St Luke's Roosevelt
Hosp Ctr, New York, NY 81; *SI: Eyelid Surgery;
Facial Rejuvenation;* **HMO:** US Hlthcre CIGNA Aetna
Hlth Plan

⬚ 🔲 🏠 💲 🔲 4+ Weeks ▦ **VISA** 💮

Cutting, Court (MD)　　PlS
New York University Med Ctr

550 1st Ave; New York, NY 10016; (212) 263-
5502; **BDCERT:** PlS 86; **MS:** U Chicago-Pritzker Sch
Med 75; **RES:** Oto, U IA Hosp, Iowa City, IA 76-80;
PlS, New York University Med Ctr, New York, NY
80-83; **FEL:** Craniofacial S, New York University
Med Ctr, New York, NY 83-84; **FAP:** Prof NYU Sch
Med; **HOSP:** Manhattan Eye, Ear & Throat Hosp; *SI:
Cleft Lip and Palate; Facial Cosmetic Surgery*

⬚ 🔲 🔲 🏠 💲 🔲 🔲 🔲 2-4 Weeks ▦ **VISA** 💮

Diktaban, Theodore (MD)　　PlS
Lenox Hill Hosp

203 E 69th St; New York, NY 10021; (212) 988-
5656; **BDCERT:** PlS 88; **MS:** NY Med Coll 76; **RES:**
Oto, Mount Sinai Med Ctr, New York, NY 78-81;
PlS, Lenox Hill Hosp, New York, NY 81-83; **FEL:** U
Louisville Hosp, Louisville, KY 84; **HOSP:** Beth
Israel North; *SI: Liposuction; Eyelid and Nasal
Surgery;* **HMO:** Blue Choice CIGNA United
Healthcare Oxford +

⬚ 🔲 🔲 🏠 💲 🔲 🔲 1 Week ▦ **VISA** 💮
🔲

Engler, Alan (MD)　　PlS
Beth Israel Med Ctr

122 E 64th St; New York, NY 10021; (212) 308-
7000; **BDCERT:** PlS 88; **MS:** Columbia P&S 80;
RES: S, Montefiore Med Ctr, Bronx, NY 80-84; **FEL:**
PlS, Montefiore Med Ctr, Bronx, NY 84-86; **FAP:**
Asst Clin Prof Albert Einstein Coll Med; **HOSP:**
Montefiore Med Ctr; *SI: Cosmetic Surgery;
Liposuction*

LANG: Fr; 🔲 🏠 💲 2-4 Weeks ▦ **VISA** 💮

Foster, Craig Allen (MD)　　PlS
Manhattan Eye, Ear & Throat Hosp

850 Park Ave; New York, NY 10021; (212) 744-
5746; **BDCERT:** PlS 82; Oto 80; **MS:** U Minn 74;
RES: PlS, New York University Med Ctr, New York,
NY 80-82; Oto, U MN Med Ctr, Minneapolis, MN
76-80; *SI: Facial Aesthetic Surgery; Body Contouring*

LANG: Swd, Fin, Ger, Itl; 🔲 🔲 🏠 4+ Weeks ▦
VISA 💮 🔲

Gayle, Lloyd (MD)　　PlS
NY Hosp-Cornell Med Ctr

1315 York Ave Fl 2; New York, NY 10021; (212)
746-5540; **BDCERT:** PlS 93; **MS:** NYU Sch Med 83;
RES: S, New York University Med Ctr, New York,
NY 83-88; MicS/HS- NY Hosp-Cornell Med Ctr,
New York, NY 88-90; **FEL:** Microsurgery, Davies
Med Ctr, San Francisco, CA 90-91; **FAP:** Asst Prof S
Cornell U; **HOSP:** NY Hosp Med Ctr of Queens; *SI:
Breast Reconstruction; Body Contouring-Liposuction;*
HMO: Oxford Blue Choice US Hlthcre PHCS PHS +

⬚ 🔲 🔲 🏠 💲 🔲 🔲 🔲 🔲 1 Week **VISA**

Ginsberg, Gerald (MD)　　PlS
NYU Downtown Hosp

170 William St 7th FL; New York, NY 10038;
(212) 312-5555; **BDCERT:** PlS 84; S 83; **MS:**
Northwestern U 74; **RES:** S, New York University
Med Ctr, New York, NY; PlS, New York University
Med Ctr, New York, NY; **FEL:** HS, New York
University Med Ctr, New York, NY; **HOSP:** New
York University Med Ctr; **HMO:** Oxford

LANG: Sp, Fr; 🔲

Godfrey, Norman (MD)　　PlS
St Vincents Hosp & Med Ctr NY

58 E 66th St; New York, NY 10021; (212) 772-
7700; **BDCERT:** PlS 84; **MS:** Harvard Med Sch 73;
RES: S, Bellevue Hosp Ctr, New York, NY 73-78;
PlS, Bellevue Hosp Ctr, New York, NY 78-80; **FEL:**
Bellevue Hosp Ctr, New York, NY 80-81; **FAP:**
Assoc Clin Prof NY Med Coll; **HOSP:** NY Hosp Med
Ctr of Queens; *SI: Rhinoplasty; Hair Replacement;*
HMO: Oxford PHS United Healthcare Blue Choice

LANG: Sp; ⬚ 🔲 🏠 🏠 💲 🔲 🔲 🔲 🔲
A Few Days ▦ **VISA** 💮 🔲

Godfrey, Philip (MD) PlS
St Vincents Hosp & Med Ctr NY

New York Plastic Associates, 58 E 66th St; New York, NY 10021; (212) 772-7700; **BDCERT:** PlS 88; **MS:** Univ Penn 81; **RES:** S, Hartford Hosp, Hartford, CT 84; PlS, NY Hosp-Cornell Med Ctr, New York, NY 86; **FEL:** S, Mem Sloan Kettering Cancer Ctr, New York, NY 86; **HOSP:** NY Hosp Med Ctr of Queens; *SI: Breast and Abdominal Surgery; Liposculpture*; **HMO:** Prucare Oxford PHS PHCS Cost Care +

LANG: Sp; ♿ 🔟 📷 🎬 💲 Mcr Mcd WC NFI 2-4 Weeks
▦ *VISA* ● 🅿️

Haher, Jane (MD) PlS
St Vincents Hosp & Med Ctr NY

5 E 83rd St; New York, NY 10028; (212) 744-1828; **BDCERT:** PlS 79; **MS:** NY Med Coll 67; **RES:** Lenox Hill Hosp, New York, NY 67-68; PlS, Univ Hosp SUNY Bklyn, Brooklyn, NY 73-75; **FAP:** Asst Clin Prof PlS NY Med Coll; *SI: Breast Surgery*

♿ 🔟 📷 🎬 🎬 💲 Mcr WC NFI Immediately

Herman, Steven (MD) PlS
New York Eye & Ear Infirmary

800 B 5th Ave; New York, NY 10021; (212) 249-7000; **BDCERT:** PlS 75; S 72; **MS:** NYU Sch Med 66; **RES:** S, New York University Med Ctr, New York, NY 67-71; PlS, Mount Sinai Med Ctr, New York, NY 71-74; **FAP:** Instr Albert Einstein Coll Med; **HOSP:** Montefiore Med Ctr-Weiler/Einstein Div; *SI: Breast Enlargement; Face Lifts*

♿ 📷 🎬 🎬 WC NFI 2-4 Weeks ▦ *VISA* ●

Hidalgo, David (MD) PlS
Mem Sloan Kettering Cancer Ctr

655 Park Ave Fl 1; New York, NY 10021; (212) 639-8991; **BDCERT:** PlS 87; **MS:** Georgetown U 78; **RES:** S, New York University Med Ctr, New York, NY 78-83; PlS, New York University Med Ctr, New York, NY 84-85; **FEL:** Microsurgery, New York University Med Ctr, New York, NY 86-87; **HOSP:** Manhattan Eye, Ear & Throat Hosp

📷 🎬 💲 A Few Days ▦ *VISA* ●

Hoffman, Lloyd (MD) PlS
New York University Med Ctr

Cornell University Medical College, 525 E 68th St; New York, NY 10021; (212) 776-5511; **BDCERT:** PlS 89; **MS:** Northwestern U 78; **RES:** S, NY Hosp-Cornell Med Ctr, New York, NY 78-83; PlS, New York University Med Ctr, New York, NY 83-86; **FEL:** HS, New York University Med Ctr, New York, NY 86-87; **HOSP:** NY Hosp-Cornell Med Ctr; *SI: Cosmetic Surgery; Breast Reconstruction*; **HMO:** Oxford US Hlthcre PHCS United Healthcare CIGNA +

LANG: Sp; ♿ 📞 🎬 💲 Mcr Immediately ▦ *VISA* ● 🅿️

Hoffman, Saul (MD) PlS
Mount Sinai Med Ctr

102 E 78th St; New York, NY 10021; (212) 734-9266; **BDCERT:** PlS 64; S 63; **MS:** U Alberta 55; **RES:** Mount Sinai Med Ctr, New York, NY 59-62; **FEL:** Mount Sinai Med Ctr, New York, NY 62-63; **FAP:** Prof S Mt Sinai Sch Med; **HOSP:** Beth Israel Med Ctr; *SI: Cosmetic Surgery; Breast Surgery*; **HMO:** Oxford Multiplan Premier PHS

♿ 📷 🎬 🎬 💲 Mcr WC NFI 2-4 Weeks

Hunter, John G (MD) PlS
Mount Sinai Med Ctr

47 E 63rd St; New York, NY 10021; (212) 751-4444; **BDCERT:** PlS 91; **MS:** SUNY Downstate 83; **RES:** S, Mount Sinai Med Ctr, New York, NY 84-86; **FEL:** PlS, Univ Hosp SUNY Bklyn, Brooklyn, NY 86-88; **FAP:** Asst Clin Prof S Cornell U; **HOSP:** New York Methodist Hosp

Imber, Gerald (MD) PlS
NY Hosp-Cornell Med Ctr

1009 5th Ave; New York, NY 10028; (212) 472-1800; **BDCERT:** PlS 76; **MS:** SUNY Downstate 66; **RES:** S, Long Island Jewish Med Ctr, New Hyde Park, NY 67-72; PlS, NY Hosp-Cornell Med Ctr, New York, NY 72-74; **FAP:** Asst Prof PlS Cornell U; *SI: Facelift*

LANG: Sp, Fr; ♿ 🎬 4+ Weeks ▦ *VISA*

Jacobs, Elliot (MD)   PlS
Beth Israel Med Ctr

815 Park Ave FL1; New York, NY 10021; (212) 570-6080; **BDCERT:** PlS 82; **MS:** Mt Sinai Sch Med 70; **RES:** S, Mount Sinai Med Ctr, New York, NY 70-74; PlS, Mount Sinai Med Ctr, New York, NY 74-77; **HOSP:** New York Eye & Ear Infirmary; **SI:** *Facial Cosmetic Surgery; Breast / Body Contouring*

LANG: Fr, Sp, Grk; ♿ 📷 💉 🏥   1 Week 💳 **VISA** 💳

Jelks, Glenn (MD)   PlS
New York University Med Ctr

875 Park Ave; New York, NY 10021; (212) 988-3303; **BDCERT:** PlS 82; Oph 79; **MS:** Mich St U 73; **RES:** Oph, UCLA Reconstructive Eye Institute, Los Angeles, CA 75-78; **FEL:** PlS, New York University Med Ctr, New York, NY 78-80; **HOSP:** Manhattan Eye, Ear & Throat Hosp

♿ 📷 💉 🏥 💲   1 Week **VISA** 💳

Karpinski, Richard (MD)   PlS
St Luke's Roosevelt Hosp Ctr

200 Central Park South; New York, NY 10019; (212) 977-9797; **BDCERT:** PlS 83; S 78; **MS:** Harvard Med Sch 71; **RES:** S, Boston Med Ctr, Boston, MA 72-73; SM, New England Deaconess Hosp, Boston, MA 73-77; **FEL:** PlS, New York University Med Ctr, New York, NY 79-81; **FAP:** Instr PlS Columbia P&S; **SI:** *Rhinoplasty; Breast Surgery;* **HMO:** Blue Cross & Blue Shield Chubb PHS Oxford CIGNA +

♿ 📷 💉 🏥 Mc Md   2-4 Weeks **VISA** 💳

Kasabian, Armen (MD)   PlS
Bellevue Hosp Ctr

530 1st Ave 8T; New York, NY 10016; (212) 263-8034; **BDCERT:** PlS 92; S 88; **MS:** Cornell U 82; **RES:** S, New York University Med Ctr, New York, NY 82-87; **FEL:** PlS, New York University Med Ctr, New York, NY 87-89; Microsurgery, New York University Med Ctr, New York, NY 89-90; **HOSP:** New York University Med Ctr; **SI:** *Reconstructive Surgery; Microsurgery;* **HMO:** Oxford Aetna Hlth Plan United Healthcare PHCS GHI +

♿ 📷 💉 🏥 💲 Mc WC NfI   1 Week

Keen, Monte (MD)   PlS
Columbia-Presbyterian Med Ctr

161 Fort Washington Ave 513; New York, NY 10032; (212) 305-1428; **BDCERT:** Oto 86; PlS 91; **MS:** UC San Francisco 81; **RES:** S, Lenox Hill Hosp, New York, NY 81-83; Oto, Columbia-Presbyterian Med Ctr, New York, NY 83-86; **FEL:** PlS, Mercy Hosp, Pittsburgh, PA 86-87; **SI:** *Rhinoplasty; Eye Lid Surgery;* **HMO:** Oxford Aetna Hlth Plan PM Care Blue Cross

♿ 💉 🏥 💲 Mc WC NfI   A Few Days 💳 **VISA** 💳

La Trenta, Gregory (MD)   PlS
NY Hosp-Cornell Med Ctr

1150 Park Ave 1A; New York, NY 10128; (212) 369-5300; **BDCERT:** PlS 90; **MS:** NY Med Coll 80; **RES:** New York University Med Ctr, New York, NY 80-87; **FEL:** New York University Med Ctr, New York, NY 88; **HMO:** None

♿ 📷 💉 🏥   A Few Days 💳 **VISA** 💳

Lesesne, Cap (MD)   PlS
Manhattan Eye, Ear & Throat Hosp

International Cosmetic Surgery, 620 Park Ave; New York, NY 10021; (914) 666-9494; **BDCERT:** PlS 87; **MS:** Duke U 80; **RES:** Stanford Med Ctr, Stanford, CA; NY Hosp-Cornell Med Ctr, New York, NY; **FEL:** PlS, Mem Sloan Kettering Cancer Ctr, New York, NY; **FAP:** Assoc Prof NYU Sch Med; **HOSP:** Northern Westchester Hosp Ctr; **SI:** *Facial Cosmetic; Liposuction;* **HMO:** +

LANG: Fr, Itl, Rus; ♿ 🏥 🔌 📷 💉 🏥 💲 NfI   A Few Days 💳 **VISA** 💳

Matarasso, Alan (MD)   PlS
Manhattan Eye, Ear & Throat Hosp

1009 Park Ave; New York, NY 10028; (212) 249-7500; **BDCERT:** PlS 86; **MS:** U Miami Sch Med 79; **RES:** S, Albert Einstein Med Ctr, Bronx, NY 79-83; PlS, Albert Einstein Med Ctr, Bronx, NY 83-85; **FEL:** PlS, Manhattan Eye, Ear & Throat Hosp, New York, NY; **FAP:** Assoc Clin Prof PlS Albert Einstein Coll Med; **HOSP:** New York Eye & Ear Infirmary; **SI:** *Liposuction; Rhinoplasty, Eye Lid Surgery*

LANG: Sp; ♿ 💉 🏥 💲   2-4 Weeks 💳

Ofodile, Ferdinand (MD) PlS
St Luke's Roosevelt Hosp Ctr
133 E 73rd St; New York, NY 10021; (212) 861-9000; **BDCERT:** S 74; PlS 76; **MS:** Northwestern U 68; **RES:** Harlem Hosp Ctr, New York, NY; Columbia-Presbyterian Med Ctr, New York, NY; **FEL:** Mayo Clinic, Rochester, MN; **HOSP:** Harlem Hosp Ctr; *SI: Plastic Surgery for Blacks; Plastic Surgery for Hispanics;* **HMO:** Oxford Blue Shield GHI

♿ 📞 📷 ⬛ ⬛ ⬛ Mcr WC NFl A Few Days

Pearlman, Steven (MD) PlS
St Luke's Roosevelt Hosp Ctr
Head & Neck Surgical Group, 425 W 59th St 4E; New York, NY 10019; (212) 262-3434; **BDCERT:** Oto 87; PlS 91; **MS:** Mt Sinai Sch Med 82; **RES:** Oto, Mount Sinai Med Ctr, New York, NY 82-87; **FEL:** Facial Plastic & Reconstructive S, St Luke's Roosevelt Hosp Ctr, New York, NY 87-88; **FAP:** Assoc Prof Columbia P&S; *SI: Facial Cosmetic; Otic And Nasal Surgery;* **HMO:** Oxford CIGNA PHCS Blue Cross & Blue Shield NYLCare +

LANG: Sp; ♿ 📞 📷 ⬛ ⬛ Mcr WC NFl A Few Days
■ *VISA* ●

Pitman, Gerald (MD) PlS
New York University Med Ctr
170 E 73rd St Fl 1; New York, NY 10021; (212) 517-2600; **BDCERT:** PlS 78; S 78; **MS:** Univ Penn 68; **RES:** S, Columbia-Presbyterian Med Ctr, New York, NY 68-69; PlS, New York University Med Ctr, New York, NY 75-77; **FEL:** Microsurgery, New York University Med Ctr, New York, NY; **HOSP:** Manhattan Eye, Ear & Throat Hosp

📷 ⬛ ⬛ ⬛ 2-4 Weeks

Razaboni, Rosa (MD) PlS
Manhattan Eye, Ear & Throat Hosp
14 E 68th St A; New York, NY 10021; (212) 772-0200; **BDCERT:** PlS 93; **MS:** Brazil 75; **RES:** S, St Vincents Hosp & Med Ctr NY, New York, NY 83-85; PlS, New York University Med Ctr, New York, NY 86-88; **FEL:** Hosp Trousseau, Paris, France 85-86
WC

Reed, Lawrence S (MD) PlS
NY Hosp-Cornell Med Ctr
45 E 85th St A1; New York, NY 10028; (212) 772-8300; **BDCERT:** PlS 78; **MS:** SUNY Hlth Sci Ctr 69; **RES:** S, Jacobi Med Ctr, Bronx, NY 69-72; Hosp of U Penn, Philadelphia, PA 72-75; **FEL:** PlS, NY Hosp-Cornell Med Ctr, New York, NY 75-77; **FAP:** Asst Prof S Cornell U; **HOSP:** Beth Israel Med Ctr

1 Week *VISA* ●

Romita, Mauro C (MD) PlS
St Vincents Hosp & Med Ctr NY
58 E 66th St; New York, NY 10021; (212) 772-7700; **BDCERT:** PlS 83; **MS:** U Miami Sch Med 73; **RES:** S, New York University Med Ctr, New York, NY 73-78; PlS, New York University Med Ctr, New York, NY 78-80; **FEL:** New York University Med Ctr, New York, NY; Craniofacial S, New York University Med Ctr, New York, NY; **FAP:** Asst Prof S NY Med Coll; **HOSP:** NY Hosp Med Ctr of Queens; *SI: Aesthetic Facial Surgery; Aesthetic Body Contouring*

LANG: Itl, Sp; ♿ 📷 ⬛ ⬛ ⬛ Mcr WC NFl 2-4 Weeks
■ *VISA* ●

Romo III, Thomas (MD) PlS
New York Eye & Ear Infirmary
150 Broadway 616; New York, NY 10038; (212) 619-3501; **BDCERT:** Oto 85; **MS:** Baylor 79; **RES:** PlS, New York Eye & Ear Infirmary, New York, NY 84-85; Oto, New York Eye & Ear Infirmary, New York, NY 82-84; **FEL:** PlS, Tampa Gen Hosp, Tampa, FL 85; **HOSP:** Lenox Hill Hosp; **HMO:** Aetna Hlth Plan CIGNA Empire Multiplan Oxford +
LANG: Sp; ♿ ⬛ ⬛ ⬛ Mcr WC NFl ■ *VISA* ●

Rosenblatt, William B (MD) PlS
Lenox Hill Hosp
308 E 79th St; New York, NY 10021; (212) 570-6100; **BDCERT:** Oto 77; PlS 80; **MS:** NY Med Coll 73; **RES:** S, Lenox Hill Hosp, New York, NY 73-74; Oto, Manhattan Eye, Ear & Throat Hosp, New York, NY 74-77; **FEL:** HS (PlS), Lenox Hill Hosp, New York, NY 77-79; **HOSP:** Manhattan Eye, Ear & Throat Hosp; *SI: Cosmetic Facial Surgery; Liposuction*

♿ 📷 ⬛ ⬛ ⬛ WC NFl Immediately ■ *VISA* ●
■

Rothaus, Kenneth (MD)   PlS
Hosp For Special Surgery

325 E 72nd St; New York, NY 10021; (212) 737-0770; **BDCERT:** PlS 82; **MS:** Harvard Med Sch 75; **RES:** Columbia-Presbyterian Med Ctr, New York, NY 75-78; NY Hosp-Cornell Med Ctr, New York, NY 78-80; **FEL:** Microsurgery, U Louisville Hosp, Louisville, KY 81; **FAP:** Asst Clin Prof Cornell U; **HOSP:** NY Hosp-Cornell Med Ctr; *SI: Laser Surgery; Facial Plastic Surgery*

♿ 📷 🧑 📅 Mcr Wc Nfi 1 Week ▨ **VISA** 💳

Schulman, Norman (MD)   PlS
Lenox Hill Hosp

799 Park Ave; New York, NY 10021; (212) 861-5004; **BDCERT:** PlS 76; S 73; **MS:** Tufts U 65; **RES:** S, Jacobi Med Ctr, Bronx, NY 65-72; PlS, Lenox Hill Hosp, New York, NY 72-74; **FEL:** Head & Neck S, Roswell Park Cancer Inst, Buffalo, NY 74-75; *SI: Facelift, Eyelid Surgery; Breast Surgery*

♿ 📷 🧑 📅 S Mcr Wc Nfi A Few Days

Schwager, Robert (MD)   PlS
NY Hosp-Cornell Med Ctr

927 5th Ave; New York, NY 10021; (212) 249-7900; **BDCERT:** PlS 76; **MS:** Cornell U 67; **RES:** NY Hosp-Cornell Med Ctr, New York, NY 71-72; **FEL:** PlS, NY Hosp-Cornell Med Ctr, New York, NY 72-74; **HOSP:** Beth Israel North; *SI: Melanoma;* **HMO:** Oxford 32BJ Aetna Hlth Plan United Healthcare +

LANG: Sp; ♿ 📷 🧑 📅 S Mcr Wc Nfi A Few Days ▨ **VISA** 💳 💳

Ship, Arthur G (MD)   PlS
Beth Israel Med Ctr

1049 5th Ave; New York, NY 10028; (212) 861-8000; **BDCERT:** PlS 63; **MS:** Harvard Med Sch 54; **RES:** Montefiore Med Ctr, Bronx, NY 57-59; St Louis U Hosp, St Louis, MO 59-61; **FAP:** Clin Prof Albert Einstein Coll Med; **HOSP:** Montefiore Med Ctr; *SI: Facial Aesthetics; Breast Deformities;* **HMO:** None

♿ 📷 🧑 📅 Mcr 1 Week **VISA** 💳

Siebert, John (MD)   PlS
Manhattan Eye, Ear & Throat Hosp

799 Park Ave; New York, NY 10021; (212) 737-8300; **BDCERT:** S 87; PlS 91; **MS:** U Wisc Med Sch 81; **RES:** S, Mass Gen Hosp, Boston, MA 81-86; PlS, New York University Med Ctr, New York, NY 86-88; **FEL:** Microsurgery, New York University Med Ctr, New York, NY 88-89; **FAP:** Assoc Prof S NYU Sch Med; **HOSP:** New York University Med Ctr; *SI: Aesthetic Surgery; Facial Reconstructive Surgery;* **HMO:** None

LANG: Sp, Prt; ♿ 📷 🧑 📅 2-4 Weeks **VISA** 💳

Silver, Lester (MD)   PlS
Mount Sinai Med Ctr

Mt Sinai Medical Ctr, 1 Gustave Levy Pl Box 1263; New York, NY 10029; (212) 241-5873; **BDCERT:** PlS 78; **MS:** U Hlth Sci/Chicago Med Sch 60; **RES:** S, Albert Einstein Med Ctr, Bronx, NY 63-66; PlS, Mount Sinai Med Ctr, New York, NY 66; **HOSP:** Hosp For Joint Diseases; **HMO:** Blue Cross & Blue Shield HealthNet Oxford PHCS PHS +

♿ 📷 🧑 📅 S Mcr A Few Days ▨ **VISA** 💳

Skolnik, Richard A (MD)   PlS
Mount Sinai Med Ctr

21 E 87th St; New York, NY 10128; (212) 722-1977; **BDCERT:** PlS 83; **MS:** Cornell U 76; **RES:** Mount Sinai Med Ctr, New York, NY 76-79; **FEL:** PlS, Mount Sinai Med Ctr, New York, NY 79-82; **FAP:** Asst Clin Prof Mt Sinai Sch Med; **HOSP:** Beth Israel Med Ctr; *SI: Cosmetic Surgery; Breast Surgery*

📷 🧑 📅 Mcr 2-4 Weeks **VISA** 💳

Spinelli, Henry M (MD)   PlS
New York Eye & Ear Infirmary

875 5th Ave; New York, NY 10021; (212) 570-6235; **BDCERT:** PlS 93; **MS:** NYU Sch Med 81; **RES:** S, Columbia-Presbyterian Med Ctr, New York, NY 85-88; PlS, Bellevue Hosp Ctr, New York, NY 89; **FEL:** Oph Craniofacial S, New York University Med Ctr, New York, NY 90-91; Manhattan Eye, Ear & Throat Hosp, New York, NY 82-85; **FAP:** Assoc Prof Cornell U; **HOSP:** Manhattan Eye, Ear & Throat Hosp; *SI: Aesthetic Facial Surgery; Occuloplastic;* **HMO:** Oxford PHS

📞 📷 🧑 📅 S 1 Week ▨ **VISA** 💳 💳

Striker, Paul (MD)　　　PlS
New York Eye & Ear Infirmary

660 Park Ave; New York, NY 10021; (212) 744-4265; **BDCERT:** PlS 72; **MS:** U Colo Sch Med 63; **RES:** Columbia Presbyterian Med Ctr, New York, NY 63-71; **HOSP:** NYU Downtown Hosp; *SI: Laser Surgery; Eyelid Surgery*

Sultan, Mark (MD)　　　PlS
Beth Israel Med Ctr

425 W 59th St Ste 7A; New York, NY 10019; (212) 523-7277; **BDCERT:** PlS 92; **MS:** Columbia P&S 82; **RES:** Columbia-Presbyterian Med Ctr, New York, NY 82-87; **FEL:** Columbia-Presbyterian Med Ctr, New York, NY 87-89; Microsurgery, Emory U Hosp, Atlanta, GA 89-90; **HOSP:** Beth Israel Med Ctr; **HMO:** None

🚹 📷 🚻 🏙 $ 1 Week

Tabbal, Nicolas (MD)　　　PlS
Manhattan Eye, Ear & Throat Hosp

521 Park Ave; New York, NY 10021; (212) 644-5800; **BDCERT:** S 77; PlS 80; **MS:** Lebanon 72; **RES:** S, Am U Med Ctr, Beirut, Lebanon 72-76; PlS, Akron City Hosp, Akron, OH 76-77; **FEL:** S, Upstate Med Ctr, Syracuse, NY 77-79; PlS, NYU Med Ctr, New York, NY 79-80; **FAP:** Clin Instr PlS NYU Sch Med

📷 🚻 🏙 $ 2-4 Weeks

Thorne, Charles (MD)　　　PlS
Manhattan Eye, Ear & Throat Hosp

812 Park Ave; New York, NY 10021; (212) 794-0044; **BDCERT:** PlS 91; S 87; **MS:** UCLA 81; **RES:** S, Mass Gen Hosp, Boston, MA 81-86; PlS, New York University Med Ctr, New York, NY 86-88; **FEL:** Craniofacial S, New York University Med Ctr, New York, NY 88-89; **FAP:** Assoc Prof NYU Sch Med; **HOSP:** New York University Med Ctr; *SI: Aesthetic Surgery; Ear Reconstuction;* **HMO:** Chubb Oxford HIP Network

🚹 🆑 📷 🚻 🏙 Mcr WC NFI 2-4 Weeks *VISA* 💳

Tornambe, Robert (MD)　　　PlS
Cabrini Med Ctr

Madison Plastic Surgery, 46 E 82nd St; New York, NY 10028; (212) 628-7600; **BDCERT:** PlS 90; **MS:** Dominican Republic 80; **RES:** S, Cabrini Medical Center, New York, NY 81-82; PlS, Cabrini Medical Center, New York, NY 83; **HMO:** Independent Health Plan 1199 Empire Blue Choice Chubb

Verga, Michelle (MD)　　　PlS
Mount Sinai Med Ctr

1010 5th Ave; New York, NY 10028; (212) 535-0470; **BDCERT:** S 82; PlS 84; **MS:** Italy 74; **RES:** S, Mount Sinai Med Ctr, New York, NY 75-78; S, Lutheran Med Ctr, Brooklyn, NY 78-80; **FEL:** PlS, Mount Sinai Med Ctr, New York, NY 80-83; **HOSP:** Beth Israel Med Ctr; *SI: Facial Cosmetic Surgery; Liposuction*

LANG: Itl, Fr, Sp; 🆑 📷 🚻 🏙 $ Immediately

Vickery, Carlin (MD)　　　PlS
Mount Sinai Med Ctr

102 E 78th St; New York, NY 10029; (212) 288-9800; **BDCERT:** PlS 87; S 83; **MS:** NYU Sch Med 77; **RES:** S, New York University Med Ctr, New York, NY 77-82; **FEL:** Microsurgery, New York University Med Ctr, New York, NY 85

🚹 📷 🚻 🏙 $ Mcr A Few Days 💳 *VISA*

Weinberg, Hubert (MD)　　　PlS
Mount Sinai Med Ctr

5 E 98th St; New York, NY 10029; (212) 241-3699; **BDCERT:** PlS 82; **MS:** Cornell U 75; **RES:** S, Mount Sinai Med Ctr, New York, NY 75-81; PlS, Mount Sinai Med Ctr, New York, NY 78-81; **FAP:** Prof Mt Sinai Sch Med; *SI: Cosmetic and Reconstructive Surgery; Microsurgery;* **HMO:** Oxford GHI Blue Choice CIGNA Chubb +

LANG: Sp, Fr, Heb, Yd; 🚹 🆑 📷 🚻 🏙 $ Mcr WC NFI A Few Days 💳 *VISA* 💳

Guide to symbols and abbreviations can be found on pages 110-113.

339

Wood-Smith, Donald (MD)　PlS
New York Eye & Ear Infirmary
830 Park Ave; New York, NY 10021; (212) 744-2224; **BDCERT:** PlS 70; **MS:** Australia 54; **RES:** New York University Med Ctr, New York, NY 60-63; Stanford Med Ctr, Stanford, CA 67-68; **FEL:** Craniofacial S, New York University Med Ctr, New York, NY 64-68; **FAP:** Prof S Columbia P&S; **HOSP:** Columbia-Presbyterian Med Ctr; *SI: Cosmetic Surgery; Reconstruction Trauma;* **HMO:** PHS

▣ ▣ ▦ Mcr NfI　A Few Days ▦ *VISA* ▦ ▦

Zevon, Scott (MD)　　PlS
St Luke's Roosevelt Hosp Ctr
75 Central Park West; New York, NY 10021; (212) 496-6600; **BDCERT:** PlS 89; **MS:** Boston U 79; **RES:** St Luke's Roosevelt Hosp Ctr, New York, NY 79-84; Nassau County Med Ctr, East Meadow, NY 84-86; **FEL:** Craniofacial S, Mayo Clinic, Rochester, MN; **HOSP:** Long Island Coll Hosp

▣ ▣ ▣ ▣ ▦ ▣ Mcr WC NfI　A Few Days ▦ ▦

Zide, Barry (MD)　　　PlS
New York University Med Ctr
420 E 55th St 1D; New York, NY 10022; (212) 421-2424; **BDCERT:** PlS 81; **MS:** Tufts U 73; **RES:** Stanford Med Ctr, Stanford, CA 73-76; U NC Hosp, Chapel Hill, NC 76-78; **FEL:** Roswell Park Cancer Inst, Buffalo, NY 78; UC San Francisco Med Ctr, San Francisco, CA 79; **FAP:** Assoc Prof NYU Sch Med; **HOSP:** Manhattan Eye, Ear & Throat Hosp; **HMO:** Chubb

▣ ▣ ▣ ▦　A Few Days ▦ *VISA* ▦

PREVENTIVE MEDICINE

Cahill, Kevin Michael (MD)　PrM
Lenox Hill Hosp
850 5th Ave; New York, NY 10021; (212) 879-2607; **BDCERT:** PrM 70; **MS:** Cornell U 61; **RES:** US Navy Med Res Unit, Cairo, Egypt 62-65; *SI: Tropical Diseases;* **HMO:** None

Landrigan, Philip (MD)　　PrM
Mount Sinai Med Ctr
Mt Sinai Sch MedEnvironmental Medicine, 1 Gustave Levy Pl; New York, NY 10029; (212) 241-6500; **BDCERT:** Ped 73; PrM 79; **MS:** Harvard Med Sch 67; **RES:** Med, Cleveland Metro Gen Hosp, Cleveland, OH 67-68; Ped, Children's Hosp, Boston, MA 68-70; **FEL:** EDM, Centers for Disease Control, Atlanta, GA 70-73; OM, U of London, London, England 76-77; **FAP:** Chrmn Mt Sinai Sch Med; *SI: Pediatric Environmental Disease; Occupational Disease;* **HMO:** Oxford

LANG: Sp, Fr, Ger, Heb, Yd; ▣ WC

PSYCHIATRY

Abramowicz, Helen (MD)　Psyc
NY Hosp-Cornell-Westchester
19 Central Park West Ste 16L; New York, NY 10023; (212) 757-3519; **BDCERT:** Psyc 80; Ped 80; **MS:** Albert Einstein Coll Med 68; **RES:** Ped, Jacobi Med Ctr, Bronx, NY 68-70; Psyc, Montefiore Med Ctr, Bronx, NY 75-77; **FEL:** ChAP, Jacobi Med Ctr, Bronx, NY 70-72; NY Hosp-Cornell-Westchester, White Plains, NY; **HMO:** None
LANG: Fr, Sp; ▣ ▣ ▣ ▣ ▣ ▦　A Few Days

Abrams, Samuel (MD) Psyc
New York University Med Ctr

25 E 83rd St 2D; New York, NY 10028; (212) 628-1071; **MS:** SUNY Downstate 53; **RES:** Psyc, Univ Hosp SUNY Bklyn, Brooklyn, NY 54-55; Psyc, Univ Hosp SUNY Bklyn, Brooklyn, NY 57-59; **FAP:** Clin Prof NYU Sch Med; **SI:** *Psychoanalysis; Psychoanalysis of Children;* **HMO:** None

♿ 📷 📹 📺 1 Week

Alger, Ian (MD) Psyc
NY Hosp-Cornell Med Ctr

500 E 77th St 132; New York, NY 10162; (212) 861-3707; **MS:** Canada 49; **RES:** Bellevue Hosp Ctr, New York, NY 50-53; **FEL:** Psyc & PMR, New York University Med Ctr, New York, NY 51-53; **FAP:** Clin Prof Psyc Cornell U; **SI:** *Couples and Marital Therapy; Psychodynamic Psychotherapy*

♿ ☽ 📷 📹 📺 A Few Days

Angrist, Burton (MD) Psyc
VA Med Ctr-Manh

423 E 23rd St; New York, NY 11010; (212) 686-7500; **BDCERT:** Psyc 73; **MS:** Albert Einstein Coll Med 62; **RES:** Kings County Hosp Ctr, Brooklyn, NY 63-64; Hillside Hosp, Glen Oaks, NY 64-66; **FEL:** Psychopharmacology, Bellevue Hosp Ctr, New York, NY 66-68; **FAP:** Prof Psyc NYU Sch Med; **SI:** *Central Nervous System Stimulants; Schizophrenia;* **HMO:** Champus

Arkow, Stan (MD) Psyc
Columbia-Presbyterian Med Ctr

305 West End Ave Ste 908; New York, NY 10023; (212) 799-5185; **BDCERT:** Psyc 85; **MS:** Columbia P&S 77; **RES:** Psyc, Columbia-Presbyterian Med Ctr, New York, NY 78-81; **FAP:** Assoc Clin Prof Psyc Columbia P&S; **SI:** *Psychotherapy of Character Disorders; Psychopharmacology;* **HMO:** Oxford

♿ ☽ 📷 📹 📺 🇸 🇲 2-4 Weeks

Aronoff, Michael (MD) Psyc
Lenox Hill Hosp

60 Riverside Dr 16E; New York, NY 10024; (212) 799-8257; **BDCERT:** Psyc 77; **MS:** Univ Penn 66; **RES:** Columbia-Presbyterian Med Ctr, New York, NY 72; **FEL:** Psychoanalysis, Columbia-Presbyterian Med Ctr, New York, NY 72; **FAP:** Clin Prof NYU Sch Med; **SI:** *Stress Management-Sleep Problems; Couples- Family- Legal*

♿ ☽ 📷 📹 📺 A Few Days

Attia, Evelyn (MD) Psyc
NYS Psychiatric Institute

239 Central Park West; New York, NY 10024; (212) 721-2850; **BDCERT:** Psyc 92; **MS:** Columbia P&S 86; **RES:** Hosp of U Penn, Philadelphia, PA 86-87; Psyc, NYS Psychiatric Institute, New York, NY 87-90; **FAP:** Asst Clin Prof Psyc Columbia P&S; **SI:** *Eating Disorders; Mood Disorders*

☽ 📹 📺 2-4 Weeks

Auchincloss, Elizabeth (MD) Psyc
Columbia-Presbyterian Med Ctr

15 W 81st St; New York, NY 10024; (212) 874-0070; **BDCERT:** Psyc 82; **MS:** Columbia P&S 77; **RES:** NY Hosp-Cornell Med Ctr, New York, NY 77-82; **FEL:** Columbia-Presbyterian Med Ctr, New York, NY 80-86; **FAP:** Asst Prof Cornell U

📷 Immediately

Barbuto, Joseph (MD) Psyc
Mem Sloan Kettering Cancer Ctr

6 W 77th St 1A; New York, NY 10024; (212) 724-7366; **BDCERT:** Psyc 83; **MS:** Albert Einstein Coll Med 78; **RES:** NY Hosp-Cornell Med Ctr, New York, NY 79-82; **FEL:** Psyc Onc, Mem Sloan Kettering Cancer Ctr, New York, NY 82-86; **SI:** *Psychiatric Treatment of Cancer Patients;* **HMO:** Blue Cross & Blue Shield Oxford

♿ 📷 📹 📺 🇸 🇲 1 Week

Basch, Samuel (MD) Psyc
Mount Sinai Med Ctr

9 E 96th St; New York, NY 10128; (212) 427-0344; **BDCERT:** Psyc 70; **MS:** Hahnemann U 61; **RES:** Mount Sinai Med Ctr, New York, NY 62-65; **HMO:** None

Baurdy, Francis (MD)   Psyc
Mount Sinai Med Ctr

9 E 96th St; New York, NY 10128; (212) 289-5024; **BDCERT:** Psyc 63; **MS:** NYU Sch Med 55; **RES:** Bellevue Hosp Ctr, New York, NY 57-59; Staten Island Mental Health Ctr, Staten Island, NY 59-60; **FAP:** Assoc Prof Albert Einstein Coll Med; **HOSP:** Montefiore Med Ctr; *SI: Psychoanalysis for French Speakers; Problems of Creativity*

LANG: Fr; 🚹 🔲 👶 🎴 Immediately

Becker, Ted (MD)   Psyc
Jacobi Med Ctr

27 W 96th St; New York, NY 10025; (212) 749-4585; **BDCERT:** Psyc 52; **MS:** Vanderbilt U Sch Med 46; **RES:** Colorado Psychiatric Hosp, Denver, CO 47-48; USPHS Hosp, Fort Worth, TX 48-50; **FEL:** NYS Psychiatric Institute, New York, NY 51-57; *SI: Child and Adolescent Psychoanalysis*; **HMO:** None

🚹 🔲 👶 🎴 1 Week

Bezahler, Harvey (MD)   Psyc
New York University Med Ctr

14 E 4th St 601; New York, NY 10012; (212) 777-8015; **BDCERT:** Psyc 63; **MS:** NYU Sch Med 56; **RES:** Menninger Clinic, Topeka, KS 57-60; **FAP:** Assoc Prof NYU Sch Med

🚹 🔲 👶 🎴 Mcr 1 Week

Birger, Daniel (MD)   Psyc
Mount Sinai Med Ctr

155 E 91st St; New York, NY 10128; (212) 831-3837; **BDCERT:** Psyc 72; **MS:** Israel 60; **RES:** Psyc, McLean Hosp, Belmont, MA 66-68; Psyc, Albert Einstein Med Ctr, Bronx, NY 68-69; **FEL:** Psychoanalysis, NYS Psychiatric Institute, New York, NY 68-73; **FAP:** Asst Clin Prof Mt Sinai Sch Med; *SI: Psychotherapy; Psychoanalysis*

LANG: Heb; 🔲 👶 🎴 A Few Days

Bone, Stanley (MD)   Psyc
Columbia-Presbyterian Med Ctr

1155 Park Ave; New York, NY 10128; (212) 831-0917; **BDCERT:** Psyc 79; **MS:** Mt Sinai Sch Med 74; **RES:** Metropolitan Hosp Ctr, New York, NY 74-75; Psyc, Columbia-Presbyterian Med Ctr, New York, NY; **FEL:** Columbia-Presbyterian Med Ctr, New York, NY 78-84

🌙 🔲 👶 🎴 1 Week

Borbely, Antal (MD)   Psyc
Metropolitan Hosp Ctr

675 W End Ave; New York, NY 10025; (212) 222-1678; **BDCERT:** Psyc 76; **MS:** Switzerland 68; **RES:** Psyc, NY State Psychiatric Institute, 70-72; Albert Einstein Med Ctr, Bronx, NY 72-73; **FEL:** Community Psyc, Albert Einstein Med Ctr, Bronx, NY 73-75; **FAP:** Asst Prof NY Med Coll; *SI: Psychodynamic Treatment*

LANG: Ger, Fr; 🌙 🔲 👶 🎴 💲 A Few Days

Breitbart, William (MD)   Psyc
Mem Sloan Kettering Cancer Ctr

Dept of Psychiatry and Behavioral Sciences, 1275 York Ave Box 421; New York, NY 10021; (212) 639-8704; **BDCERT:** Psyc 86; IM 82; **MS:** Albert Einstein Coll Med 78; **RES:** Psyc, Bronx Municipal Hosp Ctr, Bronx, NY 79-80; Psyc, Bronx Muncipal Hosp Ctr, Bronx, NY 82-84; **FEL:** Psyc Onc, Mem Sloan Kettering Cancer Ctr, New York, NY 84-86; **FAP:** Asst Lecturer Psyc Cornell U; *SI: Cancer Psychiatry and Pain Management; AIDS Psychiatry*

LANG: Yd; 🚹 🔲 🔲 👶 🎴 Immediately 💳 **VISA** 🍴 🍴

Brodie, Jonathan (MD)   Psyc
New York University Med Ctr

155 E 38th St; New York, NY 10016; (212) 986-6693; **BDCERT:** Psyc 79; **MS:** NYU Sch Med 75; **RES:** New York University Med Ctr, New York, NY 75-78; **FAP:** Prof Psyc NYU Sch Med; *SI: Psychopharmacology; Depression/Anxiety*

🚹 🌙 🔲 🎴 💲 Mcr 2-4 Weeks

Bronheim, Harold (MD)   Psyc
Mount Sinai Med Ctr

1155 Park Ave; New York, NY 10028; (212) 996-5777; **BDCERT:** Psyc 85; IM 86; **MS:** SUNY Hlth Sci Ctr 80; **RES:** Mount Sinai Med Ctr, New York, NY 80-84; Beth Israel Med Ctr, New York, NY 84-85; **FAP:** Assoc Psyc Mt Sinai Sch Med; *SI: Medical Psychiatry; Psychoanalysis*

🔲 🎴 💲   1 Week

Brook, David W (MD)   Psyc
Mount Sinai Med Ctr

330 E 79th St; New York, NY 10021; (212) 831-3388; **BDCERT:** Psyc 69; AdP 96; **MS:** Yale U Sch Med 61; **RES:** U Chicago Hosp, Chicago, IL 61-62; Mount Sinai Med Ctr, New York, NY 62-65; **FAP:** Prof Mt Sinai Sch Med; *SI: Substance Abuse; Psychopharmacology*

🔲 🔳 🔲 🔲 🔲 🎴

Brown, Richard (MD)   Psyc
Columbia-Presbyterian Med Ctr

30 East End Ave 1B; New York, NY 10028; (212) 737-0821; **BDCERT:** Psyc 83; **MS:** Columbia P&S 77; **RES:** NY Hosp-Cornell Med Ctr, New York, NY 77-82; **FEL:** Psyc, NY Hosp-Cornell Med Ctr, New York, NY 82-84; *SI: Psychopharmacology*

🔲 🔲 🎴 💲   4+ Weeks

Bukberg, Judith (MD)   Psyc
St Vincents Hosp & Med Ctr NY

3 E 10th St 1A; New York, NY 10003; (212) 614-0312; **BDCERT:** Psyc 79; **MS:** Mt Sinai Sch Med 74; **RES:** Mount Sinai Med Ctr, New York, NY 75-78; **FEL:** Mem Sloan Kettering Cancer Ctr, New York, NY 78-80

🔲 🔲 🎴 💲   Immediately

Call, Pamela (MD)   Psyc
St Vincents Hosp & Med Ctr NY

80 5th Ave; New York, NY 10011; (212) 727-8520; **BDCERT:** Psyc 89; **MS:** NY Med Coll 83; **RES:** St Vincents Hosp & Med Ctr NY, New York, NY 83-87; **FEL:** Mem Sloan Kettering Cancer Ctr, New York, NY 88; **HMO:** Empire Blue Cross & Shield PHS Oxford Most

LANG: Swa; 🔲 🔲 🔲   1 Week

Campion, Robert E (MD)   Psyc
St Clare's Hosp & Health Ctr

426 W 52nd St; New York, NY 10019; (212) 459-8004; **BDCERT:** Psyc 79; **MS:** Spain 73; **RES:** St Vincents Hosp & Med Ctr NY, New York, NY 74-77; **FAP:** Asst Clin Prof NY Med Coll; **HOSP:** St Vincents Hosp & Med Ctr NY; **HMO:** Oxford Empire Blue Cross & Shield Network Behavorial Hlth

🔲 🔲 🔲 🔲 🔲 💲 🔲   2-4 Weeks

Cancro, Robert (MD)   Psyc
Bellevue Hosp Ctr

550 1st Ave; New York, NY 10016; (212) 263-6214; **BDCERT:** Psyc 62; **MS:** SUNY Hlth Sci Ctr 55; **RES:** Kings County Hosp Ctr, Brooklyn, NY 56-59; **FAP:** Prof Psyc NYU Sch Med; **HOSP:** Lenox Hill Hosp; *SI: Schizophrenia; Depression*; **HMO:** Oxford

🔲 🔲 🔲 🔲 🔲   1 Week

Canino, Ian (MD)   Psyc
Columbia-Presbyterian Med Ctr

28 W 71st St; New York, NY 10023; (212) 877-4180; **BDCERT:** Psyc 77; ChAP 78; **MS:** U Puerto Rico 70; **RES:** Psyc, USC Med Ctr, Los Angeles, CA 70-72; ChAP, Albert Einstein Med Ctr, Bronx, NY 72-75; **FAP:** Clin Prof Psyc Columbia P&S; *SI: Attention Deficit Disorders; Learning Disabled*; **HMO:** None

LANG: Sp; 🔲 🔲 💲   1 Week

Caracci, Giovanni (MD)   Psyc
Cabrini Med Ctr

227 E 19th St; New York, NY 10003; (212) 995-6032; **BDCERT:** Psyc 90; **MS:** Italy 78; **RES:** Psyc, Metropolitan Hosp Ctr, New York, NY 79-83; *SI: Psychiatric Problems of Elderly; Medication of Psych*; **HMO:** PHCS Oxford

LANG: Itl, Sp; 🔲 🔲 🔲 🔲 🔲 💲 🔲 🔲 🔲 🔲
A Few Days

Guide to symbols and abbreviations can be found on pages 110-113.

343

Chou, James (MD) Psyc
New York University Med Ctr
550 1st Ave 22 FL; New York, NY 10016; (212) 562-7310; **BDCERT:** Psyc 89; N 89; **MS:** Tulane U 83; **RES:** Psyc, New York University Med Ctr, New York, NY 83-87; **FEL:** Nat Inst Mental Health, Bethesda, MD 85-87; **HOSP:** Bellevue Hosp Ctr; *SI: Bipolar Disorder*

💠 💠 💠 💠 Mcr Mcd 1 Week

Chung, Henry (MD) Psyc
NYU Downtown Hosp
Chinatown Health Ctr, 125 Walker St; New York, NY 10013; (212) 226-8866; **BDCERT:** Psyc 94; **MS:** SUNY Buffalo 89; **RES:** Psyc, NY Hosp-Cornell-Westchester, White Plains, NY 90-93; **FEL:** Psyc, NY Hosp-Cornell Med Ctr, New York, NY 94-95; **FAP:** Asst Prof Psyc NYU Sch Med; **HOSP:** Bellevue Hosp Ctr; *SI: Depression Disorders; Anxiety Disorders*; **HMO:** Oxford

LANG: Can, Chi; 💠 💠 💠 💠 💠 S Mcr Mcd 2-4 Weeks

Cohen, Arnold (MD) Psyc
Mount Sinai Med Ctr
64 E 94th St 1A; New York, NY 10128; (212) 289-6800; **BDCERT:** Psyc 69; **MS:** SUNY Hlth Sci Ctr 63; **RES:** Psyc, Mount Sinai Med Ctr, New York, NY 94-96; **FEL:** ChAP, Mount Sinai Med Ctr, New York, NY; **FAP:** Asst Clin Prof Mt Sinai Sch Med; *SI: Psychotherapy; Attention Deficit Disorder*; **HMO:** Blue Cross & Blue Shield

💠 💠 💠 💠 💠 Mcr A Few Days

Collins, Allen H (MD) Psyc
Lenox Hill Hosp
130 E 77th St Ste B304; New York, NY 10021; (212) 472-0220; **BDCERT:** Psyc 75; **MS:** Tufts U 68; **RES:** NYS Psychiatric Institute, New York, NY; **FEL:** Psychoanalysis, William A White Inst, New York, NY 75-80; Columbia-Presbyterian Med Ctr, New York, NY 69-74; **FAP:** Clin Prof Psyc NYU Sch Med; *SI: Depression; Anxiety Disorders*

💠 💠 💠 💠 Mcr A Few Days

Cooper, Arnold (MD) Psyc
NY Hosp-Cornell Med Ctr
50 E 78th St 1C; New York, NY 10021; (212) 879-7182; **BDCERT:** Psyc 60; **MS:** U Utah 47; **RES:** Columbia-Presbyterian Med Ctr, New York, NY 48-50; Bellevue Hosp Ctr, New York, NY 50-53; **FEL:** Harvard Med Sch, Cambridge, MA 47-48; Psychoanalysis, Columbia-Presbyterian Med Ctr, New York, NY 52-56; **FAP:** Prof Cornell U; *SI: Psychotherapy; Psychoanalysis*

💠 💠 1 Week

Coplan, Jeremy (MD) Psyc
160 Westend Ave 25E; New York, NY 10023; (212) 543-5422; **BDCERT:** Psyc 90; **MS:** South Africa 83; **RES:** Psyc, Univ Hosp SUNY Bklyn, Brooklyn, NY 86-89; **FEL:** Psychopharmacology, Columbia-Presbyterian Med Ctr, New York, NY; **FAP:** Assoc Prof Columbia P&S; *SI: Panic Disorders; Bipolar Disease*

💠 💠 💠 💠 S A Few Days

Cournos, Francine (MD) Psyc
Columbia-Presbyterian Med Ctr
ColumbiaPresby Hosp, 622 W 168th St; New York, NY 10032; (212) 543-5412; **BDCERT:** Psyc 78; **MS:** NYU Sch Med 71; **RES:** Med, Montefiore Med Ctr, Bronx, NY 71-73; Psyc, NYS Psychiatric Institute, New York, NY 73-76; **FAP:** Prof Psyc Columbia P&S; *SI: Couples Therapy; Individual Psychotherapy*; **HMO:** None

💠 💠 💠 💠 💠 S 1 Week

Curtis, James (MD) Psyc
Harlem Hosp Ctr
Columbia Harlem Hospital of Psychiatry,; New York, NY 10037; (212) 939-1000; **BDCERT:** Psyc 52; **MS:** U Mich Med Sch 46; **RES:** Psyc, Wayne Cnty Gen Hosp, Detroit, MI 49-50; State University of NY, 51; **FAP:** Clin Prof Psyc Columbia P&S; *SI: General Psychiatry; Addiction Psychiatry*

Davis, Kenneth (MD) **Psyc**
Mount Sinai Med Ctr
1 Gustave Levy Pl; New York, NY 10029; (212) 824-7008; **BDCERT:** Psyc 80; N 80; **MS:** Mt Sinai Sch Med 73; **RES:** Psyc, Stanford Med Ctr, Stanford, CA 73-76; **FEL:** PsyPharm, Stanford Med Ctr, Stanford, CA 74-76; **FAP:** Chrmn Mt Sinai Sch Med; ***SI:** Psychopharmacology; Neuropsychiatry;* **HMO:** None
LANG: Sp; ♿ ☎ 👤 📅 $ [WC] 1 Week

Douglas, Carolyn (MD) **Psyc**
Columbia-Presbyterian Med Ctr
345 E 84th St; New York, NY 10028; (212) 439-0542; **BDCERT:** Psyc 85; **MS:** Harvard Med Sch 80; **RES:** NY Hosp-Cornell Med Ctr, New York, NY 84; **FAP:** Assoc Clin Prof Columbia P&S; **HMO:** Oxford
☾ ☎ 👤 📅 2-4 Weeks

Druss, Richard (MD) **Psyc**
Columbia-Presbyterian Med Ctr
180 E End Ave; New York, NY 10128; (212) 772-8383; **BDCERT:** Psyc 70; **MS:** Columbia P&S 59; **RES:** Psyc, Columbia-Presbyterian Med Ctr, New York, NY 60-63; ***SI:** Psychotherapy/Psychoanalysis*
♿ ☎ 📅 [WC] 2-4 Weeks

English, Joseph T (MD) **Psyc**
St Vincents Hosp & Med Ctr NY
203 W 12th St Rm 627; New York, NY 10011; (212) 604-8252; **MS:** Jefferson Med Coll 58; **RES:** Psyc, Institute of Penn Hospital, Philadelphia, PA 59-61; Psyc, Nat Inst of Mental Health, Bethesda, MD 61-62

Esman, Aaron H (MD) **Psyc**
NY Hosp-Cornell Med Ctr
1100 Park Ave; New York, NY 10128; (212) 860-8767; **BDCERT:** Psyc 54; ChAP 60; **MS:** Cornell U 47; **RES:** Bellevue Hosp Ctr, New York, NY 47-50; **FEL:** ChAP, Bellevue Hosp Ctr, New York, NY 50-51; **FAP:** Prof Cornell U; ***SI:** Psychoanalysis; Adolescence*
♿ ☎ 📅 [Mcr] A Few Days

Fabian, Christopher (MD) **Psyc**
St Vincents Hosp & Med Ctr NY
33 Fifth Ave; New York, NY 10003; (212) 673-5230; **BDCERT:** Psyc 89; **MS:** Georgetown U 83; **RES:** Psyc, St Vincents Hospital, New York, NY 84-87; **FEL:** St Vincents Hospital, New York, NY 83-84

Ferran, Ernesto (MD) **Psyc**
New York University Med Ctr
1 Washington Square Village; New York, NY 10012; (212) 614-1517; **BDCERT:** Psyc 83; ChAP 86; **MS:** Albert Einstein Coll Med 76; **RES:** Psyc, Bellevue Hosp Ctr, New York, NY 76-79; **FEL:** ChAP, Bellevue Hosp Ctr, New York, NY 79-81; New York University Med Ctr, New York, NY 79-81; **FAP:** Asst Prof NYU Sch Med; **HOSP:** Bellevue Hosp Ctr; ***SI:** Marital Issues; Cultural Issues;* **HMO:** CIGNA Blue Choice
LANG: Sp; ☾ ☎ 👤 📅 $ A Few Days

Finkel, Jay (MD) **Psyc**
Mount Sinai Med Ctr
108 E 91st St; New York, NY 10128; (212) 289-2077; **BDCERT:** Psyc 85; **MS:** NY Med Coll 80; **RES:** Psyc, Mount Sinai Med Ctr, New York, NY; ***SI:** Anxiety Disorders; Depression*
☾ ☎ 📅 $ 4+ Weeks

Foster, Jeffrey (MD) **Psyc**
New York University Med Ctr
155 E 29th St Ste 31D; New York, NY 10016; (212) 686-9668; **BDCERT:** Psyc 80; 91; **MS:** NY Med Coll 70; **RES:** Mount Sinai Hosp, Cleveland, OH 74; **HMO:** Oxford
♿ ☾ ☎ 👤 $ [Mcr] Immediately

Fox, Herbert (MD) **Psyc**
Gracie Square Hosp
20 E 9th St; New York, NY 10003; (212) 674-8622; **BDCERT:** Psyc 76; GerPsy 94; **MS:** Albert Einstein Coll Med 69; **RES:** Psyc, Jacobi Med Ctr, Bronx, NY 70-73; **FAP:** Asst Prof Psyc Cornell U; **HOSP:** Lenox Hill Hosp; ***SI:** Psychotherapy; Pharmacotherapy;* **HMO:** Oxford
♿ ☾ ☎ 👤 📅 [Mcr] [Mcd] 1 Week

Guide to symbols and abbreviations can be found on pages 110-113.

Friedman, David (MD) Psyc
New York University Med Ctr
20 Park Ave; New York, NY 10016; (212) 683-
6071; BDCERT: Psyc 52; MS: NYU Sch Med 45;
RES: Bellevue Hosp Ctr, New York, NY 48-51;
HOSP: Bellevue Hosp Ctr
🄲 🄰 🄼 🄼 Immediately

Friedman, Lawrence (MD) Psyc
NY Hosp-Cornell Med Ctr
129B E 71st St; New York, NY 10021; (212) 861-
8732; BDCERT: Psyc 63; MS: Temple U 55; RES:
VA Ct Healthcare Sys-West Haven, West Haven, CT
56-57; Yale-New Haven Hosp, New Haven, CT 57-
58; FEL: Yale-New Haven Hosp, New Haven, CT
58-59; FAP: Clin Prof Psyc Cornell U; HMO: None
🄰 4+ Weeks

Friedman, Richard Alan (MD)Psyc
NY Hosp-Cornell Med Ctr
NY HospitalCornell Medical Ctr, 525 E 68th St;
New York, NY 10021; (212) 821-0769; BDCERT:
Psyc 89; MS: UMDNJ-RW Johnson Med Sch 83;
RES: Psyc, Mount Sinai Med Ctr, New York, NY 83-
87; FAP: Assoc Prof Psyc Cornell U; SI:
Psychopharmacology; Depression; HMO: None
🄰 🄲 🄰 🄼 🄼 🄼 1 Week

Friedman, Stanley (MD & PhD)Psyc
Mount Sinai Med Ctr
9 E 96th St; New York, NY 10128; (212) 722-
4466; BDCERT: Psyc 63; MS: NYU Sch Med 54;
RES: Hillside Hosp, Glen Oaks, NY 55-57; FEL: Psyc,
Mount Sinai Med Ctr, New York, NY 57-60; FAP:
Assoc Clin Prof Mt Sinai Sch Med; SI: Sex-Abuse;
Psychoanalytic Therapy; HMO: None
🄰 🄰 🄼 🄼 Immediately

Frosch, William (MD) Psyc
NY Hosp-Cornell Med Ctr
525 E 68th St; New York, NY 10021; (212) 746-
3667; BDCERT: Psyc 64; N 64; MS: NYU Sch Med
57; RES: Psyc, Bellevue Hosp Ctr, New York, NY
57-61; SI: Addiction Psychiatry
🄰 🄰 🄼 1 Week

Fullilove, Mindy (MD) Psyc
NYS Psychiatric Institute
722 W 168th St; New York, NY 10032; (212)
740-7292; BDCERT: Psyc 84; MS: Columbia P&S
78; RES: NY Hosp-Cornell-Westchester, White
Plains, NY; Montefiore Med Ctr, Bronx, NY 81-82;
SI: Addiction Psychiatry
🄰 A Few Days

Fyer, Minna R (MD) Psyc
NY Hosp-Cornell Med Ctr
242 E 72nd St; New York, NY 10021; (212) 861-
2586; BDCERT: Psyc 85; MS: SUNY Hlth Sci Ctr
80; RES: NY Hosp-Cornell Med Ctr, New York, NY
80-84; FEL: Psyc, Columbia-Presbyterian Med Ctr,
New York, NY; SI: Anxiety Disorders; Mood
Disorders; HMO: None
🄰 🄲 🄰 🄼 🄼 🄢 🄦 🄽 Immediately 🄼

Galanter, Marc (MD) Psyc
New York University Med Ctr
285 Central Park West; New York, NY 10024;
(212) 877-4093; BDCERT: Psyc 74; AdP 93; MS:
Albert Einstein Coll Med 67; RES: UCLA Med Ctr,
Los Angeles, CA 67-68; Psyc, Albert Einstein Med
Ctr, Bronx, NY 68-71; HOSP: Bellevue Hosp Ctr; SI:
Addiction Psychiatry; General Psychiatry; HMO:
None
🄰 🄲 🄰 🄼 🄼 🄢 A Few Days

Gaylin, Willard (MD) Psyc
Columbia-Presbyterian Med Ctr
20 E 63rd St Flr4; New York, NY 10021; (212)
752-8382; BDCERT: Psyc 59; MS: Case West Res U
51; RES: VA Med Ctr-Bronx, Bronx, NY 52-54;
FAP: Clin Prof Psyc Columbia P&S; SI:
Psychoanalysis; Psychotherapy
🄰 🄼 1 Week

Gershell, William J (MD)   Psyc
Mount Sinai Med Ctr
1100 Madison Ave 2 C; New York, NY 10028;
(212) 737-9300; **BDCERT:** Psyc 75; GerPsy 91;
MS: Switzerland 65; **RES:** Psyc, Mount Sinai Med
Ctr, New York, NY 66-68; **FEL:** ChAP, Mount Sinai
Med Ctr, New York, NY 68-70; **FAP:** Asst Clin Prof
Mt Sinai Sch Med; **SI:** *Psychopharmacology; Geriatric
Psychiatry*
LANG: Fr; 🦽 🔊 🏢 A Few Days

Glass, Richard (MD)   Psyc
NY Hosp-Cornell Med Ctr
65 E 76th St; New York, NY 10021; (212) 988-
7616; **BDCERT:** Psyc 62; **MS:** Johns Hopkins U 56;
RES: Jacobi Med Ctr, Bronx, NY 57-59; **FEL:** AM,
Jacobi Med Ctr, Bronx, NY; **HMO:** Blue Cross & Blue
Shield
🔊 🏢 Mcr Immediately

Glassman, Alexander (MD) Psyc
NYS Psychiatric Institute
722 W 168th St; New York, NY 10032; (212)
543-5000; **BDCERT:** Psyc 75; **MS:** Univ IL Coll Med
58; **RES:** DC Gen Hosp, Washington, DC 59; Jacobi
Med Ctr, Bronx, NY 62; **FEL:** Psyc, USPHS, New
York, NY 63-64; **HOSP:** Columbia-Presbyterian
Med Ctr; **SI:** *Psychopharmacology*; **HMO:** Oxford
🅲 🔊 $

Glick, Robert A (MD)   Psyc
Columbia-Presbyterian Med Ctr
125 E 84th St; New York, NY 10028; (212) 472-
2223; **BDCERT:** Psyc 72; **MS:** Columbia P&S 66;
RES: Psyc, NYS Psychiatric Institute, New York, NY
67-70; **FAP:** Prof Psyc Columbia P&S; **SI:**
Psychoanalysis; Psychotherapy
🅲 🔊 🏢 2-4 Weeks

Goldberg, Eugene L (MD & PhD)Psyc
Columbia-Presbyterian Med Ctr
903 Park Ave; New York, NY 10021; (212) 879-
8850; **BDCERT:** Psyc 68; **MS:** Columbia P&S 54;
RES: Psyc, Jacobi Med Ctr, Bronx, NY 58-60; **FEL:**
Psyc, Albert Einstein Med Ctr, Bronx, NY 60; **FAP:**
Assoc Clin Prof Psyc Albert Einstein Coll Med;
HOSP: Montefiore Med Ctr; **SI:** *Psychoanalysis,
Psychiatry; Post-Traumatic Stress Syndrome*; **HMO:**
Empire MDHealth
🦽 🔊 👪 🏢 Mcr A Few Days

Goldberger, Marianne (MD) Psyc
New York University Med Ctr
1130 Park Ave; New York, NY 10128; (212) 534-
3070; **BDCERT:** ChAP 79; Psyc 71; **MS:** NY Med
Coll 58; **RES:** Psyc, U of WI Hosp, Madison, WI 59-
61; **FEL:** ChAP, Children's Hosp Nat Med Ctr,
Washington, DC 61-63; **FAP:** Prof of Clin Psyc NYU
Sch Med; **HOSP:** NY Hosp-Cornell Med Ctr; **SI:**
Individual Psychotherapy
LANG: Ger; 🔊 Mcr 1 Week

Goldin, Gurston (MD)   Psyc
Columbia-Presbyterian Med Ctr
166 E 63rd St; New York, NY 10021; (212) 838-
7223; **BDCERT:** Psyc 65; **MS:** Columbia P&S 55;
RES: Psyc, Columbia-Presbyterian Med Ctr, New
York, NY 58-61; Psyc, NYS Psychiatric Institute,
New York, NY 58-61; **FEL:** Psyc, Columbia-
Presbyterian Med Ctr, New York, NY 61-63; **FAP:**
Assoc Columbia P&S; **HOSP:** NY Hosp-Cornell Med
Ctr; **SI:** *Psychotherapy; Forensic Psychiatry*; **HMO:**
Oxford
🦽 🔊 🏢 Mcr A Few Days

Goldman, David S (MD)   Psyc
New York University Med Ctr
35 E 85th St; New York, NY 10028; (212) 288-
2620; **BDCERT:** Psyc 76; **MS:** Duke U 65; **RES:**
Bellevue Hosp Ctr, New York, NY 66-69; **FEL:**
Columbia-Presbyterian Med Ctr, New York, NY 68-
75; **HOSP:** Gracie Square Hosp; **HMO:** Oxford
🦽 🅲 🔊 Mcr Immediately

Goldman, Neil S (MD) Psyc
St Vincents Hosp & Med Ctr NY
36 7th Ave Ste 412; New York, NY 10011; (212) 929-4395; **BDCERT:** Psyc 81; **MS:** U Hlth Sci/Chicago Med Sch 70; **RES:** Brookdale Univ Hosp Med Ctr, Brooklyn, NY 71-74; **FEL:** AdP, St Vincents Hosp & Med Ctr NY, New York, NY 77-79; **FAP:** Asst Prof NY Med Coll; *SI: Addictions; Mood Disorders*

⬛ ⬛ ⬛ ⬛ ⬛ ⬛ ⬛ ⬛ Immediately

Goodman, Berney (MD) Psyc
Mount Sinai Med Ctr
11 E 68th St; New York, NY 10021; (212) 535-0111; **BDCERT:** Psyc 71; GerPsy 94; **MS:** South Africa 57; **RES:** IM, Mount Sinai Med Ctr, New York, NY 62-64; Psyc, Jacobi Med Ctr, Bronx, NY 66-69; **FEL:** IM, Mount Sinai Med Ctr, New York, NY 61; **FAP:** Asst Clin Prof Mt Sinai Sch Med; **HOSP:** Lenox Hill Hosp; *SI: Treatment of Medically Ill; Psychosomatic Illness*

LANG: Itl, Yd; ⬛ ⬛ ⬛ ⬛ ⬛

Gorman, Jack (MD) Psyc
Columbia-Presbyterian Med Ctr
15 W 81st St; New York, NY 10028; (212) 543-5000; **BDCERT:** Psyc 79; **MS:** Columbia P&S 77; **RES:** Columbia-Presbyterian Med Ctr, New York, NY; **FEL:** Columbia-Presbyterian Med Ctr, New York, NY; **HOSP:** New York University Med Ctr; **HMO:** Oxford

⬛ ⬛ ⬛ ⬛ ⬛ ⬛ 2-4 Weeks

Gruen, Peter (MD) Psyc
Lenox Hill Hosp
18 E 77th St B; New York, NY 10021; (212) 249-2720; **BDCERT:** Psyc 75; **MS:** UC San Francisco 65; **RES:** Albert Einstein Med Ctr, Bronx, NY 69-72; **FEL:** Montefiore Med Ctr, Bronx, NY 72-73; **HOSP:** New York University Med Ctr; *SI: Depression; Anxiety Disorders*

⬛ ⬛ ⬛ ⬛ ⬛ A Few Days

Gusmorino, Paul (MD) Psyc
Hosp For Joint Diseases
300 E 59th St 701; New York, NY 10022; (212) 598-6204; **BDCERT:** Psyc 80; ChAP 82; **MS:** Italy 74; **RES:** Kings County Hosp Ctr, Brooklyn, NY 78; **FEL:** ChAP, NY Hosp-Cornell Med Ctr, New York, NY 80; **FAP:** Asst Clin Prof NYU Sch Med; **HOSP:** Beth Israel Med Ctr; *SI: Chronic Pain; Acute Pain Mgmt;* **HMO:** Oxford Maxiplan

LANG: Itl; ⬛ ⬛ ⬛ ⬛ ⬛ ⬛ 2-4 Weeks

Heiman, Peter (MD) Psyc
Beth Israel Med Ctr
1148 5th Ave; New York, NY 10128; (212) 410-9381; **BDCERT:** Psyc 75; **MS:** Albert Einstein Coll Med 68; **RES:** Montefiore Med Ctr, Bronx, NY 69-72; **FAP:** Asst Prof Psyc Albert Einstein Coll Med; **HOSP:** Montefiore Med Ctr; **HMO:** GHI

⬛ ⬛ ⬛ ⬛ 1 Week

Heller, Stanley (MD) Psyc
St Luke's Roosevelt Hosp Ctr
4 E 89th St; New York, NY 10128; (212) 831-5919; **BDCERT:** Psyc 75; **MS:** Columbia P&S 60; **RES:** Columbia-Presbyterian Med Ctr, New York, NY 63-66; **FAP:** Assoc Clin Prof Psyc Columbia P&S; *SI: Psychiatry & Heart Problems; Panic and Depression*

⬛ ⬛ ⬛ ⬛ 1 Week

Hendin, Herbert (MD) Psyc
Westchester Med Ctr
1045 Park Ave 3C; New York, NY 10028; (212) 348-4035; **BDCERT:** Psyc 55; **MS:** NYU Sch Med 49; **RES:** Psyc, Bellevue Hosp Ctr, New York, NY 50-52; Psyc, VA Med Ctr-Manh, New York, NY 52-53; **FEL:** Psyc, Bellevue Hosp Ctr, New York, NY 53-56; **FAP:** Lecturer NY Med Coll; *SI: Suicide; Post Traumatic Stress Disorder*

⬛ ⬛ ⬛ ⬛ A Few Days

Hoffman, Joel (MD)   Psyc
Lenox Hill Hosp

1236 Park Ave; New York, NY 10128; (212) 722-3004; **BDCERT:** Psyc 77; **MS:** Columbia P&S 63; **RES:** IM, U Mich Med Ctr, Ann Arbor, MI 64-67; Psyc, NYS Psychiatric Institute, New York, NY 69-72; **FEL:** Clin Pharmacology, Univ Hospital, Ann Arbor, MI 67; **FAP:** Asst Clin Prof Columbia P&S; **HOSP:** Columbia-Presbyterian Med Ctr; *SI: Treatment Resistant Illness; Depression*

⬛ ⬛ ⬛ ⬛ ⬛

Holland, Jimmie (MD)   Psyc
Mem Sloan Kettering Cancer Ctr

1275 York Ave 421; New York, NY 10021; (212) 639-7051; **BDCERT:** Psyc 67; **MS:** Baylor 52; **RES:** Malcolm Bliss, St Louis, MO; Mass Gen Hosp, Boston, MA; *SI: Cancer; Bereavement*

⬛

Hollander, Eric (MD)   Psyc
Mount Sinai Med Ctr

300 Central Park West 1C; New York, NY 10024; (212) 873-4051; **BDCERT:** Psyc 87; **MS:** SUNY Hlth Sci Ctr 82; **RES:** IM, Mount Sinai Med Ctr, New York, NY 82-83; Psyc, Mount Sinai Med Ctr, New York, NY 83-86; **FEL:** Psychopharmacology, Columbia-Presbyterian Med Ctr, New York, NY; NYS Psychiatric Institute, New York, NY; **FAP:** Prof Mt Sinai Sch Med; *SI: Obsessive-Compulsive Disorder; Autism*

⬛ ⬛ ⬛ ⬛ ⬛ 2-4 Weeks

Isay, Richard A (MD)   Psyc
NY Hosp-Cornell Med Ctr

55 E End Ave 1G; New York, NY 10028; (212) 535-1863; **BDCERT:** Psyc 69; **MS:** U Rochester 61; **RES:** IM, U Hosp of Cleveland, Cleveland, OH 61-62; Psyc, Yale-New Haven Hosp, New Haven, CT 62-65; **FAP:** Clin Prof Cornell U; *SI: Psychotherapy for Gay Men*

⬛ ⬛ ⬛ ⬛ ⬛ 2-4 Weeks

Jacobs, Theodore (MD)   Psyc
Montefiore Med Ctr

170 E 77th St; New York, NY 10021; (212) 879-3002; **BDCERT:** Psyc 68; **MS:** U Chicago-Pritzker Sch Med 57; **RES:** Psyc, Bronx Muncipal Hosp Ctr, Bronx, NY 58-61; **FAP:** Clin Prof Albert Einstein Coll Med; *SI: Adolescents & Young Adults; Creativity;* **HMO:** Blue Cross & Blue Shield

⬛ ⬛ ⬛ ⬛ ⬛ ⬛ ⬛ ⬛ 1 Week

Kafka, Ernest (MD)   Psyc
NY Hosp-Cornell Med Ctr

23 E 92nd St; New York, NY 10128; (212) 876-5781; **MS:** Washington U, St Louis 58; **RES:** Psyc, Albert Einstein Med Ctr, Bronx, NY 59-62; **FEL:** Albert Einstein Med Ctr, Bronx, NY 62-64

⬛ ⬛ 1 Week

Kahn, David Allen (MD)   Psyc
St Vincents Hosp & Med Ctr NY

31 W 12th St 1B; New York, NY 10011; (212) 255-4029; **BDCERT:** Psyc 93; ChAP 95; **MS:** Univ Texas, Houston 87; **RES:** Psyc, St Vincents Hosp & Med Ctr NY, New York, NY 87-90; **FEL:** ChAP, St Vincents Hosp & Med Ctr NY, New York, NY 90-92; **FAP:** Asst Clin Prof NY Med Coll; *SI: Group Psychotherapy*

⬛ ⬛ ⬛ 1 Week

Kalinich, Lila J (MD)   Psyc
Columbia-Presbyterian Med Ctr

333 Central Park West Apt 12; New York, NY 10025; (212) 866-0200; **BDCERT:** Psyc 75; **MS:** Northwestern U 69; **RES:** Columbia-Presbyterian Med Ctr, New York, NY 70-73; **FAP:** Assoc Clin Prof Psyc Columbia P&S; **HOSP:** NYS Psychiatric Institute; *SI: Psychoanalysis; Adolescent Psychiatry;* **HMO:** None

LANG: Fr, Crt; ⬛ ⬛ ⬛ 2-4 Weeks

Karasu, T Byram (MD)   Psyc
Montefiore Med Ctr
2 E 88th St; New York, NY 10128; (212) 426-
5208; **BDCERT:** Psyc 72; **MS:** Turkey 59; **RES:**
Fairfield Hills Hosp, Newton, CT 66-67; Psyc, Yale-
New Haven Hosp, New Haven, CT 67-68; **FAP:** Prof
Psyc Albert Einstein Coll Med; **HOSP:** Montefiore
Med Ctr-Weiler/Einstein Div; **SI:** *Depression;*
Personality Disorder

🄲 🎟 2-4 Weeks

Kaufmann, Charles (MD)   Psyc
Columbia-Presbyterian Med Ctr
161 Ft Washington Ave; New York, NY 10032;
(212) 305-5341; **BDCERT:** Psyc 82; **MS:** Columbia
P&S 77; **RES:** NY Hosp-Cornell Med Ctr, New York,
NY 77-81; **FEL:** Psyc, Nat Inst Health, Bethesda,
MD 81-85; Molecular N, Ctr for Neurobio and
Behavr, New York, NY 86-88; **FAP:** Assoc Prof
Columbia P&S; **SI:** *Schizophrenia; Bipolar Disease*

🅖 🄰 🔣 🎟 🅂 ⊠ 2-4 Weeks

Kleber, Herbert (MD)   Psyc
Columbia-Presbyterian Med Ctr
722 W 168th St; New York, NY 10032; (212)
543-5570; **MS:** Jefferson Med Coll 60; **RES:** Psyc,
Yale-New Haven Hosp, New Haven, CT 61-64;
FAP: Prof Columbia P&S; **SI:** *Addiction Psychiatry*

🅖 🄰 🔣 🎟 🄽🄵🄸 2-4 Weeks

Klein, Donald (MD)   Psyc
Columbia-Presbyterian Med Ctr
182 E 79th St; New York, NY 10021; (212) 737-
4166; **BDCERT:** Psyc 59; **MS:** SUNY Hlth Sci Ctr
52; **RES:** Creedmore Psych Ctr, Queens Village, NY
53-54; **HOSP:** NYS Psychiatric Institute

🄲 🄰 🔣 🎟 🅂 2-4 Weeks

Klein, Israel (MD)   Psyc
New York University Med Ctr
155 E 31st St 25L; New York, NY 10016; (212)
685-1535; **BDCERT:** Psyc 91; **MS:** SUNY Hlth Sci
Ctr 83; **RES:** Bellevue Hosp Ctr, New York, NY 83-
87; **FEL:** New York University Med Ctr, New York,
NY 87-89; **FAP:** Clin Instr Psyc NYU Sch Med; **SI:**
Psychoanalysis; Psychotherapy; **HMO:** Oxford

LANG: Heb, Yd; 🅖 🄲 🄰 🔣 🎟 🅂 ⊠ 1 Week

Kleyman, Felix (MD)   Psyc
St Vincent's Med Ctr-Westchester
161 W 54th St Ste 204; New York, NY 10019;
(212) 541-4428; **BDCERT:** Psyc 89; **MS:** Russia
72; **RES:** Psyc, Univ Hosp SUNY Bklyn, Brooklyn,
NY 82-85; **FEL:** GerPsy, NY Hosp-Cornell Med Ctr,
New York, NY 85-86; **HOSP:** Gracie Square Hosp;
HMO: Oxford

LANG: Rus; 🅖 🄲 🄰 🔣 🎟 🅂 ⊠ 🄽🄵🄸 A Few Days

Kocsis, James (MD)   Psyc
NY Hosp-Cornell Med Ctr
425 E 61st St; New York, NY 10021; (212) 821-
0723; **BDCERT:** Psyc 77; **MS:** Cornell U 68; **RES:**
NY Hosp-Cornell Med Ctr, New York, NY 69-70;
FAP: Prof Cornell U; **SI:** *Psychopharmacology;*
Affective Disorders; **HMO:** NYH Health Plan Sel Pro
Empire Blue Cross & Shield Blue Select +

🅖 🄰 🎟 🅂 ⊠ A Few Days

Kornfeld, Donald S (MD)   Psyc
Columbia-Presbyterian Med Ctr
622 W 168th St Box 427; New York, NY 10032;
(212) 305-9985; **BDCERT:** Psyc 62; **MS:** Yale U
Sch Med 54; **RES:** Columbia-Presbyterian Med Ctr,
New York, NY 57-60; **SI:** *Geriatric Psychiatry*

LANG: Sp, Can, Rus; 🅖 🎟 ⊠ Immediately

Kowallis, George (MD)   Psyc
St Vincents Hosp & Med Ctr NY
162 W 56th St 407; New York, NY 10019; (212)
757-0324; **BDCERT:** Psyc 77; ChAP 78; **MS:** Univ
Penn 69; **RES:** ChAP, St Luke's Roosevelt Hosp Ctr,
New York, NY 72-74; **SI:** *Anxiety; Depression;* **HMO:**
Aetna Hlth Plan Blue Cross & Blue Shield GHI
Mental Behavioral Care

🅖 🄲 🄰 🔣 🎟 🅂 2-4 Weeks

Koz, Gabriel (MD)   Psyc
168 W 86th St; New York, NY 10024; (212) 799-
6770; **BDCERT:** Psyc 65; FP 91; **MS:** South Africa
58; **RES:** Psyc, St Clements Hosp, London, England
61-62; Psyc, Boston Med Ctr, Boston, MA 62-64;
FAP: Clin Prof NYU Sch Med; **SI:** *General Psychiatry;*
Geriatrics

🅖 🄲 🄰 🔣 🎟 🅂 ⊠ ⊠ ⊠ 🄽🄵🄸 1 Week

Kranzler, Elliot (MD)   Psyc
Columbia-Presbyterian Med Ctr
451 West End Ave; New York, NY 10024; (212)
580-9758; **BDCERT:** Psyc 84; ChAP 86; **MS:** Albert
Einstein Coll Med 78; **RES:** Psyc, NY Hosp-Cornell
Med Ctr, New York, NY; **FEL:** ChAP, Columbia-
Presbyterian Med Ctr, New York, NY; *SI: Depression
and Bereavement; Anxiety Disorders*
⟨symbols⟩ Immediately

Kremberg, M Roy (MD)   Psyc
St Luke's Roosevelt Hosp Ctr
2109 Broadway Ste 1454; New York, NY 10023;
(212) 875-8568; **BDCERT:** Psyc 80; ChAP 82; **MS:**
Columbia P&S 76; **RES:** St Luke's Roosevelt Hosp
Ctr, New York, NY 76-78; **FEL:** ChAP, St Luke's
Roosevelt Hosp Ctr, New York, NY 78-80; **FAP:**
Instr Psyc Columbia P&S; *SI: Anxiety; Mood
Disorders*; **HMO:** Blue Cross Oxford NYLCare
Magnacare
LANG: Fr, Sp, Rus, Yd; ⟨symbols⟩
A Few Days

Lane, Fredrick M (MD)   Psyc
125 E 87th St 4E; New York, NY 10128; (212)
876-0841; **BDCERT:** Psyc 66; **MS:** Yale U Sch Med
53; **RES:** Psyc, Yale-New Haven Hosp, New Haven,
CT 54-55; Psyc, Yale-New Haven Hosp, New
Haven, CT 57-58; **FEL:** Psyc, Yale-New Haven
Hosp, New Haven, CT 58-59; **FAP:** Clin Prof Psyc
Columbia P&S
⟨symbols⟩ A Few Days

Lang, Enid (MD)   Psyc
Mount Sinai Med Ctr
1158 5th Ave 1C; New York, NY 10029; (212)
348-2066; **BDCERT:** Psyc 79; **MS:** USC Sch Med
70; **RES:** Columbia-Presbyterian Med Ctr, New
York, NY; **FEL:** Psyc, Columbia-Presbyterian Med
Ctr, New York, NY; **FAP:** Assoc Clin Prof Mt Sinai
Sch Med
⟨symbols⟩ 2-4 Weeks

Lederberg, Marguerite (MD) Psyc
Mem Sloan Kettering Cancer Ctr
Department of Psychiatry, 1275 York Ave; New
York, NY 10021; (212) 639-8705; **BDCERT:** Psyc
80; Ped 80; **MS:** Yale U Sch Med 61; **RES:** Ped,
Stanford Med Ctr, Stanford, CA 64; Psyc, Stanford
Med Ctr, Stanford, CA 72-77; **FAP:** Clin Prof Cornell
U; *SI: Psychiatric Support for Cancer; Patients and
Families.*
LANG: Fr; ⟨symbols⟩

Leeman, Cavin P (MD)   Psyc
Univ Hosp SUNY Bklyn
344 W 23rd St 1B; New York, NY 10011; (212)
675-0890; **BDCERT:** Psyc 66; **MS:** Harvard Med
Sch 59; **RES:** Mass Mental Hlth Ctr, Boston, MA 60-
62; Beth Israel Med Ctr, Boston, MA 62-64; **FEL:** U
of VA Health Sci Ctr, Charlottesville, VA; **FAP:** Clin
Prof SUNY Hlth Sci Ctr; *SI: Psychotherapy;
Psychopharmacology*; **HMO:** Oxford GHI Blue Shield
Empire MBC +
⟨symbols⟩ 1 Week

Lefer, Jay (MD)   Psyc
Beth Israel Med Ctr
200 East End Ave Suite 9J; New York, NY 10128;
(212) 427-0427; **BDCERT:** Psyc 62; **MS:**
Switzerland 55; **RES:** Yale-New Haven Hosp, New
Haven, CT 62; **FEL:** Psych, Grace New Haven Hosp,
New Haven, CT; **FAP:** Assoc Clin Prof NY Med Coll;
HOSP: Montefiore Med Ctr-Weiler/Einstein Div; *SI:
Psychosomatics; Psychoanalysis*
LANG: Fr; ⟨symbols⟩
Immediately

Leibowitz, Michael D (MD) Psyc
VA Med Ctr-Manh
75 Irving Pl Ste 1A; New York, NY 10003; (212)
732-6472; **BDCERT:** Psyc 80; **MS:** Tufts U 74; **RES:**
Psyc, Beth Israel Med Ctr, New York, NY 75-78;
FEL: Psychosomatic Medicine, Univ Hosp SUNY
Bklyn, Brooklyn, NY 78-79; **FAP:** Asst Clin Prof
Psyc NYU Sch Med; **HOSP:** New York University
Med Ctr

Levitan, Stephan (MD)   Psyc
Columbia-Presbyterian Med Ctr

185 E 85th St 29J; New York, NY 10028; (212) 722-4311; **BDCERT:** Psyc 74; **MS:** SUNY Buffalo 65; **RES:** Hillside Hosp, Glen Oaks, NY 66-69; **FEL:** NYS Psychiatric Institute, New York, NY 73; *SI: Psychotherapy; Psychopharmacology*

 ⚕ ♿ ☎ 🅰 🚾 ⊞ 1 Week

Liebowitz, Michael R (MD) Psyc
Columbia-Presbyterian Med Ctr

722 W 168th St; New York, NY 10032; (212) 543-5366; **BDCERT:** Psyc 78; **MS:** Yale U Sch Med 69; **RES:** Psyc, Med Ctr Hosp of VT, Burlington, VT 74-75; Psyc, NYS Psychiatric Institute, New York, NY 75-77; **FEL:** Psyc, NYS Psychiatric Institute, New York, NY 77-79; **FAP:** Clin Prof Psyc Columbia P&S; *SI: Anxiety Disorders*; **HMO:** None

LANG: Sp; ♿ ☎ 🚾 ⊞ 💲 1 Week

Lindenmayer, Jean- Pierre (MD) Psyc
Manh Psych Ctr-Ward's Is

18 E 77th St B; New York, NY 10021; (212) 249-2720; **BDCERT:** Psyc 75; **MS:** Switzerland 67; **RES:** Psyc, Univ Hosp SUNY Bklyn, Brooklyn, NY 70-73; **FEL:** Univ Hosp SUNY Bklyn, Brooklyn, NY 74-75; **FAP:** Clin Prof Psyc NYU Sch Med; **HOSP:** Gracie Square Hosp; *SI: Psychopharmacology; Schizophrenia*; **HMO:** Empire Blue Cross & Blue Shield Independent Health Plan

LANG: Fr, Ger; ♿ ☎ 🚾 ⊞ 💲 Mcr WC 1 Week

Lipton, Brian (MD)   Psyc
Lenox Hill Hosp

1111 Park Ave 1A; New York, NY 10128; (212) 427-4499; **BDCERT:** Psyc 70; **MS:** SUNY Hlth Sci Ctr 64; **RES:** Hillside Hosp, Glen Oaks, NY 65-68; **FAP:** Asst Clin Prof Psyc NYU Sch Med; *SI: Psychological Aspects of Infertility; Substance Abuse. Depression.*; **HMO:** Blue Cross & Blue Shield

 ⚕ ♿ ☎ 🅰 ⊞ Mcr A Few Days

Lowinson, Joyce (MD)   Psyc
Montefiore Med Ctr

111 E 56th St; New York, NY 10022; (718) 409-1916; **MS:** Albert Einstein Coll Med 62; **RES:** Psyc, Albert Einstein Med Ctr, Bronx, NY 68; **FAP:** Prof Albert Einstein Coll Med; **HOSP:** Montefiore Med Ctr-Weiler/Einstein Div; *SI: Substance Abuse; Pain Management*

 ⚕ ☎ ⊞ 💲 A Few Days

Mahon, Eugene (MD)   Psyc

Psychoanalysis Adult & Child, 6 E 96th St; New York, NY 10128; (212) 831-1414; **BDCERT:** Psyc 93; **MS:** Ireland 64; **RES:** Psyc, Columbia-Presbyterian Med Ctr, New York, NY 78; **FAP:** Asst Clin Prof Psyc Columbia P&S; *SI: Psychoanalysis of Adults and Children*

 ☎ ⊞ 1 Week

Manevitz, Alan (MD)   Psyc
NY Hosp-Cornell Med Ctr

60 Sutton Place South 1CN; New York, NY 10022; (212) 746-3834; **BDCERT:** Psyc 87; **MS:** Columbia P&S 84; **RES:** NY Hosp-Cornell Med Ctr, New York, NY; **FEL:** Psychopharmacology, NY Hosp-Cornell Med Ctr, New York, NY; Sex Therapy, NY Hosp-Cornell Med Ctr, New York, NY; **FAP:** Assoc Clin Prof Cornell U; **HOSP:** Lenox Hill Hosp; *SI: Marital/Family/Sex Therapy; Complex Medication Issues*; **HMO:** Most

 ⚕ 🆘 ♿ ☎ 🅰 ⊞ Mcr WC A Few Days 🏧 *VISA* 💳

Marcus, Eric R (MD)   Psyc
Columbia-Presbyterian Med Ctr

4 E 89th St 1D; New York, NY 10128; (212) 427-0543; **BDCERT:** Psyc 77; **MS:** U Wisc Med Sch 69; **RES:** Psyc, Columbia-Presbyterian Med Ctr, New York, NY 72-75; **FEL:** Psyc, NYS Psychiatric Institute, New York, NY 82-87; **FAP:** Clin Prof Psyc Columbia P&S; *SI: Depression; Personality Disorders*

 ♿ ☎ 🅰 ⊞ 1 Week

Marin, Deborah B (MD)   Psyc
Mount Sinai Med Ctr
1 Gustave Levy Pl Box 1230; New York, NY
10029; (212) 241-6630; **BDCERT:** Psyc 90; **MS:**
Mt Sinai Sch Med 84; **RES:** Mount Sinai Med Ctr,
New York, NY; **FEL:** NY Hosp-Cornell Med Ctr, New
York, NY; **FAP:** Assoc Prof Psyc Mt Sinai Sch Med;
SI: *Alzheimer's Disease; Geriatric Psychiatry*

♿ ♿ ♿

Markowitz, John (MD)   Psyc
NY Hosp-Cornell Med Ctr
525 E 68th St; New York, NY 10021; (212) 746-
3774; **BDCERT:** Psyc 87; **MS:** Columbia P&S 82;
RES: Psyc, NY Hosp-Cornell Med Ctr, New York,
NY; **FEL:** NY Hosp-Cornell Med Ctr, New York, NY;
FAP: Assoc Prof Psyc Cornell U; **SI:** *Interpersonal
psychotherapy; Cognitive Therapy*

♿ ♿ ♿ ♿ ♿ ♿ Immediately

McGowan, James M (MD)   Psyc
NY Hosp-Cornell Med Ctr
49 E 78th St; New York, NY 10021; (212) 876-
5028; **BDCERT:** Psyc 74; **MS:** Univ Ky Coll Med 64;
RES: Psyc, Albert Einstein Med Ctr, Bronx, NY 68-
71; IM, Bellevue Hosp Ctr, New York, NY 67-68;
FEL: Psyc, Albert Einstein Med Ctr, Bronx, NY 71-
72; **FAP:** Asst Clin Prof Psyc Cornell U; **HOSP:** St
Vincent's Med Ctr-Westchester; **SI:** *Alcoholism; Drug
Addiction*

♿ ♿ A Few Days

McGrath, Patrick (MD)   Psyc
NYS Psychiatric Institute
161 Fort Washington Ave; New York, NY 10032;
(212) 543-5764; **BDCERT:** Psyc 75; **MS:** Columbia
P&S 74; **RES:** Columbia-Presbyterian Med Ctr, New
York, NY 74-75; Psyc, NYS Psychiatric Institute,
New York, NY 75-78; **FAP:** Assoc Prof Psyc
Columbia P&S; **HOSP:** Columbia-Presbyterian Med
Ctr; **SI:** *Psychopharmacology; Depression*

♿ ♿ ♿ ♿ ♿ ♿ 2-4 Weeks

McMullen, Robert (MD)   Psyc
Columbia-Presbyterian Med Ctr
171 W 79th St; New York, NY 10024; (212) 362-
9635; **BDCERT:** Psyc 82; **MS:** Georgetown U 76;
RES: Psyc, Columbia-Presbyterian Med Ctr, New
York, NY; **HOSP:** St Luke's Roosevelt Hosp Ctr; **SI:**
Depression; Panic Disorders

♿ ♿ ♿ ♿ 1 Week ♿ **VISA** ♿

Mellman, Lisa (MD)   Psyc
Columbia-Presbyterian Med Ctr
ColumbiaPresbyterian Med Ctr, 161 Ft Washington
Ave; New York, NY 10032; (212) 305-5341;
BDCERT: Psyc 86; **MS:** Case West Res U 81; **RES:**
Columbia-Presbyterian Med Ctr, New York, NY 82-
85; **FEL:** NYS Psychiatric Institute, New York, NY;
FAP: Assoc Clin Prof Columbia P&S; **HOSP:** NYS
Psychiatric Institute; **SI:** *Depression; Relationship
Problems*; **HMO:** Oxford

♿ ♿ ♿ A Few Days

Michels, Robert (MD)   Psyc
NY Hosp-Cornell Med Ctr
418 E 71st St; New York, NY 10021; (212) 746-
6001; **BDCERT:** Psyc 64; **MS:** Northwestern U 58;
RES: Psyc, Columbia-Presbyterian Med Ctr, New
York, NY 59-62; **FAP:** Prof Psyc Cornell U

Millman, Robert B (MD)   Psyc
NY Hosp-Cornell Med Ctr
411 E 69th St; New York, NY 10021; (212) 746-
1248; **BDCERT:** Psyc 78; **MS:** SUNY Hlth Sci Ctr
65; **RES:** IM, Bellevue Hosp Ctr, New York, NY;
Psyc, NY Hosp-Cornell Med Ctr, New York, NY;
FEL: AdP, Rockefeller Univ Hosp, New York, NY

♿ ♿ ♿ ♿ ♿ ♿ ♿ Immediately

Moore, Joanne (MD)   Psyc
Columbia-Presbyterian Med Ctr
161 Ft Washington Ave; New York, NY 10032;
(212) 305-5341; **BDCERT:** Psyc 88; AdP 94; **MS:**
Harvard Med Sch 82; **RES:** Columbia-Presbyterian
Med Ctr, New York, NY 82-87; **FEL:** Psyc,
Columbia-Presbyterian Med Ctr, New York, NY;
FAP: Asst Prof Columbia P&S; **SI:** *Depression;
Anxiety*

♿ ♿ ♿ ♿ ♿ ♿ 1 Week

Guide to symbols and abbreviations can be found on pages 110-113.

353

Muskin, Philip (MD)   Psyc
Columbia-Presbyterian Med Ctr
1700 York Ave; New York, NY 10128; (212) 722-8438; **BDCERT:** Psyc 79; **MS:** NY Med Coll 74; **RES:** NYS Psychiatric Institute, New York, NY 75-78; **FEL:** Columbia-Presbyterian Med Ctr, New York, NY 78-79; Therapeutics, NYS Psychiatric Institute, New York, NY 78-79; **FAP:** Assoc Prof Columbia P&S; **SI:** *Depression; Anxiety;* **HMO:** Oxford
🄲 🄰 🎟 💲   1 Week

Myers, Wayne A (MD)   Psyc
NY Hosp-Cornell Med Ctr
60 Sutton Place South Ste 10N; New York, NY 10022; (212) 838-2325; **BDCERT:** Psyc 59; **MS:** Columbia P&S 56; **RES:** Psyc, NY Hosp-Cornell Med Ctr, New York, NY 57-62; **FAP:** Clin Instr Psyc Cornell U; **SI:** *Marital Counseling; Psychotherapy (Individual)*
🄰 🎟 💲 🄼🄲🅁   A Few Days

Nersessian, Edward (MD)   Psyc
NY Hosp-Cornell Med Ctr
72 E 91st St; New York, NY 10128; (212) 876-1537; **BDCERT:** Psyc 75; **MS:** Belgium 70; **RES:** Hillside Hosp, Glen Oaks, NY 70-72; NY Hosp-Cornell Med Ctr, New York, NY 72-73
LANG: Fr; 🄲 🄰 🎟 💲   Immediately

Nessel, Mark (MD)   Psyc
Gracie Square Hosp
167 E 67th St; New York, NY 10021; (212) 535-5247; **BDCERT:** Psyc 78; **MS:** Wayne State U Sch Med 57; **RES:** Creedmoor State Hosp, New York, NY 58; Hillside Hosp, Glen Oaks, NY 59

Neubauer, Peter B (MD)   Psyc
NY Hosp-Cornell Med Ctr
33 E 70th St; New York, NY 10021; (212) 288-2348; **MS:** Switzerland 38; **RES:** Bellevue Hosp Ctr, New York, NY; **FEL:** Bellevue Hosp Ctr, New York, NY; **FAP:** Clin Prof Psyc NYU Sch Med; **SI:** *Child Psychoanalysis*
LANG: Ger; 🄰 🆂🄰 🄲 🄰 🎟 💲 🄼🄲🅁   A Few Days

Nininger, James (MD)   Psyc
NY Hosp-Cornell Med Ctr
17 E 76th St; New York, NY 10021; (212) 879-8338; **BDCERT:** Psyc 78; GerPsy 91; **MS:** U Cincinnati 74; **RES:** Psyc, Mount Sinai Med Ctr, New York, NY 74-77; **FAP:** Assoc Clin Prof Psyc Cornell U
🄲 🄰 🎟 💲 🄼🄲🅁   1 Week

Nir, Yehuda (MD)   Psyc
NY Hosp-Cornell Med Ctr
903 Park Ave 11C; New York, NY 10021; (212) 744-8615; **BDCERT:** Psyc 79; **MS:** Israel 58; **RES:** Mount Sinai Med Ctr, New York, NY 61; **FEL:** Jewish Mem Hosp, New York, NY 61-63; **FAP:** Assoc Clin Prof Cornell U; **SI:** *Trauma; Holocaust Survivors*
LANG: Heb, Yd, Czc, Rus, Ger; 🄰 🄲 🄰 🎟 💲 🄼🄲🅁   A Few Days ▨

Nunberg, Henry (MD)   Psyc
NY Hosp-Cornell-Westchester
315 W 84th St; New York, NY 10024; (212) 501-7308; **BDCERT:** Psyc 77; **MS:** Albert Einstein Coll Med 62; **RES:** Mt Auburn Hosp, Cambridge, MA 62-63; Psyc, Mass Mental Hlth Ctr, Boston, MA 63-65; **FAP:** Asst Clin Prof Cornell U; **SI:** *Psychological Problems*
LANG: Ger, Fr; 🄰 🄲 🄰 🎟 💲   A Few Days

Nunes, Edward (MD)   Psyc
NYS Psychiatric Institute
722 W 168th St; New York, NY 10032; (212) 543-5000; **BDCERT:** Psyc 93; **MS:** U Conn Sch Med 81; **RES:** NYS Psychiatric Institute, New York, NY 82-95; Columbia-Presbyterian Med Ctr, New York, NY 92-95; **FEL:** NYS Psychiatric Institute, New York, NY 85-88; **HMO:** Oxford
🄲 🄰 🎟 💲 🄼🄲🅁   A Few Days

Oberfield, Richard (MD)　　Psyc
New York University Med Ctr
200 E 33rd St; New York, NY 10016; (212) 684-0148; **BDCERT:** Psyc 79; ChAP 80; **MS:** Mt Sinai Sch Med 74; **RES:** Psyc, Bellevue Hosp Ctr, New York, NY 74-76; **FEL:** AdP, Bellevue Hosp Ctr, New York, NY 76-78; **SI:** *Attention Deficit Disorders; Divorce;* **HMO:** Oxford

🚹 🏧 🄲 🄰 🄰 ▦ 1 Week

Oldham, John (MD)　　Psyc
NYS Psychiatric Institute
NY State Psychiatric Inst, 722 W 168th St; New York, NY 10032; (212) 543-5300; **BDCERT:** Psyc 73; **MS:** Baylor 67; **RES:** NYS Psychiatric Inst, , NY 71; **FAP:** Prof Columbia P&S; **HOSP:** Columbia-Presbyterian Med Ctr

Olds, David (MD)　　Psyc
Columbia-Presbyterian Med Ctr
2211 Broadway 1H; New York, NY 10024; (212) 362-3860; **BDCERT:** Psyc 75; **MS:** Columbia P&S 67; **RES:** NYS Psychiatric Institute, New York, NY; **FAP:** Assoc Clin Prof Columbia P&S; **SI:** *Psychoanalysis; Personality Mood Disorders*

🄲 🄰 🄰 ▦ 1 Week

Opler, Lewis (MD)　　Psyc
Columbia-Presbyterian Med Ctr
161 Fort Washington Ave; New York, NY 10032; (212) 305-5341; **BDCERT:** Psyc 83; **MS:** Albert Einstein Coll Med 76; **RES:** Psyc, Jacobi Med Ctr, Bronx, NY 76-79; **FAP:** Clin Prof Cornell U; **SI:** *Psychopharmacology; Psychotherapy*

🚹 🄲 ⓜ 4+ Weeks

Pareja, N John (MD)　　Psyc　　PCP
Mount Sinai Med Ctr
125 E 87th St; New York, NY 10128; (212) 831-6666; **BDCERT:** Psyc 69; **MS:** Harvard Med Sch 61; **RES:** Psyc, Albert Einstein Med Ctr, Bronx, NY 62-65; NYS Psychiatric Institute, New York, NY 69-73; **FAP:** Lecturer Psyc Mt Sinai Sch Med; **SI:** *Psychotherapy and Analysis; Couples Therapy*

🚹 🄲 ▦ 1 Week

Pawel, Michael (MD)　　Psyc
St Luke's Roosevelt Hosp Ctr
15 W 72nd St LJ; New York, NY 10023; (212) 873-9170; **BDCERT:** Psyc 77; **MS:** Albert Einstein Coll Med 71; **RES:** Montefiore Med Ctr, Bronx, NY 71-74; **FAP:** Asst Prof Columbia P&S; **SI:** *Adolescents; Young Adults*

🚹 🄲 🄰 🄰 ▦ 🅂 1 Week

Perry, Richard (MD)　　Psyc
New York University Med Ctr
55 W 74th St; New York, NY 10023; (212) 595-0116; **BDCERT:** Psyc 76; ChAP 85; **MS:** Belgium 70; **RES:** Bellevue Hosp Ctr, New York, NY 73; **FEL:** ChAP, Bellevue Hosp Ctr, New York, NY 74; **FAP:** Clin Prof Psyc NYU Sch Med; **HOSP:** Bellevue Hosp Ctr; **SI:** *Pervasive Develop Disorder; Behavior Disorders;* **HMO:** Oxford

🄲 🄰 ▦ 🅂 1 Week

Person, Ethel (MD)　　Psyc
Columbia-Presbyterian Med Ctr
135 Central Park West 11 So; New York, NY 10023; (212) 873-2700; **MS:** NYU Sch Med 60; **RES:** Bellevue Hosp Ctr, New York, NY 60-61; NYS Psychiatric Institute, New York, NY 61-63; **FAP:** Prof of Clin Psyc Columbia P&S; **SI:** *Psychoanalysis*

🄰 ▦ 🅂 2-4 Weeks

Peyser, Ellen (MD)　　Psyc
NY Hosp-Cornell Med Ctr
108 E 96th St; New York, NY 10128; (212) 722-5988; **BDCERT:** Psyc 79; **MS:** Albert Einstein Coll Med 74; **RES:** Mount Sinai Med Ctr, New York, NY 74-77; **FEL:** NY Hosp-Cornell Med Ctr, New York, NY 77-78; **FAP:** Asst Clin Prof Psyc NYU Sch Med; **HOSP:** Columbia-Presbyterian Med Ctr; **SI:** *Psychoanalysis;* **HMO:** Blue Cross & Blue Shield

🚹 🄲 ▦ 1 Week

Peyser, Herbert (MD)　　Psyc
Mount Sinai Med Ctr
110 E 87th St 1F; New York, NY 10128; (212) 876-6778; **BDCERT:** Psyc 63; **MS:** Columbia P&S 48; **RES:** Psyc, VA Med Ctr-Bronx, Bronx, NY 50-52; **FEL:** Psyc, Mount Sinai Med Ctr, New York, NY 62-63

Guide to symbols and abbreviations can be found on pages 110-113.

355

Pfeffer, Cynthia (MD)   Psyc
NY Hosp-Cornell Med Ctr
1100 Madison Ave; New York, NY 10128; (212)
717-2334; **BDCERT:** Psyc 75; ChAP 76; **MS:** NYU
Sch Med 68; **RES:** Albert Einstein Med Ctr, Bronx,
NY 69-73; **FEL:** ChAP, Albert Einstein Med Ctr,
Bronx, NY 71-73; **FAP:** Prof Psyc Cornell U; **HOSP:**
New York University Med Ctr; *SI: Depression;
Attention Deficit Disorder*
🛇 🔃 🔂 🎴 💲   A Few Days

Pines, Jeffrey (MD)   Psyc
Columbia-Presbyterian Med Ctr
Columbia Presb Medical Center, 161 Fort
Washington Ave; New York, NY 10032; (212)
305-5341; **BDCERT:** Psyc 82; **MS:** Columbia P&S
73; **RES:** IM, Columbia-Presbyterian Med Ctr, New
York, NY 73-76; Psyc, NYS Psychiatric Institute,
New York, NY 77-80; **FEL:** Rhu, Hosp For Special
Surgery, New York, NY 76-77; Columbia-
Presbyterian Med Ctr, New York, NY 80-81; **FAP:**
Assoc Clin Prof Psyc Columbia P&S
🛇 🔂 🎴   1 Week

Porder, Michael (MD)   Psyc
Mount Sinai Med Ctr
327 Central Park West; New York, NY 10025;
(212) 663-9479; **BDCERT:** Psyc 73; **MS:** Columbia
P&S 58; **RES:** Jacobi Med Ctr, Bronx, NY 59-62;
FAP: Assoc Clin Prof Mt Sinai Sch Med; *SI:
Psychoanalysis*
🔂 💲   2-4 Weeks

Preven, David (MD)   Psyc
Montefiore Med Ctr
52 Riverside Dr; New York, NY 10024; (718) 799-
4907; **BDCERT:** Psyc 69; **MS:** Harvard Med Sch 63;
RES: Jacobi Med Ctr, Bronx, NY 74-76; *SI:
Psychopharmacology Clinical; Forensic;* **HMO:** None
🔃 🔂 🎴 💲   1 Week

Quitkin, Frederic (MD)   Psyc
Columbia-Presbyterian Med Ctr
2 Cornelia St; New York, NY 10014; (212) 989-
8287; **BDCERT:** Psyc 70; **MS:** SUNY Hlth Sci Ctr
62; **RES:** Psyc, Long Island Jewish Med Ctr, New
Hyde Park, NY 96; **FEL:** Univ Hosp SUNY Bklyn,
Brooklyn, NY 70; **FAP:** Prof of Clin Psyc Columbia
P&S; *SI: Bipolar Depression; Anxiety*
🛇 🔃 🔂 🎴 🎴 💲   1 Week

Raskin, Raymond (MD)   Psyc
Harlem Hosp Ctr
200 E 89th St 15G; New York, NY 10128; (212)
534-1844; **BDCERT:** Psyc 57; **MS:** NYU Sch Med
46; **RES:** Ped, Beth Israel Med Ctr, New York, NY
49-50; Psyc, Bellevue Hosp Ctr, New York, NY 53-
54; **FEL:** Ped, Bellevue Hosp Ctr, New York, NY 52-
53; Columbia-Presbyterian Med Ctr, New York, NY
54-59; **FAP:** Asst Clin Prof Columbia P&S; *SI:
Psychotherapy; Psychoanalysis-Sexual Abuse*
🛇 🔂 🎴 🅼   A Few Days

Resnick, Richard (MD)   Psyc
New York University Med Ctr
Center for Psychiatry & Family Therapy, 43 W
94th St; New York, NY 10025; (212) 662-1899;
BDCERT: Psyc 65; **MS:** NY Med Coll 58; **RES:** Psyc,
Hillside Hosp, Glen Oaks, NY 59-61; Psyc,; **FAP:**
Clin Prof NYU Sch Med; **HOSP:** Bellevue Hosp Ctr;
SI: Addiction Medicine; Psychopharmacology; **HMO:**
GHI Empire Blue Cross & Blue Shield VBH Mental
Behavioral Care +
🆘 🔂 🎴 🎴 💲 🅼 🅼   A Few Days ▦

Rice, Emanuel (MD)   Psyc
Mount Sinai Med Ctr
19 E 88th St 11C; New York, NY 10128; (212)
427-3967; **BDCERT:** Psyc 69; **MS:** Howard U 61;
RES: Manhattan State Hosp, New York, NY 62-65;
FEL: Psyc, Mount Sinai Med Ctr, New York, NY;
FAP: Clin Prof Psyc Mt Sinai Sch Med; **HMO:** Aetna
Hlth Plan Blue Cross & Blue Shield Oxford
LANG: Yd; 🛇 🎴 🅼   A Few Days

Richards, Arnold (MD)   Psyc
Mount Sinai Med Ctr
200 E 89th St; New York, NY 10128; (212) 722-
0223; **BDCERT:** Psyc 65; **MS:** SUNY Hlth Sci Ctr
58; **RES:** Menninger Clinic, Topeka, KS; **FAP:** Asst
Prof NYU Sch Med
🔲 🔲 🔲 🔲 🔲 🔲 Immediately

Roose, Steven (MD)   Psyc
Columbia-Presbyterian Med Ctr
1155 Park Ave; New York, NY 10128; (212) 831-
8644; **BDCERT:** Psyc 79; **MS:** Mt Sinai Sch Med 74;
RES: Columbia-Presbyterian Med Ctr, New York,
NY 75-78; **FEL:** Depression, Columbia-Presbyterian
Med Ctr, New York, NY; Psyc, Columbia-
Presbyterian Med Ctr, New York, NY 79-84; **FAP:**
Prof
🔲 2-4 Weeks

Rosen, Arnold M (MD)   Psyc
Gracie Square Hosp
200 E 78th St; New York, NY 10021; (212) 288-
6380; **BDCERT:** Psyc 76; **MS:** U Tex SW, Dallas 68;
RES: Metropolitan Hosp Ctr, New York, NY 69-70;
Metropolitan Hosp Ctr, New York, NY 72-74; **FEL:**
Metropolitan Hosp Ctr, New York, NY 74-75;
HOSP: Lenox Hill Hosp; **SI:** Depression;
Psychopharmacology; **HMO:** Multiplan Empire Blue
Cross PHCS MBC
LANG: Sp; 🔲 🔲 🔲 🔲 🔲 🔲 A Few Days 🔲
VISA 🔲

Rosenbloom, Charles (MD)   Psyc
Gracie Square Hosp
50 E 86th St Apt 2A; New York, NY 10028; (212)
472-8673; **BDCERT:** Psyc 77; **MS:** Italy 64; **RES:** St
Vincents Hosp, New York, NY 65-66; Hillside Hosp,
Glen Oaks, NY 67-68

Rosenfeld, Alvin (MD)   Psyc
St Luke's Roosevelt Hosp Ctr
4 E 89th St 1F; New York, NY 10128; (212) 348-
5900; **BDCERT:** Psyc 76; ChAP 78; **MS:** Harvard
Med Sch 70; **RES:** Psyc, Harvard Med Sch,
Cambridge, MA 71-73; **FEL:** ChAP, Harvard Med
Sch, Cambridge, MA 73-75; Beth Israel Med Ctr,
New York, NY; **SI:** Psychotherapy
🔲 🔲 🔲 🔲 Immediately

Rosenthal, Jesse (MD)   Psyc
Beth Israel Med Ctr
21 E 93rd St; New York, NY 10128; (212) 876-
3080; **BDCERT:** Psyc 78; **MS:** Geo Wash U Sch Med
73; **RES:** Mount Sinai Hosp, Cleveland, OH 76; **SI:**
Depression and Anxiety; Attention Deficit Disorder
🔲 🔲 🔲 🔲 🔲 🔲 1 Week 🔲 **VISA** 🔲

Rosenthal, Richard N (MD) Psyc
Beth Israel Med Ctr
317 E 17th St 9th Flr; New York, NY 10003; (212)
420-2421; **BDCERT:** Psyc 85; AdP 93; **MS:** SUNY
Hlth Sci Ctr 80; **RES:** Mount Sinai Med Ctr, New
York, NY 80-84; **FAP:** Assoc Prof Albert Einstein
Coll Med; **SI:** Addictions; Mood Disorders
🔲 🔲 🔲 🔲 🔲 1 Week

Rosner, Richard (MD)   Psyc
New York University Med Ctr
140 E 83rd St 6A; New York, NY 10028; (212)
988-6014; **BDCERT:** Psyc 74; **MS:** NYU Sch Med
66; **RES:** Psyc, Mount Sinai Med Ctr, New York, NY
67-70; **HOSP:** Bronx Lebanon Hosp Ctr; **SI:**
Adolescent Psychiatry; Forensic Psychiatry
🔲 🔲 🔲 🔲 🔲 A Few Days

Sacks, Michael (MD)   Psyc
NY Hosp-Cornell Med Ctr
525 E 68th St; New York, NY 10021; (212) 746-
3710; **BDCERT:** Psyc 72; **MS:** NYU Sch Med 67;
RES: Psyc, NYS Psychiatric Institute, New York, NY
68-71; **FAP:** Prof Psyc Cornell U; **SI:** Psychotherapy;
Psychoanalysis
🔲 🔲 A Few Days

Guide to symbols and abbreviations can be found on pages 110-113.

357

Sadock, Benjamin (MD)   Psyc
New York University Med Ctr

4 E 89th St 1E; New York, NY 10128; (212) 427-0884; **BDCERT:** Psyc 66; **MS:** NY Med Coll 59; **RES:** Bellevue Hosp Ctr, New York, NY 60-63; **FAP:** Prof Psyc NYU Sch Med; **HOSP:** Lenox Hill Hosp; *SI: Anxiety and Depression; Sexual Dysfunction*

🗓 💲 1 Week

Sadock, Virginia (MD)   Psyc
New York University Med Ctr

4 E 89th St; New York, NY 10128; (212) 427-0885; **BDCERT:** Psyc 75; **MS:** NY Med Coll 70; **RES:** Metropolitan Hosp Ctr, New York, NY 70-73; *SI: Psychotherapy; Sex Therapy*

🔒 🗓 2-4 Weeks

Salkin, Paul (MD)   Psyc
Lenox Hill Hosp

200 East End Ave 6H; New York, NY 10128; (212) 427-3170; **BDCERT:** Psyc 62; **MS:** NYU Sch Med 56; **RES:** Jacobi Med Ctr, Bronx, NY 57-60; **FAP:** Asst Clin Prof Psyc NY Med Coll; **HOSP:** Beth Israel Med Ctr; *SI: Depression; Anxiety*

LANG: Fr, Sp, Ger, Heb, Yd; ♿ 🏥 📞 🔒 🚗 🗓 Mcr WC NfI Immediately

Samberg, Eslee (MD)   Psyc
NY Hosp-Cornell Med Ctr

2211 Broadway 1DS; New York, NY 10024; (212) 874-7725; **BDCERT:** Psyc 83; **MS:** Cornell U 78; **RES:** Psyc, NY Hosp-Cornell Med Ctr, New York, NY 79-82; **FAP:** Asst Clin Prof Cornell U; *SI: Psychoanalysis*

🔒 🗓

Samuels, Steven (MD)   Psyc
Mount Sinai Med Ctr

One Gustave Levy Pl Box 1230; New York, NY 10029; (212) 241-4607; **BDCERT:** Psyc 94; GerPsy 96; **MS:** SUNY Buffalo 89; **RES:** Psyc, St Vincents Hosp & Med Ctr NY, New York, NY 89-93; **FEL:** GerPsy, Hosp of U Penn, Philadelphia, PA 93-95; **FAP:** Asst Prof Psyc Mt Sinai Sch Med; *SI: Alzheimer's Disease; Depression*

♿ 🔒 🚗 🗓 Mcr Mcd 1 Week

Sawyer, David (MD)   Psyc
NY Hosp-Cornell Med Ctr

1 W 64th St 1C; New York, NY 10023; (212) 787-8260; **BDCERT:** Psyc 82; ChAP 84; **MS:** NY Med Coll 77; **RES:** Psyc, NY Hosp-Cornell-Westchester, White Plains, NY 77-80; **FEL:** ChAP, NY Hosp-Cornell-Westchester, White Plains, NY 80-82; **FAP:** Clin Instr Psyc Cornell U; *SI: Psychoanalysis/Psychosomatic Illnesses*

📞 🔒 🗓 Immediately

Scharf, Robert (MD)   Psyc
St Luke's Roosevelt Hosp Ctr

207 E 74th St 1L; New York, NY 10021; (212) 988-4145; **BDCERT:** Psyc 76; **MS:** Albert Einstein Coll Med 60; **RES:** IM, Straight Ward Med, St Louis, MO 60; Psyc, Kings County Hosp Ctr, Brooklyn, NY 61-64; **FEL:** Psychoanalysis, NYS Psychiatric Institute, New York, NY 65-73; **FAP:** Asst Clin Prof Psyc Columbia P&S; *SI: Psychotherapy; Psychopharmacology;* **HMO:** PHCS Oxford Empire Blue Cross CIGNA Prudential +

📞 🔒 🚗 🗓 1 Week

Schein, Jonah (MD)   Psyc
NY Hosp-Cornell Med Ctr

1349 Lexington Ave 1E; New York, NY 10128; (212) 876-2324; **BDCERT:** Psyc 75; **MS:** NYU Sch Med 69; **RES:** Bellevue Hosp Ctr, New York, NY 69-70; NYS Psychiatric Institute, New York, NY 70; **FAP:** Asst Clin Prof Cornell U; *SI: Depression; Anxiety*

📞 🔒 🚗 🗓 💲 A Few Days

Schore, Arthur (MD & PhD) Psyc
NY Hosp-Cornell Med Ctr

905 5th Ave; New York, NY 10021; (212) 535-6070; **BDCERT:** Psyc 79; **MS:** U Hlth Sci/Chicago Med Sch 65; **RES:** Columbia-Presbyterian Med Ctr, New York, NY 66-69; **FEL:** NYS Psychiatric Institute, New York, NY 75; **FAP:** Asst Clin Prof Psyc Cornell U

🏥 📞 🔒 🗓 WC A Few Days

Schulman, David (MD)　　Psyc
Mount Sinai Med Ctr

152 E 94th St; New York, NY 10128; (212) 876-5228; **BDCERT:** Psyc 65; **MS:** U Hlth Sci/Chicago Med Sch 53; **RES:** Kings County Hosp Ctr, Brooklyn, NY 52-54; Psyc, Mount Sinai Med Ctr, New York, NY; **FAP:** Assoc Prof Mt Sinai Sch Med; **HOSP:** NYU Downtown Hosp; **SI:** *Neuroses Anxiety; Depression;* **HMO:** Oxford Aetna Hlth Plan Blue Cross

◖ ▣ ▥ ▦ ▤ ᴹᶜ ᵂᶜ　A Few Days

Segura-Bustamante, Alina (MD) Psyc
Long Island Coll Hosp

476 Broadway 6M; New York, NY 10013; (212) 841-0994; **BDCERT:** Psyc 89; **MS:** Spain 79; **RES:** Psyc, Univ Hosp SUNY Bklyn, Brooklyn, NY 80-83; **FEL:** Psyc, Univ Hosp SUNY Bklyn, Brooklyn, NY 83; **FAP:** Clin Instr Psyc SUNY Downstate; **SI:** *Psychological Aspects of Chronic Illness; Adolescent Psychiatry;* **HMO:** Empire Blue Cross & Shield United Healthcare PHS Oxford

LANG: Sp; ◖ ▣ ▦ ▤　1 Week

Shapiro, Peter (MD)　　Psyc
Columbia-Presbyterian Med Ctr

239 Central Park West; New York, NY 10024; (212) 874-6030; **BDCERT:** Psyc 85; **MS:** Columbia P&S 80; **RES:** Psyc, NYS Psychiatric Institute, New York, NY 81-84; **FEL:** Columbia-Presbyterian Med Ctr, New York, NY 84-86; **FAP:** Assoc Clin Prof Psyc Columbia P&S

▥ ▣ ▤　4+ Weeks

Shapiro, Theodore (MD)　　Psyc
NY Hosp-Cornell Med Ctr

525 E 68trh St Box 147; New York, NY 10021; (212) 821-0724; **BDCERT:** Psyc 65; **MS:** Cornell U 57; **RES:** Bellevue Hosp Ctr, New York, NY 58-61; **FEL:** ChAP, Bellevue Hosp Ctr, New York, NY 61-63; **HOSP:** Columbia-Presbyterian Med Ctr

▥ ◖　A Few Days

Shaw, Ronda R (MD)　　Psyc
NY Hosp-Cornell Med Ctr

35 E 85th St Ste 2; New York, NY 10028; (212) 772-0321; **BDCERT:** Psyc 77; **MS:** Wayne State U Sch Med 66; **RES:** Psyc, Jacobi Med Ctr, Bronx, NY 66-70; **FAP:** Lecturer Mt Sinai Sch Med; **SI:** *Psychoanalysis; Dynamic Psychotherapy;* **HMO:** None

▣ ▥ ▦ ▤　A Few Days

Shinbach, Kent (MD)　　Psyc
Gracie Square Hosp

435 E 79th St 1C; New York, NY 10021; (212) 744-7100; **BDCERT:** Psyc 70; **MS:** Jefferson Med Coll 63; **RES:** NY Med Coll, New York, NY 68; **HOSP:** Beth Israel Med Ctr; **SI:** *Psychopharmacology; Geriatric Psychiatry*

LANG: Fr, Itl; ▣ ▥ ▦ ᴹᶜ ᵂᶜ ᴺᶠᴵ　1 Week

Siever, Larry J (MD)　　Psyc
Mount Sinai Med Ctr

1 Gustave Levy Pl; New York, NY 10021; (212) 517-1021; **BDCERT:** Psyc 80; **MS:** Stanford U 75; **RES:** McLean Hosp, Belmont, MA 75-78; **FEL:** Nat Inst Mental Health, Bethesda, MD 78-82; **FAP:** Prof Mt Sinai Sch Med; **HOSP:** VA Med Ctr-Bronx; **SI:** *Neuropsychopharmacology; Personality Disorders*

LANG: Fr; ▨ ◖ ▣ ▥ ▦ ▤　1 Week

Silber, Austin (MD)　　Psyc
New York University Med Ctr

1199 Park Ave 1C; New York, NY 10128; (212) 369-7851; **BDCERT:** Psyc 60; **MS:** SUNY Hlth Sci Ctr 51; **RES:** Kings County Hosp Ctr, Brooklyn, NY 52-55; **FEL:** Psychoanalysis, Univ Hosp SUNY Bklyn, Brooklyn, NY 53-59; **FAP:** Clin Prof Psyc NYU Sch Med; **HMO:** None

▣ ▦

Silver, Jonathan M (MD)　　Psyc
Columbia-Presbyterian Med Ctr

1430 2nd Ave Ste 103; New York, NY 10021; (212) 434-3405; **BDCERT:** Psyc 84; **MS:** Albert Einstein Coll Med 79; **RES:** NYS Psychiatric Institute, New York, NY 80-83; **FEL:** NY Psyc Inst/NIMH/Creedmoor, New York, NY 83-85; **FAP:** Clin Prof Psyc NYU Sch Med; **SI:** *Neuropsychiatry; Psychopharmacology*

▨ ▣ ▦ ▤　2-4 Weeks

Guide to symbols and abbreviations can be found on pages 110-113.

359

Singer, Paul (MD)   Psyc
Westchester Med Ctr

1045 Park Ave; New York, NY 10028; (212) 348-0635; **BDCERT:** Psyc 76; **MS:** Switzerland 59; **RES:** Brooklyn State Hosp, Brooklyn, NY 60-63; **FEL:** NYS Psychiatric Institute, New York, NY 66-72; **FAP:** Prof NY Med Coll; **HOSP:** Metropolitan Hosp Ctr; **SI:** *Depression; Anxiety*

♿ 🖻 📷 🎞 1 Week

Skeist, Loren (MD)   Psyc
Lenox Hill Hosp

19 E 88th St 1E; New York, NY 10128; (212) 722-2746; **BDCERT:** Psyc 77; **MS:** Mt Sinai Sch Med 72; **RES:** Psyc, Mount Sinai Med Ctr, New York, NY 73-76; **HMO:** None

♿ 🎞 Immediately

Snyder, Stephen (MD)   Psyc
Mount Sinai Med Ctr

Mt Sinai Medical Center Box 1228, 1 Gustave Levy Pl; New York, NY 10029; (212) 241-2155; **BDCERT:** Psyc 89; **MS:** UC San Francisco 83; **RES:** Mt Zion Hosp, San Francisco, CA 83-84; NY Hosp-Cornell Med Ctr, New York, NY 84-87; **FEL:** Mount Sinai Med Ctr, New York, NY 87-89; **FAP:** Asst Clin Prof Psyc Mt Sinai Sch Med; **SI:** *Sexual Dysfunction; Psychotherapy*; **HMO:** Aetna Hlth Plan Oxford

♿ 🖻 📷 🎞 Ⓢ &#x1F3 A; 1 Week

Spitz, Henry (MD)   Psyc
Columbia-Presbyterian Med Ctr

101 Central Park West Ste 1C; New York, NY 10023; (212) 873-1415; **BDCERT:** Psyc 73; **MS:** NYU Sch Med 65; **RES:** Psyc, NY Med Coll, New York, NY 65-69; **FEL:** Group Psychotherapy, NY Med Coll, New York, NY 69-70; **FAP:** Clin Prof Psyc Columbia P&S; **SI:** *Family/Marriage Counseling; Addiction-Substance Abuse*; **HMO:** None

♿ 🌙 🖻 📷 🎞 Ⓢ A Few Days

Stein, Stefan (MD)   Psyc
NY Hosp-Cornell Med Ctr

New York Hospital, 525 E 68th St Ste 1501; New York, NY 10021; (212) 746-3845; **BDCERT:** Psyc 70; **MS:** NYU Sch Med 63; **RES:** Boston Med Ctr, Boston, MA 63-64; Albert Einstein Med Ctr, Bronx, NY 65-68; **FEL:** Mass Gen Hosp, Boston, MA 64-65; NYS Psychiatric Institute, New York, NY 68-74; **FAP:** Clin Prof Psyc Cornell U; **SI:** *General Psychiatry; Individual and Couples*

♿ 🖻 📷 🎞 1 Week

Steinglass, Peter (MD)   Psyc
Beth Israel Med Ctr

Ackerman Institute Family Thrpy, 149 E 78th St; New York, NY 10021; (212) 879-4900; **BDCERT:** Psyc 71; **MS:** Harvard Med Sch 65; **RES:** Psyc, Jacobi Med Ctr, Bronx, NY 66-69; **FAP:** Clin Prof Cornell U; **SI:** *Family Therapy; Alcoholism/Substance Abuse*

♿ 🌙 🖻 📷 🎞 Ἲ 1 Week

Stone, Michael (MD)   Psyc
Columbia-Presbyterian Med Ctr

225 Central Park West; New York, NY 10024; (212) 758-2000; **BDCERT:** Psyc 71; **MS:** Cornell U 58; **RES:** Psyc, NYS Psychiatric Institute, New York, NY 63-66; **FAP:** Prof Psyc Columbia P&S; **SI:** *Personality Disorders*

LANG: Fr, Ger, Itl; ♿ Ἲ 🌙 🎞 A Few Days

Strain, James (MD)   Psyc
Mount Sinai Med Ctr

Mt Sinai Sch of Med, Box1228 Gustave Levy Pl Bx 1228; New York, NY 10029; (212) 241-9560; **BDCERT:** Psyc 69; **MS:** Case West Res U 62; **RES:** Psyc, U Chicago Hosp, Chicago, IL 63-66; **FEL:** Psyc, U Chicago Hosp, Chicago, IL 66-67; **FAP:** Prof/Director Psyc Mt Sinai Sch Med; **SI:** *Psychiatric Care of Medically Ill; Psychoanalysis/Psychotherapy*; **HMO:** None

♿ 🌙 🖻 📷 🎞 Ἲ 2-4 Weeks

Sulkowicz, Kerry (MD)   Psyc
New York University Med Ctr

151 E 80th St Ste 1B; New York, NY 10028; (212) 737-1950; **BDCERT:** Psyc 91; **MS:** U Tex Med Br, Galveston 85; **RES:** Psyc, New York University Med Ctr, New York, NY 85-89; **FEL:** NYS Psychiatric Institute, New York, NY 86-92; **FAP:** Asst Clin Prof NYU Sch Med; **SI:** *Psychoanalysis; Personality Disorders*

♿ 🖻 📷 🎞 1 Week

Sullivan, Ann Marie (MD)　Psyc
Elmhurst Hosp Ctr
Box 1228, 1160 5th Ave; New York, NY 10029;
(212) 686-0430; **BDCERT:** Psyc 78; **MS:** NYU Sch
Med 74; **RES:** Psyc, Bellevue Hosp Ctr, New York,
NY 74-78; **HOSP:** Mount Sinai Med Ctr; **SI:** *Brief
Psychotherapy*

 ♿ 🔳 📷 📧 🏥 💲　2-4 Weeks

Sussman, Norman (MD)　Psyc
New York University Med Ctr
20 E 68th Ste 204; New York, NY 10021; (212)
737-7946; **BDCERT:** Psyc 80; **MS:** NY Med Coll 75;
RES: Psyc, Metropolitan Hosp Ctr, New York, NY
75-77; **FAP:** Clin Prof NYU Sch Med; **SI:** *Anxiety
Disorders; Mood Disorders*

LANG: Sp; ♿ 🔳 📷 🏥 💲 Mcr　2-4 Weeks

Swiller, Hillel (MD)　Psyc
Mount Sinai Med Ctr
108 E 96th St Ste 9F; New York, NY 10128; (212)
534-5588; **BDCERT:** Psyc 72; **MS:** Cornell U 65;
RES: Psyc, Albert Einstein Med Ctr, Bronx, NY 66-
69; **FAP:** Assoc Prof Mt Sinai Sch Med; **SI:**
Psychotherapy; Group Psychotherapy; **HMO:** None

 ♿ 📷 🏥　2-4 Weeks

Taintor, Zebulon C (MD)　Psyc
New York University Med Ctr
19 E 93rd St; New York, NY 10128; (212) 426-
7645; **BDCERT:** Psyc 70; **MS:** Cornell U 62; **RES:**
Psyc, NY Hosp-Cornell Med Ctr, New York, NY 63-
66; **FAP:** Prof Psyc NYU Sch Med; **HOSP:** Manh
Psych Ctr-Ward's Is; **SI:** *Addiction Psychiatry;
Psychiatric Rehabilitation*

LANG: Ger, Fr, Mly; ♿ 🔳 📷 📧 🏥 WC NFI
A Few Days

Tancredi, Laurence R (MD)　Psyc
New York University Med Ctr
129B E 71st St; New York, NY 10021; (212) 288-
5197; **BDCERT:** Psyc 79; **MS:** Univ Penn 66; **RES:**
NYS Psychiatric Institute, New York, NY 74-75;
Psyc, Yale-New Haven Hosp, New Haven, CT 75-
77; **FAP:** Clin Prof Psyc NYU Sch Med; **SI:** *Forensic
Psychiatry; Depression*

 ♿ 🔳 📷 📧 🏥　A Few Days

Tardiff, Kenneth (MD)　Psyc
NY Hosp-Cornell Med Ctr
Payne Whitney Clinic, NY Hosp, Dept of Psychiatry,
525 E 68th St PsyBox140; New York, NY 10021;
(212) 821-0765; **BDCERT:** Psyc 76; **MS:** Tulane U
69; **RES:** Mass Gen Hosp, Boston, MA 73; **FAP:** Clin
Prof Psyc Cornell U; **SI:** *Psychotherapy; Depression,
Anxiety*

 ♿ 📷 📧 🏥 Mcr　A Few Days

Taylor, Noel (MD)　Psyc
Beth Israel Med Ctr
255 E 49th St 12D; New York, NY 10017; (212)
420-4233; **BDCERT:** Psyc 85; **MS:** Johns Hopkins U
80; **RES:** Johns Hopkins Hosp, Baltimore, MD 80-84

 ♿ 📷 📧 🏥 💲 Mcr　A Few Days

Teusink, J Paul (MD)　Psyc
Beth Israel Med Ctr
1st Ave & 16th St; New York, NY 10003; (212)
420-4680; **BDCERT:** Psyc 76; **MS:** U Mich Med Sch
69; **RES:** Allentown Gen Hosp, Allentown, PA 69-
70; Menninger Clinic, Topeka, KS 70-73; **SI:**
Geriatric Psychiatry; Depression; **HMO:** Blue Choice

 ♿ 📷 📧 🏥 Mcr　1 Week

Thomashow, Peter (MD)　Psyc
Hosp For Joint Diseases
301 E 17th St; New York, NY 10003; (212) 598-
6000; **BDCERT:** Psyc 93; **MS:** NYU Sch Med 82;
RES: New York University Med Ctr, New York, NY
82-83; Psyc, New York University Med Ctr, New
York, NY 83-86; **FAP:** Asst Clin Prof NYU Sch Med;
HOSP: New York University Med Ctr; **SI:** *Chronic
Illnesses/Chronic Pain; Stress Management*; **HMO:**
Oxford

LANG: Sp; ♿ 📷 🏥 💲 Mcr WC　2-4 Weeks

Tolchin, Joan G (MD)　Psyc
NY Hosp-Cornell Med Ctr
35 E 84th St; New York, NY 10028; (212) 744-
1446; **BDCERT:** Psyc 79; **ChAP** 82; **MS:** NYU Sch
Med 72; **RES:** Psyc, Jacobi Med Ctr, Bronx, NY 72-
75; **FEL:** ChAP, NY Hosp-Cornell Med Ctr, New
York, NY 75-77; **FAP:** Asst Clin Prof Cornell U

 ♿ 🔳 📷 🏥 💲　A Few Days

Guide to symbols and abbreviations can be found on pages 110-113.

361

Viederman, Milton (MD)   Psyc
NY Hosp-Cornell Med Ctr

525 E 68th St; New York, NY 10021; (212) 746-3919; **BDCERT:** Psyc 66; **MS:** Harvard Med Sch 55; **RES:** Psyc, NYS Psychiatric Institute, New York, NY 56-57; Psyc, NYS Psychiatric Institute, New York, NY 60-62; **FAP:** Clin Prof Psyc Cornell U; *SI: Psychoanalysis; Psychosomatic Medicine*

LANG: Fr; 🄲 🗗 👪 🏧 📠   2-4 Weeks

Wachtel, Alan (MD)   Psyc
New York University Med Ctr

Family Health Associates, 201 E 87th St 16J; New York, NY 10128; (212) 348-0175; **BDCERT:** Psyc 72; **MS:** Mt Sinai Sch Med 72; **RES:** Mount Sinai Med Ctr, New York, NY 72-76; **FEL:** NY Hosp-Cornell Med Ctr, New York, NY; **HMO:** None

🦽 🗗 👪 🏧 💲 📠   1 Week ▦ **VISA** 💳

Wager, Steven (MD)   Psyc
St Luke's Roosevelt Hosp Ctr

145 W 86th St; New York, NY 10024; (212) 769-9620; **BDCERT:** Psyc 86; **MS:** Case West Res U 80; **RES:** U Hosp of Cleveland, Cleveland, OH 80-81; Psyc, Columbia-Presbyterian Med Ctr, New York, NY 81-84; **FEL:** Psyc, Columbia-Presbyterian Med Ctr, New York, NY 84-86; **FAP:** Assoc Clin Prof Psyc Columbia P&S; *SI: Psychopharmacology*

🦽 🄲 🗗 👪 🏧 💲   2-4 Weeks

Wallack, Joel (MD)   Psyc
Cabrini Med Ctr

227 E 19th St; New York, NY 10003; (212) 995-6762; **BDCERT:** Psyc 79; **MS:** UMDNJ-NJ Med Sch, Newark 74; **RES:** Med, St Vincents Hosp & Med Ctr NY, New York, NY 74-75; Psyc, St Luke's Roosevelt Hosp Ctr, New York, NY 75-78; **FEL:** Psyc, Montefiore Med Ctr, Bronx, NY 78-79; Psyc, Mount Sinai Med Ctr, New York, NY 79-80; **FAP:** Assoc Prof Psyc NYU Sch Med; **HOSP:** Beth Israel Med Ctr; *SI: Psychopharmacology; Psych Care of Medically Ill;* **HMO:** Oxford Blue Cross & Blue Shield Empire

🦽 🄲 🗗 👪 🏧 💲 📠   A Few Days

Walsh, B Timothy (MD)   Psyc
NYS Psychiatric Institute

NYSPT- Unit 98, 722 W 168th St Ste 922; New York, NY 10032; (212) 543-5752; **BDCERT:** Psyc 78; **MS:** Harvard Med Sch 72; **RES:** IM, Dartmouth Hitchcock Med Ctr, Lebanon, NH 73; Psyc, Albert Einstein Med Ctr, Bronx, NY 77; **FAP:** Prof Columbia P&S; **HOSP:** Columbia-Presbyterian Med Ctr; *SI: Anorexia Nervosa; Bulimia;* **HMO:** None

🦽 🗗 👪 💲

Weill, Terry (MD)   Psyc
Mount Sinai Med Ctr

350 Central Park West; New York, NY 10023; (212) 316-5818; **BDCERT:** Psyc 85; GerPsy 92; **MS:** Hahnemann U 80; **RES:** Psyc, Mount Sinai Med Ctr, New York, NY 81-84; **FAP:** Asst Prof Mt Sinai Sch Med; **HOSP:** Beth Israel Med Ctr; *SI: Bipolar Illness; People with Med Illness;* **HMO:** Aetna Hlth Plan

🦽 🄲 🗗 👪 🏧 💲   1 Week

Weissberg, Josef (MD)   Psyc
Columbia-Presbyterian Med Ctr

103 E 86th St 2A; New York, NY 10028; (212) 722-5521; **BDCERT:** Psyc 61; **MS:** Albany Med Coll 52; **RES:** St Luke's Roosevelt Hosp Ctr, New York, NY 52-54; NYS Psychiatric Institute, New York, NY 56-59; **FAP:** Assoc Prof Columbia P&S; **HOSP:** St Luke's Roosevelt Hosp Ctr; *SI: Brief Focal Psychotherapy; Psychopharmacology;* **HMO:** GHI Blue Choice Anthem Health Empire Columbia-Cornell Care +

🦽 🗗 👪 🏧 💲 📠 WC NFl   A Few Days

Welsh, Howard (MD)   Psyc
New York University Med Ctr

27 W 86th St C; New York, NY 10024; (212) 362-5846; **BDCERT:** Psyc 76; **MS:** Albert Einstein Coll Med 71; **RES:** Kings County Hosp Ctr, Brooklyn, NY 71-74; **FAP:** Clin Prof NYU Sch Med; **HOSP:** St Luke's Roosevelt Hosp Ctr

🄲 🗗 👪 🏧   A Few Days

Wilner, Philip (MD)   Psyc
NY Hosp-Cornell Med Ctr
Payne Whitney Clinic, 525 E 68th St; New York, NY 10021; (212) 821-0725; **BDCERT:** Psyc 89; **MS:** Columbia P&S 83; **RES:** Psyc, NY Hosp-Cornell Med Ctr, New York, NY 83-87; Psyc, NY Hosp-Cornell Med Ctr, New York, NY 87-88; **FEL:** Psychopharmacology, NY Hosp-Cornell Med Ctr, New York, NY; **FAP:** Assoc Prof Cornell U; **HMO:** Blue Choice Blue Cross & Blue Shield

⬡ 🄲 🅂 ᴹᶜʳ 2-4 Weeks

Winters, Richard (MD)   Psyc
Metropolitan Hosp Ctr
35 E 85th St; New York, NY 10028; (212) 744-1346; **BDCERT:** Psyc 77; **MS:** NY Med Coll 72; **RES:** Metropolitan Hosp Ctr, New York, NY 72-75; **FAP:** Asst Prof NY Med Coll; **HOSP:** Hackensack Univ Med Ctr; **SI:** *Psychopharmacology; Psychotherapy*; **HMO:** Oxford Medichoice

🄲 🗗 🔧 🎚 🅂 2-4 Weeks

Zimberg, Sheldon (MD)   Psyc
St Luke's Roosevelt Hosp Ctr
245 A E 61st St; New York, NY 10021; (212) 988-5139; **BDCERT:** Psyc 94; **MS:** SUNY Hlth Sci Ctr 61; **RES:** Columbia-Presbyterian Med Ctr, New York, NY 62-63; NYS Psychiatric Institute, New York, NY 63-65; **FEL:** Columbia-Presbyterian Med Ctr, New York, NY 63-66; NYS Psychiatric Institute, New York, NY; **FAP:** Clin Prof Columbia P&S; **HOSP:** Beth Israel Med Ctr

⬡ 🄲 🗗 🔧 🎚 🅂 ᴹᶜʳ ᴹᵒᵈ Immediately

Zimmerman, Zeva (MD)   Psyc
New York University Med Ctr
139 W 13th St 6; New York, NY 10011; (212) 647-0200; **BDCERT:** Psyc 75; **MS:** Tufts U 62; **RES:** Bellevue Hosp Ctr, New York, NY 63-66; **FEL:** Bontine Institute Radcliffe, Boston, MA; **HOSP:** Bellevue Hosp Ctr; **SI:** *Psychotherapy - Adult*

⬡ 🄲 🗗 🔧 🎚 🅂 ᴹᶜʳ ᴺᶠᴵ Immediately

PULMONARY DISEASE

Adams, Francis (MD)   Pul
New York University Med Ctr
650 1st Ave FL 7; New York, NY 10016; (212) 447-0088; **BDCERT:** IM 74; Pul 76; **MS:** Cornell U 71; **RES:** Georgetown U Hosp, Washington, DC 71-73; **FEL:** Pul, Bellevue Hosp Ctr, New York, NY 73-75; **FAP:** Asst Clin Prof Med NYU Sch Med; **SI:** *Chronic Obstructive Lung Disease; Asthma*; **HMO:** Oxford Chubb

⬡ 🄲 🗗 🔧 🎚 🅂 ᴹᶜʳ A Few Days *VISA* ⬤

Adler, Jack (MD)   Pul
Mount Sinai Med Ctr
AHB Pulmonary Assoc, 19 E 80th St; New York, NY 10021; (212) 535-3622; **BDCERT:** IM 70; Pul 71; **MS:** U Chicago-Pritzker Sch Med 62; **RES:** Philadelphia Gen Hosp, Philadelphia, PA 63; Michael Reese Hosp Med Ctr, Chicago, IL 65-67; **FEL:** Pul, Bronx Muncipal Hosp Ctr, Bronx, NY; **FAP:** Assoc Prof Mt Sinai Sch Med; **HOSP:** Beth Israel Med Ctr; **SI:** *Asthma; Breathing Problems*; **HMO:** Oxford Aetna Hlth Plan PHS PHCS Blue Choice +

⬡ 🗗 🔧 🎚 🅂 ᴹᶜʳ ᴺᶠᴵ Immediately

Baskin, Martin (MD)   Pul
St Luke's Roosevelt Hosp Ctr
Manhattan West Medical PC, 185 W End Ave M; New York, NY 10023; (212) 595-7701; **BDCERT:** IM 95; Pul 85; **MS:** Mt Sinai Sch Med 81; **RES:** IM, Beth Israel Med Ctr, New York, NY 81-84; **FEL:** Pul, St Luke's Roosevelt Hosp Ctr, New York, NY 86-88; CCM, St Luke's Roosevelt Hosp Ctr, New York, NY 88-89; **FAP:** Asst Clin Prof Columbia P&S; **SI:** *Asthma; Respiratory Infections*; **HMO:** Aetna Hlth Plan Choicecare Prucare Guardian Magnacare +

LANG: Sp; ⬡ 🄲 🗗 🔧 🎚 🅂 ᴹᶜʳ Immediately

Blair, Lester (MD)　　　Pul
New York University Med Ctr

NY Downtown Med Assoc Inc, 170 William St;
New York, NY 10038; (212) 238-0101; **BDCERT:**
IM 77; Pul 80; **MS:** Columbia P&S 74; **RES:** IM,
Columbia-Presbyterian Med Ctr, New York, NY 74-
77; **FEL:** Pul, Bellevue Hosp Ctr, New York, NY 77-
79; **FAP:** Asst Clin Prof NYU Sch Med; **SI:** *Asthma;*
Sarcoidosis; **HMO:** Aetna Hlth Plan HealthNet Blue
Choice Metlife Oxford +

🔽 🗿 🔳 🏢 💲 Mcr Mod 1 Week 💳 **VISA** 💳 💳

Braun, Norma (MD)　　　Pul　　**PCP**
St Luke's Roosevelt Hosp Ctr

1090 Amsterdam Ave 5F; New York, NY 10025;
(212) 523-3655; **BDCERT:** IM 73; Pul 74; **MS:**
Columbia P&S 63; **RES:** Bellevue Hosp Ctr, New
York, NY 63-65; **FEL:** St Luke's Roosevelt Hosp Ctr,
New York, NY 67-69; **FAP:** Columbia P&S; **SI:**
Breathing Disorders; Neuromuscular Disorders; **HMO:**
Aetna Hlth Plan Blue Cross & Blue Shield PHS
Oxford Prucare +

🔽 🔳 🗿 🔳 🏢 💲 Mcr 2-4 Weeks

Bregman, Zachary (MD)　　　Pul　　**PCP**
Beth Israel Med Ctr

247 3rd Ave Suite 401; New York, NY 10010;
(212) 505-6663; **BDCERT:** IM 86; Pul 94; **MS:**
Univ Penn 80; **RES:** Beth Israel Med Ctr, New York,
NY 82-84; **FEL:** New York University Med Ctr, New
York, NY 81-82; **FAP:** Asst Clin Prof Ped Albert
Einstein Coll Med; **HOSP:** Cabrini Med Ctr; **SI:** *Lung*
Disease; HIV Medicine; **HMO:** United Healthcare
Blue Choice Oxford PHS Aetna Hlth Plan +

🔽 🔳 🏢 💲 Mcr A Few Days **VISA** 💳

Cooke, Joseph T (MD)　　　Pul
NY Hosp-Cornell Med Ctr

520 E 70th St 505; New York, NY 10021; (212)
746-2250; **BDCERT:** Pul 91; CCM 92; **MS:** SUNY
Downstate 85; **RES:** NY Hosp-Cornell Med Ctr, New
York, NY 85-88; **FEL:** NY Hosp-Cornell Med Ctr,
New York, NY 88-91; **FAP:** Assoc Prof Cornell U;
SI: *Asthma; Lung Cancer;* **HMO:** US Hlthcre Oxford
PHS Blue Choice

🔽 🗿 🏢 💲 Mcr Mod 2-4 Weeks

Eden, Edward (MD)　　　Pul
Columbia-Presbyterian Med Ctr

University Med Practice Assoc, 425 W 59th St Ste
8C; New York, NY 10019; (212) 523-7090;
BDCERT: IM 80; Pul 82; **MS:** England 75; **RES:**
Med, Wayne Cnty Gen Hosp, Detroit, MI 77-78;
Med, Univ Hosp SUNY Stony Brook, Stony Brook,
NY 78-80; **FEL:** Pul, Mount Sinai Med Ctr, New
York, NY 80-82; Pul, Columbia-Presbyterian Med
Ctr, New York, NY 82-85; **FAP:** Assoc Prof of Clin
Med Columbia P&S; **HOSP:** St Luke's Roosevelt
Hosp Ctr; **SI:** *Emphysema; Asthma;* **HMO:** CIGNA
Oxford Prucare Blue Choice Multiplan +

LANG: Sp; 🔽 🔳 🗿 🔳 🏢 Mcr A Few Days 💳
VISA 💳

Gagliardi, Anthony (MD)　　　Pul
St Vincents Hosp & Med Ctr NY

32 W 18th St; New York, NY 10011; (212) 647-
6420; **BDCERT:** IM 84; Pul 84; **MS:** UMDNJ-NJ Med
Sch, Newark 81; **RES:** St Vincents Hosp & Med Ctr
NY, New York, NY 81-84; **FEL:** Pul, Mem Sloan
Kettering Cancer Ctr, New York, NY; **HOSP:** St
Clare's Hosp & Health Ctr; **SI:** *Asthma; Emphysema;*
HMO: US Hlthcre Oxford PHCS PHS Blue Cross &
Blue Shield +

🔽 🗿 🔳 🏢 💲 Mcr 1 Week

Garay, Stuart (MD)　　　Pul
New York University Med Ctr

New York Pulmonary Associates, 436 3rd Ave Fl 2;
New York, NY 10016; (212) 685-6001; **BDCERT:**
Pul 80; IM 77; **MS:** Harvard Med Sch 74; **RES:**
Mount Sinai Med Ctr, New York, NY 74-77; **FEL:**
Pul, Bellevue Hosp Ctr, New York, NY 77-79; **SI:**
Asthma; **HMO:** Aetna Hlth Plan Oxford CIGNA
Aetna-US Healthcare Prudential +

🔽 🗿 🔳 🏢 💲 Mcr A Few Days 💳 **VISA** 💳

Gribetz, Allen (MD)　　　Pul
Mount Sinai Med Ctr

927 Park Ave; New York, NY 10028; (212) 517-
8680; **BDCERT:** Pul 78; **MS:** NYU Sch Med 71; **RES:**
Mount Sinai Med Ctr, New York, NY 71-74; **FEL:**
Pul, Mount Sinai Med Ctr, New York, NY 76-78;
FAP: Asst Clin Prof Med Mt Sinai Sch Med; **SI:**
Sarcoidosis; Asthma; **HMO:** Oxford Blue Choice
Aetna Hlth Plan CIGNA Empire +

LANG: Sp, Heb; 🔽 🗿 🔳 🏢 💲 Mcr Mod A Few Days

Kamelhar, David (MD)   Pul   `PCP`
New York University Med Ctr
436 3rd Ave; New York, NY 10016; (212) 685-6006; **BDCERT:** IM 77; Pul 80; **MS:** NYU Sch Med 74; **RES:** NY City VA Hospital, New York, NY 75-78; **FEL:** Pul, New York University Med Ctr, New York, NY 78-80; **HOSP:** Hosp For Joint Diseases; **HMO:** Oxford Chubb Aetna Hlth Plan Blue Cross & Blue Choice CIGNA +

🔊 📷 🚗 🏥 Mcr WC Immediately ▨ *VISA* 💳

Klapholz, Ari (MD)   Pul
Cabrini Med Ctr
Cabrini Med Ctr, 227 E 19th St Rm 502D; New York, NY 10003; (212) 995-6658; **BDCERT:** IM 87; Pul 90; **MS:** NY Med Coll 84; **RES:** IM, Beth Israel Med Ctr, New York, NY 84-87; **FEL:** Pul, Beth Israel Med Ctr, New York, NY 87-89; CCM, Mount Sinai Med Ctr, New York, NY 89-90; **FAP:** Asst Prof Med Mt Sinai Sch Med; **HOSP:** Beth Israel Med Ctr; *SI: Asthma; Emphysema;* **HMO:** Blue Cross & Blue Shield Oxford GHI Aetna-US Healthcare HIP Network +

LANG: Sp, Rus, Heb; 🔊 📞 📷 🚗 🏥 $ Mcr Mod A Few Days

Kolodny, Erwin (MD)   Pul   `PCP`
New York University Med Ctr
650 1st Ave; New York, NY 10016; (212) 213-0090; **BDCERT:** IM 77; Pul 78; **MS:** NYU Sch Med 73; **RES:** IM, Bellevue Hosp Ctr, New York, NY 73-76; **FEL:** Pul, New York University Med Ctr, New York, NY 76-78; **FAP:** Clin Instr NYU Sch Med; *SI: Asthma; Emphysema*

🔊 📷 🏥 A Few Days

Kutnick, Robert (MD)   Pul   `PCP`
Lenox Hill Hosp
14 E 90th St 1D; New York, NY 10128; (212) 427-4700; **BDCERT:** IM 77; Pul 80; **MS:** Albert Einstein Coll Med 74; **RES:** Med, Montefiore, Bronx, NY 75-77; **FEL:** Pul, Montefiore, Bronx, NY 77-79

Libby, Daniel (MD)   Pul
NY Hosp-Cornell Med Ctr
407 E 70th St FL5; New York, NY 10021; (212) 628-6611; **BDCERT:** IM 77; Pul 80; **MS:** Baylor 74; **RES:** NY Hosp-Cornell Med Ctr, New York, NY 74-77; **FEL:** Pul, NY Hosp-Cornell Med Ctr, New York, NY 77-79
VISA

Lowy, Joseph (MD)   Pul
New York University Med Ctr
436 3rd Ave; New York, NY 10016; (212) 685-6002; **BDCERT:** IM 83; Pul 86; **MS:** U Rochester 80; **RES:** Bellevue Hosp Ctr, New York, NY 80-83; **FEL:** Pul, USC Med Ctr, Los Angeles, CA 83-86; **FAP:** Asst Prof NYU Sch Med; **HOSP:** Hosp For Joint Diseases; *SI: Asthma; Critical Care;* **HMO:** Oxford Chubb Metlife

LANG: Sp, Itl; 🔊 📷 🚗 🏥 $ Mcr Mod 1 Week *VISA* 💳

Marks Jr, Clement E (MD)   Pul
New York University Med Ctr
530 1st Ave; New York, NY 10016; (212) 263-7450; **BDCERT:** Pul 74; Ger 94; **MS:** Columbia P&S 62; **RES:** IM, Bellevue Hosp Ctr, New York, NY 62-63; IM, Bellevue Hosp Ctr, New York, NY 65-69; **FEL:** Pul, Bellevue Hosp Ctr, New York, NY 69-73; *SI: Chronic Obstructive Lung Disease; Asthma;* **HMO:** Oxford NYU CIGNA

🔊 📞 📷 🚗 🏥 $ Immediately

Maxfield, Roger (MD)   Pul
Columbia-Presbyterian Med Ctr
16 E 60th St Suite 320; New York, NY 10022; (212) 326-8415; **BDCERT:** IM 80; Pul 86; **MS:** Brown U 77; **RES:** Georgetown U Hosp, Washington, DC 77-80; **FEL:** Bellevue Hosp Ctr, New York, NY 83-85; New York University Med Ctr, New York, NY 83-85; **FAP:** Assoc Clin Prof Med Columbia P&S; *SI: Asthma and Emphysema; Asbestosis, Lung Cancer;* **HMO:** Oxford

🔊 📷 🚗 🏥 1 Week *VISA* 💳

Guide to symbols and abbreviations can be found on pages 110-113.

365

Plottel, Claudia (MD) Pul
New York University Med Ctr
530 1st Ave 4A; New York, NY 10016; (212) 263-7015; **BDCERT:** IM 87; Pul 92; **MS:** Med Coll PA 84; **RES:** New York University Med Ctr, New York, NY 84-88; **FEL:** Pul, New York University Med Ctr, New York, NY 88-90; CCM (Anes),; **FAP:** Clin Prof NYU Sch Med; *SI: Chronic Obstructive Pulmonary Disease; Asthma;* **HMO:** Aetna Hlth Plan Oxford US Hlthcre Health Source CIGNA +

♿ ⬛ 🕅 $ Mcr 1 Week

Posner, David (MD) Pul PCP
Lenox Hill Hosp
Avenue Medical Associates, 178 E 85th St; New York, NY 10028; (212) 861-8976; **BDCERT:** IM 84; Pul 88; **MS:** NY Med Coll 81; **RES:** IM, Lenox Hill Hosp, New York, NY 81-84; Lenox Hill Hosp, New York, NY 84-85; **FEL:** Long Island Jewish Med Ctr, New Hyde Park, NY 85-87; **FAP:** Asst Prof Med NYU Sch Med; **HOSP:** Beth Israel Med Ctr; *SI: Asthma; Sleep Apnea;* **HMO:** Oxford United Healthcare Blue Choice

LANG: Sp, Dut; ♿ ⬛ 🕅 🕅 $ Mcr 1 Week 🔲
VISA 💳

Prager, Kenneth (MD) Pul
Columbia-Presbyterian Med Ctr
161 Fort Washington Ave Rm 312; New York, NY 10032; (212) 305-5535; **BDCERT:** IM 73; **MS:** Harvard Med Sch 68; **RES:** Columbia-Presbyterian Med Ctr, New York, NY 71-72; U Chicago Hosp, Chicago, IL 72-73; **FAP:** Assoc Clin Prof Med Columbia P&S; *SI: Asthma; Pulmonary Sarcoidosis;* **HMO:** None

LANG: Heb, Fr; ♿ ⬛ 🕅 🕅 $ A Few Days

Raskin, Jonathan (MD) Pul
Beth Israel Med Ctr
1000 Park Ave; New York, NY 10028; (212) 288-4600; **BDCERT:** IM 82; Pul 85; **MS:** Mexico 78; **RES:** Beth Israel Med Ctr, New York, NY 79-82; **FEL:** Mount Sinai Med Ctr, New York, NY; **HOSP:** Mount Sinai Med Ctr; *SI: Asthma; Cardiopulmonary Rehabilitation*

LANG: Sp; ♿ ⬛ 🕅 🕅 $ Mcr A Few Days

Rom, William N (MD) Pul PCP
Bellevue Hosp Ctr
550 1st Ave; New York, NY 10016; (212) 263-6479; **BDCERT:** IM 75; Pul 76; **MS:** U Minn 71; **RES:** IM, UC Davis Med Ctr, Sacramento, CA 71-72; UC Davis Med Ctr, Sacramento, CA 73-75; **FEL:** OM, Mount Sinai Med Ctr, New York, NY; Harvard Med Sch, Cambridge, MA; **HOSP:** New York University Med Ctr; **HMO:** Oxford

♿ 🕅 Mcr Mcd WC NFI Immediately

Rosen, Mark J (MD) Pul
Beth Israel Med Ctr
Beth Israel Med Ctr, 1st Ave & 16th St; New York, NY 10003; (212) 420-2697; **BDCERT:** IM 78; Pul 80; **MS:** Brown U 75; **RES:** Mount Sinai Med Ctr, New York, NY 75-78; **FEL:** CCM, Mount Sinai Med Ctr, New York, NY 78-80; St Vincents Hosp & Med Ctr NY, New York, NY 80; **HMO:** Oxford Multiplan Preferred Hlth

LANG: Sp; 🌙 ⬛ 🕅 🕅 $ Mcr A Few Days 🔲
VISA 💳

Sanders, Abraham (MD) Pul
NY Hosp-Cornell Med Ctr
525 E 68th St; New York, NY 10021; (212) 746-2250; **BDCERT:** IM 79; Pul 83; **MS:** SUNY Hlth Sci Ctr 76; **RES:** IM, Kings County Hosp Ctr, Brooklyn, NY 76-80; IM, Univ Hosp SUNY Bklyn, Brooklyn, NY 76-80; **FEL:** Pul, Kings County Hosp Ctr, Brooklyn, NY 79-80; Pul, Royal Postgraduate Sch Med, London, England 80-81; **FAP:** Assoc Prof Pul Cornell U; *SI: Asthma; Lung Cancer*

♿ 🌙 ⬛ 🕅 🕅 Mcr Immediately 🔲 *VISA*

Schultz, Barbara (MD) Pul
Mount Sinai Med Ctr
927 Park Ave; New York, NY 10028; (212) 517-8680; **BDCERT:** IM 86; Pul 88; **MS:** Mt Sinai Sch Med 83; **RES:** Mount Sinai Med Ctr, New York, NY 83-86; **FEL:** Mount Sinai Med Ctr, New York, NY 86-88; **FAP:** Mt Sinai Sch Med

♿ ⬛ 🕅 🕅 $ Mcr 1 Week

Smith, Anthony (MD)   Pul
St Vincents Hosp & Med Ctr NY
32 W 18th St; New York, NY 10011; (212) 647-6420; **BDCERT:** IM 90; Pul 95; **MS:** NY Med Coll 86

Smith, James (MD)   Pul
NY Hosp-Cornell Med Ctr
170 E 77th St; New York, NY 10021; (212) 879-2180; **BDCERT:** IM 67; Pul 68; **MS:** Georgetown U 60; **RES:** NY Hosp-Cornell Med Ctr, New York, NY 60-62; NY Hosp-Cornell Med Ctr, New York, NY 64-65; **FEL:** Pul, NY Hosp-Cornell Med Ctr, New York, NY 64-66; **HOSP:** Hosp For Special Surgery
🔲 🆂 A Few Days

Stover-Pepe, Diane E (MD)   Pul
Mem Sloan Kettering Cancer Ctr
1275 York Ave; New York, NY 10021; (212) 639-8380; **BDCERT:** IM 75; Pul 78; **MS:** Albert Einstein Coll Med 70; **RES:** Harlem Hosp Ctr, New York, NY 71-72; NY Hosp-Cornell Med Ctr, New York, NY 74-75; **FEL:** Pul, Albert Einstein Med Ctr, Bronx, NY 75; **FAP:** Prof Med Cornell U; **SI:** *Lung Infections; Lung Cancer*; **HMO:** Empire Blue Cross & Shield
🔲 🔲 🔲 🔲 🔲 🔲 1 Week▓ *VISA* 💳 🔲

Sukumaran, Muthiah (MD) Pul
NYU Downtown Hosp
67 Hudson St Ste 1B; New York, NY 10013; (212) 732-7260; **BDCERT:** IM 76; Pul 80; **MS:** India 73; **RES:** Med, Elmhurst Hosp Ctr, Elmhurst, NY 74-76; **FEL:** Pul, Elmhurst Hosp Ctr, Elmhurst, NY 76-77; **FAP:** Asst Clin Prof NY Med Coll; **HOSP:** St Vincents Hosp & Med Ctr; **SI:** *Bronchial Asthma; Lung Cancer*; **HMO:** Aetna-US Healthcare Oxford Blue Cross & Blue Shield
LANG: Chi, Sp, Hin; 🔲 🔲 🔲 🔲 🔲 🆂 🔲
A Few Days *VISA* 💳

Talavera, Wilfredo (MD)   Pul
Cabrini Med Ctr
227 E 19th St 301; New York, NY 10003; (212) 995-6629; **BDCERT:** IM 79; Pul 82; **MS:** Mt Sinai Sch Med 76; **RES:** IM, Beth Israel Med Ctr, New York, NY 76-79; Beth Israel Med Ctr, New York, NY 79-80; **FAP:** Assoc Prof NY Med Coll; **SI:** *Asthma; Pulmonary Infections*; **HMO:** Oxford NYLCare Blue Choice
LANG: Sp; 🔲 🔲 🔲 🔲 🆂 🔲 A Few Days

Teirstein, Alvin (MD)   Pul
Mount Sinai Med Ctr
5 E 98th St 10th Flr; New York, NY 10029; (212) 241-5656; **BDCERT:** IM 61; Pul 69; **MS:** SUNY Downstate 53; **RES:** Mount Sinai Med Ctr, New York, NY 55-57; **FEL:** Pul, Mount Sinai Med Ctr, New York, NY 53-54; Pul, VA Med Ctr-Bronx, Bronx, NY 54-56; **FAP:** Prof Med Mt Sinai Sch Med; **HOSP:** VA Med Ctr-Bronx; **HMO:** Aetna Hlth Plan Blue Choice Oxford PHS

Thomashow, Byron (MD)   Pul
Columbia-Presbyterian Med Ctr
161 Fort Washington Ave; New York, NY 10032; (212) 305-5261; **BDCERT:** Pul 80; IM 77; **MS:** Columbia P&S 74; **RES:** St Luke's Roosevelt Hosp Ctr, New York, NY 74-78; **FEL:** Pul, St Luke's Roosevelt Hosp Ctr, New York, NY 77-78; Harlem Hosp Ctr, New York, NY 78-79; **FAP:** Assoc Clin Prof Med Columbia P&S; **SI:** *Emphysema; Asthma*
🔲 🔲 🔲 🆂 2-4 Weeks

White, Dorothy (MD)   Pul
Mem Sloan Kettering Cancer Ctr
1275 York Ave; New York, NY 10021; (212) 639-8022; **BDCERT:** Pul 84; CCM 87; **MS:** SUNY Hlth Sci Ctr 77; **RES:** NY Hosp-Cornell Med Ctr, New York, NY 77-81; **FEL:** Pul, Yale-New Haven Hosp, New Haven, CT 82-84; **FAP:** Assoc Cornell U; **SI:** *Lung Cancer; Pulmonary Infection*; **HMO:** Blue Cross & Blue Shield
🔲 🔲 🔲 🔲 🔲 🔲 A Few Days

Yip, Chun (MD)　　　　**Pul**
Columbia-Presbyterian Med Ctr
161 Fort Washington Ave 311; New York, NY
10032; (212) 305-8548; **BDCERT:** IM 79; Pul 84;
MS: Albert Einstein Coll Med 76; **RES:** IM,
Columbia-Presbyterian Med Ctr, New York, NY 76-
79; **FEL:** Pul, Bellevue Hosp Ctr, New York, NY 79-
81; **FAP:** Assoc Clin Prof Med Columbia P&S; **SI:**
Asthma; **HMO:** Oxford Empire Blue Choice
Prudential
LANG: Chi; ♿ ⬛ ⬛ $ 4+ Weeks

RADIATION ONCOLOGY

Berson, Anthony (MD)　　**RadRO**
St Vincents Hosp & Med Ctr NY
Chairman Radiation Oncology Saint Vincents
Comprehensive Cancer Center, 153 W 11th St;
New York, NY 10011; (212) 604-8700; **BDCERT:**
RadRO 90; **MS:** Hahnemann U 84; **RES:** RadRO,
University of California, , CA 85-89; **FEL:** Lawrence
Berkeley Lab, Berkeley, CA 86-87; **FAP:** Assoc Prof
NY Med Coll; **SI:** *Prostate Seed Implants; Breast
Radiotherapy*; **HMO:** Oxford GHI United Healthcare
Prucare +
LANG: Sp, Chi, Rus, Fr, Ger; ♿ ⬛ ⬛ ⬛ Mcr Mcd
Immediately ⬛ **VISA** ⬛ ⬛

Cooper, Jay (MD)　　　　**RadRO**
New York University Med Ctr
Radiation Oncology Associates, PC, 566 1st Ave;
New York, NY 10016; (212) 263-5055; **BDCERT:**
RadRO 77; **MS:** NYU Sch Med 73; **RES:** New York
University Med Ctr, New York, NY; **SI:** *Mouth or
Throat Tumors; Skin Tumors*; **HMO:** Oxford
LANG: Sp, Rus, Chi; ♿ ⬛ ⬛ Mcr A Few Days

Fuks, Zvi (MD)　　　　　**RadRO**
Mem Sloan Kettering Cancer Ctr
1275 York Ave H201; New York, NY 10021;
(212) 639-5868; **BDCERT:** RadRO 73; **MS:** Israel
60; **RES:** RadRO, Hassadah Hosp, Jerusalem, Israel
64-69; **SI:** *Prostate*
2-4 Weeks

Harrison, Louis (MD)　　**RadRO**
Beth Israel Med Ctr
Dept of Rad Oncology, Beth Israel Hlth Care System,
10 Union Square East; New York, NY 10003; (212)
844-8087; **BDCERT:** RadRO 86; **MS:** SUNY Hlth
Sci Ctr 82; **RES:** Mount Sinai Med Ctr, New York,
NY 82-83; Yale-New Haven Hosp, New Haven, CT
83-86; **FAP:** Prof Albert Einstein Coll Med; **HOSP:**
St Luke's Roosevelt Hosp Ctr; **SI:** *Head
Brachytherapy; Neck Brachytherapy*; **HMO:** Oxford
Blue Choice Multiplan
LANG: Sp, Fr, Chi; ♿ ⬛ ⬛ ⬛ $ Mcr Mcd WC
A Few Days ⬛ **VISA** ⬛ ⬛

Isaacson, Steven (MD)　　**RadRO**
Columbia-Presbyterian Med Ctr
622 W 168th St Bhn BsmtRm 11; New York, NY
10032; (212) 305-2611; **BDCERT:** RadRO 88; Oto
78; **MS:** Jefferson Med Coll 73; **RES:** Oto, Hosp of U
Penn, Philadelphia, PA 75-78; RadRO, Univ Hosp
SUNY Bklyn, Brooklyn, NY 85-88; **FAP:** Assoc Prof
Columbia P&S; **SI:** *Head and Neck Cancers; Central
Nervous System Cancer*; **HMO:** Oxford Anthem
Health CIGNA Empire Blue Cross Multiplan +
LANG: Sp, Man, Can; ♿ ⬛ ⬛ ⬛ $ Mcr Mcd NFl
A Few Days **VISA** ⬛

Leibel, Steven A (MD)　　**RadRO**
Mem Sloan Kettering Cancer Ctr
Meml SloanKettering Canc Ctr, 1275 York Ave;
New York, NY 10021; (212) 639-6024; **BDCERT:**
Rad 76; **MS:** UC San Francisco 72; **RES:** RadRO, UC
San Francisco Med Ctr, San Francisco, CA 73-76;
SI: *Prostate Cancer; Brain Tumors*; **HMO:** None
♿ ⬛ ⬛ Mcr Mcd 2-4 Weeks ⬛ **VISA** ⬛ ⬛

Mandell, Lynda (MD & PhD)RadRO
Mount Sinai Med Ctr
Radiation Oncology Associates of Mt Sinai, 1184
5th Ave; New York, NY 10029; (212) 241-7503;
BDCERT: Rad 85; **MS:** Med Coll Va 81; **RES:** Johns
Hopkins Hosp, Baltimore, MD 81-82; Mem Sloan
Kettering Cancer Ctr, New York, NY 82-85; **FAP:**
Prof Mt Sinai Sch Med; **SI:** *Radiosurgery/Brain
Tumors; Pediatric Malignancies*; **HMO:** Aetna Hlth
Plan Oxford United Healthcare Chubb GHI +
LANG: Sp, Chi, Fr; ♿ ⬛ ⬛ ⬛ $ Mcr Mcd NFl
Immediately ⬛ **VISA** ⬛

McCormick, Beryl (MD) RadRO
Mem Sloan Kettering Cancer Ctr

1275 York Ave; New York, NY 10021; (212) 639-6828; **BDCERT:** RadRO 77; **MS:** UMDNJ-NJ Med Sch, Newark 73; **RES:** Mem Sloan Kettering Cancer Ctr, New York, NY 74-77; **SI:** *Breast Cancer; Eye Cancer*

[symbols] 2-4 Weeks **VISA**

Minsky, Bruce (MD) RadRO
Mem Sloan Kettering Cancer Ctr

1275 York Ave; New York, NY 10021; (212) 639-6817; **BDCERT:** RadRO 87; **MS:** Univ Mass Sch Med 82; **RES:** Harvard Joint Ctr Radiation Therapy, Boston, MA; **SI:** *Gastrointestinal Cancer*

[symbols] 2-4 Weeks **VISA**

Nisce, Lourdes (MD) RadRO
NY Hosp-Cornell Med Ctr

Cornell Radiation Oncology Associates, 525 E 68th St; New York, NY 10021; (212) 746-3612; **BDCERT:** RadRO 62; **MS:** Philippines 46; **RES:** Rad, NY Hosp-Cornell Med Ctr, New York, NY 57-61; **FEL:** RadRO, Mem Sloan Kettering Cancer Ctr, New York, NY 62; RadRO, USPHS Hosp, Baltimore, MD 63; **SI:** *Hodgkin's Lymphoma Leukemia; Karposi's Skin Cancer—AIDS*; **HMO:** Multiplan Empire Blue Cross & Shield NYLCare United Healthcare Oxford +

LANG: Sp; [symbols] Immediately **VISA**

Nori, Dattatreyudu (MD) RadRO
NY Hosp-Cornell Med Ctr

525 E 68th St; New York, NY 11355; (212) 746-3679; **BDCERT:** RadRO 79; **MS:** India 70; **RES:** RadRO, Mem Sloan Kettering Cancer Ctr, New York, NY 73-75; **FEL:** RadRO, Mem Sloan Kettering Cancer Ctr, New York, NY 76-77; **FAP:** Asst Prof Cornell U; **HOSP:** NY Hosp Med Ctr of Queens; **SI:** *Brachytherapy; Cancer- Abdominal, Breast*; **HMO:** Blue Cross Blue Shield Magnacare Oxford PHS +

LANG: Chi, Fil, Sp, Hin, Heb; [symbols] A Few Days [symbols] **VISA**

Rosenbaum, Alfred (MD) RadRO
Mount Sinai Med Ctr

945 5th Ave; New York, NY 10021; (212) 744-5538; **BDCERT:** RadRO 73; Rad 73; **MS:** Germany 66; **RES:** Rad, Maimonides Med Ctr, Brooklyn, NY 68-69; RadRO, Mount Sinai Med Ctr, New York, NY 69-72; **FEL:** Rad, Montefiore Med Ctr, Bronx, NY 72-73; **FAP:** Asst Clin Prof Mt Sinai Sch Med; **HOSP:** Lenox Hill Hosp; **SI:** *Breast Cancer; Prostate Cancer*; **HMO:** Aetna Hlth Plan NYLCare Oxford PHS Empire +

LANG: Ger, Flm, Sp, Hun, Itl; [symbols] Immediately **VISA**

Sadarangani, Gurmukh J (MD)RadRO
Cabrini Med Ctr

Radiation Oncology, 227 E 19th St; New York, NY 10003; (212) 995-6700; **BDCERT:** Rad 85; **MS:** India 78; **RES:** RadRO, Montefiore Med Ctr, Bronx, NY 81-85; **FAP:** Dir; **SI:** *Implants for Prostate Cancer*; **HMO:** Oxford CIGNA GHI Multiplan 1199 +

LANG: Sp, Rus, Hin, Heb; [symbols] Immediately

Schiff, Peter B (MD & PhD)RadRO
Columbia-Presbyterian Med Ctr

622 W 168th St; New York, NY 10032; (212) 305-2991; **BDCERT:** RadRO 90; **MS:** Albert Einstein Coll Med 84; **RES:** RadRO, Mem Sloan Kettering Cancer Ctr, New York, NY 84-85; RadRO, Mem Sloan Kettering Cancer Ctr, New York, NY 85-88; **FAP:** Prof Columbia P&S; **SI:** *Prostate Cancer; Gynecologic Cancer*; **HMO:** Oxford Chubb CIGNA Anthem Health Prudential +

LANG: Sp, Rus, Itl, Dut, Chi; [symbols] A Few Days **VISA**

Guide to symbols and abbreviations can be found on pages 110-113.

369

Shank, Brenda (MD) RadRO
Mount Sinai Med Ctr
Radiation Oncology Associates, 1184 5th Ave;
New York, NY 10029; (212) 241-7500; **BDCERT:**
Rad 80; **MS:** UMDNJ-RW Johnson Med Sch 76;
RES: Mem Sloan Kettering Cancer Ctr, New York,
NY 76-79; **FEL:** RadRO & Immunology, Mem Sloan
Kettering Cancer Ctr, New York, NY 79-80; **FAP:**
Chrmn Mt Sinai Sch Med; **SI:** *Breast Cancer; Total
Body Irradiation;* **HMO:** Aetna-US Healthcare
Oxford Empire Blue Choice CIGNA Prudential +

LANG: Sp, Kor, Fr, Heb, Afr; 🔊 📷 🚹 🏥 🅼🅲🆁 🅼🅲🅳
A Few Days 🔲 **VISA** 💳 💳

Steinfeld, Alan (MD) RadRO
New York University Med Ctr
Radiation Oncology Assoc, PC, 560 1st Ave
HC107; New York, NY 10016; (212) 263-5055;
BDCERT: Rad 75; **MS:** U Cincinnati 71; **RES:** Rad,
New England Med Ctr, Boston, MA 72-75; **FAP:**
Prof NYU Sch Med; **SI:** *Prostate Cancer; Lung Cancer;*
HMO: Oxford

LANG: Sp, Rus; 🔊 🏥 🅼🅲🆁 🅼🅲🅳 A Few Days

Stock, Richard (MD) RadRO
Mount Sinai Med Ctr
1184 5th Ave; New York, NY 10029; (212) 241-
7502; **BDCERT:** RadRO 93; **MS:** Mt Sinai Sch Med
88; **RES:** Beth Israel Med Ctr, New York, NY 88-89;
Mem Sloan Kettering Cancer Ctr, New York, NY
89-92; **HOSP:** Columbia-Presbyterian Med Ctr; **SI:**
Prostate Brachytherapy; **HMO:** Aetna Hlth Plan
Oxford

🔊 📷 🚹 🏥 🆂 🅼🅲🆁 🅼🅲🅳 Immediately 🔲 **VISA** 💳

Vallejo, Alvaro (MD) RadRO
NY Hosp-Cornell Med Ctr
525 E 68th St; New York, NY 10021; (212) 746-
3641; **BDCERT:** Rad 72; **MS:** Colombia 67; **RES:**
Mem Sloan Kettering Cancer Ctr, New York, NY
68-71; **FEL:** Thomas Jefferson U Hosp, Philadelphia,
PA 71-73; **FAP:** Asst Clin Prof Rad Columbia P&S;
HMO: Oxford PHS Blue Cross

Yahalom, Joachim (MD) RadRO
Mem Sloan Kettering Cancer Ctr
1275 York Ave; New York, NY 10021; (212) 639-
5999; **BDCERT:** RadRO 88; **MS:** Israel 76; **RES:**
Med, Hadassah Hosp, Jerusalem, Israel; Onc,
Hadassah Hosp, Jerusalem, Israel; **FEL:** RadRO,
Mem Sloan Kettering Cancer Ctr, New York, NY;
FAP: Assoc Prof Cornell U; **SI:** *Lymphoma; Hodgkin's
Disease;* **HMO:** Blue Cross

LANG: Heb, Sp; 🔊 📷 🚹 🏥 🅼🅲🆁 🅼🅲🅳 1 Week 🔲
VISA 💳 💳

Zelefsky, Michael (MD) RadRO
Mem Sloan Kettering Cancer Ctr
Meml Sloan Kett Cancer Ctr, 1275 York Ave; New
York, NY 10021; (212) 639-6802; **BDCERT:**
RadRO 91; **MS:** Albert Einstein Coll Med 86; **RES:**
RadRO, Mem Sloan Kettering Cancer Ctr, New
York, NY 87-89; **FAP:** Assoc Prof Cornell U; **SI:**
Prostate Cancer; Brachytherapy; **HMO:** Blue Cross &
Blue Shield

🔊 📷 🚹 🏥 4+ Weeks

RADIOLOGY

Alderson, Philip (MD) Rad
Columbia-Presbyterian Med Ctr
622 W 168th St; New York, NY 10032; (212)
305-8994; **BDCERT:** Rad 76; NuM 74; **MS:**
Washington U, St Louis 70; **RES:** RadRO, Barnes
Hosp, St Louis, MO 71-75; **FAP:** Prof & Chrmn Rad
Columbia P&S; **SI:** *Pulmonary Embolism; Lung
Cancer;* **HMO:** Oxford Aetna Hlth Plan Prucare US
Hlthcre Empire +

🔊 🆂🅰🆂🅾 🏥 🅼🅲🆁 🅼🅲🅳 🆆🅲 A Few Days 🔲 **VISA** 💳 💳

Baer, Jeanne (MD) Rad
St Luke's Roosevelt Hosp Ctr
West Side Radiology Assoc, 1090 Amsterdam Ave;
New York, NY 10025; (212) 523-1783; **BDCERT:**
Rad 71; **MS:** Columbia P&S 64; **RES:** St Luke's
Roosevelt Hosp Ctr, New York, NY 64-65; Geo
Wash U Med Ctr, Washington, DC 66-67; **FEL:** Rad,
St Luke's Roosevelt Hosp Ctr, New York, NY 67-70;
FAP: Assoc Clin Prof Columbia P&S; *SI:*
Gastrointestinal Imaging; CT Scans; **HMO:** Oxford
PHS GHI Blue Cross & Blue Shield
LANG: Fr; ♿ 📷 🏥 **S** Mcr WC NFI Immediately ***VISA***
💳

Balthazar, Emil J (MD) Rad
New York University Med Ctr
New Bellevue Hospital - Professor of Radiology, 462
1st Ave 3FL - W37-42; New York, NY 10016;
(212) 263-6372; **BDCERT:** Rad 68; **MS:** Romania
59; **RES:** Rad, Univ Hosp SUNY Bklyn, Brooklyn,
NY 64-67; **FEL:** Rad, Univ Hosp SUNY Bklyn,
Brooklyn, NY 67-69; Flower Fifth Ave Hosp, New
York, NY 69-78; **FAP:** Prof NYU Sch Med; **HOSP:**
Bellevue Hosp Ctr; *SI: GI Radiology;* **HMO:** Most
LANG: Rom; ♿ 📷 🏥 **S** Mcr WC NFI
Immediately ■ ***VISA*** 💳

Berson, Barry (MD) Rad
Mount Sinai Med Ctr
1 E 82nd St; New York, NY 10028; (212) 535-
9770; **BDCERT:** DR 90; NRad 95; **MS:** Mt Sinai Sch
Med 84; **RES:** Rad, Mount Sinai Med Ctr, New York,
NY 86-90; **FEL:** Nrad, New York University Med
Ctr, New York, NY 90-92; **FAP:** Asst Clin Prof Mt
Sinai Sch Med; *SI: Mammography; Bone*
Densitometry; **HMO:** Oxford United Healthcare
PHCS Blue Cross CIGNA +
LANG: Sp, Fr, Heb; ♿ 📷 🏥 **S** Mcr WC NFI
A Few Days ■ ***VISA*** 💳 💳

Bloch, Claude (MD) Rad
Mount Sinai Med Ctr
30 E 60th St Ste 703; New York, NY 10022; (212)
755-7656; **BDCERT:** Rad 60; **MS:** Yale U Sch Med
53; **RES:** Rad, Mount Sinai Med Ctr, New York, NY
57-60; **FEL:** Path, Mount Sinai Med Ctr, New York,
NY 54-55; **FAP:** Assoc Clin Instr Rad Mt Sinai Sch
Med; *SI: Mammography; GI Radiology;* **HMO:** Oxford
PHCS Beech Street Blue Choice PPO
LANG: Sp, Fr, Ger, Yd; ♿ 📷 🏥 🏥 **S** Mcr WC NFI
Immediately ■ ***VISA*** 💳 💳

Bosniak, Morton (MD) Rad
New York University Med Ctr
550 1st Ave; New York, NY 10016; (212) 263-
5216; **BDCERT:** Rad 61; **MS:** SUNY Hlth Sci Ctr 55;
RES: Rad, NY Hosp-Cornell Med Ctr, New York, NY
56-57; Rad, NY Hosp-Cornell Med Ctr, New York,
NY 59-61; **FAP:** Prof Rad NYU Sch Med; **HOSP:**
Bellevue Hosp Ctr; *SI: Kidney Tumors & Cysts;*
Urinary Tract Radiology
♿ 📷 🏥 Mcr Immediately ■ ***VISA*** 💳 💳

Brady, James (MD) Rad
Mercy Med Ctr
121A E 83rd St; New York, NY 10028; (212) 879-
6200; **BDCERT:** Rad 85; **MS:** Italy 77; **RES:** Mount
Sinai Med Ctr, New York, NY 79-82; **HMO:** Oxford
Aetna-US Healthcare NYLCare Blue Cross & Blue
Choice
LANG: Sp; ♿ 📷 🏥 **S** Mcr WC NFI Immediately ■
VISA 💳 💳

Castellino, Ronald A (MD) Rad
Mem Sloan Kettering Cancer Ctr
1275 York Ave; New York, NY 10021; (212) 639-
7284; **BDCERT:** DR 69; **MS:** Creighton U 62; **RES:**
Stanford Med Ctr, Stanford, CA 65-68; **FAP:** Prof
Cornell U; **HMO:** None

Guide to symbols and abbreviations can be found on pages 110-113.

371

Deck, Michael (MD)   Rad
NY Hosp-Cornell Med Ctr

525 E 68th St; New York, NY 10021; (212) 746-2575; **BDCERT:** DR 69; **MS:** Australia 61; **RES:** Rad, Sydney Hosp, Sydney, Australia 63-65; **FAP:** Prof Rad Cornell U; **HMO:** Affordable Hlth Plan Oxford PHCS

♿ 📷 ⛶ Mcr Mcd   1 Week

Feldman, Frieda (MD)   Rad
Columbia-Presbyterian Med Ctr

Dept of Radiology, Columbia-Presbyterian Med Ctr, 622 W 168th St 2121; New York, NY 10032; (212) 305-2986; **BDCERT:** Rad 62; **MS:** NYU Sch Med 57; **RES:** Beth Israel Med Ctr, New York, NY; Bellevue Hosp Ctr, New York, NY; **FEL:** Columbia-Presbyterian Med Ctr, New York, NY; **FAP:** Prof Rad Columbia P&S

Ghossein, Nemetallah A (MD)Rad
Beth Israel Med Ctr

10 Union Square E Dept RadOnc Bsmt Level, 227 E 19th St; New York, NY 10003; (212) 844-8020; **BDCERT:** Rad 63; **MS:** Egypt 57; **RES:** RadRO, Francis Delafield Hosp, New York, NY 59-61; Mem Sloan Kettering Cancer Ctr, New York, NY 61-63; **FEL:** Path CP, Columbia-Presbyterian Med Ctr, New York, NY 61-63; **FAP:** Prof RadRO Albert Einstein Coll Med; **HOSP:** Westchester Square Med Ctr; **SI:** *Radiation Oncology;* **HMO:** Oxford Empire Blue Choice Metlife Aetna Hlth Plan HIP Network +

♿ 📷 ⛶ Mcr Mcd   Immediately ■ *VISA* ⓘ ⓘ

Grunther, Howard (MD)   Rad
Mount Sinai Med Ctr

1 E 82nd St; New York, NY 10028; (212) 535-9770; **BDCERT:** Rad 69; **MS:** NY Med Coll 62; **RES:** Rad, Mount Sinai Med Ctr, New York, NY 65-68; **FAP:** Asst Clin Prof Rad Mt Sinai Sch Med; **SI:** *Mammography; Nuclear Medicine;* **HMO:** Oxford Aetna Hlth Plan PHCS Blue Choice Metlife +

LANG: Sp, Yd, Fr, Rus, Heb; ♿ SA/SO 📷 ⛶ S Mcr WC NFI A Few Days ■ *VISA* ⓘ ⓘ

Hamilton, Richard H (MD)   Rad
New York University Med Ctr

Executive Health Group, 10 Rockefeller Plaza; New York, NY 10020; (212) 332-3028; **BDCERT:** Rad 54; **MS:** NY Med Coll 47; **RES:** S, City Hosp, New York, NY 49-51; Rad, Post Grad Hosp, New York, NY 51-53; **FAP:** Assoc Clin Prof NYU Sch Med; **SI:** *CT Scans; Pulmonary Radiology;* **HMO:** None

LANG: Sp, Fr; ♿ 📷 ♿ ⛶ Mcr Mcd NFI Immediately

Hayes, Mary (MD)   Rad
NY Hosp-Cornell Med Ctr

Cornell Radiation Oncology Associates, 525 E 68th St; New York, NY 10021; (212) 746-3610; **BDCERT:** RadRO 88; **MS:** Canada 84; **RES:** RadRO, Mem Sloan Kettering Cancer Ctr, New York, NY 85-88; **HOSP:** Columbia-Presbyterian Med Ctr; **SI:** *Breast Cancer; Marrow Transplant;* **HMO:** Oxford Aetna-US Healthcare Blue Cross CIGNA US Hlthcre +

LANG: Sp, Rus, Chi; ♿ 📷 ⛶ Mcr Mcd

Held, Barry (MD)   Rad
NY Hosp-Cornell Med Ctr

New York Hosp-Cornell Med Ctr, 525 E 68th St; New York, NY 11021; (212) 746-2522; **BDCERT:** Rad 61; **MS:** SUNY Downstate 56; **RES:** Rad, Long Island Coll Hosp, Brooklyn, NY 57-60; **FAP:** Assoc Clin Prof Rad Cornell U; **SI:** *Diagnostic Radiology*

♿ C ♿ ⛶ Mcr Mcd WC NFI A Few Days ■ *VISA* ⓘ ⓘ

Kaye, Jeremy J (MD)   Rad
St Vincents Hosp & Med Ctr NY

St Vincent's Hospital, 153 W 11th St Link-251; New York, NY 10011; (212) 604-8717; **BDCERT:** Rad 70; **MS:** Cornell U 65; **RES:** Cornell Med Ctr, New York, NY 66-69; **FAP:** Prof Rad NY Med Coll

♿ SA/SO 📷 ⛶ S Mcr Mcd WC NFI A Few Days

Kazam, Elias (MD)   Rad
NY Hosp-Cornell Med Ctr

525 E 68th St; New York, NY 10021; (212) 746-2563; **BDCERT:** DR 74; NuM 76; **MS:** Albert Einstein Coll Med 66; **RES:** Med, Jacobi Med Ctr, Bronx, NY 69-70; Rad, Peter Bent Brigham Hosp, Boston, MA 70-72

♿ SA/SO C 📷 ♿ ⛶ Mcr Mcd WC Immediately

Lefkovitz, Zvi (MD)   **Rad**
Mount Sinai Med Ctr

Mt Sinai Medical Center-Dept Radiology, 1 Gustave
L Levy Place Pl Box 1234; New York, NY 10029;
(212) 241-8730; **BDCERT:** Rad 83; **MS:** U Chicago-
Pritzker Sch Med 82; **RES:** DR, Maimonides Med
Ctr, Brooklyn, NY 83-86; **FEL:** Univ Hosp SUNY
Bklyn, Brooklyn, NY 74-78; **FAP:** Chrmn Rad Mt
Sinai Sch Med; **HOSP:** Queens Hosp Ctr; *SI:*
Interventional Radiology

⬥ 🛏 Mcr Mcd WC

Mitty, Harold (MD)   **Rad**
Mount Sinai Med Ctr

1 Gustave Levy Pl; New York, NY 10029; (212)
241-7417; **BDCERT:** Rad 66; **MS:** SUNY
Downstate 58; **RES:** Mount Sinai Med Ctr, New
York, NY 62-65; **FAP:** Prof Rad Mt Sinai Sch Med;
SI: Arterial Angioplasty; Embolization of Fibroids;
HMO: Oxford Aetna Hlth Plan Prucare US Hlthcre
PHS +

LANG: Sp, Fr, Rus; ⬥ 🗃 🛏 Mcr Mcd WC Immediately
▓ **VISA** ⬤

Naidich, David P (MD)   **Rad**
New York University Med Ctr

175 E 74th St; New York, NY 10016; (212) 263-
5229; **BDCERT:** DR 80; **MS:** NYU Sch Med 75; **RES:**
DR, Johns Hopkins Hosp, Baltimore, MD 76-79;
FEL: Cross Sectional Imaging, Johns Hopkins Hosp,
Baltimore, MD 79-80; **FAP:** Prof NYU Sch Med;
HOSP: Bellevue Hosp Ctr; *SI: Chest Disease*; **HMO:**
Metlife Aetna Hlth Plan Oxford First Option

⬥ 🛏 S Mcr WC A Few Days

Newhouse, Jeffrey (MD)   **Rad**
Columbia-Presbyterian Med Ctr

177 Fort Washington Ave; New York, NY 10032;
(212) 305-7898; **BDCERT:** Rad 72; **MS:** Harvard
Med Sch 67; **RES:** Mass Gen Hosp, Boston, MA 68-
72; **FAP:** Prof Columbia P&S; *SI: Abdominal*
Radiology; **HMO:** Oxford CIGNA Multiplan PHS
PHCS +

⬥ SA/SU C Mcd WC Immediately **VISA** ⬤

Ostrovsky, Paul (MD)   **Rad**
Mount Sinai Med Ctr

121A E 83rd St; New York, NY 10028; (212) 879-
6200; **BDCERT:** Rad 82; **MS:** NY Med Coll 78; **RES:**
Mount Sinai Med Ctr, New York, NY 79-82; **HMO:**
Aetna Hlth Plan Oxford Metlife PHCS Multiplan +

⬥ SA/SU 🗃 🛏 S Mcr WC NFI ▓ **VISA** ⬤

Panicek, David (MD)   **Rad**
Mem Sloan Kettering Cancer Ctr

Memorial Sloan Kettering Cancer Center, 1275
York Ave; New York, NY 10021; (212) 639-5825;
BDCERT: Rad 84; **MS:** Cornell U 80; **RES:** Rad, NY
Hosp-Cornell Med Ctr, New York, NY 81-84; **FAP:**
Assoc Prof Rad Cornell U; *SI: Bone Tumors; Soft*
Tissue Tumors

⬥ SA/SU C 🗃 🛏 Mcr Mcd A Few Days

Pile-Spellman, John (MD)   **Rad**
Columbia-Presbyterian Med Ctr

Interventional Neuroradiology, 177 Fort
Washington Ave MHB 85; New York, NY 10032;
(212) 305-6384; **BDCERT:** Rad 86; **MS:** Tufts U
78; **RES:** New England Med Ctr, Boston, MA 79-81;
Mass Gen Hosp, Boston, MA 81-84; **FEL:** Mass Gen
Hosp, Boston, MA 84-86; New York University Med
Ctr, New York, NY 86; **FAP:** Prof Rad Columbia
P&S; **HOSP:** NY Hosp-Cornell Med Ctr; *SI:*
Aneurysms; Strokes and Carotid Disease

LANG: Fr, Sp, Vn; ⬥ 🗃 🔧 🛏 Mcr Mcd WC NFI 2-
4 Weeks **VISA** ⬤

Rabinowitz, Jack G (MD)   **Rad**
Mount Sinai Med Ctr

Radiology Associates, 1 Gustave Levy Pl; New York,
NY 10029; (212) 241-7427; **BDCERT:** Rad 60;
MS: Switzerland 55; **RES:** Rad, Kings County Hosp
Ctr, Brooklyn, NY 57-59; **FAP:** Prof & Chrmn Mt
Sinai Sch Med; **HMO:** Oxford Aetna Hlth Plan Blue
Shield 32BJ

LANG: Fr, Sp; ⬥ SA/SU 🗃 🔧 🛏 S Mcr Mcd WC NFI
Immediately ▓ **VISA** ⬤ ⬤ 🖼

Guide to symbols and abbreviations can be found on pages 110-113.

373

Rosenblatt, Ruth (MD)   Rad
Montefiore Med Ctr

New York Hospital - Cornell Radiology, 525 E 68th St; New York, NY 10021; (212) 746-2697; **BDCERT:** Rad 69; **MS:** Med Coll PA 64; **RES:** Rad, Montefiore Med Ctr, Bronx, NY 69; **FAP:** Prof of Clin Rad NY Med Coll; **HOSP:** NY Hosp-Cornell Med Ctr; **SI:** *Breast Cancer/Breast Biopsy; Breast Ultrasound;* **HMO:** Oxford Sel Pro Aetna-US Healthcare PHS Prestige +

🚹 🔒 🚼 🛏 Mar Med WC NFI Immediately

Rosenfeld, Stanley (MD)   Rad
Mount Sinai Med Ctr

945 5th Ave; New York, NY 10021; (212) 744-5538; **BDCERT:** Rad 78; **MS:** Albert Einstein Coll Med 74; **RES:** Montefiore Med Ctr, Bronx, NY 75-78; **HOSP:** Beth Israel North; **SI:** *Mammography; Ultrasonography;* **HMO:** Oxford Aetna Hlth Plan Magnacare PHCS United Healthcare +

🚹 🔒 🛏 Mar NFI Immediately 🔳 **VISA** 💳

Schlaeger, Ralph (MD)   Rad
Columbia-Presbyterian Med Ctr

Atchley Pavilion 1-119A, 161 Ft Washington Ave; New York, NY 10032; (212) 305-5170; **BDCERT:** Rad 53; **MS:** U Wisc Med Sch 45; **RES:** Rad, Hosp of U Penn, Philadelphia, PA 48-49; RadRO, Temple U Hosp, Philadelphia, PA 50-53; **FAP:** Prof Columbia P&S

A Few Days

Sostman, H Dirk (MD)   Rad
NY Hosp-Cornell Med Ctr

1300 E York Ave; New York, NY 10021; (212) 746-2520; **BDCERT:** DR 80; NuM 96; **MS:** Yale U Sch Med 76; **RES:** Med, Yale-New Haven Hosp, New Haven, CT 77-80; RadRO,; **FEL:** NuM, Yale-New Haven Hosp, New Haven, CT 79-80; Chest Imaging,; **FAP:** Prof & Chairman Cornell U; **SI:** *Pulmonary Embolism; Cardiovascular Imaging;* **HMO:** Most

🚹 SA SU 🛏 💲 Mar Med WC NFI A Few Days 🔳 **VISA** 💳 💳

Stassa, George (MD)   Rad
NY Hosp-Cornell Med Ctr

519 E 72nd St 103; New York, NY 10021; (212) 288-1575; **BDCERT:** Rad 65; **MS:** Columbia P&S 60; **RES:** Rad, Columbia-Presby Med Ctr, New York, NY 61-64; **FAP:** Assoc Clin Prof Rad Cornell U; **SI:** *Gastrointestinal Diseases; Dental Scanning;* **HMO:** Aetna Hlth Plan Blue Choice Prucare Oxford

LANG: Sp; 🚹 🅲 🔒 🛏 💲 Mar WC NFI A Few Days 🔳 **VISA** 💳

REPRODUCTIVE ENDOCRINOLOGY

Berkeley, Alan S (MD)   RE
New York University Med Ctr

NYU Program for IVF, Reproductive Surgery & Infertility, 660 1st Ave 5th Fl; New York, NY 10016; (212) 263-7629; **BDCERT:** ObG 80; **MS:** NY Med Coll 73; **RES:** Med, Geo Wash U Med Ctr, Washington, DC 73-74; ObG, Yale-New Haven Hosp, New Haven, CT 74-77; **FEL:** GO, Yale-New Haven Hosp, New Haven, CT 77-79; **EDM,** Yale-New Haven Hosp, New Haven, CT 77-79; **FAP:** Prof NYU Sch Med; **SI:** *In Vitro Fertilization; Gynecologic Surgery*

LANG: Sp, Chi; 🚹 SA SU 🔒 🚼 🛏 Mar 4+ Weeks 🔳 **VISA** 💳

David, Sami (MD)   RE
Mount Sinai Med Ctr

1047 Park Ave; New York, NY 10028; (212) 831-0430; **BDCERT:** ObG 80; **MS:** Columbia P&S 71; **RES:** IM, NY Hosp-Cornell Med Ctr, New York, NY 71-72; ObG, NY Hosp-Cornell Med Ctr, New York, NY 72-76; **FAP:** Prof RE Mt Sinai Sch Med; **SI:** *Recurrent Miscarriages; Late Pregnancies;* **HMO:** None

SA SU 🔒 🚼 🛏 💲 4+ Weeks 🔳 **VISA** 💳

Grifo, James (MD)   RE
New York University Med Ctr

660 1st Ave Fl 5; New York, NY 10016; (212)
263-7978; **BDCERT:** ObG 91; RE 94; **MS:** Case
West Res U 82; **RES:** ObG, NY Hosp-Cornell Med
Ctr, New York, NY 85-88; **FEL:** RE, Yale-New
Haven Hosp, New Haven, CT 88-90; **FAP:** Prof RE
Yale U Sch Med; **SI:** *Infertility; Reproductive
Endocrinology*

LANG: Sp, Chi, Tam, Slv, Ger; 🚻 📷 🏨   4+ Weeks
▨ **VISA** 💳

Kelly, Amalia (MD)   RE
Columbia-Presbyterian Med Ctr

860 5th Ave; New York, NY 10021; (212) 639-
9122; **BDCERT:** ObG 86; RE 89; **MS:** Tufts U 79;
RES: ObG, Columbia-Presbyterian Med Ctr, New
York, NY 79-83; **FEL:** RE, Columbia-Presbyterian
Med Ctr, New York, NY 83-85; **FAP:** Assoc Prof
Columbia P&S; **SI:** *Laparoscopy; Infertility*

🚻 📷 🏨 💲 ▨   2-4 Weeks **VISA** 💳

Lobo, Rogerio (MD)   RE
Columbia-Presbyterian Med Ctr

Dept of Obstetrics & Gynecology, 622 W 168th St;
New York, NY 10032; (212) 305-2377; **BDCERT:**
RE 82; ObG 94; **MS:** Georgetown U 74; **RES:** ObG, U
Chicago Hosp, Chicago, IL 75-78; **FEL:** RE, USC
Med Ctr, Los Angeles, CA 80; **FAP:** Prof ObG
Columbia P&S

Reyniak, Victor (MD)   RE
Mount Sinai Med Ctr

1107 5th Ave; New York, NY 10128; (212) 410-
4080; **BDCERT:** ObG 69; RE 75; **MS:** Poland 60;
RES: Brooklyn Womens Hosp, Brooklyn, NY 64-67;
FEL: EDM, NY Med Coll, New York, NY 69-70; **FAP:**
Clin Prof ObG Mt Sinai Sch Med; **HOSP:** Lenox Hill
Hosp; **SI:** *Infertility Laser Surgery; Endometriosis;*
HMO: None

LANG: Pol; 📷 🏨 🏨 💲   1 Week **VISA** 💳

Rosenwaks, Zev (MD)   RE   **PCP**
NY Hosp-Cornell Med Ctr

The Center for Reproductive Medicine and
Infertility, 505 E 70th St HT326a; New York, NY
10021; (212) 746-1743; **BDCERT:** ObG 78; RE 81;
MS: SUNY Downstate 72; **RES:** ObG, Long Island
Jewish Med Ctr, New Hyde Park, NY 72-76; **FEL:**
RE, Johns Hopkins Hosp, Baltimore, MD 76-78;
FAP: Prof ObG Cornell U; **SI:** *Infertility; Reproductive
Disorders;* **HMO:** None

LANG: Heb, Sp, Alb, Itl, Fr; 🚻 📷 🏨 🏨 💲
A Few Days ▨ **VISA** 💳 🔹

Sauer, Mark (MD)   RE
Columbia-Presbyterian Med Ctr

630 W 168th St PH 1628; New York, NY 10032;
(212) 305-9175; **BDCERT:** ObG 87; RE 88; **MS:**
Univ IL Coll Med 80; **RES:** U IL Med Ctr, Chicago, IL
80-84; **FEL:** RE, UCLA Med Ctr, Los Angeles, CA 84-
86; **FAP:** Prof Columbia P&S; **SI:** *Oocyte Donation;
Infertility*

LANG: Slv, Itl, Chi; 🚻 📷 🏨 🏨   A Few Days ▨
VISA 💳 🔹

Schmidt-Sarosi, Cecilia (MD)   RE
New York University Med Ctr

Offices for Fertility & Reproductive Medicine, PC,
251 E 33rd St 2S; New York, NY 10016; (212)
263-7566; **BDCERT:** ObG 93; RE 93; **MS:** NYU Sch
Med 76; **RES:** New York University Med Ctr, New
York, NY 76-80; **FEL:** RE, New York University Med
Ctr, New York, NY 80-82; **FAP:** Prof ObG NYU Sch
Med; **HOSP:** Beth Israel Med Ctr; **SI:** *Infertility; IVF
Egg Donation;* **HMO:** Oxford US Hlthcre Prudential
CIGNA Blue Select +

LANG: Sp, Hun; 🚻 📷 🏨 🏨 💲   4+ Weeks ▨
VISA 💳

Warren, Michelle (MD)   RE
Columbia-Presbyterian Med Ctr

134 E 73rd St; New York, NY 10021; (212) 737-
4664; **BDCERT:** IM 72; **MS:** Cornell U 65; **RES:**
Med, Bellevue Hosp Ctr, New York, NY 66-68; Mem
Sloan Kettering Cancer Ctr, New York, NY 66-68;
FEL: EDM, Columbia-Presbyterian Med Ctr, New
York, NY 68-71; **FAP:** Prof ObG Columbia P&S

RHEUMATOLOGY

Abramson, Steven B (MD)   Rhu
Hosp For Joint Diseases
Hospital for Joint Diseases, 301 E 17th St; New York, NY 10003; (212) 598-6119; **BDCERT:** IM 78; Rhu 80; **MS:** Harvard Med Sch 74; **RES:** Bellevue Hosp Ctr, New York, NY 74-77; IM, Bellevue Hosp Ctr, New York, NY 77-78; **FEL:** Rhu, Bellevue Hosp Ctr, New York, NY 78-80; Rhu, New York University Med Ctr, New York, NY 80-83; **FAP:** Prof Med NYU Sch Med; **HOSP:** New York University Med Ctr; **SI:** Rheumatoid Arthritis; **HMO:** Oxford

🦽 🔒 🏧 💲 Mcr 2-4 Weeks 💳 VISA 💳

Adlersberg, Jay (MD)   Rhu
Lenox Hill Hosp
220 E 69th St; New York, NY 10021; (212) 570-1800; **BDCERT:** IM 72; Rhu 80; **MS:** Univ Penn 69; **RES:** Bellevue Hosp Ctr, New York, NY 70-72; **FEL:** Rhu, Bellevue Hosp Ctr, New York, NY 72-74; **FAP:** Asst Prof Mt Sinai Sch Med; **HOSP:** Beth Israel Med Ctr; **SI:** Joint Pain; Back Pain; **HMO:** United Healthcare Oxford Blue Cross & Blue Shield

🦽 🔒 🧑 🏧 💲 Mcr Immediately VISA 💳

Agus, Bertrand (MD)   Rhu
New York University Med Ctr
251 E 33rd St Fl 4; New York, NY 10016; (212) 779-8421; **BDCERT:** IM 72; Rhu 72; **MS:** NYU Sch Med 65; **RES:** New York University Med Ctr, New York, NY 68-70; **FEL:** Rhu, New York University Med Ctr, New York, NY 70-72; **SI:** Systemic Lupus Erythematosus; Sarcoidosis

LANG: Fr, Sp, Heb; 🦽 🔒 🧑 🏧 💲 Immediately

Aisen, Paul (MD)   Rhu
Mount Sinai Med Ctr
133 E 95th St; New York, NY 10128; (212) 860-3331; **BDCERT:** Rhu 84; Ger 92; **MS:** Columbia P&S 79; **RES:** Med, U Hosp of Cleveland, Cleveland, OH 79-81; Med, Mount Sinai Med Ctr, New York, NY 84-85; **FEL:** Rhu, New York University Med Ctr, New York, NY 82-84; **FAP:** Assoc Prof Mt Sinai Sch Med; **SI:** Alzheimer's Disease; **HMO:** None

🔒 🧑 🏧 💲

Argyros, Thomas (MD)   Rhu
Lenox Hill Hosp
122 E 76th St; New York, NY 10021; (212) 988-7680; **BDCERT:** IM 61; **MS:** NYU Sch Med 54; **RES:** Lenox Hill Hosp, New York, NY 57-58; **FEL:** Arthritis, New York University Med Ctr, New York, NY 64-65; **FAP:** Clin Prof Med NYU Sch Med; **SI:** Lyme Disease; Lupus; **HMO:** Multiplan Magnacare PHCS US Hlthcre +

LANG: Grk, Tag, Sp; 🦽 🔒 🧑 🏧 💲 Mcr NFI 1 Week

Belmont, H Michael (MD)   Rhu
New York University Med Ctr
Rheumatology Assoc, 305 2nd Ave 16; New York, NY 10003; (212) 598-6516; **BDCERT:** IM 83; Rhu 86; **MS:** Univ Pittsburgh 80; **RES:** IM, Mount Sinai Med Ctr, New York, NY 80-83; **FEL:** Rhu, New York University Med Ctr, New York, NY 83-85; **HOSP:** Hosp For Joint Diseases; **SI:** Lupus; Rheumatoid Arthritis; **HMO:** Oxford CIGNA

🦽 🔒 🧑 🏧 💲 A Few Days 💳 VISA 💳

Blume, Ralph (MD)   Rhu
Columbia-Presbyterian Med Ctr
161 Fort Washington Ave 537; New York, NY 10032; (212) 305-5512; **BDCERT:** IM 72; Rhu 74; **MS:** Columbia P&S 64; **RES:** IM, Columbia-Presbyterian Med Ctr, New York, NY 68-69; **FEL:** Arthritis, Columbia-Presbyterian Med Ctr, New York, NY 68-70; **HMO:** PHS Prucare Chubb Oxford Metlife +

🦽 🔒 🏧 💲 1 Week

Buyon, Jill P (MD)   Rhu   `PCP`
Hosp For Joint Diseases
305 2nd Ave; New York, NY 10010; (212) 598-
6516; **BDCERT:** IM 81; Rhu 84; **MS:** Albert
Einstein Coll Med 78; **RES:** Albert Einstein Med Ctr,
Bronx, NY 78-81; **FEL:** Rhu, New York University
Med Ctr, New York, NY 81-83; **FAP:** Assoc Prof
NYU Sch Med; **HMO:** None
♿ 📷 💲 Mc Immediately ▤ **VISA** ●

Crane, Richard (MD)   Rhu   `PCP`
Mount Sinai Med Ctr
1088 Park Ave; New York, NY 10128; (212) 860-
4000; **BDCERT:** IM 84; Rhu 86; **MS:** Mt Sinai Sch
Med 81; **RES:** Mount Sinai Med Ctr, New York, NY
81-84; **FEL:** Rhu, Mount Sinai Med Ctr, New York,
NY 84-86; **FAP:** Clin Instr Mt Sinai Sch Med; *SI:*
Rheumatoid Arthritis; Lupus
♿ 📷 📷 📷 Mc A Few Days

Eberle, Mark Allen (MD)   Rhu
New York University Med Ctr
333 E 34th Street Rm1C; New York, NY 10016;
(212) 889-7217; **BDCERT:** IM 88; Rhu 94; **MS:** Mt
Sinai Sch Med 84; **RES:** IM, New York University
Med Ctr, New York, NY 87-88; IM, New York
University Med Ctr, New York, NY 84-87; **FEL:**
Rhu, New York University Med Ctr, New York, NY
88; **HOSP:** Bellevue Hosp Ctr

Faller, Jason (MD)   Rhu
St Luke's Roosevelt Hosp Ctr
333 W 57th St 104; New York, NY 10019; (212)
307-6880; **BDCERT:** IM 80; Rhu 82; **MS:** Univ
Penn 77; **RES:** IM, Rush Presbyterian-St Lukes Med
Ctr, Chicago, IL 78-80; **FEL:** Rhu, U Mich Med Ctr,
Ann Arbor, MI 80-82; **FAP:** Instr Columbia P&S; *SI:*
Lyme Disease; Rheumatoid Arthritis; **HMO:** Oxford
Aetna Hlth Plan PHS PHCS Health Source +
LANG: Sp, Fr, Heb; 📷 📿 📿 💲 1 Week ▤ **VISA**
●

Fields, Theodore (MD)   Rhu
Hosp For Special Surgery
Hospital for Special Surgery Faculty Practice, 535 E
70th St 7th Fl; New York, NY 10021; (212) 606-
1286; **BDCERT:** IM 79; Rhu 82; **MS:** SUNY
Downstate 76; **RES:** IM, Nassau County Med Ctr,
East Meadow, NY 77-79; **FEL:** Rhu, Univ Hosp
SUNY Stony Brook, Stony Brook, NY 79-82; **FAP:**
Assoc Prof Cornell U; **HOSP:** NY Hosp-Cornell Med
Ctr; *SI: Rheumatoid Arthritis; Gout & Pseudogout*
♿ 📿 📷 💲 1 Week ▤ **VISA** ●

Fischer, Harry (MD)   Rhu
Beth Israel Med Ctr
10 Union Square East 3D; New York, NY 10003;
(212) 844-8101; **BDCERT:** IM 83; Rhu 90; **MS:**
Sinai Sch Med 79; **RES:** IM, Beth Israel Med Ctr,
New York, NY 79-83; **FEL:** Rhu, Hosp For Joint
Diseases, New York, NY 83-85; **FAP:** Asst Clin Prof
Albert Einstein Coll Med; *SI: Rheumatoid Arthritis;*
Lupus; **HMO:** Oxford PHS
♿ 📷 📿 📿 Mc Mc 1 Week ▤ **VISA** ●

Golden, Brian (MD)   Rhu
Hosp For Joint Diseases
Dept of Rheum, 305 Second Ave Ste 16; New York,
NY 10003; (212) 598-6516; **BDCERT:** IM 94; Rhu
96; **MS:** Mt Sinai Sch Med 91; **RES:** Mount Sinai
Med Ctr, New York, NY 92-94; **FEL:** Hosp For Joint
Diseases, New York, NY 94-96; **FAP:** Clin Instr Med
NYU Sch Med

Goodman, Susan (MD)   Rhu
Hosp For Special Surgery
535 E 70th St; New York, NY 10021; (212) 606-
1163; **BDCERT:** IM 80; Rhu 82; **MS:** U Cincinnati
77; **RES:** IM, Lenox Hill Hosp, New York, NY 78-80;
FEL: Columbia-Presbyterian Med Ctr, New York,
NY 80-83; *SI: Lupus; Rheumatoid Arthritis;* **HMO:**
Oxford NYLCare PHS PHCS Corporate Care +
♿ 📷 📿 📿 💲 Mc A Few Days ▤ **VISA** ● ■

Guide to symbols and abbreviations can be found on pages 110-113.

377

Greisman, Stewart (MD)   Rhu
St Luke's Roosevelt Hosp Ctr
457 W 57th St; New York, NY 10019; (212) 265-1471; **BDCERT:** IM 84; Rhu 86; **MS:** Yale U Sch Med 81; **RES:** Yale-New Haven Hosp, New Haven, CT 81-84; **FEL:** Rhu, Hosp For Special Surgery, New York, NY 84-86; **FAP:** Asst Columbia P&S; **HOSP:** Hosp For Special Surgery; **SI:** *Lupus; Rheumatoid Arthritis*; **HMO:** Oxford Aetna Hlth Plan Blue Choice

🔾 🏥 💲 Mcr 2-4 Weeks

Honig, Stephen (MD)   Rhu
Hosp For Joint Diseases
Hospital for Joint Diseases, 301 E 17th St Ste 16; New York, NY 10003; (212) 598-6516; **BDCERT:** IM 75; Rhu 78; **MS:** U Tenn Ctr Hlth Sci, Memphis 72; **RES:** Rhu, St Vincents Hosp & Med Ctr NY, New York, NY 73-75; **FEL:** Rhu, New York University Med Ctr, New York, NY 75-77; **FAP:** Asst Prof NYU Sch Med; **HOSP:** New York University Med Ctr; **SI:** *Osteoporosis; Rheumatoid Arthritis*

LANG: Sp, Chi; 🔾 🏥 💲 Mcr 1 Week 🏧 **VISA** 🔾 🔾

Horowitz, Mark D (MD)   Rhu
Mount Sinai Med Ctr
21 E 90th St; New York, NY 10128; (212) 860-3077; **BDCERT:** IM 86; Rhu 90; **MS:** NE Ohio U 83; **RES:** Med, Mt Sinai Med Ctr, New York, NY 84-86; **FEL:** Rhu, Mt Sinai Med Ctr, New York, NY 87-89; **FAP:** Clin Instr Mt Sinai Sch Med; **HOSP:** Beth Israel North; **HMO:** Oxford Blue Choice PHCS PHS

Mcr

Jaffe, Israeli A (MD)   Rhu
Columbia-Presbyterian Med Ctr
161 Ft Washington Ave 410; New York, NY 10032; (212) 305-5213; **BDCERT:** IM 58; Rhu 72; **MS:** Columbia P&S 50; **RES:** Columbia-Presbyterian Med Ctr, New York, NY 51-53; Nat Inst Health, Bethesda, MD 53-55; **FEL:** Beth Israel North, New York, NY; **FAP:** Clin Prof Med Columbia P&S; **HOSP:** Beth Israel North; **SI:** *Severe Rheumatoid Arthritis; Systemic Lupus*; **HMO:** +

🔾 🔾 👤 🏥 Immediately

Kagen, Lawrence (MD)   Rhu
Hosp For Special Surgery
535 E 70th St Fl 3; New York, NY 10021; (212) 606-1449; **BDCERT:** IM 67; Rhu 74; **MS:** NYU Sch Med 60; **RES:** Columbia-Presbyterian Med Ctr, New York, NY 60-65; **FEL:** Columbia-Presbyterian Med Ctr, New York, NY; **HOSP:** NY Hosp-Cornell Med Ctr; **SI:** *Muscle Disease; Arthritis*

LANG: Sp; 🔾 🔾 👤 🏥 Mcr 2-4 Weeks 🏧 **VISA** 🔾

Kramer, Sara (MD)   Rhu   PCP
New York University Med Ctr
436 3rd Ave Fl 2; New York, NY 10016; (212) 889-3911; **BDCERT:** IM 81; Rhu 84; **MS:** SUNY Hlth Sci Ctr 78; **RES:** IM, U Hosp of Cleveland, Cleveland, OH 78-81; U Hosp of Cleveland, Cleveland, OH 78-81; **FEL:** Rhu, New York University Med Ctr, New York, NY; **HOSP:** Hosp For Joint Diseases; **SI:** *Lupus; Rheumatoid Arthritis*; **HMO:** Aetna Hlth Plan Health Source United Healthcare CIGNA Oxford +

🔾 👤 🏥 💲 A Few Days 🏧 **VISA** 🔾

Lahita, Robert (MD)   Rhu
St Luke's Roosevelt Hosp Ctr
University Medical Practice, 432 W 58th St 509; New York, NY 10019; (212) 523-7545; **BDCERT:** IM 93; Rhu 97; **MS:** Jefferson Med Coll 73; **RES:** NY Hosp-Cornell Med Ctr, New York, NY 73-76; **FEL:** Rhu, Rockefeller Univ Hosp, New York, NY 76-78; **FAP:** Assoc Prof Columbia P&S; **SI:** *Lupus Erythematosus; Autoimmune Related Diseases*; **HMO:** Oxford Aetna Hlth Plan Blue Cross & Blue Shield Magnacare 1199 +

🔾 🔾 🏥 💲 Mcr 4+ Weeks 🏧 **VISA** 🔾

Lee, Sicy H (MD)   Rhu
Hosp For Joint Diseases
305 2nd Ave Ste 16; New York, NY 10003; (212) 598-6516; **BDCERT:** PS 82; Rhu 84; **MS:** U Cincinnati 79; **RES:** Good Samaritan Hosp, Cincinnati, OH 79-82; **FEL:** Rhu, Hosp For Joint Diseases, New York, NY

🔾 🆂 🔾 🏥 💲 Mcr A Few Days 🏧 **VISA**

Lipschitz, Robin (MD) Rhu
St Luke's Roosevelt Hosp Ctr

Manhattan Medical Group, 4337 Broadway; New York, NY 10033; (212) 568-6300; **BDCERT:** IM 89; Rhu 92; **MS:** South Africa 80; **RES:** IM, Albert Einstein Med Ctr, Philadelphia, PA 83-86; **FEL:** Rhu/A&I, Univ Hosp SUNY Stony Brook, Stony Brook, NY 86-88; **HMO:** Blue Cross & Blue Shield CIGNA HIP Network

Lockshin, Michael Dan (MD)Rhu
Hosp For Special Surgery

523 E 72nd St 4th Fl; New York, NY 10012; (212) 774-2661; **BDCERT:** IM 69; Rhu 72; **MS:** Harvard Med Sch 63; **RES:** Med, Bellevue Hosp Ctr, New York, NY 66-68; **FEL:** Rhu, Columbia-Presbyterian Med Ctr, New York, NY 68-70; **FAP:** Prof Cornell U; **HOSP:** NY Hosp-Cornell Med Ctr; *SI: Lupus; Pregnancy & Rheumatoid Disease*

LANG: Sp, Fr; ♿ 🔟 🔟 🔟 🔟 🔟 2-4 Weeks

Magid, Steven K (MD) Rhu
Hosp For Special Surgery

535 E 70th St; New York, NY 10021; (212) 606-1141; **BDCERT:** IM 79; Rhu 84; **MS:** Cornell U 76; **RES:** NY Hosp-Cornell Med Ctr, New York, NY 76-79; **FEL:** Rhu, Hosp For Special Surgery, New York, NY; **FAP:** Assoc Prof Med Cornell U; **HOSP:** Mem Sloan Kettering Cancer Ctr; *SI: Lyme Disease*; **HMO:** Most

LANG: Sp, Fr; ♿ 🔟 🔟 🔟 🔟 🔟 🔟 2-4 Weeks 🔟
VISA

Marchetta, Paula (MD) Rhu
New York University Med Ctr

40 Park Ave; New York, NY 10016; (212) 696-5415; **BDCERT:** IM 86; Rhu 90; **MS:** NYU Sch Med 83; **RES:** IM, New York University Med Ctr, New York, NY 84-87; **FEL:** Rhu, New York University Med Ctr, New York, NY 87-89; **FAP:** Asst Prof of Clin Med NYU Sch Med; **HMO:** Oxford Health Source Guardian PHS

♿ 🔟 🔟 🔟 🔟 🔟 A Few Days 🔟

Meed, Steven D (MD) Rhu
Lenox Hill Hosp

Mid Manhattan Medical Associates, 270 W End Ave I N; New York, NY 10023; (212) 496-5508; **BDCERT:** IM 79; Rhu 86; **MS:** NYU Sch Med 75; **RES:** IM, Brookdale Univ Hosp Med Ctr, Brooklyn, NY 75-77; IM, Barnes Hosp, St Louis, MO 77-78; **FEL:** Rhu, Barnes Hosp, St Louis, MO 78-79; Rhu, New York University Med Ctr, New York, NY 84-87; **FAP:** Instr NYU Sch Med; **HOSP:** St Luke's Roosevelt Hosp Ctr; *SI: Lyme Disease; Medical Acupuncture*; **HMO:** Oxford Chubb US Hlthcre CIGNA PHS +

LANG: Sp, Yd, Rus; ♿ 🔟 🔟 🔟 🔟 🔟 🔟 🔟

Merrill, Joan T (MD) Rhu
St Luke's Roosevelt Hosp Ctr

425 W 59th St; New York, NY 10019; (212) 523-7090; **BDCERT:** IM 88; Rhu 94; **MS:** Cornell U 85; **RES:** IM, St Luke's Roosevelt Hosp Ctr, New York, NY 85-88; **FEL:** Rhu, New York University Med Ctr, New York, NY 88; **FAP:** Asst Prof Columbia P&S; *SI: Lupus; Rheumatoid Arthritis*; **HMO:** Oxford

🔟 🔟 🔟 🔟 🔟 🔟 2-4 Weeks

Mitnick, Hal J (MD) Rhu
New York University Med Ctr

333 E 34th St 1C; New York, NY 10016; (212) 889-7217; **BDCERT:** IM 76; Rhu 78; **MS:** NYU Sch Med 72; **RES:** Bellevue Hosp Ctr, New York, NY 72-76; **FEL:** New York University Med Ctr, New York, NY 76-78; **FAP:** Clin Prof Med NYU Sch Med; **HOSP:** Bellevue Hosp Ctr; *SI: Arthritis; Osteoporosis*

🔟 🔟 🔟 🔟 🔟 🔟 1 Week

Mundheim, Marshall (MD) Rhu
New York University Med Ctr

121 E 60th St; New York, NY 10022; (212) 838-8890; **BDCERT:** IM 70; Rhu 72; **MS:** SUNY Hlth Sci Ctr 64; **RES:** Bellevue Hosp Ctr, New York, NY 64-67; **FEL:** Rhu, Bellevue Hosp Ctr, New York, NY 67-69; **FAP:** Assoc Prof NYU Sch Med; **HOSP:** Hosp For Joint Diseases; *SI: Rheumatoid Arthritis; Lupus Back Pain Bursitis*

LANG: Sp, Fr; ♿ 🔟 🔟 🔟 🔟 A Few Days 🔟

Nickerson, Katherine (MD) Rhu
Columbia-Presbyterian Med Ctr
161 Fort Washington Ave 221; New York, NY
10032; (212) 305-8039; **BDCERT:** IM 84; Rhu 86;
MS: UC San Francisco 81; **RES:** Columbia-
Presbyterian Med Ctr, New York, NY; Beth Israel
Med Ctr, Boston, MA; **FEL:** Rhu, Columbia-
Presbyterian Med Ctr, New York, NY

♿ ⛶ **S** Immediately

Paget, Stephen (MD) Rhu
Hosp For Special Surgery
535 E 70th St; New York, NY 10021; (212) 606-
1845; **BDCERT:** IM 74; Rhu 76; **MS:** SUNY Hlth Sci
Ctr 71; **RES:** Johns Hopkins Hosp, Baltimore, MD
72-73; **SI:** *Rheumatoid Arthritis; Systemic Lupus*

♿ 📷 Mcr Mcd

Parrish, Edward (MD) Rhu
Columbia-Presbyterian Med Ctr
Hospital for Special Surgery, 523 E 72nd St 4th Flr.;
New York, NY 10021; (212) 606-1743; **BDCERT:**
IM 83; Rhu 86; **MS:** Bowman Gray 80; **RES:** IM,
Columbia-Presbyterian Med Ctr, New York, NY 81-
83; **FEL:** Rhu, Columbia-Presbyterian Med Ctr, New
York, NY 83-85; **SI:** *Immunology*; **HMO:** Oxford
United Healthcare NYLCare Multiplan

LANG: Fr; ♿ 📷 ⛶ Mcr Mcd

Rackoff, Paula (MD) Rhu
Beth Israel Med Ctr
Beth Israel Medical Center, 10 Union Square East
3D; New York, NY 10003; (212) 844-8101;
BDCERT: IM 86; Rhu 94; **MS:** Yale U Sch Med 86;
RES: Yale-New Haven Hosp, New Haven, CT 86-
89; **FEL:** Yale-New Haven Hosp, New Haven, CT
90-92; **SI:** *Osteoporosis; Sjogren's Syndrome*; **HMO:**
Oxford Aetna Hlth Plan Blue Cross & Blue Shield
Health Source PHS +

♿ 📷 👤 ⛶ **S** Mcr Immediately 📷 **VISA** 💳 💳

Radin, Allen (MD) Rhu
Lenox Hill Hosp
1085 Park Ave; New York, NY 10128; (212) 289-
6855; **BDCERT:** IM 80; Rhu 82; **MS:** NYU Sch Med
77; **RES:** Univ Hosp SUNY Stony Brook, Stony
Brook, NY 77-80; **FEL:** Rhu, New York University
Med Ctr, New York, NY 80-82; **FAP:** Clin Instr Med
Cornell U; **HOSP:** NY Hosp-Cornell Med Ctr; **SI:**
Lupus; Rheumatoid Arthritis; **HMO:** Aetna Hlth Plan
CIGNA Independent Health Plan Oxford Prucare +

📷 👤 ⛶ **S** Mcr A Few Days

Salmon, Jane (MD) Rhu
Hosp For Special Surgery
535 E 70th St; New York, NY 10021; (212) 606-
1171; **BDCERT:** IM 81; Rhu 84; **MS:** Columbia P&S
78; **RES:** IM, NY Hosp-Cornell Med Ctr, New York,
NY 79-81; **FEL:** Rhu, Hosp For Special Surgery,
New York, NY 81-83; **FAP:** Prof Cornell U; **HOSP:**
NY Hosp-Cornell Med Ctr; **SI:** *Lupus; Rheumatoid
Arthritis*; **HMO:** Oxford NYLCare Chubb Multiplan

♿ 📷 ⛶ **S** 2-4 Weeks

Schwartzman, Sergio (MD) Rhu
Hosp For Special Surgery
535 E 70th St Rm715W; New York, NY 10021;
(212) 606-1557; **BDCERT:** IM 85; **MS:** Mt Sinai
Sch Med 82; **RES:** Long Island Jewish Med Ctr, New
Hyde Park, NY 82-88; **FEL:** NY Hosp-Cornell Med
Ctr, New York, NY; Hosp For Special Surgery, New
York, NY; **FAP:** Cornell U; **HOSP:** NY Hosp-Cornell
Med Ctr; **SI:** *Lupus; Vasculitis*

LANG: Sp; ♿ 📷 👤 ⛶ **S** Mcr 4+ Weeks 📷 **VISA**

Smiles, Stephen (MD) Rhu
New York University Med Ctr
333 E 34th St; New York, NY 10016; (212) 889-
7217; **BDCERT:** IM 77; Rhu 79; **MS:** SUNY Buffalo
73; **RES:** IM, Bellevue Hosp Ctr, New York, NY; **FEL:**
Rhu, Bellevue Hosp Ctr, New York, NY; **FAP:** Asst
Clin Prof Med NYU Sch Med; **SI:** *Rheumatoid
Arthritis; Osteoporosis*

📷 ⛶ **S** 1 Week

Smith, Margaret D (MD)   Rhu
St Vincents Hosp & Med Ctr NY
121 W 11th St; New York, NY 10011; (212) 924-
1157; **BDCERT:** IM 72; Rhu 74; **MS:** Georgetown U
65; **RES:** Med, Johns Hopkins Hosp, Baltimore, MD
66-68; **FEL:** Nep, UC San Francisco Med Ctr, San
Francisco, CA 69-70; **HMO:** Oxford Blue Choice
PHS

Solomon, Gary (MD)   Rhu
Hosp For Joint Diseases
Rheumatology Associate, 305 2nd Ave Ste 16;
New York, NY 10003; (212) 598-6516; **BDCERT:**
IM 80; Rhu 82; **MS:** Mt Sinai Sch Med 77; **RES:** IM,
Mount Sinai Med Ctr, New York, NY 77-80; Albert
Einstein Med Ctr, Bronx, NY 80-82; **FAP:** Asst Prof
NYU Sch Med; **HOSP:** Beth Israel Med Ctr; **SI:**
Silicone Associated Disorders; Arthritis; **HMO:** Oxford
Prudential PHS

LANG: Sp, Chi; 🔲 🏥 🔲 🔲 🔲 🔲 1 Week **VISA**
🔲

Spiera, Harry (MD)   Rhu
Mount Sinai Med Ctr
1088 Park Ave; New York, NY 10128; (212) 860-
4000; **BDCERT:** IM 65; Rhu 72; **MS:** NYU Sch Med
58; **RES:** Mount Sinai Med Ctr, New York, NY 58-
59; VA Med Ctr-Brooklyn, Brooklyn, NY 59-60;
FEL: Columbia-Presbyterian Med Ctr, New York,
NY 61-63; **FAP:** Clin Prof Mt Sinai Sch Med; **SI:**
Lupus; Scleroderma; **HMO:** Oxford

🔲 🔲 🔲 🔲 🔲 🔲 2-4 Weeks

Spiera, Robert (MD)   Rhu
Hosp For Special Surgery
523 E 72nd St; New York, NY 10021; (212) 606-
1309; **BDCERT:** IM 92; Rhu 94; **MS:** Yale U Sch
Med 89; **RES:** IM, NY Hosp-Cornell Med Ctr, New
York, NY 89-92; **FEL:** Rhu, Hosp For Special
Surgery, New York, NY 92-95; **FAP:** Asst Prof
Cornell U; **HOSP:** NY Hosp-Cornell Med Ctr

🔲 🔲 🔲 🔲 🔲 2-4 Weeks

Stern, Richard (MD)   Rhu
Hosp For Special Surgery
1385 York Ave P1; New York, NY 10021; (212)
879-2282; **BDCERT:** IM 73; Rhu 76; **MS:** Tufts U
70; **RES:** NY Hosp-Cornell Med Ctr, New York, NY
71-73; **FEL:** Rockefeller Univ Hosp, New York, NY
73-75; Hosp For Special Surgery, New York, NY;
FAP: Assoc Clin Prof Med Cornell U; **HOSP:** NY
Hosp-Cornell Med Ctr; **SI:** *Rheumatoid Arthritis;*
Osteoarthritis; **HMO:** None

🔲 🔲 🔲 🔲 1 Week

SPORTS MEDICINE

Fleiss, David (MD)   SM
Beth Israel Med Ctr
901 5th Ave; New York, NY 10021; (212) 988-
9400; **BDCERT:** OrS 81; **MS:** Columbia P&S 75;
RES: OrS, Hosp For Special Surgery, New York, NY
76-79; S, St Luke's Roosevelt Hosp Ctr, New York,
NY 75-76; **FEL:** Trauma, St Vincents Hosp & Med
Ctr NY, New York, NY 79-80; **HOSP:** St Vincents
Hosp & Med Ctr NY; **SI:** *Shoulder Injuries; Knee*
Injuries; **HMO:** Blue Choice Prucare CIGNA PHCS
United Healthcare +

LANG: Sp; 🔲 🔲 🔲 🔲 🔲 🔲 🔲 🔲 A Few Days
🔲 **VISA** 🔲

Henry, Jack (MD)   SM
Columbia-Presbyterian Med Ctr
161 Ft Washington Ave R 236; New York, NY
10032; (212) 305-6959; **BDCERT:** OrS 71; **MS:** U
Tex Med Br, Galveston 64; **RES:** S, Pennsylvania
Hosp, Philadelphia, PA 65-66; **FEL:** OrS, Columbia-
Presbyterian Med Ctr, New York, NY 66-69; **FAP:**
Adjct Prof U North Tx Hlth Sci Ctr, Coll Osteo Med;
SI: *Knee Ligament Injuries; Joint Replacement;* **HMO:**
Aetna Hlth Plan Blue Choice Multiplan Oxford
Prudential +

🔲 🔲 🔲 🔲 🔲 🔲 🔲 🔲 Immediately **VISA** 🔲

Guide to symbols and abbreviations can be found on pages 110-113.

381

Rokito, Andrew (MD)   **SM**
Hosp For Joint Diseases

305 2nd Ave Ste 4; New York, NY 10003; (212)
598-6008; **BDCERT:** OrS 96; **MS:** Boston U 88;
RES: S, New York University Med Ctr, New York,
NY 88-89; OrS, Hosp For Joint Diseases, New York,
NY 89-93; **FEL:** SM, Kerlan-Jobe Ortho Clinic,
Inglewood, CA 93-94; **FAP:** Asst Prof OrS NYU Sch
Med; **HOSP:** New York University Med Ctr; **SI:**
Shoulder and Elbow Surgery; **HMO:** Oxford GHI
Prucare Aetna-US Healthcare Chubb +

LANG: Sp, Rus; 🔲 🔲 🔲 🔲 🔲 🔲 🔲 🔲 1 Week
🔲 *VISA* 🔲 🔲

SURGERY

Ansanelli, Vincent (MD)   **S**
N Shore Univ Hosp-Manhasset

927 Park Ave; New York, NY 10028; (212) 396-
1565; **BDCERT:** S 60; **MS:** SUNY Hlth Sci Ctr 54;
RES: Columbia-Presbyterian Med Ctr, New York,
NY 55-59; **FEL:** Columbia-Presbyterian Med Ctr,
New York, NY; **HOSP:** Lenox Hill Hosp; **SI:** *Breast
Diseases; Breast Surgery w/ Lasers;* **HMO:** Oxford
Vytra US Hlthcre United Healthcare Empire Blue
Cross & Shield +

LANG: Itl, Sp; 🔲 🔲 🔲 🔲 🔲 🔲 Immediately 🔲
VISA 🔲 🔲

Antonacci, Anthony (MD)   **S**
Beth Israel Med Ctr

170 East End Ave Ste 400; New York, NY 10128;
(212) 794-5000; **BDCERT:** S 84; **MS:** Geo Wash U
Sch Med 77; **RES:** NY Hosp-Cornell Med Ctr, New
York, NY; **FEL:** Mem Sloan Kettering Cancer Ctr,
New York, NY; **HOSP:** NY Hosp-Cornell Med Ctr;
HMO: Aetna Hlth Plan Oxford PHS

🔲 🔲 🔲 🔲 🔲 🔲 🔲 Immediately

Attiyeh, Fadi (MD)   **S**
St Luke's Roosevelt Hosp Ctr

1755 York Ave; New York, NY 10128; (212) 996-
1500; **BDCERT:** S 75; CRS 82; **MS:** Lebanon 69;
RES: S, Amer Univ Med Ctr, Beirut, Lebanon 69-73;
FEL: S Onc, Mem Sloan Kettering Cancer Ctr, New
York, NY 73-76; **FAP:** Assoc Clin Prof Columbia
P&S; **HOSP:** Beth Israel North; **SI:** *Colon and Rectal
Cancer; Hepatobiliary Surgery;* **HMO:** Oxford

LANG: Ar, Fr; 🔲 🔲 🔲 A Few Days

Aufses, Arthur (MD)   **S**
Mount Sinai Med Ctr

5 E 98th St Box 1259; New York, NY 10021; (212)
241-7646; **BDCERT:** S 56; **MS:** Columbia P&S 48;
RES: Mount Sinai Med Ctr, New York, NY 54-56;
HMO: Aetna Hlth Plan

Axelrod, Deborah (MD)   **S**
Beth Israel Med Ctr

10 Union Square East Ste 4E; New York, NY
10003; (212) 844-8212; **BDCERT:** S 89; **MS:** Israel
82; **RES:** Beth Israel Med Ctr, New York, NY 82-85;
Beth Israel Med Ctr, New York, NY 86-88; **FEL:**
Mem Sloan Kettering Cancer Ctr, New York, NY
85-86; **FAP:** Asst Prof Albert Einstein Coll Med; **SI:**
Breast Cancer; Oncology; **HMO:** NYLCare Aetna Hlth
Plan Oxford CIGNA United Healthcare +

LANG: Heb, Yd, Sp, Fr, Itl; 🔲 🔲 🔲 🔲 🔲 2-
4 Weeks 🔲 *VISA* 🔲 🔲

Barie, Philip (MD)   **S**
NY Hosp-Cornell Med Ctr

Cornell Surgical Associates, 525 E 68th St L384;
New York, NY 10021; (212) 746-5401; **BDCERT:**
S 85; SCC 87; **MS:** Boston U 77; **RES:** S, NY Hosp-
Cornell Med Ctr, New York, NY 78-84; **FEL:**
Trauma, Surg-Albany Med Coll, Albany, NY 79-
81; **FAP:** Assoc Prof S Cornell U; **HOSP:** Catholic
Med Ctr Bklyn & Qns

LANG: Sp; 🔲 🔲 🔲 🔲 🔲 🔲 🔲 🔲 🔲
Immediately 🔲 *VISA* 🔲

Bauer, Joel (MD)   S
Mount Sinai Med Ctr
25 E 69th St; New York, NY 10021; (212) 517-
8600; **BDCERT:** S 74; **MS:** NYU Sch Med 67; **RES:**
Mount Sinai Med Ctr, New York, NY 67-73; **FAP:**
Prof Mt Sinai Sch Med; *SI: Gastrointestinal Surgery;*
Laparoscopy; **HMO:** Aetna Hlth Plan Oxford Blue
Cross & Blue Shield

LANG: Sp, Fr; ▣ ▣ ▣ ▣ ▣ ▣ ▣   A Few Days
▣ **VISA** ▣

Beaton, Howard L (MD)   S
NYU Downtown Hosp
170 William Street; New York, NY 10038; (212)
312-5373; **BDCERT:** S 82; **MS:** U Rochester 76;
RES: S, NY Hosp-Cornell Med Ctr, New York, NY
76-81; **FAP:** Assoc Prof Cornell U; **HOSP:** New York
University Med Ctr; **HMO:** Oxford US Hlthcre
CIGNA Prudential NYLCare +

LANG: Sp, Chi; ▣ ▣ ▣ ▣ ▣ ▣ ▣ ▣ ▣
A Few Days ▣ **VISA** ▣ ▣

Bebawi, Magdi (MD)   S
North General Hosp
Madison Avenue Physcian Practice, 1824 Madison
Ave; New York, NY 10035; (212) 423-4900;
BDCERT: S 88; **MS:** Egypt 63; **RES:** S, North
General Hosp, New York, NY 81-86; **FAP:** Asst Clin
Prof Mt Sinai Sch Med; *SI: Hernia; Stomach & Colon*
Surgery; **HMO:** US Hlthcre GHI Aetna Hlth Plan
1199 Blue Cross & Blue Shield +

LANG: Sp, Ar; ▣ ▣ ▣ ▣ ▣ ▣ ▣   Immediately
VISA ▣ ▣

Bertagnolli, Monica (MD)   S
NY Hosp-Cornell Med Ctr
525 E 68th St; New York, NY 10021; (212) 746-
2195; **BDCERT:** S 93; **MS:** U Utah 85; **RES:** S,
Brigham & Women's Hosp, Boston, MA 86-92;
FAP: Asst Prof Cornell U; *SI: Gastrointestinal*
Surgery; Oncology; **HMO:** Aetna Hlth Plan
Magnacare CIGNA United Healthcare Oxford +

LANG: Sp; ▣ ▣ ▣ ▣ ▣ ▣ ▣   A Few Days
▣ **VISA** ▣ ▣

Bloom, Norman (MD)   S
Cabrini Med Ctr
240 1st Ave Mh; New York, NY 10009; (212) 505-
6167; **BDCERT:** S 79; **MS:** SUNY Downstate 74;
RES: S, Maimonides Med Ctr, Brooklyn, NY 74-78;
FEL: S Onc, Mem Sloan Kettering Cancer Ctr, New
York, NY 78-79; **FAP:** Asst Clin Prof Mt Sinai Sch
Med; **HOSP:** Mount Sinai Med Ctr; *SI: Surgical*
Oncology; Breast Surgery; **HMO:** Prucare Oxford
CIGNA NYLCare Magnacare +

LANG: Pol, Sp, Rus, Yd; ▣ ▣ ▣ ▣ ▣ ▣
A Few Days

Blumgart, Leslie H (MD)   S
Mem Sloan Kettering Cancer Ctr
1275 York Ave; New York, NY 10021; (212) 639-
5526; **MS:** England; **RES:** United Sheffield Hosp,
England 64-66; S, Nottingham Gen Hosp, England
66-70; **FEL:** Royal Coll of Surgeons, England; **FAP:**
Prof Cornell U; *SI: Liver and Biliary Cancer; Pancreatic*
Cancer; **HMO:** Blue Cross & Blue Shield

LANG: Ger, Fr, Sp; ▣ ▣ ▣ ▣ ▣ ▣ ▣ ▣
A Few Days

Borgen, Patrick (MD)   S
Mem Sloan Kettering Cancer Ctr
205 E 64th St; New York, NY 10021; (212) 639-
5248; **BDCERT:** S 91; **MS:** LSU Sch Med, New
Orleans 84; **RES:** Ochsner Fdn Hosp, New Orleans,
LA; **FEL:** S, Mem Sloan Kettering Cancer Ctr, New
York, NY; *SI: Breast Surgery*

▣

Bossart, Peter (MD)   S
St Luke's Roosevelt Hosp Ctr
16 E 90th St; New York, NY 10128; (212) 876-
0202; **BDCERT:** S 58; **MS:** Cornell U 51; **RES:** S, St
Luke's Roosevelt Hosp Ctr, New York, NY 52-56;
FAP: Asst Clin Prof S Columbia P&S; **HMO:** Aetna-
US Healthcare Blue Shield CIGNA Oxford

LANG: Ger; ▣ ▣ ▣ ▣ ▣ ▣ ▣ ▣   Immediately

Brennan, Murray (MD)   **S**
Mem Sloan Kettering Cancer Ctr

1275 York Ave; New York, NY 10021; (212) 639-6586; **BDCERT:** S 75; **MS:** New Zealand 64; **RES:** Harvard Med Sch, Cambridge, MA 70-75; **FEL:** Peter Bent Brigham Hosp, Boston, MA 72-75; Harvard Med Sch, Cambridge, MA 70-72; **FAP:** Prof Cornell U; **HOSP:** NY Hosp-Cornell Med Ctr; *SI: Soft Tissue-Sarcoma; Pancreatic Cancer*

LANG: Sp; 🔲 🔲 🔲 🔲 🔲

Brower, Steven (MD)   **S**
Mount Sinai Med Ctr

Surgical Oncology AssociatesMt Sinai Med Ctr, 5 E 98th St; New York, NY 10029; (212) 241-3699; **BDCERT:** S 87; **MS:** SUNY Buffalo 78; **RES:** Boston U Med Ctr, Boston, MA 80-81; **FEL:** Cancer S, Nat Cancer Inst, Bethesda, MD 81-83; Boston U Med Ctr, Boston, MA 84-86; **FAP:** Prof S Mt Sinai Sch Med; *SI: Pancreatic Cancer; Gastrointestinal Cancer*; **HMO:** Oxford Aetna Hlth Plan PHS

🔲 🔲 🔲 🔲 🔲 🔲 🔲 🔲 Immediately 🔲 *VISA* 🔲 🔲

Buda, Joseph A (MD)   **S**
Columbia-Presbyterian Med Ctr

161 Fort Washington Ave; New York, NY 10032; (212) 305-5311; **BDCERT:** S 64; **MS:** Cornell U 55; **RES:** S, Columbia-Presbyterian Med Ctr, New York, NY 59-64; **FAP:** Clin Prof S Columbia P&S; **HOSP:** Englewood Hosp & Med Ctr; *SI: Vascular Surgery; General Surgery*; **HMO:** Blue Cross & Blue Shield

LANG: Sp, Itl, Fr; 🔲 🔲 🔲 🔲 🔲 🔲 1 Week

Burchell, Albert (MD)   **S**
St Vincents Hosp & Med Ctr NY

2 5th Ave 9; New York, NY 10011; (212) 254-4242; **BDCERT:** S 64; **MS:** Cornell U 58; **RES:** S, St Vincents Hosp & Med Ctr NY, New York, NY 59-63; **FEL:** S, St Vincents Hosp & Med Ctr NY, New York, NY 63-65; **FAP:** Assoc Prof S NY Med Coll; **HMO:** Oxford Blue Choice United Healthcare US Hlthcre Prucare +

🔲 🔲 🔲 🔲 🔲 🔲 🔲 A Few Days

Burrows, Lewis (MD)   **S**
Mount Sinai Med Ctr

5 E 98th St; New York, NY 10029; (212) 241-8086; **BDCERT:** S 65; **MS:** NYU Sch Med 56; **RES:** Ohio State U Hosp, Columbus, OH 56-57; Mount Sinai Med Ctr, New York, NY 57-63; *SI: Kidney Transplant; GI Surgery*; **HMO:** Oxford Aetna-US Healthcare HIP Network Blue Cross & Blue Shield US Hlthcre +

LANG: Sp; 🔲 🔲 🔲 🔲 🔲 🔲 🔲 🔲 1 Week 🔲 *VISA* 🔲

Cahan, Anthony (MD)   **S**
Beth Israel Med Ctr

531 E 88th St; New York, NY 10128; (212) 861-4101; **BDCERT:** S 88; **MS:** Cornell U 82; **RES:** NY Hosp-Cornell Med Ctr, New York, NY 82-87; **FAP:** Asst Clin Prof S NY Med Coll; **HOSP:** St Agnes Hosp; *SI: Breast Surgery*; **HMO:** Aetna Hlth Plan Blue Choice Oxford US Hlthcre

🔲 🔲 🔲 🔲 🔲 Immediately

Cahan, William George (MD)   **S**
Mem Sloan Kettering Cancer Ctr

1275 York Ave; New York, NY 10021; (212) 737-4734; **BDCERT:** S 50; **MS:** Columbia P&S 39; **RES:** Mem Sloan Kettering Cancer Ctr, New York, NY 41-42; **FEL:** Mem Sloan Kettering Cancer Ctr, New York, NY 45-48; **FAP:** Sr Prof S Cornell U; *SI: Lung Cancer*

🔲 🔲 🔲

Cammarata, Angelo (MD)   **S**
Cabrini Med Ctr

55 E 87th; New York, NY 10128; (212) 427-2131; **BDCERT:** S 68; **MS:** NY Med Coll 62; **RES:** Metropolitan Hosp Ctr, New York, NY 63-67; **FEL:** Mem Sloan Kettering Cancer Ctr, New York, NY 67-68; **FAP:** Assoc Prof S NY Med Coll; **HOSP:** Beth Israel North; *SI: Diseases & Cancer of the Breast*; **HMO:** Oxford CIGNA Aetna Hlth Plan Blue Cross & Blue Shield

LANG: Itl, Sp; 🔲 🔲 🔲 🔲 1 Week

Cassell, Lauren (MD)　　　　S
Lenox Hill Hosp

114 E 78th St A; New York, NY 10021; (212) 535-4040; **BDCERT:** S 83; **MS:** NY Med Coll 77; **RES:** Lenox Hill Hosp, New York, NY 77-82; *SI: Breast Surgery*

🎥 🎥 🎞 💲 Mcr　Immediately

Chabot, John A (MD)　　　　S
Columbia-Presbyterian Med Ctr

161 Ft Washington Ave; New York, NY 10032; (212) 305-2500; **BDCERT:** S 90; **MS:** Dartmouth Med Sch 83; **RES:** Columbia-Presbyterian Med Ctr, New York, NY 83-90; *SI: Liver Bile Duct Gallbladder; Pancreas*

LANG: Sp; 🖐 🎥 🎥 🎞 💲 Mcr NFI　1 Week **VISA** 💳

Cioroiu, Michael (MD)　　　　S
Cabrini Med Ctr

247 3rd Ave Ste L 3; New York, NY 10010; (212) 995-8099; **BDCERT:** S 86; **MS:** Romania 71; **RES:** Cabrini Med Ctr, New York, NY 80-85; **FEL:** S Endoscopy, Mount Sinai Hosp, Cleveland, OH 84; **HOSP:** Metropolitan Hosp Ctr; *SI: Breast Surgery; Surgical Endoscopy*; **HMO:** Oxford US Hlthcre Blue Cross & Blue Shield 32BJ GHI +

LANG: Sp, Hun, Rom, Fr; 🖐 🎥 📞 🎥 🎥 🎞 Mcr Mod WC NFI　A Few Days

Clarke, James (MD)　　　　S
NY Hosp-Cornell Med Ctr

517 E 71st St; New York, NY 10021; (212) 737-2050; **BDCERT:** S 87; **MS:** Cornell U 81; **RES:** S, NY Hosp-Cornell Med Ctr, New York, NY 81-86

Cleary, Joseph (MD)　　　　S
Beth Israel North

133 E 73rd St; New York, NY 10021; (212) 570-0133; **BDCERT:** S 79; **MS:** NY Med Coll 73; **RES:** NY Med Coll, New York, NY 73-78; **HS,** St Luke's Roosevelt Hosp, New York, NY 79; **FEL:** PlS, Columbia Presbyterian Med Ctr, New York, NY 78-80; **FAP:** Asst Clin Prof S NY Med Coll; **HMO:** None

🖐 🎥 🎥 🎥 🎞 Mcr WC　1 Week

Cody, Hiram (MD)　　　　S
Mem Sloan Kettering Cancer Ctr

205 E 64th St Level 1; New York, NY 10021; (212) 639-5244; **BDCERT:** S 80; **MS:** Columbia P&S 74; **RES:** St Luke's Roosevelt Hosp Ctr, New York, NY 74-79; **FEL:** S Onc, Mem Sloan Kettering Cancer Ctr, New York, NY 79-81; **HOSP:** St Luke's Roosevelt Hosp Ctr; *SI: Surgical Oncology; Breast Surgery*; **HMO:** Blue Cross & Blue Shield

🖐 🎥 🎥 🎞 Mcr Mod　Immediately ▨ **VISA** 💳

Coit, Daniel (MD)　　　　S
Mem Sloan Kettering Cancer Ctr

1275 York Ave; New York, NY 10021; (212) 639-8411; **BDCERT:** S 84; **MS:** U Cincinnati 76; **RES:** Med, New England Deaconess Hosp, Boston, MA 76-77; S, New England Deaconess Hosp, Boston, MA 77-83; **FEL:** S, Mem Sloan Kettering Cancer Ctr, New York, NY 83-85; **FAP:** Assoc Prof S Cornell U; *SI: Melanoma; Sarcoma; Gastric Pancreatic Surgery*

🖐 🎥 🎥 🎞 Mcr Mod　Immediately ▨ **VISA** 💳 ▨

Cortese, Armand (MD)　　　　S
NY Hosp-Cornell Med Ctr

50 E 69th St Fl 5; New York, NY 10021; (212) 879-9799; **BDCERT:** S 67; TS 68; **MS:** Cornell U 58; **RES:** S, NY Hosp-Cornell Med Ctr, New York, NY 58-66; **FEL:** NY Hosp-Cornell Med Ctr, New York, NY 67-70; **FAP:** Assoc Clin Prof S Cornell U; *SI: Breast Surgery*; **HMO:** Oxford American Health Plan Blue Cross & Blue Shield PHS

🖐 🎥 🎥 🎞 💲 Mcr　A Few Days

Cunningham, John (MD)　　　　S
Mount Sinai Med Ctr

Mt Sinai Hosp, 5 E 98th St; New York, NY 10029; (212) 241-3699; **BDCERT:** S 92; **MS:** U Wisc Med Sch 85; **RES:** Temple U Hosp, Philadelphia, PA 85-91; **FEL:** Mem Sloan Kettering Cancer Ctr, New York, NY 91-93; **FAP:** Asst Prof Mt Sinai Sch Med; *SI: Breast Surgery; Stomach Surgery*; **HMO:** GHI Blue Cross & Blue Shield US Hlthcre Oxford Aetna Hlth Plan +

🖐 🎥 🎥 🎞 💲 Mcr Mod　A Few Days ▨ **VISA** 💳 ▨

Daliana, Maurizion (MD) S
Cabrini Med Ctr

247 3rd Ave 504; New York, NY 10010; (212)
995-9790; **BDCERT:** S 69; **MS:** Italy 61; **RES:** S,
Columbus Hosp, Newark, NJ 64-68; **FAP:** Asst Prof
S NY Med Coll; **HOSP:** Beth Israel Med Ctr; **HMO:**
Aetna Hlth Plan Blue Cross & Blue Shield
Independent Health Plan

LANG: Sp, Itl; 🚫 🄲 🔲 🛏 Mcr Mod WC NFI
A Few Days

Daly, John M (MD) S
NY Hosp-Cornell Med Ctr

New York HospitalCornell Med Ctr; Dept of Surgery,
525 E 68th St RmF739; New York, NY 10021;
(212) 746-6006; **BDCERT:** S 79; **MS:** Temple U 73;
RES: S, U of Texas Med Sch, Houston, TX 74-78;
FAP: Chrmn S Cornell U; *SI: Surgical Oncology;
Colorectal & Breast Surgery*

🚫 🔲 🛏 Mcr A Few Days ▦ **VISA** ⬤

Decosse, Jerome (MD) S
NY Hosp-Cornell Med Ctr

525 E 68th St Ste F1917; New York, NY 10021;
(212) 746-5414; **BDCERT:** S 61; **MS:** U Minn 52;
RES: St Luke's Roosevelt Hosp Ctr, New York, NY
53-55; **FEL:** Mem Sloan Kettering Cancer Ctr, New
York, NY 55-56

Eng, Kenneth (MD) S
New York University Med Ctr

530 1st Ave; New York, NY 10016; (212) 263-
7301; **BDCERT:** S 73; **MS:** NYU Sch Med 67; **RES:**
New York University Med Ctr, New York, NY 68-
72; **FAP:** Prof S NYU Sch Med; *SI: Colon and Rectal;
Liver Pancreas Gallbladder*; **HMO:** Aetna Hlth Plan
Blue Cross & Blue Shield CIGNA Prucare Oxford +

🚫 🔲 🛏 🍴 S Mcr WC A Few Days ▦ **VISA** ⬤

Enker, Warren (MD) S
Beth Israel Med Ctr

350 E 17th St BH1622; New York, NY 10003;
(212) 420-3960; **BDCERT:** S 73; **MS:** SUNY Hlth
Sci Ctr 67; **RES:** S, U Chicago Hosp, Chicago, IL 67-
72; **FEL:** U Chicago Hosp, Chicago, IL 72-73; U MN
Med Ctr, Minneapolis, MN 73-74; **FAP:** Prof Med
Albert Einstein Coll Med; *SI: Rectal Cancer; Liver
Resections*; **HMO:** Blue Cross & Blue Shield Oxford
Aetna-US Healthcare CIGNA PHCS +

LANG: Fr, Sp, Heb, Yd; 🚫 🔲 🛏 S Mcr A Few Days
▦ **VISA** ⬤

Estabrook, Alison (MD) S
St Luke's Roosevelt Hosp Ctr

425 W 59th St 7A; New York, NY 10032; (212)
523-7500; **BDCERT:** S 85; **MS:** NYU Sch Med 78;
RES: Columbia-Presbyterian Med Ctr, New York,
NY 78-84; **FAP:** Prof S Columbia P&S; *SI: Breast
Diseases*; **HMO:** Oxford Chubb Sanus Empire Blue
Cross & Shield

LANG: Fr, Sp; 🚫 🄲 🔲 🍴 🛏 S Mcr Immediately
VISA ⬤

Fischer, Murry (MD) S
Beth Israel Med Ctr

1st Ave & 16th St; New York, NY 10003; (212)
420-4344; **BDCERT:** S 50; **MS:** U Ark Sch Med 44;
RES: NY Med Coll, New York, NY 47; Montefiore
Med Ctr, Bronx, NY 47-48; **FEL:** Gouverneur Hosp,
New York, NY 48-50; **FAP:** Prof S Albert Einstein
Coll Med; *SI: Gall Bladder Surgery; Colon Surgery*

🚫 🔲 🍴 🛏 S Mcr 1 Week

Flogaites, Theodore (MD) S
St Clare's Hosp & Health Ctr

445 W 23rd St; New York, NY 10011; (212) 889-
8433; **BDCERT:** S 70; **MS:** Greece 58; **RES:** French
Hosp, New York, NY 60-64; Bellevue Hosp Ctr,
New York, NY 64-65; **FEL:** GVS, Methodist Hosp,
Houston, TX 64-65; **HMO:** None

SA/SU 🄲 🔲 🍴 🛏 S WC NFI Immediately

Fondacaro, Paul (MD)   **S**
Lenox Hill Hosp

Madison Medical LLP, 110 E 59th St 10C; New York, NY 10022; (212) 583-2910; **BDCERT:** S 87; **MS:** NYU Sch Med 81; **RES:** Univ Hosp SUNY Bklyn, Brooklyn, NY 81-86; **FAP:** Asst Prof Cornell U; **SI:** *Laparoscopic Surgery;* **HMO:** Chubb Oxford CIGNA US Hlthcre +

LANG: Sp, Itl; 🚫 🔟 🔟 🔟 🔟 🔟 🔟
Immediately 🔲 **VISA** 🔲 🔲

Forde, Kenneth (MD)   **S**
Columbia-Presbyterian Med Ctr

161 Fort Washington Ave; New York, NY 10032; (212) 305-5394; **BDCERT:** S 67; **MS:** Columbia P&S 59; **RES:** Bellevue Hosp Ctr, New York, NY; Columbia-Presbyterian Med Ctr, New York, NY; **SI:** *Colon Polyps; Stomach Tumors;* **HMO:** PHS Metlife Oxford Blue Shield Blue Choice +

🚫 🔟 🔟 🔟 🔟 2-4 Weeks

Freeman, Harold (MD)   **S**
St Luke's Roosevelt Hosp Ctr

133 E 73rd St; New York, NY 10021; (212) 988-4800; **BDCERT:** S 65; **MS:** Howard U 58; **RES:** S, Howard U Hosp, Washington, DC 59-64; Mem Sloan Kettering Cancer Ctr, New York, NY 64-67; **HOSP:** Columbia-Presbyterian Med Ctr; **SI:** *Breast Surgery;* **HMO:** GHI Blue Choice Oxford Multiplan PHS +

🔟 🔟 🔟 🔟 🔟 🔟 A Few Days

Friedman, Eugene W (MD)   **S**
Mount Sinai Med Ctr

715 Park Ave; New York, NY 10021; (212) 737-8757; **BDCERT:** S 52; S 85; **MS:** NYU Sch Med 43; **RES:** S, Morrisania City Hosp, New York, NY 43-45; S, Mount Sinai Med Ctr, New York, NY 47-49; **FEL:** S, Mem Sloan Kettering Cancer Ctr, New York, NY 49-52; **FAP:** Clin Prof S Mt Sinai Sch Med; **HOSP:** Lenox Hill Hosp; **SI:** *Tumors Head & Neck; Tumors of the Breast;* **HMO:** PHCS Oxford Affordable Hlth Plan

LANG: Fr, Ger, Yd; 🚫 🔟 🔟 🔟 🔟 A Few Days 🔲

Friedman, Ira (MD)   **S**
Beth Israel Med Ctr

Park Avenue Surgical Associates, PC, 1175 Park Ave 1C; New York, NY 10128; (212) 369-2222; **BDCERT:** S 64; **MS:** NYU Sch Med 57; **RES:** S, Beth Israel Med Ctr, New York, NY 58-59; S, Beth Israel Med Ctr, New York, NY 61-63; **FEL:** S, New York University Med Ctr, New York, NY 59-61; **FAP:** Assoc Clin Prof Albert Einstein Coll Med; **SI:** *Hernia; Gall Bladder & GI Surgery;* **HMO:** Oxford PHS CIGNA GHI +

LANG: Yd, Man, Sp; 🚫 🔟 🔟 🔟 🔟 🔟 🔟
Immediately

Geller, Peter (MD)   **S**
Columbia-Presbyterian Med Ctr

161 Ft Washington Ave; New York, NY 10032; (212) 305-6657; **BDCERT:** S 86; SCC 89; **MS:** Columbia P&S 80; **RES:** S, Columbia-Presbyterian Med Ctr, New York, NY 80-81; S, Columbia-Presbyterian Med Ctr, New York, NY 85-86; **FAP:** Asst Clin Prof S; **SI:** *Hernia Repair; Laparoscopic Cholecystectomy;* **HMO:** Aetna Hlth Plan Oxford Prudential US Hlthcre Chubb +

LANG: Ger; 🚫 🔟 🔟 🔟 🔟 A Few Days

Goldfarb, Alisan B (MD)   **S**
Mount Sinai Med Ctr

1185 Park Ave; New York, NY 10128; (212) 987-5000; **BDCERT:** S 81; **MS:** Mt Sinai Sch Med 75; **RES:** S, Mount Sinai Med Ctr, New York, NY 75-80; **SI:** *Breast Cancer*

🚫 🔟 🔟 🔟 🔟 A Few Days **VISA** 🔲

Golomb, Frederick (MD)   **S**
New York University Med Ctr

910 5th Ave; New York, NY 10021; (212) 535-8050; **BDCERT:** S 56; **MS:** U Rochester 49; **RES:** Johns Hopkins Hosp, Baltimore, MD 49-50; Bellevue Hosp Ctr, New York, NY 50-56; **FAP:** Prof S NYU Sch Med; **HOSP:** Beth Israel Med Ctr; **SI:** *Melanoma Surgery;* **HMO:** Health Source

🚫 🔟 🔟 Immediately

Gouge, Thomas (MD) **S**
New York University Med Ctr

530 1st Ave 6b; New York, NY 10016; (212) 263-7301; **BDCERT:** S 77; **MS:** Yale U Sch Med 70; **RES:** New York University Med Ctr, New York, NY 70-75; **SI:** *Esophageal Surgery; Stomach Surgery;* **HMO:** Aetna Hlth Plan Oxford Prudential PHS CIGNA +

🔲 🔲 🔲 🔲 🔲 Mcr Mcd WC NFI A Few Days ▓▓ *VISA* 🔲

Greenstein, Adrian (MD) **S**
Mount Sinai Med Ctr

Mount Sinai Medical Center, 5 E 98th St 11th; New York, NY 10029; (212) 241-7646; **BDCERT:** S 69; **MS:** South Africa 56; **RES:** Boston U Med Ctr, Boston, MA 65-68; Royal Postgraduate Sch Med, London, England 63-64; **FAP:** Prof S Mt Sinai Sch Med; **HMO:** Oxford PHCS 1199 Empire Blue Choice

🔲 🔲 🔲 Mcr Immediately

Grossi, Robert (MD) **S**
St Vincents Hosp & Med Ctr NY

20 W 13th St; New York, NY 10011; (212) 838-3055; **BDCERT:** S 87; GVS 89; **MS:** UMDNJ-NJ Med Sch, Newark 81; **RES:** S, St Vincents Hosp & Med Ctr NY, New York, NY 81-86; **FEL:** GVS, Temple U Hosp, Philadelphia, PA 86-87; **FAP:** Clin Instr S Mt Sinai Sch Med; **HOSP:** Cabrini Med Ctr

Hardy, Mark (MD) **S**
Columbia-Presbyterian Med Ctr

161 Fort Washington Ave; New York, NY 10032; (212) 305-5502; **BDCERT:** S 72; **MS:** Albert Einstein Coll Med 62; **RES:** Strong Mem Hosp, Rochester, NY; Albert Einstein Med Ctr, Bronx, NY; **FEL:** Harvard Med Sch, Cambridge, MA; Beth Israel Med Ctr, Boston, MA; **FAP:** Prof S Cornell U; **SI:** *Renal Transplantation; Parathyroid Surgery;* **HMO:** Oxford Blue Cross Aetna Hlth Plan GHI Champus +

LANG: Fr, Pol; 🔲 🔲 🔲 🔲 Mcr Mcd A Few Days

Harris, Matthew N (MD) **S**
New York University Med Ctr

530 1st Ave Ste 6E; New York, NY 10016; (212) 263-7330; **BDCERT:** S 64; **MS:** U Hlth Sci/Chicago Med Sch 56; **RES:** S, Bellevue Hosp Ctr, New York, NY 56-63; **FEL:** Bellevue Hosp Ctr, New York, NY 61-63; **FAP:** Prof S NYU Sch Med; **HOSP:** Bellevue Hosp Ctr; **SI:** *Breast Cancer; Malignant Melanoma;* **HMO:** Oxford

🔲 🔲 🔲 Mcr Immediately

Hecht, Pauline (MD) **S**
NYU Downtown Hosp

201 E 19th St 2H; New York, NY 10003; (212) 477-1660; **BDCERT:** S 61; **MS:** NYU Sch Med 54; **RES:** S, Bellevue Hosp Ctr, New York, NY 55-59; **FAP:** Asst Clin Prof Mt Sinai Sch Med; **SI:** *Breast Surgery;* **HMO:** US Hlthcre PHS Oxford Prudential CIGNA +

Heimann, Tomas (MD) **S**
Mount Sinai Med Ctr

5 E 98th St 11th Fl; New York, NY 10029; (212) 241-3336; **BDCERT:** S 78; **MS:** SUNY Syracuse 71; **RES:** Mount Sinai Med Ctr, New York, NY 72-77; **SI:** *Inflammatory Bowel Disease; Rectal Cancer;* **HMO:** Oxford CIGNA Metlife Aetna Hlth Plan

LANG: Sp; 🔲 🔲 🔲 🔲 Mcr Immediately ▓▓ *VISA* 🔲

Heymann, A Douglas (MD) **S**
Lenox Hill Hosp

Surgical Associates of New York, LLP, 122 E 76th St Ste 1B; New York, NY 10021; (212) 249-0469; **BDCERT:** S 71; **MS:** Albert Einstein Coll Med 65; **RES:** S, Yale-New Haven Hosp, New Haven, CT 65-66; S, Lenox Hill Hosp, New York, NY 67-69; **SI:** *Laparoscopic & Breast Surgery; Biliary Tract & Hernias;* **HMO:** Oxford United Healthcare

🔲 🔲 🔲 🔲 🔲 Mcr WC A Few Days *VISA* 🔲

Hofstetter, Stephen (MD)   S
New York University Med Ctr
530 1st Ave Ste 6C; New York, NY 10016; (212) 263-7302; **BDCERT:** S 77; **MS:** SUNY Hlth Sci Ctr 71; **RES:** S, Bellevue Hosp Ctr, New York, NY 71-76; **FAP:** Assoc Prof S NYU Sch Med; *SI: Laparoscopic Surgery; Hernia Repair;* **HMO:** Aetna Hlth Plan Oxford US Hlthcre Prucare

♿ 🔒 🚗 📷 Mcr Mcd WC   A Few Days *VISA* 💳

Kandalaft, Souheil (MD)   S
St Clare's Hosp & Health Ctr
408 W 57th St; New York, NY 10019; (212) 765-2031; **BDCERT:** S 69; **MS:** Syria 58; **RES:** St Clare's Hosp & Health Ctr, New York, NY 62-66; **HOSP:** St Luke's Roosevelt Hosp Ctr; **HMO:** Aetna Hlth Plan Blue Cross & Blue Shield Oxford CIGNA GHI +

♿ 📞 🔒 🚗 📷 Mcr Mcd WC NFI   Immediately

Katz, L Brian (MD)   S
Mount Sinai Med Ctr
1088 Park Ave; New York, NY 10128; (212) 722-6100; **BDCERT:** S 91; **MS:** South Africa 75; **RES:** Mount Sinai Med Ctr, New York, NY 77-82; **FAP:** Asst Prof Mt Sinai Sch Med; **HOSP:** Lenox Hill Hosp; *SI: Laparoscopic Gallbladder; Laparoscopic Hernia Surgery*

LANG: Heb; ♿ 🔒 🚗 📷 S Mcr   A Few Days 💳

Kemeny, Margaret Mary (MD) S
N Shore Univ Hosp-Manhasset
36 Perry St; New York, NY 10014; **BDCERT:** S 93; **MS:** Columbia P&S 72; **RES:** S, Columbia-Presbyterian Med Ctr, New York, NY 72-74; S, U CO Hosp, Denver, CO 74-76; **FEL:** S Onc, Mem Sloan Kettering Cancer Ctr, New York, NY 76-78; S Onc, Nat Cancer Inst, Bethesda, MD 79-81; **FAP:** Prof NYU Sch Med; **HOSP:** St Vincents Hosp & Med Ctr NY; *SI: Liver Metastases; Breast Cancer*

♿ 🔒 🚗 📷 Mcr Mcd WC NFI   A Few Days

Kent, K Craig (MD)   S
NY Hosp-Cornell Med Ctr
525 E 68th St Flr1911; New York, NY 10021; (212) 746-5192; **BDCERT:** S 92; **MS:** UC San Francisco 81; **RES:** S, UC San Francisco Med Ctr, San Francisco, CA 81-86; **FEL:** GVS, Brigham & Women's Hosp, Boston, MA 86-88; **FAP:** Asst Prof S

Kimmelstiel, Fred (MD)   S
St Luke's Roosevelt Hosp Ctr
225 W 71st St; New York, NY 10024; (212) 362-6060; **BDCERT:** S 95; **MS:** NY Med Coll 80; **RES:** S, St Luke's Roosevelt Hosp Ctr, New York, NY 80-85; **FEL:** Renal Transplantation, Univ Hosp SUNY Stony Brook, Stony Brook, NY; **FAP:** Asst Clin Prof Columbia P&S; **HOSP:** Beth Israel North; *SI: Breast Surgery; Laparoscopic Surgery;* **HMO:** Blue Cross Aetna Hlth Plan Oxford Prudential GHI +

LANG: Sp, Ger; ♿ 📞 🔒 🚗 📷 S Mcr WC
A Few Days

Kinne, David W (MD)   S
Columbia-Presbyterian Med Ctr
16 E 60th St 460; New York, NY 10022; (212) 326-8550; **BDCERT:** S 71; **MS:** SUNY Hlth Sci Ctr 64; **RES:** Columbia-Presbyterian Med Ctr, New York, NY 64-70; **FEL:** Transplant, U MN Med Ctr, Minneapolis, MN

♿ 🔒 🚗 📷 Mcr   A Few Days

Kreel, Isadore (MD)   S
Mount Sinai Med Ctr
25 E 69th St; New York, NY 10021; (212) 517-8600; **BDCERT:** S 60; **MS:** U Toronto 54; **RES:** Mount Sinai Med Ctr, New York, NY 55-60; **HMO:** Oxford

🔒 🚗 📷 S Mcr WC   Immediately 💳 *VISA* 💳

Guide to symbols and abbreviations can be found on pages 110-113.

389

Krieger, Karl (MD) S
NY Hosp-Cornell Med Ctr

525 E 68th St F2103; New York, NY 10021; (212) 746-5151; **BDCERT:** S 85; **MS:** Johns Hopkins U 75; **RES:** S, Johns Hopkins Hosp, Baltimore, MD 75-76; Bellevue Hosp Ctr, New York, NY 76-79; **FEL:** TS, New York University Med Ctr, New York, NY 79-81; **FAP:** Prof Cornell U; **SI:** *Mini Invasive Adult Surgery; Bloodless Adult Surgery;* **HMO:** Aetna Hlth Plan CIGNA HIP Network Metlife Travelers +

LANG: Sp; 👤 📷 🛏 Mcr Mcd WC NFI 1 Week 💳 **VISA** 💳 💳

Laraja, Raymond (MD) S
Cabrini Med Ctr

227 E 19th St Rm 446; New York, NY 10003; (212) 995-6717; **BDCERT:** S 70; **MS:** NYU Sch Med 63; **RES:** Bellevue Hosp Ctr, New York, NY 63-68; **SI:** *Breast Surgery*

LANG: Itl, Sp; 👤 📷 🛏 🏥 💲 Mcr WC 1 Week

Liang, Howard (MD) S
New York University Med Ctr

530 1st Ave 6C; New York, NY 10016; (212) 263-7302; **BDCERT:** S 84; **MS:** Washington U, St Louis 74; **RES:** S, New York University Med Ctr, New York, NY 79-82; **FAP:** Asst Prof NYU Sch Med; **HOSP:** Bellevue Hosp Ctr; **SI:** *Laparoscopic Surgery; Abdominal Surgery;* **HMO:** Oxford First Option Aetna Hlth Plan Prucare Health Source +

👤 📷 🏥 🛏 💲 Mcr Mcd WC NFI 1 Week

Lo Gerfo, Paul L (MD) S
Columbia-Presbyterian Med Ctr

161 Fort Washington Ave; New York, NY 10032; (212) 305-0444; **BDCERT:** S 75; **MS:** SUNY Syracuse 67; **RES:** Columbia-Presbyterian Med Ctr, New York, NY 67-72; **SI:** *Endocrine Surgery; Thyroid and Parathyroid*

LANG: Sp; 👤 📷 🏥 🛏 💲 A Few Days 💳 **VISA** 💳

Lugo, Raul (MD) S
Lenox Hill Hosp

Lenox Hill Surgical, PC, 870 Park Ave; New York, NY 10021; (212) 517-5701; **BDCERT:** S 86; **MS:** NY Med Coll 79; **RES:** S, Lenox Hill Hosp, New York, NY 79-84; **FEL:** S Onc, MD Anderson Cancer Ctr, Houston, TX 84-86; **SI:** *Laparoscopic Laser Surgery; Gastrointestinal Endoscopy;* **HMO:** Prucare CIGNA Blue Choice US Hlthcre Oxford +

LANG: Sp; 👤 💳 📷 🏥 🛏 💲 Mcr 1 Week 💳 **VISA** 💳 💳

Marks, Richard (MD) S
St Luke's Roosevelt Hosp Ctr

125 E 87th St; New York, NY 10128; (212) 247-6575; **BDCERT:** S 74; **MS:** Harvard Med Sch 68; **RES:** St Luke's Roosevelt Hosp Ctr, New York, NY 68-73; **FEL:** GVS, Baylor Coll Med, Houston, TX 75-76; **FAP:** Assoc Clin Prof S Columbia P&S; **SI:** *Laparoscopic Surgery; Hernia Surgery;* **HMO:** None

👤 📷 🏥 🛏 💲 Mcr Immediately

McSherry, Charles K (MD) S
NY Hosp-Cornell Med Ctr

1755 York Ave; New York, NY 10128; (212) 348-0200; **BDCERT:** S 65; **MS:** Cornell U 57; **RES:** NY Hosp-Cornell Med Ctr, New York, NY 57-64; **FEL:** NY Hosp-Cornell Med Ctr, New York, NY 64-65; **FAP:** Clin Prof Cornell U; **HOSP:** Beth Israel Med Ctr; **SI:** *Laparoscopic Surgery; Gastrointestinal Surgery;* **HMO:** Oxford Prucare Blue Cross & Blue Shield Blue Choice +

👤 📷 🏥 🛏 💲 Mcr Mcd WC A Few Days

Miller, Charles (MD) S
Mount Sinai Med Ctr

Recanati/Miller Transplantation Inst, Mt Sinai Med Ctr, 5 E 98th St 14th Fl; New York, NY 10029; (212) 241-8035; **BDCERT:** S 94; **MS:** Mt Sinai Sch Med 78; **RES:** S, Mount Sinai Med Ctr, New York, NY 79-82; S, Mount Sinai Med Ctr, New York, NY 82-83; **FEL:** Transplant, Mount Sinai Med Ctr, New York, NY 80-81; GVS, Mount Sinai Med Ctr, New York, NY 83-84; **FAP:** Prof S Mt Sinai Sch Med; **SI:** *Liver Transplant; Hepatobiliary Surgery;* **HMO:** Most

👤 📷 🛏 💲 Mcr Mcd WC NFI 1 Week 💳 **VISA** 💳

Mills, Christopher B (MD)   S
St Vincents Hosp & Med Ctr NY

31 W 9th St; New York, NY 10011; (212) 473-8633; **BDCERT:** S 79; **MS:** UMDNJ-NJ Med Sch, Newark 73; **RES:** St Vincents Hosp & Med Ctr NY, New York, NY 73-78; **FEL:** Metabolic Support, Ravenswood Hosp Med Ctr, Chicago, IL; **HOSP:** St Joseph's Hosp-Queens; **HMO:** Blue Choice Blue Cross & Blue Shield GHI Prucare Oxford +

🚗 📅 💲 Mcr WC NFI A Few Days 💳 **VISA** 💳 💳

Mizrachy, Benjamin (MD)   S
Mount Sinai Med Ctr

1120 5th Ave; New York, NY 10128; (212) 410-1110; **BDCERT:** S 67; **MS:** South Africa 58; **RES:** S, Mount Sinai Med Ctr, New York, NY 61-62; S, Mount Sinai Med Ctr, New York, NY 62-65; **FEL:** S, Mount Sinai Med Ctr, New York, NY 66-72; **FAP:** Asst Clin Prof Mt Sinai Sch Med; **HOSP:** Beth Israel North; **SI:** *Breast Surgery*; **HMO:** Oxford

LANG: Sp; ♿ 🔌 🚗 🅿 📅 💲 Mcr Immediately

Morrissey, Kevin (MD)   S
NY Hosp-Cornell Med Ctr

50 E 69th St; New York, NY 10021; (212) 744-0060; **BDCERT:** S 72; **MS:** Cornell U 65; **RES:** S, NY Hosp-Cornell Med Ctr, New York, NY 66-71; NY Hosp-Cornell Med Ctr, New York, NY 65-66; **FEL:** Ge, NY Hosp-Cornell Med Ctr, New York, NY 71-73

Nowak, Eugene (MD)   S
NY Hosp-Cornell Med Ctr

325 E 79th St; New York, NY 10021; (212) 517-6693; **BDCERT:** S 82; **MS:** UMDNJ-NJ Med Sch, Newark 75; **RES:** NY Hosp-Cornell Med Ctr, New York, NY 75-80

♿ 🚗 🅿 📅 💲 Mcr WC Immediately **VISA** 💳

Nunez, Domingo (MD)   S
Lenox Hill Hosp

110 E 59th St; New York, NY 10022; (212) 583-2910; **BDCERT:** S 87; **MS:** Columbia P&S 80; **RES:** S, Lenox Hill Hosp, New York, NY; **FEL:** Toronto Gen Hosp, Toronto, Canada; **HOSP:** Beth Israel Med Ctr; **HMO:** CIGNA

♿ 🚗 🅿 📅 💲 Mcr WC Immediately

Nussbaum, Moses (MD)   S
Beth Israel Med Ctr

1st Ave & 16th St; New York, NY 10003; (212) 420-4044; **BDCERT:** S 63; **MS:** NYU Sch Med 55; **RES:** S, Bellevue Hosp Ctr, New York, NY 56-57; S, Beth Israel Med Ctr, New York, NY 57-62; **FEL:** Head & Neck S, Beth Israel Med Ctr, New York, NY 62-63; **FAP:** Lecturer S Albert Einstein Coll Med; **SI:** *Thyroid Surgery; Parathyroid Surgery*; **HMO:** Oxford Aetna PPO PHCS US Hlthcre HealthNet +

LANG: Yd, Heb, Sp; ♿ 🚗 📅 💲 Mcr 2-4 Weeks 💳 **VISA** 💳

Osborne, Michael (MD)   S
NY Hosp-Cornell Med Ctr

428 E 72nd St 100; New York, NY 10021; (212) 794-6085; **MS:** England 70; **RES:** Charing Cross Hosp, London, England 74-77; Royal Marsden Hosp, London, England 77-80; **FEL:** Mem Sloan Kettering Cancer Ctr, New York, NY

♿ 🅿 💲 Mcr A Few Days 💳 **VISA** 💳 💳

Pachter, H Leon (MD)   S
New York University Med Ctr

530 1st Ave 6C; New York, NY 10016; (212) 263-7302; **BDCERT:** S 77; **MS:** NYU Sch Med 71; **RES:** Bellevue Hosp Ctr, New York, NY 71-76; **FEL:** Trauma S, Bellevue Hosp Ctr, New York, NY

♿ 🚗 🅿 📅 💲 Mcr WC NFI A Few Days 💳 **VISA** 💳

Paglia, Michael (MD)   S
St Vincent's Med Ctr-Richmond

1275 York Ave; New York, NY 10021; (212) 639-8679; **BDCERT:** S 63; **MS:** NYU Sch Med 53; **RES:** New York University Med Ctr, New York, NY; **FEL:** S Onc, Mem Sloan Kettering Cancer Ctr, New York, NY; **SI:** *Breast Surgery*; **HMO:** Blue Cross & Blue Shield

♿ 🚗 🅿 📅 Mcr A Few Days

Guide to symbols and abbreviations can be found on pages 110-113.

391

Pertsemlidis, Demetrius (MD) S
Mount Sinai Med Ctr

1199 Park Ave 1A; New York, NY 10128; (212) 860-1056; **BDCERT:** S 66; **MS:** Germany 59; **RES:** Mount Sinai Med Ctr, New York, NY 61-65; **FEL:** Mount Sinai Med Ctr, New York, NY 65-66; **FAP:** Clin Prof S Mt Sinai Sch Med; *SI: Adrenal Tumors; Biliary Tract;* **HMO:** Aetna Hlth Plan Blue Choice Blue Cross & Blue Shield Oxford CIGNA +

LANG: Grk, Ger, Trk; 🚻 📷 👥 🏥 ꔰ Immediately

Petrek, Jeanne (MD) S
Mem Sloan Kettering Cancer Ctr

205 E 64th St; New York, NY 10021; (212) 639-5246; **BDCERT:** S 78; **MS:** Case West Res U 73; **RES:** Peter Bent Brigham Hosp, Boston, MA 73; **FEL:** Cancer S, Mem Sloan Kettering Cancer Ctr, New York, NY 78-80; *SI: Sentinel Lymph Node Biopsy; Premenopausal Breast Cancer;* **HMO:** Blue Cross & Blue Shield Empire Blue Cross & Shield

LANG: Sp; 🚻 📷 👥 🏥 ꔰ ꔰ 1 Week 🔳 **VISA** 🔵

Pilnik, Samuel (MD) S
Lenox Hill Hosp

155 E 72nd St; New York, NY 10021; (212) 249-4200; **BDCERT:** S 68; **MS:** Argentina 55; **RES:** S, Brooklyn Jewish Hosp, Brooklyn, NY 57-60; S, Brookdale Univ Hosp Med Ctr, Brooklyn, NY 56-57; **FAP:** Assoc Clin Prof NY Med Coll; *SI: Breast Oncology*

LANG: Sp; 📷 👥 🏥 ꔰ ꔰ Immediately 🔳 **VISA** 🔵

Pressman, Peter (MD) S
Beth Israel Med Ctr

787 Park Ave; New York, NY 10021; (212) 249-8040; **BDCERT:** S 67; **MS:** Columbia P&S 59; **RES:** S, Columbia-Presbyterian Med Ctr, New York, NY 59-61; Columbia-Presbyterian Med Ctr, New York, NY 61-63; **FAP:** Clin Prof S Albert Einstein Coll Med; **HOSP:** Lenox Hill Hosp; *SI: Breast Cancer*

🚻 📷 👥 🏥 ꔰ ꔰ Immediately 🔳 **VISA** 🔵

Reader, Robert (MD) S
NYU Downtown Hosp

170 William St; New York, NY 10038; (212) 312-5255; **BDCERT:** S 81; **MS:** Univ Penn 75; **RES:** SM, New York University Med Ctr, New York, NY 75-80; **HOSP:** New York University Med Ctr; *SI: Breast Surgery; Intestinal and Hernia Surgery;* **HMO:** Oxford Aetna-US Healthcare United Healthcare 1199 Blue Shield +

LANG: Sp; 🚻 📷 👥 🏥 ꔰ ꔰ A Few Days

Reiner, Mark (MD) S
Mount Sinai Med Ctr

1010 5th Ave; New York, NY 10028; (212) 879-6677; **BDCERT:** S 80; **MS:** SUNY Hlth Sci Ctr 74; **RES:** S, Mount Sinai Med Ctr, New York, NY 74-79; **HOSP:** Lenox Hill Hosp; *SI: Laparoscopic Surgery*

🚻 📷 👥 🏥 ꔰ ꔰ 1 Week 🔳 **VISA** 🔵

Rosenberg, Vladimir (MD) S
Mount Sinai Med Ctr

114 E 72nd St 1D; New York, NY 10021; (212) 772-2331; **BDCERT:** S 78; **MS:** Argentina 65; **RES:** S, Mount Sinai Med Ctr, New York, NY 72-77; **FEL:** S, MD Anderson Cancer Ctr, Houston, TX 77-78; **FAP:** Asst Clin Prof S Mt Sinai Sch Med; **HOSP:** Beth Israel Med Ctr; *SI: Breast Cancer; Melanoma*

📷 👥 🏥 ꔰ Immediately

Roses, Daniel F (MD) S
New York University Med Ctr

530 1st Ave; New York, NY 10016; (212) 263-7330; **BDCERT:** S 75; **MS:** NYU Sch Med 69; **RES:** Bellevue Hosp Ctr, New York, NY 69-74; **FAP:** Whitehill Prof S NYU Sch Med; *SI: Breast Cancer and Melanoma; Thyroid & Parathyroid Surgery;* **HMO:** Oxford

🚻 📷 🏥 ꔰ A Few Days

Rudick, Jack (MD)　　S
Mount Sinai Med Ctr

1060 5th Ave; New York, NY 10128; (212) 534-8148; **BDCERT:** S 61; **MS:** South Africa 57; **RES:** Baragwanath Gen Hosp, Johannesberg, South Africa 58; Royal Infirmary, Glasgow, Scotland 59-64; **FEL:** U WA Med Ctr, Seattle, WA; **FAP:** Prof S Mt Sinai Sch Med; **HOSP:** Beth Israel Med Ctr; *SI: Laparoscopic Surgery; Gastrointestinal Surgery*; **HMO:** Oxford US Hlthcre CIGNA PHCS Prucare +

LANG: Sp, Dut, Ger; 🚹 🔒 📹 🏧 Mcr Mcd NFI Immediately

Salky, Barry (MD)　　S
Mount Sinai Med Ctr

1010 5th Ave; New York, NY 10028; (212) 987-0410; **BDCERT:** S 79; **MS:** U Tenn Ctr Hlth Sci, Memphis 70; **RES:** Mount Sinai Med Ctr, New York, NY 71-73

🚹 🔒 📹 🏧 S Mcr WC　A Few Days AMEX **VISA** 💳

Schnabel, Freya (MD)　　S
Columbia-Presbyterian Med Ctr

161 Fort Washington Ave Ste 1011; New York, NY 10032; (212) 305-1534; **BDCERT:** S 88; **MS:** NYU Sch Med 82; **RES:** New York University Med Ctr, New York, NY 82-87; **FEL:** Univ Hosp SUNY Bklyn, Brooklyn, NY 87-88; **FAP:** Assoc Prof of Clin Columbia P&S; **HOSP:** South Nassau Comm Hosp; *SI: Breast Surgery*

LANG: Sp; 🚹 🔒 📹 🏧 S Mcr　1 Week **VISA** 💳

Sekons, David (MD)　　S
Beth Israel Med Ctr

41 5th Ave; New York, NY 10003; (212) 228-3001; **BDCERT:** S 85; **MS:** Israel 76; **RES:** S, Beth Israel Med Ctr, New York, NY 77-78; S, Beth Israel Med Ctr, New York, NY 78-82; **FEL:** GI Endoscopy, Beth Israel Med Ctr, New York, NY 82-83; **FAP:** Asst Clin Prof Albert Einstein Coll Med; **HOSP:** St Vincents Hosp & Med Ctr NY; *SI: Breast Diseases; Abdominal Surgery*; **HMO:** Oxford Aetna-US Healthcare Prucare NYLCare GHI +

LANG: Heb, Sin, Yd, Itl, Rus; 🚹 📢 🔒 📹 🏧 S Mcr Mcd WC NFI　A Few Days

Shah, Jatin (MD)　　S
Mem Sloan Kettering Cancer Ctr

1275 York Ave C979; New York, NY 10021; (212) 639-7604; **BDCERT:** S 75; **MS:** India 64; **RES:** GVS, NY Infirmary, New York, NY 72-74; **FEL:** S Onc, Mem Sloan Kettering Cancer Ctr, New York, NY; *SI: Head & Neck Surgery; Tumors-Cancer of Head Neck*; **HMO:** Blue Shield

LANG: Sp, Chi, Hin; 🚹 🔒 📹 🏧 S Mcr　1 Week

Slater, Gary (MD)　　S
Mount Sinai Med Ctr

Mount Sinai Medical Center, 5 E 98th St; New York, NY 10029; (212) 241-7646; **BDCERT:** S 75; **MS:** NYU Sch Med 68; **RES:** Mount Sinai Med Ctr, New York, NY 68-74; *SI: Inflammatory Bowel Disease; Colorectal Surgery*

🚹 🔒 📹 🏧 S Mcr WC　Immediately AMEX **VISA**

Smith, Aloysius G (MD)　　S
St Vincents Hosp & Med Ctr NY

5 E 83rd St; New York, NY 10028; (212) 288-0450; **BDCERT:** S 80; **PlS** 85; **MS:** Jamaica 73; **RES:** S, Metropolitan Hosp Ctr, New York, NY 74-79; PS, Mayo Clinic, Rochester, MN 80-82; **FEL:** HS, Metropolitan Hosp Ctr, New York, NY 79-80; **HOSP:** Our Lady of Mercy Med Ctr; **HMO:** 1199 GHI Sanus Oxford US Hlthcre +

🚹 SA/SD 📢 🔒 📹 🏧 S Mcr Mcd WC NFI　Immediately **VISA** 💳

Spiro, Ronald H (MD)　　S
Mem Sloan Kettering Cancer Ctr

425 E 67th St; New York, NY 10021; (212) 639-6062; **BDCERT:** S 62; **MS:** SUNY Hlth Sci Ctr 55; **RES:** VA Med Ctr-Bronx, Bronx, NY 56-60; **FEL:** S Onc, Mem Sloan Kettering Cancer Ctr, New York, NY 62-65; **FAP:** Prof of Clin S Cornell U; *SI: Head & Neck Surgery*

🚹 🔒 📹 🏧 Mcr Mcd　A Few Days

Strong, Elliot (MD)   S
Mem Sloan Kettering Cancer Ctr

425 E 67th St C975; New York, NY 10021; (212) 639-5840; **BDCERT:** S 63; **MS:** Tufts U 56; **RES:** Hartford Hosp, Hartford, CT 57-61; **FEL:** S Onc, Mem Sloan Kettering Cancer Ctr, New York, NY 61-63; **FAP:** Prof S Cornell U; **HMO:** Empire Blue Cross & Shield

LANG: Sp, Rus, Grk, Itl, Prt; 🅑 🎦 📷 🏥 📅 Mcr A Few Days 🔲 *VISA* 💳 🔲

Strong, Leslie (MD)   S
Beth Israel Med Ctr

28 W 12th St; New York, NY 10011; (212) 645-0052; **BDCERT:** S 75; **MS:** UCLA 67; **RES:** Kings County Hosp Ctr, Brooklyn, NY 69-73; Harlem Hosp Ctr, New York, NY 68-69; **FAP:** Prof; *SI: Breast Surgery; Breast Cancer*

🅑 🅲 📷 🏥 📅 🆂 Mcr 2-4 Weeks 🔲

Swistel, Alexander (MD)   S
St Luke's Roosevelt Hosp Ctr

530 E 70th St M104; New York, NY 10021; (212) 988-8007; **BDCERT:** S 84; **MS:** Brown U 75; **RES:** St Luke's Roosevelt Hosp Ctr, New York, NY 75-76; St Luke's Roosevelt Hosp Ctr, New York, NY 76-81; **FEL:** S Onc, Mem Sloan Kettering Cancer Ctr, New York, NY; **HOSP:** St Luke's Roosevelt Hosp Ctr; **HMO:** Oxford Aetna Hlth Plan Prucare Chubb PHS +

🅑 🏥 📅 🆂 Mcr Immediately 🔲 *VISA* 💳

Tartter, Paul (MD)   S
Mount Sinai Med Ctr

5 E 94th St; New York, NY 10128; (212) 410-6399; **BDCERT:** S 83; **MS:** Brown U 77; **RES:** S, Mount Sinai Med Ctr, New York, NY 77-82; **FAP:** Assoc Prof Mt Sinai Sch Med; *SI: Breast Cancer Surgery;* **HMO:** Oxford GHI Empire Blue Cross & Shield

LANG: Sp, Yd; 📷 🏥 📅 🆂 Mcr 1 Week 🔲

Todd, George (MD)   S
Columbia-Presbyterian Med Ctr

161 Fort Washington Ave; New York, NY 10032; (212) 305-5505; **BDCERT:** S 80; GVS 86; **MS:** Penn State U-Hershey Med Ctr 74; **RES:** GVS, Columbia-Presbyterian Med Ctr, New York, NY 75-79; **FEL:** GVS, Columbia-Presbyterian Med Ctr, New York, NY 79-80; **FAP:** Assoc Prof of Clin S Columbia P&S; **HOSP:** Valley Hosp; *SI: Carotid Artery Surgery; Aneurysm;* **HMO:** Oxford Aetna Hlth Plan PHS Multiplan Blue Cross & Blue Shield +

LANG: Sp; 🅑 🎦 🅲 📷 🏥 📅 Mcr NfI Immediately *VISA* 💳

Turnbull, Alan (MD)   S
Mem Sloan Kettering Cancer Ctr

1275 York Ave; New York, NY 10021; (212) 639-7562; **BDCERT:** S 69; **MS:** McGill U 61; **RES:** Royal Victoria Hosp, Montreal, Canada 61-67; **FEL:** S Onc, Mem Sloan Kettering Cancer Ctr, New York, NY 67-69; Thoracic Oncology, NY Hosp-Cornell Med Ctr, New York, NY 69-71; *SI: Stomach and Esophageal Cancer; Colon Sarcoma;* **HMO:** Empire Blue Cross & Shield

LANG: Fr; 🅑 📷 🏥 📅 Mcr A Few Days

Wallack, Marc (MD)   S
St Vincents Hosp & Med Ctr NY

St Vincent's Hosp - Dept of Surgery, 153 W 11th St; New York, NY 10011; (212) 604-8344; **BDCERT:** S 79; **MS:** Univ Pittsburgh 70; **RES:** S, Hosp of U Penn, Philadelphia, PA 71-77; **FEL:** Onc, Wistar Inst Anatomy & Biology, Philadelphia, PA 73-77; **FAP:** Prof S NY Med Coll; **HOSP:** NY Hosp-Cornell Med Ctr; *SI: Melanoma; Breast Surgery;* **HMO:** Aetna Hlth Plan GHI Oxford Prudential United Healthcare +

🅑 🏥 📅 🆂 Mcr 1 Week

Wantz, George (MD)   S
NY Hosp-Cornell Med Ctr

310 E 72nd St; New York, NY 10021; (212) 249-2415; **BDCERT:** S 54; **MS:** U Mich Med Sch 46; **RES:** Rush Presbyterian-St Lukes Med Ctr, Chicago, IL; NY Hosp-Cornell Med Ctr, New York, NY; *SI: Abdominal Wall Hernias;* **HMO:** PHCS

🅑 📷 🏥 📅 Mcr WC 1 Week

Weiss, Marshall (MD)   **S**
Mount Sinai Med Ctr

785 Park Ave; New York, NY 10021; (212) 861-7755; **BDCERT:** S 63; **MS:** Northwestern U 57; **RES:** SM, Mount Sinai Med Ctr, New York, NY 58-62; **FAP:** Assoc Clin Prof Mt Sinai Sch Med; **HOSP:** Beth Israel North; **SI:** *Breast Surgery*; **HMO:** PHCS PHS Premier

🦽 📷 👪 🛏 💲 A Few Days 🖼 **VISA** 💳

Yurt, Roger (MD)   **S**
NY Hosp-Cornell Med Ctr

525 E 68th St L706; New York, NY 10021; (212) 746-5410; **BDCERT:** S 80; **MS:** U Miami Sch Med 72; **RES:** Parkland Mem Hosp, Dallas, TX 72-74; NY Hosp-Cornell Med Ctr, New York, NY 78-80; **FEL:** Harvard Med Sch, Cambridge, MA; **SI:** *Burn Injury; Wound Problems*

🦽 📷 👪 🛏 Mcr Mcd WC NFI A Few Days

THORACIC SURGERY

Altorki, Nasser (MD)   **TS**
NY Hosp-Cornell Med Ctr

525 E 68th St; New York, NY 10021; (212) 746-5156; **BDCERT:** S 86; TS 88; **MS:** Egypt 78; **RES:** U Chicago Hosp, Chicago, IL 81-85; **FEL:** U Chicago Hosp, Chicago, IL 85-87; **SI:** *Esophageal Cancer; Lung Cancer*; **HMO:** Oxford US Hlthcre ABC Health Blue Choice +

LANG: Ar, Itl; 🦽 📷 👪 🛏 Mcr Mcd WC NFI
Immediately 🖼 **VISA** 💳

Bains, Manjit (MD)   **TS**
Mem Sloan Kettering Cancer Ctr

1275 York Ave; New York, NY 10021; (212) 639-7450; **BDCERT:** TS 72; **MS:** India 63; **RES:** Rochester Gen Hosp, Rochester, NY 66-70; **HMO:** Most

🦽 📷 🛏 Mcr 🖼 **VISA** 💳 💳

Bonfils-Roberts, Enrique (MD) TS
St Vincents Hosp & Med Ctr NY

36 7th Ave 518; New York, NY 10011; (212) 675-7677; **BDCERT:** TS 71; S 71; **MS:** Argentina 62; **RES:** S, Geo Wash U Med Ctr, Washington, DC 64-66; S, St Vincents Hosp & Med Ctr NY, New York, NY 66-69; **FEL:** TS, Mayo Clinic, Rochester, MN 69-71; **FAP:** Assoc Clin Prof S NY Med Coll; **SI:** *Lung & Esophageal Cancer*; **HMO:** Aetna Hlth Plan Blue Choice Blue Cross & Blue Shield Oxford Empire +

LANG: Sp, Fr; 🦽 📷 🛏 💲 Mcr Mcd 1 Week

Boyd, Arthur D (MD)   **TS**
New York University Med Ctr

NYU Medical Ctr, 530 1st Ave Ste 6D; New York, NY 10016; (212) 263-7287; **BDCERT:** S 66; TS 67; **MS:** Univ Pittsburgh 57; **RES:** S, Johns Hopkins Hosp, Baltimore, MD 58-60; S, Cincinnati Gen Hosp, Cincinnati, OH 60-65; **FEL:** S, Johns Hopkins Hosp, Baltimore, MD 58-59; Cincinnati Gen Hosp, Cincinnati, OH 62-63; **FAP:** Prof NYU Sch Med; **HOSP:** Bellevue Hosp Ctr; **SI:** *Carcinoma of Lung; Mediastinal Chest Wall*; **HMO:** Blue Choice CIGNA Oxford HIP Network Aetna Hlth Plan +

🦽 📷 👪 🛏 💲 Mcr Mcd NFI Immediately

Camunas, Jorge (MD)   **TS**
Mount Sinai Med Ctr

Mount Sinai HospitalCardiothoracic Surgery Associates, 5 E 98th St FL12; New York, NY 10029; (212) 241-8181; **BDCERT:** TS 82; **MS:** Georgetown U 70; **RES:** S, Harlem Hosp Ctr, New York, NY 70-76; TS, Mount Sinai Med Ctr, New York, NY 78-80; **FAP:** Assoc Prof Mt Sinai Sch Med; **SI:** *Pacemakers & Defibrillators; Lung Tumors*; **HMO:** Oxford US Hlthcre

LANG: Sp, Itl, Fr, Kor; 🦽 📷 👪 🛏 Mcr Mcd WC NFI

Connery, Cliff (MD)   TS
St Luke's Roosevelt Hosp Ctr

St Lukes Roosevelt Hospital Center Div Cardithor Surg, 1111 Amsterdam Ave; New York, NY 10025; (212) 523-2798; **BDCERT:** TS 93; CCM 93; **MS:** Eastern VA Med Sch, Norfolk 84; **RES:** S, Univ Hosp SUNY Stony Brook, Stony Brook, NY 84-89; TS, Strong Mem Hosp, Rochester, NY 90-92; **FEL:** Strong Mem Hosp, Rochester, NY 89-90; **FAP:** Asst Prof Columbia P&S; **HOSP:** North General Hosp; **HMO:** HIP Network Oxford Prucare Aetna-US Healthcare

LANG: Ger, Sp; 🅰 🅰 🅰 🅰 🆂 Mcr Mod   1 Week

Crawford, Bernard (MD)   TS
New York University Med Ctr

530 1st Ave 3A; New York, NY 10016; (212) 263-7365; **BDCERT:** S 89; TS 89; **MS:** Geo Wash U Sch Med 80; **RES:** New York University Med Ctr, New York, NY 80-85; **FEL:** TS, New York University Med Ctr, New York, NY 85-87; **HOSP:** NYU Downtown Hosp; **SI:** *Lung Cancer; Mediastinal Tumors;* **HMO:** Oxford Aetna Hlth Plan CIGNA

LANG: Sp; 🅰 🅰 🅰 Mcr   Immediately

Ergin, M Arisan (MD & PhD)   TS
Mount Sinai Med Ctr

Box 1028, 1 Gustave Levy Pl; New York, NY 10029; (212) 241-8181; **BDCERT:** TS 79; **MS:** Turkey 68; **RES:** S, Kings County Hosp Ctr, Brooklyn, NY 71-73; **FEL:** TS, Kings County Hosp Ctr, Brooklyn, NY 74-76; **FAP:** Prof Mt Sinai Sch Med; **SI:** *Cardiac Surgery;* **HMO:** Oxford US Hlthcre Aetna Hlth Plan

🅰 🅰 🅰 Mcr Mod   2-4 Weeks ▦ *VISA* 💳 ▦

Galloway, Aubrey (MD)   TS
New York University Med Ctr

530 1st Ave 9V; New York, NY 10016; (212) 263-7185; **BDCERT:** TS 87; **MS:** Tulane U 78; **RES:** S, U CO Hosp, Denver, CO 83; **FEL:** TS, New York University Med Ctr, New York, NY 85; **HOSP:** Bellevue Hosp Ctr; **SI:** *Minimally Invasive;* **HMO:** Oxford Prucare Chubb

LANG: Sp; 🅰 🅰 🅰 🅰 Mcr Mod WC NFI   1 Week

Ginsberg, Robert (MD)   TS
Mem Sloan Kettering Cancer Ctr

Chief Thoracic Service Memorial Sloan Kettering, 1275 York Ave; New York, NY 10021; (212) 639-2806; **MS:** U Toronto 63; **RES:** S, U Toronto Gen Hosp, Toronto, Canada 63-68; TS, U Toronto Gen Hosp, Toronto, Canada 69; **FEL:** TS, Baylor Med Ctr, Dallas, TX 70; Pul, University Birmingham, Birmingham, England 71; **FAP:** Prof S Cornell U; **SI:** *Lung Cancer; Esophageal Cancer*

🅰 🅰 🅰 🅰 Mcr Mod WC   A Few Days

Ginsburg, Mark (MD)   TS
Columbia-Presbyterian Med Ctr

Columbia Thoracic Assoc, 161 Ft Washington Ave 310; New York, NY 10032; (212) 305-3408; **BDCERT:** S 96; TS 97; **MS:** Tufts U 80; **RES:** S, Strong Mem Hosp, Rochester, NY 80-85; **FEL:** TS, Strong Mem Hosp, Rochester, NY 85-87; **FAP:** Asst Clin Prof S Columbia P&S; **HMO:** Oxford Aetna-US Healthcare HIP Network Blue Choice Independent Health Plan +

🅰 🅰 🅰 🅰 🆂 Mcr WC NFI   Immediately

Griepp, Randall (MD)   TS
Mount Sinai Med Ctr

Annenberg Building Room 754, 1 Gustave Levy Pl; New York, NY 10029; (212) 241-8181; **BDCERT:** TS 78; **MS:** Stanford U 67; **RES:** TS, Stanford Med Ctr, Stanford, CA 68-73; **FEL:** TS, Stanford Med Ctr, Stanford, CA 71-72; **HMO:** Aetna Hlth Plan Oxford US Hlthcre

Isom, O Wayne (MD)   TS
NY Hosp-Cornell Med Ctr

525 E 68th St; New York, NY 10021; (212) 746-5151; **BDCERT:** TS 72; **MS:** Univ Texas, Houston 65; **RES:** Parkland Mem Hosp, Dallas, TX 65-70; **FEL:** TS, New York University Med Ctr, New York, NY 70-72; **FAP:** Prof CRS Cornell U; **SI:** *Coronary Artery Disease; Valvular Heart Disease;* **HMO:** Aetna Hlth Plan HIP Network CIGNA Metlife

LANG: Sp, Chi; 🅰 🅲 🅰 🅰 🅰 Mcr WC NFI   A Few Days ▦ *VISA* 💳 ▦

Keller, Steven M (MD)　　　**TS**
Beth Israel Med Ctr

350 E 17th St Fl 15; New York, NY 10003; (212) 420-4459; **BDCERT:** S 86; TS 88; **MS:** Albany Med Coll 77; **RES:** Med, Long Island Jewish Med Ctr, New Hyde Park, NY 77; S, Mount Sinai Med Ctr, New York, NY 79-85; **FEL:** S Onc, Nat Cancer Inst, Bethesda, MD 81-83; TS, Mem Sloan Kettering Cancer Ctr, New York, NY 85-87; **FAP:** Assoc Prof Albert Einstein Coll Med; *SI: Lung Cancer; Esophageal Cancer;* **HMO:** Oxford HIP Network GHI Aetna Hlth Plan US Hlthcre +

🔲 🔲 🔲 🔲 **S** 🔲 🔲 🔲 🔲 A Few Days ▨ **VISA** 🔲 🔲

Kirschner, Paul A (MD)　　　**TS**
Mount Sinai Med Ctr

Mt Sinai Med Center, 1 Gustave Levy Pl Box1028; New York, NY 10029; (212) 241-5421; **BDCERT:** S 50; TS 51; **MS:** Columbia P&S 41; **RES:** TS, VA Med Ctr-Bronx, Bronx, NY 47-48; **FAP:** Prof Mt Sinai Sch Med; *SI: Mediastinal Tumors; Thymus*

🔲 🔲 🔲 A Few Days

Krellenstein, Daniel (MD)　　　**TS**
Mount Sinai Med Ctr

16 E 98th St 1F; New York, NY 10029; (212) 423-9311; **BDCERT:** TS 77; S 74; **MS:** SUNY Buffalo 64; **HMO:** PHS Oxford HealthNet

Lajam, Fouad E (MD)　　　**TS**
Mount Sinai Med Ctr

150 E 77th St; New York, NY 10021; (212) 772-8091; **BDCERT:** S 71; TS 74; **MS:** Dominican Republic 62; **RES:** TS, Mount Sinai Med Ctr, New York, NY 70-72; S, Mt Sinai, New York, NY 64-69; **FEL:** TS, Mount Sinai Med Ctr, New York, NY 69-70; **FAP:** Asst Lecturer TS Mt Sinai Sch Med; **HMO:** Most

LANG: Sp; 🔲 🔲 🔲 🔲 🔲 🔲 🔲 🔲 Immediately

Lansman, Steven (MD)　　　**TS**
Mount Sinai Med Ctr

1 Gustave Levy Pl; New York, NY 10029; (212) 241-8181; **BDCERT:** TS 86; **MS:** SUNY Hlth Sci Ctr 77; **RES:** S, Montefiore Med Ctr, Bronx, NY 77-82; **FEL:** TS, Univ Hosp SUNY Bklyn, Brooklyn, NY 82-84; **FAP:** Assoc Prof Mt Sinai Sch Med; *SI: Coronary Bypass; Heart Transplant*

🔲 🔲 🔲 🔲 🔲 2-4 Weeks

Michler, Robert (MD)　　　**TS**
Columbia-Presbyterian Med Ctr

177 Fort Washington Ave; New York, NY 10032; (212) 305-5933; **BDCERT:** TS 90; S 88; **MS:** Dartmouth Med Sch 81; **RES:** Columbia-Presbyterian Med Ctr, New York, NY; **FEL:** Columbia-Presbyterian Med Ctr, New York, NY; Harvard Med Sch, Cambridge, MA; **HMO:** Blue Cross & Blue Shield Oxford Aetna Hlth Plan PHS GHI +

🔲 🔲 🔲 🔲 🔲 🔲 🔲 Immediately ▨ **VISA** 🔲 🔲

Raskin, Noel (MD)　　　**TS**
Cabrini Med Ctr

117 E 18th St; New York, NY 10003; (212) 254-7886; **BDCERT:** TS 86; **MS:** NY Med Coll 77; **RES:** St Vincents Hosp & Med Ctr NY, New York, NY 77-78; Univ Hosp SUNY Stony Brook, Stony Brook, NY 78-82; **FEL:** U Miami Hosp, Miami, FL 82-84; Thoracic Oncology, U Miami Hosp, Miami, FL 84-85; **HOSP:** Beth Israel Med Ctr; *SI: Lung Cancer; Video Assisted Chest Surgery;* **HMO:** Aetna Hlth Plan CIGNA Oxford Blue Cross HIP Network +

LANG: Fr, Sp; 🔲 🔲 🔲 🔲 **S** 🔲 🔲 🔲 🔲
A Few Days

Rosengart, Todd (MD)　　　**TS**
NY Hosp-Cornell Med Ctr

525 E 68th St; New York, NY 10021; (212) 746-5151; **BDCERT:** S 90; TS 92; **MS:** Northwestern U 83; **RES:** New York University Med Ctr, New York, NY 89; **FEL:** TS, NY Hosp-Cornell Med Ctr, New York, NY; Mem Sloan Kettering Cancer Ctr, New York, NY; **FAP:** Assoc Prof Cornell U; *SI: Bloodless Surgery; Gene Therapy;* **HMO:** Oxford

LANG: Sp; 🔲 🔲 🔲 🔲 🔲 🔲 A Few Days

Rusch, Valerie (MD) TS
Mem Sloan Kettering Cancer Ctr
Memorial Sloan Kettering Cancer Ctr, 1275 York Ave Ste 867; New York, NY 10021; (212) 639-5873; **BDCERT:** TS 83; S 81; **MS:** Columbia P&S 75; **RES:** S, U WA Med Ctr, Seattle, WA 75-80; Cv, U WA Med Ctr, Seattle, WA 80-82; **FAP:** Prof S Cornell U; **SI:** *Lungs & Esophageal Cancer; Mesothelioma*

LANG: Fr, Sp; ▭ ▭ ▭ Immediately

Skinner, David B (MD) TS
Columbia-Presbyterian Med Ctr
525 E 68th St; New York, NY 10021; (212) 746-4004; **BDCERT:** TS 66; S 66; **MS:** Yale U Sch Med 59; **RES:** TS, Frenchay Hosp, Bristol, MA 63-64; TS, Mass Gen Hosp, Boston, MA 64-65; **FAP:** Prof S Columbia P&S; **SI:** *Esophageal Diseases; Esophageal and Lung Cancer;* **HMO:** Aetna-US Healthcare Blue Cross Oxford United Healthcare PHS +

▭ ▭ ▭ ▭ ▭ ▭ ▭ 2-4 Weeks

Smith, Craig R (MD) TS
Columbia-Presbyterian Med Ctr
161 Ft Washington Ave; New York, NY 10032; (212) 305-8312; **BDCERT:** TS 86; **MS:** Case West Res U 77; **RES:** Strong Mem Hosp, Rochester, NY 78-82; **HMO:** Aetna Hlth Plan Blue Choice Chubb Oxford

Spencer, Frank C (MD) TS
Bellevue Hosp Ctr
530 1st Ave Ste 6D; New York, NY 10016; (212) 263-6382; **BDCERT:** S 56; TS 57; **MS:** Vanderbilt U Sch Med 47; **RES:** S, Johns Hopkins Hosp, Baltimore, MD; UCLA Med Ctr, Los Angeles, CA; **HOSP:** VA Med Ctr-Manh; **HMO:** Oxford Blue Choice Aetna Hlth Plan Chubb Metlife +

▭ ▭ ▭ ▭ ▭ ▭ ▭ ▭ ▭ A Few Days

Spotnitz, Henry (MD) TS
Columbia-Presbyterian Med Ctr
444 E 86th St 31G; New York, NY 10028; (212) 305-6191; **BDCERT:** S 74; TS 76; **MS:** Columbia P&S 66; **RES:** IM, Bellevue Hosp Ctr, New York, NY 66-67; Cv, Columbia-Presbyterian Med Ctr, New York, NY 69-73; **FEL:** TS, Columbia-Presbyterian Med Ctr, New York, NY 73-75; **FAP:** Prof Columbia P&S; **SI:** *Pacemaker & Defibrillator; Surgery;* **HMO:** Oxford Blue Cross & Blue Shield GHI Prudential 1199 +

LANG: Sp; ▭ ▭ ▭ ▭ ▭ ▭ A Few Days

Steinglass, Kenneth (MD) TS
Columbia-Presbyterian Med Ctr
161 Fort Washington Ave 310; New York, NY 10032; (212) 305-3408; **BDCERT:** TS 80; GVS 86; **MS:** Harvard Med Sch 72; **RES:** Columbia-Presbyterian Med Ctr, New York, NY 72-77; **FEL:** TS, Mayo Clinic, Rochester, MN 77-79; **FAP:** Clin Prof S Columbia P&S; **HOSP:** Nyack Hosp; **SI:** *Lung Cancer; Esophageal Disease;* **HMO:** Oxford Aetna Hlth Plan CIGNA

▭ ▭ ▭ ▭ ▭ ▭ 1 Week

Stelzer, Paul (MD) TS
Beth Israel Med Ctr
317 E 17th St 11th Fl; New York, NY 10003; (212) 420-2584; **BDCERT:** TS 82; S 79; **MS:** Columbia P&S 72; **RES:** St Luke's Roosevelt Hosp Ctr, New York, NY 73-77; NY Hosp-Cornell Med Ctr, New York, NY 79-81; **HMO:** US Hlthcre United Healthcare Oxford

▭ ▭

Subramanian, Valavanur (MD) TS
Lenox Hill Hosp
130 E 77th St Fl 4; New York, NY 10021; (212) 737-9131; **BDCERT:** TS 74; **MS:** India 62; **RES:** NY Hosp-Cornell Med Ctr, New York, NY 68-72; **HMO:** Most

▭ ▭ ▭ ▭ ▭ ▭ A Few Days

Tortolani, Anthony (MD)　　TS
NY Hosp-Cornell Med Ctr

Dept of Cardiothoracic Surgery at NY Hospital, 525 E 68th St F2103; New York, NY 11021; (212) 746-5121; **BDCERT:** S 79; TS 88; **MS:** Geo Wash U Sch Med 69; **RES:** S, N Shore Univ Hosp-Manhasset, Manhasset, NY 69-74; **FEL:** Cardio TS, New York University Med Ctr, New York, NY 76-78; **HOSP:** NY Hosp Med Ctr of Queens; **SI:** *Minimally Invasive Cardiac Surgery; Coronary Artery Bypass;* **HMO:** Oxford Blue Cross & Blue Shield GHI Aetna-US Healthcare

🔲 🔲 🔲 🔲 🔲 🔲 🔲 🔲 Immediately

Tranbaugh, Robert (MD)　　TS
Beth Israel Med Ctr

10 Nathan D Perlman Pl; New York, NY 10003; (212) 420-2584; **BDCERT:** TS 86; **MS:** Univ Penn 76; **RES:** S, UC San Francisco Med Ctr, San Francisco, CA 76-83; TS, UC San Francisco Med Ctr, San Francisco, CA 83-85; **FAP:** Assoc Prof Albert Einstein Coll Med; **SI:** *Coronary Artery Bypass; Valvular Heart Disease;* **HMO:** HIP Network US Hlthcre Aetna Hlth Plan Blue Cross Oxford +

🔲 🔲 🔲 🔲 🔲 🔲 Immediately

Whitsell, John (MD)　　TS
NY Hosp-Cornell Med Ctr

449 E 68th St; New York, NY 10021; (212) 535-1514; **BDCERT:** S 62; TS 64; **MS:** Washington U, St Louis 54; **RES:** NY Hosp-Cornell Med Ctr, New York, NY 55-61

🔲 🔲 🔲 Immediately

UROLOGY

Benson, Mitchell C (MD)　　U
Columbia-Presbyterian Med Ctr

161 Ft Washington Ave; New York, NY 10032; (212) 305-5201; **BDCERT:** U 84; **MS:** Columbia P&S 77; **RES:** Mount Sinai Med Ctr, New York, NY 77-79; Columbia-Presbyterian Med Ctr, New York, NY 79-82; **FEL:** Onc, Johns Hopkins Hosp, Baltimore, MD 82-84; **SI:** *Continent Urinary Diversion; Radical Prostatectomy;* **HMO:** Oxford

LANG: Sp; 🔲 🔲 🔲 🔲 🔲 🔲 2-4 Weeks **VISA** 💳

Berman, Steven (MD)　　U
Beth Israel Med Ctr

55 E 9th St; New York, NY 10003; (212) 673-7300; **BDCERT:** U 88; **MS:** SUNY Downstate 81; **RES:** Montefiore Med Ctr, Bronx, NY 77-81; **HOSP:** Montefiore Med Ctr; **HMO:** Oxford PHS Guardian CIGNA NYLCare +

LANG: Sp, Itl; 🔲 🔲 🔲 🔲 🔲 🔲 A Few Days 🔲
VISA 💳 🔲

Birkhoff, John (MD)　　U
Columbia-Presbyterian Med Ctr

161 Fort Washington Ave; New York, NY 10032; (212) 305-5421; **BDCERT:** U 76; **MS:** Columbia P&S 69; **RES:** U, Columbia-Presbyterian Med Ctr, New York, NY 70-75; **FAP:** Asst Prof Columbia P&S; **SI:** *Cancer; Stones, Urinary;* **HMO:** Oxford Prudential Aetna Hlth Plan Anthem Health Multiplan +

🔲 🔲 🔲 🔲 🔲 A Few Days

Birns, Douglas (MD)　　U
Mount Sinai Med Ctr

157 E 72nd St; New York, NY 10021; (212) 744-8700; **BDCERT:** U 88; **MS:** SUNY Downstate 81; **RES:** U, Mount Sinai Med Ctr, New York, NY 82-86; **HOSP:** Beth Israel Med Ctr; **HMO:** CIGNA Oxford United Healthcare PHCS Magnacare +

LANG: Sp; 🔲 🔲 🔲 🔲 🔲 Immediately **VISA** 💳

Blaivas, Jerry G (MD)　　U
NY Hosp-Cornell Med Ctr

400 E 56th St; New York, NY 10022; (212) 308-6565; **BDCERT:** U 78; **MS:** Tufts U 68; **RES:** S, Boston Med Ctr, Boston, MA 71; U, New England Med Ctr, Boston, MA 76; **FAP:** Clin Prof Cornell U; **HOSP:** Beth Israel Med Ctr; **SI:** *Urogynecology; Prostate Problems*

🔲 🔲 🔲 🔲 🔲 🔲 Immediately 🔲 **VISA**

Boczko, Stanley (MD)　　　U
Montefiore Med Ctr
23 E 79th St; New York, NY 10021; (212) 628-1800; **BDCERT:** U 80; **MS:** Albert Einstein Coll Med 73; **RES:** Montefiore Med Ctr, Bronx, NY 73-79; **FEL:** Montefiore Med Ctr, Bronx, NY 75; **FAP:** Albert Einstein Coll Med; **HOSP:** Lenox Hill Hosp; **SI:** *Impotence; Prostate Cancer;* **HMO:** Oxford Aetna Hlth Plan NYLCare CIGNA GHI +

LANG: Sp, Heb; ♿ 🕐 🎥 👣 🛏 💲 Ⓜ Immediately

Brodherson, Michael (MD)　　U
Lenox Hill Hosp
4 E 76th St; New York, NY 10021; (212) 794-2749; **BDCERT:** U 81; **MS:** SUNY Downstate 73; **RES:** U, Lenox Hill Hosp, New York, NY 74-79; **HOSP:** Cabrini Med Ctr; **HMO:** CIGNA Aetna Hlth Plan Oxford

♿ 🎥 🛏 💲 Immediately ▓

Brown, Jordan (MD)　　　U
New York University Med Ctr
NYU Medical Ctr, 530 1st Ave Fl 3; New York, NY 10016; (212) 263-7318; **BDCERT:** U 64; **MS:** NYU Sch Med 54; **RES:** S, Bellevue Hosp Ctr, New York, NY 54-56; U, Bellevue Hosp Ctr, New York, NY 58-61; **FAP:** Clin Prof U NYU Sch Med; **SI:** *Oncology; Prostate Diseases;* **HMO:** Oxford Aetna Hlth Plan PHS United Healthcare NYLCare +

♿ 🎥 👣 🛏 💲 Ⓜ 1 Week

Cohen, Elliot L (MD)　　　U
Mount Sinai Med Ctr
103 E 80th St; New York, NY 10021; (212) 288-0056; **BDCERT:** U 76; **MS:** U Hlth Sci/Chicago Med Sch 67; **RES:** S, Bellevue Hosp Ctr, New York, NY 68-69; U, NY Med Coll, Valhalla, NY 71-74; **SI:** *Prostate Disorders; Impotence;* **HMO:** Oxford GHI Aetna Hlth Plan Blue Cross & Blue Shield Sanus +

LANG: Sp, Fr; ♿ 🕐 🎥 👣 🛏 💲 Ⓜ ♿ Immediately

Coleman, John (MD)　　　U
NY Hosp-Cornell Med Ctr
53 E 70th St; New York, NY 10021; (212) 535-4545; **BDCERT:** U 76; **MS:** Georgetown U 64; **RES:** U, NY Hosp-Cornell Med Ctr, New York, NY 64-66; U, NY Hosp-Cornell Med Ctr, New York, NY 68-72; **SI:** *Prostate and Bladder; Kidney-Stones;* **HMO:** Oxford US Hlthcre CIGNA Anthem Health Blue Choice +

LANG: Man, Can; ♿ 🍽 🎥 🛏 💲 Ⓜ Immediately
VISA 💳 💳

Davis, Joseph (MD)　　　U
Cabrini Med Ctr
595 Madison Ave Ste 2100; New York, NY 10022; (212) 421-8143; **BDCERT:** U 64; **MS:** NY Med Coll 53; **RES:** Flower Fifth Ave Hosp, New York, NY 54-55; Bellevue Hosp Ctr, New York, NY 57-60; **FAP:** Clin Prof NYU Sch Med; **SI:** *Indigo Laser Prostatectomy;* **HMO:** Blue Choice Aetna-US Healthcare Oxford CIGNA Magnacare +

LANG: Sp; ♿ 🎥 👣 🛏 💲 Ⓜ Ⓜ Ⓦ Ⓝ
Immediately **VISA** 💳

Dillon, Robert (MD)　　　U
Mount Sinai Med Ctr
157 E 72nd St; New York, NY 10021; (212) 794-9000; **BDCERT:** U 80; **MS:** NY Med Coll 73; **RES:** S, Mount Sinai Med Ctr, New York, NY 73-75; U, Mount Sinai Med Ctr, New York, NY 75-78; **FAP:** Asst Clin Prof Mt Sinai Sch Med; **HOSP:** Lenox Hill Hosp; **SI:** *Infertility; Urologic Malignancies*

♿ 🎥 👣 🛏 💲 Ⓜ 1 Week ▓ **VISA** 💳

Droller, Michael J (MD)　　U
Mount Sinai Med Ctr
Urology Associates, 5 E 98th St Box 1272; New York, NY 10029; (212) 241-4812; **BDCERT:** U 79; **MS:** Harvard Med Sch 68; **RES:** S, Peter Bent Brigham Hosp, Boston, MA 70; U, Stanford Med Ctr, Stanford, CA 76; **FAP:** Prof Mt Sinai Sch Med; **SI:** *Prostate Cancer; Bladder Cancer;* **HMO:** Oxford Aetna-US Healthcare Vytra Blue Choice

♿ 🎥 👣 🛏 💲 Ⓜ A Few Days ▓ **VISA** 💳

Eid, Francois (MD)   U
NY Hosp-Cornell Med Ctr
428 E 72nd Street Ste 400; New York, NY 10021;
(212) 746-5473; **BDCERT:** U 90; **MS:** Cornell U 82;
RES: S, NY Hosp-Cornell Med Ctr, New York, NY
83-84; U, NY Hosp-Cornell Med Ctr, New York, NY
84-87; **SI:** *Impotence*; **HMO:** Blue Choice Sel Pro

Etra, William (MD)   U
Beth Israel Med Ctr
461 Park Ave S; New York, NY 10016; (212) 679-
6464; **BDCERT:** U 76; **MS:** NY Med Coll 69; **RES:** U,
Beth Israel Med Ctr, New York, NY 69-74; **FEL:** U
Onc, Roswell Park Cancer Inst, Buffalo, NY 74-75;
FAP: Clin Instr Albert Einstein Coll Med; **HOSP:**
Hosp For Joint Diseases; **SI:** *Urologic Oncology*; **HMO:**
Aetna Hlth Plan Blue Cross & Blue Shield PHS GHI
Oxford +

♿ ☾ 🔒 💧 🛏 $ Mcr   Immediately

Fine, Eugene M (MD)   U
Mount Sinai Med Ctr
12 E 86th St; New York, NY 10028; (212) 517-
9555; **BDCERT:** U 87; U 95; **MS:** Mexico 78; **RES:**
IM, Univ Hosp SUNY Bklyn, Brooklyn, NY 79-80; S,
Univ Hosp SUNY Bklyn, Brooklyn, NY 80-81; **FEL:**
U, Mount Sinai Med Ctr, New York, NY 81-85;
FAP: Asst Clin Prof U Mt Sinai Sch Med; **HOSP:**
Beth Israel North; **SI:** *Prostate Cancer; Kidney Stones*;
HMO: Oxford Blue Choice Blue Cross & Blue Shield
Aetna Hlth Plan GHI +

LANG: Sp; ♿ ☾ 🔒 💧 🛏 $ Mcr   A Few Days

Fisch, Harry (MD)   U
Columbia-Presbyterian Med Ctr
944 Park Ave Ste 1C; New York, NY 10028; (212)
879-0800; **BDCERT:** U 91; **MS:** Mt Sinai Sch Med
83; **RES:** S, Montefiore Med Ctr, Bronx, NY 83-85;
U, Montefiore Med Ctr, Bronx, NY 85-89; **FAP:** Asst
Prof U Columbia P&S; **SI:** *Male Infertility*; **HMO:**
Aetna Hlth Plan Oxford

♿ 🔒 💧 🛏 $ 2-4 Weeks

Fracchia, John (MD)   U
Lenox Hill Hosp
880 5th Ave; New York, NY 10021; (212) 570-
6800; **BDCERT:** U 81; S 81; **MS:** UMDNJ-NJ Med
Sch, Newark 73; **RES:** NY Hosp-Cornell Med Ctr,
New York, NY 75-79; N Shore Univ Hosp-
Manhasset, Manhasset, NY 73-75; **HOSP:** NY
Hosp-Cornell Med Ctr; **HMO:** CIGNA Metlife Chubb
US Hlthcre HIP Network +

♿ 🔒 💧 🛏 $ Immediately ■ *VISA* ⬤

Furey, Robert J (MD)   U
St Vincents Hosp & Med Ctr NY
61 Irving Pl LLB; New York, NY 10003; (212) 533-
6411; **BDCERT:** U 78; **MS:** NY Med Coll 62; **RES:**
S/Rad, St Vincents Hosp & Med Ctr NY, New York,
NY 65-67; U, St Luke's Roosevelt Hosp Ctr, New
York, NY 67-70; **FAP:** Asst Clin Prof NY Med Coll;
HMO: Oxford Blue Cross & Blue Shield Aetna Hlth
Plan

♿ ☾ 🔒 💧 🛏 $ Mcr Mcr   A Few Days

Georgsson, Sverrir (MD)   U
St Vincents Hosp & Med Ctr NY
36 7th Ave 505; New York, NY 10011; (212) 675-
5828; **BDCERT:** U 72; **MS:** Iceland 62; **RES:** NY
Hosp-Cornell Med Ctr, New York, NY 68; U, Yale-
New Haven Hosp, New Haven, CT 69; **HMO:**
Oxford Blue Choice Choicecare PHS Prucare +

🔒 💧 🛏 $ Mcr   Immediately ■

Goldstein, Marc (MD)   U
NY Hosp-Cornell Med Ctr
Center for Male Reproductive Medicine and
Microsurgery, 525 E 68th St; New York, NY
10021; (212) 746-5470; **BDCERT:** U 82; **MS:**
SUNY Hlth Sci Ctr 72; **RES:** S, Columbia-
Presbyterian Med Ctr, New York, NY 72-74; U,
Univ Hosp SUNY Bklyn, Brooklyn, NY 77-80; **FEL:**
Rockefeller Univ Hosp, New York, NY 80-82;
Rockefeller Univ Hosp, New York, NY 80-82; **FAP:**
Prof Cornell U; **SI:** *Male Infertility; Vasectomy and
Reversal*; **HMO:** PHS American Health Plan
Random House

♿ 🔒 💧 🛏 $ Mcr WC ■ *VISA* ⬤

Golimbu, Mircea (MD)　U
New York University Med Ctr

530 1st Ave Rm 3D; New York, NY 10016; (212) 263-7327; **BDCERT:** U 75; **MS:** Romania 63; **RES:** U, New York University Med Ctr, New York, NY 70-73; **FEL:** U, NY Academy of Med, New York, NY 74-75; **FAP:** Clin Prof U NYU Sch Med; **HOSP:** Cabrini Med Ctr; **SI:** *Urinary Stones; Prostate;* **HMO:** Oxford Blue Shield 1199 Aetna Hlth Plan +

LANG: Itl, Sp, Rom; ♿ 📷 🅿 🏨 $ Mcr Mod A Few Days

Gribetz, Michael (MD)　U
Mount Sinai Med Ctr

1155 Park Ave; New York, NY 10128; (212) 831-1300; **BDCERT:** U 80; **MS:** Albert Einstein Coll Med 73; **RES:** U, Mount Sinai Med Ctr, New York, NY 75-78; SM, Montefiore Med Ctr, Bronx, NY 73-75; **FAP:** Asst Clin Prof U Mt Sinai Sch Med; **SI:** *Prostate Diseases; Erectile Dysfunction;* **HMO:** Aetna Hlth Plan Oxford HealthNet CIGNA PHS +

LANG: Heb, Yd, Sp, Itl; ♿ 📷 🅿 🏨 $ Mcr Immediately ▩ **VISA** ●

Hensle, Terry (MD)　U
Columbia-Presbyterian Med Ctr

3959 Broadway 219N; New York, NY 10032; (212) 305-8510; **BDCERT:** U 78; **MS:** Cornell U 68; **RES:** Boston Med Ctr, Boston, MA 68-73; Mass Gen Hosp, Boston, MA 73-76; **FEL:** Ped, Mass Gen Hosp, Boston, MA 76-77; Great Ormond St Hosp, London, England 77-78; **FAP:** Lecturer U Columbia P&S; **HOSP:** Hackensack Univ Med Ctr; **SI:** *Reconstructive Urology; Intersex;* **HMO:** Oxford Multiplan Blue Choice First Option Prucare +

♿ 🆘 📷 🅿 🏨 Mcr Mod A Few Days

Herr, Harry W (MD)　U
Mem Sloan Kettering Cancer Ctr

1275 York Ave; New York, NY 10021; (212) 639-8264; **BDCERT:** U 76; **MS:** UC Irvine 69; **RES:** UC Irvine Med Ctr, Orange, CA 70-74; **FEL:** U Onc, Mem Sloan Kettering Cancer Ctr, New York, NY 74-76; **FAP:** Assoc Prof S Cornell U; **HOSP:** NY Hosp-Cornell Med Ctr; **HMO:** Empire Blue Cross & Blue Shield HealthNet

♿ 📷 🏨 Mcr Mod WC NFI Immediately

Kaminetsky, Jed (MD)　U
New York University Med Ctr

Park Ave Urologic Ctr, 30 Park Ave; New York, NY 10016; (212) 686-9015; **BDCERT:** U 92; **MS:** NYU Sch Med 84; **RES:** New York University Med Ctr, New York, NY 90; **HOSP:** St Vincents Hosp & Med Ctr NY; **SI:** *Prostate Cancer; Sexual Dysfunction;* **HMO:** Aetna Hlth Plan Oxford GHI Magnacare CIGNA +

LANG: Sp; ◖ 📷 🅿 🏨 $ Mcr A Few Days **VISA**

Kirschenbaum, Alexander (MD)U
Mount Sinai Med Ctr

5 E 98th St; New York, NY 10029; (212) 241-8711; **BDCERT:** U 97; **MS:** Mt Sinai Sch Med 80; **RES:** S, Mount Sinai Med Ctr, New York, NY 80-82; U, Mt Sinai Med Ctr, New York, NY 82-85; **FEL:** U Onc, Mount Sinai Med Ctr, New York, NY 85-87; **FAP:** Assoc Prof U Mt Sinai Sch Med; **SI:** *Radical Prostatectomy; Cystectomy;* **HMO:** Oxford Blue Cross & Blue Shield Aetna Hlth Plan

♿ 📷 🅿 🏨 $ Mcr WC NFI

Klein, George (MD)　U
Mount Sinai Med Ctr

157 E 72nd St; New York, NY 10021; (212) 744-8700; **BDCERT:** U 81; **MS:** Cornell U 76; **RES:** Mount Sinai Med Ctr, New York, NY; Mount Sinai Med Ctr, New York, NY; **FEL:** Mount Sinai Med Ctr, New York, NY; **FAP:** Mt Sinai Sch Med; **SI:** *Sexual Dysfunction; Prostatectomy;* **HMO:** Aetna Hlth Plan Blue Choice Blue Cross & Blue Shield

LANG: Hun, Sp, Tag; ♿ 📷 🅿 🏨 $ Mcr Immediately **VISA** ●

Lepor, Herbert (MD)　U
New York University Med Ctr

NYU Urology Associates, 550 1st Ave Ste 10R; New York, NY 10016; (212) 263-6420; **BDCERT:** U 87; U 97; **MS:** Johns Hopkins U 79; **RES:** S, Johns Hopkins Hosp, Baltimore, MD 80-81; U, Johns Hopkins Hosp, Baltimore, MD 81-85; **FAP:** Chrmn U NYU Sch Med; **SI:** *Prostate Cancer; Benign Prostatic Hyperplasia;* **HMO:** Aetna-US Healthcare Prudential CIGNA Blue Shield

LANG: Sp, Itl; ♿ 🅿 🏨 $ Mcr Mod ▩ **VISA** ● ▦

Loo, Marcus (MD)   U
NY Hosp-Cornell Med Ctr

53 E 70th St; New York, NY 10021; (212) 535-4545; **BDCERT:** U 90; **MS:** Cornell U 81; **RES:** NY Hosp-Cornell Med Ctr, New York, NY 81-88; **FEL:** U, NY Hosp-Cornell Med Ctr, New York, NY 83-84; **SI:** *Prostate Disease; Kidney Stones*; **HMO:** Oxford Blue Choice 1199 Aetna Hlth Plan Prudential +

LANG: Chi; ♿ 🈂 🅲 📷 👤 🏥 💲 Mcr Immediately
VISA 💳 📠

Lowe, Franklin (MD)   U
St Luke's Roosevelt Hosp Ctr

425 W 59th St 3A; New York, NY 10019; (212) 523-7790; **BDCERT:** U 87; **MS:** Columbia P&S 79; **RES:** S, Johns Hopkins Hosp, Baltimore, MD 79-81; U, Johns Hopkins Hosp, Baltimore, MD 81-84; **FAP:** Assoc Clin Prof U Columbia P&S; **HOSP:** NY Hosp-Cornell Med Ctr; **SI:** *Prostate Cancer; Prostate Disorders*; **HMO:** Oxford GHI PHS Multiplan

LANG: Sp; ♿ 📷 👤 🏥 Mcr 1 Week ***VISA*** 💳

Marans, Hillel (MD)   U
St Vincents Hosp & Med Ctr NY

36 7th Ave 514; New York, NY 10011; (212) 206-9130; **BDCERT:** U 88; **MS:** Cornell U 80; **RES:** S, St Vincents Hosp & Med Ctr NY, New York, NY 80-82; U, Montefiore Med Ctr, Bronx, NY 82-85; **FAP:** Asst Clin Prof U NY Med Coll; **SI:** *Urinary Tract Infection Recurrent; Urologic Cancers*; **HMO:** Oxford Aetna-US Healthcare Prucare 1199 +

LANG: Sp, Heb; ♿ 📷 🏥 💲 Mcr A Few Days ***VISA*** 💳

Marks, Jon (MD)   U
Beth Israel Med Ctr

Metropolitan Urological Associates, 55 E 9th St; New York, NY 10003; (212) 673-7300; **BDCERT:** U 83; **MS:** NY Med Coll 76; **RES:** U, Lenox Hill Hosp, New York, NY 78-81; **FAP:** Clin Instr Albert Einstein Coll Med; **HOSP:** Cabrini Med Ctr; **SI:** *Kidney Stones; Interstitial Cystitis*; **HMO:** Oxford US Hlthcre Sanus CIGNA Blue Cross & Blue Shield +

LANG: Sp; ♿ 📷 👤 🏥 💲 Mcr Immediately 🏧
VISA 💳

McGovern, Thomas P (MD)   U
NY Hosp-Cornell Med Ctr

927 5th Ave; New York, NY 10021; (212) 772-7411; **BDCERT:** U 83; **MS:** Cornell U 74; **RES:** Mass Gen Hosp, Boston, MA 74-76; NY Hosp-Cornell Med Ctr, New York, NY 76-80; **HOSP:** Lenox Hill Hosp; **SI:** *Bladder Tumors; Prostate Cancer*

♿ 📷 👤 🏥 💲 4+ Weeks

Melman, Arnold (MD)   U
Montefiore Med Ctr

Montefiore Medical Center, 969 Park Ave Ste 1G; New York, NY 10028; (212) 639-1561; **BDCERT:** U 76; **MS:** U Rochester 66; **RES:** U, Strong Mem Hosp, Rochester, NY 66-68; U, UCLA Med Ctr, Los Angeles, CA 70-74; **FEL:** Nep, Cedars-Sinai Med Ctr, Los Angeles, CA 71-72; **FAP:** Chrmn Albert Einstein Coll Med; **SI:** *Sexual Dysfunction; Prostate Cancer*; **HMO:** GHI US Hlthcre Oxford PHS Blue Cross & Blue Shield +

LANG: Sp; ♿ 🏥 💲 Mcr Mcd WC 1 Week ***VISA*** 💳

Muecke, Edward (MD)   U
NY Hosp-Cornell Med Ctr

NY Urological Assoc, 880 5th Ave; New York, NY 10021; (212) 570-6800; **BDCERT:** U 68; **MS:** Cornell U 57; **RES:** NY Hosp-Cornell Med Ctr, New York, NY 60-65; **FEL:** Carnegie Institute, Washington, DC 61; **FAP:** Prof Cornell U; **HOSP:** Lenox Hill Hosp; **SI:** *Prostatic & Kidney Cancers; General Diagnostic Urology*; **HMO:** Guardian NYLCare Aetna-US Healthcare United Healthcare Oxford +

LANG: Sp, Grk, Ger; ♿ 📷 🏥 💲 Mcr 1 Week 🏧
VISA 💳

Nagler, Harris M (MD)   U
Beth Israel Med Ctr

10 Union Square East; New York, NY 10003; (212) 844-8900; **BDCERT:** U 82; **MS:** Temple U 75; **RES:** Columbia-Presbyterian Med Ctr, New York, NY 76-80; **FEL:** RE, Columbia-Presbyterian Med Ctr, New York, NY; **FAP:** Prof Albert Einstein Coll Med; **SI:** *Infertility; Impotence*; **HMO:** Oxford CIGNA US Hlthcre Blue Choice NYLCare +

LANG: Sp, Rus; ♿ 🅲 📷 👤 🏥 💲 Mcr Immediately 🏧 ***VISA*** 💳 📠

Olsson, Carl (MD) U
Columbia-Presbyterian Med Ctr
161 Ft Washington Ave; New York, NY 10032;
(212) 305-0100; **BDCERT:** U 72; **MS:** Boston U 63;
RES: U, Boston VA Med Ctr, Boston, MA 66-69;
FEL: Cleveland Clinic Hosp, Cleveland, OH 67-68;
FAP: Chrmn U; *SI: Urologic Oncology*
🚻 📷 👥 🏥 Mcr 1 Week

Peng, Benjamin (MD) U
NYU Downtown Hosp
168 Canal St 510; New York, NY 10013; (212)
226-2200; **BDCERT:** U 92; **MS:** Columbia P&S 84;
RES: S, Mount Sinai Med Ctr, New York, NY 84-86;
U, Columbia-Presbyterian Med Ctr, New York, NY
86-90; **FAP:** Asst Prof NYU Sch Med; *SI: Prostate
Diseases; Urinary Tract Stones;* **HMO:** Oxford Aetna-
US Healthcare Blue Cross & Blue Shield GHI United
Healthcare +
LANG: Chi, Sp; 🚻 💳 📷 👥 🏥 $ Mcr A Few Days

Provet, John (MD) U
New York University Med Ctr
530 1st Ave 7S; New York, NY 10016; (212) 263-
7092; **BDCERT:** U 91; **MS:** NYU Sch Med 83; **RES:**
S, NY VA Med Ctr/Bellevue/NYU Med Ctr, New
York, NY 83-85; U, NY VA/Bellevue/NYU Med Ctr,
New York, NY 85-89; **FEL:** U Onc, NY Academy of
Med, New York, NY 89-90; **FAP:** Asst Prof U NYU
Sch Med; *SI: Oncology; Prostatic Hyperplasia;* **HMO:**
Oxford Chubb Blue Cross & Blue Shield
🚻 📷 👥 🏥 Mcr Immediately

Reckler, Jon Michael (MD) U
NY Hosp-Cornell Med Ctr
NY Urological Associates, PC, 880 5th Ave; New
York, NY 10021; (212) 535-1950; **BDCERT:** U 76;
MS: Harvard Med Sch 66; **RES:** S, U Hosp of
Cleveland, Cleveland, OH 66-68; U, Peter Bent
Brigham Hosp, Boston, MA 74; **HOSP:** Lenox Hill
Hosp
🚻 📷 🏥 $ Mcr 1 Week ▨ *VISA* ●

Romas, Nicholas A (MD) U
St Luke's Roosevelt Hosp Ctr
1000 10th Ave; New York, NY 10019; (212) 523-
7788; **BDCERT:** U 74; **MS:** Columbia P&S 62; **RES:**
S, NY Hosp-Cornell Med Ctr, New York, NY 62-64;
U, Columbia-Presbyterian Med Ctr, New York, NY
64-68; **FEL:** Nat Inst Health, Bethesda, MD 66;
FAP: Clin Prof U Columbia P&S; **HOSP:** Columbia-
Presbyterian Med Ctr; **HMO:** CIGNA Aetna Hlth
Plan Oxford Empire PHS +
LANG: Grk, Rus, Sp; 🚻 📷 👥 🏥 $ Mcr 1 Week

Russo, Paul (MD) U
Mem Sloan Kettering Cancer Ctr
1275 York Ave; New York, NY 10021; (212) 639-
5944; **BDCERT:** U 95; **MS:** Columbia P&S 79; **RES:**
S Onc, Barnes Hosp, St Louis, MO 79-84; **FEL:** U
Onc, Mem Sloan Kettering Cancer Ctr, New York,
NY 84-88; *SI: Prostate Cancer Surgery; Continent
Urinary Diversion*
🚻 👥 🏥 Mcr Mcd ▨ *VISA* ● ●

Sawczuk, Ihor S (MD) U
Columbia-Presbyterian Med Ctr
161 Fort Washington Ave; New York, NY 10032;
(212) 305-0103; **BDCERT:** U 86; **MS:** Med Coll PA
79; **RES:** St Vincents Hosp & Med Ctr NY, New
York, NY 79-81; Columbia-Presbyterian Med Ctr,
New York, NY 81-84; **FEL:** U Onc, Columbia-
Presbyterian Med Ctr, New York, NY 84-86; **FAP:**
Prof Columbia P&S; *SI: Kidney Cancer; Bladder
Cancer;* **HMO:** Oxford Blue Choice Bronx Health
CIGNA Prudential +
🚻 📷 👥 🏥 $ Mcr 1 Week *VISA* ●

Schiff, Howard (MD) U
Mount Sinai Med Ctr
1120 Park Ave 1E; New York, NY 10128; (212)
996-6660; **BDCERT:** U 82; **MS:** W Va U Sch Med
75; **RES:** S, Montefiore Med Ctr, Bronx, NY 75-77;
U, Mount Sinai Med Ctr, New York, NY 77-80;
FAP: Asst Clin Prof Mt Sinai Sch Med; **HOSP:** Beth
Israel Med Ctr; *SI: Prostate Diseases; Incontinence*
LANG: Sp; 🚻 📷 👥 🏥 $ Mcr NFI Immediately
VISA ● ●

Schlegel, Peter (MD)   U
NY Hosp-Cornell Med Ctr

525 E 68th St F905A; New York, NY 10021; (212) 746-5491; **BDCERT:** U 93; **MS:** Univ Mass Sch Med 83; **RES:** S, Johns Hopkins Hosp, Baltimore, MD 83-85; U, Johns Hopkins Hosp, Baltimore, MD 85-89; **FEL:** Onc, Johns Hopkins Hosp, Baltimore, MD 86-87; Male Reproduction, NY Hosp-Cornell Med Ctr, New York, NY 89-91; **FAP:** Assoc Prof Cornell U; *SI: Male Infertility; Radical Prostatectomy;* **HMO:** Blue Choice Amerihealth NYLCare PHS

🦽 📷 👤 🏥 Mcr A Few Days 🎫 **VISA** 💳

Shabsigh, Ridwan (MD)   U
Columbia-Presbyterian Med Ctr

161 Fort Washington Ave 11th Fl; New York, NY 10032; (212) 305-0123; **BDCERT:** U 92; **MS:** Syria 76; **RES:** U, Baylor Med Ctr, Dallas, TX 87-90; **FEL:** Impotence Protheses, Baylor Med Ctr, Dallas, TX 84-87; *SI: Impotence;* **HMO:** Oxford PHS Blue Cross & Blue Shield CIGNA Bronx Health +

🦽 📷 👤 🏥 S Mcr Immediately

Silva, Jose (MD)   U
St Luke's Roosevelt Hosp Ctr

345 W 58th St; New York, NY 10019; (212) 582-3421; **BDCERT:** U 83; **MS:** India 70; **RES:** S, Beth Israel Med Ctr, New York, NY 77-78; U, St Luke's Roosevelt Hosp Ctr, New York, NY 78-81; **FEL:** S, Mem Sloan Kettering Cancer Ctr, New York, NY 81-82; **FAP:** Clin Instr Columbia P&S; **HOSP:** Montefiore Med Ctr; *SI: Urologic Oncology;* **HMO:** Oxford US Hlthcre CIGNA Chubb Blue Cross +

LANG: Prt, Sp, Hin; 🦽 📲 📷 👤 🏥 Mcr Immediately

Sogani, Pramod (MD)   U
Mem Sloan Kettering Cancer Ctr

1275 York Ave; New York, NY 10021; (212) 639-7704; **BDCERT:** U 76; **MS:** India 60; **RES:** New York University Med Ctr, New York, NY 68-69; Geo Wash U Med Ctr, Washington, DC 69-71; **FEL:** U Onc, Mem Sloan Kettering Cancer Ctr, New York, NY 71; **FAP:** Prof U Cornell U; *SI: Prostatectomy; Kidney and Bladder Cancer*

🦽 📊 📷 🏥 S Mcr A Few Days 🎫 **VISA** 💳

Sosa, R Ernest (MD)   U
NY Hosp-Cornell Med Ctr

Brady Urology Associates, 525 E 68th St; New York, NY 10021; (212) 746-5362; **BDCERT:** U 86; **MS:** Cornell U 78; **RES:** S, NY Hosp-Cornell Med Ctr, New York, NY 78; U, NY Hosp-Cornell Med Ctr, New York, NY 80-84; **FEL:** Renal Physiology, NY Hosp-Cornell Med Ctr, New York, NY 84-86; **FAP:** Assoc Prof U Cornell U; *SI: Stones, Urinary; Prostatic Diseases;* **HMO:** Aetna Hlth Plan CIGNA Oxford

🦽 🅲 📷 👤 🏥 S Mcr Mcd A Few Days 🎫 **VISA** 💳

Sperber, Alan B (MD)   U
New York University Med Ctr

257 Lexington Ave; New York, NY 10016; (212) 889-5256; **BDCERT:** U 77; **MS:** NYU Sch Med 67; **RES:** Albert Einstein Med Ctr, Bronx, NY 67-69; NYU Med Ctr, New York, NY 71-75; **FAP:** Assoc Clin Prof NYU Sch Med; **HOSP:** Cabrini Med Ctr; *SI: Urological Tumors; Prostate Disorders;* **HMO:** Oxford United Healthcare Blue Choice Blue Choice Aetna Hlth Plan +

LANG: Sp, Fr, Ger; 🦽 📷 👤 🏥 S Mcr Immediately

Tessler, Arthur (MD)   U
New York University Med Ctr

NYU Medical Ctr, 530 1st Ave 3D; New York, NY 10016; (212) 263-7300; **BDCERT:** U 63; **MS:** NYU Sch Med 52; **RES:** Maimonides Med Ctr, Brooklyn, NY 52-54; Bellevue Hosp Ctr, New York, NY 56-59; **FAP:** Prof of Clin U NYU Sch Med; **HOSP:** Bellevue Hosp Ctr; *SI: Urological Tumors; Prostate Diseases;* **HMO:** Oxford

🦽 📷 👤 🏥 S Mcr 1 Week

Vapnek, Jonathon M (MD)   U
Mount Sinai Med Ctr

Mt Sinai Medical Ctr, 5 E 98th St 6fl.; New York, NY 10029; (212) 241-4812; **BDCERT:** U 95; **MS:** UC San Diego 86; **RES:** S, UC San Diego Med Ctr, San Diego, CA 87-88; U, UC San Francisco Med Ctr, San Francisco, CA 88-92; **FEL:** N, UC Davis Med Ctr, Sacramento, CA 92-93; **FAP:** Asst Prof Mt Sinai Sch Med; **HOSP:** VA Med Ctr-Bronx; *SI: Urinary Incontinence; Urology (Female);* **HMO:** Oxford Aetna Hlth Plan Vytra CIGNA Blue Choice +

🦽 📷 👤 🏥 Mcr Mcd WC NFI Immediately 🎫 **VISA** 💳

Vaughan, Edwin D (MD)   U
NY Hosp-Cornell Med Ctr

Cornell Physician Organization, 525 E 68th St;
New York, NY 10021; (212) 746-5480; **BDCERT:**
U 86; **MS:** U Va Sch Med 65; **RES:** Vanderbilt U Med
Ctr, Nashville, TN; U of VA Health Sci Ctr,
Charlottesville, VA; **FEL:** U, Vanderbilt U Med Ctr,
Nashville, TN; U of VA Health Sci Ctr,
Charlottesville, VA; **HOSP:** Mem Sloan Kettering
Cancer Ctr; **SI:** *Urologic Tumors; Prostate Benign &*
Malignant; **HMO:** Blue Cross & Blue Shield Aetna
Hlth Plan Oxford PHS +

♿ 📷 🗃 🏥 Mcr   2-4 Weeks 💳 **VISA** 💳 💳

Wechsler, Michael (MD)   U
Columbia-Presbyterian Med Ctr

911 Park Ave; New York, NY 10021; (212) 861-
9310; **BDCERT:** U 75; **MS:** St Louis U 65; **RES:**
UCLA Med Ctr, Los Angeles, CA 68; Columbia-
Presbyterian Med Ctr, New York, NY 69-73; **HMO:**
Oxford PHS Multiplan CIGNA

♿ 📷 🗃 🏥 S Mcr   Immediately

Williams, John (MD)   U
NY Hosp-Cornell Med Ctr

820 Park Ave; New York, NY 10021; (212) 861-
1100; **BDCERT:** U 76; **MS:** Georgetown U 66; **RES:**
S, Strong Mem Hosp, Rochester, NY 66-68; NY
Hosp-Cornell Med Ctr, New York, NY 70-74; **HOSP:**
Lenox Hill Hosp; **SI:** *Prostate Surgery; Kidney &*
Bladder Cancer

📷 🏥 S   A Few Days 💳 **VISA** 💳 💳

VASCULAR & INTERVENTIONAL RADIOLOGY

Bakal, Curtis (MD)   VIR
St Luke's Roosevelt Hosp Ctr

St Luke's Hosp Rsvelt Div Dept of Radiology, 1000
10th Ave; New York, NY 10019; (212) 523-6384;
BDCERT: Rad 84; VIR 95; **MS:** Harvard Med Sch
76; **RES:** Mass Gen Hosp, Boston, MA 81-84; **FEL:**
VIR, NY Med Coll, Valhalla, NY 84-85; **FAP:** Prof
Albert Einstein Coll Med; **SI:** *Peripheral Vascular*
Disease; Angioplasty; **HMO:** Most

♿ 📷 🏥 Mcr Mcd WC NFI

Martin, Eric C (MD)   VIR
Columbia-Presbyterian Med Ctr

622 W 168th St St; New York, NY 10032; (212)
305-5123; **BDCERT:** Rad 75; VIR 94; **MS:** England
67; **RES:** St Bartholomew's Hosp, London, England
70-74; Nat Heart Hosp, London, England 68-70;
FEL: Cv, Peter Bent Brigham Hosp, Boston, MA 74-
75; **FAP:** Prof Rad Columbia P&S; **SI:** *Interventional*
Radiology; **HMO:** Oxford

📷 🏥 🏥 Mcr Mcd WC   1 Week 💳 **VISA** 💳 💳

Rosen, Robert J (MD)   VIR
New York University Med Ctr

560 1st Ave; New York, NY 10016; (212) 263-5898; **BDCERT:** DR 80; Rad 96; **MS:** Hahnemann U 76; **RES:** Hahnemann U Hosp, Philadelphia, PA 77-79; **FEL:** VIR, Hosp of U Penn, Philadelphia, PA 79-80; **FAP:** Assoc Prof NYU Sch Med; **HOSP:** Bellevue Hosp Ctr; **SI:** *Peripheral Vascular Disease; Vascular Malformations*

LANG: Fr, Sp; 🦽 📷 🚘 🏨 Mcr Mcd WC NFi   1 Week

VASCULAR SURGERY (GENERAL)

Adelman, Mark (MD)   GVS
New York University Med Ctr

530 1st Ave Ste 6F; New York, NY 10016; (212) 263-7311; **BDCERT:** S 91; GVS 93; **MS:** NYU Sch Med 85; **RES:** New York University Med Ctr, New York, NY 86-90; **FEL:** GVS, New York University Med Ctr, New York, NY 90-91; **HOSP:** Bellevue Hosp Ctr; **HMO:** Aetna Hlth Plan Chubb Oxford Metlife

🦽 📷 🚘 🏨 💲 Mcr   A Few Days

Ahmed, Maher (MD)   GVS
Lenox Hill Hosp

110 E 59th St 10C; New York, NY 10022; (212) 583-2910; **BDCERT:** S 79; **MS:** Egypt 70; **RES:** S, Lenox Hill Hosp, New York, NY 74-78; Nazareth Hospital, Nazareth, PA 73-74; **FEL:** GVS, Cumberland Med Ctr, Brooklyn, NY 78-79; TS, St Vincents Hosp & Med Ctr NY, New York, NY 78-79

🦽 🚘 🏨 💲 Mcr Mcd   2-4 Weeks 🖃 **VISA** 💳 💳

Benvenisty, Alan (MD)   GVS
Columbia-Presbyterian Med Ctr

161 Fort Washington Ave; New York, NY 10032; (212) 305-8055; **BDCERT:** S 84; GVS 91; **MS:** Columbia P&S 78; **RES:** Columbia-Presbyterian Med Ctr, New York, NY 79-83; **FEL:** Columbia-Presbyterian Med Ctr, New York, NY 83-84; **HMO:** Oxford Empire Blue Cross & Blue Shield

🦽 📷 🏨 Mcr Mcd WC NFi   A Few Days

Blumenthal, Jesse (MD)   GVS
St Vincents Hosp & Med Ctr NY

36 7th Ave 422; New York, NY 10011; (212) 337-0600; **BDCERT:** S 67; **MS:** Columbia P&S 60; **RES:** S, St Luke's Roosevelt Hosp Ctr, New York, NY 61-65; **FAP:** Asst Clin Prof S Mt Sinai Sch Med; **SI:** *Varicose Veins; Occlusive Arterial Disease;* **HMO:** Oxford

🦽 📷 🏨 💲 Mcr Mcd WC NFi   A Few Days

Bush Jr, Harry (MD)   GVS
NY Hosp-Cornell Med Ctr

NY Hosp Cornell Med Ctr, 525 E 68th St 2003; New York, NY 10021; (212) 746-5392; **BDCERT:** S 79; **MS:** Columbia P&S 68; **RES:** S, Columbia-Presbyterian Med Ctr, New York, NY 68-69; **FEL:** S, Columbia-Presbyterian Med Ctr, New York, NY 69-70; **FAP:** Instr S Columbia P&S

Chideckel, Norman (MD)   GVS
Beth Israel Med Ctr

306 E 15th St; New York, NY 10003; (212) 529-2407; **BDCERT:** S 89; **MS:** SUNY Downstate 79; **RES:** Beth Israel Med Ctr, New York, NY 79-84; **FEL:** Lutheran Med Ctr, Brooklyn, NY 84-85; **FAP:** Clin Instr Albert Einstein Coll Med; **SI:** *Varicose Veins; Circulation Abnormalities;* **HMO:** Aetna Hlth Plan Blue Choice Oxford CIGNA HIP Network +

LANG: Sp, Heb, Yd; 🦽 📷 🚘 🏨 💲 Mcr Mcd WC NFi   Immediately

Fantini, Gary (MD)   GVS
NY Hosp-Cornell Med Ctr

170 E End Ave; New York, NY 10128; (212) 870-7200; **BDCERT:** S 90; GVS 92; **MS:** Albert Einstein Coll Med 83; **RES:** S, NY Hosp-Cornell Med Ctr, New York, NY 83-89; **FEL:** GVS, UC San Francisco Med Ctr, San Francisco, CA 89-90; **FAP:** Assoc Prof Cornell U; **HOSP:** Beth Israel North; **SI:** *Carotid Artery; Thoracic Outlet;* **HMO:** Oxford Aetna Hlth Plan CIGNA Blue Choice Multiplan +

LANG: Sp; 🦽 📷 🚘 🏨 💲 Mcr Mcd WC NFi   Immediately 🖃 **VISA** 💳

Giangola, Gary (MD)　　　GVS
St Luke's Roosevelt Hosp Ctr
St Lukes-Roosevelt Hosp Ctr, 425 W 59th St 7B; New York, NY 10019; (212) 523-8700; **BDCERT:** GVS 86; **MS:** NYU Sch Med 80; **RES:** IM, New York University Med Ctr, New York, NY 80-81; S, New York University Med Ctr, New York, NY 81-85; **FEL:** GVS, New York University Med Ctr, New York, NY 85-86; **FAP:** Asst Prof of Clin S NYU Sch Med; *SI: Carotid Artery; Aortic Aneurysm;* **HMO:** Oxford Aetna Hlth Plan US Hlthcre Chubb

LANG: Sp; 🔲 🔲 🔲 🔲 🔲 🔲　Immediately

Haimov, Moshe (MD)　　　GVS
Mount Sinai Med Ctr
12 E 97th St 1C; New York, NY 10029; (212) 289-3180; **BDCERT:** S 69; GVS 83; **MS:** Israel 62; **RES:** Mount Sinai Med Ctr, New York, NY 64-68; **FAP:** Clin Prof Mt Sinai Sch Med; **HOSP:** Beth Israel Med Ctr; *SI: Carotid Aneurysm; Vascular Reconstruction;* **HMO:** Aetna Hlth Plan CIGNA Oxford

LANG: Sp, Itl, Bul; 🔲 🔲 🔲 🔲 🔲 🔲 🔲 🔲　A Few Days

Harrington, Elizabeth (MD)　GVS
Mount Sinai Med Ctr
Mount Sinai Medical Ctr, 5 E 98th St; New York, NY 10029; (212) 241-7646; **BDCERT:** S 81; GVS 89; **MS:** NY Med Coll 75; **RES:** Mount Sinai Med Ctr, New York, NY 75-80; **FEL:** GVS, Mount Sinai Med Ctr, New York, NY 80-81; **FAP:** Assoc Prof S Mt Sinai Sch Med; *SI: Carotid Endarterectomy*

LANG: Sp, Heb, Rus; 🔲 🔲 🔲 🔲 🔲 🔲 🔲　Immediately ▬ *VISA* 💳 💳

Harrington, Martin (MD)　　　GVS
Mount Sinai Med Ctr
Mt Sinai Med Ctr, 5 E 98th St; New York, NY 10029; (212) 241-7646; **BDCERT:** S 85; GVS 90; **MS:** Harvard Med Sch 75; **RES:** S, Mount Sinai Med Ctr, New York, NY 80-84; IM, St Luke's Roosevelt Hosp Ctr, New York, NY 75-79; **FEL:** Mount Sinai Med Ctr, New York, NY 88-89; S Onc, Mem Sloan Kettering Cancer Ctr, New York, NY 80-84; *SI: Vascular Surgery; Aneurysm Abdominal Aortic*

🔲 🔲 🔲 🔲 🔲 🔲 🔲　Immediately

Haveson, Stephen (MD)　　　GVS
Beth Israel Med Ctr
306 E 15th St; New York, NY 10003; (212) 529-2407; **BDCERT:** S 76; **MS:** Albert Einstein Coll Med 65; **RES:** S, Beth Israel Med Ctr, New York, NY 69-72; **FEL:** GVS, New York University Med Ctr, New York, NY 72-73; **HOSP:** Cabrini Med Ctr; **HMO:** Aetna Hlth Plan Blue Choice Blue Cross & Blue Shield CIGNA HealthNet +

Hollier, Larry (MD)　　　GVS
Mount Sinai Med Ctr
5 E 98th St Box 1259; New York, NY 10029; (212) 241-7646; **BDCERT:** S 76; **MS:** LSU Sch Med, New Orleans 68; **RES:** S, Charity Hosp, New Orleans, LA 68-75; **FEL:** GVS, Baylor Med Ctr, Dallas, TX 73-74; **FAP:** Prof Mt Sinai Sch Med; *SI: Aneurysms; Carotid Disease*

LANG: Fr, Sp, Heb, Rus, Grk; 🔲 🔲 🔲 🔲 🔲 🔲 🔲　A Few Days

Lamparello, Patrick (MD)　　GVS
New York University Med Ctr
Universal Vascular Assoc, 530 1st Ave 6F; New York, NY 10016; (212) 263-7311; **BDCERT:** S 81; GVS 84; **MS:** Albert Einstein Coll Med 76; **RES:** Montefiore Med Ctr, Bronx, NY 76-80; **FEL:** VIR, New York University Med Ctr, New York, NY 80-81; **FAP:** Assoc Prof NYU Sch Med; **HOSP:** Bellevue Hosp Ctr; *SI: Vascular Diseases; Aneurysms*

🔲 🔲 🔲 🔲 🔲 🔲 🔲　A Few Days

Mendes, Donna (MD)　　　GVS
St Luke's Roosevelt Hosp Ctr
1090 Amsterdam Ave 8F; New York, NY 10025; (212) 636-4990; **BDCERT:** S 84; GVS 91; **MS:** Columbia P&S 77; **RES:** S, St Luke's Roosevelt Hosp Ctr, New York, NY 77-82; **FEL:** S, Englewood Hosp, Englewood, NJ 82-84; **FAP:** Asst Clin Prof S Columbia P&S; *SI: Bypass Surgery; Aneurysm Surgery;* **HMO:** Aetna-US Healthcare PHS Magnacare Blue Choice

LANG: Sp; 🔲 🔲 🔲 🔲　A Few Days

Moore, Eric (MD) GVS
St Luke's Roosevelt Hosp Ctr
30 W 60th St; New York, NY 10023; (212) 247-6575; **BDCERT:** S 81; **MS:** Columbia P&S 75; **RES:** St Luke's Roosevelt Hosp Ctr, New York, NY 75-80; **FEL:** GVS, Mem Sloan Kettering Cancer Ctr, New York, NY 80-82; Newark Beth Israel Med Ctr, Newark, NJ 82-83; *SI: Breast Surgery; Carotid Artery Surgery;* **HMO:** CIGNA United Healthcare US Hlthcre Oxford Prucare +

♿ 📷 🅿 🎬 💲 Mcr Immediately ⬤

Nowygrod, Roman (MD) GVS
Columbia-Presbyterian Med Ctr
161 Ft Washington Ave; New York, NY 10032; (212) 305-5374; **BDCERT:** GVS 78; **MS:** Columbia P&S 70; **RES:** Columbia-Presbyterian Med Ctr, New York, NY 76; **FEL:** Columbia-Presbyterian Med Ctr, New York, NY 72; *SI: Aortic Aneurysm Surgery; Carotid Artery;* **HMO:** Aetna Hlth Plan Blue Choice US Hlthcre Oxford Blue Cross & Blue Shield +

♿ 🆂🆄 🅲 📷 🅿 🎬 Mcr A Few Days

Riles, Thomas (MD) GVS
New York University Med Ctr
Universal Vascular Assoc, 550 1st Ave 6F; New York, NY 10016; (212) 263-7311; **BDCERT:** S 77; GVS 83; **MS:** Baylor 69; **RES:** S, New York University Med Ctr, New York, NY 70-76; **FEL:** GVS, New York University Med Ctr, New York, NY 76-77; **FAP:** Prof S NYU Sch Med; **HOSP:** Bellevue Hosp Ctr; *SI: Carotid Artery Surgery; Aneurysm Surgery;* **HMO:** Aetna Hlth Plan Oxford US Hlthcre Prucare United Healthcare +

LANG: Sp, Itl; ♿ 📷 🎬 💲 Mcr Immediately

Rossi, Giuseppi (MD) GVS
St Vincents Hosp & Med Ctr NY
20 W 13th St; New York, NY 10011; (212) 838-3055; **BDCERT:** TS 63; GVS 93; **MS:** Italy 51; **RES:** Aultman Hosp, Canton, OH 54-58; Med Coll of GA Hosp, Augusta, GA 58-61; **HOSP:** Cabrini Med Ctr; *SI: Vascular Surgery; Thoracic Surgery;* **HMO:** GHI Oxford Aetna Hlth Plan US Hlthcre

LANG: Itl, Fr; ♿ 📷 🎬 Mcr Mcd WC Nfl Immediately

Schanzer, Harry (MD) GVS
Mount Sinai Med Ctr
993 Park Ave; New York, NY 10028; (212) 423-0510; **BDCERT:** S 77; **MS:** Chile 68; **RES:** Mount Sinai Med Ctr, New York, NY 71-76; **FAP:** Clin Prof S Mt Sinai Sch Med; **HMO:** Oxford HealthNet Guardian Sanus

Silane, Michael F (MD) GVS
Beth Israel Med Ctr
170 East End Ave 400; New York, NY 10128; (212) 861-2200; **BDCERT:** S 78; GVS 83; **MS:** Georgetown U 69; **RES:** NY Hosp-Cornell Med Ctr, New York, NY 69-72; NY Hosp-Cornell Med Ctr, New York, NY 74-76; **FEL:** GVS, UC San Francisco Med Ctr, San Francisco, CA 77-78; Harvard Med Sch, Cambridge, MA 78-79; **FAP:** Assoc Clin Prof S Cornell U; **HOSP:** NY Hosp-Cornell Med Ctr; *SI: Aortic Aneurysms; Carotid Surgery;* **HMO:** United Healthcare Blue Cross & Blue Shield Oxford CIGNA ABC Health +

LANG: Sp; ♿ 📷 🅿 🎬 Mcr Nfl Immediately

Stein, Jeffrey S (MD) GVS
Mount Sinai Med Ctr
Surgical Associates, 5 E 98th St 14th Fl; New York, NY 10029; (212) 241-7646; **BDCERT:** S 89; GVS 94; **MS:** Washington U, St Louis 82; **RES:** S, Mount Sinai Med Ctr, New York, NY 82-88; **FEL:** SCC, Mount Sinai Med Ctr, New York, NY 88-89; GVS, Mount Sinai Med Ctr, New York, NY 89-91; **FAP:** Asst Prof Mt Sinai Sch Med; *SI: Aneurysms; Varicose Veins;* **HMO:** Oxford Blue Cross & Blue Shield PHS Aetna Hlth Plan

LANG: Sp, Fr; ♿ 📷 🅿 🎬 💲 Mcr Mcd Immediately
VISA ⬤

Guide to symbols and abbreviations can be found on pages 110-113.

409

BRONX
COUNTY

UR LADY OF MERCY MEDICAL CENTER

OUR LADY OF MERCY MEDICAL CENTER
*A University Hospital of New York Medical College
and a Member of the Catholic Health Care Network.*

600 EAST 233rd STREET
BRONX, NY 10466
(718) 920-9000 OR FAX 920-9245
1870 PELHAM PARKWAY SOUTH
BRONX, NY 10461
(718) 430-6000 OR FAX 430-6071

onsorship	Not-for-Profit; Sponsored by the Archdiocese of New York
ds	612
creditation	Joint Commission on Accreditation of Healthcare Organizations, Association of American Medical Colleges, New York State Department of Health

MEMBER OF OUR LADY OF MERCY HEALTHCARE SYSTEM

rving the northeast Bronx and lower Westchester County from its locations at 600 East 233rd Street and e Florence D'Urso Pavilion at 1870 Pelham Parkway South, Our Lady of Mercy Medical Center is a ember of Our Lady of Mercy Healthcare System. The system is comprised of three hospitals (Our Lady Mercy Medical Center, the Florence D'Urso Pavilion and Saint Agnes Hospital), an ambulatory care vilion, six Medical Villages (physician office sites), senior citizen housing, a physician-hospital ganization, a residence for unwed mothers, and a home health agency.

ır Lady of Mercy Medical Center has fully equipped chronic and acute hemodialysis units, inpatient d outpatient psychiatric services, alcoholism services, ambulatory surgery centers, intensive care units, ophthalmology unit, a maternity and newborn unit with NICU, specialized geriatric units, a full-ser-:e dental department and numerous ambulatory care services.

UNIVERSITY HOSPITAL OF NEW YORK MEDICAL COLLEGE

ır Lady of Mercy boasts of twelve departments headed by full-time board certified physicians who pro-de significant educational and research programs. The medical center is one of two University ospitals of New York Medical College, which sponsors most of OLM's residency programs. The niversity Hospital designation came as a reflection of a substantially increased graduate medical lucation program that now includes 17 residencies and 5 fellowships, along with an increased focus on search. Our Lady of Mercy Medical Center offers approved residency programs in anesthesiology, mmunity medicine, dentistry, dermatology, emergency medicine, ENT, internal medicine, obstetrics d gynecology, ophthalmology, orthopedics, pediatrics, physical medicine and rehabilitation, podiatry, rgery and urology.

ENTERS OF EXCELLENCE

eriatric Medicine	One of the largest acute care geriatric programs in the region.
ncology	Services include the Center for Breast Diseases and Stereotactic Radiosurgery.
aternal and Child Health	The Roy Rogers & Dale Evans Children's Center.
ome Health Care	Preventative and supportive home care services.
astroenterology	More than 3,000 procedures are performed each year.
ardiology	Nuclear cardiology services and cutting-edge equipment.

ur Lady of Mercy Medical Center operates a toll-free, 7 days a week, 24 hours a day physician referral service -800-628-1008). Multilingual operators are available, with computerized access to more than 600 staff and affil-ted physicians. More than 80 percent of the physicians are board certified in their fields.

Specialties in capital letters indicate Primary Care Specialties. However, many doctors will be certified in subspecialty, but will practice predominantly primary care medicine. In our lists this will be indicated.

*Oncologists deal with Cancer

ADDICTION PSYCHIATRY

Kierszenbaum, Hugo (MD) AdP
Our Lady of Mercy Med Ctr
Our Lady of Mercy Medical Center, 4401 Bronx
Blvd; Bronx, NY 10470; (718) 920-9100;
BDCERT: AdP 77; **MS:** Argentina 63; **RES:** Psyc,
Kings County Hosp Ctr, Brooklyn, NY 73-76; **FAP:**
Assoc Clin Prof NY Med Coll; **HOSP:** Westchester
Med Ctr; *SI: Substance Disorders*
LANG: Sp; ⓖ 🏧 Ⓒ 🔲 🏧 Ⓢ Ⓜ Ⓜ Ⓦ
A Few Days

ADOLESCENT MEDICINE

Coupey, Susan (MD) AM
Montefiore Med Ctr
111 E 210th St; Bronx, NY 10467; (718) 920-
6783; **BDCERT:** Ped 79; **MS:** Canada 75; **RES:**
Montreal Gen Hosp, Montreal, Canada 75-76;
Montreal Children's Hosp, Montreal, Canada 76-
78; **FEL:** AM, Montefiore Med Ctr, Bronx, NY 78-
79; **FAP:** Prof Albert Einstein Coll Med; *SI:*
Adolescent Gynecology; Eating Disorders; **HMO:** Blue
Cross & Blue Shield
ⓖ 🔲 Ⓜ Ⓝ 2-4 Weeks **VISA** 💳

ALLERGY & IMMUNOLOGY

Kaufman, Alan (MD) A&I
Westchester Square Med Ctr
3626 E Tremont Ave; Bronx, NY 10465; (718)
597-9000; **BDCERT:** A&I 89; IM 88; **MS:** West
Indies 84; **RES:** IM, Metropolitan Hosp Ctr, New
York, NY 84-87; **FEL:** A&I, Albert Einstein Med Ctr,
Bronx, NY 87-89; **HOSP:** Our Lady of Mercy Med
Ctr; *SI: Asthma; Sinusitis*; **HMO:** Blue Cross CIGNA
Oxford Prucare United Healthcare +
LANG: Itl; ⓖ 🏧 Ⓒ 🔲 🏧 🏧 Ⓢ Ⓜ A Few Days

Lehach, Joan (MD) A&I
St Barnabas Hosp-Bronx
1488 Metropolitan Ave; Bronx, NY 10462; (718)
918-1991; **BDCERT:** A&I 90; **MS:** Chile 85; **RES:**
IM, St Barnabas Med Ctr, Bronx, NY 85-88; **FEL:**
A&I, Albert Einstein Med Ctr, Bronx, NY 88-90

Resnick, David (MD) A&I
Columbia-Presbyterian Med Ctr
Columbia University Dept Pedtrc & Allergy, 3765
Riverdale Ave 7; Bronx, NY 10463; (718) 796-
9393; **BDCERT:** A&I 91; **MS:** SUNY Hlth Sci Ctr 86;
RES: Brookdale Univ Hosp Med Ctr, Brooklyn, NY
86-89; **FEL:** A&I, Columbia-Presbyterian Med Ctr,
New York, NY 89-91; **FAP:** Asst Lecturer Ped
Columbia P&S; **HOSP:** NYU Downtown Hosp; *SI:*
Asthma; Allergic Rhinitis; **HMO:** Oxford Blue Cross &
Blue Shield Prucare Aetna Hlth Plan
ⓖ Ⓒ 🏧 🏧 Ⓢ 1 Week

Rosenstreich, David (MD) A&I
Montefiore Med Ctr
Albert Einstein College of Medicine Faculty Practice,
1575 Blondell Ave; Bronx, NY 10461; (718) 405-
8308; **BDCERT:** A&I 75; **MS:** NYU Sch Med 67;
RES: Med, Albert Einstein Med Ctr, Bronx, NY 68-
69; **FEL:** A&I, Nat Inst Health, Bethesda, MD 69-72;
FAP: Prof Albert Einstein Coll Med; *SI: Urticaria;*
Sinusitis; **HMO:** NYLCare Oxford US Hlthcre GHI
HealthNet +
LANG: Sp, Rus; ⓖ Ⓒ 🔲 🏧 🏧 Ⓢ Ⓜ Ⓜ Ⓦ Ⓝ 🏧
VISA 💳

Rubinstein, Arye (MD) A&I
Montefiore Med Ctr
1300 Morris Park Ave; Bronx, NY 10461; (718)
430-2319; **BDCERT:** A&I 77; Ped 76; **MS:**
Switzerland 62; **RES:** Tel Hashomer Hosp, Tel Aviv,
Israel 63-67; **FEL:** A&I, U of Bern, Bern, Switzerland
67-69; Harvard Med Sch, Cambridge, MA 71-73;
FAP: Prof Albert Einstein Coll Med; **HOSP:**
Montefiore Med Ctr-Weiler/Einstein Div; *SI:*
Immunodeficiencies; Allergies—Asthma; **HMO:** Blue
Cross & Blue Shield Blue Choice United Healthcare
CIGNA Oxford +
LANG: Ger, Heb, Rus, Sp; ⓖ Ⓒ 🔲 🏧 🏧 Ⓢ Ⓜ Ⓜ
2-4 Weeks 🏧 **VISA** 💳

ANESTHESIOLOGY

Saubermann, Albert J (MD) Anes
Montefiore Med Ctr

111 E 210th St; Bronx, NY 10467; (718) 920-2802; **BDCERT:** Anes 72; **MS:** UC San Francisco 68; **RES:** Anes, Beth Israel Med Ctr, Boston, MA 69-72; **FEL:** Anes, Harvard Med Sch, Cambridge, MA 72-73; **FAP:** Prof Albert Einstein Coll Med; **HMO:** CIGNA Empire Blue Cross & Shield HIP Network Metlife

CARDIOLOGY (CARDIOVASCULAR DISEASE)

Bhalodkar, Narendra (MD)   Cv
Bronx Lebanon Hosp Ctr

Dept of Medicine, 1650 Selwyn Ave 8C; Bronx, NY 10457; (718) 960-2086; **BDCERT:** IM 77; Cv 79; **MS:** India 70; **RES:** IM, Bronx Lebanon Hosp Ctr, Bronx, NY 74-76; **FEL:** Cv, Bronx Lebanon Hosp Ctr, Bronx, NY 76-78; **HMO:** Blue Cross & Blue Shield HealthNet US Hlthcre Oxford Bronx Health +

LANG: Sp, Hin, Guj, Mar; ⑤ ⓒ ⓐ ⓧ ⬛ ⑤ Mcr Mod WC 2-4 Weeks

Chiaramida, Salvatore (MD)   Cv
Our Lady of Mercy Med Ctr

600 E 233rd St; Bronx, NY 10466; (718) 920-9257; **BDCERT:** IM 77; Cv 79; **MS:** NY Med Coll 74; **RES:** IM, NY Med Coll, New York, NY; **FEL:** Cv, NY Hosp-Cornell Med Ctr, New York, NY; N Shore Univ Hosp-Manhasset, Manhasset, NY; **SI:** *Congestive Heart failure; Angina;* **HMO:** Prucare US Hlthcre Blue Choice Empire Oxford +

LANG: Sp, Rus; ⑤ ⓐ ⬛ Mcr Mod NFl Immediately

Fisher, John D (MD)   Cv
Montefiore Med Ctr

Arrhythmia Service, 111 E 210th St; Bronx, NY 10461; (718) 920-4291; **BDCERT:** IM 72; Cv 75; **MS:** Wayne State U Sch Med 69; **RES:** Boston Med Ctr, Boston, MA; NY Hosp-Cornell Med Ctr, New York, NY; **FEL:** Cv, Montefiore Med Ctr, Bronx, NY; Hammersmith Hosp, London, England; **FAP:** Prof Albert Einstein Coll Med; **HOSP:** North Central Bronx Hosp; **SI:** *Pacemaker Implantation; Radio Frequency Ablation;* **HMO:** GHI Aetna Hlth Plan Empire Blue Cross & Shield Bronx Health CIGNA +

LANG: Sp, Rus; ⑤ ⓐ ⓧ ⬛ Mcr Mod 2-4 Weeks

Goldberg, Jack (MD)   Cv
Montefiore Med Ctr

3201 Grand Concourse 1J; Bronx, NY 10468; (718) 933-2244; **BDCERT:** Cv 57; **MS:** SUNY Downstate 57; **RES:** IM, Montefiore Med Ctr, Bronx, NY 60-62; **FEL:** Cv, Mt Zion Hosp, San Francisco, CA 62-63; **HMO:** Oxford Blue Cross & Blue Shield Blue Cross & Blue Shield GHI

LANG: Sp, Alb; ⑤ ⓐ ⬛ Mcr Mod 1 Week

Gordon, Garet M (MD)   Cv
Montefiore Med Ctr

111 E 210th St; Bronx, NY 10467; (718) 920-7638; **BDCERT:** IM 65; Cv 68; **MS:** SUNY Hlth Sci Ctr 58; **RES:** IM, Montefiore Med Ctr, Bronx, NY 58-61; **FEL:** Cv, Montefiore Med Ctr, Bronx, NY 61-62; **FAP:** Assoc Prof Albert Einstein Coll Med; **SI:** *Clinical Cardiology; Noninvasive Cardiology;* **HMO:** Oxford US Hlthcre HIP Network Magnacare Blue Choice +

LANG: Sp; ⑤ ⓐ ⬛ Mcr Mod WC NFl Immediately
VISA 💳

Keller, Peter Karl (MD)   Cv
Montefiore Med Ctr-Weiler/Einstein Div

1578 Williamsbridge Rd; Bronx, NY 10461; (718) 892-7817; **BDCERT:** IM 88; Cv 91; **MS:** Mt Sinai Sch Med 85; **RES:** IM, Bronx Muncipal Hosp Ctr, Bronx, NY 86-88; **FEL:** Cv, Bronx Muncipal Hosp Ctr, Bronx, NY 88-91; **FAP:** Assoc Clin Prof Albert Einstein Coll Med; **HOSP:** Westchester Square Med Ctr; **SI:** *Congestive Heart Failure; Coronary Artery Disease;* **HMO:** GHI Oxford US Hlthcre CIGNA

⑤ ⓒ ⓐ ⓧ ⬛ ⑤ Mcr Mod WC A Few Days

Lucariello, Richard (MD) Cv
Our Lady of Mercy Med Ctr
Our Lady Mercy, 600 E 233 St; Bronx, NY 10466; (718) 920-9256; **BDCERT:** IM 87; Cv 91; **MS:** NY Med Coll 84; **RES:** IM, Westchester Med Ctr, Valhalla, NY 85-87; **FEL:** Cv, St Vincent's, New York, NY 87-89; Cv, Westchester Med Ctr, Valhalla, NY 89-90; *SI: Congestive Heart Failure; Angina;* **HMO:** Oxford Blue Choice US Hlthcre GHI Prucare +

    Immediately

Menegus, Mark (MD) Cv
Montefiore Med Ctr
Div of Urol/ Montefiore Med Ctr, 111 E 210th St; Bronx, NY 10467; (718) 920-5528; **BDCERT:** Cv 87; IM 84; **MS:** UMDNJ-RW Johnson Med Sch 81; **RES:** IM, Montefiore Med Ctr, Bronx, NY 81-84; **FEL:** Cv, Montefiore Med Ctr, Bronx, NY 85-87; **FAP:** Assoc Prof Albert Einstein Coll Med; *SI: Coronary Angioplasty; Lipid Management*

LANG: Sp, Rus;   1 Week

Monrad, E Scott (MD) Cv
Montefiore Med Ctr-Weiler/Einstein Div
1825 Eastchester Ave; Bronx, NY 10461; (718) 904-2927; **BDCERT:** IM 82; Cv 85; **MS:** McGill U 79; **RES:** New England Med Ctr, Boston, MA 79-82; **FEL:** Cv, Beth Israel Med Ctr, Boston, MA 82-85; **HOSP:** Jacobi Med Ctr; *SI: Angioplasty; Stents;* **HMO:** Oxford Aetna-US Healthcare US Hlthcre

LANG: Sp, Itl, Ger, Fr;   Immediately

Nisi, Rudolph (MD) Cv
Westchester Square Med Ctr
1625 St Peter's Ave; Bronx, NY 10461; (718) 824-8693; **MS:** Italy 58; **RES:** New Rochelle Hosp Med Ctr, New Rochelle, NY; **HMO:** Oxford

    Immediately

Phillips, Malcolm (MD) Cv
St Barnabas Hosp-Bronx
4422 3rd Ave; Bronx, NY 10457; (718) 960-6205; **BDCERT:** IM 80; Cv 82; **MS:** Columbia P&S 76; **RES:** NY Hosp-Cornell Med Ctr, New York, NY; **FEL:** Cv, NYU Med Ctr, New York, NY

Scheuer, James (MD) Cv
Montefiore Med Ctr
1300 E Morris Park Ave; Bronx, NY 10461; (718) 430-8560; **BDCERT:** IM 63; Cv 74; **MS:** Yale U Sch Med 56; **RES:** Bellevue Hosp Ctr, New York, NY 56-57; Mount Sinai Med Ctr, New York, NY 57-58; **FEL:** Mount Sinai Med Ctr, New York, NY 58-59; NY Hosp-Cornell Med Ctr, New York, NY 62-63; *SI: Arteriosclerotic Heart Disease; Congestive Heart Failure;* **HMO:** Aetna Hlth Plan CIGNA GHI Health First NYLCare +

    2-4 Weeks **VISA**

Schick, David (MD) Cv
Montefiore Med Ctr
3201 Grand Concourse 1J; Bronx, NY 10468; (718) 933-2244; **BDCERT:** IM 72; Cv 75; **MS:** Albert Einstein Coll Med 66; **RES:** Cv, Montefiore Med Ctr, Bronx, NY 71-73; Med, Montefiore Med Ctr, Bronx, NY 69-71; **FAP:** Asst Clin Prof Albert Einstein Coll Med; **HMO:** Aetna Hlth Plan Oxford Blue Choice Blue Cross Blue Shield +

LANG: Sp, Itl;   2-4 Weeks

Silverman, Rubin (MD) Cv
Montefiore Med Ctr-Weiler/Einstein Div
Park Medical Associates, 1180 Morris Park Ave Fl 2; Bronx, NY 10461; (718) 409-3335; **BDCERT:** IM 81; **MS:** Albert Einstein Coll Med 78; **RES:** Jacobi Med Ctr, Bronx, NY 78-81; **FEL:** Cv, Montefiore Med Ctr, Bronx, NY 81-83; **FAP:** Asst Prof Med Albert Einstein Coll Med; **HOSP:** St Barnabas Hosp-Bronx; *SI: Echocardiography;* **HMO:** Oxford Aetna Hlth Plan CIGNA GHI Magnacare +

LANG: Yd, Heb;   A Few Days

Ware, J Anthony (MD) Cv
Montefiore Med Ctr
Montefiore Medical Center, 1300 Morris Park Ave; Bronx, NY 10461; (718) 920-7049; **BDCERT:** IM 81; Cv 85; **MS:** Univ Kans Sch Med 77; **RES:** Baylor Coll Med, Houston, TX 78-79; Cv, Baylor Coll Med, Houston, TX 79-81; **FAP:** Prof Med Albert Einstein Coll Med; *SI: Angiogenesis; Vascular Biology*

CHILD NEUROLOGY

Kang, Harriet (MD)   ChiN
Montefiore Med Ctr
111 E 210th St; Bronx, NY 10467; (718) 920-
4378; **BDCERT:** ChiN 81; Ped 79; **MS:** Johns
Hopkins U 74; **RES:** Ped, Johns Hopkins Hosp,
Baltimore, MD 74-76; N, U MN Med Ctr,
Minneapolis, MN 76-79; **FEL:** C/Nph, U MN Med
Ctr, Minneapolis, MN 79-80; **FAP:** Assoc Prof
Albert Einstein Coll Med; **HMO:** Aetna Hlth Plan
Blue Choice CIGNA HealthNet Metlife +
🚫 🔟 🖼 🛏 💲 Mcr A Few Days **VISA** 💳

Rapin, Isabelle (MD)   ChiN
Montefiore Med Ctr
1165 Morris Park Ave 325; Bronx, NY 10461;
(718) 430-3814; **BDCERT:** N 60; ChiN 68; **MS:**
Switzerland 52; **RES:** N, Columbia-Presbyterian
Med Ctr, New York, NY 54-57; **FEL:** ChiN,
Columbia-Presbyterian Med Ctr, New York, NY 57-
58; **FAP:** Prof Albert Einstein Coll Med; **SI:** *Autism;
Developmental Disorders;* **HMO:** None
LANG: Fr; 🚫 🛏 💲 4+ Weeks **VISA** 💳

Shinnar, Shlomo (MD)   ChiN
Montefiore Med Ctr
Montefiore/Einstein Epilepsy Management Ctr, 111
E 210th St; Bronx, NY 10467; (718) 920-4378;
BDCERT: N 84; Ped 84; **MS:** Albert Einstein Coll
Med 78; **RES:** Ped, Johns Hopkins Hosp, Baltimore,
MD 78-80; N, Johns Hopkins Hosp, Baltimore, MD
80-83; **SI:** *Epilepsy & Seizure Disorders;* **HMO:**
Oxford CIGNA US Hlthcre Metlife PHCS +
LANG: Sp, Heb; 🚫 📞 🔟 🖼 🛏 💲 Mcr NFl 1 Week

Spiro, Alfred (MD)   ChiN
Montefiore Med Ctr
1165 Morris Park Ave 3rd Fl; Bronx, NY 10461;
(718) 430-3814; **BDCERT:** N 68; ChiN 69; **MS:**
Switzerland 55; **RES:** Hosp of U Penn, Philadelphia,
PA 63-64; Children's Hosp of Philadelphia,
Philadelphia, PA 64-66; **FAP:** Lecturer ChiN Albert
Einstein Coll Med; **SI:** *Muscle Diseases; Muscle
Biopsies*
🚫 🔟 🖼 🛏 💲 Mcr A Few Days

COLON & RECTAL SURGERY

Foxx, Martin (MD)   CRS
Montefiore Med Ctr
3224 Grand Concourse E2; Bronx, NY 10458;
(718) 584-6531; **BDCERT:** S 71; **MS:** U Hlth
Sci/Chicago Med Sch 65; **RES:** S, Kings County
Hosp Ctr, Brooklyn, NY 65-66; S, Montefiore Med
Ctr, Bronx, NY 67-71; **FAP:** Asst Clin Prof S Albert
Einstein Coll Med; **SI:** *Hernia Repair Colorectal;
Laparoscopic Gallbladder*
LANG: Sp; 🔟 🖼 🛏 💲 Mcr WC NFl A Few Days

CRITICAL CARE MEDICINE

Halpern, Neil (MD)   CCM
VA Med Ctr-Bronx
VA Medical Center, 130 W Kingsbridge Rd; Bronx,
NY 10468; (718) 584-9000; **BDCERT:** IM 84; CCM
89; **MS:** Mt Sinai Sch Med 81; **RES:** IM, Mount Sinai
Med Ctr, New York, NY 82-84; **FEL:** CCM, U of
Pittsburgh Med Ctr, Pittsburgh, PA 84-85; **FAP:**
Assoc Prof Mt Sinai Sch Med; **HOSP:** Mount Sinai
Med Ctr; **SI:** *Critical Illness*
🚫 📞 🔟 🖼 🛏

DERMATOLOGY

Alaghabend, Mehran (MD)   D
Our Lady of Mercy Med Ctr
Faculty Dermatology, 600 E 233rd St; Bronx, NY
10466; (718) 324-7546; **BDCERT:** D 96; **MS:** NY
Med Coll 91; **FAP:** Asst Prof NY Med Coll; **HOSP:**
Westchester Square Med Ctr; **SI:** *Skin Cancer;
Pediatric Dermatology;* **HMO:** Blue Cross Oxford US
Hlthcre GHI Magnacare +
LANG: Sp, Per; 🚫 📞 🔟 🖼 🛏 💲 Mcr

Berger, Joshua (MD) D
Montefiore Med Ctr

3333 Henry Hudson Pkwy 1B; Bronx, NY 10463;
(718) 543-0900; **BDCERT:** D 77; **MS:** SUNY
Downstate 72; **RES:** D, Albert Einstein Med Ctr,
Bronx, NY 74-77; **HMO:** Oxford

🔲 🔲 🔲 🔲 🔲 A Few Days

Burk, Peter (MD) D
Montefiore Med Ctr

2600 Netherland Ave; Bronx, NY 10463; (718)
543-7711; **BDCERT:** D 74; **MS:** Duke U 66; **RES:** U
of Pittsburgh Med Ctr, Pittsburgh, PA 66-67;
Eugene Talmadge Hosp, Augusta, GA 67-68; **FEL:**
D, Harvard Med Sch, Cambridge, MA 71-73; **FAP:**
Assoc Clin Prof Med Albert Einstein Coll Med;
HOSP: Montefiore Med Ctr-Weiler/Einstein Div;
HMO: Blue Choice US Hlthcre United Healthcare
GHI

Don, Philip (MD & PhD) D
Metropolitan Hosp Ctr

295 W 231st St; Bronx, NY 10463; (718) 549-
1300; **BDCERT:** D 87; **MS:** Israel 82; **RES:** U Hosp of
Cleveland, Cleveland, OH 84-87; **FEL:** Hassadah
Hosp, Jerusalem, Israel 75; **FAP:** Assoc Prof NY Med
Coll; **SI:** *Eczema; Acne;* **HMO:** Prucare Oxford
Magnacare GHI US Hlthcre +

LANG: Chi, Rus, Sp, Heb, Yd; 🔲 🔲 🔲 🔲 🔲 🔲 🔲
🔲 🔲 🔲 Immediately

Fisher, Michael (MD) D
Montefiore Med Ctr-Weiler/Einstein Div

1575 Blondell Ave; Bronx, NY 10461; (718) 405-
8306; **BDCERT:** D 70; **MS:** SUNY Hlth Sci Ctr 63;
RES: Mass Gen Hosp, Boston, MA 66-69; **HOSP:**
Montefiore Med Ctr

Katz, Susan (MD) D
Montefiore Med Ctr

1578 Williamsbridge Rd; Bronx, NY 10461; (718)
518-8888; **BDCERT:** D 83; **MS:** NYU Sch Med 77;
RES: IM, St Luke's Roosevelt Hosp Ctr, New York,
NY 77-79; D, Montefiore Med Ctr, Bronx, NY 80-
83; **FAP:** Asst Prof Med Albert Einstein Coll Med; **SI:**
Psoriasis; Skin Cancer; **HMO:** Oxford Blue Choice
HealthNet

LANG: Itl, Ger, Sp; 🔲 🔲 🔲 🔲 🔲 🔲 🔲 2-
4 Weeks 🔲 **VISA** 🔲 🔲

Liteplo, Ronald (MD) D
Montefiore Med Ctr

3176 Bainbridge Ave; Bronx, NY 10467; (718)
515-0200; **BDCERT:** D 78; **IM** 75; **MS:** NYU Sch
Med 72; **RES:** IM, Univ Hosp SUNY Buffalo, Buffalo,
NY 72-75; D, Univ Hosp SUNY Buffalo, Buffalo, NY
76-78; **FEL:** IM, Univ Hosp SUNY Buffalo, Buffalo,
NY 75-76; **FAP:** Asst Clin Prof Albert Einstein Coll
Med; **SI:** *Connective Tissue Disease and Immunology;
Scabies. Infestations.;* **HMO:** Blue Choice PHS GHI
IPA

LANG: Ukr, Sp; 🔲 🔲 🔲 🔲 🔲 🔲 🔲 🔲
A Few Days

Mermelstein, Harold (MD) D
New York University Med Ctr

3333 Henry Hudson Pkwy 1L; Bronx, NY 10463;
(718) 601-2504; **BDCERT:** D 79; **MS:** NY Med Coll
75; **RES:** D, New York University Med Ctr, New
York, NY 76-79; **FEL:** Dermatologic S, New York
University Med Ctr, New York, NY 79-80; **FAP:**
Asst Clin Prof NYU Sch Med; **HOSP:** Lawrence
Hosp; **HMO:** Oxford

🔲 🔲 🔲 🔲 🔲 🔲 🔲 🔲 A Few Days

O'Connor, Kathleen (MD) D
Montefiore Med Ctr

1578 Williamsbridge Rd; Bronx, NY 10461; (718)
518-8888; **BDCERT:** D 75; **MS:** Ireland 65; **RES:**
Med, Elmhurst Hosp Ctr, Elmhurst, NY 66-68; D,
Albert Einstein Med Ctr, Bronx, NY 74; **HOSP:**
Montefiore Med Ctr-Weiler/Einstein Div; **SI:** *Skin
Cancer; Eczema;* **HMO:** Oxford Blue Choice PHS
United Healthcare

🔲 🔲 🔲 🔲 🔲 🔲 🔲 1 Week 🔲 **VISA** 🔲

Guide to symbols and abbreviations can be found on pages 110-113.

419

DIAGNOSTIC RADIOLOGY

Lang, Jeffrey (MD) DR
Our Lady of Mercy Med Ctr

Dept of Radiology Our Lady of Mercy Med Ctr, 600 E 23th St; Bronx, NY 10466; (718) 920-9188; **BDCERT:** Rad 84; NR 96; **MS:** Emory U Sch Med 80; **RES:** DR, St Vincents Hosp & Med Ctr NY, New York, NY 80-84; **FEL:** NR, New York University Med Ctr, New York, NY 84-85; **FAP:** Asst Clin Prof NY Med Coll; **SI:** *Neuroradiology; MRI; CT Scanning;* **HMO:** Most

[symbols] A Few Days

Morehouse, Helen (MD) DR
Jacobi Med Ctr

Bronx Lebanon Hosp Ctr,; Bronx, NY 10461; (718) 518-5633; **BDCERT:** DR 76; **MS:** Univ Ky Coll Med 71; **RES:** Rochester Gen Hosp, Rochester, NY 71-72

EMERGENCY MEDICINE

Haydock, Timothy (MD) EM
Our Lady of Mercy Med Ctr

Our Lady of Mercy Med Ctr, 600 E 2 33rd St; Bronx, NY 10466; (718) 920-9135; **BDCERT:** EM 94; **MS:** Case West Res U 79

Osborn, Harold (MD) EM
St Barnabas Hosp-Bronx

LI College Hospital - ER, 600 Minnieford Ave; Bronx, NY 10464; (718) 780-4764; **BDCERT:** EM 82; IM 79; **MS:** Columbia P&S 70; **RES:** Ped, Lincoln Med & Mental Hlth Ctr, Bronx, NY; IM, Lincoln Med & Mental Hlth Ctr, Bronx, NY; **SI:** *Asthma; Sickle Cell Anemia;* **HMO:** Most Plans

[symbols] Immediately

Sunderwirth-Bailly, Ramona (MD) EM
Bronx Lebanon Hosp Ctr

Bronx Lebanon Hospital Center, Dept of Emergency Medicine, 1650 Grand Concourse; Bronx, NY 10457; (718) 518-5760; **BDCERT:** Ped 89; EM 96; **MS:** France 85; **RES:** Ped, Bronx Lebanon Hosp Ctr, Bronx, NY 86-89; **FEL:** Columbia-Presbyterian Med Ctr, New York, NY 90-91; **FAP:** Asst Prof Albert Einstein Coll Med; **SI:** *Child Abuse Neglect;* **HMO:** HIP Network Oxford Health First Bronx Health

LANG: Fr, Prt, Sp; [symbols] Immediately

ENDOCRINOLOGY, DIABETES & METABOLISM

Allen, Carol (MD) EDM
VA Med Ctr-Bronx

130 W Kingsbridge Rd; Bronx, NY 10468; (718) 584-9000; **BDCERT:** IM 82; **MS:** Univ Penn 79; **RES:** VA Med Ctr-Bronx, Bronx, NY 82; **FEL:** EDM, VA Med Ctr-Bronx, Bronx, NY 84

[symbols] 1 Week

Cohen, Charmian (MD) EDM **PCP**
Montefiore Med Ctr-Weiler/Einstein Div

1578 Williamsbridge Rd; Bronx, NY 10461; (718) 892-7033; **BDCERT:** IM 87; EDM 89; **MS:** South Africa 77; **FEL:** EDM, Albert Einstein Med Ctr, Bronx, NY; **HOSP:** Westchester Square Med Ctr; **SI:** *Diabetes; Obesity;* **HMO:** Oxford GHI Aetna-US Healthcare Blue Choice

LANG: Sp, Afk; [symbols] Immediately

Fleischer, Norman (MD)   EDM
Montefiore Med Ctr

1575 Blondell Ave 200; Bronx, NY 10461; (718) 405-8260; **BDCERT:** IM 68; EDM 73; **MS:** Vanderbilt U Sch Med 61; **RES:** Albert Einstein Med Ctr, Bronx, NY 61-64; **FEL:** Vanderbilt U Med Ctr, Nashville, TN 64-66; **FAP:** Dir EDM Albert Einstein Coll Med; **HOSP:** Montefiore Med Ctr-Weiler/Einstein Div; **SI:** *Thyroid; Pituitary and Adrenal;* **HMO:** Oxford Blue Choice PHS NYLCare US Hlthcre +

♿ 🔆 🔒 🚹 🏥 🆂 🅼 2-4 Weeks **VISA** 💳

Freeman, Ruth (MD)   EDM
Montefiore Med Ctr-Weiler/Einstein Div

1300 Morris Park Ave; Bronx, NY 10461; (718) 405-8214; **BDCERT:** EDM 72; **MS:** Albert Einstein Coll Med 60; **RES:** Mount Sinai Med Ctr, New York, NY 63-64; **FEL:** EDM, Mount Sinai Med Ctr, New York, NY 64-65; **HOSP:** Bronx Lebanon Hosp Ctr; **HMO:** Blue Choice HealthNet GHI Oxford US Hlthcre +

♿ 🔆 🔒 🏥 🆂 🅼 4+ Weeks

Guzman, Rodolpho (MD)   EDM
Bronx Lebanon Hosp Ctr

Bronx Lebanon Hospital, 860 Grand Concourse Ste 1I; Bronx, NY 10451; (718) 585-5060; **BDCERT:** IM 91; EDM 95; **MS:** Dominican Republic 79; **RES:** EDM, Lincoln Med & Mental Hlth Ctr, Bronx, NY 90-92; **HMO:** 32BJ 1199 Aetna-US Healthcare Empire Corporate Care +

LANG: Sp; 🔒 🏥 🆂 🅼 2-4 Weeks

Hupart, Kenneth (MD)   EDM
Montefiore Med Ctr

Montefiore Medical Center, 111 E 210th St; Bronx, NY 10467; (718) 920-4819; **BDCERT:** EDM 89; IM 85; **MS:** SUNY Hlth Sci Ctr 82; **RES:** IM, Montefiore Med Ctr, Bronx, NY 82-86; IM, Montefiore Med Ctr, Bronx, NY 85-86; **FEL:** EDM, Montefiore Med Ctr, Bronx, NY 86-88; **FAP:** Assoc Prof Albert Einstein Coll Med; **SI:** *Thyroid Disease; Lipid Disorders & Diabetes*

♿ 🏥 🆂 🅼 4+ Weeks ▦ **VISA** 💳

Schwartz, Ernest (MD)   EDM
Our Lady of Mercy Med Ctr

600 E 233rd Rd; Bronx, NY 10466; (718) 220-2188; **BDCERT:** IM 56; EDM 72; **MS:** Columbia P&S 51; **RES:** UC San Francisco Med Ctr, San Francisco, CA 51-53; Wadsworth VA Hosp, Los Angeles, CA 53-54; **FEL:** EDM, Mem Sloan Kettering Cancer Ctr, New York, NY 56-57; **HOSP:** VA Med Ctr-Bronx; **SI:** *Endocrinology & Diabetes; Thyroid Disease;* **HMO:** Blue Choice GHI

🆂🅂 🔆 🔒 🚹 🏥 🅼 1 Week

Shamoon, Harry (MD)   EDM
Montefiore Med Ctr

Endocrinology & Diabetes Faculty Practice, 1575 Blondell Ave 200; Bronx, NY 10461; (718) 405-8271; **BDCERT:** IM 77; EDM 79; **MS:** Yale U Sch Med 74; **RES:** Jacobi Med Ctr, Bronx, NY 75-77; **FEL:** EDM, Yale-New Haven Hosp, New Haven, CT 78-79; **FAP:** Prof Albert Einstein Coll Med; **SI:** *Diabetes;* **HMO:** CIGNA Oxford Blue Cross & Blue Shield Multiplan US Hlthcre +

♿ 🔆 🔒 🏥 🆂 🅼 2-4 Weeks **VISA** 💳

Surks, Martin (MD)   EDM
Montefiore Med Ctr

111 E 210th St; Bronx, NY 10467; (718) 920-4331; **BDCERT:** IM 67; EDM 77; **MS:** NYU Sch Med 60; **RES:** Montefiore Med Ctr, Bronx, NY 60-62; VA Med Ctr-Bronx, Bronx, NY 62-63; **FEL:** Montefiore Med Ctr, Bronx, NY 63-64; **FAP:** Prof Med Albert Einstein Coll Med; **HOSP:** North Central Bronx Hosp; **SI:** *Thyroid, Pituitary Disorders,; Calcium Disorders;* **HMO:** Oxford Aetna Hlth Plan Empire 1199 Sel Pro +

♿ 🔆 🔒 🚹 🏥 🆂 🅼 🅼 A Few Days **VISA** 💳

Zonszein, Joel (MD)   EDM
Montefiore Med Ctr

1575 Blondell Ave 200; Bronx, NY 10461; (718) 405-8260; **BDCERT:** EDM 77; IM 77; **MS:** Mexico 69; **RES:** Maimonides Med Ctr, Brooklyn, NY 70-72; Jacobi Med Ctr, Bronx, NY 72-73; **FEL:** Northwestern Mem Hosp, Chicago, IL 73-74; Georgetown U Hosp, Washington, DC 74-75; **FAP:** Assoc Prof Albert Einstein Coll Med; **SI:** *Diabetes Mellitus; Thyroid Disease*

LANG: Sp, Heb; ♿ 🆂🅂 🔆 🏥 🆂 🅼 1 Week

Guide to symbols and abbreviations can be found on pages 110-113.

421

FAMILY PRACTICE

Biagiotti, Wendy (MD)   FP   PCP
Westchester Square Med Ctr

3167 E Tremont Ave; Bronx, NY 10461; (718) 863-7925; **BDCERT:** FP 95; **MS:** Mexico 88; **RES:** St Joseph's Med Ctr-Stamford, Stamford, CT 92-94; **HMO:** Oxford Magnacare Chubb Pomco

LANG: Itl, Sp; [symbols] 1 Week

Cahill, John (MD)   FP   PCP
Westchester Square Med Ctr

4000 Seton Ave; Bronx, NY 10466; (718) 324-5408; **BDCERT:** FP 72; **MS:** Georgetown U 60; **RES:** Kings County Hosp Ctr, Brooklyn, NY 60-61; **HMO:** GHI Oxford NYLCare Blue Cross CIGNA +

[symbols] A Few Days

Cordero, Evelyn (MD)   FP   PCP
Our Lady of Mercy Med Ctr

941 Castle Hill Ave; Bronx, NY 10473; (718) 792-3117; **BDCERT:** FP 82; **MS:** SUNY Hlth Sci Ctr 79; **RES:** FP, St Joseph's Med Ctr-Yonkers, Yonkers, NY 79-82; **HOSP:** St Barnabas Hosp-Bronx; **HMO:** Aetna-US Healthcare Oxford Prucare United Healthcare GHI +

LANG: Sp; [symbols] A Few Days

D'Angelo, Enrico (MD)   FP   PCP
Westchester Square Med Ctr

1803 Mahan Ave; Bronx, NY 10461; (718) 409-2762; **BDCERT:** FP 95; **MS:** Mexico 82; **RES:** FP, Brookdale Univ Hosp, Brooklyn, NY; Univ Hosp SUNY Brooklyn, Brooklyn, NY

Deblasio, Maria (MD)   FP   PCP
Our Lady of Mercy Med Ctr

3065 Grand Concourse; Bronx, NY 10468; (718) 295-3898; **MS:** Italy 67; **RES:** S, Misericordia Hosp, Bronx, NY 68; Path CP, Misericordia Hosp, Bronx, NY 69; **FEL:** Oph, Misericordia Hosp, Bronx, NY 70; **FAP:** Asst S; **SI:** *Diabetes Mellitus; Thyroid Hypertension;* **HMO:** GHI US Hlthcre Blue Cross PPO Aetna Hlth Plan +

LANG: Itl, Fr, Sp; [symbols] Immediately

Delaney, Brian (MD)   FP   PCP
St Barnabas Hosp-Bronx

Belmont Medical Associates, 2371 Arthur Ave; Bronx, NY 10458; (718) 364-6199; **BDCERT:** FP 86; Ger 93; **MS:** Albert Einstein Coll Med 83; **RES:** Montefiore Med Ctr, Bronx, NY 83-86; **FAP:** Asst Prof Albert Einstein Coll Med; **HOSP:** Montefiore Med Ctr; **SI:** *Geriatric Problems;* **HMO:** Oxford GHI Blue Cross & Blue Shield US Hlthce CIGNA +

LANG: Sp, Itl, Alb; [symbols] 1 Week

Dietrich, Marianne (DO)   FP   PCP
Montefiore Med Ctr

Montefiore Medical GroupValentine Lane Family Practice, 503 S Broadway; Yonkers, NY 10705; (914) 965-9771; **BDCERT:** FP 92; **MS:** NY Coll Osteo Med 88; **RES:** FP, Peninsula Hosp Ctr, Far Rockaway, NY 89-91; **HMO:** US Hlthcre 1199 CIGNA Prucare

LANG: Sp; [symbols] A Few Days

Franzetti, Carl (DO)   FP   PCP
St Joseph's Med Ctr-Yonkers

Riverdale Family Practice, 3125 Tibbett Ave; Bronx, NY 10463; (718) 543-2700; **BDCERT:** FP 93; **MS:** NY Coll Osteo Med 84; **RES:** FP, Saddlebrook Hosp, Saddlebrook, NJ 85; FP, Warren Hosp, Phillipsburg, NJ 85-87; **FAP:** Assoc Columbia P&S; **HOSP:** Columbia-Presbyterian Med Ctr; **HMO:** Oxford NYLCare CIGNA GHI Aetna Hlth Plan +

LANG: Sp, Itl, Rus, Alb, Pol; [symbols] 2-4 Weeks *VISA* [symbols]

Guilbe, Rose (MD)   FP   PCP
Montefiore Med Ctr

Dept Family Medicine, 3544 Jerome Ave; Bronx, NY 10467; (718) 920-4678; **BDCERT:** FP 94; **MS:** U del Caribe Escuela Med 87; **RES:** Montefiore Med Ctr, New York, NY

Lurio, Joseph (MD)   FP   **PCP**
Montefiore Med Ctr
Family Ctr Montefiore Med Ctr, 360 E 193rd St;
Bronx, NY 10458; (718) 933-2400; **BDCERT:** FP
83; Rad 90; **MS:** Columbia P&S 80; **RES:** FP,
Montefiore Med Ctr, Bronx, NY 80-83; **HMO:**
HealthNet Sanus

♿ ♿ ♿ Mcr Mcd WC NFI

Maselli, Frank (MD)   FP   **PCP**
St Joseph's Med Ctr-Yonkers
Riverdale Family Practice, 3125 Tibbett Ave;
Bronx, NY 10463; (718) 543-2700; **BDCERT:** FP
86; **MS:** Israel 83; **RES:** Univ Hosp SUNY Bklyn,
Brooklyn, NY; **HOSP:** Columbia-Presbyterian Med
Ctr; **SI:** *Diving Medicine; Hyperbaric Medicine;* **HMO:**
GHI US Hlthcre Oxford Blue Choice Prucare +

LANG: Sp, Rus; ♿ ♿ ♿ ♿ ♿ ♿ ♿ Mcr WC NFI 2-
4 Weeks *VISA* 💳

McKee, Melissa Diane (MD)   FP   **PCP**
Montefiore Med Ctr
503 S Broadway Ste 210; Yonkers, NY 10705;
(914) 965-9771; **BDCERT:** FP 92; **MS:** U Tenn Ctr
Hlth Sci, Memphis 89

Mcr

Morrow, Robert (MD)   FP   **PCP**
St Joseph's Med Ctr-Yonkers
5997 Riverdale Ave; Bronx, NY 10471; (718) 884-
9803; **BDCERT:** FP 77; Ge 88; **MS:** Mt Sinai Sch
Med 74; **RES:** FP, Montefiore Med Ctr, Bronx, NY
74-77; **SI:** *Geriatrics; Adolescent Medicine;* **HMO:** US
Hlthcre Beech Street Blue Cross Oxford Bronx
Health +

LANG: Sp, Rus; ♿ ♿ ♿ ♿ ♿ ♿ ♿ Mcr WC NFI
A Few Days

O'Connell, Daniel (MD)   FP   **PCP**
Montefiore Med Ctr
West Farms Family Practice, 1055 E Tremont Ave;
Bronx, NY 10460; (718) 842-8040; **BDCERT:** FP
94; **MS:** Univ Mass Sch Med 91; **RES:** FP,
Montefiore Med Ctr, Bronx, NY 91-94; *SI:*
Community Medicine; **HMO:** Blue Cross & Blue
Shield Bronx Health Health First CIGNA US Hlthcre
+

LANG: Sp; ♿ ♿ ♿ ♿ ♿ ♿ Mcr Mcd 2-4 Weeks

Pringle, Sheryl (MD)   FP   **PCP**
Montefiore Med Ctr
Montefiore Fordham Family Practice, 1 Fordham
Plaza; Bronx, NY 10458; (718) 405-4010;
BDCERT: FP 95; **MS:** Temple U 92; **HMO:** Aetna
Hlth Plan US Hlthcre Blue Cross Blue Shield GHI
PPO +

LANG: Sp; ♿ ♿ ♿ ♿ ♿ ♿ Mcr Mcd 4+ Weeks

Soloway, Bruce (MD)   FP   **PCP**
Bronx Lebanon Hosp Ctr
BronxLebanon Family Practice Center, 1265
Franklin Ave Fl 3; Bronx, NY 10456; (718) 901-
8236; **BDCERT:** FP 94; **MS:** Albert Einstein Coll
Med 85; **RES:** FP, Montefiore Med Ctr, Bronx, NY
85-88; **FAP:** Asst Prof Albert Einstein Coll Med; *SI:*
HIV Infection; **HMO:** ABC Health Oxford US Hlthcre
Bronx Health Health First +

♿ ♿ ♿ ♿ ♿ ♿ Mcr Mcd 2-4 Weeks

Townsend, Janet (MD)   FP   **PCP**
Montefiore Med Ctr
Montefiore Medical CenterFamily Medical, 3412
Bainbridge Ave; Bronx, NY 10467; (718) 920-
5523; **BDCERT:** FP 96; **MS:** Harvard Med Sch 78

Weinstein, Joshua (MD)   FP   **PCP**
Montefiore Med Ctr-Weiler/Einstein Div
2157 Tomlinson Ave; Bronx, NY 10461; (718)
828-2560; **BDCERT:** FP 75; **MS:** SUNY Downstate
72; **RES:** Med, Mount Sinai Med Ctr, New York, NY
74; Med, Maimonides Med Ctr, Brooklyn, NY 73;
FEL: Albert Einstein Med Ctr, Bronx, NY 74; **FAP:**
Asst Prof Med Albert Einstein Coll Med; **HMO:**
Aetna Hlth Plan Blue Choice Sanus Travelers

♿ ♿ ♿ ♿ Mcr

GASTROENTEROLOGY

Antony, Michael (MD)   Ge   PCP
Jacobi Med Ctr
1577 Hone Ave; Bronx, NY 10461; (718) 828-0100; **BDCERT:** IM 85; Ge 89; **MS:** SUNY Hlth Sci Ctr 82; **RES:** Albert Einstein Med Ctr, Bronx, NY 82-86; IM, Jacobi Med Ctr, Bronx, NY; **FEL:** Ge, Montefiore Med Ctr, Bronx, NY 86-88; **FAP:** Asst Prof Med Albert Einstein Coll Med; **HOSP:** Montefiore Med Ctr-Weiler/Einstein Div; *SI: Colon Cancer Screening; Colonoscopy and Endoscopy*; **HMO:** 1199 GHI Oxford Blue Cross +

LANG: Grk; 🚻 🆘 🈁 ☎ 🔧 🛏 Mcr Mcd   Immediately
VISA 💳 💳

Bloom, Alan (MD)   Ge
Bronx Lebanon Hosp Ctr
Gastroenterology Dept, 1650 Grand Concourse; Bronx, NY 10457; (718) 518-5550; **BDCERT:** IM 63; Ge 73; **MS:** U Hlth Sci/Chicago Med Sch 56; **RES:** Montefiore Med Ctr, Bronx, NY 57-59

LANG: Sp; 🚻 🈁 🔧 🛏 Mcr Mcd   2-4 Weeks

Brandt, Lawrence (MD)   Ge
Montefiore Med Ctr
111 E 210th St; Bronx, NY 10467; (718) 920-4476; **BDCERT:** IM 72; Ge 75; **MS:** SUNY Downstate 68; **RES:** IM, Mount Sinai Med Ctr, New York, NY 68-72; **FEL:** Ge, Mount Sinai Med Ctr, New York, NY 71-72; **FAP:** Prof Med Albert Einstein Coll Med; *SI: Colitis; Colonoscopy*; **HMO:** Oxford CIGNA Sanus GHI Health First +

LANG: Sp; 🚻 🈁 🛏 💲 Mcr   2-4 Weeks 🈁 *VISA* 💳 💳

Buiumsohn, Arno (MD)   Ge
Bronx Lebanon Hosp Ctr
Bronx Lebanon Hospital Center, 1650 Grand Concourse; Bronx, NY 10457; (718) 960-1049; **BDCERT:** Ped 75; **MS:** Romania 54; **RES:** Pge, Bronx Lebanon Hosp Ctr, Bronx, NY 68-69; **FEL:** PGe, Bronx Lebanon Hosp Ctr, Bronx, NY 69-71; **FAP:** Asst Prof Ped Albert Einstein Coll Med

Carvajal, Simeon (MD)   Ge   PCP
Bronx Lebanon Hosp Ctr
674 E 220th St; Bronx, NY 10467; (718) 652-4178; **MS:** Philippines 65; **RES:** Bronx Lebanon Hosp Ctr, Bronx, NY 67-71; Bronx Lebanon Hosp Ctr, Bronx, NY 70; **FEL:** Bronx Lebanon Hosp Ctr, Bronx, NY 71-73; Bronx Lebanon Hosp Ctr, Bronx, NY 72; **HOSP:** Our Lady of Mercy Med Ctr; *SI: Peptic Ulcer Disease; Colon Cancer Early Detect*; **HMO:** CIGNA US Hlthcre Blue Choice Prucare Health First +

LANG: Sp, Chi, Fil; 🆘 ☎ 🈁 🔧 🛏 💲 Mcr Mcd   Immediately

Fleischner, Gerald (MD)   Ge
Montefiore Med Ctr
Tenbroeck Medical Assoc, 1180 Morris Park Ave; Bronx, NY 10461; (718) 863-8465; **BDCERT:** IM 74; **MS:** Geo Wash U Sch Med 63; **RES:** IM, DC Gen Hosp, Washington, DC 63-64; IM, DC Gen Hosp, Washington, DC 67-68; **FEL:** Ge, Albert Einstein Med Ctr, Bronx, NY 68-71; **FAP:** Asst Prof Albert Einstein Coll Med; **HOSP:** Westchester Square Med Ctr; *SI: Inflammatory Bowel Disease; Irritable Bowel Disease*; **HMO:** Oxford Aetna Hlth Plan Empire GHI Blue Choice +

🚻 🆘 ☎ 🈁 🔧 🛏 💲 Mcr Mcd   1 Week *VISA*

Frager, Joseph (MD)   Ge
Montefiore Med Ctr
2600 Netherland Ave Ste 114; Bronx, NY 10463; (718) 884-5837; **BDCERT:** Ge 85; IM 83; **MS:** Univ Penn 80; **RES:** Montefiore Med Ctr, Bronx, NY 83; **FEL:** Montefiore Med Ctr, Bronx, NY; **FAP:** Asst Clin Prof Med Albert Einstein Coll Med; *SI: Colon Cancer Screening; Peptic Ulcer Disease*; **HMO:** Blue Choice Oxford GHI US Hlthcre

🚻 🈁 🔧 🛏 Mcr   Immediately *VISA* 💳

Frank, Michael (MD)   Ge   PCP
Lenox Hill Hosp
1600 Hering Ave; Bronx, NY 10461; (718) 931-4700; **BDCERT:** Ge 77; **MS:** Albert Einstein Coll Med 74; **RES:** Jacobi Med Ctr, Bronx, NY; **FEL:** Montefiore Med Ctr, Bronx, NY; **HMO:** Chubb Aetna Hlth Plan

🈁 🔧 🛏 💲   Immediately 🈁 *VISA* 💳

Gupta, Sanjeev (MD)　　　Ge
Montefiore Med Ctr

1575 Blondell Ave; Bronx, NY 10461; (718) 430-2098; **BDCERT:** IM 89; Ge 93; **MS:** India 77; **RES:** IM, Hammersmith Hosp, London, England 81-82; IM, Albert Einstein Coll Med, Bronx, NY 88-89; **FEL:** Ge, Hammersmith Hosp, London, England 82-85; Hepatology, USC Med Ctr, Los Angeles, CA 85-87; **FAP:** Assoc Prof Med Albert Einstein Coll Med; **HOSP:** Jacobi Med Ctr; *SI: Liver Problems; Gastrointestinal Problems;* **HMO:** Blue Choice US Hlthcre Oxford GHI PHCS +

LANG: Hin, Itl, Sp, Ur, Pun; 🅰 🔅 🎗 🏥 💲 Mcr NFI A Few Days 🏧 **VISA** ● ▦

Gutwein, Isadore (MD)　　　Ge
Montefiore Med Ctr

Riverdale Gastroenterology, 3765 Riverdale Ave 8; Bronx, NY 10463; (718) 549-4267; **BDCERT:** IM 76; Ge 79; **MS:** Albert Einstein Coll Med 73; **RES:** IM, Montefiore Med Ctr, Bronx, NY 74-75; IM, Montefiore Med Ctr, Bronx, NY 75-76; **FEL:** Ge, St Luke's Roosevelt Hosp Ctr, New York, NY 76-77; Ge, St Luke's Roosevelt Hosp Ctr, New York, NY 77-78; **HOSP:** St Joseph's Med Ctr-Yonkers; **HMO:** Oxford US Hlthcre Aetna Hlth Plan GHI +

LANG: Yd, Sp; 🅰 🌙 🔅 🎗 🏥 💲 Mcr 1 Week **VISA** ●

Hertan, Hilary (MD)　　　Ge
Our Lady of Mercy Med Ctr

Dept of Gastroenterology - Our Lady of Mercy Med Ctr, 600 E 233rd St; Bronx, NY 10466; (718) 920-9887; **BDCERT:** IM 86; **MS:** NY Med Coll 82; **RES:** IM, N Shore Univ Hosp-Cornell, Manhasset, NY 82-85; **FEL:** Nutrition, Our Lady of Mercy Med Ctr, Bronx, NY 87-88; Ge, Our Lady of Mercy Med Ctr, Bronx, NY 88-90; **FAP:** Asst Prof Med NY Med Coll; *SI: Endoscopic Ultrasound; General Gastroenterology;* **HMO:** Blue Choice Oxford Aetna-US Healthcare GHI

LANG: Heb, Fr, Sp, Thai, Hin; 🅰 🔅 🎗 🏥 💲 Mcr Mcd A Few Days

Manzione, Nancy (MD)　　　Ge
Montefiore Med Ctr-Weiler/Einstein Div

1575 Blondell Ave 101; Bronx, NY 10461; (718) 405-8301; **BDCERT:** IM 81; Ge 83; **MS:** SUNY Downstate 78; **RES:** Jacobi Med Ctr, Bronx, NY 78-81; **FEL:** Jacobi Med Ctr, Bronx, NY 81-84; **FAP:** Assoc Prof Med Albert Einstein Coll Med; **HOSP:** Montefiore Med Ctr; *SI: Endoscopy;* **HMO:** US Hlthcre Oxford GHI Blue Cross & Blue Shield

🅰 🔅 🎗 🏥 💲 Mcr Immediately **VISA** ●

Pitchumoni, Capecomo (MD)　Ge
Our Lady of Mercy Med Ctr

600 E 233rd St; Bronx, NY 10466; (718) 920-9692; **BDCERT:** IM 70; Ge 71; **MS:** India 60; **RES:** Med Coll Hosp, Trivandrum, India 60-65; Norwalk Hosp, Norwalk, CT 67-68; **FEL:** Yale-New Haven Hosp, New Haven, CT 68-69; Metropolitan Hosp Ctr, New York, NY 69-71; **HMO:** GHI Prucare Oxford Blue Cross & Blue Shield

🅰 🌙 🔅 🎗 🏥 Mcr Mcd Immediately

Remy, Prospere (MD)　　　Ge
Bronx Lebanon Hosp Ctr

860 Grand Concourse Ste 1A; Bronx, NY 10451; (718) 585-5060; **BDCERT:** IM 91; **MS:** Mexico 84; **RES:** IM, Bronx Lebanon Hosp Ctr, Bronx, NY 88-89; IM, Bronx Lebanon Hosp Ctr, Bronx, NY 89-90; **FEL:** Ge, Bronx Lebanon Hosp Ctr, Bronx, NY 90-92; *SI: Liver;* **HMO:** Aetna Hlth Plan Blue Cross & Blue Shield CIGNA

🅰 🌙 🔅 🎗 🏥 💲 Mcr Mcd 2-4 Weeks

Sable, Robert (MD)　　　Ge
Montefiore Med Ctr

3765 Riverdale Ave 8; Bronx, NY 10463; (718) 549-4267; **BDCERT:** IM 76; Ge 79; **MS:** Albert Einstein Coll Med 73; **RES:** IM, Montefiore Med Ctr, Bronx, NY 73-76; **FEL:** Ge, NY Med Coll, Valhalla, NY 76-78; **FAP:** Instr Albert Einstein Coll Med; **HOSP:** Columbia-Presbyterian Med Ctr; *SI: Inflammatory Bowel Disease; Liver Disease;* **HMO:** Oxford Prucare Blue Cross & Blue Shield United Healthcare Aetna Hlth Plan +

LANG: Sp; 🅰 🌙 🔅 🏥 💲 Mcr 2-4 Weeks **VISA** ●

Schweitzer, Philip (MD) Ge
Montefiore Med Ctr

3184 Grand Concourse 2D; Bronx, NY 10458;
(718) 584-0404; **BDCERT:** IM 72; Ge 77; **MS:**
Cornell U 67; **RES:** St Luke's Roosevelt Hosp Ctr,
New York, NY 70-72; **FEL:** Ge, Mount Sinai Med
Ctr, New York, NY 72-74; **HOSP:** Our Lady of
Mercy Med Ctr; **HMO:** Aetna Hlth Plan Blue Choice
HealthNet Prucare

LANG: Sp, Ger; 🦽 📷 👤 🎫 💲 Mcr Mcd Immediately

Sherman, Howard (MD) Ge
Montefiore Med Ctr

1625 St Peters Ave; Bronx, NY 10461; (718) 863-
7397; **BDCERT:** IM 76; Ge 79; **MS:** Albert Einstein
Coll Med 73; **RES:** IM, Emory U Hosp, Atlanta, GA
73-74; IM, Emory U Hosp, Atlanta, GA 74-76; **FEL:**
Ge, Emory U Hosp, Atlanta, GA; **FAP:** Assoc Clin
Prof Med Albert Einstein Coll Med; **HOSP:**
Westchester Square Med Ctr; **SI:** *Gastrointestinal
Endoscopy; Hepatobiliary Diseases*; **HMO:** United
Healthcare Blue Cross & Blue Shield Oxford CIGNA
GHI +

🦽 📞 📷 🎫 💲 Mcr A Few Days

Zimetbaum, Marcel (MD) Ge
Montefiore Med Ctr

3333 Henry Hudson Pkwy; Riverdale, NY 10463;
(718) 796-1000; **BDCERT:** Ge 65; **MS:** NYU Sch
Med 58; **RES:** Ge, Montefiore Med Ctr, Bronx, NY
61-62; IM, Montefiore Med Ctr, Bronx, NY 58-61;
FAP: Asst Clin Prof Albert Einstein Coll Med; **SI:**
Inflammatory Bowel Disease; Esophageal Disease;
HMO: Oxford Aetna Hlth Plan Prudential CIGNA
GHI +

LANG: Pat, Prt, Flm, Yd; 🦽 📷 🎫 Mcr Mcd 1 Week

GERIATRIC MEDICINE

Jacobs, Laurie (MD) Ger PCP
Montefiore Med Ctr

111 E 210th St; Bronx, NY 10467; (718) 920-
6723; **BDCERT:** IM 88; Ger 92; **MS:** Columbia P&S
85; **RES:** IM, Montefiore Med Ctr, Bronx, NY 85-88;
FEL: Ger, Montefiore Med Ctr, Bronx, NY 88-91;
Albert Einstein Med Ctr, Bronx, NY 88-91; **FAP:**
Assoc Prof of Clin Med Albert Einstein Coll Med; **SI:**
Osteoporosis; Incontinence; **HMO:** Oxford US Hlthcre

LANG: Sp, Rus; 🦽 📷 👤 🎫 Mcr Mcd 2-4 Weeks 🏧
VISA 💳

Kessler, Joseph (MD) Ger
Montefiore Med Ctr

2925 Grand Concourse; Bronx, NY 10468; (718)
933-8282; **BDCERT:** IM 68; **MS:** NY Med Coll 62;
RES: IM, Lenox Hill Hosp, New York, NY 66-68

Malik, Rubina (MD) Ger PCP
Montefiore Med Ctr

Sair Clinic/Montefiore Hosp, 111 E 210th St;
Bronx, NY 10467; (718) 920-6721; **BDCERT:** IM
95; **MS:** SUNY Stony Brook 92; **RES:** IM, Univ Hosp
SUNY Stony Brook, Stony Brook, NY 92-93; Ge,
Univ Hosp SUNY Stony Brook, Stony Brook, NY 95-
96; **FAP:** Clin Instr Albert Einstein Coll Med; **SI:**
Osteoporosis; **HMO:** Oxford

🦽 📷 👤 🎫 💲 Mcr Mcd 2-4 Weeks

Nichols, Jeffrey (MD) Ger
Cabrini Med Ctr

2975 Independence Ave; Bronx, NY 10463; (212)
358-6255; **BDCERT:** IM 79; Ger 88; **MS:** Cornell U
76; **RES:** IM, St Vincents Hosp & Med Ctr NY, New
York, NY 76-77; Ger, St Vincents Hosp & Med Ctr
NY, New York, NY 77-79; **FAP:** Asst Clin Prof Ger
Cornell U; **SI:** *Home Care; Decision Making Capacity*;
HMO: Fidelis PHS Oxford Mt Sinai Hlth

🦽 📷 👤 🎫 Mcr Mcd WC 2-4 Weeks

Russell, Robin (MD)　　　Ger　[PCP]
Our Lady of Mercy Med Ctr

YDR Medical Associates, 4141 Carpenter Ave;
Bronx, NY 10466; (718) 920-9040; **BDCERT:** IM
74; Ger 90; **MS:** U New Mexico 71; **RES:** IM, Harlem
Hosp Ctr, New York, NY 71-72; IM, Harlem Hosp
Ctr, New York, NY 72-74; **FEL:** Renal Disease,
Harlem Hosp Ctr, New York, NY 74-76; **FAP:** Asst
Prof Med NY Med Coll; **SI:** *Geriatrics; Renal Disease in
the Aged*; **HMO:** Blue Cross & Blue Shield Oxford
CIGNA GHI

🚻 📷 🏧 💲 Mcr Mcd　1 Week

Thomas, Rogelio (MD)　　　Ger
Bronx Lebanon Hosp Ctr

Bronx Lebanon Hosp, 1265 Fulton Ave; Bronx, NY
10456; (718) 579-7060; **BDCERT:** IM 94; **MS:**
Harvard Med Sch 83; **RES:** IM, Brigham &
Women's Hosp, Boston, MA 83-84; IM, Mount
Sinai Med Ctr, New York, NY 84-87; **FAP:** Asst
Lecturer Albert Einstein Coll Med

LANG: Sp; 🚻 🏧 🏧

GERIATRIC PSYCHIATRY

Weisblatt, Steven (MD)　　GerPsy
Montefiore Med Ctr

2445 Woodhull Ave; Bronx, NY 10469; (718)
405-0494; **BDCERT:** Psyc 90; Psyc 96; **MS:** SUNY
Hlth Sci Ctr 84; **RES:** Psyc, Albert Einstein Med Ctr,
Bronx, NY 84-88; **FAP:** Asst Prof of Clin Psyc Albert
Einstein Coll Med; **SI:** *Mental Retardation*

🚻 ♿ 📷 🏧 🏧 💲 Mcr WC NFI　Immediately

GYNECOLOGIC ONCOLOGY

Fields, Abbie (MD)　　　GO
Montefiore Med Ctr

AECOM 7 Montefiore Med Ctr, 1695 Eastchester Rd
Ste L2; Bronx, NY 10461; (718) 405-8200;
BDCERT: ObG 94; GO 96; **MS:** Ohio State U 87;
RES: ObG, Northwestern Mem Hosp, Chicago, IL
87-91; **FEL:** GO, Johns Hopkins Hosp, Baltimore,
MD 91-93; **FAP:** Asst Prof Albert Einstein Coll Med;
SI: *Investigational Chemotherapy; Familial Cancers*

LANG: Sp, Rus, Heb; 🚻 📷 🏧 🏧 💲 Mcr Mcd
A Few Days **VISA** 💳

Goldberg, Gary L (MD)　　GO
Montefiore Med Ctr

AECOM 7 Montefiore Medical Center, 1695
Eastchester Rd Ste L2; Bronx, NY 10461; (718)
405-8200; **BDCERT:** ObG 88; GO 96; **MS:** South
Africa 75; **RES:** ObG, Groote Schuur Hosp, Cape
Town, South Africa 78-81; **FEL:** GO, Groote Schuur
Hosp, Cape Town, South Africa 82-83; **FAP:** Asst
Prof Albert Einstein Coll Med; **HMO:** Aetna Hlth
Plan Oxford GHI CIGNA Multiplan +

LANG: Sp, Rus, Heb; 🚻 📷 🏧 🏧 💲 Mcr Mcd
A Few Days **VISA** 💳 💳

HAND SURGERY

Kulick, Roy (MD)　　　HS
Montefiore Med Ctr

75 E Gun Hill Rd; Bronx, NY 10467; (718) 515-
3333; **BDCERT:** OrS 80; HS 90; **MS:** Cornell U 73;
RES: S, St Luke's Roosevelt Hosp Ctr, New York, NY
73-75; OrS, Columbia-Presbyterian Med Ctr, New
York, NY 75-77; **FEL:** HS, Hosp For Special Surgery,
New York, NY; **FAP:** Asst Clin Prof Albert Einstein
Coll Med; **HOSP:** Our Lady of Mercy Med Ctr; **SI:**
Carpal Tunnel Syndrome; Arthritis of the Hand; **HMO:**
Oxford Blue Choice NYLCare

🚻 📷 🏧 🏧 💲 Mcr WC NFI　1 Week **VISA** 💳

Guide to symbols and abbreviations can be found on pages 110-113.

427

HEMATOLOGY

Billett, Henny (MD) Hem
Montefiore Med Ctr-Weiler/Einstein Div
Dir Clin Hemat - Albert Einstein Med Ctr, 1300 Morris Park Ave; Bronx, NY 10461; (718) 920-7763; **BDCERT:** IM 79; Hem 82; **MS:** Mt Sinai Sch Med 74; **RES:** Med, Montefiore Med Ctr, Bronx, NY 74-76; Med, Montefiore Med Ctr, Bronx, NY 77-79; **FEL:** Hem, Montefiore Med Ctr, Bronx, NY 79-81; **FAP:** Assoc Prof Albert Einstein Coll Med; **HOSP:** Montefiore Med Ctr; ***SI:*** *Bleeding Problems; Clotting Problems*; **HMO:** Aetna Hlth Plan Oxford Select PPO Prucare Health First +
LANG: Fr, Ger; ♿ 📅 $ [Mcr] 1 Week

Camacho, Fernando (MD) Hem
Montefiore Med Ctr
3130 Grand Concourse 1H; Bronx, NY 10458; (718) 220-4900; **BDCERT:** Hem 78; Onc 81; **MS:** SUNY Buffalo 73; **RES:** Med, Montefiore Med Ctr, Bronx, NY 74-76; Montefiore Med Ctr, Bronx, NY 73-74; **FEL:** Hem, Montefiore Med Ctr, Bronx, NY 76-77; Onc, Mem Sloan Kettering Cancer Ctr, New York, NY 77-79; **FAP:** Asst Clin Prof Med Albert Einstein Coll Med; **HOSP:** St Joseph's Med Ctr-Yonkers; ***SI:*** *Oncology*; **HMO:** US Hlthcre Oxford GHI HealthNet
LANG: Sp; ♿ ☎ 📅 $ [Mcr] [Mcd] 1 Week

Guy, Roscoe Bruce (MD) Hem
Our Lady of Mercy Med Ctr
4141 Carpenter Ave; Bronx, NY 10466; (718) 920-9202; **BDCERT:** Hem 72; Onc 85; **MS:** Cornell U 63; **RES:** IM, Univ Hosp SUNY Syracuse, Syracuse, NY 63-64; **FEL:** IM, Univ Hosp SUNY Syracuse, Syracuse, NY 64-66; Hem, NY Hosp-Cornell Med Ctr, New York, NY 67-69; **HOSP:** Westchester Med Ctr

Landau, Leon (MD) Hem
Montefiore Med Ctr
75 E Gun Hill Rd; Bronx, NY 10467; (718) 655-3932; **BDCERT:** Hem 78; Onc 81; **MS:** Albert Einstein Coll Med 71; **RES:** IM, Montefiore Med Ctr, Bronx, NY 72-73; IM, Metropolitan Hosp, New York, NY 73-74; **FEL:** Onc, Albert Einstein Med Ctr, Bronx, NY 74-76; Montefiore Med Ctr, Bronx, NY 76-78; **HOSP:** Community Hosp At Dobbs Ferry; **HMO:** Oxford Aetna Hlth Plan Blue Cross & Blue Shield
LANG: Sp; ♿ [SA SU] ☾ ☎ 📅 $ [Mcr] [Mcd] A Few Days

Levine, Shirley (MD) Hem
Montefiore Med Ctr
111 E 210th St; Bronx, NY 10467; (718) 920-7388; **BDCERT:** IM 73; Hem 76; **MS:** Med Coll PA 69; **RES:** IM, U Chicago Hosp, Chicago, IL 69-71; IM, UC San Diego Med Ctr, San Diego, CA 71-72; **FEL:** Hem, UC San Diego Med Ctr, San Diego, CA 72-75; **FAP:** Prof Albert Einstein Coll Med; ***SI:*** *Platelet Disorders; Thrombosis*
♿ ☎ 👤 📅 $ [Mcr] [Mcd] 1 Week

Muhlfelder, Thomas (MD) Hem
VA Med Ctr-Bronx
360 W 245th St; Bronx, NY 10471; (718) 549-4706; **BDCERT:** Hem 74; IM 71; **MS:** Jefferson Med Coll 66; **RES:** IM, Montefiore Hosp, Bronx, NY 67-69; Hem, Montefiore Hosp, Bronx, NY 69-70; **FEL:** Hem, Montefiore Hosp, Bronx, NY 72-73; **FAP:** Asst Clin Prof Mt Sinai Sch Med; **HOSP:** Mount Sinai Med Ctr
♿ ☎ 👤 📅 2-4 Weeks

Nagel, Ronald (MD) Hem
Montefiore Med Ctr-Weiler/Einstein Div
1300 Morris Park Ave Ull 921; Bronx, NY 10461; (718) 430-2186; **MS:** Chile 60; **RES:** IM, JJ Aguirre, Santiago, Chile 60-61; **FEL:** Hem, Albert Einstein Med Ctr, Bronx, NY 63-66; **FAP:** Prof Albert Einstein Coll Med; **HOSP:** Montefiore Med Ctr; ***SI:*** *Sickle Cell Anemia; Thalassemia*; **HMO:** PHS Oxford
LANG: Sp; ♿ ☎ 👤 📅 [Mcr] [Mcd] [WC] [NFI] 1 Week

Guide to symbols and abbreviations can be found on pages 110-113.

Schreiber, Zwi (MD) Hem
Bronx Lebanon Hosp Ctr

1650 Selwyn Ave 3C; Bronx, NY 10457; (718)
960-1078; BDCERT: IM 74; Hem 76; MS: Israel
62; RES: Queens Hosp Ctr, Jamaica, NY 65-66;
Bronx Lebanon Hosp Ctr, Bronx, NY 73-74; FEL:
Hem, Maimonides Med Ctr, Brooklyn, NY 67-69;
HOSP: Westchester Square Med Ctr; SI: Lymphoma;
Anemia; HMO: Oxford Aetna Hlth Plan Magnacare
Bronx Health

LANG: Sp, Fr; 🔱 📷 🏧 💲 Mcr Mcd 1 Week

INFECTIOUS DISEASE

Berger, Judith (MD) Inf
St Barnabas Hosp-Bronx

216 Bronxville Ave; Bronx, NY 10462; (718) 822-
1515; BDCERT: IM 84; Hem 86; MS: Mt Sinai Sch
Med 80; RES: Brookdale Univ Hosp Med Ctr,
Brooklyn, NY 81-84

LANG: Sp, Fr; 🔱 📷 🏧

Corpuz, Marilou (MD) Inf
Our Lady of Mercy Med Ctr

Our Lady of Mercy Medical Center, Dept of
Infectious Disease, 600 E 233rd St; Bronx, NY
10466; (718) 920-9889; BDCERT: IM 88; Inf 92;
MS: 85; RES: IM, Griffin Hosp, Derby, CT 85-88;
FEL: Inf, Long Island Jewish Med Ctr, New Hyde
Park, NY 89-91; FAP: Asst Prof NY Med Coll;
HMO: Blue Cross & Blue Shield Oxford GHI 1199
CIGNA +

LANG: Sp, Fil; 🔱 📷 🚹 🏧 💲 Mcr A Few Days

Justman, Jessica (MD) Inf PCP
Bronx Lebanon Hosp Ctr

Dept of Internal Medicine, 1650 Grand Concourse
8th; Bronx, NY 10457; (718) 590-1800; BDCERT:
IM 88; Inf 92; MS: U Rochester 85; RES: IM, N
Shore Univ Hosp-Manhasset, Manhasset, NY 85-
86; IM, Montefiore Med Ctr, Bronx, NY 86-88; FEL:
Inf, Montefiore Med Ctr, Bronx, NY 89-93; FAP:
Asst Lecturer Med Albert Einstein Coll Med; SI: HIV;
Hepatitis

LANG: Sp, Fr; 🔱 🆘 🚹 🏧 Mcr Mcd WC NFI
A Few Days

Robbins, Noah (MD) Inf PCP
Montefiore Med Ctr

Montefiore Med Group, 3400 Bainbridge Ave;
Bronx, NY 10467; (718) 920-8888; BDCERT: IM
74; MS: McGill U 69; RES: Albany Med Ctr, Albany,
NY 73-75; FEL: Albert Einstein Med Ctr, Bronx, NY
75-76; FAP: Assoc Prof Med Albert Einstein Coll
Med; SI: AIDS; Sexually Transmitted Diseases; HMO:
Blue Choice GHI US Hlthcre Montecare Blue Cross
& Blue Shield +

🔱 🆘 🅲 📷 🚹 🏧 💲 Mcr Mcd WC NFI 2-4 Weeks 📧
VISA 💳

Saltzman, Simone (MD) Inf PCP
Montefiore Med Ctr-Weiler/Einstein Div

Internal Medicine/Infectious Disease, 1575
Blondell Ave 200; Bronx, NY 10461; (718) 405-
8309; BDCERT: IM 77; MS: SUNY Downstate 73;
FEL: Inf, Montefiore Med Ctr, Bronx, NY 80; FAP:
Asst Prof Albert Einstein Coll Med; HMO: Oxford US
Hlthcre Blue Choice

LANG: Sp, Itl; 🔱 🅲 📷 🏧 💲 Mcr 2-4 Weeks

Soeiro, Ruy (MD) Inf
Montefiore Med Ctr-Weiler/Einstein Div

1300 Morris Park Ave 200; Bronx, NY 10461;
(718) 430-2371; MS: Tufts U 58; RES: Med, Boston
Med Ctr, Boston, MA 59; Med, New England Med
Ctr, Boston, MA 61; FAP: Prof Med Albert Einstein
Coll Med

🔱 📷 🚹 🏧 Mcr NFI 1 Week VISA 💳

Steigbigel, Neal H (MD) Inf
Montefiore Med Ctr

Montefiore Medical Center, 111 E 210th St; Bronx,
NY 10467; (718) 920-5439; BDCERT: IM 67; Inf
72; MS: Harvard Med Sch 60; RES: IM, Harvard
Med Sch, Cambridge, MA 60-65; FEL: Inf, Harvard
Med Sch, Cambridge, MA 65-67; FAP: Dir Inf
Albert Einstein Coll Med

LANG: Sp; 🔱 📷 🏧 💲 Mcr Mcd 1 Week VISA 💳

Tanowitz, Herbert (MD) Inf
Montefiore Med Ctr-Weiler/Einstein Div
Montefiore Medical Park, 1575 Blondell Ave; Bronx, NY 10461; (718) 405-8309; **BDCERT:** IM 74; Inf 76; **MS:** Albert Einstein Coll Med 67; **RES:** Med, Lincoln Med & Mental Hlth Ctr, Bronx, NY 68-71; **FEL:** Inf, Albert Einstein Med Ctr, Bronx, NY 71-73; **FAP:** Prof Albert Einstein Coll Med; *SI: Tropical Medicine;* **HMO:** HealthNet Blue Choice Metlife NYLCare

LANG: Itl, Sp, Yd; 🚫 📞 🔚 🏧 Mcr Mcd NFI Immediately ▦ **VISA** 💳 ▦

Telzak, Edward E (MD) Inf
Bronx Lebanon Hosp Ctr
Bronx Lebanon Hospital Center, Dept of Infectious Disease, 1650 Grand Concourse; Bronx, NY 10457; (718) 518-5811; **BDCERT:** IM 83; Inf 88; **MS:** Albert Einstein Coll Med 80; **RES:** IM, New England Med Ctr, Boston, MA 81-83; **FEL:** Inf, New England Med Ctr, Boston, MA 85-86; Inf, Brigham & Women's Hosp, Boston, MA 84-85; **FAP:** Assoc Prof Albert Einstein Coll Med; *SI: AIDS; Tuberculosis*
LANG: Sp; 🚫 📞 🔚 🏧 Mcr Mcd WC NFI 1 Week

Weiss, Louis (MD) Inf
Montefiore Med Ctr
1575 Blondell Ave Rm 200; Bronx, NY 10461; (718) 405-8310; **BDCERT:** IM 85; Inf 88; **MS:** Johns Hopkins U 82; **RES:** IM, U Chicago Hosp, Chicago, IL 82-85; **FEL:** Inf, Montefiore Med Ctr, Bronx, NY 85-89; **HOSP:** Jacobi Med Ctr; *SI: Tropical Medicine; AIDS*

🚫 📞 🔚 🏧 🏧 $ Mcr Mcd NFI 1 Week **VISA** 💳

INTERNAL MEDICINE

Baker, Barry (MD) IM `PCP`
Westchester Square Med Ctr
3665 E Tremont Ave; Bronx, NY 10465; (718) 863-7755; **BDCERT:** IM 92; **MS:** Philippines 78; **RES:** New York University Med Ctr, New York, NY 79; **FEL:** New York University Med Ctr, New York, NY

🚫 📞 🏧 🏧 $ Mcr Immediately

Berger, Matthew (MD) IM
Montefiore Med Ctr-Weiler/Einstein Div
EinsteinMontefiore Faculty Practice, 1575 Blondell Ave Ste 200; Bronx, NY 10461; (718) 405-8300; **BDCERT:** IM 86; **MS:** Univ Penn 82; **RES:** IM, Jacobi Med Ctr, Bronx, NY 82-86; **FAP:** Assoc Prof Albert Einstein Coll Med; **HOSP:** Montefiore Med Ctr

Bernanke, Harold (MD) IM
Montefiore Med Ctr
201 E Mosholu Pkwy; Bronx, NY 10467; (718) 547-7310; **BDCERT:** IM 54; **MS:** SUNY Hlth Sci Ctr 54; **RES:** VA Med Ctr-Brooklyn, Brooklyn, NY 55-56; Beth Israel Med Ctr, New York, NY 58-59; **HMO:** GHI Magnacare United Healthcare Prudential PHCS +

🏧 📞 🏧 🏧 $ Mcr 2-4 Weeks

Bernstein, Leslie (MD) IM
Montefiore Med Ctr
111 E 210th St; Bronx, NY 10467; (718) 920-4846; **BDCERT:** IM 67; Ge 75; **MS:** KY Med Sch, Louisville 58; **RES:** IM, Jacobi Med Ctr, Bronx, NY 58-62; **FEL:** New York University Med Ctr, New York, NY 62-63; GI, Albert Einstein Med Ctr, Bronx, NY 63-65; **FAP:** Prof Med Albert Einstein Coll Med; **HOSP:** Jacobi Med Ctr; *SI: Bowel Disease; Malabsorption;* **HMO:** Most

🚫 🏧 Mcr Mcd WC 4+ Weeks ▦ **VISA** 💳 ▦

Biagiotti, Emilio (MD) IM `PCP`
Westchester Square Med Ctr
Family Medical Center, 3167 E Tremont Ave; Bronx, NY 10461; (718) 863-7925; **MS:** NY Med Coll 89; **RES:** Stamford Hosp, Stamford, CT; **HMO:** GHI Oxford Magnacare Multiplan
LANG: Itl, Sp; 🚫 📞 🏧 🏧 $ Mcr A Few Days

Blaufox, M Donald (MD & PhD) IM
Montefiore Med Ctr-Weiler/Einstein Div
Montefiore Medical Park, 1695A Eastchester Rd;
Bronx, NY 10461; (718) 405-8454; **BDCERT:** IM
66; NuM 72; **MS:** SUNY Hlth Sci Ctr 59; **RES:**
Jewish Mem Hosp, New York, NY 59-60; Mayo
Clinic, Rochester, MN 60-64; **FEL:** Med & Rad, Peter
Bent Brigham Hosp, Boston, MA 64-65; **FAP:**
Chrmn Albert Einstein Coll Med; **HOSP:** Montefiore
Med Ctr; **SI:** *High Blood Pressure; Kidney Disease;*
HMO: Blue Cross & Blue Shield HealthNet Oxford
⌖ ⌂ 🎦 Mcr Mod WC NFI A Few Days ▦ 🖵 🖵

Buatti, Elizabeth (MD) IM
Montefiore Med Ctr
Department of Medicine Faculty Practice, 111 E
210th St; Bronx, NY 10467; (718) 920-7763;
BDCERT: IM 81; **MS:** Georgetown U 78; **RES:** IM, St
Vincents Hosp & Med Ctr NY, New York, NY 79-81;
FAP: Assoc Prof Med Albert Einstein Coll Med;
HMO: CIGNA
⌖ 🎦 NFI

Casey, Joan (MD) IM
Montefiore Med Ctr
111 E 210th St; Bronx, NY 10467; (718) 920-
1700; **BDCERT:** IM 71; **MS:** Canada 66; **RES:** IM,
Boston Med Ctr, Boston, MA 67-70; **FEL:** Inf,
Boston Med Ctr, Boston, MA 66-69; **FAP:** Prof Med
Albert Einstein Coll Med; **HOSP:** North Central
Bronx Hosp; **SI:** *Infectious Diseases*
⌖ ⌂ S Mcr Mod Immediately

Chernaik, Richard (MD) IM **PCP**
Montefiore Med Ctr
100 Elgan Pl; Bronx, NY 10475; (718) 320-2188;
BDCERT: IM 68; **MS:** Jefferson Med Coll 60; **RES:**
Jersey City Med Ctr, Jersey City, NJ 64-65; VA Med
Ctr-Brooklyn, Brooklyn, NY 65-67; **FAP:** Asst Clin
Prof Med Albert Einstein Coll Med
⌖ ⌂ 🚘 🎦 S Mcr Mod A Few Days

Cimino, James E (MD) IM **PCP**
Calvary Hosp
1740 Eastchester Rd; Bronx, NY 10461; (718)
518-2202; **BDCERT:** IM 61; Nep 72; **MS:** NYU Sch
Med 54; **RES:** IM, EJ Meyer Mem Hosp, Buffalo, NY
54-57; **FEL:** Physiology, Univ Hosp SUNY Buffalo,
Buffalo, NY 57-58; **FAP:** Adjct Prof N NYU Sch
Med; **SI:** *Palliative Care; Nutrition*
LANG: Sp, Itl, Fr; ⌖ ⌂ 🚘 🎦 Mcr Mod Immediately
VISA 🖵

Coco, Maria (MD) IM
Montefiore Med Ctr
Montefiore Medical Center, 111 E 210th St;
Amawalk, NY 10467; (718) 920-4136; **BDCERT:**
IM 85; **MS:** Italy 82; **RES:** IM, Bronx Lebanon Hosp
Ctr, Bronx, NY 82-85; **FEL:** Nep, Montefiore Med
Ctr, Bronx, NY 85-88; **FAP:** Asst Prof; **SI:** *Kidney
Disease; Hypertension*
LANG: Sp, Itl; ⌖ ⌂ 🚘 🎦 S Mcr ▦ **VISA** 🖵 🖵

Comfort, Christopher P (MD) IM **PCP**
Montefiore Med Ctr-Weiler/Einstein Div
3517 E Tremont Ave; Bronx, NY 10465; (718)
822-4262; **BDCERT:** IM 86; Ger 93; **MS:** St Louis U
82; **RES:** Albert Einstein Med Ctr, Bronx, NY 85-88;
Jacobi Med Ctr, Bronx, NY 88-89; **HOSP:**
Westchester Square Med Ctr
LANG: Sp; ⌖ 🔳 C ⌂ 🎦 S Mcr 2-4 Weeks

Diaz, Maria (MD) IM **PCP**
Montefiore Med Ctr
Montefiore Medical Group, 105 W 188th St; Bronx,
NY 10451; (718) 563-0757; **BDCERT:** IM 87; **MS:**
Albert Einstein Coll Med 90; **RES:** IM, Jacobi Med
Ctr, Bronx, NY 93
LANG: Sp; ⌖ 🔳 C ⌂ 🎦 S Mcr Mod 2-4 Weeks

Ehrlich, Elyse (MD) IM
Montefiore Med Ctr
2100 White Plains Rd; Bronx, NY 10462; (718)
892-1626; **MS:** NY Med Coll 91; **RES:** IM, Mount
Sinai Med Ctr, New York, NY; **HOSP:** Montefiore
Med Ctr-Weiler/Einstein Div; **HMO:** Blue Choice
Oxford CIGNA Prucare
⌖ 🔳 C ⌂ 🚘 🎦 S Mcr WC

Ehrlich, Martin (MD)   IM   **PCP**
Montefiore Med Ctr

111 E 210th St; Bronx, NY 10467; (718) 920-6097; **BDCERT:** IM 88; **MS:** Columbia P&S 85; **RES:** Harlem Hosp Ctr, New York, NY 85-88; *SI: Preventive Medicine;* **HMO:** CIGNA PHS GHI US Hlthcre Oxford +

LANG: Sp; ♿ ☾ ⬛ ⬛ ⬛ $ ⬛ ⬛

Fojas, Antonio (MD)   IM   **PCP**
Our Lady of Mercy Med Ctr

Medical Village, Bronx River, 600 E 233rd St; Bronx, NY 10466; (718) 920-9600; **BDCERT:** IM 93; **MS:** Philippines 84; **RES:** Our Lady of Mercy Med Ctr, Bronx, NY 84-87; **FEL:** Med, Our Lady of Mercy Med Ctr, Bronx, NY 87-88; **HMO:** Blue Choice Oxford

♿ ⬛ ⬛ ⬛ $ ⬛   A Few Days

Gabbay, Mona (MD)   IM   **PCP**
Our Lady of Mercy Med Ctr

Our Lady of Mercy/Dept of Medicine, 600 E 233rd St; Bronx, NY 10466; (718) 920-9889; **BDCERT:** IM 95; **MS:** Mt Sinai Sch Med 92; **RES:** Mount Sinai Med Ctr, New York, NY 93-95; **FAP:** Asst Prof NY Med Coll; *SI: Women's Health;* **HMO:** +

♿ ⬛ ⬛ ⬛ ⬛ ⬛ ⬛   1 Week

Gold, Jay (MD)   IM   **PCP**
Beth Israel Med Ctr

Pelham Bay Medical Group, 2809 Middleton Rd; Bronx, NY 10461; (718) 931-4551; **BDCERT:** IM 87; Onc 89; **MS:** SUNY Hlth Sci Ctr 84; **RES:** Beth Israel Med Ctr, New York, NY 84-87; **FEL:** Hem Onc, Beth Israel Med Ctr, New York, NY 87-89; Hem Onc, Beth Israel Med Ctr, New York, NY 89-90; *SI: Asthma; Diabetetic Nutrition;* **HMO:** Oxford Aetna-US Healthcare GHI PHS Magnacare +

LANG: Sp, Itl; ♿ ☾ ⬛ ⬛ ⬛ $ ⬛   A Few Days ⬛ **VISA** ⬛ ⬛

Gorkin, Janet (MD)   IM   **PCP**
Montefiore Med Ctr

Montefiore Faculty Practice, 3400 Bainbridge Ave; Bronx, NY 10467; (718) 920-7763; **BDCERT:** IM 76; Nep 80; **MS:** Mt Sinai Sch Med 73; **RES:** IM, Mount Sinai Med Ctr, New York, NY 73-76; **FEL:** Nep, Mount Sinai Med Ctr, New York, NY 76-78; **FAP:** Prof Albert Einstein Coll Med; *SI: Hypertension; Kidney Disease;* **HMO:** Oxford CIGNA PHS NYLCare 32BJ +

LANG: Sp; ♿ ⬛ ⬛ ⬛ $ ⬛   A Few Days **VISA** ⬛

Grajower, Martin (MD)   IM   **PCP**
Montefiore Med Ctr

Riverdale Medical Associates, 3736 Henry Hudson Pkwy; Riverdale, NY 10463; (718) 549-6268; **BDCERT:** IM 76; EDM 81; **MS:** Albert Einstein Coll Med 73; **RES:** IM, Montefiore Med Ctr, Bronx, NY 74-75; IM, Boston Med Ctr, Boston, MA 75-76; **FEL:** EDM, Montefiore Med Ctr, Bronx, NY 76-78; *SI: Diabetes; Endocrinology;* **HMO:** 32BJ

♿ ☾ ⬛ ⬛ ⬛ $ ⬛   A Few Days ⬛ **VISA** ⬛

Irwin, Michael (MD)   IM
Montefiore Med Ctr

1000 S Pelham Pkwy; Bronx, NY 10461; (718) 409-8200; **BDCERT:** IM 79; **MS:** Univ Texas, Houston 75; **RES:** St Luke's Roosevelt Hosp Ctr, New York, NY 77-79; *SI: Geriatrics*

Kaplan, Deborah (MD)   IM   **PCP**
Montefiore Med Ctr

111 E 210th St; Bronx, NY 10467; (718) 920-6666; **BDCERT:** IM 95; **MS:** Albert Einstein Coll Med 91; **RES:** IM, Mount Sinai Med Ctr, New York, NY 91-94; **FAP:** Instr Med Albert Einstein Coll Med; *SI: Thyroid; Hypertension;* **HMO:** United Healthcare US Hlthcre CIGNA Montecare

LANG: Fr; ♿ ⬛ ⬛ ⬛ ⬛ ⬛   2-4 Weeks

Kelly, Carol (MD)   IM   **PCP**
Montefiore Med Ctr

Tenbroeck Medical Assoc, 1180 Morris Park Ave; Bronx, NY 10461; (718) 863-8465; **BDCERT:** IM 82; **MS:** Brown U 79; **RES:** Duke U Med Ctr, Durham, NC 79-82; **HOSP:** Westchester Square Med Ctr; **HMO:** Blue Choice Aetna Hlth Plan Blue Cross & Blue Shield Oxford GHI +

⬧ 🅢 📷 🔳 🔲 🅢 Mc Md 2-4 Weeks **VISA**

Laitman, Robert (MD)   IM
Montefiore Med Ctr-Weiler/Einstein Div

1525 Blondell Ave Ste 101; Bronx, NY 10461; (718) 518-1276; **BDCERT:** IM 86; Nep 88; **MS:** Washington U, St Louis 83; **RES:** Jacobi Med Ctr, Bronx, NY 83-86; **FEL:** Nep, Montefiore Med Ctr, Bronx, NY

⬧ 🅢 🅲 📷 🔳 🔲 Mc Immediately ▦ **VISA**

Lief, Philip (MD)   IM
Montefiore Med Ctr

Einstein Hospital, 1825 Eastchester Rd 7NW; Bronx, NY 10461; (718) 904-2500; **BDCERT:** IM 74; Nep 74; **MS:** Univ Penn 65; **RES:** IM, Montefiore Med Ctr, Bronx, NY 65-68; **FEL:** Nep, New England Med Ctr, Boston, MA 68-70; **FAP:** Prof Med Albert Einstein Coll Med; *SI: Hypertension; Kidney Disease;* **HMO:** Blue Choice Blue Cross & Blue Shield CIGNA Prucare Sanus +

LANG: Sp, Itl; ⬧ 📷 🔳 🔲 🅢 Mc 1 Week ▦ **VISA** ⬤ ▦

Lucariello, Ralph (MD)   IM   **PCP**
Our Lady of Mercy Med Ctr

4141 Carpenter Ave Fl 4; Bronx, NY 10466; (718) 655-4222; **BDCERT:** IM 60; **MS:** Georgetown U 51; **RES:** IM, Metropolitan Hosp Ctr, New York, NY 52-54; IM, VA Med Ctr-Manh, New York, NY 56-57; **FAP:** Asst Clin Prof NY Med Coll; *SI: Diabetes;* **HMO:** Prucare Oxford

LANG: Itl; ⬧ 📷 🔲 🅢 Mc 2-4 Weeks

McGinn, Thomas (MD)   IM   **PCP**
Montefiore Med Ctr

Montefiore Med Ctr-Dept of Medicine, 3400 Bainbridge Ave 2nd Fl; Bronx, NY 10467; (718) 920-7763; **BDCERT:** IM 93; **MS:** SUNY Downstate 89; **RES:** IM, Albert Einstein Med Ctr, Bronx, NY 89-92; Albert Einstein Med Ctr, Bronx, NY 92-93; **FAP:** Asst Prof Albert Einstein Coll Med; **HOSP:** Montefiore Med Ctr-Weiler/Einstein Div; *SI: Low Back Pain; Primary Care;* **HMO:** US Hlthcre Oxford Most ~

LANG: Sp; ⬧ 📷 🔳 🔲 🅢 Mc A Few Days ▦ **VISA** ⬤

Menon, Latha (MD)   IM   **PCP**
Bronx Lebanon Hosp Ctr

Eara Pulmonary Associates, 1770 Grand Concourse 2G; Bronx, NY 10456; (718) 518-5581; **BDCERT:** IM 79; CCM 90; **MS:** India 72; **RES:** IM, Flushing Hosp Med Ctr, Flushing, NY 75-78; **FEL:** Pul, Albert Einstein Med Ctr, Bronx, NY 78-80; **FAP:** Assoc Prof Albert Einstein Coll Med; *SI: Asthma; Critical Care;* **HMO:** Health First Oxford US Hlthcre

⬧ 📷 🔳 🔲 Mc Md Immediately

Mojtabai, Shaparak (MD)   IM
St Barnabas Hosp-Bronx

2371 Arthur Ave; Bronx, NY 10458; (718) 364-6199; **BDCERT:** IM 89; **MS:** Iran 89; **RES:** St Barnabas Hosp-Bronx, Bronx, NY 85-88; **FEL:** St Barnabas Hosp-Bronx, Bronx, NY 88-89; **FAP:** Assoc Clin Prof NY Coll Osteo Med; *SI: Primary Care;* **HMO:** US Hlthcre Oxford Prucare First Option GHI +

LANG: Frs, Sp, Itl, Alb; ⬧ 📷 🔳 🔲 🅢 Mc 1 Week

Nyer, Kenneth (MD)   IM   **PCP**
Montefiore Med Ctr

1931 Williamsbridge Rd; Bronx, NY 10461; (718) 409-6400; **BDCERT:** IM 88; Ger 88; **MS:** Albert Einstein Coll Med 84; **RES:** N Shore Univ Hosp-Manhasset, Manhasset, NY 84-87; **HOSP:** Westchester Square Med Ctr; **HMO:** Magnacare Blue Choice GHI Oxford Medichoice +

Immediately

Pintauro, Frank (MD) IM
Westchester Square Med Ctr
1750 Seminole Ave Main Office; Bronx, NY 10461; (718) 863-3079; **MS:** Italy 78; **RES:** IM, Norwalk Hosp, Norwalk, CT 82; **HOSP:** Our Lady of Mercy Med Ctr; **HMO:** Oxford Blue Choice Magnacare PHCS Guardian +
LANG: Itl; ♿ [SA SU] ☾ ☎ 👤 📅 $ [WC] [NFI] A Few Days

Pintauro, Robert (MD) IM [PCP]
Westchester Square Med Ctr
2138 Continental Ave; Bronx, NY 10461; (718) 824-5525; **MS:** West Indies 81; **RES:** Norwalk Hosp, Norwalk, CT 81-84; **HOSP:** Our Lady of Mercy Med Ctr; ***SI:*** *Nutrition/Preventive Med.; Diabetes*; **HMO:** Aetna Hlth Plan Oxford Prudential Blue Cross & Blue Shield Magnacare +
LANG: Sp; ♿ [SA SU] ☾ ☎ 👤 📅 [Mcr] [WC] [NFI] A Few Days

Pulle, Dunstan (MD) IM [PCP]
Our Lady of Mercy Med Ctr
2410 Barker Ave; Bronx, NY 10467; (718) 547-5880; **BDCERT:** IM 70; Pul 71; **MS:** Sri Lanka 62; **RES:** VA Med Ctr-Brooklyn, Brooklyn, NY 66-69; **HOSP:** Community Hosp At Dobbs Ferry; ***SI:*** *Asthma; Hypertension Cholesterol*; **HMO:** US Hlthcre CIGNA Oxford Blue Choice United Healthcare +
♿ ☎ 👤 📅 [Mcr] [Mcd] [WC] [NFI] Immediately

Reed, Louis Juden (MD) IM
Westchester Square Med Ctr
Tenbroeck Medical Assoc, 1180 Morris Park Ave; Bronx, NY 10461; (718) 863-8465; **BDCERT:** IM 73; **MS:** Washington U, St Louis 59; **RES:** Jacobi Med Ctr, Bronx, NY 59-60; Jacobi Med Ctr, Bronx, NY 60-62; **FEL:** Jacobi Med Ctr, Bronx, NY; Hammersmith Hosp, London, England; **HOSP:** Montefiore Med Ctr-Weiler/Einstein Div; **HMO:** Oxford Blue Choice Blue Cross & Blue Shield US Hlthcre
♿ [SA SU] ☾ ☎ 👤 📅 [Mcr] Immediately VISA 💳

Ricci, Mario (MD) IM
Our Lady of Mercy Med Ctr
841 Burke Ave; Bronx, NY 10467; (718) 654-1726; **MS:** NYU Sch Med 47; **RES:** VA Med Ctr-Brooklyn, Brooklyn, NY 53-56; **HMO:** Blue Choice Chubb

Rogg, Gary (MD) IM [PCP]
Montefiore Med Ctr-Weiler/Einstein Div
1575 Blondell Ave; Bronx, NY 10461; (718) 405-8312; **BDCERT:** IM 91; **MS:** NYU Sch Med 88; **RES:** IM, Jacobi Med Ctr, Bronx, NY 88-91; **FAP:** Asst Dir Med Albert Einstein Coll Med; ***SI:*** *Cardiac; GI*; **HMO:** Oxford Blue Choice US Hlthcre CIGNA
LANG: Sp, Bul, Itl, Rus, Fr; ♿ ☾ ☎ 👤 📅 $ [Mcr] [Mcd] [WC] [NFI] 2-4 Weeks VISA 💳

Rosendorf, Clive (MD) IM
Mount Sinai Med Ctr
Mt Sinai/VA Medical CenterBronx, Dept of Internal Medicine, 130 W Kingsbridge Rd; Bronx, NY 10468; (718) 579-1695; **MS:** South Africa 62; **RES:** St Thomas Hosp, London, England 64-67; **HOSP:** VA Med Ctr-Bronx; ***SI:*** *High Blood Pressure; Cardiology*
♿ ☎ 👤 📅 A Few Days

Ross, Lawrence (MD) IM [PCP]
Montefiore Med Ctr
Tenbroeck Medical Assoc, 1180 Morris Park Ave; Bronx, NY 10461; (718) 863-8983; **BDCERT:** IM 75; Nep 78; **MS:** Albert Einstein Coll Med 72; **RES:** Jacobi Med Ctr, Bronx, NY 72-75; **FEL:** Nep, Jacobi Med Ctr, Bronx, NY 75-77; **FAP:** Asst Clin Prof Med Albert Einstein Coll Med; **HOSP:** Westchester Square Med Ctr; **HMO:** Oxford Aetna Hlth Plan Blue Choice CIGNA Prucare +
LANG: Sp, Itl, Heb, Yd; ♿ [SA SU] ☾ ☎ 👤 📅 [Mcr] [WC] [NFI] 1 Week [AMERICAN EXPRESS]

Sander, Norbert (MD) IM [PCP]
Sound Shore Med Ctr-Westchester
340 City Island Ave; Bronx, NY 10028; (718) 885-0333; **BDCERT:** IM 81; **MS:** Albert Einstein Coll Med 71; **RES:** IM, Metropolitan Hosp Ctr, New York, NY 71-74; Lincoln Med & Mental Hlth Ctr, Bronx, NY; ***SI:*** *Preventive Medicine; Sports Medicine*; **HMO:** Oxford CIGNA GHI Aetna Hlth Plan Blue Cross +
LANG: Fr, Itl; ♿ [SA SU] ☾ ☎ 👤 📅 $ [Mcr] [WC] Immediately

Guide to symbols and abbreviations can be found on pages 110-113.

Shah, Mahendra (MD)   **IM**
Bronx Lebanon Hosp Ctr

3184 Grand Concourse Ste 2E; Bronx, NY 10458;
(718) 561-7290; **BDCERT:** IM 81; **MS:** India 61;
RES: IM, Jersey City Med Ctr, Jersey City, NJ 67; IM,
VA Med Ctr-Bronx, Bronx, NY 68-69; **FEL:** Hem
Onc, VA Med Ctr-Bronx, Bronx, NY 69; Onc, Bronx
Lebanon Hosp Ctr, Bronx, NY 70; **FAP:** Instr Med
Albert Einstein Coll Med; **SI:** *Treatment for Cancer;*
HMO: 1199 GHI US Hlthcre

⬥ 🅂🅂 🅲 📷 🅟 🎞 🅂 Mcr Mcl 1 Week

Shapiro, Lawrence (MD)   **IM**
Montefiore Med Ctr

111 E 210th St; Bronx, NY 10467; (718) 579-
5886; **BDCERT:** IM 75; **MS:** SUNY Hlth Sci Ctr 71;
RES: IM, Bellevue Hosp Ctr, New York, NY 72-74;
HOSP: Lincoln Med & Mental Hlth Ctr

Shoreibah, Ahmed (MD)   **IM**   **PCP**
St Barnabas Hosp-Bronx

Bronx Park Medical Pavillion, 2016 Bronxdale Ave
302; Bronx, NY 10462; (718) 822-1515; **BDCERT:**
IM 95; **MS:** U Fla Coll Med 91; **RES:** U Miami Hosp,
Miami, FL 91-92; Jackson Mem Hosp, Miami, FL
92-94; **FAP:** Clin Instr Cornell U; **SI:** *Asthma; Heart
Failure;* **HMO:** GHI Oxford Blue Cross First Option
Health Source +

⬥ 📷 🅟 🎞 🅂 Mcr Mcl A Few Days

Solomon, Gregory (MD)   **IM**   **PCP**
Montefiore Med Ctr

Montefiore Medical Center Faculty Practice, 3400
Bainbridge Ave 2nd; Bronx, NY 10467; (718) 920-
7763; **BDCERT:** IM 95; **MS:** NYU Sch Med 91; **RES:**
IM, Montefiore Med Ctr, Bronx, NY 91-94; **FAP:**
Assoc Prof Med Albert Einstein Coll Med; **SI:** *General
Internal Medicine; Preventative Medicine*

⬥ 🅲 📷 🅟 🎞 🅂 Mcr A Few Days *VISA* 💳

Sonnenblick, Edmund (MD)   **IM**
Montefiore Med Ctr-Weiler/Einstein Div

1300 Morris Park Ave; Bronx, NY 10461; (718)
904-2932; **BDCERT:** IM 68; **MS:** Harvard Med Sch
58; **RES:** IM, Columbia-Presbyterian Med Ctr, New
York, NY 59-63; **FEL:** Columbia - Presbyterian
Hosp, New York, NY 58-59; **FAP:** Prof Med Albert
Einstein Coll Med; **HOSP:** Mount Sinai Med Ctr

⬥ 📷 🅟 🎞 Mcr Mcl Immediately 💳 *VISA* 💳

Sparano, Joseph (MD)   **IM**
Montefiore Med Ctr

Montefiore Medical Center, 111 E 210th St 100;
Bronx, NY 10467; (718) 920-6706; **BDCERT:** IM
86; **MS:** NY Med Coll 82; **RES:** St Vincents Hosp &
Med Ctr NY, New York, NY 82-86; **FEL:** Onc, Albert
Einstein Med Ctr, Bronx, NY 86-88; **FAP:** Assoc
Prof Med Albert Einstein Coll Med; **SI:** *Breast Cancer;
Lymphoma;* **HMO:** Blue Cross & Blue Shield US
Hlthcre

⬥ 📷 🅟 🎞 🅂 Mcr Mcl A Few Days

Teffera, Fassil (MD)   **IM**   **PCP**
Our Lady of Mercy Med Ctr

Dept of Medicine, 600 E 233rd St; Bronx, NY
10466; (718) 920-9889; **BDCERT:** IM 93; **MS:**
Ethiopia 76; **RES:** IM, Our Lady of Mercy Med Ctr,
Bronx, NY 91-93; **FAP:** Asst Clin Prof Med NY Med
Coll; **SI:** *Preventive Medicine; Hypertension;* **HMO:** US
Hlthcre Blue Choice Chubb Oxford CIGNA +

LANG: Sp; ⬥ 🅂🅂 🅲 📷 🅟 🎞 🅂 Mcr Mcl NFl
Immediately

Uday, Kalpana (MD)   **IM**   **PCP**
Bronx Lebanon Hosp Ctr

NephrologyInternal Medicine, 1650 Grand
Concourse DIALYSIS 10th FL; Bronx, NY 10457;
(718) 518-5232; **BDCERT:** IM 89; **Nep** 92; **MS:**
India 80; **RES:** IM, Jamaica Med Ctr, Jamaica, NY
86-89; **FEL:** Nep, Montefiore Med Ctr, Bronx, NY
89-91; **FAP:** Asst Prof Med Albert Einstein Coll
Med; **SI:** *High Blood Pressure; Kidney Diseases;* **HMO:**
1199 Oxford Aetna-US Healthcare MHS Blue Cross
& Blue Shield +

LANG: Fr, Sp; ⬥ 🅂🅂 📷 🅟 🎞 🅂 Mcr Mcl
A Few Days

Walker, Yvette (MD)   IM   **PCP**
Bronx Lebanon Hosp Ctr
Avalon Medical Assocs, 1770 Grand Concourse;
Bronx, NY 10457; (718) 518-5581; **BDCERT:** IM
86; **MS:** SUNY Downstate 83; **RES:** IM, Kings
County Hosp Ctr, Brooklyn, NY 83-84; IM, Kings
County Hosp Ctr, Brooklyn, NY 84-86; **FAP:** Assoc
Prof Albert Einstein Coll Med; **SI:** *Diabetes Mellitus;*
Hypertension; **HMO:** Oxford HealthNet

LANG: Sp; ⬥ ☎ 🚹 🏧 Mcr Mcd NFI   A Few Days

MATERNAL & FETAL MEDICINE

Chazotte, Cynthia (MD)   MF   **PCP**
Montefiore Med Ctr-Weiler/Einstein Div
Weiler Hosp of Albert Einstein College of Med, 1825
Eastchester Rd Rm701; Bronx, NY 10461; (718)
918-6312; **BDCERT:** ObG 96; MF 96; **MS:** NY Med
Coll 81; **RES:** ObG, Albert Einstein Med Ctr, Bronx,
NY 81-84; ObG, Albert Einstein Med Ctr, Bronx, NY
84-85; **FEL:** Albert Einstein Med Ctr, Bronx, NY 85-
87; **FAP:** Assoc Prof Albert Einstein Coll Med;
HOSP: Montefiore Med Ctr; **SI:** *Pregnancy—Medical*
Complications; Asthma During Pregnancy; **HMO:**
Montefiore IPA Oxford PHCS Aetna Hlth Plan
CIGNA +

LANG: Sp, Rus; ⬥ 🅒 ☎ 🚹 🏧 $ Mcr Mcd NFI
A Few Days *VISA* 💳

MEDICAL GENETICS

Gross, Susan (MD)   MG
Montefiore Med Ctr
Division of Reproductive GeneticsMontefiore
Medical Center, 1695 Eastchester Rd Ste 301;
Bronx, NY 10461; (718) 547-4864; **BDCERT:** MG
96; ObG 95; **MS:** U Toronto 85; **RES:** ObG, U
Toronto Gen Hosp, Ontario, Canada 87-91; **FEL:**
MF, U Toronto Gen Hosp, Toronto, Canada 91-92;
MG, U Tenn Hosp, Memphis, TN 92-94; **FAP:** Asst
Prof Albert Einstein Coll Med; **SI:** *Prenatal Genetic*
Testing; Prenatal Ultrasound; **HMO:** CIGNA United
Healthcare Oxford PHS +

LANG: Sp; ⬥ ☎ 🚹 🏧 $ Mcr Mcd   A Few Days

Marion, Robert (MD)   MG
Montefiore Med Ctr
111 E 210th St; Bronx, NY 10467; (718) 920-
4300; **BDCERT:** Ped 85; MG 87; **MS:** Albert
Einstein Coll Med 79; **RES:** New England Med Ctr,
Boston, MA 79-80; Albert Einstein Med Ctr, Bronx,
NY 80-82; **FEL:** MG, Albert Einstein Med Ctr,
Bronx, NY 82-84; **FAP:** Prof Ped Albert Einstein
Coll Med; **HOSP:** Blythedale Children's Hosp; **SI:**
Birth Defects; Spinal Bifida; **HMO:** Oxford Blue Cross
& Blue Shield GHI

LANG: Sp; ⬥ ☎ 🚹 🏧 $ Mcd WC NFI   1 Week

Nitowsky, Harold (MD)   MG
Montefiore Med Ctr
1695 Eastchester Rd 301; Bronx, NY 10461; (718)
405-8150; **BDCERT:** Ped 56; MG 82; **MS:** NYU Sch
Med 47; **RES:** U CO Hosp, Denver, CO 47-50; **FEL:**
Ped, U CO Hosp, Denver, CO; **FAP:** Prof MG Albert
Einstein Coll Med; **SI:** *Prenatal Diagnosis; Clinical*
Genetics; **HMO:** Aetna Hlth Plan HIP Network Blue
Choice CIGNA Prucare +

LANG: Sp; ⬥ ☎ 🏧 $ Mcr Mcd   1 Week *VISA* 💳

MEDICAL ONCOLOGY

Brescia, Michael J (MD)   Onc
Calvary Hosp
1740 Eastchester Rd; Bronx, NY 10461; (718)
518-2219; **BDCERT:** IM 89; **MS:** Georgetown U 58;
RES: IM, VA Med Ctr-Bronx, Bronx, NY 59-62;
FAP: Asst Clin Prof Med NY Med Coll; **SI:** *Advanced*
Cancer; Palliative Care; **HMO:** Aetna Hlth Plan Blue
Choice Blue Cross & Blue Choice +
1 Week

Dutcher, Janice P (MD)   Onc
Montefiore Med Ctr
111 E 210th St; Bronx, NY 10467; (718) 920-4674; **BDCERT:** IM 78; Onc 83; **MS:** UC Davis 75; **RES:** IM, Rush Presbyterian-St Lukes Med Ctr, Chicago, IL 75-78; **FEL:** Onc, Nat Cancer Inst, Bethesda, MD 78-81; **FAP:** Prof Albert Einstein Coll Med; **HOSP:** Jacobi Med Ctr; **SI:** *Renal Cell Cancer; Melanoma;* **HMO:** GHI US Hlthcre Magnacare Oxford Prucare +

LANG: Sp, Rus, Trk; 🅰 📷 🔧 🏛 💲 Mcr Mcd WC NFI A Few Days 💳 **VISA** 💳

Fuks, Joachim (MD)   Onc
Montefiore Med Ctr
Advanced Oncology Associates, 1578 Williamsbridge Rd Fl 2; Bronx, NY 10461; (718) 931-2290; **BDCERT:** IM 81; Onc 83; **MS:** Spain 75; **RES:** Mount Sinai Med Ctr, New York, NY 76-78; **FEL:** Onc, Nat Cancer Inst, Bethesda, MD; **FAP:** Asst Clin Prof Albert Einstein Coll Med; **HOSP:** Our Lady of Mercy Med Ctr; **SI:** *Breast Cancer; Lung Cancer;* **HMO:** Oxford Empire Blue Cross & Shield Aetna Hlth Plan Chubb GHI +

LANG: Sp, Pol; 🅰 📷 🔧 🏛 💲 Mcr Mcd A Few Days

Greenwald, Edward (MD)   Onc
Montefiore Med Ctr
111 E 210th St; Bronx, NY 10467; (718) 920-4816; **BDCERT:** IM 60; Onc 73; **MS:** NYU Sch Med 52; **RES:** Montefiore Med Ctr, Bronx, NY 55-56; Jacobi Med Ctr, Bronx, NY 56-57; **FEL:** Onc, Montefiore Med Ctr, Bronx, NY 57-58; **FAP:** Prof Med Albert Einstein Coll Med; **HOSP:** Our Lady of Mercy Med Ctr; **HMO:** Aetna Hlth Plan Blue Choice Blue Cross & Blue Shield CIGNA Metlife +

LANG: Sp; 🅰 📷 🔧 🏛 💲 Mcr Mcd Immediately

Hoffman, Anthony (MD)   Onc
Montefiore Med Ctr-Weiler/Einstein Div
Sciode Med Plc, 2330 Eastchester 3A; Bronx, NY 10469; (718) 881-7111; **BDCERT:** IM 92; Onc 97; **MS:** Geo Wash U Sch Med 89; **RES:** Med, Albert Einstein Med Ctr, Bronx, NY 85-89; **FEL:** Onc, Mem Sloan Kettering Cancer Ctr, New York, NY 89-92; **HOSP:** Westchester Square Med Ctr; **SI:** *Breast Cancer; Prostate Cancer;* **HMO:** Oxford US Hlthcre CIGNA PHS

LANG: Itl, Sp, Rus; 🅰 SA SD 🅲 📷 🔧 🏛 💲 Mcr

Ramirez, Mark A (MD)   Onc
Montefiore Med Ctr
3130 Grand Concourse 1H; Bronx, NY 10458; (718) 220-4900; **BDCERT:** Hem 92; Onc 89; **MS:** Cornell U 82; **RES:** Med, Montefiore Med Ctr, Bronx, NY 82-85; **FEL:** Hem, Montefiore Med Ctr, Bronx, NY 85-86; Onc, Montefiore Med Ctr, Bronx, NY 86-88; **FAP:** Asst Clin Prof Med Albert Einstein Coll Med; **HOSP:** St Joseph's Med Ctr-Yonkers; **SI:** *Non-Hodgkin's Lymphoma; Breast Cancer;* **HMO:** Oxford Sanus CIGNA Well Care

LANG: Sp; 🅰 📷 🏛 💲 Mcr Mcd A Few Days

Reed, Mary K (MD)   Onc
Bronx Lebanon Hosp Ctr
165 Grand Concourse; Bronx, NY 11432; (718) 518-5806; **BDCERT:** Hem 94; Onc 91; **MS:** Boston U 80; **RES:** Henry Ford Hosp, Detroit, MI 80-83; **FEL:** Hem, Long Island Jewish Med Ctr, New Hyde Park, NY 85

Reilly, John Patrick (MD)   Onc
Our Lady of Mercy Med Ctr
600 E 233rd St; Bronx, NY 10466; (718) 920-9260; **BDCERT:** Hem 94; Onc 91; **MS:** West Indies 84; **RES:** IM, St John's Epis Hosp-S Shore, Far Rockaway, NY 84-87; **FEL:** Hem, Coney Island Hosp, Brooklyn, NY 87-88; Onc, Montefiore Med Ctr, Bronx, NY 88-90; **FAP:** Asst Prof Med NY Med Coll; **SI:** *Pain Management; Breast Cancer*

LANG: Sp; 🅰 📷 🔧 🏛 Mcr Mcd A Few Days 💳 **VISA** 💳 💳

Vogl, Steven Edward (MD)   Onc
Montefiore Med Ctr-Weiler/Einstein Div
2220 Tiemann Ave; Bronx, NY 10469; (718) 519-7774; **BDCERT:** IM 75; Onc 75; **MS:** Cornell U 70; **RES:** IM, Jacobi Med Ctr, Bronx, NY; **FEL:** Onc, Mount Sinai Med Ctr, New York, NY; **FAP:** Assoc Clin Prof Albert Einstein Coll Med; **SI:** *Breast Cancer; Lung Cancer*

📷 🔧 🏛 Mcr Mcd Immediately

Wadler, Scott (MD)   Onc
Montefiore Med Ctr
Montefiore Medical Ctr, 111 E 210th St; Bronx, NY
10467; (718) 920-4830; BDCERT: IM 84; Onc 87;
MS: NYU Sch Med 80; RES: Bellevue Hosp Ctr, New
York, NY 81-83; FEL: Onc, Mount Sinai Med Ctr,
New York, NY; New York University Med Ctr, New
York, NY; HMO: Empire Blue Cross & Shield GHI US
Hlthcre Blue Choice Aetna Hlth Plan +

LANG: Sp, Itl; 🔣 🔣 🔣 🔣 🔣 2-4 Weeks

Wiernik, Peter H (MD)   Onc
Montefiore Med Ctr
Montefiore Medical Ctr, 111 E 210th St; Bronx, NY
10467; (718) 920-4826; BDCERT: IM 73; Onc 73;
MS: U Va Sch Med 65; RES: Med, Cleveland Metro
Gen Hosp, Cleveland, OH 66-67; Med, Johns
Hopkins Hosp, Baltimore, MD 69-71; FEL: Onc, Nat
Cancer Inst, Bethesda, MD 68-70; FAP: Prof Albert
Einstein Coll Med; SI: Leukemia; Lymphoma; HMO:
GHI GHI US Hlthcre Blue Cross & Blue Shield Oxford
+

LANG: Srb, Heb, Itl; 🔣 🔣 🔣 🔣 🔣 🔣 🔣
A Few Days

NEONATAL-PERINATAL MEDICINE

Brion, Luc (MD)   NP
Montefiore Med Ctr-Weiler/Einstein Div
Neonatology Associates, 1825 Eastchester 715;
Bronx, NY 10461; (718) 904-4105; BDCERT: Ped
87; NP 87; MS: Belgium 76; RES: Ped, Hosp St
Pierre, Brussells, Belgium 76-81; Ped, Montefiore
Med Ctr, Bronx, NY 85-86; FEL: NP, Hosp For Sick
Children, Toronto, Canada 81-82; NP, Montefiore
Med Ctr, Bronx, NY 83-85; FAP: Assoc Prof Albert
Einstein Coll Med; HOSP: Montefiore Med Ctr; SI:
Kidney; Growth; HMO: Aetna Hlth Plan GHI Empire
Blue Cross & Shield Prudential US Hlthcre +

LANG: Sp, Fr, Heb, Flm, Dut; 🔣 🔣 🔣 🔣 🔣 🔣 🔣
🔣 Immediately ▦ *VISA* ⬤ 🔳

Campbell, Deborah (MD)   NP
Montefiore Med Ctr
1825 Eastchester Ave; Bronx, NY 10461; (718)
904-4105; BDCERT: Ped 83; NP 83; MS: SUNY
Buffalo 78; RES: Ped, Montefiore Med Ctr, Bronx,
NY 78-81; FEL: NP, Montefiore Med Ctr, Bronx, NY
81-83; FAP: Assoc Prof Ped Albert Einstein Coll
Med; HOSP: North Central Bronx Hosp; SI:
Developmental Follow-up; HMO: Oxford Montecare
Sanus CIGNA US Hlthcre +

🔣 🔣 🔣 🔣 🔣 🔣 🔣 🔣

Reinersman, Gerold (MD)   NP
North Central Bronx Hosp
1825 Eastchester Rd Rm 75-25; Bronx, NY 10461;
(718) 519-3820; BDCERT: Ped 80; NP 85; MS:
Univ Ky Coll Med 74; RES: Ped, Oregon Health Sci U
Hosp, Portland, OR 77-79; FEL: NP, U UT Hosp, Salt
Lake City, UT 83-85; FAP: Asst Prof Ped Albert
Einstein Coll Med; HOSP: Montefiore Med Ctr; SI:
Nutrition Problems
LANG: Sp;

Vega-Rich, Carlos (MD)   NP
Montefiore Med Ctr
13 Agnes Cir; Ardsley, NY 10502; (718) 904-
4105; BDCERT: Ped 89; MS: Panama 78; RES: Ped,
Hosp for Mothers and Infants, David, Panama 80-
83; FEL: NP, Albert Einstein Med Ctr, Bronx, NY
84-87; FAP: Asst Prof Ped Albert Einstein Coll Med;
SI: Newborns-Sick, Premature; HMO: US Hlthcre HIP
Network GHI Blue Cross PHS +

LANG: Sp, Fr, Heb, Itl; 🔣 🔣 🔣 🔣 🔣 🔣 🔣
Immediately ▦ *VISA* ⬤ 🔳

NEPHROLOGY

Charytan, Chaim (MD)   Nep
NY Hosp Med Ctr of Queens
Nephrology Associates, 1874 Pelham Pkwy South
LR; Bronx, NY 10461; (718) 931-5800; BDCERT:
Nep 69; MS: Albert Einstein Coll Med 64; RES:
Bronx Muncipal Hosp Ctr, Bronx, NY 65-67; HOSP:
Montefiore Med Ctr-Weiler/Einstein Div; SI:
Hypertension; Nephrology; HMO: Oxford GHI CIGNA
Blue Cross

🔣 🔣 🔣 🔣 🔣 🔣 🔣 1 Week

Croll, James (MD)   Nep
St Barnabas Hosp-Bronx
4422 3rd Ave; Bronx, NY 10457; (718) 960-6295; **BDCERT:** IM 78; Nep 82; **MS:** Belgium 75; **RES:** Genesee Hosp, Rochester, NY 75-78; **FEL:** Nep, VA Med Ctr-Bronx, Bronx, NY 79-81; *SI: Hemodialysis; Peritoneal Dialysis;* **HMO:** Oxford Aetna-US Healthcare Prucare

♿ 🆂🅄 📷 🚹 🏧 Mcr Mod NFI

Dave, Mahendraray (MD)   Nep
Bronx Lebanon Hosp Ctr
Hemo Dialysis Unit, 1650 Grand Concourse; Bronx, NY 10457; (718) 518-5232; **BDCERT:** Nep 82; **MS:** India 71; **RES:** Bronx Lebanon Hosp Ctr, Bronx, NY 76-78; **HMO:** Blue Choice Blue Cross & Blue Shield HealthNet US Hlthcre

♿ 🆂🅄 🌙 📷 🚹 🏧 Mcr Mod NFI   Immediately

Dharmarajin, T S (MD)   Nep   PCP
Our Lady of Mercy Med Ctr
4141 Carpenter Ave; Bronx, NY 10466; (718) 920-9041; **BDCERT:** Ger 88; Nep 80; **MS:** India 68; **RES:** IM, Our Lady of Mercy Med Ctr, Bronx, NY; **FEL:** Nep, Our Lady of Mercy Med Ctr, Bronx, NY 77-79; **HMO:** Blue Cross & Blue Shield HealthNet US Hlthcre

♿ 📷 🚹 🏧 🅂 Mcr   A Few Days

Folkert, Vaughn W (MD)   Nep
Montefiore Med Ctr
1575 Blondell Ave; Bronx, NY 10461; (718) 405-8304; **BDCERT:** IM 77; Nep 84; **MS:** Mich St U 74; **RES:** IM, Hartford Hosp, Hartford, CT 74-77; **FEL:** Nep, Albert Einstein Med Ctr, Bronx, NY; **FAP:** Assoc Prof Albert Einstein Coll Med; *SI: Kidney Stones; Dialysis*

LANG: Sp; ♿ 📷 🚹 🏧 🅂 Mcr Mod   A Few Days

Lynn, Robert (MD)   Nep
Montefiore Med Ctr
1525 Blondell Ave; Bronx, NY 10461; (718) 518-1276; **BDCERT:** IM 77; Nep 80; **MS:** Columbia P&S 74; **RES:** Columbia-Presbyterian Med Ctr, New York, NY 74-77; **FEL:** Yale-New Haven Hosp, New Haven, CT 77-79; **FAP:** Assoc Prof Albert Einstein Coll Med; **HOSP:** Sound Shore Med Ctr-Westchester; *SI: Dialysis; Chronic Kidney Disorder;* **HMO:** GHI 1199 Oxford Blue Choice

LANG: Sp; ♿ 🆂🅄 🌙 📷 🏧 Mcr Mod   A Few Days **VISA** 💳

Schuster, Victor L (MD)   Nep
Montefiore Med Ctr
1300 Morris Park Ave; Bronx, NY 10461; (718) 430-3158; **BDCERT:** IM 80; Nep 84; **MS:** Washington U, St Louis 77; **RES:** IM, U WA Med Ctr, Seattle, WA 77-81; **FEL:** Nep, U Texas SW Med Ctr, Dallas, TX 81-83; **FAP:** Prof Med Albert Einstein Coll Med; **HOSP:** Montefiore Med Ctr-Weiler/Einstein Div; **HMO:** CIGNA HealthNet Sanus-NYLCare Oxford

LANG: Sp; ♿ 🅂 Mcr WC ▦ **VISA** 💳 💳

Weiner, Bernard M (MD)   Nep
Montefiore Med Ctr
Tenbroeck Medical Associates, PC, 1180 Morris Park Ave; Bronx, NY 10461; (718) 863-8465; **BDCERT:** IM 76; Nep 78; **MS:** Albert Einstein Coll Med 73; **RES:** Med, Jacobi Med Ctr, Bronx, NY 73-74; Med, Albert Einstein Med Ctr, Bronx, NY 74-76; **FEL:** Hosp of U Penn, Philadelphia, PA 76-78; **FAP:** Asst Clin Prof Med Albert Einstein Coll Med; **HOSP:** Westchester Square Med Ctr

♿ 📷 🚹 🏧 🅂 Mcr

Yoo, Jinil (MD)   Nep
Our Lady of Mercy Med Ctr
Medical Village, 4170 Bronx Blvd; Bronx, NY 10466; (718) 920-9600; **BDCERT:** Nep 76; Ger 88; **MS:** South Korea 67; **RES:** Joslin Diabetic Clinic, Boston, MA; Metropolitan Hosp Ctr, New York, NY; **FEL:** Diabetes Mellitus, Joslin Diabetic Clinic, Boston, MA; NY Med Coll, Valhalla, NY; **HOSP:** Westchester Med Ctr; *SI: Diabetes;* **HMO:** HealthNet HIP Network

♿ 🚹 🏧 🅂 Mcr Mod   A Few Days ▦ **VISA** 💳

NEUROLOGICAL SURGERY

Goodrich, James (MD)   NS
Montefiore Med Ctr
111 E 210th St NW800; Bronx, NY 10467; (718) 920-4197; **BDCERT:** NS 89; PS 96; **MS:** Columbia P&S 80; **RES:** Columbia-Presbyterian Med Ctr, New York, NY 80-81; Columbia-Presbyterian Med Ctr, New York, NY 81-86; **FAP:** Assoc Prof Albert Einstein Coll Med; **HOSP:** Jacobi Med Ctr; *SI: Pediatric Neurosurgery; Craniofacial Surgery;* **HMO:** US Hlthcre Bronx Health Oxford Prucare United Healthcare +
LANG: Sp; ♿ 🅟 ♿ 🏠 Ⓢ Mcr Mcd WC NFI A Few Days **VISA** 💳

Lasala, Patrick (MD)   NS
Montefiore Med Ctr
Montefiore Medical Ctr, 3316 Rochambeau Ave; Bronx, NY 10467; (718) 920-7466; **BDCERT:** NS 91; **MS:** Columbia P&S 80; **RES:** NS, Columbia-Presbyterian Med Ctr, New York, NY 82-87; **FEL:** Columbia-Presbyterian Med Ctr, New York, NY
♿ 🅟 ♿ 🏠 Mcr Mcd WC NFI Immediately

Michelsen, W Jost (MD)   NS
Montefiore Med Ctr
111 E 210th St; Bronx, NY 10467; (718) 920-4196; **BDCERT:** NS 71; **MS:** Columbia P&S 63; **RES:** NS, Columbia-Presbyterian Med Ctr, New York, NY 65-69
♿ 🅒 🅟 ♿ 🏠 Mcr Mcd WC NFI Immediately 🔲 **VISA**

Tabaddor, Kamran (MD)   NS
Our Lady of Mercy Med Ctr
4170 Bronx Blvd; Bronx, NY 10467; (718) 655-9111; **BDCERT:** NS 79; **MS:** Iran 67; **RES:** NS, Albert Einstein Med Ctr, Bronx, NY 69-70; S, Greater Baltimore Med Ctr, Baltimore, MD 70-71; **FEL:** Albert Einstein Med Ctr, Bronx, NY 72-75; **FAP:** Prof Albert Einstein Coll Med; **HOSP:** Montefiore Med Ctr; **HMO:** Aetna Hlth Plan Prucare Blue Choice CIGNA Sanus +
LANG: Sp, Itl; ♿ 🅟 🏠 Ⓢ Mcr Mcd WC NFI 2-4 Weeks

Torres Gluck, Jose (MD)   NS
Our Lady of Mercy Med Ctr
NY Neurosurg Assocs PC, 4170 Bronx Blvd; Bronx, NY 10466; (718) 655-9111; **MS:** Coll Physicians & Surgeons 87; **RES:** NS, Albert Einstein Med Ctr, Bronx, NY 88-93; **FEL:** NS Onc, Mem Sloan Kettering Cancer Ctr, New York, NY 93-95; **HOSP:** St Agnes Hosp; **HMO:** Oxford US Hlthcre NYLCare PHS Magnacare +
LANG: Sp; ♿ 🅟 🏠 Ⓢ Mcr Mcd WC NFI 1 Week

Waltz, Joseph (MD)   NS
St Barnabas Hosp-Bronx
4422 3rd Ave; Bronx, NY 10457; (718) 960-6544; **BDCERT:** NS 74; **MS:** U Oreg/Hlth Sci U, Portland 56; **RES:** S, U Mich Med Ctr, Ann Arbor, MI 56-58; **FAP:** Asst Prof Coll Of Osteo Med-Pacific; **HOSP:** Englewood Hosp & Med Ctr; *SI: Cerebral Palsy; Movement Disorders;* **HMO:** Blue Shield GHI US Hlthcre HIP Network
LANG: Sp; ♿ 🅟 🏠 Ⓢ Mcr Mcd WC NFI 2-4 Weeks

NEUROLOGY

Cohen, Joel (MD)   N
Montefiore Med Ctr-Weiler/Einstein Div
Montefiore Medical Park, 1575 Blondell Ave 225; Bronx, NY 10461; (718) 405-8259; **BDCERT:** N 92; **MS:** Albert Einstein Coll Med 83; **RES:** IM, Univ Hosp SUNY Bklyn, Brooklyn, NY 83-84; N, Albert Einstein Med Ctr, Bronx, NY 84-87; **FEL:** Albert Einstein Med Ctr, Bronx, NY 87-88; **FAP:** Asst Prof N Albert Einstein Coll Med; *SI: Epilepsy; Headache*
♿ 🅟 🏠 Mcr WC NFI A Few Days

Crystal, Howard (MD)   N
Montefiore Med Ctr
1165 Morris Park Ave; Bronx, NY 10461; (718) 430-3832; **BDCERT:** N 81; **MS:** Univ Penn 76; **RES:** N, Albert Einstein Med Ctr, Bronx, NY 77-80; Med, Hosp Med College of PA, Philadelphia, PA; **FEL:** Albert Einstein Med Ctr, Bronx, NY; **HOSP:** Montefiore Med Ctr-Weiler/Einstein Div; *SI: Alzheimer's Disease; Memory Disorders*
♿

Elkin, Rene (MD) N
Bronx Lebanon Hosp Ctr

1650 Grand Concourse; Bronx, NY 10457; (718) 960-1335; **BDCERT:** NR 94; **MS:** Africa 75; **RES:** Groote Schuur Hosp, Cape Town, South Africa 77-80; N, Albert Einstein Med Ctr, Bronx, NY 89-92; **FEL:** Neuroimmunology, Groote Schuur Hosp, Cape Town, South Africa 83-85; **FAP:** Asst Prof NR Unknown/other New York Sch ool; **HOSP:** St Agnes Hosp; *SI: Multiple Sclerosis; Headache*

LANG: Sp; ⌖ 🄲 🄰 🄷 🅂 Mcr Mcd 2-4 Weeks

Freddo, Lorenza (MD) N
St Barnabas Hosp-Bronx

2371 Arthur Ave; Bronx, NY 10458; (718) 364-6199; **BDCERT:** N 92; **MS:** Italy 80; **RES:** N, Italy, 80-84; N, Colum Presb Med Ctr, New York, NY 87-90; **FEL:** Colum Presb Med Ctr, New York, NY 83-85

Grenell, Steven (MD) N
Montefiore Med Ctr

3765 Riverdale Ave 7; Bronx, NY 10463; (718) 796-6055; **BDCERT:** N 89; IM 90; **MS:** UMDNJ-RW Johnson Med Sch 77; **RES:** IM, Montefiore Med Ctr, Bronx, NY 77-80; N,; **FAP:** Asst Clin Prof N Albert Einstein Coll Med; *SI: Pain; Headache;* **HMO:** None

⌖ 🄲 🄰 🄴 🄷 Mcr NFl 1 Week

Herskovitz, Steven (MD) N
Montefiore Med Ctr

Montefiore Medical Center, 111 E 210th St; Bronx, NY 10467; (718) 920-4930; **BDCERT:** N 87; **MS:** Cornell U 80; **RES:** IM, Montefiore Med Ctr, Bronx, NY 80-83; N, Montefiore Med Ctr, Bronx, NY 83-86; **FEL:** N, Montefiore Med Ctr, Bronx, NY; **FAP:** Assoc Prof N Albert Einstein Coll Med; **HOSP:** Beth Israel Med Ctr; *SI: Electromyography; Neuromuscular Disorders;* **HMO:** Oxford US Hlthcre Bronx Health

⌖ 🄰 🄷 🅂 Mcr Mcd WC NFl Immediately 🅰 *VISA* 💳

Kaplan, Jerry (MD) N
Montefiore Med Ctr

Montefiore Medical Park, 1575 Blondell Ave Suite 225; Bronx, NY 10461; (718) 405-8258; **BDCERT:** N 80; **MS:** Albert Einstein Coll Med 75; **RES:** Albert Einstein Med Ctr, Bronx, NY 75; **FEL:** Electromyography, Mass Gen Hosp, Boston, MA; **FAP:** Assoc Prof Albert Einstein Coll Med; **HMO:** Oxford US Hlthcre

⌖ 🄷 Mcr A Few Days

Kaufman, David (MD) N
Montefiore Med Ctr

3400 Bainbridge Ave; Bronx, NY 10467; (718) 920-4730; **BDCERT:** N 76; Psyc 76; **MS:** U Chicago-Pritzker Sch Med 68; **RES:** Montefiore Med Ctr, Bronx, NY; Albert Einstein Med Ctr, Bronx, NY; **HOSP:** Montefiore Med Ctr-Weiler/Einstein Div; **HMO:** CIGNA Oxford Prucare Blue Cross & Blue Shield US Hlthcre +

⌖ 🅂 Mcr A Few Days 🅰 *VISA* 💳

Kazmi, Mahmood Mehdi (MD) N
Montefiore Med Ctr

Montefiore Hospital, 111 E 210th St; Bronx, NY 10467; (718) 920-4636; **BDCERT:** Psyc 95; N 95; **MS:** Egypt 84; **RES:** Psyc, Albert Einstein Med Ctr, Bronx, NY 89-95; N, Albert Einstein Med Ctr, Bronx, NY 89-95; **FAP:** Asst Clin Prof NP Albert Einstein Coll Med; **HOSP:** Community Hosp At Dobbs Ferry; *SI: Headache; Neuropsychiatry;* **HMO:** PHS Blue Cross & Blue Choice PHCS

LANG: Ur, Ar, Pun, Hin, Sp; ⌖ 🅂🄰 🄲 🄰 🄴 🄷 Mcr 1 Week 🅰 *VISA* 💳

Lombard, Jay (MD) N
Westchester Square Med Ctr

3175 E Tremont Ave; Bronx, NY 10706; (718) 597-6925; **BDCERT:** N 95; **MS:** U South Fla Coll Med 88; **RES:** Psyc, Long Island Jewish Med Ctr, New Hyde Park, NY 89-91; N, Long Island Jewish Med Ctr, New Hyde Park, NY 91-95; **FAP:** Asst Clin Prof N Cornell U; **HOSP:** Montefiore Med Ctr-Weiler/Einstein Div; *SI: Autism; Neuropsychiatry;* **HMO:** Oxford Aetna-US Healthcare Blue Cross & Blue Shield

⌖ 🄰 🄴 🄷 Mcr Mcd A Few Days *VISA* 💳

Miller, Ann (MD) **N**
Montefiore Med Ctr
3765 Riverdale Ave 7; Bronx, NY 10463; (718) 549-4629; **BDCERT:** Psyc 86; **MS:** SUNY Downstate 81; **RES:** IM, Long Island Jewish Med Ctr, New Hyde Park, NY 81; N, Albert Einstein Med Ctr, Bronx, NY 82-85; **FAP:** Asst Clin Prof N Albert Einstein Coll Med; ***SI:*** *Parkinson's Disease; Headache*; **HMO:** Blue Cross & Blue Shield Empire 32BJ Anthem Health United Healthcare +
♿ ☾ ☎ 👥 📅 $ [Mcr] [NFI] A Few Days

Moshe, Solomon (MD) **N**
Montefiore Med Ctr
1165 Morris Park Ave; Bronx, NY 10461; (718) 430-3814; **BDCERT:** N 79; ChiN 79; **MS:** Greece 72; **RES:** Ped, U MD Hosp, Baltimore, MD 73-75; N, Albert Einstein Med Ctr, Bronx, NY 75-78; **FEL:** N, Albert Einstein Med Ctr, Bronx, NY 78-79; **FAP:** Prof N Albert Einstein Coll Med; ***SI:*** *Epilepsy*; **HMO:** Aetna Hlth Plan Blue Choice Blue Cross & Blue Shield CIGNA Metlife +
LANG: Grk, Fr, Sp; ♿ ☎ 👥 📅 $ [Mcr] [Mcd] [NFI] 1 Week VISA MasterCard

Newman, Lawrence C (MD) **N**
Montefiore Med Ctr
Montefiore Head Unit, 111 E 210th St; Bronx, NY 10467; (718) 920-2797; **BDCERT:** N 94; **MS:** Mexico 83; **RES:** IM, Elmhurst Hosp Ctr, Elmhurst, NY 85-86; N, Albert Einstein Med Ctr, Bronx, NY 86-89; **FEL:** Montefiore Med Ctr, Bronx, NY 89-90; **FAP:** Asst Prof Albert Einstein Coll Med; ***SI:*** *Headache*
☎ 👥 📅 $ [Mcr] 4+ Weeks VISA MasterCard

Rosenbaum, Daniel (MD) **N**
Montefiore Med Ctr
Montefiore Med Ctr, 111 E 210th St Stern Stroke Ctr; Bronx, NY 10467; (718) 920-6402; **BDCERT:** N 88; **MS:** Albert Einstein Coll Med 82; **RES:** IM, Brookdale Univ Hosp Med Ctr, Brooklyn, NY 82-83; N, Albert Einstein Med Ctr, Bronx, NY 83-86; **FEL:** Stroke, U of Texas Med Sch, Houston, TX 86-88; **FAP:** Assoc Prof Albert Einstein Coll Med; ***SI:*** *Stroke*; **HMO:** Blue Choice GHI Montefiore IPA United Healthcare PHS +
♿ ☎ 👥 📅 [Mcr] 1 Week

Schaumburg, Herbert (MD) **N**
Montefiore Med Ctr
616 King Ave; Bronx, NY 10464; (718) 430-3166; **BDCERT:** N 66; **MS:** Washington U, St Louis 60; **RES:** N, Albert Einstein Med Ctr, Bronx, NY 61-64; **FEL:** N Path, Mass Gen Hosp, Boston, MA 69-71; **FAP:** Chrmn N Albert Einstein Coll Med; ***SI:*** *Peripheral Nerve Injury; Neurotoxicology*
♿ ☎ 📅 [Mcr] 2-4 Weeks American Express VISA

Smith, Charles (MD) **N**
Bronx Lebanon Hosp Ctr
1650 Selwyn Ave Ste 11F; Bronx, NY 10457; (718) 960-1335; **BDCERT:** N 84; **MS:** Canada 76; **RES:** Toronto Western Hosp, Toronto, Canada 77-78; Toronto Gen Hosp, Toronto, Canada 78-81; **FEL:** Albert Einstein Med Ctr, Bronx, NY 81-83; **HOSP:** St Agnes Hosp; **HMO:** Aetna Hlth Plan Blue Choice Blue Cross & Blue Shield US Hlthcre Premier +
♿ ☾ ☎ 👥 📅 $ [Mcr] [Mcd] Immediately

Solomon, Seymour (MD) **N**
Montefiore Med Ctr
111 E 210th St; Bronx, NY 10467; (718) 920-4203; **BDCERT:** N 55; **MS:** Med Coll Wisc 47; **RES:** Mt Sinai Med Ctr, Milwaukee, WI 48-50; Montefiore Med Ctr, Bronx, NY 50-52; **FAP:** Prof Albert Einstein Coll Med; ***SI:*** *Headache; Migraine*
☎ 👥 📅 $ [Mcr] 1 Week American Express VISA MasterCard 💳

Guide to symbols and abbreviations can be found on pages 110-113.

Sparr, Steven (MD)   **N**
Montefiore Med Ctr
Stern Stroke Center, 111 E 210th St; Bronx, NY
10467; (718) 920-6402; **BDCERT:** IM 87; **MS:**
SUNY Buffalo 80; **RES:** IM, Boston Med Ctr, Boston,
MA 80-83; N, Albert Einstein Med Ctr, Bronx, NY
83-86; **FEL:** NeuroRehab, Burke Rehabilitation
Hosp, White Plains, NY 86-87; **FAP:** Assoc Prof N
Albert Einstein Coll Med; **SI:** *Stroke;* **HMO:** Blue
Cross & Blue Shield Metlife Sanus

🔲 🔲 🔲 🔲 🔲 🔲 A Few Days **VISA** 💳

Swerdlow, Michael (MD)   **N**
Montefiore Med Ctr
Neurological Assoc, 111 E 210th St A 200; Bronx,
NY 10467; (718) 920-4178; **BDCERT:** N 75; **MS:**
Univ Penn 67; **RES:** Med, Mount Sinai Med Ctr,
New York, NY 67-69; N, Albert Einstein Med Ctr,
Bronx, NY 69-72; **FEL:** Nat Inst Health, Bethesda,
MD 72-74; **FAP:** Prof Albert Einstein Coll Med; **SI:**
Myasthenia Gravis; Spine Disorders; **HMO:** Oxford
Aetna-US Healthcare Prucare CIGNA NYLCare +

LANG: Sp, Fr; 🔲 🔲 🔲 🔲 🔲 🔲 A Few Days **VISA**
💳

NUCLEAR MEDICINE

Freeman, Leonard M (MD) NuM
Montefiore Med Ctr
Nuclear Medicine Associates, 111 E 210th St;
Bronx, NY 10400; (718) 920-6060; **BDCERT:**
NuM 72; Rad 66; **MS:** U Hlth Sci/Chicago Med Sch
61; **RES:** Rad, Bronx Muncipal Hosp Ctr, Bronx, NY
62-65; **FAP:** Prof NuM Albert Einstein Coll Med; **SI:**
Gastrointestinal/Nuclear Medicine; Nuclear Oncology;
HMO: GHI Blue Choice United Healthcare

LANG: Sp, Itl, Hin, Pak; 🔲 🔲 🔲 🔲 🔲 🔲 🔲 🔲
🔲 Immediately 💳 **VISA** 💳

Milstein, David (MD)   **NuM**
Montefiore Med Ctr
1825 Chester Rd; Bronx, NY 10461; (718) 904-
4058; **BDCERT:** NuM 72; DR 72; **MS:** Albert
Einstein Coll Med 67; **RES:** DR/Rad, Bronx Muni
Hosp Ctr, Bronx, NY 68-72; **FAP:** Prof NRad Albert
Einstein Coll Med; **HOSP:** Montefiore Med Ctr-
Weiler/Einstein Div; **HMO:** Most

🔲 🔲 🔲 🔲 🔲 🔲 🔲 Immediately 💳 **VISA** 💳
🔲

OBSTETRICS & GYNECOLOGY

Afif, Juan Simon (MD)   **ObG**
Our Lady of Mercy Med Ctr
1214 Pelham Pkwy South; Bronx, NY 10461;
(718) 824-2200; **BDCERT:** ObG 79; **MS:** Argentina
70; **RES:** ObG, Misericordia Hosp, Bronx, NY 73-77;
S, Albert Einstein Med Ctr, Bronx, NY 73-74;
HOSP: Westchester Square Med Ctr; **SI:** *Laparoscopic
Surgery; Hysteroscopy*

🔲 🔲 🔲 🔲 🔲 🔲 🔲 🔲 A Few Days

Aro, Dominic (DO)   **ObG**   **PCP**
Westchester Med Ctr
603 187th St; Bronx, NY 10457; (718) 561-2881;
BDCERT: ObG 95; **MS:** Kirksville Coll Osteo Med 88;
RES: ObG, Westchester County Med Ctr, Valhalla,
NY 89-93; **FAP:** Assoc Prof NY Med Coll; **HOSP:** St
Agnes Hosp; **SI:** *Menopause Education; Chronic Pain;*
HMO: Aetna-US Healthcare Prucare Oxford GHI
PHS +

🔲 🔲 🔲 🔲 🔲 🔲 🔲 🔲 🔲 🔲 🔲 A Few Days

Dyson, Robert (MD)   **ObG**
Westchester Square Med Ctr
1072 Esplanade Ave; Bronx, NY 10461; (718)
829-6335; **BDCERT:** ObG 62; **MS:** Albany Med Coll
55; **RES:** Columbia-Presbyterian Med Ctr, New
York, NY 56-59; **FAP:** Asst Prof ObG Albert
Einstein Coll Med; **HOSP:** Montefiore Med Ctr-
Weiler/Einstein Div; **HMO:** Aetna-US Healthcare
Oxford Empire Prudential GHI +

LANG: Itl; 🔲 🔲 🔲 🔲 🔲 🔲 🔲 A Few Days

Katz, Nadine (MD) ObG
Montefiore Med Ctr-Weiler/Einstein Div

1695 Eastchester Rd Ste L2; Bronx, NY 10461; (718) 405-8200; **MS:** Albert Einstein Coll Med 87; **RES:** Jacobi Med Ctr, Bronx, NY 87-91; **HOSP:** Jacobi Med Ctr; **HMO:** Health One Blue Cross & Blue Shield US Hlthcre GHI Oxford +

Levie, Mark (MD) ObG PCP
Montefiore Med Ctr

Montefiore Medical Center, Dept of Obstetrics & Gynecology, 111 E 210th St; Bronx, NY 10467; (718) 405-8200; **BDCERT:** ObG 95; **MS:** Albert Einstein Coll Med 89; **RES:** ObG, Albert Einstein Med Ctr, Bronx, NY 89-93; **SI:** *Laparoscopic Surgery; Hysteroscopic Surgery;* **HMO:** US Hlthcre Oxford Empire United Healthcare Multiplan +

🌙 📷 🛏 Mcr WC Immediately

Levy, Judith (MD) ObG PCP
Montefiore Med Ctr

1695 Eastchester Rd L2; Bronx, NY 10461; (718) 405-8200; **BDCERT:** ObG 88; **MS:** Albert Einstein Coll Med 81; **RES:** ObG, Albert Einstein Med Ctr, Bronx, NY 81-85; **FAP:** Asst Prof Albert Einstein Coll Med; **HOSP:** Montefiore Med Ctr-Weiler/Einstein Div; **SI:** *Abnormal Pap Smears; Diabetes in Pregnancy;* **HMO:** Oxford Aetna Hlth Plan PHS NYLCare +

LANG: Sp; ♿ 📷 🛏 🛏 💲 Mcr 2-4 Weeks 🔳 **VISA** ⬤

Lim, Aquillina (MD) ObG
Our Lady of Mercy Med Ctr

1920 Benedict Ave; Bronx, NY 10462; (718) 863-4421; **BDCERT:** ObG 73; **MS:** Philippines 61; **RES:** ObG, Baltimore City Hosp, Baltimore, MD 64-69; ObG, Sisters of Charity Hosp, Buffalo, NY 64-66; **FEL:** ObG, EJ Meyer Mem Hosp, Buffalo, NY 66-67; **SI:** *Infertility; Maternity;* **HMO:** US Hlthcre United Healthcare GHI Oxford

LANG: Fil, Chi, Sp; 🕍 🌙 📷 🛏 🛏 💲 Mcr Mcd
A Few Days 🔳 **VISA** ⬤

Merkatz, Irwin R (MD) ObG
Montefiore Med Ctr

1300 Morris Park Ave Rm B502; Bronx, NY 10461; (718) 430-4192; **BDCERT:** ObG 67; **MS:** Cornell U 58; **RES:** NY Hosp-Cornell-Westchester, White Plains, NY

Muscillo, George (MD) ObG PCP
Montefiore Med Ctr-Weiler/Einstein Div

1072 Esplanade Ave; Bronx, NY 10461; (718) 829-6335; **BDCERT:** ObG 66; **MS:** NY Med Coll 58; **RES:** ObG, Metropolitan Hosp Ctr, New York, NY 59-67; **HOSP:** Westchester Square Med Ctr; **HMO:** US Hlthcre Oxford Blue Choice PHCS Empire +

LANG: Itl, Sp; 🌙 📷 🛏 🛏 💲 Immediately

Packer, Paul (MD) ObG
Jacobi Med Ctr

Jacobi Medical Center, 1400 Pelham Pkwy South; Bronx, NY 10461; (718) 918-6320; **BDCERT:** ObG 63; **MS:** NYU Sch Med 55; **RES:** ObG, Jacobi Med Ctr, Bronx, NY 55-60; **FAP:** Assoc Prof Albert Einstein Coll Med; **SI:** *Pelvic Reconstruction Surgery*

♿ 📷 🛏 🛏 💲 Mcr Mcd NFl Immediately 🔳 **VISA** ⬤ ⬤

Reilly, Kevin D (MD) ObG
Our Lady of Mercy Med Ctr

600 E 233rd St; Bronx, NY 10466; (718) 920-9649; **BDCERT:** ObG 76; **MS:** U Mich Med Sch 69; **RES:** ObG, St Vincents Hosp & Med Ctr NY, New York, NY 70-74; **FAP:** Asst Clin Prof NY Med Coll; **SI:** *Menopause;* **HMO:** US Hlthcre 1199 Oxford Aetna Hlth Plan Sanus +

♿ 📷 🛏 🛏 💲 Mcr Mcd 1 Week

Runowicz, Carolyn (MD) ObG
Montefiore Med Ctr

1695 Eastchester Rd L2; Bronx, NY 10461; (718) 405-8210; **BDCERT:** ObG 84; **MS:** Jefferson Med Coll 77; **RES:** ObG, Mount Sinai Med Ctr, New York, NY 77-81; **FEL:** GO, Mount Sinai Med Ctr, New York, NY 81-83; **SI:** *Cervical Cancer; Ovarian Cancer;* **HMO:** CIGNA Prucare GHI Blue Choice HealthNet +

♿ 📷 🛏 💲 Mcr Mcd 2-4 Weeks **VISA** ⬤

Santoro, Nanette (MD)   ObG
Montefiore Med Ctr

1300 Morris Park Ave; Bronx, NY 10461; (718) 430-3152; **BDCERT:** ObG 87; **MS:** Albany Med Coll 79; **RES:** Beth Israel Med Ctr, New York, NY 79-83; **FEL:** RE, Mass Gen Hosp, Boston, MA 83-86; **FAP:** Assoc Prof UMDNJ New Jersey Sch Osteo Med; *SI: Menopause; Amenorrhea*

Shulman, Joanna (MD)   ObG
Montefiore Med Ctr

Montefiore Med Ctr, 60 E 208th St; Bronx, NY 10467; (718) 515-0299; **BDCERT:** ObG 86; **MS:** NY Med Coll 80; **RES:** ObG, Bronx Muncipal Hosp Ctr, Bronx, NY 80-84; **FAP:** Asst Prof ObG Albert Einstein Coll Med; **HOSP:** North Central Bronx Hosp

LANG: Sp, Fr; ♿ 🔲 🔳 🔳 🔳 🔲 🔲 🔲 1 Week

OPHTHALMOLOGY

Burde, Ronald (MD)   Oph
Montefiore Med Ctr

3400 Bainbridge Ave; Bronx, NY 10467; (718) 920-2020; **BDCERT:** Oph 70; **MS:** Jefferson Med Coll 64; **RES:** Barnes Hosp, St Louis, MO 65-68; **FEL:** N/Oph & Glaucoma, Barnes Hosp, St Louis, MO 68-70; **HMO:** Multiplan Aetna-US Healthcare CIGNA Prudential Blue Cross & Blue Shield +

♿ 🔲 🔳 🔳 🔲 🔲 🔲 🔲 Immediately **VISA** 💳

Fleischman, Jay (MD)   Oph
Montefiore Med Ctr

111 E 210th St Floor 3; Bronx, NY 10467; (718) 920-2020; **BDCERT:** Oph 80; **MS:** Columbia P&S 75; **RES:** Johns Hopkins Hosp, Baltimore, MD 76-79; **FAP:** Assoc Prof Albert Einstein Coll Med

LANG: Sp, Kor; ♿ 🔳 🔳 🔲 🔲 🔲 🔲 🔲
Immediately 🔲 **VISA** 💳 🔲

Gurland, Judith (MD)   Oph
Montefiore Med Ctr

3332 Rochambeau Ave; Bronx, NY 10467; (718) 920-6244; **BDCERT:** Oph 74; **MS:** SUNY Downstate 68; **RES:** Univ Hosp SUNY Bklyn, Brooklyn, NY; **FEL:** N Oph, Kingsbrook Jewish Med Ctr, Brooklyn, NY; Motility, Columbia-Presbyterian Med Ctr, New York, NY; **HOSP:** Bronx Lebanon Hosp Ctr; **HMO:** Most

♿ 🔲 🔳 🔳 🔲 A Few Days

Hayworth, Robin (MD)   Oph
Manhattan Eye, Ear & Throat Hosp

787 Lydig Ave; Bronx, NY 10462; (718) 863-7774; **BDCERT:** Oph 85; **MS:** Cornell U 78; **RES:** NY Hosp-Cornell Med Ctr, New York, NY 78-80; Manhattan Eye, Ear & Throat Hosp, New York, NY 80-83; **HOSP:** Montefiore Med Ctr-Weiler/Einstein Div; *SI: Cataract; Glaucoma*; **HMO:** Oxford US Hlthcre Prudential 32BJ Blue Choice +

LANG: Sp, Rus; ♿ 🔳 🔲 🔳 🔳 🔲 Immediately

Juechter, Kenneth (MD)   Oph
Our Lady of Mercy Med Ctr

4141 Carpenter Ave 215; Bronx, NY 10466; (718) 231-3200; **BDCERT:** Oph 79; **MS:** NY Med Coll 68; **RES:** Metropolitan Hosp Ctr, New York, NY 69-73; **FEL:** Oph, Armed Forces Inst Path, Washington, DC 70-71; **FAP:** Asst Clin Prof NY Med Coll

Mayers, Martin (MD)   Oph
Montefiore Med Ctr

111 E 210th St; Bronx, NY 10467; (718) 920-2020; **BDCERT:** Oph 85; **MS:** Albert Einstein Coll Med 79; **RES:** Oph, Univ Hosp SUNY Bklyn, Brooklyn, NY 80-83; **FEL:** Cornea/Veins, UC San Francisco Med Ctr, San Francisco, CA 83-84; **FAP:** Assoc Prof Albert Einstein Coll Med; **HOSP:** Bronx Lebanon Hosp Ctr; *SI: Cataract Surgery; Corneal Transplant Surgery*; **HMO:** Blue Cross Prucare US Hlthcre Oxford CIGNA +

LANG: Sp, Itl, Rus; ♿ 🔲 🔳 🔳 🔲 🔲 2-4 Weeks
VISA 💳

Nirenberg, Jason (MD)   Oph
New York Eye & Ear Infirmary

1101 Pelham Pkwy N; Bronx, NY 10469; (718) 519-1000; **BDCERT:** Oph 87; **MS:** U Miami Sch Med 81; **RES:** U Texas, Houston, TX 82-85

Rosenbaum, Pearl (MD)   Oph
Montefiore Med Ctr

111 E 210th St FL3; Bronx, NY 10467; (718) 920-2020; **BDCERT:** Oph 88; **MS:** Albert Einstein Coll Med 82; **RES:** Albert Einstein Med Ctr, Bronx, NY 83-86

♿ 🔲 🔳 🔳 🔲 🔲 4+ Weeks 🔲 **VISA** 💳 🔲

Guide to symbols and abbreviations can be found on pages 110-113.

445

Schneider, Karen (MD)   Oph
Montefiore Med Ctr

Riverdale Eye Assoc, 2600 Netherland Ave Ste 101; Bronx, NY 10463; (718) 548-5500; **BDCERT:** Oph 87; **MS:** Cornell U 80; **RES:** Oph, Montefiore Med Ctr, Bronx, NY 81-84; **FAP:** Asst Clin Prof Albert Einstein Coll Med; **HOSP:** St Joseph's Med Ctr-Yonkers; **SI:** *Glaucoma; Comprehensive Eye Care*; **HMO:** Oxford US Hlthcre GHI United Healthcare Prucare +

LANG: Sp, Ger, Fr; ♿ ☎ 📷 📅 💵 Mcr Mcd   2-4 Weeks

Slamovits, Thomas (MD)   Oph
Montefiore Med Ctr

111 E 210th St Fl3; Bronx, NY 10467; (718) 920-5223; **BDCERT:** Oph 80; N 80; **MS:** Ohio State U 75; **RES:** Eye & Ear Hosp, Pittsburgh, PA 79; **FEL:** Barnes Hosp, St Louis, MO 80; **FAP:** Prof Oph Albert Einstein Coll Med; **SI:** *Optic Nerve Diseases*; **HMO:** Blue Cross & Blue Shield HealthNet HIP Network

LANG: Fr, Sp, Ger; ♿ 📅 💵 Mcr   Immediately ***VISA*** ●

Tiwari, Ram (MD)   Oph
Our Lady of Mercy Med Ctr

1739 Williamsbridge Rd; Bronx, NY 10461; (718) 824-1560; **BDCERT:** Oph 77; **MS:** India 66; **RES:** Oph, Maulana Azad Med Coll, New Delhi, India 68-71; **FEL:** Oph/Retina, Columbia-Presbyterian Med Ctr, New York, NY 76-78; **FAP:** Asst Clin Prof Columbia P&S; **HOSP:** Columbia-Presbyterian Med Ctr; **SI:** *Diabetic Retinopathy; Cataract*; **HMO:** Prucare Oxford PHS United Healthcare CIGNA +

LANG: Hin, Rus, Sp; ♿ 🏥 ☎ 📅 💵 Mcr   1 Week

Wolf, Kenneth (MD)   Oph
Montefiore Med Ctr

1180 Morris Park Ave Fl 2; Bronx, NY 10461; (718) 892-6110; **BDCERT:** Oph 80; **MS:** Albert Einstein Coll Med 74; **RES:** Oph, Montefiore Med Ctr, Bronx, NY 75-78; **FAP:** Asst Clin Prof Albert Einstein Coll Med; **HMO:** Aetna Hlth Plan Oxford PHS

♿ ☎ 📷 📅 Mcr   A Few Days

ORTHOPAEDIC SURGERY

Adler, Melvin (MD)   OrS
Montefiore Med Ctr

Central Bronx Orthopedic Group, 75 E Gun Hill Rd; Bronx, NY 10467; (718) 798-1000; **BDCERT:** OrS 78; **MS:** SUNY Syracuse 71; **RES:** OrS, Montefiore Med Ctr, Bronx, NY 74-77; **FAP:** Clin Instr OrS Albert Einstein Coll Med

Dyal, Cherise M (MD)   OrS
Montefiore Med Ctr

3400 Bainbridge Ave; Bronx, NY 10467; (718) 920-2061; **BDCERT:** OrS 97; **MS:** Yale U Sch Med 89; **RES:** OrS, Columbia-Presbyterian Med Ctr, New York, NY 90-94; **FEL:** OrS, Hosp For Special Surgery, New York, NY 94-95; **FAP:** Asst Prof Albert Einstein Coll Med; **SI:** *Foot; Ankle*; **HMO:** Blue Cross & Blue Shield Oxford Aetna-US Healthcare Prudential

LANG: Sp; ♿ ☎ 📷 📅 💵 Mcr Mcd WC NFi   2-4 Weeks

Flink, Elisheva (MD)   OrS
Bronx Lebanon Hosp Ctr

Bronx Lebanon Hospital Center, Dept of Orthopedic Surgery, 2432 Grand Concourse; Bronx, NY 10457; **MS:** U Mich Med Sch 79; **RES:** OrS, Phoenix Mem Hosp, Phoenix, AZ 89-94; **FEL:** Rancho Los Amigos Med Ctr, Downey, CA 88-89; **HS:** Los Angeles Cty Hosp, Los Angeles, CA 94-95; **SI:** *Hand Surgery; Trauma/Fractures*; **HMO:** GHI Magnacare US Hlthcre Oxford Health First +

LANG: Sp, Heb, Fr; ♿ 📷 📅 💵 Mcr Mcd WC NFi   A Few Days

Habermann, Edward (MD) OrS
Montefiore Med Ctr

Montefiore Hospital, 111 E 210th St 200; Bronx, NY 10467; (718) 920-4961; **BDCERT:** OrS 94; **MS:** SUNY Syracuse 59; **RES:** S, Hosp For Joint Diseases, New York, NY 62-63; OrS, Hosp for Joint Dis, New York, NY 63-66; **FEL:** Hip Reconstr, Wrightington Hosp, Wrightington, England 67; **FAP:** Prof & Chrmn OrS Albert Einstein Coll Med; *SI: Hip Joint; Knee Joint*; **HMO:** Aetna Hlth Plan Blue Choice Blue Cross & Blue Shield CIGNA GHI +

[⌖] [☏] [⌂] [♿] [⊞] [Mcr] [WC] [NFI] A Few Days [AMEX] **VISA** [●]

Hirsh, David M (MD) OrS
Montefiore Med Ctr

University Orthopaedic Speciality Associates, 1180 Morris Park Ave; Bronx, NY 10461; (718) 863-3400; **BDCERT:** OrS 70; **MS:** Albert Einstein Coll Med 63; **RES:** S, Albert Einstein Med Ctr, Bronx, NY 64-65; OrS, Albert Einstein Med Ctr, Bronx, NY 65-68; **FEL:** S, United Kingdom; **FAP:** Assoc Clin Prof Albert Einstein Coll Med; **HOSP:** Westchester Square Med Ctr; *SI: Total Hip Replacement; Total Knee Replacement*; **HMO:** Empire Blue Cross & Shield Anthem Health Prucare CIGNA Oxford +

[⌖] [♿] [⊞] [S] [Mcr] [WC] [NFI] A Few Days **VISA** [●]

Hoppenfeld, Stanley (MD) OrS
Montefiore Med Ctr

1180 Morris Park Ave; Bronx, NY 10461; (718) 863-1608; **BDCERT:** OrS 69; **MS:** U Hlth Sci/Chicago Med Sch 59; **RES:** Hosp For Joint Diseases, New York, NY 61-64; **HOSP:** Our Lady of Mercy Med Ctr; *SI: Scoliosis; Spinal Deformities*; **HMO:** HIP Network Oxford CIGNA Blue Choice United Healthcare +

[⌖] [⌂] [⊞] [S] [Mcr] [Mcd] [WC] [NFI] 1 Week

Insler, Harvey (MD) OrS
White Plains Hosp Ctr

Orthopaedic Associates Bronx, 1650 Selwyn Ave 5C; Bronx, NY 10457; (718) 960-1300; **BDCERT:** OrS 82; **MS:** Geo Wash U Sch Med 74; **RES:** S, Hartford Hosp, Hartford, CT 74-75; OrS, U Conn Hlth Ctr, Farmington, CT 76-79; **FEL:** OrS, London Hosp, London, England 79-80; OrS, Charnley, London, England, UK 80-81; **HOSP:** Bronx Lebanon Hosp Ctr; *SI: Joint Replacement; Arthritis Surgery*; **HMO:** Oxford Chubb Aetna Hlth Plan Sanus-NYLCare Metlife +

LANG: Sp; [⌖] [☏] [⌂] [♿] [⊞] [Mcr] [Mcd] [WC] [NFI] A Few Days **VISA** [●]

Kaphan, Mitchell (MD) OrS
Westchester Square Med Ctr

3612 E Tremont Ave; Bronx, NY 10465; (718) 409-9494; **MS:** Mexico 77; **RES:** OrS, Bronx Lebanon Hosp Ctr, Bronx, NY 80-84; **HOSP:** Mount Vernon Hosp; *SI: Arthroscopic Surgeries; Total Joint Replacements*; **HMO:** CIGNA Aetna Hlth Plan Pomco US Hlthcre Prucare +

LANG: Sp, Itl; [⌖] [⊞] [S] [Mcr] [Mcd] [WC] [NFI] 2-4 Weeks

Kleinman, Paul (MD) OrS
Lincoln Med & Mental Hlth Ctr

234 E 149th St; Bronx, NY 10451; (718) 579-5918; **BDCERT:** OrS 88; **MS:** Stanford U 79; **RES:** Columbia-Presbyterian Med Ctr, New York, NY 82-85; **FEL:** HS, Allegheny Gen Hosp, Pittsburgh, PA; Ped OrS, Hosp For Joint Diseases, New York, NY; *SI: Pediatric Orthopedics; Hand Surgery*; **HMO:** Empire

LANG: Sp; [⌖] [⌂] [♿] [⊞] [S] [Mcr] [WC] [NFI] 1 Week

Rose, Louis (MD) OrS
Our Lady of Mercy Med Ctr

3058 E Tremont Rd; Bronx, NY 10595; (718) 409-5000; **MS:** UMDNJ-NJ Med Sch, Newark 82; **RES:** NY Hosp-Cornell-Westchester, White Plains, NY 86; **FEL:** HS, Westchester County Med Ctr, Valhalla, NY 87; *SI: Hand Surgery*; **HMO:** Blue Choice Pomco US Hlthcre Oxford Independent Health Plan +

LANG: Sp; [⌖] [☏] [⌂] [♿] [⊞] [S] [Mcr] [Mcd] [WC] [NFI] 1 Week [AMEX] **VISA** [●] [◻]

Guide to symbols and abbreviations can be found on pages 110-113.

447

Sadler, Arthur (MD)   OrS
Montefiore Med Ctr

Montefiore Medical Center, Dept of Orthopaedic Surgery, 1500 Blondell Ave; Bronx, NY 10461; (718) 405-8433; **BDCERT:** OrS 65; **MS:** SUNY Downstate 55; **RES:** OrS, Hosp For Joint Diseases, New York, NY 58-62; **FAP:** Assoc Prof Albert Einstein Coll Med; **HOSP:** Montefiore Med Ctr-Weiler/Einstein Div; *SI: Joint Replacement; Fractures;* **HMO:** GHI Magnacare Prudential Blue Cross & Blue Shield

  🔶 🔶 🔶 🔶 🔶 🔶 🔶 🔶 🔶   A Few Days

Weinstein, Richard (MD)   OrS
Bronx Lebanon Hosp Ctr

Bronx Lebanon Hosp, 1650 Grand Concourse 5 C; Bronx, NY 10457; (718) 960-1300; **BDCERT:** SM 97; **MS:** NYU Sch Med 91; **RES:** S, N Shore Univ Hosp-Manhasset, Manhasset, NY 91-92; OrS, Bronx Lebanon Hosp Ctr, Bronx, NY 92-96; **FEL:** SM, U Conn Hlth Ctr, Farmington, CT 96-97; **FAP:** Albert Einstein Coll Med; *SI: Knee Injuries; Shoulder Injuries;* **HMO:** US Hlthcre Oxford CIGNA Health First Bronx Health +

LANG: Sp; 🔶 🔶 🔶 🔶 🔶 🔶 🔶 🔶   Immediately

OTOLARYNGOLOGY

Berkower, Alan (MD & PhD) Oto
Our Lady of Mercy Med Ctr

3250 Westchester Ave; Bronx, NY 10461; (718) 597-6099; **BDCERT:** Oto 90; **MS:** Columbia P&S 84; **RES:** S, Mount Sinai Med Ctr, New York, NY 84-86; Oto, Mount Sinai Med Ctr, New York, NY 86-89; **FAP:** Asst Prof NY Med Coll; **HOSP:** Westchester Med Ctr; *SI: Head & Neck Surgery; Sinus Surgery;* **HMO:** Oxford Aetna Hlth Plan Prucare Empire Blue Choice +

LANG: Sp; 🔶 🔶 🔶 🔶 🔶 🔶 🔶   1 Week

Daniello, Nicholas (MD)   Oto
Westchester Square Med Ctr

3594 Tremont Ave; Bronx, NY 10465; (718) 863-4366; **BDCERT:** Oto 78; **MS:** NY Med Coll 74; **RES:** Oto, Manhattan Eye, Ear & Throat Hosp, New York, NY 75-78; Metropolitan Hosp Ctr, New York, NY 74-75; **HOSP:** St John's Riverside Hosp; *SI: Facial Plastic Surgery; Sinus Surgery;* **HMO:** Aetna Hlth Plan Oxford Blue Choice Pomco Anthem Health +

LANG: Itl; 🔶 🔶 🔶 🔶 🔶 🔶   A Few Days 🔶
VISA 💳

Eviatar, Abraham (MD)   Oto
Montefiore Med Ctr-Weiler/Einstein Div

1578 Williamsbridge Rd 150; Bronx, NY 10461; (718) 822-1103; **BDCERT:** Oto 73; **MS:** Israel 61; **RES:** Med, Tel Hashomer Hosp, Tel Aviv, Israel 61-63; Oto, Tel Hashomer Hosp, Tel Aviv, Israel 63-66; **FEL:** UCLA Med Ctr, Los Angeles, CA 66-69; Ont, UCLA Med Ctr, Los Angeles, CA 66-69; **HOSP:** Montefiore Med Ctr; **HMO:** Oxford Blue Cross & Blue Shield Sanus Travelers Magnacare +

  🔶 🔶 🔶 🔶 🔶 🔶   A Few Days **VISA** 💳

Feghali, Joseph (MD)   Oto
Beth Israel Med Ctr

159 E Gunhill Rd; Bronx, NY 10467; (718) 881-3277; **BDCERT:** Oto 90; **MS:** Lebanon 78; **RES:** Oto, Albert Einstein Med Ctr, Bronx, NY; **FEL:** Oto, House Ear Inst, Los Angeles, CA 82-83; Mem Sloan Kettering Cancer Ctr, New York, NY 83-84; **FAP:** Prof Albert Einstein Coll Med; **HOSP:** Montefiore Med Ctr; *SI: Acoustic Neuromas; Ear Surgery*

  🔶 🔶 🔶 🔶 🔶 🔶 🔶 🔶 🔶   A Few Days

Mayers, Martin (MD)   Oto
Montefiore Med Ctr

111 E 210th St; Bronx, NY 10467; (718) 920-2020; **BDCERT:** Oph 85; **MS:** Albert Einstein Coll Med 79; **RES:** Oph, Univ Hosp SUNY Bklyn, Brooklyn, NY 80-83; **FEL:** Cornea/Veins, UC San Francisco Med Ctr, San Francisco, CA 83-84; **FAP:** Assoc Prof Albert Einstein Coll Med; **HOSP:** Bronx Lebanon Hosp Ctr; *SI: Cataract Surgery; Corneal Transplant Surgery;* **HMO:** Blue Cross Prucare US Hlthcre Oxford CIGNA +

LANG: Sp, Itl, Rus; 🔶 🔶 🔶 🔶 🔶 🔶   2-4 Weeks
VISA 💳

Mehta, Dinesh (MD)   Oto
Montefiore Med Ctr

1575 Blondell Ave 150; Bronx, NY 10461; (718)
405-8350; **BDCERT:** Oto 79; **MS:** India 60; **RES:** St
Thomas Hosp, Akron, OH; **FEL:** Oto, Jacobi Med Ctr,
Bronx, NY

♿ 🚗 Mcr   Immediately ■ **VISA** 💳

Moulin, Nicole (MD)   Oto
Bronx Lebanon Hosp Ctr

Bronx Lebanon Hospital Center, Dept of
NeonatalPerinatal Medicine, 1650 Grand
Concourse; Bronx, NY 10457; (718) 518-5159;
BDCERT: Oto 82; **MS:** France 74; **RES:** Oto,
Montefiore Med Ctr, Bronx, NY 79-82; **FAP:** Assoc
Prof; **SI:** *Allergic Rhinitis; Chronic Otitis-Hearing Loss*

LANG: Sp, Fr; ♿ 📷 🚗 🛏 Mcr Mcd   Immediately

Ruben, Robert (MD)   Oto
Montefiore Med Ctr

Montefiore Medical Center / Gold Zone, 3400
Bainbridge Ave Fl 3; Bronx, NY 10467; (718) 920-
2991; **BDCERT:** Oto 65; **MS:** Johns Hopkins U 59;
RES: S, Johns Hopkins Hosp, Baltimore, MD 59-61;
Oto, Johns Hopkins Hosp, Baltimore, MD 60-64;
FEL: S, Baltimore City Hosp, Baltimore, MD 62-63;
Oto, Johns Hopkins Hosp, Baltimore, MD 63-64;
FAP: Prof Albert Einstein Coll Med; **HOSP:** Jacobi
Med Ctr; **SI:** *Ear, Nose & Throat Problems Pediatric;
Speech Language Problems*; **HMO:** Oxford CIGNA
Blue Shield Aetna-US Healthcare Blue Cross +

LANG: Sp; ♿ 🌙 📷 🚗 🛏 💲 Mcr Mcd   2-4 Weeks
VISA 💳

Rubin, Robert (MD)   Oto
Montefiore Med Ctr

3400 Bainbridge Ave 3rd Fl; Bronx, NY 10467;
(718) 920-2991; **BDCERT:** Oto 65; **MS:** Johns
Hopkins U 59; **RES:** S, John Hopkins Univ,
Baltimore, MD 59-64; Oto, John Hopkins Univ,
Baltimore, MD 58-64; **FEL:** N, Nat Inst Mental
Health, Bethesda, MD 64-66; **FAP:** Chmn and Prof
Oto Albert Einstein Coll Med; **HOSP:** Montefiore
Med Ctr-Weiler/Einstein Div; **SI:** *Pediatric
Otolaryngology*; **HMO:** Most

LANG: Sp; ♿ 📷 🚗 🛏 💲 Mcr Mcd   4+ Weeks **VISA**
💳

Yankelowitz, Stanley (MD)   Oto
Montefiore Med Ctr

2310 Eastchester Rd; Bronx, NY 10469; (718)
547-1000; **BDCERT:** Oto 86; **MS:** Africa 74; **RES:** U
Cape Town, Cape Town, South Africa; **FEL:** Royal
Coll of Surgeons, Edinburgh, Scotland; Oto, Albert
Einstein Med Ctr, Bronx, NY; **HOSP:** Westchester
Square Med Ctr; **SI:** *Sinus and Nasal Surgery;
Pediatric Otolaryngology*

♿ 📷 🚗 🛏 💲 Mcr   1 Week **VISA** 💳

PAIN MANAGEMENT

Agin, Carole (MD)   PM
Montefiore Med Ctr

3400 Bainbridge Ave Ste 400; Bronx, NY 10467;
(718) 920-7246; **BDCERT:** Anes 91; PM 93; **MS:** U
Hlth Sci/Chicago Med Sch 86; **RES:** Anes, Beth
Israel Med Ctr, New York, NY 87-90; **FEL:** Anes,
Mem Sloan Kettering Cancer Ctr, New York, NY
90-91; **FAP:** Asst Prof Anes Albert Einstein Coll
Med; **HOSP:** Montefiore Med Ctr-Weiler/Einstein
Div; **SI:** *Acupuncture*; **HMO:** Oxford Aetna Hlth Plan
GHI Empire Blue Cross PHS +

♿ 📷 🛏 💲 Mcr Mcd WC NFI   2-4 Weeks **VISA** 💳

Correoso, Lyla J (MD)   PM
Calvary Hosp

1740 Eastchester Rd; Bronx, NY 10461; (718)
518-2218; **MS:** Meharry Med Coll 80; **RES:** IM, LI
College Hospital, Long Island, NY 80-83; **FEL:**
Hem/Onc, LI College Hospital, Long Island, NY 83-
86; **FAP:** Clin Instr NY Med Coll; **SI:** *Palliative Care*;
HMO: Oxford Blue Cross & Blue Shield of NJ Aetna
Hlth Plan HIP Network +

Mcr Mcd

Guide to symbols and abbreviations can be found on pages 110-113.

449

PEDIATRIC CARDIOLOGY

Eisenberg, Robert (MD)   PCd
Montefiore Med Ctr
111 E 210th St; Bronx, NY 10467; (718) 920-
4431; **BDCERT:** Ped 60; PCd 62; **MS:** NYU Sch Med
53; **RES:** Childrens Hosp Med Ctr, San Francisco,
CA 53-54; Ped, Long Island Coll Hosp, Brooklyn,
NY 54-55; **FEL:** Cv, Stanford Med Ctr, Stanford, CA
56-58; **FAP:** Asst Prof Albert Einstein Coll Med; *SI:*
Pediatric Cardiology; **HMO:** Most

🔲 🏠 💲 Mcr Mcd 2-4 Weeks

Greenberg, Mark (MD)   PCd
Montefiore Med Ctr
111 E 210th St; Bronx, NY 10467; (718) 920-
4212; **BDCERT:** IM 73; Cv 79; **MS:** Univ IL Coll Med
73; **RES:** Med, Montefiore Med Ctr, Bronx, NY 73-
76; **FEL:** Cv, Montefiore Med Ctr, Bronx, NY 76-78;
FAP: Prof of Clin Med Albert Einstein Coll Med; *SI:*
Intervention Cardiology; **HMO:** Blue Shield Bronx
Health CIGNA GHI 1199 +

LANG: Sp; 🔲 🏠 👨 🏠 💲 Mcr Mcd A Few Days

Issenberg, Henry (MD)   PCd
Montefiore Med Ctr
111 E 210th St; Bronx, NY 10467; (718) 920-
4793; **BDCERT:** Ped 79; PCd 79; **MS:** Emory U Sch
Med 74; **RES:** Jacobi Med Ctr, Bronx, NY 74-77;
FEL: Cv, Children's Hosp, Boston, MA 77-80; **FAP:**
Assoc Prof Albert Einstein Coll Med; *SI: Cardiac*
Catheterization; Fetal Echogram; **HMO:** Sanus Blue
Choice Blue Cross & Blue Shield CIGNA HealthNet
+

🔲 🏠 👨 🏠 💲 Mcr Mcd A Few Days ▨▨ *VISA* 💳

Steeg, Carl (MD)   PCd
Montefiore Med Ctr
Montefiore Medical Center, 111 E 210th St; Bronx,
NY 10467; (718) 920-4793; **BDCERT:** Ped 68;
PCd 71; **MS:** NY Med Coll 62; **RES:** Ped, Long Island
Jewish Med Ctr, New Hyde Park, NY 63-67; **FEL:**
PCd, Columbia-Presbyterian Med Ctr, New York,
NY 67-69; **FAP:** Assoc Prof Albert Einstein Coll
Med; *SI: Congenital Heart Disease; Sports Evaluation*;
HMO: Oxford Blue Shield Prucare CIGNA United
Healthcare +

🔲 🏠 👨 🏠 💲 NFI A Few Days

Walsh, Christine A (MD)   PCd
Montefiore Med Ctr
111 E 210th St; Bronx, NY 10467; (718) 920-
4793; **BDCERT:** PCd 83; PCCM 87; **MS:** Yale U Sch
Med 73; **RES:** Ped, Columbia-Presbyterian Med Ctr,
New York, NY 73-76; **FEL:** PCd, Columbia-
Presbyterian Med Ctr, New York, NY 76-80; **FAP:**
Assoc Prof Albert Einstein Coll Med; **HOSP:**
Montefiore Med Ctr-Weiler/Einstein Div; *SI: Heart*
Rhythm Abnormalities; Heart Defects in Children;
HMO: US Hlthcre Oxford Metlife PHS Blue Choice +

🔲 🏠 👨 🏠 💲 Mcr Mcd 2-4 Weeks

PEDIATRIC CRITICAL CARE MEDICINE

Lopez, Deborah (MD)   PCCM
Montefiore Med Ctr
3103 Fairfield Ave 11A; Bronx, NY 10463; (718)
920-4999; **BDCERT:** Ped 95; **MS:** West Indies 90;
RES: Ped, Cabell Huntingon Hosp, Huntington, WV
90-94; **FEL:** CCM, Montefiore Med Ctr, Bronx, NY
94-97; **FAP:** Asst Prof Albert Einstein Coll Med
LANG: Sp; 🔲

Singer, Lewis (MD) PCCM
Montefiore Med Ctr
Montefiore Medical Center, 111 E 210th St; Bronx, NY 10467; (718) 920-4999; **BDCERT:** Ped 81; PCCM 90; **MS:** UMDNJ-NJ Med Sch, Newark 77; **RES:** Ped, Montefiore Med Ctr, Bronx, NY 77-80; Ped, Montefiore Med Ctr, Bronx, NY 80-81; **FEL:** NP, Montefiore Med Ctr, Bronx, NY 81-83; **FAP:** Prof Ped Albert Einstein Coll Med; *SI: Respiratory Failure; Airway Obstruction;* **HMO:** Health One HIP Network Empire Health First Magnacare +

🔲 🔲 🔲 🔲 🔲 🔲 🔲 🔲 🔲

PEDIATRIC ENDOCRINOLOGY

Markowitz, Morri (MD) PEn
Montefiore Med Ctr
Montefiore Med Ctr Peds, 111 E 210th St; Bronx, NY 10467; (718) 920-5016; **BDCERT:** Ped 80; PEn 97; **MS:** Albert Einstein Coll Med 74; **RES:** Ped, Montefiore Med Ctr, Bronx, NY 75-78; **FEL:** PEn, Montefiore Med Ctr, Bronx, NY 79-81; **FAP:** Lecturer Ped Albert Einstein Coll Med; *SI: Lead Poisoning; Bone Mineral Disorders*

LANG: Sp, Ger, Fr, Yd; 🔲 🔲 🔲 🔲 🔲 🔲 🔲
1 Week

Saenger, Paul (MD) PEn
Montefiore Med Ctr
Division of Pediatric Endocrinology, 111 E 210th St; Bronx, NY 10467; (718) 920-4664; **BDCERT:** Ped 73; PEn 78; **MS:** Germany 69; **RES:** Ped, Montefiore Medical Center, New York, NY 69-71; **FEL:** Ped, NYU Medical Center, New York, NY 71-75

🔲 🔲 🔲 🔲 🔲 🔲 A Few Days

PEDIATRIC HEMATOLOGY-ONCOLOGY

Bestak, Marc (MD) PHO
Montefiore Med Ctr
111 E 210th St NW556; Bronx, NY 10467; (718) 920-7844; **BDCERT:** Ped 77; PHO 80; **MS:** SUNY Hlth Sci Ctr 72; **RES:** Ped, NY Hosp-Cornell Med Ctr, New York, NY 72-75; NY Hosp-Cornell Med Ctr, New York, NY 75-76; **FEL:** PHO, NY Hosp-Cornell Med Ctr, New York, NY 76-79; **FAP:** Assoc Prof Albert Einstein Coll Med; **HOSP:** Montefiore Med Ctr-Weiler/Einstein Div; *SI: Acute Leukemia; Lymphoma;* **HMO:** Prudential US Hlthcre Blue Cross & Blue Choice Metlife CIGNA +

LANG: Sp; 🔲 🔲 🔲 🔲 Immediately

Dasgupta, Indira (MD) PHO
Our Lady of Mercy Med Ctr
600 E 233rd St; Bronx, NY 10466; (718) 920-9014; **BDCERT:** Ped 81; PHO 84; **MS:** India 66; **RES:** New York Methodist Hosp, Brooklyn, NY; **FEL:** Mem Sloan Kettering Cancer Ctr, New York, NY; PEn, Mount Sinai Med Ctr, New York, NY; **HMO:** Empire Blue Cross & Shield Magnacare 1199 Aetna-US Healthcare Oxford +

🔲 🔲 🔲 🔲 A Few Days

Radel, Eva (MD) PHO
Montefiore Med Ctr
111 E 210th St; Bronx, NY 10467; (718) 920-7844; **BDCERT:** Ped 64; PHO 74; **MS:** NYU Sch Med 58; **RES:** Ped, Jacobi Med Ctr, Bronx, NY 58-61; **FEL:** PHO, Albert Einstein Med Ctr, Bronx, NY 61-63; **FAP:** Prof Albert Einstein Coll Med; *SI: Pediatric Cancer; Childhood Blood Disorders;* **HMO:** HIP Network US Hlthcre Oxford GHI Empire Blue Cross & Shield +

🔲 🔲 🔲 🔲 Immediately

PEDIATRIC NEPHROLOGY

Greifer, Ira (MD)   PNep
Montefiore Med Ctr

Einstein Coll Med, 111 E 210th St; Bronx, NY 10467; (718) 655-1120; **BDCERT:** Ped 61; **MS:** Univ Vt Coll Med 56; **RES:** Ped, Bronx Muncipal Hosp Ctr, Bronx, NY 56-59; **FEL:** PNep, Albert Einstein Med Ctr, Bronx, NY 61-65; **FAP:** Ped Albert Einstein Coll Med; **HOSP:** Montefiore Med Ctr-Weiler/Einstein Div; **SI:** *Blood and Protein in the Urine;* **HMO:** Blue Choice Health First Oxford Bronx Health GHI +

LANG: Sp, Heb; 🦽 🔲 🏢 $ Mcr Mcd Immediately **VISA** 💳

Mortiz, Michael (MD)   PNep
Montefiore Med Ctr

Montefiore Med Center, Dept of Ped Neph, 111 E 210th St; Bronx, NY 10467; (718) 920-4321; **BDCERT:** Ped 94; **MS:** U Chicago-Pritzker Sch Med 91; **RES:** Ped, Childrens Mem Med Ctr, Chicago, IL 91-94; **FEL:** PNep, Texas Children's Hosp, Houston, TX 94-97; **FAP:** Asst Dir Ped Albert Einstein Coll Med; **SI:** *Dialysis; Transplantation*

LANG: Fr, Sp; 🦽 🔲 🏢 $ Mcr Mcd 1 Week

Spitzer, Adrian (MD)   PNep
Montefiore Med Ctr

111 E 210th St; Bronx, NY 10467; (718) 655-1120; **BDCERT:** PNep 66; **MS:** Romania 52; **RES:** Hosp Med College of PA, Philadelphia, PA 64-66; **FEL:** Nep, Albert Einstein Med Ctr, Bronx, NY 66-67; Nep, , NY; **FAP:** Prof Ped Albert Einstein Coll Med; **HOSP:** Jacobi Med Ctr; **HMO:** Empire Blue Cross & Shield Oxford Bronx Health GHI

LANG: Rom, Fr; 🦽 🔲 🏢 $ Mcr Mcd WC 2-4 Weeks

PEDIATRIC PULMONOLOGY

Perez, Iris (MD)   PPul
Montefiore Med Ctr

Montefiore Medical Center, Dept of Pediatric Pulmonology, 111 E 210th St; Bronx, NY 10467; (718) 920-2178; **BDCERT:** Ped 94; **MS:** Philippines 84; **RES:** Ped, Montefiore Med Ctr, Bronx, NY 90-94; **FEL:** PPul, Children's Hosp of Los Angeles, Los Angeles, CA 94-97; **FAP:** Asst Prof Albert Einstein Coll Med; **SI:** *Asthma; Sleep Apnea;* **HMO:** PHS PHCS PPAC Health First

LANG: Tag; 🦽 🔲 🏢 🏢 $ Mcr Mcd A Few Days

PEDIATRIC SURGERY

Boley, Scott (MD)   PS
Montefiore Med Ctr

111 E 210th St; Bronx, NY 10467; (718) 920-4758; **BDCERT:** S 57; PS 75; **MS:** Jefferson Med Coll 49; **RES:** Queens Hosp Ctr, Jamaica, NY 50-51; Kingsbrook Jewish Med Ctr, Brooklyn, NY 53-56; **FAP:** Prof S Albert Einstein Coll Med; **SI:** *Hirschsprung's Disease; Inflammatory Bowel Disease;* **HMO:** US Hlthcre Blue Choice Bronx Health Multiplan United Healthcare +

LANG: Sp; 🔲 🏢 $ Mcr Mcd 1 Week

Kleinhaus, Sylvain (MD)   PS
Montefiore Med Ctr

3355 Bainbridge Ave FL2; Bronx, NY 10467; (718) 920-4214; **BDCERT:** S 69; PS 69; **MS:** Switzerland 62; **RES:** Brooklyn Jewish Hosp, Brooklyn, NY 63-67; **FEL:** PdS, St Justines Childrens Hosp, Montreal, Canada 68-69; **FAP:** Prof S Albert Einstein Coll Med; **SI:** *Minimally Invasive Surgery; Endoscopy*

LANG: Fr; 🏢 🏢 $ A Few Days

Weinberg, Gerard (MD)   PS
Montefiore Med Ctr

1575 Blondell Ave 125; Bronx, NY 10461; (718) 405-8241; **BDCERT:** S 80; **MS:** Albert Einstein Coll Med 73; **RES:** Albert Einstein Med Ctr, Bronx, NY 73-76; Children's Hosp, Boston, MA 76-77; **FEL:** U Miami Hosp, Miami, FL 78-79; **FAP:** Assoc Prof Albert Einstein Coll Med; **HOSP:** Jacobi Med Ctr; *SI: Hernias; GI Tract Surgical Disorder;* **HMO:** Oxford CIGNA PHS Blue Cross & Blue Shield GHI +

🚫 🔟 🏧 💲 🅼 🅼 A Few Days **VISA** 💳

Zitsman, Jeffrey (MD)   PS
Our Lady of Mercy Med Ctr

Medical Village, 3250 Westchester Ave; Bronx, NY 10461; **BDCERT:** SCC 94; PS 95; **MS:** Tufts U 76; **RES:** S, New England Med Ctr, Boston, MA 77-81; **FEL:** PdS, Babies Hosp, New York, NY 83-85; **FAP:** Asst Prof S Columbia P&S; **HOSP:** Bronx Lebanon Hosp Ctr

PEDIATRICS

Alderman, Elizabeth (MD)   Ped   PCP
Montefiore Med Ctr

111 E 210th St Ste 674; Bronx, NY 10467; (718) 920-6614; **BDCERT:** Ped 90; AM 94; **MS:** SUNY Stony Brook 87; **RES:** Ped, Montefiore Med Ctr, Bronx, NY 87-90; **FEL:** AM, Montefiore Med Ctr, Bronx, NY 90-92; **FAP:** Asst Prof Albert Einstein Coll Med; *SI: Gynecology; Eating Disorders*

LANG: Sp; 🔟 🅼 🏧 💲 1 Week

Andrade, Joseph (MD)   Ped   PCP
Our Lady of Mercy Med Ctr

1163 Mannor Ave; Bronx, NY 10472; (718) 589-3501; **BDCERT:** Ped 92; **MS:** Ecuador 81; **RES:** IM, Our Lady of Mercy, Bronx, NY 86-88; Ped, Our Lady of Mercy, Bronx, NY 83-86; **HMO:** Blue Choice Chubb

LANG: Sp; 🚫 🏧 🔟 🅼 🏧 💲 🅼 Immediately
VISA 💳

Arnstein, Ellis (MD)   Ped   PCP
Montefiore Med Ctr

Montefiore Medical Group Morris Park, 1621 Eastchester Rd; Bronx, NY 10461; (718) 405-8040; **BDCERT:** Ped 75; **MS:** SUNY Downstate 69; **RES:** IM, USPHS Hosp, Baltimore, MD 69-70; Ped, U WA Med Ctr, Seattle, WA 71-73; **FEL:** ChAP, New England Med Ctr, Boston, MA 73-74; **FAP:** Asst Prof Albert Einstein Coll Med; **HOSP:** St Vincents Hosp & Med Ctr NY; *SI: Developmental Disabilities;* **HMO:** Bronx Health US Hlthcre Health First

LANG: Sp, Rus; 🚫 🅲 🔟 🅼 🏧 💲 🅼 🅼 2-4 Weeks

Bailey, Michelle (MD)   Ped   PCP
Our Lady of Mercy Med Ctr

120-1 Dekruif Place; Bronx, NY 10475; (718) 320-7401; **BDCERT:** Ped 94; **MS:** West Indies 89; **RES:** Ped, Lincoln Med & Mental Hlth Ctr, Bronx, NY 91-94; **FAP:** Asst Clin Prof Ped NY Med Coll; *SI: Well Care & Immunization; Acute Illness & Asthma;* **HMO:** Magnacare Fidelis GHI NYLCare Empire Blue Cross +

LANG: Sp; 🚫 🅲 🔟 🅼 🏧 💲 🅼 NFI A Few Days

Balk, Sophie (MD)   Ped
Montefiore Med Ctr

Bronx Muni Hosp Ctr, Pelham Pkwy South BS46; Bronx, NY 10461; (718) 918-4076; **BDCERT:** Ped 79; **MS:** Albert Einstein Coll Med 74; **RES:** Ped, Montefiore Med Ctr, Bronx, NY 74-77; **FAP:** Assoc Prof Ped Albert Einstein Coll Med

Cohen, Herbert J (MD)   Ped
Jacobi Med Ctr

1410 Pelham Pkwy South; Bronx, NY 10461; (718) 430-8522; **BDCERT:** Ped 64; **MS:** SUNY Hlth Sci Ctr 59; **RES:** Bellevue Hosp Ctr, New York, NY 59-60; NY Hosp-Cornell Med Ctr, New York, NY 60-62; **FEL:** N, Albert Einstein Med Ctr, Bronx, NY 64-66; **FAP:** Prof Ped Albert Einstein Coll Med; **HOSP:** Montefiore Med Ctr-Weiler/Einstein Div; *SI: Developmental Pediatrics;* **HMO:** Most

LANG: Chi, Sp, Fr, Itl, Pol; 🚫 🔟 🏧 🅼 2-4 Weeks

Easton, Lon (MD) Ped `PCP`
Montefiore Med Ctr

3620 E Tremont Ave; Bronx, NY 10465; (718) 863-1050; **BDCERT:** Ped 83; **MS:** NY Med Coll 78; **RES:** Ped, Metropolitan Hosp Ctr, New York, NY 78-81; **HMO:** Oxford Aetna Hlth Plan PHCS Magnacare Travelers +

🏨 📞 📷 🏧 🎂 💲 A Few Days **VISA** 💳

Esteban, Nora (MD) Ped
Montefiore Med Ctr

Albert Einstein Med CtrBronx Muni Hosp, Pediatrics Dept; Bronx, NY 10461; (718) 920-4321; **BDCERT:** Ped 93; **MS:** Argentina 79; **RES:** Ped, Albert Einstein Med Ctr, Bronx, NY 92-93; Ped, Italion Hosp, Buenos Aires, Argentina 81-83; **FEL:** Nat Inst Health, Bethesda, MD 84-91; **FAP:** Asst Prof Albert Einstein Coll Med; **HOSP:** Montefiore Med Ctr-Weiler/Einstein Div

Haber, Patricia (MD) Ped `PCP`
Montefiore Med Ctr

1500 Astor Ave; Bronx, NY 10469; (718) 881-0100; **BDCERT:** Ped 81; Ped Rhu 97; **MS:** Johns Hopkins U 76; **RES:** Ped, Johns Hopkins Hosp, Baltimore, MD 76-79; **FEL:** Ped Immunology, U of Alabama Hosp, Birmingham, AL 79-82; Ped Rhu, U of Alabama Hosp, Birmingham, AL 82-84; **FAP:** Asst Prof Albert Einstein Coll Med; **HMO:** US Hlthcre 1199 Oxford NYLCare CIGNA +

♿ 📷 🎂 🏧 💲 Mcr Mcd A Few Days

Hirschman, Alan (MD) Ped `PCP`
Montefiore Med Ctr

Pediatric Associates, 3765 Riverdale Ave; Bronx, NY 10463; (718) 548-7300; **BDCERT:** Ped 81; **MS:** UMDNJ-NJ Med Sch, Newark 76; **RES:** Ped, Montefiore Med Ctr, Bronx, NY 76-79; **FEL:** Montefiore Med Ctr, Bronx, NY 79-80; **FAP:** Asst Clin Prof Albert Einstein Coll Med; **SI:** *Asthma*; **HMO:** Oxford Aetna Hlth Plan CIGNA NYLCare Blue Choice +

♿ 📞 📷 🎂 🏧 💲 Immediately 📇 **VISA** 💳 💳

Huberman, Harris (MD) Ped `PCP`
Montefiore Med Ctr

230 E 162nd St; Bronx, NY 10451; (718) 579-2500; **BDCERT:** Ped 93; **MS:** Albert Einstein Coll Med 83; **RES:** Montefiore Med Ctr, Bronx, NY 89-93; **HMO:** Blue Cross & Blue Shield CIGNA

♿ 📷 🎂 Mcr Mcd **VISA**

Igel, Gerard (MD) Ped `PCP`
Montefiore Med Ctr

1613 Tenbroeck Ave; Bronx, NY 10461; (718) 828-9060; **BDCERT:** Ped 86; **MS:** Israel 81; **RES:** Jacobi Med Ctr, Bronx, NY 81-84; **HMO:** None

LANG: Heb, Pol; ♿ 📞 📷 🎂 🏧 A Few Days

Kaskel, Frederick (MD) Ped
Montefiore Med Ctr •

Montefiore Medical Ctr, Pediatric Nephrology Div, 111 E 210th St; Bronx, NY 10467; (718) 655-1120; **BDCERT:** Ped 80; Nep 82; **MS:** U Cincinnati 75; **RES:** Montefiore Med Ctr, Bronx, NY; **FEL:** PNep, Albert Einstein Med Ctr, Bronx, NY; **HOSP:** Winthrop Univ Hosp; **SI:** *Nephritic Syndrome; Urinary Tract Abnormality*; **HMO:** CIGNA HIP Network US Hlthcre

LANG: Sp; ♿ 📞 📷 🎂 🏧 Mcr Mcd WC Immediately 📇 **VISA** 💳 💳

Korin, Daniel (MD) Ped
Lincoln Med & Mental Hlth Ctr

234 E 149th St Rm1B1; Bronx, NY 10451; (718) 579-5723; **BDCERT:** Ped 82; **MS:** Argentina 67; **RES:** Montefiore Med Ctr, Bronx, NY 77-79

Litman, Nathan (MD) Ped
Montefiore Med Ctr

Dept of Peds, 111 E 210th St; Bronx, NY 10467; (718) 920-5947; **BDCERT:** Ped 78; **MS:** Albert Einstein Coll Med 71; **RES:** Ped, Montefiore Med Ctr, Bronx, NY 71-74; **FEL:** Inf, Montefiore Med Ctr, Bronx, NY 76-78; **FAP:** Prof Ped Albert Einstein Coll Med; **HMO:** Blue Cross & Blue Shield Bronx Health GHI Health First Oxford +

📷 🎂 Mcr Mcd 1 Week

London, Ronald (MD)   Ped   **PCP**
Montefiore Med Ctr

Throgs Neck Pediatrics, 3594 E Tremont Ave;
Bronx, NY 10465; (718) 863-1050; **BDCERT:** Ped
88; **MS:** Israel 84; **RES:** Montefiore Med Ctr, Bronx,
NY 84-87; **FEL:** Albert Einstein Med Ctr, Bronx, NY
87-88; **HOSP:** Montefiore Med Ctr-Weiler/Einstein
Div; **HMO:** Oxford Magnacare PHCS Metlife CIGNA
+

LANG: Itl; ♿ 🅂🄰 🌙 ⏰ 🈂 🎴 💲 1 Week **VISA** 💳

Maseda, Nelly (MD)   Ped   **PCP**
Montefiore Med Ctr

5525 Broadway; Bronx, NY 10463; (718) 884-
0279; **BDCERT:** Ped 91; **MS:** Albert Einstein Coll
Med 88; **RES:** Ped, Columbia-Presbyterian Med Ctr,
New York, NY 88-90; **FAP:** Asst Clin Prof Albert
Einstein Coll Med; *SI: Asthma; Obesity;* **HMO:**
CIGNA Aetna-US Healthcare Blue Cross & Blue
Shield Bronx Health Health First +

LANG: Sp; ♿ 🅂🄰 🌙 ⏰ 🎴 🈂 💲 Ⓜ Ⓜ 1 Week

Masella, Peter A (MD)   Ped
St Barnabas Hosp-Bronx

603 E 187th St; Bronx, NY 10457; (718) 733-
3873; **MS:** Italy 72; **RES:** Ped, Metropolitan Hosp
Ctr, New York, NY 74-76; **FEL:** Ped, Metropolitian
Hosp Ctr,, New York, NY 76-77; **HOSP:** Lenox Hill
Hosp

Mayers, Marguerite (MD)   Ped   **PCP**
Montefiore Med Ctr

Dept Primary Care, Montefiore Medical Center, 111
E 210th St; Bronx, NY 10467; (718) 920-5871;
BDCERT: Ped 77; Inf 94; **MS:** Albert Einstein Coll
Med 71; **RES:** Ped, Montefiore Med Ctr, Bronx, NY
71-74; **FEL:** Inf, Montefiore Med Ctr, Bronx, NY 74-
76; **FAP:** Assoc Prof Ped Albert Einstein Coll Med;
SI: Tuberculosis; Pediatric Aids; **HMO:** Bronx Health
Montefiore IPA

LANG: Sp; ♿ 🅂🄰 🌙 ⏰ 🎴 🈂 Ⓜ Ⓜ Ⓝ 1 Week 🈵
VISA 💳

Mezey, Andrew (MD)   Ped   **PCP**
Jacobi Med Ctr

1300 Morris Park Ave; Bronx, NY 10461; (718)
430-4282; **BDCERT:** Ped 66; **MS:** NYU Sch Med
60; **RES:** Ped, Jacobi Med Ctr, Bronx, NY 60-64;
FAP: Prof Albert Einstein Coll Med; **HOSP:**
Montefiore Med Ctr; **HMO:** None
♿ 🈂

Okun, Alex (MD)   Ped   **PCP**
Montefiore Med Ctr

Pediatric Academic Associates, 1621 Eastchester
Rd; Bronx, NY 10461; (718) 405-8040; **BDCERT:**
Ped 87; **MS:** Columbia P&S 83; **RES:** Ped,
Columbia-Presbyterian Med Ctr, New York, NY 83-
86; **FEL:** ChAP, Jacobi Med Ctr, Bronx, NY 88-90;
Albert Einstein Med Ctr, Bronx, NY; **FAP:** Assoc
Prof of Clin Ped Albert Einstein Coll Med; *SI: Chronic
Illnesses;* **HMO:** Bronx Health NYLCare US Hlthcre
1199

LANG: Sp; ♿ ⏰ 🎴 🈂 Ⓜ 1 Week

Oppedisano, Carlyn (MD)   Ped   **PCP**
Columbia-Presbyterian Med Ctr

Riverdale Pediatrics PC, 2600 Netherland Ave 125;
Bronx, NY 10463; (718) 796-3580; **BDCERT:** Ped
86; **MS:** Columbia P&S 81; **RES:** Ped, Babies Hosp,
New York, NY 81-84; Ped, Babies Hosp, New York,
NY 84-85; **FAP:** Assoc Clin Prof Ped Columbia P&S;
HMO: Oxford

LANG: Sp; ♿ 🅂🄰 ⏰ 🎴 🈂 💲 1 Week 🈵 **VISA**
💳

Ozuah, Philip (MD)   Ped
Montefiore Med Ctr

Montefiore Medical Ctr, 111 E 210th St; Bronx, NY
10467; (718) 579-2500; **BDCERT:** Ped 92; **MS:**
Nigeria 85; **RES:** Ped, Montefiore Med Ctr, Bronx,
NY 89; **FEL:** USC Med Ctr, Los Angeles, CA 87-8;
FAP: Assoc Prof of Clin Ped Albert Einstein Coll Med

Santorineou, Maria (MD) Ped
Jacobi Med Ctr

Jacobi Medical Center, Pelham Pkwy South Rd Rm 815; Bronx, NY 10461; (718) 918-6966; **BDCERT:** Ped 64; Hem 74; **MS:** Greece 58; **RES:** Ped, St Louis Children's Hosp, St Louis, MO 60-62; **FEL:** PHO, Children's Hosp, Boston, MA 62-64; **FAP:** Lecturer Ped Albert Einstein Coll Med; **HOSP:** Montefiore Med Ctr-Weiler/Einstein Div; **HMO:** None

LANG: Grk; ♿ 🕐 📋 🏧 📠 A Few Days 📇 ●

Schechter, Miriam (MD) Ped PCP
Montefiore Med Ctr

Pediatric Academic Associates at Montefiore Medical Group, 1621 Eastchester Rd; Bronx, NY 10461; (718) 405-8040; **BDCERT:** Ped 92; **MS:** NYU Sch Med 89; **RES:** Ped, Mount Sinai Med Ctr, New York, NY; Ped, Mount Sinai Med Ctr, New York, NY; **FAP:** Asst Prof Albert Einstein Coll Med; *SI: Teenage Mothers*

LANG: Sp; ♿ 🕐 📋 🏧 💲 📠 Immediately

Schonberg, Samuel Kenneth (MD) Ped
Montefiore Med Ctr

111 E 210th St; Bronx, NY 10467; (718) 920-6781; **BDCERT:** Ped 71; **MS:** U Chicago-Pritzker Sch Med 65; **RES:** Ped, Montefiore Med Ctr, Bronx, NY 66-68; **FEL:** AM, Montefiore Med Ctr, Bronx, NY 70-71; **FAP:** Prof Ped Albert Einstein Coll Med

Shookoff, Charlene (MD) Ped
Our Lady of Mercy Med Ctr

4141 Carpenter Ave; Bronx, NY 10466; (718) 920-9014; **BDCERT:** Ped 93; **MS:** Dominican Republic 85; **FEL:** Albert Einstein Med Ctr, Bronx, NY

Stein, Ruth (MD) Ped
Montefiore Med Ctr

111 E 210th St; Bronx, NY 10467; (718) 920-6490; **BDCERT:** Ped 71; **MS:** Albert Einstein Coll Med 66; **RES:** Ped, Bronx Municipal Hosp`, Bronx, NY 67-68; Ped, Children's Hosp Nat Med Ctr, Washington, DC 68-69; **FEL:** Ped, Children's Hosp Nat Med Ctr, Washington, DC 68-69; **FAP:** Prof Albert Einstein Coll Med; **HOSP:** Montefiore Med Ctr-Weiler/Einstein Div; *SI: Chronic Childhood Ilness*

Strassberg, Barbara (MD) Ped PCP
Columbia-Presbyterian Med Ctr

Riverdale Pediatrics, 2600 Netherland Ave 125; Bronx, NY 10463; (718) 796-3580; **BDCERT:** Ped 86; **MS:** SUNY Syracuse 81; **RES:** Columbia-Presbyterian Med Ctr, New York, NY 82-84; **FAP:** Assoc Prof of Clin Ped Columbia P&S; *SI: Developmental Pediatrics*; **HMO:** Oxford Blue Cross & Blue Shield

LANG: Sp; ♿ 🕐 📋 🏧 💲 A Few Days 📇 **VISA** ●

Tolchin, Deborah (MD) Ped PCP
Montefiore Med Ctr-Weiler/Einstein Div

1500 Astor Ave; Bronx, NY 10469; (718) 881-0100; **BDCERT:** Ped 70; **MS:** SUNY Hlth Sci Ctr 66; **RES:** Kings County Hosp Ctr, Brooklyn, NY 66-67; Jacobi Med Ctr, Bronx, NY 67-69; **FAP:** Assoc Prof Albert Einstein Coll Med; **HOSP:** Jacobi Med Ctr; *SI: General Pediatrics; Adolescents*

♿ 🕐 📋 🏧 💲 🚾 📠 2-4 Weeks **VISA** ● 📇

Uy, Rodolfo (MD) Ped PCP
Our Lady of Mercy Med Ctr

4409 Byron Ave; Bronx, NY 10466; (718) 994-6755; **BDCERT:** Ped 97; **MS:** Philippines 79; **RES:** Ped, Our Lady of Mercy Med Ctr, Bronx, NY 83-86; **HMO:** Aetna-US Healthcare Blue Cross & Blue Shield GHI 1199 +

LANG: Chi, Slv, Fil; 🏧 🅲 🕐 🏧 💲 Mcr Med
A Few Days 📇 **VISA** ●

Weiner, Richard (MD) Ped PCP
Montefiore Med Ctr

University Pediatrics, 1500 Astor Ave; Bronx, NY 10469; (718) 881-0100; **BDCERT:** Ped 79; **MS:** Albert Einstein Coll Med 75; **RES:** Ped, Jacobi Med Ctr, Bronx, NY 75-78; **FAP:** Assoc Prof Ped Albert Einstein Coll Med; *SI: Adolescent Medicine*; **HMO:** Oxford US Hlthcre Blue Choice

♿ 🕐 📋 🏧 💲 1 Week **VISA**

Wong, Martha (MD)   Ped
Bronx Lebanon Hosp Ctr
Bronx Associate In Pediatric, 1770 Grand
Concourse 1M; Bronx, NY 10457; (718) 294-
1104; **BDCERT:** Ped 72; PHO 78; **MS:** Taiwan 66;
RES: Ped, Kings County Hosp Ctr, Brooklyn, NY 67-
68; Ped, Kings County Hosp Ctr, Brooklyn, NY 68-
70; **FEL:** PHO, Albert Einstein Med Ctr, Bronx, NY
70-72; **SI:** *Sickle Cell Anemia; Hemophilia, Leukemia;*
HMO: Health One GHI Blue Cross & Blue Shield
Health First Benefit Plan +

LANG: Sp, Chi; 🚻 ⬛ 🔲 🔲 🔲 🔲 🔲   Immediately

Zoltan, Irving (MD)   Ped   `PCP`
Montefiore Med Ctr
1613 Tenbroeck Ave; Bronx, NY 10461; (718)
828-9060; **BDCERT:** Ped 79; **MS:** Albert Einstein
Coll Med 74; **RES:** Ped, Jacobi Med Ctr, Bronx, NY
74-78; **FAP:** Asst Prof Albert Einstein Coll Med; **SI:**
Premature & Hi-Risk Infant

🔲 🔲 🔲 🔲 🔲 🔲   A Few Days

PHYSICAL MEDICINE & REHABILITATION

De Araujo, Maria (MD)   PMR
Our Lady of Mercy Med Ctr
Our Lady of Mercy Med Ctr, 600 E 233rd St; Bronx,
NY 10466; (718) 920-9171; **BDCERT:** PMR 89;
MS: Brazil 72; **RES:** PMR, St Vincents Hosp & Med
Ctr NY, New York, NY 79-80; PMR, St Vincents
Hosp & Med Ctr NY, New York, NY 87-88; **FEL:**
PMR/EMG, Westchester County Med Ctr, Valhalla,
NY 88-89; **FAP:** Assoc Prof NY Med Coll; **SI:** *Low
Back Pain; Arthritis;* **HMO:** Prudential Oxford
Independent Health Plan

LANG: Prt, Sp, Fr; 🔲 🔲 🔲 🔲 🔲 🔲 🔲 🔲 🔲
A Few Days

Gladstone, Lenore (MD)   PMR
Montefiore Med Ctr
Rehabilitation Medicine Associates, 3435 Dekalb
Ave; Bronx, NY 10467; (718) 547-8899; **BDCERT:**
PMR 75; **MS:** South Africa 56; **RES:** PMR,
Montefiore Med Ctr, Bronx, NY 69-71; PMR,
Columbia-Presbyterian Med Ctr, New York, NY 71-
73; **FAP:** Asst Prof Albert Einstein Coll Med; **HOSP:**
St Barnabas Hosp-Bronx; **SI:** *Sports Medicine;
Geriatrics;* **HMO:** 1199 US Hlthcre United
Healthcare Oxford CIGNA +

LANG: Srb, Rus; 🚻 🔲 🔲 🔲 🔲 🔲 🔲 🔲 🔲
A Few Days

Greenbaum, Mark (MD)   PMR
Montefiore Med Ctr
3010 Grand Concourse L3; Bronx, NY 10458;
(718) 933-0271; **BDCERT:** PMR 89; **MS:** Mexico
80; **RES:** Booth Mem Hosp, Flushing, NY 82; Albert
Einstein Med Ctr, Bronx, NY 85-87

🔲 🔲 🔲 🔲 🔲 🔲 🔲   Immediately 💳 **VISA** 💳
💳

Levin, Sheryl (MD)   PMR
Montefiore Med Ctr
3435 Dekalb Ave; Bronx, NY 10467; (718) 547-
8899; **BDCERT:** PMR 89; **MS:** Cornell U 84; **RES:**
NY Hosp-Cornell Med Ctr, New York, NY 85-88; St
Luke's Roosevelt Hosp Ctr, New York, NY 84-85;
FAP: Assoc Prof Albert Einstein Coll Med; **HOSP:**
NY Hosp-Cornell Med Ctr; **SI:** *Musculoskeletal Pain;*
HMO: Aetna Hlth Plan CIGNA Oxford United
Healthcare GHI +

LANG: Sp, Rus; 🔲 🔲 🔲 🔲 🔲 🔲 🔲 🔲
Immediately

Roussan, Matei S (MD)   PMR
Montefiore Med Ctr
1500 Blondell Ave; Bronx, NY 10464; (718) 405-
8410; **BDCERT:** PMR 60; **MS:** France 51; **RES:**
Knickerbocker Hosp, New York, NY 52-53; Long
Island Jewish Med Ctr, New Hyde Park, NY 54-55;
FEL: Bellevue Hosp Ctr, New York, NY 56-58

🔲 🔲 🔲 🔲 🔲 🔲 🔲 🔲   A Few Days 💳 **VISA**
💳

PLASTIC SURGERY

Dolich, Barry (MD) PlS
Montefiore Med Ctr-Weiler/Einstein Div

1578 Williamsbridge Rd; Bronx, NY 10461; (718) 430-0942; **BDCERT:** PlS 75; **MS:** SUNY Syracuse 66; **RES:** S, Albert Einstein Med Ctr, Bronx, NY 66-70; PlS, Albert Einstein Med Ctr, Bronx, NY 70-73; **FEL:** France; Microsurgery, Vienna, Austria 73; **FAP:** Assoc Prof Albert Einstein Coll Med; **HOSP:** New York Eye & Ear Infirmary; *SI: Cosmetic Surgery; Hand Surgery;* **HMO:** Oxford CIGNA Blue Cross & Blue Shield Guardian

LANG: Sp; ⬡ 🅲 🔳 🔳 🔳 🅂 Mcr Mcd WC NFI A Few Days **VISA** ⬤ ▨

Goldstein, Robert (MD) PlS
Montefiore Med Ctr

1625 Poplar St 200; Bronx, NY 10461; (718) 405-8444; **BDCERT:** PlS 85; **HS** 90; **MS:** Univ Penn 77; **RES:** Montefiore Med Ctr, Bronx, NY 77-81; **FEL:** HS, Albert Einstein Med Ctr, Bronx, NY 81-82; **FAP:** Assoc Prof Albert Einstein Coll Med; **HOSP:** Montefiore Med Ctr-Weiler/Einstein Div; *SI: Breast Surgery; Cosmetic Surgery;* **HMO:** GHI Oxford Aetna Hlth Plan

LANG: Sp, Itl; ⬡ 🆂🆄 🔳 🔳 🔳 🅂 Mcr WC NFI 1 Week **VISA** ⬤

Patel, Mahendrakumar (MD) PlS
Montefiore Med Ctr

1625 Poplar St 200; Bronx, NY 10461; (718) 405-8333; **BDCERT:** PlS 78; **MS:** India 58; **RES:** Med Coll Hosp, Trivandrum, India 58-64; Montefiore U Hosp, Pittsburgh, PA 64-67; **FEL:** Montefiore Med Ctr, Bronx, NY 67-69; Roswell Park Cancer Inst, Buffalo, NY 69; **HOSP:** Jacobi Med Ctr; *SI: Breast Reconstruction; Burns;* **HMO:** HIP Network Bronx Health US Hlthcre Oxford Prudential +

LANG: EIn, Sp, Itl; ⬡ 🔳 🔳 🔳 🅂 Mcr Mcd WC NFI Immediately

Rubinstein, Joshua (MD) PlS
Bronx Lebanon Hosp Ctr

1650 Grand Concourse; Bronx, NY 10457; (718) 960-2004; **BDCERT:** PlS 95; **HS** 96; **MS:** Case West Res U 84; **RES:** PlS, Univ of Med & Dent NJ Hosp, Newark, NJ 89-91; S, Univ Hosp SUNY Bklyn, Brooklyn, NY 85-89; **FEL:** HS, New York University Med Ctr, New York, NY 91-92; **FAP:** Asst Prof S Albert Einstein Coll Med; *SI: Breast Surgery; Face Lifts*

LANG: Sp; ⬡ 🔳 🔳 🔳 🅂 Mcr Mcd 2-4 Weeks **VISA** ⬤

Strauch, Berish (MD) PlS
Montefiore Med Ctr

3331 Bainbridge Ave; Bronx, NY 10467; (718) 920-5551; **BDCERT:** PlS 70; S 65; **MS:** Columbia P&S 59; **RES:** S, Montefiore Med Ctr, Bronx, NY 60-64; PlS, Stanford Med Ctr, Stanford, CA 66-68; **FEL:** Hand, St Luke's Roosevelt Hosp Ctr, New York, NY; **FAP:** Chrmn PlS Albert Einstein Coll Med; *SI: Breast Surgery Aesthetic*

🔳 🔳 🔳 🅂 Mcr WC NFI 1 Week ▦ **VISA** ⬤

PSYCHIATRY

Asnis, Gregory (MD) Psyc
Montefiore Med Ctr

111 E 210th St; Bronx, NY 10467; (718) 920-4287; **BDCERT:** Psyc 78; Ger 97; **MS:** Hahnemann U 72; **RES:** Mount Sinai Med Ctr, New York, NY 76; **FEL:** Psyc, Columbia-Presbyterian Med Ctr, New York, NY 80; **HOSP:** Phelps Mem Hosp Ctr; **HMO:** CIGNA UBA PHS Pomco

⬡ 🆂🆄 🔳 🔳 🔳 🅂 Mcr Immediately

Bluestone, Harvey (MD) Psyc
Bronx Lebanon Hosp Ctr

Bronx Lebanon Hosp, 1285 Fulton Ave; Bronx, NY 10456; (718) 817-7117; **BDCERT:** Psyc 60; **MS:** England 47; **RES:** Psyc, Rockland State, Orangeburg, SC 59-60; Psyc, Overbrook Hosp, Cedar Grove, NJ 55-57; **FEL:** Psyc, Hosp For Joint Diseases, New York, NY 54; **FAP:** Sr Prof Psyc Albert Einstein Coll Med; **HMO:** Health One Bronx Health

Gelfand, Janice (MD)　　Psyc
Columbia-Presbyterian Med Ctr
3765 Riverdale Ave; Bronx, NY 10463; (718) 361-3482; **BDCERT:** Psyc 90; **MS:** NYU Sch Med 85; **RES:** New York University Med Ctr, New York, NY 85-89; **FEL:** Beth Israel Med Ctr, New York, NY; **FAP:** Asst Prof Columbia P&S; *SI: Depression; Anxiety*

⬚ ⬚ ⬚ ⬚ ⬚ ⬚ 2-4 Weeks

Gerbino-Rosen, Ginny (MD) Psyc
Bronx Children's Psych Ctr
Bronx Children's Psych Ctr, 1000 Waters Pl; Bronx, NY 10461; (718) 892-0808; **BDCERT:** Psyc 81; ChAP 87; **MS:** Creighton U 76; **RES:** Bellevue Hosp Ctr, New York, NY 76-79; **FEL:** ChAP, Bellevue Hosp Ctr, New York, NY 79-81; **HMO:** None

⬚ ⬚ ⬚

Gorman, Lauren (MD)　　Psyc
Columbia-Presbyterian Med Ctr
2700 Arlington Ave; Bronx, NY 10463; (718) 548-0568; **BDCERT:** Psyc 83; **MS:** Columbia P&S 77; **RES:** Psyc, Mount Sinai Med Ctr, New York, NY 82; **FEL:** Montefiore Med Ctr, Bronx, NY 82-84; **HMO:** None

⬚ ⬚ ⬚ ⬚ ⬚ ⬚ ⬚ ⬚ 2-4 Weeks

Hirschowitz, Jack (MD)　　Psyc
VA Med Ctr-Bronx
VA Medical Ctr, 130 W Kingsbridge Rd; Bronx, NY 10468; (718) 579-1627; **MS:** South Africa 69; **RES:** Psyc, Groote Schuur Hosp, Cape Town, South Africa 73-76; **FAP:** Sr Prof Psyc Mt Sinai Sch Med; *SI: Biological Psychiatry; Schizophrenia*

⬚ ⬚ ⬚ ⬚

Kennedy, Gary (MD)　　Psyc
Montefiore Med Ctr
Geriatric Associates Practice, 111 E 210th St; Bronx, NY 10467; (718) 920-4236; **BDCERT:** Psyc 80; **MS:** U Tex San Antonio 75; **RES:** U Hosp-S TX Med Ctr, San Antonio, TX 75-79; **FEL:** Ger, Montefiore Med Ctr, Bronx, NY 79-83; **FAP:** Prof Albert Einstein Coll Med; *SI: Depression; Dementia*

⬚ ⬚ ⬚ ⬚ ⬚ 2-4 Weeks

Lebinger, Martin (MD)　　Psyc
Bronx Psych Ctr
1540 Pelham Pkwy South 1A; Bronx, NY 10461; (718) 518-0222; **BDCERT:** Psyc 80; **MS:** Albert Einstein Coll Med 76; **RES:** Psyc, Montefiore Med Ctr, Bronx, NY 76-79; **FEL:** Psychotherapy, Long Island Jewish Med Ctr, New Hyde Park, NY 79-81; **FAP:** Assoc Clin Prof Albert Einstein Coll Med; *SI: Depression; Panic Disorder & Anxiety*

LANG: Yd; ⬚ ⬚ ⬚ ⬚ ⬚ ⬚ 1 Week

Meyers, Donald (MD)　　Psyc
Columbia-Presbyterian Med Ctr
4560 Delafield Ave; Bronx, NY 10471; (718) 548-7979; **BDCERT:** Psyc 70; **MS:** Jefferson Med Coll 50; **RES:** Bellevue Hosp Ctr, New York, NY 54; **FEL:** Psychoanalysis, Columbia-Presbyterian Med Ctr, New York, NY 68; **FAP:** Clin Prof Columbia P&S; *SI: Psychoanalysis; Psychotherapy*

⬚ ⬚ ⬚ A Few Days

Meyers, Helen (MD)　　Psyc
Columbia-Presbyterian Med Ctr
4560 Delafield Ave; Riverdale, NY 10471; (718) 548-7979; **MS:** NYU Sch Med 49; **RES:** Bellevue Hosp Ctr, New York, NY 51-54; **FAP:** Prof Psyc Columbia P&S

⬚ ⬚ 2-4 Weeks

Muhlbauer, Helen (MD)　　Psyc
Bronx Lebanon Hosp Ctr
Bronx Lebanon Hospital Center, 1276 Franklin Ave; Bronx, NY 10456; (718) 901-8222; **BDCERT:** Psyc 91; **MS:** Albert Einstein Coll Med 77; **RES:** Psyc, Albert Einstein Med Ctr, Bronx, NY 78-81; **FAP:** Asst Prof Albert Einstein Coll Med; **HOSP:** Beth Israel Med Ctr; *SI: Women's Issues; Emergency Psychiatry*

LANG: Yd, Heb; ⬚ ⬚ ⬚ ⬚ ⬚ ⬚ ⬚

Osei-Tutu, John (MD)　　Psyc
Bronx Lebanon Hosp Ctr
1276 Fulton Ave; Bronx, NY 10451; (718) 901-6133; **BDCERT:** Psyc 90; AdP 93; **MS:** Ghana 76; **HMO:** Aetna Hlth Plan Blue Cross & Blue Shield

Guide to symbols and abbreviations can be found on pages 110-113.

459

Smith, Michael O (MD)   Psyc
Lincoln Med & Mental Hlth Ctr

349 E 140th St; Bronx, NY 10454; (718) 993-3100; **MS:** UC San Francisco 68; **RES:** Psyc, Albert Einstein Med Ctr, Bronx, NY 72; **FAP:** Asst Prof NY Med Coll; **SI:** *Addiction Medicine; Acupuncture*

LANG: Sp; 🦽 🈸 🔲 ♿ 🏨 Mcr Mcd   Immediately

PULMONARY DISEASE

Aldrich, Thomas (MD)   Pul
Montefiore Med Ctr

111 E 210th St; Bronx, NY 10467; (718) 920-6087; **BDCERT:** IM 78; Pul 80; **MS:** U Minn 75; **RES:** IM, UC Irvine Med Ctr, Orange, CA 75-78; **FEL:** A&I/Pul, U of VA Health Sci Ctr, Charlottesville, VA 78-80; Respiratory Physiology, U of VA Health Sci Ctr, Charlottesville, VA 78-80; **FAP:** Prof & Dir Pul Albert Einstein Coll Med; **SI:** *Asthma/Chronic Obstructive Pulmonary Disease; Sickle Cell Lung Disease;* **HMO:** Prucare Oxford US Hlthcre PHS GHI +

🦽 🔲 ♿ 🏨 S Mcr   A Few Days 💳 **VISA** 💳

Casper, Theodore (MD)   Pul
Westchester Square Med Ctr

1180 Morris Park Ave; Bronx, NY 10461; (718) 892-1200; **BDCERT:** IM 83; Pul 83; **MS:** Columbia P&S 80; **RES:** St Luke's Roosevelt Hosp Ctr, New York, NY 80-83; **FEL:** Pul, St Luke's Roosevelt Hosp Ctr, New York, NY 83; **FAP:** Albert Einstein Coll Med; **HOSP:** Montefiore Med Ctr-Weiler/Einstein Div; **HMO:** US Hlthcre Blue Choice HealthNet

🦽 🔲 ♿ 🏨 Mcr   Immediately

Ernst, Jerome (MD)   Pul
Bronx Lebanon Hosp Ctr

1770 Grand Concourse; Bronx, NY 10457; (718) 590-1800; **BDCERT:** IM 78; Pul 82; **MS:** Israel 69; **RES:** Med, Montefiore Med Ctr, Bronx, NY 70-72; **FEL:** Pul, Montefiore Med Ctr, Bronx, NY 75-77; **FAP:** Assoc Prof Med Albert Einstein Coll Med; **SI:** *AIDS;* **HMO:** Most

LANG: Sp, Heb, Itl, Fr; 🦽 🔲 ♿ 🏨 Mcr Mcd   2-4 Weeks

Klapper, Philip (MD)   Pul
Montefiore Med Ctr

3777 Independence Ave; Riverdale, NY 10463; (718) 884-2000; **BDCERT:** IM 86; Pul 90; **MS:** Albert Einstein Coll Med 83; **RES:** Montefiore Med Ctr, Bronx, NY 83-86; **FEL:** Pul, Univ Hosp SUNY Bklyn, Brooklyn, NY 88-90; CCM, Montefiore Med Ctr, Bronx, NY 90-91; **FAP:** Clin Instr Albert Einstein Coll Med; **HOSP:** Lawrence Hosp; **SI:** *Asthma; Emphysema;* **HMO:** Oxford US Hlthcre GHI Prucare

LANG: Sp; 🦽 ♿ 🏨 S Mcr   A Few Days

Marino, William (MD)   Pul
Our Lady of Mercy Med Ctr

600 E 233rd St; Bronx, NY 10466; (718) 920-9268; **BDCERT:** Pul 84; CCM 97; **MS:** Albert Einstein Coll Med 77; **RES:** IM, Montefiore Med Ctr, Bronx, NY 77-80; **FEL:** Pul, Columbia-Presbyterian Med Ctr, New York, NY 80-82; **FAP:** Assoc Prof Med NY Med Coll; **SI:** *Emphysema; Asthma;* **HMO:** US Hlthcre Oxford CIGNA

🦽 🔲 Mcr Mcd WC NFI   2-4 Weeks

Pinsker, Kenneth (MD)   Pul
Montefiore Med Ctr

Montefiore Medical Center, 111 E 210th St 423; Bronx, NY 10467; (718) 920-6095; **BDCERT:** IM 72; Pul 76; **MS:** U Hlth Sci/Chicago Med Sch 68; **RES:** IM, Montefiore Med Ctr, Bronx, NY 68-70; IM, Jacobi Med Ctr, Bronx, NY 71; **FEL:** Pul, Montefiore Med Ctr, Bronx, NY 71-72; Pul, Montefiore Med Ctr, Bronx, NY 74-75; **FAP:** Prof Albert Einstein Coll Med; **SI:** *Asthma; Lung Cancer;* **HMO:** Oxford US Hlthcre GHI 1199 Bronx Health +

LANG: Sp; 🦽 🔲 ♿ 🏨 Mcr   A Few Days

Prezant, David (MD)   Pul
Montefiore Med Ctr

111 E 210th St Rm 423; Bronx, NY 10467; (718) 920-6054; **BDCERT:** IM 84; Pul 86; **MS:** Albert Einstein Coll Med 81; **RES:** Med, Harlem Hosp Ctr, New York, NY 81-84; **FEL:** PPul, Montefiore Med Ctr, Bronx, NY 84-85; **FAP:** Assoc Prof Albert Einstein Coll Med; **SI:** *Asthma; Smoke Inhalation;* **HMO:** GHI

🦽 S Mcr Mcd

Reichel, Joseph (MD)   **Pul**
Montefiore Med Ctr-Weiler/Einstein Div
1825 Eastchester Rd; Bronx, NY 10461; (718) 904-2983; **BDCERT:** IM 63; **MS:** NYU Sch Med 56; **RES:** Bellevue Hosp Ctr, New York, NY 56-58; Mount Sinai Med Ctr, New York, NY 58-59; **FEL:** Pul, Montefiore Med Ctr, Bronx, NY 59-60; **FAP:** Prof Albert Einstein Coll Med; **HOSP:** Jacobi Med Ctr; **SI:** *Obstructive Lung Diseases; Cough;* **HMO:** Oxford GHI Blue Choice HealthNet United Healthcare +

LANG: Yd, Sp; 🔲 🔲 🔲 🔲 🔲 🔲 🔲   A Few Days

Sender, Joel (MD)   **Pul**
St Barnabas Hosp-Bronx
2016 Bronxdale Ave 301; Bronx, NY 10462; (718) 409-2222; **BDCERT:** Pul 80; **MS:** Albany Med Coll 75; **RES:** Mount Sinai Med Ctr, New York, NY 75-78; **FEL:** Pul, Mount Sinai Med Ctr, New York, NY 78-80; **SI:** *Asthma; Sarcoidosis;* **HMO:** Oxford GHI Aetna-US Healthcare United Healthcare Magnacare +

LANG: Sp; 🔲 🔲 🔲 🔲 🔲   1 Week

RADIATION ONCOLOGY

Beitler, Jonathan (MD)   **RadRO**
Montefiore Med Ctr
Dept of Radiology/Oncology, 111 E 210th St; Bronx, NY 10467; (718) 920-4942; **BDCERT:** RadRO 90; **MS:** Med Coll PA 82; **RES:** S, Univ Hosp SUNY Bklyn, Brooklyn, NY 82-85; RadRO, Mem Sloan Kettering Cancer Ctr, New York, NY 85-88; **HOSP:** Montefiore Med Ctr-Weiler/Einstein Div; **SI:** *Head and Neck Cancer; Gynecologic Cancers;* **HMO:** Oxford HIP Network US Hlthcre

LANG: Sp; 🔲 🔲 🔲 🔲 🔲 🔲   A Few Days *VISA* 🔲

Bodner, William (MD)   **RadRO**
Our Lady of Mercy Med Ctr
Our Lady of Mercy Med Ctr, 600 E 233rd St; Bronx, NY 10466; (718) 920-9204; **BDCERT:** RadRO 96; **MS:** Bowman Gray 87

Del Rowe, John (MD)   **RadRO**
Montefiore Med Ctr
111 E 210th St; Bronx, NY 10467; (718) 920-4140; **BDCERT:** RadRO 84; **MS:** Hahnemann U 79; **RES:** Path CP, New York University Med Ctr, New York, NY 79-80; RadRO, New York University Med Ctr, New York, NY 80; **SI:** *Lung Cancer;* **HMO:** Oxford HIP Network GHI Aetna Hlth Plan US Hlthcre +

LANG: Sp; 🔲 🔲 🔲 🔲 🔲 🔲 🔲   Immediately 🔲 *VISA* 🔲 🔲

Hilaris, Basil (MD)   **RadRO**
Our Lady of Mercy Med Ctr
Radiation Oncology & Clinical Research Associates, 600 E 233rd St; Bronx, NY 10466; (718) 920-9750; **BDCERT:** RadRO 68; **MS:** Greece 55; **RES:** Rad, Mem Sloan Kettering Cancer Ctr, New York, NY 57-59; **FAP:** Chrmn NY Med Coll; **HOSP:** St Agnes Hosp; **SI:** *Prostate Implants; Stereotactic Radiosurgery;* **HMO:** Oxford US Hlthcre Blue Choice

LANG: Grk, Fr, Sp, Chi, Ar; 🔲 🔲 🔲 🔲 🔲 🔲   Immediately

Vikram, Bhadrasain (MD)RadRO
Montefiore Med Ctr
3335 Steuben Ave; Bronx, NY 10467; (718) 920-5280; **BDCERT:** Rad 78; **MS:** India 79; **RES:** Mem Sloan Kettering Cancer Ctr, New York, NY 75-78; **HOSP:** Maimonides Med Ctr

🔲 🔲 🔲 🔲 🔲 🔲 🔲 🔲   Immediately 🔲 *VISA* 🔲 🔲

RADIOLOGY

Amis Jr, E Stephen (MD)   **Rad**
Montefiore Med Ctr
111 E 210th St; Bronx, NY 10467; (718) 920-5113; **BDCERT:** U 75; Rad 79; **MS:** Northwestern U 67; **RES:** U, Naval Med Ctr, San Diego, CA 68-72; DR, Naval Med Ctr, San Diego, CA 75-78; **FEL:** U Rad, Mass Gen Hosp, Boston, MA 80-81; **FAP:** Prof Rad Albert Einstein Coll Med; **HOSP:** Jacobi Med Ctr; **SI:** *Radiology of urinary tract*

🔲 🔲 🔲 🔲 🔲 🔲 🔲 🔲

Guide to symbols and abbreviations can be found on pages 110-113.

461

Bello, Jacqueline A (MD)   Rad
Montefiore Med Ctr

111 E 210th St; Bronx, NY 10467; (718) 920-4030; **BDCERT:** Rad 84; NRad 97; **MS:** Columbia P&S 80; **RES:** Rad, Columbia-Presbyterian Med Ctr, New York, NY 81-84; **FAP:** Prof Albert Einstein Coll Med; **HMO:** GHI Oxford Blue Cross Mastercare Magnacare +

🦽 🆂🅾 🅲 📷 🎬 🆂 Mcr Mcd WC NFi A Few Days **VISA** 💳 📇

Bernstein, Robert (MD)   Rad
Montefiore Med Ctr-Weiler/Einstein Div

Albert Einstein Hospital ——Radiology Dept, 1825 Eastchester Rd; Bronx, NY 10461; (718) 904-2965; **BDCERT:** Rad 65; **MS:** Albert Einstein Coll Med 60; **RES:** NY Hosp-Cornell Med Ctr, New York, NY 61-64; Hosp of U Penn, Philadelphia, PA 60-61; **FAP:** Chf Rad Albert Einstein Coll Med

🦽 Immediately

Buchbinder, Shalom (MD)   Rad
Montefiore Med Ctr

Montefiore Medical Center, 1625 Poplar St 100; Bronx, NY 10461; (718) 405-8440; **BDCERT:** Rad 86; **MS:** Albert Einstein Coll Med 81; **RES:** Albert Einstein Med Ctr, Bronx, NY 82-85; **FAP:** Assoc Prof Albert Einstein Coll Med; *SI: Mammography; Breast Disease*; **HMO:** Oxford Blue Choice GHI PHS US Hlthcre +

🦽 📷 🎬 🆂 Mcr Mcd WC NFi A Few Days **VISA** 💳

Geffen, Merwin (MD)   Rad
Our Lady of Mercy Med Ctr

600 E 233rd St; Bronx, NY 10466; (718) 920-9056; **BDCERT:** Rad 61; **MS:** Switzerland 55; **RES:** Rad, Montefiore Med Ctr, Bronx, NY 58-59; **FEL:** Rad, Montefiore Med Ctr, Bronx, NY; Our Lady of Mercy Med Ctr, Bronx, NY

Haramati, Linda (MD)   Rad
Jacobi Med Ctr

Pelham Pkwy South; Bronx, NY 10461; (718) 918-4595; **BDCERT:** DR 90; **MS:** Albert Einstein Coll Med 85; **RES:** IM, Maimonides Med Ctr, Brooklyn, NY 85; DR, Montefiore Med Ctr, Bronx, NY 86-90; **FEL:** Rad, Columbia-Presbyterian Med Ctr, New York, NY 90-91; **FAP:** Assoc Prof Rad Albert Einstein Coll Med; **HOSP:** Montefiore Med Ctr; *SI: Chest CT; Lung Cancer*

🦽 📷 🎬 Mcr Mcd WC Immediately

Haramati, Nogah (MD)   Rad
Montefiore Med Ctr

11 E 210th St; Bronx, NY 10467; (718) 920-4626; **BDCERT:** DR 90; **MS:** SUNY Hlth Sci Ctr 85; **RES:** Montefiore Med Ctr, Bronx, NY 86-90; **FEL:** Rad, Columbia-Presbyterian Med Ctr, New York, NY 90-91; **FAP:** Assoc Prof Albert Einstein Coll Med; **HOSP:** Jacobi Med Ctr; *SI: Orthopaedics; Rheumatology*; **HMO:** Empire Aetna Hlth Plan Oxford CIGNA US Hlthcre +

LANG: Sp, Fr, Ger, Ar, Chi; 🦽 🆂🅾 🅲 🎬 🆂 Mcr Mcd WC NFi Immediately ▦ **VISA** 💳 📇

Koenigsberg, Mordecai (MD) Rad
Montefiore Med Ctr

Einstein Radiology Group, 1825 Eastchester Rd; Bronx, NY 10461; (718) 904-2322; **BDCERT:** NuM 73; DR 74; **MS:** Albert Einstein Coll Med 63; **RES:** Ped, Jacobi Med Ctr, Bronx, NY 64-66; DR, Jacobi Med Ctr, Bronx, NY 70-74; **FAP:** Prof Albert Einstein Coll Med; *SI: Ultrasound*; **HMO:** Most

LANG: Sp; 🦽 📷 🎬 Mcr Mcd WC NFi A Few Days ▦ **VISA** 💳

Pritzker, Henry (MD)   Rad
Montefiore Med Ctr

111 E 210th St; Bronx, NY 10467; (718) 920-4865; **BDCERT:** Rad 68; **MS:** Albert Einstein Coll Med 60; **RES:** Rad, Montefiore Med Ctr, Bronx, NY 64-67; **FEL:** PR, Columbia-Presbyterian Med Ctr, New York, NY; **FAP:** Assoc Prof PR Albert Einstein Coll Med; *SI: Pediatric Radiology; Neonatal Radiology*

LANG: Sp, Ger; 🦽 🎬 Mcr Mcd WC A Few Days

Radparvar, Dariush (MD)   Rad
Bronx Lebanon Hosp Ctr

1650 Selwyn Ave; Bronx, NY 10457; (718) 960-1276; **BDCERT:** Rad 84; **MS:** Iran 77; **RES:** RadRO, Kings County Hosp Ctr, Brooklyn, NY 78-81; **FEL:** RadRO, Univ Hosp SUNY Bklyn, Brooklyn, NY 81-84

Rozenblit, Alla (MD)   Rad
Montefiore Med Ctr

111 E 210th St; Bronx, NY 10467; (718) 920-4396; **BDCERT:** Rad 84; **MS:** Russia 71; **RES:** Long Island Jewish Med Ctr, New Hyde Park, NY 81-84; **FEL:** Rad, Long Island Jewish Med Ctr, New Hyde Park, NY; **FAP:** Assoc Prof Albert Einstein Coll Med; *SI: CT and Angiography of Aorta; CT—MRI Liver;* **HMO:** Health First GHI Blue Cross & Blue Shield PHCS Sanus +

LANG: Sp, Rus, Chi, Itl, Sgn; 🚹 💲 Mcr Mcd WC NFI
1 Week **VISA** 💳 💳

Spindola-Franco, Hugo (MD) Rad
Montefiore Med Ctr

Radiology/Cardiac Radiology, 111 E 210th St; Bronx, NY 10467; (718) 920-4852; **BDCERT:** Rad 70; **MS:** Mexico 62; **RES:** Rad, Montefiore Med Ctr, Bronx, NY 67-70; **FEL:** Cv, Peter Bent Brigham Hosp, Boston, MA 70-71; **FAP:** Prof Rad Albert Einstein Coll Med; *SI: Cardiac MRI, Coronary Arteriography; Congenital Heart Diseases*

LANG: Sp; 🚹 📷 🎥 🏠 Mcr Mcd WC NFI Immediately
💳 **VISA** 💳 💳

Stern, Harvey (MD)   Rad
Bronx Lebanon Hosp Ctr

1650 Grand Concourse; Bronx, NY 10457; (718) 518-5030; **BDCERT:** Rad 75; **MS:** Albert Einstein Coll Med 71; **RES:** RadRO, Bronx Muncipal Hosp Ctr, Bronx, NY 72-75; **FAP:** Asst Prof Rad Albert Einstein Coll Med; *SI: Nuclear Medicine;* **HMO:** Health First ABC Health Bronx Health Aetna-US Healthcare Blue Cross & Blue Shield +

LANG: Sp, Rus; 🚹 🚿 🌙 📷 🎥 🏠 💲 Mcr Mcd WC NFI
A Few Days

Wolf, Ellen L (MD)   Rad
Montefiore Med Ctr

111 E 210th St; Bronx, NY 10467; (718) 920-4851; **BDCERT:** Rad 76; **MS:** Mt Sinai Sch Med 72; **RES:** Columbia-Presbyterian Med Ctr, New York, NY 73-74; Johns Hopkins Hosp, Baltimore, MD 74-76; **FEL:** PR, Columbia-Presbyterian Med Ctr, New York, NY 76-78; **FAP:** Assoc Lecturer Rad Albert Einstein Coll Med; **HMO:** Oxford US Hlthcre Sanus Blue Choice Magnacare +

LANG: Sp; 🚹 🚿 🌙 📷 🏠 Mcr Mcd WC NFI
Immediately

Zelefsky, Melvin (MD)   Rad
Jacobi Med Ctr

1400 Pelham Pkwy South; Bronx, NY 10461; (718) 918-4595; **BDCERT:** Rad 65; NuM 74; **MS:** Albert Einstein Coll Med 60; **RES:** Rad, Jacobi Med Ctr, Bronx, NY 61-63; **FEL:** Pul Rad, Jacobi Med Ctr, Bronx, NY; **FAP:** Prof Rad Albert Einstein Coll Med; *SI: Pulmonary Radiology*

🚹 📷 🏠 Mcr Mcd WC NFI Immediately

REPRODUCTIVE ENDOCRINOLOGY

Koren, Zeev (MD)   RE
Montefiore Med Ctr-Weiler/Einstein Div

1695 Eastchester Rd Ste L2; Bronx, NY 10461; (718) 904-2797; **BDCERT:** ObG 72; **MS:** Israel 53; **RES:** Hadassah Med Sch, 54-55; Hadassah Med Sch, 58-60; **FEL:** ObG, Univ of Michigan, , MI 66-68; **FAP:** Prof Albert Einstein Coll Med

Guide to symbols and abbreviations can be found on pages 110-113.

463

RHEUMATOLOGY

Barland, Peter (MD)   Rhu
Montefiore Med Ctr
111 E 210th St; Bronx, NY 10467; (718) 920-5455; **BDCERT:** IM 67; Rhu 72; **MS:** Albert Einstein Coll Med 59; **RES:** Strong Mem Hosp, Rochester, NY 59-60; IM, Jacobi Med Ctr, Bronx, NY 61-63; **FEL:** Albert Einstein Med Ctr, Bronx, NY 60-61; **FAP:** Prof Med Albert Einstein Coll Med; *SI: Vasculitis; Lupus;* **HMO:** Oxford Empire Blue Cross & Shield Health First Carpenters NYLCare +

🚹 🔒 🛏 Mcr   2-4 Weeks ▩ **VISA** ●

Cavaliere, Ludovico (MD)   Rhu
Lincoln Med & Mental Hlth Ctr
234 E 149th St; Bronx, NY 10451; (718) 579-4769; **BDCERT:** IM 93; Rhu 94; **MS:** Italy 85; **RES:** Metropolitan Hosp Ctr, New York, NY 86-89; **FEL:** RE, Metropolitan Hosp Ctr, New York, NY 89-91; **HOSP:** Westchester Square Med Ctr

🚹 🔒 🛏 Mcr Mcd   2-4 Weeks

Diamond, Betty A (MD)   Rhu
Montefiore Med Ctr-Weiler/Einstein Div
1300 Morris Park Ave Rm 405; Bronx, NY 10461; (718) 430-2811; **BDCERT:** IM 76; **MS:** Harvard Med Sch 73; **RES:** IM, Colum-Presby Hosp, New York, NY 73-76; **HOSP:** Montefiore Med Ctr; *SI: Lupus*

🚹

Fomberstein, Barry (MD)   Rhu
Our Lady of Mercy Med Ctr
600 E 233rd St; Bronx, NY 10466; (718) 920-9168; **BDCERT:** IM 79; Rhu 82; **MS:** Albert Einstein Coll Med 76; **RES:** Med, Long Island Jewish Med Ctr, New Hyde Park, NY 76-79; **FEL:** Rhu, Long Island Jewish Med Ctr, New Hyde Park, NY 79-81; **FAP:** Asst Prof Med NY Med Coll; **HMO:** Aetna Hlth Plan Oxford Chubb CIGNA 1199 +

LANG: Sp; 🚹 🔒 🛏 🛏 $ Mcr   A Few Days

Keiser, Harold (MD)   Rhu
Montefiore Med Ctr
1575 Blondell Ave Ste 200; Bronx, NY 10461; (718) 405-8309; **BDCERT:** IM 72; **MS:** NYU Sch Med 64; **RES:** IM, Cleveland Metro Gen Hosp, Cleveland, OH 64-68; **FEL:** Rhu, Albert Einstein Med Ctr, Bronx, NY; **HOSP:** Jacobi Med Ctr; **HMO:** Blue Choice CIGNA HealthNet Sanus US Hlthcre +

🚹 🔒 🛏 🛏 $ Mcr   A Few Days ▩ **VISA** ● ▪

SURGERY

Agarwal, Nanakram (MD)   S
Our Lady of Mercy Med Ctr
600 E 233rd St; Bronx, NY 10466; (718) 920-9143; **BDCERT:** S 82; **MS:** India 89; **RES:** Our Lady of Mercy Med Ctr, Bronx, NY; **FEL:** Westchester County Med Ctr, Valhalla, NY; **HOSP:** Westchester Med Ctr

Balsano, Nicholas (MD)   S
Our Lady of Mercy Med Ctr
Our Lady of Mercy Hosp, Dept of Surgery, 600 E 233rd St; Bronx, NY 10466; (718) 823-1014; **BDCERT:** S 72; **MS:** Geo Wash U Sch Med 65; **RES:** Our Lady of Mercy Med Ctr, Bronx, NY 66-69; **FEL:** GVS, Our Lady of Mercy Med Ctr, Bronx, NY 69-70; **HMO:** Oxford HealthNet Chubb

🚹 🅲 🔒 🛏 🛏 Mcr Mcd WC NFI   A Few Days

Berlin, Arnold (MD)   S
North Central Bronx Hosp
Montefiore Medical Ctr, 111 E 210th St; Bronx, NY 10467; (718) 920-4321; **BDCERT:** S 88; **MS:** NYU Sch Med 72; **RES:** S, Montefiore Med Ctr, Bronx, NY 72-74; S, U Conn Hlth Ctr, Farmington, CT 75-78; **FAP:** Assoc Albert Einstein Coll Med; **HOSP:** Montefiore Med Ctr; *SI: Geriatrics; Colorectal Surgery;* **HMO:** Aetna Hlth Plan Oxford Blue Cross & Blue Shield CIGNA Bronx Health +

LANG: Sp; 🚹 🔒 🛏 🛏 $ Mcr Mcd WC NFI
A Few Days

Burger, Steven (MD)   S
Westchester Square Med Ctr
1803 Mahan Ave; Bronx, NY 10461; (718) 863-3722; **BDCERT:** S 88; **MS:** Albert Einstein Coll Med 81; **RES:** Jacobi Med Ctr, Bronx, NY 81-86; **FAP:** Asst Prof Albert Einstein Coll Med; **HOSP:** Montefiore Med Ctr; **SI:** *Laparoscopic Surgery;* **HMO:** Oxford Aetna-US Healthcare GHI Blue Cross & Blue Shield +

♿ 📷 📆 S Mcr WC NFI   1 Week

Carnevale, Nino (MD)   S
Montefiore Med Ctr-Weiler/Einstein Div
1695 Easchester Rd Ste 304; Bronx, NY 10461; (718) 824-2001; **BDCERT:** S 71; **MS:** UMDNJ-NJ Med Sch, Newark 63; **RES:** S, Montefiore Med Ctr, Bronx, NY 64-68; **FAP:** Assoc Prof S Albert Einstein Coll Med; **HOSP:** Westchester Square Med Ctr; **HMO:** Aetna-US Healthcare CIGNA Oxford GHI Most +

Cayten, C Gene (MD)   S
Our Lady of Mercy Med Ctr
600 E 233rd St Fl 4; Bronx, NY 10466; (718) 920-9522; **BDCERT:** S 75; **MS:** NY Med Coll 67; **RES:** S, Hosp of U Penn, Philadelphia, PA 67-73; **FAP:** Prof S NY Med Coll; **HOSP:** Westchester Med Ctr; **SI:** *Biliary Disease; Breast Surgery;* **HMO:** GHI Oxford US Hlthcre Empire Blue Cross & Shield Prucare +

LANG: Sp; ♿ 📷 🚗 📆 Mcr Mcd WC NFI   A Few Days

Curras, Ernesto (MD)   S
St Barnabas Hosp-Bronx
St Barnabas Surgical Group PC, 4422 3rd Ave; Bronx, NY 10457; (718) 960-6493; **BDCERT:** S 85; **MS:** Spain 78; **RES:** Bronx Lebanon Hosp Ctr, Bronx, NY 79-84; **FAP:** Asst Prof NY Coll Osteo Med; **SI:** *Breast Diseases; Hernia Surgery;* **HMO:** Oxford Aetna Hlth Plan US Hlthcre

LANG: Sp, Itl; ♿ 📷 🚗 📆 S Mcr Mcd WC NFI
A Few Days

Delany, Harry (MD)   S
Montefiore Med Ctr-Weiler/Einstein Div
1575 Blondell Ave 125; Bronx, NY 10461; (718) 918-5565; **BDCERT:** S 64; **MS:** Columbia P&S 58; **RES:** Bellevue Hosp Ctr, New York, NY 60; Montefiore Med Ctr, Bronx, NY 61-63; **HOSP:** Jacobi Med Ctr

♿ 📷 🚗 📆 S Mcr Mcd WC NFI   Immediately

Deluca, Frank Ross (MD)   S
Westchester Square Med Ctr
1874 Pelham Pkwy South Lk; Bronx, NY 10461; (718) 824-4300; **BDCERT:** S 54; **MS:** NYU Sch Med 47; **RES:** Harlem Hosp Ctr, New York, NY 50; Harlem Hosp Ctr, New York, NY 52; **HOSP:** Montefiore Med Ctr-Weiler/Einstein Div; **HMO:** Aetna Hlth Plan Blue Choice Blue Cross & Blue Shield CIGNA Metlife +

📷 📆 S Mcr WC   Immediately

Flax, Herschel (MD)   S
Montefiore Med Ctr
1575 Blondell Ave Ste 100; Bronx, NY 10461; (718) 405-8244; **BDCERT:** S 97; **MS:** South Africa 64; **RES:** U of London, London, England 66-74; Albert Einstein Med Ctr, Bronx, NY 74-75; **FAP:** Clin Prof S Albert Einstein Coll Med; **HOSP:** N Shore Univ Hosp-Manhasset; **SI:** *Breast Cancer; Colorectal Cancer;* **HMO:** Oxford Empire Prucare NYLCare Aetna Hlth Plan +

LANG: Sp, Prt, Itl, Heb, Yd; ♿ 📷 🚗 📆 S Mcr Mcd WC   A Few Days

Gliedman, Marvin L (MD)   S
Montefiore Med Ctr
111 E 210th St; Bronx, NY 10467; (718) 920-4716; **BDCERT:** S 63; **MS:** SUNY Downstate 54; **RES:** S, Kings County Hosp Ctr, Brooklyn, NY 55-56; S, US Naval Hosp, Brooklyn, NY 56-58; **FEL:** Kings County Hosp Ctr, Brooklyn, NY 58-60; **FAP:** Prof S Albert Einstein Coll Med; **SI:** *Biliary Tract Disease; Pancreatic Disease;* **HMO:** Aetna-US Healthcare Blue Shield HIP Network GHI Oxford +

📷 🚗 📆 S Mcr Mcd NFI   A Few Days

Greenstein, Stuart (MD)   S
Montefiore Med Ctr

111 E 210th St; Bronx, NY 10467; (718) 920-
4321; **BDCERT:** S 85; **MS:** Harvard Med Sch 79;
RES: New York University Med Ctr, New York, NY
79-80; Univ of Med & Dent NJ Hosp, Newark, NJ
80-84; **FEL:** GVS, Hosp of U Penn, Philadelphia, PA
84-85; Transplant S, Univ Hosp SUNY Bklyn,
Brooklyn, NY 85-86; **FAP:** Assoc Prof Albert
Einstein Coll Med; **SI:** *Kidney Transplants; Dialysis
Surgery;* **HMO:** US Hlthcre CIGNA Aetna Hlth Plan
Prucare Oxford +

LANG: Sp, Heb; 🖔 🖭 🖩 🏛 🆂 Mcr Mcd WC NFl
Immediately

Gumbs, Milton (MD)   S
Bronx Lebanon Hosp Ctr

1650 Grand Concourse; Bronx, NY 10457; (718)
960-1256; **BDCERT:** S 74; **MS:** Italy 67; **RES:**
Bronx Lebanon Hosp Ctr, Bronx, NY 69-73; **FAP:**
Assoc Lecturer Albert Einstein Coll Med; **SI:** *Breast
Surgery; Gastrointestinal Surgery;* **HMO:** Oxford US
Hlthcre GHI Empire Blue Cross & Shield ABC Health
+

LANG: Sp, Itl; 🖔 🖭 🖩 🏛 🆂 Mcr Mcd WC NFl
A Few Days

Hodgson, W John B (MD)   S
Montefiore Med Ctr

Montefiore Medical Center, Dept of Surgery, 1575
Blondell Ave Ste 125; Bronx, NY 10461; (718)
405-8239; **BDCERT:** S 75; **MS:** England 64; **RES:** S,
U of London, London, England 64-73; **FEL:** GI S,
Mount Sinai Med Ctr, New York, NY 73-74; **FAP:**
Prof S NY Med Coll; **HOSP:** Montefiore Med Ctr-
Weiler/Einstein Div; **SI:** *Laparoscopic Surgery;
Colorectal & Liver Cancer;* **HMO:** Aetna Hlth Plan
GHI Oxford Prucare US Hlthcre +

LANG: Sp, Prt; 🖔 🖭 🖩 🏛 🆂 Mcr Mcd WC NFl
A Few Days **VISA** 💳 💳

Kaleya, Ronald (MD)   S
Montefiore Med Ctr

111 E 210th St; Bronx, NY 10467; (718) 920-
4327; **BDCERT:** S 87; **MS:** Cornell U 80; **RES:** S,
Albert Einstein Med Ctr, Bronx, NY 80-85; **FEL:** S
Onc, Mem Sloan Kettering Cancer Ctr, New York,
NY 85-87; **FAP:** Assoc Prof S Albert Einstein Coll
Med; **SI:** *Breast Cancer; Liver & Pancreatic Tumors;*
HMO: Most

LANG: Sp; 🖔 🖭 🖩 🏛 🆂 Mcr Mcd WC NFl 1 Week

Keolamphu, Narong (MD)   S
Our Lady of Mercy Med Ctr

280 Bedford Park Blvd; Bronx, NY 10458; (718)
365-9499; **BDCERT:** S 79; **MS:** Thailand 62

Lan, Sam (MD)   S
Montefiore Med Ctr-Weiler/Einstein Div

1180 Morris Park Ave; Bronx, NY 10461; (718)
655-9099; **BDCERT:** S 76; **MS:** South Africa 66;
RES: St Luke's Roosevelt Hosp Ctr, New York, NY
71-72; **HOSP:** Montclair Comm Hosp; **HMO:** Blue
Cross & Blue Shield HIP Network Travelers

LANG: Sp, Heb, Fr; 🖭 🖩 🏛 🆂 Mcr Mcd WC
Immediately

McElhinney, A James (MD)   S
VA Med Ctr-Bronx

VA Medical Center, 130 W Kingsbridge Rd; Bronx,
NY 10468; (718) 579-1605; **BDCERT:** S 70; **MS:**
Cornell U 54; **RES:** S, St Vincents Hosp & Med Ctr
NY, New York, NY 57-59; TS, VA Med Ctr-Bronx,
Bronx, NY 59-63; **FAP:** Prof S Mt Sinai Sch Med; **SI:**
Esophageal Disease; Cancer Surgery

🖔 🖭 🖩 🏛 Immediately

Pai, Narayan (MD)   S
Bronx Lebanon Hosp Ctr

1650 Selwyn Ave 5A; Bronx, NY 10457; (718)
960-1320; **BDCERT:** S 69; **MS:** India 61; **RES:**
Bronx Lebanon Hosp Ctr, Bronx, NY 64-68; **FEL:**
GVS, New York University Med Ctr, New York, NY
69; **SI:** *Poor Circulation-Bypass; Fistula-Grafts-
Dialysis;* **HMO:** Oxford Empire Oxford

🖔 🖭 🏛 🆂 Mcr Mcd WC NFl 1 Week

Plummer, Robert (MD)   S
Lincoln Med & Mental Hlth Ctr

4769 White Plains Rd; Bronx, NY 10470; (718)
324-2296; **BDCERT:** S 89; **MS:** UMDNJ-RW
Johnson Med Sch 83; **RES:** S, Harlem Hosp Ctr, New
York, NY 84-88; **FEL:** S, Harlem Hosp Ctr, New
York, NY 88-89; **FAP:** Asst Prof S NY Med Coll;
HOSP: St Joseph's Med Ctr-Yonkers

Porreca, Francis (MD)   S
Our Lady of Mercy Med Ctr

3219 E Tremont Ave; Bronx, NY 10461; (718)
792-8115; **BDCERT:** S 84; **MS:** Albert Einstein Coll
Med 78; **RES:** Montefiore Med Ctr, Bronx, NY 78-
83; **FEL:** GVS, Pennsylvania Hosp, Philadelphia, PA
83-84; **HOSP:** Westchester Square Med Ctr; **HMO:**
GHI Prucare Sanus Magnacare Blue Choice +

[symbols] Immediately [symbols] **VISA** [symbols]

Reynolds, Benedict (MD)   S
Westchester Square Med Ctr

1578 Williamsbridge Rd Fl 2; Bronx, NY 10461;
(718) 933-3366; **BDCERT:** S 56; **MS:** NYU Sch Med
48; **RES:** Bellevue Hosp Ctr, New York, NY 51-55;
FEL: NY Academy of Med, New York, NY; **HOSP:**
Our Lady of Mercy Med Ctr; *SI: Breast Surgery; Colon
Surgery;* **HMO:** GHI Blue Cross & Blue Shield Aetna
Hlth Plan Oxford

[symbols] Immediately

Sas, Norman (MD)   S
Montefiore Med Ctr

3220 Fairfield Ave; Riverdale, NY 10463; (718)
549-0700; **BDCERT:** S 80; **MS:** NY Med Coll 74;
RES: S, Montefiore Med Ctr, Bronx, NY 74-78;
HOSP: St Joseph's Med Ctr-Yonkers

Schechner, Richard (MD)   S
Montefiore Med Ctr

Transplant Surgery Department, 111 E 210th St;
Bronx, NY 10467; (718) 920-4718; **BDCERT:** S
91; **MS:** NY Med Coll 83; **RES:** Montefiore Med Ctr,
Bronx, NY 84-88; **FEL:** Pan-Transplantation,
University of Minnesota, Minneapolis, MN 88-89;
HOSP: Montefiore Med Ctr-Weiler/Einstein Div; *SI:
Transplant Surgery*

[symbols] Immediately [symbols] **VISA** [symbols]

Schwartz, Aaron (MD)   S
Montefiore Med Ctr

Montefiore Medical Ctr, 3400 Bainbridge Ave;
Bronx, NY 10467; (718) 920-5436; **BDCERT:** S
58; **MS:** NY Med Coll 50; **RES:** Beth Israel Med Ctr,
New York, NY 50-52; Montefiore Med Ctr, Bronx,
NY 54-57; **FEL:** S, Roswell Park Cancer Inst,
Buffalo, NY 57-58; **FAP:** Assoc Prof S Albert
Einstein Coll Med; *SI: Breast;* **HMO:** Oxford US
Hlthcre GHI Magnacare Travelers +

LANG: Sp, Ger, Yd; [symbols]
Immediately

Shapiro, Nella (MD)   S
Montefiore Med Ctr-Weiler/Einstein Div

1515 Jarret Pl; Bronx, NY 10461; (718) 409-
1155; **BDCERT:** S 80; Rad 89; **MS:** Albert Einstein
Coll Med 72; **RES:** S, Montefiore Med Ctr, Bronx, NY
72-76; **FAP:** Asst Prof Albert Einstein Coll Med;
HOSP: Montefiore Med Ctr; *SI: Breast Cancer;
Laparoscopic Surgery;* **HMO:** Metlife GHI Oxford
HealthNet US Hlthcre +

LANG: Sp, Fr; [symbols] Immediately
VISA [symbols]

Silver, Carl (MD)   S
Montefiore Med Ctr

111 E 210th St; Bronx, NY 10467; (718) 920-
4308; **BDCERT:** S 66; **MS:** SUNY Hlth Sci Ctr 59;
RES: IM, Montefiore Med Ctr, Bronx, NY 60-61; S,
Montefiore Med Ctr, Bronx, NY 61-65; **FAP:**
Lecturer S Albert Einstein Coll Med; **HMO:** Aetna
Hlth Plan CIGNA Empire HIP Network Metlife +

[symbols] Immediately

Tellis, Vivian (MD) S
Montefiore Med Ctr

Montefiore Medical Center, 111 E 210th St; Bronx, NY 10467; (718) 920-4718; **BDCERT:** S 69; **MS:** India 60; **RES:** Jersey City Med Ctr, Jersey City, NJ 63-65; Montefiore Med Ctr, Bronx, NY 66-68; **FEL:** Montefiore Med Ctr, Bronx, NY 68-70; **FAP:** Prof S Albert Einstein Coll Med; *SI: Kidney Transplantation; Dialysis;* **HMO:** US Hlthcre Prudential PHS

♿ 📷 🦽 🛏 Mcr Mcd WC NFI A Few Days

Veith, Frank (MD) S
Montefiore Med Ctr

Montefiore Med Ctr, 111 E 210th St; Bronx, NY 10467; (718) 920-4757; **BDCERT:** TS 68; **MS:** Cornell U 55; **RES:** Peter Bent Brigham Hosp, Boston, MA 55-60; **FEL:** Harvard Med Sch, Cambridge, MA 62-63; **FAP:** Prof S Albert Einstein Coll Med; **HOSP:** Long Island Coll Hosp; *SI: Abdominal Aortic Aneurysms; Carotid Disease;* **HMO:** Oxford Aetna Hlth Plan GHI Blue Cross & Blue Shield US Hlthcre +

LANG: Sp; ♿ 📷 🛏 S Mcr Mcd WC NFI 2-4 Weeks

THORACIC SURGERY

Attai, Lari (MD) TS
Montefiore Med Ctr

Montefiore Med Ctr, 3316 Rochambeau Ave 2nd Fl; Bronx, NY 10467; (718) 655-4900; **BDCERT:** TS 67; **MS:** Iran 57; **RES:** S, Morrisania City Hosp, New York, NY 59-62; TS, Montefiore Med Ctr, Bronx, NY 63-65; **FEL:** GVS, Newark Beth Israel Med Ctr, Newark, NJ; **FAP:** Assoc Lecturer S Albert Einstein Coll Med; *SI: Cardiac Surgery;* **HMO:** Oxford US Hlthcre HIP Network

📷 🦽 🛏 Mcr Mcd Immediately

Brodman, Richard (MD) TS
Montefiore Med Ctr

171 E Gunhill Rd; Bronx, NY 10467; (718) 920-1000; **BDCERT:** TS 78; S 76; **MS:** U Fla Coll Med 72; **RES:** S, Montefiore Med Ctr, Bronx, NY 72-76; TS, Montefiore Med Ctr, Bronx, NY 76-78; **FEL:** U FL Shands Hosp, Gainesville, FL 69-70; **FAP:** Prof Albert Einstein Coll Med; **HOSP:** Montefiore Med Ctr-Weiler/Einstein Div; *SI: Cardiac-Bypass Surgery; Lung Procedures;* **HMO:** Aetna Hlth Plan Oxford Blue Cross & Blue Shield GHI PHS +

LANG: Sp; ♿ 📷 🛏 S Mcr Mcd Immediately

Frater, Robert (MD) TS
Montefiore Med Ctr

1575 Blondell Ave 125; Bronx, NY 10461; (718) 405-8249; **BDCERT:** S 64; TS 66; **MS:** South Africa 52; **RES:** South Africa 53-54; Lewisham Hosp, London, England 54-55; **FEL:** TS, U MN Med Ctr, Minneapolis, MN 55-61; **FAP:** Prof Albert Einstein Coll Med; **HOSP:** Westchester Square Med Ctr; *SI: Valvular Heart Disease; Repair & Replacement;* **HMO:** Oxford US Hlthcre

♿ 📷 🦽 🛏 Mcr Mcd WC NFI A Few Days

Furman, Seymour (MD) TS
Montefiore Med Ctr

111 E 210th St; Bronx, NY 10467; (718) 920-4776; **BDCERT:** S 64; Cv 86; **MS:** SUNY Downstate 55; **RES:** S, Montefiore Med Ctr, Bronx, NY 56-60; TS, Baylor Coll Med, Houston, TX 62-63; **FAP:** Prof Albert Einstein Coll Med; *SI: Cardiac Pacemakers; Implantable Defibrillation;* **HMO:** United Payors Premier Blue Shield Montefiore IPA GHI +

LANG: Sp, Rus, Yd, Heb, Pol; ♿ 📷 🛏 Mcr Mcd
A Few Days **VISA** 💳

Gerst, Paul (MD) TS
Bronx Lebanon Hosp Ctr

1650 Grand Concourse; Bronx, NY 10457; (718) 588-5330; **BDCERT:** TS 62; **MS:** Columbia P&S 52; **RES:** S, Columbia-Presbyterian Med Ctr, New York, NY 56-60; TS, Columbia-Presbyterian Med Ctr, New York, NY 60-62; **FAP:** Lecturer S Albert Einstein Coll Med; *SI: Pacemakers*

♿ 📷 Mcr Mcd

Gold, Jeffrey P (MD)   TS
Montefiore Med Ctr

3400 Bainbridge Ave Flr5; Bronx, NY 10467;
(718) 920-7000; **BDCERT:** TS 86; S 85; **MS:**
Cornell U 74; **RES:** S, NY Hosp-Cornell Med Ctr,
New York, NY 78-83; TS, Brigham & Women's
Hosp, Boston, MA 83-84; **FEL:** PdS, Children's
Hosp, Boston, MA 84-85; **FAP:** Chrmn Cv Albert
Einstein Coll Med; *SI: Coronary Bypass; Birth Defects*;
HMO: Blue Cross & Blue Shield Oxford US Hlthcre
Sanus GHI +

LANG: Sp, Rus, Itl; ♿ 🏧 📞 📷 🐦 🏥 💲 Mcr Mcd WC
NFI A Few Days 💳 **VISA** 💳 💳

Merav, Avraham (MD)   TS
Montefiore Med Ctr

3316 Rochambeau Ave; Bronx, NY 10467; (718)
652-0100; **BDCERT:** TS 95; S 74; **MS:** Switzerland
64; **RES:** S, Montefiore Med Ctr, Bronx, NY 69-73;
FEL: TS, Montefiore Med Ctr, Bronx, NY 73-75;
FAP: Assoc Clin Prof TS Mt Sinai Sch Med

Rohman, Michael (MD)   TS
Lincoln Med & Mental Hlth Ctr

234 E 149th St; Bronx, NY 10451; (718) 579-
5900; **BDCERT:** TS 59; S 56; **MS:** Boston U 50; **RES:**
S, Mass Gen Hosp, Boston, MA 50-55; TS, Jacobi
Med Ctr, Bronx, NY 55-58; **FEL:** TS, Jacobi Med Ctr,
Bronx, NY 56-58; **FAP:** Prof S NYU Sch Med;
HOSP: Westchester Med Ctr; *SI: Lung Cancer; Cancer
of Esophagus*

♿ 📷 🐦 🏥 Mcr Mcd WC NFI Immediately

Sisto, Donato (MD)   TS
Montefiore Med Ctr

1575 Blondell Ave; Bronx, NY 10461; (718) 405-
8375; **BDCERT:** TS 84; **MS:** Italy 74; **RES:** S,
Montefiore Med Ctr, Bronx, NY 76-77; S, Mount
Sinai Med Ctr, New York, NY 78-81; **FEL:** TS,
Montefiore Med Ctr, Bronx, NY 81-83; **HMO:** Blue
Cross & Blue Shield CIGNA Metlife PHS

♿ 📷 🐦 🏥 Mcr Mcd Immediately

UROLOGY

Bekirov, Huseyin (MD)   U
Montefiore Med Ctr-Weiler/Einstein Div

1578 Williamsbridge Rd Fl 2; Bronx, NY 10461;
(718) 892-2100; **BDCERT:** U 77; **MS:** Bulgaria 61;
RES: U, Albert Einstein Med Ctr, Bronx, NY 72-75;
S, Albert Einstein Med Ctr, Bronx, NY 71-72;
HOSP: Westchester Square Med Ctr; **HMO:** Blue
Choice Oxford NYLCare

LANG: Bul, Trk, Rus, Itl, Sp; ♿ 📷 Mcr A Few Days

Cea, Philip (MD)   U
Westchester Square Med Ctr

1625 St Peters Ave; Bronx, NY 10461; (718) 822-
1152; **BDCERT:** U 80; **MS:** NY Med Coll 70; **RES:** S,
Metropolitan Hosp Ctr, New York, NY 70-72; U, St
Luke's Roosevelt Hosp Ctr, New York, NY 72-76;
HOSP: Our Lady of Mercy Med Ctr; **HMO:** Oxford
US Hlthcre GHI

♿ 📷 🐦 🏥 💲 Mcr A Few Days

Geisler, Edward (MD)   U
Bronx Lebanon Hosp Ctr

1770 Grand Concourse Ste 1F; Bronx, NY 10457;
(718) 901-8173; **BDCERT:** U 87; **MS:** Jefferson Med
Coll 78; **RES:** S, Beth Israel Hosp, New York, NY 78-
80; U, NYU, New York, NY 80-84; **FAP:** Asst Prof U
Albert Einstein Coll Med; *SI: Tumors; Impotence*;
HMO: US Hlthcre Oxford Health One Bronx Health

Gentile, Ralph (MD)   U
Montefiore Med Ctr

3130 Grand Concourse 1S; Bronx, NY 10458;
(718) 295-9400; **BDCERT:** U 64; **MS:** Columbia
P&S 56; **RES:** Columbia-Presbyterian Med Ctr, New
York, NY 58; Montefiore Med Ctr, Bronx, NY 61;
HOSP: Our Lady of Mercy Med Ctr; **HMO:** US
Hlthcre Oxford Blue Cross & Blue Shield

♿ 📞 📷 🐦 🏥 💲 Mcr Mcd 1 Week

Kahan, Norman (MD)   U
Montefiore Med Ctr

Montefiore Medical Ctr University Urology Faculty
Practice, 3400 Bainbridge Ave 5F; Bronx, NY
10467; (718) 920-4031; **BDCERT:** U 75; **MS:** NYU
Sch Med 66; **RES:** U, Montefiore Med Ctr, Bronx, NY
70-73; S, Montefiore Med Ctr, Bronx, NY 67-68;
FAP: Asst Prof Albert Einstein Coll Med; **HOSP:**
Community Hosp At Dobbs Ferry; **SI:** *Prostate
Cancer;* **HMO:** GHI US Hlthcre PHS CIGNA Health
First +

LANG: Sp; ♿ 📷 👍 💲 ▣ ▣ ▣ ▣   1 Week **VISA**
●

Laor, Eliahu (MD)   U
Montefiore Med Ctr-Weiler/Einstein Div
1695 Eastchester Rd 501; Bronx, NY 10461; (718)
904-1720; **BDCERT:** U 82; **MS:** France 74; **RES:**
Albert Einstein Med Ctr, Bronx, NY 75-77; Albert
Einstein Med Ctr, Bronx, NY 77-78; **FEL:** U, Albert
Einstein Med Ctr, Bronx, NY; **HOSP:** Westchester
Square Med Ctr; **HMO:** 1199 Blue Cross & Blue
Shield GHI

LANG: Fr, Yd, Ger; ♿ 📷 👍 ▦ 💲 ▣ ▣
Immediately **VISA**

Reid, Roberto (MD)   U
Montefiore Med Ctr
Assoceated Advanced Urology, 1695 Eastchester
Rd 306; Bronx, NY 10461; (718) 904-0222;
BDCERT: U 65; **MS:** Case West Res U 58; **RES:** VA
Med Ctr, Cleveland, OH 59-60; Jacobi Med Ctr,
Bronx, NY 60-63; **FAP:** Clin Prof U Albert Einstein
Coll Med; **HOSP:** Columbia-Presbyterian Med Ctr;
SI: *Female Urology; Urethral Stricture*

LANG: Sp, Ur, Heb; ♿ 📷 👍 ▦ 💲 ▣ ▣ ▣
Immediately **VISA**

Stein, Mark (MD)   U
Montefiore Med Ctr
171 E Gun Hill Rd; Bronx, NY 10467; (718) 518-
1108; **BDCERT:** U 92; **MS:** Yale U Sch Med 84; **RES:**
U, Montefiore Med Ctr, Bronx, NY 84-90; **HOSP:**
Beth Israel Med Ctr; **SI:** *Incontinence; Impotence;*
HMO: Aetna Hlth Plan Oxford Metlife GHI CIGNA
+

LANG: Sp, Rus; ♿ ▣ ☾ 📷 👍 ▦ 💲 ▣
A Few Days ▣ **VISA** ●

VASCULAR SURGERY (GENERAL)

Lyon, Ross (MD)   GVS
Montefiore Med Ctr
111 E 210th St; Bronx, NY 10467; (718) 920-
8861; **BDCERT:** S 90; GVS 93; **MS:** U Chicago-
Pritzker Sch Med 81; **RES:** S, Barnes Hosp, St Louis,
MO 82-83; S, UC San Diego Med Ctr, San Diego, CA
85-89; **FEL:** GVS, U Chicago Hosp, Chicago, IL 83-
85; Med Ctr LA U, New Orleans, LA 89-90; **FAP:**
Asst Prof Albert Einstein Coll Med; **HOSP:**
Montefiore Med Ctr-Weiler/Einstein Div; **SI:** *Arterial
and Venous Surgery; Endovascular Surgery;* **HMO:**
Aetna Hlth Plan Blue Cross & Blue Shield CIGNA
Oxford HealthNet +

LANG: Sp; ♿ 📷 👍 💲 ▣   1 Week

Rivers, Steven P (MD)   GVS
Montefiore Med Ctr
1575 Blondell Ave; Bronx, NY 10461; (718) 405-
8232; **BDCERT:** S 84; GVS 89; **MS:** U Md Sch Med
75; **RES:** S, Oregon Health Sci U Hosp, Portland, OR
83; **FEL:** GVS, Montefiore Med Ctr, Bronx, NY 83-
84; **FAP:** Assoc Prof Albert Einstein Coll Med;
HOSP: Jacobi Med Ctr; **HMO:** HIP Network Oxford
Aetna Hlth Plan GHI Prudential +

LANG: Sp; ♿ 📷 👍 ▦ 💲 ▣ ▣   A Few Days

Suggs, William (MD)   GVS
Montefiore Med Ctr
Montefiore Med Ctr-Vascular Surgery, 111 E 210th
St; Bronx, NY 10467; (718) 920-6338; **BDCERT:** S
90; GVS 93; **MS:** Bowman Gray 83; **RES:** Geo Wash
U Med Ctr, Washington, DC 83-89; **FEL:** GVS,
Emory U Hosp, Atlanta, GA 89-90; Emory U Hosp,
Atlanta, GA 90-91; **HOSP:** North Central Bronx
Hosp; **SI:** *Limb Salvage; Carotid Surgery*

LANG: Sp; ♿ 📷 ▦ 💲 ▣ ▣ ▣ ▣   Immediately

KINGS (BROOKLYN) COUNTY

THE BROOKLYN HOSPITAL CENTER

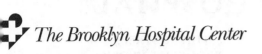 *The Brooklyn Hospital Center*

121 DEKALB AVENUE
BROOKLYN, NY 11201
PHONE (718) 855-TBHC

onsorship	Voluntary Not-for-Profit
eds	653 acute 48 bassinet
ccreditation	Joint Commission on Accreditation of Healthcare Organizations (JCAHO), Accreditation Councils for Graduate Medical Education and Continuing Medical Education

XCELLENCE

ie Brooklyn Hospital Center is a leading hospital and dynamic presence in New York City's largest rough. It is a member of The New York and Presbyterian Hospital Care Network and the academic id clinical affiliate of The New York Hospital-Cornell Medical Center.

UALITY

ie Hospital Center has a medical staff of 900 doctors who possess the highest quality of medical educa- n, certification, training, and skill. The physicians represent an impressive range of specialty care and e largest complement of primary care practitioners in the borough.

IGH STANDARDS IN MEDICAL EDUCATION

ist-graduate medical education is available in dentistry, emergency medicine, family practice, internal edicine, obstetrics/gynecology, oral and maxillofacial surgery, pathology, pediatrics, and surgery. Post- ictoral training is offered in numerous specialty areas.

ENTERS OF EXCELLENCE

ancer Care

Exemplary among the comprehensive cancer care services is the bone marrow trans- plantation program, a leading, regional center for both autologous and allogenic trans- plants.

bstetrics/Gynecology

A leading choice for delivery among women in the region, the highly-regarded Perinatal Diagnostic Center offers diagnosis and treatment for high-risk pregnancies. The Fertility Institute offers supportive and sophisticated services for men and women.

ardiology

A certified emergency cardiac-care facility, the Cardiology Department offers non- invasive treatment in renovated facilities equipped with state-of-the-art technology.

iildren's Health Institute

The Children's Health Institute offers a regional neonatal intensive care unit, advanced programs in sickle cell and development disorders, and extensive specialty services.

rooklyn Health Network

The Brooklyn Health Network is dedicated to making primary care more accessible to Brooklyn neighborhoods through location, community involvement, culture, and lan- guage. The Network includes 14 family health centers, clinics, physician's offices, and school-based health clinics.

nysician Referral

4-CHOICE (718) 424-6423, the physicians' referral line of The Brooklyn Hospital Center, provides 24 hour, 7 days a week, in-depth information about and direct contact with highly qualified doctors who are attending or affiliated physicians.

THE LONG ISLAND COLLEGE HOSPITAL

Continuum Health Partners, Inc.

Primary Clinical Teaching
Affiliate of SUNY—
Health Science Center
at Brooklyn

339 HICKS STREET
BROOKLYN, NY 11201
(718) 780-1000

Sponsorship	Voluntary Not-for-Profit
Beds	516
Accreditation	Joint Commission on Accreditation of Healthcare Organizations (JCAHO)

The Long Island College Hospital has served the residents of Brooklyn and the wider metropolitan ar
since 1858. Today, LICH combines the best features of a major medical center, through teaching ar
research, with the personal approach of a community-centered hospital. Its mission–to provide the hig
est quality care in a caring environment–is emphasized every day throughout the hospital. As prima
teaching affiliate of the SUNY Health Science Center at Brooklyn, The Long Island College Hospital offe
training programs for resident physicians in more than 20 medical specialties.

The Long Island College Hospital is especially renowned for its many clinical areas of excellence, includir

Asthma/Allergies	Comprehensive services for asthma, allergies and immunology, and pulmona medicine.
Bloodless Medicine	Features The New York Center for Bloodless Medicine and Surgery, with round-th clock, on-site coordinators.
Cancer	Offers comprehensive cancer care, including extensive support services.
Dentistry	Offers high quality dental care with a wide range of leading edge services, includir a Special Patient Care Center that provides dental care to physically and mental challenged patients.
Nephrology	Established one of the largest renal dialysis programs in the country.
Neurology	Complete services for children and adults, including a comprehensive stroke center ar the Stanley S. Lamm Institute for Child Neurology and Developmental Disabilities–or of the first centers in the nation for the treatment of neurological disabilities.
Ophthalmology	Features Brooklyn's only 24-hour ophthalmic trauma center with state-of-the-a equipment as well as the only facility in Brooklyn for the treatment of ocular cancer
Otolaryngology	Comprehensive services include treatment for communicative disorders as well head and neck surgery.
Pediatrics	Comprehensive, accessible pediatric medical and surgical services, includir Brooklyn's only Cystic Fibrosis Center, treatment for digestive disorders and the bo ough's only Thalassemia treatment program.
Psychiatry	Full range of psychiatric services, including geriatric services and Brooklyn's only parti hospitalization program.
Urology	Features the New York Stone Center, the region's most comprehensive source for kidne stone treatment and prevention. Pioneered techniques for radical prostate surgery.
Women's Health	Provides a full range of women's health services, including a midwifery program ar a hospital-based rape crisis intervention program.
Physician Referral	With more than 1,700 physicians in a wide range of specialties, The Referral Servic can help you find a primary care physician or specialist affiliated with Beth Isra Medical Center, St. Luke's-Roosevelt Hospital Center or Long Island College Hospita The Referral Staff is available Monday through Friday, from 8:30 a.m. to 6:00 p.n Eastern Standard Time. A member of its multilingual staff can assist you in findir information about specialty care, convenient locations, insurance plans accepted an more. For a great doctor in your neighborhood, call (800) 420-4004.

LUTHERAN MEDICAL CENTER

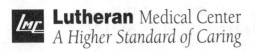

Lutheran Medical Center
A Higher Standard of Caring

150 55TH STREET
BROOKLYN, NY 11220
PHONE (718) 630-7000
FAX (718) 492-5948

Sponsorship	Voluntary, not-for-profit, teaching
Beds	501, including Rehabilitation and Detoxification
Accreditation <u>with</u> <u>Commendation</u>	Joint Commission on Accreditation of Healthcare Organizations
Other Accreditation:	College of American Pathologists

Lutheran Medical Center (LMC), founded in 1883, is one of Brooklyn's leading health care providers. A voluntary, not-for-profit hospital, LMC is the heart of the LMC Health System, a comprehensive system of health and human services. The system includes: Lutheran Medical Center; the Sunset Park Family Health Center Network, a major provider of ambulatory care; Augustana Lutheran Home; Shore Hill and Harbor Hill housing for older adults, Community Care Organization, Inc. (home care); and HEALTH-PLUS and Child Health Plus managed health plan.

Lutheran Medical Center has 544 active attending physicians, over 77% of whom are Board certified. Residency programs include medicine, family practice, obstetrics and gynecology, podiatry and dentistry. Pediatrics and surgery are shared residencies.

Lutheran Medical Center was the first winner of the Foster G. McGaw Prize of the American Hospital Association for Excellence in Community Service and the C. Everett Koop National Health Award (1997).

Medical/Surgical/ and Intensive Care/ Ob/Gyn/Pediatrics	Medical/surgical and intensive care services; maternity including birthing suites neonatal and newborn nurseries; new pediatrics unit and playroom.
Rehabilitation Services	Physical, occupational and speech therapy on our NOR (Neurological, Orthopedic and Rehabilitation) unit, as well as sports medicine and an extensive outpatient program. We also offer cardiac rehabilitation.
Center for Behavioral Health	Inpatient psychiatric and chemical dependency detoxification care; outpatient services include mental health and substance abuse counseling.
State of the Art Technology	CT scans, MRI and Lithotripsy, ABBI™ breast biopsy, bone densitometry, linear accelerator, mammography, sonography and vascular testing.
Ambulatory Surgery/ Ambulatory Oncology	Newly renovated ambulatory surgery suite; ambulatory oncology provides chemotherapy and transfusion services for cancer patients.

Sunset Park Family Health Center Network	A comprehensive ambulatory care system serving some 70,000 patients with nearly 400,000 visits annually at the main site, satellite facilities and schools throughout Brooklyn.
Women's Health Initiatives	Women's Health Partnership, a health resource and education center, menopause education, mature women's clinic and extensive prenatal care.
Services for Older Adults	Support services in four senior housing facilities, adult day services, a bus transportation system, meals on wheels, caregivers support and a wellness program.

Physician Referral	718/630-7979 Mon-Fri 7AM to 10PM; Sat 9AM to 6PM; Sun 10AM to 5PM
Website	www.lmcmc.com

ABBI is a registered trademark of United States Surgical Corporation.

MAIMONIDES MEDICAL CENTER

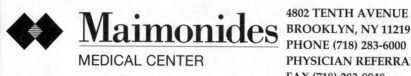

Maimonides
MEDICAL CENTER

4802 TENTH AVENUE
BROOKLYN, NY 11219
PHONE (718) 283-6000
PHYSICIAN REFERRAL (888) MMC-DOC
FAX (718) 283-8848

Sponsorship	Voluntary Not-for-Profit
Beds	705 acute 70 psych
Accreditation	Joint Commission on Accreditation of Healthcare Organizations (JCAHO Accreditation, Council of Graduate Medical Education (ACGME)

GENERAL DESCRIPTION

Maimonides Medical Center is the nation's third largest independent teaching hospital. A nonsectaria institution under Jewish auspices, it serves patients from the New York metropolitan area. Maimonides i a major teaching affiliate of the State University of New York's Health Science Center at Brooklyn.

MEDICAL STAFF

Maimonides Medical Center has 848 active doctors. It recently expanded its distinguished medical sta by recruiting internationally renowned specialists to chair major departments.

TEACHING PROGRAMS

The hospital offers 24 residency programs in the following areas: Anesthesiology, Internal Medicin Ob/Gyn, Pediatrics, Psychiatry, Radiology, Surgery, Urology, Osteopathic Medicine, and various subspe cialties of Internal Medicine and Surgery. The hospital's resident staff is composed of 380 residents.

SPECIAL PROGRAMS

Cardiac Institute	World renowned for excellence in cardiac surgery (1,000+ procedures annually) an for pioneering many new angiographic techniques (e.g., atherectomy and percuta neous transmyocardial revascularization)
Orthopaedics	Performs various complex procedures (e.g., limb-lengthening techniques, correction o congenital deformities, cutting-edge endoscopic spinal surgery, delicate hand surgery and repair of traumatic sports injuries)
Pediatrics	Provides a wide range of subspecialty services, including adolescent medicine, allergy behavioral, cardiology, ear, nose & throat, endocrinology, gastroenterology, genetics hematology/oncology, infectious disease, neonatology, and surgery
Obstetrics/Gynecology	Offers a full range of women's services, including comprehensive prenatal care, preg nancy screening, perinatal testing, infertility services, menopause counseling, high risk pregnancy care, and gynecologic cancer care

OTHER SERVICES

Ambulatory Health Network	A network of more than 20 office-based primary and specialty care services, including a cardiac rehabilitation program, one-stop health care for women at Brooklyn Women' Services, and technically sophisticated infertility treatments at Brooklyn IVF.
Payson Birthing Center	The birthing center is staffed with 40 doctors and 10 midwives and provides a warm environment for giving birth without sacrificing life-saving technology.
Weinberg Emergency Center	About 60,000 cases annually can be treated in the newly expanded emergency center The X-ray, cardiac, and trauma facilities have been updated to speed up treatment, and a separate pediatric area provides emergency services for children from infants to teens.
Physician Referral	The hospital has a free, seven-day, 24-hour telephone service that offers referrals to more than 400 Maimonides-affiliated physicians.

NEW YORK METHODIST HOSPITAL

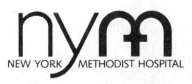

NEW YORK METHODIST HOSPITAL

506 SIXTH STREET
BROOKLYN, N.Y. 11215
PHONE: (718) 780-3000
FAX: (718) 780-3770
http://www.nym.org

Sponsorship	Voluntary, Not-for-Profit
Beds	485 acute 50 psych 25 rehab 42 bassinets
Accreditation	Joint Commission on Accreditation of Healthcare Organizations (JCAHO), American College of Surgeons, American Medical Association, American Association of Blood Banks

GENERAL DESCRIPTION

New York Methodist Hospital (NYM), a member of the New York and Presbyterian Healthcare Network, has served the neighborhoods of Brooklyn for nearly 120 years. NYM's medical programs have recently expanded significantly and the hospital's campus facilities in Park Slope have been extensively renovated. In addition, NYM maintains satellite outpatient health centers throughout Brooklyn.

MEDICAL STAFF

NYM has nearly 700 physicians on staff; 90% are board certified or board eligible. Many physicians at NYM are known for the outstanding work they have done in their individual fields.

TEACHING PROGRAMS

NYM offers medical residency programs in internal medicine, surgery, pediatrics, obstetrics/gynecology, radiation oncology, diagnostic radiology, nuclear medicine, anesthesiology, emergency medicine and podiatry and fellowships in several medical subspecialties.

SPECIAL PROGRAMS

Cancer Program	A full range of diagnostic services (including a Women's Diagnostic Center) and state-of-the-art treatment programs, which include surgery, radiation therapy (administered in our regional radiation oncology center) and chemotherapy.
Cardiology Services	A wide variety of cardiology services, from screening and diagnostic modalities (including cardiac catheterization) to emergency and ongoing treatment of heart attacks and chronic heart disease (718/780-3622).
Emergency Medicine	An EMS 911 Receiving Hospital, the Emergency Department houses a Chest Pain Emergency Center, a Stroke Early Warning Program and a dedicated Pediatric Emergency Service (718/780-3136).
Home Care	The largest hospital-based certified home health agency in Brooklyn. (718/780-5166).
The Brooklyn Spine and Arthritis Center	Diagnosis and treatment of arthritis and spine-related disorders (718/780-3104). (See Centers of Excellence section)
The Sleep/Wake Disorders Center	Diagnosis and treatment for insomnia, snoring, narcolepsy and other sleeping problems (718/780-3017).
The Parkinson's Disease Program	The only comprehensive diagnostic and treatment program for Parkinson's and other tremor disorders in Brooklyn (718/780-5320). (See Centers of Excellence section)
The Sickle Cell/ Thalassemia Program	Comprehensive health care and treatment for pediatric, adolescent and adult patients with sickle cell disease and thalassemia (718/857-5643).
Physician Referral	The Hospital has a free seven-day, 24-hour telephone and computer on-line physician referral service. The public is welcome to use the service to find a doctor in any specialty with a convenient office location, area of specialization and insurance and billing policies (718)499-CARE or http://www.nym.org).

STATEN ISLAND UNIVERSITY HOSPITAL

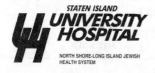

STATEN ISLAND UNIVERSITY HOSPITAL
NORTH SHORE-LONG ISLAND JEWISH HEALTH SYSTEM

475 SEAVIEW AVENUE
STATEN ISLAND, NY 10305
PHONE: (718) 226-9000
FAX: (718) 226-2734

Sponsorship	Voluntary not-for-profit
Beds	Multi-site hospital, 633 acute beds
Accreditation	Joint Commission on the Accreditation of Healthcare Organizations with Commendation (JCAHO); Commission on Accreditation of Rehabilitation Facilities (CARF); American College of Radiology.

GENERAL DESCRIPTION

Staten Island University Hospital, founded in 1861, was selected among America's Top 100 Hospitals for both 1996 and 1997 in an independent survey of more than 3,500 hospitals in the US. A Level 1 trauma center, it is part of the North Shore-Long Island Jewish Health System, and a major teaching affiliate of SUNY Health Science Center at Brooklyn. A multi-site facility, it has two major hospital locations and an extensive primary care network throughout the five boroughs of New York City. A cardiac surgery center begins construction in 1998.

MEDICAL STAFF AND FACULTY

Staten Island University Hospital has 912 attending staff, 72% of which are board certified. Many of the medical staff are nationally and internationally recognized. The hospital has residency programs in internal medicine, surgery, pediatrics, and Ob/Gyn, and yearly trains more than 300 residents.

SPECIAL PROGRAMS

Cancer Care	University Hospital is known internationally for its leadership program in Stereotactic Radiosurgery using three advanced linear accelerators for both brain and body tumors. A freestanding ambulatory cancer institute supports the hospital's commitment to treating all cancers, and gives access to advanced treatment protocols.
Diabetic Foot	A national Center of Excellence for its Hansen's Disease center, therapies developed are used successfully in treating Diabetic Foot disorders and difficult-healing wounds associated with diabetes.
Prostate Health	Treating both benign and cancerous prostate conditions with a variety of therapies, including cutting-edge Radiation Seed Implants, advanced forms of surgeries, and state-of-the-art laser treatment.
Burn Center	Featuring recognized specialists in the treatment of burns, University Hospital opened its 10-bed Regional Burn Center in 1998.

OTHER SERVICES

Women's Center	Emphasizing well care, the Center for Women's Health provides primary care, mammography, gynecology, obstetrics and osteoporosis. The hospital also has a birthing suite with a Jacuzzi tub and spacious facilities.
Bariatric Surgery	A highly specialized treatment for patients who are more than 100 pounds overweight, and for whom their obesity causes other serious medical problems.
RK/PRK	The Advanced Vision Care program is designed to correct near and farsightedness, and astigmatism using state-of-the-art laser surgery.
Physician referral	The hospital provides free access to more than 900 physicians and dentists through a a referral service available 70 hours a week (7 days).Call 718-226-2880.

UNIVERSITY HOSPITAL OF BROOKLYN

450 CLARKSON AVENUE
BROOKLYN, NY 11203
PHONE 718-270-1000
FAX 718-270-1628

Sponsorship	State University of New York hospital
Beds	376 beds, 20 bassinets
Accreditation	Joint Commission on Accreditation of Healthcare Organization

PROFILE

University Hospital of Brooklyn is the primary teaching hospital of the State University of New York Health Science Center at Brooklyn, or Downstate, Brooklyn's only academic medical center. Medical staff: University Hospital has 655 attending physicians; 72 percent are board certified.

PIONEERING MEDICINE

University Hospital physicians performed the first successful kidney-pancreas transplant in the state, employ the most sophisticated intensity-modulated radiation therapy system in the world, and lead a national study of a new stent-graft revolutionizing the repair of abdominal aneurysms.

SPECIAL PROGRAMS

Cardiovascular	The hospital is one of only two certified cardiovascular centers in Brooklyn and the only one performing pediatric heart surgery. Its angioplasty and open heart surgery programs consistently rank among the state's best.
Nephrology, Urology, and Transplantation	The hospital has one of the largest pediatric dialysis programs in the country, and its pediatric urologists are nationally recognized. University Hospital has performed more kidney transplants than any other New York hospital and performs liver transplantation.
Neurology and Neurosurgery	The hospital has experts in all fields of neurology, including epilepsy and Alzheimer's. Our neurosurgeons are recognized for their innovative treatment of syringomyelia and other malformations of the brain.
Primary Care	University Hospital's primary care programs emphasize patient education and wellness. Ambulatory care is available at the hospital and its satellite, Family Health Services, located at 840 Lefferts Avenue.
Women and Children	University Hospital leads in managing high-risk pregnancies and treating infertility, caring for premature babies, and assisting children who are physically or developmentally delayed. It also offers stereotactic breast imaging, a lupus clinic, chronic back pain management, breast reconstruction, and an osteoporosis center.

NEW SERVICES

Acute Care Center	Patients suffering from chest pain and asthma receive immediate treatment 24 hours a day.
Bloodless Surgery	The center offers education and medical alternatives to blood therapy for those patients desiring medical management without the use of blood products.
Diabetes and Vascular Center	The center provides comprehensive care for people suffering from diabetes and its complications.

Physician Referral	University Physicians of Brooklyn provide outstanding medical care in virtually every medical specialty. For a referral, call toll-free, 24 hours a day: 1-888-270-SUNY.

SPECIALTY & SUBSPECIALTY	ABBREVIATION	PAGE(S)	SPECIALTY & SUBSPECIALTY	ABBREVIATION	PAGE(S)
Adolescent Medicine	AM	481	Pediatric Cardiology	PCd	528
Allergy & Immunology	A&I	481-482	Pediatric Endocrinology	PEn	528
Anesthesiology	Anes	482	Pediatric Gastroenterology	PGe	529-530
Cardiology (Cardiovascular Disease)	Cv	482-485	Pediatric Hematology–Oncology*	PHO	530
Child & Adolescent Psychiatry	ChAP	485	Pediatric Infectious Disease	PInf	530
Child Neurology	ChiN	486	Pediatric Nephrology	PNep	531
Colon & Rectal Surgery	CRS	486	Pediatric Pulmonology	PPul	531
Critical Care Medicine	CCM	487	Pediatric Radiology	PR	531
Dermatology	D	487-489	Pediatric Rheumatology	PRhu	531
Diagnostic Radiology	DR	489	Pediatric Surgery	PS	532
Emergency Medicine	EM	489	PEDIATRICS (GENERAL)	Ped	532-536
Endocrinology, Diabetes & Metabolism	EDM	490-491	Physical Medicine & Rehabilitation	PMR	536-537
FAMILY PRACTICE	FP	491-494	Plastic Surgery	PlS	537-538
Gastroenterology	Ge	494-497	Psychiatry	Psyc	538-539
Geriatric Medicine	Ger	497	Pulmonary Disease	Pul	539-541
Geriatric Psychiatry	GerPsy	497	Radiation Oncology*	RadRO	541-542
Gynecologic Oncology*	GO	497	Radiology	Rad	542-543
Hand Surgery	HS	498	Reproductive Endocrinology	RE	543-544
Hematology	Hem	498-500	Rheumatology	Rhu	544-545
Infectious Disease	Inf	500-501	Sports Medicine	SM	545
INTERNAL MEDICINE	IM	501-508	Surgery	S	545-549
Medical Genetics	MG	508	Thoracic Surgery (includes open heart surgery)	TS	550
Medical Oncology*	Onc	508-509	Urology	U	551-553
Neonatal-Perinatal Medicine	NP	510	Vascular Surgery (General)	GVS	553-554
Nephrology	Nep	510-513			
Neurological Surgery	NS	513-514			
Neurology	N	514-516			
Nuclear Medicine	NuM	516-517			
OBSTETRICS & GYNECOLOGY	ObG	517-520			
Ophthalmology	Oph	520-524			
Orthopaedic Surgery	OrS	524-526			
Otolaryngology	Oto	526-527			
Pain Management	PM	528			

Specialties in capital letters indicate Primary Care Specialties. However, many doctors will be certified in a subspecialty, but will practice predominantly primary care medicine. In our lists this will be indicated.

*Oncologists deal with Cancer

ADOLESCENT MEDICINE

Hayes-McKenzie, Leslie (MD)AM
Brooklyn Hosp Ctr-Downtown
121 Dekalb Ave 9th Fl; Brooklyn, NY 11201; (718) 940-5246; **BDCERT:** Ped 91; **MS:** Mt Sinai Sch Med 86; **RES:** Children's Hosp Nat Med Ctr, Washington, DC; **FEL:** AM, Univ of Med & Dent NJ Hosp, Newark, NJ; **HMO:** Most US Hlthcre

Sacker, Ira (MD)   AM
Brookdale Univ Hosp Med Ctr
Brookdale Hospital Medical Center, 9620 Church Ave FL2; Brooklyn, NY 11212; (718) 240-6451; **BDCERT:** Ped 82; **MS:** USC Sch Med 64; **RES:** Ped, NYU Med Ctr, New York, NY 69-72; **FEL:** AM, Children's Hosp of Los Angeles, Los Angeles, CA 71-72; **FAP:** Assoc Prof Ped SUNY Downstate; **SI:** *Eating Disorders, Anorexia, Bulimia;* **HMO:** Aetna Hlth Plan Blue Choice Blue Cross & Blue Shield Choicecare CIGNA +

🏳 📞 📷 ♿ ⌚ 💲 A Few Days

ALLERGY & IMMUNOLOGY

Greeley, Norman (MD)   A&I   PCP
Long Island Coll Hosp
140 Clinton St Fl 1; Brooklyn, NY 11201; (718) 624-4465; **BDCERT:** IM 85; A&I 87; **MS:** Mexico 80; **RES:** Med, Long Island Coll Hosp, Brooklyn, NY 82-85; **FEL:** Univ Hosp SUNY Bklyn, Brooklyn, NY 85-87; **SI:** *Asthma*

LANG: Sp; 🏳 📞 📷 ♿ ⌚ 💲 ⌚ Immediately

Herzlich, Barry (MD)   A&I
Maimonides Med Ctr
Maimonides Primary Care, 47-02 Fort Hamilton Pkwy; Brooklyn, NY 11219; (718) 283-6101; **BDCERT:** IM 79; A&I 81; **MS:** U Wisc Med Sch 76; **RES:** IM, Kings County Hosp Ctr, Brooklyn, NY 76-79; **FEL:** A&I, Kings County Hosp Ctr, Brooklyn, NY 79-81; Hem, VA Med Ctr-Bronx, Bronx, NY 81-83; **FAP:** Assoc Lecturer Med SUNY Hlth Sci Ctr; **SI:** *Allergies; Asthma;* **HMO:** Oxford Health First US Hlthcre 1199

📞 ♿ ⌚ ⌚ 1 Week

Josephson, Alan S (MD)   A&I
Univ Hosp SUNY Bklyn
450 Clarkson Ave Bx 50; Brooklyn, NY 11203; (718) 270-2156; **BDCERT:** IM 65; A&I 75; **MS:** NYU Sch Med 56; **RES:** Bellevue Hosp Ctr, New York, NY 60-61; **FEL:** IM, New York University Med Ctr, New York, NY 58-60; **FAP:** Prof Med SUNY Hlth Sci Ctr

Kalanadhabhatta, Vivekannad (MD) A&I
Univ Hosp SUNY Bklyn
450 Clarkson Ave; Brooklyn, NY 11203; (718) 270-1082; **BDCERT:** IM 90; **MS:** India 81; **RES:** IM, Kingsbrook Jewish Med Ctr, Brooklyn, NY 87-90; **FEL:** A&I, Univ Hosp SUNY Bklyn, Brooklyn, NY 90-92; **FAP:** Asst Prof Med SUNY Hlth Sci Ctr; **HOSP:** Kingsbrook Jewish Med Ctr; **SI:** *Bronchial Asthma; Sinus Problems;* **HMO:** Aetna-US Healthcare CIGNA Oxford 1199 Blue Cross & Blue Choice +

♿ 📞 📷 ⌚ 💲 ⌚ A Few Days

Klein, Norman (MD)   A&I
Brookdale Univ Hosp Med Ctr
1648 E 14th St; Brooklyn, NY 11229; (718) 627-0183; **BDCERT:** A&I 83; **MS:** SUNY Hlth Sci Ctr 76; **RES:** Ped, Brookdale Univ Hosp Med Ctr, Brooklyn, NY 76-79; **FEL:** A&I, Albert Einstein Med Ctr, Bronx, NY; **SI:** *Asthma; Food Allergies;* **HMO:** Blue Cross GHI Oxford Aetna Hlth Plan PM Care +

♿ 📞 📷 ⌚ 💲 ⌚ A Few Days **VISA** 💳

Schneider, Arlene (MD)   A&I
Long Island Coll Hosp

Allergy & Asthma Care Ctr, 159 Clinton St; Brooklyn, NY 11201; (718) 624-6495; **BDCERT:** A&I 74; Ped 74; **MS:** SUNY Downstate 68; **RES:** Ped, Long Island Coll Hosp, Brooklyn, NY 70-72; **FEL:** A&I, Long Island Coll Hosp, Brooklyn, NY 72-74; **FAP:** Asst Clin Prof SUNY Hlth Sci Ctr; **SI:** *Asthma; Sinus Problems;* **HMO:** Aetna-US Healthcare Oxford GHI Prudential PHCS +

LANG: Czc, Rus, Ger; 📞 🔒 👥 🏥 💲 Mcr
A Few Days

Snyder, Richard (MD)   A&I
Maimonides Med Ctr

2632 E 21st St; Brooklyn, NY 11235; (718) 332-9728; **MS:** Bowman Gray 58; **RES:** Kings County Hosp Ctr, Brooklyn, NY 58-60; Children's Hosp of Los Angeles, Los Angeles, CA 60-61; **FEL:** U CO Hosp, Denver, CO 61-62; **SI:** *Asthma;* **HMO:** GHI Blue Shield Magnacare PHS

📞 🔒 👥 🏥 💲 Mcr   A Few Days

ANESTHESIOLOGY

Schianodicola, Joseph (MD) Anes
New York Methodist Hosp

Park Slope Anesthesia Associates, 506 6th St 3003; Brooklyn, NY 11215; (718) 780-3279; **BDCERT:** Anes 91; PM 93; **MS:** Grenada 85; **RES:** Anes, New York Methodist Hosp, Brooklyn, NY 85-89; **HOSP:** Maimonides Med Ctr; **SI:** *Regional Anesthesia; Acute Pain Management;* **HMO:** Aetna Hlth Plan Blue Choice PPO Elderplan GHI PPO US Hlthcre +

LANG: Itl, Rus; ♿ 🔒 🏥 💲 Mcr Mod WC NFI   1 Week

Shevde, Ketan (MD)   Anes
Maimonides Med Ctr

Anesthesiology Associates of Boro Park, LLP, 931 48th St; Brooklyn, NY 11219; (718) 283-8816; **BDCERT:** Anes 93; CCM (Anes) 89; **MS:** India 68; **RES:** IM, Brooklyn Jewish Hosp, Brooklyn, NY 70-71; Anes, Mount Sinai Med Ctr, New York, NY 71-73; **FEL:** Mount Sinai Med Ctr, New York, NY 73-74; **HOSP:** Coney Island Hosp; **HMO:** Aetna Hlth Plan HIP Network Oxford Empire GHI +

LANG: Sp, Rus, Chi, Pol; ♿ 🏧 🔒 🏥 Mcr Mod WC NFI
Immediately **VISA** 💳

CARDIOLOGY (CARDIOVASCULAR DISEASE)

Buscaino, Giacomo (MD)   Cv
Victory Memorial Hosp

149 Battery Ave; Brooklyn, NY 11209; (718) 748-2900; **BDCERT:** Cv 81; CCM 87; **MS:** SUNY Downstate 78; **RES:** Med, Kings County Hosp Ctr, Brooklyn, NY 79-81; **FEL:** Cv, Kings County Hosp Ctr, Brooklyn, NY 81-83; **HMO:** CIGNA US Hlthcre

Charnoff, Judah (MD)   Cv
Maimonides Med Ctr

813 Quentin Rd 203; Brooklyn, NY 11223; (718) 645-8376; **BDCERT:** IM 87; Cv 95; **MS:** NYU Sch Med 84; **RES:** IM, Brookdale Univ Hosp Med Ctr, Brooklyn, NY 85-87; **FEL:** Cv, Maimonides Med Ctr, Brooklyn, NY 87-89; **HOSP:** New York Methodist Hosp; **SI:** *Congestive Heart Failure; Coronary Artery Disease;* **HMO:** Oxford GHI US Hlthcre CIGNA Magnacare +

♿ 📞 🔒 👥 🏥 💲 Mcr Mod   A Few Days

Clark, Luther T (MD)   Cv
Univ Hosp SUNY Bklyn

Downstate Cardiology Associates, 450 Clarkson Ave Bx1199; Brooklyn, NY 11203; (718) 270-1568; **BDCERT:** IM 78; Cv 81; **MS:** Harvard Med Sch 75; **RES:** IM, St Luke's Roosevelt Hosp Ctr, New York, NY 75-78; IM, St Luke's Roosevelt Hosp Ctr, New York, NY 78-79; **FEL:** Cv, St Luke's Roosevelt Hosp Ctr, New York, NY 78-80; **FAP:** Prof SUNY Hlth Sci Ctr; **SI:** *Heart Disease; Hypertension Prevention;* **HMO:** Empire CIGNA Oxford Metlife US Hlthcre +

LANG: Fr, Itl, Chi, Sp; ♿ 🔒 🏥 💲 Mcr WC
A Few Days

Gelbfish, Joseph (MD)　　　　Cv
New York Methodist Hosp

2500 Avenue I; Brooklyn, NY 11210; (718) 951-0100; **BDCERT:** IM 86; Cv 90; **MS:** NYU Sch Med 80; **RES:** S, Maimonides Med Ctr, Brooklyn, NY 82-84; IM, Maimonides Med Ctr, Brooklyn, NY 84-85; **FEL:** Cv, Maimonides Med Ctr, Brooklyn, NY 86-88; Cv, Beth Israel Med Ctr, Boston, MA 88-89; **HOSP:** Maimonides Med Ctr; *SI: Diagnosis of Chest Symptoms; Prevention of Heart Disease;* **HMO:** Oxford Blue Cross & Blue Shield GHI Aetna-US Healthcare

LANG: Heb, Yd; 🔟 🔟 🔟 🔟 🔟 1 Week

Gupta, Prem (MD)　　　　Cv
Maimonides Med Ctr

4709 Fort Hamilton Pkwy; Brooklyn, NY 11219; (718) 633-4244; **BDCERT:** IM 71; Cv 73; **MS:** India 64; **RES:** IM, VA Med Ctr-Manh, New York, NY 67-68; IM, VA Med Ctr-Bronx, Bronx, NY 68-69; **FEL:** Cv, VA Med Ctr-Bronx, Bronx, NY 69-71; **FAP:** Clin Prof Med SUNY Hlth Sci Ctr; *SI: Cardiac Risk Reduction; Echo and Stress Testing;* **HMO:** Aetna Hlth Plan Prucare PHS CIGNA Oxford +

LANG: Hin, Ur, Itl, Pun; 🔟 🔟 🔟 🔟 🔟 1 Week

Hanley, Gerard (MD)　　　　Cv
Beth Israel Med Ctr

University Heart Assoc, 3131 Kings Hwy Suite B1; Brooklyn, NY 11234; (718) 253-9511; **BDCERT:** IM 89; Cv 91; **MS:** SUNY Stony Brook 84; **RES:** IM, Univ Hosp SUNY Bklyn, Brooklyn, NY 85-87; **FEL:** Cv, Univ Hosp SUNY Bklyn, Brooklyn, NY 88-90; Cv, Westchester County Med Ctr, Valhalla, NY 90-91; **FAP:** Asst Prof SUNY Downstate; **HOSP:** New York Methodist Hosp; *SI: Acute Invasive Cardiology;* **HMO:** Blue Choice Oxford CIGNA United Healthcare US Hlthcre +

LANG: Sp, Itl, Rus, Rom; 🔟 🔟 🔟 🔟 🔟 🔟 🔟 A Few Days

Jacobowitz, Israel (MD)　　　　Cv
Lenox Hill Hosp

3131 Kings Hwy; Brooklyn, NY 11234; (212) 472-3129; **BDCERT:** TS 82; S 82; **MS:** SUNY Buffalo 73; **RES:** S, New York University Med Ctr, New York, NY; **FEL:** Cv, New York University Med Ctr, New York, NY; **HOSP:** Maimonides Med Ctr; **HMO:** HIP Network GHI Blue Cross Oxford Aetna Hlth Plan +

LANG: Yd; 🔟 🔟 🔟 🔟 🔟 🔟

Kleeman, Harris J (MD)　　　　Cv
Maimonides Med Ctr

1660 E 14th St Ste LL3; Brooklyn, NY 11229; (718) 375-6969; **BDCERT:** IM 82; Cv 85; **MS:** SUNY Hlth Sci Ctr 79; **RES:** IM, Staten Island Univ Hosp, Staten Island, NY 79-83; **FEL:** Cv, Maimonides Med Ctr, Brooklyn, NY 83-85; *SI: Heart Artery & Valve Disease; Chest Discomfort Hypertension;* **HMO:** GHI Empire

🔟 🔟 🔟 🔟 🔟 🔟 Immediately

Lazar, Eliot (MD)　　　　Cv
Brooklyn Hosp Ctr-Caledonian

121 Dekalb Ave; Brooklyn, NY 11201; (718) 250-6925; **BDCERT:** IM 84; Cv 87; **MS:** SUNY Hlth Sci Ctr 81; **RES:** Albert Einstein Med Ctr, Bronx, NY 81-85; **FEL:** Cv, Mount Sinai Med Ctr, New York, NY 85-87; **HMO:** Oxford Aetna Hlth Plan

🔟 🔟 🔟 🔟 A Few Days

Leff, Sanford (MD)　　　　Cv
New York Methodist Hosp

Park Slope Cardiac, 47 Plaza St West; Brooklyn, NY 11217; (718) 789-4332; **BDCERT:** IM 74; Cv 79; **MS:** SUNY Buffalo 68; **RES:** Albert Einstein Med Ctr, Bronx, NY; Lincoln Med & Mental Hlth Ctr, Bronx, NY 72-74; **FEL:** Cv, St Luke's Roosevelt Hosp Ctr, New York, NY 77; **FAP:** Clin Prof SUNY Downstate; **HOSP:** Interfaith Med Ctr-St John's; *SI: Preventive Cardiology;* **HMO:** Oxford Empire GHI 1199

LANG: Sp, Pol; 🔟 🔟 🔟 🔟 🔟 🔟 A Few Days

Lichstein, Edgar (MD)　　　　Cv
Maimonides Med Ctr

4802 10th Ave; Brooklyn, NY 11219; (718) 283-7074; **BDCERT:** IM 69; Cv 73; **MS:** SUNY Hlth Sci Ctr 61; **RES:** IM, Lenox Hill Hosp, New York, NY 61-63; IM, New York University Med Ctr, New York, NY 63-64; **FEL:** Cv, New York University Med Ctr, New York, NY 64-66; **FAP:** Prof Med SUNY Hlth Sci Ctr; **HOSP:** Univ Hosp SUNY Bklyn; *SI: Heart Failure; Coronary Heart Disease;* **HMO:** Oxford US Hlthcre GHI Mt Sinai Hlth

🔟 🔟 🔟 🔟 🔟 🔟 A Few Days

Lotongkhum, Vichai (MD)   Cv
Wyckoff Heights Med Ctr

361 Stockholm St; Brooklyn, NY 11237; (718) 381-2121; **BDCERT:** IM 75; Cv 77; **MS:** Thailand 70; **RES:** Wyckoff Heights Med Ctr, Brooklyn, NY 72-74; **FEL:** Cv, Cumberland Med Ctr, Brooklyn, NY 74-76; **SI:** *Chest Pain; Palpitations;* **HMO:** Blue Choice Oxford US Hlthcre GHI

LANG: Ger, Thai; 🌙 📞 ♿ 🏥 Med A Few Days

Lyon, Alan (MD)   Cv
Brookdale Univ Hosp Med Ctr

Brookdale Hospital, Brookdale Plaza; Brooklyn, NY 11212; (718) 240-5753; **BDCERT:** IM 61; **MS:** NYU Sch Med 54; **RES:** IM, Bellevue Hosp Ctr, New York, NY 54-56; IM, VA Med Ctr-Bronx, Bronx, NY 56-57; **FEL:** Cv, VA Med Ctr-Bronx, Bronx, NY 57-58; **FAP:** Prof SUNY Hlth Sci Ctr; **SI:** *Electrocardiography; Heart Failure;* **HMO:** Oxford US Hlthcre PHS Independent Health Plan Well Care +

♿ 📞 ♿ 🏥 Mcr WC NFI A Few Days

Nozad, Steve (MD)   Cv
New York Comm Hosp of Bklyn

2513 E 12th St; Brooklyn, NY 11235; (718) 332-5009; **MS:** Iran 73; **RES:** St Vincents Hosp & Med Ctr NY, New York, NY; **FEL:** Cv, Mount Sinai Med Ctr, New York, NY

♿ 🌙 📞 ♿ 🏥 💲 Mcr 2-4 Weeks

Rafii, Shahrokh (MD)   Cv
Brookdale Univ Hosp Med Ctr

Brookdale University Hospital Medical Center, One Brookdale Plaza; Brooklyn, NY 11212; (718) 240-5000; **BDCERT:** IM 73; Cv 75; **MS:** Iran 67; **RES:** Cv, Coney Island Hospital, Brooklyn, NY 70-73; Med, Brookdale Univ Hosp, Brooklyn, NY 73-75

Reddy, Chatla (MD)   Cv
New York Methodist Hosp

New York Methodist Hosp—CV Diseases, 506 6th St; Brooklyn, NY 11215; (718) 780-3622; **BDCERT:** IM 72; Cv 75; **MS:** India 66; **RES:** IM, Misericordia Hosp, Bronx, NY 69-72; FEL: Misericordia Hosp, Bronx, NY 72-74; **FAP:** Assoc Clin Prof Med Cornell U; **HOSP:** NY Hosp-Cornell Med Ctr; **SI:** *Heart Catheterization; Angioplasty;* **HMO:** Oxford GHI United Healthcare Blue Shield +

LANG: Sp, Hin, Rus; ♿ 📞 ♿ 🏥 Mcr Mcd WC NFI 2-4 Weeks

Sacchi, Terrence J (MD)   Cv
Long Island Coll Hosp

339 Hicks St; Brooklyn, NY 11201; (718) 780-4626; **BDCERT:** IM 79; Cv 81; **MS:** Albany Med Coll 76; **RES:** IM, St Vincents Hosp & Med Ctr NY, New York, NY 77-79; **FEL:** Cv, Georgetown U Hosp, Washington, DC 79-81; **HOSP:** Maimonides Med Ctr; **HMO:** Oxford US Hlthcre Blue Cross & Blue Shield Prucare

LANG: Itl, Sp; ♿ 📞 ♿ 🏥 2-4 Weeks

Shani, Jacob (MD)   Cv
Maimonides Med Ctr

4802 10th Ave; Brooklyn, NY 11219; (718) 283-7480; **BDCERT:** IM 81; Cv 83; **MS:** Israel 77; **RES:** Maimonides Med Ctr, Brooklyn, NY 77-81; **FEL:** Cv, Beth Israel Med Ctr, Boston, MA 81-83; Harvard Med Sch, Cambridge, MA; **HOSP:** Columbia-Presbyterian Med Ctr; **SI:** *Interventional Cardiology; Catheterization Angioplasty;* **HMO:** Oxford Blue Cross HIP Network Elderplan Aetna Hlth Plan +

LANG: Itl, Sp, Rus, Heb; ♿ 🌙 📞 🏥 Mcr Mcd WC A Few Days **VISA** 💳

Traube, Charles (MD)   Cv
Beth Israel Med Ctr-Kings Hwy
2270 Kimball St 101; Brooklyn, NY 11234; (718) 692-2700; **BDCERT:** IM 78; Ger 92; **MS:** Albert Einstein Coll Med 75; **RES:** IM, Brookdale Univ Hosp Med Ctr, Brooklyn, NY 75-78; **FEL:** Cv, Brookdale Univ Hosp Med Ctr, Brooklyn, NY 78-80; **FAP:** Asst Clin Prof SUNY Downstate; **HOSP:** Brookdale Univ Hosp Med Ctr; **SI:** *Cardiac Disease Prevention*; **HMO:** Oxford Guardian Aetna-US Healthcare

LANG: Yd, Heb; 🔲 🔲 🔲 🔲 🔲 🔲 🔲 Immediately

Vasavada, Balendu (MD)   Cv
Long Island Coll Hosp
339 Hicks St; Brooklyn, NY 11201; (718) 780-2944; **BDCERT:** IM 77; Cv 79; **MS:** India 72; **RES:** Lincoln Med & Mental Hlth Ctr, Bronx, NY 74-77; **FEL:** Cv, Brooklyn Hosp Ctr, Brooklyn, NY 77-79; **FAP:** Asst Clin Prof SUNY Downstate; **SI:** *Transesophageal Echo; Stress Echo*; **HMO:** Oxford Aetna Hlth Plan US Hlthcre HIP Network

🔲 🔲 🔲 🔲 🔲 🔲 🔲 A Few Days

Wein, Paul (MD)   Cv
Beth Israel Med Ctr-Kings Hwy
3131 Kings Hwy D6; Brooklyn, NY 11234; (718) 338-2283; **BDCERT:** IM 77; Cv 83; **MS:** SUNY Hlth Sci Ctr 76; **RES:** IM, Norwalk Hosp, Norwalk, CT 76-79; **FEL:** Cv, Long Island Jewish Med Ctr, New Hyde Park, NY 79-81; **HOSP:** St Francis Med Ctr

🔲 🔲 🔲 🔲 🔲 🔲 🔲 🔲 Immediately

Zaloom, Robert (MD)   Cv
Lutheran Med Ctr
217 Ovington Ave; Brooklyn, NY 11209; (718) 238-0098; **BDCERT:** IM 86; Cv 89; **MS:** France 83; **RES:** IM, Lutheran Med Ctr, Brooklyn, NY 83-86; **FEL:** Cv, Univ Hosp SUNY Bklyn, Brooklyn, NY 86-88; **HOSP:** St Vincents Hosp & Med Ctr NY; **SI:** *Cardiac Catheterization*; **HMO:** US Hlthcre Oxford HealthNet Blue Choice CIGNA +

LANG: Sp, Fr, Ar; 🔲 🔲 🔲 🔲 🔲 🔲 A Few Days

CHILD & ADOLESCENT PSYCHIATRY

Holzer, Barry D (MD)   ChAP
NY Hosp Med Ctr of Queens
Center for Attention Deficits and Behavoir Disorders, 1801 Avenue M; Brooklyn, NY 11230; (718) 421-2400; **BDCERT:** Psyc 90; ChAP 95; **MS:** Albert Einstein Coll Med 84; **RES:** IM, Maimonides Med Ctr, Brooklyn, NY 84-85; **FEL:** Hillside Hosp, Glen Oaks, NY 86-88; Schneider Children's Hosp, New Hyde Park, NY 88-90; **HOSP:** Long Island Jewish Med Ctr; **SI:** *Attention Deficit Disorders; Behavior Disorders*; **HMO:** Aetna Hlth Plan GHI

LANG: Heb; 🔲 🔲 🔲 🔲 🔲 A Few Days 🔲 **VISA** 🔲

Shabry, Fryderyka (MD)   ChAP
Coney Island Hosp
1014 E 24th St; Brooklyn, NY 11210; (718) 377-6045; **BDCERT:** Psyc 83; ChAP 86; **MS:** Poland 63; **RES:** Ped, Brookdale Univ Hosp Med Ctr, Brooklyn, NY; Psyc, Brookdale Univ Hosp Med Ctr, Brooklyn, NY; **FEL:** ChAP, Brookdale Univ Hosp Med Ctr, Brooklyn, NY

🔲 🔲 🔲 🔲 Immediately

Welch, John (MD)   ChAP
New York Methodist Hosp
808 Carroll St; Brooklyn, NY 11215; (718) 622-4700; **BDCERT:** Psyc 73; **MS:** Univ Kans Sch Med 64; **RES:** Psyc, Univ Hosp SUNY Bklyn, Brooklyn, NY 67-69; **FEL:** ChAP, Univ Hosp SUNY Bklyn, Brooklyn, NY 69; **SI:** *Psychopharmacology; Psychopharmacology-Children*; **HMO:** None

🔲 🔲 🔲 🔲 🔲 🔲 A Few Days

CHILD NEUROLOGY

Bender-Cracco, Joan (MD)   ChiN
Univ Hosp SUNY Bklyn
450 Clarkson Ave; Brooklyn, NY 11203; (718)
270-2035; **BDCERT:** Ped 69; N 72; **MS:** UMDNJ-NJ
Med Sch, Newark 63; **RES:** Ped, Mayo Clinic,
Rochester, MN 64-66; N, Thomas Jefferson U Hosp,
Philadelphia, PA 66-69; **FAP:** Prof SUNY Hlth Sci
Ctr; **HOSP:** Kings County Hosp Ctr; **SI:** *Spina Bifida*
 ♿ 🚪

Bennett, Harvey S (MD)   ChiN
Long Island Coll Hosp
110 Amity St; Brooklyn, NY 11201; (718) 780-
2848; **BDCERT:** Ped 79; ChiN 91; **MS:** Albert
Einstein Coll Med 76; **RES:** Ped, St Christopher's
Hosp for Children, Philadelphia, PA 76-78; ChiN,
Albert Einstein Med Ctr, Bronx, NY 78-81; **FAP:**
Assoc Clin Prof NP SUNY Hlth Sci Ctr; **HOSP:**
Maimonides Med Ctr; **SI:** *Cerebral Palsy; Tic
Disorders;* **HMO:** Oxford US Hlthcre Blue Cross &
Blue Shield CIGNA Prucare +

LANG: Heb, Sp, Fr, Rus; ♿ 🚪 🧑 🏥 $ 2-4 Weeks

Rose, Arthur L (MD)   ChiN
Univ Hosp SUNY Bklyn
450 Clarkson Ave Rm B4330; Brooklyn, NY
11203; (718) 270-2042; **BDCERT:** Ped 63; N 69;
MS: England 57; **RES:** N, Columbia-Presbyterian
Med Ctr, New York, NY 61-63; **HOSP:** Kings
County Hosp Ctr; **HMO:** Chubb Oxford US Hlthcre

Tepperberg, Jerome (MD)   ChiN
Maimonides Med Ctr
745 64th St; Brooklyn, NY 11220; (718) 283-
1924; **BDCERT:** Ped 68; ChiN 78; **MS:** U Fla Coll
Med 63; **RES:** Bellevue Hosp Ctr, New York, NY 63-
65; Beth Israel Med Ctr-Kings Hwy, Brooklyn, NY
65-66; **FEL:** ChiN, Columbia-Presbyterian Med Ctr,
New York, NY 66-69; **FAP:** Assoc Clin Prof N SUNY
Hlth Sci Ctr; **HMO:** Blue Choice Independent Health
Plan Travelers HealthNet +

♿ 🚪 🏥 Mcr Mcd   Immediately

COLON & RECTAL SURGERY

Bopaiah, Vinod (MD)   CRS
Staten Island Univ Hosp-South
Coney Island Medical Group, 1616 Voorhies Ave;
Brooklyn, NY 11235; (718) 769-5158; **BDCERT:**
CRS 91; S 92; **MS:** India 76; **RES:** Interfaith Med
Ctr, Brooklyn, NY 76-80; **FEL:** Sacred Heart Hosp,
Allentown, PA 80-81; **HOSP:** New York Methodist
Hosp; **HMO:** Oxford US Hlthcre GHI Aetna Hlth
Plan

LANG: Rus, Hin; ♿ SA/SU ☾ 🚪 🧑 🏥 $ Mcr Mcd
A Few Days

Charnoff, Judah (MD)   CRS
Maimonides Med Ctr
813 Quentin Rd 203; Brooklyn, NY 11223; (718)
645-8376; **BDCERT:** IM 87; Cv 95; **MS:** NYU Sch
Med 84; **RES:** IM, Brookdale Univ Hosp Med Ctr,
Brooklyn, NY 85-87; **FEL:** Cv, Maimonides Med Ctr,
Brooklyn, NY 87-89; **HOSP:** New York Methodist
Hosp; **SI:** *Congestive Heart Failure; Coronary Artery
Disease;* **HMO:** Oxford GHI US Hlthcre CIGNA
Magnacare +

♿ ☾ 🚪 🧑 🏥 $ Mcr Mcd   A Few Days

Fleischer, Marian (MD)   CRS
Maimonides Med Ctr
9707 4th Ave; Brooklyn, NY 11209; (718) 836-
3603; **BDCERT:** CRS 84; S 83; **MS:** Italy 72; **RES:** S,
Maimonides Med Ctr, Brooklyn, NY 77-81; CRS,
Baltimore Med Ctr, Baltimore 81-82; **HOSP:** Beth
Israel Med Ctr-Kings Hwy; **HMO:** Oxford Blue
Choice HealthNet United Healthcare

♿ ☾ 🧑 🏥 Mcr   A Few Days

Golub, Richard (MD)   CRS
Univ Hosp SUNY Bklyn
Colon & Rectal Surgical Assoc, 470 Clarkson Ave
H; Brooklyn, NY 11203; (718) 270-3349;
BDCERT: S 92; CRS 92; **MS:** Albert Einstein Coll
Med 84; **RES:** Univ Hosp SUNY Stony Brook, Stony
Brook, NY 84-90; **FEL:** Grant Hosp, Columbus, OH
90-91; **FAP:** Asst Prof SUNY Downstate; **HOSP:**
Long Island Coll Hosp; **SI:** *Colon and Rectal Cancer;*
HMO: Empire CIGNA Oxford US Hlthcre

♿ 🚪 🧑 🏥 $ Mcr Mcd WC NFI   A Few Days

CRITICAL CARE MEDICINE

Demetis, Spiro (MD)   CCM
Univ Hosp SUNY Bklyn
9001 Fort Hamilton Pkwy; Brooklyn, NY 11209;
(718) 748-4446; **BDCERT:** IM 89; Pul 90; **MS:**
Mexico 83; **RES:** Univ Hosp SUNY Bklyn, Brooklyn,
NY 84-87; Univ Hosp SUNY Bklyn, Brooklyn, NY;
FEL: Pul, Univ Hosp SUNY Bklyn, Brooklyn, NY 88-
90; CCM, Univ Hosp SUNY Bklyn, Brooklyn, NY
90-91; **FAP:** Asst Prof SUNY Downstate; **HOSP:**
Lutheran Med Ctr; **SI:** *Asthma and Emphysema; Lung
Cancer Sarcoidosis;* **HMO:** GHI Blue Cross & Blue
Shield CIGNA US Hlthcre

LANG: Sp, Grk; 🚹 🔲 🔳 🔲 🔲 🔳 🔳 🔳
A Few Days

Tessler, Sidney (MD)   CCM
Maimonides Med Ctr
953 49th St; Brooklyn, NY 11219; (718) 283-
8380; **BDCERT:** IM 77; Pul 80; **MS:** SUNY Hlth Sci
Ctr 70; **RES:** IM, Maimonides Med Ctr, Brooklyn,
NY 74-75; IM, Coney Island Hosp, Brooklyn, NY
71-72; **FEL:** Coney Island Hosp, Brooklyn, NY 75-
77; Maimonides Med Ctr, Brooklyn, NY 70-71;
FAP: Clin Prof Med SUNY Hlth Sci Ctr; **SI:** *Chronic
Lung Disease; Asthma;* **HMO:** Oxford US Hlthcre Blue
Choice Aetna Hlth Plan Prucare +

LANG: Itl, Heb, Rus, Yd; 🚹 🔲 🔳 🔳   A Few Days

DERMATOLOGY

Baldwin, Hilary (MD)   D
Univ Hosp SUNY Bklyn
142 Joralemon St; Brooklyn, NY 11201; (718)
797-3340; **BDCERT:** D 88; **MS:** Boston U 84; **RES:**
New York University Med Ctr, New York, NY 85-
88; **HOSP:** Kings County Hosp Ctr; **SI:** *Keloids; Spider
Veins;* **HMO:** GHI Empire CIGNA Oxford 1199 +

🚹 🔳 🔳 🔳 🔳 🔳 🔳   Immediately

Berry, Richard (MD)   D
Univ Hosp SUNY Bklyn
2820 Ocean Pkwy; Brooklyn, NY 11235; (718)
996-3000; **BDCERT:** D 78; **MS:** SUNY Hlth Sci Ctr
74; **RES:** SUNY Health Sci Ctr, Brooklyn, NY; **FAP:**
Asst Clin Prof SUNY Hlth Sci Ctr; **HMO:** HealthNet
Blue Choice US Hlthcre Oxford Metlife +

LANG: Sp, Fr, Heb, Rus; 🚹 🔲 🔳 🔳 🔳 🔳 🔳
Immediately

Biro, Laszlo (MD)   D
Victory Memorial Hosp
9921 4th Ave; Brooklyn, NY 11209; (718) 833-
7616; **BDCERT:** D 63; **MS:** Hungary 53; **RES:** D,
New York University Med Ctr, New York, NY 58-
60; **FEL:** D, New York University Med Ctr, New
York, NY 58-60; **FAP:** Clin Prof D SUNY Hlth Sci
Ctr; **HOSP:** Lutheran Med Ctr; **SI:** *Cryosurgery; Laser
Surgery;* **HMO:** Aetna Hlth Plan Blue Choice Blue
Cross & Blue Shield

LANG: Hun, Itl, Fr, Rus, Nwg; 🚹 🔲 🔳 🔳 🔳
🔳 🔳 🔳

Brancaccio, Ronald R (MD)   D
Lutheran Med Ctr
Bay Ridge Dermatology Assocs, 7901 4th Ave;
Brooklyn, NY 11209; (718) 491-5800; **BDCERT:** D
77; **MS:** Geo Wash U Sch Med 72; **RES:** IM, Lenox
Hill Hosp, New York, NY 72-73; D, Oregon Health
Sci U Hosp, Portland, OR 73-76; **FEL:** Tropical
Disease, Univ of Sao Paulo, Sao Paulo, Brazil 76;
Leprosy, Lauro de Souza Lima, Lima, Peru; **FAP:**
Clin Prof NYU Sch Med; **HOSP:** New York
University Med Ctr; **SI:** *Contact Dermatitis; Cosmetic
Dermatology;* **HMO:** Oxford Blue Choice CIGNA

LANG: Itl, Sp, Fr, Rus, Ger; 🚹 🔲 🔳 🔳 🔳 🔳 🔳
🔳 🔳   Immediately 🔳 **VISA** 🔳

Carr, Elizabeth (MD)   D
Univ Hosp SUNY Bklyn
Bay Ridge Skin Cancer Dermatology, 9921 4th
Ave; Brooklyn, NY 11209; (718) 833-7616;
BDCERT: D 90; **MS:** Albany Med Coll 86; **RES:** IM,
Albany Med Ctr, Albany, NY 86-87; D, Univ Hosp
SUNY Bklyn, Brooklyn, NY 87-90; **SI:** *Cosmetic
Dermatology; Skin Cancer;* **HMO:** Oxford GHI Sanus
Prucare

LANG: Sp, Fr, Ar, Hun; 🚹 🔲 🔳 🔳 🔳 🔳 🔳
Immediately **VISA** 🔳 🔳

Deitz, Marcia (MD) D
Coney Island Hosp

1486 Ocean Pkwy; Brooklyn, NY 11230; (718) 627-3024; **BDCERT:** D 84; **MS:** SUNY Hlth Sci Ctr 80; **RES:** IM, Brookdale Univ Hosp Med Ctr, Brooklyn, NY 80-81; D, NY Med Coll, New York, NY 81-84; **HMO:** GHI Blue Choice Oxford Atlantis

▨ ▣ ▥ ▤ ▦ A Few Days

Feldman, Philip (MD) D
Long Island Coll Hosp

142 Joralemon St 4B; Brooklyn, NY 11201; (718) 237-0404; **BDCERT:** D 70; **MS:** Switzerland 63; **RES:** Columbia-Presbyterian Med Ctr, New York, NY 64-67; **FAP:** Asst Clin Prof; **HOSP:** Brooklyn Hosp Ctr-Downtown; **SI:** *Drug Allergy*; **HMO:** United Healthcare Oxford US Hlthcre GHI Empire Blue Choice +

LANG: Yd, Ger; ▨ ▣ ▥ ▤ ▦ ▩ 2-4 Weeks

Felman, Yehudi (MD) D
Univ Hosp SUNY Bklyn

8100 Bay Pkwy; Brooklyn, NY 11214; (718) 256-2600; **BDCERT:** D 68; **MS:** Albert Einstein Coll Med 63; **RES:** Colum Presb Med Ctr, New York, NY 64-67; **FAP:** Clin Prof D SUNY Hlth Sci Ctr; **HOSP:** Maimonides Med Ctr; **SI:** *Sexually Transmitted Diseases*; **HMO:** Prucare GHI Blue Choice Oxford Magnacare +

LANG: Sp, Heb, Rus; ▨ ▧ ▣ ▥ ▤ ▦ Immediately ▨ *VISA* ⬤

Gereme, Sebahat (MD) D
Brookdale Univ Hosp Med Ctr

Dermatology, 625 Rockaway Pkwy; Brooklyn, NY 11212; (718) 240-5855; **BDCERT:** D 82; **MS:** Pakistan 65; **RES:** Brookdale Univ Hosp Med Ctr, Brooklyn, NY 73-74; Brookdale Univ Hosp Med Ctr, Brooklyn, NY 77-78; **FEL:** New York University Med Ctr, New York, NY 74-77; **HMO:** 1199 GHI US Hlthcre

▨ ▣ ▥ ▤ ▦ ▩ A Few Days

Laude, Teresita A (MD) D
Kings County Hosp Ctr

450 Clarkson Ave Box 46; Brooklyn, NY 11203; (718) 270-1230; **BDCERT:** D 93; **MS:** Philippines 60; **RES:** D, Univ Hosp SUNY Bklyn, Brooklyn, NY 89-93; Kings County Hosp Ctr, Brooklyn, NY 65-67; **HOSP:** Univ Hosp SUNY Bklyn

▨ ▣ ▥ ▤ ▦ ▩ 4+ Weeks

Milburn, Peter (MD) D
Lutheran Med Ctr

8026 5th Ave; Brooklyn, NY 11209; (718) 680-2800; **BDCERT:** D 81; **MS:** Albert Einstein Coll Med 77; **RES:** Univ Hosp SUNY Bklyn, Brooklyn, NY 77-78; D, Columbia-Presbyterian Med Ctr, New York, NY 78-81; **HMO:** Aetna Hlth Plan Blue Choice Blue Cross & Blue Shield Choicecare CIGNA +

▨ ▧ ▣ ▥ ▤ ▦ ▩ Immediately *VISA* ⬤

Shalita, Alan (MD) D
Univ Hosp SUNY Bklyn

Downstate Dermatology Associates PC, 450 Clarkson Ave 46; Brooklyn, NY 11203; (718) 270-1229; **BDCERT:** D 71; **MS:** Bowman Gray 64; **RES:** New York University Med Ctr, New York, NY 67-70; **FEL:** D, New York University Med Ctr, New York, NY 70-73; **FAP:** Chrmn SUNY Hlth Sci Ctr; **HOSP:** Kings County Hosp Ctr; **SI:** *Acne; Rosacea*; **HMO:** Oxford GHI Empire

LANG: Fr; ▨ ▣ ▤ ▦ ▩ 2-4 Weeks

Simon, Steven (MD) D
Brookdale Univ Hosp Med Ctr

2270 Kimball St 201; Brooklyn, NY 11234; (718) 253-4550; **BDCERT:** D 81; **MS:** Mexico 75; **RES:** Brookdale Univ Hosp Med Ctr, Brooklyn, NY 76-78; Univ Hosp SUNY Bklyn, Brooklyn, NY 78-81; **HMO:** Empire Blue Cross & Shield Oxford CIGNA

▨ ▧ ▣ ▥ ▤ ▦ 2-4 Weeks

Westfried, Morris (MD)   **D**
Maimonides Med Ctr
532 Neptune Ave 209; Brooklyn, NY 11224; (718) 449-8860; **BDCERT:** D 80; **MS:** Yale U Sch Med 75; **RES:** Maimonides Med Ctr, Brooklyn, NY 76-77; D, Univ Hosp SUNY Bklyn, Brooklyn, NY 77-80; **FEL:** Chemosurgery, Henry Ford Hosp, Detroit, MI 80-86; **FAP:** Asst Clin Prof NY Med Coll; **HOSP:** Brooklyn Hosp Ctr-Downtown; **SI:** *Hair Removal - Laser; Spider Veins - Laser;* **HMO:** Oxford GHI 1199 Multiplan Magnacare +

LANG: Yd, Sp, Rus; ♿ 🆘 🅲 🄰 🄼 🄸 🅂 🄼🄲
A Few Days 💳 **VISA** 💳 💳

DIAGNOSTIC RADIOLOGY

Cohen, Harris L (MD)   **DR**
Univ Hosp SUNY Bklyn
University Hosp of Brooklyn University Hosp Associates, 450 Clarkson Ave Box 1208; Brooklyn, NY 11203; (718) 270-2916; **BDCERT:** DR 80; **PR** 95; **MS:** SUNY Downstate 76; **RES:** IM, Nassau County Med Ctr, East Meadow, NY 76-77; DR, Univ Hosp SUNY Bklyn, Brooklyn, NY 77-80; **FEL:** PR, Children's Hosp Nat Med Ctr, Washington, DC 80-81; **FAP:** Prof Rad SUNY Hlth Sci Ctr; **SI:** *Fetal Ultrasound; Pediatric/Adolescent OS/CT;* **HMO:** GHI US Hlthcre Oxford

LANG: Sp; ♿ 🄸 🅂 🄼🄲 🄼🄳 🅆🄲 🄽🄵🄸 A Few Days **VISA** 💳

Gerard, Perry (MD)   **DR**
Maimonides Med Ctr
4802 10th Ave; Brooklyn, NY 11219; (718) 283-8355; **BDCERT:** DR 87; NuM 89; **MS:** Rush Med Coll 80; **RES:** DR, Maimonides Med Ctr, Brooklyn, NY 81-84; **FEL:** Diagnostic Imaging, Maimonides Med Ctr, Brooklyn, NY 84-85; **FAP:** Asst Clin Prof Rad SUNY Downstate

LANG: Sp; ♿ 🆘 🅲 🄰 🄸 🄼🄲 🄼🄳 🅆🄲 🄽🄵🄸
Immediately 💳 **VISA** 💳

Gregoire, Clyde (MD)   **DR**
Wyckoff Heights Med Ctr
Wyckoff Radiological, 418 Stanhope St; Brooklyn, NY 11237; (718) 366-9492; **BDCERT:** DR 76; **MS:** Howard U 70; **RES:** ObG, Nassau County Med Ctr, East Meadow, NY 71-72; **FEL:** Rad, Nassau County Med Ctr, East Meadow, NY 73-75

LANG: Sp; 🅂 🄼🄲 🄼🄳 🅆🄲 🄽🄵🄸 Immediately

EMERGENCY MEDICINE

Bove, Joseph (MD)   **EM**
New York Methodist Hosp
Park Slope Emerg Phys PC NY Methodist Emerg Dpt, 506 6th St; Brooklyn, NY 11215; (718) 780-3159; **BDCERT:** EM 90; **MS:** Georgetown U 81; **RES:** S, Bellevue Hosp Ctr, New York, NY 81-83; **FAP:** Asst Prof EM Cornell U; **SI:** *Stroke-Emergency Care; Environmental Injuries;* **HMO:** Oxford Sel Pro Genesis US Hlthcre Aetna Hlth Plan +

LANG: Sp, Rus, Chi; ♿ 🆘 🅲 🄰 🄸 🄼🄲 🄼🄳 🅆🄲 🄽🄵🄸
Immediately 💳 **VISA** 💳 💳

Davidson, Steven (MD)   **EM**
Maimonides Med Ctr
Maimonides Med Ctr Emergency Med Facility Practice, 4802 10th Ave; Brooklyn, NY 11219; (718) 283-6030; **BDCERT:** EM 90; **MS:** Temple U 75; **RES:** EM, Hosp Med College of PA, Philadelphia, PA 75-78; **FAP:** Prof of Clin EM SUNY Downstate; **SI:** *Emergency Cardiac Care; Emergency Pediatric Care;* **HMO:** Oxford GHI HIP Network

LANG: Rus, Yd, Sp, Can, Man; ♿ 🆘 🅲 🄰 🄸 🄼🄲 🄼🄳 🅆🄲 🄽🄵🄸 Immediately **VISA** 💳

Van Amerongen, Robert (MD)EM
New York Methodist Hosp
New York Methodist Hospital, 506 6th St; Brooklyn, NY 11215; (718) 780-5040; **BDCERT:** Ped 96; EM 96; **MS:** Albert Einstein Coll Med 86; **RES:** Ped, N Shore Univ Hosp-Manhasset, Manhasset, NY 86; **FEL:** PEn, Bellevue Hosp Ctr, New York, NY 87; **SI:** *Pediatric Emergency Medical Services; Sedation for Procedures*

LANG: Sp, Rus, Heb; ♿ 🆘 🅲 🄰 🄸 🄼🄳 🅆🄲 🄽🄵🄸 Immediately

ENDOCRINOLOGY, DIABETES & METABOLISM

Banerji, Mary (MD) EDM
Univ Hosp SUNY Bklyn
450 Lenox Rd; Brooklyn, NY 11203; (718) 270-1000; **BDCERT:** IM 79; EDM 89; **MS:** Temple U 76; **RES:** Med, Univ Hosp SUNY Brooklyn, Brooklyn, NY 76-80; **FEL:** IM, Univ Hosp SUNY Brooklyn, Brooklyn, NY 80-81; EDM, Univ Hosp SUNY Brooklyn, Brooklyn, NY 81-83; *SI: Diabetes (Type II); Diabetes, Adult Onset;* **HMO:** Blue Cross & Blue Shield

♿ 🚻 🕗 Mcr Mcd 1 Week

Brickman, Alan (MD) EDM
Maimonides Med Ctr
1318 52nd St; Brooklyn, NY 11219; (718) 436-9898; **BDCERT:** IM 79; EDM 81; **MS:** Albert Einstein Coll Med 76; **RES:** Maimonides Med Ctr, Bronx, NY 76-79; **FEL:** EDM, Yale-New Haven Hosp, New Haven, CT 79-81; **HMO:** Oxford

🔌 📷 🕗 S Mcr 2-4 Weeks

Chaiken, Rochelle (MD) EDM
Univ Hosp SUNY Bklyn
SUNYHSC Brooklyn, 450 Clarkson Ave; Brooklyn, NY 11203; (718) 270-3052; **BDCERT:** IM 82; EDM 85; **MS:** SUNY Hlth Sci Ctr 78; **RES:** IM, Univ Hosp SUNY Bklyn, Brooklyn, MA 78-82; **FEL:** EDM, Beth Israel Med Ctr, Boston, MA 82; **FAP:** Assoc Prof SUNY Hlth Sci Ctr; *SI: Diabetes; Thyroid;* **HMO:** Empire GHI

♿ 📷 🚻 🕗 S Mcr A Few Days

Giegerich, Edmund (MD) EDM
Long Island Coll Hosp
Long Island College Hosptil, 340 Henry St; Brooklyn, NY 11201; (718) 780-4671; **BDCERT:** IM 80; EDM 83; **MS:** SUNY Downstate 77; **RES:** Rhode Island Hosp, Providence, RI 77-80; **FEL:** EDM, Mount Sinai Med Ctr, New York, NY 80-82; **FAP:** Assoc Clin Prof SUNY Hlth Sci Ctr

♿ 🔌 🚻 🕗 S Mcr 2-4 Weeks

Goldman, Joel (MD) EDM
Brookdale Univ Hosp Med Ctr
555 Rockaway; Brooklyn, NY 11212; (718) 240-5378; **BDCERT:** IM 76; EDM 79; **MS:** U Ariz Coll Med 73; **RES:** IM, Univ of Med & Dent NJ Hosp, Newark, NJ 73-75; IM, Albert Einstein Med Ctr, Bronx, NY 75-76; **FEL:** EDM, Nat Inst Health, Bethesda, MD 76-79; **FAP:** Assoc Prof SUNY Downstate; **HOSP:** Beth Israel Med Ctr; *SI: Diabetes; Thyroid Biopsies;* **HMO:** Oxford Blue Choice United Healthcare Magnacare US Hlthcre +

LANG: Yd; ♿ 🔌 📷 🚻 🕗 S Mcr Mcd WC 2-4 Weeks

Khan, Farida (MD) EDM
New York Methodist Hosp
NY Methodist Hosp, 506 6th St; Brooklyn, NY 11215; (718) 246-8500; **BDCERT:** IM 77; EDM 81; **MS:** India 62; **RES:** IM, Brooklyn Jewish Hosp, Brooklyn, NY 70-73; **FEL:** EDM, Brooklyn Jewish Hosp, Brooklyn, NY 71-73; **FAP:** Assoc Prof Cornell U; *SI: Diabetes; Thyroid Diseases;* **HMO:** Oxford GHI 1199 Blue Cross & Blue Shield NYLCare +

LANG: Sp, Hin, Rus; ♿ 📷 🚻 🕗 Mcr Mcd 2-4 Weeks

Lebovitz, Harold (MD) EDM
Univ Hosp SUNY Bklyn
450 Clarkson Ave; Brooklyn, NY 11203; (718) 270-1698; **MS:** Univ Pittsburgh 56; **RES:** Univ Pittsburgh, Pittsburgh, PA 56-59

Mann, David (MD) EDM
Long Island Coll Hosp
340 Henry St; Brooklyn, NY 11201; (718) 780-4672; **BDCERT:** IM 80; EDM 83; **MS:** Cornell U 77; **RES:** IM, Beth Israel Med Ctr, New York, NY 77-80; **FEL:** EDM, Montefiore Med Ctr, Bronx, NY 80-83; **FAP:** Asst Prof SUNY Hlth Sci Ctr; *SI: General Endocrinology;* **HMO:** Prucare Aetna-US Healthcare GHI NYLCare Atlantis +

LANG: Fr; ♿ 🕗 S Mcr 4+ Weeks

Pepper, Gary (MD)   EDM
Brooklyn Hosp Ctr-Caledonian
121 Dekalb Ave; Brooklyn, NY 11201; (718) 240-
6391; **BDCERT:** IM 79; EDM 81; **MS:** Tufts U 76;
RES: Montefiore Med Ctr, Bronx, NY; **FEL:** EDM,
Mount Sinai Med Ctr, New York, NY; **HMO:** Oxford
Aetna Hlth Plan Blue Cross & Blue Shield

Schussler, George (MD)   EDM
Univ Hosp SUNY Stony Brook
450 Clarkson Ave Box 57; Brooklyn, NY 11203;
(718) 270-2159; **BDCERT:** IM 63; EDM 73; **MS:**
Cornell U 56; **RES:** IM, Univ Hosp SUNY Syracuse,
Syracuse, NY 56-58; **FEL:** EDM, Boston Med Ctr,
Boston, MA 58-60; **FAP:** Prof SUNY Hlth Sci Ctr;
HOSP: Kings County Hosp Ctr; **SI:** *Thyroid; Calcium
Metabolism;* **HMO:** GHI HealthNet US Hlthcre
CIGNA Oxford +

🦽 🏠 🎞 $ Mcr Mcd   Immediately

Silverberg, Arnold (MD)   EDM
Maimonides Med Ctr
908 48th St; Brooklyn, NY; (718) 283-6200;
BDCERT: IM 68; EDM 77; **MS:** Albert Einstein Coll
Med 61; **RES:** IM, Montefiore Med Ctr, Bronx, NY
62-63; IM, Mount Sinai Med Ctr, New York, NY 64-
65; **FEL:** Physiology, Mem Sloan Kettering Cancer
Ctr, New York, NY 65-66; EDM, Mount Sinai Med
Ctr, New York, NY 66-68; **FAP:** Assoc Clin Prof
SUNY Downstate; **SI:** *Thyroid Disorders;
Osteoporosis;* **HMO:** Oxford PHCS Blue Choice
Elderplan
LANG: Yd; 🏠 🚹 🎞 Mcr   2-4 Weeks

Spergel, Gabriel (MD)   EDM
Lutheran Med Ctr
135 Ocean Pkwy; Brooklyn, NY 11218; (718)
853-3702; **MS:** Albert Einstein Coll Med 61; **RES:**
IM, Kings County Hosp Ctr, Brooklyn, NY 61-62;
IM, Kings County Hosp Ctr, Brooklyn, NY 62-64;
FEL: EDM, Kings County Hosp Ctr, Brooklyn, NY
64-65; EDM, Long Island Jewish Med Ctr, Glen
Oaks, NY 65-67; **FAP:** Assoc Clin Prof Cornell U;
HOSP: New York Comm Hosp of Bklyn; **SI:** *Diabetes;
Thyroid Disease;* **HMO:** Blue Choice PHS 1199
LANG: Rus, Sp, Yd; 🦽 🏠 🎞 WC NFI   1 Week

Wheeler, Mary (MD)   EDM
Coney Island Hosp
2601 Ocean Pkwy YN98; Brooklyn, NY 11235;
(718) 616-3897; **BDCERT:** IM 69; EDM 78; **MS:**
Cornell U 60; **RES:** Kings County Hosp Ctr,
Brooklyn, NY 60-63; **FEL:** EDM, Maimonides Med
Ctr, Brooklyn, NY 63-65; **FAP:** Assoc Prof of Clin
Med SUNY Hlth Sci Ctr; **HMO:** Oxford CIGNA
Metroplus Elderplan Health Plus +

🦽 🌙 🏠 🎞 $ Mcr Mcd WC NFI   2-4 Weeks 🖼 **VISA**

FAMILY PRACTICE

Athanail, Steven (MD)   FP   PCP
Lutheran Med Ctr
268 Bay Ridge Pkwy 1B; Brooklyn, NY 11209;
(718) 748-7272; **BDCERT:** FP 83; **MS:** Howard U
79; **RES:** Montefiore Med Ctr, Bronx, NY 81-83; **SI:**
Sports Medicine; **HMO:** CIGNA GHI Blue Choice
Child Health Plus +
LANG: Grk; 🌙 🏠 🚹 🎞 $ A Few Days

Candelaria, Luis (MD)   FP   PCP
Brooklyn Hosp Ctr-Caledonian
121 Dekalb Ave; Brooklyn, NY 11201; (718) 250-
8560; **BDCERT:** FP 84; FP 92; **MS:** U Puerto Rico
78; **RES:** U Puerto Rico, Caguas Regional Hosp,
Puerto Rico; **HMO:** Blue Cross & Blue Shield Chubb
GHI NYLCare
LANG: Sp, Fr, Rus; 🦽 🌙 🏠 🚹 🎞 $ Mcr Mcd WC   2-
4 Weeks

Caruana, Joseph (DO)   FP   PCP
Victory Memorial Hosp
Dyker Heights Family Med, 8413 13th Ave Fl 1;
Brooklyn, NY 11228; (718) 234-0826; **BDCERT:**
FP 90; FP 96; **MS:** NY Coll Osteo Med 87; **RES:** New
York Methodist Hosp, Brooklyn, NY 87-88; FP,
Lutheran Med Ctr, Brooklyn, NY 88-90; **HOSP:**
Lutheran Med Ctr; **SI:** *Well Child Care; Preventive
Care;* **HMO:** Oxford US Hlthcre NYLCare Aetna Hlth
Plan United Healthcare +
LANG: Itl; 🦽 🈯 🌙 🏠 🚹 🎞 Mcr   2-4 Weeks

De Caprariis, Pascal (MD)   FP   PCP
Univ Hosp SUNY Bklyn

450 Clarkson Ave Box 1240; Brooklyn, NY 11203; (718) 270-4180; **BDCERT:** FP 83; **MS:** Italy 78; **RES:** Luth Med Ctr, Brooklyn, NY 80-82; **FEL:** Inf, Qns Hosp Ctr, Jamaica, NY 82-84; **FAP:** Asst Prof Med SUNY Hlth Sci Ctr; **SI:** *AIDS; Infectious Diseases*

⬡ 🔲 🔲 🔲 🔲 🔲 🔲 A Few Days

de Larosa, Maritza (MD)   FP   PCP
Brooklyn Hosp Ctr-Caledonian

121 Dekalb Ave; Brooklyn, NY 11201; (718) 250-8621; **MS:** U del Caribe Escuela Med 80; **RES:** Lutheran Med Ctr, Brooklyn, NY 80-83; **HMO:** Oxford US Hlthcre Health First Chubb

🔲 🔲

Falkow, Seymour (MD)   FP   PCP
Brookdale Univ Hosp Med Ctr

1 Brookdale Plaza 324; Brooklyn, NY 11212; (718) 240-5984; **BDCERT:** FP 98; Ge 88; **MS:** Switzerland 56; **RES:** IM, Brookdale Univ Hosp Med Ctr, Brooklyn, NY 57; VA Med Ctr-Brooklyn, Brooklyn, NY 60; **FAP:** Asst Prof FP SUNY Hlth Sci Ctr; **SI:** *Geriatrics; Metabolism and Diabetes*

LANG: Fr, Ger, Yd; ⬡ 🔲 🔲 🔲

Gradler, Thomas (MD)   FP   PCP
Lutheran Med Ctr

234 Ovington Ave; Brooklyn, NY 11209; (718) 745-0309; **BDCERT:** FP 76; **MS:** SUNY Hlth Sci Ctr 73; **RES:** St Vincents Hosp & Med Ctr NY, New York, NY 73-74; FP, Lutheran Med Ctr, Brooklyn, NY 74-76; **HMO:** GHI Blue Choice HealthNet Metlife

🔲 🔲 🔲 🔲 🔲 🔲 🔲 2-4 Weeks

Holden, David (MD)   FP   PCP
Long Island Coll Hosp

Family Care Center, 165 Cadman Plaza East; Brooklyn, NY 11201; (718) 522-1099; **BDCERT:** FP 92; Ped 68; **MS:** Yale U Sch Med 63; **RES:** Ped, Yale-New Haven Hosp, New Haven, CT 63-64; Ped, Babies Hosp, New York, NY 64-66; **FAP:** Prof FP SUNY Hlth Sci Ctr; **HMO:** US Hlthcre Oxford HIP Network

LANG: Sp, Fr; ⬡ 🔲 🔲 🔲 🔲 🔲 🔲 🔲 🔲 1 Week

Jaffe, Kenneth (MD)   FP   PCP
New York Methodist Hosp

60 8th Ave; Brooklyn, NY 11217; (718) 638-1722; **BDCERT:** FP 80; **MS:** SUNY Buffalo 75; **RES:** U Mass Med Ctr, Worcester, MA 75-76; Brookdale Univ Hosp Med Ctr, Brooklyn, NY 78-80

🔲 🔲 🔲 🔲 Immediately **VISA** 💳

Liu, Kang (MD)   FP   PCP
Long Island Coll Hosp

397 Clinton St; Brooklyn, NY 11251; (718) 624-2776; **MS:** China 70; **RES:** Hackensack U Med Ctr, Hackensack, NJ 71; **HOSP:** Winthrop Univ Hosp; **HMO:** Oxford Aetna Hlth Plan GHI Blue Choice Empire +

LANG: Chi; 🔲 🔲 🔲 🔲 🔲 Immediately

Lopez, Clark (MD)   FP   PCP
New York Methodist Hosp

52 8th Ave; Brooklyn, NY 11217; (718) 783-3919; **BDCERT:** FP 76; **MS:** SUNY Downstate 72; **RES:** IM, Kings County Hosp Ctr, Brooklyn, NY; FP, Kings County Hosp Ctr, Brooklyn, NY; **FEL:** ObG, Kings County Hosp Ctr, Brooklyn, NY; **FAP:** Instr SUNY Downstate; **HOSP:** Lutheran Med Ctr; **HMO:** Oxford Blue Choice Aetna Hlth Plan Metlife Multiplan +

LANG: Sp, Fr; ⬡ 🔲 🔲 🔲 🔲 🔲 🔲 🔲 Immediately

Moskowitz, George (MD)   FP   PCP
Kings County Hosp Ctr

1318 42nd St; Brooklyn, NY 11219; (718) 436-2496; **BDCERT:** FP 78; **MS:** Belgium 73; **RES:** U Med Ctr, Jacksonville, FL; Med U of SC Med Ctr, Charleston, SC; **HOSP:** Maimonides Med Ctr; **SI:** *Women's Health; Heart Disease Prevention;* **HMO:** Oxford Empire

LANG: Yd, Fr, Heb, Rus; 🔲 🔲 🔲 🔲 🔲 🔲 🔲 🔲 Immediately

Purpura, Anthony (MD) FP **PCP**
Victory Memorial Hosp

8684 15th Ave; Brooklyn, NY 11228; (718) 232-0703; **MS:** Geo Wash U Sch Med 63; **RES:** Meadowbrook Hospital, East Meadow, NY 64; Maine Corp, 64-66; **HOSP:** Staten Island Univ Hosp-South; **HMO:** United Healthcare CIGNA Blue Cross & Blue Shield

LANG: Itl; 🗎 🕻 🔊 🖬 🛏 💲 Mcr Mcd WC NFI Immediately ▦ *VISA* ⬤

Reich, J Douglas (MD) FP **PCP**
Brooklyn Hosp Ctr-Downtown

Dept of Family Practice, 121 Dekalb Ave; Brooklyn, NY 11201; (718) 940-5910; **MS:** Mexico 81; **RES:** U Mass Med Ctr, Worcester, MA 82-83; Univ Hosp SUNY Stony Brook, Stony Brook, NY 83-84; **FEL:** UC San Francisco Med Ctr, San Francisco, CA; **HMO:** Blue Cross & Blue Shield GHI Oxford US Hlthcre

---

Rudorfer, Alvin (DO) FP **PCP**
New York Comm Hosp of Bklyn

2300 E 13th St; Brooklyn, NY 11229; (718) 743-1234; **BDCERT:** FP 74; **MS:** Chicago Coll Osteo Med 62; **RES:** Detroit Osteopathic Hosp, Detroit, MI 62-63; **HMO:** GHI Empire PHCS Blue Shield Oxford +

🔊 🖬 🛏 💲 Mcr Immediately

Sadovsky, Richard (MD) FP **PCP**
Univ Hosp SUNY Bklyn

450 Clarkson Ave; Brooklyn, NY 11203; (718) 270-2441; **BDCERT:** FP 77; **MS:** SUNY Hlth Sci Ctr 74; **RES:** FP, Univ Hosp SUNY Bklyn, Brooklyn, NY 74-77; **FAP:** Assoc Prof SUNY Hlth Sci Ctr; **SI:** *Preventive Heath Care*; **HMO:** Oxford CIGNA Blue Cross GHI

LANG: Sp; 🗎 🔊 🖬 🛏 💲 Mcr Mcd 2-4 Weeks

Schiowitz, Emanuel (DO) FP **PCP**
Maimonides Med Ctr

1701 59th St; Brooklyn, NY 11204; (718) 259-0222; **BDCERT:** FP 68; **MS:** Philadelphia Coll Osteo Med 63; **RES:** Interboro Gen Hosp, Brooklyn, NY 63-64; **FAP:** Adjct Clin Instr FP; **HOSP:** New York Methodist Hosp; **HMO:** Oxford Blue Choice Aetna Hlth Plan Independent Health Plan NYLCare +

LANG: Yd, Itl; 🗎 🕻 🔊 🖬 🛏 💲 Mcr 1 Week *VISA* ⬤

Scott, Norman (MD) FP **PCP**
Brookdale Univ Hosp Med Ctr

1381B Linden Blvd; Brooklyn, NY 11212; (718) 498-3104; **BDCERT:** FP 92; **MS:** Tulane U 76; **RES:** FP, Brookdale Univ Hosp Med Ctr, Brooklyn, NY 76-79

🗎 🗎 🕻 🔊 🛏 💲 Mcr Mcd Immediately

Shachner, Arthur (MD) FP **PCP**
Kings County Hosp Ctr

6910 Avenue U; Brooklyn, NY 11234; (718) 251-1200; **BDCERT:** FP 78; **MS:** Howard U 57; **RES:** Naval Hosp, Newport, RI; **HOSP:** New York Comm Hosp of Bklyn; **SI:** *Internal Medicine-Asthma; Cardiology—Diabetes*; **HMO:** Oxford Blue Cross & Blue Shield Blue Choice

🗎 🕻 🔊 🖬 🛏 💲 Mcr 1 Week ▦ *VISA* ⬤

Smith, Alford (MD) FP **PCP**
Kings County Hosp Ctr

322 Linden Blvd 1A; Brooklyn, NY 11226; (718) 282-1570; **MS:** SUNY Buffalo 82

Vincent, Miriam (MD) FP **PCP**
Univ Hosp SUNY Bklyn

470 Clarkson Ave; Brooklyn, NY 11203; (718) 270-2697; **BDCERT:** FP 88; **MS:** SUNY Hlth Sci Ctr 85; **RES:** Univ Hosp SUNY Bklyn, Brooklyn, NY 85-88; **HOSP:** Kings County Hosp Ctr; **SI:** *Dermatology; Pediatrics*; **HMO:** CIGNA GHI Health First Oxford Empire +

🗎 🕻 🔊 🖬 🛏 💲 Mcr Mcd A Few Days

Zachary, Mary (MD)   FP   `PCP`
Long Island Coll Hosp

Brooklyn Family Practice Associates, 165 Cadman Plaza; Brooklyn, NY 11201; (718) 522-1099; **BDCERT:** FP 88; **MS:** Mt Sinai Sch Med 85; **RES:** FP, Montefiore Med Ctr, Bronx, NY 85-88; **FAP:** Asst Clin Prof SUNY Hlth Sci Ctr; **SI:** *Women's Health; Alternative Medicine;* **HMO:** Oxford US Hlthcre Sanus United Healthcare HIP Network +

🦽 📞 🔒 👤 🏫 Mcr Mcd WC NFI   1 Week

Zimmerman, Saul (MD)   FP   `PCP`
New York Comm Hosp of Bklyn

202 W End Ave; Brooklyn, NY 11235; (718) 332-5447; **BDCERT:** FP 92; Anes 62; **MS:** U Hlth Sci/Chicago Med Sch 54; **RES:** Anes, VA Med Ctr-Brooklyn, Brooklyn, NY 55-57; **HMO:** Blue Cross & Blue Shield Metlife

GASTROENTEROLOGY

Albert, Joel (MD)   Ge
Maimonides Med Ctr

9707 4th Ave; Brooklyn, NY 11209; (718) 833-3700; **MS:** Mexico 73; **RES:** Maimonides, Brooklyn, NY 74-79

LANG: Sp; 🦽 📞 🔒 🏫 S Mcr   1 Week

Arya, Yashpal (MD)   Ge
Wyckoff Heights Med Ctr

Gastrointestinal Diagnostic, 372 Stanhope St; Brooklyn, NY 11237; (718) 821-0643; **BDCERT:** IM 72; **MS:** India 66; **RES:** IM, Wyckoff Heights Med Ctr, Brooklyn, NY 68-69; IM, Jewish Hosp Med Ctr, Brooklyn, NY 69-71; **FEL:** Ge, Queens Hosp Ctr, Jamaica, NY 71-73; **HOSP:** St John's Queens Hosp; **SI:** *Colon Cancer; Gastric Ulcer;* **HMO:** Blue Cross & Blue Shield Oxford GHI Aetna-US Healthcare MHS +

LANG: Sp, Hin, Itl; 🦽 SA/SU 📞 🔒 👤 🏫 S Mcr Mcd NFI
A Few Days

Bigajer, Charles (MD)   Ge
Brookdale Univ Hosp Med Ctr

1 Brookdale Plaza Rm 323R; Brooklyn, NY 11212; (718) 240-6385; **BDCERT:** Ge 81; IM 77; **MS:** Albert Einstein Coll Med 74; **RES:** IM, Brookdale Univ Hosp Med Ctr, Brooklyn, NY 74-77; **FEL:** Ge, New York University Med Ctr, New York, NY 78-80; **FAP:** Asst Clin Prof Ge SUNY Downstate; **HOSP:** Beth Israel Med Ctr-Kings Hwy; **SI:** *Endoscopy; Liver Diseases;* **HMO:** GHI Oxford Aetna-US Healthcare Prucare Blue Cross & Blue Shield +

LANG: Heb, Sp, Rus, Fr; 🦽 📞 🔒 👤 🏫 S Mcr
A Few Days

Cerulli, Maurice (MD)   Ge
Brooklyn Hosp Ctr-Caledonian

121 Dekalb Ave; Brooklyn, NY 11201; (718) 250-6945; **BDCERT:** IM 75; Ge 77; **MS:** SUNY Hlth Sci Ctr 72; **RES:** Kings County Hosp Ctr, Brooklyn, NY 72-75; **FEL:** Ge, Johns Hopkins Hosp, Baltimore, MD 75-77; **FAP:** Assoc Prof NYU Sch Med; **SI:** *Gastric & Colonic Diseases; Liver Disease & Nutrition;* **HMO:** Blue Choice Oxford Aetna Hlth Plan GHI

LANG: Sp, Chi, Rus, Itl, Fr; 🦽 🔒 👤 🏫 Mcr
A Few Days 📧

Cohen, Paul (MD)   Ge
Univ Hosp SUNY Bklyn

450 Clarkson Ave; Brooklyn, NY 11203; (718) 270-1112; **BDCERT:** IM 89; Ge 91; **MS:** Grenada 86; **RES:** Kings County Hosp Ctr, Brooklyn, NY 86-89; **FEL:** Ge, Kings County Hosp Ctr, Brooklyn, NY 89-91; **FAP:** Asst Prof Med SUNY Hlth Sci Ctr; **HMO:** CIGNA Oxford US Hlthcre Empire GHI +

🦽 SA/SU 📞 🔒 👤 🏫 Mcr Mcd   Immediately

Erber, William (MD)   Ge
Maimonides Med Ctr

591 Ocean Pkwy; Brooklyn, NY 11218; (718) 972-8500; **BDCERT:** Ge 79; IM 75; **MS:** U Hlth Sci/Chicago Med Sch 67; **RES:** Med, Maimonides Med Ctr, Brooklyn, NY 67; **FEL:** Ge, Albert Einstein Med Ctr, Bronx, NY 73-75; **FAP:** Asst Clin Prof SUNY Downstate; **HOSP:** Beth Israel Med Ctr; **SI:** *Ulcer Disease; Gastrointestinal Cancer;* **HMO:** Blue Cross & Blue Shield Oxford Aetna Hlth Plan United Healthcare CIGNA +

LANG: Rus, Fr, Heb, Yd, Ger; 🦽 SA/SU 📞 🔒 👤 🏫 S Mcr   Immediately

Geders, Jane (MD & PhD)   Ge
New York Methodist Hosp
Dep't of Medicine, 506 6th St; Brooklyn, NY
11215; (718) 780-5246; **BDCERT:** IM 90; Ge 93;
MS: U South Fla Coll Med 87; **RES:** IM, NY Hosp-
Cornell Med Ctr, New York, NY 87-88; IM, N Shore
Univ Hosp-Manhasset, Manhasset, NY 88-89; *SI:*
Hepatology Specialist
🔣 🔣 🔣 1 Week **VISA** 🔣

Gettenberg, Gary (MD)   Ge
Maimonides Med Ctr
813 Quentin Rd 104; Brooklyn, NY 11223; (718)
339-0391; **BDCERT:** IM 87; Ge 89; **MS:** NY Med
Coll 83; **RES:** IM, Maimonides Med Ctr, Brooklyn,
NY 84-86; **FEL:** Ge, Maimonides Med Ctr, Brooklyn,
NY 86-88; *SI: Gastrointestinal Endoscopy; Cancer*
Screening; **HMO:** US Hlthcre Oxford Aetna Hlth
Plan Prudential
LANG: Yd, Heb, Rus, Sp; 🔣 🔣 🔣 🔣 🔣 🔣 🔣 🔣
🔣 1 Week

Grosman, Irwin (MD)   Ge
Long Island Coll Hosp
339 Hicks St; Brooklyn, NY 11201; (718) 780-
1468; **BDCERT:** IM 87; Ge 89; **MS:** SUNY Stony
Brook 84; **RES:** IM, Montefiore Med Ctr, Bronx, NY
85-87; **FEL:** Ge, Montefiore Med Ctr, Bronx, NY 87-
89; **FAP:** Asst Prof SUNY Hlth Sci Ctr; **HMO:** Oxford
US Hlthcre GHI Blue Shield
🔣 🔣 🔣 🔣 🔣 🔣 🔣 🔣 A Few Days

Gusset, George (MD)   Ge
Beth Israel Med Ctr-Kings Hwy
2815 Ocean Pky; Brooklyn, NY 11235; (718) 769-
9595; **BDCERT:** IM 75; Ge 79; **MS:** KY Med Sch,
Louisville 60; **RES:** IM, VA Med Ctr-Brooklyn,
Brooklyn, NY 61-62; IM, Brooklyn Jewish Hosp,
Brooklyn, NY 62-63; **FEL:** Ge, Brooklyn Jewish
Hosp, Brooklyn, NY 63-64
🔣 🔣 🔣 🔣 🔣 🔣 🔣 🔣 A Few Days

Iswara, Kadirawel (MD)   Ge
Maimonides Med Ctr
2560 Ocean Ave Ste 3A; Brooklyn, NY 11229;
(718) 615-0400; **BDCERT:** IM 74; Ge 75; **MS:** Sri
Lanka 68; **RES:** IM, Coney Island Hosp, Brooklyn,
NY 71-72; Med, Bronx VA Hospital, Bronx, NY 72-
73; **FEL:** Ge, Maimonides Med Ctr, Bronx, NY 73-
76; *SI: Colon and Rectal Cancer; Gallstone—*
Nonsurgical Removal; **HMO:** GHI US Hlthcre Oxford
Blue Cross & Blue Shield Aetna Hlth Plan +
LANG: Rus, Tam, Heb, Yd; 🔣 🔣 🔣 🔣 🔣 🔣 🔣
🔣 Immediately

Kodsi, Baroukh (MD)   Ge
Maimonides Med Ctr
925 48th St; Brooklyn, NY 11219; (718) 851-
6767; **BDCERT:** Ge 63; **MS:** Egypt 45; **RES:** Boston
Med Ctr, Boston, MA 59-61; **FEL:** Ge, Boston Med
Ctr, Boston, MA 61-63; *SI: GI Cancer, Stomach &*
Colon-Cancer; Polypectomy & Reflux Disease; **HMO:**
Oxford Aetna-US Healthcare CIGNA Guardian GHI
+
LANG: Rus, Yd, Fr, Itl; 🔣 🔣 🔣 🔣 🔣 Immediately

Leb, Alvin (MD)   Ge
Beth Israel Med Ctr-Kings Hwy
2985 Quentin Rd; Brooklyn, NY 11229; (718)
336-2218; **BDCERT:** Ge 85; IM 85; **MS:** SUNY
Downstate 82; **RES:** IM, Brookdale Univ Hosp Med
Ctr, Brooklyn, NY 82-85; **FEL:** Ge, Brookdale Univ
Hosp Med Ctr, Brooklyn, NY 85-88; **HOSP:**
Brookdale Univ Hosp Med Ctr; *SI: Gastrointestinal*
Diseases; Cancer Prevention; **HMO:** United
Healthcare Magnacare Oxford Multiplan Blue
Choice +
LANG: Yd; 🔣 🔣 🔣 🔣 🔣 Immediately

Levendoglu, Hulya (MD)   Ge
Brookdale Univ Hosp Med Ctr
Brookdale Hosp, 580 Rockaway Pkwy 337;
Brooklyn, NY 11212; (718) 240-6025; **BDCERT:**
Ge 79; **MS:** Turkey 72; **RES:** Med, Cook Cty Hosp,
Chicago, IL 73-76; **FEL:** Ge, Cook Cty Hosp,
Chicago, IL 76-78; **FAP:** Assoc Prof of Clin Med
SUNY Hlth Sci Ctr; *SI: Hepatitis; Gastrointestinal*
Motility; **HMO:** US Hlthcre Oxford Blue Cross & Blue
Shield GHI 1199 +
LANG: Trk, Chi; 🔣 🔣 🔣 🔣 🔣 🔣 🔣

Guide to symbols and abbreviations can be found on pages 110-113.

495

Maizel, Barry (MD)　　Ge
New York Methodist Hosp
90 8th Ave; Brooklyn, NY 11215; (718) 622-
8255; **BDCERT:** IM 79; Ge 81; **MS:** Italy 75; **RES:**
Jewish Hosp Med Ctr, Brooklyn, NY 75-78; **FEL:** Ge,
New York University Med Ctr, New York, NY 78-
80; **HOSP:** Catholic Med Ctr Bklyn & Qns; **HMO:**
Magnacare CIGNA Oxford Multiplan PHS +

🚿 🔲 🔳 🏧 💲 Mcr A Few Days

Mayer, Ira (MD)　　Ge
Maimonides Med Ctr
2560 Ocean Ave 2A; Brooklyn, NY 11229; (718)
891-0100; **BDCERT:** IM 78; Ge 81; **MS:** NY Med
Coll 75; **RES:** Metropolitan Hosp Ctr, New York, NY
75-78; **FEL:** Ge, Emory U Hosp, Atlanta, GA 78-80;
HMO: Oxford CIGNA HealthNet Prucare Sanus +

🚿 🔲 🔳 🔳 🏧 💲 Mcr Immediately

Moskowitz, Sam (MD)　　Ge
Beth Israel Med Ctr-Kings Hwy
GastroBiliary Associates, PC, 1901 Utica Ave;
Brooklyn, NY 11375; (718) 520-0857; **BDCERT:**
IM 79; Ge 81; **MS:** Albert Einstein Coll Med 76; **RES:**
IM, Brookdale Univ Hosp Med Ctr, Brooklyn, NY
76-79; **FEL:** Ge, VA Med Ctr-Manh, New York, NY
79-81; **SI:** Colon Cancer Screening; Liver Diseases;
HMO: Oxford Blue Choice PPO Aetna-US
Healthcare Magnacare Prucare +

LANG: Yd, Heb; 🚿 🔲 🔳 🔳 🏧 Mcr Immediately
VISA 💳

Piccione, Paul (MD)　　Ge
Lutheran Med Ctr
466 Bay Ridge Pkwy; Brooklyn, NY 11209; (718)
748-5219; **BDCERT:** IM 85; Ge 87; **MS:** Italy 81;
RES: Lutheran Med Ctr, Brooklyn, NY 83-85; **FEL:**
Ge, St Luke's Roosevelt Hosp Ctr, New York, NY 85-
86; **HOSP:** Victory Memorial Hosp; **SI:**
Gastroenterology; Liver Disease; **HMO:** Oxford US
Hlthcre GHI Blue Choice

LANG: Itl, Rus, Sp; 🔲 🏧 Mcr Mcd 1 Week

Rezk, George (MD)　　Ge　 PCP
Long Island Coll Hosp
7906 4th Ave; Brooklyn, NY 11209; (718) 745-
8269; **BDCERT:** IM 81; Ge 83; **MS:** Italy 76; **RES:**
Long Island Coll Hosp, Brooklyn, NY 76-79; **FEL:**
Ge, Long Island Coll Hosp, Brooklyn, NY 79-81;
HOSP: New York Methodist Hosp; **HMO:** Oxford
Aetna Hlth Plan PHS Prucare United Healthcare +

LANG: Itl; 🚿 🔲 🔳 🔳 🏧 💲 Mcr Mcd 2-4 Weeks

Sorra, Toomas (MD)　　Ge
Long Island Coll Hosp
166 Clinton St; Brooklyn, NY 11201; (718) 834-
0100; **BDCERT:** IM 81; Ge 83; **MS:** Mexico 75; **RES:**
IM, Long Island Coll Hosp, Brooklyn, NY 77-80;
FEL: GO, Long Island Coll Hosp, Brooklyn, NY 80-
82; **FAP:** Clin Instr SUNY Downstate; **SI:** Colon
Cancer; Chronic Hepatitis; **HMO:** Oxford Blue Choice
Aetna Hlth Plan Magnacare GHI +

LANG: Sp, Est; 🚿 🔲 🔳 🔳 🏧 💲 Mcr 2-4 Weeks

Tracer, Robert (MD)　　Ge
Brookdale Univ Hosp Med Ctr
3131 Kings Hwy D7; Brooklyn, NY 11234; (718)
377-9011; **BDCERT:** IM 83; Ge 87; **MS:** SUNY Hlth
Sci Ctr 80; **RES:** IM, Kings County Hosp Ctr,
Brooklyn, NY 80-83; **FEL:** Ge, Brookdale Univ Hosp
Med Ctr, Brooklyn, NY 83-85; **FAP:** Clin Instr
SUNY Hlth Sci Ctr; **HOSP:** Beth Israel Med Ctr-
Kings Hwy; **HMO:** Oxford US Hlthcre Prucare
CIGNA GHI +

🚿 🔲 🔳 🔳 🏧 💲 Mcr Immediately

Wolfson, David (MD)　　Ge
Maimonides Med Ctr
801 Avenue N; Brooklyn, NY 11230; (718) 627-
6800; **BDCERT:** IM 79; Ge 81; **MS:** Harvard Med
Sch 76; **RES:** Mount Sinai Med Ctr, New York, NY
76; Mount Sinai Med Ctr, New York, NY 77-79;
FEL: Ge, Mount Sinai Med Ctr, New York, NY 79-
81; **HOSP:** New York Methodist Hosp; **SI:** Colon
Polyps; Ulcers; **HMO:** Oxford Blue Choice CIGNA
HealthNet Sanus +

LANG: Heb, Yd; 🔲 🔳 🔳 🏧 💲 Mcr Immediately
💳 **VISA** 💳

Zimbalist, Eliot (MD)   Ge
Maimonides Med Ctr
4802 10th Ave; Brooklyn, NY 11219; (718) 851-
1618; **BDCERT:** IM 83; Ge 85; **MS:** Mt Sinai Sch
Med 80; **RES:** Maimonides Med Ctr, Brooklyn, NY
80-83; **FEL:** Ge, Mem Sloan Kettering Cancer Ctr,
New York, NY; **FAP:** Assoc Prof SUNY Downstate;
SI: Gastrointestinal Endoscopy; Colon Cancer; **HMO:**
Oxford Aetna Hlth Plan CIGNA Premier Empire +

LANG: Sp, Fr, Rus, Chi; ▣ ▣ ▣ ▦ ▦ ▦
Immediately ▨ **VISA** ▧

GERIATRIC MEDICINE

Siegler, Eugenia (MD)   Ger
Brooklyn Hosp Ctr-Caledonian
Brooklyn Hosp Center, 121 Dekalb Ave; Brooklyn,
NY 11201; (718) 250-6131; **BDCERT:** IM 86; Ger
90; **MS:** Johns Hopkins U 83; **RES:** IM, Bellevue
Hosp Ctr, New York, NY 83-86; IM, Bellevue Hosp
Ctr, New York, NY 86-87; **FEL:** Ger, Hosp of U
Penn, Philadelphia, PA 87-89; **FAP:** Assoc Prof of
Clin Med NYU Sch Med; *SI: Dementia*

GERIATRIC PSYCHIATRY

Cohen, Carl (MD)   GerPsy
Univ Hosp SUNY Bklyn
SUNY Heath Sci Ctr Assoc, 370 Lenox Rd;
Brooklyn, NY 11226; (718) 287-4806; **BDCERT:**
Psyc 77; Psyc 91; **MS:** SUNY Buffalo 71; **RES:** Psyc,
Bellevue Hosp Ctr, New York, NY 72-74; Psyc,
Hosp Med College of PA, Philadelphia, PA 71-72;
FEL: Community Psyc, New York University Med
Ctr, New York, NY 74-75; **FAP:** Prof Psyc SUNY
Hlth Sci Ctr; *SI: Mental Disorders in Aged; Alzheimer's
Disease;* **HMO:** Oxford
▣ ▣ ▣ ▦ ▦ ▦ ▦ 1 Week

Samuelly, Israel (MD)   GerPsy
Maimonides Med Ctr
928 Albemarle Rd; Brooklyn, NY 11218; (718)
282-1981; **BDCERT:** Psyc 69; GerPsy 96; **MS:**
Israel 61; **RES:** Brooklyn Jewish Hosp, Brooklyn, NY
62-65; **FAP:** Assoc Clin Prof SUNY Downstate; *SI:
Geriatric Psychiatry*

LANG: Heb, Rom; ▣ ▣ ▣ ▣ ▦ ▦ ▦ 1 Week

GYNECOLOGIC ONCOLOGY

Boyce, John G (MD)   GO   `PCP`
Univ Hosp SUNY Bklyn
450 Clarkson Ave 24; Brooklyn, NY 11203; (718)
270-2081; **BDCERT:** ObG 69; GO 74; **MS:** U British
Columbia Fac Med 62; **RES:** ObG, Kings County
Hosp Ctr, Brooklyn, NY 63-67; **FEL:** GO, Kings
County Hosp Ctr, Brooklyn, NY 67-69; **HOSP:**
Kings County Hosp Ctr; **HMO:** US Hlthcre Aetna
Hlth Plan CIGNA Blue Cross & Blue Choice

▣ ▣ ▣ ▦ ▦ ▦ ▦ ▦ Immediately ▨ **VISA**
▧

Vardi, Joseph R (MD)   GO
Maimonides Med Ctr
941 48th St; Brooklyn, NY 11219; (718) 871-
3737; **BDCERT:** ObG 76; GO 79; **MS:** Israel 67;
RES: UC Davis Med Ctr, Sacramento, CA 72-74;
FEL: New England Med Ctr, Boston, MA 78; **HOSP:**
Lutheran Med Ctr; *SI: Ovarian Cancer; Cervix
Abnormality*

LANG: Fr, Heb, Sp; ▣ ▣ ▣ ▦ ▦ ▦ Immediately

HAND SURGERY

Monsanto, Enrique (MD)   HS
New York Methodist Hosp

Hand & Shoulder Institute, 519 6th St Rm B7308; Brooklyn, NY 11215; (718) 771-1765; **BDCERT:** OrS 86; **MS:** Columbia P&S 78; **RES:** OrS, Columbia-Presbyterian Med Ctr, New York, NY 80-83; **FEL:** HS, Columbia-Presbyterian Med Ctr, New York, NY 80-83; **FAP:** Asst Clin Prof OrS SUNY Downstate; **HOSP:** Long Island Coll Hosp; *SI: Nerve Entrapments; Rotator Cuff Disease*; **HMO:** Oxford United Healthcare Magnacare Premier Anthem Health +

LANG: Sp, Itl; [symbols] Immediately

Patel, Mukund (MD)   HS
Maimonides Med Ctr

Orthopedic Surgical Assoc, 4901 Fort Hamilton Pkwy; Brooklyn, NY 11219; (718) 435-4944; **BDCERT:** OrS 72; **MS:** India 81; **RES:** Hosp of U Penn, Philadelphia, PA 67-68; Maimonides Med Ctr, Brooklyn, NY 68-70; **FEL:** Mass Gen Hosp, Boston, MA 70-71; **FAP:** Assoc Clin Prof SUNY Downstate; **HOSP:** Staten Island Univ Hosp-South; *SI: Arthritis; Carpal Tunnel Syndrome*; **HMO:** Oxford US Hlthcre United Healthcare Blue Choice GHI +

LANG: Rus, Yd, Sp, Hin; [symbols] Immediately [VISA symbols]

Solomon, Ronald (MD)   HS
Long Island Coll Hosp

142 Joralemon St Ste 12A; Brooklyn, NY 11201; (718) 625-4975; **BDCERT:** S 96; HS 94; **MS:** U Rochester 72; **RES:** S, Univ Hosp SUNY Bklyn, Brooklyn, NY 77-79; S, Metropolitan Hosp Ctr, New York, NY 79; **FEL:** HS, NY Med Coll, New York, NY 82; **HOSP:** Brooklyn Hosp Ctr-Caledonian; *SI: Disorders of the Hand*; **HMO:** Aetna Hlth Plan US Hlthcre CIGNA HIP Network +

LANG: Sp; [symbols] 1 Week

HEMATOLOGY

Bashevkin, Michael (MD)   Hem
Maimonides Med Ctr

MMC Hematology/Oncology FPP, 6323 7th Ave; Brooklyn, NY 11220; (718) 283-6900; **BDCERT:** Hem 78; Onc 79; **MS:** SUNY Downstate 73; **RES:** IM, VA Med Ctr-Manhattan, New York, NY 74-76; Hem Onc-Maim Med Ctr, Brooklyn, NY 76-79; **FAP:** Instr Med SUNY Downstate; *SI: Oncology*

LANG: Sp, Rus, Heb; [symbols] 2-4 Weeks

Bradley, Thomas (MD)   Hem
Univ Hosp SUNY Bklyn

450 Clarkson Ave Box 50; Brooklyn, NY 11203; (718) 270-1573; **BDCERT:** IM 87; Onc 91; **MS:** Mexico 82; **RES:** IM, Univ Hosp SUNY Bklyn, Brooklyn, NY 84-87; Univ Hosp SUNY Bklyn, Brooklyn, NY 87-88; **FEL:** Hem Onc, Univ Hosp SUNY Bklyn, Brooklyn, NY 89-91; **FAP:** Asst Prof SUNY Hlth Sci Ctr; *SI: Lymphoma*; **HMO:** CIGNA Oxford GHI Health First

[symbols] 1 Week

Daya, Rami (MD)   Hem
New York Methodist Hosp

Hematology & Medical Oncology, 457 Bay Ridge Pkwy; Brooklyn, NY 11209; (718) 921-1672; **BDCERT:** IM 87; **MS:** Syria 81; **RES:** IM, New York Methodist Hosp, Brooklyn, NY 83-84; IM, New York Methodist Hosp, Brooklyn, NY 84-86; **FEL:** Onc, Univ of Med & Dent NJ Hosp, Newark, NJ 86-89; Hem, Univ of Med & Dent NJ Hosp, Newark, NJ; **HOSP:** Lutheran Med Ctr; *SI: Breast Cancer; Colon Cancer*; **HMO:** Blue Cross & Blue Shield Oxford Aetna Hlth Plan GHI Magnacare +

[symbols] Immediately

Dipillo, Frank (MD)   Hem
Long Island Coll Hosp

339 Hicks St; Brooklyn, NY 11201; (718) 780-1555; **BDCERT:** IM 63; Hem 72; **MS:** SUNY Downstate 56; **RES:** Long Island Coll Hosp, Brooklyn, NY 57-60; **FEL:** Hem, Montefiore Med Ctr, Bronx, NY

[symbols] 1 Week

Dosik, Harvey (MD)   Hem
New York Methodist Hosp

5016 6th St 1J; Brooklyn, NY 11215; (718) 891-9055; **BDCERT:** IM 70; Hem 76; **MS:** NYU Sch Med 63; **RES:** IM, Kings County Hosp Ctr, Brooklyn, NY 63-64; IM, Kings County Hosp Ctr, Brooklyn, NY 66-67; **FEL:** Hem, Maimonides Med Ctr, Brooklyn, NY 67-69; **FAP:** Prof Med Cornell U; **SI:** *Leukemia-Lymphoma; Genetics*; **HMO:** Oxford US Hlthcre Blue Choice PHS Multiplan +

LANG: Rus, Sp, Itl; ⚕ 📷 🏥 🛏 💲 Mcr WC
A Few Days

Friedberg, Neal (MD)   Hem
Brookdale Univ Hosp Med Ctr

Hemoncare PC, 2558 E 18th St; Brooklyn, NY 11234; (718) 616-0801; **BDCERT:** Hem 72; Onc 75; **MS:** SUNY Syracuse 66; **RES:** IM, Montefiore Med Ctr, Bronx, NY 66-68; **FEL:** Hem, Montefiore Med Ctr, Bronx, NY 68-70; **FAP:** Asst Prof Med SUNY Downstate; **HOSP:** New York Methodist Hosp; **SI:** *Lung Cancer; Breast Cancer*; **HMO:** Oxford Blue Cross Travelers Anthem Health Well Care +

LANG: Fr, Heb, Ur, Rus, Sp; ⚕ 📷 🛏 🏥 💲 Mcr
Immediately

Hyde, Phyllis (MD)   Hem
Long Island Coll Hosp

46 Livingston St; Brooklyn, NY 11201; (718) 855-1124; **BDCERT:** Hem 86; Onc 87; **MS:** SUNY Downstate 80; **RES:** IM, Columbia-Presbyterian Med Ctr, New York, NY 81-83; Onc, New York University Med Ctr, New York, NY 83-86; **HMO:** Oxford Aetna-US Healthcare United Healthcare GHI CIGNA +

LANG: Sp; ⚕ 📷 🏥 Mcr   A Few Days

Kopel, Samuel (MD)   Hem
Maimonides Med Ctr

MMC Hemotology & Oncology, 6323 7th Ave; Brooklyn, NY 11220; (718) 283-6900; **BDCERT:** Hem 78; Onc 79; **MS:** Italy 72; **RES:** IM, Jewish Hosp Med Ctr, Brooklyn, NY 73-75; Jewish Hosp Med Ctr, Brooklyn, NY 74-76; **FEL:** Hem, Jewish Hosp Med Ctr, Brooklyn, NY 75-76; Hem Onc, Mount Sinai Med Ctr, New York, NY 76-78; **FAP:** Asst Prof of Clin Med SUNY Downstate; **HMO:** GHI Aetna Hlth Plan US Hlthcre

LANG: Itl, Sp, Heb, Rus, Yd; ⚕ 📷 🏥 💲 Mcr Mcd WC NFI   1 Week

Lee, Stanley (MD)   Hem
Brookdale Univ Hosp Med Ctr

Brookdale Hospital, 580 Rockaway Pky 175; Brooklyn, NY 11212; (718) 240-6207; **BDCERT:** IM 52; Hem 74; **MS:** Harvard Med Sch 43; **RES:** Mount Sinai Med Ctr, New York, NY 43-44; IM, Mount Sinai Med Ctr, New York, NY 46-48; **FEL:** Path, Mount Sinai Med Ctr, New York, NY 48-49; Hem, Mount Sinai Med Ctr, New York, NY 49-53; **FAP:** Sr Prof SUNY Hlth Sci Ctr; **SI:** *Leukemia; Systemic Lupus*

⚕ 📷 🏥 Mcr Mcd WC NFI   Immediately

Levin, Mark (MD) Hem
Brookdale Univ Hosp Med Ctr

1 Brookdale Plaza; Brooklyn, NY 11212; (718) 240-6147; **BDCERT:** Onc 89; Hem 90; **MS:** SUNY Downstate 84; **RES:** IM, Hahnemann U Hosp, Philadelphia, PA 84-86; IM, NY Infirm/Beekman Dwntn Hosp, New York, NY 86-87; **FEL:** Hem/Onc, Long Island Jewish Med Ctr, New Hyde Park, NY 87-90

LANG: Rus; ⓢ ◙ Ⓢ Ⓜ Ⓜ 1 Week

Nawabi, Ismat (MD) Hem
Maimonides Med Ctr

MMC Hematology/Oncology FPP, 6323 7th Ave; Brooklyn, NY 11220; (718) 283-6900; **BDCERT:** IM 71; Hem 74; **MS:** Afghanistan 60; **RES:** IM, Cumberland Med Ctr, Brooklyn, NY 66-69; **FEL:** Hem, Maimonides Med Ctr, Brooklyn, NY 69-71; **FAP:** Asst Prof Med SUNY Downstate; **HMO:** GHI Aetna Hlth Plan US Hlthcre

LANG: Sp, Heb, Itl, Rus, Yd; ⓢ ◙ Ⓜ Ⓢ Ⓜ Ⓜ Ⓦ Ⓝ 1 Week

Rieder, Ronald (MD) Hem
Univ Hosp SUNY Bklyn

450 Clarkson Ave 20; Brooklyn, NY 11203; (718) 270-1500; **BDCERT:** IM 72; Hem 72; **MS:** NYU Sch Med 58; **RES:** IM, Bellevue Hosp Ctr, New York, NY 58-60; IM, Bellevue Hosp Ctr, New York, NY 64-65; **FEL:** Hem, Johns Hopkins Hosp, Baltimore, MD 62-64; **FAP:** Prof Med SUNY Hlth Sci Ctr; **SI:** *Anemia; Sickle Cell Disease*

LANG: Fr; ⓢ ◙ Ⓜ Ⓜ Ⓜ Ⓦ Ⓝ 1 Week

INFECTIOUS DISEASE

Berkowitz, Leonard B (MD) Inf
Brooklyn Hosp Ctr-Downtown

121 DeKalb Ave; Brooklyn, NY 11201; (718) 250-6141; **BDCERT:** IM 80; Inf 84; **MS:** SUNY Hlth Sci Ctr 77; **RES:** IM, Univ Hosp SUNY Bklyn, Brooklyn, NY 77-81; **FEL:** Inf, Univ Hosp SUNY Bklyn, Brooklyn, NY 81-83; **FAP:** Asst Prof SUNY Hlth Sci Ctr; **HOSP:** Long Island Coll Hosp; **SI:** *HIV; AIDS*; **HMO:** Prucare US Hlthcre Oxford Blue Cross NYLCare +

ⓢ ◙ Ⓜ Ⓜ Ⓜ 1 Week

Chapnick, Edward (MD) Inf
Maimonides Med Ctr

4802 10th Ave; Brooklyn, NY 11219; (718) 283-7492; **BDCERT:** IM 88; Inf 92; **MS:** SUNY Hlth Sci Ctr 85; **RES:** IM, Maimonides Med Ctr, Brooklyn, NY 85-88; IM, Maimonides Med Ctr, Brooklyn, NY 88-89; **FEL:** Inf, Maimonides Med Ctr, Brooklyn, NY 89-91; **FAP:** Asst Prof SUNY Hlth Sci Ctr; **SI:** *HIV/AIDS*; **HMO:** Oxford Aetna Hlth Plan CIGNA GHI Blue Choice +

ⓢ Ⓒ ◙ Ⓨ Ⓜ Ⓢ Ⓜ Ⓜ A Few Days **VISA** ●

Cofsky, Richard (MD) Inf
Brookdale Univ Hosp Med Ctr

1 Brookdale Plaza; Brooklyn, NY 11212; (718) 240-5096; **BDCERT:** IM 81; Inf 84; **MS:** U Md Sch Med 78; **RES:** Maimonides Med Ctr, Brooklyn, NY 78-81; **FEL:** Univ Hosp SUNY Bklyn, Brooklyn, NY 82-84; **FAP:** SUNY Downstate; **HOSP:** Beth Israel Med Ctr-Kings Hwy; **HMO:** Blue Choice Blue Cross & Blue Shield HealthNet Prucare Travelers +

ⓢ ◙ Ⓜ Ⓜ Ⓝ Immediately

Colby, Steven (MD) Inf
New York Methodist Hosp

NY Methodist Hosp—Inf Dis/Int Med Dept, 506 6th St; Brooklyn, NY 11238; (718) 246-8500; **BDCERT:** IM 81; Inf 83; **MS:** Loyola U-Stritch Sch Med, Maywood 75; **RES:** IM, Boston Med Ctr, Boston, MA 76-79; **FEL:** Inf, Naval Med Ctr, San Diego, CA 79-81; **FAP:** Asst Prof SUNY Hlth Sci Ctr; **SI:** *AIDS; Sexually Transmitted Disease*; **HMO:** GHI Empire Blue Cross

ⓢ ◙ Ⓨ Ⓜ Ⓜ Ⓜ A Few Days

Cortes, Hiram (MD) Inf 🅿🅲🅿
New York Methodist Hosp

115 Prospect Park West; Brooklyn, NY 11215; (718) 369-3555; **BDCERT:** IM 97; **MS:** West Indies 84; **RES:** IM, New York Methodist Hosp, Brooklyn, NY 84-88; Inf, Cabrini Med Ctr, New York, NY 88-90; **HOSP:** Bayley Seton Hosp; **SI:** *Lyme Disease,; AIDS, Hepatitis*; **HMO:** PHS United Healthcare Oxford NYLCare HIP Network +

LANG: Sp; ⓢ Ⓒ ◙ Ⓨ Ⓜ Ⓢ Ⓜ Ⓜ A Few Days

Lutwick, Larry Irwin (MD)   Inf
Maimonides Med Ctr

369 93rd St; Brooklyn, NY 11209; (718) 680-6000; **BDCERT:** Med 75; Inf 76; **MS:** SUNY Downstate 72; **RES:** Barnes Hosp, St Louis, MO 72-74; **FEL:** Stanford Med Ctr, Stanford, CA 74-76; **FAP:** Prof Med SUNY Downstate; **SI:** *Hepatitis*; **HMO:** Most

▦ ☏ ⚕ ⊞ Mcr Mcl WC NFl A Few Days▨ **VISA**
◉ ▤

McCormack, William M (MD)Inf
Univ Hosp SUNY Bklyn

Box 56, 450 Clarkson Ave RmB5302; Brooklyn, NY 11203; (718) 270-1432; **BDCERT:** IM 71; Inf 72; **MS:** SUNY Hlth Sci Ctr 63; **RES:** IM, Columbia-Presbyterian Med Ctr, New York, NY 64-65; IM, Mass Gen Hosp, Boston, MA 68-69; **FEL:** Inf, Beth Israel Med Ctr, Boston, MA 69-71; **FAP:** Prof SUNY Downstate; **SI:** *Vaginitis & Vulvitis; Sexually Transmitted Diseases*; **HMO:** Oxford CIGNA Empire Blue Cross & Shield Aetna Hlth Plan GHI +

♿ ☏ ⚕ ⊞ S Mcr 1 Week

Sepkowitz, Douglas (MD)   Inf   PCP
Long Island Coll Hosp

149 Congress St; Brooklyn, NY 11201; (718) 797-4684; **BDCERT:** IM 82; Inf 86; **MS:** U Okla Coll Med 79; **RES:** Maimonides Med Ctr, Brooklyn, NY 79-82; **FEL:** Inf, Long Island Coll Hosp, Brooklyn, NY 84-86; **SI:** *AIDS*; **HMO:** Most

LANG: Fr; ☏ ⊞ S Mcr Mcl 1 Week

Stein, Alan (MD)   Inf
New York Methodist Hosp

Infectious Diseases Associated of Brooklyn, 263 7th Ave Suite F; Brooklyn, NY 11201; (718) 369-8010; **BDCERT:** IM 76; Inf 78; **MS:** NY Med Coll 72; **RES:** IM, Lenox Hill Hosp, New York, NY; Metropolitan Hosp Ctr, New York, NY 1; **FEL:** Inf, New York University Med Ctr, New York, NY; **FAP:** Assoc Clin Prof NYU Sch Med; **HOSP:** Brooklyn Hosp Ctr-Downtown; **SI:** *AIDS/HIV; Travel Medicine*; **HMO:** Oxford US Hlthcre CIGNA GHI

♿ ▦ ☏ ⚕ ⊞ S Mcr Mcl Immediately

INTERNAL MEDICINE

Abott, Michael (MD)   IM   PCP
New York Methodist Hosp

The Chest Medical Group of Brooklyn, 7501 16th Ave; Brooklyn, NY 11214; (718) 234-3333; **BDCERT:** IM 83; Pul 86; **MS:** Mexico 78; **RES:** Med, Coney Island Hosp, Brooklyn, NY 79-80; IM, Coney Island Hosp, Brooklyn, NY 80-82; **FEL:** Pul, Albert Einstein Med Ctr, Bronx, NY 82-84; **FAP:** Clin Prof Cornell U; **HOSP:** Victory Memorial Hosp; **SI:** *Asthma; Emphysema*; **HMO:** Blue Cross & Blue Shield Oxford Aetna Hlth Plan CIGNA US Hlthcre +

LANG: Sp, Itl, Fr, Per; ☏ ⚕ ⊞ S Mcr 2-4 Weeks

Baccash, Emil (MD)   IM   PCP
New York Methodist Hosp

20 8th Ave; Brooklyn, NY 11217; (718) 622-7000; **BDCERT:** IM 81; Ger 94; **MS:** Italy 78; **RES:** IM, New York Methodist Hosp, Brooklyn, NY 78-81; **FAP:** Clin Instr SUNY Hlth Sci Ctr; **HMO:** Oxford US Hlthcre CIGNA 1199 Blue Choice +

LANG: Itl; ☏ ⚕ ⊞ S Mcr Mcl 2-4 Weeks

Behm, Dutsi (MD)   IM
New York Methodist Hosp

1128 Foster Ave; Brooklyn, NY 11230; (718) 859-8600; **MS:** Ukraine 73

Bharathan, Thayyulla (MD) IM   PCP
New York Methodist Hosp

263 7th Ave; Brooklyn, NY 11215; (718) 246-8500; **BDCERT:** IM 76; Ger 88; **MS:** India 62; **RES:** New York Methodist Hosp, Brooklyn, NY 69-72; **FAP:** Asst Clin Prof Cornell U; **SI:** *Geriatric Medicine*; **HMO:** US Hlthcre Oxford Blue Cross GHI 1199 +

LANG: Hin; ♿ ☏ ⚕ ⊞ S Mcr NFl A Few Days

Bloom, Jerry (MD)   IM   PCP
Brookdale Univ Hosp Med Ctr

1 Brookdale Plaza; Brooklyn, NY 11212; (718) 240-5818; **BDCERT:** IM 71; **MS:** SUNY Downstate 62; **RES:** Med, Maimonides Med Ctr, Brooklyn, NY 63-65; Med, Maimonides Med Ctr, Brooklyn, NY; **FAP:** Assoc Clin Prof Med SUNY Downstate; *SI: Infectious Diseases*; **HMO:** Oxford GHI

LANG: Fr, Ger, Yd; ⬧ 📷 🚹 🛏 Mcr   A Few Days

Brown, Lawrence S (MD)   IM   PCP
Columbia-Presbyterian Med Ctr

22 Chapel St; Brooklyn, NY 11201; (718) 260-2917; **BDCERT:** IM 92; **MS:** NYU Sch Med 79; **RES:** IM, Harlem Hosp Ctr, New York, NY 79-82; **FEL:** EDM, Columbia-Presbyterian Med Ctr, New York, NY 83-86; **FAP:** Asst Clin Prof Med Columbia P&S; *SI: Addiction Medicine; HIV*

⬧ 📶 📷 🚹 🛏 Mcr Mcd WC   2-4 Weeks

Cohen, Barry (MD)   IM   PCP
New York Methodist Hosp

2 West End Ave; Brooklyn, NY 11235; (718) 934-1222; **BDCERT:** IM 86; **MS:** Dominican Republic 82; **RES:** Elmhurst Hosp Ctr, Elmhurst, NY 83-84; **HOSP:** New York Comm Hosp of Bklyn; *SI: High Blood Pressure; Diabetes*; **HMO:** United Healthcare Oxford PHS Prucare CIGNA +

⬧ 🅒 📷 🚹 🛏 🆂 Mcr   Immediately

Cohn, Steven (MD)   IM   PCP
Kings County Hosp Ctr

470 Clarkson Ave; Brooklyn, NY 11203; (718) 270-1531; **BDCERT:** IM 83; **MS:** Mexico 78; **RES:** Univ Hosp SUNY Bklyn, Brooklyn, NY 79-82; **FAP:** Assoc Prof Med SUNY Hlth Sci Ctr; *SI: Preoperative Consultation; Hypertension*; **HMO:** Oxford US Hlthcre HIP Network

⬧ 📷 🛏 🆂 Mcr   2-4 Weeks

De Rose, Joseph J (MD)   IM   PCP
Univ Hosp SUNY Bklyn

7606 7th Avenue; Brooklyn, NY 11209; (718) 492-5518; **MS:** SUNY Downstate 63; **RES:** Med, Kings County Hosp Ctr, Brooklyn, NY 64-65; Med, Kings County Hosp Ctr, Brooklyn, NY 65-66; **FEL:** Med, Univ Hosp SUNY Bklyn, Brooklyn, NY 66-67; **FAP:** Assoc Prof SUNY Hlth Sci Ctr; *SI: Paget's Disease of Bone; Cardiology-Echocardiography*; **HMO:** United Healthcare Empire

⬧ 📷 🛏 WC   2-4 Weeks

Dooley, Evelyn (MD)   IM   PCP
Brookdale Univ Hosp Med Ctr

555 Rockaway Pkwy Ste 105; Brooklyn, NY 11212; (718) 240-5105; **BDCERT:** IM 72; Ger 92; **MS:** UMDNJ-NJ Med Sch, Newark 64; **RES:** IM, St Luke's Roosevelt Hosp Ctr, New York, NY 65-67; **FEL:** Cv, St Luke's Roosevelt Hosp Ctr, New York, NY 67; **FAP:** Asst Clin Prof Med SUNY Downstate; *SI: Urinary Incontinence; Feeding Disorders of Elderly*; **HMO:** 1199 Blue Cross & Blue Shield Sanus-NYLCare Oxford

⬧ 📷 🚹 🛏 🆂 Mcr   2-4 Weeks

Dunst, Maurice (MD)   IM
Brooklyn Hosp Ctr-Caledonian

2281 Ocean Pky; Brooklyn, NY 11223; (718) 375-1010; **BDCERT:** IM 60; Ger 88; **MS:** NYU Sch Med 52; **RES:** Med, Mount Sinai Med Ctr, New York, NY 56-57; MF, Montefiore Med Ctr, Bronx, NY 55-56; **FEL:** Cv, Mount Sinai Med Ctr, New York, NY 57-58; **HMO:** Aetna Hlth Plan Blue Cross & Blue Shield Metlife

Ellis, Earl A (MD)   IM   PCP
Catholic Med Ctr Bklyn & Qns

66 Rutland Rd; Brooklyn, NY 11225; (718) 282-4412; **BDCERT:** IM 84; Ger 90; **MS:** Howard U 80; **RES:** Elmhurst Hosp Ctr, Elmhurst, NY 80-83; **HOSP:** St Mary's Hosp; *SI: Geriatrics*; **HMO:** Empire Blue Cross & Shield Aetna-US Healthcare 1199 Oxford United Healthcare +

📶 🅒 📷 🚹 🛏 🆂 Mcr   Immediately

Ginsberg, Donald (MD)   IM   **PCP**
Beth Israel Med Ctr-Kings Hwy

3131 Kings Hwy; Brooklyn, NY 11234; (718) 252-2300; **BDCERT:** IM 65; **MS:** SUNY Buffalo 58; **RES:** IM, Brookdale Univ Hosp Med Ctr, Brooklyn, NY 59-61; IM, VA Med Ctr-Brooklyn, Brooklyn, NY 61-62; *SI: Hyperlipidemia;* **HMO:** Oxford Blue Choice

⬚ ⬚ ⬚ ⬚   A Few Days

Goldberg, Richard (MD)   IM   **PCP**
Beth Israel Med Ctr

3131 Kings Hwy D10; Brooklyn, NY 11234; (718) 377-4860; **BDCERT:** IM 94; **MS:** Italy 72; **RES:** IM, Brooklyn Jewish Hosp, Brooklyn, NY 73-76; **HOSP:** New York Methodist Hosp; *SI: Geriatrics;* **HMO:** NYLCare Oxford GHI

LANG: Sp, Itl, Rus; ⬚ ⬚ ⬚ ⬚ ⬚ ⬚ ⬚ ⬚ Immediately

Grob, David (MD)   IM
Maimonides Med Ctr

4802 10th Ave; Brooklyn, NY 11219; (718) 283-7969; **BDCERT:** IM 51; **MS:** Johns Hopkins U 42; **RES:** Johns Hopkins Hosp, Baltimore, MD 45-46; **FEL:** Johns Hopkins Hosp, Baltimore, MD 47-48; **FAP:** Prof Med SUNY Hlth Sci Ctr; **HOSP:** Univ Hosp SUNY Bklyn; *SI: Myasthenia Gravis; Autoimmune Diseases*

LANG: Ger, Fr; ⬚ ⬚ ⬚ ⬚ ⬚ ⬚ ⬚   1 Week

Grunzweig, Milton (MD)   IM   **PCP**
Brookdale Univ Hosp Med Ctr

2044 Ocean Ave A6; Brooklyn, NY 11230; (718) 998-2222; **BDCERT:** IM 89; **MS:** SUNY Hlth Sci Ctr 86; **RES:** Brookdale Univ Hosp Med Ctr, Brooklyn, NY 89; **HOSP:** Beth Israel Med Ctr; **HMO:** Oxford US Hlthcre Blue Cross Prucare GHI +

LANG: Heb, Yd, Fr, Rus; ⬚ ⬚ ⬚ ⬚ ⬚ ⬚ ⬚ ⬚ ⬚ ⬚ Immediately

Hollander, Gerald (MD)   IM
Maimonides Med Ctr

4802 10th Ave; Brooklyn, NY 11219; (718) 283-7489; **BDCERT:** IM 76; Cv 79; **MS:** SUNY Downstate 73; **RES:** IM, Brookdale Univ Hosp Med Ctr, Brooklyn, NY 73-76; **FEL:** Cv, Brookdale Univ Hosp Med Ctr, Brooklyn, NY 76-78; **FAP:** Assoc Clin Prof Med SUNY Hlth Sci Ctr

LANG: Yd, Heb; ⬚ ⬚ ⬚ ⬚ ⬚   2-4 Weeks

Husney, Joseph (MD)   IM   **PCP**
New York Comm Hosp of Bklyn

2579 Ocean Ave; Brooklyn, NY 11229; (718) 934-1234; **BDCERT:** IM 76; **MS:** France 70; **RES:** IM, Beekman Downtown Hosp, New York, NY 71-72; IM, Beekman Downtown Hosp, New York, NY 72-73; **FEL:** Cv, Kingsbrook Jewish Med Ctr, Brooklyn, NY 73-74; **HOSP:** Beth Israel Med Ctr-Kings Hwy; *SI: High Pressure Diabetes; Heart Disease/Lung Disease;* **HMO:** Oxford Blue Choice Prudential CIGNA PHS +

LANG: Fr, Heb, Ar, Sp; ⬚ ⬚ ⬚ ⬚ ⬚ ⬚ ⬚ 1 Week

Imperato, Pascal James (MD)   IM   **PCP**
Univ Hosp SUNY Bklyn

450 Clarkson Ave; Brooklyn, NY 11203; (718) 270-1056; **BDCERT:** PrM 72; **MS:** SUNY Hlth Sci Ctr 62; **RES:** IM, Long Island Coll Hosp, Brooklyn, NY 62-65; **FEL:** Tropical Medicine, Tulane U Med Ctr, New Orleans, LA 65-66; **FAP:** Prof SUNY Downstate; **HOSP:** Kings County Hosp Ctr; *SI: Urination Problems; Non Operative Urology*

LANG: Sp; ⬚ ⬚ ⬚   A Few Days

Jonas, Murray (MD)   IM
Beth Israel Med Ctr-Kings Hwy

1569 E 18th St; Brooklyn, NY 11230; (718) 375-6500; **BDCERT:** IM 85; Inf 96; **MS:** SUNY Downstate 77; **RES:** IM, Metropolitan Hosp Ctr, New York, NY 77-78; IM, Nassau County Med Ctr, East Meadow, NY 78-80; **FEL:** Inf, Winthrop Univ Hosp, Mineola, NY 80-83; **HOSP:** New York Methodist Hosp; **HMO:** Oxford Blue Cross GHI Multiplan

LANG: Sp, Rus, Heb, Yd; ⬚ ⬚ ⬚ ⬚ ⬚ ⬚ ⬚ Immediately

Jones, Vann (MD)   IM   PCP
Brooklyn Hosp Ctr-Caledonian
10 Plaza St E E1; Brooklyn, NY 11238; (718) 638-
3434; **BDCERT:** IM 72; **MS:** Howard U 66; **RES:**
Kings County Hosp Ctr, Brooklyn, NY 66-68;
Montefiore Med Ctr, Bronx, NY 68-70; **FAP:** Asst
Clin Prof SUNY Hlth Sci Ctr; **HMO:** Metlife US
Hlthcre Chubb Blue Cross & Blue Shield

🦽 🌓 📷 🏥 💲   A Few Days

Kaiser, Stephen (MD)   IM   PCP
Maimonides Med Ctr
465 Ocean Pkwy; Brooklyn, NY 11218; (718)
941-5600; **BDCERT:** IM 72; **MS:** SUNY Buffalo 64;
RES: EJ Meyer Mem Hosp, Buffalo, NY 64-65; Kings
County Hosp Ctr, Brooklyn, NY 65-67; **FEL:** Hem,
Maimonides Med Ctr, Brooklyn, NY 67-69; *SI:*
Diabetes Mellitus; Hypertension; **HMO:** HealthNet
Oxford Blue Choice PHS US Hlthcre +

🦽 🛏 📷 🏥 💲 ⛐ ⛐   A Few Days

Katzenelenbogen, Moshe (MD) IM   PCP
Beth Israel Med Ctr
2992 Avenue Z; Brooklyn, NY 11235; (718) 646-
1422; **BDCERT:** IM 84; Ger 92; **MS:** Romania 80;
RES: IM, Coney Island Hosp, Brooklyn, NY 83-84;
HMO: Oxford Multiplan GHI Magnacare

LANG: Heb, Yd, Rom; 🦽 🌓 📷 🏥 🏥 💲 ⛐
1 Week

Kazdin, Hal (MD)   IM   PCP
New York Comm Hosp of Bklyn
90 Brighton 11th St; Brooklyn, NY 11235; (718)
332-7770; **BDCERT:** IM 82; **MS:** Philippines 77;
RES: Elmhurst Hosp Ctr, Elmhurst, NY 78;
Elmhurst Hosp Ctr, Elmhurst, NY 79-81; **FEL:** Rhu,
Long Island Jewish Med Ctr, New Hyde Park, NY
81-83; **HOSP:** Beth Israel Med Ctr-Kings Hwy; *SI:*
Rheumatoid Arthritis; Osteoarthritis Pain Control;
HMO: Independent Health Plan PHS GHI
Magnacare Oxford +

LANG: Rus, Sp; 🛏 🌓 📷 🏥 🏥 💲 ⛐ ⛐
A Few Days

Kelter, Robert (MD)   IM   PCP
Victory Memorial Hosp
346 77th St; Brooklyn, NY 11209; (718) 745-
1064; **BDCERT:** IM 95; **MS:** Dominica 84; **RES:** IM,
St Vincent's Med Ctr-Richmond, Staten Island, NY
84-87; **HOSP:** Lutheran Med Ctr; *SI: High Blood*
Pressure; Diabetes Mellitus; **HMO:** Oxford GHI United
Healthcare Blue Choice Prucare +

🦽 🌓 📷 🏥 🏥 💲 ⛐ ⛐   Immediately ▨ **VISA**
💳 💳

Konka, Sudarsanam (MD)   IM
Long Island Coll Hosp
142 Joralemon St #11D; Brooklyn, NY 11201;
(718) 935-9837; **BDCERT:** IM 74; Cv 77; **MS:** India
70; **RES:** Long Island Coll Hosp, Brooklyn, NY 71-
74; **FEL:** Nassau Cty Med Ctr, East Meadow, NY 74-
75; Long Island Coll Hosp, East Meadow, NY 75-
76; **HOSP:** Long Island Jewish Med Ctr

Kurz, Larry (MD)   IM   PCP
New York Methodist Hosp
54 8th Ave Fl 1; Brooklyn, NY 11217; (718) 638-
2551; **BDCERT:** IM 77; **MS:** Washington U, St
Louis 70; **RES:** IM, Univ Hosp SUNY Bklyn,
Brooklyn, NY 74-77; *SI: General Medicine;* **HMO:**
PHS United Healthcare Oxford

📷 🏥 🏥 ⛐ ⛐ ⛐   A Few Days

Levey, Robert (MD)   IM   PCP
Long Island Coll Hosp
8672 Bay Pkwy; Brooklyn, NY 11214; (718) 372-
2234; **BDCERT:** IM 77; **MS:** U Mich Med Sch 70;
RES: New York University Med Ctr, New York, NY
70-71; Long Island Coll Hosp, Brooklyn, NY 75-77;
SI: Geriatrics; **HMO:** Oxford Prucare Blue Choice
Magnacare

LANG: Yd; 🌓 📷 🏥 🏥 💲 ⛐   A Few Days

Levin, Nathan (MD)   IM   PCP
Cabrini Med Ctr
500 Brightwater Ct; Brooklyn, NY 11235; (718)
743-7700; **BDCERT:** IM 93; **MS:** Ukraine 60; **RES:**
St Vincents Hosp & Med Ctr NY, New York, NY 90;
HOSP: Beth Israel Med Ctr; **HMO:** Blue Cross & Blue
Shield Oxford Aetna Hlth Plan GHI

🦽 🛏 🌓 📷 🏥 🏥 ⛐ ⛐ ⛐   Immediately

Lifshitz, Benjamin (MD)   **IM**
Maimonides Med Ctr
3043 Ocean Ave; Brooklyn, NY 11235; (718) 856-8600; **BDCERT:** IM 88; **MS:** Cornell U 85; **RES:** Maimonides Med Ctr, Brooklyn, NY 85-88

Louis, Bertin Magloi (MD)   **IM**
Maimonides Med Ctr
953 43rd St Rm 611; Brooklyn, NY 11219; (718) 283-7903; **BDCERT:** IM 75; Nep 82; **MS:** Haiti 64; **RES:** IM, Washington, DC 66-67; IM, VA Med Ctr-Brooklyn, Brooklyn, NY 67-70; **FEL:** Nep, Maimonides Med Ctr, Bronx, NY 70-72; *SI: Kidney Disease; Hypertension;* **HMO:** Blue Cross & Blue Shield Oxford GHI Prudential
LANG: Fr, Sp; ♿ ⌂ ⚕ ⏰ $ Mcr Mod WC   2-4 Weeks

Malik, Asim (MD)   **IM**   **PCP**
New York Methodist Hosp
1224 8th Ave 203; Brooklyn, NY 11215; (718) 788-5588; **BDCERT:** IM 94; **MS:** Pakistan 76; **RES:** S, New York Methodist Hosp, Brooklyn, NY 77-78; Med, New York Methodist Hosp, Brooklyn, NY 78-81; **FEL:** Ge, Wayne Cnty Gen Hosp, Detroit, MI; **HOSP:** Maimonides Med Ctr; *SI: Stomach Problems; Digestive Problems;* **HMO:** Metlife Magnacare GHI Blue Cross & Blue Shield Sanus +
LANG: Hin, Ur, Pun, Sp; ♿ ☾ ⌂ ⚕ ⏰ $ Mcr
A Few Days

Marrone, Vincent (MD)   **IM**
Brooklyn Hosp Ctr-Downtown
155 Henry St; Brooklyn, NY 11201; (718) 852-2241; **BDCERT:** IM 65; **MS:** Italy 57; **RES:** Mt Sinai Med Ctr, New York, NY; City Hospital, New York, NY; **FAP:** Asst Clin Prof SUNY Hlth Sci Ctr; *SI: Cardiology; Diabetes;* **HMO:** Aetna Hlth Plan
☾ ⌂ ⏰ $ Mcr   1 Week

Marush, Arthur (MD)   **IM**
Brookdale Univ Hosp Med Ctr
2270 Kimball St; Brooklyn, NY 11234; (718) 692-2700; **BDCERT:** IM 81; **MS:** Albert Einstein Coll Med 78; **RES:** Brookdale Hosp Ctr, Brooklyn, NY 78

Massad, Susan (MD)   **IM**   **PCP**
Long Island Coll Hosp
Long Island Coll Primary Care Internal Med Assoc, 340 Henry St 3rd Fl; Brooklyn, NY 11209; (718) 780-1473; **BDCERT:** IM 73; **MS:** UC San Francisco 62; **RES:** IM, Bellevue Hosp Ctr, New York, NY 62-64; IM, VA Med Ctr, San Francisco, CA 67-68; **FEL:** UC San Francisco Med Ctr, San Francisco, CA 69-70; **FAP:** Assoc Inf SUNY Downstate; *SI: Chronic Illness;* **HMO:** Oxford US Hlthcre Genesis Blue Cross & Blue Shield PHS +
LANG: Sp, Kor, Brm; ♿ ☾ ⌂ ⚕ ⏰ $ Mcr Mod WC
A Few Days [AMEX] *VISA* ●

Moskowitz, Robert (MD)   **IM**   **PCP**
Maimonides Med Ctr
1353 49th St; Brooklyn, NY 11219; (718) 972-9227; **BDCERT:** IM 85; Ger 90; **MS:** U Miami Sch Med 82; **RES:** Maimonides Med Ctr, Brooklyn, NY 82-85; **HMO:** Oxford Prucare
LANG: Sp, Yd; ⌂ ⚕ ⏰ $ Mcr

Nacier, Paul (MD)   **IM**
St Mary's Hosp
124 E 43rd St 1; Brooklyn, NY 11203; (718) 940-6166; **BDCERT:** IM 85; Ge 85; **MS:** Spain 77; **RES:** Harlem Hosp Ctr, New York, NY; **FEL:** Harley Hosp, New York, NY; **FAP:** Asst Clin Prof Med SUNY Downstate; *SI: Liver Disease; Stomach Pain;* **HMO:** Oxford United Healthcare Blue Cross CIGNA Magnacare +
LANG: Sp, Fr, Cre; ⚿ ☾ ⌂ ⚕ ⏰ $ Mcr
Immediately

Newhouse, Stanley (MD)   **IM**   **PCP**
Beth Israel Med Ctr-Kings Hwy
2525 Batchelder St; Brooklyn, NY 11235; (718) 891-1500; **BDCERT:** IM 66; EDM 82; **MS:** Holland 57; **RES:** IM, Brooklyn Jewish Hosp, Brooklyn, NY 59-60; EDM, Jewish Hosp Med Ctr, Brooklyn, NY 60-62; **FEL:** EDM, Jewish Hosp Med Ctr, Brooklyn, NY 61-62; **HOSP:** Kingsbrook Jewish Med Ctr; *SI: Diabetes; Thyroid Problems;* **HMO:** Oxford Aetna Hlth Plan CIGNA Blue Choice +
♿ ☾ ⌂ ⚕ ⏰ $ Mcr   1 Week

Ong, Kenneth (MD) IM
Brooklyn Hosp Ctr-Caledonian

121 Dekalb Ave; Brooklyn, NY 11201; (718) 250-8265; **BDCERT:** IM 86; Cv 88; **MS:** SUNY Hlth Sci Ctr 83; **RES:** IM, Winthrop Univ Hosp, Mineola, NY 86; **FEL:** Cv, Winthrop Univ Hosp, Mineola, NY 86-88; **FAP:** Asst Prof Med; **SI:** *Coronary Disease; Heart Failure;* **HMO:** Blue Cross & Blue Shield US Hlthcre Chubb Oxford

♿ 📷 🏨 Mcr Mcd A Few Days

Press, Joseph H (MD) IM PCP
New York University Med Ctr

2350 Ocean Ave; Brooklyn, NY 11229; (718) 627-9322; **BDCERT:** IM 53; **MS:** NYU Sch Med 41; **RES:** Brookdale Univ Hosp Med Ctr, Brooklyn, NY 41; Kingsbrook Jewish Med Ctr, Brooklyn, NY 42-43; **HOSP:** Bellevue Hosp Ctr

♿ 📷 🏨 💲 A Few Days

Rayner, Martha (MD) IM
Long Island Coll Hosp

142 Joralemon St 4A; Brooklyn, NY 11201; (718) 624-8300; **BDCERT:** IM 74; **MS:** Argentina 64; **RES:** IM, St John's Epis Hosp-S Shore, Far Rockaway, NY 66-69; **FEL:** Long Island Coll Hosp, Brooklyn, NY 69-71; **HMO:** Aetna Hlth Plan Blue Choice United Healthcare Multiplan PHS +

LANG: Sp; ♿ 📷 🅿 🏨 💲 Mcr 4+ Weeks

Saxena, Anil (MD) IM PCP
Kingsbrook Jewish Med Ctr

Brooklyn Endocrine, Diabetes & Metabolic Ctr, 1700 Flatbush Ave; Brooklyn, NY 11210; (718) 951-6495; **BDCERT:** IM 75; **MS:** India 71; **RES:** IM, St Clare's Hosp & Health Ctr, New York, NY 72-73; IM, Kingsbrook Jewish Med Ctr, Brooklyn, NY 73-75; **FEL:** EDM, Univ Hosp SUNY Bklyn, Brooklyn, NY 75-77; **HOSP:** Beth Israel Med Ctr-Kings Hwy; **SI:** *Diabetes; Thyroid Disorders;* **HMO:** 1199 Blue Choice GHI Empire +

LANG: Hin, Pun; ♿ 📞 🏨 💲 Mcr A Few Days

Schiff, Carl (MD) IM
Maimonides Med Ctr

Maimonides Medical Ctr, 4802 10th Ave 326; Brooklyn, NY 11219; (718) 283-8519; **BDCERT:** IM 83; **MS:** Yale U Sch Med 80; **RES:** Mount Sinai Med Ctr, New York, NY 81-83; **FEL:** Rhu, Columbia-Presbyterian Med Ctr, New York, NY 84-86; **FAP:** Asst Clin Prof SUNY Hlth Sci Ctr; **HOSP:** Long Island Coll Hosp

Schlecker, Austin (MD) IM PCP
Maimonides Med Ctr

2560 Ocean Ave 3B; Brooklyn, NY 11229; (718) 646-4003; **BDCERT:** IM 60; **MS:** NYU Sch Med 50; **RES:** IM, Maimonides Med Ctr, Brooklyn, NY 50-51; IM, Goldwater Mem Hosp, New York, NY 51-52; **FEL:** IM, Maimonides Med Ctr, Brooklyn, NY 53-55; Rhu, Maimonides Med Ctr, Brooklyn, NY 55-57; **FAP:** Assoc Clin Prof SUNY Downstate; **SI:** *Rheumatology; Geriatrics;* **HMO:** GHI Oxford Blue Cross & Blue Shield

LANG: Yd; ♿ 📷 🏨 💲 Mcr A Few Days

Schmidt, Philip (MD) IM
Beth Israel Med Ctr-Kings Hwy

3043 Ocean Ave 102; Brooklyn, NY 11235; (718) 648-9200; **BDCERT:** IM 77; **MS:** Albert Einstein Coll Med 60; **RES:** IM, Jewish Hosp Med Ctr, Brooklyn, NY 60-62; IM, Jewish Hosp Med Ctr, Brooklyn, NY 64-65; **FEL:** EDM, Jewish Hosp Med Ctr, Brooklyn, NY 65-66; **FAP:** Asst Clin Prof SUNY Hlth Sci Ctr; **HOSP:** New York Methodist Hosp; **SI:** *Diabetes and Complications; Thyroid Diseases;* **HMO:** Blue Cross PPO Oxford

LANG: Yd, Heb, Ger, Sp; ♿ 📞 📷 🏨 💲 1 Week

Shah, Jitendra (MD) IM
Victory Memorial Hosp

8502 Ft Hamilton Pkwy; Brooklyn, NY 11209; (718) 748-4274; **BDCERT:** IM 80; PM 94; **MS:** India 74; **RES:** IM, Kingsbrook Jewish Med Ctr, Brooklyn, NY; **FEL:** IM, VA Med Ctr-Brooklyn, Brooklyn, NY; Kingsbrook Jewish Med Ctr, Brooklyn, NY; **HOSP:** New York Comm Hosp of Bklyn; **HMO:** Aetna Hlth Plan CIGNA Oxford

♿ 📞 📷 🅿 🏨 Mcr A Few Days

Sherbell, Stanley (MD)   **IM**
New York Methodist Hosp
62 Rugby Rd; Brooklyn, NY 11226; (718) 462-4499; **BDCERT:** IM 72; **MS:** SUNY Downstate 57; **RES:** IM, Jewish Hosp Med Ctr, Brooklyn, NY 57-61; **FEL:** Pul, Kings County Hosp Ctr, Brooklyn, NY 71-72; **FAP:** Clin Prof Cornell U; **SI:** *Asthma;* **HMO:** Oxford Blue Cross & Blue Shield Aetna Hlth Plan
▨ ◖ ▧ ▨ ▥ ▤ ▨ A Few Days

Sherman, Frederic (MD)   **IM**   **PCP**
Long Island Coll Hosp
8672 Bay Pkwy; Brooklyn, NY 11214; (718) 372-2234; **BDCERT:** IM 76; Ger 88; **MS:** NYU Sch Med 72; **RES:** Mount Sinai Med Ctr, New York, NY 74; Long Island Coll Hosp, Brooklyn, NY 75-76; **FEL:** Cv, Long Island Coll Hosp, Brooklyn, NY 76-77; **HOSP:** Victory Memorial Hosp; **HMO:** Oxford Prucare United Healthcare GHI
LANG: Hun, Yd; ◖ ▧ ▥ ▤ ▨ ▨

Tal, Avraham (MD)   **IM**   **PCP**
Coney Island Hosp
University Medical Associates, PC, 2601 Ocean Pkwy 4N38; Brooklyn, NY 11235; (718) 616-3000; **BDCERT:** IM 83; **MS:** Italy 75; **RES:** IM, Long Island Coll Hosp, Brooklyn, NY 76-77; IM, Kingsbrook Jewish Med Ctr, Brooklyn, NY 77-78; **FAP:** Clin Instr SUNY Downstate; **SI:** *Hypertension;* **HMO:** Metroplus CIGNA Oxford
LANG: Itl, Heb, Rus; ▧ ◖ ▧ ▨ ▥ ▤ ▨ ▨
A Few Days **VISA** ⬤

Turovsky, Leon (MD)   **IM**
New York Comm Hosp of Bklyn
2912 Avenue X; Brooklyn, NY 11235; (718) 615-0162; **BDCERT:** IM 84; **MS:** Russia 70; **RES:** Cabrini Med Ctr, New York, NY 84; **HOSP:** Beth Israel Med Ctr-Kings Hwy; **SI:** *Heart Illnesses; Lipid Disorders Management*
LANG: Rus, Fr; ▧ ◖ ▧ ▥ ▤ ▨ ▨ ▨ ▨ ▨
A Few Days

Tutino, Jody (MD)   **IM**
New York Methodist Hosp
10 Plaza St East; Brooklyn, NY 11238; (718) 636-2050; **BDCERT:** IM 82; Ger 96; **MS:** Italy 77; **RES:** IM, Mount Sinai Med Ctr, New York, NY 76-80; **FEL:** Ge, Univ Hosp SUNY Stony Brook, Stony Brook, NY 81-83; **SI:** *Digestive Diseases; Chronic Hepatitis;* **HMO:** Oxford CIGNA Blue Cross & Blue Shield PHS GHI +
LANG: Itl, Sp, Fr; ▨ ◖ ▧ ▨ ▥ ▤ ▨ 1 Week

Viera, Jeffery (MD)   **IM**   **PCP**
Long Island Coll Hosp
340 Henry St; Brooklyn, NY 11201; (718) 780-2996; **BDCERT:** IM 80; **MS:** NY Med Coll 77; **FEL:** Inf, Univ Hosp SUNY Bklyn, Brooklyn, NY; **HOSP:** New York Methodist Hosp; **SI:** *HIV AIDS; Infectious Diseases;* **HMO:** CIGNA Oxford GHI NYLCare
LANG: Fr; ▨ ▧ ◖ ▧ ▨ ▥ ▤ ▨ ▨ ▨ A Few Days

Youn, Hyung Joong (MD)   **IM**   **PCP**
Wyckoff Heights Med Ctr
149 Saint Nicholas Ave; Brooklyn, NY 11237; (718) 366-1583; **BDCERT:** IM 72; **MS:** South Korea 65; **RES:** Med, Wyckoff Heights Med Ctr, Brooklyn, NY 68-71; Psyc, Traverse City State Hosp, Traverse City, MI 67
LANG: Kor, Sp; ▧ ▧ ▤ ▨ ▨ ▨ Immediately

Ziemba, David (MD)   **IM**   **PCP**
Long Island Coll Hosp
1458 47th St; Brooklyn, NY 11219; (718) 438-0600; **BDCERT:** IM 83; **MS:** SUNY Downstate 79; **RES:** Coney Island Hosp, Brooklyn, NY 80-83; **FAP:** Instr Med SUNY Downstate; **HOSP:** Beth Israel Med Ctr-Kings Hwy; **HMO:** Oxford Blue Choice
LANG: Yd, Heb; ▧ ◖ ▧ ▥ ▤ ▨ ▨ Immediately

Guide to symbols and abbreviations can be found on pages 110-113.

507

Zupnick, Henry (MD)   **IM**
Brookdale Univ Hosp Med Ctr
AHB Pulmonary Assoc, 1275 Linden Blvd;
Brooklyn, NY 11212; (718) 240-5236; **BDCERT:**
IM 83; Pul 88; **MS:** Albert Einstein Coll Med 80;
RES: IM, Brookdale Univ Hosp Med Ctr, Brooklyn,
NY 80-83; **FEL:** Pul, Columbia-Presbyterian Med
Ctr, New York, NY 83-85; CCM, Mount Sinai Med
Ctr, New York, NY 85-87; **FAP:** Asst Clin Prof
SUNY Downstate; *SI: Asthma; Coughs;* **HMO:** US
Hlthcre GHI Oxford United Healthcare
LANG: Heb; 🦽 📷 👤 🛏 Mcr A Few Days

MEDICAL GENETICS

Lieber, Ernest (MD)   **MG**
New York Methodist Hosp
Methodist Hospital—Med Genetics Dept, 506 6th
St; Brooklyn, NY 11215; (718) 780-3264;
BDCERT: MG 84; **MS:** Austria 63; **RES:** Med, VA
Med Ctr-Bronx, Bronx, NY 64-65; Med, VA Med
Ctr-Manh, New York, NY 65-66; **FEL:** MG, New
York University Med Ctr, New York, NY 67-69; UC
San Francisco Med Ctr, San Francisco, CA 69-70;
FAP: Assoc Prof SUNY Hlth Sci Ctr; *SI: Infertility;
Birth Defects;* **HMO:** US Hlthcre Oxford PHS Empire
LANG: Fr, Ger; 🦽 📷 👤 🛏 Mcr Mcd WC NFI
A Few Days 🔲 **VISA** 🔲

MEDICAL ONCOLOGY

Ahmed, Fakhiuddin (MD)   **Onc**
Brookdale Univ Hosp Med Ctr
Hemoncare, PC, 2558 E 18th St; Brooklyn, NY
11234; (718) 616-0801; **BDCERT:** IM 72; **MS:**
India 66; **RES:** Brookdale Univ Hosp Med Ctr,
Brooklyn, NY 68-70; **FEL:** Hem Onc, Brookdale
Univ Hosp Med Ctr, Brooklyn, NY 70-73; **FAP:**
Assoc Prof Med SUNY Hlth Sci Ctr; **HOSP:** New
York Methodist Hosp; *SI: Breast Cancer; Lung Cancer;*
HMO: GHI Empire Blue Cross & Shield Oxford 1199
Prudential +
LANG: Sp, Rus, Fr, Ur; 🦽 📷 👤 🛏 S Mcr
Immediately **VISA**

Chandra, Pradeep (MD)   **Onc**
Wyckoff Heights Med Ctr
Chairman, Dept of Medicine, Wyckoff Hts Hosp,
374 Stockholm St; Brooklyn, NY 11237; (718)
963-7585; **BDCERT:** IM 72; Onc 83; **MS:** India 66;
RES: IM, Wyckoff Heights Med Ctr, Brooklyn, NY
68-69; IM, Bronx Lebanon Hosp Ctr, Bronx, NY 69-
71; **FEL:** Hem Onc, Long Island Jewish Med Ctr,
New Hyde Park, NY 71-73; **FAP:** Clin Prof Med
SUNY Downstate; *SI: Breast Cancer; Leukemia;*
HMO: GHI Oxford Blue Cross & Blue Shield
Magnacare 1199 +
🦽 📷 🛏 S Mcr Mcd NFI A Few Days

Colella, Frank (MD)   **Onc**
New York Methodist Hosp
455 Bay Ridge Pkwy; Brooklyn, NY 11209; (718)
833-3836; **BDCERT:** Onc 89; Hem 92; **MS:** Italy
78; **RES:** IM, New York Methodist Hosp, Brooklyn,
NY 78-81; **FEL:** Hem Onc, Hahnemann U Hosp,
Philadelphia, PA 81-84; *SI: Breast Cancer;
Lymphoma;* **HMO:** Oxford Blue Cross GHI Blue
Choice
LANG: Itl; 📞 📷 👤 🛏 S Mcr Mcd NFI Immediately

Cook, Perry (MD)   **Onc**
Brooklyn Hosp Ctr-Caledonian
121 Dekalb Ave; Brooklyn, NY 11201; (718) 250-
6960; **BDCERT:** IM 90; Hem 82; **MS:** U Iowa Coll
Med 77; **RES:** St Luke's Roosevelt Hosp Ctr, New
York, NY 77-79; Columbia-Presbyterian Med Ctr,
New York, NY 79-80; **FEL:** Hem Onc, Columbia-
Presbyterian Med Ctr, New York, NY 80-83; *SI:
Breast Surgery;* **HMO:** Aetna Hlth Plan Blue Choice
Oxford US Hlthcre

Friscia, Philip (MD)   **Onc**
Long Island Coll Hosp
University Physician Oncology/Hematology Group,
149 Congress St; Brooklyn, NY 11201; (718) 246-
4281; **BDCERT:** Onc 81; **MS:** Italy 72; **RES:** Long
Island Coll Hosp, Brooklyn, NY 74-76; **FEL:** Hem
Onc, Long Island Coll Hosp, Brooklyn, NY 76-79;
HOSP: Victory Memorial Hosp; *SI: Hematology;
Oncology;* **HMO:** Oxford US Hlthcre GHI NYLCare
LANG: Itl; 🦽 📷 🛏 S Mcr Mcd A Few Days

Feldman, Alan (MD)   Onc
Coney Island Hosp

Coney Island Hospital, Division of
Hematology/Oncology, 2601 Ocean Pkwy;
Brooklyn, NY 11235; (718) 616-3183; **BDCERT:**
IM 85; **MS:** Univ Penn 80; **RES:** Kaiser Foundation
Hosp, San Francisco, CA 80-83; **FEL:** Hem, Coney
Island Hosp, Brooklyn, NY 85-87; Onc,
Maimonides Med Ctr, Brooklyn, NY 87-88; **FAP:**
Asst Prof SUNY Hlth Sci Ctr; **HMO:** Oxford Aetna
Hlth Plan HIP Network

LANG: Sp; 🔲 🔲 🔲 🔲 🔲 🔲 🔲 🔲 🔲
A Few Days 🔲 **VISA**

Geraghty, Michael (MD)   Onc
Long Island Coll Hosp

9920 4th Ave; Brooklyn, NY 11209; (718) 833-
0215; **BDCERT:** IM 72; Hem 74; **MS:** Georgetown
U 66; **RES:** Georgetown U Hosp, Washington, DC
66-68; Bellevue Hosp Ctr, New York, NY 70-71;
FEL: Hem, Bellevue Hosp Ctr, New York, NY 71-73;
FAP: Asst Clin Prof SUNY Hlth Sci Ctr; **HOSP:**
Victory Memorial Hosp; *SI: Chemotherapy*

LANG: Sp, Tag; 🔲 🔲 🔲 🔲 🔲 🔲 🔲 🔲 1 Week

Lebowicz, Joseph (MD)   Onc
Maimonides Med Ctr

MMC Hematology/Oncolgy, FPP, 6323 7th Ave;
Brooklyn, NY 11220; (718) 283-6900; **BDCERT:**
IM 78; Onc 81; **MS:** Albert Einstein Coll Med 75;
RES: IM, Maimonides Med Ctr, Brooklyn, NY 76-
78; **FEL:** Hem Onc, Maimonides Med Ctr, Brooklyn,
NY 78-81; **FAP:** Instr Med SUNY Downstate; **HMO:**
GHI US Hlthcre Aetna Hlth Plan

LANG: Yd, Heb, Rus; 🔲 🔲 🔲 🔲 🔲 🔲 🔲 🔲
A Few Days

Lichter, Stephen M (MD)   Onc
Brookdale Univ Hosp Med Ctr

Hemoncare PC, 2558 E 18th St; Brooklyn, NY
11235; (718) 616-0801; **BDCERT:** IM 78; Onc 81;
MS: U Hlth Sci/Chicago Med Sch 75; **RES:** Med,
Brookdale Univ Hosp Med Ctr, Brooklyn, NY 75-78;
FEL: Onc, Brookdale Univ Hosp Med Ctr, Brooklyn,
NY 78-80; **FAP:** Asst Clin Prof Med SUNY Hlth Sci
Ctr; **HOSP:** Beth Israel Med Ctr-Kings Hwy; **HMO:**
NYLCare GHI US Hlthcre 1199 Magnacare +

LANG: Sp, Rus, Ur, Chi, Heb; 🔲 🔲 🔲 🔲 🔲
Immediately **VISA** 🔲

Novetsky, Allan (MD)   Onc
Brookdale Univ Hosp Med Ctr

Hem On Care, PC, 2558 E 18th St; Brooklyn, NY
11235; (718) 616-0801; **BDCERT:** IM 75; **MS:**
Albert Einstein Coll Med 70; **RES:** IM, Brookdale
Univ Hosp Med Ctr, Brooklyn, NY 73-75; **FEL:** Onc,
Brookdale Univ Hosp Med Ctr, Brooklyn, NY 75-77;
Hem, Brookdale Univ Hosp Med Ctr, Brooklyn, NY
77-78; **FAP:** Assoc Prof SUNY Hlth Sci Ctr; **HOSP:**
Beth Israel Med Ctr-Kings Hwy; *SI: Breast Cancer;*
Lung Cancer; **HMO:** Most

LANG: Sp, Heb, Ur; 🔲 🔲 🔲 🔲 🔲 🔲 Immediately
VISA 🔲

Rosenthal, C Julian (MD)   Onc
Long Island Coll Hosp

3131 Kings Hwy; Brooklyn, NY 11234; (718) 377-
7629; **BDCERT:** IM 72; Onc 77; **MS:** Italy 67; **RES:**
Mount Sinai Med Ctr, New York, NY 68-69; IM,
Albert Einstein Med Ctr, Bronx, NY 69-71; **FEL:**
Onc, Mount Sinai Med Ctr, New York, NY 71-72;
New York University Med Ctr, New York, NY 72-
74; **FAP:** Prof Med SUNY Hlth Sci Ctr; **HOSP:** Beth
Israel Med Ctr-Kings Hwy; *SI: Solid Tumors, Breast*
Lung; Leukemia Lymphoma Myeloma; **HMO:** Oxford
Empire Blue Cross & Shield Aetna Hlth Plan Metlife

LANG: Itl, Fr, Rom, Rus; 🔲 🔲 🔲 🔲 🔲 🔲 🔲 🔲
🔲 🔲 1 Week

Rothenberg, Sheldon (MD)   Onc
Univ Hosp SUNY Bklyn

450 Clarkson Ave Box 20; Brooklyn, NY 11208;
(718) 270-2785; **BDCERT:** Hem 72; Onc 77; **MS:** U
Hlth Sci/Chicago Med Sch 55; **RES:** IM, VA Med
Ctr-Bronx, Bronx, NY 59-60; **FEL:** Hem, Long
Island Jewish Med Ctr, New Hyde Park, NY 60-61

NEONATAL-PERINATAL MEDICINE

Grieg, Adolfo (DO) NP
Wyckoff Heights Med Ctr
Wyckoff Neonatal Services, PC, 374 Stockholm St; Brooklyn, NY 11237; (718) 963-6479; **BDCERT:** Ped 91; NP 95; **MS:** NY Coll Osteo Med 87; **RES:** Ped, Brookdale Univ Hosp Med Ctr, Brooklyn, NY 89-91; **FEL:** NP, Montefiore Med Ctr, Bronx, NY 91-94; **SI:** *Neonatal Neurology*; **HMO:** US Hlthcre Well Care GHI Blue Cross & Blue Choice

LANG: Sp; 🔊 📷 🔧 🎬 Mod 2-4 Weeks

Gudavalli, Madhu R (MD) NP
New York Methodist Hosp
506 6th St WP5; Brooklyn, NY 11215; (718) 780-5261; **BDCERT:** Ped 80; NP 83; **MS:** India 72; **RES:** Ped, NY Infirmary, New York, NY 74; Ped, Booth Mem Hosp, Flushing, NY 76; **FEL:** NP, Bellevue Hosp Ctr, New York, NY 77; **FAP:** Adjct Prof Ped NYU Sch Med; **SI:** *Premature Babies; Special Problems Of Newborns*

🔊 📷 🎬 S Mcr Mod Immediately

Mehta, Rajeev (MD) NP
Maimonides Med Ctr
Maimonides Med Ctr Dept Peds, 4802 10th Ave; Brooklyn, NY 11219; (718) 283-7780; **BDCERT:** Ped 90; NP 93; **MS:** India 79; **RES:** Ped, QPH StMarys Hospital, Dudley Road, England 81-83; Ped, Univ Hosp SUNY Bklyn, Brooklyn, NY 89-90; **FEL:** Ped, Bradford Royal Infirmary, England 87-89; **HOSP:** Lutheran Med Ctr; **SI:** *Prematurity Extreme; Neonates-Unstable*

LANG: Sp, Heb, Chi, Itl, Rus; 🔊 📱 🔧 🎬 Mod NFI 💳 **VISA** 💳

Sokal, Myron (MD) NP
Brookdale Univ Hosp Med Ctr
1 Brookdale Plaza; Brooklyn, NY 11212; (718) 240-5629; **BDCERT:** Ped 72; NP 75; **MS:** Albert Einstein Coll Med 67; **RES:** Ped, Yale-New Haven Hosp, New Haven, CT 67-69; **FEL:** NP, Columbia-Presbyterian Med Ctr, New York, NY 69-71; **FAP:** Prof Ped SUNY Hlth Sci Ctr; **SI:** *Care for Newborns*; **HMO:** Aetna Hlth Plan Blue Choice Blue Cross & Blue Shield Prucare Sanus +

🔊 📱 📷 🔧 🎬 Mcr Mod Immediately

Varada, Koteswar (MD) NP
Maimonides Med Ctr
Maimonides HospPed Dept, 4802 10th Ave; Brooklyn, NY 11219; (718) 283-8260; **BDCERT:** Ped 92; **MS:** India 78; **RES:** Ped, Hahnemann U Hosp, Philadelphia, PA 87-90; **FEL:** NP, N Shore Univ Hosp-Manhasset, Manhasset, NY 90-93; **FAP:** Asst Prof Ped SUNY Hlth Sci Ctr

NEPHROLOGY

Avram, Morrell M (MD) Nep
Long Island Coll Hosp
Heights Nephrology Medical Group, 115 1/2 Remsen St; Brooklyn, NY 11201; (718) 858-4949; **MS:** Switzerland 59; **RES:** Nep, Long Island Coll Hosp, Brooklyn, NY 59; Nep, Long Island Coll Hosp, Brooklyn, NY 60; **FEL:** Nep, Long Island Coll Hosp, Brooklyn, NY 61; Nep, Long Island Coll Hosp, Brooklyn, NY 62; **FAP:** Prof Med; **SI:** *Diabetic Kidney Disease; Dialysis*; **HMO:** Aetna-US Healthcare GHI United Healthcare

📷 📱 🔧 🎬 S Mcr Mod Immediately

Chou, Shyan-yih (MD) Nep
Brookdale Univ Hosp Med Ctr
1 Brookdale Plaza 169HC; Brooklyn, NY 11212; (718) 240-5615; **BDCERT:** IM 72; Nep 74; **MS:** Taiwan 66; **RES:** IM, Brookdale Univ Hosp Med Ctr, Brooklyn, NY 68-69; IM, Brookdale Univ Hosp Med Ctr, Brooklyn, NY 69-70; **FEL:** Nep, Brookdale Univ Hosp Med Ctr, Brooklyn, NY 70-73; **FAP:** Prof Med SUNY Hlth Sci Ctr; **SI:** *Hypertension; Kidney Failure;* **HMO:** Blue Cross & Blue Shield CIGNA Oxford Prucare PHS +

LANG: Chi, Twn; ⬛ ⬛ ⬛ ⬛ ⬛ ⬛ ⬛ 1 Week

Del Monte, Mary (MD) Nep
Brooklyn Hosp Ctr-Caledonian
121 Dekalb Ave; Brooklyn, NY 11201; (718) 250-8160; **BDCERT:** IM 72; Nep 72; **MS:** Boston U 67; **RES:** St Eliz Hosp, Boston, MA 67-71; **FEL:** Nep, St Vinct Hosp, New York, NY 70-71; Nep, SUNY Health Scie Ctr, Brooklyn, NY 71-73; **FAP:** Asst Clin Prof Med NYU Sch Med; **SI:** *Renal Disease; Hypertension;* **HMO:** Aetna Hlth Plan Blue Cross & Blue Shield HIP Network

LANG: Sp; ⬛ ⬛ ⬛ ⬛ ⬛ A Few Days

Delano, Barbara (MD) Nep
Univ Hosp SUNY Bklyn
450 Clarkson Ave; Brooklyn, NY 11203; (718) 270-1584; **MS:** SUNY Hlth Sci Ctr 65; **RES:** Kings County Hosp Ctr, Brooklyn, NY 65-66; Nep, Univ Hosp SUNY Bklyn, Brooklyn, NY 66-67; **FEL:** Nep, Univ Hosp SUNY Bklyn, Brooklyn, NY 67-69; **FAP:** Prof SUNY Hlth Sci Ctr; **HOSP:** Kings County Hosp Ctr; **SI:** *Peritoneal Dialysis; Home Hemodialysis;* **HMO:** Blue Cross US Hlthcre Blue Shield Empire

⬛ ⬛ ⬛ ⬛ ⬛ ⬛ A Few Days

Friedman, Eli A (MD) Nep
Univ Hosp SUNY Bklyn
Downstate Renal Associates, 450 Clarkson Ave Box 52; Brooklyn, NY 11203; (718) 270-1584; **BDCERT:** IM 65; Nep 74; **MS:** SUNY Downstate 57; **RES:** IM, Peter Bent Brigham Hosp, Boston, MA 57-59; **FEL:** Nep, Peter Bent Brigham Hosp, Boston, MA 61-62; **FAP:** Prof Med SUNY Downstate; **HOSP:** Kings County Hosp Ctr; **SI:** *Diabetic Kidney Disease; Hypertension;* **HMO:** Oxford CIGNA Aetna-US Healthcare Blue Cross PPO GHI +

LANG: Sp, Fr, Rus; ⬛ ⬛ ⬛ ⬛ ⬛ ⬛ ⬛ ⬛ A Few Days ⬛ **VISA** ⬛ ⬛

Lipner, Henry (MD) Nep
Maimonides Med Ctr
4802 10th Ave; Brooklyn, NY 11219; (718) 270-7054; **BDCERT:** Nep 76; IM 74; **MS:** NYU Sch Med 68; **RES:** IM, Jewish Hosp Med Ctr, Brooklyn, NY 68-71; **FEL:** Nep, Montefiore Med Ctr, Bronx, NY 71-72; **FAP:** Asst Prof Med SUNY Downstate; **HOSP:** Beth Israel Med Ctr; **SI:** *Kidney Disease; Hypertension;* **HMO:** GHI Oxford US Hlthcre Aetna Hlth Plan

⬛ ⬛ ⬛ ⬛ ⬛ ⬛

Markell, Mariana (MD) Nep
Univ Hosp SUNY Bklyn
Downstate Renal Associates, 450 Clarkson Ave Box 52; Brooklyn, NY 11203; (718) 270-1584; **BDCERT:** IM 84; Nep 86; **MS:** NY Med Coll 81; **RES:** Med, Columbia-Presbyterian Med Ctr, New York, NY 81-84; **FEL:** Nep, Columbia-Presbyterian Med Ctr, New York, NY 84-85; NS, UCLA Med Ctr, Los Angeles, CA 85-86; **FAP:** Assoc Prof Nep SUNY Hlth Sci Ctr; **SI:** *Renal Transplant; Alternative Medicine;* **HMO:** Oxford CIGNA US Hlthcre GHI

LANG: Sp; ⬛ ⬛ ⬛ ⬛ ⬛ ⬛ 2-4 Weeks

Mittman, Neal (MD)   Nep
Long Island Coll Hosp

Heights Nephrology Medical Group, 115 1/2
Remsen St; Brooklyn, NY 11201; (718) 852-4949;
BDCERT: IM 80; Nep 82; **MS:** NY Med Coll 77; **RES:**
IM, Metropolitan Hosp Ctr, New York, NY 77-80;
FEL: Nep, Albert Einstein Med Ctr, Bronx, NY 80-
82; **FAP:** Assoc Clin Prof Med SUNY Hlth Sci Ctr; *SI:
Dialysis; Lupus Nephritis*; **HMO:** Oxford Aetna-US
Healthcare Empire Blue Cross & Shield HIP
Network Sanus +

LANG: Sp, Itl; 🔲 🔲 🔲 🔲 🔲 🔲 🔲   A Few Days

Neelakantappa, Kotresha (MD)Nep
New York Methodist Hosp

9920 4th Ave Ste 309; Brooklyn, NY 11209; (718)
745-3079; **BDCERT:** IM 77; **MS:** India 69; **RES:**
New York Methodist Hosp, Brooklyn, NY 71-74;
FEL: N, New York University Med Ctr, New York,
NY 74-76; **FAP:** Asst Clin Prof Med NYU Sch Med;
SI: Kidney Diseases; Dialysis; **HMO:** Most

🔲 🔲 🔲 🔲 🔲 🔲 🔲   1 Week

Parnes, Eliezer (MD)   Nep
Beth Israel Med Ctr-Kings Hwy

3131 Kings Hwy Suite D5; Brooklyn, NY 11234;
(718) 338-2283; **BDCERT:** IM 89; Nep 92; **MS:**
SUNY Downstate 86; **RES:** IM, Brookdale Univ Hosp
Med Ctr, Brooklyn, NY 86-89; **FEL:** Nep, Brookdale
Univ Hosp Med Ctr, Brooklyn, NY 89-92; *SI:
Hypertension; Dialysis*; **HMO:** Oxford US Hlthcre GHI
United Healthcare Blue Cross +

LANG: Yd, Sp, Itl; 🔲 🔲 🔲 🔲 🔲 🔲 🔲 🔲 🔲 🔲 🔲
A Few Days

Porush, Jerome (MD)   Nep
Brookdale Univ Hosp Med Ctr

Brookdale Plaza Nephrology Associates, 1
Brookdale Plz 169HC; Brooklyn, NY 11212; (718)
240-5615; **BDCERT:** IM 62; Nep 74; **MS:** SUNY
Hlth Sci Ctr 55; **RES:** IM, Maimonides Med Ctr,
Brooklyn, NY 61-62; IM, Mount Sinai Med Ctr,
New York, NY 59-60; **FEL:** Nep, Mount Sinai Med
Ctr, New York, NY 60-61; **FAP:** Prof SUNY Hlth Sci
Ctr; *SI: Chronic Kidney Failure; High Blood Pressure*;
HMO: US Hlthcre HIP Network GHI Empire Blue
Cross & Shield Prudential +

LANG: Sp, Fr, Yd; 🔲 🔲 🔲 🔲 🔲 🔲 🔲 🔲
Immediately

Reiser, Ira (MD)   Nep
Brookdale Univ Hosp Med Ctr

Brookdale HospitalPlaza Nephrology Assocs, 1
Brookdale Plza; Brooklyn, NY 11212; (718) 240-
5615; **BDCERT:** IM 83; Nep 86; **MS:** Mt Sinai Sch
Med 80; **RES:** IM, Brookdale Univ Hosp Med Ctr,
Brooklyn, NY 81-83; **FEL:** Nep, Brookdale Univ
Hosp Med Ctr, Brooklyn, NY 83-86; **FAP:** Asst
Lecturer Med SUNY Hlth Sci Ctr; *SI: Hypertension;
Lupus*; **HMO:** Oxford Aetna-US Healthcare GHI
CIGNA Prucare +

🔲 🔲 🔲 🔲 🔲 🔲   2-4 Weeks

Rosen, Herman (MD)   Nep
Coney Island Hosp

2601 Ocean Pkwy; Brooklyn, NY 11235; (718)
616-4233; **BDCERT:** IM 77; Nep 72; **MS:** SUNY
Downstate 59; **RES:** Boston U Med Ctr, Boston, MA
59-61; **FEL:** New England Med Ctr, Boston, MA 61-
65; **FAP:** Clin Prof Med Cornell U; *SI: Hypertension;
Kidney Failure*

🔲 🔲 🔲 🔲 🔲   2-4 Weeks

Sari Markell, Marian (MD)   Nep
Univ Hosp SUNY Bklyn

450 Clarkson Ave; Brooklyn, NY 11203; (718)
270-1584; **BDCERT:** IM 84; Nep 86; **MS:** NY Med
Coll 81; **RES:** IM, Colum Presb Med Ctr, New York,
NY 81-84; **FEL:** Nep, Colum Presb Med Ctr, New
York, NY 84-85; UCLA Med Ctr, Los Angeles, CA
85-86; **FAP:** Assoc Prof Med SUNY Hlth Sci Ctr;
HOSP: Kings County Hosp Ctr; *SI:
Hypertension/Dialysis; Kidney Transplantation*; **HMO:**
Oxford US Hlthcre CIGNA

LANG: Sp; 🔲 🔲 🔲 🔲 🔲 🔲 🔲   A Few Days

Shapiro, Warren (MD)   Nep
Brookdale Univ Hosp Med Ctr

Brookdale Hosp, 1 Brookdale Plaza 169 HC;
Brooklyn, NY 11212; (718) 240-5615; **BDCERT:**
IM 72; **MS:** U Hlth Sci/Chicago Med Sch 66; **RES:**
San Francisco Gen Hosp, San Francisco, CA 66-67;
NY Med Coll, Valhalla, NY 68-70; **FEL:** Nep, NY
Med Coll, Valhalla, NY 70-71; *SI: Hypertension &
Lupus; Nephritis, Nephrosis, Dialysis*; **HMO:** Oxford
Aetna-US Healthcare US Hlthcre GHI CIGNA +

LANG: Fr, Sp, Ger, Yd, Man; 🔲 🔲 🔲 🔲 🔲 🔲
1 Week

Shein, Leon (MD)   Nep   `PCP`
New York Methodist Hosp

New York Methodist Hospital, 446 McDonald Ave; Brooklyn, NY 11218; (718) 972-4200; **BDCERT:** IM 89; Nep 92; **MS:** Philippines 83; **RES:** Med, Interfaith Med Ctr, Brooklyn, NY 83-84; Med, Woodhull Med Ctr, Brooklyn, NY 84-86; **FEL:** Nep, Brookdale Univ Hosp Med Ctr, Brooklyn, NY 86-88; **FAP:** Asst Prof SUNY Buffalo; **HOSP:** Interfaith Med Ctr-Bklyn Jewish Div; **SI:** *Kidney Diseases; Hypertension;* **HMO:** Blue Cross & Blue Shield Oxford Health Source US Hlthcre GHI +

LANG: Rus, Hun, Hin, Sp, Ar; 🚻 🆘 💳 🔒 🚲 🛏 Mcr Mcd WC NFI Immediately *VISA* 💳

Spitalewitz, Samuel (MD)   Nep
Brookdale Univ Hosp Med Ctr

One Brookdale Plaza 169CHC; Brooklyn, NY 11212; (718) 240-5615; **BDCERT:** IM 78; Nep 80; **MS:** NYU Sch Med 75; **RES:** IM, Brookdale Univ Hosp Med Ctr, Brooklyn, NY 75-78; **FEL:** Nep, Brookdale Univ Hosp Med Ctr, Brooklyn, NY 78-81; **FAP:** Asst Prof Med SUNY Hlth Sci Ctr; **SI:** *Diabetic Kidney Disease; Hypertension;* **HMO:** Empire Blue Cross & Shield Sanus CIGNA Prucare Oxford +

LANG: Fr, Heb, Sp; 🚻 🔒 🛏 💲 Mcr WC   A Few Days

Stam, Lawrence (MD)   Nep
New York Methodist Hosp

506 6th St; Brooklyn, NY 11215; (718) 830-7109; **BDCERT:** IM 82; Nep 84; **MS:** SUNY Stony Brook 78; **RES:** St Elizabeth's Med Ctr, Boston, MA 78-81; **FEL:** Jewish Hosp Med Ctr, Brooklyn, NY 81-82; **FAP:** Asst Clin Prof Cornell U; **SI:** *Hemodialysis; Plasmapheresis;* **HMO:** Aetna Hlth Plan Oxford GHI CIGNA Magnacare +

🚻 🆘 🔒 🚲 🛏 Mcr Mcd   Immediately

NEUROLOGICAL SURGERY

Anant, Ashok (MD)   NS
Maimonides Med Ctr

Neuroscience Associates Of NY, 9920 4th Ave 207; Brooklyn, NY 11209; (718) 238-0878; **BDCERT:** NS 84; **MS:** India 73; **RES:** S, Maimonides Med Ctr, Brooklyn, NY 75-77; NS, Univ Hosp SUNY Bklyn, Brooklyn, NY 77-82; **FAP:** Assoc Clin Prof NYU Sch Med; **HOSP:** New York Methodist Hosp; **SI:** *Spinal Surgery; Brain Tumors;* **HMO:** Aetna Hlth Plan CIGNA US Hlthcre Metlife GHI +

🚻 🔒 🚲 🛏 💲 Mcr WC NFI   Immediately 💳 *VISA* 💳 💳

Andersen, Bruce J (MD)   NS
Brooklyn Hosp Ctr-Caledonian

121 Dekalb Ave; Brooklyn, NY 11201; (718) 250-8103; **BDCERT:** NS 96; **MS:** Northwestern U 82; **RES:** NS, Med Coll VA Hosp, Richmond, VA 83-88; **FEL:** NS, VA Commonwealth U, Richmond, VA 89-90; NS, U of South FL, Tampa, FL 89-90; **FAP:** Asst Prof NS NYU Sch Med; **HOSP:** New York University Med Ctr; **SI:** *Cerebrovascular Disease; Complex Spine Disease;* **HMO:** Blue Cross & Blue Shield NYLCare Oxford HIP Network US Hlthcre +

LANG: Sp, Fr; 🚻 🔒 🛏 💲 Mcr Mcd WC NFI   4+ Weeks

Cardoso, Erico R (MD)   NS
Wyckoff Heights Med Ctr

Wyckoff Heights Medical Ctr, 374 Stockholm St; Brooklyn, NY 11237; (718) 963-7266; **BDCERT:** PM 93; NS 94; **MS:** Brazil 73; **RES:** S, Ottawa Civic Hospital, Ottawa, Canada 75-76; NS, Ottawa Civic Hospital, Ottawa, Canada 76-80; **FEL:** NS, Clinical Research Fellowship University Hospital, Onatario 80-81; NS, Institute of Neurological Sciences, Glasgow, Scotland 81-82; **FAP:** Assoc Prof Cornell U; **HOSP:** New York Methodist Hosp; **SI:** *Diseases of Spinal Cord; Diseases of Brain;* **HMO:** GHI Oxford US Hlthcre Blue Choice PHS +

LANG: Prt, Sp; 🚻 🔒 🚲 🛏 💲 Mcr Mcd WC NFI   2-4 Weeks

Milhorat, Thomas H (MD)   NS
Long Island Coll Hosp

Dept of Neurosurgery, SUNY Health Sciences
Center-Brooklyn, 450 Clarkson Ave Box 1189;
Brooklyn, NY 11203; (718) 270-2111; **BDCERT:**
NS 72; **MS:** Cornell U 61; **RES:** S, NY Hosp-Cornell
Med Ctr, New York, NY 61-63; NS, NY Hosp-
Cornell Med Ctr, New York, NY 65-69; **FEL:** NS, Nat
Inst Health, Bethesda, MD 63-65; **FAP:** Chrmn NS
SUNY Downstate; **HOSP:** Univ Hosp SUNY Bklyn;
HMO: HIP Network GHI Oxford US Hlthcre United
Healthcare +

LANG: Sp, Rus, Ger, Fr; 🚗 🔟 📷 Mcr Mcd WC NFI
1 Week ▦ **VISA** 💳 💳

NEUROLOGY

Bodis-Wollner, Ivan (MD)   N
Univ Hosp SUNY Bklyn

470 Clarkson Ave; Brooklyn, NY 11203; (718)
270-2502; **BDCERT:** N 77; **MS:** Austria 65; **RES:**
Mount Sinai Med Ctr, New York, NY 71-74; **FEL:**
Neurobiology, Mass Gen Hosp, Boston, MA 74;
FAP: Prof N SUNY Downstate; **HOSP:** Beth Israel
Med Ctr; **SI:** *Parkinson's Disease; Non-Ocular Visual
Disorders;* **HMO:** None

🚗 📷 📶 🔟 💲 Mcr 2-4 Weeks

Consiglio, Michael (MD)   N
Maimonides Med Ctr

415 Albemarle Rd; Brooklyn, NY 11218; (718)
853-3400; **BDCERT:** Psyc 89; N 89; **MS:** UMDNJ-
NJ Med Sch, Newark 67; **RES:** N, Bellevue Hosp Ctr,
New York, NY 68-73; **FAP:** Instr N SUNY
Downstate; **HOSP:** New York Methodist Hosp; **SI:**
Head & Neck Pain; Behavioral Problems; **HMO:** Blue
Choice Guardian Sanus NYLCare

SA SU 📷 📶 🔟 💲 WC NFI A Few Days

Drexler, Ellen (MD)   N
Maimonides Med Ctr

Maimonides Neurological Associates, 4802 10th
Ave; Brooklyn, NY 11219; (718) 283-7470;
BDCERT: N 83; **MS:** SUNY Hlth Sci Ctr 78; **RES:** St
Vincents Hosp & Med Ctr NY, New York, NY 78-79;
Albert Einstein Med Ctr, Bronx, NY 79-82; **FAP:**
Assoc Clin Prof N SUNY Hlth Sci Ctr; **SI:** *Headache;*
HMO: Aetna-US Healthcare Prucare Blue Choice
Oxford United Healthcare +

LANG: Sp, Rus, Heb, Est; 🚗 📷 📶 🔟 💲 Mcr 2-
4 Weeks **VISA**

Gropen, Toby Ira (MD)   N
Long Island Coll Hosp

L I C HNeurocare PC, 399 Hicks St; Brooklyn, NY
11201; (718) 780-1124; **BDCERT:** N 93; **MS:** Univ
Texas, Houston 87; **RES:** N, Columbia-Presbyterian
Med Ctr, New York, NY 88-91; **FEL:** N, Columbia-
Presbyterian Med Ctr, New York, NY 92-93; **FAP:**
Asst Prof NR SUNY Hlth Sci Ctr; **SI:** *Stroke;* **HMO:**
Empire Blue Cross & Shield Oxford CIGNA Aetna-
US Healthcare MHS +

LANG: Sp; 🚗 📷 📶 🔟 💲 Mcr 1 Week

Hirschenstein, Eva (MD)   N
Brooklyn Hosp Ctr-Downtown

121 Dekalb Ave; Brooklyn, NY 11201; (718) 250-
6940; **BDCERT:** N 71; **MS:** Italy 60; **RES:** IM,
Kingsbrook Jewish Med Ctr, Brooklyn, NY 63; N,
Boston VA Med Ctr, Boston, MA 64-65; **FEL:** N, VA
Med Ctr-Manhattan, New York, NY 65-67; **FAP:**
Assoc Clin Prof NYU Sch Med; **HMO:** US Hlthcre
Oxford Blue Cross & Blue Shield Chubb

LANG: Itl, SCr, Sp, Fr, Ger; 🚗 📷 🔟 💲 Mcr 2-
4 Weeks

Kay, Arthur (MD)   N
Brookdale Univ Hosp Med Ctr

Neurological Associates of Brookdale, One Brookdale Plaza St 400; Brooklyn, NY 11212; (718) 240-5622; **BDCERT:** N 83; **MS:** SUNY Downstate 78; **RES:** IM, Brookdale Univ Hosp Med Ctr, Brooklyn, NY 78-79; N, Mount Sinai Med Ctr, New York, NY 79-82; **FEL:** Nat Inst Health, Bethesda, MD 82-84; **FAP:** Assoc Prof N SUNY Hlth Sci Ctr; *SI: Stroke; Parkinson's Disease;* **HMO:** Aetna Hlth Plan Blue Choice Blue Cross & Blue Shield HealthNet GHI +

LANG: Sp, Heb; ⬛ ⬛ ⬛ ⬛ ⬛   A Few Days

Keilson, Marshall (MD)   N
Maimonides Med Ctr

4802 10th Ave; Brooklyn, NY 11219; (718) 283-7470; **BDCERT:** N 82; **MS:** Albert Einstein Coll Med 77; **RES:** Montefiore Med Ctr, Bronx, NY; Albert Einstein Med Ctr, Bronx, NY; **FEL:** C/Nph, Univ Hosp SUNY Bklyn, Brooklyn, NY; **FAP:** Assoc Prof; *SI: Epilepsy; Alzheimer's Disease;* **HMO:** Prucare Travelers Blue Cross & Blue Shield HealthNet CIGNA +

LANG: Sp, Rus, Heb; ⬛ ⬛ ⬛ ⬛ ⬛ ⬛   1 Week
VISA ⬛

Kula, Roger W (MD)   N
Long Island Coll Hosp

LICH NeuroCare, PC, 339 Hicks St; Brooklyn, NY 11201; (718) 780-1124; **BDCERT:** N 77; IM 75; **MS:** Johns Hopkins U 70; **RES:** IM, NY Hosp-Cornell Med Ctr, New York, NY 70-72; N, UC San Francisco Med Ctr, San Francisco, CA 72-74; **FEL:** Nat Inst Health, Bethesda, MD 74-77; **FAP:** Assoc Clin Prof SUNY Hlth Sci Ctr; **HOSP:** Univ Hosp SUNY Bklyn; *SI: Neuromuscular Diseases; Spinal Cord Disorders;* **HMO:** Blue Cross & Blue Shield Empire Oxford GHI

LANG: Sp; ⬛ ⬛ ⬛ ⬛ ⬛ ⬛   1 Week

Maccabee, Paul J (MD)   N
Univ Hosp SUNY Stony Brook

450 Clarkson Ave; Brooklyn, NY 11203; (718) 270-2430; **BDCERT:** N 77; **MS:** Boston U 70; **RES:** N, Boston U Med Ctr, Boston, MA 76; **FEL:** CNph, Mass Gen Hosp, Boston, MA 76-78; **FAP:** Assoc Prof SUNY Downstate; *SI: Neuropathy; Cervical-Lumbar -Sacroiliac;* **HMO:** Empire Oxford US Hlthcre CIGNA +

⬛ ⬛ ⬛ ⬛ ⬛ ⬛   2-4 Weeks

Maniscalco, Anthony (MD)   N
Maimonides Med Ctr

Neurology Associates, 117 70th St; Brooklyn, NY 11209; (718) 836-8800; **BDCERT:** IM 82; N 88; **MS:** Italy 78; **RES:** IM, Maimonides Med Ctr, Brooklyn, NY 78-81; N, St Vincents Hosp & Med Ctr NY, New York, NY 81-84; **FAP:** Asst Clin Prof N SUNY Downstate; **HOSP:** St Vincents Hosp & Med Ctr NY; *SI: Movement Disorders; Cerebrovascular Disease;* **HMO:** Oxford US Hlthcre Aetna Hlth Plan

LANG: Itl, Yd, Sp, Grk; ⬛ ⬛ ⬛ ⬛ ⬛ ⬛ ⬛ ⬛ ⬛   2-4 Weeks

Miller, Aaron (MD)   N
Maimonides Med Ctr

4802 10th Ave; Brooklyn, NY 11219; (718) 283-7470; **BDCERT:** IM 72; N 77; **MS:** NYU Sch Med 68; **RES:** Jacobi Med Ctr, Bronx, NY 68-70; Albert Einstein Med Ctr, Bronx, NY 70-75; **FEL:** EDM, Johns Hopkins Hosp, Baltimore, MD 75-77; Microbiology/Immunology, Albert Einstein Med Ctr, Bronx, NY 77-78; **FAP:** Clin Prof N SUNY Hlth Sci Ctr; **HOSP:** Long Island Coll Hosp; *SI: Multiple Sclerosis; Alzheimer's Disease;* **HMO:** Oxford Aetna Hlth Plan PHS United Healthcare CIGNA +

LANG: Sp, Rus; ⬛ ⬛ ⬛ ⬛ ⬛ ⬛   1 Week ***VISA*** ⬛

Pincas, Martin (MD)   N
New York Methodist Hosp
115 Prospect Park West; Brooklyn, NY 11215;
(718) 768-8442; **BDCERT:** Psyc 80; N 80; **MS:**
Hahnemann U 75; **RES:** N, Mount Sinai Med Ctr,
New York, NY 76-79; Med, Beth Israel Med Ctr,
New York, NY 75-76; **FAP:** Clin Prof N Cornell U;
HOSP: Brooklyn Hosp Ctr-Downtown; *SI:*
Parkinson's; Headache; **HMO:** Oxford Aetna Hlth
Plan CIGNA Blue Cross & Blue Shield Elderplan +
LANG: Sp, Fr; 🔣 🔣 🔣 🔣 🔣 🔣 🔣 🔣
Immediately

Pitem, Michael (DO)   N
Brookdale Univ Hosp Med Ctr
Brookdale Hospital, 1275 Linden Blvd 400;
Brooklyn, NY 11212; (718) 240-5622; **BDCERT:**
Psyc 90; N 90; **MS:** NY Coll Osteo Med 85; **RES:**
Metropolitan Hosp, Philadelphia, PA 85-86; Albert
Einstein Med Ctr, Bronx, NY 86-89; **FAP:** Asst Clin
Prof; **HMO:** US Hlthcre Oxford CIGNA 32BJ 1199 +
LANG: Heb, Yd; 🔣 🔣 🔣 🔣 🔣 🔣 2-4 Weeks

Slotwiner, Paul (MD)   N
St Vincents Hosp & Med Ctr NY
Neurology Associates, 117 70th St; Brooklyn, NY
11209; (718) 836-8800; **BDCERT:** N 68; **MS:** U
Chicago-Pritzker Sch Med 59; **RES:** N, Mount Sinai
Med Ctr, New York, NY 60-63; **HOSP:** Beth Israel
Med Ctr-Kings Hwy; **HMO:** Aetna-US Healthcare
Sanus-NYLCare US Hlthcre Oxford PHS +
🔣 🔣 🔣 🔣 🔣 🔣 🔣 🔣 🔣 2-4 Weeks

Sobol, Norman (MD)   N
Beth Israel Med Ctr-Kings Hwy
Neurology Associates, 3131 Kings Hwy Ste C7;
Brooklyn, NY 11234; (718) 677-0020; **BDCERT:**
Psyc 80; **MS:** U Chicago-Pritzker Sch Med 74;
HOSP: Maimonides Med Ctr; *SI: Geriatric Neurology*
LANG: Heb; 🔣 🔣 🔣 🔣 🔣 🔣 A Few Days

Somasundaram, Mahend (MD)N
Univ Hosp SUNY Bklyn
Downstate Neurological Associates, 450 Clarkson
Ave; Brooklyn, NY 11203; (718) 270-2502;
BDCERT: N 75; **MS:** Sri Lanka 59; **RES:** St James
Hosp, England 63-65; NY Hosp-Cornell Med Ctr,
New York, NY 72-73; **FEL:** U WA Med Ctr, Seattle,
WA 67-68; **FAP:** Prof SUNY Hlth Sci Ctr; **HOSP:**
Kings County Hosp Ctr; *SI: Stroke; Epilepsy;* **HMO:**
GHI Empire Blue Cross & Blue Shield Oxford
LANG: Hun; 🔣 🔣 🔣 🔣 🔣 🔣 🔣 A Few Days

Vas, George A (MD)   N
Univ Hosp SUNY Bklyn
450 Clarkson Ave 35; Brooklyn, NY 11203; (718)
270-1950; **BDCERT:** N 77; IM 73; **MS:** Univ
Pittsburgh 70; **RES:** IM, NY Hosp-Cornell Med Ctr,
New York, NY 71-72; N, NY Hosp-Cornell Med Ctr,
New York, NY 72-75; **FAP:** Prof SUNY Downstate;
HMO: GHI CIGNA Health First US Hlthcre Oxford +
🔣 🔣 🔣 🔣 🔣 🔣 2-4 Weeks

Yellin, Joseph (DO)   N
New York Methodist Hosp
2502 Kings Hwy; Brooklyn, NY 11229; (718) 377-
2223; **BDCERT:** N 88; **MS:** Univ Osteo Med & Hlth
Sci 78; **RES:** Kings County Hosp Ctr, Brooklyn, NY
79-82; **HOSP:** New York Comm Hosp of Bklyn; *SI:*
Headaches; Dementia; **HMO:** Blue Cross & Blue Shield
Aetna Hlth Plan Oxford Magnacare
🔣 🔣 🔣 🔣 🔣 🔣 🔣 🔣 A Few Days

NUCLEAR MEDICINE

Strashun, Arnold M (MD)   NuM
Univ Hosp SUNY Bklyn
450 Clarkson Ave; Brooklyn, NY 11203; (718)
245-3692; **BDCERT:** IM 77; NuM 79; **MS:** Baylor
74; **RES:** Baylor Med Ctr, Dallas, TX 75; IM, Texas
Med Ctr, Houston, TX 77; **FEL:** NuM, VA Med Ctr-
Bronx, Bronx, NY; Mount Sinai Med Ctr, New York,
NY; **FAP:** Prof Rad SUNY Downstate; **HOSP:** Kings
County Hosp Ctr; *SI: Coronary Artery Disease; Lung
Cancer;* **HMO:** Oxford US Hlthcre Aetna Hlth Plan
United Healthcare CIGNA +
LANG: Sp, Rus, Chi, Yd, Cre; 🔣 🔣 🔣 🔣 🔣 🔣 🔣
🔣 Immediately *VISA* 💳

Sy, Wilfrido M (MD) NuM
Brooklyn Hosp Ctr-Downtown
The Brooklyn Hospital Ctr, 121 Dekalb Ave;
Brooklyn, NY 11201; (718) 250-8225; **BDCERT:**
NuM 72; **MS:** Philippines 62; **RES:** St Mary's Hosp,
Tucson, AZ 63-64; Coney Island Hosp, Brooklyn,
NY 64-67; **FEL:** MD Anderson Cancer Ctr, Houston,
TX 67; Maimonides Med Ctr, Brooklyn, NY 67; **SI:**
Nuclear Medicine; MRI; **HMO:** Blue Cross GHI Fidelis
Health First HIP Network +

LANG: Sp, Kor, Rus, Can, Tag; 🖑 🖂 🏧 Mcr Mcd WC
NFI Immediately

OBSTETRICS & GYNECOLOGY

Barzegar, Hooshang (MD) ObG **PCP**
Brookdale Univ Hosp Med Ctr
1636 E 14th St Ste 124; Brooklyn, NY 11229;
(718) 998-3500; **BDCERT:** ObG 79; **MS:** Iran 60;
RES: ObG, Brooklyn-Cumberland Hosp, Brooklyn,
NY 67-68; ObG, Montefiore Med Ctr, Bronx, NY
68-69; **FEL:** Montefiore Med Ctr, Bronx, NY 69-70;
FAP: Asst Clin Prof SUNY Downstate; **HOSP:** Long
Island Coll Hosp; **SI:** *Laser Surgery;* **HMO:** Oxford
United Healthcare US Hlthcre GHI Blue Choice +

SA/SU 🖂 🖂 🏧 🏧 🖂 Mcr A Few Days 🖂 **VISA** 🖂

Brennan, John P (MD) ObG **PCP**
Long Island Coll Hosp
Long Island Coll Hosp, Hicks St & Atlantic Ave;
Brooklyn, NY 11201; (718) 780-2855; **BDCERT:**
ObG 92; **MS:** Columbia P&S 85; **RES:** Albert
Einstein Med Ctr, Bronx, NY 84-88; **HMO:** Aetna
Hlth Plan Oxford CIGNA Blue Cross & Blue Shield
Metlife +

Cabbad, Michael (MD) ObG
Brooklyn Hosp Ctr-Caledonian
121 Dekalb Ave 3D; Brooklyn, NY 11201; (718)
250-8302; **BDCERT:** ObG 88; MF 91; **MS:** Mexico
79; **RES:** ObG, Brooklyn Hosp Ctr, Brooklyn, NY 80-
84; **FEL:** MF, Univ Hosp SUNY Bklyn, Brooklyn, NY
84-86; **FAP:** Asst Prof NYU Sch Med; **HOSP:**
Lutheran Med Ctr; **HMO:** Aetna Hlth Plan Blue
Choice None Oxford United Healthcare +

LANG: Sp, Grk, Ar, Rus, Fr; 🖑 🖂 🖂 🏧 🏧 🖂 Mcr
1 Week

Camilien, Louis (MD) ObG
New York Methodist Hosp
506 6th St; Brooklyn, NY 11215; (718) 780-3272;
BDCERT: ObG 88; **MS:** Haiti 77; **RES:** Kings County
Hosp Ctr, Brooklyn, NY 81-83; ObG, Kings County
Hosp Ctr, Brooklyn, NY 83-86; **HOSP:** Univ Hosp
SUNY Bklyn; **SI:** *Colposcopy;* **HMO:** US Hlthcre
United Healthcare GHI CIGNA Magnacare +

LANG: Fr, Sp; 🖑 🖂 🖂 🏧 🏧 🖂 Mcr Mcd
A Few Days 🖂 **VISA** 🖂

Chandra, Prasanta C (MD) ObG **PCP**
Wyckoff Heights Med Ctr
Wyckoff Heights Medical Center, Dept of Obstetrics
& Gynecology, 374 Stockholm St; Brooklyn, NY
11237; (718) 963-7331; **BDCERT:** ObG 79; MF
80; **MS:** India 69; **RES:** S, Bronx Muncipal Hosp Ctr,
Bronx, NY 71-72; ObG, Bronx Muncipal Hosp Ctr,
Bronx, NY 73-76; **FEL:** MF, Bronx Muncipal Hosp
Ctr, Bronx, NY 76-78; **FAP:** Assoc Prof
Hahnemann U; **SI:** *Obstetrics High Risk; Premature
Labor;* **HMO:** US Hlthcre Oxford Multiplan Aetna
Hlth Plan CIGNA +

LANG: Bng, Hin, Ar, Grk; 🖑 🖂 🖂 🏧 🏧 🖂 Mcr Mcd
1 Week

Cohen, Lawrence (MD) ObG **PCP**
Maimonides Med Ctr
1624 E 14th St; Brooklyn, NY 11229; (718) 376-
2220; **BDCERT:** ObG 78; **MS:** Ind U Sch Med 71;
RES: U MN Med Ctr, Minneapolis, MN 72-76; **HMO:**
Aetna Hlth Plan US Hlthcre Prucare CIGNA Sanus
+

🖂 🖂 🏧 🏧 🖂 Mcr 1 Week **VISA** 🖂

Comrie, Millicent (MD)   ObG
Long Island Coll Hosp
115 Pacific St Bsmt; Brooklyn, NY 11201; (718) 852-9180; **BDCERT:** ObG 83; **MS:** SUNY Hlth Sci Ctr 76; **RES:** Long Island Coll Hosp, Brooklyn, NY 76-80; MF, Columbia-Presbyterian Med Ctr, New York, NY; **HMO:** Aetna Hlth Plan
▨ ◖ ⚲ ▣ ⏣ ⑂ ⓜ

Dor, Nathan (MD)   ObG
Maimonides Med Ctr
943 48th St; Brooklyn, NY 11219; (718) 853-1535; **BDCERT:** ObG 80; **MS:** Israel 73; **RES:** ObG, Albert Einstein Med Ctr, Bronx, NY 73-77; **FEL:** NY Med Coll, New York, NY 77-79; **FAP:** Asst Prof SUNY Downstate; **SI:** *High Risk Obstetrics*
LANG: Heb, Yd; ⚲ ▣ ⏣ ⑂   A Few Days

Fuchs, Yael (DO)   ObG
New York Methodist Hosp
263 7th Ave; Brooklyn, NY 11215; (718) 246-8500; **MS:** SUNY Hlth Sci Ctr 90; **RES:** ObG, Univ Hosp SUNY Bklyn, Brooklyn, NY 91-?; **HOSP:** Long Island Coll Hosp; **SI:** *Abnormal Pap Smears; Obstetrics;* **HMO:** Oxford CIGNA US Hlthcre NYCCARE
LANG: Heb, Sp; ♿ ◖ ⚲ ▣ ⏣ ⑂ ⓜ   2-4 Weeks

Gallousis, Spiro (MD)   ObG
Long Island Coll Hosp
9 Pierrepont St; Brooklyn, NY 11201; (718) 852-5810; **BDCERT:** ObG 69; **MS:** Switzerland 62; **RES:** Long Island Coll Hosp, Brooklyn, NY 64-67; **FEL:** Univ Hosp SUNY Bklyn, Brooklyn, NY; **SI:** *Laparoscopic Surgery; Laser Surgery;* **HMO:** Aetna Hlth Plan CIGNA HealthNet Prucare Sanus-NYLCare +
♿ ⚲ ▣ ⏣ ⑂   A Few Days 🖼 **VISA** 💳

Guirguis, Fayez (MD)   ObG
New York Methodist Hosp
464 77th St; Brooklyn, NY 11209; (718) 768-8500; **BDCERT:** ObG 91; **MS:** Egypt 60; **RES:** ObG, Brooklyn Hosp Ctr-Caledonian, Brooklyn, NY 75-80; **HOSP:** Lutheran Med Ctr; **SI:** *Obstetrics; Laparoscopic Surgery;* **HMO:** GHI CIGNA Blue Choice Unicare Primary Plus
LANG: Sp, Ar; ♿ ◖ ⚲ ▣ ⏣ ⑂   A Few Days

Kerr, Angela (MD)   ObG
Brooklyn Hosp Ctr-Caledonian
121 Dekalb Ave; Brooklyn, NY 11201; (718) 250-8318; **BDCERT:** ObG 89; **MS:** SUNY Downstate 83; **RES:** Kings County Hosp Ctr, Brooklyn, NY 83-87; **SI:** *Colposcopy;* **HMO:** Blue Cross & Blue Choice Aetna-US Healthcare Magnacare Oxford PHS +
LANG: Rus, Sp; ♿ ◖ ⚲ ▣ ⑂ ⓜ   2-4 Weeks

Kliot, David (MD)   ObG
New York Methodist Hosp
225 Marlborough Rd; Brooklyn, NY 11226; (718) 693-1011; **BDCERT:** ObG 67; **MS:** SUNY Downstate 59; **RES:** ObG, Brookdale Univ Hosp Med Ctr, Brooklyn, NY 60-64; **FAP:** + Clin Prof SUNY Downstate; **HOSP:** Maimonides Med Ctr; **SI:** *MIDWIVES Available;* **HMO:** Oxford Empire Blue Cross & Shield GHI Aetna-US Healthcare +
LANG: Yd, Heb, Rus; ◖ ⚲ ▣ ⏣ ⑂ ⓜ   2-4 Weeks

Kofinas, Alexander (MD)   ObG
Brooklyn Hosp Ctr-Caledonian
Perinatal Diagnostic Center, 240 Willoughby St 7A; Brooklyn, NY 11201; (718) 250-8123; **BDCERT:** ObG 89; MF 90; **MS:** Greece 76; **RES:** S, Good Samaritan Hosp, Cincinnati, OH 81; ObG, Brooklyn Hosp Ctr, Brooklyn, NY 85; **FEL:** MF, Wake Forest U, Winston-Salem, NC 85-87; **FAP:** Assoc Prof NYU Sch Med; **HOSP:** Victory Memorial Hosp; **SI:** *High Risk Obstetrics; Fetal Diagnosis & Treatment;* **HMO:** Aetna Hlth Plan Oxford Blue Cross & Blue Choice US Hlthcre GHI +
LANG: Fr, Rus, Sp; ♿ ◖ ⚲ ⏣ ⑂   1 Week

Kofinas, George (MD)   ObG
Brooklyn Hosp Ctr-Caledonian
Fertility Institute, 161 Ashland Pl; Brooklyn, NY 11201; (718) 643-6307; **BDCERT:** ObG 87; RE 88; **MS:** Greece 75; **RES:** New York Methodist Hosp, Brooklyn, NY 80-82; Brooklyn Hosp Ctr, Brooklyn, NY 82-84; **FEL:** RE, Univ Hosp SUNY Bklyn, Brooklyn, NY 84-86; **FAP:** Asst Prof SUNY Hlth Sci Ctr; **HOSP:** New York Methodist Hosp; **SI:** *Infertility; Fibroids;* **HMO:** United Healthcare Oxford US Hlthcre
LANG: Sp, Rus, Grk, Pol; ♿ ◖ ⚲ ▣ ⏣ ⑂ ⓜ   2-4 Weeks

Lamarque, Madeleine (MD) ObG
Univ Hosp SUNY Bklyn
601 E 18th St Suite 109; Brooklyn, NY 11226; (718) 434-5373; **BDCERT:** ObG 83; **MS:** Haiti 70; **RES:** ObG, Catholic Med Ctr, Brooklyn, NY 75-79; **FAP:** Clin Instr Albert Einstein Coll Med; **HOSP:** St Mary's Hosp; ***SI:*** *High Risk Obstetrics; Adolescent Gynecology*; **HMO:** Aetna-US Healthcare Oxford CIGNA GHI Blue Cross +

LANG: Fr, Sp, Cre; ♿ [SA SU] ☾ ☎ 👤 📅 $ [Mcr] Immediately

Lederman, Sanford (MD) ObG
Long Island Coll Hosp
9 Pierrepont St; Brooklyn, NY 11201; (718) 852-5810; **BDCERT:** ObG 82; **MS:** Mexico 73; **RES:** ObG, Long Island Coll Hosp, Brooklyn, NY 75-79; **FEL:** Med, U Cailf—Irvine Meml H, Long Beach, CA 79-81; ***SI:*** *Perinatology*; **HMO:** Sanus Prucare Oxford US Hlthcre

☎ 👤 📅 $ 2-4 Weeks [AMEX] VISA [MasterCard]

Ligouri, Lorene (MD) ObG
Lutheran Med Ctr
7111 5th Ave; Brooklyn, NY 11209; (718) 238-6778; **BDCERT:** ObG 87; **MS:** Mt Sinai Sch Med 80; **RES:** Staten Island Univ Hosp, Staten Island, NY 80-82; Beth Israel Med Ctr, New York, NY 82-85; **HOSP:** New York Methodist Hosp; ***SI:*** *Laparoscopic Gynecologic Surgery; Vulvar Dystrophies*; **HMO:** GHI Empire Blue Choice CIGNA Oxford +

LANG: Sp, Rus, Heb, Grk; ♿ [SA SU] ☾ ☎ 👤 📅 $ [Mcr] A Few Days VISA [MasterCard]

Mitchell, Janet L (MD) ObG [PCP]
St Mary's Hosp
Woodhull Medical Ctr, 760 Broadway; Brooklyn, NY 11206; (718) 963-8533; **BDCERT:** ObG 83; **MS:** Howard U 76; **RES:** ObG, Harlem Hosp Ctr, New York, NY 76-80; **FEL:** MF, Albert Einstein Med Ctr, Bronx, NY 80-82; ***SI:*** *Maternal & Fetal Medicine*; **HMO:** Blue Cross & Blue Shield Chubb

♿ ☎ 👤 📅 $ [Mcr] [Mcd] [WC] A Few Days [AMEX] VISA [MasterCard] [Discover]

Molson, Robert (MD) ObG
Victory Memorial Hosp
660 92nd St; Brooklyn, NY 11228; (718) 836-1585; **BDCERT:** ObG 82; **MS:** Italy 70; **RES:** ObG, Westchester County Med Ctr, Valhalla, NY 71-72; ObG, Brooklyn Hosp Ctr-Caledonian, Brooklyn, NY 72-76; **FAP:** Dir ObG; ***SI:*** *Director of OB-GYN*; **HMO:** GHI Aetna Hlth Plan Blue Cross & Blue Shield CIGNA Oxford +

LANG: Itl, Rus; ♿ ☾ ☎ 👤 📅 $ A Few Days [MasterCard]

Motahedeh, Faraj (MD) ObG
New York Methodist Hosp
3302 Avenue N; Brooklyn, NY 11234; (718) 252-4466; **BDCERT:** ObG 78; **MS:** Iran 67; **RES:** New York Methodist Hosp, Brooklyn, NY 70-74; **HMO:** Blue Choice CIGNA GHI Oxford United Healthcare +

[SA SU] ☎ 👤 📅 $ Immediately

Reizis, Igal (MD) ObG
Maimonides Med Ctr
Boro Park OB/GYN, 401 Ditmas Ave; Brooklyn, NY 11218; (718) 972-2700; **BDCERT:** ObG 84; **MS:** Israel 77; **RES:** ObG, Maimonides Med Ctr, Brooklyn, NY 82; **HMO:** Oxford Aetna Hlth Plan PHCS PHS Multiplan +

☾ ☎ 👤 📅 $ [Mcr] A Few Days

Reyes, Francisco I (MD) ObG
Long Island Coll Hosp
Fertility & Hormone Ctr of New York, 161 Atlantic Ave 202; Brooklyn, NY 11201; (718) 237-2727; **BDCERT:** ObG 74; RE 76; **MS:** Mexico 59; **RES:** U Manitoba, Winnipeg, Canada 67-70; **FEL:** U Manitoba, Winnipeg, Canada; Columbia-Presbyterian Med Ctr, New York, NY; ***SI:*** *Infertility; Menstrual Abnormalities*; **HMO:** Blue Choice Empire GHI Aetna Hlth Plan US Hlthcre +

LANG: Sp; [SA SU] ☾ ☎ 👤 📅 $ A Few Days VISA [MasterCard]

Rosenblum, Neal (MD)　　ObG
Brookdale Univ Hosp Med Ctr
6410 Veterans Ave 203; Brooklyn, NY 11234;
(718) 209-0966; **BDCERT:** ObG 86; **MS:** NY Med
Coll 79; **RES:** ObG, Brookdale Univ Hosp Med Ctr,
Brooklyn, NY 79-83; **FEL:** Colposcopy, Brookdale
Univ Hosp Med Ctr, Brooklyn, NY 83-84; **HMO:**
Oxford Empire Blue Cross US Hlthcre GHI PHCS +

⬤ 🔋 📷 📺 🏠 💲 Mcr　1 Week

Rubenstein, Janet (MD)　　ObG
Maimonides Med Ctr
4506 12th Ave; Brooklyn, NY 11219; (718) 633-
3131; **BDCERT:** ObG 97; **MS:** Med Coll PA 78; **RES:**
Maimonides Med Ctr, Brooklyn, NY 78-82; **HMO:**
Most

SA SU 🔋 📷 📺 🏠 💲 Mcr　1 Week

Shiffman, Rebecca (MD)　　ObG
New York Methodist Hosp
506 6th St; Brooklyn, NY 11215; (718) 780-3272;
BDCERT: ObG 87; **MF** 88; **MS:** Belgium 80; **RES:**
ObG, Jewish Hosp Med Ctr, Brooklyn, NY 80-84;
FEL: MF, Nassau County Med Ctr, East Meadow, NY
84-86; **FAP:** Asst Prof Cornell U; **SI:** *Recurrent
Pregnancy Loss; High Risk Pregnancy*

LANG: Sp, Fr, Heb, Yd; ⬤ 📷 🏠 Mcr Mcd
Immediately

Slatkin, Richard (MD)　　ObG
Long Island Coll Hosp
97 Amity St FL4; Brooklyn, NY 11201; (718) 643-
0007; **BDCERT:** ObG 84; **MS:** Italy 70; **RES:** ObG,
Brookdale Univ Hosp Med Ctr, Brooklyn, NY 77-79;
ObG, Brookdale Univ Hosp Med Ctr, Brooklyn, NY
79-80; **SI:** *Obstetrics; Colposcopies*; **HMO:** Oxford
CIGNA US Hlthcre NYLCare Metlife +

LANG: Sp, Itl, Ger; ⬤ 🔋 📷 📺 🏠 💲 Mcr　1 Week

Weinstock, Judith (MD)　　ObG
Long Island Coll Hosp
9 Pierrpont St; Brooklyn, NY 11201; (718) 852-
5810; **BDCERT:** ObG 88; ObG 97; **MS:** Baylor 82;
RES: ObG, Long Island Coll Hosp, Brooklyn, NY 82-
86; **FAP:** Assoc Clin Prof SUNY Downstate; **SI:**
Pregnancy; Menopause; **HMO:** CIGNA Aetna-US
Healthcare Oxford PHCS NYLCare +

⬤ 📷 📺 🏠 💲 NfI　4+ Weeks ▦ **VISA** ⬤

OPHTHALMOLOGY

Ackerman, Jacob (MD)　　Oph
Brookdale Univ Hosp Med Ctr
Brook Plaza Ophthalmology Associates, PC, 1901
Utica Ave Fl 1; Brooklyn, NY 11234; (718) 968-
8700; **BDCERT:** Oph 76; **MS:** Albert Einstein Coll
Med 71; **RES:** Oph, Long Island Jewish Med Ctr,
New Hyde Park, NY 72-75; **FAP:** Asst Prof Oph
SUNY Hlth Sci Ctr; **HOSP:** New York Comm Hosp of
Bklyn; **SI:** *Glaucoma; Ophthalmic Plastic Surgery*;
HMO: United Healthcare Blue Cross & Blue Shield
CIGNA Sanus Oxford +

LANG: Fr, Heb, Yd, Rus, Sp; ⬤ 🌙 📷 📺 🏠 💲 Mcr
Mcd　Immediately ▦

Brecher, Rubin (MD)　　Oph
Maimonides Med Ctr
736 Ocean Pkwy; Brooklyn, NY 11230; (718)
851-1186; **BDCERT:** Oph 91; **MS:** Albert Einstein
Coll Med 84; **RES:** Albert Einstein Med Ctr, Bronx,
NY; **FEL:** Albert Einstein Med Ctr, Bronx, NY 85-88;
Moorefields Eye Hosp, London, England 88-89;
HOSP: Montefiore Med Ctr; **SI:** *Diabetic Retinopathy;
Macular Degeneration*; **HMO:** Oxford US Hlthcre
1199 Blue Choice Magnacare +

LANG: Heb, Yd; ⬤ SA SU 🌙 📷 📺 🏠 💲 Mcr
Immediately

Deutsch, James A (MD)　　Oph
Long Island Coll Hosp
110 Remsen St; Brooklyn, NY 11201; (718) 855-
8700; **BDCERT:** Oph 89; **MS:** NYU Sch Med 84;
RES: Oph, Mount Sinai Med Ctr, New York, NY 85-
88; **FEL:** Ped Oph, Wills Eye Hosp, Philadelphia, PA
88-89; **FAP:** Asst Clin Prof Mt Sinai Sch Med;
HOSP: Brooklyn Hosp Ctr-Downtown; **SI:**
Strabismus; Cataract Surgery; **HMO:** GHI US Hlthcre
Oxford United Healthcare

LANG: Sp, Fr; SA SU 🌙 📷 📺 🏠 💲 Mcr　2-4 Weeks
VISA ⬤

Feinstein, Neil (MD)   Oph
Maimonides Med Ctr
919 48th St; Brooklyn, NY 11219; (718) 435-1800; **BDCERT:** Oph 79; **MS:** Albert Einstein Coll Med 74; **RES:** Univ Hosp SUNY Brooklyn, Brooklyn, NY 75-78; **FEL:** Manhattan Eye, Ear & Throat Hosp, New York, NY; **HOSP:** Manhattan Eye, Ear & Throat Hosp

Freedman, Jeffrey (MD & PhD)Oph
Long Island Coll Hosp
161 Atlantic Ave 203; Brooklyn, NY 11201; (718) 596-9086; **BDCERT:** Oph 75; **MS:** South Africa 64; **RES:** Baragwanath Gen Hosp, Johannesberg, South Africa 64-66; Transvaal Mem Hosp, Johannesberg, South Africa 66-67; *SI: Glaucoma; Cornea*; **HMO:** Oxford GHI Blue Choice 1199

♿ 📷 🚗 🏨 **S** Mcr   A Few Days

Greenidge, Kevin (MD)   Oph
Long Island Coll Hosp
University Ophthalmic Consultants, PC, 339 Hicks St; Brooklyn, NY; (718) 780-2600; **BDCERT:** Oph 82; **MS:** SUNY Buffalo 77; **RES:** Oph, Emory U Hosp, Atlanta, GA 78-81; **FEL:** Glaucoma, Wills Eye Hosp, Philadelphia, PA 81-82; **FAP:** Chrmn SUNY Downstate; **HOSP:** Univ Hosp SUNY Bklyn; *SI: Glaucoma; Poor Vision*; **HMO:** 1199 Aetna-US Healthcare Blue Cross & Blue Shield CIGNA GHI +

LANG: Sp, Rus; ♿ 📷 🚗 🏨 **S** Mcr Mod   A Few Days

Hyman, George (MD)   Oph
Brookdale Univ Hosp Med Ctr
Brookdale Eye Institute, 2460 Flatbush Ave 1; Brooklyn, NY 11234; (718) 332-3030; **BDCERT:** Oph 76; **MS:** U Md Sch Med 68; **RES:** Univ Hosp SUNY Bklyn, Brooklyn, NY 71-74; **FEL:** Anterior Segment S, U of Witswatersand, Johannesburg, S Africa; **FAP:** Asst Prof SUNY Hlth Sci Ctr; *SI: Refractive Surgery; Cataract*; **HMO:** Oxford US Hlthcre Aetna Hlth Plan Sanus GHI +

♿ SA/SU **C** 📷 🚗 🏨 **S** Mcr   A Few Days

Jaffe, Herbert (MD)   Oph
Beth Israel Med Ctr-Kings Hwy
2128 Ocean Ave; Brooklyn, NY 11229; (718) 339-7469; **BDCERT:** Oph 83; **MS:** Belgium 68; **RES:** Nassau County Med Ctr, East Meadow, NY 69; Univ Hosp SUNY Bklyn, Brooklyn, NY 71; **HOSP:** Univ Hosp SUNY Bklyn; *SI: Cataract; Glaucoma*; **HMO:** GHI Blue Cross & Blue Shield Aetna-US Healthcare Oxford PHS +

C 📷 🚗 🏨 **S** Mcr WC NFI   A Few Days **VISA** 💳

Langone, Daniel (MD)   Oph
Lutheran Med Ctr
9602 4th Ave; Brooklyn, NY 11209; (718) 836-3456; **BDCERT:** Oph 82; **MS:** Spain 74; **RES:** Metropolitan Hosp Ctr, New York, NY 75-77; Catholic Med Ctr Bklyn & Qns, Jamaica, NY 77-80; **HOSP:** Catholic Med Ctr Bklyn & Qns; **HMO:** GHI Oxford US Hlthcre Blue Cross & Blue Shield

LANG: Sp; ♿ SA/SU **C** 📷 🚗 🏨 Mcr Mod   A Few Days

Lazzaro, E Clifford (MD)   Oph
New York Eye & Ear Infirmary
7901 4th Ave A4; Brooklyn, NY 11209; (718) 748-1334; **BDCERT:** Oph 73; **MS:** SUNY Hlth Sci Ctr 65; **RES:** Oph, Brooklyn Eye & Ear Hosp, Brooklyn, NY 68-71; *SI: Glaucoma; Systemic Diseases of the Eye*; **HMO:** US Hlthcre Metlife Prudential CIGNA Blue Choice +

LANG: Itl, Sp, Grk; ♿ SA/SU 📷 🚗 🏨 **S** Mcr WC   A Few Days

Lebowitz, Mark (MD)   Oph
New York Eye & Ear Infirmary
1301 Ave J; Brooklyn, NY 11230; (718) 284-1921; **BDCERT:** Oph 87; **MS:** NYU Sch Med 82; **RES:** Oph, Univ Hosp SUNY, Brooklyn, NY 83-86; **FEL:** Manh Eye, Ear & Throat Hosp, New York, NY; **HOSP:** Maimonides Med Ctr

Lieberman, David M (MD) Oph
New York Methodist Hosp
9 Prospect Park West 1B; Brooklyn, NY 11215; (718) 622-8900; **BDCERT:** Oph 73; **MS:** SUNY Downstate 65; **RES:** Univ Hosp SUNY Bklyn, Brooklyn, NY 66-70; **FAP:** Chf Oph; *SI: Cornea Research*; **HMO:** Most

⬤ ⬤ ⬤ ⬤ ⬤ ⬤ ⬤ 1 Week

Lombardo, James (MD) Oph
New York Eye & Ear Infirmary
7801 4th Ave; Brooklyn, NY 11209; (718) 836-6661; **BDCERT:** Oph 82; **MS:** NYU Sch Med 76; **RES:** St Vincents Hosp & Med Ctr, New York, NY 76-77; New York Eye & Ear Infirmary, New York, NY 77-80

Lombardo, John (MD) Oph
New York Eye & Ear Infirmary
7801 4th Ave; Brooklyn, NY 11209; (718) 836-6661; **BDCERT:** Oph 83; Psyc 81; **MS:** Columbia P&S 73; **RES:** Manhattan Eye, Ear & Throat Hosp, New York, NY 79-82; Columbia-Presbyterian Med Ctr, New York, NY 74-77; **HOSP:** Victory Memorial Hosp; *SI: Cataract Implants; Laser Surgery For Myopia*; **HMO:** Oxford US Hlthcre GHI HealthNet Aetna Hlth Plan +

LANG: Sp, Fr, Itl; ⬤ ⬤ ⬤ ⬤ ⬤ ⬤ ⬤ ⬤ ⬤ Immediately *VISA* ⬤

Mc Groarty, James (MD) Oph
New York Methodist Hosp
140 Joralemon St; Brooklyn, NY 11201; (718) 780-3000; **BDCERT:** Oph 76; **MS:** NY Med Coll 68; **RES:** Oph, Hollywood Presbyterian Medical Center, Los Angeles, CA 72-74; **FEL:** Good Samaritan Hosp, Los Angeles, CA 75-76; *SI: Diabetic Eye Disease; Retinal Surgery*; **HMO:** Oxford US Hlthcre Empire GHI CIGNA +

LANG: Sp; ⬤ ⬤ ⬤ ⬤ ⬤ A Few Days

Pearlstein, Eric (MD) Oph
Long Island Coll Hosp
Ophthalmology Associates of Bay Ridge, 8721 4th Ave; Brooklyn, NY 11209; (718) 680-1500; **BDCERT:** Oph 88; **MS:** SUNY Hlth Sci Ctr 83; **RES:** Oph, Long Island Jewish Med Ctr, New Hyde Park, NY 84-87; **FEL:** Cataract, U MN-Duluth Sch Med, Duluth, MN 87-88; *SI: Cataract; Cornea*; **HMO:** Oxford Prucare GHI Magnacare US Hlthcre +

LANG: Sp, Itl, Grk; ⬤ ⬤ ⬤ ⬤ ⬤ ⬤ ⬤ ⬤ ⬤ A Few Days *VISA* ⬤

Reich, Raymond (MD) Oph
Long Island Coll Hosp
118 West End Ave; Brooklyn, NY 11235; (718) 332-6200; **BDCERT:** Oph 78; **MS:** Albert Einstein Coll Med 73; **RES:** Oph, Univ Hosp SUNY Bklyn, Brooklyn, NY 74-77; **FEL:** Oph, Harvard Med Sch, Cambridge, MA 78; **FAP:** Asst Prof SUNY Hlth Sci Ctr; **HOSP:** Maimonides Med Ctr; *SI: Cataract Laser Surgery; Plastic Surgery*; **HMO:** Oxford Prucare Aetna Hlth Plan Elderplan Metlife +

LANG: Rus, Heb, Yd, Fr; ⬤ ⬤ ⬤ ⬤ ⬤ ⬤ ⬤ ⬤ ⬤ ⬤ A Few Days

Rosenthal, J Robert (MD) Oph
New York Eye & Ear Infirmary
2613 E 16th St; Brooklyn, NY 11235; (718) 332-1313; **BDCERT:** Oph 64; **MS:** U Hlth Sci/Chicago Med Sch 58; **RES:** New York Eye & Ear Infirmary, New York, NY 58-60; **FEL:** Oph, Castroviejo Hosp, New York, NY 61-62; **FAP:** Asst Prof Oph NY Med Coll; **HMO:** Blue Cross & Blue Shield CIGNA Sanus-NYLCare Oxford United Healthcare +

LANG: Sp, Rus; ⬤ ⬤ ⬤ ⬤ ⬤ 2-4 Weeks

Rothman, Harold (MD) Oph
Interfaith Med Ctr-St John's
2911 Kings Hwy; Brooklyn, NY 11229; (718) 252-3356; **BDCERT:** Oph 50; **MS:** England 38; **RES:** Oph, Goldwater Mem Hosp, New York, NY 47-48; Oph, Precept-Dr SW Smith, New York, NY 46-47; **HOSP:** Beth Israel Med Ctr-Kings Hwy; **HMO:** GHI Blue Shield Multiplan NYLCare Magnacare +

LANG: Yd; ⬤ ⬤ ⬤ ⬤ ⬤ ⬤ ⬤ ⬤ ⬤ Immediately

Saffra, Norman (MD)   Oph
Maimonides Med Ctr
921 49th St; Brooklyn, NY 11219; (718) 283-8000; **BDCERT:** Oph 94; **MS:** Albert Einstein Coll Med 88; **RES:** IM, Maimonides Med Ctr, Brooklyn, NY 88-89; Oph, Montefiore Med Ctr, Bronx, NY 89-92; **FEL:** Retina Vitreous, Univ Hosp SUNY Bklyn, Brooklyn, NY 93; **FAP:** Asst Clin Prof Oph SUNY Hlth Sci Ctr; **HOSP:** New York Eye & Ear Infirmary; **HMO:** Oxford Empire Blue Cross & Shield Empire Blue Cross & Shield GHI

LANG: Rus, Yd, Heb; [symbols] Immediately
VISA [symbol]

Schechter, Ronald (MD)   Oph
Univ Hosp SUNY Bklyn
9 Prospect Park West 1B; Brooklyn, NY 11215; (718) 783-7200; **BDCERT:** Oph 82; **MS:** Albert Einstein Coll Med 69; **RES:** US Public Health Svc Hospital, Staten Island, NY 77-80; **FEL:** Ped, Downstate Medical Ctr, Brooklyn, NY 81-82; **HMO:** Aetna-US Healthcare Blue Cross & Blue Shield

Sciortino, Patrick (MD)   Oph
Long Island Coll Hosp
914 Bay Ridge Pkwy; Brooklyn, NY 11228; (718) 748-5700; **MS:** NY Med Coll 78; **RES:** St Vincents Hosp & Med Ctr NY, New York, NY 79-80; Oph, Catholic Med Ctr Bklyn & Qns, Jamaica, NY 80; **FEL:** N Oph, Univ Hosp SUNY Bklyn, Brooklyn, NY 83-84; **HOSP:** New York Comm Hosp of Bklyn; *SI: Laser Surgery; Cataract Surgery;* **HMO:** Blue Choice Blue Cross GHI PHCS PHS +

LANG: Itl, Sp; [symbols] Immediately
[symbols] **VISA** [symbol]

Sherman, Steven (DO)   Oph
New York Methodist Hosp
671 Flatbush Ave; Brooklyn, NY 11235; (718) 693-8200; **BDCERT:** Oph 90; **MS:** Univ Hlth Sci Coll -Osteo Med 77; **RES:** USPHS Hosp, Baltimore, MD 79-82; **FEL:** Univ Hosp SUNY Bklyn, Brooklyn, NY 82-83; **FAP:** Clin Instr SUNY Downstate; **HOSP:** Long Island Coll Hosp; *SI: Cataract; Glaucoma;* **HMO:** Elderplan US Hlthcre Oxford Aetna Hlth Plan

LANG: Yd, Sp; [symbols]
A Few Days **VISA** [symbols]

Silberman, Deborah (MD)   Oph
Brookdale Univ Hosp Med Ctr
1 Brookdale Plz # 104; Brooklyn, NY 11212; (718) 240-5557; **BDCERT:** Oph 90; **MS:** SUNY Buffalo 84; **RES:** IM, St Luke's Roosevelt Hosp, New York, NY 84-85; Oph, Brookdale Univ Hosp, Brooklyn, NY 85-88; **HOSP:** Maimonides Med Ctr

Smith, Edward (MD)   Oph
Univ Hosp SUNY Bklyn
Downstate Ophthalmology Associates, 11 Plaza St West; Brooklyn, NY 11217; (718) 638-2020; **BDCERT:** Oph 89; **MS:** SUNY Downstate 84; **RES:** Oph, Univ Hosp SUNY Bklyn, Brooklyn, NY; **FEL:** N Oph, Univ Hosp SUNY Bklyn, Brooklyn, NY; **FAP:** Asst Prof SUNY Downstate; *SI: Cataract; Optic Nerve Disorders;* **HMO:** Aetna Hlth Plan US Hlthcre Metlife Oxford GHI +

LANG: Sp, Fr, Prt, Yd, Rus; [symbols]
[symbols] 1 Week

Stein, Arnold (MD)   Oph
Long Island Jewish Med Ctr
1000 Ocean Pky LA1; Brooklyn, NY 11230; (718) 692-0400; **BDCERT:** Oph 87; **MS:** SUNY Downstate 82; **RES:** Med, Brookdale Univ Hosp Med Ctr, Brooklyn, NY 82-83; Oph, Long Island Jewish Med Ctr, New Hyde Park, NY 83-86; **HOSP:** Beth Israel Med Ctr-Kings Hwy; **HMO:** Oxford Blue Choice Magnacare Aetna Hlth Plan Prudential +

Unterricht, Sam (MD)   Oph
New York Methodist Hosp
20 Plaza Street; Brooklyn, NY 11238; (718) 622-5800; **BDCERT:** Oph 82; **MS:** SUNY Downstate 76; **RES:** Oph, Univ Hosp SUNY Bklyn, Brooklyn, NY 77-80; **FEL:** Nph, Kingsbrook Jewish Med Ctr, Brooklyn, NY 80-81; Retina Vitreous, Univ Hosp SUNY Bklyn, Brooklyn, NY 81-82; **FAP:** Asst Clin Prof SUNY Hlth Sci Ctr; **HOSP:** Univ Hosp SUNY Bklyn; *SI: Diabetes/Macular Diseases; Retinal & Nerve Problems;* **HMO:** Aetna Hlth Plan Oxford MHS Blue Shield GHI +

LANG: Yd, Sp, Can, Fr, Heb; [symbols]
[symbols] A Few Days

Weseley, Alan (MD) Oph
New York Eye & Ear Infirmary
2626 E 14th St; Brooklyn, NY 11235; (718) 332-7932; **BDCERT:** Oph 62; **MS:** NY Med Coll 56; **RES:** New York Eye & Ear Infirmary, New York, NY 57-60; **HOSP:** Lenox Hill Hosp; **HMO:** Blue Cross & Blue Shield CIGNA Aetna Hlth Plan US Hlthcre GHI +

🔲 🧑 🏠 💲 Mcr WC NFI A Few Days

Wolintz, Arthur (MD) Oph
Univ Hosp SUNY Bklyn
100 Ocean Pkwy; Brooklyn, NY 11218; (718) 854-7360; **BDCERT:** Oph 73; N 70; **MS:** SUNY Hlth Sci Ctr 62; **RES:** N, Mount Sinai Med Ctr, New York, NY 65-66; Oph, Univ Hosp SUNY Bklyn, Brooklyn, NY 69-71; **FEL:** N Path, Columbia-Presbyterian Med Ctr, New York, NY 67-68; **FAP:** Prof SUNY Hlth Sci Ctr; **HOSP:** Kingsbrook Jewish Med Ctr; *SI: Eye Diseases re: the Brain*; **HMO:** US Hlthcre Aetna Hlth Plan CIGNA Chubb PHS +

LANG: Heb, Yd, Sp; ♿ 📞 🔲 🧑 🏠 💲 WC
A Few Days

Zellner, James (MD) Oph
New York Eye & Ear Infirmary
454 Bay Ridge Pkwy; Brooklyn, NY 11209; (718) 748-2020; **BDCERT:** Oph 82; **MS:** Albert Einstein Coll Med 77; **RES:** Univ Hosp SUNY Bklyn, Brooklyn, NY 81; **HOSP:** Lutheran Med Ctr; *SI: Cataracts; Glaucoma*; **HMO:** GHI Oxford Aetna Hlth Plan CIGNA US Hlthcre +

♿ 🔲 📞 🏠 🏠 💲 Mcr 2-4 Weeks

ORTHOPAEDIC SURGERY

Gordon, Stanley (MD) OrS
Univ Hosp SUNY Bklyn
PO Box 30; Brooklyn, NY 11203; (718) 270-2179; **BDCERT:** OrS 72; **MS:** Univ Pittsburgh 64; **RES:** OrS, U of Pittsburgh Med Ctr, Pittsburgh, PA 68-71; **FEL:** HS, Israel; **FAP:** Prof SUNY Hlth Sci Ctr; *SI: Orthopaedic Surgery; Hand Surgery*; **HMO:** CIGNA Oxford GHI

LANG: Fr, Man; ♿ 🔲 🧑 🏠 💲 Mcr WC NFI 1 Week
💳 *VISA* 💳 💳

Mani, John (MD) OrS
Long Island Coll Hosp
161 Atlantic Ave; Brooklyn, NY 11201; (718) 855-0088; **BDCERT:** OrS 77; **MS:** India 70; **RES:** SM, Brookdale Univ Hosp Med Ctr, Brooklyn, NY 72-76; **FEL:** Arthritis, Hosp For Special Surgery, New York, NY 77-78; **FAP:** Assoc Clin Prof SUNY Hlth Sci Ctr; **HOSP:** Lenox Hill Hosp; *SI: Hip and Knee Replacement*; **HMO:** Oxford Prucare Aetna Hlth Plan Blue Choice +

♿ 🔲 🧑 🏠 💲 Mcr A Few Days

Menezes, Placido (MD) OrS
New York Methodist Hosp
543 2nd St; Brooklyn, NY 11215; (718) 788-7600; **BDCERT:** OrS 80; **MS:** India 70; **RES:** S, New York Methodist Hosp, Brooklyn, NY 71-75; OrS, Brooklyn Jewish Hosp, Brooklyn, NY 76-78; **HOSP:** Brooklyn Hosp Ctr-Caledonian; *SI: Trauma; Joint Replacement*; **HMO:** Oxford Blue Choice CIGNA US Hlthcre GHI +

♿ 📞 🔲 🧑 🏠 💲 Mcr WC NFI A Few Days

Pearlman, Hubert (MD) OrS
Maimonides Med Ctr
Orthopedic Surgical Assoc, 4901 Ft Hamilton Pkwy; Brooklyn, NY 11219; (718) 435-4944; **BDCERT:** OrS 60; **MS:** Univ IL Coll Med 50; **RES:** Kings County Hosp Ctr, Brooklyn, NY 54-57; Walter Reed Army Med Ctr, Washington, DC 53-54; **FAP:** Clin Prof U of Hlth Sci, Coll Osteo Med; **HOSP:** New York Methodist Hosp; *SI: Sports Med; Trauma*; **HMO:** Oxford Aetna Hlth Plan United Healthcare Empire Blue Cross & Shield GHI +

LANG: Itl, Rus, Sp, Fr, Hin; ♿ 🔲 🧑 🏠 💲 Mcr Mcd WC NFI 1 Week 💳 *VISA* 💳 💳

Sclafani, Salvatore (MD) OrS
Lutheran Med Ctr
435 Bay Ridge Pkwy; Brooklyn, NY 11209; (718) 833-1808; **BDCERT:** OrS 67; **MS:** SUNY Hlth Sci Ctr 57; **RES:** S, VA Med Ctr-Brooklyn, Brooklyn, NY 58-59; OrS, VA Med Ctr-Brooklyn, Brooklyn, NY 61-64; **FAP:** Asst Clin Prof SUNY Downstate; **HOSP:** Victory Memorial Hosp; *SI: Sports Medicine; Joint Replacement*; **HMO:** GHI US Hlthcre Blue Cross & Blue Shield Oxford

LANG: Itl; 📞 🔲 🧑 🏠 Mcr WC NFI A Few Days

Splain, Shepard (DO)   OrS
Brookdale Univ Hosp Med Ctr

Linden Blvd & Rockaway Pkwy; Brooklyn, NY 11212; (718) 240-5888; **BDCERT:** OrS 80; **MS:** Mich St U 73; **RES:** Brookdale Univ Hosp Med Ctr, Brooklyn, NY 74-78; **FEL:** Sm, Univ Hosp, Oklahoma City, OK; **FAP:** Asst Clin Prof OrS SUNY Downstate; **HOSP:** Long Island Coll Hosp; *SI: Arthroscopic Surgery; Sports Medicine*; **HMO:** Oxford GHI Blue Cross & Blue Shield CIGNA 1199 +

⌖ ⌖ ⌖ ⌖ ⌖ ⌖ ⌖ ⌖ 1 Week

Strongwater, Allan (MD)   OrS
Maimonides Med Ctr

927 49th St; Brooklyn, NY 11219; (718) 283-7400; **BDCERT:** OrS 86; **MS:** Rush Med Coll 78; **RES:** Yale-New Haven Hosp, New Haven, CT 78-83; **FEL:** Ped OrS, Hosp For Joint Diseases, New York, NY 83-84; **HOSP:** Hosp For Joint Diseases; *SI: Clubfoot; Hip Dysplasia*

⌖ ⌖ ⌖ ⌖ ⌖ A Few Days ▦ **VISA** ●

Teicher, Joel (MD)   OrS
Brookdale Univ Hosp Med Ctr

Brookdale Orthopedics, 1275 Linden Blvd; Brooklyn, NY 11212; (718) 240-5442; **BDCERT:** OrS 69; **MS:** NYU Sch Med 60; **RES:** VA Med Ctr-Manh, New York, NY 61-62; Mount Sinai Med Ctr, New York, NY 64-67; *SI: Total Joint Replacement; Fracture Treatment*; **HMO:** Prucare Oxford Prucare 1199

⌖ ⌖ ⌖ ⌖ ⌖ ⌖ ⌖ ⌖ ⌖ A Few Days

Tepler, Melvin (MD)   OrS
Maimonides Med Ctr

1412 E 9th St; Brooklyn, NY 11230; (718) 627-6000; **BDCERT:** OrS 88; **MS:** NY Med Coll 80; **RES:** Maimonides Med Ctr, Brooklyn, NY 85; **HOSP:** Beth Israel Med Ctr; **HMO:** Blue Choice Oxford Magnacare PHCS

LANG: Heb, Yd; ⌖ ⌖ ⌖ ⌖ ⌖ ⌖ ⌖ ⌖ ⌖
Immediately

Tischler, Henry (MD)   OrS
Univ Hosp SUNY Bklyn

Brooklyn Spine and Arthritis Ctr, 519 6th St; Brooklyn, NY 11203; (718) 780-3104; **BDCERT:** OrS 95; **MS:** SUNY Downstate 85; **RES:** S, Univ Hosp SUNY Bklyn, Brooklyn, NY 85-86; OrS, Univ Hosp SUNY Bklyn, Brooklyn, NY 86-90; **FEL:** Tampa Gen Hosp, Tampa, FL 90-91; **FAP:** Asst Prof SUNY Hlth Sci Ctr; **HOSP:** New York Methodist Hosp; *SI: Total Joint Replacements; Hip and Knee Surgery*; **HMO:** CIGNA US Hlthcre Oxford GHI Blue Cross & Blue Shield +

⌖ ⌖ ⌖ ⌖ ⌖ ⌖ ⌖ ⌖ ⌖ 2-4 Weeks **VISA** ●

Verde, Robert (MD)   OrS
Lutheran Med Ctr

Orthopedic Surgical Cnslnts, 9921 4th Ave; Brooklyn, NY 11209; (718) 238-5565; **BDCERT:** OrS 91; **MS:** Italy 79; **RES:** S, Lutheran Med Ctr, Brooklyn, NY 81-83; OrS, Elyria Mem Hosp, Elyria, OH 81-84; **FEL:** S, Dallas Hosp, Dallas, TX 85; **HOSP:** Bayley Seton Hosp; *SI: Knee Surgery; Reconstructive Surgery*; **HMO:** Blue Cross & Blue Shield CIGNA Metlife Oxford GHI +

LANG: Itl, Sp; ⌖ ⌖ ⌖ ⌖ ⌖ ⌖ ⌖

Wert, Sanford (MD)   OrS
New York Comm Hosp of Bklyn

3075 Brighton 13th St; Brooklyn, NY 11235; (718) 332-4747; **BDCERT:** OrS 85; **MS:** Mexico 74; **RES:** OrS, Long Island Jewish Med Ctr, New Hyde Park, NY 76-79; Maimonides Med Ctr, Brooklyn, NY 74-75

LANG: Rus, Sp, Fr; ⌖ ⌖ ⌖ ⌖ ⌖ ⌖ ⌖ ⌖
A Few Days

Weseley, Martin (MD)   OrS
Victory Memorial Hosp

478 Bay Ridge Pkwy; Brooklyn, NY 11209; (718) 238-2661; **BDCERT:** OrS 64; **MS:** NY Med Coll 56; **RES:** Lenox Hill Hosp, New York, NY 56-57; Hosp For Joint Diseases, New York, NY 57-58; **FEL:** Hosp For Joint Diseases, New York, NY 58-61; **HOSP:** Maimonides Med Ctr; **HMO:** GHI Oxford Blue Choice PHCS

LANG: Sp, Itl, Grk; ⌖ ⌖ ⌖ ⌖ ⌖ ⌖ ⌖ ⌖
A Few Days **VISA** ●

Wolpin, Martin (MD)   OrS
Maimonides Med Ctr
1301 57th St; Brooklyn, NY 11219; (718) 438-6400; **BDCERT:** OrS 71; **MS:** SUNY Hlth Sci Ctr 63; **RES:** S, Mather AFB Hosp, Sacramento, CA 64-66; OrS, Univ Hosp SUNY Bklyn, Brooklyn, NY 66-69; **FAP:** Asst Prof SUNY Downstate; **HOSP:** Beth Israel Med Ctr-Kings Hwy; **SI:** *Scoliosis; Spinal Pathology;* **HMO:** Oxford Empire Prucare Multiplan Blue Choice +

⬥ 🖻 🏥 💲 Mcr WC NFI 1 Week *VISA* 💳

OTOLARYNGOLOGY

Brownstein, Howard (MD)   Oto
Lutheran Med Ctr
9602 4th Ave; Brooklyn, NY 11209; (718) 748-5225; **BDCERT:** Oto 69; **MS:** England 61; **RES:** S, Meadowbrook Hosp, East Meadow, NY 62-63; Oto, New York Eye & Ear Infirmary, New York, NY 63-66; **HOSP:** Hempstead Gen Hosp Med Ctr; **HMO:** Aetna Hlth Plan Blue Choice Blue Cross & Blue Shield HealthNet GHI +

⬥ ☾ 🖻 🏥 Mcr WC NFI A Few Days

Chaudhry, Rashid M (MD)   Oto
Brookdale Univ Hosp Med Ctr
1 Brookdale Plza Ste 157; Brooklyn, NY 11212; (718) 240-6366; **BDCERT:** Oto 78; **HS** 78; **MS:** Pakistan 69; **RES:** Oto, Univ Hosp SUNY Bklyn, Brooklyn, NY 74-78; **SI:** *Facial Plastic Surgery; Sinus Surgery;* **HMO:** US Hlthcre Oxford GHI Blue Cross & Blue Shield 32BJ +

LANG: Sp, Ur, Bng, Hin; ⬥ ☾ 🖻 🏥 💲 Mcr NFI
A Few Days

Cohen, Maurice (MD)   Oto
Long Island Coll Hosp
34 Plaza St E 106; Brooklyn, NY 11238; (718) 622-0505; **BDCERT:** Oto 65; **MS:** Canada 59; **RES:** Kings County Hosp Ctr, Brooklyn, NY 60-64; **HOSP:** Kingsbrook Jewish Med Ctr; **HMO:** GHI Empire Oxford 1199

⬥ ☾ 🖻 🏥 💲 Mcr A Few Days

Goldsmith, Ari (MD)   Oto
Long Island Coll Hosp
University Otolaryngologists, 134 Atlantic Ave; Brooklyn, NY 11201; (718) 780-1498; **BDCERT:** Ped 94; Oto 93; **MS:** Albert Einstein Coll Med 88; **RES:** Oto, Long Island Jewish Med Ctr, New Hyde Park, NY 93; **FEL:** Ped Oto, Children's Hosp, Boston, MA 93-94; **FAP:** Asst Prof SUNY Hlth Sci Ctr; **HOSP:** Univ Hosp SUNY Stony Brook; **SI:** *Airway Anomalies Pediatric; Otitis Media;* **HMO:** Oxford GHI US Hlthcre Prucare CIGNA +

LANG: Heb, Rus, Sp; ⬥ ☾ 🖻 🏥 🏥 💲 Mcr Mcr NFI
2-4 Weeks *VISA* 💳

Habib, Mohsen (MD)   Oto
Victory Memorial Hosp
7333 6th Ave; Brooklyn, NY 11209; (718) 833-0515; **BDCERT:** Oto 83; **MS:** Egypt 69; **RES:** Brookdale Univ Hosp Med Ctr, Brooklyn, NY 79; New York Eye & Ear Infirmary, New York, NY 83; **FEL:** Oto N, Lenox Hill Hosp, New York, NY; **HOSP:** New York Methodist Hosp; **SI:** *Head & Neck Surgery;* **HMO:** Oxford US Hlthcre Empire GHI

LANG: Itl, Sp, Ar, Chi, Fr; ⬥ ☾ 🏥 🏥 💲 Mcr WC NFI
A Few Days *VISA* 💳

Har-El, Gady (MD)   Oto
Long Island Coll Hosp
University Otolaryngologists, 134 Atlantic Ave; Brooklyn, NY 11201; (718) 780-1498; **BDCERT:** Oto 92; **MS:** Israel 83; **RES:** Univ Hosp SUNY Bklyn, Brooklyn, NY 86-91; **FAP:** Prof SUNY Hlth Sci Ctr; **HOSP:** Univ Hosp SUNY Bklyn; **SI:** *Head and Neck Cancer; Sinus Surgery;* **HMO:** GHI CIGNA US Hlthcre Blue Choice Oxford +

LANG: Sp, Rus, Heb, Itl; ⬥ ☾ 🖻 🏥 🏥 💲 Mcr
1 Week *VISA* 💳

Huh, Chung-ho (MD)   Oto
Wyckoff Heights Med Ctr
Kingsbridge Jewish Medical Center;DMR Building 3rd Floor, 585 Schenectady Ave 3353; Brooklyn, NY 11203; (718) 756-9025; **MS:** South Korea 64
Mcr

Lucente, Frank (MD) Oto
Long Island Coll Hosp
University Otolaryngologists, 445 Lenox Rd J; Brooklyn, NY 11203; (718) 780-1498; **BDCERT:** Oto 74; **MS:** Yale U Sch Med 68; **RES:** Oto, Barnes Hosp, St Louis, MO 74; **FAP:** Chrmn Oto SUNY Downstate; **HOSP:** Univ Hosp SUNY Bklyn; *SI: Rhinology*; **HMO:** US Hlthcre Oxford Prucare GHI Empire +

LANG: Sp, Rus, Heb; ⚕ 🔁 🔅 🛏 🅂 Mcr
A Few Days ▨ **VISA** ⬤

Rosenfeld, Richard M (MD) Oto
Long Island Coll Hosp
University Otolaryngologists, 134 Atlantic Ave; Brooklyn, NY 11201; (718) 780-1498; **BDCERT:** Oto 89; **MS:** SUNY Buffalo 84; **RES:** Oto, Mount Sinai Med Ctr, New York, NY 84-89; **FEL:** Ped Oto, Children's Hosp of Pittsburgh, Pittsburgh, PA 89-91; **FAP:** Assoc Prof SUNY Hlth Sci Ctr; **HOSP:** Univ Hosp SUNY Bklyn; *SI: Pediatric Sinusitis; Middle Ear Problems*; **HMO:** Empire United Healthcare CIGNA Oxford Multiplan +

LANG: Sp, Rus; ⚕ 🔁 🛏 🅂 Mcr 2-4 Weeks **VISA** ⬤

Shulman, Abraham (MD) Oto
Brooklyn Hosp Ctr-Downtown
SUNY Tinnintus Research Center, 450 Clarkson Ave Box 1235; Brooklyn, NY 11203; (718) 773-8888; **BDCERT:** Oto 62; **MS:** Switzerland 55; **RES:** Kings County Hosp Ctr, Brooklyn, NY 56-60; **FEL:** Lempert Institute Otology, New York, NY 60; **FAP:** Prof Oto SUNY Hlth Sci Ctr; **HOSP:** Kings County Hosp Ctr; *SI: Hearing Loss; Tinnitus/Vertigo*; **HMO:** Metlife US Hlthcre CIGNA

⚕ 🏥 🔁 🔅 🛏 🅂 Mcr 2-4 Weeks

Sperling, Neil Michael (MD) Oto
Long Island Coll Hosp
University Otolaryngologists, 134 Atlantic Ave; Brooklyn, NY 11201; (718) 780-1498; **BDCERT:** Oto 90; **MS:** NY Med Coll 85; **RES:** S, Beth Israel Med Ctr, New York, NY 85-86; Oto, New York Eye & Ear Infirmary, New York, NY 86-90; **FEL:** Oto, Minnesota Ear Clinic, Minneapolis, MN; **FAP:** Asst Prof SUNY Hlth Sci Ctr; **HOSP:** Univ Hosp SUNY Bklyn; *SI: Hearing Loss; Skull Base Tumors*; **HMO:** Oxford US Hlthcre GHI CIGNA Magnacare +

LANG: Fr, Sp, Rus, Itl; ⚕ 📞 🔁 🔅 🛏 🅂 Mcr NFl
1 Week **VISA** ⬤

Vastola, A Paul (MD) Oto
Maimonides Med Ctr
919 49th St; Brooklyn, NY 11219; (718) 283-6260; **BDCERT:** Med 90; Oto 95; **MS:** Boston U 88; **RES:** Manhattan Eye, Ear & Throat Hosp, New York, NY 90-93; **FEL:** Ped Oto, Texas Children's Hosp, Houston, TX 93-94; **FAP:** Asst Prof of Clin Oto SUNY Hlth Sci Ctr; **HOSP:** St Vincents Hosp & Med Ctr NY

Weiss, Michael H (MD) Oto
Maimonides Med Ctr
919 49th St; Brooklyn, NY 11219; (718) 283-6260; **BDCERT:** Oto 87; **MS:** Albert Einstein Coll Med 82; **RES:** New York University Med Ctr, New York, NY 84-89; **FAP:** Assoc Prof SUNY Downstate; *SI: Head & Neck Surgery*; **HMO:** Oxford CIGNA Magnacare GHI Blue Choice +

LANG: Sp; 📞 🔁 🔅 🛏 🅂 Mcr WC NFl 2-4 Weeks **VISA** ⬤

Guide to symbols and abbreviations can be found on pages 110-113.

527

PAIN MANAGEMENT

Lefkowitz, Matthew (MD)   PM
Long Island Coll Hosp
164 Clinton St; Brooklyn, NY 11201; (718) 625-4244; **BDCERT:** PM 94; Anes 93; **MS:** Belgium 83; **RES:** Mount Sinai Med Ctr, New York, NY 84-86; Lenox Hill Hosp, New York, NY 83-84; **FEL:** Mount Sinai Med Ctr, New York, NY 86-87; **FAP:** Assoc Clin Prof SUNY Downstate; **HOSP:** New York Methodist Hosp; **SI:** *Pain Management; Low Back Pain;* **HMO:** GHI Oxford Prucare Empire

LANG: Itl, Sp, Fr, Rus; 🦽 📷 🎫 $ Mcr Mcd WC NFI

Weissman, Allan Mark (MD) PM
Long Island Coll Hosp
Long Island College Hosp, 350 Henry St; Brooklyn, NY 11201; (718) 780-1663; **BDCERT:** Anes 95; PM 96; **MS:** Albert Einstein Coll Med 90; **RES:** Anes, Montefiore Med Ctr, Bronx, NY 91-94; **FEL:** Pain Management, Univ Hosp SUNY Bklyn, Brooklyn, NY 94-95; **FAP:** Asst Clin Prof SUNY Hlth Sci Ctr; **HOSP:** Univ Hosp SUNY Bklyn; **SI:** *Low Back Pain; Nerve Pain;* **HMO:** GHI Oxford Aetna Hlth Plan US Hlthcre Magnacare +

LANG: Vn, Sp; 🦽 🅲 📷 ♿ 🎫 Mcr Mcd WC NFI
A Few Days

PEDIATRIC CARDIOLOGY

Kaplovitz, Harry (MD)   PCd
Maimonides Med Ctr
Maimonides Med Ctr—Div of Pediatric Cardiology, 4802 10th Ave; Brooklyn, NY 11219; (718) 283-8260; **BDCERT:** Ped 88; PCd 92; **MS:** Albert Einstein Coll Med 81; **RES:** Ped, N Shore Univ Hosp-Manhasset, Manhasset, NY 81-84; **FEL:** PCd, New York University Med Ctr, New York, NY 84-86; **FAP:** Asst Prof SUNY Hlth Sci Ctr; **HOSP:** Lutheran Med Ctr; **SI:** *Heart Murmur; Arrhythmia;* **HMO:** Aetna Hlth Plan Blue Cross & Blue Shield CIGNA GHI Oxford +

LANG: Rus, Yd, Heb, Sp; 🦽 📷 ♿ 🎫 $ Mcr Mcd
1 Week *VISA* 💳

La Corte, Michael (MD)   PCd
Brooklyn Hosp Ctr-Caledonian
121 Dekalb Ave; Brooklyn, NY 11201; (718) 250-6935; **BDCERT:** Ped 75; PCd 77; **MS:** NYU Sch Med 71; **RES:** Bellevue Hosp Ctr, New York, NY 71-73; **FEL:** Children's Hosp, Boston, MA; **HMO:** US Hlthcre Oxford Aetna Hlth Plan Chubb

🦽 📷 🎫 Mcr Mcd   1 Week

Presti, Salvatore (MD)   PCd
Long Island Coll Hosp
Long Island College Hosp, 340 Henry St; Brooklyn, NY 11201; (718) 780-1025; **BDCERT:** Ped 84; PCd 88; **MS:** Italy 78; **RES:** Univ Hosp SUNY Bklyn, Brooklyn, NY 79-80; Lenox Hill Hosp, New York, NY 80-82; **FEL:** Cv, New York University Med Ctr, New York, NY 82-84; **HOSP:** Lenox Hill Hosp; **HMO:** Oxford Metlife Blue Choice CIGNA US Hlthcre +

🦽 📷 🎫 $ Immediately

Schmer, Veronica (MD)   PCd
New York Methodist Hosp
Methodist Hosp, 506 6th St; Brooklyn, NY 11215; (718) 780-5260; **BDCERT:** Ped 89; **MS:** Belgium 82; **RES:** Ped, Bellevue Hospital, New York, NY 81-84; **FEL:** PCd, Bellevue Hospital, New York, NY 84-87

PEDIATRIC ENDOCRINOLOGY

Anhalt, Henry (DO)   PEn
Maimonides Med Ctr
Maimonides Children's Center, 977 48 St; Brooklyn, NY 11219; (718) 283-8143; **BDCERT:** Ped 92; PEn 97; **MS:** NY Coll Osteo Med 88; **RES:** Brookdale Univ Hosp Med Ctr, Brooklyn, NY 88; Ped, Winthrop Univ Hosp, Mineola, NY 89-92; **FEL:** PEn, Stanford Med Ctr, Stanford, CA 92-95; **HOSP:** Lutheran Med Ctr; **SI:** *Diabetes, Thyroid Disorders; Obesity;* **HMO:** Blue Cross & Blue Shield Oxford Aetna-US Healthcare CIGNA Health First +

LANG: Sp, Heb, Rus, Yd, Czc; 🦽 📷 🎫 $ Mcr Mcd   2-4 Weeks *VISA* 💳

Avruskin, Theodore W (MD) PEn
Brookdale Univ Hosp Med Ctr

Brookdale Medical Center, 1 Brookdale Plaza 300;
Brooklyn, NY 11212; (718) 240-5244; **BDCERT:**
Ped 65; EDM 65; **MS:** Canada 60; **RES:** Ped,
Montreal Children's Hosp, Montreal, Canada 60-
63; Ped, Children's Hosp, Boston, MA 63-64; **FEL:**
EDM, Children's Hosp, Boston, MA 64-70; **FAP:**
Prof Ped SUNY Downstate; **SI:** *Growth Disorders;
Diabetes;* **HMO:** HIP Network US Hlthcre Prucare
HealthNet Oxford +

LANG: Fr, Sp, Yd, Rus; ⬡ 🕐 🔒 🏛 💲 Mcr Mcd
A Few Days

Fennoy, Ilene (MD) PEn PCP
Brooklyn Hosp Ctr-Caledonian

Pediatric Faculty Practice, 121 Dekalb Ave;
Brooklyn, NY 11201; (718) 250-8762; **BDCERT:**
Ped 79; PEn 80; **MS:** UC San Francisco 73; **RES:**
Montefiore Med Ctr, Bronx, NY 74-75; **FEL:**
Columbia-Presbyterian Med Ctr, New York, NY 76-
77; Nat Inst Health, Bethesda, MD 78-79; **FAP:**
Assoc Clin Prof Ped NYU Sch Med; **SI:** *Growth;
Diabetes;* **HMO:** Aetna-US Healthcare Blue Cross &
Blue Shield Oxford GHI CIGNA +

LANG: Sp; ⬡ 🔒 🏛 💲 Mcd NFI 4+ Weeks

Lifshitz, Fima (MD) PEn
Maimonides Med Ctr

4802 10th Ave; Brooklyn, NY 11219; (718) 283-
7906; **BDCERT:** Ped 67; PEn 78; **MS:** Mexico 61;
RES: Ped, Children's Mercy Hosp, Kansas City, MO
61-62; Ped, U KS Med Ctr, Kansas City, KS 62-64;
FEL: EDM, Johns Hopkins Hosp, Baltimore, MD;
HMO: US Hlthcre Aetna Hlth Plan GHI Oxford
CIGNA +

🔲 💲 1 Week *AMERICAN* **VISA** 💳

PEDIATRIC GASTROENTEROLOGY

Fisher, Stanley (MD) PGe
Univ Hosp SUNY Bklyn

Pediatrics Box 49, 450 Clarkson Ave; Brooklyn, NY
11203; (718) 270-1625; **BDCERT:** Ped 74; PGe
90; **MS:** Johns Hopkins U 69; **RES:** Children's Hosp
of Pittsburgh, Pittsburgh, PA 70; **FEL:** Ge, U of
Pittsburgh Med Ctr, Pittsburgh, PA 74-77; **FAP:**
Prof Ped NYU Sch Med; **HOSP:** Kings County Hosp
Ctr; **HMO:** Aetna Hlth Plan Blue Cross & Blue Shield
CIGNA

Jelin, Abraham (MD) PGe
Brooklyn Hosp Ctr-Caledonian

121 Dekalb Ave; Brooklyn, NY 11201; (718) 250-
6277; **BDCERT:** Ped 77; PGe 97; **MS:** NYU Sch Med
72; **RES:** Grady Mem Hosp, Atlanta, GA 72-73;
Montefiore Med Ctr, Bronx, NY 73-74; **FEL:** PGe,
Emory U Hosp, Atlanta, GA 75-77; **FAP:** Asst Prof
of Clin Ped NYU Sch Med; **HOSP:** St Vincent's Med
Ctr-Richmond; **SI:** *Nutrition;* **HMO:** Oxford Blue
Choice GHI US Hlthcre CIGNA +

⬡ 🔒 🕎 🏛 💲 Mcd 1 Week

Rabinowitz, Simon (MD) PGe
Staten Island Univ Hosp-North

450 Clarkson Ave; Brooklyn, NY 11203; (718)
270-1647; **BDCERT:** Ped 88; PGe 92; **MS:** U Miami
Sch Med 83; **RES:** Ped, Mount Sinai Med Ctr, New
York, NY 83-85; **FEL:** Ge, Mount Sinai Med Ctr,
New York, NY 85-87; **FAP:** Clin Prof SUNY Hlth Sci
Ctr; **HOSP:** Univ Hosp SUNY Bklyn; **SI:**
Inflammatory Bowel Disease; Hepatitis; **HMO:** Blue
Cross & Blue Shield GHI Aetna Hlth Plan Oxford
CIGNA +

⬡ 🔒 🏛 💲 Mcr Mcd WC NFI 1 Week

Guide to symbols and abbreviations can be found on pages 110-113.

529

Schwarz, Steven M (MD)   PGe
Long Island Coll Hosp
LI Coll Hosp - Chairman, Dept of Pediatrics, 339
Hicks St; Brooklyn, NY 11201; (718) 780-1146;
BDCERT: Ped 79; PGe 97; **MS:** Columbia P&S 74;
RES: Ped, Columbia-Presbyterian Med Ctr, New
York, NY 74-77; **FEL:** PGe, Stanford Med Ctr,
Stanford, CA 77-80; PGe, Columbia-Presbyterian
Med Ctr, New York, NY 78-80; **FAP:** Prof Ped
SUNY Hlth Sci Ctr; *SI: Nutrition-Inflammatory Bowel
Disease; Gastroesophageal Reflux;* **HMO:** Oxford
Aetna-US Healthcare Blue Cross & Blue Shield
Prucare CIGNA +

LANG: Sp; 🔲 🔲 🔲 🔲 🔲 Immediately

PEDIATRIC HEMATOLOGY-ONCOLOGY

Guarini, Ludovico (MD)   PHO
Maimonides Med Ctr
997 48th St; Brooklyn, NY 11219; (718) 283-
8260; **BDCERT:** PHO 92; Ped 84; **MS:** Italy 74;
RES: Ped, Beth Israel Med Ctr, New York, NY 78-
81; **FEL:** PHO, Columbia-Presbyterian Med Ctr,
New York, NY 81-84; **FAP:** Assoc Prof SUNY
Downstate; *SI: Leukemia; Low Platelets;* **HMO:** Aetna
Hlth Plan Blue Choice Blue Cross & Blue Shield

LANG: Itl, Sp, Rus; 🔲 🔲 🔲 🔲 🔲 🔲 🔲

Kulpa, Jolanta (MD)   PHO
Long Island Coll Hosp
Long Island College Hosp, 340 Henry St; Brooklyn,
NY 11201; (718) 780-1025; **BDCERT:** Ped 83;
PHO 84; **MS:** Med Coll PA 72; **RES:** Ped, Lenox Hill
Hosp, New York, NY 72-75; **FEL:** PHO, NY Hosp-
Cornell Med Ctr, New York, NY 78-79; PHO, Mem
Sloan Kettering Cancer Ctr, New York, NY 79-80;
FAP: Asst Clin Prof PHO SUNY Hlth Sci Ctr; *SI:
Anemia/Thalassemia; Sickle Cell Anemia; Hemophilia;*
HMO: Blue Cross & Blue Shield US Hlthcre Oxford
GHI Premier +

LANG: Pol; 🔲 🔲 🔲 🔲 🔲 🔲 🔲 🔲 🔲
Immediately

Sadanandan, Swayam (MD)   PHO
Brooklyn Hosp Ctr-Caledonian
121 Dekalb Ave; Brooklyn, NY 11201; (718) 250-
6074; **BDCERT:** Ped 80; PHO 84; **MS:** India 72;
RES: LTMG Hosp, Bombay, India; St Vincents Hosp
& Med Ctr NY, New York, NY; **FEL:** New York
University Med Ctr, New York, NY; **FAP:** Asst Clin
Prof Ped NYU Sch Med; *SI: Pediatric Cancers;
Pediatric Blood Disorders*

LANG: Hin, Mly, Tam, Crt, Mar; 🔲 🔲 🔲 🔲 🔲 🔲
Immediately

Sundaram, Revathy (MD)   PHO
Long Island Coll Hosp
339 Hicks St; Brooklyn, NY 11201; (718) 780-
1025; **BDCERT:** Ped 80; PHO 84; **MS:** India 73;
RES: Ped, Long Island Coll Hosp, Brooklyn, NY 78;
Ped, Rutgers U Med Ctr, New Brunswick, NJ 77-8;
FEL: PHO, Long Island Coll Hosp, Brooklyn, NY 80;
FAP: Asst Prof Ped SUNY Hlth Sci Ctr; *SI:
Thalassemia; Sickle Cell Anemia;* **HMO:** Aetna-US
Healthcare Oxford GHI Blue Cross & Blue Shield
HIP Network +

LANG: Hin, Tam, Pol, Tel; 🔲 🔲 🔲 🔲 🔲 🔲
Immediately

PEDIATRIC INFECTIOUS DISEASE

Mendez, Hermann (MD)   Ped Inf   PCP
Univ Hosp SUNY Bklyn
450 Clarkson Ave; Brooklyn, NY 11203; (718)
270-3825; **BDCERT:** Ped 85; 94; **MS:** El Salvador
77; **RES:** Children's Med Ctr, Brooklyn, NY 80-83;
FEL: Inf, Univ Hosp SUNY Bklyn, Brooklyn, NY 83-
88; **FAP:** Assoc Prof SUNY Hlth Sci Ctr; **HOSP:**
Kings County Hosp Ctr; *SI: HIV-AIDS Pediatric;
Infections in Children;* **HMO:** Most

LANG: Sp, Fr; 🔲 🔲 🔲 🔲 🔲 Immediately **VISA**
🔲

PEDIATRIC NEPHROLOGY

Schoeneman, Morris J (MD)PNep
Brooklyn Hosp Ctr-Caledonian

121 Dekalb Ave; Brooklyn, NY 11205; (718) 250-6857; **BDCERT:** Ped 74; PNep 74; **MS:** Georgetown U 69; **RES:** U NC Hosp, Chapel Hill, NC 69-70; U MD Hosp, Baltimore, MD 70-72; **FEL:** NP, Albert Einstein Med Ctr, Bronx, NY 72-75; **FAP:** Prof SUNY Hlth Sci Ctr; **HOSP:** St Vincents Hosp & Med Ctr NY

LANG: Fr, Ger, Slv, Heb; ♿ 🅰 🏧 💲 Mcr Mcd NFI
A Few Days

Sen, Dilip (MD)   PNep   PCP
New York Methodist Hosp

6 Sutter Ave; Brooklyn, NY 11212; (718) 756-1355; **BDCERT:** Ped 95; **MS:** India 72; **RES:** PNep, New York Methodist Hosp, Brooklyn, NY 78-81; **FEL:** Ped, Univ Hosp SUNY Bklyn, Brooklyn, NY 81-83; **FAP:** Asst Prof Ped SUNY Downstate; **HMO:** CIGNA GHI Empire Blue Cross & Shield Fidelis CarePlus +

LANG: Bng, Ur, Hin; ♿ 🆂🆄 🅰 🅿 🏧 💲 Mcd
Immediately

PEDIATRIC PULMONOLOGY

Emre, Umit Berk (MD)   PPul
Long Island Coll Hosp

Long Island College Hospital, 340 Henry St; Brooklyn, NY 11201; (718) 780-1025; **BDCERT:** Ped 93; PPul 96; **MS:** Other Foreign Country 84; **RES:** Ped, Univ Hosp SUNY Bklyn, Brooklyn, NY; **FEL:** PPul, Univ Hosp SUNY Bklyn, Brooklyn, NY; **FAP:** Asst Prof Ped SUNY Downstate; **SI:** Asthma; Apnea; **HMO:** Oxford Aetna-US Healthcare PHS HIP Network GHI +

♿ 🅰 🏧 💲 Mcr Mcd NFI Immediately

Giusti, Robert (MD)   PPul
Long Island Coll Hosp

Long Island Coll Hosp, 97 Amity St; Brooklyn, NY 11201; (718) 780-1025; **BDCERT:** Ped 87; PPul 96; **MS:** SUNY Downstate 81; **RES:** Ped, Bellevue Hosp Ctr, New York, NY 81-85; **FAP:** Clin Instr NYU Sch Med; **HOSP:** New York University Med Ctr; **SI:** Cystic Fibrosis; **HMO:** Oxford Blue Cross GHI Aetna Hlth Plan US Hlthcre +

LANG: Itl, Sp; ♿ 🅒 🅰 🅿 🏧 💲 Mcr Mcd WC NFI
1 Week

Rao, Madu (MD)   PPul
Univ Hosp SUNY Bklyn

450 Clarkson Ave; Brooklyn, NY 11203; (718) 270-1524; **BDCERT:** Ped 68; PPul 92; **MS:** India 61; **RES:** Ped, Kings County Hosp Ctr, Brooklyn, NY 65-67; **FEL:** PPul, Kings County Hosp Ctr, Brooklyn, NY 67-69; **FAP:** Prof Ped SUNY Hlth Sci Ctr; **HOSP:** Kings County Hosp Ctr; **SI:** Asthma; **HMO:** Most

LANG: Sp; ♿ 🅒 🅰 🅿 🏧 💲 Mcd WC NFI 1 Week

PEDIATRIC RADIOLOGY

Haller, Jack (MD)   PR
Kings County Hosp Ctr

450 Clarkson Ave; Brooklyn, NY 11203; (718) 270-2670; **BDCERT:** Rad 75; PR 95; **MS:** SUNY Downstate 69; **RES:** PR, Columbia-Presbyterian Med Ctr, New York, NY; **FEL:** PR, Columbia-Presbyterian Med Ctr, New York, NY; **FAP:** Prof SUNY Downstate; **HOSP:** Univ Hosp SUNY Bklyn

LANG: Sp, Heb, Yd; ♿ 🆂🆄 🅰 🅿 🏧 💲 Mcr Mcd
Immediately 🏧 **VISA** 💳 💳

PEDIATRIC RHEUMATOLOGY

Liebling, Anne (MD)   Ped Rhu
Univ Hosp SUNY Bklyn

450 Clarkson Ave Box 42; Brooklyn, NY 11203; (718) 270-1662; **BDCERT:** Ped 90; 94; **MS:** SUNY Downstate 86; **RES:** U, Chicago Hosp, Chicago, IL 87-90

♿ 🅰 🏧 Mcr

PEDIATRIC SURGERY

Cohen, Bertram (MD)   PS
Maimonides Med Ctr

8420 Ridge Blvd; Brooklyn, NY 11209; (718) 748-1313; **BDCERT:** S 57; **MS:** NYU Sch Med 48; **RES:** Maimonides Med Ctr, Bronx, NY 49-50; Montreal Children's Hosp, Montreal, Canada 50-55; **HOSP:** Staten Island Univ Hosp-South

♿ 🆂🅰 🅲 🅶 🅺 🎟 🆂 Mcr WC NFI   Immediately

Gilcrist, Brien (MD)   PS
Univ Hosp SUNY Bklyn

SUNYDiv Ped Surg, 450 Clarkson Ave Box 40; Brooklyn, NY 11203; (718) 270-1386; **BDCERT:** PS 93; **MS:** Tufts U 84; **RES:** S, Oregon Health Sci U Hosp, Portland, OR 86-90; PdS, St Jude Children's Hosp, Memphis, TN 90-92; **FEL:** Transplant S, Harvard Med Sch, Cambridge, MA 92-93; PdS, Rhode Island Hosp, Providence, RI 93-95; **FAP:** Asst Prof SUNY Downstate; *SI: Inflammatory Bowel Disease; Tumors;* **HMO:** Oxford Health First

LANG: Fr, Arm; ♿ 🅲 🅺   Immediately 💳 *VISA* 💳 💳

Klotz, Donald (MD)   PS
Brookdale Univ Hosp Med Ctr

450 Clarkson Ave; Brooklyn, NY 11203; (718) 270-1386; **BDCERT:** Ped 71; **MS:** Ohio State U 60; **RES:** PS, Kings County Hosp Ctr, Brooklyn, NY 62-68; **HOSP:** Long Island Coll Hosp; **HMO:** Aetna Hlth Plan Blue Cross & Blue Shield Blue Choice CIGNA HealthNet +

1 Week

Ramenofsky, Max (MD)   PS
Univ Hosp SUNY Bklyn

Brooklyn Pediatric Surgical, 450 Clarkson Ave Box 40; Brooklyn, NY 11203; (718) 270-1386; **BDCERT:** S 72; PS 75; **MS:** U Tenn Ctr Hlth Sci, Memphis 65; **RES:** John Gaston Hosp, Memphis, TN 65-66; **FEL:** S, Cook Cty Hosp, Chicago, IL 66-71; PdS, Children's Hosp of Pittsburgh, Pittsburgh, PA 72-74; **FAP:** Prof PS SUNY Downstate; **HOSP:** St Vincent's Med Ctr-Richmond; *SI: Surgery of the Newborn; Childhood Injury;* **HMO:** GHI Aetna Hlth Plan US Hlthcre CIGNA HIP Network +

LANG: Sp, Rus, Fr; ♿ 🆂🅰 🅶 🅺 🎟 🆂 Mcr Mcd WC NFI   Immediately

PEDIATRICS

Annavajjhala, Durga (MD)   Ped
Brookdale Univ Hosp Med Ctr

Linden Blvd & Rockaway Pky; Brooklyn, NY 11212; (718) 240-5627; **BDCERT:** Ped 98; NP 91; **MS:** India 81; **RES:** Ped, Harlem Hosp Ctr, New York, NY 84-87; **FEL:** NP, New York University Med Ctr, New York, NY 87-88; NP, Maine Med Ctr, Portland, ME 88-90; **FAP:** Assoc NP

♿ 🆂🅰 🅲 🅺 Mcd

Bromberg, Kenneth (MD)   Ped   🆁🅲🅿
Univ Hosp SUNY Bklyn

450 Clarkson Ave BSB4333; Brooklyn, NY 11203; (718) 245-2957; **BDCERT:** Ped 80; Inf 94; **MS:** SUNY Buffalo 75; **RES:** NY Hosp-Cornell Med Ctr, New York, NY 75-78; **FEL:** Rhode Island Hosp, Providence, RI 78-80; **FAP:** Assoc Clin Prof SUNY Hlth Sci Ctr; *SI: Congenital Infections; Vaccines;* **HMO:** Metlife GHI United Healthcare Oxford

LANG: Fr; ♿ 🅶 🅺 🎟 Mcd   A Few Days

Bulmash, Max (MD)   Ped   `PCP`
New York Methodist Hosp

3904 16th Ave; Brooklyn, NY 11218; (718) 851-8080; **BDCERT:** Ped 87; **MS:** U Md Sch Med 78; **RES:** Sheppard Pratt Hosp, Baltimore, MD 79-80; Maimonides Med Ctr, Brooklyn, NY 80-84; **FAP:** Assoc Clin Instr SUNY Downstate; **HOSP:** Maimonides Med Ctr; **SI:** *Diabetes; Down's Syndrome*; **HMO:** Oxford Empire 1199 GHI Blue Choice +

LANG: Heb, Yd, Rus; ♿ 🏥 🌙 📷 👪 🎫 💲 🩺 🔬 Immediately

Chen, Hua Chin (MD)   Ped
Kingsbrook Jewish Med Ctr

7406 Avenue U; Brooklyn, NY 11234; (718) 763-1636; **BDCERT:** Ped 61; **MS:** Taiwan 54; **RES:** Philadelphia Gen Hosp, Philadelphia, PA 56-58; **FEL:** Pul, Univ Hosp SUNY Bklyn, Brooklyn, NY 58-65; **FAP:** Asst Clin Prof SUNY Downstate; **SI:** *Asthma; Pulmonary Function Testing*; **HMO:** GHI Blue Cross 1199 United Healthcare PHS +

LANG: Chi; ♿ 🌙 📷 👪 🎫 🚾 A Few Days

Comes, Bina (MD)   Ped   `PCP`
Long Island Coll Hosp

6410 Veterans Ave 201; Brooklyn, NY 11234; (718) 531-4600; **BDCERT:** Ped 89; **MS:** Spain 84; **RES:** Long Island Coll Hosp, Brooklyn, NY 84-87; **HMO:** Oxford PHCS Magnacare Blue Choice CIGNA +

LANG: Sp, Itl; ♿ 🏥 🌙 📷 👪 🎫 Immediately

Fernandes, David R (MD)   Ped   `PCP`
Long Island Coll Hosp

126 95th St; Brooklyn, NY 11209; (718) 238-7842; **BDCERT:** Ped 80; **MS:** SUNY Downstate 72; **RES:** Kings County Hosp Ctr, Brooklyn, NY 72-74; N Shore Univ Hosp-Manhasset, Manhasset, NY 75; **FEL:** Bellevue Hosp Ctr, New York, NY 75-77; **HMO:** Oxford PHS Beech Street PHCS

LANG: Prt; 🏥 🌙 📷 🎫 💲 Immediately

Fikrig, Senih (MD)   Ped   `PCP`
Kings County Hosp Ctr

450 Clarkson Ave; Brooklyn, NY 11203; (718) 270-1908; **BDCERT:** Ped 59; A&I 79; **MS:** Turkey 52; **RES:** Bellevue Hosp Ctr, New York, NY 55-56; Bronx Muncipal Hosp Ctr, Bronx, NY 56-58; **FEL:** Kings County Hosp Ctr, Brooklyn, NY 58-59; **HOSP:** Univ Hosp SUNY Bklyn; **HMO:** Blue Cross & Blue Shield CIGNA HealthNet Prucare

♿ 📷 👪 🎫 💲 🩺 🚾 Immediately

Finkelman, Martin (MD)   Ped   `PCP`
Long Island Coll Hosp

46 Livingston St; Brooklyn, NY 11201; (718) 858-4924; **BDCERT:** Ped 73; **MS:** Albert Einstein Coll Med 67; **RES:** Montefiore Med Ctr, Bronx, NY 67-68

♿ 🏥 📷 👪 🎫 💲 A Few Days

Gabriel, Michael (MD)   Ped   `PCP`
New York Methodist Hosp

1 Harbor Ln; Brooklyn, NY 11209; (718) 833-5858; **BDCERT:** Ped 62; **MS:** Greece 54; **RES:** Lincoln Med & Mental Hlth Ctr, Bronx, NY 58-59; Kings County Hosp Ctr, Brooklyn, NY 59-61; **FEL:** Good Samaritan Hosp, Cincinnati, OH; **HOSP:** Lutheran Med Ctr; **HMO:** GHI Sanus CIGNA Oxford Metlife +

♿ 🏥 🌙 📷 👪 🎫 💲 2-4 Weeks

Gately, Adrian (MD)   Ped   `PCP`
New York Methodist Hosp

62 8th Ave; Brooklyn, NY 11217; (718) 622-0469; **BDCERT:** Ped 83; **MS:** Albert Einstein Coll Med 75; **RES:** Jacobi Med Ctr, Bronx, NY 75-78; **HMO:** Oxford

LANG: Sp; ♿ 🏥 📷 👪 🎫 💲 A Few Days

Glaser, Amy (MD)   Ped   `PCP`
Long Island Coll Hosp

44 8th Ave; Brooklyn, NY 11217; (718) 636-0999; **BDCERT:** Ped 85; **MS:** Mt Sinai Sch Med 79; **RES:** Ped, Montefiore Med Ctr, Bronx, NY; **HOSP:** New York University Med Ctr; **SI:** *Adolescent Medicine*; **HMO:** Oxford Aetna Hlth Plan PHS US Hlthcre Blue Choice +

LANG: Sp; 🏥 🌙 📷 👪 🎫 💲 1 Week

Guide to symbols and abbreviations can be found on pages 110-113.

533

Glass, Leonard (MD)   Ped
New York Methodist Hosp
New York Methodist Hosp, 506 6th Ave; Brooklyn, NY 11215; (718) 780-5260; **BDCERT:** Ped 64; **MS:** SUNY Downstate 58; **RES:** Ped, Jewish Hosp Med Ctr, Brooklyn, NY 59-60; NY Hosp-Cornell Med Ctr, New York, NY 60-61; **HMO:** Most

Koenig, Eli (MD)   Ped
Long Island Coll Hosp
340 Henry St; Brooklyn, NY 11201; (718) 780-1025; **BDCERT:** Ped 86; **MS:** Italy 79; **RES:** Bronx Lebanon Hosp Ctr, Bronx, NY 79-80; Beth Israel Med Ctr, New York, NY 80-82; **FEL:** NP, Babies Hosp, New York, NY 82; **FAP:** Asst Prof SUNY Buffalo; **SI:** *Newborn Intensive Care*

LANG: Sp, Itl, Guj, Pol; 🚹 🔊 👥 🛏 Ⓜ
Immediately

Krieger, Ben-Zion (MD)   Ped   PCP
Maimonides Med Ctr
1365 48th St; Brooklyn, NY 11219; (718) 435-6700; **BDCERT:** Ped 86; **MS:** Italy 78; **RES:** Ped, Maimonides Med Ctr, Brooklyn, NY 80-83; **FEL:** A&I, Albert Einstein Med Ctr, Bronx, NY 83-85; **FAP:** Assoc Clin Prof SUNY Hlth Sci Ctr; **HMO:** Blue Choice Oxford Aetna Hlth Plan HealthNet

LANG: Itl, Heb, Yd; 🆘 🅲 🔊 👥 🛏 🅢   Immediately

Lew, Mark (MD)   Ped
New York Methodist Hosp
2704 Glenwood Rd; Brooklyn, NY 11210; (718) 859-6440; **BDCERT:** Ped 83; **MS:** Belgium 76; **RES:** Ped, Brkdle Univ Hosp, Brooklyn, NY 77; Ped, Emory U Sch Med, Atlanta, GA 78-80; **FEL:** Ped, Kingsbrk Jewish Med Ctr, Brooklyn, NY; **HOSP:** Brookdale Univ Hosp Med Ctr

Mogilner, Leonard (MD)   Ped   PCP
Maimonides Med Ctr
Ocean Parkway Pediatric Group, 515 Avenue I; Brooklyn, NY 11230; (718) 377-8800; **BDCERT:** Ped 65; **MS:** Albert Einstein Coll Med 59; **RES:** Ped, Jacobi Med Ctr, Bronx, NY 59-61; **FEL:** Interfaith Med Ctr, Brooklyn, NY 61-62; **FAP:** Asst Clin Prof Ped SUNY Downstate; **HOSP:** Lutheran Med Ctr; **HMO:** Aetna Hlth Plan Oxford Blue Cross & Blue Shield GHI US Hlthcre +

LANG: Heb, Yd, Fr, Itl, Sp; 🆘 🔊 👥 🛏 🅢 Ⓜ
Immediately

Nudel, Dov (MD)   Ped
Univ Hosp SUNY Bklyn
SUNY HSC Hosp—Div of Pediatric Cardiology, 450 Clarkson Ave; Brooklyn, NY 11203; (718) 270-2881; **BDCERT:** Ped 75; PCd 78; **MS:** Israel 69; **RES:** Ped, Hartford Hosp, Hartford, CT 71-73; Ped A&I, Tel Hashomer Hosp, Tel Aviv, Israel 70-71; **FEL:** PCd, Yale-New Haven Hosp, New Haven, CT 73-76; **FAP:** Prof PCd SUNY Hlth Sci Ctr; **HOSP:** Maimonides Med Ctr; **SI:** *Congenital and Acquired; Hear Disease in Pediatrics*

LANG: Heb, Ger; 🚹 🔊 👥 🛏 🅢 Ⓜ Ⓜ Ⓦ Ⓝ
1 Week 💳 **VISA** 💳

Nussbaum, Arnold (MD)   Ped
Maimonides Med Ctr
2462 65th St; Brooklyn, NY 11204; (718) 376-6600; **BDCERT:** Ped 61; **MS:** SUNY Hlth Sci Ctr 54; **RES:** Ped, Jewish Hosp, Brooklyn, NY

Oghia, Hady (MD)   Ped   PCP
St Vincents Hosp & Med Ctr NY
8411 13th Ave; Brooklyn, NY 11228; (718) 331-3166; **MS:** Mexico 79; **RES:** St Vincents Hosp & Med Ctr NY, New York, NY 80-83; **HOSP:** Victory Memorial Hosp; **HMO:** GHI Aetna Hlth Plan Magnacare 1199 PHS +

LANG: Sp, Fr, Ar; 🚹 🆘 🔊 👥 🛏 🅢   Immediately
VISA 💳 💳

Preis, Oded (MD)   Ped   `PCP`
Maimonides Med Ctr

1742 E 13th St; Brooklyn, NY 11229; (718) 339-4919; **BDCERT:** Ped 78; **NP** 78; **MS:** Israel 71; **RES:** Ped, Maimonides Med Ctr, Brooklyn, NY 73-75; **FEL:** NP, Univ Hosp SUNY Bklyn, Brooklyn, NY 75-77; **HOSP:** New York Methodist Hosp; **SI:** *Critical Care Medicine; Prematurity;* **HMO:** Prucare NYLCare GHI CIGNA Oxford +

LANG: Heb, Ger, Fr, Yd; ▨ ◖ ▣ ▨ ▥ ▤ ▨
A Few Days ▨ *VISA* ●

Roth, Olitsa (MD)   Ped
Maimonides Med Ctr

5117 15th Ave; Brooklyn, NY 11219; (718) 851-7444; **BDCERT:** Ped 86; **MS:** Russia 72; **RES:** Maimonides Med Ctr, Brooklyn, NY 79-82

Santilli, Veronica (MD)   Ped   `PCP`
Maimonides Med Ctr

BrookIsland Pediatrics Group, 2462 65th St; Brooklyn, NY 11204; (718) 376-6600; **BDCERT:** Ped 72; **MS:** Med Coll PA 66; **RES:** Ped, Maimonides Medical Center, Brooklyn, NY 66-69; **FAP:** Clin Instr Ped SUNY Hlth Sci Ctr; **HMO:** Blue Choice Blue Cross & Blue Shield CIGNA

Saraiya, Narendra (MD)   Ped   `PCP`
New York Methodist Hosp

1545 Atlantic Ave; Brooklyn, NY 11213; (718) 604-6335; **BDCERT:** Ped 88; **PHO** 94; **MS:** India 71; **RES:** Ped, New York Methodist Hosp, Brooklyn, NY 77-80; **FEL:** PHO, Maimonides Med Ctr, Brooklyn, NY 80-82; **PHO,** Roswell Park Cancer Inst, Buffalo, NY 82-84; **FAP:** Asst Clin Prof Ped SUNY Hlth Sci Ctr; **HOSP:** Maimonides Med Ctr; **SI:** *Sickle Cell Anemia; Cooley's Anemia;* **HMO:** Aetna-US Healthcare Empire Blue Cross Health First Health Plus GHI +

LANG: Hin, Guj; ▨ ▨ ▣ ▨ ▥ ▤ ▨ ▨ ▨ 1 Week

Schaeffer, Henry (MD)   Ped   `PCP`
Maimonides Med Ctr

Maimonides Medical Ctr Dept of Pediatrics, 4802 10th Ave; Brooklyn, NY 11219; (718) 283-8918; **BDCERT:** Ped 69; **MS:** NYU Sch Med 63; **RES:** Bellevue Hosp Ctr, New York, NY 63-64; Bellevue Hosp Ctr, New York, NY 66-68; **FAP:** Clin Prof SUNY Hlth Sci Ctr; **HOSP:** Coney Island Hosp

▣ ▨ ▨ A Few Days

Schulman, Susan (MD)   Ped   `PCP`
Maimonides Med Ctr

901 48th St; Brooklyn, NY 11219; (718) 436-3705; **BDCERT:** Ped 79; **MS:** Geo Wash U Sch Med 71; **RES:** Ped, Maimonides Med Ctr, Bronx, NY 71-76; **FAP:** Assoc Clin Prof Ped SUNY Downstate; **SI:** *Breast Feeding;* **HMO:** Oxford

LANG: Yd, Heb, Rus; ▨ ▣ ▨ ▨ Immediately

Schwimmer, Richard (MD)   Ped
Brookdale Univ Hosp Med Ctr

2635 Nostrand Ave; Brooklyn, NY 11210; (718) 252-3622; **BDCERT:** Ped 76; **MS:** Jefferson Med Coll 71; **RES:** Montefiore Med Ctr, Bronx, NY

Sergiou, Harry (MD)   Ped   `PCP`
Long Island Coll Hosp

554 Henry St; Brooklyn, NY 11231; (718) 625-5591; **BDCERT:** Ped 97; **MS:** Greece 79; **RES:** Long Island Coll Hosp, Brooklyn, NY 80; Ped, Long Island Coll Hosp, Brooklyn, NY; **SI:** *Developmental Pediatrics; Infectious Disease;* **HMO:** GHI Oxford Blue Cross & Blue Shield PHS Magnacare +

LANG: Grk, Sp; ▨ ▨ ◖ ▣ ▨ ▥ ▨ A Few Days

Shelov, Steven (MD)   Ped
Maimonides Med Ctr

Maimonides Med Ctr Dept of Pediatrics, Chairman, 4802 10th Ave; Brooklyn, NY 11219; (718) 283-7502; **BDCERT:** Ped 76; **MS:** Med Coll Wisc 71; **RES:** Ped, Montefiore Med Ctr, Bronx, NY; **FAP:** Prof SUNY Downstate; **HOSP:** Lutheran Med Ctr

Shulman, Susan (MD)   Ped   `PCP`
Maimonides Med Ctr

Schulman Med Assoc, 901 48th St; Brooklyn, NY 11219; (718) 436-3705; **BDCERT:** Ped 79; **MS:** Geo Wash U Sch Med 71; **HMO:** Oxford

[icons] 2-4 Weeks

Strominger, Mitchell (MD)   Ped
Maimonides Med Ctr

921 49th St; Brooklyn, NY 11219; (718) 283-8000; **BDCERT:** Oph 94; **MS:** Washington U, St Louis 86; **RES:** IM, Strong Mem Hosp, Rochester, NY 86-89; Oph, Albert Einstein Med Ctr, Bronx, NY 89-92; **FEL:** N Oph, Bascom Palmer Eye Inst, Miami, FL 92-93; Ped Oph, Manhattan Eye, Ear & Throat Hosp, New York, NY 93-94; **FAP:** Asst Prof SUNY Hlth Sci Ctr; **HOSP:** Univ Hosp SUNY Bklyn; **SI:** *Eye Movement Disorders; Optic Nerve Disorders*; **HMO:** Most

LANG: Sp, Rus; [icons] A Few Days [VISA logos]

Trainin, Eugene (MD)   Ped   `PCP`
New York Methodist Hosp

1909 Quentin Rd; Brooklyn, NY 11229; (718) 627-1999; **BDCERT:** Ped 75; **MS:** SUNY Hlth Sci Ctr 70; **RES:** Kings County Hosp Ctr, Brooklyn, NY 70-73; **FEL:** NP, Albert Einstein Med Ctr, Bronx, NY 75-76; **HOSP:** Maimonides Med Ctr; **SI:** *Asthma*; **HMO:** Oxford CIGNA Sanus US Hlthcre United Healthcare +

[icons] Immediately

Vinas, Sonia (MD)   Ped
Brooklyn Hosp Ctr-Caledonian

121 Dekalb Ave; Brooklyn, NY 11201; (718) 250-8671; **BDCERT:** Ped 91; **MS:** U Puerto Rico 84; **RES:** Bayamon U Hosp, Puerto Rico 84; **FEL:** NP, Bklyn Hosp Ctr, Brooklyn, NY; **SI:** *Premature Infants; Neonatology*; **HMO:** Oxford US Hlthcre Health First Blue Choice Aetna Hlth Plan

Viswanathan, Kusum (MD) Ped
Brookdale Univ Hosp Med Ctr

1 Brookdale Plz; Brooklyn, NY 11212; (718) 240-5904; **BDCERT:** PHO 87; Ped 86; **MS:** India 80; **RES:** Ped, Long Island Coll Hosp, Brooklyn, NY 81-84; **FEL:** PHO, Long Island Coll Hosp, Brooklyn, NY 84-86; **SI:** *Sickle Cell Anemia; Cancer in Children*; **HMO:** Oxford MHS Blue Cross & Blue Shield Empire US Hlthcre +

LANG: Hin, Sp, Fr; [icons] Immediately

Wolk, Joel (MD)   Ped
Brookdale Univ Hosp Med Ctr

1275 Linden Blvd 801; Brooklyn, NY 11212; (718) 240-5904; **BDCERT:** Ped 72; PHO 75; **MS:** SUNY Syracuse 68; **RES:** Children's Hosp of Philadelphia, Philadelphia, PA 69-70; **FEL:** Univ Hosp SUNY Syracuse, Syracuse, NY 73-85; Univ Hosp SUNY Syracuse, Syracuse, NY 72-73; **FAP:** Asst Prof Ped SUNY Downstate

[icons] A Few Days

PHYSICAL MEDICINE & REHABILITATION

Atakent, Pinar (MD)   PMR
Long Island Coll Hosp

Long Island College Hosp, 339 Hicks St; Brooklyn, NY 11201; (718) 780-4685; **BDCERT:** PMR 82; **MS:** Turkey 71; **RES:** Jacobi Med Ctr, Bronx, NY 78-81; **SI:** *Pain Management; Physical Disabilities*; **HMO:** GHI Oxford Aetna Hlth Plan US Hlthcre

LANG: Itl, Rus, Sp, Trk; [icons] Immediately

Bernstein, Lawrence J (MD) PMR
Brookdale Univ Hosp Med Ctr

Brookdale Univ Hosp Med Ctr, 1 Brookdale Plz; Brooklyn, NY 11212; (718) 240-6126; **BDCERT:** PMR 68; IM 65; **MS:** NYU Sch Med 58; **RES:** IM, Bellevue Hosp Ctr, New York, NY 59-61; **FEL:** Rhu, New York University Med Ctr, New York, NY 61-62; **HMO:** Oxford

[icons] [VISA logos]

Gifford, Irina (MD)   PMR
Kingsbrook Jewish Med Ctr

585 Schenectady Ave 333; Brooklyn, NY 11203;
(718) 604-5369; **BDCERT:** PMR 90; **MS:** Romania
60; **RES:** Mount Sinai Med Ctr, New York, NY 86-
89; **FEL:** PMR, Albert Einstein Med Ctr, Bronx, NY
89-90; *SI: Pain Management; Neuro-Muscular Rehab;*
HMO: 1199 Blue Choice Blue Cross & Blue Shield
GHI Oxford +

LANG: Fr, Itl, Ger, Rom; ⬥ 🄲 📷 🄿 🎬 🅂 Mcr WC
NFI A Few Days

Stein, Perry (MD)   PMR
New York Methodist Hosp

383 Ocean Pkwy; Brooklyn, NY 11218; (718)
941-6000; **BDCERT:** PMR 91; **MS:** Mexico 85; **RES:**
Univ Hosp SUNY Bklyn, Brooklyn, NY 87-90;
HMO: Most

Vallarino, Ramon (MD)   PMR
New York Methodist Hosp

119 70th St; Brooklyn, NY 11209; (718) 680-
7229; **BDCERT:** PMR 77; **MS:** Peru 66; **RES:** PMR,
Mt Sinai Hosp, New York, NY 67-68; NYU Med Ctr,
New York, NY 75; **FEL:** Rhu, Mount Sinai Med Ctr,
New York, NY 67-68; **FAP:** Asst Clin Prof SUNY
Hlth Sci Ctr; **HOSP:** Victory Memorial Hosp; **HMO:**
Oxford Prucare NYLCare Blue Choice Magnacare +

Yhu, Hyung Harry (MD)   PMR
New York Methodist Hosp

506 6th St 806; Brooklyn, NY 11215; (718) 622-
8000; **BDCERT:** PMR 78; **MS:** South Korea 65;
RES: Univ Hosp SUNY Bklyn, Brooklyn, NY; **HOSP:**
Kingsbrook Jewish Med Ctr; **HMO:** Oxford

⬥ 📷 🎬 Mcr Mod A Few Days

PLASTIC SURGERY

Feldman, David (MD)   PlS
Maimonides Med Ctr

925 49th St; Brooklyn, NY 11219; (718) 283-
7022; **BDCERT:** S 90; PlS 94; **MS:** Duke U 84; **RES:**
S, St Luke's Roosevelt Hosp Ctr, New York, NY 84-
89; PlS, Duke U Med Ctr, Durham, NC 89-92; **FEL:**
HS, Kleinert Inst, Louisville, KY; **FAP:** Asst Lecturer
S SUNY Hlth Sci Ctr; **HOSP:** Lutheran Med Ctr; *SI:*
Laser Surgery; Cosmetic Surgery; **HMO:** GHI Oxford
Aetna Hlth Plan Blue Choice CIGNA +

⬥ 📷 🎬 🅂 Mcr WC NFI A Few Days 🔲 **VISA** 💳
💳

Fleischer, Arie (MD)   PlS
Maimonides Med Ctr

112 Prospect Park West; Brooklyn, NY 11215;
(718) 369-3000; **BDCERT:** PlS 85; **MS:** Romania
69; **RES:** PlS, Manhattan Eye, Ear & Throat Hosp,
New York, NY; PlS, Columbia-Presbyterian Med
Ctr, New York, NY; **HOSP:** New York Methodist
Hosp; *SI: Facial Cosmetic Surgery; Breast Surgery;*
HMO: Oxford HIP Network Blue Cross & Blue Shield

LANG: Ger, Fr, Yd; 🄿 🎬 🅂 Mcr WC NFI 2-4 Weeks
VISA 💳

Roth, Malcolm (MD)   PlS
Brookdale Univ Hosp Med Ctr

580 Rockaway Pkwy 145; Brooklyn, NY 11212;
(718) 240-5799; **BDCERT:** PlS 91; **MS:** NY Med
Coll 82; **RES:** S, Beth Israel Med Ctr, New York, NY
82-85; PlS, NY Hosp-Cornell Med Ctr, New York,
NY 85-87; **FEL:** HS, Hosp For Special Surgery, New
York, NY 87-88; **FAP:** Asst Clin Prof SUNY Hlth Sci
Ctr; **HOSP:** Beth Israel Med Ctr; *SI: Cosmetic Surgery;*
Hand Surgery; **HMO:** GHI

⬥ 📷 🄿 🎬 🅂 Mcr WC NFI **VISA** 💳

Schiller, Carl (MD)   **PlS**
Maimonides Med Ctr

9920 4th Ave 313; Brooklyn, NY 11209; (718) 287-3900; **BDCERT:** PlS 77; **MS:** NYU Sch Med 36; **RES:** S, Coney Island Hosp, Brooklyn, NY 39-42; SM, Coney Island Hosp, Brooklyn, NY 36-37; **FEL:** PlS, McGill Teaching Hosp, Montreal, Canada 49-50; PlS, Royal Victoria Hosp, Montreal, Canada 49-52; **HOSP:** Lutheran Med Ctr; **SI:** *Breast Augmentation and Reduction; Cosmetic Surgery;* **HMO:** Blue Shield HIP Network GHI Oxford Prucare +

♿ ⌂ ⏰ $ Mcr WC NFI   A Few Days

PSYCHIATRY

Berkowitz, Howard (MD)   **Psyc**
Maimonides Med Ctr

4715 Fort Hamilton Pkwy; Brooklyn, NY 11219; (718) 633-2025; **BDCERT:** Psyc 77; GerPsy 94; **MS:** Albert Einstein Coll Med 72; **RES:** Beth Israel Med Ctr, New York, NY 72-73; Psyc, Kings County Hosp Ctr, Brooklyn, NY 73-76; **FEL:** Psyc, Kings County Hosp Ctr, Brooklyn, NY 76-77; **FAP:** Assoc Clin Prof SUNY Downstate; **SI:** *Geriatric Psychiatry, Anxiety; Consultation-Depression;* **HMO:** Empire Beech Street First Health Preferred Hlth

♿ ⌂ ♿ ⏰ $ 1 Week

Berman, Sheldon (MD)   **Psyc**
Brookdale Univ Hosp Med Ctr

Brookdale HospChrm Dept Psych, 1 Brookdale Plaza; Brooklyn, NY 11212; (718) 240-5644; **BDCERT:** Psyc 79; **MS:** U Hlth Sci/Chicago Med Sch 69; **RES:** Psyc, Brookdale Univ Hosp Med Ctr, Brooklyn, NY 70-73; **FAP:** Asst Clin Prof Psyc SUNY Downstate; **SI:** *Psychotherapy for Cancer Patients and Families;* **HMO:** None

♿ ⌂ ⏰ $ Mcr   A Few Days

Breen, Charles (MD)   **Psyc**
New York Methodist Hosp

808 Carroll St Grnd Flr.; Brooklyn, NY 11215; (718) 622-4024; **BDCERT:** Psyc 82; **MS:** Albert Einstein Coll Med 66; **RES:** Psyc, CT Mental Health Ctr, New Haven, CT 67-69; VA Ct Healthcare Sys-West Haven, West Haven, CT 69-70; **SI:** *College Student Health;* **HMO:** Empire Blue Cross & Shield

SA/SD ℂ ⌂ ⏰ $ Mcr WC NFI

Feigelson, Eugene (MD)   **Psyc**
Univ Hosp SUNY Bklyn

450 Clarkson Ave; Brooklyn, NY 11203; (718) 270-2022; **BDCERT:** Psyc 74; **MS:** Washington U, St Louis 56; **RES:** Columbia-Presbyterian Med Ctr, New York, NY; NYS Psychiatric Institute, New York, NY; **HOSP:** VA Med Ctr-Brooklyn

♿ ⌂ ⏰ Mcr   Immediately

Fine, James (MD)   **Psyc**
Kings County Hosp Ctr

Kings County Addict Dis Hosp-Bldg K, 600 Albany Ave; Brooklyn, NY 11203; (212) 627-2650; **BDCERT:** Psyc 84; AdP 93; **MS:** UMDNJ-NJ Med Sch, Newark 78; **RES:** Psyc, St Vincents Hosp & Med Ctr NY, New York, NY 79-82; **FAP:** Assoc Clin Prof SUNY Hlth Sci Ctr; **HMO:** Blue Cross & Blue Shield

Gannon, Fredric (MD)   **Psyc**
St Vincents Hosp & Med Ctr NY

142 Joralemon St 10F; Brooklyn, NY 11201; (718) 858-3200; **BDCERT:** Psyc 67; **MS:** Georgetown U 60; **RES:** St Vincents Hosp & Med Ctr NY, New York, NY 61-64; **HOSP:** Long Island Coll Hosp; **HMO:** Blue Choice Empire

♿ ⌂ ♿ ⏰ $ WC NFI   1 Week

Goldberg, Jeffrey (DO)   **Psyc**
Maimonides Med Ctr

5025 Fort Hamilton Pkwy; Brooklyn, NY 11219; (718) 633-8183; **BDCERT:** Psyc 86; GerPsy 96; **MS:** NY Coll Osteo Med 81; **RES:** Maimonides Med Ctr, Brooklyn, NY 82-85; **FAP:** Asst Prof SUNY Downstate; **SI:** *Geriatric Psychiatry; Anxiety Disorders*

ℂ ⌂ ⏰ $ 2-4 Weeks

Idupuganti, Sudharam (MD)Psyc
Maimonides Med Ctr
448 74th St; Brooklyn, NY 11209; (718) 921-
1001; **BDCERT:** Psyc 81; **MS:** India 74; **RES:** India
76; Maimonides Med Ctr, Brooklyn, NY 76-79;
FAP: Asst Prof SUNY Downstate; **HOSP:** Victory
Memorial Hosp; *SI: Psychotherapy;*
Psychopharmacology; **HMO:** Aetna Hlth Plan
▨ ◖ ▣ ▨ ▥ ▤

Licht, Arnold (MD)   Psyc
Long Island Coll Hosp
339 Hicks St; Brooklyn, NY 11201; (718) 935-
0986; **BDCERT:** Psyc 75; GerPsy 92; **MS:** SUNY
Hlth Sci Ctr 69; **RES:** Psyc, Albert Einstein Med Ctr,
Bronx, NY 70-73; *SI: Geriatric Psychiatry; Mood*
Disorders; **HMO:** Oxford Prudential US Hlthcre
Aetna Hlth Plan Empire Blue Cross & Shield +
LANG: Rus, Sp, Hin; ▨ ◖ ▨ ▥ ▤ ▥ ▥ ▥ ▥
A Few Days

Lipkowitz, Marvin (MD)   Psyc
Maimonides Med Ctr
920 48th St; Brooklyn, NY 11219; (718) 283-
8163; **BDCERT:** Psyc 63; **MS:** Temple U 56; **RES:**
Kings County Hosp Ctr, Brooklyn, NY 56-57; Psyc,
Kings County Hosp Ctr, Brooklyn, NY 57-60; *SI:*
Depression; Geriatric Problems; **HMO:** None
LANG: Yd; ▨ ◖ ▣ ▤   2-4 Weeks

Nayak, Devdutt (MD)   Psyc
New York Methodist Hosp
506 6th St; Brooklyn, NY 11215; (718) 780-3771;
BDCERT: Psyc 77; **MS:** India 69; **RES:** Psyc, Long
Island Jewish Med Ctr, New Hyde Park, NY 72-76;
HMO: GHI Oxford Empire Blue Choice PHS

Nieporent, Hans (MD)   Psyc
Maimonides Med Ctr
2623 E 16th St; Brooklyn, NY 11235; (718) 934-
2424; **BDCERT:** Psyc 64; **MS:** Switzerland 56; **RES:**
Brooklyn State Hosp, Brooklyn, NY 57-62; *SI:*
Psychopharmacology; Forensic (Legal)Psychiatry;
HMO: GHI
▨ ◖ ▣ ▨ ▥ ▤ ▥   A Few Days

Rosen, Evelyn (MD)   Psyc
New York Methodist Hosp
New York Methodist Hospital, 460 6th St;
Brooklyn, NY 11215; (212) 813-9410; **BDCERT:**
GerPsy 94; Psyc 92; **MS:** Mexico 86; **RES:** Univ
Hosp SUNY Bklyn, Brooklyn, NY 87-91; **FEL:** Univ
Hosp SUNY Bklyn, Brooklyn, NY 91-92; **FAP:** Asst
Clin Prof SUNY Hlth Sci Ctr; **HOSP:** Univ Hosp
SUNY Bklyn; *SI: Depression; Geriatrics*
◖ ▤ ▥

Sultan, Joseph (MD)   Psyc
Maimonides Med Ctr
913 49th St; Brooklyn, NY 11219; (718) 851-
1144; **BDCERT:** Psyc 77; **MS:** Albert Einstein Coll
Med 68; **RES:** Psyc, Montefiore Med Ctr, Bronx, NY
71-72; Psyc, Bronx Psych Ctr, Bronx, NY 72-74;
HMO: Blue Cross & Blue Shield HealthNet
◖ ▣ ▤   1 Week

Viswanathan, Ramasmy (MD)Psyc
Univ Hosp SUNY Bklyn
450 Clarkson Ave # 127; Brooklyn, NY 11203;
(718) 270-2352; **BDCERT:** Psyc 78; IM 89; **MS:**
India 72; **RES:** IM, Qns Hosp Ctr, Jamaica, NY 73-
74; Kings Cty Hosp, Brooklyn, NY 74-77; **FEL:**
Kings Cty Hosp, Brooklyn, NY; **FAP:** Assoc Prof
SUNY Hlth Sci Ctr; **HOSP:** Kings County Hosp Ctr;
SI: Depression; Anxiety; **HMO:** VBH Oxford
▨ ▨ ◖ ▣ ▨ ▥   1 Week

PULMONARY DISEASE

Bergman, Michael I (MD)   Pul
Long Island Coll Hosp
339 Hicks St; Brooklyn, NY 11201; (718) 780-
1416; **BDCERT:** IM 81; Pul 84; **MS:** Albert Einstein
Coll Med 78; **RES:** IM, Brookdale Univ Hosp Med
Ctr, Brooklyn, NY 78-81; **FEL:** Pul, Mount Sinai
Med Ctr, New York, NY 82-84; **FAP:** Asst Prof
SUNY Hlth Sci Ctr; *SI: Asthma; Chronic Lung Disease;*
HMO: Oxford Prucare GHI NYLCare +
▨ ▣ ▨ ▥ ▤ ▥ ▥ ▥   2-4 Weeks

Bernstein, Chaim (MD)   Pul
Beth Israel Med Ctr-Kings Hwy

Kings Pulmonary Associates, 3131 Kings Hwy
D10; Brooklyn, NY 11234; (718) 252-3590;
BDCERT: IM 77; Pul 82; **MS:** NYU Sch Med 74;
RES: Brookdale Univ Hosp Med Ctr, Brooklyn, NY
75-77; **FEL:** Pul, New York University Med Ctr,
New York, NY 77-79; **FAP:** Asst Clin Prof SUNY
Hlth Sci Ctr; *SI: Asthma; Pneumonia;* **HMO:** Oxford
Magnacare Choicecare CIGNA US Hlthcre +

LANG: Yd, Rus; 🔵 🔘 📷 🎫 💲 Mcr A Few Days
VISA 💳

Bernstein, Martin (MD)   Pul
Maimonides Med Ctr

2107 Avenue N; Brooklyn, NY 11210; (718) 434-
3320; **BDCERT:** IM 63; Pul 74; **MS:** SUNY Hlth Sci
Ctr 56; **RES:** Med, Maimonides Med Ctr, Brooklyn,
NY 57-58; Med, Maimonides Med Ctr, Brooklyn,
NY 58-59; **FEL:** Pul, Kings County Hosp Ctr,
Brooklyn, NY 60; Pul, Columbia-Presbyterian Med
Ctr, New York, NY 61; **FAP:** Asst Clin Prof Med
SUNY Downstate; **HOSP:** Beth Israel Med Ctr-Kings
Hwy; *SI: Bronchial Asthma; Lung Cancer;* **HMO:**
Magnacare Oxford Multiplan PHCS PHS +

LANG: Sp, Yd, Fr; 🔵 🔘 📷 🎫 💲 Mcr A Few Days
VISA 💳 💰

Bondi, Elliott (MD)   Pul
Brookdale Univ Hosp Med Ctr

2460 Flatbush Ave; Brooklyn, NY 11234; (718)
240-5236; **BDCERT:** IM 74; Pul 82; **MS:** U Md Sch
Med 71; **RES:** Med, Maimonides Med Ctr, Brooklyn,
NY 71-73; Med, Bronx Muncipal Hosp Ctr, Bronx,
NY 73-74; **FEL:** Pul, Bronx Muncipal Hosp Ctr,
Bronx, NY 74-76; **FAP:** Assoc Prof SUNY
Downstate; *SI: Chronic Obstructive Lung Disease;
Asthma Tuberculosis;* **HMO:** Oxford Blue Cross
Aetna-US Healthcare Prucare CIGNA +

LANG: Yd, Hun; 🔵 🔘 📷 🎫 💲 Mcr NFI A Few Days

Dhar, Santi (MD)   Pul
Coney Island Hosp

2601 Ocean Pkwy; Brooklyn, NY 11235; (718)
616-3171; **BDCERT:** IM 72; Pul 74; **MS:** India 58;
RES: IM, French Hosp, New York, NY 68-69; IM,
NY Med Coll, New York, NY 70-71; **FEL:** Chest Med,
Coney Island Hosp, Brooklyn, NY 72-73; Chest
Med, Albert Einstein Med Ctr, Bronx, NY 72; **FAP:**
Assoc Clin Prof SUNY Downstate; **HOSP:** Beth
Israel Med Ctr-Kings Hwy; *SI: Asthma; Lung Cancer;*
HMO: Oxford Empire Blue Cross & Shield CIGNA

LANG: Hun; 🔵 🔘 📷 🎫 💲 Mcr WC A Few Days

Efferen, Linda S (MD)   Pul
Kings County Hosp Ctr

451 Clarkson Ave; Brooklyn, NY 11203; (718)
270-1770; **BDCERT:** Pul 90; CCM 91; **MS:** Israel
83; **RES:** Kings County Hosp Ctr, Brooklyn, NY 83-
87; **FEL:** Albert Einstein Med Ctr, Bronx, NY 87-89;
CCM, Albert Einstein Med Ctr, Bronx, NY 89-90;
HOSP: Univ Hosp SUNY Bklyn; *SI: Sarcoidosis*
🔵 📷 🎫 Mcr Mcd WC 1 Week

Groopman, Jacob (MD)   Pul
Maimonides Med Ctr

953 49th St; Brooklyn, NY 11219; (718) 283-
8380; **BDCERT:** IM 79; Pul 80; **MS:** SUNY Hlth Sci
Ctr 74; **RES:** IM, Maimonides Med Ctr, Brooklyn,
NY 74-78; **FEL:** Pul, New York University Med Ctr,
New York, NY 78-80; *SI: Asthma; Emphysema;*
HMO: Multiplan Oxford Blue Cross US Hlthcre
🔵 🔘 🎫 💲 Mcr Immediately

Gulrajani, Ramesh (MD)   Pul   PCP
Brooklyn Hosp Ctr-Caledonian

121 Dekalb Ave 7F; Brooklyn, NY 11201; (718)
250-6950; **BDCERT:** IM 79; Pul 84; **MS:** India 74;
RES: Cumberland Med Ctr, Brooklyn, NY 76-79;
FEL: Pul, Cumberland Med Ctr, Brooklyn, NY 79-
81; **FAP:** Asst Prof of Clin Med NYU Sch Med; *SI:
Asthma; Sarcoidosis;* **HMO:** Aetna-US Healthcare
GHI United Healthcare Oxford

LANG: Sp, Rus, Hin; 🔵 🔘 📷 🎫 💲 Mcr Mcd 2-
4 Weeks

Kamholz, Stephan (MD)   Pul
Univ Hosp SUNY Bklyn

SUNY Health Sci Ctr, 450 Clarkson Ave; Brooklyn, NY 11203; (718) 270-2030; **BDCERT:** IM 75; CCM 87; **MS:** NY Med Coll 72; **RES:** IM, Montefiore Med Ctr, Bronx, NY 72-75; **FEL:** Pul, Montefiore Med Ctr, Bronx, NY 75-77; **FAP:** Chrmn Med SUNY Hlth Sci Ctr; **HOSP:** Kings County Hosp Ctr; **SI:** *Tuberculosis; Lung Transplant Evaluation*

LANG: Fr; 🔲 🔲 🔲 🔲   1 Week

Lombardo, Gerard (MD)   Pul
New York Methodist Hosp

7702 4th Ave; Brooklyn, NY 11220; (718) 745-1156; **BDCERT:** IM 84; Pul 86; **MS:** Grenada 81; **RES:** IM, New York Methodist Hosp, Brooklyn, NY 81-82; IM, New York Methodist Hosp, Brooklyn, NY 82-84; **FEL:** Pul, New York Methodist Hosp, Brooklyn, NY 84-86; **SI:** *Lung Diseases; Sleep Disorders;* **HMO:** Blue Cross PPO Aetna Hlth Plan NYLCare US Hlthcre

LANG: Sp; 🔲 🔲 🔲 🔲 🔲 🔲   Immediately

Miarrostami, M Rameen (MD)Pul   **PCP**
New York Methodist Hosp

The Chest Medical Group of Brooklyn, PC, 7501 16th Ave; Brooklyn, NY 11214; (718) 234-3333; **MS:** Dominican Republic 85; **FEL:** Pul, Long Island Coll Hosp, Brooklyn, NY; **FAP:** Clin Prof Cornell U; **HOSP:** Victory Memorial Hosp; **SI:** *Asthma; Emphysema;* **HMO:** Oxford Empire Blue Cross & Shield CIGNA Elderplan

LANG: Frs, Itl, Sp; 🔲 🔲 🔲 🔲 🔲   2-4 Weeks

Saleh, Anthony (MD)   Pul
New York Methodist Hosp

7510 4th Ave; Brooklyn, NY 11209; (718) 745-1156; **BDCERT:** Pul 90; IM 88; **MS:** West Indies 85; **RES:** New York Methodist Hosp, Brooklyn, NY 85-88; **FEL:** Pul, New York Methodist Hosp, Brooklyn, NY 88-90; **SI:** *Asthma;* **HMO:** Blue Cross & Blue Shield Blue Choice PHS 32BJ NYLCare +

LANG: Sp; 🔲 🔲 🔲 🔲 🔲   A Few Days

Schwartz, Marlene (MD)   Pul
Brooklyn Hosp Ctr-Downtown

The Brooklyn Hospital Center, 121 DeKalb Ave; Brooklyn, NY 11201; (718) 250-6100; **BDCERT:** IM 91; Pul 94; **MS:** SUNY Downstate 88; **RES:** IM, Brookdale Univ Hosp Med Ctr, Brooklyn, NY 89-91; **FEL:** PCCM, Long Island Jewish Med Ctr, New Hyde Park, NY 91; **FAP:** Dir CCM; **SI:** *Critical Care Medicine; Sleep Problems*

🔲 🔲 🔲 🔲 🔲 🔲   Immediately

Smith, Peter (MD)   Pul
Long Island Coll Hosp

339 Hicks St; Brooklyn, NY 11201; (718) 780-2905; **BDCERT:** IM 73; Pul 74; **MS:** Columbia P&S 64; **RES:** Jacobi Med Ctr, Bronx, NY 70-71; SUNY Health Science Ctr-Bklyn, Brooklyn, NY 71-72; **FEL:** Pul, Univ Hosp SUNY Bklyn, Brooklyn, NY 72-74; **FAP:** Assoc Prof Med SUNY Hlth Sci Ctr; **SI:** *Asthma; Emphysema;* **HMO:** Aetna Hlth Plan Blue Choice GHI

LANG: Sp; 🔲 🔲 🔲 🔲 🔲 🔲   1 Week

RADIATION ONCOLOGY

Huh, Sun (MD)   RadRO
Brooklyn Hosp Ctr-Downtown

Brooklyn Hospital Center-Downtown, 121 Dekalb Ave; Brooklyn, NY 11201; (718) 250-8248; **BDCERT:** Rad 74; **MS:** South Korea 64; **RES:** RadRO, Mem Sloan Kettering Cancer Ctr, New York, NY 71-74; S, Jamaica Med Ctr, Jamaica, NY 70-71; **FEL:** RadRO, Mem Sloan Kettering Cancer Ctr, New York, NY 74-75; **FAP:** Asst Prof Rad Mt Sinai Sch Med; **HOSP:** Kingsbrook Jewish Med Ctr; **SI:** *Prostate Cancer;* **HMO:** HIP Network Oxford GHI Blue Cross & Blue Shield Aetna-US Healthcare +

LANG: Kor, Ger, Chi, Sp, Rus; 🔲 🔲 🔲 🔲 🔲 🔲 🔲   Immediately 🔲 *VISA* 🔲 🔲

Rafia, Sameer (MD)　　RadRO
New York Methodist Hosp
506 6th St; Brooklyn, NY 11215; (718) 780-3677;
BDCERT: RadRO 76; MS: England 63; RES: Royal
Cancer Hosp, London, England 63; Cairo Univ
Hosp, Cairo, Egypt; FEL: Royal Marsden Hosp, 64;
FAP: Clin Prof Cornell U; HOSP: Maimonides Med
Ctr; HMO: Oxford Aetna-US Healthcare GHI CIGNA
NYLCare +

LANG: Sp, Ar, Rus, Hin; 🚹 🔟 🅿 🏧 Mcr Mcd
A Few Days 💳 **VISA**

Rafla, Sameer Demetrious (MD)RadRO
New York Methodist Hosp
NY Methodist Hosp, 506 6th St; Brooklyn, NY
11215; (718) 780-3677; BDCERT: Rad 76; MS:
Egypt 54; RES: Rad, Cairo U Hosp, Egypt 54-56;
RadRO, Royal Marsden Hosp, London, England 61-
65; FEL: RadRO, Royal Marsden Hosp, London,
England 65-67; FAP: Clin Prof RadRO SUNY
Downstate; HOSP: Wyckoff Heights Med Ctr

Rotman, Marvin (MD)　　RadRO
Univ Hosp SUNY Bklyn
Brooklyn Radiation PC: Metropolitan Radiation PC,
Box 1211; Brooklyn, NY 11203; (718) 270-2181;
BDCERT: Rad 66; MS: Jefferson Med Coll 58; RES:
IM, Albert Einstein Med Ctr, Philadelphia, PA 59-
60; RadRO, Montefiore Med Ctr, Bronx, NY 62-65;
FAP: Chrmn SUNY Downstate; HOSP: Long Island
Coll Hosp; SI: GYN Oncology-Cervix; Prostate-
Bladder-Uterus; HMO: US Hlthcre Empire HIP
Network Magnacare Oxford +

LANG: Rus, Yd, Sp, Itl; 🚹 🔟 🅿 🏧 Mcr Mcd WC
Immediately 💳 **VISA** 💳

RADIOLOGY

Aziz, Hassan (MD)　　Rad
Long Island Coll Hosp
SUNY Downstate Med Ctr, 450 Clarkson St Box
1211; Brooklyn, NY 11201; (718) 270-2181;
BDCERT: Rad 78; MS: Pakistan 62; RES: RadRO,
England, UK; FAP: Clin Prof SUNY Downstate;
HOSP: Univ Hosp SUNY Bklyn; HMO: Oxford
CIGNA HIP Network

LANG: Itl, Sp, Rus, Hin, Yd; 🚹 🔟 🏧 Mcr Mcd

Becker, Joshua (MD)　　Rad
Univ Hosp SUNY Bklyn
450 Clarkson Ave; Brooklyn, NY 11203; (718)
270-1603; BDCERT: Rad 61; MS: Temple U 57;
RES: Temple U Hosp, Philadelphia, PA 58-61;
HOSP: Kings County Hosp Ctr

🚹 🔟 🏧 Mcr Mcd WC NFI　A Few Days **VISA**

Bryk, David (MD)　　Rad
Maimonides Med Ctr
Maimonides Radiology Associates PC, 4802 10th
Ave; Brooklyn, NY 11219; (718) 283-7115;
BDCERT: Rad 59; MS: SUNY Downstate 53; RES:
Rad, Mount Sinai Med Ctr, New York, NY 54-55;
Rad, Mount Sinai Med Ctr, New York, NY 57-59;
FAP: Prof Rad SUNY Downstate; SI: Intestinal
Obstruction; Swallowing Problems; HMO: Oxford
Elderplan GHI Health One Empire +

🚹 🔟 🏧 💲 Mcr Mcd WC NFI　A Few Days **VISA** 💳

Garner, Steven (MD)　　Rad
Catholic Med Ctr Bklyn & Qns
Catholic Medical Center of Radiology Department,
187 Marlborough Rd; Brooklyn, NY 11226; (718)
558-7248; BDCERT: DR 84; EM 87; MS: U
Chicago-Pritzker Sch Med 76; RES: Rad, Mount
Sinai Med Ctr, New York, NY 80-83; FAP: Clin Instr
Albert Einstein Coll Med; HOSP: St Joseph's Hosp-
Queens; SI: Mammography Breast Biopsy; Non-
Invasive Vascular Lap

LANG: Sp, Kor, Rus, Yd, Cre; 🚹 🔟 🅲 🔟 🏧 🏧 Mcr
Mcd WC NFI 💳 **VISA** 💳

Kassner, E George (MD) Rad
Univ Hosp SUNY Bklyn
4802 10th Ave; Brooklyn, NY 11219; (718) 283-7478; **BDCERT:** Rad 68; **MS:** U Wisc Med Sch 60; **RES:** Rad, Columbia-Presbyterian Med Ctr, New York, NY 64-67; **FAP:** Prof of Clin Rad SUNY Downstate; *SI: Pediatric Radiology*; **HMO:** Oxford GHI Prudential US Hlthcre CIGNA +

⟨symbols⟩ *VISA* ⟨symbols⟩

Ramanathan, Kumudha (MD)Rad
New York Comm Hosp of Bklyn
Professional Radiology Svcs PC & RLP Imaging PC, 142 Joralemon St 5C; Brooklyn, NY 11201; (718) 624-2222; **BDCERT:** Rad 82; **MS:** India 76; **RES:** S, Mount Sinai Med Ctr, New York, NY 78-79; Rad, Long Island Coll Hosp, Brooklyn, NY 79-82; *SI: Mammography; Ultrasounds*; **HMO:** Oxford Prucare GHI NYLCare US Hlthcre +

LANG: Sp, Ger, Itl, Can; ⟨symbols⟩ Immediately *VISA* ⟨symbols⟩

Rosenthal, David (MD) Rad
Beth Israel Med Ctr-Kings Hwy
Highway Imaging Associate, 3131 Kings Hwy A3; Brooklyn, NY 11234; (718) 338-6868; **BDCERT:** NuM 87; **MS:** Mt Sinai Sch Med 81; **RES:** DR, St Vincents Hosp & Med Ctr NY, New York, NY 82-85; NuM, St Vincents Hosp & Med Ctr NY, New York, NY 85-87; **HMO:** Oxford NYLCare United Healthcare GHI Magnacare +

LANG: Rus, Sp, Itl; ⟨symbols⟩ 1 Week

Yaghoobian, Jahangui (MD) Rad
Victory Memorial Hosp
699 92nd St; Brooklyn, NY 11228; (718) 567-1245; **BDCERT:** Rad 74; **MS:** Iran 66; **RES:** Long Island Coll Hosp, Brooklyn, NY 68-69; **HMO:** Most

LANG: Rus, Itl; ⟨symbols⟩ Immediately

Youssef, Ezzat (MD) Rad
New York Methodist Hosp
Radiation Dept, 506 6th St; Brooklyn, NY 11215; (718) 780-3677; **BDCERT:** Rad 75; **MS:** Egypt 60; **RES:** RadRO, Albert Einstein Med Ctr, Bronx, NY 72; **FAP:** Asst Clin Prof Cornell U; *SI: Head & Neck Malignancy; Gastrointestinal Malignancy*; **HMO:** GHI Oxford US Hlthcre Aetna Hlth Plan Blue Choice +

LANG: Fr, Sp, Rus, Ar, Itl; ⟨symbols⟩ Immediately

REPRODUCTIVE ENDOCRINOLOGY

Bray, Mary (MD) RE
Long Island Coll Hosp
Fertility & Hormone Ctr, 161 Atlantic Ave 202; Brooklyn, NY 11201; (718) 237-2727; **BDCERT:** ObG 89; RE 91; **MS:** SUNY Downstate 81; **RES:** Univ Hosp SUNY Bklyn, Brooklyn, NY 81-85; **FEL:** Univ Hosp SUNY Bklyn, Brooklyn, NY 85-87; *SI: Infertility; Painful Periods*; **HMO:** PHCS Aetna Hlth Plan GHI Beech Street

LANG: Sp; ⟨symbols⟩ A Few Days *VISA* ⟨symbols⟩

Grazi, Richard (MD) RE
Maimonides Med Ctr
1355 84th St; Brooklyn, NY 11228; (718) 283-6565; **BDCERT:** ObG 88; RE 89; **MS:** SUNY Buffalo 81; **RES:** New York University Med Ctr, New York, NY 81-85; **FEL:** RE, New York University Med Ctr, New York, NY 85-87; **HOSP:** St Vincent's Med Ctr-Richmond; **HMO:** Aetna Hlth Plan CIGNA Oxford US Hlthcre Metlife +

⟨symbols⟩ 2-4 Weeks *VISA* ⟨symbols⟩

Guide to symbols and abbreviations can be found on pages 110-113.

543

Lobell, Susan M (MD) RE
Maimonides Med Ctr
Brooklyn IVF, 1355 84th St; Brooklyn, NY 11228;
(718) 283-8600; **BDCERT:** RE 94; ObG 92; **MS:**
Harvard Med Sch 85; **RES:** ObG, Brigham &
Women's Hosp, Boston, MA 85-89; **FEL:** RE,
Brigham & Women's Hosp, Boston, MA 89-91;
FAP: Asst Prof SUNY Downstate; **HOSP:** St
Vincent's Med Ctr-Richmond; **SI:** *In Vitro
Fertilization; Infertility;* **HMO:** Oxford US Hlthcre
GHI Prucare Blue Choice +

LANG: Heb, Rus, Sp, Ar, Yd; 🚭 🗂 🔧 🏭 💲 2-
4 Weeks ▨ **VISA** ▨

Oktay, Kutluk (MD) RE
New York Methodist Hosp
Park Slope OB/GYN, PC, 263 7th Ave Fl 3;
Brooklyn, NY 11215; (718) 246-8500; **BDCERT:**
ObG 97; **MS:** Turkey 86; **RES:** IM, Cook Cty Hosp,
Chicago, IL 86-89; ObG, U Conn Hlth Ctr,
Farmington, CT 89-93; **FEL:** RE, Univ Texas HSC,
San Antonio, TX 93-95; RE, U Leeds HSC, Leeds,
England 95-96; **FAP:** Asst Prof RE Cornell U; **HOSP:**
NY Hosp-Cornell Med Ctr; **SI:** *Unexplained Infertility;
Anovulation;* **HMO:** Blue Cross & Blue Shield Oxford
1199 US Hlthcre

LANG: Fr, Sp, Itl, Rus, Scr; 🚭 🗂 🔧 🏭 💲 🔧 🔧
🔧 Immediately

RHEUMATOLOGY

Bienenstock, Harry (MD) Rhu
Hosp For Special Surgery
Center For Arthritis, 4013 Avenue U; Brooklyn, NY
11234; (718) 252-8181; **BDCERT:** IM 65; **MS:** U
Hlth Sci/Chicago Med Sch 57; **RES:** IM, VA Med
Ctr-Brooklyn, Brooklyn, NY 58-60; **FEL:** Rhu, Hosp
For Special Surgery, New York, NY 60-62; **FAP:**
Assoc Clin Prof Med Cornell U; **HOSP:** Coney Island
Hosp; **SI:** *Rheumatoid Arthritis; Musculoskeletal
Diseases;* **HMO:** Empire Blue Cross Multiplan Oxford
PHS PHCS +

LANG: Sp, Yd, Heb; 🚭 🗂 🔧 🏭 💲 🔧

Chahrouri, Joseph (MD) Rhu
New York Methodist Hosp
2818 Ocean Ave 9; Brooklyn, NY 11235; (718)
743-9642; **BDCERT:** IM 85; Rhu 88; **MS:** France
80; **RES:** Univ Hosp SUNY Bklyn, Brooklyn, NY 82-
85; **FEL:** Rhu, Univ Hosp SUNY Bklyn, Brooklyn,
NY 85-87; **SI:** *Rheumatoid Arthritis; Osteoporosis;*
HMO: Oxford Aetna Hlth Plan CIGNA Magnacare
Blue Choice +

LANG: Fr, Ar, Sp, Itl; 🚭 🗂 🔧 🏭 💲 🔧 2-
4 Weeks

Garner, Bruce (MD) Rhu
Lutheran Med Ctr
7901 4th Ave Ste A5; Brooklyn, NY 11209; (718)
921-5239; **BDCERT:** IM 87; Rhu 88; **MS:** Mexico
81; **RES:** Brookdale Univ Hosp Med Ctr, Brooklyn,
NY 82-83; Lutheran Med Ctr, Brooklyn, NY 83-85;
FEL: Rhu, Washington Hosp Ctr, Washington, DC;
SI: *Lupus; Rheumatoid Arthritis;* **HMO:** GHI Oxford
Blue Choice 1199

LANG: Sp, Itl; 🚭 🗂 🔧 🏭 🔧 2-4 Weeks

Ginzler, Ellen (MD) Rhu
Univ Hosp SUNY Bklyn
PO Box 42; Brooklyn, NY 11203; (718) 270-1662;
BDCERT: IM 72; Rhu 74; **MS:** Case West Res U 69;
RES: Kings County Hosp Ctr, Brooklyn, NY;
Bellevue Hosp Ctr, New York, NY; **FEL:** Rhu, Univ
Hosp SUNY Bklyn, Brooklyn, NY; **FAP:** Prof SUNY
Hlth Sci Ctr; **HOSP:** Kings County Hosp Ctr

🚭 🏭 🔧 🔧 2-4 Weeks

Green, Stuart (MD) Rhu
Brooklyn Hosp Ctr-Caledonian
121 Dekalb Ave FL4; Brooklyn, NY 11201; (718)
250-6921; **BDCERT:** Rhu 86; IM 82; **MS:**
Georgetown U 79; **RES:** St Luke's Roosevelt Hosp
Ctr, New York, NY 79-82; **FEL:** Univ Hosp SUNY
Bklyn, Brooklyn, NY 83-85; **SI:** *Rheumatoid
Arthritis; Lupus;* **HMO:** Oxford US Hlthcre Blue
Choice Aetna-US Healthcare

🚭 🗂 🔧 🏭 💲 🔧

Lesser, Robert (MD)   Rhu
Brookdale Univ Hosp Med Ctr

Brookdale Hospital, 1 Brookdale Plaza; Brooklyn,
NY 11212; (718) 240-6130; **BDCERT:** IM 85; Rhu
88; **MS:** U Hlth Sci/Chicago Med Sch 82; **RES:**
Hahnemann U Hosp, Philadelphia, PA 82-85; **FEL:**
Rhu, Hahnemann U Hosp, Philadelphia, PA 85-87;
HOSP: Beth Israel Med Ctr-Kings Hwy; *SI:
Inflammatory Arthritis; Degenerative Arthritis*; **HMO:**
Blue Choice Oxford CIGNA United Healthcare US
Hlthcre +

LANG: Fr, Heb; ♿ 🌙 📷 🔧 📅 💲 Mcr WC NFI
A Few Days

Patel, Jitendra K (MD)   Rhu
Kingsbrook Jewish Med Ctr

3131 Kings Hwy B8; Brooklyn, NY 11234; (718)
258-7019; **BDCERT:** IM 79; Rhu 82; **MS:** India 75;
RES: IM, Mem U Newfoundland, St Johns, Canada
76-79; **FEL:** Rhu, Georgetown U Hosp,
Washington, DC 80-82

♿ 🏥 🌙 📷 🔧 📅 Mcr Mcd   2-4 Weeks

Ricciardi, Daniel (MD)   Rhu
Long Island Coll Hosp

164 Clinton St; Brooklyn, NY 11201; (718) 834-
0070; **BDCERT:** IM 97; Rhu 98; **MS:** Grenada 81;
RES: IM, Long Island Coll Hosp, Brooklyn, NY 81-
84; **FEL:** Rhu, Long Island Coll Hosp, Brooklyn, NY
84-86; *SI: Rheumatoid Arthritis; Lupus*; **HMO:** ABC
Health GHI Oxford Prudential United Healthcare +

🌙 📷 🔧 📅 💲 Mcr   2-4 Weeks **VISA** 💳

SPORTS MEDICINE

Manning, Reginald (MD)   SM
Long Island Coll Hosp

97 Amity St; Brooklyn, NY 11201; (718) 522-
2121; **BDCERT:** OrS 86; **MS:** Columbia P&S 78;
RES: S, St Luke's Roosevelt Hosp Ctr, New York, NY
79-80; OrS, Lenox Hill Hosp, New York, NY 80-83;
FEL: SM, Lenox Hill Hosp, New York, NY 83-84;
FAP: Asst Prof SUNY Downstate

SURGERY

Adler, Harry (MD)   S
Maimonides Med Ctr

4802 10th Ave; Brooklyn, NY 11219; (718) 283-
7952; **BDCERT:** S 94; SCC 88; **MS:** NYU Sch Med
80; **RES:** Bellevue Hosp Ctr, New York, NY 80-85;
FEL: S, Maimonides Med Ctr, Brooklyn, NY 85-86;
FAP: Asst Clin Prof SUNY Downstate; *SI: Colon
Surgery; Gall Bladder Surgery*; **HMO:** Prucare Oxford
GHI Aetna Hlth Plan Magnacare +

LANG: Sp, Ger, Heb; ♿ 📷 🔧 📅 💲 Mcr WC NFI
1 Week

Alfonso, Antonio (MD)   S
Long Island Coll Hosp

100 Amity St FL1; Brooklyn, NY 11201; (718)
875-3244; **BDCERT:** S 73; **MS:** Philippines 68;
RES: Temple U Hosp, Philadelphia, PA 68-72; **FEL:**
S Onc, Mem Sloan Kettering Cancer Ctr, New York,
NY 72-74; NY Hosp-Cornell Med Ctr, New York,
NY; **FAP:** Prof S SUNY Hlth Sci Ctr; **HOSP:** Univ
Hosp SUNY Bklyn; *SI: Breast Surgery; Thyroid
Surgery*; **HMO:** Aetna Hlth Plan Oxford CIGNA US
Hlthcre Blue Cross & Blue Shield +

♿ 🌙 📷 🔧 📅 💲 Mcr Mcd WC NFI   A Few Days

Amiruddin, Qamar (MD)   S
Coney Island Hosp

Coney Island Hosp, 2601 Ocean Pkwy; Brooklyn,
NY 11235; (718) 616-3440; **BDCERT:** S 88; **MS:**
Pakistan 66; **RES:** Maimonides Med Ctr, Brooklyn,
NY 72-77; **FEL:** Kings County Hosp Ctr, Brooklyn,
NY; *SI: Breast Surgery*

♿ 📷 📅 Mcr Mcd WC NFI   Immediately

Angus, L D George (MD)   S
Brookdale Univ Hosp Med Ctr

1 Linden Blvd; Brooklyn, NY 11226; (718) 240-
6391; **BDCERT:** S 89; CCM 90; **MS:** Albert Einstein
Coll Med 82; **RES:** Long Island Jewish Med Ctr, New
Hyde Park, NY 83-86; **FEL:** MD Institute For
Emergency Med Services, Baltimore, MD 86-87

Bernstein, Michael (MD)   S
Long Island Coll Hosp
350 Henry St; Brooklyn, NY 11201; (718) 780-1563; **BDCERT:** S 72; CCM 90; **MS:** Penn State U-Hershey Med Ctr 83; **RES:** S, Univ Hosp SUNY Bklyn, Brooklyn, NY 83-88; **FAP:** Asst Prof SUNY Downstate; *SI: Abdominal Surgery; Tumor & Breast Surgery;* **HMO:** Aetna Hlth Plan United Healthcare Oxford Blue Cross & Blue Choice Premier +

LANG: Sp, Rus; ⬛ ⬛ ⬛ ⬛ ⬛ ⬛ ⬛ ⬛
A Few Days

Borriello, Raffaele (MD)   S
Long Island Coll Hosp
350 Henry St; Brooklyn, NY 11201; (718) 780-1562; **BDCERT:** S 87; **MS:** SUNY Downstate 81; **RES:** Kings County Hosp Ctr, Brooklyn, NY 81; *SI: Breast Laparoscopic Surgery; Hernia Repair;* **HMO:** Oxford US Hlthcre United Healthcare Prucare

LANG: Itl, Sp; ⬛ ⬛ ⬛ ⬛ ⬛ ⬛ ⬛ ⬛
A Few Days

Brevetti, Gregorio (MD)   S
New York Methodist Hosp
8318 4th Ave; Brooklyn, NY 11209; (718) 748-0500; **BDCERT:** TS 69; S 63; **MS:** Italy 48; **RES:** S, New York Methodist Hosp, Brooklyn, NY 55-59; **FEL:** TS, Kings County Hosp Ctr, Brooklyn, NY 59-61; *SI: Gastrointestinal Surgery; Thoracic Surgery;* **HMO:** Aetna-US Healthcare GHI Oxford Blue Choice CIGNA +

LANG: Itl; ⬛ ⬛ ⬛ ⬛ ⬛ ⬛ ⬛ ⬛   A Few Days

Choe, Dai-sun (MD)   S
Victory Memorial Hosp
7501 4th Ave; Brooklyn, NY 11209; (718) 238-6116; **BDCERT:** S 74; **MS:** South Korea 58; **RES:** S, Lutheran Med Ctr, Brooklyn, NY 68-71; **FEL:** S, Lahey Clinic, Burlington, MA 72-73; **HOSP:** Lutheran Med Ctr; *SI: Breast Cancer Surgery; Hernia Surgery;* **HMO:** Magnacare Oxford Blue Choice GHI

LANG: Kor; ⬛ ⬛ ⬛ ⬛ ⬛ ⬛ ⬛ ⬛ ⬛
Immediately

Duncan, Albert (MD)   S
Brooklyn Hosp Ctr-Caledonian
50 E 40th St; Brooklyn, NY 11203; (718) 778-6898; **BDCERT:** S 90; **MS:** MC Ohio, Toledo 80; **RES:** Univ Hosp SUNY Bklyn, Brooklyn, NY 80; **FEL:** Kings County Hosp Ctr, Brooklyn, NY; **HOSP:** Kings County Hosp Ctr; *SI: Breast Laparoscopy;* **HMO:** US Hlthcre 1199 GHI Oxford Health One +

LANG: Sp; ⬛ ⬛ ⬛ ⬛ ⬛ ⬛ ⬛ ⬛ ⬛
Immediately

Fahoum, Bashar (MD)   S
New York Methodist Hosp
Methodist HospitalDept of Surgery, 506 6th St; Brooklyn, NY 11215; (718) 780-3288; **BDCERT:** S 94; **MS:** Syria 87; **RES:** New York Methodist Hosp, Brooklyn, NY 89-93; *SI: Laparoscopy; Critical Care;* **HMO:** Oxford Blue Cross & Blue Shield GHI Aetna Hlth Plan Prudential +

LANG: Fr, Ar; ⬛ ⬛ ⬛ ⬛ ⬛ ⬛ ⬛ ⬛ ⬛   1 Week
VISA ⬛ ⬛ ⬛

Fogler, Richard (MD)   S
Brookdale Univ Hosp Med Ctr
1 Brookdale Plaza Rm122; Brooklyn, NY 11212; (718) 240-5437; **BDCERT:** S 73; **MS:** NY Med Coll 68; **RES:** Brookdale Univ Hosp Med Ctr, Brooklyn, NY 73; **HMO:** Blue Choice Blue Cross & Blue Shield HealthNet Metlife Prucare +

⬛ ⬛ ⬛ ⬛ ⬛ ⬛ ⬛ ⬛   Immediately

Genato, Romulo (MD)   S
Brooklyn Hosp Ctr-Caledonian
121 Dekalb Ave Fl 8; Brooklyn, NY 11201; (718) 250-8970; **BDCERT:** S 80; **MS:** Philippines 72; **RES:** Brooklyn Hosp Ctr, Brooklyn, NY 74-79; **FAP:** Assoc Clin Prof S NYU Sch Med; *SI: Breast Surgery; Laparoscopic Surgery;* **HMO:** Aetna Hlth Plan Oxford US Hlthcre Blue Cross & Blue Shield Chubb +

LANG: Sp, Fil; ⬛ ⬛ ⬛ ⬛ ⬛ ⬛ ⬛ ⬛
Immediately

Hedayati, Hossein (MD)　　S
New York Methodist Hosp
9920 4th Ave 311; Brooklyn, NY 11209; (718)
833-2600; **BDCERT:** S 69; **MS:** Iran 62; **RES:** New
York Methodist Hosp, Brooklyn, NY 67-68; Mem
Sloan Kettering Cancer Ctr, New York, NY 66-67;
FEL: Univ Hosp SUNY Bklyn, Brooklyn, NY 68-70;
HOSP: Victory Memorial Hosp; **HMO:** Aetna Hlth
Plan Blue Cross & Blue Shield Magnacare Oxford
CIGNA +

Hong, Joon (MD)　　S
Stony Lodge Hosp
450 Clarkson Ave Box 40; Brooklyn, NY 11203;
(718) 270-2386; **BDCERT:** S 81; **MS:** South Korea
67; **RES:** Univ Hosp SUNY Bklyn, Brooklyn, NY;
FEL: Univ Hosp SUNY Bklyn, Brooklyn, NY; **SI:**
Kidney Transplant; Liver Transplant; **HMO:** Oxford US
Hlthcre Most GHI

LANG: Fr, Ar, Sp, Kor; 🅰 🚹 🏢 Mcr Mcd　A Few Days

Horovitz, Joel (MD)　　S
Maimonides Med Ctr
953 49th St Fl 4; Brooklyn, NY 11219; (718) 283-
8461; **BDCERT:** S 74; **MS:** McGill 67; **RES:** McGill
Teaching Hosp, Montreal, Canada 68-73; **HMO:**
GHI CIGNA

Khafif, Rene (MD)　　S
Lutheran Med Ctr
2219 Ocean Ave; Brooklyn, NY 11229; (718) 376-
6580; **BDCERT:** S 64; **MS:** France 56; **RES:** S,
Maimonides Med Ctr, Brooklyn, NY 57-62; **FEL:** S,
USPHS, New York, NY 59-60; **FAP:** Clin Prof SUNY
Downstate; **HOSP:** Maimonides Med Ctr; **SI:** *Head &
Neck Surgery-Thyroid; Breast-Melanoma-Skin Cancer;*
HMO: CIGNA HealthNet Metlife Blue Cross & Blue
Shield

LANG: Fr, Ar, Heb, Sp; 🅲 🔒 🚹 🏢 💲 Mcr Mcd
A Few Days

Kumar, Sampath (MD)　　S
Lutheran Med Ctr
7517 6th Ave; Brooklyn, NY 11209; (718) 630-
5777; **BDCERT:** S 83; **MS:** India 75; **RES:** Lutheran
Med Ctr, Brooklyn, NY; **FEL:** GVS, Lutheran Med
Ctr, Brooklyn, NY; **HOSP:** Victory Memorial Hosp;
SI: *Laparoscopic Procedures; Breast Surgery: Non
Invasive;* **HMO:** US Hlthcre Empire Blue Cross &
Shield GHI United Healthcare

🅰 🈺 🅲 🔒 🚹 🏢 💲 Mcr Mcd WC NfI　Immediately

Lacqua, Frank (MD)　　S
Victory Memorial Hosp
7513 Ft Hamilton Pkwy; Brooklyn, NY 11228;
(718) 680-6604; **BDCERT:** S 91; CRS 92; **MS:**
SUNY Buffalo 85; **SI:** *Colon & Rectal Diseases*
🅲 🔒 🏢 💲 Mcr　Immediately

Lamaute, Henry (MD)　　S
St Mary's Hosp
170 Buffalo Ave; Brooklyn, NY 11213; (718) 221-
3318; **BDCERT:** S 75; **MS:** Haiti 66; **RES:** S,
Brooklyn Jewish Hosp, Brooklyn, NY 69-73; **FAP:**
Asst Prof Cornell U; **SI:** *Digestive Diseases; Glandular
Disorders;* **HMO:** 1199 Blue Cross Oxford MHS
LANG: Fr, Pat, Sp; 🈺 🔒 🚹 🏢 Mcr Mcd　Immediately

Lois, William (MD)　　S
Kingsbrook Jewish Med Ctr
Wound Care Assoc Of Brooklyn, 2035 Ralph Ave
B5; Brooklyn, NY 11234; (718) 251-1111;
BDCERT: S 88; **MS:** Spain 82; **RES:** S, Interfaith
Med ctr, Brooklyn, NY 82-87; **HMO:** Oxford Blue
Choice Sanus

Mohaideen, A Hassan (MD)　　S
Victory Memorial Hosp
Island Surgical Group, 705 86th St M4; Brooklyn,
NY 11228; (718) 238-6100; **BDCERT:** S 77; S 96;
MS: India 65; **RES:** Long Island Coll Hosp,
Brooklyn, NY; **FAP:** Asst Clin Prof SUNY Hlth Sci
Ctr; **HOSP:** Brooklyn Hosp Ctr-Caledonian; **SI:**
Vascular Surgery; **HMO:** Aetna Hlth Plan United
Healthcare Oxford US Hlthcre Prucare +
LANG: Tam; 🅰 🅲 🔒 🏢 Mcr WC NfI　A Few Days

Nicolas, Fred (MD)   S
Brookdale Univ Hosp Med Ctr
903 E 85th St; Brooklyn, NY 11236; (718) 209-0600; **BDCERT:** S 77; **EM** 90; **MS:** Egypt 65; **RES:** S, Jewish Hosp, Brooklyn, NY 70-74; **FEL:** S, Brookdale Med Ctr, Brooklyn, NY

Oloumi, Mohammad (MD)   S
New York Methodist Hosp
258 85th St; Brooklyn, NY 11209; (718) 833-5994; **BDCERT:** S 78; **MS:** Iran 68; **RES:** S, New York Methodist Hosp, Brooklyn, NY 72; S, New York Methodist Hosp, Brooklyn, NY 77; **FEL:** S Onc, Univ Hosp SUNY Bklyn, Brooklyn, NY 77-78; **SI:** *Breast Surgery; Thyroid Surgery;* **HMO:** PHS Oxford Guardian Blue Choice NYLCare +

LANG: Frs; ♿ 🔒 👶 🏥 Med WC Immediately

Padilla, Crisologo (MD)   S
New York Comm Hosp of Bklyn
2413 Ocean Ave; Brooklyn, NY 11229; (718) 332-6767; **BDCERT:** S 70; **MS:** Philippines 62; **RES:** S, Knickerbocker Hosp, New York, NY 64-65; S, Jewish Hosp Med Ctr, Brooklyn, NY 66-69; **HMO:** GHI Magnacare United Healthcare Multiplan PHS +

🌙 🔒 👶 🏥 S Mcr WC NFI Immediately

Panetta, Thomas F (MD)   S
Univ Hosp SUNY Bklyn
450 Clarkson Ave; Brooklyn, NY 11203; (718) 270-1035; **BDCERT:** S 92; **GVS** 95; **MS:** SUNY Hlth Sci Ctr 77; **RES:** S, Univ Hosp SUNY Bklyn, Brooklyn, NY 77-82; **FEL:** GVS, Baylor Med Ctr, Dallas, TX 82-83; **FAP:** Prof S SUNY Downstate; **HOSP:** St Vincent's Med Ctr-Richmond; **HMO:** Blue Choice GHI US Hlthcre Oxford

♿ 🌙 🔒 👶 🏥 Mcr Med WC NFI Immediately

Raju, Ramanathan (MD)   S
Lutheran Med Ctr
7517 6th Ave; Brooklyn, NY 11209; (718) 630-5777; **BDCERT:** S 88; **MS:** India 76; **RES:** S, Lutheran Med Ctr, Brooklyn, NY 82-87; GVS, Lutheran Med Ctr, Brooklyn, NY 87-88; **FEL:** Royal Coll of Surgeons, Edinburgh, England; **FAP:** Asst Clin Prof S SUNY Hlth Sci Ctr; **HOSP:** Victory Memorial Hosp; **SI:** *Minimally Invasive Breast Surgery; Laparoscopic Surgery;* **HMO:** GHI CIGNA US Hlthcre Oxford Blue Choice +

LANG: Sp, Itl; ♿ SA SD 🌙 🔒 👶 🏥 Mcr Med WC NFI Immediately

Rao, Addagada (MD)   S
Wyckoff Heights Med Ctr
145 Saint Nicholas Ave; Brooklyn, NY 11237; (718) 443-1500; **BDCERT:** S 74; **MS:** India 65; **RES:** S, Wyckoff Heights Med Ctr, Brooklyn, NY 67-72; **HMO:** Oxford Aetna Hlth Plan CIGNA Blue Choice United Healthcare +

Richter, Robert (MD)   S
New York Methodist Hosp
1 Hanson Pl 1511; Brooklyn, NY 11243; (718) 783-6222; **BDCERT:** S 66; **MS:** Albany Med Coll 58; **RES:** S, Mount Sinai Med Ctr, New York, NY 58-64; **FAP:** Assoc Clin Prof S SUNY Downstate; **HOSP:** Brooklyn Hosp Ctr-Downtown; **SI:** *Gastrointestinal Diseases; Endoscopy;* **HMO:** US Hlthcre Blue Choice 1199 CIGNA Oxford +

LANG: Sp; ♿ 🔒 👶 🏥 S Mcr Med WC A Few Days

Schwartzman, Alexander (MD) S
Long Island Coll Hosp
350 Henry St; Brooklyn, NY 11201; (718) 330-0405; **BDCERT:** S 89; **MS:** Dominican Republic 83; **RES:** Brooklyn Hosp Ctr, Brooklyn, NY 83-88; **FAP:** Asst Prof S SUNY Hlth Sci Ctr; **SI:** *Laparoscopic Surgery; Tumor Surgery;* **HMO:** US Hlthcre Aetna Hlth Plan Oxford GHI Blue Cross & Blue Shield +

LANG: Rus, Sp, Pol, Ukr; ♿ 🌙 🔒 👶 🏥 S NFI
A Few Days **VISA** 💳

Siegman, Felix (MD)   **S**
Maimonides Med Ctr
4802 10th Ave; Brooklyn, NY 11219; (718) 283-6299; **BDCERT:** S 52; **MS:** Tulane U 44; **RES:** S, Israel Zion Hosp, Brooklyn, NY 45-46; S, Maimonides Med Ctr, Brooklyn, NY 48-52; **FAP:** Asst Prof SUNY Downstate; **SI:** *Hernia; Vein Problems*; **HMO:** Oxford US Hlthcre GHI NYLCare Empire Blue Cross & Shield +

LANG: Yd, Rus, Pol; ♿ 📷 👪 🛏 Mcr WC NFi
A Few Days

Sommer, Bruce (MD)   **S**
Univ Hosp SUNY Bklyn
450 Clarkson Ave; Brooklyn, NY 11203; (718) 270-1898; **BDCERT:** S 82; S 91; **MS:** U Minn 74; **RES:** U MN Med Ctr, Minneapolis, MN 74-81; U MN Med Ctr, Minneapolis, MN 82; **FAP:** Prof S SUNY Hlth Sci Ctr; **HOSP:** Kings County Med Ctr; **SI:** *Solid Organ Transplantation; Vascular Access*; **HMO:** Oxford CIGNA US Hlthcre HIP Network

LANG: Sp, Fr, Kor, Ar, Rus; ♿ 📷 👪 🛏 Mcr Mcd WC
A Few Days

Steiner, Henry (MD)   **S**
Maimonides Med Ctr
8105 Bay Pkwy; Brooklyn, NY 11214; (718) 331-7314; **BDCERT:** S 82; **MS:** SUNY Downstate 76; **RES:** Maimonides Med Ctr, Brooklyn, NY 76-80; Coney Island Hosp, Brooklyn, NY 76-80; **FEL:** GVS, Maimonides Med Ctr, Brooklyn, NY 80-81; **HOSP:** Peninsula Hosp Ctr

Tanchajja, Supoj (MD)   **S**
Long Island Coll Hosp
142 Joralemon St; Brooklyn, NY 11201; (718) 852-6450; **BDCERT:** S 81; **MS:** Thailand 72; **RES:** Brooklyn Hosp Ctr, Brooklyn, NY 74; New York Methodist Hosp, Brooklyn, NY 75; **FEL:** Long Island Coll Hosp, Brooklyn, NY 77; **FAP:** Instr SUNY Downstate; **HOSP:** Victory Memorial Hosp; **HMO:** Blue Cross & Blue Shield CIGNA HealthNet
♿ 📷 👪 🛏 Mcr WC   A Few Days

Wait, Richard B (MD)   **S**
Univ Hosp SUNY Bklyn
SUNY Hlth Sci Ctr Box 140, 450 Clarkson Ave; Brooklyn, NY 11203; (718) 270-1421; **BDCERT:** S 84; **MS:** Univ Vt Coll Med 78; **RES:** S, Med Ctr Hosp of VT, Burlington, VT; **FEL:** S, Med Ctr Hosp of VT, Burlington, VT; **HOSP:** Kings County Hosp Ctr
♿ 📷 🛏 Mcr Mcd WC NFi   A Few Days

Wise, Leslie (MD)   **S**
New York Methodist Hosp
506 6th St; Brooklyn, NY 11215; (718) 780-3288; **BDCERT:** S 70; **MS:** Australia 58; **RES:** Hammersmith Hosp, London, England 62; St Mark's Hosp, London, England; **FEL:** Johns Hopkins Hosp, Baltimore, MD 67; Barnes Hosp, St Louis, MO; **HOSP:** Long Island Jewish Med Ctr
♿ 📷 👪 🛏 Mcr Mcd WC   Immediately

Woloszyn, Thomas T (MD)   **S**
Maimonides Med Ctr
953 49th St Fl 4; Brooklyn, NY 11219; (718) 283-8631; **BDCERT:** S 93; PlS 97; **MS:** U Hlth Sci/Chicago Med Sch 86; **RES:** S, Maimonides Med Ctr, Brooklyn, NY 86-92; PlS, Nassau County Med Ctr, East Meadow, NY 93-95; **FEL:** HS, Hand Surgery Ctr of Texas, Houston, TX 92-93; **HOSP:** Lutheran Med Ctr; **SI:** *Hand Reconstruction; Scar Revision*; **HMO:** Aetna-US Healthcare GHI Oxford Health Plus +

LANG: Sp, Pol; ♿ 📷 🛏 S Mcr WC NFi   A Few Days

Wright, Albert (MD)   **S**
Interfaith Med Ctr-St John's
1 Plaza St West; Brooklyn, NY 11217; (718) 638-1971; **BDCERT:** S 81; **MS:** England 70; **RES:** S, Mount Sinai Med Ctr, New York, NY; **HOSP:** Brooklyn Hosp Ctr-Downtown; **SI:** *Breast Diseases; Laparoscopic Procedures*; **HMO:** CIGNA Aetna-US Healthcare MHS Sanus-NYLCare +

♿ 🅲 📷 👪 🛏 Mcr Mcd WC NFi   Immediately

THORACIC SURGERY

Ahmed, Nafis (MD)   TS
Victory Memorial Hosp
1722 85th St; Brooklyn, NY 11214; (718) 259-5533; **BDCERT:** S 91; **MS:** India 72; **RES:** S, Univ Hosp SUNY Bklyn, Brooklyn, NY 72-73; S, VA Med Ctr-Brooklyn, Brooklyn, NY 73-76; **FEL:** TS, VA Med Ctr-Brooklyn, Brooklyn, NY 76-78; *SI: Lung Cancer; Leg Blood Vessel Bypass*; **HMO:** Blue Choice GHI Oxford Aetna-US Healthcare United Healthcare +

LANG: Hin, Itl; 🦽 🌙 📷 👤 🏥 💲 Mcr WC NFI Immediately

Burack, Joshua H (MD)   TS
Brooklyn Hosp Ctr-Downtown
SUNY Health Sci Ctr, 450 Clarkson Ave Box 40; Brooklyn, NY 11203; **BDCERT:** TS 91; S 88; **MS:** Albert Einstein Coll Med 82; **RES:** S, Albert Einstein Med Ctr, Bronx, NY 84-87; **FEL:** TS, Univ Hosp SUNY Bklyn, Brooklyn, NY 87-89; **FAP:** Asst Prof S SUNY Downstate; **HMO:** Elderplan Aetna-US Healthcare GHI Blue Cross & Blue Choice Mayan +

🦽 🌙 📷 🏥 💲 Mcr Mcd WC NFI Immediately

Connolly, Mark (MD)   TS
Maimonides Med Ctr
4802 10th Ave; Brooklyn, NY 11219; (718) 283-7686; **BDCERT:** TS 89; **MS:** Northwestern U 79; **RES:** S, NYU Medical Center, New York, NY 83-88; TS, Emory Univ, Atlanta, GA 88-91; **FEL:** S, Maimonides Medical Center, Brooklyn, NY 84-86

Cunningham, Joseph (MD)   TS
Maimonides Med Ctr
4802 10th Ave; Brooklyn, NY 11219; (718) 283-7686; **BDCERT:** TS 75; S 73; **MS:** U Ala Sch Med 66; **RES:** S, Parkland Mem Hosp, Dallas, TX 67-72; **FEL:** Cv, New York University Med Ctr, New York, NY 72-74; **FAP:** Prof S SUNY Downstate; **HMO:** Oxford Aetna Hlth Plan CIGNA Blue Choice United Healthcare +

Mathur, Ambrish P (MD)   TS
Brookdale Univ Hosp Med Ctr
984 50th St; Brooklyn, NY 11219; (718) 438-8600; **BDCERT:** TS 74; **MS:** India 60; **RES:** Baltimore City Hosp, Baltimore, MD 64-67; Kingsbrook Jewish Med Ctr, Brooklyn, NY 67-71; **FEL:** Jewish Hosp Med Ctr, Brooklyn, NY 69-70; Long Island Coll Hosp, Brooklyn, NY 71-72; **HOSP:** Long Island Coll Hosp; **HMO:** Aetna Hlth Plan Blue Cross & Blue Shield HIP Network Prucare

📷 🏥 Mcr Mcd Immediately

Okadigwe, Chukuma (MD)   TS
New York Methodist Hosp
191 Ocean Ave; Brooklyn, NY 11225; (718) 287-0505; **BDCERT:** TS 79; **MS:** U Colo Sch Med 68; **RES:** S, Kings County Hosp Ctr, Brooklyn, NY 74; TS, Univ Hosp SUNY Bklyn, Brooklyn, NY 74-76; **FAP:** Asst Prof SUNY Stony Brook; **HOSP:** Brookdale Univ Hosp Med Ctr; *SI: Lung Cancer; Thorascopic Surgery*; **HMO:** United Healthcare GHI Oxford Aetna Hlth Plan

SA/SU 🌙 📷 👤 🏥 💲 Mcr Mcd WC NFI Immediately

Plantilla, Eduardo (MD)   TS
Maimonides Med Ctr
Solomon Ciprut MD PC, 2560 Ocean Ave 2A; Brooklyn, NY 11229; (718) 891-5595; **BDCERT:** TS 81; S 77; **MS:** Philippines 68; **RES:** S, Maimonides Med Ctr, Brooklyn, NY 75-76; TS, Maimonides Med Ctr, Brooklyn, NY 77-78; **FEL:** PCd S, Children's Hosp Med Ctr, Cincinnati, OH 80; **FAP:** Asst Instr S; **HOSP:** Lutheran Med Ctr; **HMO:** GHI Oxford CIGNA NYLCare US Hlthcre +

🦽 🌙 📷 👤 🏥 Mcr WC NFI 1 Week

UROLOGY

Abbate, Anthony (MD)   U
Beth Israel Med Ctr-Kings Hwy

455 Ocean Pkwy; Brooklyn, NY 11218; (718) 941-2002; **BDCERT:** Ge 72; **MS:** Italy 64; **RES:** Long Island Coll Hosp, Brooklyn, NY 64-67; Maimonides Med Ctr, Brooklyn, NY 68-69; **FAP:** Clin Instr SUNY Downstate; **HOSP:** Maimonides Med Ctr; *SI: Prostate Disease-Sexual Dysfunction; Urinary Stone Disease*

Barbera, Jude (MD)   U
Maimonides Med Ctr

2519 Avenue U; Brooklyn, NY 11229; (718) 332-4080; **BDCERT:** U 90; **MS:** Dominican Republic 81; **RES:** S, Maimonides Med Ctr, Brooklyn, NY 82-84; **FEL:** U, Maimonides Med Ctr, Brooklyn, NY 84-88; **HOSP:** St John's Queens Hosp; *SI: Prostate Cancer; Kidney Stones;* **HMO:** CIGNA PHCS Oxford Elderplan GHI +

LANG: Sp, Rus, Itl; ♿ 🅒 📷 🚺 🏧 🅢 Mcr Immediately

Florio, Francis (MD)   U
New York Methodist Hosp

355 Ovington Ave; Brooklyn, NY 11209; (718) 238-1818; **BDCERT:** U 83; **MS:** NY Med Coll 75; **RES:** U, New York University Med Ctr, New York, NY 77-81; **FAP:** Instr U Cornell U; *SI: Urinary Incontinence; Benign Prostatic Hypertrophy;* **HMO:** Oxford Aetna Hlth Plan Blue Choice CIGNA

♿ 🅒 📷 🚺 🏧 🅢 Mcr 📇 *VISA* 🔴 💳

Friedman, Steven (MD)   U
Maimonides Med Ctr

Pediatric Urology Associates, 909 49th St Fl 2; Brooklyn, NY 11219; (718) 283-7743; **BDCERT:** U 91; **MS:** SUNY Downstate 83; **RES:** S, Beth Israel Med Ctr, New York, NY 83-85; U, Maimonides Med Ctr, Brooklyn, NY 85-88; **FEL:** Ped U, Children's Hosp of MI, Detroit, MI 90-91; **HOSP:** Schneider Children's Hosp; *SI: Genital Abnormalities; Undescended Testes;* **HMO:** Oxford GHI Blue Cross & Blue Shield US Hlthcre Magnacare +

LANG: Sp; ♿ 📷 🚺 🏧 Mcr A Few Days 📇 *VISA*

Glassberg, Kenneth (MD)   U
Univ Hosp SUNY Bklyn

450 Clarkson Ave; Brooklyn, NY 11203; (718) 270-1958; **BDCERT:** U 77; **MS:** SUNY Downstate 68; **RES:** S, Montefiore Med Ctr, Bronx, NY 71-72; U, Univ Hosp SUNY Bklyn, Brooklyn, NY 72-75; **FEL:** England; **FAP:** Prof SUNY Hlth Sci Ctr; *SI: Pediatric Urology;* **HMO:** Oxford Empire Blue Cross & Shield US Hlthcre CIGNA Blue Cross & Blue Shield +

LANG: Heb, Yd; ♿ 📷 🚺 🏧 🅢 Mcr Mcd 1 Week

Godec, Ciril (MD)   U
Long Island Coll Hosp

Long Island College Urology, 339 Hicks St Fl 7; Brooklyn, NY 11201; (718) 780-1520; **BDCERT:** U 79; **MS:** Yugoslavia 83; **RES:** U MN Med Ctr, Minneapolis, MN 72-76; **HOSP:** Univ Hosp SUNY Bklyn; *SI: Prostate Cancer; Erectile Dysfunction;* **HMO:** GHI Oxford 1199 US Hlthcre

LANG: Sp, Fr, Slv; ♿ 📷 🏧 🅢 Mcr WC NFl 1 Week

Grunberger, Ivan (MD)   U
Long Island Coll Hosp

Brooklyn Heights Urology Associates, 339 Hicks St; Brooklyn, NY 11201; (718) 780-1520; **BDCERT:** U 88; **MS:** NYU Sch Med 80; **RES:** S, N Shore Univ Hosp-Manhasset, Manhasset, NY 80-82; U, New York University Med Ctr, New York, NY 82-86; **FAP:** Assoc Prof U SUNY Hlth Sci Ctr; *SI: Impotence; Kidney Stones;* **HMO:** Aetna-US Healthcare Oxford NYLCare Prucare CIGNA +

LANG: Sp, Rus, Czc, Slv; ♿ 📷 🚺 🏧 🅢 Mcr Mcd WC A Few Days

Hashmat, Aizid (MD)   U
Brooklyn Hosp Ctr-Caledonian

Brooklyn Hosp Ctr, 121 Dekalb Ave; Brooklyn, NY 11201; (718) 250-6880; **BDCERT:** U 82; **MS:** Pakistan 64; **RES:** Univ Hosp SUNY Bklyn, Brooklyn, NY 77-80; **FEL:** Ped, U London, London, England; *SI: Erectile Dysfunction;* **HMO:** Oxford US Hlthcre NYLCare Blue Cross & Blue Shield

LANG: Ur, Tam; ♿ 📷 🚺 🏧 🅢 Mcr Mcd A Few Days

Irwin, Mark (MD) U
Univ Hosp SUNY Bklyn
339 Hicks St; Brooklyn, NY 11201; (718) 780-1520; **BDCERT:** U 91; **MS:** Med Coll Wisc 82; **RES:** U, Kings County Hosp Ctr, Brooklyn, NY 85-88; St Luke's Roosevelt Hosp Ctr, New York, NY 77-79; **HOSP:** Long Island Coll Hosp

Kim, Hong (MD) U
Brookdale Univ Hosp Med Ctr
Urology Suites, 1 Brookdale Plaza Rm5C4; Brooklyn, NY 11212; (718) 240-5323; **BDCERT:** U 76; **MS:** South Korea 65; **RES:** Brookdale Univ Hosp Med Ctr, Brooklyn, NY 69; U NE Med Ctr, Omaha, NE 74; **FEL:** NY Academy of Med, New York, NY; **HMO:** Aetna Hlth Plan Blue Choice Blue Cross & Blue Shield CIGNA HealthNet +

 ⬧ 🔲 🚹 🏠 🍴 💲 Mcr Immediately

Lindsay, Gaius K (MD) U
Coney Island Hosp
Coney Island Medical Group, 1616 Voorhies Ave Ste B; Brooklyn, NY 11235; (718) 769-5158; **BDCERT:** U 76; **MS:** India 67; **RES:** S, New York Methodist Hosp, Brooklyn, NY 69-70; U, Maimonides Med Ctr, Brooklyn, NY 70-73; **FAP:** Asst Clin Prof SUNY Downstate; **HOSP:** Maimonides Med Ctr; **HMO:** Oxford CIGNA NYLCare Empire GHI +

 ⬧ 🆑 🌙 🏠 🍴 💲 Mcr A Few Days

Macchia, Richard (MD) U
Kings County Hosp Ctr
445 Lenox Rd; Brooklyn, NY 11203; (718) 270-2554; **BDCERT:** U 77; **MS:** NY Med Coll 69; **RES:** S, St Vincents Hosp & Med Ctr NY, New York, NY 70; U, Univ Hosp SUNY Bklyn, Brooklyn, NY 71-74; **FEL:** U Onc, Mem Sloan Kettering Cancer Ctr, New York, NY 75-76; **FAP:** Prof U SUNY Hlth Sci Ctr; **HOSP:** Univ Hosp SUNY Bklyn; **SI:** *Urination Problems; Non Operative Urology;* **HMO:** GHI Blue Cross & Blue Shield CIGNA HIP Network +

 ⬧ 🏠 🚹 🍴 💲 Mcr Mcd A Few Days

Mandel, Edmund (MD) U
New York Comm Hosp of Bklyn
Advanced Urology Assoc, 2460 Flatbush Ave 8; Brooklyn, NY 11234; (718) 692-0020; **BDCERT:** U 88; **MS:** Temple U 81; **RES:** U, Mount Sinai Med Ctr, New York, NY 82-86; **FAP:** Asst Clin Prof Mt Sinai Sch Med; **SI:** *Incontinence; Renal Stones;* **HMO:** Oxford GHI Blue Cross US Hlthcre

LANG: Sp, Rus, Fr, Yd; ⬧ 🏠 🍴 💲 Mcr WC
A Few Days **VISA** 💳 💳

Mazzarino, Aldo (MD) U
Lutheran Med Ctr
468 77th St; Brooklyn, NY 11209; (718) 745-0771; **BDCERT:** U 68; **MS:** Italy 59; **RES:** New York Methodist Hosp, Brooklyn, NY 60; NY Med Coll, Valhalla, NY 61; **FAP:** Assoc Prof SUNY Buffalo; **HOSP:** New York Methodist Hosp; **SI:** *Collagen Implant for Urinary Incontinence; Lithotripsy Kidney Stones;* **HMO:** Magnacare Aetna Hlth Plan Blue Choice Oxford CIGNA +

LANG: Itl, Sp; 🏠 🍴 💲 Mcr WC Immediately

Meisenberg, Eugene (MD) U
New York Methodist Hosp
New York Methodist Hospital, 263 7th Ave Ste 5C; Brooklyn, NY 11215; (718) 369-8030; **MS:** Russia 88; **RES:** U, RWJ Univ Hosp-New Brunswick, New Brunswick, NJ 93-94; S, Beth Israel Med Ctr, New York, NY 92-93; **HOSP:** Long Island Coll Hosp; **SI:** *Prostate Care Impotence; Kidney Stones;* **HMO:** Blue Cross & Blue Shield Aetna-US Healthcare Prudential 1199 CIGNA +

LANG: Rus; ⬧ 🆑 🌙 🏠 🚹 🍴 Mcr Mcd WC NFl
A Few Days

Raju, Samanthi (MD) U
Brooklyn Hosp Ctr-Caledonian
121 Dekalb Ave; Brooklyn, NY 11201; (718) 250-6880; **MS:** India 75; **RES:** Crawley Hosp, England 80-81; The London Hosp, England 82; **FEL:** Univ Hosp SUNY, Brooklyn, NY; **SI:** *Interstitial Cystitis; Pediatric Urology; Congenital Adrenal Hyperplasia*

 ⬧ 🆑 🏠 🚹 🍴 💲 Mcr Mcd Immediately

Rosenthal, Sheldon (MD)   U
Wyckoff Heights Med Ctr
359 Stockholm St FL1; Brooklyn, NY 11237; (718) 821-3200; **BDCERT:** U 77; **MS:** U Hlth Sci/Chicago Med Sch 67; **RES:** S, Albert Einstein Med Ctr, Bronx, NY 68-70; U, NY Med Coll, New York, NY 70-73; **HOSP:** St John's Queens Hosp; *SI: Kidney Stones; Bladder & Prostate Disease;* **HMO:** GHI US Hlthcre Blue Choice PPO 32BJ NY Hosp Hlth +

LANG: Sp, Itl, Rus; ♿ 🌙 🔒 💉 🏥 💲 Mcr Mcd WC NFI
Immediately

Saada, Simon (MD)   U
Victory Memorial Hosp
705 86th St M2; Brooklyn, NY 11228; (718) 238-1075; **BDCERT:** U 81; **MS:** Egypt 70; **RES:** U, Charleston Area Med Ctr, Charleston, WV 76-77; S, Long Island Coll Hosp, Brooklyn, NY 73-74; **FAP:** Asst Clin Prof Columbia P&S; *SI: Stone Disease-Lithotripsy; Prostrate/Kidney Cancer;* **HMO:** Aetna Hlth Plan Blue Choice Blue Cross & Blue Shield

LANG: Fr, Itl, Ar, Rus; ♿ 🌙 🔒 💉 🏥 Mcr Mcd
A Few Days

Tunis, Leonard (MD)   U
Maimonides Med Ctr
3043 Ocean Ave 203; Brooklyn, NY 11235; (718) 934-2525; **BDCERT:** U 66; **MS:** Tulane U 55; **RES:** Maimonides Med Ctr, Brooklyn, NY 61; **HOSP:** Beth Israel Med Ctr-Kings Hwy; *SI: Prostatectomy; Prostate Cancer;* **HMO:** Empire Blue Cross & Blue Shield Oxford US Hlthcre Metlife +

🔒 💉 🏥 💲 Mcr   A Few Days

Wainstein, Sasha (MD)   U
Maimonides Med Ctr
Urologic Surgical Assoc, 4711 12th Ave; Brooklyn, NY 11219; (718) 436-3900; **BDCERT:** U 77; **MS:** Colombia 69; **RES:** Maimonides Med Ctr, Brooklyn, NY 70-75; **FAP:** Clin Instr SUNY Downstate; **HOSP:** Victory Memorial Hosp; *SI: Cancer; Impotence;* **HMO:** Oxford Blue Choice US Hlthcre CIGNA United Healthcare +

LANG: Sp, Yd, Itl; ♿ 🌙 🔒 💉 🏥 💲 Mcr
Immediately *VISA* 💳

Wise, Gilbert (MD)   U
Maimonides Med Ctr
953 49th St Fl 3; Brooklyn, NY 11219; (718) 438-3475; **BDCERT:** U 69; **MS:** Johns Hopkins U 57; **RES:** U Hosp of Cleveland, Cleveland, OH 57-59; Montefiore Med Ctr, Bronx, NY 61-65

♿ 🔒 💉 🏥 💲 Mcr Mcd   A Few Days

VASCULAR SURGERY (GENERAL)

Ascher, Enrico (MD)   GVS
Maimonides Med Ctr
903 49th St; Brooklyn, NY 11219; (718) 283-7957; **BDCERT:** S 84; GVS 85; **MS:** Brazil 74; **RES:** S, NY Med Coll, Valhalla, NY 76-81; **FEL:** GVS, Montefiore Med Ctr, Bronx, NY 81-82; **FAP:** Prof S NYU Sch Med; **HOSP:** Lutheran Med Ctr; *SI: Stroke Prevention; Limb Salvage;* **HMO:** GHI HIP Network Blue Cross Blue Shield Elderplan +

LANG: Sp, Rus; ♿ 🌙 🔒 🏥 💲 Mcr WC NFI
A Few Days

Ilkhani, Rahman (MD)   GVS
New York Methodist Hosp
263 7th Ave 5E; Brooklyn, NY 11215; (718) 768-3560; **BDCERT:** S 94; **MS:** Iran 74; **RES:** S, New York Methodist Hosp, Brooklyn, NY 77-82; **FEL:** GVS, Texas Heart Inst, Houston, TX 82-83; *SI: Venous Conditions; Aneurysms*

♿ 🌙 🔒 💉 🏥 Mcr   A Few Days

Levowitz, Bernard (MD)   GVS
Brooklyn Hosp Ctr-Caledonian
6410 Veterans Ave # 103; Brooklyn, NY 11234; (718) 209-1400; **BDCERT:** S 63; **MS:** NY Med Coll 49; **RES:** Kings Cty Hosp Ctr, Brooklyn, NY 52-59; **FEL:** TS, U Pittsbrgh, Pittsburg, PA; **FAP:** Prof SUNY Hlth Sci Ctr; **HOSP:** Brookdale Univ Hosp Med Ctr; *SI: Non-invasive Vascular Diagnosis; Vascular Surgery;* **HMO:** Metlife Sanus Prucare Oxford US Hlthcre +

♿ 🌙 🔒 💉 🏥 💲 Mcr Mcd WC NFI   Immediately *VISA* 💳 💳

Shin, Choon (MD) GVS
New York Comm Hosp of Bklyn
2525 Kings Hwy; Brooklyn, NY 11229; (718) 692-
5315; **BDCERT:** TS 94; GVS 96; **MS:** South Korea
65; **RES:** S, New York Methodist Hosp, Brooklyn,
NY 66-70; **FEL:** TS/VS, Brooklyn Jewish Hosp,
Brooklyn, NY 70-72; **FAP:** Assoc Clin Prof S Cornell
U; **HOSP:** New York Methodist Hosp; *SI: Bypass
Surgery—Angioplasty; Thoracoscopy-Aneurysm;*
HMO: Empire Blue Cross & Shield GHI CIGNA
Oxford United Healthcare +

LANG: Kor, Itl, Sp; 🔲 🏧 📞 🔳 🔳 🔳 💲 Mcr Mod wc
Immediately

Weiser, Robert (MD) GVS
Long Island Coll Hosp
107 Joralemon St FL1; Brooklyn, NY 11201; (718)
797-1101; **BDCERT:** S 84; **MS:** Albert Einstein Coll
Med 77; **RES:** S, Albert Einstein Med Ctr, Bronx, NY
77-82; **FEL:** GVS, Albert Einstein Med Ctr, Bronx,
NY 82-83; **FAP:** Assoc SUNY Hlth Sci Ctr; **HMO:**
Oxford Prucare NYLCare CIGNA HIP Network +

LANG: Itl, Sp; 📞 🔳 🔳 🔳 💲 Mcr A Few Days

QUEENS COUNTY

CATHOLIC MEDICAL CENTER OF BROOKLYN AND QUEENS

88-25 153 STREET
JAMAICA, NEW YORK 11432
PHONE (718) 558-6900 • FAX (718) 558-7286

ponsorship	Voluntary Not-for-Profit
eds	1,104 acute – 603 long-term care
ccreditation	Joint Commission on Accreditation of Healthcare Organizations (JCAHO)

Ve, the healthcare arm of the Roman Catholic Diocese of Brooklyn, own and manage four acute care hos-
itals, three long-term care facilities and an extensive network of family health centers. We operate one
f the largest hospital-based home health agencies in the country.

he acute care hospitals include: Mary Immaculate Hospital in Jamaica, St. Joseph's Hospital in Flushing,
t. John's Queens Hospital in Elmhurst and St. Mary's Hospital of Brooklyn. Nursing homes include:
ishop Mugavero Center for Geriatric Care and Holy Family Home in Brooklyn and Monsignor
itzpatrick Skilled Nursing Pavilion in Queens. Some 1,600 physicians, both voluntary and salaried, are
ffiliated with CMC.

MC serves as the Brooklyn and Queens campus of the Albert Einstein College of Medicine and offers
esidency programs in eight areas of medical specialty. Over 240 physicians are currently training in these
esidency and fellowship programs. We also operate a school of nursing, an emergency medical services
nstitute and sponsor physician assistant, radiography, medical technologist, and pathologist's assistant
raining programs.

rimary Care	Our Family Health Care Network delivers comprehensive primary care services to residents of Brooklyn and Queens within their own neighborhoods, close to their homes and offices. We are committed to extending high quality medical services in underserved areas.
mergency	Mary Immaculate Hospital serves as a Regional Level I Trauma Center for central Queens and regularly treats the most critical emergencies with skill and compassion. The emergency department at St. John's Queens Hospital is a certified cardiac care center. Both hospitals offer Family Med Express units to "fast track" patients who are not too seriously ill or injured.
ancer Care	Mary Immaculate Hospital also houses the CMC Cancer Institute, a facility that delivers technologically advanced therapy.
adiology	CMC houses the only Radiology Department in a NYC hospital to enjoy full accreditation by the American College of Radiology and among the first in the country to obtain certification of stereotactic breast biopsy. Its accredited vascular lab permits the non-invasive assessment of veins and arteries, and its MRI unit at St. John's Queens Hospital can perform specialized brain sequences in addition to standard examinations.
phthalmology	St. Joseph's Hospital houses a highly acclaimed Eye Care Center offering the most advanced diagnostic and treatment services.
rthopedics	St. John's Queens Hospital offers a multidiscipline care plan for hip and knee replacement elective surgery, proven to help accelerate the rehabilitation process.
ong Term Care	Our reputation for delivering outstanding long-term care has been well earned. Residents at these facilities receive the highest quality care in a supportive environment.
hysician Referral	(888) 262-4433

Specialties in capital letters indicate Primary Care Specialties. However, many doctors will be certified in a subspecialty, but will practice predominantly primary care medicine. In our lists this will be indicated.

*Oncologists deal with Cancer

ADOLESCENT MEDICINE

Jacobson, Marc S (MD) AM
Long Island Jewish Med Ctr

Schneider Children's Hospital, 269-01 76th Ave;
New Hyde Park, NY 11040; (718) 470-3274;
BDCERT: Ped 83; **MS:** Univ Kans Sch Med 73; **RES:**
U Kansas, Kansas City, KS 73-77; **FEL:** U MD Hosp,
Baltimore, MD 77-79; **FAP:** Prof Albert Einstein
Coll Med; *SI: Cholesterol; Obesity and Nutrition*

🔲 🔲 🔲 🔲 🔲 🔲 A Few Days 🔲 *VISA* 🔲

ALLERGY & IMMUNOLOGY

Bernstein, Larry (MD) A&I
Montefiore Med Ctr

110-55 72nd Rd L1; Flushing, NY 11375; (718)
544-6641; **BDCERT:** A&I 85; **MS:** Albert Einstein
Coll Med 58; **RES:** Ped, Jacobi Med Ctr, Bronx, NY
77-81; **FEL:** A&I, Albert Einstein Med Ctr, Bronx,
NY 81-83; **FAP:** Assoc Clin Prof; **HOSP:** NY Hosp
Med Ctr of Queens; *SI: Asthma; Recurrent Sinusitis;*
HMO: GHI Blue Choice Oxford US Hlthcre +

🔲 🔲 🔲 🔲 🔲 🔲 🔲 A Few Days

Bonagura, Vincent R (MD) A&I
Long Island Jewish Med Ctr

Long Island Jewish Med Ctr, 269-01 76th Ave;
New Hyde Park, NY 11040; (718) 470-3300;
BDCERT: Ped 80; A&I 81; **MS:** Columbia P&S 75;
RES: Ped, Columbia-Presbyterian Med Ctr, New
York, NY 78; **FEL:** A&I, Columbia-Presbyterian Med
Ctr, New York, NY 81; **HMO:** Guardian Magnacare
Multiplan Blue Choice Aetna-US Healthcare +

🔲 🔲 🔲 🔲 🔲 🔲 🔲 🔲 Immediately *VISA* 🔲

Fine, Stanley (MD) A&I
Flushing Hosp Med Ctr

37-31 149th St; Flushing, NY 11354; (718) 358-
5565; **BDCERT:** A&I 72; **MS:** Columbia P&S 57;
RES: Jacobi Med Ctr, Bronx, NY 57-59; Montefiore
Med Ctr, Bronx, NY 61-62; **FEL:** St Luke's Roosevelt
Hosp Ctr, New York, NY 62-63; **FAP:** Assoc Clin
Prof Med Cornell U; **HOSP:** NY Hosp Med Ctr of
Queens; *SI: Asthma; Drug Reactions;* **HMO:** Blue
Cross & Blue Shield CIGNA US Hlthcre Prucare US
Hlthcre +

🔲 🔲 🔲 🔲 🔲 🔲 🔲 A Few Days

Lo Galbo, Peter (MD) A&I
Long Island Jewish Med Ctr

269-01 76th Ave; New Hyde Park, NY 11040;
(718) 470-3300; **BDCERT:** A&I 72; **MS:** SUNY
Hlth Sci Ctr 78; **RES:** Mount Sinai Med Ctr, New
York, NY 78-80; **FEL:** A&I, Duke U Med Ctr,
Durham, NC 80-82; **FAP:** Asst Prof Albert Einstein
Coll Med; **HOSP:** Pascack Valley Hosp; *SI: Asthma;*
Immunodeficiency; **HMO:** US Hlthcre Oxford GHI
Aetna Hlth Plan Blue Cross & Blue Shield +

🔲 🔲 🔲 🔲 🔲 🔲 🔲 A Few Days

Menchell, David (MD) A&I
NY Hosp Med Ctr of Queens

73-03 198th St; Fresh Meadow, NY 11366; (718)
465-4100; **BDCERT:** IM 80; A&I 83; **MS:** NYU Sch
Med 77; **RES:** IM, NY Hosp Med Ctr of Queens,
Flushing, NY 77-80; **FEL:** A&I, NY Hosp Med Ctr of
Queens, Flushing, NY 81-83; **HMO:** GHI
Magnacare Blue Choice Aetna Hlth Plan Oxford +

🔲 🔲 🔲 🔲 🔲 🔲 🔲 🔲 Immediately

Novick, Brian (MD) A&I
Lenox Hill Hosp

Allergy Testing Center, 118-21 Queens Blvd; Forest
Hills, NY 11375; (718) 261-3663; **BDCERT:** A&I
89; Ped 84; **MS:** Mexico 78; **RES:** Ped, Albert
Einstein Med Ctr, Bronx, NY 79-82; Ped, Albert
Einstein Med Ctr, Bronx, NY 80-82; **FEL:** A&I,
Albert Einstein Med Ctr, Bronx, NY 82-84; **FAP:**
Asst Clin Prof Albert Einstein Coll Med; **HOSP:**
Montefiore Med Ctr; *SI: Asthma; Hay Fever;* **HMO:**
Oxford United Healthcare Aetna-US Healthcare
CIGNA Magnacare +

LANG: Sp; 🔲 🔲 🔲 🔲 🔲 🔲 🔲 Immediately 🔲
VISA 🔲 🔲

Guide to symbols and abbreviations can be found on pages 110-113.

559

Siegal, Frederick P (MD) A&I
Long Island Jewish Med Ctr

Division of Hem/Onc, Long Island Jewish Hospital Med Ctr,; New Hyde Park, NY 11040; (718) 470-8930; **BDCERT:** IM 71; A&I 74; **MS:** Columbia P&S 65; **RES:** IM, Mount Sinai Med Ctr, New York, NY 65-67; IM, Mount Sinai Med Ctr, New York, NY 69-70; **FEL:** Immunology, Rockefeller Univ Hosp, New York, NY 70-73; **FAP:** Prof Med Albert Einstein Coll Med; **SI:** *Primary Immunodeficiencies; AIDS and HIV Infection;* **HMO:** Oxford US Hlthcre Aetna-US Healthcare 1199 Blue Choice +

🚺 📷 🏥 💲 Mcr Mcd WC 2-4 Weeks ▨ **VISA** 💳

CARDIOLOGY (CARDIOVASCULAR DISEASE)

Boal, Bernard (MD) Cv
Catholic Med Ctr Bklyn & Qns

88-25 153rd St 5H; Jamaica, NY 11432; (718) 657-7208; **BDCERT:** IM 70; Cv 75; **MS:** Canada 62; **RES:** IM, Winnipeg Gen Hosp, Winnipeg, Canada 62-63; IM, U UT Hosp, Salt Lake City, UT 64-66; **FEL:** Cv, Bellevue Hosp Ctr, New York, NY 66-68; **FAP:** Assoc Prof Med Albert Einstein Coll Med; **HOSP:** Long Island Jewish Med Ctr; **SI:** *Pacemakers; Heart Disease;* **HMO:** Blue Cross & Blue Choice GHI 32BJ Fidelis

🚺 📷 🚹 🏥 💲 Mcr WC 2-4 Weeks

Bodenheimer, Monty (MD) Cv
Long Island Jewish Med Ctr

LI Jewish Hospital, 270-05 76th Ave Rm 2135; New Hyde Park, NY 11040; (516) 470-7331; **BDCERT:** IM 72; Cv 75; **MS:** U Manitoba 69; **RES:** Sinai Hosp of Baltimore, Baltimore, MD 7-73; **FEL:** Cv, Mt Sinai Med Ctr, New York, NY 72-73

Hsueh, John Tzu-Lang (MD) Cv
NY Hosp Med Ctr of Queens

43-45 Parsons Blvd; Flushing, NY 11355; (718) 886-6400; **BDCERT:** IM 75; Cv 79; **MS:** Taiwan 70; **RES:** IM, Flushing Hosp Med Ctr, Flushing, NY 72-76; **FEL:** Cv, Wayne Cnty Gen Hosp, Detroit, MI 76-78; **FAP:** Clin Instr SUNY Stony Brook; **HOSP:** Flushing Hosp Med Ctr

Jaitly, Sharad (MD) Cv
NY Hosp Med Ctr of Queens

132-26 Booth Memorial Ave; Flushing, NY 11355; (718) 463-5874; **BDCERT:** IM 87; Cv 91; **MS:** India 77; **RES:** Cv, NY Hosp-Cornell Med Ctr, New York, NY 86-88; Cv, Mem Sloan Kettering Cancer Ctr, New York, NY 86-88; **FEL:** Cv, Kingsbrook Jewish Med Ctr, Brooklyn, NY 85-86

Koss, Jerome (MD) Cv
Long Island Jewish Med Ctr

Cardiology, 270-05 76th Ave; New Hyde Park, NY 11040; (718) 470-7340; **BDCERT:** IM 77; Cv 81; **MS:** Albert Einstein Coll Med 74; **RES:** Jacobi Med Ctr, Bronx, NY; **FEL:** Montefiore Med Ctr, Bronx, NY; **HMO:** Blue Cross & Blue Shield PHS US Hlthcre Oxford

🚺 📷 🏥 1 Week

Robbins, Michael (MD) Cv
Mount Sinai Med Ctr

94-36 58th Ave Ste G4; Rego Park, NY 11373; (718) 760-0011; **BDCERT:** IM 84; Cv 87; **MS:** Cornell U 81; **RES:** IM, Albert Einstein Med Ctr, Bronx, NY 81-85; **FEL:** Cv, Mount Sinai Med Ctr, New York, NY 85-87; **FAP:** Asst Clin Prof Mt Sinai Sch Med; **HOSP:** St John's Queens Hosp; **SI:** *Echocardiography;* **HMO:** Blue Cross & Blue Shield Oxford Aetna-US Healthcare GHI +

🚺 📷 🏥 💲 Mcr 1 Week

Rydzinski, Mayer (MD) **Cv**
Parkway Hosp
70-31 108th St Suite 7; Forest Hills, NY 11375; (718) 268-7633; **BDCERT:** IM 79; Cv 81; **MS:** Albert Einstein Coll Med 76; **RES:** Metropolitan Hosp Ctr, New York, NY 76-77; Montefiore Med Ctr, Bronx, NY 77-79; **FEL:** Cv, Long Island Jewish Med Ctr, New Hyde Park, NY 79-81; **HOSP:** St Francis Hosp-Roslyn; **HMO:** Oxford GHI US Hlthcre

♿ ☎ 👤 📅 $ [Mcr] 2-4 Weeks

Siskind, Steven Jay (MD) **Cv**
NY Hosp Med Ctr of Queens
56-45 Main St; Flushing, NY 11355; (718) 670-1234; **BDCERT:** Cv 81; **MS:** Albert Einstein Coll Med 76; **RES:** Jacobi Med Ctr, Bronx, NY 76-79; **FEL:** Cv, Albert Einstein Med Ctr, Bronx, NY 79-81; **FAP:** Asst Prof Cornell U; **HOSP:** NY Hosp-Cornell Med Ctr; ***SI:*** *Angina; Congenital Heart Failure*; **HMO:** Blue Choice Blue Cross & Blue Shield Oxford Aetna Hlth Plan GHI +

LANG: Sp, Rus; ♿ ☾ ☎ 👤 📅 [Mcr] [WC] Immediately

Tenet, William (MD) **Cv**
NY Hosp Med Ctr of Queens
Cardiovascular Associates of New York, 200-12 44th Ave; Flushing, NY 11361; (718) 423-3355; **BDCERT:** IM 83; Cv 87; **MS:** Italy 80; **RES:** NY Hosp Med Ctr of Queens, Flushing, NY 80-84; **FEL:** Cv, U Conn Hlth Ctr, Farmington, CT 84-86; **FAP:** Asst Clin Prof Med Cornell U; **HOSP:** NY Hosp-Cornell Med Ctr; ***SI:*** *Congestive Heart Failure; Coronary Artery Disease*; **HMO:** CIGNA NYLCare Oxford Blue Cross & Blue Shield Aetna Hlth Plan +

LANG: Grk, Itl, Sp; ♿ ☾ ☎ 👤 📅 [Mcr] [Mcd] 1 Week

Termine, Charles (MD) **Cv**
St Joseph's Hosp-Queens
87-47 Myrtle Ave; Glendale, NY 11385; (718) 849-8609; **BDCERT:** IM 64; **MS:** SUNY Downstate 54; **RES:** Brooklyn Hosp Ctr, Brooklyn, NY 55-58

☾ ☎ 👤 📅 $ [WC]

Visco, Ferdinand (MD) **Cv**
St John's Queens Hosp
90-02 Queens Blvd; Elmhurst, NY 11373; (718) 558-1830; **BDCERT:** IM 73; Cv 77; **MS:** Italy 69; **RES:** Flushing Hosp Med Ctr, Flushing, NY 69-70; IM, Queens Hosp Ctr, Jamaica, NY 70-72; **FEL:** Cv, Nassau County Med Ctr, East Meadow, NY 72-74; **HOSP:** Catholic Med Ctr Bklyn & Qns; **HMO:** Independent Health Plan Blue Choice Blue Cross & Blue Shield Metlife

LANG: Itl, Sp; ♿ ☾ ☎ 👤 📅 $ [Mcr] [Mcd] 1 Week

Weg, Ira (MD) **Cv**
Long Island Jewish Med Ctr
270-01 76th Ave; New Hyde Park, NY 11040; (718) 470-7331; **BDCERT:** IM 79; Cv 81; **MS:** SUNY Hlth Sci Ctr 76; **RES:** IM, Kings County Hosp Ctr, Brooklyn, NY 76-79; **FEL:** Cv, Montefiore Med Ctr, Bronx, NY 79-81; **FAP:** Asst Prof Albert Einstein Coll Med; **HMO:** Oxford US Hlthcre Magnacare

♿ ☎ 📅 $ [Mcr] Immediately ***VISA***

CHILD & ADOLESCENT PSYCHIATRY

Foley, Carmel (MD) **ChAP**
Long Island Jewish Med Ctr
Div of Child & Adolescent Psychiatry, 269-01 76th Ave; New Hyde Park, NY 11040; (718) 470-3510; **BDCERT:** Psyc 79; ChAP 81; **MS:** Ireland 72; **RES:** Ireland 73-76; Lafayette Clin, Detroit, MI 76-78; **FEL:** ChAP, Long Island Jewish Med Ctr, New Hyde Park, NY; **HMO:** Oxford PHS

CHILD NEUROLOGY

Novak, Gerald P (MD)   ChiN
Long Island Jewish Med Ctr
76th Ave Rm 261; New Hyde Park, NY 11040;
(718) 470-3450; **BDCERT:** Ped 82; ChiN 86; **MS:**
Albert Einstein Coll Med 77; **RES:** Ped, Children's
Hosp of Philadelphia, Philadelphia, PA; **FEL:** ChiN,
Albert Einstein Med Ctr, Bronx, NY 80-83; Clinical
Neurophysiology, Albert Einstein Med Ctr, Bronx,
NY 83-85; **FAP:** Asst Prof Albert Einstein Coll Med;
SI: Epilepsy; Attention Deficit Disorder; **HMO:** US
Hlthcre Oxford GHI Blue Choice CIGNA +

LANG: Rus, Chi, Heb; ⬛ ⬛ ⬛ ⬛ 2-4 Weeks ⬛
VISA ⬛ ⬛

COLON & RECTAL SURGERY

Golub, Robert (MD)   CRS
Flushing Hosp Med Ctr
Flushing Surgical PC, 146-01 45th Ave 211;
Flushing, NY 11355; (718) 670-3137; **BDCERT:**
CRS 88; **MS:** Albert Einstein Coll Med 81; **RES:**
Montefiore Med Ctr, Bronx, NY 81-83; Westchester
County Med Ctr, Valhalla, NY 83-86; **FEL:** CRS,
Grant Hosp, Columbus, OH 86-87; **FAP:** Asst Prof S
Cornell U; **HOSP:** NY Hosp Med Ctr of Queens; *SI:*
Colon Cancer; Hemorrhoids; **HMO:** US Hlthcre Oxford
Multiplan GHI Guardian +

⬛ ⬛ ⬛ ⬛ ⬛ ⬛ ⬛ ⬛ ⬛ A Few Days

Tiszenkel, Howard (MD)   CRS
NY Hosp Med Ctr of Queens
56-45 Main St; Flushing, NY 11355; (718) 445-
0220; **BDCERT:** CRS 88; S 96; **MS:** NY Med Coll 81;
RES: S, St Luke's Roosevelt Hosp Ctr, New York, NY
81-86; CRS, U IL Med Ctr, Chicago, IL 86-87

CRITICAL CARE MEDICINE

Brady, Terence (MD)   CCM
NY Hosp Med Ctr of Queens
56-45 Main St; Flushing, NY 11355; (718) 670-
1072; **BDCERT:** IM 87; CCM 89; **MS:** West Indies
83; **RES:** IM, NY Hosp Med Ctr of Queens, Flushing,
NY 84-87; **FEL:** CCM, NY Hosp Med Ctr of Queens,
Flushing, NY 87-88; **FAP:** Asst Clin Prof Med
Cornell U; **HMO:** Aetna Hlth Plan Blue Cross & Blue
Shield

⬛ ⬛ ⬛ ⬛ ⬛ ⬛ 2-4 Weeks

DERMATOLOGY

Beyda, Bernadette (MD)   D
NY Hosp Med Ctr of Queens
141-23 59th Ave; Flushing, NY 11355; (718)
445-0566; **BDCERT:** D 82; **MS:** France 76; **RES:**
IM, NY Hosp Med Ctr of Queens, Flushing, NY 77-
78; D, NY Hosp-Cornell Med Ctr, New York, NY 79-
82; **HOSP:** NY Hosp-Cornell Med Ctr; **HMO:** Aetna
Hlth Plan Empire Blue Cross & Shield Blue Cross &
Blue Shield GHI Oxford +

LANG: Fr, Sp, Rus, Tag; ⬛ ⬛ ⬛ ⬛ ⬛ ⬛ ⬛
A Few Days

Hisler, Barbara (MD)   D
Long Island Jewish Med Ctr
270-05 76th Ave; New Hyde Park, NY 11040;
(718) 470-4426; **BDCERT:** D 89; IM 86; **MS:** NY
Med Coll 83; **RES:** Long Island Jewish Med Ctr, New
Hyde Park, NY 83-85; **FEL:** Detroit Med Ctr, Detroit,
MI 86-88; **FAP:** Assoc Lecturer Med Albert Einstein
Coll Med; **HMO:** Oxford Blue Cross & Blue Shield
Empire Sel Pro

⬛ ⬛ ⬛ ⬛ ⬛ ⬛ 1 Week *VISA* ⬛

Pereira, Frederick (MD)   **D**
NY Hosp Med Ctr of Queens
51-14 Kissena Blvd; Flushing, NY 11355; (718)
359-4425; **BDCERT:** D 75; **MS:** UMDNJ-NJ Med
Sch, Newark 68; **RES:** Mount Sinai Med Ctr, New
York, NY 72-74; Metropolitan Hosp Ctr, New York,
NY 74-75; **HOSP:** Flushing Hosp Med Ctr; **SI:** *Skin
Cancer and Growths; Herpes and Venereal Disease*;
HMO: Oxford Aetna Hlth Plan GHI MDNY Blue
Cross +

⬧ ▣ ▣ ▦ ▣ ▨ ▨   2-4 Weeks

DIAGNOSTIC RADIOLOGY

Herman, Peter (MD)   **DR**
Long Island Jewish Med Ctr
21 Beverly Rd; Great Neck, NY 11021; (718) 470-
7175; **BDCERT:** Rad 62; **MS:** Hungary 55; **RES:**
Kings County Hosp Ctr, Brooklyn, NY 57-58; Rad,
Kings County Hosp Ctr, Brooklyn, NY 58-61; **FAP:**
Prof Rad Albert Einstein Coll Med

Mollin, Joel (MD)   **DR**
Elmhurst Hosp Ctr
79-01 Broadway;Elmhurst, NY 11373; (718) 334-
2062; **BDCERT:** Psyc 76; Rad 85; **MS:** SUNY
Downstate 69; **RES:** DR, Mount Sinai Med Ctr, New
York, NY 81-83; DR, USPHS Hosp, Baltimore, MD
79-81

EMERGENCY MEDICINE

Sixsmith, Diane (MD)   **EM**
NY Hosp Med Ctr of Queens
Emergency Practice Plan/NY HospQueens, 56-45
Main St; Flushing, NY 11355; (718) 670-1426;
BDCERT: EM 96; IM 76; **MS:** Univ Pittsburgh 73;
RES: IM, Harlem Hosp Ctr, New York, NY 73-76;
FAP: Asst Clin Prof Cornell U; **HOSP:** Flushing Hosp
Med Ctr; **HMO:** Oxford NYLCare Aetna Hlth Plan
US Hlthcre GHI +

ENDOCRINOLOGY, DIABETES & METABOLISM

Arevalo, Carlos (MD)   **EDM**
Mary Immaculate Hosp
40-45 78th St Fl 1; Garden City, NY 11530; (718)
446-2626; **BDCERT:** IM 79; EDM 87; **MS:** Peru 74;
RES: IM, Elmhurst Hosp Ctr, Elmhurst, NY 75-78;
IM, Elmhurst Hosp Ctr, Elmhurst, NY 75-78; **FEL:**
EDM, New York University Med Ctr, New York, NY
79-80; **FAP:** Asst Clin Prof Med Albert Einstein Coll
Med; **HOSP:** St John's Queens Hosp; **SI:** *Osteoporosis;
Thyroid Disorders*; **HMO:** Blue Choice United
Healthcare Oxford US Hlthcre Multiplan +

LANG: Sp; ▣ ▣ ▣ ▦ ▦ ▣ ▨   A Few Days

Kukar, Narinder (MD)   **EDM**
Wyckoff Heights Med Ctr
68-15 Central Ave; Flushing, NY 11385; (718)
497-0060; **BDCERT:** IM 77; EDM 81; **MS:** India 60;
RES: IM, Wycoff Heights, Brooklyn, NY 66-69; **FEL:**
EDM, SUNY Downstate, Brooklyn, NY 69-71; **FAP:**
Asst Prof Med SUNY Hlth Sci Ctr; **HOSP:** Jamaica
Med Ctr; **SI:** *Diabetes; Thyroid Diseases*; **HMO:** Oxford
Blue Cross & Blue Choice Chubb

LANG: Hin, Ur, Rom, Sp; ▣ ▣ ▣ ▦ ▦ ▣ ▨
A Few Days

Lorber, Daniel (MD)   **EDM**
NY Hosp Med Ctr of Queens
59-45 161st St; Flushing, NY 11365; (718) 762-
3111; **BDCERT:** IM 75; EDM 77; **MS:** Albert
Einstein Coll Med 72; **RES:** Jacobi Med Ctr, Bronx,
NY 72-75; Albert Einstein Med Ctr, Bronx, NY 72-
75; **FEL:** EDM, Vanderbilt U Med Ctr, Nashville, TN
75-77; **FAP:** Assoc Clin Prof Cornell U; **HOSP:**
Flushing Hosp Med Ctr; **SI:** *Diabetes; Thyroid Disease*;
HMO: Oxford Prudential CIGNA Blue Shield
Magnacare +

LANG: Sp; ⬧ ▣ ▣ ▦ ▦ ▣ ▨   2-4 Weeks **VISA**
▣

Rosman, Lawrence (MD)   EDM
Parkway Hosp
Osteoporosis Center Of Queens, 112-03 Queens Blvd 207; Flushing, NY 11375; (718) 263-3718; **BDCERT:** IM 78; EDM 83; **MS:** NYU Sch Med 75; **RES:** IM, New York University Med Ctr, New York, NY 76-77; IM, New York University Med Ctr, New York, NY 77-78; **FEL:** EDM, New York University Med Ctr, New York, NY 78; **FAP:** Asst Clin Prof Med NYU Sch Med; **SI:** *Thyroid Disease; Osteoporosis;* **HMO:** GHI Magnacare Multiplan

LANG: Sp, Prt, Rom, Yd, Ger; 🔾 🔾 🔾 🔾 🔾 🔾 🔾 1 Week

Tibaldi, Joseph (MD)   EDM
Flushing Hosp Med Ctr
59-45 161st St; Flushing, NY 11365; (718) 762-3111; **BDCERT:** IM 82; EDM 85; **MS:** Mt Sinai Sch Med 79; **RES:** Nassau County Med Ctr, East Meadow, NY 80-81; Mount Sinai Med Ctr, New York, NY 81-82; **FEL:** EDM, Montefiore Med Ctr, Bronx, NY 82-83; **HOSP:** NY Hosp Med Ctr of Queens; **SI:** *Thyroid; Diabetes;* **HMO:** NYLCare Oxford Magnacare CIGNA Blue Choice +

LANG: Sp; 🔾 🔾 🔾 🔾 🔾 🔾 🔾 2-4 Weeks

FAMILY PRACTICE

Birrer, Richard (MD)   FP   PCP
Catholic Med Ctr Bklyn & Qns
88-25 153rd St; Jamaica, NY 11432; (718) 558-6929; **BDCERT:** EM 82; FP 83; **MS:** Cornell U 75; **RES:** FP, Univ Hosp SUNY Bklyn, Brooklyn, NY 79-81; **FAP:** Assoc Prof Albert Einstein Coll Med; **SI:** *Emergency Medicine; Sports Medicine*

🔾 🔾 🔾 🔾 🔾 🔾 🔾 🔾 🔾 Immediately

Ciuffo, Joseph (MD)   FP   PCP
St John's Queens Hosp
73-01 Grand Ave; Flushing, NY 11378; (718) 457-5900; **BDCERT:** FP 98; **MS:** SUNY Downstate 83; **RES:** Brookdale Univ Hosp Med Ctr, Brooklyn, NY 83-86; **HOSP:** NY Hosp Med Ctr of Queens; **SI:** *General Family Practice;* **HMO:** Oxford Aetna Hlth Plan GHI US Hlthcre

🔾 🔾 🔾 🔾 🔾 🔾 🔾 🔾 🔾 1 Week

Di Scala, Reno (MD)   FP   PCP
Western Queens Comm Hosp
Steinway Medical Group, 22-02 Steinway St; Long Island City, NY 11105; (718) 721-3330; **BDCERT:** FP 88; FP 94; **MS:** Italy 82; **RES:** FP, Community Hosp, Glen Cove, NY 85-87; S, Catholic Med Ctr Bklyn & Qns, Jamaica, NY 82-85; **HOSP:** N Shore Univ Hosp-Forest Hills; **HMO:** Oxford Aetna-US Healthcare Magnacare PHS GHI +

LANG: Itl, Sp; 🔾 🔾 🔾 🔾 🔾 🔾 🔾 1 Week

Douglas, Montgomery (MD) FP   PCP
Mary Immaculate Hosp
258-11 147th Ave Fl 1; Rosedale, NY 11422; (718) 276-4036; **BDCERT:** FP 89; **MS:** Cornell U 86; **RES:** FP, Rochester Gen Hosp, Rochester, NY 86-89; **FAP:** Instr FP Albert Einstein Coll Med; **HOSP:** St John's Queens Hosp; **SI:** *Obstetrics in Family Practice;* **HMO:** Oxford Aetna Hlth Plan PHCS CIGNA 1199 +

LANG: Sp, Fr; 🔾 🔾 🔾 🔾 🔾 🔾 A Few Days 🔾 *VISA* 🔾 🔾

Fisher, George (MD)   FP   PCP
Western Queens Comm Hosp
22-33 33rd St; Long Island City, NY 11106; (718) 726-1000; **BDCERT:** FP 93; **MS:** England 79; **RES:** FP, St Joseph Medical Center-Yonkers, Yonkers, NY 90-93

Istrico, Richard A (DO)   FP   PCP
Long Island Jewish Med Ctr
158-01 Crossbay Blvd; Jamaica, NY 11414; (718) 738-9115; **BDCERT:** FP 81; SM 95; **MS:** Philadelphia Coll Osteo Med 78; **RES:** Interboro Gen Hosp, Brooklyn, NY; Baptist Med Ctr, Brooklyn, NY; **FAP:** Adjct Clin Prof NY Coll Osteo Med; **HOSP:** Parkway Hosp; **SI:** *Sports Injuries;* **HMO:** Oxford CIGNA Select Prudential Merit Behavioral Health Plans +

🔾 🔾 🔾 🔾 🔾 🔾 Immediately

Langman, Ronald (DO)   FP   **PCP**
Parkway Hosp
74-01 Myrtle Ave; Glendale, NY 11385; (718) 821-5500; **BDCERT:** FP 95; **MS:** Univ Osteo Med & Hlth Sci 92; **RES:** Peninsula Hosp Ctr, Far Rockaway, NY 93-95; **HOSP:** Peninsula Hosp Ctr; *SI: Preventive Medicine; Weight Loss;* **HMO:** GHI Aetna-US Healthcare Oxford

LANG: Sp, Grk; 🔲 🔲 🔲 🔲 🔲 🔲 🔲 🔲 🔲 Immediately ▦ **VISA** 💳

Molnar, Thomas (MD)   FP   **PCP**
NY Hosp Med Ctr of Queens
83-39 Daniels St; Jamaica, NY 11435; (718) 291-5151; **BDCERT:** FP 88; FP 95; **MS:** Hungary 82; **RES:** S, Flushing Hosp Med Ctr, Flushing, NY 82-85; FP, Univ Hosp SUNY Bklyn, Brooklyn, NY 85-88; **HOSP:** Flushing Hosp Med Ctr; *SI: Hypertension; Diabetes;* **HMO:** Oxford US Hlthcre CIGNA Blue Shield Aetna Hlth Plan +

LANG: Hun; 🔲 🔲 🔲 🔲 🔲 🔲 🔲 🔲 A Few Days

Muraca, Glenn (DO)   FP   **PCP**
Parkway Hosp
Woodhaven Medical Ctr, 86-18 Jamaica Ave; Woodhaven, NY 11421; (718) 805-0037; **MS:** NY Coll Osteo Med 90; **RES:** Peninsula Hosp Ctr, Far Rockaway, NY; **HOSP:** Catholic Med Ctr Bklyn & Qns; *SI: Sports Medicine; Nutritional Medicine;* **HMO:** NYLCare CIGNA GHI US Hlthcre Oxford +

LANG: Itl, Rus, Sp, Grk; 🔲 🔲 🔲 🔲 🔲 🔲 🔲 🔲 🔲 🔲 Immediately **VISA** 💳 💳

Patton-Greenidge, Loretta (MD) FP   **PCP**
Catholic Med Ctr Bklyn & Qns
88-25 153rd; Jamaica, NY 11432; (718) 558-7160; **BDCERT:** FP 94; **MS:** Albany Med Coll 78; **RES:** FP, Brookdale Univ Hosp Med Ctr, Brooklyn, NY 79-81; **HOSP:** Mary Immaculate Hosp; **HMO:** US Hlthcre CIGNA Oxford GHI NYLCare +

Reddy, Malikar Juna (MD)   FP   **PCP**
St Joseph's Hosp-Queens
Flushing Primary Care, 72-18 164th St; Flushing, NY 11365; (718) 969-6640; **BDCERT:** FP 96; **MS:** India 82; **RES:** FP, Mary Immaculate Hospital, New York, NY 86-90; *SI: Geriatrics*

LANG: Hin, Tel; 🔲 🔲 🔲 🔲 🔲 🔲 🔲 A Few Days

GASTROENTEROLOGY

Bank, Simmy (MD)   Ge
Long Island Jewish Med Ctr
270-05 76th Ave; New Hyde Park, NY 11040; (718) 470-4692; **MS:** South Africa 54; **RES:** Cape Town, South Africa; London, England; **FEL:** Cape Town, South Africa; **HMO:** Oxford US Hlthcre Empire Sanus-NYLCare

LANG: Heb, Grk; 🔲 🔲 🔲 🔲 🔲 🔲 🔲 A Few Days

Blumstein, Meyer (MD)   Ge
Long Island Jewish Med Ctr
270-05 76th Ave; New Hyde Park, NY 11040; (718) 470-7281; **BDCERT:** IM 89; Ge 91; **MS:** SUNY Hlth Sci Ctr 86; **RES:** Long Island Jewish Med Ctr, New Hyde Park, NY 86-89; **FEL:** Long Island Jewish Med Ctr, New Hyde Park, NY 89-91; *SI: Endoscopy; Liver Disease;* **HMO:** Oxford GHI Blue Choice US Hlthcre Empire +

🔲 🔲 🔲 🔲 🔲 🔲 🔲 🔲 🔲 A Few Days **VISA** 💳

Greenberg, Ronald (MD)   Ge
Long Island Jewish Med Ctr
Long Island Jewish Med Ctr—Dept of Medicine, Rm 8205; New Hyde Park, NY 11040; (718) 470-7281; **BDCERT:** IM 82; Ge 85; **MS:** Hahnemann U 79; **RES:** Albany Med Ctr, Albany, NY 79-82; **FEL:** Ge, St Luke's Roosevelt Hosp Ctr, New York, NY 82-85; **FAP:** Assoc Clin Prof Med Albert Einstein Coll Med; *SI: Inflammatory Bowel Disease; Peptic Ulcer Disease;* **HMO:** Oxford Multiplan US Hlthcre NYLCare Magnacare +

LANG: Grk; 🔲 🔲 🔲 🔲 🔲 2-4 Weeks ▦ **VISA** 💳

Harooni, Robert (MD)   Ge
NY Hosp Med Ctr of Queens
55-16 Main St 1; Flushing, NY 11355; (718) 461-6161; **BDCERT:** IM 81; Ge 85; **MS:** Iran 73; **RES:** IM, Booth Mem Hosp, Flushing, NY 81-82; IM, Booth Mem Hosp, Flushing, NY 82-83; **FEL:** Ge, Booth Mem Hosp, Flushing, NY 83-84; Ge,; **FAP:** Clin Instr Med Cornell U; **SI:** *Prevention of Colon Cancer; Prevention of Peptic Ulcer;* **HMO:** Aetna-US Healthcare Oxford Vytra Blue Choice GHI +

LANG: Per, Trk, Chi; 🕎 💳 🔲 👤 🏠 💲 Mcr Mcd WC NFI A Few Days

Lowy, Robert (MD)   Ge
Long Island Jewish Med Ctr
44-20 Douglaston Pkwy; Douglaston, NY 11363; (718) 478-0330; **BDCERT:** IM 71; Ge 74; **MS:** SUNY Hlth Sci Ctr 59; **RES:** Montefiore Med Ctr, Bronx, NY 60-61; VA Med Ctr-Brooklyn, Brooklyn, NY 61-62; **FEL:** Ge, Montefiore Med Ctr, Bronx, NY 62-63; **FAP:** Asst Prof Med Albert Einstein Coll Med; **HOSP:** NY Hosp Med Ctr of Queens; **SI:** *Liver Disease; Gastrointestinal Endoscopy;* **HMO:** GHI Empire Magnacare US Hlthcre Oxford +

🕎 💳 🔲 👤 🏠 Mcr A Few Days 🔲 **VISA**

Martin, George (MD)   Ge
NY Hosp Med Ctr of Queens
56-28 Main St; Flushing, NY 11355; (718) 939-1800; **BDCERT:** IM 74; Ger 88; **MS:** NYU Sch Med 71; **RES:** Bellevue Hosp Ctr, New York, NY 71-75; **FEL:** Peter Bent Brigham Hosp, Boston, MA 75-76; Bellevue Hosp Ctr, New York, NY 76-77; **FAP:** Asst Prof Cornell U

🔲 👤 🏠 💲 1 Week

Nussbaum, Michel (MD)   Ge
NY Hosp Med Ctr of Queens
142-43 Booth Memorial Ave; Flushing, NY 11355; (718) 886-1919; **BDCERT:** IM 81; Ge 92; **MS:** Belgium 77; **RES:** IM, NY Hosp Med Ctr of Queens, Flushing, NY 77-80; **FEL:** Ge, NY Hosp Med Ctr of Queens, Flushing, NY 80-82; **FAP:** Clin Instr Cornell U; **HOSP:** Flushing Hosp Med Ctr; **SI:** *Gastrointestinal Endoscopy; Inflammation Bowel Disease;* **HMO:** Prucare Empire Blue Choice Aetna Hlth Plan Oxford GHI +

LANG: Fr; 🔲 👤 🏠 💲 Mcr Mcd 1 Week

Ramgopal, Mekala (MD)   Ge   PCP
St John's Epis Hosp-S Shore
21-24 Camp Rd; Far Rockaway, NY 11691; (718) 327-0207; **BDCERT:** Ge 79; Ger 88; **MS:** India 74; **RES:** IM, Jersey City Med Ctr, Jersey City, NJ 75-76; IM, VA Med Ctr-Bronx, Bronx, NY 76-77; **FEL:** Ge, Univ of Med & Dent NJ Hosp, Newark, NJ 77-79; **HOSP:** Peninsula Hosp Ctr; **HMO:** Blue Choice Oxford NYLCare 1199 GHI +

🕎 🍴 💳 🔲 👤 🏠 💲 Mcr Immediately

Rand, James (MD)   Ge
Flushing Hosp Med Ctr
Solo Practition, 200-12 44th Ave; Bayside, NY 11361; (718) 224-7454; **BDCERT:** IM 78; Ge 81; **MS:** Albert Einstein Coll Med 75; **RES:** Med, Strong Mem Hosp, Rochester, NY 76-77; Med, Columbia-Presbyterian Med Ctr, New York, NY 77-78; **FEL:** Ge, Montefiore Med Ctr, Bronx, NY 78-80; **HOSP:** NY Hosp Med Ctr of Queens; **HMO:** Aetna Hlth Plan Blue Choice Blue Cross & Blue Shield Oxford GHI +

🕎 💳 🔲 🏠 💲 Mcr Immediately **VISA** 🔲

Rosman, Sidney (MD)   Ge
Parkway Hosp
112-03 Queens Blvd 207; Flushing, NY 11375; (718) 544-7077; **BDCERT:** Ge 80; **MS:** Albert Einstein Coll Med 78; **RES:** VA Med Ctr-Manh, New York, NY; **FEL:** Ge, VA Med Ctr-Manh, New York, NY; **HOSP:** Catholic Med Ctr Bklyn & Qns

🕎 💳 🔲 🏠 Mcr 1 Week

Safier, Henry L (MD)   Ge
NY Hosp Med Ctr of Queens
71-46 110th St; Forest Hills, NY 11375; (718) 261-2500; **BDCERT:** IM 76; Ge 79; **MS:** Switzerland 60; **RES:** IM, VA Med Ctr-Brooklyn, Brooklyn, NY 63-64; IM, Long Island Jewish Med Ctr, New Hyde Park, NY 64-65; **FEL:** VA Med Ctr-Brooklyn, Brooklyn, NY 65-66; Liver Disease, VA Med Ctr-Brooklyn, Brooklyn, NY 70; **HOSP:** Parkway Hosp

Weg, Arnold (MD)   Ge   `PCP`
NYU Downtown Hosp
71-36 110th St 1G; Flushing, NY 11375; (718)
520-2210; **BDCERT:** IM 85; **MS:** NYU Sch Med 82;
RES: Columbia-Presbyterian Med Ctr, New York,
NY 83-85; **FEL:** Ge, NY Hosp-Cornell Med Ctr, New
York, NY 85; **FAP:** Instr Med Cornell U; **HMO:** Blue
Choice Empire Oxford GHI

LANG: Sp; 🔲 🔲 💲 4+ Weeks ▦

GERIATRIC PSYCHIATRY

Greenwald, Blaine (MD) GerPsy
Long Island Jewish Med Ctr
75-59 263rd St; Glen Oaks, NY 11004; (718) 470-
8159; **BDCERT:** Psyc 83; GerPsy 91; **MS:** NY Med
Coll 78; **RES:** Psyc, Mount Sinai Med Ctr, New York,
NY 79-82; **FEL:** GerPsy, Mount Sinai Med Ctr, New
York, NY 82-83; **FAP:** Assoc Prof Psyc Albert
Einstein Coll Med; **SI:** *Late Life Depression; Dementia*

🔲 🔲 🔲 ▦ 2-4 Weeks

Shelley, Gabriella (MD) GerPsy
Western Queens Comm Hosp
Senior Health Care Center, 27-15 30th Ave; Long
Island City, NY 11102; (718) 932-0007; **BDCERT:**
Psyc 96; GerPsy 97; **MS:** Albert Einstein Coll Med
89; **RES:** Yale Univ Hosp, New Haven, CT 90-93;
FEL: GerPsy, McLean Hosp-Harvard, Belmont, MA
93-94; **FAP:** Asst Prof Psyc Mt Sinai Sch Med; **SI:**
Post Traumatic Stress Disorders

🔲 🔲 🔲 ▦ 1 Week

GYNECOLOGIC ONCOLOGY

Serur, Eli (MD)   GO
Brooklyn Hosp Ctr-Caledonian
30-94 Judith Drive; Bellmore, NY 11710; (718)
250-8106; **BDCERT:** ObG 92; GO 97; **MS:** NYU Sch
Med 85; **RES:** ObG, Kings County Hosp Ctr,
Brooklyn, NY 85-89; ObG, Kings County Hosp Ctr,
Brooklyn, NY 89-91; **FAP:** Assoc Prof Cornell U;
HOSP: St Vincents Hosp & Med Ctr NY; **SI:**
Endometrial Cancer; Laparoscopy; **HMO:** Oxford GHI
US Hlthcre HIP Network CIGNA +

🔲 🔲 🔲 ▦ ▦ ▦ ▦ 1 Week

HAND SURGERY

Eswar, Sounder (MD)   HS
Mary Immaculate Hosp
157-48 85th St; Howard Beach, NY 11414; (718)
738-6223; **BDCERT:** OrS 75; **MS:** India 70; **RES:**
New York Methodist Hosp, Brooklyn, NY 69-70;
Mary Immaculate Hosp, Jamaica, NY 70-73; **FEL:**
HS, Hosp For Joint Diseases, New York, NY; **HOSP:**
St Joseph's Hosp-Queens; **SI:** *Joint Replacements;
Hand Surgery*; **HMO:** Oxford US Hlthcre Blue Choice
Prucare CIGNA +

🔲 🔲 🔲 🔲 💲 ▦ ▦ ▦ A Few Days ***VISA*** 💳 💳

Roger, Ignatius Daniel (MD) HS
St John's Queens Hosp
69-40 108th St; Forest Hills, NY 11375; (718)
544-3590; **BDCERT:** PlS 93; HS 95; **MS:** Mt Sinai
Sch Med 80; **RES:** Staten Island Univ Hosp, Staten
Island, NY 81-84; Catholic Med Ctr Bklyn & Qns,
Jamaica, NY 84-85; **FEL:** Albany Med Ctr, Albany,
NY 85-87; **HOSP:** St Mary's Hosp; **SI:** *Carpal Tunnel
Syndrome; Hand and Wrist Trauma*; **HMO:** US
Hlthcre Blue Choice Oxford Magnacare United
Healthcare +

LANG: Sp, Pol; 🔲 🔲 🔲 🔲 ▦ 💲 ▦ ▦ ▦
Immediately

Zweig, Julian (MD)   HS
Flushing Hosp Med Ctr

112-47 Queens Blvd; Forest Hills, NY 11375; (718) 268-3322; **BDCERT:** S 69; **MS:** Switzerland 61; **RES:** Beth-El Hosp, Brooklyn, NY 62-63; Brookdale Univ Hosp Med Ctr, Brooklyn, NY 63-67; **FEL:** HS, Grace Hosp, Detroit, MI 67; **HOSP:** Parkway Hosp; **HMO:** CIGNA Magnacare Oxford GHI US Hlthcre +

♿ 🔂 📠 🕭 $ Mcr WC NFI Immediately

HEMATOLOGY

Rai, Kanti (MD)   Hem
Long Island Jewish Med Ctr

Long Island Jewish Medical Center, 76th Ave; New Hyde Park, NY 11042; (718) 470-7135; **BDCERT:** Ped 61; **MS:** India 55; **RES:** Lincoln Med & Mental Hlth Ctr, Bronx, NY 57-58; N Shore Univ Hosp-Manhasset, Manhasset, NY 58-59; **FEL:** NuM & Hem, Long Island Jewish Med Ctr, New Hyde Park, NY 59; **SI:** *Leukemias; Lymphomas;* **HMO:** Oxford Blue Choice NYLCare GHI CIGNA +

♿ 🕭 $ Mcr Mcd WC Immediately **VISA** 💳

INFECTIOUS DISEASE

Donnelly, Harrison (MD)   Inf
St Joseph's Hosp-Queens

158-40 79th Ave; Flushing, NY 11366; (718) 558-6200; **MS:** Mexico 74; **RES:** VA Med Ctr-Manh, New York, NY 76-79; St Clare's Hosp & Health Ctr, New York, NY 79-81; **FEL:** Inf, Mem Sloan Kettering Cancer Ctr, New York, NY 81-84; **HOSP:** Catholic Med Ctr Bklyn & Qns; **HMO:** PHS Oxford

♿ SA C 🔂 🕭 Mcr A Few Days

Rahal, James (MD)   Inf
NY Hosp Med Ctr of Queens

56-45 Main St 609S; Flushing, NY 11355; (718) 670-1525; **BDCERT:** IM 68; Inf 72; **MS:** Tufts U 59; **RES:** Bellevue Hosp Ctr, New York, NY 59-61; New England Med Ctr, Boston, MA 61-62; **FEL:** Inf, New England Med Ctr, Boston, MA 62-65; **FAP:** Clin Prof Med Cornell U; **SI:** *Antibiotic Resistance; Hospital Infections;* **HMO:** Oxford Blue Shield Prudential

🔂 🕭 Mcr Mcd NFI Immediately 💳 **VISA** 💳 💳

Singer, Carol (MD)   Inf
Long Island Jewish Med Ctr

270-05 76th Ave FP333; New Hyde Park, NY 11040; (718) 470-7290; **BDCERT:** IM 73; Inf 78; **MS:** Cornell U 70; **RES:** U Mich Med Ctr, Ann Arbor, MI 70-72; NY Hosp-Cornell Med Ctr, New York, NY 72-73; **FEL:** Inf, Mem Sloan Kettering Cancer Ctr, New York, NY 73-75; **FAP:** Assoc Prof Med Albert Einstein Coll Med; **SI:** *Fever Unknown Etiology; Immunocompromised Patient;* **HMO:** Oxford US Hlthcre United Healthcare Sel Pro PHS +

♿ 🔂 📠 🕭 $ Mcr Mcd 1 Week **VISA** 💳

INTERNAL MEDICINE

Albertini, Francis (MD)   IM   **PCP**
Parkway Hosp

Yellowstone Medical Associates, 112-47 Queens Blvd 20; Forest Hills, NY 11375; (718) 268-1750; **BDCERT:** IM 91; **MS:** SUNY Stony Brook 86; **RES:** IM, Flushing Hosp Med Ctr, Flushing, NY 86-89; **SI:** *Primary Care;* **HMO:** Oxford US Hlthcre Aetna Hlth Plan Blue Cross & Blue Shield GHI +

LANG: Hin; SA 🔂 📠 🕭 Mcr WC A Few Days

Amin, Mahendra (MD)   IM   **PCP**
NY Hosp Med Ctr of Queens

89-02 Springfield Blvd; Queens Village, NY 11427; (718) 776-4444; **BDCERT:** IM 84; **MS:** India 78; **RES:** Metropolitan Hosp Ctr, New York, NY 81-84; **HOSP:** Long Island Jewish Med Ctr; **HMO:** GHI Oxford Magnacare US Hlthcre United Healthcare +

LANG: Hin; SA C 🔂 📠 🕭 Mcd Immediately

Ankobiah, William (MD)   IM   **PCP**
Franklin Hosp Med Ctr

Rosedale Medical Office PLLC, 253-02 147th Ave; Jamaica, NY 11422; (718) 341-3535; **BDCERT:** IM 87; Pul 92; **MS:** Ghana 78; **RES:** IM, Woodhull Med Ctr, Brooklyn, NY 83-87; **FEL:** Pul, Univ Hosp SUNY Bklyn, Brooklyn, NY; **FAP:** Asst Prof SUNY Hlth Sci Ctr; **HOSP:** St John's Epis Hosp-S Shore; **SI:** *Asthma; Tuberculosis;* **HMO:** Prudential CIGNA Oxford Blue Cross Aetna-US Healthcare +

LANG: Ash, Pol; ♿ SA C 🔂 📠 🕭 Mcr Mcd WC NFI Immediately 💳 **VISA** 💳 💳

Bader, Paul (MD)   IM   `PCP`
Parkway Hosp
108-37 71st Ave; Forest Hills, NY 11375; (718)
263-7766; **BDCERT:** IM 82; Onc 85; **MS:** Wayne
State U Sch Med 79; **RES:** Harlem Hosp Ctr, New
York, NY 80-82; Metropolitan Hosp Ctr, New York,
NY 79-80; **FEL:** Hem Onc, Columbia-Presbyterian
Med Ctr, New York, NY 82-84; **HOSP:** Long Island
Jewish Med Ctr; **HMO:** Blue Cross NYLCare Oxford
Aetna-US Healthcare Chubb +

⬛ ⬛ ⬛ ⬛ ⬛ Immediately

Beyda, Allan (MD)   IM   `PCP`
NY Hosp Med Ctr of Queens
141-23 59th Ave; Flushing, NY 11355; (718)
359-7406; **BDCERT:** IM 79; **MS:** France 76; **RES:**
IM, NY Hosp Med Ctr of Queens, Flushing, NY 76-
79; **HOSP:** Long Island Jewish Med Ctr; **HMO:**
Aetna Hlth Plan Blue Choice Blue Cross & Blue
Shield Choicecare Oxford +

LANG: Fr; ⬛ ⬛ ⬛ ⬛ ⬛ 4+ Weeks **VISA**

Brewer, Marlon (MD)   IM
Elmhurst Hosp Ctr
79-01 Broadway Rm D124; Elmhurst, NY 11373;
(718) 334-2490; **BDCERT:** IM 94; **MS:** Spain 88;
RES: Elmhurst Hosp Ctr, Elmhurst, NY 89-92; **FAP:**
Asst Clin Prof Mt Sinai Sch Med; **SI:** *Diabetes;
Hypertension*; **HMO:** Blue Cross & Blue Choice
Metroplus

LANG: Sp; ⬛ ⬛ ⬛ ⬛ ⬛ ⬛ ⬛ ⬛

Foley, Conn J (MD)   IM   `PCP`
Long Island Jewish Med Ctr
Parker Jewish Institute for Health Care &
Rehabilitation, 271-11 76th Ave; New Hyde Park,
NY 11040; (718) 289-2277; **BDCERT:** IM 79; Ger
88; **MS:** Ireland 72; **RES:** IM, Ireland 73-75; Ger,
Ireland 76; **FEL:** Ger, Long Island Jewish Med Ctr,
New Hyde Park, NY 78-79; **FAP:** Assoc Prof Med
Albert Einstein Coll Med; **SI:** *Health Care of the
Elderly; Alzheimer's*

⬛ ⬛ ⬛ ⬛ ⬛ ⬛ ⬛ ⬛ ⬛ A Few Days

Joseph, John (MD)   IM   `PCP`
Parkway Hosp
66-20 108th St; Flushing, NY 11375; (718) 896-
8920; **BDCERT:** IM 83; **MS:** Mexico 77; **RES:** IM,
Coney Island Hosp, Brooklyn, NY 80-82; **FEL:** Rhu,
Long Island Coll Hosp, Brooklyn, NY 82-84; **HOSP:**
NY Hosp Med Ctr of Queens; **HMO:** Aetna Hlth Plan
Blue Choice Blue Cross & Blue Shield Choicecare
CIGNA +

⬛ ⬛ ⬛ ⬛ ⬛ ⬛ A Few Days

Kumar, Dharamjit (MD)   IM   `PCP`
St John's Queens Hosp
103-14 Lefferts Blvd; Richmond Hill, NY 11419;
(718) 843-2244; **BDCERT:** IM 90; **MS:** India 80;
RES: IM, Wyckoff Heights, Brooklyn, NY 81-83;
FEL: Nep, Lenox Hill, New York, NY 83-85; **HOSP:**
Mary Immaculate Hosp; **HMO:** Most

LANG: Hin; ⬛ ⬛ ⬛ ⬛ ⬛ A Few Days

Lempel, Herbert (MD)   IM   `PCP`
NY Hosp Med Ctr of Queens
112-47 Queens Blvd 109; Flushing, NY 11375;
(718) 544-9023; **BDCERT:** IM 84; **MS:** NY Med
Coll 81; **RES:** NY Hosp Med Ctr of Queens, Flushing,
NY 81-84; **HOSP:** Long Island Jewish Med Ctr;
HMO: Aetna Hlth Plan Prucare US Hlthcre CIGNA
Choicecare +

⬛ ⬛ ⬛ ⬛ ⬛ ⬛ ⬛ A Few Days **VISA** ⬛

Lichtenstein, David (MD)   IM   `PCP`
Peninsula Hosp Ctr
121-05 Rockaway Beach Blvd; Far Rockaway, NY
11694; (718) 318-3434; **BDCERT:** IM 89; **MS:** Mt
Sinai Sch Med 83; **RES:** IM, Mount Sinai Med Ctr,
New York, NY 84-87; **FAP:** Assoc Med NY Med
Coll; **HMO:** Oxford GHI Prucare CIGNA

LANG: Sp; ⬛ ⬛ ⬛ ⬛ ⬛ ⬛ ⬛ ⬛ ⬛ ⬛
Immediately ⬛ **VISA**

Messana, Ida (MD)   IM   PCP
Long Island Jewish Med Ctr
109-33 71st Rd 2E; Forest Hills, NY 11375; (718)
263-4345; **BDCERT:** IM 88; Ger 90; **MS:** SUNY
Stony Brook 84; **RES:** IM, Montefiore Med Ctr,
Bronx, NY 84-87; **FEL:** Ger, Montefiore Med Ctr,
Bronx, NY 87-89; **HOSP:** N Shore Univ Hosp-Forest
Hills; **SI:** *Primary Care;* **HMO:** Oxford
⬡ ⬡ ⬡ ⬡ ⬡ ⬡ A Few Days

Mohrer, Jonathan (MD)   IM   PCP
Long Island Jewish Med Ctr
114-06 Queens Blvd A8; Flushing, NY 11375;
(718) 575-9787; **BDCERT:** IM 83; **MS:** U Conn Sch
Med 80; **RES:** IM, Long Island Jewish Med Ctr, New
Hyde Park, NY 80-83; **HOSP:** NY Hosp Med Ctr of
Queens; **HMO:** Oxford US Hlthcre Vytra Prudential
GHI +
⬡ ⬡ ⬡ ⬡ ⬡ ⬡ A Few Days **VISA** ⬤

Munoz, Jose (MD)   IM   PCP
Parkway Hosp
37-45 89th St; Jackson Heights, NY 11372; (718)
779-1155; **MS:** West Indies 58; **RES:**
Knickerbocker Hosp, New York, NY 64-65; Lincoln
Med & Mental Hlth Ctr, Bronx, NY 65-67; **HOSP:**
Western Queens Comm Hosp; **HMO:** PHS Blue
Choice American Health Plan Choicecare
⬡ ⬡ ⬡ ⬡ ⬡ ⬡ ⬡ ⬡ A Few Days **VISA** ⬤ ⬤

Patel, Sunil (MD)   IM   PCP
Parkway Hosp
112-47 Queens Blvd 206; Forest Hills, NY 11375;
(718) 268-1750; **BDCERT:** IM 89; **MS:** India 81;
RES: IM, Flushing Hosp Med Ctr, Flushing, NY 86-
89; **SI:** *Primary Care;* **HMO:** Oxford US Hlthcre GHI
Blue Cross & Blue Shield
LANG: Hin; ⬡ ⬡ ⬡ ⬡ ⬡ ⬡

Qadir, Shuja (MD)   IM   PCP
Mary Immaculate Hosp
98-10 Metropolitan Ave; Forest Hills, NY 11375;
(718) 575-0639; **BDCERT:** IM 84; Cv 87; **MS:**
SUNY Hlth Sci Ctr 77; **RES:** IM, Catholic Med Ctr
Bklyn & Qns, Jamaica, NY 82-85; **FEL:** Cv, Catholic
Med Ctr Bklyn & Qns, Jamaica, NY 85-87; **HOSP:** N
Shore Univ Hosp-Forest Hills; **SI:** *Palpitations; Chest
Pains;* **HMO:** Blue Choice United Healthcare Oxford
NYLCare Aetna Hlth Plan +
LANG: Afr; ⬡ ⬡ ⬡ ⬡ ⬡ ⬡ ⬡ ⬡ ⬡
A Few Days

Reilly, Thomas (MD)   IM   PCP
St John's Queens Hosp
86-27 Forest Pkwy; Woodhaven, NY 11421; (718)
805-2404; **BDCERT:** IM 84; **MS:** SUNY Hlth Sci Ctr
84; **RES:** Staten Island Univ Hosp, Staten Island, NY
79-82; **FEL:** Hem, St Vincents Hosp & Med Ctr NY,
New York, NY 82-85; **FAP:** Clin Instr NY Med Coll;
HOSP: St Vincents Hosp & Med Ctr NY; **HMO:** Blue
Choice Oxford Metlife GHI +
⬡ ⬡ ⬡ ⬡ ⬡ 1 Week

Rose, David (MD)   IM   PCP
Mount Sinai Med Ctr
Long Island Jewish Medical Center, 410 Lakeville
Rd Ste 105; New Hyde Park, NY 10042; (516)
437-9180; **BDCERT:** IM 84; PrM 84; **MS:** NY Med
Coll 73; **RES:** IM, Beth Israel Med Ctr, New York,
NY 73-76; PMR, Mount Sinai Med Ctr, New York,
NY 79-81; **FAP:** Asst Prof Med; **HMO:** Oxford Aetna
Hlth Plan
⬡ ⬡ ⬡ ⬡ 1 Week

Rosenberg, Peter (MD)   IM   PCP
NY Hosp Med Ctr of Queens
26-19 212th St; Bayside, NY 11360; (718) 224-2022; **BDCERT:** IM 77; Cv 79; **MS:** SUNY Hlth Sci Ctr 74; **RES:** Jacobi Med Ctr, Bronx, NY 74-77; **FEL:** Cv, Montefiore Med Ctr, Bronx, NY; **HOSP:** N Shore Univ Hosp-Manhasset; *SI: Cardiology;* **HMO:** Aetna Hlth Plan Blue Cross & Blue Shield CIGNA Metlife Prucare +

🚹 📞 📷 🚹 🛏 Mcr Mcd WC NFI   Immediately

Sciales, John (MD)   IM   PCP
NY Hosp Med Ctr of Queens
New York Primary Care, 163-03 Oak Ave; Flushing, NY 11358; (718) 445-2298; **BDCERT:** IM 87; Ger 94; **MS:** SUNY Hlth Sci Ctr 84; **RES:** Med, NY Hosp Med Ctr of Queens, Flushing, NY 84-87; **FAP:** Clin Instr Med Cornell U; *SI: Health Prevention; Geriatrics;* **HMO:** Aetna-US Healthcare Vytra Oxford United Healthcare CIGNA +

LANG: Itl; 📞 📷 🚹 🛏 S Mcr NFI   2-4 Weeks

Shanies, Harvey (MD)   IM
Elmhurst Hosp Ctr
79-01 Broadway; Flushing, NY 11373; (718) 334-3298; **BDCERT:** IM 76; CCM 87; **MS:** NYU Sch Med 73; **RES:** Med, Bronx Muncipal Hosp Ctr, Bronx, NY 73-75; Med, Bronx Muncipal Hosp Ctr, Bronx, NY 75-77; **FAP:** Asst Prof Med Mt Sinai Sch Med; *SI: Asthma; Emphysema;* **HMO:** Multiplan United Payors Health First Oxford

LANG: Sp, Ur, Chi, Hin, Itl; 🚹 📞 📷 🚹 🛏 Mcr Mcd WC NFI *VISA* ⬤

Sossi, Anthony (MD)   IM
Catholic Med Ctr Bklyn & Qns
88-25 153rd St; Jamaica, NY 11432; (718) 558-7150; **BDCERT:** IM 67; **MS:** UMDNJ-NJ Med Sch, Newark 60; **RES:** IM, Montefiore Med Ctr, Bronx, NY 64-65; **HOSP:** Mary Immaculate Hosp

Talor, Zvi (MD)   IM
Queens Hosp Ctr
90-02 Queens Blvd; Elmhurst, NY 11373; (718) 558-1977; **BDCERT:** IM 87; **MS:** Israel 72; **RES:** Rambam Haifalisrael, Israel 78-79; **FEL:** Nep, Rambam Haifalisrael, Israel 72-77; U Chicago Hosp, Chicago, IL 80-81; **HOSP:** Mary Immaculate Hosp; *SI: Renal Diseases; Hypertension*

LANG: Heb, Sp; 🚹 📷 🛏 Mcr Mcd   2-4 Weeks *VISA* ⬤

Tumminello, Calogero (MD)   IM   PCP
Wyckoff Heights Med Ctr
3378 Parkway Drive; Baldwin Harbor, NY 11510; (718) 497-1399; **BDCERT:** IM 96; **MS:** Dominica 86; **RES:** IM, Wyckoff Heights Med Ctr, Brooklyn, NY; **FAP:** Cornell U; **HMO:** US Hlthcre GHI Oxford United Healthcare

LANG: Itl, Sp, Fr; SA/50 📞 🚹 🛏 S Mcr   Immediately

MEDICAL ONCOLOGY

Benisovich, Vladimir I (MD)   Onc
Elmhurst Hosp Ctr
79-01 Broadway; Elmhurst, NY 11373; (718) 334-3723; **BDCERT:** Hem 84; Onc 85; **MS:** Russia 66; **RES:** Bronx Lebanon Hosp Ctr, Bronx, NY 79-80; Wyckoff Heights Med Ctr, Brooklyn, NY 77-78; **FEL:** Mount Sinai Med Ctr, New York, NY 82-83; New York University Med Ctr, New York, NY 80-82; **FAP:** Instr Onc Mt Sinai Sch Med; **HOSP:** Mount Sinai Med Ctr

🚹 📷 Mcr Mcd   1 Week

Cortes, Engracio P (MD)   Onc
NY Hosp Med Ctr of Queens
51-06 Kissena Blvd; Flushing, NY 11355; (718) 886-2911; **BDCERT:** IM 76; Onc 77; **MS:** Philippines 64; **RES:** Lemuel Shattuck Hosp, Boston, MA 69; **FEL:** Onc, Roswell Park Cancer Inst, Buffalo, NY; **FAP:** Clin Prof Albert Einstein Coll Med; **HOSP:** Long Island Jewish Med Ctr; *SI: Breast Cancer; Lung Cancer;* **HMO:** GHI Oxford Magnacare PHS CIGNA +

LANG: Tag; 🚹 📷 🛏 S Mcr   Immediately

Kaplan, Barry (MD)   Onc
NY Hosp Med Ctr of Queens

56-45 Main St; Flushing, NY 11355; (718) 460-2300; **BDCERT:** IM 70; Onc 75; **MS:** Johns Hopkins U 62; **RES:** Johns Hopkins Hosp, Baltimore, MD 62; Bronx Muncipal Hosp Ctr, Bronx, NY 66-67; **FEL:** Hem, Johns Hopkins Hosp, Baltimore, MD 63-64; Bronx Muncipal Hosp Ctr, Bronx, NY 67-68; **HMO:** Aetna Hlth Plan Blue Choice Metlife Oxford Travelers +

🚹 📷 🚼 🛏 Mcr   Immediately

Shum, Kee (MD)   Onc
NY Hosp Med Ctr of Queens

136-25 Maple Ave 205; Flushing, NY 11355; (718) 463-2245; **BDCERT:** IM 84; Onc 87; **MS:** Cornell U 81; **RES:** IM, Kings County Hosp Ctr, Brooklyn, NY 81-85; **FEL:** Onc, Mem Sloan Kettering Cancer Ctr, New York, NY 85-87; **HOSP:** Flushing Hosp Med Ctr; *SI: Breast Cancer; Lung Cancer;* **HMO:** Oxford Aetna Hlth Plan Magnacare

🚹 SA SU 🅲 📷 🛏 $ Mcr   Immediately

NEONATAL-PERINATAL MEDICINE

Lipsitz, Philip (MD)   NP
Long Island Jewish Med Ctr

270-05 76th Ave; New Hyde Park, NY 11040; (718) 470-3440; **BDCERT:** Ped 71; NP 75; **MS:** South Africa 52; **RES:** Ped, England; **FEL:** Cleveland Metro Gen Hosp, Cleveland, OH; Children's Hosp, Boston, MA; **FAP:** Prof Ped Albert Einstein Coll Med; *SI: High-Risk Newborns; Jaundice of the Newborn*

LANG: Sp, Heb, Chi, Rus; 📷 🛏   Immediately ▨
VISA 💳

NEPHROLOGY

Epstein, Edward (MD)   Nep
St John's Queens Hosp

110-42 72nd Rd; Forest Hills, NY 11375; (718) 263-0059; **BDCERT:** IM 80; Nep 82; **MS:** NYU Sch Med 77; **RES:** IM, Brookdale Univ Hosp Med Ctr, Brooklyn, NY 78-80; **FEL:** Nep, Brookdale Univ Hosp Med Ctr, Brooklyn, NY 80-82; *SI: Renal Diseases; High Blood Pressure;* **HMO:** CIGNA Blue Cross & Blue Shield PHS Multiplan PHCS +

🅲 📷 🛏 $ Mcr NFI   1 Week

Galler, Marilyn (MD)   Nep
NY Hosp Med Ctr of Queens

Nephrology Associates, 56-45 Main St; Flushing, NY 11355; (718) 670-1151; **BDCERT:** IM 80; Nep 84; **MS:** NYU Sch Med 75; **RES:** Bronx Muncipal Hosp Ctr, Bronx, NY 75-79; **FEL:** Albert Einstein Med Ctr, Bronx, NY 78-81; **HOSP:** Montefiore Med Ctr-Weiler/Einstein Div; *SI: High Blood Pressure; Kidney Diseases*

LANG: Heb, Itl; 🚹 📷 🛏 $ Mcr

Kostadaras, Ari (MD)   Nep
Western Queens Comm Hosp

Hellenic Medical Center, 30-16 30th Dr; Astoria, NY 11102; (718) 721-4440; **BDCERT:** IM 93; **MS:** Grenada 89; **RES:** IM, LaGuardia Hosp, Forest Hills, NY 89-92; **FEL:** Nep, Nassau Cty Med Ctr, East Meadow, NY 92-94

Mattoo, Nirmal (MD)   Nep
Wyckoff Heights Med Ctr

385 Seneca Ave; Flushing, NY 11385; (718) 545-3617; **BDCERT:** IM 74; Nep 78; **MS:** India 67; **HOSP:** N Shore Univ Hosp-Forest Hills

LANG: Sp, Hin, Ur, Kan; 🚹 SA SU 🅲 🛏 $ Mcr Mcr
Immediately

Neff, Martin (MD) Nep
Elmhurst Hosp Ctr
79-01 Broadway; Elmhurst, NY 11373; (718) 334-3927; **BDCERT:** IM 70; Nep 72; **MS:** NY Med Coll 63; **RES:** Hahnemann U Hosp, Philadelphia, PA 66-68; **FEL:** Nep, Hahnemann U Hosp, Philadelphia, PA 68-70; **FAP:** Prof Mt Sinai Sch Med; **SI:** *Hemodialysis; Hypertension;* **HMO:** Oxford Metroplus Well Care

⬦ 🔲 🎫 Mcr Mcd 2-4 Weeks

Singhal, Pravin (MD) Nep **PCP**
Long Island Jewish Med Ctr
Kidney Disease & Hypertension Long Island Jewish, 270-05 76th Ave 228; New Hyde Park, NY 11040; (718) 470-7360; **BDCERT:** IM 83; Nep 86; **MS:** India 70; **RES:** IM, Brigham & Women's Hosp, Boston, MA 82; **FEL:** Nep, Albert Einstein Med Ctr, Bronx, NY 85; **SI:** *Hypertension; Diabetic Kidney Disease;* **HMO:** Blue Choice Blue Cross & Blue Shield HealthNet Oxford US Hlthcre +

LANG: Hin; ⬦ 🄲 🔲 🎫 🎫 Mcr Mcd NFi Immediately
VISA 💳

Spinowitz, Bruce (MD) Nep
NY Hosp Med Ctr of Queens
56-45 Main St; Flushing, NY 11355; **BDCERT:** IM 76; Nep 78; **MS:** NYU Sch Med 73; **RES:** Med, Bellevue Hosp Ctr, New York, NY 74-76; Nep, Bellevue Hosp Ctr, New York, NY 76-78; **FAP:** Assoc Clin Prof Med Cornell U; **HOSP:** Montefiore Med Ctr-Weiler/Einstein Div; **SI:** *Diabetic Kidney Disease; Kidney Stones;* **HMO:** Blue Cross & Blue Shield Oxford CIGNA HIP Network Guardian +

LANG: Heb, Sp; ⬦ 🔲 🎫 💲 Mcr A Few Days

NEUROLOGICAL SURGERY

Khatib, Reza (MD) NS
Catholic Med Ctr Bklyn & Qns
90-02 Queens Blvd; Elmhurst, NY 11373; (718) 464-4600; **BDCERT:** NS 69; **MS:** Iran 56; **RES:** Path, Barnert Hosp, Paterson, NJ 59; N, Brooklyn Jewish Hosp, Brooklyn, NY 60; **HOSP:** Long Island Jewish Med Ctr; **HMO:** GHI Blue Cross & Blue Shield US Hlthcre Sanus Prucare +

⬦ 🔲 🎫 🎫 💲 Mcr Mcd WC NFi Immediately

Miller, John I (MD) NS
Catholic Med Ctr Bklyn & Qns
95-25 Queens Blvd; Rego Park, NY 11374; (718) 459-7700; **BDCERT:** NS 92; PEn 97; **MS:** Georgetown U 79; **RES:** Children's Hosp Nat Med Ctr, Washington, DC 80-82; Kings County Hosp Ctr, Brooklyn, NY 82-87; **HOSP:** N Shore Univ Hosp-Forest Hills; **HMO:** US Hlthcre 32BJ Blue Cross & Blue Choice HIP Network Oxford +

⬦ 🔲 🎫 💲 Mcr Mcd WC NFi A Few Days

NEUROLOGY

Casson, Ira (MD) N
Parkway Hosp
112-03 Queens Blvd; Forest Hills, NY 11375; (718) 544-6633; **BDCERT:** N 80; **MS:** NYU Sch Med 75; **RES:** N, New York University Med Ctr, New York, NY 76-79; **HOSP:** Long Island Jewish Med Ctr; **SI:** *Sports Neurology; Head Injuries;* **HMO:** Oxford US Hlthcre GHI Magnacare

⬦ 🔲 🎫 💲 Mcr WC NFi A Few Days

Eviatar, Lydia (MD) N
Long Island Jewish Med Ctr
269-01 76th Ave 267; New Hyde Park, NY 11040; (718) 470-3451; **BDCERT:** Ped 68; N 77; **MS:** Israel 61; **RES:** Ped, Israel 61-66; **FEL:** UCLA Med Ctr, Los Angeles, CA 66-67; N, UCLA Med Ctr, Los Angeles, CA 67-69; **HMO:** Magnacare Multiplan US Hlthcre Blue Choice GHI +

LANG: Fr, Heb, Rom, Rus; ⬦ 🔲 🎫 🎫 💲 2-4 Weeks 💳 *VISA* 💳 💳

Gordon, Marc L (MD) N
Long Island Jewish Med Ctr

270-05 76th Avenue Room 222; New Hyde Park,
NY 11040; (718) 470-7366; **BDCERT:** N 90; **MS:**
Columbia P&S 85; **RES:** Lenox Hill Hosp, New York,
NY 85-86; Albert Einstein Med Ctr, Bronx, NY 86-
89; **FEL:** Neuropsychopharmacology, Albert
Einstein Med Ctr, Bronx, NY 89-90; **FAP:** Asst Prof
Med Albert Einstein Coll Med; **HOSP:** Montefiore
Med Ctr; **SI:** *Botox Treatment; Dystonia;* **HMO:**
Oxford Sel Pro Empire Blue Cross & Shield PHS
United Healthcare +

LANG: Sp, Fr, Rus; ⚹ 🕿 🏥 💲 Mcr Mod 1 Week 🌐
VISA 💳

Kanner, Ronald (MD) N
Long Island Jewish Med Ctr

270-05 76th Ave; New Hyde Park, NY 11040;
(718) 470-7311; **BDCERT:** N 80; **MS:** Spain 75;
RES: Med, Hosp of U Penn, Philadelphia, PA 75; N,
Albert Einstein Med Ctr, Bronx, NY 76-79; **FEL:** N
Onc/Pain, Mem Sloan Kettering Cancer Ctr, New
York, NY 79-81; **SI:** *Pain Management;* **HMO:** US
Hlthcre Aetna Hlth Plan Oxford

LANG: Sp, Itl, Yd; ⚹ 🕿 🏥 💲 Mcr 2-4 Weeks **VISA**
💳

Libman, Richard (MD) N
Long Island Jewish Med Ctr

270-05 76th Ave 222; New Hyde Park, NY 11040;
(718) 470-7260; **BDCERT:** N 91; **MS:** McGill U 86;
RES: Albert Einstein Med Ctr, Bronx, NY 87-90;
FEL: Cerebrovascular Disease, Columbia-
Presbyterian Med Ctr, New York, NY 80-82; **FAP:**
Asst Clin Prof Albert Einstein Coll Med; **SI:** *Stroke
Treatment*

⚹ 🕿 🏥 💲 Mcr A Few Days 🌐 **VISA** 💳

Schaul, Neil (MD) N
Long Island Jewish Med Ctr

270-05 76th Ave; New Hyde Park, NY 11040;
(718) 470-7310; **BDCERT:** N 76; **MS:** SUNY Hlth
Sci Ctr 66; **RES:** Montreal Neur Inst, Montreal,
Canada 71-74; **FEL:** Montreal Neur Inst, Montreal,
Canada 74-77; **FAP:** Assoc Prof Albert Einstein Coll
Med; **HOSP:** Catholic Med Ctr Bklyn & Qns; **SI:**
Epilepsy; **HMO:** US Hlthcre Oxford NYLCare
Multiplan US Hlthcre +

LANG: Heb; ⚹ 🕿 🏥 🏥 Mcr Mod WC 1 Week 🌐
VISA 💳

NEURORADIOLOGY

Patel, Mahendra (MD) NRad
Long Island Jewish Med Ctr

Dept of Radiology Long Island Jewish Medical
Center, 270-05 76th Ave; New Hyde Park, NY
11040; (718) 470-7175; **BDCERT:** DR 84; N 95;
MS: India 71; **RES:** Rad, St Thomas Hosp, London,
England 74-77; Fellow of Royal College of
Radiologists, London, England 79; **FEL:** NR, Albert
Einstein Med Ctr, Bronx, NY 81; Musculoskeletal
Radiology, Hosp For Joint Diseases, New York, NY
82; **FAP:** Assoc Prof Albert Einstein Coll Med;
HOSP: Jamaica Med Ctr; **SI:** *Brain/Head and Neck
Diseases; Spinal Cord;* **HMO:** Aetna-US Healthcare
Empire Oxford

LANG: Hin, Sp, Fr; ⚹ 🆘 🕿 🏥 Mcr Mod WC NFI
A Few Days 🌐 **VISA** 💳

NUCLEAR MEDICINE

Palestro, Christopher (MD) NuM
Long Island Jewish Med Ctr

LI Jewish Med Ctr, 270-05 76th Ave; New Hyde
Park, NY 11040; (718) 470-7080; **BDCERT:** NuM
82; **MS:** Mexico 75; **RES:** DR, St Luke's Roosevelt
Hosp Ctr, New York, NY 77-80; **FEL:** NuM, Mem
Sloan Kettering Cancer Ctr, New York, NY 80-82;
FAP: Prof NR Albert Einstein Coll Med; **SI:** *AIDS;
Joint Replacements;* **HMO:** Oxford US Hlthcre PHS
1199 Magnacare +

⚹ 🆘 🌙 🕿 🏥 🏥 💲 Mcr Mod WC NFI Immediately
VISA 💳

OBSTETRICS & GYNECOLOGY

Bracero, Louis (MD)   ObG
Catholic Med Ctr Bklyn & Qns
Catholic Med Ctr Dept of Women's Health Services, 88-25 153rd St Ste 4G; Jamaica, NY 11432; (718) 558-7295; **BDCERT:** ObG 94; MF 94; **MS:** Mt Sinai Sch Med 78; **RES:** ObG, Columbia-Presbyterian Med Ctr, New York, NY 79-82; **FEL:** MF, Jacobi Med Ctr, Bronx, NY 83-84; MF, Winthrop Univ Hosp, Mineola, NY 84-85; **FAP:** Assoc Prof ObG NY Med Coll; **HOSP:** Maimonides Med Ctr; **SI:** *High-Risk Obstetrics*

LANG: Sp; ⓑ ⓐ ⓨ ⊞ $ Mcr Mcd   2-4 Weeks

Concannon, Patrick (MD)   ObG
N Shore Univ Hosp-Manhasset
140-55 34th Ave; Flushing, NY 11354; (718) 445-1716; **BDCERT:** ObG 65; **MS:** NYU Sch Med 55; **RES:** ObG, Flushing Hosp Med Ctr, Flushing, NY 59-62; Path CP, Kings County Hosp Ctr, Brooklyn, NY 59; **FEL:** ObG, St Albans Naval Hosp, St Albans, VT 57-58; **HOSP:** St Francis Hosp-Roslyn; **SI:** *Menopause; Vaginal Delivery After C/S*; **HMO:** GHI Aetna-US Healthcare Empire Magnacare +

LANG: Sp; ⓑ Ⓒ ⓐ ⓨ ⊞ $ Mcr   A Few Days

Finley, Maria (MD)   ObG
NY Hosp Med Ctr of Queens
136-12 59th Ave; Flushing, NY 11355; (718) 961-1891; **BDCERT:** ObG 87; **MS:** SUNY Buffalo 77; **RES:** ObG, Bellevue Hosp Ctr, New York, NY 77-81; **HMO:** Aetna Hlth Plan Metlife

Georgis, Michael (MD)   ObG
Wyckoff Heights Med Ctr
25-40 30th Rd A1; Astoria, NY 11102; (718) 728-2626; **BDCERT:** ObG 85; **MS:** Greece 73; **RES:** S, Beekman Downtown Hosp, New York, NY 75-77; ObG, Brooklyn Jewish Hosp, Brooklyn, NY 77-81

Ghosh, Snehanshu (MD)   ObG
St John's Epis Hosp-S Shore
327 Beach 19 St; Far Rockaway, NY 11691; (718) 868-7382; **BDCERT:** ObG 77; **MS:** India 68; **RES:** Albert Einstein Med Ctr, Bronx, NY 72-75; **SI:** *Osteoporosis; Infertility*; **HMO:** Oxford GHI 1199 Empire

ⓑ ⓢ Ⓒ ⓐ ⓨ ⊞ $ Mcr   1 Week

Guarnaccia, Gary (MD)   ObG   **PCP**
Parkway Hosp
Assn of University Physicians, 11203 Queens Blvd Ste 200; Forest Hills, NY 11375; (718) 268-8383; **BDCERT:** ObG 80; **MS:** UMDNJ-NJ Med Sch, Newark 74; **RES:** Bellevue Hosp Ctr, New York, NY 74-78; **FAP:** Asst Clin Prof NYU Sch Med; **HOSP:** Long Island Jewish Med Ctr; **SI:** *Colposcopy; Laparoscopy*; **HMO:** GHI Empire Blue Cross & Shield

ⓑ Ⓒ ⓐ ⓨ ⊞ $ Mcr   Immediately ▨ **VISA** ⊛ ▨

Hakim-Elahi, Enayat (MD)   ObG
N Shore Univ Hosp-Forest Hills
Choices Women's Medical Ctr, 97-77 Queens Blvd; Forest Hills, NY 11375; (718) 275-6020; **BDCERT:** ObG 77; **MS:** Iran 59; **RES:** ObG, Queens Hosp Ctr, Jamaica, NY 60-64; GO, Francis Delafield Hosp, New York, NY 64-65; **FEL:** Cancer Gyn, Queens Hosp Ctr, Jamaica, NY 65; **FAP:** Assoc Prof Columbia P&S; **SI:** *Colposcopy and Contraception; Fertility Management*; **HMO:** GHI HIP Network Aetna-US Healthcare Oxford

LANG: Ger; ⓑ ⓢ Ⓒ ⓐ ⓨ ⊞ $ Mcr Mcd A Few Days ▨ **VISA** ⊛

Mandeville, Edgar (MD)   ObG   **PCP**
NY Hosp Med Ctr of Queens
177-14 Wexford Ter; Jamaica, NY 11432; (718) 523-4422; **BDCERT:** ObG 76; **MS:** Meharry Med Coll 67; **RES:** ObG, Harlem Hosp Ctr, New York, NY 71-74; **HOSP:** Long Island Jewish Med Ctr; **HMO:** Aetna Hlth Plan Choicecare HealthNet Metlife Oxford +

ⓑ Ⓒ ⓐ ⓨ ⊞ $ Mcr   A Few Days

Nerenberg, Alan (MD) ObG
Flushing Hosp Med Ctr

45-18 Parsons Blvd; Flushing, NY 11355; (718) 762-6622; **BDCERT:** ObG 83; **MS:** Wayne State U Sch Med 76; **RES:** Flushing Hosp Med Ctr, Flushing, NY 76-81; **HOSP:** Long Island Jewish Med Ctr; **HMO:** Magnacare US Hlthcre PHCS Oxford +

♿ 📟 📱 🖥 💻 💵 A Few Days

Pellettieri, John (MD) ObG `PCP`
Flushing Hosp Med Ctr

30-49 36th St; Long Island City, NY 11103; (718) 278-2126; **BDCERT:** ObG 70; **MS:** NYU Sch Med 63; **RES:** ObG, St Vincents Hosp & Med Ctr NY, New York, NY 64-68; **FAP:** Asst Clin Prof Albert Einstein Coll Med; **HOSP:** Long Island Jewish Med Ctr; **HMO:** Oxford Blue Choice PPO Multiplan

📱 🖥 💻 💵 1 Week

Pennisi, Joseph (MD) ObG
Flushing Hosp Med Ctr

Flushing Ob/Gyn, 146-01 45th Ave; Flushing, NY 11355; (718) 461-2277; **BDCERT:** ObG 62; **MS:** SUNY Downstate 53; **RES:** Flushing Hosp, Flushing, NY 56-59

Post, Robert (MD) ObG `PCP`
NY Hosp Med Ctr of Queens

NY Queens OB/GYN PC, 56-26 Main St; Flushing, NY 11355; (718) 539-4483; **BDCERT:** ObG 66; **MS:** KY Med Sch, Louisville 58; **RES:** ObG, Bellevue Hosp Ctr, New York, NY 59-63; *SI: High Risk Obstetrics; Benign Gynecologic Surgery*; **HMO:** US Hlthcre GHI Oxford United Healthcare Prucare +

📱 🖥 💻 💵 💳 1 Week

Schiavello, Henry (MD) ObG `PCP`
Wyckoff Heights Med Ctr

Intercounty Obstetrics & Gynecology Assoc, 146-01 45th Ave 201; Flushing, NY 11355; (718) 358-8944; **BDCERT:** ObG 70; **MS:** Italy 60; **RES:** ObG, Flushing Hosp Med Ctr, Flushing, NY 62-65; **FAP:** Asst Clin Prof Albert Einstein Coll Med; *SI: High Risk Pregnancies*; **HMO:** US Hlthcre Oxford GHI Magnacare Blue Choice +

LANG: Itl, Sp; ♿ 📱 🖥 💻 💵 Immediately

Schuster, Stephen (MD) ObG
NY Hosp Med Ctr of Queens

58-34 Main St; Flushing, NY 11355; (718) 939-0111; **BDCERT:** ObG 74; **MS:** NYU Sch Med 67; **RES:** New York University Med Ctr, New York, NY 68-72; Bellevue Hosp Ctr, New York, NY 68-72; **HOSP:** New York University Med Ctr; *SI: Pelvic Infection; Vulvovaginal Disease*; **HMO:** Oxford Blue Choice Prucare Aetna Hlth Plan

LANG: Sp, Itl; 📱 💻 🏥 💵 💳 1 Week

Seiler, Jerome (MD) ObG
NY Hosp Med Ctr of Queens

NY Queens OB/GYN, PC, 56-26 Main St; Flushing, NY 11355; (718) 539-4483; **BDCERT:** ObG 71; Rad 91; **MS:** U Hlth Sci/Chicago Med Sch 64; **RES:** Bellevue Hosp Ctr, New York, NY 65-69; **FAP:** Assoc Clin Prof Cornell U; *SI: Pelvic Support Defects; Operative Laparoscopy*; **HMO:** Oxford Vytra NYLCare US Hlthcre Blue Choice +

LANG: Ger, Heb; ♿ 📱 🖥 💻 🏥 💵 💳 1 Week

Toles, Allen (MD) ObG `PCP`
Long Island Jewish Med Ctr

Ann & Jules Gottlies Women's Comprehensive Health Center, 1554 Northern Blvd; Manhasset, NY 11030; (516) 390-9242; **BDCERT:** ObG 92; **MS:** Meharry Med Coll 86; **RES:** Howard U Hosp, Washington, DC 86-90; **FAP:** Asst Prof Albert Einstein Coll Med; *SI: High Risk Obstetrics; Low Risk Obstetrics*; **HMO:** US Hlthcre Oxford Magnacare 1199 CIGNA +

LANG: Sp; ♿ 📱 🖥 💻 🏥 💵 💳 Immediately 💳
VISA 💳 💳

Tsin, Daniel (MD) ObG
Western Queens Comm Hosp

37-42 77th St; Flushing, NY 11372; (718) 898-0913; **BDCERT:** ObG 76; **MS:** Argentina 65; **RES:** St Luke's Roosevelt Hosp Ctr, New York, NY 74; **HOSP:** NY Hosp Med Ctr of Queens; *SI: Laparoscopy; Laser ObG*; **HMO:** Prucare GHI CIGNA Magnacare Blue Cross & Blue Shield +

LANG: Sp; ♿ 📟 📱 🖥 💻 🏥 💵 💳 A Few Days

Younus, Bazaga (MD)   ObG   **PCP**
Catholic Med Ctr Bklyn & Qns
Obstetric & Gynecology, 42-66 Kissena Blvd;
Flushing, NY 11355; (718) 353-1223; **BDCERT:**
ObG 95; **MS:** India 78; **RES:** ObG, Catholic Med Ctr
Bklyn & Qns, Jamaica, NY 75-79; **HOSP:** St John's
Queens Hosp; **HMO:** CIGNA Oxford US Hlthcre PHS
Aetna Hlth Plan +

LANG: Sp, Ur, Hin; ♿ 🏥 🌙 📷 🚗 🏠 💲 Mcr
A Few Days

OPHTHALMOLOGY

Aharon, Raphael (MD)   Oph
Parkway Hosp
108-37 71st Ave; Flushing, NY 11375; (718) 268-
6120; **BDCERT:** Oph 87; **MS:** Albert Einstein Coll
Med 80; **RES:** Brookdale Univ Hosp Med Ctr,
Brooklyn, NY 80-81; Oph, Albert Einstein Med Ctr,
Bronx, NY 81-84; **HOSP:** NY Hosp Med Ctr of
Queens; **HMO:** Oxford CIGNA Aetna Hlth Plan
United Healthcare Magnacare +

♿ 🌙 📷 🚗 🏠 💲 Mcr NFI   Immediately

Boniuk, Vivien (MD)   Oph
Long Island Jewish Med Ctr
82-68 164th St; Jamaica, NY 11432; (718) 883-
2020; **BDCERT:** Oph 69; **MS:** Dalhousie U 64; **RES:**
Barnes Hosp, St Louis, MO 64-67; **FEL:** Oph, Baylor
Coll Med, Houston, TX 67-68; **FAP:** Assoc Prof Oph
Albert Einstein Coll Med; **HMO:** Blue Choice CIGNA
Oxford US Hlthcre

Fisch, Robert (MD)   Oph
New York Eye & Ear Infirmary
43-33 42nd St; Long Island City, NY 11104; (718)
784-4932; **BDCERT:** Oph 77; **MS:** Italy 71; **RES:**
Oph, Kingsbrook Jewish Med Ctr, Brooklyn, NY 72-
75

Fishman, Allen (MD)   Oph
Parkway Hosp
92-29 Queens Blvd 2I; Flushing, NY 11374; (718)
261-7007; **BDCERT:** Oph 81; **MS:** U Hlth
Sci/Chicago Med Sch 76; **RES:** Brookdale Univ Hosp
Med Ctr, Brooklyn, NY 77-80; **HOSP:** New York
Eye & Ear Infirmary; **SI:** *Cataract Surgery—Stitchless*;
HMO: Oxford US Hlthcre GHI 1199 Blue Cross &
Blue Shield +

LANG: Sp, Yd; ♿ 🌙 📷 🚗 🏠 💲 Mcr Mcd
Immediately **VISA** 💳

Goldberg, Robert T (MD)   Oph
NY Hosp Med Ctr of Queens
142-10 Roosevelt Ave B; Flushing, NY 11354;
(718) 539-2992; **BDCERT:** Oph 64; **MS:** NYU Sch
Med 56; **RES:** Oph, New York University Med Ctr,
New York, NY 59-60; Oph, Univ Hosp SUNY Bklyn,
Brooklyn, NY 60-63; **FEL:** Oph, New York
University Med Ctr, New York, NY 63-65; **FAP:**
Assoc Clin Prof Oph NYU Sch Med; **HOSP:** Long
Island Jewish Med Ctr; **SI:** *Glaucoma; Diabetic
Retinopathy*; **HMO:** Aetna Hlth Plan Blue Shield
Oxford Prudential NYH Health Plan +

LANG: Sp, Ger, Yd; ♿ 📷 🚗 🏠 💲 Mcr   2-4 Weeks

Grasso, Cono M (MD)   Oph
Catholic Med Ctr Bklyn & Qns
83-05 Grand Ave; Elmhurst, NY 11373; (718)
429-0300; **BDCERT:** Oph 79; **MS:** NYU Sch Med
74; **RES:** Wills Eye Hosp, Philadelphia, PA 75-78;
HOSP: Manhattan Eye, Ear & Throat Hosp; **HMO:**
Blue Choice GHI Aetna-US Healthcare Oxford
United Healthcare +

♿ 📷 🚗 🏠 Mcr Mcd WC NFI   A Few Days

Kaufmann, Cheryl (MD)   Oph
NY Hosp Med Ctr of Queens
43-44 Kissena Blvd; Flushing, NY 11355; (718)
353-5970; **BDCERT:** Oph 77; **MS:** NYU Sch Med
72; **RES:** Manhattan Eye, Ear & Throat Hosp, New
York, NY 73-76; Bellevue Hosp Ctr, New York, NY
72-73; **HOSP:** Manhattan Eye, Ear & Throat Hosp;
HMO: Sanus Oxford Prucare Aetna Hlth Plan 1199
+

♿ 🌙 📷 🚗 🏠 Mcr NFI   Immediately

Mackool, Richard (MD)   Oph
New York Eye & Ear Infirmary
31-27 41st St; Astoria, NY 11103; (718) 728-
3400; **BDCERT:** Oph 75; **MS:** Boston U 68; **RES:**
Oph, New York Eye & Ear Infirmary, New York, NY
70-73; **SI:** Cataract; **HMO:** Aetna Hlth Plan US
Hlthcre Oxford United Healthcare Prudential +
LANG: Sp, Ilo, Chi, Fr, Ar; ♿ 🔒 ⚕ 🏧 💲 Mcr 2-
4 Weeks **VISA** 💳

Seidenfeld, Andrew (MD)   Oph
New York Eye & Ear Infirmary
73-09 Myrtle Ave; Glendale, NY 11385; (718)
456-9500; **BDCERT:** Oph 82; **MS:** U Hlth
Sci/Chicago Med Sch 76; **RES:** Oph, New York Eye
& Ear Infirmary, New York, NY 80; **HOSP:** Wyckoff
Heights Med Ctr; **SI:** Cataract; Glaucoma; **HMO:**
Oxford Aetna Hlth Plan GHI Magnacare US Hlthcre
+
LANG: Sp, Fr, Ger, Yd; ♿ 🌙 🔒 ⚕ 🏧 💲 Mcr
1 Week **VISA** 💳 💳

Slavin, Michael (MD)   Oph
Long Island Jewish Med Ctr
600 Northern Blvd; Great Neck, NY 11021; (516)
470-2020; **BDCERT:** Oph 81; **MS:** Albert Einstein
Coll Med 76; **RES:** Univ Hosp SUNY Bklyn,
Brooklyn, NY 77-80; **FEL:** Bascom Palmer Eye Inst,
Miami, FL 80; Retina, Moorefields Eye Hosp,
London, England 90; **HMO:** Sanus US Hlthcre
♿ 🔒 🏧 💲 Immediately **VISA** 💳

Zaffuto, Stephen (MD)   Oph
Flushing Hosp Med Ctr
16-20 157th St; Flushing, NY 11357; (718) 746-
3021; **BDCERT:** Oph 72; **MS:** Univ Pittsburgh 64;
RES: Oph, Lenox Hill Hosp, New York, NY 64-68;
FEL: Oph, Lenox Hill Hosp, New York, NY 68-69;
HOSP: Lenox Hill Hosp; **SI:** Cataract; Glaucoma;
HMO: Oxford
♿ 🔒 ⚕ 🏧 💲 Mcr WC NFI 2-4 Weeks

ORTHOPAEDIC SURGERY

Denton, John (MD)   OrS
Catholic Med Ctr Bklyn & Qns
88-25 153rd St; Jamaica, NY 11432; (718) 558-
7241; **BDCERT:** OrS 73; **MS:** U Ala Sch Med 67;
RES: OrS, New York Orthopaedic Hosp, New York,
NY 69-73; S, St Luke's Roosevelt Hosp Ctr, New
York, NY 67-69; **FEL:** OrS, New York Orthopaedic
Hosp, New York, NY 72-73; **HOSP:** Mary
Immaculate Hosp

Goldman, Arnold (MD)   OrS
Parkway Hosp
113-13 76th Rd; Flushing, NY 11375; (718) 263-
7300; **BDCERT:** OrS 90; **MS:** SUNY Syracuse 81;
RES: SM, New York University Med Ctr, New York,
NY 82-86; **FEL:** Arthroscopy/SM, New York
University Med Ctr, New York, NY 87; Foot/Ankle
S, New York University Med Ctr, New York, NY 87;
FAP: Asst NY Med Coll; **HOSP:** NY Hosp Med Ctr of
Queens; **SI:** Arthroscopy; Foot & Ankle Surgery;
HMO: Blue Choice Blue Cross & Blue Shield
Choicecare CIGNA HealthNet +
LANG: Sp, Heb, Yd; ♿ SA 🌙 🔒 🏧 💲 Mcr WC NFI
A Few Days

Handelsman, John (MD)   OrS
Schneider Children's Hosp
Schneider Children's Hospital, Division of Pediatric
Orthopaedic Surgery, 269-01 76th Ave CH158;
New Hyde Park, NY 11040; (718) 470-3570;
BDCERT: OrS 78; **MS:** South Africa 53; **RES:** Med,
South Africa 54-58; OrS, Nuffield Orthopaedic
Centre, Oxford, England 58-61; **FEL:** OrS, Walton
Hospital, Liverpool, England 62-63; **FAP:** Prof Ped
Albert Einstein Coll Med; **SI:** Clubfoot and Hip
Torsions; CP Spina Bifida Dystrophies; **HMO:** Aetna-
US Healthcare United Healthcare NYLCare PHS
Vytra +
LANG: Sp, Rus, Yd, Kor, Chi; ♿ 🔒 ⚕ 🏧 💲 Mcr Mcd
NFI 4+ Weeks

Katz, Michael (MD)   OrS
Long Island Jewish Med Ctr
146-53 Delaware Ave; Flushing, NY 11355; (718) 353-3131; **BDCERT:** OrS 85; **MS:** SUNY Hlth Sci Ctr 64; **RES:** OrS, Hosp of U Penn, Philadelphia, PA 81-85; **FAP:** Instr OrS Univ Penn; **HOSP:** Hosp For Joint Diseases; **SI:** *Sports Medicine; Work Injuries*; **HMO:** United Healthcare 1199 US Hlthcre Multiplan NYLCare +

🦽 🐌 📶 📷 🛏 Mcr WC NFI Immediately 💳 *VISA*

Schwartz, Evan (MD)   OrS
Catholic Med Ctr Bklyn & Qns
90-02 Queens Blvd; Flushing, NY 11373; (718) 457-9231; **BDCERT:** OrS 89; **MS:** SUNY Buffalo 81; **RES:** OrS, Montefiore Med Ctr, Bronx, NY 82-86; **FEL:** SM, Hosp For Special Surgery, New York, NY 86-87; **FAP:** Asst Prof OrS Albany Med Coll; **HOSP:** Montefiore Med Ctr-Weiler/Einstein Div; **SI:** *Sports Medicine; Shoulder Surgery*; **HMO:** US Hlthcre Oxford Most Aetna Hlth Plan Blue Choice +

🦽 📶 📷 🛏 🛏 $ Mcr WC NFI Immediately

Toriello, Edward (MD)   OrS
Wyckoff Heights Med Ctr
78-15 Eliot Ave; Middle Village, NY 11379; (718) 458-8944; **BDCERT:** OrS 97; **MS:** SUNY Buffalo 85; **RES:** OrS, Univ Hosp SUNY Bklyn, Brooklyn, NY 80-85; **HOSP:** St John's Queens Hosp; **SI:** *Joint Replacement; Sports Medicine*; **HMO:** Oxford CIGNA Blue Cross

🦽 📷 🛏 🛏 $ Mcr WC NFI A Few Days

OTOLARYNGOLOGY

Kahn, Alvin (MD)   Oto
Western Queens Comm Hosp
37-44 90th St; Flushing, NY 11372; (718) 424-1444; **BDCERT:** Oto 74; S 58; **MS:** Bowman Gray 46; **RES:** IM, Touro Infirmary, New Orleans, LA 48-50; S, Jersey City Med Ctr, Jersey City, NJ 52-54; **FAP:** Asst Clin Prof SUNY Downstate; **HMO:** Blue Cross & Blue Shield CIGNA Metlife

La Marca, Charles (MD)   Oto
St John's Queens Hosp
75-06 Eliot Ave; Middle Village, NY 11379; (718) 335-2224; **BDCERT:** Oto 84; **MS:** Mexico 77; **RES:** Oto, Kings County Hosp Ctr, Brooklyn, NY; **HOSP:** N Shore Univ Hosp-Forest Hills; **HMO:** Oxford Blue Cross CIGNA GHI

📶 📷 🛏 🛏 $ Mcr

Moscoso, Juan (MD)   Oto
Elmhurst Hosp Ctr
Department of Otolaryngology, 79-01 Broadway Room H269; Elmhurst, NY 11373; (718) 334-3391; **BDCERT:** Oto 92; **MS:** Columbia P&S 85; **RES:** S, Mount Sinai Med Ctr, New York, NY 85-87; Oto, Columbia-Presbyterian Med Ctr, New York, NY 87-91; **FEL:** Head & Neck Reconstructive S, Mount Sinai Med Ctr, New York, NY 91-93; **FAP:** Assoc Clin Prof Mt Sinai Sch Med; **SI:** *Head and Neck Cancer; Ear, Nose & Throat Surgery*

LANG: Sp; 🦽 📷 🛏 🛏 $ Mcr Med WC A Few Days

Myssiorek, David (MD)   Oto
Long Island Jewish Med Ctr
270-05 76th Ave; New Hyde Park, NY 11040; (718) 470-7552; **BDCERT:** Oto 85; **MS:** NYU Sch Med 80; **RES:** Bellevue Hosp Ctr, New York, NY 81-84; VA Med Ctr-Manh, New York, NY 81-84; **FEL:** Head & Neck S, Montefiore Med Ctr, Bronx, NY 84-85; **FAP:** Asst Prof Med Albert Einstein Coll Med; **HOSP:** Schneider Children's Hosp; **SI:** *Thyroid Cancer; Salivary Gland Tumors*; **HMO:** Oxford US Hlthcre Magnacare GHI NYLCare +

LANG: Sp; 🦽 📷 🛏 🛏 $ Mcr NFI 2-4 Weeks 📧

Shikowitz, Mark (MD)   Oto
Long Island Jewish Med Ctr
270-05 76th Ave; New Hyde Park, NY 11040; (718) 470-7557; **BDCERT:** Oto 87; **MS:** Dominican Republic 81; **RES:** Long Island Jewish Med Ctr, New Hyde Park, NY 82-86; **FAP:** Assoc Prof Albert Einstein Coll Med; **HMO:** Oxford US Hlthcre Sel Pro CIGNA Blue Choice +

LANG: Sp; 🦽 📷 🛏 🛏 $ Mcr NFI 2-4 Weeks

Snyder, Gary (MD)   Oto
Flushing Hosp Med Ctr
26-01 Corporal Kennedy St FL 1; Bayside, NY
11360; (718) 423-4091; **BDCERT:** Oto 83; **MS:** NY
Med Coll 79; **RES:** S, N Shore Univ Hosp-
Manhasset, Manhasset, NY 79-80; Oto, Manhattan
Eye, Ear & Throat Hosp, New York, NY 80-83;
HOSP: N Shore Univ Hosp-Plainview; **SI:** *Facial
Cosmetic Surgery; Endoscopic Sinus Surgery;* **HMO:**
Oxford Aetna Hlth Plan CIGNA GHI

LANG: Sp, Itl, Fr; 🈂 🌙 ⏰ 🚻 🏧 💲 Mcr WC NFI
Immediately 🔲 **VISA** 💳

Zahtz, Gerald (MD)   Oto
Long Island Jewish Med Ctr
270-05 76th Ave; New Hyde Park, NY 11040;
(718) 470-7554; **BDCERT:** Oto 81; **MS:** St Louis U
77; **RES:** Oto, Long Island Jewish Med Ctr, New
Hyde Park, NY 77-81; **FAP:** Assoc Prof Albert
Einstein Coll Med; **SI:** *Pediatrics Otolaryngology;
Sinus Disease;* **HMO:** Oxford CIGNA NYLCare PHS
US Hlthcre +

LANG: Heb, Sp; ⏰ 🔒 🚻 🏧 💲 Mcr Mcd   2-4 Weeks

PAIN MANAGEMENT

Kaplan, Bruce (MD)   PM
NY Hosp Med Ctr of Queens
NY Hosp Med Ctr of Queens, Booth Memorial Ave;
Flushing, NY 11355; (718) 670-1081; **BDCERT:**
Anes 85; PM 90; **MS:** U Rochester 78; **RES:** S,
Albert Einstein Med Ctr, Bronx, NY 78-81; **FEL:**
Anes, Bellevue Hosp Ctr, New York, NY 82-84; TS,
Cleveland Clinic Hosp, Cleveland, OH 85-86; **FAP:**
Asst Clin Prof Anes Cornell U; **SI:** *Pain Management;
End of Life Care;* **HMO:** Most

LANG: Fr, Sp, Rus; ⏰ 🌙 🔒 🚻 🏧 Mcr Mcd WC NFI
1 Week 🔲 **VISA** 💳 💳

Kudowitz, Paul (MD)   PM
Western Queens Comm Hosp
Queens Pain Management, PC, 23-22 30th Rd 1H;
Astoria, NY 11102; (718) 545-5000; **BDCERT:**
Anes 88; PM 94; **MS:** Dominican Republic 82; **RES:**
Anes, Nassau County Med Ctr, East Meadow, NY
82-85; **FEL:** PM, Nassau County Med Ctr, East
Meadow, NY 85-86; **SI:** *Chronic Pain; Cancer Pain;*
HMO: Oxford Magnacare Heritage Genesis

LANG: Sp, Rus, Yd, Heb; ⏰ 🔒 🚻 🏧 💲 Mcr WC NFI
A Few Days 🔲 **VISA** 💳

PEDIATRIC CARDIOLOGY

Bierman, Fredrick Z (MD)   PCd
Long Island Jewish Med Ctr
26-01 76th Ave; New Hyde Park, NY 11040;
(718) 470-7350; **BDCERT:** Ped 78; **MS:** SUNY Hlth
Sci Ctr 76; **RES:** Ped, Mount Sinai Med Ctr, New
York, NY 73-76; **FEL:** PCd, Children's Hosp, Boston,
MA 76-79; **HOSP:** Schneider Children's Hosp

LANG: Rus, Sp; ⏰ 🔒 🚻 🏧 💲 Mcd   Immediately
VISA

Kern, Jeffrey H (MD)   PCd
Flushing Hosp Med Ctr
146-01 45th Ave; Flushing, NY 11354; (718)
670-3022; **BDCERT:** Ped 92; **MS:** Albert Einstein
Coll Med 89; **RES:** Ped, Mount Sinai Med Ctr, New
York, NY 89-92; **FEL:** PCd, Babies Hosp, New York,
NY 93-96; **FAP:** Asst Clin Prof Cornell U; **HOSP:** NY
Hosp-Cornell Med Ctr

LANG: Heb; ⏰ 🌙 🔒 🚻 🏧 Mcr Mcd WC NFI
Immediately

Rutkovsky, Lisa Rosner (MD) PCd
NY Hosp Med Ctr of Queens
56-45 Main St; Flushing, NY 11355; (718) 670-
1945; **BDCERT:** Ped 89; PCd 92; **MS:** NYU Sch Med
86; **RES:** Ped, N Shore Univ Hosp-Manhasset,
Manhasset, NY 87-89; **FEL:** PCd, NYU-Bellevue
Hosp, New York, NY 89; **FAP:** Asst Clin Prof NYU
Sch Med; **HMO:** GHI 1199 Oxford CIGNA
Magnacare +

LANG: Sp; ⏰ 🌙 🔒 🚻 🏧 💲 Mcr Mcd WC NFI
A Few Days

Shapir, Yehuda (MD)   **PCd**
Schneider Children's Hosp

LI Jewish Med Ctr, 269-01 76th Ave Rm 2104;
New Hyde Park, NY 11042; (718) 470-7350;
BDCERT: Ped 89; **MS:** Israel 77; **RES:** Ped, Rambam
Medical Center, Haifa, Israel 77-81; **FEL:** Ped, UCLA
Med Ctr, Los Angeles, CA 82-85; **FAP:** Assoc Prof
Albert Einstein Coll Med; *SI: Congenital Heart
Disease; Echocardiography*; **HMO:** Oxford Blue Cross
& Blue Shield US Hlthcre Aetna Hlth Plan Guardian
+

LANG: Heb, Pol, Itl; 🚻 🆘 🔟 📠 🏧 $ Mcr Mcd WC NFI
Immediately ▨ **VISA** ●

Steinberg, L Gary (MD)   **PCd**
Elmhurst Hosp Ctr

Elmhurst Hospital Center, 79-01 Broadway A7-34;
Elmhurst, NY 11373; (718) 334-3380; **BDCERT:**
Ped 91; **MS:** Philippines 85; **RES:** Ped, Elmhurst
Hosp Ctr, Elmhurst, NY 85-88; Ped, Elmhurst Hosp
Ctr, Elmhurst, NY 88-89; **FEL:** PCd, Mount Sinai
Med Ctr, New York, NY 89-92; Cardiology Medical
Center, New York, NY 89-92; **FAP:** Asst Prof Mt
Sinai Sch Med; *SI: Cardiac Murmur Evaluation;
Congenital Heart Disease*; **HMO:** Oxford Health First
Well Care Quest More Neighborhood Hlth +

LANG: Sp; 🚻 🔟 🏧 $ Mcd 2-4 Weeks

PEDIATRIC CRITICAL CARE MEDICINE

Sagy, Meyer (MD)   **PCCM**
Long Island Jewish Med Ctr

The Schneider Children Hospital, 269-01 76th
Ave; New Hyde Park, NY 11040; (718) 470-3330;
BDCERT: Ped 90; PCCM 92; **MS:** Israel 72; **RES:**
Chaim Sheba Med Ctr, Israel 77-82; **FEL:** PCCM,
Children Hosp of Philadelphia, Philadelphila, PA
82-84; **HOSP:** Schneider Children's Hosp; **HMO:**
Aetna Hlth Plan Blue Choice Child Health Plus GHI
CIGNA +

LANG: Heb, Sp; 🚻 🔟 📠 🏧 Mcd A Few Days

PEDIATRIC ENDOCRINOLOGY

Carey, Dennis (MD)   **PEn**
Long Island Jewish Med Ctr

Sneider Childrens Hospital, 269-01 76th Ave Rm
234; New Hyde Park, NY 11042; (718) 470-3290;
BDCERT: Ped 79; PEn 83; **MS:** SUNY Downstate
73; **RES:** St Vincents Hosp & Med Ctr NY, New
York, NY 73-74; Ped, Long Island Jewish Med Ctr,
New Hyde Park, NY 74-76; **FEL:** UC San Diego Med
Ctr, San Diego, CA 77-80; **FAP:** Assoc Prof Albert
Einstein Coll Med; **HOSP:** Schneider Children's
Hosp; *SI: Calcium Metabolism; Diabetes*

🚻 📠 🏧 $ Mcr Mcd 2-4 Weeks ▨ **VISA** ●

Frank, Graeme (MD)   **PEn**
Schneider Children's Hosp

Schneiders Chldns Hosp LI Jewish Hosp, 271-16
76th Ave; New Hyde Park, NY 11042; (718) 470-
3290; **BDCERT:** Ped 98; EDM 95; **MS:** South Africa
82; **RES:** Ped, Schneider Children's Hosp, New Hyde
Park, NY 88-91; **FEL:** PEn, Children's Hosp Med
Ctr, Cincinnati, OH 91-94; **FAP:** Assoc Prof Ped
Albert Einstein Coll Med; *SI: Disorders of Puberty;
Disorders of Growth*; **HMO:** Oxford GHI US Hlthcre
Empire Magnacare +

🚻 🔟 📠 🏧 Mcr Mcd 2-4 Weeks ▨ **VISA** ● ▨

Kreitzer, Paula (MD)   **PEn**
Schneider Children's Hosp

Schneider Children's Hospital, 269-01 76th Ave;
New Hyde Park, NY 11040; (718) 470-3290;
BDCERT: Ped 87; PEn 89; **MS:** U NC Sch Med 82;
RES: PEn, Schneider Children's Hosp, New Hyde
Park, NY; **HMO:** Most

🔟 🏧 Mcd 4+ Weeks **VISA** ●

PEDIATRIC GASTROENTEROLOGY

Kessler, Brad (MD)   PGe
Long Island Jewish Med Ctr
Long Island Jewish Med Ctr.; New Hyde Park, NY
11042; (718) 470-3430; **BDCERT:** Ped 88; Ge 90;
MS: SUNY Downstate 82; **RES:** Ped, N Shore Univ
Hosp-Manhasset, Manhasset, NY 82-85; **FAP:**
Assoc Prof Albert Einstein Coll Med; **HOSP:**
Schneider Children's Hosp; *SI: Inflammatory Bowel
Disease;* **HMO:** Oxford Aetna Hlth Plan HealthNet
🚹 🏥 💲 Ⓜ️   Immediately

Pettei, Michael (MD)   PGe
Long Island Jewish Med Ctr
269-01 76th Ave; New Hyde Park, NY 11040;
(718) 470-3430; **BDCERT:** Ped 86; PGe 90; **MS:** U
Miami Sch Med 80; **RES:** Ped, Mount Sinai Med Ctr,
New York, NY 80-82; **FEL:** PGe & Nutrition,
Columbia-Presbyterian Med Ctr, New York, NY 82-
84; **FAP:** Assoc Prof Ped Albert Einstein Coll Med;
HOSP: Schneider Children's Hosp; *SI: Inflammatory
Bowel Disease; Pediatric Nutrition;* **HMO:** Oxford US
Hlthcre Empire Blue Cross & Shield Empire Vytra +
🚹 📞 🔒 🏥 💲 Ⓜ️ Ⓜ️   A Few Days ▦ **VISA** 💳

PEDIATRIC HEMATOLOGY-ONCOLOGY

Karayalcin, Gungor (MD)   PHO
Schneider Children's Hosp
269-01 76th Ave; New Hyde Park, NY 11040;
(718) 470-3460; **BDCERT:** Ped 72; **MS:** Turkey 59;
RES: Queens Hosp Ctr, Jamaica, NY 62-65; **FEL:**
PHO, Queens Hosp Ctr, Jamaica, NY 65-66; PHO,
Queens Hosp Ctr, Jamaica, NY 68; **FAP:** Assoc Prof
SUNY Stony Brook; **HMO:** Blue Choice United
Healthcare Oxford GHI

PEDIATRIC NEPHROLOGY

Gauthier, Bernard (MD)   PNep
Schneider Children's Hosp
269-01 76th Ave 365; New Hyde Park, NY 11040;
(718) 470-3491; **BDCERT:** Ped 74; PNep 74; **MS:**
Australia 61; **RES:** Australia 61-62; Austria 64-68;
FEL: N, Univ Hosp SUNY Bklyn, Brooklyn, NY 70-
72; **FAP:** Prof Ped Albert Einstein Coll Med; *SI:
Blood in the Urine; Protein in the Urine;* **HMO:** Oxford
US Hlthcre CIGNA GHI Blue Choice +
LANG: Fr; 🚹 🔒 🅿️ 🏥 💲 Ⓜ️ Ⓜ️ NFI   2-4 Weeks ▦
VISA 💳 💳

Trachtman, Howard (MD)   PNep
Long Island Jewish Med Ctr
269-01 76th Ave 365; New Hyde Park, NY 11040;
(718) 470-3491; **BDCERT:** Ped 83; **MS:** Univ Penn
78; **RES:** New England Med Ctr, Boston, MA 78-80;
Jacobi Med Ctr, Bronx, NY 80-81; **FEL:** PNep,
Albert Einstein Med Ctr, Bronx, NY; **FAP:** Prof
Albert Einstein Coll Med; **HOSP:** Schneider
Children's Hosp; *SI: Hypertension; Hemolytic Uremic
Syndrome;* **HMO:** Oxford US Hlthcre Child Health
Plus CIGNA Blue Choice +
LANG: Sp, Heb, Fr; 🚹 🔒 🅿️ 🏥 Ⓜ️ Ⓜ️ WC
A Few Days ▦ **VISA** 💳 💳

PEDIATRIC RADIOLOGY

Leonidas, John (MD)   PR
Long Island Jewish Med Ctr
269-05 76th Ave; New Hyde Park, NY 11040;
(718) 470-3404; **BDCERT:** Rad 69; Ped 65; **MS:**
Greece 55; **RES:** Kingsbrook Jewish Med Ctr,
Brooklyn, NY 61-63; Columbia-Presbyterian Med
Ctr, New York, NY 65-68; **FEL:** PCd, Kings County
Hosp Ctr, Brooklyn, NY 63-64; **FAP:** Prof Albert
Einstein Coll Med
LANG: Grk; 🚹 🔒 🏥 Ⓜ️ Ⓜ️ NFI   Immediately **VISA**
💳

PEDIATRIC SURGERY

Pena, Alberto (MD)   **PS**
Long Island Jewish Med Ctr
269-01 76th Ave 158; New Hyde Park, NY 11040;
(718) 470-3637; **MS:** Mexico 62; **RES:** Military
Hosp, Mexico City, Mexico 63-66; **FEL:** PdS,
Children's Hosp, Boston, MA 69-71; **FAP:** Prof Ped
Albert Einstein Coll Med; **SI:** *Anorectal Malformation;
Colorectal Problems;* **HMO:** Oxford CIGNA Empire
Blue Choice 1199 Multiplan +

LANG: Sp; ⧉ ⧉ ⧉ ⧉ ⧉ ⧉ Immediately

PEDIATRICS

Abularrage, Joseph (MD)   **Ped**   **PCP**
NY Hosp Med Ctr of Queens
56-34 Main St; Flushing, NY 11355; (718) 670-
1813; **BDCERT:** Ped 81; **MS:** NYU Sch Med 75;
RES: Bellevue Hosp Ctr, New York, NY 75-78;
Bellevue Hosp Ctr, New York, NY 78-79; **FEL:** EDM,
Columbia-Presbyterian Med Ctr, New York, NY;
Child Dev, Columbia-Presbyterian Med Ctr, New
York, NY; **FAP:** Assoc Prof Cornell U; **HMO:** Oxford
CIGNA GHI Magnacare

⧉ ⧉ ⧉ ⧉ ⧉ ⧉ ⧉ Immediately

Azizirad, Hassan (MD)   **Ped**
Catholic Med Ctr Bklyn & Qns
152-11 89th Ave; Jamaica, NY 11432; (718) 692-
6490; **BDCERT:** Ped 72; **MS:** Iran 65; **RES:** Coney
Island Hosp, Brooklyn, NY 68-71; **HOSP:** Mary
Immaculate Hosp

D'Arienzo, Nicholas (MD)   **Ped**   **PCP**
St John's Epis Hosp-S Shore
70-04 Kissel St; Forest Hills, NY 11375; (718) 544-
7770; **BDCERT:** Ped 63; **MS:** Italy 58; **RES:** Ped, St
Catherine's Hosp, Brooklyn, NY 59-61; **FEL:** Cv, St
Francis Hosp-Roslyn, Roslyn, NY; **HOSP:** Long
Island Jewish Med Ctr; **HMO:** Blue Cross & Blue
Shield GHI Oxford CIGNA PHCS +

LANG: Itl; ⧉ ⧉ ⧉ A Few Days

Dilello Sr, Edmund (MD)   **Ped**   **PCP**
Catholic Med Ctr Bklyn & Qns
83-21 57th Ave; Elmhurst, NY 11373; (718) 429-
1373; **BDCERT:** Ped 68; **MS:** Middlesex U Sch Med
45; **RES:** Ped, St John's Epis Hosp-S Shore, Far
Rockaway, NY 48-49; **HOSP:** Mary Immaculate
Hosp; **HMO:** Blue Cross & Blue Shield Aetna Hlth
Plan US Hlthcre PHS

⧉ ⧉ ⧉ ⧉ 1 Week

Eden, Alvin N (MD)   **Ped**   **PCP**
Wyckoff Heights Med Ctr
107-21 Queens Blvd 7; Flushing, NY 11375; (718)
261-8989; **BDCERT:** Ped 57; **MS:** Boston U 52;
RES: New York University Med Ctr, New York, NY
53-55; **FAP:** Assoc Clin Prof Ped Cornell U; **HOSP:**
NY Hosp Med Ctr of Queens; **SI:** *Pediatric Obesity;*
HMO: Aetna Hlth Plan Oxford United Healthcare
Prucare GHI +

⧉ ⧉ ⧉ ⧉ ⧉ ⧉ ⧉ ⧉ A Few Days

Friedman, Lorna (MD)   **Ped**   **PCP**
NY Hosp-Cornell Med Ctr
36-11 21st St; Long Island City, NY 11106; (718)
482-7772; **BDCERT:** Ped 94; **MS:** NY Med Coll 91;
RES: Children's Hosp of Philadelphia, Philadelphia,
PA 91-94; **FAP:** Clin Instr Ped Cornell U; **HOSP:**
Queens Hosp Ctr

LANG: Sp, Grk, Fr; ⧉ ⧉ ⧉ ⧉ ⧉ ⧉ A Few Days

Gattereau-Edwards, M (MD) **Ped**   **PCP**
St Vincents Hosp & Med Ctr NY
Gattereau and Edwards, MD, PC, 191-05 Hillside
Ave; Holliswood, NY 11423; (718) 468-8400;
BDCERT: Ped 89; **MS:** Hahnemann U 82; **RES:** Ped,
St Luke's Roosevelt Hosp Ctr, New York, NY 82-85;
HOSP: NY Hosp Med Ctr of Queens; **SI:** *Asthma; Skin
Rashes*

LANG: Sp, Fr, Dut; ⧉ ⧉ ⧉ ⧉ ⧉ ⧉ ⧉
Immediately ▨ *VISA* ▨ ▨

Goldstein, Steven J (MD)   Ped   `PCP`
Long Island Jewish Med Ctr
141-49 70th Rd; Flushing, NY 11367; (718) 268-5282; **BDCERT:** Ped 81; PEn 83; **MS:** SUNY Hlth Sci Ctr 78; **RES:** Ped, Long Island Jewish Med Ctr, New Hyde Park, NY 78-81; **HOSP:** NY Hosp Med Ctr of Queens; **SI:** *Nutrition; Asthma*; **HMO:** Oxford Blue Cross CIGNA HealthNet GHI +

LANG: Sp, Yd; ⛬ 🏥 ☎ 🅿 🛏 $ Mcr Mcd
A Few Days **VISA** ⬤

Grijnsztein, Jacob (MD)   Ped   `PCP`
Long Island Jewish Med Ctr
KGR Pediatric Assoc, 98-15 Horace Harding Expy; Flushing, NY 11368; (718) 699-8500; **BDCERT:** Ped 79; **MS:** NYU Sch Med 73; **RES:** Ped, Bellevue Hosp Ctr, New York, NY 73-76; **HOSP:** N Shore Univ Hosp-Manhasset; **SI:** *Allergies; Well Baby Care*; **HMO:** GHI Oxford Blue Cross & Blue Shield Health First Multiplan +

LANG: Sp, Rus; ⛬ 🏥 ⬤ ☎ 🅿 🛏 $ Immediately
VISA ⬤

Hankin, Dorie (MD)   Ped
Long Island Jewish Med Ctr
Schneider Children's Hosp, 269-01 76th Ave SCH139; Mineola, NY 10042; (718) 470-3540; **BDCERT:** Ped 80; **MS:** Albert Einstein Coll Med 74; **RES:** Ped, Montefiore Med Ctr, Bronx, NY 74-78; **FEL:** Child Development, Albert Einstein Med Ctr, Bronx, NY 78-80; **FAP:** Asst Clin Prof Ped Albert Einstein Coll Med; **SI:** *Child Development; Child Behavior*; **HMO:** Oxford Aetna-US Healthcare Chubb Empire Blue Cross & Shield United Healthcare +

⛬ ☎ 🅿 🛏 $ Mcr Mcd 2-4 Weeks

Nerwen, Clifford (MD)   Ped   `PCP`
Schneider Children's Hosp
Schneider Children's Hosp, 269-01 76th Ave; New Hyde Park, NY 11040; (718) 470-3281; **BDCERT:** Ped 95; **MS:** U Conn Sch Med 91; **RES:** Ped, Schneider Children's Hosp, New Hyde Park, NY 91-94; **SI:** *Inadequate Weight Gain*; **HMO:** US Hlthcre Oxford GHI Blue Cross & Blue Shield CIGNA +

LANG: Sp; ⛬ ☎ 🅿 🛏 $ Mcd WC A Few Days ▦
VISA ⬤

Reddy, Gaddam D (MD)   Ped   `PCP`
Catholic Med Ctr Bklyn & Qns
93-06 35th Ave; Jackson Heights, NY 11372; (718) 886-5680; **BDCERT:** Ped 71; **MS:** Turkey 63; **RES:** Children's Hosp, Boston, MA; **FEL:** Cv, Long Island Jewish Med Ctr, New Hyde Park, NY; **HOSP:** Long Island Jewish Med Ctr; **HMO:** Oxford Empire 1199

Resmovits, Marvin (MD)   Ped   `PCP`
Long Island Jewish Med Ctr
98-15 Horace Harding Expy; Flushing, NY 11368; (718) 699-8500; **BDCERT:** Ped 84; **MS:** SUNY Buffalo 79; **RES:** Ped, Long Island Jewish Med Ctr, New Hyde Park, NY 79-82; **HOSP:** N Shore Univ Hosp-Manhasset; **HMO:** PHS Blue Choice United Healthcare Oxford

LANG: Sp; ⛬ 🏥 ⬤ ☎ 🅿 🛏 $ A Few Days **VISA**
⬤

Rubin, Lorry (MD)   Ped
Long Island Jewish Med Ctr
Schneider Childrens Hospital, 269-01 76th Ave 365; New Hyde Park, NY 11040; (718) 470-3480; **BDCERT:** Ped 83; **MS:** Rush Med Coll 78; **RES:** Children's Hosp of Los Angeles, Los Angeles, CA 78-80; **FEL:** Ped Inf, Johns Hopkins Hosp, Baltimore, MD 80-82; **FAP:** Prof Ped Albert Einstein Coll Med; **SI:** *Lyme Disease; Tuberculosis & Fevers*; **HMO:** Oxford US Hlthcre

⛬ 🅿 🛏 $ Mcr Mcd NFI A Few Days ▦ **VISA** ⬤

Salemi, Mozafar (MD)   Ped
Mary Immaculate Hosp
88-25 153rd St Apt 2N; Jamaica, NY 11432; (718) 558-7212; **BDCERT:** Ped 72; **MS:** Iran 64; **RES:** Ped, Univ of Med & Dent NJ Hosp, Newark, NJ 67-70; **FEL:** Ped, Long Island Jewish Med Ctr, New Hyde Park, NY 70-72; **FAP:** Clin Instr Albert Einstein Coll Med; **HOSP:** St Mary's Hosp; **SI:** *Blood Disorders*; **HMO:** Most

LANG: Frs; Immediately

Villegas, Emilio (MD) Ped `PCP`
Mount Sinai Med Ctr
STAT Medical Care, 95-42 Roosevelt Ave; Jackson Heights, NY 11372; (718) 565-7900; **BDCERT:** Ped 92; **MS:** Dominican Republic 80; **RES:** Ped, Mount Sinai Med Ctr, New York, NY 89; **FAP:** Clin Instr Mt Sinai Sch Med; **HOSP:** Flushing Hosp Med Ctr; **SI:** *Developmental Pediatrics;* **HMO:** Prudential Oxford Aetna Hlth Plan PHCS Blue Cross +

LANG: Sp, Rus, Tag, Chi; ⌖ 🅂🄰 🌓 📷 📋 🎴 💲 🄼 Immediately ▒ **VISA** 💳 💳

PHYSICAL MEDICINE & REHABILITATION

Cole, Jeffrey L (MD) PMR
NY Hosp Med Ctr of Queens
56-45 Queens Blvd W403; Flushing, NY 11355; (718) 670-1290; **BDCERT:** PMR 83; **MS:** Mexico 77; **RES:** IM, NY Hosp Med Ctr of Queens, Flushing, NY 77-79; PMR, Albert Einstein Med Ctr, Bronx, NY 79-82; **FEL:** NY Hosp Med Ctr of Queens, Flushing, NY 82-83; **SI:** *Muscles & Nerves-EMG; SSEP Testing;* **HMO:** Aetna Hlth Plan Prucare CIGNA Magnacare PHS +

⌖ 📷 📋 💲 🄼 🅆🄲 🄽🄵 2-4 Weeks

Fishman, Loren (MD) PMR
Flushing Hosp Med Ctr
45-00 Parsons Blvd; Flushing, NY 11355; (718) 670-5515; **BDCERT:** PMR 86; **MS:** Harvard Med Sch 79; **RES:** New England Med Ctr, Boston, MA 79-81; **HOSP:** Little Neck Comm Hosp; **HMO:** US Hlthcre Blue Choice Oxford Magnacare

⌖ 🌓 📷 📋 🎴 🄼 🅆🄲 🄽🄵 Immediately

Gasalberti, Richard (MD) PMR
Hosp For Joint Diseases
111-20 Queens Blvd; Forest Hills, NY 11375; (718) 544-7700; **BDCERT:** PMR 94; **MS:** West Indies 84; **RES:** PMR, Mount Sinai Med Ctr, New York, NY; NY Hosp Med Ctr of Queens, Flushing, NY; **FEL:** Hosp For Joint Diseases, New York, NY; **HOSP:** Parkway Hosp; **SI:** *Pain Management; Sports Medicine;* **HMO:** Oxford Magnacare Chubb Blue Cross & Blue Shield GHI +

⌖ 🅂🄰 🌓 📷 🎴 📋 💲 🄼 🄼 🅆🄲 🄽🄵 Immediately ▒ **VISA** 💳

Gupta, Saroj (MD) PMR
Wyckoff Heights Med Ctr
180-16 Wexford Terr; Jamaica Estates, NY 11432; (718) 963-7656; **BDCERT:** PMR 85; **MS:** India 73; **RES:** Mount Sinai Med Ctr, New York, NY 79-82

Kyriakides, Christopher (DO)PMR
Parkway Hospital
38-25 Astoria Blvd; Long Island City, NY 11103; (718) 274-5207; **BDCERT:** PMR 94; **MS:** NY Coll Osteo Med 89; **RES:** New York University Med Ctr, New York, NY 90-93; **FAP:** Clin Prof NY Coll Osteo Med; **SI:** *Back Pain; Neck Pain;* **HMO:** GHI Oxford Blue Cross & Blue Shield

LANG: Sp, Grk, Itl, Man, Pol; ⌖ 🅂🄰 🌓 📷 🎴 📋 🄼 🅆🄲 🄽🄵 Immediately ▒ **VISA** 💳

PLASTIC SURGERY

Kraft, Robert (MD) PlS
N Shore Univ Hosp-Manhasset
112-03 Queens Blvd 205; Forest Hills, NY 11375; (718) 263-6868; **BDCERT:** PlS 87; **MS:** Yale U Sch Med 78; **RES:** Albert Einstein Med Ctr, Bronx, NY 78-82; Albert Einstein Med Ctr, Bronx, NY 82-84; **FEL:** Microvascular S, Montefiore Med Ctr, Bronx, NY; **HOSP:** NY Hosp Med Ctr of Queens; **SI:** *Breast Reduction; Liposuction;* **HMO:** Blue Cross & Blue Shield HealthNet Prucare United Healthcare US Hlthcre +

⌖ 🌓 📷 🎴 📋 💲 🄼 🅆🄲 🄽🄵 A Few Days ▒ **VISA** 💳

Guide to symbols and abbreviations can be found on pages 110-113.

585

Loeb, Thomas (MD)   PlS
Beth Israel North

161-03 Horace Harding Blvd; Flushing, NY 11365;
(718) 461-9400; **BDCERT:** PlS 88; **MS:**
Washington U, St Louis 80; **RES:** S, New York
University Med Ctr, New York, NY 80-82; Booth
Mem Hosp, Flushing, NY 82-84; **FEL:** PlS, Baylor
Med Ctr, Dallas, TX 84-86; **FAP:** Clin Instr Cornell
U; *SI: Facelifts; Liposuction;* **HMO:** Oxford PHS GHI
Tristate

LANG: Sp; 🚹 🔲 🔳 🛏 🅂 Mcr NFI A Few Days ▨
VISA 💳

PSYCHIATRY

Applebaum, Seymour (MD) Psyc
Jamaica Med Ctr

118-80 Metropolitan Ave 2D; Kew Gardens, NY
11415; (718) 849-1086; **BDCERT:** Psyc 75; **MS:**
Albert Einstein Coll Med 59; **RES:** Hawaii State Coll,
Honolulu, HI 60-61; Los Angeles Cty Hosp, Los
Angeles, CA 61-63; *SI: Geriatrics; Addictions;* **HMO:**
GHI VBH MHCS CMG Multiplan +

🚹 🆂 🔳 🔲 🛏 🅂 Mcr Mcd A Few Days

Cole, Steven A (MD)   Psyc
Long Island Jewish Med Ctr

75-59 263rd St; Glen Oaks, NY 11004; (718) 470-
8515; **BDCERT:** Psyc 80; **MS:** Duke U 74; **RES:** U
NC Hosp, Chapel Hill, NC 77

🚹 🔲 🛏 🅂 Mcr 1 Week

Kane, John M (MD)   Psyc
Long Island Jewish Med Ctr

75-59 263rd St; Glen Oaks, NY 11004; (718) 470-
8141; **BDCERT:** Psyc 77; **MS:** NYU Sch Med 71;
RES: Long Island Jewish Med Ctr, New Hyde Park,
NY

🚹 🔲 🛏 2-4 Weeks

Lubin, Martin (MD)   Psyc
Queens Hosp Ctr

NY Hospital Medical Ctr Queens, 56-45 Main St;
Flushing, NY 11355; (718) 670-1030; **BDCERT:**
Psyc 69; **MS:** U Miami Sch Med 61; **RES:** Psyc,
Bellevue Hosp Ctr, New York, NY 62-65; **FAP:** Asst
Clin Prof Cornell U; **HOSP:** NY Hosp Med Ctr of
Queens; **HMO:** Aetna-US Healthcare Vytra United
Healthcare GHI

🚹 🔲 🔳 🛏 🅂 Mcr A Few Days ▨ **VISA** 💳

Mendelowitz, Alan (MD)   Psyc
Long Island Jewish Med Ctr

75-59 263rd St Rm209; Glen Oaks, NY 11004;
(718) 470-8397; **BDCERT:** Psyc 92; Ger 94; **MS:**
Rutgers U 87; **RES:** Psyc, Long Island Jewish Med
Ctr, New Hyde Park, NY 88-91; **FAP:** Asst Prof Psyc
Albert Einstein Coll Med; **HMO:** Oxford GHI Premier
Beech Street

🆂 🔲 🔳 🛏 🅂 Mcr NFI Immediately **VISA** 💳

Mildener, Barry (MD)   Psyc
Long Island Jewish Med Ctr

75-59 263rd St; Glen Oaks, NY 11004; (718) 470-
8447; **BDCERT:** Psyc 93; GerPsy 95; **MS:** Mexico
85; **RES:** Psyc, Univ Hosp SUNY Bklyn, Brooklyn,
NY 87-91; **FEL:** GerPsy, Long Island Jewish Med
Ctr, New Hyde Park, NY 91-92; **FAP:** Asst Prof
Albert Einstein Coll Med; *SI: Depression and Anxiety
of Elderly; Psychopharmacology*

🚹 🔲 🔳 🛏 Mcr Mcd A Few Days

Rajput, Ashok (MD)   Psyc
Western Queens Comm Hosp

84-04 Penelope Ave; Flushing, NY 11379; (718)
894-6963; **BDCERT:** Psyc 90; **MS:** India 78; **RES:**
Amntsae, Punjab, India 79-80; Psyc, Elmhurst
Hosp Ctr, Elmhurst, NY 82-85; **FAP:** Asst Clin Prof
Mt Sinai Sch Med; **HOSP:** Jamaica Med Ctr; *SI:
Geriatric Psychiatry; Depression;* **HMO:** Oxford
Magnacare Anthem Health

LANG: Hin, Rom, Ur; 🔳 🔲 🛏 🅂 Mcr Immediately

Rifkin, Arthur (MD) Psyc
Long Island Jewish Med Ctr

75-59 263rd St; Glen Oaks, NY 11004; (718) 470-8075; **BDCERT:** Psyc 68; **MS:** SUNY Downstate 61; **RES:** Hillside Hosp, Glen Oaks, NY 62-65; **FEL:** Univ Hosp SUNY Bklyn, Brooklyn, NY 67-69; **FAP:** Prof Albert Einstein Coll Med; **HMO:** Oxford Blue Cross & Blue Shield

🚹 🕍 📞 📦 🕎 🎛 Mcr NFl   A Few Days

Selzer, Jeffrey A (MD) Psyc
Long Island Jewish Med Ctr

Long Island Jewish Medical Center, 75-59 263rd St; Glen Oaks, NY 11004; (718) 470-8023; **BDCERT:** Psyc 85; AdP 93; **MS:** U Mich Med Sch 79; **RES:** Ped, Children's Hosp of Los Angeles, Los Angeles, CA 79-80; Psyc, UCLA Med Ctr, Los Angeles, CA 80-83; **FAP:** Asst Prof Albert Einstein Coll Med; *SI: Addictions; Mood Disorders/Depressions*

🚹 📞 📦 🕎 💲 Mcr   2-4 Weeks **VISA** 💳

Siris, Samuel G (MD) Psyc
Long Island Jewish Med Ctr

75-59 263rd St; Glen Oaks, NY 11004; (718) 470-8138; **BDCERT:** Psyc 76; **MS:** Columbia P&S 70; **RES:** Med, Mount Sinai Med Ctr, New York, NY 70-71; Psyc, NYS Psychiatric Institute, New York, NY 71-74; **FEL:** Psyc, Nat Inst Mental Health, Bethesda, MD 74-76; **FAP:** Prof Psyc Albert Einstein Coll Med; *SI: Psychopharmacology; Schizophrenia*

📞 📦 🕎 💲   2-4 Weeks

Vivek, Seeth (MD) Psyc
Jamaica Med Ctr

75-58 113th St 1A; Forest Hills, NY 11375; (718) 268-9595; **BDCERT:** Psyc 80; Ger 94; **MS:** India 72; **RES:** Nat Inst Mental Health, Bethesda, MD 74-76; Mount Sinai Med Ctr, New York, NY 76-79; **FAP:** Assoc Clin Prof NY Coll Osteo Med; **HOSP:** NY Hosp Med Ctr of Queens; *SI: Depression; Panic Disorders*; **HMO:** GHI Aetna-US Healthcare US Hlthcre VBH MBC +

LANG: Sp, Hin, Tam; 🚹 📞 📦 🕎 🎛 💲 Mcr   A Few Days

PULMONARY DISEASE

Dantzker, David (MD) Pul
Long Island Jewish Med Ctr

270-05 76th Ave; New Hyde Park, NY 11040; (718) 470-7621; **BDCERT:** IM 72; Pul 74; **MS:** SUNY Buffalo 67; **RES:** Med, Univ Hosp SUNY Buffalo, Buffalo, NY 68-69; Med, EJ Meyer Mem Hosp, Buffalo, NY 69-70; **FEL:** Pul, UC San Diego Med Ctr, San Diego, CA 72-73; UC San Diego Med Ctr, San Diego, CA 73-75; **FAP:** Prof Albert Einstein Coll Med; **HMO:** Oxford

🚹 📦 💲 Mcr Med   2-4 Weeks **VISA** 💳

Donath, Joseph (MD) Pul
St John's Queens Hosp

112-41 Queens Blvd; Forest Hills, NY 11375; (718) 380-1553; **BDCERT:** IM 80; Pul 82; **MS:** Hungary 72; **RES:** IM, VA Med Ctr-Bronx, Bronx, NY 77-80; **FEL:** Pul, Mount Sinai Med Ctr, New York, NY 80-82; **FAP:** Asst Prof of Clin Med Albert Einstein Coll Med; **HOSP:** Catholic Med Ctr Bklyn & Qns; *SI: Asthma; Lung Tumors*; **HMO:** Empire Blue Choice Multiplan 32BJ GHI CIGNA +

LANG: Hun; 🚹 📞 📦 🕎 🎛 💲 Mcr Med WC   1 Week

Greenberg, Harly (MD) Pul
Long Island Jewish Med Ctr

270-05 76th Ave; New Hyde Park, NY 11040; (718) 470-7058; **BDCERT:** Pul 88; CCM 89; **MS:** NYU Sch Med 82; **RES:** N Shore Univ Hosp-Manhasset, Manhasset, NY 82-85; Mem Sloan Kettering Cancer Ctr, New York, NY 82-85; **FEL:** Pul, New York University Med Ctr, New York, NY 85-87; Bellevue Hosp Ctr, New York, NY 88; **FAP:** Asst Prof Med Albert Einstein Coll Med; **HOSP:** Montefiore Med Ctr; *SI: Sleep Disorders Medicine*; **HMO:** Well Care HIP Network Magnacare US Hlthcre

🚹 📦 🕎 🎛 💲 Mcr   2-4 Weeks 💳 **VISA** 💳

Guide to symbols and abbreviations can be found on pages 110-113.

587

Karbowitz, Stephen (MD)   Pul
NY Hosp Med Ctr of Queens
56-45 Main St M216; Flushing, NY 11355; (718) 670-1405; **BDCERT:** Pul 76; IM 74; **MS:** Albert Einstein Coll Med 71; **RES:** IM, Montefiore Med Ctr, Bronx, NY 71-74; **FEL:** Pul, Montefiore Med Ctr, Bronx, NY 74-76; **FAP:** Asst Prof Cornell U; **SI:** *Asthma; Emphysema;* **HMO:** Oxford NYLCare Aetna-US Healthcare Magnacare Blue Cross +

♿ 📷 🚽 $ Mcr

Mehra, Sunil (MD)   Pul
Western Queens Comm Hosp
41-11 30th St; Long Island City, NY 11101; (718) 726-3535; **BDCERT:** IM 82; Pul 87; **MS:** India 77; **RES:** IM, Kingsbrook Jewish Med Ctr, Brooklyn, NY 79-82; **FEL:** Pul/CCM, Long Island Jewish Med Ctr, New Hyde Park, NY; **FAP:** Asst Clin Prof Albert Einstein Coll Med; **HOSP:** St John's Queens Hosp; **SI:** *Asthma and Emphysema; Lung Diseases;* **HMO:** Oxford Blue Choice Vytra Magnacare United Healthcare +

LANG: Hin, Ur, Sp; ♿ SA SD 🚽 $ Mcr   A Few Days

Miller, Albert (MD)   Pul
Mary Immaculate Hosp
88-25 153rd St 3J; Jamaica, NY 11432; (718) 558-7227; **BDCERT:** IM 66; Pul 72; **MS:** U Wisc Med Sch 59; **RES:** IM, Mount Sinai Med Ctr, New York, NY 59-60; VA Med Ctr-Bronx, Bronx, NY 61-62; **FEL:** Pul, Mt Sinai Med Ctr, New York, NY 60-61; Mt Sinai Med Ctr, New York, NY 64-65; **FAP:** Clin Prof Med Albert Einstein Coll Med; **HOSP:** Catholic Med Ctr Bklyn & Qns; **SI:** *Asthma, Occupational; Sarcoidosis;* **HMO:** 32BJ MCI

LANG: Fr, Ger; ♿ 📷 🚽 Mcr   1 Week

Mondrow, Stanley (MD)   Pul
St Joseph's Hosp-Queens
Queens Pulmonary Diagnostic, 147-15 70th Rd; Flushing, NY 11367; (718) 544-5622; **BDCERT:** Pul 82; CCM 87; **MS:** Albert Einstein Coll Med 76; **RES:** IM, Montefiore Med Ctr, Bronx, NY 77-78; Montefiore Med Ctr, Bronx, NY 76-77; **FEL:** Pul, Montefiore Med Ctr, Bronx, NY 76-77; **HMO:** Blue Choice Blue Cross & Blue Shield CIGNA

Multz, Alan (MD)   Pul
Long Island Jewish Med Ctr
270-05 76th Ave; New Hyde Park, NY 11040; (718) 470-7230; **BDCERT:** IM 88; Pul 90; **MS:** Boston U 85; **RES:** IM, Montefiore Med Ctr, Bronx, NY 85-88; **FEL:** Pul, Albert Einstein Med Ctr, Bronx, NY 88-90; CCM, Montefiore Med Ctr, Bronx, NY 90-91; **FAP:** Asst Prof Med Albert Einstein Coll Med; **SI:** *Respiratory Distress Syndrome; Sepsis;* **HMO:** Oxford US Hlthcre CIGNA

♿ 📷 🚽 $ Mcr   Immediately 💳 **VISA** 💳

Nath, Sunil (MD)   Pul
NY Hosp Med Ctr of Queens
55-14 Main St; Flushing, NY 11355; (718) 359-3131; **BDCERT:** IM 80; Pul 82; **MS:** India 76; **RES:** NY Hosp Med Ctr of Queens, Flushing, NY 77-80; **FEL:** Pul, NY Hosp Med Ctr of Queens, Flushing, NY 80-82; **SI:** *Asthma and Emphysema; Lung Cancer;* **HMO:** Aetna Hlth Plan Oxford United Healthcare

LANG: Hin; ♿ 🌙 📷 🚽 Mcr   A Few Days

Silverman, Joel (MD)   Pul
Parkway Hosp
112-03 Queens Blvd Ste 201; Forest Hills, NY 11375; (718) 544-4600; **BDCERT:** IM 77; Pul 79; **MS:** U Okla Coll Med 74; **RES:** IM, N Shore Univ Hosp-Manhasset, Manhasset, NY; **FEL:** Pul/Chest Med, Bellevue Hosp Ctr, New York, NY 77-79; Critical Care Boards, 89; **SI:** *Emphysemia-Asthma; Pulmonary Rehabilitation;* **HMO:** Oxford US Hlthcre Aetna Hlth Plan Aetna Hlth Plan

LANG: Sp, Hin; ♿ 🌙 📷 🚽 Mcr Mcd WC NFi   Immediately

Steinberg, Harry (MD)   Pul
Long Island Jewish Med Ctr
270-05 76th Ave; New Hyde Park, NY 11040; (718) 470-7231; **MS:** Temple U 66; **RES:** Temple U Hosp, Philadelphia, PA; Long Island Jewish Med Ctr, New Hyde Park, NY 62; **FEL:** CCM, Long Island Jewish Med Ctr, New Hyde Park, NY 67-69; Hosp of U Penn, Philadelphia, PA 72-74; **FAP:** Prof Albert Einstein Coll Med; **SI:** *Emphysema; Lung Cancer;* **HMO:** Oxford Aetna Hlth Plan Vytra PHS Blue Choice +

♿ 📷 🚽 $ Mcr WC NFi   A Few Days 💳 **VISA**

RADIATION ONCOLOGY

Dalton, Jack F (MD) RadRO
Mount Sinai Med Ctr
NY Radiation Therapy Assoc, 106-14 70th Ave; Forest Hills, NY 11375; (718) 520-6620; **BDCERT:** IM 74; Hem 76; **MS:** Univ Pittsburgh 70; **RES:** Med, Geo Wash U Med Ctr, Washington, DC; Hem, Mount Sinai Med Ctr, New York, NY; **FEL:** RadRO, Mount Sinai Med Ctr, New York, NY; **HOSP:** Lenox Hill Hosp; **HMO:** Oxford

♿ 📷 🛏 Mcr Mcd WC NFI Immediately

Fazekas, John T (MD) RadRO
Mary Immaculate Hosp
Cancer Institute of CMC, 152-11 89th Ave; Jamaica, NY 11432; (718) 558-2050; **BDCERT:** RadRO 72; **MS:** Ohio State U 67; **RES:** UC San Francisco Med Ctr, San Francisco, CA 68-69; Mt Zion Hosp, San Francisco, CA 69-71; **SI:** *Combined Modality Therapy;* **HMO:** US Hlthcre GHI HIP Network Fidelis NYLCare +

LANG: Sp, Chi, Fr; ♿ 📷 🛏 🏠 Mcr Mcd A Few Days

Lipsztein, Roberto (MD) RadRO
Mount Sinai Med Ctr
NY Radiation Therapy Assoc, 106-14 70th Ave; Flushing, NY 11375; (718) 520-6620; **BDCERT:** RadRO 82; **MS:** Brazil 74; **RES:** Mount Sinai Med Ctr, New York, NY 76-79; **FEL:** RadRO, Mount Sinai Med Ctr, New York, NY 76-79; **HOSP:** Lenox Hill Hosp

LANG: Sp, Fr, Rus; ♿ 🆘 📷 🛏 💲 Mcr Mcd A Few Days **VISA**

RADIOLOGY

Doshi, Leena (MD) Rad
Flushing Hosp Med Ctr
43-55 147th St Fl 1; Flushing, NY 11355; (717) 762-7132; **BDCERT:** Rad 78; **MS:** India 73; **RES:** Lenox Hill Hosp, New York, NY 77; **FEL:** Lenox Hill Hosp, New York, NY 78; **HMO:** Aetna Hlth Plan GHI CIGNA HealthNet Blue Cross & Blue Shield +

LANG: Hin, Sp, Rus; ♿ 🆘 🅲 🏠 🛏 💲 Mcr Mcd WC NFI Immediately ▨ **VISA** 💳 🔲

Goldberg, Itzhak D (MD) Rad
Long Island Jewish Med Ctr
270-05 76th Ave; New Hyde Park, NY 11040; (718) 470-7196; **BDCERT:** Rad 82; TS 82; **MS:** Albert Einstein Coll Med 76; **RES:** Brookdale Univ Hosp Med Ctr, Brooklyn, NY 76-77; Harvard Joint Ctr Radiation Therapy, Boston, MA 79-82; **FEL:** Med, Beth Israel Med Ctr, Boston, MA 77-78; Beth Israel Med Ctr, Boston, MA 78-79; **FAP:** Prof Onc Albert Einstein Coll Med; **SI:** *Breast Cancer; Prostate Cancer;* **HMO:** Oxford CIGNA 1199 US Hlthcre +

LANG: Heb, Sp, Chi, Fr; ♿ 📷 🏠 🛏 Mcr Mcd A Few Days **VISA** 💳

Hoffman, Janet C (MD) Rad
Long Island Jewish Med Ctr
LI Jewish Med Ctr 76th Ave; New Hyde Park, NY 11040; (718) 470-7181; **BDCERT:** DR 78; **MS:** SUNY Downstate 74; **RES:** Rad, Colum Presb Med Ctr, New York, NY 75-78; **FEL:** NY Hosp, New York, NY

Lee, Won Jay (MD) Rad
Long Island Jewish Med Ctr
LIJ Radiology Priv Prac, 270-05 76th Ave; New Hyde Park, NY 11042; (718) 470-7171; **BDCERT:** Rad 70; NuM 73; **MS:** South Korea 62; **RES:** Rad, New York University Med Ctr, New York, NY 66-69; **FEL:** DR, Long Island Jewish Med Ctr, New Hyde Park, NY 69-70; **FAP:** Prof Rad Albert Einstein Coll Med; **SI:** *Genitourinary Radiology; Abdominal Radiology;* **HMO:** Oxford US Hlthcre Empire GHI United Healthcare +

♿ 📷 🛏 Mcr Mcd WC NFI A Few Days **VISA** 💳

Spreecher, Stanley (MD)   Rad
Peninsula Hosp Ctr
Peninsula Radiology Associates, 51-15 Beach
Channel Dr; Far Rockaway, NY 11691; (718) 945-
7100; **BDCERT:** Rad 82; NR 83; **MS:** Albert
Einstein Coll Med 77; **RES:** Rad, Univ Hosp SUNY
Bklyn, Brooklyn, NY; NuM, St Vincents Hosp & Med
Ctr NY, New York, NY; **HMO:** Blue Choice CIGNA
Oxford Magnacare HealthNet +

LANG: Sp, Rus, Heb, Ger; ⚕ 🏥 🌙 🔒 🏥 Mcr Mcd WC
NFI Immediately

Tartell, Jay (MD)   Rad
Western Queens Comm Hosp
Advanced Radiological Imaging Associates, PC,
89-40 56th Ave; Elmhurst, NY 11373; (718) 335-
5532; **BDCERT:** Rad 87; **MS:** NY Med Coll 82; **RES:**
Albert Einstein Med Ctr, Bronx, NY 82-86; **FEL:** N
Shore Univ Hosp-Manhasset, Manhasset, NY 86-
87; **HMO:** US Hlthcre Oxford United Healthcare
Magnacare Blue Choice +

LANG: Grk, Sp, Rus; ⚕ 🏥 🌙 🔒 🏥 S Mcr Mcd WC
NFI Immediately *VISA* 💳

Youner, Craig (MD)   Rad
Western Queens Comm Hosp
Advanced Radiological Imaging, 29-16 Astoria
Blvd; Astoria, NY 11102; (718) 204-5800;
BDCERT: Rad 78; **MS:** Albany Med Coll 73; **RES:**
Rad, N Shore Univ Hosp-Manhasset, Manhasset,
NY 75-78; IM, N Shore Univ Hosp-Manhasset,
Manhasset, NY 74-75; **FEL:** Rad, NY Hosp-Cornell
Med Ctr, New York, NY 77-78; **FAP:** Asst Clin Prof
Rad Cornell U

LANG: Sp, Grk, Itl; ⚕ 🏥 🌙 🔒 🏥 Mcr Mcd WC NFI
A Few Days *VISA* 💳

REPRODUCTIVE ENDOCRINOLOGY

Saraf, Varsha (MD)   RE
NY Hosp Med Ctr of Queens
Queens Fertility & Gynecological PC, 108-48 70th
Rd 2F; Flushing, NY 11375; (718) 793-7752;
BDCERT: ObG 86; RE 96; **MS:** India 70; **RES:** ObG,
Harlem Hosp Ctr, New York, NY 80-83; **FEL:** RE,
Columbia-Presbyterian Med Ctr, New York, NY 83-
85; **FAP:** Asst Prof ObG Cornell U; **HOSP:** N Shore
Univ Hosp-Manhasset; *SI: In Vitro Fertilization;*
Infertility; **HMO:** Blue Choice HealthNet Prucare
Sanus Travelers +

LANG: Hin, Guj; ⚕ 🏥 🌙 🐾 🏥 S Mcr   A Few Days
VISA 💳

RHEUMATOLOGY

Greenwald, Robert (MD)   Rhu
Long Island Jewish Med Ctr
Rm 337 Faculty Practice, 270-05 76th Ave; New
Hyde Park, NY 11040; (718) 470-7251; **BDCERT:**
IM 72; **MS:** Johns Hopkins U 67; **RES:** Long Island
Jewish Med Ctr, New Hyde Park, NY 67-70; **FEL:**
Univ Hosp SUNY Bklyn, Brooklyn, NY 70-72; *SI:*
Rheumatic Arthritis; Psoriatic Arthritis; **HMO:** Oxford
US Hlthcre Empire Aetna Hlth Plan Magnacare +

⚕ 🔒 🐾 🏥 S Mcr   2-4 Weeks *VISA* 💳

Hoffman, Michael L (MD)   Rhu
NY Hosp Med Ctr of Queens
Bay Rheumatology PC, 43-24 220th St; Bayside,
NY 11361; (718) 428-1400; **BDCERT:** IM 71; **MS:**
SUNY Downstate 65; **RES:** Med, Maimonides Med
Ctr, Brooklyn, NY 65-67; Med, Jacobi Med Ctr,
Bronx, NY 67-68; **FEL:** Med, Hosp For Special
Surgery, New York, NY 68-70; **FAP:** Assoc Clin
Prof Albert Einstein Coll Med; **HOSP:** Long Island
Jewish Med Ctr; *SI: Rheumatoid Arthritis; Lupus;*
HMO: Oxford

LANG: Sp, Grk; ⚕ 🌙 🔒 🐾 🏥 S   1 Week 🖼
VISA 💳

Sharon, Ezra (MD)   Rhu
Western Queens Comm Hosp
70-31 108th St; Forest Hills, NY 11375; (718)
793-6832; **BDCERT:** IM 73; Rhu 74; **MS:** Israel 67;
RES: Mount Sinai Med Ctr, New York, NY 69-71;
Rhu, SUNY Bklyn, Brooklyn, NY 71-73; **FEL:**
Mount Sinai Med Ctr, New York, NY; **HOSP:**
Parkway Hosp; *SI: Rheumatoid Arthritis; Lupus;*
HMO: Most

LANG: Itl, Sp, Ar; [symbols]
Immediately

Sonpal, Girish (MD)   Rhu
Flushing Hosp Med Ctr
149-65 24th Ave; Flushing, NY 11357; (718) 445-
0500; **BDCERT:** IM 74; Rhu 76; **MS:** India 69; **RES:**
Med, Catholic Med Ctr, Brooklyn, NY 71-74; **FEL:**
Rhu, Worcester City Hosp, Worcester, MA 74-75
[symbols] 1 Week

SPORTS MEDICINE

Gerberg, Lynda Frances (MD)SM
Schneider Children's Hosp
Schneider Children's Hospital, 269-01 76th Ave;
New Hyde Park, NY 11040; (718) 470-3281;
BDCERT: Ped 94; **MS:** Mexico 87; **RES:** Schneider
Children's Hosp, New Hyde Park, NY 91-93; **FEL:**
Children's Hosp, Boston, MA 93-94; **FAP:** Asst Prof
Albert Einstein Coll Med; **HOSP:** Long Island Jewish
Med Ctr; **HMO:** US Hlthcre Blue Cross Oxford
NYLCare CIGNA +

Silverman, Marc (MD)   SM
Hosp For Joint Diseases
97-17 64th Rd; Rego Park, NY 11374; (718) 575-
9896; **BDCERT:** OrS 94; **MS:** Albert Einstein Coll
Med 85; **RES:** OrS, NY Med Coll, Valhalla, NY 86-
90; **FEL:** SpinalS, Univ of Toronto, Toronto, Canada
90; SM, Hosp For Joint Diseases, New York, NY 91;
FAP: Instr OrS NYU Sch Med; **HOSP:** St Barnabas
Hosp-Bronx; *SI: Sports Medicine; Arthroscopic
Surgery;* **HMO:** GHI Prucare Magnacare US Hlthcre
Guardian +

LANG: Sp, Yd, Heb, Rus; [symbols]
[symbol] 1 Week

SURGERY

Benedicto, Ramon (MD)   S
Wyckoff Heights Med Ctr
58-10 Catalpa Ave; Ridgewood, NY 11385; (212)
440-1597; **BDCERT:** S 80; **MS:** Philippines 72;
RES: SM, Wyckoff Heights Med Ctr, Brooklyn, NY
74-79; **HMO:** Aetna-US Healthcare GHI Blue
Choice Oxford Magnacare +

LANG: Fil, Sp; [symbols] Immediately
VISA

Drew, Michael (MD)   S
Parkway Hosp
69-60 108th St; Flushing, NY 11375; (718) 575-
9595; **BDCERT:** S 82; **MS:** Georgetown U 76; **RES:**
Mount Sinai Med Ctr, New York, NY 76-81; **HOSP:**
Mount Sinai Med Ctr; *SI: Laparoscopy; Varicose Vein
Treatment;* **HMO:** Oxford US Hlthcre GHI Empire
Blue Cross & Shield

LANG: Sp, Tag; [symbols] A Few Days
VISA

Manolas, Panos (MD)   S
NY Hosp Med Ctr of Queens
30-16 30th Dr; Astoria, NY 11102; (718) 626-
0707; **BDCERT:** S 90; **MS:** Greece 82; **RES:** S, New
York Methodist Hosp, Brooklyn, NY 84-89; **HOSP:**
N Shore Univ Hosp-Forest Hills; *SI: Breast Surgery;
Laparoscopic Surgery;* **HMO:** Oxford GHI United
Healthcare Magnacare US Hlthcre +

LANG: Grk, Sp, Itl, Kor, Fr; [symbols]
[symbol] Immediately *VISA* [symbol]

Pace, Benjamin (MD)   S
Queens Hosp Ctr
82-68 164th St; Jamaica, NY 11432; (718) 883-
4640; **BDCERT:** S 85; **MS:** Mexico 77; **RES:** S, Long
Island Jewish Med Ctr, New Hyde Park, NY; **HOSP:**
Mount Sinai Med Ctr; *SI: Surgery of the Breast;
Breast Cancer*
[symbols] A Few Days

Rifkind, Kenneth (MD)   **S**
NY Hosp Med Ctr of Queens
56-45 Main St & Booth Memorial Ave; Flushing,
NY 11355; (718) 445-0220; **BDCERT:** S 95; **SCC**
91; **MS:** NYU Sch Med 69; **RES:** S, New York
University Med Ctr, New York, NY 70-75; **FAP:**
Asst Clin Prof Rhu NYU Sch Med; **HMO:** Oxford
Blue Choice CIGNA PHS Aetna Hlth Plan +

Savasatit, Panas (MD)   **S**
Wyckoff Heights Med Ctr
55-12 Main St; Flushing, NY 11355; (718) 460-
4668; **BDCERT:** S 75; **MS:** Thailand 65; **RES:** S,
Booth Mem Hosp, Flushing, NY 67-71; **FEL:** S,
Roswell Park Cancer Inst, Buffalo, NY 72-73;
HOSP: Flushing Hosp Med Ctr; **SI:** *Gall Bladder
Surgery; Hernia Surgery;* **HMO:** Aetna Hlth Plan
Oxford Blue Cross & Blue Shield Prucare US Hlthcre
+
LANG: Grk, Thai; 🖐 📞 📷 📠 🎬 **S** Mcr WC
A Few Days

Siddiqi, Ahmed Mutee (MD)   **S**
Peninsula Hosp Ctr
South Shore Surgical Associates, 916 Cornaga Ave;
Far Rockaway, NY 11691; (718) 337-5858;
BDCERT: S 71; **MS:** India 62; **RES:** Brookdale Univ
Hosp Med Ctr, Brooklyn, NY; **HOSP:** St John's Epis
Hosp-S Shore; **SI:** *Endoscopy;* **HMO:** Most
LANG: Fil, Hin; 🖐 📷 🎬 **S** Mcr WC NFl   A Few Days

Siegel, Beth (MD)   **S**
St Vincents Hosp & Med Ctr NY
55-12 Main St; Flushing, NY 11355; (718) 460-
3547; **BDCERT:** S 90; **MS:** Dominica 82; **RES:** NY
Hosp Med Ctr, Queens, NY; **FEL:** Brigham Women's
Hosp,; **HOSP:** NY Hosp Med Ctr of Queens; **SI:**
Breast Surgery; **HMO:** Most
📞 📷 🎬 Mcr   2-4 Weeks

Sung, Kap-jae (MD)   **S**
Catholic Med Ctr Bklyn & Qns
68-07 Eliot Ave; Middle Village, NY 11379; (718)
651-2929; **BDCERT:** S 95; **MS:** South Korea 73;
RES: Wyckoff Heights Med Ctr, Brooklyn, NY 86;
HOSP: Wyckoff Heights Med Ctr; **SI:** *Breast Cancer;
Laparoscopic Surgery;* **HMO:** Oxford US Hlthcre Blue
Choice United Healthcare CIGNA +
LANG: Itl, Kor; 🏥 📞 📷 📠 🎬 **S** Mcr WC
A Few Days

Turner, James (MD)   **S**
NY Hosp Med Ctr of Queens
CRT Surgical Associates, The New York Hospital
Medical Center of Queens; Flushing, NY 11355;
(718) 445-0220; **BDCERT:** S 76; **MS:** Eastern VA
Med Sch, Norfolk 70; **RES:** S, New York University
Med Ctr, New York, NY 70-75; **FAP:** Assoc Clin
Prof Cornell U; **HOSP:** Flushing Hosp Med Ctr; **SI:**
Laparoscopic Abdominal Surgery; Vascular Surgery;
HMO: Empire Blue Choice US Hlthcre Oxford
Prucare
LANG: Fr, Itl, Sp; 📞 📷 🎬 **S** Mcr WC NFl
A Few Days 📷 **VISA** 💳 📷

Yatco, Ruben (MD)   **S**
Mary Immaculate Hosp
177-06 Wexford Ter; Jamaica, NY 11432; (718)
262-9456; **BDCERT:** S 97; **MS:** Philippines 72;
RES: S, Catholic Med Ctr Bklyn & Qns, Jamaica, NY
75-79; S, New York Methodist Hosp, Brooklyn, NY
79-82; **FEL:** Cv, Arizona Heart Inst, Phoenix, AZ
82-83; **HOSP:** Jamaica Med Ctr; **SI:** *A-V Fistula-
Graft Surgery; Bypass Lower Extremity-Leg;* **HMO:**
Oxford CIGNA Aetna-US Healthcare GHI Blue Cross
& Blue Shield +
LANG: Tag, Sp; 🖐 📷 📠 🎬 **S** Mcr Mcl WC   1 Week

THORACIC SURGERY

Graver, L Michael (MD)   TS
Long Island Jewish Med Ctr
270-05 76th Ave; New Hyde Park, NY 11040; (718) 470-7460; **BDCERT:** TS 86; **MS:** Albany Med Coll 77; **RES:** S, St Luke's Roosevelt Hosp Ctr, New York, NY 82; Children's Hosp, Boston, MA 83; **FEL:** Cv, NY Hosp-Cornell Med Ctr, New York, NY 81; New England Deaconess Hosp, Boston, MA 83-85; **FAP:** Assoc Prof S Albert Einstein Coll Med; **SI:** *Heart Surgery; Esophageal Surgery;* **HMO:** Aetna Hlth Plan US Hlthcre Empire Blue Cross & Shield Magnacare Vytra +

LANG: Itl, Sp; ⓚ ⓐ ⓜ ⑪ Ⓢ Ⓜⓒⓡ Ⓜⓞⓓ Ⓦⓒ
A Few Days

Lajam, Frank E (MD)   TS
Parkway Hosp
140-04 58th Rd; Flushing, NY 11355; (718) 886-1512; **BDCERT:** S 71; TS 74; **MS:** Dominican Republic 62; **RES:** S, Mt Sinai Medical Ctr, New York, NY 64-69; **FEL:** Cardio-Thoracic Surgery, Mt Sinai Medical Ctr, New York, NY 69-70; **HOSP:** Western Queens Comm Hosp; **SI:** *Cardiothoracic and Lung Surgeries; Pacemakers;* **HMO:** Most

LANG: Sp; Ⓒ ⓐ ⑪ Ⓜⓒⓡ Ⓜⓞⓓ Ⓦⓒ Ⓝⓕ   Immediately

Moideen, Ahamed (MD)   TS
Wyckoff Heights Med Ctr
Queens Thoracic Vascular Surgical Associates PC, 146-01 45th Ave 406; Flushing, NY 11355; (718) 539-1261; **BDCERT:** TS 83; **MS:** India 64; **RES:** S, Flushing Hosp Med Ctr, Flushing, NY 74-79; TS, Wayne Cnty Gen Hosp, Detroit, MI 79-81; **FAP:** Assoc Prof Albert Einstein Coll Med; **HOSP:** Long Island Jewish Med Ctr; **SI:** *Peripheral Vascular Surgery*

LANG: Heb, Ar, Tam; ⓚ Ⓒ ⓐ ⓜ ⑪ Ⓢ Ⓜⓒⓡ Ⓜⓞⓓ
A Few Days

Pugkhem, Tretorn (MD)   TS
NY Hosp Med Ctr of Queens
New York Hospital Medical Center of Queens, 56-45 Main St; Flushing, NY 11355; (718) 670-5000; **BDCERT:** TS 90; S 73; **MS:** Thailand 64; **RES:** Bellevue Hosp Ctr, New York, NY 66-72; **FEL:** TS, Bellevue Hosp Ctr, New York, NY 70-72; **FAP:** Chf NYU Sch Med

UROLOGY

Badlani, Gopal (MD)   U
Long Island Jewish Med Ctr
270-05 76th Ave; New Hyde Park, NY 11042; (718) 470-7225; **BDCERT:** U 82; **MS:** India 73; **RES:** S, St Agnes, Baltimore, MD 75-80; U, Long Island Jewish Med Ctr, New Hyde Park, NY 77-80; **FEL:** N, Baylor Med Ctr, Dallas, TX 83; **FAP:** Prof Albert Einstein Coll Med; **SI:** *Incontinence; Prostate New Therapy;* **HMO:** Oxford Aetna Hlth Plan Multiplan CIGNA

LANG: Sp, Hin; ⓚ ⓐ ⓜ ⑪ Ⓢ Ⓜⓒⓡ Ⓦⓒ   2-4 Weeks
▦ *VISA* ⬤

Farrell, Robert (MD)   U
NY Hosp Med Ctr of Queens
149-06 33rd Ave; Flushing, NY 11354; (718) 539-3312; **BDCERT:** U 76; **MS:** Cornell U 66; **RES:** NY Hosp Med Ctr of Qns,, Flushing, NY 66-67; NY Hosp Med Ctr of Qns, Flushing, NY 67-68; **FEL:** NY Hosp Med Ctr of Qns, Flushing, NY 70-72; Vietnam, 68-70; **HOSP:** Flushing Hosp Med Ctr

Ginsberg, Stanley (MD)   U
Peninsula Hosp Ctr
704 Empire Ave; Far Rockaway, NY 11691; (718) 327-6434; **BDCERT:** U 68; **MS:** Columbia P&S 59; **RES:** S, VA Med Ctr-Brooklyn, Brooklyn, NY 60-61; U, Mount Sinai Med Ctr, New York, NY 61-64; **HOSP:** Long Beach Med Ctr; **HMO:** Blue Choice Blue Cross & Blue Shield Choicecare HealthNet

Ⓒ ⓐ ⑪ Ⓢ Ⓜⓒⓡ Ⓜⓞⓓ Ⓦⓒ Ⓝⓕ   A Few Days

Moldwin, Robert (MD)   U
Long Island Jewish Med Ctr

270-05 76th Ave; New Hyde Park, NY 11040;
(718) 470-7223; **BDCERT:** U 93; **MS:** U Chicago-
Pritzker Sch Med 84; **RES:** U, Long Island Jewish
Med Ctr, New Hyde Park, NY; **FEL:** Inf, Thomas
Jefferson U Hosp, Philadelphia, PA; **FAP:** Asst Prof U
Albert Einstein Coll Med; **SI:** *Interstitial Cystitis;
Infertility;* **HMO:** Blue Choice GHI US Hlthcre
Multiplan Oxford +

LANG: Sp; ⬛ ⬛ ⬛ ⬛ ⬛ ⬛ ⬛ 2-4 Weeks ▦
VISA ⬛

Sandhaus, Jeffrey (MD)   U
Western Queens Comm Hosp

36-01 31st Ave; Long Island City, NY 11106;
(718) 932-3535; **BDCERT:** U 76; **MS:** NY Med Coll
66; **RES:** U, Univ Hosp SUNY Bklyn, Brooklyn,
NY 70-73; **FEL:** Nep, Univ Hosp SUNY Bklyn, Brooklyn,
NY 69-70; **FAP:** Clin Instr Cornell U; **HOSP:** NY
Hosp-Cornell Med Ctr; **SI:** *Prostate Cancer; Stone
Disease;* **HMO:** Blue Choice Prucare PHS CIGNA US
Hlthcre +

LANG: Sp, Rus, Crt, Itl, Ukr; ⬛ ⬛ ⬛ ⬛ ⬛ ⬛
1 Week ▦

Tarasuk, Albert (MD)   U
NY Hosp Med Ctr of Queens

58-42 Main St; Flushing, NY 11355; (718) 353-
3710; **BDCERT:** U 72; **MS:** Geo Wash U Sch Med
69; **RES:** Beth Israel Med Ctr, New York, NY 64-69;
HOSP: Flushing Hosp Med Ctr; **SI:** *Prostatic Disease;
Kidney & Bladder Disease;* **HMO:** Oxford GHI US
Hlthcre Blue Choice Aetna Hlth Plan +

⬛ ⬛ ⬛ ⬛ ⬛ ⬛ ⬛ A Few Days

Weiss, Gary (MD)   U
Long Island Coll Hosp

270-05 76th Ave; New Hyde Park, NY 11040;
(718) 470-4227; **BDCERT:** U 91; **MS:** Albert
Einstein Coll Med 82; **RES:** S, Vanderbilt U Med Ctr,
Nashville, TN 82-84; U, Strong Mem Hosp,
Rochester, NY 84-88; **FEL:** U, Nat Cancer Inst,
Bethesda, MD 88-89; **FAP:** Asst Prof Albert Einstein
Coll Med; **HOSP:** NY Hosp Med Ctr of Queens; **SI:**
Prostate Cancer; Bladder Cancer; **HMO:** Aetna Hlth
Plan CIGNA Oxford US Hlthcre +

⬛ ⬛ ⬛ ⬛ ⬛ 2-4 Weeks ▦ **VISA** ⬛

VASCULAR SURGERY (GENERAL)

Chaudhry, Saqib S (MD)   GVS
Flushing Hosp Med Ctr

Queens Thoracic & Vascular Surgical Associates,
146-01 45th Ave Ste 406; Flushing, NY 11355;
(718) 539-1261; **BDCERT:** Cv 90; TS 92; **MS:** Iraq
72; **RES:** TS, Flushing Hosp Med Ctr, Flushing, NY
78-80; S, Flushing Hosp, Flushing, NY 74-78; **FEL:**
Wayne Cnty Gen Hosp, Detroit, MI; **HOSP:** N Shore
Univ Hosp-Manhasset; **SI:** *Limb Salvage and
Revascularization; Carotid Endarterectomy;* **HMO:**
Oxford US Hlthcre Blue Choice CIGNA +

LANG: Ar, Tam, Ur; ⬛ ⬛ ⬛ ⬛ ⬛ ⬛ ⬛
Immediately

Cohen, Jon (MD)   GVS
Long Island Jewish Med Ctr

Long Island Jewish Med Ctr, 270-05 76th Ave;
New Hyde Park, NY 11040; (718) 470-7377;
BDCERT: S 85; GVS 87; **MS:** U Miami Sch Med 79;
RES: NY Hosp-Cornell Med Ctr, New York, NY 79-
84; **FEL:** GVS, Brigham & Women's Hosp, Boston,
MA 84-85; **FAP:** Prof S Albert Einstein Coll Med; **SI:**
*Abdominal Aortic Aneurysms; Carotid
Endarterectomy;* **HMO:** Oxford US Hlthcre PHS
NYLCare Empire +

⬛ ⬛ ⬛ ⬛ ⬛ ⬛ 2-4 Weeks **VISA** ⬛

Flores, Lucio (MD)   GVS
Brookdale Univ Hosp Med Ctr

64-10 Veterans Ave 103; Flushing, NY 11372;
(718) 478-2767; **BDCERT:** GVS 77; **MS:** Peru 68;
RES: Kingsbrook Jewish Med Ctr, Brooklyn, NY 70-
75; **HOSP:** Brooklyn Hosp Ctr-Caledonian; **HMO:**
Aetna Hlth Plan Blue Choice US Hlthcre

⬛ ⬛ ⬛ ⬛ ⬛ ⬛ ⬛ ⬛ ⬛ ⬛ Immediately **VISA**
⬛

Kaynan, Arieh (MD)   **GVS**
Western Queens Comm Hosp
188-15 Radnor Rd; Jamaica Estates, NY 11423;
(718) 479-0582; **BDCERT:** S 78; TS 93; **MS:** 66;
RES: S, Mount Sinai Med Ctr, New York, NY 69-74;
FEL: GVS, Mount Sinai Med Ctr, New York, NY 74-
75; **FAP:** Assoc Clin Prof Mt Sinai Sch Med; *SI:*
Carotid Surgery; Revascularization of Limbs; **HMO:**
Oxford US Hlthcre CIGNA Blue Cross & Blue Choice

LANG: Heb, Sp; 🚻 🌙 📷 🕴 🎫 🆂 Mcr Mcd NFI
A Few Days

Zeitlin, Alan (MD)   **GVS**
Parkway Hosp
69-60 108th St; Forest Hills, NY 11375; (718)
544-0442; **BDCERT:** S 81; **MS:** U Miami Sch Med
74; **RES:** Albert Einstein Med Ctr, Bronx, NY 74-79;
SI: Circulation Problems of Legs; Breast Cancer; **HMO:**
US Hlthcre Oxford Empire Blue Cross & Shield
CIGNA

LANG: Sp, Tag; 📷 🎫 🆂 Mcr Mcd WC   Immediately
VISA 💳

RICHMOND (STATEN ISLAND) COUNTY

STATEN ISLAND UNIVERSITY HOSPITAL

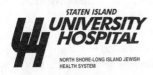

STATEN ISLAND
UNIVERSITY HOSPITAL
NORTH SHORE-LONG ISLAND JEWISH
HEALTH SYSTEM

475 SEAVIEW AVENUE
STATEN ISLAND, NY 10305
PHONE: (718) 226-9000
FAX: (718) 226-2734

Sponsorship	Voluntary not-for-profit
Beds	Multi-site hospital, 633 acute beds
Accreditation	Joint Commission on the Accreditation of Healthcare Organizations with Commendation (JCAHO); Commission on Accreditation of Rehabilitation Facilities (CARF); American College of Radiology.

GENERAL DESCRIPTION

Staten Island University Hospital, founded in 1861, was selected among America's Top 100 Hospitals for both 1996 and 1997 in an independent survey of more than 3,500 hospitals in the US. A Level 1 trauma center, it is part of the North Shore-Long Island Jewish Health System, and a major teaching affiliate of SUNY Health Science Center at Brooklyn. A multi-site facility, it has two major hospital locations and an extensive primary care network throughout the five boroughs of New York City. A cardiac surgery center begins construction in 1998.

MEDICAL STAFF AND FACULTY

Staten Island University Hospital has 912 attending staff, 72% of which are board certified. Many of the medical staff are nationally and internationally recognized. The hospital has residency programs in internal medicine, surgery, pediatrics, and Ob/Gyn, and yearly trains more than 300 residents.

SPECIAL PROGRAMS

Cancer Care	University Hospital is known internationally for its leadership program in Stereotactic Radiosurgery using three advanced linear accelerators for both brain and body tumors. A freestanding ambulatory cancer institute supports the hospital's commitment to treating all cancers, and gives access to advanced treatment protocols.
Diabetic Foot	A national Center of Excellence for its Hansen's Disease center, therapies developed are used successfully in treating Diabetic Foot disorders and difficult-healing wounds associated with diabetes.
Prostate Health	Treating both benign and cancerous prostate conditions with a variety of therapies, including cutting-edge Radiation Seed Implants, advanced forms of surgeries, and state-of-the-art laser treatment.
Burn Center	Featuring recognized specialists in the treatment of burns, University Hospital opened its 10-bed Regional Burn Center in 1998.

OTHER SERVICES

Women's Center	Emphasizing well care, the Center for Women's Health provides primary care, mammography, gynecology, obstetrics and osteoporosis. The hospital also has a birthing suite with a Jacuzzi tub and spacious facilities.
Bariatric Surgery	A highly specialized treatment for patients who are more than 100 pounds overweight, and for whom their obesity causes other serious medical problems.
RK/PRK	The Advanced Vision Care program is designed to correct near and farsightedness, and astigmatism using state-of-the-art laser surgery.
Physician referral	The hospital provides free access to more than 900 physicians and dentists through a a referral service available 70 hours a week (7 days).Call 718-226-2880.

SPECIALTY & SUBSPECIALTY	ABBREVIATION	PAGE(S)
Adolescent Medicine	AM	601
Allergy & Immunology	A&I	601
Anesthesiology	Anes	601
Cardiology (Cardiovascular Disease)	Cv	601-603
Child & Adolescent Psychiatry	ChAP	603
Dermatology	D	603
Diagnostic Radiology	DR	604
Emergency Medicine	EM	604
Endocrinology, Diabetes & Metabolism	EDM	604
FAMILY PRACTICE	FP	605
Gastroenterology	Ge	605-606
Geriatric Medicine	Ger	606
Gynecologic Oncology*	GO	606
Hematology	Hem	606
Infectious Disease	Inf	606-607
INTERNAL MEDICINE	IM	607-608
Medical Genetics	MG	609
Medical Oncology*	Onc	609
Neonatal-Perinatal Medicine	NP	609
Nephrology	Nep	609-610
Neurological Surgery	NS	610
Neurology	N	610
OBSTETRICS & GYNECOLOGY	ObG	611-612
Ophthalmology	Oph	612
Orthopaedic Surgery	OrS	612-613
Otolaryngology	Oto	614

SPECIALTY & SUBSPECIALTY	ABBREVIATION	PAGE(S)
Pediatric Cardiology	PCd	614
Pediatric Pulmonology	PPul	614
PEDIATRICS (GENERAL)	Ped	614-616
Physical Medicine & Rehabilitation	PMR	617
Plastic Surgery	PlS	617
Psychiatry	Psyc	618
Pulmonary Disease	Pul	618-619
Radiation Oncology*	RadRO	619
Radiology	Rad	619
Rheumatology	Rhu	619-620
Surgery	S	620-621
Thoracic Surgery (includes open heart surgery)	TS	621
Urology	U	621
Vascular Surgery (General)	GVS	622

Specialties in capital letters indicate Primary Care Specialties. However, many doctors will be certified in a subspecialty, but will practice predominantly primary care medicine. In our lists this will be indicated.

*Oncologists deal with Cancer

ADOLESCENT MEDICINE

Lee, April (MD) AM `PCP`
Staten Island Univ Hosp-North
475 Seaview Ave 5; Staten Island, NY 10305;
(718) 226-6294; **BDCERT:** Ped 86; AM 94; **MS:**
NYU Sch Med 80; **RES:** New York University Med
Ctr, New York, NY 80-83; **FEL:** AM, Brookdale Univ
Hosp Med Ctr, Brooklyn, NY; **FAP:** Asst Prof SUNY
Hlth Sci Ctr

⌖ ⓒ ⓐ ⓨ ⊞ Mod A Few Days

ALLERGY & IMMUNOLOGY

Krol, Kristine (MD) A&I
Staten Island Univ Hosp-South
Allercare, 4143 Richmond Ave; Staten Island, NY
10312; (718) 967-7337; **BDCERT:** IM 87; **MS:**
SUNY Hlth Sci Ctr 81; **RES:** IM, Staten Island Univ
Hosp, Staten Island, NY 81-8; Med, Staten Island
Univ Hosp, Staten Island, NY 84-85; **FEL:** A&I,
Mass Gen Hosp, Boston, MA 85-87; Children's
Hosp, Boston, MA; **FAP:** Asst Clin Prof Med
Unknown/other New York Sch ool; **SI:** *Bee Stings;
Drug Allergies;* **HMO:** PHS United Healthcare US
Hlthcre Blue Cross & Blue Shield GHI +

⌖ 🆂🆄 ⓒ ⓐ ⓨ ⊞ 🅢 Mcr Mod WC 2-4 Weeks

ANESTHESIOLOGY

Alhasan, Harith (MD) Anes
St Vincent's Med Ctr-Richmond
St Vincent's/Bayley Seton Hosp, 75 Vanderbilt Ave;
Staten Island, NY 10304; (718) 354-5960;
BDCERT: Anes 88; **MS:** Iraq 72; **RES:** Anes, Mount
Sinai Med Ctr, New York, NY 81-82; IM, Flushing
Hosp Med Ctr, Flushing, NY 82-83; **HOSP:** Bayley
Seton Hosp

LANG: Ar; ⌖ 🆂🆄 ⓒ ⓐ ⓨ ⊞ Mcr Mod WC NFl 1 Week

Stilwell, Anne Marie (MD) Anes
St Vincent's Med Ctr-Richmond
St Vincent's Medical Center, 355 Bard Ave; Staten
Island, NY 10310; (718) 876-3732; **BDCERT:**
Anes 95; PM 96; **MS:** U Rochester 90; **RES:** Anes,
NY Hosp-Cornell Med Ctr, New York, NY 91-94;
FEL: PM, NY Hosp-Cornell Med Ctr, New York, NY
95-96; **HOSP:** Bayley Seton Hosp; **SI:** *Herniated Disc,
Sciatica; Reflex Sympathetic Dystrophy;* **HMO:** Oxford
Magnacare NYLCare HIP Network +

⌖ ⓒ ⓐ ⓨ ⊞ 🅢 Mcr WC NFl A Few Days ▨ **VISA**
● 🖪

CARDIOLOGY (CARDIOVASCULAR DISEASE)

Besser, Louis (MD) Cv `PCP`
St Vincent's Med Ctr-Richmond
11 Ralph Pl 310; Staten Island, NY 10304; (718)
442-1777; **BDCERT:** IM 88; Cv 89; **MS:** Mexico 81;
RES: St Vincent's Med Ctr-Richmond, Staten Island,
NY 83-86; **FEL:** Cv, St Vincent's Med Ctr-
Richmond, Staten Island, NY 86-88; **FAP:** Asst Clin
Prof NY Med Coll; **HOSP:** Doctors Hosp of Staten
Island; **SI:** *Coronary Artery Disease; Cardiac
Arrythmias;* **HMO:** Oxford Blue Cross Blue Choice
Metlife

LANG: Itl, Sp; ⌖ 🆂🆄 ⓒ ⓐ ⓨ ⊞ 🅢 Mcr
Immediately

Bloomfield, Dennis A (MD) Cv
St Vincent's Med Ctr-Richmond
355 Bard Ave; Staten Island, NY 10310; (718)
442-5230; **MS:** Australia 56; **RES:** IM, Royal Perth
Hosp, Perth, Australia 62-63; Royal Prince Alfred
Hosp, Sydney, Australia 60-61; **FEL:** Cv, Hallstrom
Inst of Cardiology, Sydney, Australia; Vanderbilt U
Med Ctr, Nashville, TN; **FAP:** Clin Prof Med NY Med
Coll; **HOSP:** St Vincents Hosp & Med Ctr NY; **SI:**
Cardiac Catheterization; Pulmonary Embolus; **HMO:**
Aetna Hlth Plan Oxford Empire Blue Cross & Shield
Blue Choice HIP Network +

⌖ 🆂🆄 ⓒ ⓐ ⓨ ⊞ 🅢 Mcr A Few Days

Bogin, Marc (MD)   Cv
St Vincent's Med Ctr-Richmond

11 Ralph Pl Ste 108; Staten Island, NY 10304; (718) 447-7899; **BDCERT:** IM 89; Cv 93; **MS:** Mexico 85; **RES:** IM, Booth Mem Hosp, Flushing, NY 86-89; IM, Booth Mem Hosp, Flushing, NY 89-90; **FEL:** Cv, St Vincent's Med Ctr-Richmond, Staten Island, NY 90-93; **HOSP:** Staten Island Univ Hosp-North; **HMO:** Oxford GHI Magnacare Prucare Blue Choice +

♿ 🙻 🙻 🙻 🙻 🙻 Mcr WC NFI Immediately

Costantino, Thomas (MD)   Cv
Staten Island Univ Hosp-North

1870 Richmond Rd; Staten Island, NY 10306; (718) 442-4084; **BDCERT:** IM 74; Cv 74; **MS:** Georgetown U; **RES:** Geo Wash U Med Ctr, Washington, DC 67-69; IM, NY Hosp-Cornell Med Ctr, New York, NY 69; **FEL:** Cv, Georgetown U Hosp, Washington, DC 69-71; **FAP:** Asst Clin Prof SUNY Downstate; **SI:** *Congestive Heart Failure; Hypercholesterolemia;* **HMO:** Oxford Aetna-US Healthcare Blue Cross & Blue Shield NYLCare

LANG: Sp, Itl; ♿ 🙻 🙻 🙻 🙻 🙻 Mcr WC NFI A Few Days

Grodman, Richard (MD)   Cv
St Vincent's Med Ctr-Richmond

355 Bard Ave Fl 6; Staten Island, NY 10310; (718) 876-4642; **BDCERT:** IM 76; Cv 79; **MS:** SUNY Downstate 73; **RES:** IM, Univ Hosp SUNY Bklyn, Brooklyn, NY 73-76; **FEL:** CCM, Univ Hosp SUNY Bklyn, Brooklyn, NY 76-77; Cv, Rhode Island Hosp, Providence, RI 77-79; **FAP:** Asst Prof Med NY Med Coll; **SI:** *Echocardiography; Cardiac Catheterization*

♿ 🙻 🙻 Mcr NFI A Few Days

Homayuni, Ali (MD)   Cv
Staten Island Univ Hosp-South

3311 Hylan Blvd; Staten Island, NY 10306; (718) 351-3111; **BDCERT:** IM 88; Cv 91; **MS:** SUNY Downstate 85; **RES:** Staten Island Univ Hosp, Staten Island, NY 85-88; **FEL:** Cv, St Vincent's Med Ctr-Richmond, Staten Island, NY 88-91; **HOSP:** St Vincent's Med Ctr-Richmond; **SI:** *Interventional Cardiology;* **HMO:** Aetna Hlth Plan Oxford Sanus-NYLCare Metlife CIGNA +

LANG: Fr, Frs; ♿ 🙻 🙻 🙻 🙻 🙻 🙻 Mcr Mcd WC NFI A Few Days

Lafferty, James (MD)   Cv
Staten Island Univ Hosp-South

3311 Hylan Blvd; Staten Island, NY 10306; (718) 351-3111; **BDCERT:** IM 85; **MS:** SUNY Hlth Sci Ctr 82; **RES:** IM, Staten Island Univ Hosp, Staten Island, NY 82-85; **FEL:** Cv, Univ Hosp SUNY Bklyn, Brooklyn, NY 85-87; **FAP:** Assoc; **SI:** *Pacing, Cardiac; Electrophysiology*

♿ 🙻 🙻 🙻 🙻 🙻 Mcr 2-4 Weeks

Malpeso, James (MD)   Cv
Staten Island Univ Hosp-South

1870 Richmond Rd; Staten Island, NY 10306; (718) 351-2200; **BDCERT:** Cv 79; **MS:** Albert Einstein Coll Med 75; **RES:** Kings Cty Hosp Ctr, Brooklyn, NY 75-78; **FEL:** St Vincent's Hosp, New York, NY 78-80; **FAP:** Asst Prof SUNY Downstate; **HOSP:** St Vincent's Med Ctr-Richmond; **SI:** *Cardiac Catheterization; Angioplasty*

LANG: Sp; ♿ 🙻 🙻 🙻 🙻 Mcr Mcd WC NFI 1 Week

Schwartz, Charles (MD)   Cv
Staten Island Univ Hosp-North

Staten Island Heart, PC, 3710 Richmond Ave; Staten Island, NY 10312; (718) 967-6220; **BDCERT:** IM 83; Cv 85; **MS:** SUNY Downstate 80; **RES:** Staten Island Univ Hosp, Staten Island, NY 80-83; **FEL:** Cv, St Vincent's Med Ctr-Richmond, Staten Island, NY 83-85; **FAP:** Asst Clin Prof SUNY Downstate; **SI:** *Stress Echocardiography; Cardiac Catheterization;* **HMO:** Aetna-US Healthcare Oxford Choicecare GHI Prucare +

♿ 🙻 🙻 🙻 🙻 Mcr Immediately

Swamy, Samala (MD)   Cv
St Vincent's Med Ctr-Richmond

1366 Victory Blvd B; Staten Island, NY 10301; (718) 442-8351; **BDCERT:** IM 77; Cv 79; **MS:** India 72; **RES:** St Vincent's Med Ctr-Richmond, Staten Island, NY; **FEL:** Cook Cty Hosp, Chicago, IL; St Vincent's Med Ctr-Richmond, Staten Island, NY; **FAP:** Asst Prof Med NY Med Coll; **HOSP:** Doctors Hosp of Staten Island; **SI:** *Cholesterol; Heart Diseases;* **HMO:** Oxford Blue Cross & Blue Shield GHI Empire

LANG: Hin, Tel; ♿ 🙻 🙻 🙻 🙻 🙻 Mcr A Few Days

Vazzana, Thomas (MD)   Cv
St Vincent's Med Ctr-Richmond

11 Ralph Pl Ste 108; Staten Island, NY 10304; (718) 447-7899; **BDCERT:** IM 89; Cv 91; **MS:** Grenada 85; **RES:** St Joseph's Hosp-Paterson, Paterson, NJ 86-89; **FEL:** Cv, St Vincent's Med Ctr-Richmond, Staten Island, NY 89-91; **FAP:** Instr NY Med Coll; **HOSP:** Staten Island Univ Hosp-North; *SI: Cardiac Catheterization; Non-Invasive Cardiology;* **HMO:** GHI Prucare Oxford US Hlthcre

♿ 🅲 🗭 🎟 🏧 🆂 Mcr WC NFl Immediately

CHILD & ADOLESCENT PSYCHIATRY

Kaplan, William (MD)   ChAP
Long Island Jewish Med Ctr

675 Forest Ave; Staten Island, NY 10310; (718) 720-8075; **BDCERT:** Psyc 83; ChAP 84; **MS:** Brown U 77; **RES:** Psyc, U Chicago Hosp, Chicago, IL 78-80; **FEL:** ChAP, U Chicago Hosp, Chicago, IL 80-82; Columbia-Presbyterian Med Ctr, New York, NY 88; **HMO:** MCC Blue Choice Blue Cross & Blue Shield CIGNA Oxford +

🅲 🗭 🎟 🏧 🆂 1 Week

DERMATOLOGY

Bernstein, Charles (MD)   D
Staten Island Univ Hosp-South

4287 Richmond Ave; Staten Island, NY 10312; (718) 966-6601; **BDCERT:** IM 83; D 87; **MS:** SUNY Hlth Sci Ctr 80; **RES:** IM, Staten Island Univ Hosp, Staten Island, NY 80-84; D, Univ Hosp SUNY Bklyn, Brooklyn, NY 84-87; **FAP:** Assoc Clin Prof SUNY Hlth Sci Ctr; **HMO:** Blue Choice HealthNet Independent Health Plan Metlife Blue Cross & Blue Shield +

♿ 🆂🅐 🅲 🗭 🎟 🏧 🆂 Mcr 2-4 Weeks

Engber, Peter (MD)   D
St Vincent's Med Ctr-Richmond

95 New Dorp Ln; Staten Island, NY 10306; (718) 351-2303; **BDCERT:** D 78; **MS:** Italy 71; **RES:** D, NY Med Coll, Valhalla, NY 75-78; **FAP:** Asst Clin Prof D NY Med Coll; **HOSP:** Bayley Seton Hosp; *SI: Skin Surgery; Pediatric Dermatology;* **HMO:** GHI Oxford Prucare Empire Blue Cross & Shield US Hlthcre +

LANG: Itl; 🅲 🗭 🎟 🏧 🆂 Mcr 2-4 Weeks

Harris, Harriet (MD)   D
St Vincent's Med Ctr-Richmond

1545 Victory Blvd; Staten Island, NY 10314; (718) 442-1888; **BDCERT:** D 66; **MS:** SUNY Downstate 61; **RES:** New York University Med Ctr, New York, NY 62-65; **HOSP:** New York University Med Ctr; *SI: Skin Cancer; Sclerotherapy;* **HMO:** Aetna Hlth Plan Blue Choice Blue Cross & Blue Shield CIGNA HealthNet +

♿ 🗭 🎟 🏧 🆂 Mcr A Few Days

Lederman, Josiane (MD)   D
Bayley Seton Hosp

2040 Victory Blvd; Staten Island, NY 10314; (718) 370-0422; **BDCERT:** D 86; **MS:** France 81; **RES:** D, Paris, France 81-83; **FEL:** Harvard Med Sch, Cambridge, MA 83-85; **FAP:** Instr; **HOSP:** St Vincent's Med Ctr-Richmond; *SI: Skin Cancer/Screening & Treatment; Cosmetic Lasers;* **HMO:** GHI

LANG: Fr, Rus; ♿ 🆂🅐 🅲 🗭 🎟 🏧 🆂 Mcr Immediately ▨ **VISA** 💳

McCormack, Patricia (MD)   D
Bayley Seton Hosp

Bayley Seton Hospital, 75 Vanderbilt Ave; Staten Island, NY 10304; (718) 448-8828; **BDCERT:** D 85; **MS:** Rutgers U 81; **RES:** D, NY Med Coll, Valhalla, NY 82-85; **FAP:** Asst Prof D NY Med Coll; **HOSP:** St Vincent's Med Ctr-Richmond

DIAGNOSTIC RADIOLOGY

Giamo, Thomas (MD)   DR
Bayley Seton Hosp
Bailey's Radiology Dept, 75 Vanderbilt Ave; Staten Island, NY 10304; (718) 354-5734; **MS:** Italy 82; **RES:** Med, Catholic Med Ctr Bklyn & Qns, Jamaica, NY 82-84; Rad, St Vincents Hosp & Med Ctr NY, New York, NY 84-88; **HOSP:** St Vincent's Med Ctr-Richmond

🚫 📷 🏢 Mcr Mcd A Few Days

EMERGENCY MEDICINE

O'Shaughnessy, Jane (MD)   EM
St Vincent's Med Ctr-Richmond
St Vincent's Med Ctr of Richmond, 355 Bard Ave BC68; Staten Island, NY 10310; (718) 876-2054; **BDCERT:** IM 74; EM 82; **MS:** St Louis U 68; **RES:** IM, Indiana U Med Ctr, Indianapolis, IN 69-74; ObG, Mt Sinai Med Ctr, New York, NY 69-72; **FAP:** Clin Prof EM NY Med Coll

🚫 🅂🄳 🌙 📷 🅙 🏢 Mcr Mcd WC NFI Immediately
VISA 💳 AE 🔲

ENDOCRINOLOGY, DIABETES & METABOLISM

Calamia, Vincent (MD)   EDM   PCP
Staten Island Univ Hosp-South
584 Forest Ave; Staten Island, NY 10310; (718) 226-5600; **BDCERT:** IM 81; EDM 83; **MS:** U Miami Sch Med 78; **RES:** IM, Nassau County Med Ctr, East Meadow, NY 78-81; **FEL:** EDM, Nassau County Med Ctr, East Meadow, NY 81-83; **FAP:** Asst Clin Prof Med SUNY Downstate; *SI: Thyroid Disease; Diabetes Mellitus;* **HMO:** Aetna-US Healthcare Oxford GHI Prudential

🚫 🅂🄳 🌙 📷 🅙 🏢 🅢 Mcr WC NFI 2-4 Weeks

Cohen, Neil (MD)   EDM
Staten Island Univ Hosp-North
1460 Victory Blvd; Staten Island, NY 10301; (718) 442-1404; **BDCERT:** IM 93; EDM 95; **MS:** Med Coll PA 90; **RES:** IM, N Shore Univ Hosp-Forest Hills, Forest Hills, NY 90-93; **FEL:** EDM, Albert Einstein Med Ctr, Bronx, NY 93-95; *SI: Diabetes; Thyroid Disorders;* **HMO:** Oxford US Hlthcre CIGNA GHI

🚫 🅂🄳 🌙 📷 🅙 🏢 🅢 Mcr 1 Week

Das, Seshadri (MD)   EDM   PCP
St Vincent's Med Ctr-Richmond
45 Little Clove Rd; Staten Island, NY 10301; (718) 273-5522; **BDCERT:** IM 83; **MS:** England 68; **RES:** IM, North Middlesex Hosp, England; **HOSP:** Bayley Seton Hosp

LANG: Pol, Fil; 🚫 🅂🄳 🌙 📷 🅙 🏢 🅢 Mcr Mcd NFI 2-4 Weeks

Hoffman, Richard (MD)   EDM
Staten Island Univ Hosp-South
University Group Physicians - Endocrine Division, 1460 Victory Blvd; Staten Island, NY 10301; (718) 442-0300; **BDCERT:** IM 71; EDM 73; **MS:** SUNY Hlth Sci Ctr 65; **RES:** IM, Long Island Coll Hosp, Brooklyn, NY 65-67; IM, Boston Med Ctr, Boston, MA 67-68; **FEL:** IM, Boston Med Ctr, Boston, MA 68-70; IM, Harvard Med Sch, Cambridge, MA 70; **FAP:** Assoc Clin Prof SUNY Downstate; *SI: Diabetes; Thyroid Disease;* **HMO:** US Hlthcre Oxford CIGNA Sanus-NYLCare +

🚫 🅂🄳 🌙 📷 🅙 🏢 🅢 Mcr Mcd NFI Immediately

Rothman, Jeffrey (MD)   EDM
Staten Island Univ Hosp-South
University Physicians Group Endocrine Division, 1460 Victory Blvd; Staten Island, NY 10301; (718) 442-0300; **BDCERT:** IM 73; EDM 75; **MS:** SUNY Buffalo 70; **RES:** IM, Hosp of U Penn, Philadelphia, PA 70-73; **FEL:** EDM, Hosp of U Penn, Philadelphia, PA 75-77; **FAP:** Asst Clin Prof Med SUNY Hlth Sci Ctr; *SI: Thyroid/Diabetes; Osteoporosis;* **HMO:** Aetna Hlth Plan Blue Choice Blue Cross & Blue Shield Sanus-NYLCare Travelers +

LANG: Itl, Hin, Ur; 🚫 🌙 📷 🅙 🏢 🅢 Mcr 2-4 Weeks

FAMILY PRACTICE

Gianvito, Louis (MD)   FP   PCP
Staten Island Univ Hosp-North
666 Castleton Ave; Staten Island, NY 10301; (718) 447-8867; **BDCERT:** FP 70; Ger 88; **MS:** NY Med Coll 53; **RES:** Staten Island Univ Hosp, Staten Island, NY 53-54; IM, Metropolitan Hosp Ctr, New York, NY 54-55; **HOSP:** St Vincents Hosp & Med Ctr NY; **HMO:** Oxford US Hlthcre Aetna-US Healthcare Prucare

🚫 🆘 🅲 🔒 🎥 🎬 💲 Mcr Mcd WC NFl   A Few Days

La Barbera, Marianne (MD)   FP   PCP
St Vincent's Med Ctr-Richmond
1975 Hylan Blvd 201; Staten Island, NY 10306; (718) 667-1200; **BDCERT:** FP 89; **MS:** Mexico 83; **RES:** FP, Community Hosp, Glen Cove, NY 86-89; S, Flushing Hosp Med Ctr, Flushing, NY 84-86; **HOSP:** Doctors Hosp of Staten Island; **HMO:** Oxford Prucare Aetna Hlth Plan GHI Empire Blue Cross & Shield +

LANG: Sp; 🚫 🆘 🅲 🔒 🎥 🎬 💲 Mcr WC NFl

GASTROENTEROLOGY

Kalman, Jeffery (MD)   Ge
Staten Island Univ Hosp-South
129 Slosson Ave; Staten Island, NY 10314; (718) 720-5928; **BDCERT:** Ge 82; Ge 82; **MS:** SUNY Downstate 79; **RES:** Staten Island Univ Hosp, Staten Island, NY 79-82; **FEL:** Ge, Bridgeport Hosp, Bridgeport, CT; **HOSP:** St Vincent's Med Ctr-Richmond; **HMO:** US Hlthcre Magnacare Oxford

LANG: Chi, Grk; 🚫 🅲 🔒 🎬 Mcr   1 Week

Megna, Daniel (MD)   Ge
Staten Island Univ Hosp-North
360 Edison St; Staten Island, NY 10306; (718) 351-6377; **BDCERT:** IM 75; Ge 76; **MS:** Duke U 69; **RES:** IM, USPHS, Staten Island, NY 69-70; **FEL:** Ge, Yale-New Haven Hosp, New Haven, CT 72-74; Ge, USPHS, Staten Island, NY 74-75; **FAP:** Assoc Clin Prof SUNY Downstate; **SI:** *Swallowing Disorders-Biliary Disease; Colitis & Liver Disorders;* **HMO:** Oxford Blue Choice Blue Cross & Blue Shield CIGNA Prucare +

LANG: Itl; 🚫 🆘 🅲 🔒 🎥 🎬 💲   1 Week

Parikh, Divyang (MD)   Ge
St Vincents Hosp & Med Ctr NY
Digestive Liver Disease Ctr, 5 Little Clove Rd; Staten Island, NY 10301; (718) 876-9600; **BDCERT:** IM 84; **MS:** India 75; **RES:** IM, Brookdale Univ Hosp Med Ctr, Brooklyn, NY 84-86; **FEL:** Ge, Brookdale Univ Hosp Med Ctr, Brooklyn, NY 86-87; **HOSP:** Doctors Hosp of Staten Island; **SI:** *Rectal Bleeding; Laser Rx Hem; Colon Tumor;* **HMO:** GHI Blue Choice Oxford Multiplan United Healthcare +

LANG: Chi, Sp, Itl, Hin, Guj; 🅲 🔒 🎥 🎬 💲 Mcr
A Few Days 🖼️ **VISA** 💳 💳

Shaps, Jeffrey (MD)   Ge   PCP
Staten Island Univ Hosp-South
2285 Victory Blvd; Staten Island, NY 10314; (718) 761-9319; **BDCERT:** IM 80; Ge 83; **MS:** SUNY Hlth Sci Ctr 76; **RES:** SI Univ Hosp, Staten Island, NY; **FEL:** Ge, VA Hospital, Brooklyn, NY; **SI:** *Gatrointestinal Disorders; Hepatology;* **HMO:** Blue Cross & Blue Shield CIGNA HealthNet US Hlthcre Oxford +

LANG: Sp; 🚫 🆘 🅲 🔒 🎥 🎬 💲 Mcr   Immediately

Sottile, Vincent M (MD)   Ge
Staten Island Univ Hosp-South
360 Edison St; Staten Island, NY 10306; (718)
351-6377; **BDCERT:** IM 63; Ge 73; **MS:**
Georgetown U 56; **RES:** IM, Staten Island Univ
Hosp, Staten Island, NY 52-54; Ge, VA Med Ctr-
Brooklyn, Brooklyn, NY 54-55; **FEL:** Ge, VA Med
Ctr-Brooklyn, Brooklyn, NY 55-56; **FAP:** Asst Clin
Prof SUNY Downstate; *SI: Colonoscopy and
Gastroscopy; Colitis Ulcers Cancer;* **HMO:** Blue Choice
Oxford Aetna Hlth Plan

LANG: Itl; ⌖ 🅂🄰 🄶 💼 🎹 Mcr Immediately 🌐
VISA 💳 💳

Wickremesinghe, Prasanna (MD)   Ge
St Vincents Hosp & Med Ctr NY
481 Bard Ave; Staten Island, NY 10310; (718)
448-0865; **BDCERT:** IM 74; Ge 75; **MS:** Sri Lanka
68; **RES:** Med, General Hospital, Colombo, Ceylon
68-70; Med, Coney Island Hosp, Brooklyn, NY 71-
72; **FEL:** Ge, Maimonides Med Ctr, Brooklyn, NY
72-75; **FAP:** Asst Lecturer Med NY Med Coll; **HOSP:**
Bayley Seton Hosp; *SI: Inflammatory Bowel Disease;
Hepatitis-Chronic;* **HMO:** Oxford US Hlthcre Blue
Choice CIGNA GHI +

⌖ 🄶 💼 🎹 🅂 Mcr

GERIATRIC MEDICINE

Strange, Theodore (MD)   Ger   **PCP**
Staten Island Univ Hosp-South
68 Seguine Ave; Staten Island, NY 10309; (718)
356-6500; **BDCERT:** IM 88; Ger 92; **MS:** SUNY
Hlth Sci Ctr 85; **RES:** Staten Island Univ Hosp,
Staten Island, NY 85-88; **FAP:** Asst Clin Prof SUNY
Hlth Sci Ctr; **HMO:** Oxford United Healthcare
CIGNA US Hlthcre Magnacare +

⌖ 🅂🄰 🄲 🄶 💼 🎹 🅂 Mcr WC NFl Immediately

GYNECOLOGIC ONCOLOGY

Maiman, Mitchell (MD)   GO
Univ Hosp SUNY Bklyn
Center For Cancer, 256 Mason Ave; Staten Island,
NY 10305; (718) 226-6400; **BDCERT:** ObG 90;
MS: SUNY Hlth Sci Ctr 81; **RES:** ObG, Jacobi Med
Ctr, Bronx, NY 81-85; **FEL:** GO, Univ Hosp SUNY
Bklyn, Brooklyn, NY 85-87; **HOSP:** Winthrop Univ
Hosp

⌖ 🄶 💼 🎹 Mcr Mod WC Immediately

HEMATOLOGY

Forte, Frank (MD)   Hem
New York University Med Ctr
Univ Physical Oncology/Hemotology Group, 256
Mason Ave; Staten Island, NY 10305; (718) 226-
6400; **BDCERT:** IM 75; Hem 76; **MS:** Creighton U
69; **RES:** IM, Staten Island Univ Hosp, Staten Island,
NY 70-73; **HOSP:** Staten Island Univ Hosp-North
LANG: Rus, Ar, Heb; ⌖ 🄲 🄶 🅂 Mcr Mod
A Few Days

INFECTIOUS DISEASE

Glazer, Jordan (MD)   Inf   **PCP**
Staten Island Univ Hosp-South
20 Ebbitts St; Staten Island, NY 10306; (718) 273-
4199; **BDCERT:** IM 82; Inf 84; **MS:** SUNY Hlth Sci
Ctr; **RES:** IM, Staten Island Univ Hosp, Staten
Island, NY 79-80; Inf, Staten Island Univ Hosp,
Staten Island, NY 80-82; **FEL:** Inf, Univ Hosp SUNY
Bklyn, Brooklyn, NY 82-84; **HMO:** Blue Cross &
Blue Shield GHI Oxford HealthNet US Hlthcre +
⌖ 🅂🄰 🄲 🄶 💼 🎹 🅂 Mcr Mod WC NFl Immediately

Nedunchezian, Deeptha (MD) Inf
St Vincent's Med Ctr-Richmond
207 Benedict Rd; Staten Island, NY 10304; (718) 966-3405; **BDCERT:** Inf 86; IM 82; **MS:** India 75; **RES:** IM, St Vincent's Med Ctr, New York, NY 79-80; **FEL:** Inf, Downstate Med Ctr, Brooklyn, NY 80-82; **FAP:** Asst Prof Med NY Med Coll; **HOSP:** Bayley Seton Hosp; ***SI:*** *AIDS; Tuberculosis*; **HMO:** Empire Blue Cross & Shield GHI Oxford HIP Network US Hlthcre +
LANG: Hin, Tam; ♿ ☾ ☎ 👤 📅 $ [Mcr] [WC] [NFI] A Few Days

INTERNAL MEDICINE

Chen, Chia-maou (MD) IM
Bayley Seton Hosp
50 Rome Ave; Staten Island, NY 10304; (718) 273-0810; **BDCERT:** IM 80; Cv 81; **MS:** Taiwan 62; **RES:** Pawtucket Mem Hosp, Pawtucket, RI 77-79; **FEL:** Cv, USPHS Hosp, Baltimore, MD 79-81; **HOSP:** St Vincent's Med Ctr-Richmond; ***SI:*** *Thyroid Disease*; **HMO:** United Healthcare GHI Blue Choice Magnacare
LANG: Chi, Jpn; ♿ [SA SU] ☾ 📅 $ [Mcr] A Few Days

Di Maso, Gerald (MD) IM [PCP]
Staten Island Univ Hosp-South
68 Seguine Ave; Staten Island, NY 10309; (718) 356-6500; **BDCERT:** IM 90; Ger 94; **MS:** SUNY Stony Brook 86; **RES:** SI Univ Hosp, Staten Island, NY 86-89; **FAP:** Asst Prof Med SUNY Downstate; ***SI:*** *Geriatrics*; **HMO:** CIGNA Oxford Sanus-NYLCare Aetna Hlth Plan Blue Choice +
♿ [SA SU] ☾ ☎ 👤 📅 [Mcr] [WC] [NFI] A Few Days

Fazio, Richard (MD) IM
St Vincent's Med Ctr-Richmond
Medical Ctr Suite 203, 78 Todt Hill Rd; Staten Island, NY 10314; (718) 448-1122; **BDCERT:** IM 82; Ge 83; **MS:** Italy 78; **RES:** IM, Maimonides Med Ctr, Brooklyn, NY 78; IM, Maimonides Med Ctr, Brooklyn, NY 78-81; **FEL:** St Vincent's Med Ctr-Richmond, Staten Islnd, NY 81-83; **FAP:** Prof SUNY Downstate; **HOSP:** Maimonides Med Ctr; ***SI:*** *Colonoscopic Polyp removal; Endoscopic stone removal*; **HMO:** Oxford GHI Prudential US Hlthcre United Healthcare +
LANG: Itl, Ger, Sp, Chi; ♿ ☾ ☎ 👤 📅 $ [Mcr]
Immediately

Forlenza, Thomas (MD) IM
Bayley Seton Hosp
102 Hart Blvd; Staten Island, NY 10301; (718) 816-4949; **BDCERT:** IM 81; Hem 84; **MS:** Boston U 77; **RES:** U KY Hosp, Lexington, KY; **FEL:** New York University Med Ctr, New York, NY; Onc, Kings County Hosp Ctr, Brooklyn, NY; **FAP:** Asst Clin Prof NYU Sch Med; **HOSP:** Doctors Hosp of Staten Island; ***SI:*** *Hospice Care*; **HMO:** US Hlthcre CIGNA Oxford NYLCare Prucare +
LANG: Sp, Itl; ☾ ☎ 📅 $ [Mcr] 2-4 Weeks

Fulop, Robert (MD) IM [PCP]
St Vincent's Med Ctr-Richmond
476 Klondike Ave; Staten Island, NY 10314; (718) 761-1156; **BDCERT:** IM 82; Ger 94; **MS:** SUNY Syracuse 78; **RES:** Brookdale Univ Hosp Med Ctr, Brooklyn, NY 79-81; ***SI:*** *Diagnostic Specialist*; **HMO:** Oxford GHI Aetna Hlth Plan United Healthcare
[SA SU] ☾ ☎ 👤 📅 [Mcr] [WC] [NFI] Immediately

Gazzara, Paul (MD) IM [PCP]
Staten Island Univ Hosp-North
3589 Hylan Blvd; Staten Island, NY 10308; (718) 966-3700; **BDCERT:** IM 86; Ger 92; **MS:** SUNY Downstate 83; **RES:** Staten Island Univ Hosp, Staten Island, NY 86; **FAP:** Assoc SUNY Downstate; **HOSP:** Staten Island Univ Hosp-South; ***SI:*** *Geriatrics; Substance Abuse*; **HMO:** Oxford GHI 1199 US Hlthcre
LANG: Itl, Sp; ♿ [SA SU] ☾ ☎ 👤 📅 $ [Mcr]
A Few Days [AMERICAN EXPRESS] VISA [MasterCard] [DISCOVER]

Hendricks, Judith (MD)   IM   PCP
Staten Island Univ Hosp-North

1361 Hylan Blvd; Staten Island, NY 10305; (718)
667-5400; **BDCERT:** IM 78; **MS:** U Okla Coll Med
75; **RES:** Staten Island Univ Hosp, Staten Island, NY
75-78; **FAP:** Asst Clin Prof SUNY Hlth Sci Ctr; *SI:*
Medicine; **HMO:** Aetna Hlth Plan Oxford CIGNA
Blue Cross & Blue Shield US Hlthcre +

[symbols] A Few Days

Malach, Barbara (MD)   IM   PCP
Staten Island Univ Hosp-South

2627 Hylan Blvd B; Staten Island, NY 10306;
(718) 987-6000; **BDCERT:** IM 83; Ger 88; **MS:**
SUNY Hlth Sci Ctr 79; **RES:** Staten Island Univ
Hosp, Staten Island, NY 79-82

[symbols] 1 Week

McGinn, Regina (MD)   IM   PCP
Staten Island Univ Hosp-North

475 Seaview Ave; Staten Island, NY 10305; (718)
226-6158; **BDCERT:** IM 87; Ger 92; **MS:** SUNY
Hlth Sci Ctr 83; **RES:** IM, Staten Island Univ Hosp,
Staten Island, NY 84-87; **FEL:** Staten Island Univ
Hosp-North, Staten Island, NY; **FAP:** Asst Clin Prof
SUNY Hlth Sci Ctr; *SI: Geriatrics; Preventive*
Medicine; **HMO:** US Hlthcre Oxford GHI

[symbols] 2-4 Weeks

Messo, Ralph K (DO)   IM   PCP
Staten Island Univ Hosp-North

Internal Medicine Pedatrics, 1361 Hylan Blvd;
Staten Island, NY 10305; (718) 980-1729;
BDCERT: Ped 93; IM 94; **MS:** Univ N E Coll Osteo
Med Biddeford 89; **RES:** Ped, Staten Island Univ
Hosp, Staten Island, NY 89-93; **HOSP:** St Vincent's
Med Ctr-Richmond; **HMO:** Blue Choice Aetna-US
Healthcare Oxford Magnacare Multiplan +

LANG: Sp; [symbols]
Immediately **VISA**

Santiamo, Joseph (MD)   IM   PCP
Bayley Seton Hosp

4268 Richmond Ave; Staten Island, NY 10312;
(718) 967-3000; **MS:** Mexico 81; **RES:** Long Island
Coll Hosp, Brooklyn, NY 83-86; **FEL:** Ger, Long
Island Jewish Med Ctr, New Hyde Park, NY; **FAP:**
Assoc Clin Prof NY Med Coll; **HOSP:** St Vincent's
Med Ctr-Richmond; *SI: Alzheimer's Disease;* **HMO:**
US Hlthcre Sanus-NYLCare Magnacare Blue Choice
Oxford +

LANG: Sp; [symbols] Immediately

Stathopoulos, Peter (MD)   IM   PCP
St Vincent's Med Ctr-Richmond

856 Castelon Ave; Staten Island, NY 10310; (718)
720-6300; **BDCERT:** IM 95; **MS:** Greece 81; **RES:**
IM, St Vincent's Med Ctr-Richmond, Staten Island,
NY 81-84; **HOSP:** Bayley Seton Hosp; **HMO:** Oxford
Blue Choice GHI Magnacare Multiplan +

LANG: Grk; [symbols] A Few Days
VISA

Tursi, William (MD)   IM   PCP
Staten Island Univ Hosp-South

4131 Richmond Ave; Staten Island, NY 10312;
(718) 948-4523; **BDCERT:** IM 80; Ger 94; **MS:**
Italy 77; **RES:** IM, St Barnabas Med Ctr, Livingston,
NJ 78-80; **HOSP:** St Vincent's Med Ctr-Richmond;
HMO: Oxford Aetna-US Healthcare CIGNA Prucare
Metlife +

LANG: Itl; [symbols] A Few Days

Winter, Steven (MD)   IM
Staten Island Univ Hosp-South

2627 Hylan Blvd Bldg B; Staten Island, NY 10306;
(718) 351-5600; **BDCERT:** IM 79; Cv 81; **MS:**
UMDNJ-NJ Med Sch, Newark 76; **RES:** N Shore
Univ Hosp-Manhasset, Manhasset, NY 76-79; Mem
Sloan Kettering Cancer Ctr, New York, NY 76-79;
FEL: Cv, Rhode Island Hosp, Providence, RI 79-81;
HOSP: St Vincent's Med Ctr-Richmond; *SI:*
Cholesterol Management; **HMO:** Oxford GHI Blue
Choice Blue Cross & Blue Shield

LANG: Heb; [symbols] 1 Week

MEDICAL GENETICS

Sklower Brooks, Susan (MD) MG
St Vincent's Med Ctr-Richmond
NYS Institute for Basic Research, 1050 Forest Hill Rd; Staten Island, NY 10314; (718) 494-5221; **BDCERT:** Ped 79; MG 82; **MS:** Mt Sinai Sch Med 75; **RES:** Ped, Mount Sinai Med Ctr, New York, NY 75-77; **FEL:** MG, Mount Sinai Med Ctr, New York, NY 77-79; **FAP:** Assoc Clin Prof Mt Sinai Sch Med; **HOSP:** Staten Island Univ Hosp-North; *SI: Inborn Errors of Metabolism; Fragile X;* **HMO:** Oxford Anthem Health

🚻 📷 🔧 🛏 ♦ ♦ A Few Days

MEDICAL ONCOLOGY

Hamilton, Audrey (MD)   Onc
Staten Island Univ Hosp-North
Center For Cancer, 256 Mason Ave FL1; Staten Island, NY 10305; (718) 226-6400; **BDCERT:** Onc 95; Hem 94; **MS:** Harvard Med Sch 83; **RES:** IM, Brigham & Women's Hosp, Boston, MA 84-86; **FAP:** Instr Albert Einstein Coll Med

NEONATAL-PERINATAL MEDICINE

Roth, Philip (MD)   NP
Staten Island Univ Hosp-North
597 Rutland Ave; Teaneck, NJ 07666; (718) 226-9796; **BDCERT:** Ped 87; NP 89; **MS:** Columbia P&S 82; **RES:** Children's Hosp of Philadelphia, Philadelphia, PA 82-86; **FEL:** NP, Hosp of U Penn, Philadelphia, PA 86-88; **FAP:** Assoc Prof SUNY Downstate; *SI: Neonatal Infection*

🚻 📷 🔧 🛏 ♦

Siracuse, Jeffrey F (MD)   NP
St Vincent's Med Ctr-Richmond
Sisters of Charity - St Vincents Campus, 355 Bard Ave; Staten Island, NY 10310; (718) 876-4636; **BDCERT:** Ped 85; NP 85; **MS:** Italy 77; **RES:** Ped, St Vincents-Richmond, Staten Island, NY 77-80; **FEL:** NP, Columbia-Presby, New York, NY 80-82; **FAP:** Asst Clin Prof Ped NYU Sch Med; **HMO:** Most

🚻 ♦ 🔧 📷 🛏 ♦ Immediately

NEPHROLOGY

Alpert, Bertram (MD)   Nep
Staten Island Univ Hosp-South
Richmond Kidney Ctr, 1366 Victory Blvd; Staten Island, NY 10301; (718) 273-3400; **BDCERT:** IM 76; Nep 78; **MS:** NY Med Coll 72; **RES:** U Mich Med Ctr, Ann Arbor, MI 73-76; **FEL:** Nep, Albert Einstein Med Ctr, Bronx, NY 76-78; **HOSP:** St Vincent's Med Ctr-Richmond; **HMO:** Oxford US Hlthcre CIGNA GHI PHS +

LANG: Itl; 🚻 ♦ 🔧 📷 🛏 🛏 $ ♦ ♦ ♦ 2-4 Weeks *VISA* 💳

Grossman, Susan (MD)   Nep   [PCP]
St Vincent's Med Ctr-Richmond
355 Bard Ave; Staten Island, NY 10310; (718) 876-2416; **BDCERT:** IM 80; Nep 82; **MS:** UMDNJ-NJ Med Sch, Newark 77; **RES:** Univ of Med & Dent NJ Hosp, Newark, NJ 77-80; **FEL:** Nep, New England Med Ctr, Boston, MA 80-82; **FAP:** Assoc Clin Prof NY Med Coll; *SI: Nutrition;* **HMO:** Oxford Blue Choice Guardian NYLCare Aetna-US Healthcare +

🚻 🔧 📷 🛏 🛏 ♦ A Few Days

Kleiner, Morton (MD)   Nep   [PCP]
Staten Island Univ Hosp-South
Regan & McGinn, MD PC, 347 Edison St; Staten Island, NY 10306; (718) 351-1136; **BDCERT:** IM 77; Nep 82; **MS:** NY Med Coll 74; **RES:** IM, N Shore Univ Hosp-Manhasset, Manhasset, NY 75-77; **FEL:** Nep, NY Hosp-Cornell Med Ctr, New York, NY 77-79; **HOSP:** Maimonides Med Ctr; *SI: Kidney Transplants;* **HMO:** Oxford Aetna Hlth Plan Blue Cross & Blue Shield CIGNA United Healthcare +

LANG: Heb; 🚻 ♦ 🔧 📷 🛏 $ ♦ Immediately

Maniscalco, Albert (MD)   Nep
Staten Island Univ Hosp-South
1366 Victory Blvd; Staten Island, NY 10301; (718) 448-8824; **BDCERT:** IM 72; Nep 76; **MS:** NY Med Coll 66; **RES:** St Vincent's Med Ctr-Richmond, Staten Island, NY 67-70; **FEL:** Duke U Med Ctr, Durham, NC 72-74; **HOSP:** Bayley Seton Hosp; **HMO:** GHI CIGNA Metlife Oxford Prucare +

⬇ 🅲 🔂 🈁 🎚 🆂 Mcr Immediately ▦ **VISA**

Pepe, John (MD)   Nep
St Vincent's Med Ctr-Richmond
1550 Richmond Ave S103; Staten Island, NY 10314; (718) 876-9800; **BDCERT:** IM 78; **MS:** Med Coll PA 75; **RES:** IM, Univ Hosp SUNY Stony Brook, Stony Brook, NY 76-78; IM, Coney Island Hosp, Brooklyn, NY 75-76; **FEL:** Albert Einstein Med Ctr, Bronx, NY 78-80; **FAP:** Asst Prof NY Med Coll; **HOSP:** Staten Island Univ Hosp-South; **SI:** *Kidney Disease; Transplant Follow-up*

LANG: Itl, Sp; ⬇ 🆂🅂 🅲 🔂 🎚 🈁 🆂 Mcr Mod WC NFI A Few Days

NEUROLOGICAL SURGERY

Chang, Edwin (MD)   NS
St Vincent's Med Ctr-Richmond
Healthcare Associates in Medicine, 1099 Targee St; Staten Island, NY 10304; (718) 448-3210; **BDCERT:** NS 93; **MS:** U Minn-Duluth Sch Med 82; **RES:** NS, Ohio State U Hosp, Columbus, OH 83-88; **HOSP:** Staten Island Univ Hosp-South; **HMO:** Aetna Hlth Plan GHI United Healthcare US Hlthcre Oxford +

LANG: Man, Can; ⬇ 🅲 🔂 🈁 🎚 🆂 Mcr Mod WC NFI A Few Days **VISA** ● ▦

Ho, Victor (MD)   NS
Doctors Hosp of Staten Island
1551 Richmond Rd; Staten Island, NY 10304; (718) 980-5000; **BDCERT:** NS 86; **MS:** SUNY Hlth Sci Ctr 78; **RES:** NS, New York University Med Ctr, New York, NY 77-81; **HOSP:** St Vincent's Med Ctr-Richmond

Mod

NEUROLOGY

Jutkowitz, Robert (MD)   N
St Vincent's Med Ctr-Richmond
78 Todt Hill Rd 205; Staten Island, NY 10314; (718) 442-7133; **BDCERT:** Psyc 76; **MS:** Univ Ky Coll Med 68; **RES:** N, Mount Sinai Med Ctr, New York, NY 71-73; **FAP:** Asst Clin Prof NY Med Coll; **HOSP:** Bayley Seton Hosp; **SI:** *Multiple Sclerosis; Parkinson's Disease*; **HMO:** Blue Cross & Blue Shield GHI Prucare Oxford US Hlthcre +

LANG: Itl; ⬇ 🅲 🔂 🈁 🆂 Mcr NFI 1 Week

Kulick, Stephen (MD)   N
Staten Island Univ Hosp-South
Healthcare Associates in Medicine, PC, 1099 Targee St; Staten Island, NY 10304; (718) 448-3210; **BDCERT:** N 69; **MS:** Boston U 61; **RES:** Med, Boston VA Med Ctr, Boston, MA 62-63; N, Mount Sinai Med Ctr, New York, NY 63-66; **FAP:** Asst Clin Prof Mt Sinai Sch Med; **HOSP:** St Vincent's Med Ctr-Richmond; **SI:** *Parkinson's Disease; Migraine*; **HMO:** Chubb Sanus-NYLCare US Hlthcre CIGNA GHI +

LANG: Chi, Rus, Sp, Fr, Tag; ⬇ 🆂🅂 🔂 🈁 🆂 Mcr WC NFI 2-4 Weeks ▦ **VISA** ● ▦

Perel, Allan (MD)   N
Staten Island Univ Hosp-North
27 New Dorp Ln; Staten Island, NY 10306; (718) 667-3800; **BDCERT:** N 90; **MS:** SUNY Downstate 85; **RES:** N, Columbia-Presbyterian Med Ctr, New York, NY 86-89; **FAP:** Asst Clin Prof SUNY Hlth Sci Ctr; **HMO:** Aetna Hlth Plan Blue Choice US Hlthcre

OBSTETRICS & GYNECOLOGY

Gonzalez, Orlando (MD)   ObG
St Vincent's Med Ctr-Richmond
78 Todt Hill Rd # 107; Staten Island, NY 10314;
(718) 273-6034; **BDCERT:** ObG 90; ObG 98; **MS:**
Mexico 82; **RES:** ObG, St Vincent's Med Ctr-
Richmond, Staten Island, NY 84-88; **FEL:** GO, Mem
Sloan Kettering Cancer Ctr, New York, NY 85-86;
HOSP: Doctors Hosp of Staten Island; *SI:*
Laparoscopic Surgery; Alternative Hysterectomy;
HMO: Aetna Hlth Plan Oxford GHI United
Healthcare Magnacare +
🦽 📞 🔒 🖼 🏨 $ 	A Few Days

Grecco, Michael (MD)   ObG   `PCP`
Staten Island Univ Hosp-South
1984 Richmond Rd; Staten Island, NY 10306;
(718) 667-1111; **BDCERT:** ObG 92; **MS:** West
Indies 82; **RES:** Univ Hosp SUNY Buffalo, Buffalo,
NY 84-89; **HOSP:** St Vincent's Med Ctr-Richmond;
HMO: US Hlthcre Prucare Aetna Hlth Plan Metlife
HIP Network +
📞 🔒 🖼 🏨 $ Mcr 	Immediately **VISA** 💳

Herzog, David (MD)   ObG   `PCP`
St Vincent's Med Ctr-Richmond
Women's Health Care Specialists, 4855 Highland
Blvd; Staten Island, NY 10312; (718) 966-8337;
BDCERT: ObG 94; **MS:** Mexico 85; **RES:** Staten
Island Univ Hosp, Staten Island, NY 87-90; **HMO:**
US Hlthcre Sanus-NYLCare Aetna Hlth Plan Oxford
GHI +
📞 🔒 🖼 🏨 $ Mcr 	1 Week

Moretti, Michael (MD)   ObG
St Vincent's Med Ctr-Richmond
Antepartum Testing Ctr, 355 Bard Ave 208; Staten
Island, NY 10310; (718) 876-3287; **BDCERT:** ObG
89; MF 90; **MS:** Mexico 81; **RES:** ObG, Staten Island
Univ Hosp, Staten Island, NY 82-86; **FEL:** MF, U
Tenn Hosp, Memphis, TN 86-88; **HOSP:** Staten
Island Univ Hosp-North; **HMO:** GHI Oxford CIGNA
Blue Cross & Blue Shield HIP Network +
🦽 📞 🔒 🖼 🏨 $ Mcr Mcd WC NFI 	1 Week **VISA** 💳

Perry, Kathleen (MD)   ObG
Staten Island Univ Hosp-North
539 Castleton Ave; Staten Island, NY 10301; (718)
727-9700; **BDCERT:** ObG 77; **MS:** NY Med Coll 67;
RES: Staten Island Univ Hosp, Staten Island, NY; *SI:*
Cervical Disorders; Menstrual Disorders Over 35;
HMO: Aetna-US Healthcare GHI Oxford CIGNA
United Healthcare +
🦽 📞 🔒 🖼 🏨 $ Mcr 	2-4 Weeks ▨ **VISA** 💳

Pillari, Vincent (MD)   ObG
St Vincent's Med Ctr-Richmond
355 Bard Ave; Staten Island, NY 10310; (718)
876-4293; **BDCERT:** ObG 68; **MS:** Loyola U-Stritch
Sch Med, Maywood 62; **RES:** ObG, Nassau County
Med Ctr, East Meadow, NY 63-64; ObG, Univ Hosp
SUNY Syracuse, Syracuse, NY 64-66; **HMO:** Aetna
Hlth Plan Oxford Blue Cross & Blue Shield HIP
Network GHI +
🦽 🔒 🖼 🏨 Mcr 	A Few Days

Ponterio, Jane M (MD)   ObG   `PCP`
St Vincent's Med Ctr-Richmond
1583 Richmond Ave; Staten Island, NY 10314;
(718) 983-0204; **BDCERT:** ObG 97; **MS:** NY Med
Coll 81; **RES:** ObG, St Luke's Roosevelt Hosp Ctr,
New York, NY 81-85; **FAP:** Asst Prof ObG NY Med
Coll; *SI: First Pregnancy/Menopause;* **HMO:** GHI Blue
Choice Oxford PHS Magnacare +
LANG: Sp; 📞 🔒 🖼 🏨 $ 	1 Week ▨ **VISA** 💳

Rapp, Lynn (MD)   ObG
Staten Island Univ Hosp-South
2627 Hylan Blvd Bldg A; Staten Island, NY 10306;
(718) 351-6265; **BDCERT:** ObG 90; **MS:** Italy 83;
RES: Staten Island Univ Hosp, Staten Island, NY 84-
88; **FAP:** Clin Instr SUNY Hlth Sci Ctr; **HOSP:** St
Vincent's Med Ctr-Richmond; *SI: Pregnancy &*
Delivery; Gynecologic Surgery; **HMO:** Chubb PHCS
Magnacare 1199 US Hlthcre +
LANG: Itl; 🦽 📞 🔒 🖼 🏨 $ Mcr 	A Few Days

Spierer, Gary (MD)   ObG
Staten Island Univ Hosp-North

Gateway Ob/Gyn Associates, 78 Cromwell Ave; Staten Island, NY 10304; (718) 987-9175; **BDCERT:** ObG 85; **MS:** Mexico 75; **RES:** Staten Island Univ Hosp, Staten Island, NY 77-81; **FAP:** Asst Clin Instr SUNY Downstate; **HOSP:** Staten Island Univ Hosp-South; *SI: Infertility;* **HMO:** Most

LANG: Dut, Ger, Sp, Heb; 🖻 🅲 🖸 🏥 💲 Mcr 4+ Weeks

OPHTHALMOLOGY

Boozan, William (MD)   Oph
Bayley Seton Hosp

78 Todt Hill Rd 111; Staten Island, NY 10314; (718) 442-3232; **MS:** U Cincinnati 83; **RES:** St Vincents Hosp & Med Ctr NY, New York, NY 86-89; **HOSP:** St Vincent's Med Ctr-Richmond; *SI: Glaucoma; Cataracts-Sutureless Surgery;* **HMO:** Most

🖻 🅲 🖸 🏥 Mcr NFl 1 Week *VISA* 💳

Derespinis, Patrick (MD)   Oph
Staten Island Univ Hosp-South

3055 Richmond Rd; Staten Island, NY 10306; (718) 667-1010; **BDCERT:** Oph 89; **MS:** Mexico 81; **RES:** Med, Booth Mem Hosp, Flushing, NY 83; Oph, Univ of Med & Dent NJ Hosp, Newark, NJ 84-87; **FEL:** Ped Oph & Strabismus, Manhattan Eye, Ear & Throat Hosp, New York, NY 87-88; **FAP:** Assoc Clin Prof UMDNJ New Jersey Sch Osteo Med; **HOSP:** Manhattan Eye, Ear & Throat Hosp; *SI: Pediatric Ophthalmology; Eye Muscle Surgery;* **HMO:** GHI Blue Choice Blue Cross & Blue Shield CIGNA HIP Network +

🖻 🆂🆄 🖸 🏥 💲 Mcr WC NFl 4+ Weeks

Kramer, Philip (MD)   Oph
Staten Island Univ Hosp-South

Ophthalmology Associates of Staten Island, 1460 Victory Blvd; Staten Island, NY 10301; (718) 447-0022; **BDCERT:** Oph 85; **MS:** Temple U 80; **RES:** Oph, New York Eye & Ear Infirmary, New York, NY 81-84; **HOSP:** New York Eye & Ear Infirmary; *SI: Diabetic Retinopathy; Cataract & Glaucoma;* **HMO:** Oxford US Hlthcre CIGNA Blue Cross & Blue Shield GHI +

LANG: Sp; 🖻 🆂🆄 🅲 🖸 🕱 🏥 💲 Mcr WC NFl 2-4 Weeks *VISA* 💳

Zerykier, Abraham (MD)   Oph
Staten Island Univ Hosp-South

16 Ross Ave; Staten Island, NY 10306; (718) 667-4444; **BDCERT:** Oph 80; **MS:** Hahnemann U 75; **RES:** IM, Brookdale Univ Hosp Med Ctr, Brooklyn, NY 75-76; Oph, Interfaith Med Ctr-Bklyn Jewish Div, Brooklyn, NY 76-79; **HOSP:** Beth Israel Med Ctr; *SI: Cataract Surgery, No Stitches; Diabetic Eye Laser Surgery;* **HMO:** GHI Oxford US Hlthcre Empire

LANG: Itl, Sp, Heb, Yd; 🖻 🅲 🖸 🕱 🏥 💲 Mcr WC NFl 2-4 Weeks *VISA* 💳

ORTHOPAEDIC SURGERY

Accettola, Albert (MD)   OrS
Staten Island Univ Hosp-South

Healthcare Associates in Medicine PC, 3311 Hylan Blvd; Staten Island, NY 10306; (718) 667-7500; **BDCERT:** OrS 82; **MS:** Belgium 74; **RES:** S, Staten Island Univ Hosp, Staten Island, NY 75-76; OrS, Bellevue Hosp Ctr, New York, NY 76-79; **FAP:** Asst Clin Prof NYU Sch Med; **HOSP:** Doctors Hosp of Staten Island; *SI: Trauma;* **HMO:** Aetna Hlth Plan Empire Blue Cross & Shield Oxford United Healthcare GHI +

LANG: Itl, Fr; 🖻 🆂🆄 🅲 🖸 🕱 🏥 💲 Mcr WC NFl A Few Days *VISA* 💳

Bonamo, Joel (MD)   OrS
Staten Island Univ Hosp-South

1551 Richmond Rd; Staten Island, NY 10304; (718) 351-6500; **MS:** Italy 76; **RES:** OrS, NYU Med Center, New York, NY 78-81; S, Staten Island Hospital, Staten Island, NY 77-78; **HMO:** Amerihealth Health Plus 1199 Magnacare

LANG: Sp; ⬛ 🔲 🔲 Mcr Mcd   1 Week ▨ *VISA* ⬤

Drucker, David (MD)   OrS
Staten Island Univ Hosp-South

Staten Island Orthopaedics, 1460 Victory Blvd Ste D; Staten Island, NY 10301; (718) 447-0182; **BDCERT:** OrS 93; **MS:** U Chicago-Pritzker Sch Med 83; **RES:** Univ of Med & Dent NJ Hosp, Newark, NJ 85-89; **FEL:** Indiana U Med Ctr, Indianapolis, IN 89-90; **HOSP:** Univ of Med & Dent NJ Hosp; **SI:** *Total Hip and Knee Replacements*; **HMO:** US Hlthcre Oxford CIGNA Aetna Hlth Plan Multiplan +

LANG: Sp; ⬛ ⬛ 🔲 🔲 🔲 Mcr WC NFI   Immediately *VISA* ⬤

Flynn, Maryirene (MD)   OrS
Bayley Seton Hosp

Staten Island Orthopaedics & Sports Medicine, 1551 Richmond Rd; Staten Island, NY 10304; (718) 351-6500; **BDCERT:** OrS 94; **MS:** Albert Einstein Coll Med 86; **RES:** S, Montefiore Med Ctr, Bronx, NY 86-87; OrS, Montefiore Med Ctr, Bronx, NY 87-91; **FEL:** SM, Staten Island Univ Hosp, Staten Island, NY 91-93; **HOSP:** Staten Island Univ Hosp-South; **SI:** *Arthroscopic Surgery; Sports Medicine*; **HMO:** Oxford CIGNA Empire Blue Cross Magnacare Anthem Health +

LANG: Itl; ⬛ 🔲 🔲 🔲 S Mcr WC NFI   A Few Days ▨ *VISA* ⬤

Jayaram, Nadubetthi (MD)   OrS
St Vincent's Med Ctr-Richmond

Richmond Orthopaedics, 11 Ralph Pl Ste 102; Staten Island, NY 10304; (718) 447-6545; **BDCERT:** OrS 90; S 84; **MS:** India 73; **RES:** S, Univ Hosp SUNY Bklyn, Brooklyn, NY 76-81; OrS, Univ Hosp SUNY Bklyn, Brooklyn, NY 82-85; **FEL:** GVS, Lutheran Med Ctr, Brooklyn, NY 81-82; Hand Microsurgery, U of Alabama Hosp, Birmingham, AL 87-88; **HOSP:** Bayley Seton Hosp; **SI:** *Hand Specialist*; **HMO:** Oxford CIGNA Chubb Prudential +

⬛ 🔲 🔲 🔲 Mcr WC NFI   2-4 Weeks *VISA* ⬤ ▨

Reilly, John (MD)   OrS
Staten Island Univ Hosp-South

Healthcare Associates in Medicine, PC, 3311 Hylan Blvd; Staten Island, NY 10306; (718) 667-7500; **BDCERT:** OrS 89; **MS:** SUNY Hlth Sci Ctr 81; **RES:** OrS, Lenox Hill Hosp, New York, NY 82-86; OrS, Children's Hosp, Boston, MA 83; **FEL:** OrS, U MD Hosp, Baltimore, MD 86-87; **HOSP:** Beth Israel North; **SI:** *Sports Medicine; Trauma*; **HMO:** Aetna-US Healthcare Oxford GHI Empire Blue Cross & Shield United Healthcare +

LANG: Itl, Fr; ⬛ ⬛ ⬛ 🔲 🔲 🔲 S Mcr Mcd WC NFI
A Few Days *VISA* ⬤ ▨

Sherman, Mark (MD)   OrS
Bayley Seton Hosp

1551 Richmond Rd; Staten Island, NY 10304; (718) 351-6500; **BDCERT:** OrS 81; **MS:** NYU Sch Med 75; **RES:** S, Bellevue Hosp Ctr, New York, NY 75-76; OrS, Bellevue Hosp Ctr, New York, NY 76-79; **FEL:** SM, Hosp For Special Surgery, New York, NY 79-80; **HMO:** Most

⬛ 🔲 🔲 🔲 S Mcr WC NFI   A Few Days ▨ *VISA* ⬤

Suarez, Joseph (MD)   OrS
Staten Island Univ Hosp-South

3311 Hylan Blvd; Staten Island, NY 10306; (718) 667-7500; **BDCERT:** OrS 77; **MS:** Italy 68; **RES:** Hosp For Joint Diseases, New York, NY 73-76; **FAP:** Clin Instr OrS Mt Sinai Sch Med; **HOSP:** Doctors Hosp of Staten Island; **SI:** *Sports Medicine-Orthopaedics*; **HMO:** CIGNA Aetna Hlth Plan CHN Blue Cross & Blue Shield GHI

⬛ ⬛ ⬛ 🔲 🔲 🔲 Mcr WC NFI   Immediately *VISA* ⬤ ▨

OTOLARYNGOLOGY

Castellano, Bartolomeo (MD) Oto
St Vincent's Med Ctr-Richmond
Richmond Otolarynology Group, 78 Todt Hill Rd
204; Staten Island, NY 10314; (718) 273-2626;
BDCERT: Oto 85; **MS:** Mexico 79; **RES:** Oto, New
York University Med Ctr, New York, NY 81-84;
FEL: PlS, Mount Sinai Med Ctr, New York, NY 84-
85; **FAP:** Asst NYU Sch Med; **HOSP:** Staten Island
Univ Hosp-North; **HMO:** Oxford Blue Choice CIGNA
Prucare Multiplan +

Macatangay, Angelo (MD)   Oto
Staten Island Univ Hosp-South
3635 Richmond Ave; Staten Island, NY 10312;
(718) 948-5222; **MS:** Virgin Islands 60; **RES:**
Bellevue Hosp Ctr, New York, NY 69-71; Albert
Einstein Coll Med, Bronx, NY 66-68; **HOSP:** St
Vincent's Med Ctr-Richmond; **HMO:** GHI
Magnacare Metlife Chubb Oxford +

LANG: Sp, Tag; ♿ 🏥 📞 📅 👤 🏨 💲 Immediately
▨ VISA ●

Sinnreich, Abraham (MD)   Oto
Staten Island Univ Hosp-North
161 Lily Pond Ave; Staten Island, NY 10305; (718)
442-3030; **BDCERT:** Oto 84; **MS:** Albert Einstein
Coll Med 79; **RES:** Maimonides Med Ctr, Brooklyn,
NY 79-80; Mount Sinai Med Ctr, New York, NY 80-
83; **HOSP:** Mount Sinai Med Ctr; **SI:** *Sinus Disorders;*
Snoring and Sleep Apnea

♿ 📞 👤 🏨 💲 Mcr WC NFI 1 Week

Wooh, Kenneth (MD)   Oto
Staten Island Univ Hosp-North
1460 Victory Blvd; Staten Island, NY 10301; (718)
447-1261; **BDCERT:** Oto 78; **MS:** South Korea 67;
RES: S, Staten Island Univ Hosp, Staten Island, NY
73; Oto, Med Coll VA Hosp, Richmond, VA 76;
FAP: Asst Clin Prof SUNY Downstate; **SI:** *Middle Ear*
Surgery; Cancer of Head & Neck; **HMO:** GHI Oxford
US Hlthcre

♿ 📞 📅 👤 🏨 💲 Mcr NFI 1 Week

PEDIATRIC CARDIOLOGY

Ritter, Sam (MD)   PCd
Staten Island Univ Hosp-North
Staten Island Univ Hosp-North, 475 Seaview Ave;
Staten Island, NY 10305; (718) 226-9360;
BDCERT: Ped 81; **PCd** 83; **MS:** USC Sch Med 76;
RES: Ped, Columbia-Presbyterian Med Ctr, New
York, NY 77-79; **FEL:** PCd, Columbia-Presbyterian
Med Ctr, New York, NY 79-82; **FAP:** Prof Ped
Cornell U

PEDIATRIC PULMONOLOGY

Marcus, Michael (MD)   PPul
Staten Island Univ Hosp-North
401 Seaview Ave C; Staten Island, NY 10305;
(718) 980-5864; **BDCERT:** Ped 87; **MS:** SUNY Hlth
Sci Ctr 80; **RES:** Ped, Nassau County Med Ctr, East
Meadow, NY 80-83; **FEL:** A&I/Pul, Children's Hosp
of Philadelphia, Philadelphia, PA 83-85; **HOSP:** St
Vincent's Med Ctr-Richmond; **HMO:** Multiplan
Champus Oxford Magnacare

📞 📅 👤 🏨 💲 Mcr Immediately

PEDIATRICS

Bastawros, Mary (MD)   Ped   PCP
St Vincent's Med Ctr-Richmond
81 Hylan Blvd; Staten Island, NY 10305; (718)
727-1200; **BDCERT:** Ped 85; **MS:** Egypt 66; **RES:**
Ped, New York Methodist Hosp, Brooklyn, NY 73-
74; **FAP:** Asst SUNY Downstate; **SI:** *Well Baby Care;*
Growth and Development; **HMO:** Oxford Empire Blue
Cross & Shield GHI CIGNA United Healthcare +

LANG: Ar; ♿ 📞 📅 👤 🏨 💲 Mcr Mcd NFI
A Few Days

Corpus, Marina (MD) **Ped** [PCP]
St Vincent's Med Ctr-Richmond
491 Henderson Ave; Staten Island, NY 10310; (718) 816-0640; **BDCERT:** Ped 64; **MS:** Virgin Islands 58; **RES:** N Shore Univ Hosp-Plainview, Plainview, NY 60-61; St Vincent's Med Ctr-Richmond, Staten Island, NY 62-64; **FEL:** Albert Einstein Med Ctr, Bronx, NY 67-73; **HOSP:** Staten Island Univ Hosp-North; ***SI:** Pediatric Heart Problems*
LANG: Fil, Cey; ♿ [SA SU] ☾ ☎ 👤 📅 [$] Immediately
DISCOVER

Duchnowska, Alicja (MD) **Ped** [PCP]
Staten Island Univ Hosp-South
934 Ionia Ave; Staten Island, NY 10309; (718) 984-5255; **BDCERT:** Ped 85; **MS:** Poland 65; **RES:** Ped, Nat Inst of Mother & Child, Warsaw, Poland 67-70; Ped, Staten Island Univ Hosp, Staten Island, NY 80-82; **FEL:** Ped, Staten Island Univ Hosp, Staten Island, NY 82-84; **HMO:** Aetna Hlth Plan Blue Cross & Blue Shield Travelers Magnacare +
LANG: Rus, Pol; [SA SU] ☾ ☎ 👤 📅 [$] A Few Days

Faraci, Nick (MD) **Ped** [PCP]
Staten Island Univ Hosp-South
Comprehensive Pediatrics, 2889 Amboy Rd; Staten Island, NY 10306; (718) 667-2020; **BDCERT:** Ped 89; **MS:** West Indies 81; **RES:** Univ Hosp SUNY Bklyn, Brooklyn, NY 81-83; Staten Island Univ Hosp, Staten Island, NY 83-84; **HOSP:** New York Methodist Hosp; ***SI:** Asthma; Dermatology*; **HMO:** GHI Blue Cross & Blue Shield HealthNet Oxford United Healthcare +
LANG: Itl, Sp, Tag, Rus; ♿ [SA SU] ☾ ☎ 👤 📅 [$] [Mcr] [Mcd] [WC] [NFI] Immediately AMERICAN EXPRESS VISA MasterCard

Harin, Anantham (MD) **Ped** [PCP]
St Vincent's Med Ctr-Richmond
37 Greta Pl; Staten Island, NY 10301; (718) 876-5777; **BDCERT:** Ped 75; NP 77; **MS:** Sri Lanka 70; **RES:** Ped, Kings County Hosp Ctr, Brooklyn, NY 72-73; **FEL:** NP, N Shore Univ Hosp-Manhasset, Manhasset, NY; **FAP:** Clin Prof Ped NYU Sch Med; ***SI:** Neonatology*; **HMO:** GHI Blue Cross Oxford Prucare US Hlthcre +
LANG: Tam; [SA SU] ☾ ☎ 👤 📅 [Mcd] Immediately

Lazar, Emanuel (MD) **Ped** [PCP]
Staten Island Univ Hosp-South
211 Richmond Hill Rd; Staten Island, NY 10314; (718) 494-4646; **BDCERT:** Ped 89; **MS:** Romania 81; **RES:** Staten Island Univ Hosp, Staten Island, NY 84-87; **HOSP:** St Vincent's Med Ctr-Richmond
[SA SU] ☎ 👤 📅 [$] [NFI]

Mevs, Clifford (MD) **Ped** [PCP]
St Vincent's Med Ctr-Richmond
Pediatrics Health Care PC, 101 3rd St; Staten Island, NY 10306; (718) 980-5437; **BDCERT:** Ped 87; **MS:** U Puerto Rico 81; **RES:** Ped, St Vincent's Med Ctr-Richmond, Staten Island, NY 82-85; **FEL:** Ped, Rhode Island Hosp, Providence, RI; **FAP:** Asst Clin Prof NYU Sch Med; **HOSP:** Staten Island Univ Hosp-North; ***SI:** Developmental Disabilities*
LANG: Sp, Fr; ♿ [SA SU] ☾ ☎ 👤 📅 [$] A Few Days
VISA MasterCard

Pang, Kenneth (MD) **Ped** [PCP]
Staten Island Univ Hosp-South
160 Todt Hill Rd; Staten Island, NY 10314; (718) 698-8576; **BDCERT:** Ped 73; **MS:** South Korea 64; **RES:** Ped, Wyckoff Heights Med Ctr, Brooklyn, NY 69-70; Ped, Coney Island Hosp, Brooklyn, NY 70-71; **FEL:** PHO, Coney Island Hosp, Brooklyn, NY 71-73; **HMO:** Aetna-US Healthcare CIGNA Oxford United Healthcare Blue Cross & Blue Shield +
LANG: Kor; [SA SU] ☾ ☎ 👤 📅 [$] Immediately

Patrick, Albert (MD) **Ped**
Staten Island Univ Hosp-South
219 3rd St; Staten Island, NY 10306; (718) 351-1004; **BDCERT:** Ped 52; **MS:** SUNY Downstate 46; **RES:** Cv, Shapin Hosp, Providence, RI; **HOSP:** St Vincent's Med Ctr-Richmond; ***SI:** Adolescent Medicine*; **HMO:** CIGNA
♿ ☎ 👤 📅 [$] Immediately

Potaznik, Daniel (MD)   Ped
Staten Island Univ Hosp-South
Nalitt Inst for Cancer and Blood related Dis, 256
Mason Ave; Staten Island, NY 10305; (718) 226-
6435; **BDCERT:** Ped 87; PHO 87; **MS:** Belgium 70;
RES: Ped A&I, Sheba Med Ctr, Tel Hashomer, Israel
70-75; **FEL:** PHO, Mem Sloan Kettering Cancer Ctr,
New York, NY 80-83; **FAP:** Asst Clin Prof Ped
SUNY Hlth Sci Ctr; **SI:** *Cancer Pediatric*; **HMO:** Blue
Choice US Hlthcre Metlife CIGNA HIP Network +

[symbols] A Few Days

Purow, Henry (MD)   Ped   PCP
Staten Island Univ Hosp-South
1326 Clove Rd; Staten Island, NY 10301; (718)
727-7272; **BDCERT:** Ped 74; NP 75; **MS:** SUNY
Buffalo 68; **RES:** Columbia-Presbyterian Med Ctr,
New York, NY 69-70; Staten Island Univ Hosp,
Staten Island, NY; **FEL:** NP, Univ Hosp SUNY Bklyn,
Brooklyn, NY; **HOSP:** St Vincent's Med Ctr-
Richmond; **HMO:** Oxford Blue Choice Blue Cross &
Blue Shield CIGNA HealthNet +

[symbols] A Few Days

Short, Joan (MD)   Ped   PCP
St Vincent's Med Ctr-Richmond
32 2nd St; Staten Island, NY 10306; (718) 979-
7472; **BDCERT:** Ped 82; **MS:** U Tenn Ctr Hlth Sci,
Memphis 66; **RES:** City of Memphis Hosp, Memphis,
TN; St Jude Children's Hosp, Memphis, TN; **FEL:** Ped
Onc, St Jude Children's Hosp, Memphis, TN; **HOSP:**
Staten Island Univ Hosp-North; **SI:** *Developmental*
Medicine; *Asthma*; **HMO:** Oxford Blue Cross & Blue
Shield Prucare GHI United Healthcare +

[symbols] 1 Week *VISA*

Vadde, Nirmala (MD)   Ped
St Vincent's Med Ctr-Richmond
355 Bard Ave Fl 3; Staten Island, NY 10310; (718)
876-4634; **BDCERT:** Ped 77; **MS:** India 69; **RES:** St
Vincent's Med Ctr-Richmond, Staten Island, NY 73-
76; **FAP:** Adjct Clin Instr Ped NY Med Coll; **SI:**
Asthma
LANG: Fil;

Visconti, Ernest (MD)   Ped
Lutheran Med Ctr
81 Hylan Blvd; Staten Island, NY 10305; (718)
727-1200; **BDCERT:** Ped 76; Ped 92; **MS:** SUNY
Downstate 71; **RES:** NY Hosp-Cornell Med Ctr, New
York, NY 71-74; **FEL:** Rhode Island Hosp,
Providence, RI 76-78; **HOSP:** St Vincent's Med Ctr-
Richmond; **SI:** *Pediatrics; Tick Related Diseases*;
HMO: GHI Blue Cross Oxford United Healthcare
Anthem Health +

[symbols] A Few Days

Volpe, Salvatore (MD)   Ped   PCP
Staten Island Univ Hosp-South
2760 Amboy Rd; Staten Island, NY 10306; (718)
351-2222; **BDCERT:** Ped 90; IM 90; **MS:** SUNY
Hlth Sci Ctr 86; **RES:** Staten Island Univ Hosp,
Staten Island, NY 90; **SI:** *Holistic Medicine;*
Adolescent Medicine; **HMO:** US Hlthcre Oxford GHI
Aetna Hlth Plan United Healthcare +

[symbols] Immediately *VISA*

Wu, Bernard (MD)   Ped   PCP
Staten Island Univ Hosp-South
105 Byrne Ave; Staten Island, NY 10314; (718)
698-7220; **BDCERT:** Ped 70; **MS:** Burma 61; **RES:**
Ped, Queen Mary Children's Hosp, Stockton,
England 63; **FEL:** Ped Chest Disease, Yale-New
Haven Hosp, New Haven, CT 68-71; **HOSP:** St
Vincent's Med Ctr-Richmond; **SI:** *Asthma; Noisy*
Breathing; **HMO:** Oxford HMO Blue
LANG: Chi, Brm; [symbols]
Immediately

PHYSICAL MEDICINE & REHABILITATION

Stickevers, Susan (MD)   PMR
Bayley Seton Hosp
Bayley Seton Hosp, 75 Vanderbilt Ave; Staten
Island, NY 10304; (718) 354-5943; **BDCERT:**
PMR 91; **MS:** Albert Einstein Coll Med 86; **RES:**
PMR, Columbia-Presbyterian Med Ctr, New York,
NY 87-90; **SI:** *Electromyography; Sports Medicine;*
HMO: Aetna Hlth Plan Blue Cross & Blue Shield
Amerihealth US Hlthcre GHI +

LANG: Fr, Sp; 🦽 🚹 🛏 Mcr Mod WC NFI   A Few Days

Weinberg, Jeffrey (MD)   PMR
Staten Island Univ Hosp-North
Staten Island Rehab Medicine, PC, 475 Seaview
Ave; Staten Island, NY 10305; (718) 226-6362;
BDCERT: PMR 85; **MS:** NY Med Coll 80; **RES:**
Hackensack U Med Ctr, Hackensack, NJ 80-81;
PMR, New York University Med Ctr, New York, NY
81-83; **FEL:** Ger, New York University Med Ctr,
New York, NY 84; **FAP:** Asst Clin Prof PMR NYU
Sch Med; **SI:** *Geriatric Rehabilitation; Musculoskeletal
Disorders;* **HMO:** Aetna Hlth Plan CIGNA GHI
Magnacare Oxford +

🦽 📞 🔲 🚹 🛏 Mcr Mod WC NFI   A Few Days **VISA** 💳

PLASTIC SURGERY

Cherofsky, Alan (MD)   PlS
Staten Island Univ Hosp-South
4546 Hyland Blvd; Staten Island, NY 10312; (718)
967-3300; **BDCERT:** PlS 93; **MS:** SUNY Hlth Sci Ctr
82; **RES:** PlS, U MO Kansas City Sch Med, Kansas
City, MO 87-89; S, Staten Island Univ Hosp, Staten
Island, NY 82-87; **FAP:** Dir PlS; **HOSP:** St Vincent's
Med Ctr-Richmond; **SI:** *Breast Reconstruction and
Enlargement; Pediatric Plastic Surgery;* **HMO:** GHI
Oxford Blue Cross & Blue Shield United Healthcare
PHCS +

📞 🔲 🚹 🛏 💲 Mcr NFI   Immediately **VISA** 💳 💳

Cutolo Jr, Louis C (MD)   PlS
Staten Island Univ Hosp-South
3710 Richmond Ave; Staten Island, NY 10312;
(718) 984-8910; **BDCERT:** PlS 61; **MS:** SUNY Hlth
Sci Ctr 85; **RES:** S, Staten Island Univ Hosp, Staten
Island, NY 85-90; **FEL:** PlS, U FL Shands Hosp,
Gainesville, FL 90; **HOSP:** Long Island Coll Hosp; **SI:**
Cosmetic Surgery; **HMO:** GHI

🦽 📠 🔲 🚹 🛏 Mcr WC NFI   Immediately 💳 **VISA**
💳 📠

Decorato, John (MD)   PlS
Bayley Seton Hosp
1122 Richmond Rd; Staten Island, NY 10304;
(718) 980-1352; **BDCERT:** S 92; PlS 95; **MS:**
Mexico 84; **RES:** S, Brooklyn Hosp Ctr, Brooklyn,
NY 86-91; **FEL:** PlS, U NC Hosp, Chapel Hill, NC 91-
93; **HOSP:** St Vincent's Med Ctr-Richmond; **SI:**
Liposuction Body Contouring; **HMO:** Magnacare GHI
Oxford Prudential

LANG: Sp; 🦽 📞 🔲 🚹 🛏 💲 Mcr WC NFI
Immediately 💳 **VISA** 💳

Lovelle-Allen, Susan (MD)   PlS
St Vincent's Med Ctr-Richmond
105 Benton Ave; Staten Island, NY 10305; (718)
979-7070; **BDCERT:** S 94; **MS:** Coll Physicians &
Surgeons 88; **RES:** S, Columbia Presbyterian
Medical Ctr, New York, NY 88-93; PlS, Montefiore
Medical Ctr, Bronx, NY 94-96; **FEL:** Micro-Surgery,
Montefiore Medical Ctr, Bronx, NY 93-94; **HOSP:**
Bayley Seton Hosp; **SI:** *Reconstructive Surgery*

Raju, Raghava (MD)   PlS
Doctors Hosp of Staten Island
2131 Richmond Rd; Staten Island, NY 10306;
(718) 979-5553; **BDCERT:** PlS 83; **MS:** India 67;
RES: S, New York Methodist Hosp, Brooklyn, NY
72-76; PlS, St Luke's Roosevelt Hosp Ctr, New
York, NY 78-79; **FEL:** PlS, Cleveland Clinic Hosp,
Cleveland, OH 79-80; **HOSP:** St Vincent's Med Ctr-
Richmond; **HMO:** PHCS Sanus-NYLCare
Magnacare Blue Cross & Blue Shield QualCare +

📞 🔲 🚹 🛏 💲 Mcr WC NFI   Immediately

PSYCHIATRY

Di Buono, Mark (MD)   Psyc
Staten Island Univ Hosp-South
4287 Richmond Ave; Staten Island, NY 10312;
(718) 226-2440; **BDCERT:** Psyc 90; **MS:** Mexico
81; **RES:** Univ Hosp SUNY Stony Brook, Stony
Brook, NY 82-86; **FAP:** Asst Clin Prof SUNY
Downstate; *SI: Anxiety/Depression; Obsessive
Compulsive Disorder*; **HMO:** GHI Oxford
LANG: Sp; ⬥ ⬥ ⬥ ⬥ ⬥ ⬥ ⬥ ⬥   1 Week

Lee, Chol (MD)   Psyc
St Vincent's Med Ctr-Richmond
1430 Clove Rd; Staten Island, NY 10301; (718)
448-0066; **BDCERT:** Psyc 77; **MS:** South Korea 60;
RES: Medfield St Hosp, Medfield, MA 66-69; **FEL:**
Bellevue Hosp Ctr, New York, NY; NY Hosp-Cornell
Med Ctr, New York, NY; **HOSP:** Bayley Seton Hosp;
SI: Depression and Anxiety; Schizophrenia; **HMO:**
Prucare
LANG: Kor, Jpn; ⬥ ⬥ ⬥ ⬥ ⬥ ⬥   Immediately

Miller, Lawrence (MD)   Psyc
St Vincent's Med Ctr-Richmond
1430 Clove Rd; Staten Island, NY 10301; (718)
816-8322; **BDCERT:** Psyc 63; ChAP 65; **MS:**
Switzerland 55; **RES:** ChAP, Mental Health
Clinic/USPHS, Staten Is, NY 59-61; **FEL:** ChAP,
Staten Island MH Soc, Staten Is, NY 61-63; **FAP:**
Assoc Prof Psyc NY Med Coll; **HOSP:** Bayley Seton
Hosp

PULMONARY DISEASE

Castellano, Michael A (MD)   Pul
Staten Island Univ Hosp-North
SI Pulmonary Associates, 27 New Dorp Ln; Staten
Island, NY 10306; (718) 980-5700; **BDCERT:** Pul
78; CCM 87; **MS:** Italy 68; **RES:** Med, Staten Islan
Univ Hosp, Staten Island, NY 69-72; **FEL:** Pul,
NYU-Bellvue Hosp Ctr, New York, NY 73-74; **FAP:**
Asst Prof Med SUNY Downstate; *SI: Asthma;
Emphysema*; **HMO:** Oxford Aetna Hlth Plan CIGNA
United Healthcare
LANG: Itl, Sp; ⬥ ⬥ ⬥ ⬥ ⬥ ⬥ ⬥ ⬥
A Few Days

Ciccone, Ralph (MD)   Pul
Staten Island Univ Hosp-North
27 New Dorp Ln; Staten Island, NY 10306; (718)
980-5700; **BDCERT:** Pul 90; **MS:** Mexico 80; **RES:**
IM, SI Univ Hosp, Staten Island, NY 83-85; *SI: Sleep
Apnea*

Maniatis, Theodore (MD)   Pul
Staten Island Univ Hosp-North
27 New Dorp Ln; Staten Island, NY 10306; (718)
980-5700; **BDCERT:** IM 83; **MS:** SUNY Hlth Sci Ctr
80; **RES:** Staten Island Univ Hosp, Staten Island, NY
80-83; **FEL:** Univ of Med & Dent NJ Hosp, Newark,
NJ 83-85; **HMO:** Aetna Hlth Plan Blue Choice
CIGNA HealthNet Sanus-NYLCare +
⬥ ⬥ ⬥ ⬥ ⬥ ⬥ ⬥ ⬥ ⬥   A Few Days ⬥ **VISA**
⬥

Martins, Publius (MD)   Pul
St Vincent's Med Ctr-Richmond
283 Bard Ave; Staten Island, NY 10310; (718)
816-8068; **BDCERT:** IM 84; Pul 92; **MS:** Portugal
75; **RES:** IM, St Vincents Hosp & Med Ctr NY, New
York, NY 78-81; **FEL:** Pul, Pawtucket Mem Hosp,
Pawtucket, RI 81-83; **FAP:** Asst Clin Prof NY Med
Coll; **HOSP:** Doctors Hosp of Staten Island; *SI:
Asthma*; **HMO:** Oxford Blue Cross & Blue Shield
HealthNet Sanus-NYLCare GHI +
LANG: Sp, Prt, Itl; ⬥ ⬥ ⬥ ⬥ ⬥ ⬥ ⬥ ⬥ ⬥ ⬥
A Few Days ⬥

Sasso, Louis (MD)   Pul
Staten Island Univ Hosp-North

Staten Island Pulmonary Associates, 27 New Dorp Ln; Staten Island, NY 10306; (718) 980-5700; **BDCERT:** Pul 78; CCM 95; **MS:** UMDNJ-NJ Med Sch, Newark 72; **RES:** St Vincents Hosp & Med Ctr NY, New York, NY 72-74; Univ of Med & Dent NJ Hosp, Newark, NJ 74-75; **FEL:** New York University Med Ctr, New York, NY 75-77; Bellevue Hosp Ctr, New York, NY; **FAP:** Asst Clin Prof SUNY Downstate; **SI:** *Asthma/Chronic Lung Disease; Pulmonary Fibrosis;* **HMO:** Oxford CIGNA Aetna Hlth Plan Empire Blue Cross & Shield PHCS +

LANG: Itl; 🦽 🈂 🌙 🔌 🔧 🛏 🅂 Mcr   A Few Days

Tarantola, Vincent (MD)   Pul   **PCP**
Bayley Seton Hosp

78 Todt Hill Rd 206; Staten Island, NY 10314; (718) 816-0034; **BDCERT:** IM 84; **MS:** Italy 76; **RES:** St Vincents Hosp, New York, NY 77-70; **HOSP:** St Vincent's Med Ctr-Richmond; **HMO:** Prucare Oxford Blue Cross GHI

🦽 🌙 🔧 🛏 Mcr   2-4 Weeks

RADIATION ONCOLOGY

Adams, Marc (MD)   RadRO
St Vincent's Med Ctr-Richmond

Regl Rad, 360 Bard Ave; Staten Island, NY 10310; (718) 876-2000; **BDCERT:** RadRO 90; **MS:** U Ala Sch Med 85; **RES:** St Barnabas Med Ctr, Livingston, NJ 86-89; St Barnabas Med Ctr, Livingston, NJ 85-86; **HMO:** Blue Cross US Hlthcre GHI Oxford +

Lederman, Gil (MD)   RadRO
Staten Island Univ Hosp-South

475 Seaview Ave; Staten Island, NY 10305; (718) 226-8862; **BDCERT:** Rad 87; **MS:** U Iowa Coll Med 78; **RES:** IM, Michael Reese Hosp Med Ctr, Chicago, IL 78-81; RadRO, Harvard Med Sch, Cambridge, MA 84-87; **FEL:** Onc, Harvard Med Sch, Cambridge, MA 81-84; **HMO:** Most

🦽 🔌 🔧 🛏 Mcr Mcd WC   Immediately ▨ *VISA* 💳 💳

RADIOLOGY

Manfredi, Orlando (MD)   Rad
St Vincent's Med Ctr-Richmond

Regional Radiology, 243 Bard Ave; Staten Island, NY 10310; (718) 876-4189; **BDCERT:** Rad 56; **MS:** Med Coll Wisc 52; **RES:** Rad, VA Med Ctr-Bronx, Bronx, NY 53-56; **FAP:** Asst Clin Prof Rad NY Med Coll; **HOSP:** Bayley Seton Hosp; **SI:** *Nuclear Medicine Imaging;* **HMO:** Oxford US Hlthcre Prudential GHI Prucare +

LANG: Sp, Rus, Ger; 🦽 🈂 🌙 🔌 🛏 Mcr Mcd WC NFI   Immediately *VISA* 💳 💳

RHEUMATOLOGY

Garjian, Peggy Ann (MD)   Rhu
Bayley Seton Hosp

71 Todt Hill Rd; Staten Island, NY 10314; (718) 720-1030; **BDCERT:** IM 94; **MS:** Mexico 81; **RES:** Lutheran Med Ctr, Brooklyn, NY 83-85; U Conn Hlth Ctr, Farmington, CT; **FEL:** Rhu, Univ Conn, Farmington, CT 85-87; **HOSP:** St Vincent's Med Ctr-Richmond

Goldstein, Mark (MD)   Rhu
Staten Island Univ Hosp-South

1478 Victory Blvd; Staten Island, NY 10301; (718) 447-0055; **BDCERT:** IM 82; Rhu 88; **MS:** NY Med Coll 79; **RES:** IM, Montefiore Med Ctr, Bronx, NY 79-80; IM, Montefiore Med Ctr, Bronx, NY 80-82; **FEL:** CCM, Montefiore Med Ctr, Bronx, NY 82-83; Rhu, Albert Einstein Med Ctr, Bronx, NY 85-87; **FAP:** Instr SUNY Downstate; **HOSP:** St Vincent's Med Ctr-Richmond; **SI:** *Arthritis; Osteoporosis;* **HMO:** Oxford United Healthcare CIGNA GHI

🦽 🌙 🔌 🔧 🛏 🅂 Mcr NFI   A Few Days

Jarrett, Mark (MD)   Rhu
Staten Island Univ Hosp-South
1478 Victory Blvd; Staten Island, NY 10301; (718) 447-0055; **BDCERT:** IM 78; Rhu 80; **MS:** NYU Sch Med 75; **RES:** Montefiore Med Ctr, Bronx, NY 75-78; **FEL:** Rhu, Montefiore Med Ctr, Bronx, NY 78-80; **FAP:** Clin Prof Med; **HOSP:** St Vincent's Med Ctr-Richmond; **SI:** *Lupus; Rheumatoid Arthritis;* **HMO:** Aetna Hlth Plan GHI Blue Cross & Blue Shield Oxford 1199 +

⛎ 🌙 📷 💉 🏥 🅂 Mcr WC NFI 2-4 Weeks **VISA** 💳

SURGERY

D'Anna, John (MD)   S
Staten Island Univ Hosp-South
1130 Victory Blvd; Staten Island, NY 10301; (718) 447-5400; **BDCERT:** S 83; **MS:** Georgetown U 77; **RES:** St Vincents Hosp & Med Ctr NY, New York, NY 77-82; **FEL:** GVS, St Vincents Hosp & Med Ctr NY, New York, NY 82-83; **HOSP:** St Vincent's Med Ctr-Richmond; **HMO:** Oxford US Hlthcre United Healthcare GHI CIGNA +

⛎ 🌙 📷 💉 🏥 🅂 Mcr Mcd WC 2-4 Weeks

Ferzli, George (MD)   S
Staten Island Univ Hosp-North
78 Cromwell Ave; Staten Island, NY 10304; (718) 667-8100; **BDCERT:** S 93; SCC 94; **MS:** Lebanon 79; **RES:** Staten Island Univ Hosp, Staten Island, NY 80-85; **FAP:** Asst Prof of Clin SUNY Downstate; **SI:** *Laparoscopic Surgery; Breast Cancer Surgery;* **HMO:** GHI Oxford Aetna Hlth Plan CIGNA Empire +

LANG: Fr, Ar; ⛎ 🌙 📷 💉 🏥 🅂 Mcr WC NFI Immediately

Hornyak, Stephen (MD)   S
St Vincent's Med Ctr-Richmond
1130 Victory Blvd; Staten Island, NY 10301; (718) 442-3400; **BDCERT:** S 80; S 90; **MS:** SUNY Hlth Sci Ctr 74; **RES:** Kings County Hosp Ctr, Brooklyn, NY 74-79; **FEL:** Mem Sloan Kettering Cancer Ctr, New York, NY 79-80; **HOSP:** Staten Island Univ Hosp-North; **SI:** *Diseases of the Breast; Laparoscopic Surgery Laser;* **HMO:** Oxford US Hlthcre CIGNA GHI United Healthcare +

⛎ 🌙 📷 💉 🏥 🅂 Mcr Mcd WC NFI 1 Week

Lansigan, Nicholas (MD)   S
St Vincent's Med Ctr-Richmond
1366 Victory Blvd; Staten Island, NY 10301; (718) 442-4777; **BDCERT:** S 78; **MS:** Philippines 66; **RES:** St Vincent's Med Ctr-Richmond, Staten Island, NY 69-73; Philippine Gen Hosp, Manilla, Philippines 66-69; **FEL:** Ped, Mem Sloan Kettering Cancer Ctr, New York, NY; **HOSP:** Bayley Seton Hosp; **HMO:** Prucare Blue Choice Blue Cross & Blue Shield HealthNet Sanus-NYLCare +

⛎ 🌙 📷 💉 🏥 🅂 Mcr Mcd WC NFI Immediately **VISA** 💳

Pahuja, Murlidhar (MD)   S
Staten Island Univ Hosp-South
2026 Richmond Ave; Staten Island, NY 10314; (718) 351-4691; **BDCERT:** S 84; S 92; **MS:** Pakistan 71; **RES:** Med Coll Penn, 74; Stamford Hosp, Stamford, CT 75-78; **FEL:** NYU Cornell Med Ctr, New York, NY 80; **FAP:** Clin Instr S SUNY Downstate; **SI:** *Breast Cancer; Laparoscopic Surgery;* **HMO:** Sanus-NYLCare US Hlthcre Blue Cross & Blue Shield Multiplan PHS +

SA/SU 🌙 📷 💉 🏥 🅂 Mcr Mcd WC NFI Immediately

Pomper, Stuart (MD)   S
St Vincent's Med Ctr-Richmond
2691 Hylan Blvd; Staten Island, NY 10306; (718) 979-9100; **BDCERT:** S 86; **MS:** SUNY Hlth Sci Ctr 80; **RES:** S, Staten Island Univ Hosp, Staten Island, NY 81-85; **FEL:** GVS, Maimonides Med Ctr, Brooklyn, NY 85-86; **HOSP:** Bayley Seton Hosp; **HMO:** Prucare Blue Choice Aetna Hlth Plan GHI US Hlthcre +

⛎ 🌙 📷 💉 🏥 Mcr NFI Immediately

Silich, Robert (MD)   S
Staten Island Univ Hosp-South
1130 Victory Blvd; Staten Island, NY 10301; (718) 447-5400; **BDCERT:** S 75; **MS:** NY Med Coll 67; **RES:** Staten Island Univ Hosp, Staten Island, NY 67-72; **FAP:** Assoc Clin Prof S SUNY Downstate; **HOSP:** St Vincent's Med Ctr-Richmond; **SI:** *Breast Cancer; Colon Cancer;* **HMO:** Oxford US Hlthcre CIGNA GHI +

⛎ 🌙 📷 🏥 🅂 Mcr WC NFI 1 Week **VISA** 💳 💳

620

Steinbruck, Richard (MD)   S
St Vincent's Med Ctr-Richmond

1366 Victory Blvd A; Staten Island, NY 10301;
(718) 447-5211; **BDCERT:** S 87; **MS:** SUNY
Syracuse 91; **RES:** Univ Hosp SUNY Bklyn,
Brooklyn, NY 81-86; **HOSP:** Bayley Seton Hosp; *SI:
Breast Surgery; Laparoscopic Surgery*; **HMO:** Blue
Choice HealthNet Independent Health Plan Sanus-
NYLCare Oxford +

 🦽 🌙 📷 🔧 🏥 Mcr   Immediately

Tedesco, Salvatore (MD)   S
Bayley Seton Hosp

1366 Victory Blvd; Staten Island, NY 10301; (718)
442-4777; **BDCERT:** S 85; S 93; **MS:** SUNY Buffalo
78; **RES:** S, Univ Hosp SUNY Bklyn, Brooklyn, NY
78-83; **HOSP:** St Vincent's Med Ctr-Richmond;
HMO: Chubb GHI Blue Cross & Blue Shield
Travelers US Hlthcre +

 🦽 🌙 📷 🔧 🏥 $ Mcr Mcd WC NFI   Immediately **VISA**
💳

THORACIC SURGERY

Galdieri, Ralph (MD)   TS
St Vincent's Med Ctr-Richmond

1460 Victory Blvd; Staten Island, NY 10301; (718)
981-3373; **BDCERT:** TS 91; S 89; **MS:** Italy 78;
RES: TS, Univ of Med & Dent NJ Hosp, Newark, NJ
83-86; **FEL:** PCd, Children's Hosp of NJ, Newark, NJ
86-87; **FAP:** Instr Albert Einstein Coll Med; **HOSP:**
Bayley Seton Hosp

 🦽 📷 🏥 Mcr Mcd   1 Week

McGinn Jr, Joseph (MD)   TS
Staten Island Univ Hosp-South

1460 Victory Blvd; Staten Island, NY 10301; (718)
981-3373; **BDCERT:** S 87; TS 90; **MS:** SUNY Hlth
Sci Ctr 81; **RES:** S, Downstate Med Ctr, Brooklyn,
NY 81-85; S, Downstate Med Ctr, Brooklyn, NY 85-
86; **FEL:** TS, LI Jewish Med Ctr, New Hyde Park, NY
86-88; **HOSP:** St Vincent's Med Ctr-Richmond; *SI:
Cardiac Surgery; Thoracospic*; **HMO:** US Hlthcre
Metlife Blue Choice Aetna Hlth Plan HIP Network +

 🦽 📷 🔧 🏥 Mcr Mcd WC NFI   Immediately

UROLOGY

Lessing, Jeffrey (MD)   U
Staten Island Univ Hosp-South

78 Todt Hill Rd 201; Staten Island, NY 10314;
(718) 448-3880; **BDCERT:** U 82; **MS:** NYU Sch
Med 75; **RES:** S, New York University Med Ctr, New
York, NY 75-77; U, Mount Sinai Med Ctr, New
York, NY 77-80; **HOSP:** St Vincent's Med Ctr-
Richmond; *SI: Infertility-Impotency; Kidney Stone
Disease*; **HMO:** Oxford GHI Aetna Hlth Plan CIGNA
US Hlthcre +

 🦽 🌙 📷 🔧 🏥 $ Mcr WC   A Few Days **VISA** 💳

Miranda, Luis (MD)   U
Doctors Hosp of Staten Island

11 Ralph Pl 202; Staten Island, NY 10304; (718)
448-1555; **BDCERT:** U 88; **MS:** India 65; **RES:** PM,
NY Hosp-Cornell Med Ctr, New York, NY 69-72; U,
Lenox Hill Hosp, New York, NY 79-83; **HOSP:** St
Vincent's Med Ctr-Richmond; *SI: Prostate Cancer;
Impotence*; **HMO:** Oxford CIGNA GHI Aetna-US
Healthcare

 🦽 🌙 🔧 🏥 $ Mcr NFI

Raboy, Adley (MD)   U
Staten Island Univ Hosp-North

Staten Island Urological Assoc, 1460 Victory Blvd;
Staten Island, NY 10301; (718) 273-8100;
BDCERT: U 92; **MS:** SUNY Downstate 84; **RES:** S,
Staten Island Hosp, Staten Is, NY 85-86; **FEL:** U,
SUNY-HSC, Brooklyn, NY 86-90; **FAP:** Clin Instr
SUNY Hlth Sci Ctr

Savino, Michael (MD)   U
Bayley Seton Hosp

78 Todt Hill Rd 112; Staten Island, NY 10314;
(718) 448-3880; **BDCERT:** U 89; **MS:** Mexico 79;
RES: Coney Island Hosp, Brooklyn, NY 79-80;
Maimonides Med Ctr, Brooklyn, NY 80-85; **FAP:**
Instr NY Med Coll; **HOSP:** St Vincent's Med Ctr-
Richmond; *SI: Cancer; Stones, Urinary*; **HMO:** US
Hlthcre Oxford CIGNA

LANG: Sp; 🦽 🌙 📷 🔧 🏥 $ Mcr Mcd   4+ Weeks 💳

VASCULAR SURGERY (GENERAL)

Dossa, Christos (MD)   **GVS**
Staten Island Univ Hosp-North
2235 Clove Rd; Staten Island, NY 10305; (718)
981-4500; **BDCERT:** S 92; GVS 95; **MS:** Med Coll
Ga 86; **RES:** S, Henry Ford Hosp, Detroit, MI 86-87;
S, Henry Ford Hosp, Detroit, MI 87-91; **FEL:** GVS,
Henry Ford Hosp, Detroit, MI 91-93; **FAP:** Asst Clin
Prof Mt Sinai Sch Med; **HOSP:** Mount Sinai Med Ctr;
SI: Carotid Surgery; Aneurysm Surgery; **HMO:**
CIGNA US Hlthcre Oxford GHI Empire +

LANG: Grk; ♿ 🌙 🔲 🏥 💲 Mcr Mcd 1 Week

Sithian, Nedunchezia (MD) GVS
Staten Island Univ Hosp-South
1130 Victory Blvd; Staten Island, NY 10301; (718)
447-5400; **BDCERT:** S 77; GVS 87; **MS:** India 70;
RES: Luth Med Ctr, Brooklyn, NY 72-76; **FEL:** GVS,
Downstate Med Ctr, New York, NY 77-78; Luth
Med Ctr, Brooklyn, NY 77-78; **FAP:** Clin Instr S
SUNY Downstate; **HOSP:** St Vincent's Med Ctr-
Richmond; **HMO:** Affordable Hlth Plan Champus
CIGNA GHI Mastercare

♿ 🌙 🔲 ⚕ 🏥 💲 Mcr WC Immediately

NASSAU COUNTY

LONG BEACH MEDICAL CENTER

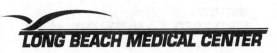

445 EAST BAY DRIVE
LONG BEACH, NY 11561
PHONE (516) 897-1000
FAX (516) 897-1214
WWW.LBMC.ORG

Sponsorship	Voluntary Not-for-Profit, A Member of The Mount Sinai Health System
Beds	164 acute, 24 short term psychiatric, 200 sub-acute & skilled care
Accreditation	Joint Commission on Accreditation of Healthcare Organizations

SERVING THE SOUTH SHORE OF LONG ISLAND SINCE 1922

Long Beach Medical Center is a clinical campus of the New York College of Osteopathic Medicine and the New York College of Podiatric Medicine, offering residencies in Family Practice Medicine and Podiatry as well as rotating internships.

Our superb Medical Staff encompasses virtually every medical specialty. More than 95% of physicians are board certified. Many have published extensively and are widely recognized.

A continuum of care. From Emergency Room Ombudsmen to Surgical Waiting Room, compassionate attention is extended to patients and families. Preventive health care programs, community screenings and workshops focus on helping people take better care of themselves.

EXCEPTIONAL CARE IN A UNIQUE SETTING

Medical Imaging	State of the art technology includes open MRI, Spiral CT, ACR accredited Mammography and a sophisticated Nuclear Medicine Center.
The Heart Station	Here is a new era in noninvasive diagnostic cardiology. Technology includes E-Cam dual digital, variable angle single photon emission computerized tomography: first in the New York area. More sensitive and accurate information is acquired in a fraction of the time used by previous technology. The Heart Station offers a full complement of noninvasive diagnostic studies.
Rehabilitation Services	Medical Rehabilitation is a mission of Long Beach Medical Center. Inpatient and out-patient services feature an integrated approach to case management, with each patient's team working to restore his or her highest levels of independent functioning.
Elder Care	The Komanoff Center for Geriatric and Rehabilitative Medicine provides sub-acute care, sub-acute and acute rehabilitation, chronic illness management, wound care, long-term skilled care, and care for the terminally ill.
Home Care	The pioneer in home health care, since 1982, Long Beach Medical Center "wrote the book" on bringing quality care to patients' homes. From short term care to long-term "nursing home without walls," Home Care helps families and patients access the help they need.
Family Care	Through every age and stage of life, The Family Care Center provides every level of health care. Free childhood immunizations, walk-in clinic after hours, and a full range of medical/surgical services is complemented by nutritional counseling and patient education.
Physician Referral	Free, 7 day, 24 hour Physician Referral Service provides access to attending and affiliated physicians in virtually every specialty. 1-800-618-6662.

SPECIALTY & SUBSPECIALTY	ABBREVIATION	PAGE(S)	SPECIALTY & SUBSPECIALTY	ABBREVIATION	PAGE(S)
Adolescent Medicine	AM	627	Pediatric Allergy & Immunology	PA&I	674
Allergy & Immunology	A&I	627-628	Pediatric Cardiology	PCd	674-675
Cardiac Electrophysiology	CE	629	Pediatric Endocrinology	PEn	675-676
Cardiology (Cardiovascular Disease)	Cv	629-635	Pediatric Gastroenterology	PGe	676-677
Child & Adolescent Psychiatry	ChAP	635	Pediatric Hematology–Oncology*	PHO	677
Child Neurology	ChiN	635	Pediatric Infectious Disease	PInf	677
Colon & Rectal Surgery	CRS	636	Pediatric Pulmonology	PPul	677-678
Dermatology	D	636-639	Pediatric Rheumatology	PRhu	678
Diagnostic Radiology	DR	639	Pediatric Surgery	PS	678-679
Emergency Medicine	EM	639	*PEDIATRICS (GENERAL)*	Ped	679-683
Endocrinology, Diabetes & Metabolism	EDM	639-641	**Physical Medicine & Rehabilitation**	PMR	683
FAMILY PRACTICE	FP	641-642	**Plastic Surgery**	PlS	684-687
Gastroenterology	Ge	642-645	**Psychiatry**	Psyc	687-689
Geriatric Medicine	Ger	645	Pulmonary Disease	Pul	689-691
Gynecologic Oncology*	GO	645-646	Radiation Oncology*	RadRO	692
Hand Surgery	HS	646	**Radiology**	Rad	692-693
Hematology	Hem	646-647	Reproductive Endocrinology	RE	693
Infectious Disease	Inf	647-648	Rheumatology	Rhu	694-695
INTERNAL MEDICINE	IM	648-654	Sports Medicine	SM	695
Maternal & Fetal Medicine	MF	654	**Surgery**	S	696-700
Medical Genetics	MG	654-655	**Thoracic Surgery** (includes open heart surgery)	TS	700-702
Medical Oncology*	Onc	655-656	**Urology**	U	702-705
Neonatal-Perinatal Medicine	NP	656	Vascular Surgery (General)	GVS	705-706
Nephrology	Nep	657			
Neurological Surgery	NS	658			
Neurology	N	659-661			
Nuclear Medicine	NuM	661			
OBSTETRICS & GYNECOLOGY	ObG	661-665			
Ophthalmology	Oph	665-668			
Orthopaedic Surgery	OrS	669-672			
Otolaryngology	Oto	672-674			
Pain Management	PM	674			

Specialties in capital letters indicate Primary Care Specialties. However, many doctors will be certified in a subspecialty, but will practice predominantly primary care medicine. In our lists this will be indicated.

*Oncologists deal with Cancer

ADOLESCENT MEDICINE

Arden, Martha (MD)   AM
Long Island Jewish Med Ctr
269-01 76th Ave; New Hyde Park, NY 11040; (718) 470-3270; **BDCERT:** Ped 88; **MS:** Yale U Sch Med 84; **RES:** Ped, Babies Hosp, New York, NY 84-87; **FEL:** Med, Schneider Children's Hosp, New Hyde Park, NY 87-90; **FAP:** Asst Prof Albert Einstein Coll Med; **SI:** *Adolescent Gynecology; Adolescent Nutrition;* **HMO:** Blue Choice PHS US Hlthcre Empire Oxford +

♿ 🅿 🏥 🛏 💲 Mcr **VISA** 💳 📧

ALLERGY & IMMUNOLOGY

Boxer, Mitchell (MD)   A&I
Long Island Jewish Med Ctr
560 Northern Blvd 209; Great Neck, NY 11021; (516) 482-0910; **BDCERT:** A&I 87; **MS:** NY Med Coll 81; **RES:** Long Island Jewish Med Ctr, New Hyde Park, NY 81-84; **FEL:** A&I, Northwestern Mem Hosp, Chicago, IL 85-87; **FAP:** Asst Clin Prof A&I Albert Einstein Coll Med; **HOSP:** Little Neck Comm Hosp; **SI:** *Asthma; Drug Allergies;* **HMO:** Blue Choice PHS Oxford CIGNA Guardian +

♿ 📞 🅿 🛏 🏥 💲 1 Week

Chiorazzi, Nicholas (MD)   A&I
N Shore Univ Hosp-Manhasset
North Shore University Hosp, 300 Community Dr 208; Manhasset, NY 11030; (516) 562-1085; **BDCERT:** IM 73; A&I 89; **MS:** Georgetown U 70; **RES:** Med, NY Hosp-Cornell Med Ctr, New York, NY 70-74; **FEL:** A&I, NY Hosp-Cornell Med Ctr, New York, NY 83-87; **FAP:** Prof Med NY Med Coll; **SI:** *Rheumatoid Arthritis; Systemic Erythematosus*

♿ 🅿 🛏 💲 Mcr Mcd **VISA** 💳

Corriel, Robert (MD)   A&I
N Shore Univ Hosp-Manhasset
Mahasset Allergy & Asthma Associates, 2110 Northern Blvd 210; Manhasset, NY 11030; (516) 365-6077; **BDCERT:** A&I 85; Ped 83; **MS:** Bowman Gray 76; **RES:** Ped, N Shore Univ Hosp-Manhasset, Manhasset, NY 76-79; **FEL:** A&I, U Hosp-S TX Med Ctr, San Antonio, TX 79-81; **FAP:** Asst Prof NYU Sch Med; **SI:** *Asthma; Sinusitis;* **HMO:** Oxford Prucare Blue Choice PHS PHCS +

LANG: Itl, Fr; ♿ 🅿 📞 🅿 🛏 🏥 💲 Mcr 1 Week
VISA 💳

Edwards, Bruce (MD)   A&I
Long Island Jewish Med Ctr
700 Old Country Rd 105; Plainview, NY 11803; (516) 933-1125; **BDCERT:** A&I 89; Ped 88; **MS:** Case West Res U 84; **RES:** Ped, Columbia-Presbyterian Med Ctr, New York, NY 84-87; **FEL:** a&I, Long Island Jewish Med Ctr, New Hyde Park, NY 87-89; **FAP:** Instr Albert Einstein Coll Med; **HOSP:** N Shore Univ Hosp-Plainview; **SI:** *Asthma and Pediatric Asthma; Food Allergy;* **HMO:** Aetna Hlth Plan Magnacare HealthNet United Healthcare Metlife +

♿ 🅿 📞 🅿 🛏 🏥 💲 A Few Days

Fonacier, Luz (MD)   A&I
Winthrop Univ Hosp
222 Station Plaza North 430; Mineola, NY 11501; (516) 663-2097; **BDCERT:** A&I 91; IM 89; **MS:** Philippines 78; **RES:** IM, Lutheran Med Ctr, Brooklyn, NY 86-89; D, Philippine Gen Hosp, Manilla, Philippines 82; **FEL:** NY Hosp-Cornell Med Ctr, New York, NY 89-91; New York University Med Ctr, New York, NY 84-86; **FAP:** Assoc Prof SUNY Stony Brook; **SI:** *Skin Allergies; Drug Allergies;* **HMO:** Vytra Oxford Empire US Hlthcre GHI +

LANG: Fil; ♿ 📞 🅿 🛏 🏥 💲 Mcr Mcd 2-4 Weeks

Frieri, Marianne (MD) A&I
Nassau County Med Ctr

2201 Hempstead Tpke; East Meadow, NY 11554; (516) 572-3214; **BDCERT:** IM 84; A&I 85; **MS:** Loyola U-Stritch Sch Med, Maywood 78; **RES:** St Joseph's Hosp, Chicago, IL 78-80; **FEL:** A&I, Nat Inst Health, Bethesda, MD 80-83; **FAP:** Assoc Lecturer SUNY Stony Brook; *SI: Asthma and Food Allergies; Autoimmune Disorders*; **HMO:** Health First Magnacare Oxford Multiplan CIGNA +

 🚫 🔌 📷 🔧 📅 💲 Mcr Mcd WC A Few Days

Goldstein, Stanley (MD) A&I
Long Island Jewish Med Ctr

Allergy & Asthma Care of Long Island, 242 Merrick Rd 401; Rockville Centre, NY 11570; (516) 536-7336; **BDCERT:** Ped 79; Pul 89; **MS:** NY Med Coll 75; **RES:** Ped, Long Island Jewish Med Ctr, New Hyde Park, NY 76-77; Long Island Jewish Med Ctr, New Hyde Park, NY 78; **FEL:** Ped A&I, Children's Hosp of Buffalo, Buffalo, NY 77; Allergy/Clinical Immunology, Univ Hosp SUNY Buffalo, Buffalo, NY 78-80; **HOSP:** Mercy Med Ctr; *SI: Asthma; Allergy*; **HMO:** Aetna-US Healthcare Oxford Vytra NYLCare Blue Cross +

LANG: Sp, Itl; 🚫 📶 🔌 📷 📅 💲 Mcr WC A Few Days **VISA**

Nicholas, William (MD) A&I
Long Island Jewish Med Ctr

44 Country Village Ln; New Hyde Park, NY 11040; (516) 354-7740; **BDCERT:** A&I 74; **MS:** SUNY Syracuse 54; **RES:** Med, Univ Hosp SUNY Syracuse, Syracuse, NY 55-58; A&I, St Luke's Roosevelt Hosp Ctr, New York, NY 60-61; **FAP:** Asst Clin Prof Albert Einstein Coll Med; **HMO:** Blue Choice Blue Cross & Blue Shield

Reiss, Joseph (MD) A&I
South Nassau Comm Hosp

1492 Wantagh Ave; Wantagh, NY 11793; (516) 221-6565; **BDCERT:** Ped 74; **MS:** SUNY Hlth Sci Ctr 65; **RES:** Ped, Brooklyn Jewish Hosp, Brooklyn, NY 66-68; **FEL:** A&I, Nassau County Med Ctr, East Meadow, NY 71-73; **HOSP:** St John's Epis Hosp-S Shore; *SI: Bronchial Asthma; Allergic Nasal & Skin*; **HMO:** GHI Oxford Empire Vytra Blue Cross & Blue Shield +

LANG: Rus, Sp; 🚫 🔌 📷 🔧 📅 💲 Mcr Mcd WC Immediately

Sicklick, Marc (MD) A&I
Montefiore Med Ctr

123 Grove Ave 110; Cedarhurst, NY 11516; (516) 569-5550; **BDCERT:** A&I 87; **MS:** Albert Einstein Coll Med 74; **RES:** Ped, Bronx Muncipal Hosp Ctr, Bronx, NY 74-77; **FEL:** A&I, Albert Einstein Med Ctr, Bronx, NY 77-79; **FAP:** Assoc Clin Prof Albert Einstein Coll Med; **HOSP:** South Nassau Comm Hosp; *SI: Asthma; Allergies*; **HMO:** GHI Blue Choice Oxford Aetna Hlth Plan +

 🚫 🔌 📷 🔧 📅 💲 Mcr A Few Days

Spina, Christopher (MD) A&I
Brooklyn Hosp Ctr-Caledonian

23 Lynwood Dr; Westbury, NY 11590; (516) 333-1055; **BDCERT:** A&I 74; IM 63; **MS:** Columbia P&S 56; **RES:** IM, Brooklyn Hosp Ctr, Brooklyn, NY 56-59; **FEL:** A&I, St Luke's Roosevelt Hosp Ctr, New York, NY 59; **HOSP:** Winthrop Univ Hosp; *SI: Rhinitis*

LANG: Itl, Sp; 🔌 📷 📅 Mcr Mcd A Few Days

Weinstock, Gary (MD) A&I
N Shore Univ Hosp-Manhasset

310 E Shore Rd 308; Great Neck, NY 11023; (516) 487-1073; **BDCERT:** A&I 85; IM 82; **MS:** Albany Med Coll 79; **RES:** IM, N Shore Univ Hosp-Manhasset, Manhasset, NY 79-82; **FEL:** Pul, Univ Hosp SUNY Stony Brook, Stony Brook, NY 82-83; A&I, Univ Hosp SUNY Stony Brook, Stony Brook, NY 83-86; **FAP:** Asst Clin Prof Med NYU Sch Med; **HOSP:** N Shore Univ Hosp-Glen Cove; *SI: Asthma; Hives*; **HMO:** Oxford United Healthcare Empire GHI Aetna Hlth Plan +

 🚫 🔌 📷 🔧 📅 💲 Mcr A Few Days

CARDIAC ELECTROPHYSIOLOGY

Levine, Joseph H (MD)   CE
St Francis Hosp-Roslyn
100 Port Washington Blvd; Roslyn, NY 11576; (516) 562-6672; **BDCERT:** IM 83; Cv 87; **MS:** U Rochester 80; **RES:** IM, Yale-New Haven Hosp, New Haven, CT 83; Cv, Johns Hopkins Hosp, Baltimore, MD 86; **HOSP:** Good Samaritan Hosp; **SI:** *Ablation of Arrhythmia; Sudden Death Prevention*; **HMO:** Oxford Aetna-US Healthcare Vytra

LANG: Heb, Fr, Sp; 🚫 📞 🔒 ▓ ⊞ Mcr Mcd WC ▦ *VISA* 💳

CARDIOLOGY (CARDIOVASCULAR DISEASE)

Abittan, Meyer H (MD)   Cv
St Francis Hosp-Roslyn
100 Port Washington Blvd; Roslyn, NY 11576; (516) 627-1155; **BDCERT:** IM 89; Cv 91; **MS:** Mt Sinai Sch Med 84; **RES:** Brkdle Univ Hosp, Brooklyn, NY 87-89

Anto, Maliakal J (MD)   Cv
Huntington Hosp
N Shore Cardiopulmonary Assoc, PC, 175 Jericho Tpke 320; Syosset, NY 11791; (516) 496-7900; **BDCERT:** IM 80; Cv 89; **MS:** India 74; **RES:** IM, Our Lady of Mercy Med Ctr, Bronx, NY 76-79; **FEL:** Cv, Nassau County Med Ctr, East Meadow, NY 79-81; **FAP:** Instr Med SUNY Stony Brook; **HOSP:** N Shore Univ Hosp-Plainview; **HMO:** Oxford CIGNA United Healthcare US Hlthcre Empire +

🚫 📞 🔒 ▓ ⊞ S Mcr Mcd WC NFl   A Few Days *VISA* 💳

Berke, Andrew D (MD)   Cv
St Francis Hosp-Roslyn
Long Island Interventional Cardiology, 100 Port Washington Blvd; Roslyn, NY 11576; (516) 365-2211; **BDCERT:** IM 82; Cv 85; **MS:** Brown U 79; **RES:** IM, Columbia-Presbyterian Med Ctr, New York, NY 80-82; **FEL:** Cv, Columbia-Presbyterian Med Ctr, New York, NY 82-85; **FAP:** Asst Prof of Clin Med Columbia P&S; **HOSP:** South Nassau Comm Hosp; **SI:** *Interventional Cardiology; Angioplasty Stent*; **HMO:** Oxford Magnacare United Healthcare US Hlthcre Blue Choice +

🚫 🔒 ▓ ⊞ Mcr Mcd WC   Immediately *VISA* 💳

Better, Donna (MD)   Cv
Winthrop Univ Hosp
259 1st St; Mineola, NY 11501; (516) 663-8535; **BDCERT:** Ped 92; PCd 97; **MS:** Albert Einstein Coll Med 89; **RES:** Mount Sinai Med Ctr, New York, NY 90-92; **FEL:** PCd, Columbia-Presbyterian Med Ctr, New York, NY 92-95; **HOSP:** Columbia-Presbyterian Med Ctr; **SI:** *Pediatric Echocardiography; Fetal Echocardiography*; **HMO:** Oxford US Hlthcre Vytra Empire Blue Cross & Shield +

LANG: Sp; 🚫 🔒 ▓ ⊞ S Mcd   Immediately

Binder, Alan (MD)   Cv
N Shore Univ Hosp-Plainview
Cardiology Consultants, 120 Bethpage Rd 102; Hicksville, NY 11801; (516) 938-3000; **BDCERT:** IM 76; Cv 79; **MS:** SUNY Syracuse 73; **RES:** IM, N Shore Univ Hosp-Manhasset, Manhasset, NY 74-76; **FEL:** Cv, N Shore Univ Hosp-Manhasset, Manhasset, NY 78; **HOSP:** N Shore Univ Hosp-Manhasset; **HMO:** PHS Aetna Hlth Plan Metlife Independent Health Plan

🚫 🔒 ▓ ⊞ S Mcr   1 Week *VISA* 💳

Breen, William (MD)   Cv
N Shore Univ Hosp-Plainview
Cardiology Consultants, 120 Bethpage Rd 102; Hicksville, NY 11801; (516) 938-3000; **BDCERT:** IM 80; Cv 83; **MS:** NY Med Coll 77; **RES:** Med, N Shore Univ Hosp-Manhasset, Manhasset, NY 79-82; **FEL:** Cv, N Shore Univ Hosp-Manhasset, Manhasset, NY 79-82; **FAP:** Assoc Prof Med Cornell U

🚫 ⊞ S Mcd   2-4 Weeks ▦ 💳

Budow, Jack (MD)   Cv   [PCP]
Winthrop Univ Hosp

975 Stewart Ave; Garden City, NY 11530; (516)
222-8680; **BDCERT:** IM 67; Cv 73; **MS:** South
Africa 56; **RES:** IM, Jewish Hosp Med Ctr, Brooklyn,
NY 58-62; **FEL:** Cv, Jewish Hosp Med Ctr, Brooklyn,
NY 62-64; **HOSP:** N Shore Univ Hosp-Glen Cove;
SI: Coronary Disease; Heart Failure; **HMO:** Vytra
Oxford Blue Choice United Healthcare GHI +

⬚ ⬚ ⬚ ⬚ ⬚ ⬚ ⬚   A Few Days

Chesner, Michael (MD)   Cv
Long Beach Med Ctr

325 W Park Ave; Long Beach, NY 11561; (516)
432-2004; **BDCERT:** IM 91; Cv 97; **MS:** Albert
Einstein Coll Med 87; **RES:** IM, Bronx Muncipal
Hosp Ctr, Bronx, NY 87-90; **FEL:** Cv, Long Island
Jewish Med Ctr, New Hyde Park, NY 90-93; **HOSP:**
South Nassau Comm Hosp; *SI: Prevention of Heart
Disease; Treatment of Heart Disease;* **HMO:** Oxford
Aetna Hlth Plan GHI Blue Cross & Blue Shield PHS
+

⬚ ⬚ ⬚ ⬚ ⬚ ⬚ ⬚ ⬚ ⬚ ⬚   Immediately

Cramer, Marvin (MD)   Cv
N Shore Univ Hosp-Manhasset

450 Plandome Rd 103; Manhasset, NY 11030;
(516) 365-5380; **BDCERT:** IM 74; Cv 77; **MS:**
Jefferson Med Coll 69; **RES:** Med, St Luke's
Roosevelt Hosp Ctr, New York, NY 69-71; Med, St
Luke's Roosevelt Hosp Ctr, New York, NY 73-74;
FEL: Cv, Columbia-Presbyterian Med Ctr, New
York, NY 74-76; **FAP:** Assoc Clin Prof NYU Sch
Med; **HOSP:** St Francis Med Ctr; *SI: Coronary
Disease; Arrythmias;* **HMO:** Oxford Blue Cross & Blue
Shield Blue Choice Sel Pro Chubb +

⬚ ⬚ ⬚ ⬚ ⬚ ⬚ ⬚ ⬚   1 Week **VISA** 💳

D'Agostino, Ronald (MD)   Cv
Long Island Jewish Med Ctr

Long Island Carrdiovascular Consultants, PC, 1129
Northern Blvd 408; Manhasset, NY 11030; (516)
627-2121; **BDCERT:** IM 89; Cv 91; **MS:** NY Med
Coll 85; **RES:** IM, Long Island Jewish Med Ctr, New
Hyde Park, NY 86-89; Long Island Jewish Med Ctr,
New Hyde Park, NY 92-93; **FEL:** Cv, Long Island
Jewish Med Ctr, New Hyde Park, NY 89-92; **HOSP:**
N Shore Univ Hosp-Manhasset; *SI: Nuclear
Cardiology;* **HMO:** Oxford Vytra GHI Aetna-US
Healthcare Blue Cross & Blue Shield +

⬚ ⬚ ⬚ ⬚ ⬚ ⬚ ⬚   1 Week

Davison, Edward (MD)   Cv
Franklin Hosp Med Ctr

300 Franklin Ave; Valley Stream, NY 11580; (516)
872-8280; **BDCERT:** Cv 77; IM 66; **MS:** Bowman
Gray 59; **RES:** IM, Maimonides Med Ctr, Brooklyn,
NY 62-63; **FEL:** Cv, Mount Sinai Med Ctr, New
York, NY 63-64; Cv, Mount Sinai Med Ctr, New
York, NY 64-65; **HOSP:** St Francis Hosp-Roslyn;
HMO: Blue Choice GHI Oxford US Hlthcre Vytra +

LANG: Sp, Itl, Grk, Yd; ⬚ ⬚ ⬚ ⬚ ⬚ ⬚ ⬚ ⬚
Immediately 📧 **VISA** 💳 💳

Dresdale, Robert (MD)   Cv
N Shore Univ Hosp-Manhasset

450 Plandome Rd 103; Manhasset, NY 11030;
(516) 365-5380; **BDCERT:** IM 75; Cv 77; **MS:**
Columbia P&S 72; **RES:** Columbia-Presbyterian
Med Ctr, New York, NY 72-74; **FEL:** Cv, Columbia-
Presbyterian Med Ctr, New York, NY; **FAP:** Assoc
Clin Prof NYU Sch Med; **HOSP:** St Francis Hosp-
Roslyn; *SI: Heart Disease in Women; High Cholesterol;*
HMO: Oxford Blue Choice CIGNA Magnacare PHS
+

⬚ ⬚ ⬚ ⬚ ⬚ ⬚   A Few Days **VISA** 💳 💳

Ezratty, Ari M (MD)   Cv
St Francis Hosp-Roslyn

100 Port Washington Blvd; Roslyn, NY 11576;
(516) 627-1155; **BDCERT:** Cv 92; IM 88; **MS:** Mt
Sinai Sch Med 85; **RES:** Mount Sinai Med Ctr, New
York, NY 86-89; **FEL:** Brigham & Women's Hosp,
Boston, MA; Inverventional Cv, Mount Sinai Med
Ctr, New York, NY; *SI: Interventional Cardiology*

Gindea, Aaron (MD)   Cv
Long Island Jewish Med Ctr
800 Community Dr; Manhasset, NY 11030; (516)
627-6622; **BDCERT:** IM 85; Cv 89; **MS:** NYU Sch
Med 82; **RES:** IM, Bellevue Hosp Ctr, New York, NY
82-85; **FEL:** Cv, Bellevue Hosp Ctr, New York, NY
85-88; **FAP:** Asst Prof of Clin Med NYU Sch Med;
HOSP: St Francis Hosp-Roslyn; **SI:** *Valvular Heart
Disease; Congenital Heart Disease;* **HMO:** GHI Blue
Cross & Blue Shield United Healthcare CIGNA 1199
+

LANG: Heb, Sp; 🔲 🔲 🔲 🔲 🔲 🔲 🔲 1 Week
VISA 🔲

Gleckel, Louis Wade (MD)   Cv   **PCP**
Long Island Jewish Med Ctr
2800 Marcus Ave; Lake Success, NY 11042; (516)
354-3344; **BDCERT:** IM 86; Cv 91; **MS:** SUNY Hlth
Sci Ctr 83; **RES:** IM, Long Island Jewish Med Ctr,
New Hyde Park, NY 83-86; Long Island Jewish Med
Ctr, New Hyde Park, NY 88-89; **FEL:** Cv, Long
Island Jewish Med Ctr, New Hyde Park, NY 86-88;
FAP: Assoc Prof Albert Einstein Coll Med; **HOSP:** N
Shore Univ Hosp-Forest Hills; **HMO:** GHI 1199
Oxford Prucare US Hlthcre +

LANG: Heb, Sp, Kor; 🔲 🔲 🔲 🔲 🔲 🔲 🔲 🔲 🔲
Immediately

Goldberg, Joel (MD)   Cv
N Shore Univ Hosp-Manhasset
310 E Shore Rd 104; Great Neck, NY 11023; (516)
829-9550; **BDCERT:** IM 81; Cv 83; **MS:** Penn State
U-Hershey Med Ctr 78; **RES:** IM, N Shore Univ
Hosp-Manhasset, Manhasset, NY 78-81; Cv, N
Shore Univ Hosp-Manhasset, Manhasset, NY 78-
81; **FEL:** IM, N Shore Univ Hosp-Manhasset,
Manhasset, NY 81-83; Cv, N Shore Univ Hosp-
Manhasset, Manhasset, NY 81-83; **HMO:** Oxford
PHS Sel Pro CIGNA

LANG: Sp, Pol, Chi; 🔲 🔲 🔲 🔲 🔲 🔲 1 Week
VISA 🔲

Goldberg, Steven (MD)   Cv
N Shore Univ Hosp-Manhasset
1010 Northern Blvd 110; Great Neck, NY 11021;
(516) 390-2430; **BDCERT:** IM 82; Cv 85; **MS:** Univ
Penn 79; **RES:** N Shore Univ Hosp-Manhasset,
Manhasset, NY 80-82; Mem Sloan Kettering
Cancer Ctr, New York, NY; **FEL:** N Shore Univ
Hosp-Manhasset, Manhasset, NY 82-84; **FAP:** Clin
Instr Med Cornell U; **HOSP:** St Francis Hosp-Roslyn;
SI: *High Cholesterol; Preventive Cardiology;* **HMO:**
Magnacare Multiplan PHS Oxford JJ Newman +

🔲 🔲 🔲 🔲 🔲 🔲 🔲 🔲 1 Week **VISA** 🔲

Goldman, George J (MD)   Cv
St Francis Hosp-Roslyn
Community Cardiology, PC, 800 Community Dr;
Manhasset, NY 11030; (516) 627-6622; **BDCERT:**
IM 79; Cv 81; **MS:** SUNY Downstate 76; **RES:** IM,
Long Island Jewish Med Ctr, New Hyde Park, NY
76-79; IM, Long Island Jewish Med Ctr, New Hyde
Park, NY 81-82; **FEL:** Cv, Mount Sinai Med Ctr,
New York, NY; **FAP:** Clin Instr NYU Sch Med;
HOSP: N Shore Univ Hosp-Manhasset; **SI:**
Echocardiography; Nuclear Cardiology; **HMO:** Oxford
Empire GHI

LANG: Sp, Heb; Immediately **VISA** 🔲

Goodman, Mark (MD)   Cv   **PCP**
N Shore Univ Hosp-Manhasset
Cardiovascular Medical Associates, PC, 975
Stewart Ave; Garden City, NY 11530; (516) 222-
8610; **BDCERT:** IM 72; Cv 73; **MS:** SUNY Hlth Sci
Ctr 67; **RES:** Montefiore Med Ctr, Bronx, NY 69-72;
Mount Sinai Med Ctr, New York, NY 70-71; **FEL:**
Cv, Montefiore Med Ctr, Bronx, NY 72-74; **FAP:**
Assoc Prof Med SUNY Hlth Sci Ctr; **HOSP:**
Winthrop Univ Hosp; **SI:** *Evaluate High Risk Heart
Disease; Congestive Heart Failure;* **HMO:** Magnacare
Aetna-US Healthcare Independent Health Plan
Vytra Oxford +

LANG: Sp, Rus, Chi; 🔲 🔲 🔲 🔲 🔲 🔲 🔲 🔲
Immediately **VISA** 🔲

Green, Stephen (MD)　　Cv
N Shore Univ Hosp-Manhasset

300 Community Dr; Manhasset, NY 11030; (516) 562-4100; **BDCERT:** IM 85; **MS:** Tufts U 80; **RES:** N Shore Univ Hosp-Manhasset, Manhasset, NY 80-83; **FEL:** Cv, N Shore Univ Hosp-Manhasset, Manhasset, NY 83-85; **FAP:** Assoc Clin Prof Med NYU Sch Med; *SI: Angioplasty; Heart Attack;* **HMO:** Aetna Hlth Plan Oxford HIP Network Chubb GHI +

 🦽 📷 🛏 Mcr Mcd　A Few Days ▨ **VISA** ⬤

Greenberg, Steven M (MD)　　Cv
St Francis Hosp-Roslyn

100 Port Washington Blvd; Roslyn, NY 11576; (516) 562-6672; **BDCERT:** Cv 89; IM 86; **MS:** Albany Med Coll 83; **RES:** Albert Einstein Coll Med, Bronx, NY 86-87; Mt Sinai Med Ctr, New York, NY 87-90

Gulotta, Stephen J (MD)　　Cv
St Francis Hosp-Roslyn

100 Port Washington Blvd; Roslyn, NY 11576; (516) 365-2900; **BDCERT:** Cv 68; IM 65; **MS:** SUNY Hlth Sci Ctr 58; **RES:** Montefiore Med Ctr, Bronx, NY 59-61; **FEL:** Cv, NY Hosp-Cornell Med Ctr, New York, NY 61-62; *SI: Coronary Angiography; Coronary Angioplasty;* **HMO:** Oxford US Hlthcre

LANG: Fr, Itl, Sp, Grk; 🦽 📷 🚼 🛏 💲 Mcr Mcd WC A Few Days **VISA**

Hamby, Robert I (MD)　　Cv
St Francis Hosp-Roslyn

NY Cardiology Group, PC, 100 Port Washington Blvd; Roslyn, NY 11576; (516) 365-5000; **BDCERT:** Cv 67; IM 66; **MS:** NYU Sch Med 59; **RES:** Cleveland Clinic Hosp, Cleveland, OH 60-61; Long Island Jewish Med Ctr, New Hyde Park, NY 63-64; **FEL:** Cv, NY Hosp-Cornell Med Ctr, New York, NY 61-62; Mount Sinai Med Ctr, New York, NY 62-63; **HOSP:** South Nassau Comm Hosp; **HMO:** Oxford GHI Aetna-US Healthcare US Hlthcre

🦽 📷 🛏 💲 Mcr Mcd NFl　A Few Days ▨ **VISA** ⬤

Hershman, Ronnie (MD)　　Cv
St Francis Hosp-Roslyn

43 Crossways Park Dr; Woodbury, NY 11797; (516) 677-0400; **BDCERT:** Cv 87; IM 85; **MS:** Mt Sinai Sch Med 82; **RES:** IM, Mt Sinai Med Ctr, New York, NY 83-85; Cv, Mt Sinai Med Ctr, New York, NY 85-87; **FEL:** Cv, Mt Sinai Med Ctr, New York, NY

Jelveh, Mansoor (MD)　　Cv
Mid-Island Hosp

Cardiovascular Diagnostic, 875 Old Country Rd 102; Plainview, NY 11803; (516) 935-8877; **BDCERT:** IM 75; Cv 77; **MS:** India 68; **RES:** IM, Nassau County Med Ctr, East Meadow, NY 72-75; **FEL:** Cv, Beth Israel Med Ctr, Boston, MA 75-77

Katz, Stanley (MD)　　Cv
Winthrop Univ Hosp

Med Offices, 35 Cornwall La; Port Washington, NY 11050; **BDCERT:** IM 76; Cv 79; **MS:** South Africa 70; **RES:** Med Ctr Hosp of VT, Burlington, VT; Cv, Boston U Med Ctr, Boston, MA; **HOSP:** N Shore Univ Hosp-Manhasset

Kirtane, Sanjay (MD)　　Cv
St John's Epis Hosp-S Shore

12 Causeway; Lawrence, NY 11559; (516) 239-7812; **BDCERT:** IM 80; Cv 83; **MS:** India 74; **RES:** St John's Epis Hosp-S Shore, Far Rockaway, NY 77-80; **FEL:** Long Island Jewish Med Ctr, New Hyde Park, NY 80-82; **HOSP:** Peninsula Hosp Ctr; *SI: Coronary Disease; Arrhythmia;* **HMO:** Oxford US Hlthcre Blue Choice NYLCare CIGNA +

LANG: Mar, Hin, Tel; 🦽 🌙 📷 🚼 🛏 💲 Mcr Mcd A Few Days

Kuslansky, Phillip (MD)   Cv
N Shore Univ Hosp-Manhasset
1000 Northern Blvd 120; Great Neck, NY 11021;
(516) 829-5609; **BDCERT:** IM 70; Cv 73; **MS:**
SUNY Downstate 65; **RES:** IM, Mount Sinai Med
Ctr, New York, NY 65-68; **FEL:** Cv, Mount Sinai
Med Ctr, New York, NY 68-69; **FAP:** Asst Clin Prof
Med NYU Sch Med; **SI:** *Stress Testing;*
Echocardiograms; **HMO:** Oxford Chubb Blue Choice
CIGNA

LANG: Itl; 🚹 🔂 🔟 🎞 🆂 🔤   1 Week

La Mendola, Christopher (MD)Cv
St Francis Hosp-Roslyn
100 Port Washington Blvd; Roslyn, NY 11576;
(516) 627-2173; **BDCERT:** S 93; **MS:** SUNY Hlth
Sci Ctr 85; **RES:** New York University Med Ctr, New
York, NY 86-92; TS, New York University Med Ctr,
New York, NY 92-94; **SI:** *Aortic Aneurysms; Mitral*
Valve Repair

🚹 🔂 🔟 🎞 🔤 🔤 🔤   1 Week

Monteleone, Bernard B (MD) Cv
St Francis Hosp-Roslyn
100 Port Washington Blvd; Roslyn, NY 11576;
(516) 627-4800; **BDCERT:** IM 74; Cv 76; **MS:** Med
Coll Wisc 69; **RES:** Lenox Hill Hosp, New York, NY
69-70; Bellevue Hosp Ctr, New York, NY 73-74;
FEL: Montefiore Med Ctr, Bronx, NY 74-76; **SI:**
Cardiology Only; **HMO:** Oxford GHI Aetna Hlth Plan
PHS Blue Cross & Blue Shield +

LANG: Frs, Sp, Rus; 🚹 🔳 🔂 🔟 🎞 🆂 🔤
Immediately

Nejat, Moosa (MD)   Cv
N Shore Univ Hosp-Manhasset
833 Northern Blvd 120; Great Neck, NY 11021;
(516) 829-0066; **BDCERT:** IM 72; Cv 75; **MS:** Iran
62; **RES:** Hosp of U Penn, Philadelphia, PA 64-67;
FEL: Cv, Mount Sinai Med Ctr, New York, NY 67-
68; Cv, Maimonides Med Ctr, Brooklyn, NY 68-69;
HOSP: Beth Israel Med Ctr-Kings Hwy; **SI:** *Heart*
Attack, Heart Failure; High Blood Pressure; **HMO:**
Blue Cross & Blue Shield GHI Oxford United
Healthcare

LANG: Frs, Rus; 🚹 🔳 🔂 🔟 🎞 🆂 🔤 🔤   1 Week

Nicosia, Thomas A (MD)   Cv
St Francis Hosp-Roslyn
1615 Northern Blvd; Manhasset, NY 11030; (516)
627-9355; **BDCERT:** IM 79; Cv 81; **MS:** U
Cincinnati 74; **RES:** IM, Mt Sinai Hosp, Hartford, CT
78; **FEL:** Cv, Bellevue Hosp Ctr, New York, NY 78-
80; **HOSP:** N Shore Univ Hosp-Manhasset; **HMO:**
Options US Hlthcre Empire Blue Choice MDNY +

🚹 🔳 🔂 🎞 🆂   2-4 Weeks

Pacienza, Vincent (MD)   Cv
St Francis Hosp-Roslyn
75 Plandome Rd; Manhasset, NY 11030; (516)
365-5151; **BDCERT:** IM 90; Cv 93; **MS:** Mexico 82;
RES: Winthrop Univ Hosp, Mineola, NY 83-86;
FEL: Cv, Metrop Hosp, New York, NY; **HOSP:**
Winthrop Univ Hosp; **SI:** *Non-invasive Cardiology;*
Stress Testing; Mitral Valve Prolapse; **HMO:**
Choicecare Empire Blue Cross Independent Health
Plan Metlife

🔤 🔤 **VISA** 💳

Pappas, Thomas W (MD)   Cv
St Francis Hosp-Roslyn
100 Port Washington Blvd; Roslyn, NY 11576;
(516) 365-2900; **BDCERT:** IM 86; Cv 89; **MS:**
Cornell U 83; **RES:** IM, NY Hosp-Cornell Med Ctr,
New York, NY 84-86; **FEL:** NY Hosp-Cornell Med
Ctr, New York 86-88; Interventional Cv, New York
Universtiy Med Ctr, New York, NY 89-90

Petrossian, George A (MD)   Cv
St Francis Hosp-Roslyn
New York Cardiology Group PC, 100 Port
Washington Blvd; Roslyn, NY 11576; (516) 365-
5000; **BDCERT:** IM 86; Cv 89; **MS:** Mt Sinai Sch
Med 83; **RES:** Columbia-Presbyterian Med Ctr, New
York, NY 84-86; Columbia-Presbyterian Med Ctr,
New York, NY 86-87; **FEL:** Columbia-Presbyterian
Med Ctr, New York, NY 87-89; Cv, Mass Gen Hosp,
Boston, MA 89-90; **FAP:** Asst Clin Prof Med
Columbia P&S; **SI:** *Angioplasty and Stents; Carotid*
Artery Disease; **HMO:** US Hlthcre GHI PHS Oxford
Blue Cross +

🚹 🔂 🔟 🎞 🆂 🔤 🔤 🔤 🔤   Immediately 🔤
VISA 💳

Ragno, Philip David (MD)   Cv
Winthrop Univ Hosp
Island Cardiac Specialists, 80 E Jerico Tpke;
Mineola, NY 11501; (516) 877-2626; **BDCERT:** IM
87; Cv 89; **MS:** SUNY Stony Brook 84; **RES:**
Winthrop Univ Hosp; **FEL:** Winthrop Univ Hosp;
HOSP: N Shore Univ Hosp-Manhasset; **HMO:**
Oxford, Vytra, Aetna-USHC, PHS, United
Healthcare +

LANG: Itl; 🚹 🅲 Mcr WC Immediately ▨ **VISA** ⬤

Reduto, Lawrence (MD)   Cv
St Francis Hosp-Roslyn
100 Port Washington Blvd; Roslyn, NY 11576;
(516) 562-6000; **BDCERT:** IM 75; Cv 77; **MS:** NY
Med Coll 72; **RES:** NY Hosp-Cornell Med Ctr, New
York, NY 75-76; **FEL:** Cv, NY Hosp-Cornell Med Ctr,
New York, NY 74-75; Cv, Yale-New Haven Hosp,
New Haven, CT 76-78; **FAP:** Assoc Clin Prof NY
Med Coll; **HOSP:** South Nassau Comm Hosp

LANG: Fr, Itl; 🚹 🖬 🎽 🎟 🅂 Mcr Mcd WC 1 Week
VISA

Rosoff, Maxine (MD)   Cv   PCP
N Shore Univ Hosp-Plainview
Mid Island Internal Medicine, 4277 Hempstead
Tpke 209; Bethpage, NY 11714; (516) 731-7770;
BDCERT: IM 78; Cv 83; **MS:** Harvard Med Sch 75;
RES: Mount Sinai Med Ctr, New York, NY 75-79;
FEL: Cv, Montefiore Med Ctr, Bronx, NY 79-81;
HOSP: Mid-Island Hosp; **SI:** *Echocardiography*;
HMO: United Healthcare Aetna Hlth Plan Prucare
Blue Cross & Blue Shield Choicecare +

🚹 🖬 🎽 🎟 🅂 Mcr WC NFI 1 Week **VISA** ⬤

Rutkovsky, Edward (MD)   Cv
N Shore Univ Hosp-Manhasset
2035 Lakeville Rd 101; New Hyde Park, NY
11040; (516) 328-9797; **BDCERT:** IM 87; Cv 89;
MS: NYU Sch Med 84; **RES:** New York University
Med Ctr, New York, NY 84-87; **FEL:** Cv, N Shore
Univ Hosp-Manhasset, Manhasset, NY 87-89; **FAP:**
Clin Instr Med NYU Sch Med; **HOSP:** St Francis
Hosp-Roslyn; **SI:** *Thallium Stress Testing;
Echocardiography*; **HMO:** Oxford United Healthcare
Aetna-US Healthcare GHI Magnacare +

LANG: Sp, Rus, Grk, Heb, Frs; 🚹 🆂🆄 🅲 🖬 🎽 🎟 🅂
Mcr WC NFI Immediately **VISA** ⬤

Schreiber, Carl (MD)   Cv
N Shore Univ Hosp-Glen Cove
North Nassau Cardiology Associates, 14 Glen Cove
Rd; Roslyn Heights, NY 11577; (516) 484-7893;
BDCERT: IM 82; Cv 85; **MS:** Med Coll Ga 79; **RES:**
Columbia-Presbyterian Med Ctr, New York, NY 79-
82; **FEL:** Cv, Westchester County Med Ctr, Valhalla,
NY 82-84; **HOSP:** N Shore Univ Hosp-Syosset;
HMO: Oxford Blue Cross US Hlthcre Chubb CIGNA
+

🚹 🆂🆄 🖬 🎽 🎟 🅂 Mcr NFI Immediately

Shlofmitz, Richard A (MD)   Cv
St Francis Hosp-Roslyn
Long Island Intervention Cardiology, 100 Port
Washington Blvd; Roslyn, NY 11576; (516) 365-
2900; **BDCERT:** IM 84; Cv 87; **MS:** NYU Sch Med
80; **RES:** N Shore Univ Hosp-Manhasset,
Manhasset, NY 80-84; Columbia-Presbyterian Med
Ctr, New York, NY 84-87; **HMO:** Oxford US Hlthcre
Aetna Hlth Plan GHI MDNY +

LANG: Sp, Fr, Grk, Yd; 🚹 🖬 🎽 🎟 🅂 Mcr Mcd WC NFI
Immediately **VISA** ⬤

Spadaro, Louise A (MD)   Cv
St Francis Hosp-Roslyn
100 Port Washington Blvd; Roslyn, NY 11576;
(516) 562-6653; **BDCERT:** IM 87; Cv 89; **MS:** NYU
Sch Med 84; **RES:** IM, Bellevue Hosp Ctr, New York,
NY 85; IM, Bellevue Hosp Ctr, New York, NY 85-
87; **FEL:** Cv, Bellevue Hosp Ctr, New York, NY 87-
89; **FAP:** Instr Columbia P&S; **SI:** *Preventive
Cardiology; Women & Heart Disease*; **HMO:** Oxford
Aetna Hlth Plan Blue Choice PPO

LANG: Sp; 🚹 🖬 🎟 🅂 Mcr Mcd 2-4 Weeks

Stahl, Jeffrey (MD)   Cv
St Francis Hosp-Roslyn
100 Port Washington Blvd; Roslyn, NY 11576;
(516) 562-6535; **BDCERT:** IM 87; Cv 87; **MS:**
Albert Einstein Coll Med 84; **RES:** Jacobi Med Ctr,
Bronx, NY 85-87; **FEL:** Cv, Mount Sinai Med Ctr,
New York, NY 87-90; **FAP:** Asst Clin Prof Columbia
P&S; **HMO:** Oxford PHS

🚹 🅲 🖬 🎽 🎟 🅂 Mcr NFI Immediately **VISA**

Weitzman, Lee (MD)   Cv
Long Beach Med Ctr
325 W Park Ave 7; Long Beach, NY 11561; (516) 432-2004; **BDCERT:** IM 81; Cv 83; **MS:** NYU Sch Med 78; **RES:** IM, New York University Med Ctr, New York, NY 78-79; IM, New York University Med Ctr, New York, NY 79-81; **FEL:** Cv, New York University Med Ctr, New York, NY 81-83; **FAP:** NYU Sch Med; **SI:** *Heart Disease; Hypertension;* **HMO:** PHS Oxford Blue Cross Independent Health Plan

♿ 🚽 📷 🔄 🏥 $ Mcr Wc NFI   Immediately

Young, Melvin (MD)   Cv
St John's Epis Hosp-S Shore
Long Island Cardiovascular Grp, 123 Grove Ave 216; Cedarhurst, NY 11516; (516) 569-5200; **BDCERT:** IM 72; Cv 74; **MS:** U Hlth Sci/Chicago Med Sch 63; **RES:** IM, Kings County Hosp Ctr, Brooklyn, NY 64-65; IM, Montefiore Med Ctr, Bronx, NY 65-66; **FEL:** Cv, Montefiore Med Ctr, Bronx, NY 69-71; Cv, Long Island Jewish Med Ctr, Glen Oaks, NY 70-71; **FAP:** Assoc Prof Med SUNY Stony Brook; **HOSP:** Long Island Jewish Med Ctr; **SI:** *Coronary Artery Disease; Cholesterol Metabolism;* **HMO:** Oxford CIGNA US Hlthcre GHI Blue Cross & Blue Shield +

LANG: Heb, Fr, Yd; ♿ 📷 🔄 🏥 Mcr Mcd Wc NFI A Few Days

CHILD & ADOLESCENT PSYCHIATRY

Fornari, Victor (MD)   ChAP
N Shore Univ Hosp-Manhasset
400 Community Dr; Manhasset, NY 11030; (516) 562-3005; **BDCERT:** Psyc 84; ChAP 85; **MS:** SUNY Hlth Sci Ctr 79; **RES:** Ped, Long Island Coll Hosp, Brooklyn, NY 79-80; Psyc, Hosp of U Penn, Philadelphia, PA 80-82; **FEL:** ChAP, Long Island Jewish Med Ctr, New Hyde Park, NY 82-84; **FAP:** Assoc Prof NYU Sch Med; **SI:** *Eating Disorders Trauma;* **HMO:** None

LANG: Sp, Itl, Fr; ♿ 🌙 📷 🔄 🏥 $ Mcr Wc NFI 1 Week

Hertz, Stanley (MD)   ChAP
Long Island Jewish Med Ctr
55 Fern Dr; Roslyn, NY 11576; (516) 484-6366; **BDCERT:** Psyc 80; ChAP 82; **MS:** NY Med Coll 75; **RES:** Psyc, Columbia-Presbyterian Med Ctr, New York, NY 76-79; **FEL:** ChAP, Columbia-Presbyterian Med Ctr, New York, NY 79-81; ChAP, Columbia-Presbyterian Med Ctr, New York, NY 81-82; **FAP:** Asst Clin Prof Albert Einstein Coll Med; **SI:** *Eating Disorders; Psychopharmacology;* **HMO:** Oxford GHI Merit Behavioral Health Plans VBH Blue Cross & Blue Shield +

♿ 🚽 🌙 📷 🔄 🏥 $ Mcr Wc NFI   1 Week

Williams, Daniel T (MD)   ChAP
Columbia-Presbyterian Med Ctr
3003 New Hyde Park Rd 204; New Hyde Park, NY 11042; (516) 488-3636; **BDCERT:** Psyc 75; ChAP 76; **MS:** Cornell U 69; **RES:** Psyc, Mount Sinai Med Ctr, New York, NY 70-72; **FEL:** ChAP, Columbia-Presbyterian Med Ctr, New York, NY 72-74; **FAP:** Clin Prof Psyc Columbia P&S; **HOSP:** Long Island Jewish Med Ctr; **SI:** *Psychosomatic Disorders; Psychopharmacology;* **HMO:** Oxford

♿ 🚽 🌙 📷 🏥 $ Mcr   A Few Days

CHILD NEUROLOGY

Maytal, Joseph (MD)   ChiN
Schneider Children's Hosp
Schneider Childrens Hospital, 26901 76th Ave; New Hyde Park, NY 11040; (718) 470-3450; **BDCERT:** Ped 86; ChiN 88; **MS:** Israel 78; **RES:** Ped, Long Island Jewish Med Ctr, New Hyde Park, NY 81; Ped, Brookdale Univ Hosp Med Ctr, Brooklyn, NY 82; **FEL:** ChiN, Albert Einstein Med Ctr, Bronx, NY 83-86; Clinical Neurophysiology, Albert Einstein Med Ctr, Bronx, NY 86-87; **FAP:** Assoc Prof Albert Einstein Coll Med; **HOSP:** Long Island Jewish Med Ctr; **SI:** *Epilepsy Seizures; Headaches Developmental;* **HMO:** Oxford Aetna Hlth Plan GHI US Hlthcre Blue Choice +

LANG: Rus, Chi, Sp, Rom, Heb; ♿ 📷 🔄 🏥 Mcd NFI 2-4 Weeks

COLON & RECTAL SURGERY

Gallo, Victor A (MD)   CRS
Winthrop Univ Hosp
1075 Franklin Ave; Garden City, NY 11530; (516) 248-7733; **BDCERT:** CRS 80; **MS:** Italy 71; **RES:** Univ Hosp SUNY Stony Brook, Stony Brook, NY 75-79; **FEL:** CRS, Suburban Hosp, Bethesda, MD; **HOSP:** Mercy Med Ctr; **HMO:** Oxford Metlife Blue Choice Magnacare Prucare +

🏥 📠 📞 🔒 🔧 🏨 $ Mcr Immediately **VISA** 💳

Greenwald, Marc (MD)   CRS
Winthrop Univ Hosp
310 E Shore Rd Ste 203; Great Neck, NY 11023; (516) 482-8657; **BDCERT:** CRS 92; **S** 91; **MS:** Albert Einstein Coll Med 85; **RES:** S, Montefiore Med Ctr, Bronx, NY 85-90; **FEL:** CRS, St Francis Hosp Med Ctr, Hartford, CT 90-91; **FAP:** Clin Instr S NYU Sch Med; **HOSP:** Long Island Jewish Med Ctr; *SI: Inflammatory Bowel Disease; Anorectal Diseases*; **HMO:** Oxford GHI United Healthcare Aetna-US Healthcare Prucare +

🏥 🔒 🔧 🏨 $ Mcr WC NFI Immediately **VISA** 💳

Hoexter, Barton (MD)   CRS
N Shore Univ Hosp-Manhasset
Colon & Rectal Surgical Assoc, 60 Cuttermill Rd 507; Great Neck, NY 11021; (516) 487-8738; **BDCERT:** CRS 72; **MS:** Geo Wash U Sch Med 62; **RES:** S, Mount Sinai Med Ctr, New York, NY 66-70; **FEL:** CRS,; **FAP:** Assoc Clin Prof Cornell U; **HOSP:** St Francis Hosp-Roslyn; *SI: Hemorrhoids; Colon & Rectal Cancer*; **HMO:** Oxford Empire GHI Blue Choice Vytra +

🏥 📞 🔒 🔧 🏨 $ Mcr Immediately **VISA** 💳

Kalafatic, Alfredo (MD)   CRS
Mid-Island Hosp
4277 Hempstead Tpke 203; Bethpage, NY 11714; (516) 735-3001; **BDCERT:** CRS 83; S 83; **MS:** Italy 70; **RES:** Long Island Jewish Med Ctr, New Hyde Park, NY 73-79; **FEL:** CRS, Mid-Island Hosp, Bethpage, NY 79-81; **HOSP:** N Shore Univ Hosp-Plainview; *SI: Colonoscopy; Rectal Cancer*; **HMO:** Aetna Hlth Plan Blue Cross & Blue Shield Metlife Prucare Sanus-NYLCare +

LANG: Sp, Itl; 🏥 📞 🔒 🔧 🏨 $ Mcr A Few Days **VISA** 💳

Procaccino, John (MD)   CRS
N Shore Univ Hosp-Manhasset
1000 Northern Blvd 130; Great Neck, NY 11021; (516) 466-5260; **BDCERT:** CRS 92; S 90; **MS:** NYU Sch Med 84; **RES:** S, N Shore Univ Hosp-Manhasset, Manhasset, NY 84-89; **FEL:** CRS, Cleveland Clinic Hosp, Cleveland, OH 89-90; **FAP:** Asst Clin Prof S Cornell U; **HOSP:** Long Island Jewish Med Ctr; *SI: Inflammatory Bowel Disease; Colorectal Cancer*; **HMO:** Oxford US Hlthcre NYLCare CIGNA PHCS +

🏥 🔒 🔧 🏨 $ WC Immediately **VISA** 💳

DERMATOLOGY

Aprile, Georgette (MD)   D
N Shore Univ Hosp-Manhasset
Lower Level, 8 Med Plz; Glen Cove, NY 11542; (516) 759-9200; **BDCERT:** D 78; **MS:** NY Med Coll 74; **RES:** NY Hosp-Cornell Med Ctr, New York, NY 75-78; **HOSP:** Long Island Jewish Med Ctr; *SI: Teenage Acne*; **HMO:** Aetna Hlth Plan Vytra Empire Blue Cross & Shield Oxford Empire +

LANG: Prt, Sp, Itl; 🏥 📠 📞 🔒 🔧 🏨 $ Mcr A Few Days 🏨 **VISA** 💳 💳

Bodian, Eugene L (MD)   **D**
N Shore Univ Hosp-Manhasset

475 Northern Blvd Ste 10; Great Neck, NY 11021;
(516) 482-2882; **BDCERT:** D 58; **MS:** SUNY
Downstate 52; **RES:** D, New York University Med
Ctr, New York, NY 53-56; **FAP:** Clin Prof NYU Sch
Med; **HOSP:** New York University Med Ctr; **SI:** *Laser
Dermatology; Liposuction*; **HMO:** GHI Oxford Aetna-
US Healthcare Prudential

LANG: Fr, Sp, Heb, Rus; ⬛ ⬛ ⬛ ⬛ ⬛ ⬛ ⬛ ⬛
⬛ ⬛ Immediately **VISA** ⬛ ⬛ ⬛

Bruckstein, Robert (MD)   **D**
Sound Shore Med Ctr-Westchester

290 Central Ave 206; Lawrence, NY 11559; (516)
239-2332; **BDCERT:** D 77; **MS:** NYU Sch Med 72;
RES: New York University Med Ctr, New York, NY
73-75; Bellevue Hosp Ctr, New York, NY 73-75;
HOSP: Peninsula Hosp Ctr; **SI:** *Acne; Skin Cancer*;
HMO: Blue Choice HealthNet Metlife Travelers
Choicecare +

⬛ ⬛ ⬛ ⬛ ⬛ ⬛ ⬛ ⬛ Immediately

De Pietro, William (MD)   **D**
N Shore Univ Hosp-Glen Cove

10 Medical Plz Ste 102; Glen Cove, NY 11542;
(516) 671-1780; **BDCERT:** D 80; **MS:** Georgetown
U 76; **FEL:** D, St Luke's Roosevelt Hosp Ctr, New
York, NY 77-80; **SI:** *Laser Surgery; Cosmetic Surgery*;
HMO: Most

⬛ ⬛ ⬛ ⬛ ⬛ ⬛ ⬛ Immediately

Demento, Frank (MD)   **D**
Winthrop Univ Hosp

520 Franklin Ave Ste 229; Garden City, NY 11530;
(516) 746-1227; **BDCERT:** D 69; **MS:** UMDNJ-NJ
Med Sch, Newark 64; **RES:** D, USPHS Hosp,
Baltimore, MD; **FEL:** D, Columbia-Presbyterian Med
Ctr, New York, NY 66-68; **HOSP:** Nassau County
Med Ctr

⬛ ⬛ ⬛ ⬛ ⬛ ⬛ ⬛ ⬛ Immediately **VISA** ⬛

Dolitsky, Charisse (MD)   **D**
Long Beach Med Ctr

Island Dermatology, 604 E Park Ave; Long Beach,
NY 11561; (516) 432-0011; **BDCERT:** D 89; **MS:**
SUNY Downstate 85; **RES:** D, Univ Hosp SUNY
Bklyn, Brooklyn, NY 86-89; **HOSP:** South Nassau
Comm Hosp; **SI:** *Acne; Laser Surgery*; **HMO:** Benefit
Plan Oxford US Hlthcre Empire GHI +

LANG: Sp, Heb; ⬛ ⬛ ⬛ ⬛ ⬛ ⬛ ⬛ ⬛
Immediately **VISA** ⬛

Falcon, Ronald (MD)   **D**
Long Beach Med Ctr

Island Dermatology, 604 E Park Ave; Long Beach,
NY 11561; (516) 432-0011; **BDCERT:** D 89; **MS:**
SUNY Downstate 85; **RES:** IM, Montefiore Med Ctr,
Bronx, NY 85-86; D, Univ Hosp SUNY Bklyn,
Brooklyn, NY 86-89; **HOSP:** South Nassau Comm
Hosp; **SI:** *Skin Cancer; Acne*; **HMO:** Aetna Hlth Plan
Empire Blue Cross & Blue Shield GHI

LANG: Sp, Heb; ⬛ ⬛ ⬛ ⬛ ⬛ ⬛ ⬛ ⬛
A Few Days **VISA** ⬛

Feinstein, Robert (MD)   **D**
Winthrop Univ Hosp

DERMEDX, 173 Mineola Blvd 203; Mineola, NY
11501; (516) 741-1730; **BDCERT:** D 72; **MS:** NYU
Sch Med 67; **RES:** D, Columbia-Presbyterian Med
Ctr, New York, NY 68-71; **FAP:** Asst Clin Prof
Columbia P&S; **HOSP:** Columbia-Presbyterian Med
Ctr; **SI:** *Acne; Skin Cancers*; **HMO:** Empire Vytra
Oxford Prucare Aetna Hlth Plan +

LANG: Sp; ⬛ ⬛ ⬛ ⬛ ⬛ ⬛ ⬛ A Few Days **VISA**
⬛

Funt, Tina (MD)   **D**
Winthrop Univ Hosp

229 7th St Ste 105; Garden City, NY 11530; (516)
747-7778; **BDCERT:** D 89; **MS:** SUNY Hlth Sci Ctr
84; **RES:** Ped, Montefiore Med Ctr, Bronx, NY 84-
86; Ped, Albert Einstein Med Ctr, Bronx, NY 84-86;
FEL: D, NY Med Coll, Valhalla, NY 86-88; **HOSP:**
Mercy Med Ctr; **HMO:** GHI Choicecare Aetna Hlth
Plan Metlife Oxford +

⬛ ⬛ ⬛ ⬛ ⬛ ⬛ ⬛ ⬛

Gladstein, Michael (MD) D
Western Queens Comm Hosp
9 Oyster Bay Rd; Locust Valley, NY 11560; (718) 728-8979; **BDCERT:** D 87; **MS:** NYU Sch Med 79; **RES:** D, NYU Med Ctr, New York, NY 83; **FAP:** Asst Prof NYU Sch Med; **HMO:** United Healthcare Empire Aetna Hlth Plan US Hlthcre GHI +

LANG: Sp; ⬛ ⬛ ⬛ ⬛ ⬛ A Few Days

Hefter, Harold (MD) D
Franklin Hosp Med Ctr
135 Rockaway Tpke 100; Lawrence, NY 11559; (516) 371-1600; **BDCERT:** D 85; **MS:** Albert Einstein Coll Med 81; **RES:** D, Albert Einstein Med Ctr, Bronx, NY 82-85; **SI:** *Cosmetic Dermatology; General & Surgical Dermatology;* **HMO:** PHS Prucare Independent Health Plan MDLI

⬛ ⬛ ⬛ ⬛ ⬛ ⬛ ⬛ Immediately *VISA* ⬛

Krivo, James (MD) D
Winthrop Univ Hosp
516 Dogwood Ave; Franklin Square, NY 11010; (516) 481-4920; **BDCERT:** D 73; **MS:** U Chicago-Pritzker Sch Med 66; **RES:** D, U Chicago Hosp, Chicago, IL 67-68; D, NY Med Coll, Valhalla, NY 70-72; **FAP:** SUNY Stony Brook; **HOSP:** Franklin Hosp Med Ctr; **SI:** *Psychocutaneous Diseases; Skin Cancer;* **HMO:** Oxford Vytra US Hlthcre GHI United Healthcare +

⬛ ⬛ ⬛ ⬛ ⬛ ⬛ ⬛ 1 Week

Levine, Laurie J (MD) D
Winthrop Univ Hosp
200 Old Country Rd 140; Mineola, NY 11501; (516) 742-6136; **BDCERT:** D 88; **MS:** SUNY Hlth Sci Ctr 84; **RES:** Thomas Jefferson U Hosp, Philadelphia, PA 85-88; **FEL:** Laser S, Thomas Jefferson U Hosp, Philadelphia, PA; **HMO:** Prucare Vytra Magnacare US Hlthcre Multiplan +

LANG: Sp, Prt; ⬛ ⬛ ⬛ ⬛ ⬛ ⬛ ⬛ ⬛ ⬛
A Few Days ⬛ *VISA* ⬛

Meyers, John H (MD) D
N Shore Univ Hosp-Glen Cove
130 Forest Ave; Glen Cove, NY 11542; (516) 671-7666; **BDCERT:** D 56; **MS:** Yale U Sch Med 50; **RES:** NY Hosp-Cornell Med Ctr, New York, NY 53-54; **HMO:** Vytra Oxford United Healthcare PHS Magnacare +

⬛ ⬛ ⬛ ⬛ ⬛ ⬛ ⬛ A Few Days

Pacernick, Lawrence (MD) D
N Shore Univ Hosp-Plainview
700 Old Country Rd 203; Plainview, NY 11803; (516) 822-9730; **BDCERT:** D 73; **MS:** U Mich Med Sch 66; **RES:** Michael Reese Hosp Med Ctr, Chicago, IL 66-68; U Chicago Hosp, Chicago, IL 70-73; **HOSP:** Nassau County Med Ctr; **HMO:** Oxford Prucare Metlife Multiplan Magnacare +

LANG: Sp; ⬛ ⬛ ⬛ ⬛ ⬛ ⬛ ⬛ ⬛ ⬛ ⬛ ⬛
1 Week *VISA* ⬛ ⬛

Paltzik, Robert (MD) D
N Shore Univ Hosp-Manhasset
2 Hillside Ave G; Williston Park, NY 11596; (516) 747-2230; **BDCERT:** D 77; **Ped** 76; **MS:** NYU Sch Med 71; **RES:** Ped, Yale-New Haven Hosp, New Haven, CT 71-73; D, Univ Hosp SUNY Bklyn, Brooklyn, NY 75-77; **HOSP:** Winthrop Univ Hosp; **SI:** *Pediatric Dermatology; Skin Cancer;* **HMO:** Oxford Aetna-US Healthcare PHCS Travelers Independent Health Plan +

⬛ ⬛ ⬛ ⬛ ⬛ ⬛ ⬛ Immediately ⬛ *VISA* ⬛

Spinowitz, Alan (MD) D
Franklin Hosp Med Ctr
877 Stewart Ave 27; Garden City, NY 11530; (516) 745-0606; **BDCERT:** D 82; **MS:** SUNY Hlth Sci Ctr 81; **RES:** D, U IL Med Ctr, Chicago, IL 82-85; **FEL:** Mohs S, U IL Med Ctr, Chicago, IL 85-87; **SI:** *Skin Cancer Surgery;* **HMO:** Oxford Aetna Hlth Plan US Hlthcre Vytra GHI +

⬛ ⬛ ⬛ ⬛ ⬛ ⬛ A Few Days *VISA* ⬛

638

Weinberg, Samuel (MD)　　　D
New York University Med Ctr

2035 Lakeville Rd 3310; New Hyde Park, NY
10016; (516) 352-6151; **BDCERT:** D 62; Ped 55;
MS: U Hlth Sci/Chicago Med Sch 48; **RES:** Beth-El
Hosp, Brooklyn, NY 48-49; Ped, NY Foundling
Hosp, Brooklyn, NY 53; **FEL:** D, New York
University Med Ctr, New York, NY 57-61; **FAP:**
Prof D NY Med Coll; **HOSP:** Long Island Jewish Med
Ctr; **SI:** *Pediatric Dermatology;* **HMO:** None

🦽 🔒 ⛨ 🎲　A Few Days

DIAGNOSTIC RADIOLOGY

Mendelsohn, Steven (MD)　　DR
N Shore Univ Hosp-Plainview

126 Hicksville Rd; Massapequa, NY 11758; (516)
798-4242; **BDCERT:** DR 84; **MS:** Jefferson Med Coll
79; **RES:** N Shore Univ Hosp-Manhasset,
Manhasset, NY 80-83

LANG: Sp; 🦽 🏥 🌙 🔒 💲 Mcr Mcd WC NFI
A Few Days ▦ **VISA** 💳

Sitron, Alan (MD)　　　DR
Mid-Island Hosp

4277 Hempstead Tpke 200; Bethpage, NY 11714;
(516) 796-4340; **BDCERT:** Rad 75; **MS:** Albany
Med Coll 71; **RES:** Rad, Albert Einstein, Bronx, NY
72-75; **HMO:** Prucare Oxford Empire

🦽 🏥 🌙 🎲 💲 Mcr WC NFI　Immediately ▦ **VISA**
💳 💳

EMERGENCY MEDICINE

Canter, Robert (MD)　　　EM
Long Beach Med Ctr

455 E Bay Dr; Long Beach, NY 11561; (516) 897-
1100; **BDCERT:** EM 90; IM 81; **MS:** SUNY Syracuse
78; **RES:** IM, Nassau County Med Ctr, East Meadow,
NY 79-81; **FEL:** Hem Onc, Nassau County Med Ctr,
East Meadow, NY 81-83

Packy, Theodore (MD)　　　EM
N Shore Univ Hosp-Plainview

Central Emergency Physicians, 46 Niagara St;
Miller Place, NY 11764; (516) 719-2484;
BDCERT: IM 87; **MS:** SUNY Downstate 83; **RES:**
IM, Booth Mem Hosp, Flushing, NY 83-86; **SI:**
Toxicology; Intensive Care; **HMO:** Oxford HIP
Network Vytra US Hlthcre Blue Cross & Blue Shield
+

LANG: Sp, Fr, Pol, Ger, Itl; 🦽 🏥 🌙 🔒 ⛨ 🎲 Mcr Mcd
WC NFI　Immediately ▦ **VISA** 💳 💳

Sama, Andrew (MD)　　　EM
N Shore Univ Hosp-Manhasset

Dept of Emerg Med, N Shore Univ Hosp Manhasset,
300 Community Dr; Manhasset, NY 11030; (516)
562-3090; **BDCERT:** IM 84; EM 89; **MS:** Cornell U
81; **RES:** IM, N Shore Univ Hosp-Manhasset,
Manhasset, NY 81-84; **FAP:** Assoc Clin Prof NYU
Sch Med; **HMO:** Most

LANG: Sp; 🦽 🏥 🌙 🔒 ⛨ 🎲 💲 Mcr Mcd WC NFI
Immediately ▦ **VISA** 💳 💳

ENDOCRINOLOGY, DIABETES & METABOLISM

Aloia, John (MD)　　　EDM
Winthrop Univ Hosp

222 Station Plaza North 350; Mineola, NY 11501;
(516) 663-3511; **BDCERT:** IM 69; **MS:** Creighton U
62; **RES:** IM, Meadowbrook Hosp, East Meadow, NY
65-66

🦽 🌙 🔒 ⛨ 🎲 💲 Mcr Mcd　2-4 Weeks ▦ **VISA** 💳
💳

Bhatt, Anjani (MD)   **EDM**
Long Beach Med Ctr

871 E Park Ave; Long Beach, NY 11561; (516) 889-8844; **BDCERT:** IM 83; EDM 85; **MS:** India 76; **RES:** IM, Brooklyn Hosp Ctr, Brooklyn, NY 78-79; **FEL:** IM, Brooklyn Hosp Ctr, Brooklyn, NY 79-81; EDM, Brooklyn Hosp Ctr, Brooklyn, NY 82-84; *SI: Diabetes; Thyroid;* **HMO:** GHI Blue Choice US Hlthcre Magnacare Multiplan +

LANG: Rom, Hin; ⛐ 🏧 📞 🔒 🅿 🎫 💲 📠
A Few Days

Friedman, Seth (MD)   **EDM**
N Shore Univ Hosp-Glen Cove

560 Northern Blvd; Great Neck, NY 11021; (516) 466-6165; **BDCERT:** IM 91; EDM 93; **MS:** Mt Sinai Sch Med 88; **RES:** IM, Long Island Jewish Med Ctr, New Hyde Park, NY 88-91; **FEL:** EDM, Albert Einstein Med Ctr, Bronx, NY 91-93; **HOSP:** Long Island Jewish Med Ctr; *SI: Thyroid Disease; Diabetes;* **HMO:** Oxford US Hlthcre CIGNA Blue Choice United Healthcare +

LANG: Heb, Sp; ⛐ 📞 🔒 🅿 🎫 💲 📠 1 Week
VISA 💳

Gordon, Jeffrey (MD)   **EDM**
St Francis Hosp-Roslyn

3 School St 306; Glen Cove, NY 11542; (516) 759-2420; **BDCERT:** IM 72; EDM 73; **MS:** Cornell U 65; **RES:** Bellevue Hosp Ctr, New York, NY 67; **FEL:** Duke U Med Ctr, Durham, NC 69-70; EDM, VA Ct Healthcare Sys-West Haven, West Haven, CT 70; **HOSP:** N Shore Univ Hosp-Manhasset; **HMO:** None

⛐ 🔒 🅿 🎫 💲 A Few Days

Goussis, Onoufrios (MD)   **EDM**   **PCP**
St Francis Hosp-Roslyn

1010 Northern Blvd 100; Great Neck, NY 11021; (516) 773-6301; **BDCERT:** EDM 93; IM 83; **MS:** Greece 72; **RES:** IM, CAMC, 76-77; IM, Cooper Hosp U, Camden, NJ 78-79; **FEL:** EDM, UHJ-UCLA, Los Angelas, CA 79-82; **FAP:** Asst Prof Med UMDNJ-NJ Med Sch, Newark; **HOSP:** N Shore Univ Hosp-Glen Cove; **HMO:** CIGNA Independent Health Plan Aetna Hlth Plan PHS Guardian +

LANG: Grk; ⛐ 📞 🔒 🎫 💲 📠 Immediately

Greenfield, Martin (MD)   **EDM**
Long Island Jewish Med Ctr

560 Northern Blvd 107; Great Neck, NY 11021; (516) 482-3433; **BDCERT:** IM 74; **MS:** SUNY Downstate 68; **RES:** Long Island Jewish Med Ctr, New Hyde Park, NY 68-71; **FEL:** Brigham & Women's Hosp, Boston, MA 73-75; **FAP:** Asst Clin Prof Albert Einstein Coll Med; **HOSP:** N Shore Univ Hosp-Manhasset; *SI: Diabetes and Complications; Thyroid Disorders;* **HMO:** Prucare Select Oxford Multiplan Sel Pro +

⛐ 📞 🔒 🎫 💲 📠 🔳 2-4 Weeks *VISA* 💳 💳

Katzeff, Harvey (MD)   **EDM**
Long Island Coll Hosp

Long Island Jewish Med Ctr, 270-05 76th Ave; New Hyde Park, NY 11040; (718) 470-7240; **BDCERT:** IM 80; EDM 83; **MS:** SUNY Downstate 76; **RES:** IM, Good Samaritan Hosp, Phoenix, AZ 76-79; **FEL:** EDM, Med Ctr Hosp of VT, Burlington, VT 79-82; **FAP:** Assoc Prof Albert Einstein Coll Med; *SI: Diabetes; Thyroid Diseases;* **HMO:** Oxford Aetna Hlth Plan

⛐ 🔒 🎫 💲 📠 2-4 Weeks *VISA* 💳

Klass, Evan (MD)   **EDM**   **PCP**
N Shore Univ Hosp-Manhasset

Endocrinology and Diabetic Associates of LI, PC, 242 Merrick Rd 403; Rockville Centre, NY 11570; (516) 536-3700; **BDCERT:** IM 79; EDM 83; **MS:** NY Med Coll 76; **RES:** IM, Long Island Jewish Med Ctr, New Hyde Park, NY 76-79; **FEL:** EDM, Geo Wash U Med Ctr, Washington, DC 80-82; **FAP:** Asst Clin Prof Albert Einstein Coll Med; **HOSP:** South Nassau Comm Hosp; *SI: Diabetes; Thyroid Diseases;* **HMO:** Oxford Empire CIGNA Multiplan

⛐ 📞 🔒 🅿 🎫 💲 📠 🔳 2-4 Weeks 🔳 *VISA* 💳

Kolodny, Howard (MD) EDM
Long Island Jewish Med Ctr

North Shore Diabetes Assoc, 3003 New Hyde Park Rd 201; New Hyde Park, NY 11042; (516) 829-3442; **BDCERT:** IM 68; EDM 73; **MS:** NYU Sch Med 59; **RES:** Cleveland Clinic Hosp, Cleveland, OH 59-60; Montefiore Med Ctr, Bronx, NY 60-61; **FEL:** EDM, Mount Sinai Med Ctr, New York, NY 61-63; **FAP:** Clin Prof Med Albert Einstein Coll Med; **HOSP:** N Shore Univ Hosp-Manhasset; **SI:** *Diabetes; Thyroid Disease*

🚻 ⬛ 🔧 👥 🏠 Mcr 1 Week 🔵

Lomasky, Steven (MD) EDM
Long Island Jewish Med Ctr

Endocrinology & Diabetes Associates of Long Island, 242 Merrick Rd; Rockville Ctr, NY 11570; (516) 536-3700; **BDCERT:** IM 85; EDM 89; **MS:** Israel 82; **RES:** IM, Montefiore Med Ctr, Bronx, NY 83-86; **FEL:** EDM, Albert Einstein Med Ctr, Bronx, NY 86-87; **FAP:** Asst Clin Prof Med Albert Einstein Coll Med; **HOSP:** South Nassau Comm Hosp; **HMO:** Most

LANG: Sp; 🚻 🌙 ⬛ 👥 🏠 💲 Mcr 2-4 Weeks 🟨
VISA 🔵

Margulies, Paul (MD) EDM
N Shore Univ Hosp-Manhasset

444 Community Dr; Manhasset, NY 11030; (516) 627-1366; **BDCERT:** IM 75; **MS:** U Chicago-Pritzker Sch Med 70; **RES:** Med, NY Hosp-Cornell Med Ctr, New York, NY 73-75; **FEL:** EDM, NY Hosp-Cornell Med Ctr, New York, NY 75-76; **FAP:** Assoc Clin Prof Med NYU Sch Med; **SI:** *Thyroid Disease; Adrenal Disease*; **HMO:** Oxford

🚻 🌙 ⬛ 👥 🏠 💲 WC 2-4 Weeks

Rosenthal, David S (MD) EDM
N Shore Univ Hosp-Plainview

Island Medical Group PC, 4150 Sunrise Hwy; Massapequa, NY 11758; (516) 541-1721; **BDCERT:** IM 69; EDM 72; **MS:** NYU Sch Med 63; **RES:** IM, Wilford Hall USAF Med Ctr, San Antonio, TX 64-67; **FEL:** EDM, Boston U Med Ctr, Boston, MA 71-72; **FAP:** Asst Clin Prof Med SUNY Stony Brook; **HOSP:** Mid-Island Hosp; **SI:** *Thyroid Disease; Pituitary Disease*; **HMO:** CIGNA Aetna Hlth Plan Blue Choice United Healthcare Oxford +

🚻 🌙 ⬛ 👥 🏠 💲 Mcr 2-4 Weeks 🟨 ***VISA*** 🔵

Vaswani, Ashok N (MD) EDM
Winthrop Univ Hosp

520 Franklin Ave; Garden City, NY 11530; (516) 739-0414; **BDCERT:** IM 77; EDM 83; **MS:** India 70; **RES:** Nassau County Med Ctr, East Meadow, NY 72-74; **FEL:** Yale-New Haven Hosp, New Haven, CT; Med Ctr Hosp of VT, Burlington, VT; **FAP:** Asst Prof Med SUNY Stony Brook; **SI:** *Osteoporosis; Obesity*; **HMO:** Choicecare Aetna Hlth Plan Empire Metlife

🚻 🌙 ⬛ 🏠 💲 Mcr A Few Days

Weinerman, Stuart (MD) EDM
N Shore Univ Hosp-Forest Hills

Division of Endocrinology, North Shore Univ Hosp, 865 Northern Blvd Ste 202; Great Neck, NY 10021; (516) 622-5200; **BDCERT:** IM 87; EDM 89; **MS:** Albert Einstein Coll Med 84; **RES:** N Shore Univ Hosp-Manhasset, Manhasset, NY 84-87; Mem Sloan Kettering Cancer Ctr, New York, NY 84-87; **FEL:** EDM, NY Hosp-Cornell Med Ctr, New York, NY 87-89; **SI:** *Osteoporosis*; **HMO:** Most

🚻 ⬛ 🏠 Mcr WC A Few Days 🟨 ***VISA*** 🔵 💳

FAMILY PRACTICE

Capobianco, Luigi (MD) FP **PCP**
N Shore Univ Hosp-Glen Cove

1 School St 203; Glen Cove, NY 11542; (516) 671-9800; **BDCERT:** FP 88; Ger 96; **MS:** Italy 84; **RES:** FP, N Shore Univ Hosp-Glen Cove, Glen Cove, NY 85-88; **FAP:** Clin Instr SUNY Stony Brook; **SI:** *Geriatrics*; **HMO:** Aetna Hlth Plan Oxford Vytra CIGNA HealthNet +

LANG: Itl, Sp; 🚻 ⬛ 🌙 ⬛ 🏠 Mcr Mod WC NFI
Immediately ***VISA*** 🔵

Edelstein, Martin (MD) FP **PCP**
N Shore Univ Hosp-Manhasset

11 Beverly Rd; Great Neck, NY 11021; (516) 487-1614; **BDCERT:** FP 76; **MS:** McGill U 71; **RES:** Jewish Gen Hosp, Montreal, Canada 71-73; **FAP:** Asst Clin Prof NYU Sch Med; **SI:** *Check-ups*; **HMO:** Oxford MDNY NSHIP

LANG: Fr; 🚻 🌙 ⬛ 👥 🏠 💲 Mcr Immediately ***VISA*** 🔵

Guide to symbols and abbreviations can be found on pages 110-113.

641

Kann, Ferdinand (MD)   FP   PCP
N Shore Univ Hosp-Glen Cove
2 Kirkwood Dr; Glen Cove, NY 11542; (516) 676-8628; **BDCERT:** FP 80; **MS:** Switzerland 55; **RES:** Path, Community Hosp, Glen Cove, NY 57-58; **FEL:** Path, Community Hosp, Glen Cove, NY 59-60; **FAP:** Asst Clin Prof SUNY Stony Brook; **SI:** Geriatrics; Cardiology; **HMO:** Empire Oxford Vytra Blue Cross & Blue Shield PHCS +

LANG: Fr, Ger; ♿ 🗓 🏥 💲 Mcr Mcd WC NFI
Immediately

Lehrfeld, Jerome (MD)   FP   PCP
N Shore Univ Hosp-Plainview
797 Merrick Ave; East Meadow, NY 11554; (516) 539-0300; **BDCERT:** FP 77; **MS:** SUNY Downstate 58; **RES:** FP, Hunterdon Med Ctr, Flemington, NJ 61-62; **SI:** Alcoholism; Adolescents; **HMO:** US Hlthcre Empire Blue Cross & Shield GHI Vytra CIGNA +

LANG: Vn; ♿ 🗓 🕐 🗓 🏥 💲 Mcr Mcd WC NFI
A Few Days ▦ **VISA** ●

Moynihan, Brian (DO)   FP   PCP
Massapequa Gen Hosp
East Meadow Family Practice Associates, 611 Newbridge Rd; East Meadow, NY 11554; (516) 781-1141; **BDCERT:** FP 85; **MS:** NY Coll Osteo Med 83; **RES:** Massapequa Gen Hosp, Seaford, NY 83-84; Kennedy Mem Hosp, Stratford, NJ 84-85; **FAP:** Adjct Prof NY Coll Osteo Med; **HOSP:** Winthrop Univ Hosp; **SI:** Skin Surgery; Cardiovascular Medicine; **HMO:** Oxford Multiplan Magnacare GHI Vytra +

🗓 🕐 🗓 🏥 💲 Mcr WC NFI   Immediately ▦
VISA ●

Sklar, Barrett (MD)   FP   PCP
Winthrop Univ Hosp
Family Medicine Specialists, 404 Jerusalem Ave; Hicksville, NY 11801; (516) 931-4285; **BDCERT:** FP 97; **MS:** Loyola U-Stritch Sch Med, Maywood 59; **RES:** Meadowbrook Hosp, East Meadow, NY 60; **FAP:** Asst Prof FP SUNY Stony Brook

♿ 🗓 🕐 🗓 🏥 💲 Mcr WC NFI   A Few Days **VISA** ●

Soskel, Neil (DO)   FP   PCP
South Nassau Comm Hosp
185 Merrick Rd; Lynbrook, NY 11563; (516) 887-0077; **BDCERT:** FP 95; **MS:** NY Coll Osteo Med 86; **RES:** FP, Community Hosp, Glen Cove, NY 87-89; **HMO:** Most

♿ 🗓 🕐 🗓 🏥 💲 Mcr   A Few Days

Turtel, Allen (MD)   FP   PCP
N Shore Univ Hosp-Plainview
1181 Old Country Rd 3; Melville, NY 11803; (516) 931-2320; **BDCERT:** FP 95; **MS:** Holland 56; **RES:** IM, Brookdale Univ Hosp Med Ctr, Brooklyn, NY 56-58; IM, Flower Fifth Ave Hosp, New York, NY 58-60; **FAP:** Asst Prof FP SUNY Stony Brook; **SI:** Primary Care; **HMO:** Aetna Hlth Plan Blue Shield US Hlthcre Oxford

LANG: Dut, Itl, Sp; ♿ 🗓 🗓 🏥 💲 Mcr WC NFI

Zackson, Ephraim (MD)   FP   PCP
Winthrop Univ Hosp
26020 81st Ave; Floral Park, NY 11004; (718) 347-4583; **BDCERT:** FP 78; FP 96; **MS:** Hahnemann U 49; **RES:** Queens Hosp Ctr, Jamaica, NY; **FAP:** Asst Clin Prof FP SUNY Stony Brook
●

GASTROENTEROLOGY

Bartolomeo, Robert (MD)   Ge
Winthrop Univ Hosp
Gastroenterology Associates, 173 Mineola Blvd 202; Mineola, NY 11501; (516) 248-3737; **BDCERT:** IM 74; Ge 77; **MS:** NY Med Coll 71; **RES:** IM, Metropolitan Hosp Ctr, New York, NY 71-73; IM, Beth Israel Med Ctr, New York, NY 73-74; **FEL:** Ge, Bridgeport Hosp, Bridgeport, CT 74-76; **HOSP:** N Shore Univ Hosp-Glen Cove; **SI:** Endoscopy & Colonoscopy; Inflammatory Bowel Disease; **HMO:** Aetna-US Healthcare Empire Oxford GHI

LANG: Sp; ♿ 🕐 🗓 🗓 🏥 💲 Mcr   A Few Days ▦
VISA ●

Caccese, William (MD)   Ge
N Shore Univ Hosp-Plainview
700 Old Country Rd Ste 206; Plainview, NY
11803; (516) 681-1200; **BDCERT:** Med 81; Ge 83;
MS: SUNY Hlth Sci Ctr 78; **RES:** IM, N Shore Univ
Hosp-Manhasset, Manhasset, NY 78-81; **FEL:** Ge, N
Shore Univ Hosp-Manhasset, Manhasset, NY 81-
83; **FAP:** Asst Clin Prof NYU Sch Med; **SI:** *GI
Endoscopy; Colon Cancer Screening*; **HMO:** Oxford US
Hlthcre Empire Blue Choice
🚫 🌙 🔒 ⏰ 💲 Mcr   2-4 Weeks

Farber, Charles (MD)   Ge
N Shore Univ Hosp-Plainview
376 S Oyster Bay Rd; Hicksville, NY 11801; (516)
822-4314; **BDCERT:** IM 81; Ge 83; **MS:** SUNY Hlth
Sci Ctr 78; **RES:** N Shore Univ Hosp-Manhasset,
Manhasset, NY 78-81; **FEL:** Ge, Albert Einstein Med
Ctr, Bronx, NY; **HOSP:** Mid-Island Hosp; **SI:** *Cancer
Prevention*
🚫 🌙 🔒 👤 ⏰ 💲 Mcr   Immediately *VISA*

Goldblum, Lester (DO)   Ge
Massapequa Gen Hosp
Massapequa Gastroenterology Associates, 535
Broadway; Massapequa, NY 11758; (516) 541-
0440; **BDCERT:** IM 83; Ge 91; **MS:** NY Coll Osteo
Med 79; **RES:** IM, Nassau County Med Ctr, East
Meadow, NY 80-83; **FEL:** Ge, Nassau County Med
Ctr, East Meadow, NY 83-85; **HOSP:** Brunswick
Hosp Ctr; **SI:** *Gastrointestinal Endoscopy; Ulcer
Disease*; **HMO:** Oxford United Healthcare US Hlthcre
GHI Vytra +
🚫 🌙 🔒 ⏰ 💲 Mcr Mcd   A Few Days *VISA* ●

Goldman, Ira (MD)   Ge
N Shore Univ Hosp-Manhasset
310 E Shore Rd Ste 206; Great Neck, NY 11023;
(516) 487-7677; **BDCERT:** IM 80; Ge 83; **MS:**
Columbia P&S 77; **RES:** IM, Columbia-Presbyterian
Med Ctr, New York, NY 77-80; **FEL:** Ge, UC San
Francisco Med Ctr, San Francisco, CA 80-83; **FAP:**
Assoc Prof of Clin Med NYU Sch Med; **HOSP:** St
Francis Hosp-Roslyn; **SI:** *Endoscopy; Liver Disease*
🚫 🅂🅄 🌙 🔒 👤 ⏰ 💲 Mcr   Immediately *VISA* ●

Gould, Perry (MD)   Ge
Winthrop Univ Hosp
Gastroenterology Associates, 173 Mineola Blvd
202; Mineola, NY 11501; (516) 248-3737;
BDCERT: IM 80; Ge 83; **MS:** NY Med Coll 77; **RES:**
Long Island Jewish Med Ctr, New Hyde Park, NY
77-80; **FEL:** NY Med Coll, Valhalla, NY 80-82; **FAP:**
Asst Clin Prof SUNY Stony Brook; **SI:** *Endoscopy*;
HMO: Empire GHI Oxford Prucare
LANG: Sp; 🚫 🌙 🔒 👤 ⏰ 💲 Mcr   A Few Days *VISA*
●

Gutman, David (MD)   Ge   **PCP**
Mid-Island Hosp
4277 Hempstead Tpke 209; Bethpage, NY 11714;
(516) 731-7770; **BDCERT:** Ge 89; IM 86; **MS:**
Baylor 83; **RES:** Baylor Med Ctr, Dallas, TX 83-86;
FEL: Ge, Presbyterian Med Ctr, Philadelphia, PA 86-
88; **HOSP:** N Shore Univ Hosp-Plainview; **SI:**
Gastroesophageal Reflux; Hepatitis C; **HMO:**
Multiplan Aetna Hlth Plan Choicecare Chubb
🚫 🌙 🔒 👤 ⏰ 💲 Mcr WC   1 Week *VISA* ●

Jacob, Harold (MD)   Ge
St John's Epis Hosp-Smithtown
Southshore Gastroenterology, 657 Central Ave;
Cedarhurst, NY 11516; (516) 374-0670; **BDCERT:**
IM 80; Ger 83; **MS:** Albert Einstein Coll Med 77;
RES: Jacobi Med Ctr, Bronx, NY 77-80; **FEL:**
Montefiore Med Ctr, Bronx, NY 80-82; **HOSP:**
South Nassau Comm Hosp; **SI:** *Pancreaticobiliary
Disease; Colonic Cancer Prevention*; **HMO:** Aetna Hlth
Plan Oxford
🚫 🅂🅄 🌙 🔒 👤 ⏰ Mcr   1 Week *VISA* ●

Katz, Seymour (MD)   Ge
N Shore Univ Hosp-Manhasset
Nassau Gastroenterology Associates, PC, 1000
Northern Blvd 140; Great Neck, NY 11021; (516)
466-2340; **BDCERT:** IM 71; Ge 72; **MS:** NYU Sch
Med 64; **RES:** Albert Einstein Med Ctr, Bronx, NY
64-66; Jacobi Med Ctr, Bronx, NY 68-69; **FEL:** NY
Hosp-Cornell Med Ctr, New York, NY 69-71; Mem
Sloan Kettering Cancer Ctr, New York, NY 69-71;
HOSP: Long Island Jewish Med Ctr; **SI:** *Inflammatory
Bowel Disease; Colon Cancer*; **HMO:** Aetna Hlth Plan
PHS Oxford PHCS Multiplan +
🚫 🅂🅄 🔒 ⏰ 💲   1 Week *VISA* ●

McKinley, Matthew (MD) Ge
N Shore Univ Hosp-Manhasset
ProHealth Care Associates, 2800 Marcus Ave; Lake Success, NY 11042; (516) 662-6076; **BDCERT:** IM 78; Ge 81; **MS:** Creighton U 75; **RES:** IM, N Shore Univ Hosp-Manhasset, Manhasset, NY 75-78; Mem Sloan Kettering Cancer Ctr, New York, NY 75-78; **FEL:** Ge, Yale-New Haven Hosp, New Haven, CT; Hosp of St Raphael, New Haven, CT 78-80; *SI: Gallstones; Barrett's Esophagitis;* **HMO:** Empire Blue Cross & Shield Aetna Hlth Plan Oxford HIP Network

⟦symbols⟧ A Few Days ⟦VISA⟧

Miller, Seth (MD) Ge
Long Beach Med Ctr
2920 Hempstead Tpk; Levittown, NY 11756; (516) 735-8860; **BDCERT:** IM 83; Ge 87; **MS:** Mt Sinai Sch Med 80; **RES:** IM, Beth Israel Med Ctr, New York, NY 81-83; Ge, Beth Israel Med Ctr, New York, NY 83-85

⟦symbols⟧ Immediately

Milman, Perry (MD) Ge
Long Island Jewish Med Ctr
2001 Marcus Ave W260; Lake Success, NY 11042; (516) 775-7770; **BDCERT:** IM 76; Ge 79; **MS:** SUNY Downstate 73; **RES:** IM, Long Island Jewish Med Ctr, New Hyde Park, NY 73-76; **FEL:** Ge, VA Med Ctr-Manh, New York, NY 76-78; **FAP:** Asst Clin Prof Med Albert Einstein Coll Med; **HOSP:** Queens Hosp Ctr; *SI: Peptic Ulcer Disease; Inflammatory Bowel Disease;* **HMO:** Oxford Magnacare Blue Choice Oxford

LANG: Sp; ⟦symbols⟧ 1 Week

Pervil, Paul (MD) Ge
N Shore Univ Hosp-Plainview
Gastrointestinal Associates, 146A Manetto Hill Rd; Plainview, NY 11803; (516) 822-4314; **BDCERT:** IM 82; **MS:** Mexico 76; **RES:** Maimonides Med Ctr, Brooklyn, NY 78-80; **FEL:** Ge, Nassau County Med Ctr, East Meadow, NY 80-82; **HOSP:** Mid-Island Hosp; **HMO:** Aetna-US Healthcare Vytra Oxford Blue Cross & Blue Shield MDNY +

LANG: Sp; ⟦symbols⟧ Immediately ⟦VISA⟧

Schmelkin, Ira (MD) Ge
N Shore Univ Hosp-Manhasset
North Shore Gastroenterology Associates, 233 E Shore Rd; Great Neck, NY 11023; (516) 487-5200; **BDCERT:** IM 87; Ge 89; **MS:** SUNY Buffalo 84; **RES:** IM, Mount Sinai Med Ctr, New York, NY 85-87; **FEL:** Ge, Mount Sinai Med Ctr, New York, NY 87-89; **HOSP:** St Francis Hosp-Roslyn; *SI: Inflammatory Bowel Disease; Endoscopy Colonoscopy;* **HMO:** MDNY Oxford GHI Blue Choice Independent Health Plan +

⟦symbols⟧ Immediately

Schwartz, Gary (MD) Ge
Winthrop Univ Hosp
Gastroenterology Associates, PC, 173 Mineola Blvd 202; Mineola, NY 11501; (516) 248-3737; **BDCERT:** IM 85; Ge 87; **MS:** Mexico 79; **RES:** Winthrop Univ Hosp, Mineola, NY 81-83; **FEL:** Univ Hosp SUNY Syracuse, Syracuse, NY 83-86; **FAP:** Clin Instr SUNY Stony Brook; *SI: Colon and Rectal Cancer; Peptic Ulcer Disease;* **HMO:** Vytra Oxford Empire Prucare

LANG: Sp; ⟦symbols⟧ 1 Week ⟦VISA⟧

Soterakis, Jack (MD) Ge
St Francis Hosp-Roslyn
Gastrointestinal Associates of Long Island, PC, 139 Plandome Rd; Manhasset, NY 11030; (516) 365-4950; **BDCERT:** IM 75; Ge 77; **MS:** Italy 68; **RES:** IM, Catholic Med Ctr Bklyn & Qns, Jamaica, NY 70-72; New England Med Ctr, Boston, MA 72-73; **FEL:** Ge, U MD Hosp, Baltimore, MD 73-74; Ge, Lemuel Shattuck Hosp, Boston, MA 72-73; **HOSP:** N Shore Univ Hosp-Glen Cove; *SI: Endoscopy Therapeutic ERCP; Liver Diseases;* **HMO:** Oxford Blue Choice Aetna Hlth Plan CIGNA PHS +

LANG: Grk, Itl, Sp; ⟦symbols⟧ A Few Days ⟦VISA⟧

Talansky, Arthur (MD)   Ge
N Shore Univ Hosp-Manhasset
North Shore Gastroenterology, 233 E Shore Rd
101; Great Neck, NY 11023; (516) 487-2444;
BDCERT: IM 80; **MS:** Mt Sinai Sch Med 77; **RES:**
IM, Mem Sloan Kettering Cancer Ctr, New York,
NY 77-80; **FEL:** Ge, Mount Sinai Med Ctr, New
York, NY 80-82; **FAP:** Asst Clin Prof Med NYU Sch
Med; **HOSP:** St Francis Hosp-Roslyn; **SI:** *Crohn's
Disease; Ulcerative Colitis;* **HMO:** Oxford Vytra Blue
Choice GHI

🔲 🔲 🔲 🔲 🔲 🔲 🔲 A Few Days **VISA** 🔲

GERIATRIC MEDICINE

Guzick, Howard (MD)   Ger   **PCP**
N Shore Univ Hosp-Manhasset
Geriatric Medical Group, 865 Northern Blvd; Great
Neck, NY 11021; (516) 622-5046; **BDCERT:** IM
85; Ger 88; **MS:** Albert Einstein Coll Med 81; **RES:**
Montefiore Med Ctr, Bronx, NY 81-84; **FEL:**
Montefiore Med Ctr, Bronx, NY 84-85; **FAP:** Assoc
Prof of Clin Med NYU Sch Med; **HMO:** Most

🔲 🔲 🔲 🔲

Lanman, Geraldine (MD)   Ger
Long Island Jewish Med Ctr
2500 Marcus Ave; Lake Success, NY 11042; (516)
354-0622; **BDCERT:** IM 83; Ger 88; **MS:** U Calgary
80; **RES:** Long Island Jewish Med Ctr, New Hyde
Park, NY 82-83; Long Island Jewish Med Ctr, New
Hyde Park, NY 85-86; **FEL:** Ger, Long Island Jewish
Med Ctr, New Hyde Park, NY; **HMO:** Sanus Oxford

🔲 🔲 🔲 🔲 🔲 🔲 🔲 🔲 2-4 Weeks

Reddy, Munagala (MD)   Ger   **PCP**
Long Beach Med Ctr
180 E Penn St; Long Beach, NY 11561; (516) 431-
2277; **BDCERT:** IM 78; Ger 90; **MS:** India 70; **RES:**
Med, New York Methodist Hosp, Brooklyn, NY 74-
77; **FEL:** Pul, Albany Med Ctr, Albany, NY 77-79;
HMO: Most
LANG: Hin; 🔲 🔲 🔲 🔲 🔲 🔲 🔲 Immediately

Wolf-Klein, Gisele (MD)   Ger
Long Island Jewish Med Ctr
Parker Jewish Geriatric Institute, 96 Wildwood Rd;
New Hyde Park, NY 11040; (718) 289-2276;
BDCERT: IM 84; **MS:** Switzerland 75; **RES:** IM,
Long Island Jewish Med Ctr, New Hyde Park, NY
76-78; **FEL:** Ger, Long Island Jewish Med Ctr, New
Hyde Park, NY 78-79; **FAP:** Assoc Prof Albert
Einstein Coll Med; **SI:** *Alzheimer's Disease; Falls*

LANG: Fr, Sp, Itl; 🔲 🔲 🔲 🔲 🔲 🔲 🔲 🔲
A Few Days

GYNECOLOGIC ONCOLOGY

Gal, David (MD)   GO
N Shore Univ Hosp-Manhasset
North Shore Hospital, 300 Community Dr;
Manhasset, NY 11030; (516) 562-4438; **BDCERT:**
ObG 84; GO 92; **MS:** Israel 72; **RES:** ObG, Rambam
Medical Center, Haifa, Israel 72-75; ObG, Brookdale
Univ Hosp Med Ctr, Brooklyn, NY 75-79; **FEL:** GO,
Mem Sloan Kettering Cancer Ctr, New York, NY
78; GO, Parkland Mem Hosp, Dallas, TX 79-83;
FAP: Prof NYU Sch Med; **SI:** *Laparoscopic Radical
Surgery; Hormones & Gynecological Onc;* **HMO:**
Oxford Vytra US Hlthcre Aetna Hlth Plan
Prudential +

LANG: Itl, Hun, Heb; 🔲 🔲 🔲 🔲 🔲 🔲 🔲 🔲
A Few Days 🔲 **VISA** 🔲 🔲

Lovecchio, John (MD)   GO
N Shore Univ Hosp-Manhasset
North Shore Hosp, 300 Community Dr; Manhasset,
NY 11030; (516) 562-4438; **BDCERT:** ObG 83; GO
83; **MS:** SUNY Buffalo 75; **RES:** ObG, U Hosp of
Cleveland, Cleveland, OH 75-79; **FEL:** GO, Jackson
Mem Hosp, Miami, FL 80-82; **FAP:** Chf GO NYU
Sch Med; **HOSP:** N Shore Univ Hosp-Glen Cove; **SI:**
Ovarian Cancer; Uterine Cancer

🔲 🔲 🔲 🔲 🔲 🔲 Immediately 🔲 **VISA** 🔲

Guide to symbols and abbreviations can be found on pages 110-113.

645

Seltzer, Vicki (MD)   GO   `PCP`
Long Island Jewish Med Ctr

Long Island Jewish Med Ctr, 1554 Northern Blvd Fl
5; New Hyde Park, NY 11040; (718) 470-7660;
BDCERT: ObG 79; GO 82; MS: NYU Sch Med 73;
RES: ObG, Bellevue Hosp Ctr, New York, NY 73-77;
FEL: GO, NY Med Coll, New York, NY 77-78; GO,
Mem Sloan Kettering Cancer Ctr, New York, NY
78-79; FAP: Prof Albert Einstein Coll Med; SI:
Women's Health; HMO: Oxford US Hlthcre
🦽 🧑 $ Mcr   2-4 Weeks

Palmieri, Thomas J (MD)   HS
Long Island Jewish Med Ctr

1901 New Hyde Park Rd; New Hyde Park, NY
11040; (516) 822-4843; BDCERT: S 71; HS 89;
MS: SUNY Hlth Sci Ctr 64; RES: IM, St Luke's
Roosevelt Hosp Ctr, New York, NY 65-66; S, Long
Island Jewish Med Ctr, New Hyde Park, NY 66-70;
FEL: Columbia-Presbyterian Med Ctr, New York,
NY 70; Hosp For Joint Diseases, New York, NY 71
🦽 🌙 📷 🧑 🏠 $ Mcr Mcd WC NFl   Immediately VISA
💳

HAND SURGERY

Kamler, Kenneth (MD)   HS
Long Island Jewish Med Ctr

410 Lakeville Rd 100; New Hyde Park, NY 11042;
(516) 326-8810; MS: France 75; RES: Long Island
Jewish Med Ctr, New Hyde Park, NY 75-80; FEL:
Columbia-Presbyterian Med Ctr, New York, NY 80-
81; HOSP: Winthrop Univ Hosp; SI: Carpal Tunnel
Syndrome; Arthritis

LANG: Fr; 🦽 📷 🧑 🏠 $ Mcr WC NFl   Immediately
VISA 💳

Lane, Lewis B (MD)   HS
Long Island Jewish Med Ctr

800 Community Dr FL2; Manhasset, NY 11030;
(516) 627-8717; BDCERT: OrS 81; HS 97; MS:
Columbia P&S 74; RES: S, NY Hosp-Cornell Med
Ctr, New York, NY 74-75; OrS, Hosp For Special
Surgery, New York, NY 76-79; FEL: OrS, Hosp For
Special Surgery, New York, NY 75-76; HS, St
Luke's Roosevelt Hosp Ctr, New York, NY 78-79;
FAP: Assoc Clin Prof OrS Albert Einstein Coll Med;
HOSP: N Shore Univ Hosp-Manhasset; SI: Carpal
Tunnel Syndrome; Thumb and Wrist Problems; HMO:
Oxford Blue Choice MDLI Empire Magnacare +

🦽 🌙 📷 🧑 🏠 $ Mcr WC NFl   1 Week

HEMATOLOGY

Allen, Steven (MD)   Hem
N Shore Univ Hosp-Manhasset

Don Monti Div of Onc, Div of Hematology, 300
Community Dr; Manhasset, NY 11030; (516) 562-
8959; BDCERT: IM 80; Hem 82; MS: Johns
Hopkins U 77; RES: Med, NY Hosp-Cornell Med Ctr,
New York, NY 77-78; FEL: Onc, NY Hosp-Cornell
Med Ctr, New York, NY 78-80; Hem, NY Hosp-
Cornell Med Ctr, New York, NY 80-83; FAP: Assoc
Clin Prof Med NYU Sch Med; SI:
Lymphoma/Leukemia; Blood Clotting; HMO: Oxford
Aetna Hlth Plan Blue Choice Chubb Metlife +

🦽 📷 🧑 🏠 $ Mcr Mcd   A Few Days 📖 VISA 💳

Dittmar, Klaus (MD)   Hem
N Shore Univ Hosp-Manhasset

North Shore Hematology/Oncology, 1201
Northern Blvd; Manhasset, NY 11030; (516) 627-
1221; BDCERT: IM 69; Onc 79; MS: Germany 57;
RES: IM, Mount Sinai Med Ctr, New York, NY 62-
64; Hem, Mount Sinai Med Ctr, New York, NY 64-
65; FAP: Asst Clin Prof Med NYU Sch Med; HOSP:
St Francis Hosp-Roslyn; SI: Lymphoma & Iron
Overload; Hemachromatosis

LANG: Ger, Itl, Fr; 🦽 🌙 📷 🧑 🏠 Mcr NFl
Immediately VISA 💳

Gartenhaus, Willa (MD)   Hem
Long Island Jewish Med Ctr

Hematology & Oncology of LI, 3003 New Hyde Park Rd 401; New Hyde Park, NY 11042; (516) 354-5700; **BDCERT:** IM 77; **MS:** SUNY Syracuse 73; **RES:** Hem, Montefiore, Bronx, NY 76-77; Med, Hillside Med Ctr, 74-76; **FEL:** Onc, Mt Sinai Med Ctr, New York, NY 77-78; **FAP:** Asst Prof Med Albert Einstein Coll Med; **HMO:** Blue Choice

♿

Kessler, Leonard (MD)   Hem
South Nassau Comm Hosp

South Shore Hematology Oncology Assoc, 242 Merrick Rd Ste 301; Rockville Centre, NY 11570; (516) 536-1455; **BDCERT:** Onc 81; Hem 82; **MS:** Albert Einstein Coll Med 75; **RES:** IM, Montefiore Med Ctr, Bronx, NY 75-77; **FEL:** Hem, Montefiore Med Ctr, Bronx, NY 78-81; Onc, Mem Sloan Kettering Cancer Ctr, New York, NY 79-80; **HOSP:** Mercy Med Ctr; **SI:** Stem Cell Transplantation; **HMO:** Oxford Aetna-US Healthcare Choicecare Magnacare PHS +

LANG: Itl, Sp, Heb; ♿ 🅿 📷 🏥 💲 Mcr Mcd NFI
1 Week **VISA** ⚫

Marsh, Jonathan (MD)   Hem
N Shore Univ Hosp-Manhasset

HematologyOncology Assoc, 3003 New Hyde Park Rd; New Hyde Park, NY 11042; (516) 354-5700; **BDCERT:** Hem 92; Onc 91; **MS:** SUNY Stony Brook 86; **RES:** Med, Winthrop Univ Hosp, Mineola, NY 86-89; **FEL:** Hem Onc, N Shore Univ Hosp-Manhasset, Manhasset, NY 89-92; **FAP:** NYU Sch Med; **HOSP:** Long Island Jewish Med Ctr; **SI:** Malignancies; Blood Disorders; **HMO:** Oxford CIGNA Magnacare Multiplan

♿ 🅿 📷 🏥 💲 Mcr   A Few Days **VISA** ⚫

Vinciguerra, Vincent (MD)   Hem
N Shore Univ Hosp-Manhasset

Northshore University Hospital, 300 Community Dr; Manhasset, NY 11030; (516) 562-8954; **BDCERT:** IM 74; Onc 75; **MS:** Georgetown U 66; **RES:** IM, NY Hosp-Cornell Med Ctr, New York, NY 68-69; IM, N Shore Univ Hosp-Manhasset, Manhasset, NY 70-71; **FAP:** Prof Med NYU Sch Med; **SI:** Solid Tumors Breast/Lung; Cancer Prevention

♿ 🅿 📷 🏥 💲 Mcr Mcd   A Few Days

Wang, Jen Chin (MD)   Hem
Long Beach Med Ctr

5 E Walnut St; Long Beach, NY 11561; (516) 889-7447; **BDCERT:** IM 76; **MS:** Taiwan 69; **RES:** Hem, Brookdale Univ Hosp Med Ctr, Brooklyn, NY 74-76; Med, Brookdale Univ Hosp Med Ctr, Brooklyn, NY 72-74; **FAP:** Assoc Prof Med SUNY Downstate; **HOSP:** N Shore Univ Hosp-Forest Hills

🅿 📷 🏥 💲 Mcr Mcd WC NFI   Immediately

INFECTIOUS DISEASE

Cunha, Burke A (MD)   Inf
Winthrop Univ Hosp

Infectious Disease Assocs, Winthrop Univ Hosp; Mineola, NY 11501; (516) 663-2507; **BDCERT:** IM 77; Inf 78; **MS:** Penn State U-Hershey Med Ctr 72; **RES:** IM, Hartford Hosp, Hartford, CT 72-75; **FEL:** Inf, Hartford Hosp, Hartford, CT 75-77; **FAP:** Prof Med SUNY Stony Brook; **SI:** Fever of Unknown Origin (FUO); Chronic Fatigue Syndrome/Lyme

♿ 🏥 💲 Mcr   2-4 Weeks

Farber, Bruce (MD)   Inf
N Shore Univ Hosp-Manhasset

300 Community Dr; Manhasset, NY 11030; (516) 562-4280; **BDCERT:** Inf 84; **MS:** Northwestern U 76; **RES:** U of VA Health Sci Ctr, Charlottesville, VA 76-80; **FEL:** Mass Gen Hosp, Boston, MA 80-82

♿ 🅿 🏥 💲 Mcr Mcd   1 Week **VISA**

Gombert, Myles (MD)   Inf   **PCP**
Long Beach Med Ctr

Island Park Medical Care, 30 Wood Rd; Pt Washington, NY 11050; (516) 897-4325; **BDCERT:** IM 78; Inf 82; **MS:** NY Med Coll 75; **RES:** IM, Westchester County Med Ctr, Valhalla, NY 75-79; **FEL:** Inf, Univ Hosp SUNY Bklyn, Brooklyn, NY 79-81; **FAP:** Clin Prof SUNY Downstate; **HMO:** Blue Choice Oxford Vytra

♿ 🅿 📷 🏥 💲 Mcr WC NFI   A Few Days

Guide to symbols and abbreviations can be found on pages 110-113.

647

Hilton, Eileen (MD)   Inf
Long Island Jewish Med Ctr
444 Lakeville Rd Ste 301; New Hyde Park, NY
11042; (516) 470-6900; **BDCERT:** IM 81; Inf 84;
MS: Columbia P&S 78; **RES:** IM, Bronx Muncipal
Hosp Ctr, Bronx, NY 79-81

Kaplan, Mark (MD)   Inf
N Shore Univ Hosp-Manhasset
300 Community Dr; Manhasset, NY 11030; (516)
562-4280; **BDCERT:** IM 72; Inf 74; **MS:** Cornell U
66; **RES:** IM, Bellevue Hosp Ctr, New York, NY 67-
68; IM, Mem Sloan Kettering Cancer Ctr, New
York, NY 70-71; **FEL:** Inf, Mem Sloan Kettering
Cancer Ctr, New York, NY 71-72; **FAP:** Clin Prof
Med NY Med Coll; **SI:** *HIV-AIDS; Infectious Diseases*;
HMO: Oxford Aetna Hlth Plan HIP Network Metlife
[symbols] Immediately [symbols] *VISA* [symbols]
[symbol]

Lipsky, William M (MD)   Inf
Long Beach Med Ctr
325 W Park Ave; Long Beach, NY 11561; (516)
432-9377; **MS:** Dominican Republic 80; **RES:** IM,
Bronx Lebanon Hosp Ctr, Bronx, NY 81-83; **FEL:**
Inf, Nassau County Med Ctr, East Meadow, NY 83-
85; **FAP:** Asst Prof NY Med Coll; **HOSP:** Parkway
Hosp; **HMO:** Most
LANG: Sp, Fr, Yd; [symbols] Immediately

Tenenbaum, Marvin J (MD)   Inf
N Shore Univ Hosp-Manhasset
North Shore Infectious Diseases Consultants,PC, 44
S Bayles Ave #216; Port Washington, NY 11050;
(516) 767-7771; **BDCERT:** IM 75; Inf 80; **MS:** Med
Coll Va 71; **RES:** Med, Med Coll VA Hosp,
Richmond, VA 72-74; **FEL:** Inf, Med Coll VA Hosp,
Richmond, VA 77-79; **FAP:** Asst Prof Med NYU Sch
Med; **HOSP:** St Francis Hosp-Roslyn; **HMO:** Aetna
Hlth Plan CIGNA Oxford PHS PHCS +
[symbols] A Few Days

Weinstein, Mark (MD)   Inf   PCP
N Shore Univ Hosp-Plainview
Island Medical Group, 4277 Hempstead Tpke Ste
209; Bethpage, NY 11714; (516) 731-7770;
BDCERT: IM 78; Inf 80; **MS:** Harvard Med Sch 75;
RES: IM, U Hosp of Cleveland, Cleveland, OH 75-78;
FEL: Inf, U Hosp of Cleveland, Cleveland, OH 78-80;
HOSP: Mid-Island Hosp; **HMO:** Aetna Hlth Plan
Blue Cross Oxford United Healthcare PHS +
[symbols] 2-4 Weeks

INTERNAL MEDICINE

Altus, Jonathan (MD)   IM   PCP
South Nassau Comm Hosp
920 Atlantic Ave; Baldwin Harbor, NY 11510;
(516) 623-8700; **BDCERT:** IM 88; **MS:** SUNY
Downstate 84; **RES:** IM, Beth Israel Med Ctr, New
York, NY 84-87; **FEL:** Pul, New York University
Med Ctr, New York, NY 87-89; **HOSP:** Franklin
Hosp Med Ctr; **SI:** *Asthma; Pulmonary Rehabilitation*;
HMO: Aetna Hlth Plan Vytra Oxford Health Source
+
[symbols] Immediately

Ammazzalorso, Michael (MD)IM   PCP
Winthrop Univ Hosp
Winthrop Int Med Assocs, 222 Station Plaza North
Ste 310; Mineola, NY 11501; (516) 663-2051;
BDCERT: IM 90; Ger 94; **MS:** SUNY Downstate 87;
RES: IM, Staten Island Univ Hosp, Staten Island, NY
87-91; **FAP:** Asst Prof Med SUNY Stony Brook; **SI:**
Hypertension; Diabetes Mellitus; **HMO:** Vytra Aetna
Hlth Plan GHI Sel Pro Blue Choice +
LANG: Itl, Sp; [symbols] 4+ Weeks

Asheld, John (MD)   IM   PCP
Mercy Med Ctr
1201 George Rd; North Bellmore, NY 11710;
(516) 781-4500; **BDCERT:** IM 78; **MS:** SUNY
Buffalo 75; **RES:** Nassau County Med Ctr, East
Meadow, NY 75-78; **HOSP:** South Nassau Comm
Hosp; **SI:** *Diabetes; Cholesterol*
[symbols] A Few Days

Ausubel, Herbert (MD)   IM   **PCP**
Franklin Hosp Med Ctr
509 W Merrick Rd; Valley Stream, NY 11580;
(516) 561-8188; **BDCERT:** IM 61; **MS:** Harvard
Med Sch 54; **RES:** Bellevue Hosp Ctr, New York, NY
57-59; Mem Sloan Kettering Cancer Ctr, New York,
NY 57-59; **FEL:** Mem Sloan Kettering Cancer Ctr,
New York, NY 59-60; **HMO:** Aetna Hlth Plan
Metlife Prucare Sanus-NYLCare Blue Cross & Blue
Shield +

🆘 🅲 🔚 🔛 🎴 Mcr Mcd WC NFI   Immediately

Berger, David (MD)   IM   **PCP**
N Shore Univ Hosp-Manhasset
900 Northern Blvd 250; Great Neck, NY 11021;
(516) 482-6250; **BDCERT:** IM 89; Ge 91; **MS:** NY
Med Coll 86; **RES:** N Shore Univ Hosp-Manhasset,
Manhasset, NY 86-89; **FEL:** Ge, N Shore Univ Hosp-
Manhasset, Manhasset, NY 89; **FAP:** Asst NYU Sch
Med; **SI:** *Colitis; Ulcer Disease*; **HMO:** Oxford HIP
Network

🔚 🆘 🅲 🔚 🎴 🔛 💲 Mcr   2-4 Weeks 🔲 **VISA** 🔵
🔳

Calio, Anthony (MD)   IM   **PCP**
Winthrop Univ Hosp
222 Station Plaza North 310; Mineola, NY 11501;
(516) 663-2057; **BDCERT:** IM 86; **MS:** Mexico 81;
RES: Winthrop Univ Hosp, Mineola, NY 83-86;
HMO: PHCS Metlife Blue Cross & Blue Shield
Prucare Choicecare +

🔚 🅲 🔚 🎴 💲 Mcr   1 Week

Condon, Edward (MD)   IM   **PCP**
N Shore Univ Hosp-Forest Hills
North Shore Diabetes & Endocrine Associates, 3003
New Hyde Park Rd 201; New Hyde Park, NY
11042; (516) 328-8822; **MS:** Mexico 73; **RES:** IM,
Mount Sinai Med Ctr, New York, NY 74-76; **FEL:**
EDM, Mount Sinai Med Ctr, New York, NY 76-78;
FAP: Asst Prof NYU Sch Med; **HOSP:** Long Island
Jewish Med Ctr; **SI:** *Diabetes Comprehensive Care*;
HMO: Magnacare GHI PHS

LANG: Sp, Heb, Frs, Itl, Fr; 🔚 🆘 🅲 🔚 🎴 🔛 💲 Mcr
A Few Days 🔲 **VISA** 🔵

Corapi, Mark (MD)   IM   **PCP**
Winthrop Univ Hosp
222 Station Plaza North 310; Mineola, NY 11501;
(516) 663-2056; **BDCERT:** IM 85; **MS:** SUNY
Downstate 82; **RES:** IM, Long Island Jewish Med
Ctr, New Hyde Park, NY 83-85; **FEL:** Med, LI
Jewish-Hillside Hosp, New Hyde Pk, NY 85-86;
FAP: Assoc Prof SUNY Stony Brook; **SI:** *Primary
Care; Perioperative Medicine*; **HMO:** Vytra Oxford
Prucare Empire GHI +

🔚 🔚 🎴 🔛 💲 Mcr Mcd   1 Week

Cusumano, Stephen (MD)   IM   **PCP**
Mid-Island Hosp
26 Blue Grass Lane; Levittown, NY 11756; (516)
735-5454; **BDCERT:** IM 88; **MS:** U Hlth
Sci/Chicago Med Sch 85; **RES:** IM, Winthrop Univ
Hosp, Mineola, NY 85-86; IM, Winthrop Univ
Hosp, Mineola, NY 86-88; **HOSP:** Winthrop Univ
Hosp; **SI:** *Hypertension; Asthma*; **HMO:** Vytra Oxford
GHI Multiplan

🔚 🅲 🔚 🎴 🔛 💲 Mcr WC NFI   Immediately

Dilorenzo, Randolph (MD)   IM   **PCP**
N Shore Univ Hosp-Syosset
99 Cold Spring Rd; Syosset, NY 11791; (516) 921-
2817; **BDCERT:** IM 91; **MS:** West Indies 87; **RES:** N
Shore Univ Hosp-Forest Hills, Forest Hills, NY 88;
HOSP: Winthrop Univ Hosp; **SI:** *High Cholesterol*;
HMO: Oxford Vytra United Healthcare MDNY Sel
Pro +

🔚 🆘 🅲 🔚 🎴 🔛 💲 Mcr WC NFI   A Few Days **VISA**
🔵

Federbush, Richard (MD)   IM   **PCP**
N Shore Univ Hosp-Plainview
175 Jericho Tpke 216; Syosset, NY 11791; (516)
364-9800; **BDCERT:** IM 90; **MS:** Mexico 85; **RES:**
IM, Univ Hosp SUNY Stony Brook, Stony Brook, NY
87-89; **HOSP:** N Shore Univ Hosp-Syosset; **SI:**
Hypertension; Hypercholesterolemia; **HMO:** Metlife
Empire US Hlthcre Oxford Prucare +

LANG: Sp; 🔚 🅲 🔚 🎴 🔛 💲 Mcr WC NFI   1 Week

Feinberg, Arthur W (MD) IM PCP
N Shore Univ Hosp-Manhasset
Geriatric Medical Group, 330 Community Dr;
Manhasset, NY 11030; (516) 622-5046; **BDCERT:**
IM 53; **MS:** Columbia P&S 45; **RES:** IM, Lenox Hill
Hosp, New York, NY 45-46; IM, Maimonides Med
Ctr, Brooklyn, NY 48-51; **FAP:** Prof of Clin Med
NYU Sch Med; *SI: Peripheral Vascular Disease;
Geriatrics*

⬚ ⬚ ⬚ ⬚ ⬚ ⬚ 2-4 Weeks

Furie, Richard (MD) IM
N Shore Univ Hosp-Manhasset
North Shore University Hosp, 300 Community Dr;
Manhasset, NY 11030; (516) 562-4392; **BDCERT:**
IM 82; Rhu 84; **MS:** Cornell U 79; **RES:** IM, NY
Hosp-Cornell Med Ctr, New York, NY 79-82; **FEL:**
Rhu, Hosp For Special Surgery, New York, NY 82-
84; **FAP:** Assoc Prof NYU Sch Med; *SI: Lupus;
Rheumatoid Arthritis*; **HMO:** Aetna Hlth Plan Oxford
GHI CIGNA Metlife +

LANG: Sp; ⬚ ⬚ ⬚ ⬚ ⬚ ⬚ ⬚ ⬚ Immediately

Garbitelli, Vincent (MD) IM
Winthrop Univ Hosp
71 E Williston Ave; Williston Park, NY 11596;
(516) 294-3332; **BDCERT:** IM 80; **MS:** Loyola U-
Stritch Sch Med, Maywood 77; **RES:** Winthrop Univ
Hosp, Mineola, NY 77-80

Gelberg, Burt (MD) IM PCP
Franklin Hosp Med Ctr
401 Franklin Ave; Franklin Square, NY 11010;
(516) 326-2255; **BDCERT:** IM 75; **MS:** SUNY Hlth
Sci Ctr 72; **RES:** IM, Lenox Hill Hosp, New York, NY
73-75; **FEL:** Ge, Lenox Hill Hosp, New York, NY 75-
77; *SI: Intestinal Disorders; GI Endoscopy*; **HMO:**
Oxford GHI PHS

⬚ ⬚ ⬚ ⬚ ⬚ ⬚ ⬚ ⬚ ⬚ Immediately

Gelfand, Mathew (MD) IM PCP
Long Beach Med Ctr
718 E Park Ave; Long Beach, NY 11561; (516)
432-0203; **BDCERT:** IM 61; **MS:** Harvard Med Sch
53; **RES:** Med, NE Ctr Hosp, Boston, MA 57-58;
Med, Beth Israel Hosp, Boston, MA 56-57; **FEL:**
Med, Harvard, Boston, MA 55-56; **HMO:** Blue
Choice Oxford Vytra Aetna-US Healthcare PHS +

⬚ ⬚ ⬚ ⬚ ⬚ ⬚ ⬚ A Few Days

Gorski, Lydia E (MD) IM PCP
Mary Immaculate Hosp
Primary & Speciality Medical Care, PC, 820 Jericho
Tpke; New Hyde Park, NY 11040; (516) 352-
0430; **BDCERT:** IM 88; Ger 92; **MS:** Poland 82;
RES: IM, Catholic Med Ctr Bklyn & Qns, Jamaica,
NY 83-86; *SI: Women's Health Issues*; **HMO:** Aetna
Hlth Plan Oxford US Hlthcre Chubb Metlife +

LANG: Pol; ⬚ ⬚ ⬚ ⬚ ⬚ ⬚ ⬚ ⬚ ⬚
Immediately *VISA* ⬚ ⬚

Gottridge, Joanne (MD) IM PCP
N Shore Univ Hosp-Manhasset
North Shore University Hosp, 865 Northern Blvd
102; Great Neck, NY 11021; (516) 662-5000;
BDCERT: IM 83; **MS:** Case West Res U 80; **RES:** IM,
N Shore Univ Hosp-Manhasset, Manhasset, NY 80-
83; **FAP:** Prof Med NYU Sch Med; **HMO:** Aetna Hlth
Plan CIGNA Anthem Health Oxford Metlife +

LANG: Sp, Itl; ⬚ ⬚ ⬚ ⬚ ⬚ ⬚ ⬚ ⬚
Immediately ⬚ *VISA* ⬚

Greenblatt, Michael (MD) IM PCP
Mid-Island Hosp
Long Island Primary Medical Care, 120 Bethpage
Rd; Hicksville, NY 11801; (516) 827-4500;
BDCERT: IM 70; **MS:** SUNY Hlth Sci Ctr 63; **RES:**
IM, Mount Sinai Med Ctr, New York, NY 63-65; IM,
Case Western Reserve U Hosp, Cleveland, OH 67-
68; **FEL:** Ge, Case Western Reserve U Hosp,
Cleveland, OH; **FAP:** Asst Clin Prof Med SUNY
Stony Brook; **HOSP:** Winthrop Univ Hosp; *SI:
Gastroenterology*; **HMO:** Oxford Aetna Hlth Plan
United Healthcare Multiplan Vytra +

⬚ ⬚ ⬚ ⬚ ⬚ ⬚ ⬚ ⬚ ⬚ ⬚ Immediately *VISA*
⬚

Hershon, Kenneth (MD)   IM
N Shore Univ Hosp-Glen Cove
North Shore Diabetes Assoc, 3003 New Hyde Park
Rd 201; New Hyde Park, NY 11042; (516) 327-
0850; **BDCERT:** IM 79; EDM 81; **MS:** Albert
Einstein Coll Med 76; **RES:** IM, Mount Sinai Med
Ctr, New York, NY 77-79; **FEL:** EDM, U WA Med
Ctr, Seattle, WA 79-81; **HOSP:** Long Island Jewish
Med Ctr; **SI:** *Diabetes; Osteoporosis*

♿ ⚇ ✆ ☎ ⚐ ⚑ $ Mcr   A Few Days **VISA** ● ▧

Holden, Melvin (MD)   IM   PCP
N Shore Univ Hosp-Plainview
Island Pulmonary Internists, 453 S Oyster Bay Rd;
Plainview, NY 11803; (516) 433-2922; **BDCERT:**
IM 66; Pul 72; **MS:** SUNY Downstate 59; **RES:** IM,
Montefiore Med Ctr, Bronx, NY 61-62; VA Med Ctr-
Bronx, Bronx, NY 62-63; **FAP:** Asst Prof of Clin
Med SUNY Stony Brook; **SI:** *Emphysema; Asthma;*
HMO: Oxford United Healthcare Aetna Hlth Plan
GHI

♿ ☎ ⚐ ⚑ $ Mcr   A Few Days **VISA** ● ▧

Hotchkiss, Edward (MD)   IM   PCP
Long Island Jewish Med Ctr
158 Hempstead Ave; Lynbrook, NY 11563; (516)
593-3541; **BDCERT:** IM 72; **MS:** SUNY Hlth Sci Ctr
65; **RES:** IM, Long Island Jewish Med Ctr, New Hyde
Park, NY 68-72; **FEL:** Psyc, Univ Hosp SUNY Bklyn,
Brooklyn, NY 70-71; **HOSP:** South Nassau Comm
Hosp; **SI:** *Relationship of Feelings to Medical Illness;*
Medical Illness; **HMO:** Oxford Chubb Blue Cross &
Blue Shield

♿ ⚇ ☎ ⚐ ⚑ $ Mcr   A Few Days **VISA** ●

Klein, Irwin (MD)   IM
N Shore Univ Hosp-Manhasset
300 Community Dr; Manhasset, NY 11030; (516)
562-4329; **BDCERT:** IM 79; EDM 85; **MS:** NYU Sch
Med 73; **RES:** IM, Hosp of U Penn, Philadelphia, PA
73-75; IM, U Miami Hosp, Miami, FL 77-78; **FEL:**
EDM, U Miami Hosp, Miami, FL 78-79; **FAP:** Prof
Med NYU Sch Med; **SI:** *Thyroid Disease*

♿ ☎ ⚑ $ Mcr Mod WC   2-4 Weeks

Kryle, Lawrence S (MD)   IM   PCP
Winthrop Univ Hosp
336 I U Willets Rd; Roslyn Heights, NY 11577;
(516) 621-3415; **BDCERT:** IM 54; **MS:** NYU Sch
Med 44; **RES:** Bellevue Hosp Ctr, New York, NY 47-
49; **FEL:** New York University Med Ctr, New York,
NY; **HOSP:** N Shore Univ Hosp-Manhasset; **SI:**
Rheumatic Fever; Cardiology; **HMO:** Oxford Aetna
Hlth Plan US Hlthcre CIGNA Blue Cross & Blue
Shield +

♿ ⚇ ✆ ☎ ⚐ ⚑ $ Mcr Mod WC NFI   Immediately

Leong, Pauline (MD)   IM   PCP
N Shore Univ Hosp-Manhasset
North Shore in Manhasset/Internal Med Dept, 865
Northern Blvd 102; Great Neck, NY 11021; (516)
622-5000; **BDCERT:** IM 88; **MS:** NYU Sch Med 83;
RES: NY Hosp-Cornell Med Ctr, New York, NY 88

♿ ☎ ⚐ ⚑ $ Mcr Mod WC NFI   Immediately

Levine, Milton (MD)   IM
Franklin Hosp Med Ctr
509 W Merrick Rd; Valley Stream, NY 11580;
(516) 561-8188; **BDCERT:** IM 61; Ge 65; **MS:**
Harvard Med Sch 54; **RES:** Bellevue Hosp Ctr, New
York, NY 57-59; **FEL:** Ge, Bellevue Hosp Ctr, New
York, NY; **HOSP:** Long Island Jewish Med Ctr; **SI:**
Esophageal Diseases; **HMO:** GHI Oxford Aetna Hlth
Plan Empire Blue Cross & Shield Chubb +

☎ ⚐ ⚑ Mcr   A Few Days

Lipstein-Kresch, Esther (MD) IM
Long Island Jewish Med Ctr
Pro Health Care Associates, 2800 Marcus Ave;
Lake Success, NY 11042; (516) 622-6090;
BDCERT: IM 82; Rhu 84; **MS:** SUNY Hlth Sci Ctr
79; **RES:** IM, Long Island Jewish Med Ctr, New Hyde
Park, NY 79-82; Long Island Jewish Med Ctr, New
Hyde Park, NY 84-85; **FEL:** Rhu, Long Island
Jewish Med Ctr, New Hyde Park, NY 82-84; **FAP:**
Asst Prof Med Mt Sinai Sch Med; **HOSP:** N Shore
Univ Hosp-Glen Cove; **SI:** *Osteoporosis; Women's
Health*

LANG: Sp; ♿ ⚇ ✆ ☎ ⚐ ⚑ $ Mcr WC NFI
A Few Days

Luciano, Anthony (MD)   IM   PCP
St Francis Hosp-Roslyn
450 Plandome Rd # 101; Manhasset, NY 11030; (516) 365-5050; **BDCERT:** IM 86; **MS:** Italy 81; **RES:** La Guardia Hosp, Forest Hills, NY 81-84; **FAP:** Clin Instr Cornell U; **HOSP:** N Shore Univ Hosp-Manhasset; **SI:** *Cardiovascular Medicine; Gastroenterology; Pulmonary; Cancer Screening*
♿ 🅢🅤 📷 🏥 🎬 🅢 🆆🅲 A Few Days **VISA** ●

Mattana, Joseph (MD)   IM
Long Island Jewish Med Ctr
27005 76th Ave; New Hyde Park, NY 11040; (718) 470-7360; **BDCERT:** IM 90; Nep 94; **MS:** SUNY Hlth Sci Ctr 87; **RES:** IM, Long Island Jewish Med Ctr, New Hyde Park, NY 87-90; **FEL:** Nep, Long Island Jewish Med Ctr, New Hyde Park, NY 90-93; **FAP:** Asst Prof Med Albert Einstein Coll Med; **SI:** *Diabetic Kidney Disease; Hypertension*; **HMO:** Oxford Aetna-US Healthcare CIGNA GHI PHS +
♿ 📷 🎬 Mcr Mcd A Few Days

Meltzer, Marc (MD)   IM   PCP
N Shore Univ Hosp-Manhasset
70 Glen Cove Rd Ste 306; Roslyn Heights, NY 11577; (516) 621-7720; **BDCERT:** IM 87; **MS:** NYU Sch Med 84; **RES:** N Shore Univ Hosp-Manhasset, Manhasset, NY 84-87; Mem Sloan Kettering Cancer Ctr, New York, NY 84-87; **FAP:** Asst Clin Prof Med NYU Sch Med; **SI:** *Hypertension*; **HMO:** Magnacare Oxford Blue Choice United Healthcare Multiplan +
♿ 🅢🅤 📷 🏥 🎬 🅢 Mcr 🆆🅲 NFI A Few Days

Mensch, Alan (MD)   IM
N Shore Univ Hosp-Plainview
Island Pulmonary Internists, 453 S Oyster Bay Rd; Plainview, NY 11803; (516) 433-2922; **BDCERT:** IM 76; Pul 78; **MS:** U Hlth Sci/Chicago Med Sch 73; **RES:** Nassau County Med Ctr, East Meadow, NY; **FEL:** Pul, Nassau County Med Ctr, East Meadow, NY; **SI:** *Asthma; Emphysema*; **HMO:** United Healthcare Sel Pro GHI Oxford
♿ 📷 🏥 🎬 🅢 Mcr 🆆🅲 NFI 1 Week **VISA** ●

Mintz, Fredric (MD)   IM   PCP
N Shore Univ Hosp-Plainview
358 S Oyster Bay Rd; Hicksville, NY 11801; (516) 935-1312; **BDCERT:** IM 82; **MS:** NY Med Coll 79; **RES:** Stamford Hosp, Stamford, CT 79-82; **HOSP:** N Shore Univ Hosp-Manhasset; **HMO:** Multiplan Oxford Blue Choice PHCS Magnacare +
♿ 🅢🅤 🌙 📷 🏥 🎬 🅢 Mcr 🆆🅲 NFI A Few Days **VISA** ● ●

Pollak, Harvey (MD)   IM   PCP
N Shore Univ Hosp-Manhasset
Great Neck Med Assoc, 900 Northern Blvd 250; Great Neck, NY 11021; (516) 482-6250; **BDCERT:** IM 75; **MS:** U Hlth Sci/Chicago Med Sch 71; **RES:** NY Hosp-Cornell Med Ctr, New York, NY 71-74; **FEL:** N Shore Univ Hosp-Manhasset, Manhasset, NY 74-75; **FAP:** Sr Prof; **HMO:** Oxford
♿ 🅢🅤 📷 🎬 🅢 Mcr NFI 2-4 Weeks **VISA** ●

Prisco, Douglas L (MD)   IM
Long Island Jewish Med Ctr
Metropolitan Pulmonary, 1575 Hillside Ave 105; New Hyde Park, NY 11040; (516) 488-2880; **BDCERT:** IM 78; **MS:** Italy 74; **RES:** IM, Elmhurst Hosp Ctr, Elmhurst, NY 74-77; **FEL:** Pul,; **HOSP:** NY Hosp Med Ctr of Queens; **SI:** *Asthma; Chronic Lung Diseases*; **HMO:** Oxford Prucare CIGNA Magnacare
LANG: Itl; ♿ 🌙 📷 🏥 🎬 🅢 Mcr Mcd NFI A Few Days **VISA** ●

Rakowitz, Frederic (MD)   IM   PCP
N Shore Univ Hosp-Manhasset
295 Northern Blvd 208; Great Neck, NY 11021; (516) 482-4940; **BDCERT:** IM 81; **MS:** Albany Med Coll 78; **RES:** N Shore Univ Hosp-Manhasset, Manhasset, NY 78-81; **SI:** *Preventive Medicine; Diet/Exercise*; **HMO:** HIP Network Oxford PHCS
♿ 🅢🅤 📷 🎬 🅢 A Few Days

Rosenberg, Alan (MD) IM **PCP**
N Shore Univ Hosp-Manhasset
North Shore Cardiology and Internal Assoc, 1010
Northern Blvd 110; Great Neck, NY 11021; (516)
487-8883; **BDCERT:** IM 71; **MS:** Albert Einstein
Coll Med 62; **RES:** IM, Montefiore Med Ctr, Bronx,
NY 65-67; **FEL:** Cv, Mount Sinai Med Ctr, New
York, NY; **HOSP:** St Francis Hosp-Roslyn; **HMO:**
Aetna-US Healthcare Empire Blue Cross & Shield
Oxford MDNY

🚫 🏥 🅲 📷 🏨 Mcr WC NFI A Few Days **VISA** 💳 💳

Rubenstein, Jack (MD) IM **PCP**
N Shore Univ Hosp-Manhasset
70 Glen Cove Rd 301; Roslyn Heights, NY 11577;
(516) 621-1502; **BDCERT:** IM 79; **MS:** NY Med
Coll 76; **RES:** IM, N Shore Univ Hosp-Manhasset,
Manhasset, NY 76-79; **FEL:** Nep, N Shore Univ
Hosp-Manhasset, Manhasset, NY 79-80; Nep, New
York University Med Ctr, New York, NY 80-81;
FAP: Assoc Clin Prof NYU Sch Med; **SI:** *Difficult
Diagnosis; Kidney Stones;* **HMO:** Oxford Chubb
NSHIP

🚫 🏥 🅲 📷 🏨 Ⓢ 4+ Weeks **VISA** 💳

Rucker, Steve (MD) IM **PCP**
Long Island Jewish Med Ctr
560 Northern Blvd 206; Great Neck, NY 11021;
(516) 482-8880; **BDCERT:** IM 86; Nep 88; **MS:**
Univ Pittsburgh 83; **RES:** IM, Long Island Jewish
Med Ctr, New Hyde Park, NY 84-86; **FEL:** Nep,
Mount Sinai Med Ctr, New York, NY; **HOSP:** St
Francis Hosp-Roslyn; **SI:** *High Blood Pressure;
Diabetes;* **HMO:** Oxford Blue Choice GHI Vytra
CIGNA +

🚫 🅲 📷 🎖 🏨 Ⓢ Mcr Mcd WC NFI Immediately

Scheer, Max (MD) IM **PCP**
N Shore Univ Hosp-Manhasset
Woodmere Medical Associates PC, 15 Irving Pl;
Woodmere, NY 11598; (516) 374-6750; **BDCERT:**
IM 79; Inf 82; **MS:** SUNY Downstate 75; **RES:** FP,
Univ Hosp SUNY Bklyn, Brooklyn, NY 78; IM, Univ
Hosp SUNY Bklyn, Brooklyn, NY 79; **FEL:** Inf,
Mount Sinai Med Ctr, New York, NY 81; **FAP:** Asst
Clin Prof Med NYU Sch Med; **HMO:** None

🚫 🏥 📷 🎖 🏨 Ⓢ Mcr 1 Week 💳 **VISA** 💳

Schulman, Nathan (MD) IM
Long Island Jewish Med Ctr
Long Island Medical and Gastroenterology, 192 E
Shore Rd; Great Neck, NY 11023; (516) 487-
4500; **BDCERT:** IM 83; **MS:** Univ Ky Coll Med 80;
RES: IM, Long Island Jewish Med Ctr, New Hyde
Park, NY 81-83; **FEL:** Ge, Long Island Jewish Med
Ctr, New Hyde Park, NY; **FAP:** Clin Instr NYU Sch
Med

Schwechter, Leon (DO) IM **PCP**
Winthrop Univ Hosp
80 E Jericho Tpke; Mineola, NY 11501; (516) 294-
9220; **BDCERT:** IM 83; Ger 88; **MS:** Univ Hlth Sci
Coll -Osteo Med 78; **RES:** IM, Winthrop Univ Hosp,
Mineola, NY 79-82; **HOSP:** St Francis Hosp-Roslyn;
SI: *Preventive Medicine;* **HMO:** Oxford

🚫 🅲 📷 🎖 🏨 Mcr A Few Days **VISA** 💳

Sood, Harish (MD) IM **PCP**
Long Beach Med Ctr
Island Int Med, 680 Merrick Rd; Baldwin, NY
11510; (516) 378-2070; **BDCERT:** IM 75; **MS:**
India 67; **RES:** Cumberland Med Ctr, Brooklyn, NY
70-71; Queens Hosp Ctr, Jamaica, NY 71-73;
HOSP: South Nassau Comm Hosp

🚫 🏥 🅲 📷 Ⓢ Mcr WC Immediately

Taubman, Lowell (MD) IM **PCP**
Long Beach Med Ctr
206 Riverside Blvd; Long Beach, NY 11561; (516)
432-5670; **BDCERT:** IM 88; **MS:** Mexico 80; **RES:**
Beekman Downtown Hosp, New York, NY 81-82;
Montefiore U Hosp, Pittsburgh, PA 82-83; **FEL:** St
Clares Hosp, New York, NY 83-84; **FAP:** Adjct Clin
Instr NY Coll Osteo Med; **SI:** *Geriatrics; Dementia;*
HMO: GHI Blue Choice Empire

🚫 Immediately

Toffler, Allan (MD)　　　IM
N Shore Univ Hosp-Glen Cove
10 Medical Plaza Ste 204; Glen Cove, NY 11542;
(516) 671-6666; **BDCERT:** IM 63; **MS:** SUNY Hlth
Sci Ctr 55; **RES:** IM, Montefiore Med Ctr, Bronx, NY
55-57; IM, Montefiore Med Ctr, Bronx, NY 59-60;
FEL: Ge, Yale-New Haven Hosp, New Haven, CT
60-62; *SI: Ulcers; Colitis;* **HMO:** MDNY HIP
Network

🚻 📷 👤 📺 💲 Mcr Mcd WC NFI　Immediately

Walerstein, Steven J (MD)　　IM　　PCP
Long Island Jewish Med Ctr
LIJ Medical Associates, 410 Lakeville Rd #105;
New Hyde Park, NY 11042; (516) 437-9184;
BDCERT: IM 82; **MS:** Albany Med Coll 79; **RES:** IM,
Geo Wash U Med Ctr, Washington, DC 79-82; **FAP:**
Assoc Chrmn Albert Einstein Coll Med; **HMO:**
Oxford GHI US Hlthcre Blue Choice

LANG: Rus, Sp, Heb; 🚻 📷 👤 📺 💲 Mcr Mcd　1 Week
VISA 💳

Wolff, Edward (MD)　　　IM　　PCP
St Francis Hosp-Roslyn
75 S Middle Neck Rd; Great Neck, NY 11021; (516)
829-6662; **BDCERT:** IM 72; **MS:** Georgetown U 66;
RES: NY Med Coll, Valhalla, NY 67-71; **FEL:** Pul,
NY Med Coll, New York, NY 70-71; **FAP:** Clin Instr
Cornell U; *SI: Asthma; Arteriosclerotic Heart Disease;*
HMO: Oxford Health Source PHS 1199 PHS +

LANG: Sp; 🚻 SA/SD 📷 👤 📺 💲 Mcr WC NFI
Immediately

MATERNAL & FETAL MEDICINE

Klein, Victor (MD)　　　MF　　PCP
N Shore Univ Hosp-Manhasset
Great Neck Obstetrics and Gynecology, 900
Northern Blvd 220; Great Neck, NY 11021; (516)
466-0778; **BDCERT:** ObG 97; **MF** 97; **MS:** SUNY
Downstate 80; **RES:** IM, Univ Hosp SUNY Bklyn,
Brooklyn, NY 80-81; ObG, Johns Hopkins Hosp,
Baltimore, MD 81-85; **FEL:** MG, U Texas SW Med
Ctr, Dallas, TX 85-88; MF, U Texas SW Med Ctr,
Dallas, TX 85-88; *SI: High Risk Pregnancies; Multiple
Births;* **HMO:** Oxford PHS Aetna Hlth Plan US
Hlthcre HIP Network +

LANG: Grk, Sp; 🚻 🌙 📷 👤 📺 💲 Mcr　1 Week

MEDICAL GENETICS

Angulo, Moris (MD)　　　MG
Winthrop Univ Hosp
Winthrop Univ Hosp, 120 Mineola Blvd 210;
Mineola, NY 11501; (516) 663-3069; **BDCERT:**
MG 84; PEn 86; **MS:** El Salvador 76; **RES:** Ped A&I,
Nassau County Med Ctr, East Meadow, NY 77-79;
FEL: MG, Nassau County Med Ctr, East Meadow,
NY 79-84; *SI: Endocrinology;* **HMO:** Aetna Hlth
Plan Blue Choice Blue Cross & Blue Shield

LANG: Sp; 🚻 📷 📺 💲 Mcr Mcd　Immediately ***VISA***
💳

Bialer, Martin G (MD)　　　MG
Huntington Hosp
North Shore U Hosp,Division of Child Development
& Human Genetics, 300 Comm Dr Peds Dpt;
Manhasset, NY 11030; (516) 365-3996; **BDCERT:**
Ped 87; 90; **MS:** Med U SC, Charleston 80; **RES:**
Ped, N Shore Univ Hosp-Manhasset, Manhasset,
NY 83-86; **FEL:** MG, U of VA Health Sci Ctr,
Charlottesville, VA 86-89; **FAP:** Asst Prof Ped
Cornell U; **HOSP:** N Shore Univ Hosp-Manhasset;
SI: Neurofibromatosis; Marfan's Syndrome

🚻 📷 👤 📺 💲 Mcr Mcd　A Few Days 📇 ***VISA*** 💳

Fox, Joyce (MD)   MG
Long Island Jewish Med Ctr
269-01 76th Ave CH009; New Hyde Park, NY
11040; (718) 470-3010; **BDCERT:** Ped 86; MG 87;
MS: Columbia P&S 80; **RES:** Ped, Case Western
Reserve U Hosp, Cleveland, OH 80-83; **FEL:** MG,
Yale-New Haven Hosp, New Haven, CT 83-86;
FAP: Assoc Prof Albert Einstein Coll Med; **HMO:**
Blue Choice Empire Blue Cross & Shield GHI PHS
Oxford +

🔲 🔲 🔲 🔲 🔲 🔲 2-4 Weeks 🔲 *VISA* 🔲 🔲

MEDICAL ONCOLOGY

Citron, Marc L (MD)   Onc
Long Island Jewish Med Ctr
LI Jewish Med Ctr Sect Med Onco, LI Jewish Med Ctr
Med Onc; New Hyde Park, NY 11042; (516) 622-
6150; **BDCERT:** IM 77; Onc 79; **MS:** Wayne State U
Sch Med 74; **RES:** Med, Georgetown U Hosp,
Washington, DC 77; Georgetown U Hosp,
Washington, DC 75-77; **FEL:** Onc, Georgetown U
Hosp, Washington, DC 77-79; **FAP:** Assoc Prof Med
Albert Einstein Coll Med

🔲 🔲 🔲 🔲 🔲 A Few Days 🔲 *VISA* 🔲 🔲

Kappel, Bruce (MD)   Onc
N Shore Univ Hosp-Plainview
Medical Oncology Associates of Long Island, 175
Jericho Tpke Ste 302; Syosset, NY 11791; (516)
921-5533; **BDCERT:** Onc 88; Hem 89; **MS:** Emory
U Sch Med 82; **RES:** Emory U Hosp, Atlanta, GA 82-
85; **FEL:** Hem Onc, Columbia-Presbyterian Med Ctr,
New York, NY 85-88; **HOSP:** Mid-Island Hosp;
HMO: Oxford Prucare CIGNA Most

LANG: Sp; 🔲 🔲 🔲 🔲 🔲 🔲 🔲 A Few Days

Marino, John (MD)   Onc
N Shore Univ Hosp-Manhasset
44 S Bayles Ave 218; Port Washington, NY 11050;
(516) 883-0122; **BDCERT:** IM 82; Onc 84; **MS:** NY
Med Coll 79; **RES:** IM, N Shore Univ Hosp-
Manhasset, Manhasset, NY; IM, Mem Sloan
Kettering Cancer Ctr, New York, NY 79-82; **FEL:**
Onc, Jacobi Med Ctr, Bronx, NY 82-83; Onc, N
Shore Univ Hosp-Manhasset, Manhasset, NY 83;
FAP: Assoc NYU Sch Med; **HOSP:** St Francis Hosp-
Roslyn; **HMO:** Oxford Guardian PHS MDNY

LANG: Sp; 🔲 🔲 🔲 🔲 🔲 🔲 1 Week

Phillips, Reed (MD)   Onc
N Shore Univ Hosp-Glen Cove
338 Glen Head Rd; Glen Head, NY 11545; (516)
671-8995; **BDCERT:** IM 76; Onc 79; **MS:** SUNY
Hlth Sci Ctr 73; **RES:** Long Island Jewish Med Ctr,
New Hyde Park, NY 73-76; **FEL:** Onc, Columbia-
Presbyterian Med Ctr, New York, NY; **HMO:** Aetna
Hlth Plan Choicecare CIGNA PHS Oxford +

🔲 🔲 🔲 🔲 🔲 🔲 1 Week

Pipala, Joseph (MD)   Onc
N Shore Univ Hosp-Glen Cove
3 School St Ste 204; Glen Head, NY 11542; (516)
674-2413; **BDCERT:** Onc 85; Ger 92; **MS:**
Georgetown U 80; **RES:** IM, N Shore Univ Hosp-
Manhasset, Manhasset, NY 80-83; **FEL:** Montefiore
Med Ctr, Bronx, NY 83-84; Hem Onc, Beth Israel
Med Ctr, New York, NY 84-85; **FAP:** Clin Instr NYU
Sch Med; **HOSP:** N Shore Univ Hosp-Manhasset;
HMO: Oxford Vytra Magnacare GHI Aetna-US
Healthcare +

🔲 🔲 🔲 🔲 🔲 🔲 🔲 A Few Days

Schwartz, Paula R (MD)   Onc
Long Island Coll Hosp
HemOnc Assoc LI, 3003 New Hyde Park Rd Ste
401; New Hyde Park, NY 11042; (516) 354-5700;
BDCERT: IM 86; Onc 91; **MS:** SUNY Downstate 80;
RES: IM, Long Island Jewish Med Ctr, New Hyde
Park, NY 80-81; IM, Long Island Jewish Med Ctr,
New Hyde Park, NY 81-83; **FEL:** Hem, Mount Sinai
Med Ctr, New York, NY 83-85; Hem, N Shore Univ
Hosp-Manhasset, Manhasset, NY 87-89; *SI: Breast
Cancer; Lymphoma*; **HMO:** Oxford CIGNA
Magnacare Multiplan

🔲 🔲 🔲 🔲 🔲 *VISA* 🔲

Stein, Alvin (MD)   Onc
Brunswick Hosp Ctr
4271 Hempstead Tpke; Bethpage, NY 11714;
(516) 796-1500; **BDCERT:** IM 71; Onc 75; **MS:**
Albert Einstein Coll Med 61; **RES:** Bellevue Hosp Ctr,
New York, NY 61-64; **FEL:** New York University
Med Ctr, New York, NY 64-65; Baltimore Cancer
Res Ctr, Baltimore, MD 65-67; **HOSP:** Mid-Island
Hosp

Tomao, Frank (MD)   Onc
N Shore Univ Hosp-Manhasset
44 S Bayles Ave 218; Port Washington, NY 11050;
(516) 883-0122; **BDCERT:** IM 74; Onc 75; **MS:**
Cornell U 65; **RES:** Onc, Mem Sloan Kettering
Cancer Ctr, New York, NY 66-67; Onc, Bellevue
Hosp Ctr, New York, NY 67-68; **FEL:** Onc, Mem
Sloan Kettering Cancer Ctr, New York, NY 68-69;
HOSP: St Francis Hosp-Roslyn; **SI:** *Chemotherapy*;
HMO: Oxford Empire PHS MDNY
⬛ 🔲 🏠 🕮 🏥 1 Week

Weiselberg, Lora (MD)   Onc
N Shore Univ Hosp-Manhasset
300 Community Dr; Manhasset, NY 11030; (516)
562-8963; **BDCERT:** Onc 81; Hem 82; **MS:** NY
Med Coll 75; **RES:** IM, Stamford Hosp, Stamford, CT
75-78; **FEL:** Hem, N Shore Univ Hosp-Manhasset,
Manhasset, NY 78; N Shore Univ Hosp-Manhasset,
Manhasset, NY 80; **FAP:** Adjct Prof Med NYU Sch
Med; **SI:** *Breast Cancer; Cancer Prevention*; **HMO:**
Oxford United Healthcare PHCS Blue Choice Vytra
+
⬛ 🔲 🏠 🅂 🕮 🏥 A Few Days ▨ **VISA** ⬤ ▨

Weiss, Rita (MD)   Onc
N Shore Univ Hosp-Manhasset
833 Northern Blvd Ste . 140; Great Neck, NY
11021; (516) 482-0080; **BDCERT:** IM 84; **MS:**
Mexico 77; **RES:** IM, Winthrop Univ Hosp, Mineola,
NY 77-80; **FEL:** Neoplastic Disease, Mount Sinai
Med Ctr, New York, NY 80-82; **HOSP:** St Francis
Hosp-Roslyn; **HMO:** Oxford PHS MDNY HIP
Network
⬛ 🔲 🏠 🅂 🕮 Immediately **VISA** ⬤

NEONATAL-PERINATAL MEDICINE

Davis, Jonathan (MD)   NP
Winthrop Univ Hosp
Winthrop U Hosp Neonatology/Newborn, 259 1st
St; Mineola, NY 11501; (516) 663-3853; **BDCERT:**
Ped 85; NP 87; **MS:** McGill U 81; **RES:** Ped,
Children's Hosp, Boston, MA 81-84; **FEL:** NP,
Children's Hosp of Philadelphia, Philadelphia, PA
84-86; **FAP:** Assoc Prof Ped SUNY Stony Brook; **SI:**
Premature Infants; Lung Problems; **HMO:** Oxford
Vytra US Hlthcre CIGNA Prucare +

Harper, Rita (MD)   NP
N Shore Univ Hosp-Manhasset
300 Community Dr; Manhasset, NY 11030; (516)
562-4665; **BDCERT:** Ped 68; **MS:** UMDNJ-NJ Med
Sch, Newark 62; **RES:** Ped, Univ Hosp SUNY Bklyn,
Brooklyn, NY 63-66; **FAP:** Prof Ped NYU Sch Med;
HMO: JJ Newman Magnacare Oxford PHCS Aetna
Hlth Plan +

LANG: Fr; ⬛ 🔲 🄲 🏠 🅿 🕮 🏥 Immediately ▨
VISA ⬤ ▨

Steele, Andrew M (MD)   NP
Long Island Jewish Med Ctr
Schneider Children's Hospital, 269-01 76th Ave;
New Hyde Park, NY 11040; (718) 470-3440;
BDCERT: Ped 81; NP 81; **MS:** SUNY Hlth Sci Ctr
76; **RES:** Ped, Long Island Jewish Med Ctr, New
Hyde Park, NY 75-78; **FEL:** NP, Long Island Jewish
Med Ctr, New Hyde Park, NY 78-80; **FAP:** Assoc
Prof Albert Einstein Coll Med; **SI:** *Infant Lung
Disorders; Infant Apnea*; **HMO:** Oxford United
Healthcare Metlife 1199 Aetna Hlth Plan +
⬛ 🏠 🕮 🅂 🏥 Immediately

NEPHROLOGY

Bellucci, Alessandro (MD)   Nep
N Shore Univ Hosp-Manhasset
100 Community Dr; Great Neck, NY 11021; (516) 465-8200; **BDCERT:** IM 79; Nep 82; **MS:** Italy 75; **RES:** IM, Cabrini Med Ctr, New York, NY 76-79; **FEL:** Nep, N Shore Univ Hosp-Manhasset, Manhasset, NY 79-82; **FAP:** Assoc Prof NYU Sch Med; **HMO:** Oxford Blue Cross Aetna Hlth Plan

LANG: Itl; 🦽 🔲 🔂 📶 💲 Mcr Mcd WC   A Few Days
▨ **VISA** 💳 🔳

Bourla, Steven (MD)   Nep
N Shore Univ Hosp-Plainview
Island Medical Group, 789 Old Country Rd; Plainview, NY 11803; (516) 433-3600; **BDCERT:** IM 79; Nep 82; **MS:** NY Med Coll 75; **RES:** IM, Long Island Jewish Med Ctr, New Hyde Park, NY 76-78; **FEL:** Nep, New York University Med Ctr, New York, NY 79-81; **HMO:** Oxford Blue Choice Magnacare

🦽 🔲 🔂 📶 💲 Mcr   Immediately **VISA** 💳

Brennan, Lawrence (MD)   Nep
Mid-Island Hosp
South Shore Renal Physicians PC, 267 W Merrick Rd; Freeport, NY 11520; (516) 379-5000; **BDCERT:** Nep 72; IM 72; **MS:** Univ Penn 65; **RES:** IM, St Luke's Roosevelt Hosp Ctr, New York, NY 65-66; **FEL:** Nep, NY Hosp-Cornell Med Ctr, New York, NY 70-72; **HOSP:** Huntington Hosp; **SI:** *Chronic Renal Failure; Hypertension;* **HMO:** Aetna Hlth Plan Chubb CIGNA Empire Blue Cross Oxford +

LANG: Fr; 🦽 🔳 🔂 📶 Mcr Mcd NFl   A Few Days

Kerpen, Howard Owen (MD) Nep
Long Island Jewish Med Ctr
New Hyde Park Intenal Medicine Specilists, PC, 1575 Hillside Ave 102; New Hyde Park, NY 11040; (516) 775-4114; **BDCERT:** IM 75; Nep 78; **MS:** Hahnemann U 72; **RES:** IM, Long Island Jewish Med Ctr, New Hyde Park, NY 77-78; Long Island Jewish Med Ctr, New Hyde Park, NY 73-75; **FEL:** N, Bellevue Hosp Ctr, New York, NY 75-77; **FAP:** Asst Prof Med Albert Einstein Coll Med; **HOSP:** Winthrop Univ Hosp; **SI:** *Hypertension; Autoimmune Renal Disease;* **HMO:** Oxford PHS PHCS Magnacare Blue Shield +

🦽 🔂 🔲 🔂 📶 💲 Mcr NFl   1 Week

Mossey, Robert (MD)   Nep
N Shore Univ Hosp-Manhasset
North Shore University Hosp, 300 Community Dr; Manhasset, NY 11030; (516) 465-8200; **BDCERT:** IM 74; Nep 78; **MS:** St Louis U 69; **RES:** N Shore Univ Hosp-Manhasset, Manhasset, NY 70-74; **FEL:** N Shore Univ Hosp-Manhasset, Manhasset, NY 74-76; **FAP:** Assoc Prof of Clin Med NYU Sch Med; **SI:** *Dialysis; High Blood Pressure*

🦽 🔂 🔲 📶 💲 Mcr Mcd   A Few Days ▨ **VISA** 💳 🔳

Thies, Harold (MD)   Nep
Long Island Jewish Med Ctr
2800 Marcus Ave; New Hyde Park, NY 11042; (516) 622-6000; **BDCERT:** IM 80; Nep 84; **MS:** Univ Mo-Columbia Sch Med 77; **RES:** Long Island Jewish Med Ctr, New Hyde Park, NY 77-78; Long Island Jewish Med Ctr, New Hyde Park, NY 78-81; **FEL:** Mount Sinai Med Ctr, New York, NY 81-83; **HMO:** Blue Choice Oxford Magnacare GHI +

🦽 🔂 🔲 📶 💲 Mcr Mcd

Wagner, John (MD)   Nep
Long Island Jewish Med Ctr
270-05 76th Ave # 228; New Hyde Park, NY 11040; (516) 470-7360; **BDCERT:** IM 81; Nep 84; **MS:** Yale U Sch Med 78; **RES:** IM, Bellevue Hosp Ctr, New York, NY 78-82; **FEL:** Nep, Bellevue Hosp Ctr, New York, NY 82-84; **FAP:** Assoc Clin Prof Albert Einstein Coll Med; **SI:** *Dialysis; Diabetic Kidney Diseases;* **HMO:** Oxford US Hlthcre Blue Choice GHI

🦽 🔂 🔲 📶 💲 Mcr   1 Week 💳

NEUROLOGICAL SURGERY

Carras, Robert (MD)   NS
N Shore Univ Hosp-Manhasset
Long Island Neurosurgical Associates PC, 410 Lakeville Rd 204; New Hyde Park, NY 11042; (516) 354-3401; **BDCERT:** NS 67; **MS:** SUNY Hlth Sci Ctr 55; **RES:** Albert Einstein Med Ctr, Bronx, NY 59-63; **HOSP:** Long Island Jewish Med Ctr; *SI: Brain Tumors; Spinal Procedures;* **HMO:** Choicecare CIGNA Aetna Hlth Plan Magnacare PHS +

🦽 ☎ 🛏 $ Mcr WC NFI   1 Week

Decker, Robert (MD)   NS
Long Island Jewish Med Ctr
Long Island Neurosurgical Associates, PC, 410 Lakeville Rd 100; New Hyde Park, NY 11042; (516) 354-3401; **BDCERT:** NS 71; **MS:** Temple U 63; **RES:** Mount Sinai Med Ctr, New York, NY 65-69; **FEL:** Connstar Hosp, Zurich, Switzerland; *SI: Pituitary Tumors; Stereotactic Radiosurgery;* **HMO:** Oxford PHS Aetna Hlth Plan US Hlthcre Blue Choice +

🦽 ☎ 🛏 $ Mcr WC NFI   1 Week

Dimancescu, Mihai (MD)   NS
South Nassau Comm Hosp
Neurological Surgery, PC, 88 S Bergen Pl Ll; Freeport, NY 11520; (516) 378-5750; **BDCERT:** NS 79; **MS:** France 68; **RES:** NS, Jackson Mem Hosp, Miami, FL 72-76; **HOSP:** Winthrop Univ Hosp; *SI: Cerebrovascular Surgery; Spine Surgery;* **HMO:** GHI Oxford Chubb Aetna-US Healthcare Blue Choice +

LANG: Fr; 🦽 ☎ 🛏 $ Mcr WC NFI   A Few Days

Mechanic, Alan (MD)   NS
Winthrop Univ Hosp
410 Lakeville Rd; New Hyde Park, NY 11042; (516) 354-3401; **BDCERT:** NS 92; **MS:** Emory U Sch Med 65; **RES:** S, Beth Israel Med Ctr, New York, NY 81-82; NS, Hahnemann U Hosp, Philadelphia, PA 82-87; *SI: Brain Tumors;* **HMO:** Affordable Hlth Plan Chubb Cost Care Empire Blue Choice CIGNA +

LANG: Sp; 🦽 🛏 $ Mcr Mcd WC NFI   1 Week

Overby, M Chris (MD)   NS
N Shore Univ Hosp-Manhasset
900 Northern Blvd; Great Neck, NY 11021; (516) 773-7737; **BDCERT:** NS 90; **MS:** Tufts U 79; **RES:** NS, Mount Sinai Med Ctr, New York, NY 81-86; **HOSP:** Queens Hosp Ctr; *SI: Spinal Reconstruction; Spinal Cord Tumors;* **HMO:** Oxford Vytra GHI Aetna-US Healthcare Empire Blue Choice +

🦽 ☎ 🛏 $ Mcr WC NFI   1 Week

Rosenthal, Alan (MD)   NS
Long Island Jewish Med Ctr
Long Island Neurosurgical Associates, PC, 410 Lakeville Rd 204; New Hyde Park, NY 11042; (516) 354-3401; **BDCERT:** NS 71; **MS:** Med Coll Va 62; **RES:** Peter Bent Brigham Hosp, Boston, MA 64-68; Children's Hosp, Boston, MA 64-68; **FEL:** NS, Harvard Med Sch, Cambridge, MA 67-68; **HOSP:** Winthrop Univ Hosp; *SI: Pediatric Brain Tumors; Arteriovenous Malformation;* **HMO:** Aetna Hlth Plan Empire Blue Cross & Shield Blue Choice Magnacare Multiplan +

🦽 ☎ 🛏 $ Mcr Mcd WC NFI   1 Week

Schneider, Steven Jack (MD)   NS
Long Island Jewish Med Ctr
410 Lakeville Rd Ste 204; New Hyde Park, NY 11042; (516) 354-3401; **BDCERT:** NS 92; **MS:** Baylor 82; **RES:** NS, Baylor Coll Med, Houston, TX 83-88; **FEL:** Ped NS, New York University Med Ctr, New York, NY 88-89; **FAP:** Asst Clin Instr NS Cornell U; **HOSP:** N Shore Univ Hosp-Manhasset; *SI: Pediatric Brain Tumors; Pediatric Spinal Cord Tumors;* **HMO:** Oxford Aetna-US Healthcare CIGNA Health Source Blue Choice +

LANG: Sp; 🦽 ☎ 🛏 $ Mcr Mcd WC NFI   1 Week

NEUROLOGY

Biddle, David (MD) N
Long Island Jewish Med Ctr
3003 New Hyde Park Rd; New Hyde Park, NY 11042; (516) 326-0669; **BDCERT:** N 79; **MS:** Jefferson Med Coll 70; **RES:** Long Island Jewish Med Ctr, New Hyde Park, NY 74-77; **HOSP:** N Shore Univ Hosp-Plainview; **SI:** *Spine; Myasthenia Gravis*; **HMO:** Oxford US Hlthcre Magnacare PHS

[⟊] [€] [🔒] [🏠] [§] [Mcr] [WC] [NFI] Immediately [▨] **VISA** [●]

Haimovic, Itzhak (MD) N
N Shore Univ Hosp-Manhasset
East Shore Neurological Associates LLP, 333 E Shore Rd 204; Manhasset, NY 11030; (516) 487-4464; **BDCERT:** N 81; **MS:** NY Med Coll 75; **RES:** N, N Shore Univ Hosp-Manhasset, Manhasset, NY 75-77; N, NY Hosp-Cornell Med Ctr, New York, NY 77-80; **FEL:** EEG & Epilepsy, Columbia-Presbyterian Med Ctr, New York, NY 80-81; **HOSP:** Long Island Jewish Med Ctr; **SI:** *Seizure Disorders; Headaches*; **HMO:** Oxford Vytra Multiplan Chubb Blue Choice +

[⟊] [SA/SU] [€] [🔒] [🏠] [§] [Mcr] [WC] [NFI] A Few Days **VISA** [●]

Hainline, Brian (MD) N
N Shore Univ Hosp-Manhasset
ProHealth Care Assocs, 2800 Marcus Ave; Lakee Success, NY 11042; (516) 622-6088; **BDCERT:** N 87; **MS:** U Chicago-Pritzker Sch Med 82; **RES:** N, NY Hosp-Cornell Med Ctr, New York, NY 83-86; **FAP:** Adjct Clin Prof NYU Sch Med; **SI:** *Chronic Pain; Headache*; **HMO:** Oxford US Hlthcre Blue Cross & Blue Shield CIGNA United Healthcare +

[⟊] [🔒] [👥] [🏠] [§] [Mcr] [WC] [NFI] A Few Days [▨] **VISA** [●]

Halperin, John (MD) N
N Shore Univ Hosp-Manhasset
300 Community Dr; Manhasset, NY 11030; (516) 562-4300; **BDCERT:** N 82; IM 78; **MS:** Harvard Med Sch 75; **RES:** IM, U Chicago Hosp, Chicago, IL 75-77; N, Mass Gen Hosp, Boston, MA 77-80; **FEL:** Neuromuscular Disease, Mass Gen Hosp, Boston, MA 80-82; **FAP:** Prof N NYU Sch Med; **SI:** *Neuromuscular Disease; Lyme Disease*; **HMO:** Aetna Hlth Plan HealthNet Oxford Multiplan PHS +

[⟊] [🔒] [🏠] [§] [Mcr] 2-4 Weeks [▨] **VISA**

Hollis, Peter (MD) N
N Shore Univ Hosp-Manhasset
900 Northern Blvd Ste 150; Great Neck, NY 11021; (516) 773-7737; **BDCERT:** N 92; **MS:** Mt Sinai Sch Med 81; **RES:** Mount Sinai Med Ctr, New York, NY; **FAP:** Asst Clin Prof NYU Sch Med; **HOSP:** NY Hosp Med Ctr of Queens; **HMO:** Chubb Aetna Hlth Plan Sanus Blue Choice Blue Cross & Blue Shield +

[⟊] [🔒] [👥] [🏠] [§] [WC] Immediately

Kelemen, John (MD) N
N Shore Univ Hosp-Plainview
824 Old Country Rd; Plainview, NY 11803; (516) 822-2230; **BDCERT:** Psyc 79; N 79; **MS:** Georgetown U 74; **RES:** Nassau County Med Ctr, East Meadow, NY 75-78; **FEL:** New England Med Ctr, Boston, MA 78-80; **FAP:** Asst Clin Prof N NYU Sch Med; **HOSP:** Mid-Island Hosp; **SI:** *Electromyography*; **HMO:** Aetna Hlth Plan Oxford US Hlthcre United Healthcare Blue Choice +

LANG: Itl, Hun; [⟊] [🔒] [👥] [🏠] [§] [Mcr] [NFI] 1 Week **VISA** [●] [▨]

Kessler, Jeffrey (MD) N
N Shore Univ Hosp-Manhasset
Neurological Associates of LI, 179 Community Dr 301; Great Neck, NY 11021; (516) 365-8086; **BDCERT:** IM 74; N 76; **MS:** Cornell U 69; **RES:** IM, NY Hosp-Cornell Med Ctr, New York, NY 69-70; Med, NY Hosp-Cornell Med Ctr, New York, NY 70-71; **FEL:** N, NY Hosp-Cornell Med Ctr, New York, NY; **HOSP:** St Francis Hosp-Roslyn; **SI:** *Parkinson's Disease; Alzheimer's Disease*; **HMO:** Blue Cross Aetna-US Healthcare Oxford Multiplan

LANG: Sp, Fr, Tag; [⟊] [🔒] [🏠] [§] [Mcr] [WC] [NFI] Immediately **VISA** [●]

Klinger, Ronald (MD)   N
Massapequa Gen Hosp

Klinger & Misra, 880 N Broadway; Massapequa,
NY 11758; (516) 541-0300; **BDCERT:** N 89; **MS:**
Bowman Gray 82; **RES:** Med, Brookdale Univ Hosp
Med Ctr, Brooklyn, NY; N, N Shore Univ Hosp-
Manhasset, Manhasset, NY; **FAP:** Clin Instr NYU
Sch Med; **HOSP:** Winthrop Univ Hosp; **SI:** *Headache
Specialist;* **HMO:** Oxford Vytra CIGNA GHI

♿ 📷 🏥 $ Mcr WC NFI   4+ Weeks

Levine, Mitchell E (MD)   N
N Shore Univ Hosp-Manhasset

900 Northern Blvd 150; Great Neck, NY 11021;
(516) 773-7737; **BDCERT:** N 87; **MS:** Mt Sinai Sch
Med 77; **RES:** S, Mount Sinai Hosp, Cleveland, OH
77-78; NS, Mount Sinai Med Ctr, New York, NY
78-83; **HOSP:** NY Hosp Med Ctr of Queens; **SI:** *Brain
Tumors; Herniated Disks Fusion;* **HMO:** Oxford GHI
Vytra United Healthcare Aetna Hlth Plan +

LANG: Sp; ♿ 📷 🚹 🏥 WC   Immediately

Levy, Lewis (MD)   N
South Nassau Comm Hosp

1705 Broadway 2A; Hewlett, NY 11557; (516)
887-3516; **BDCERT:** N 79; **MS:** SUNY Downstate
73; **RES:** N, Albert Einstein Med Ctr, Bronx, NY 74-
77; **FAP:** Asst Clin Prof N Albert Einstein Coll Med;
HOSP: Long Beach Med Ctr; **SI:** *Tourette's Syndrome;
Headache & Tourette's Syndrome;* **HMO:** Oxford Blue
Choice Multiplan Magnacare PHS +

LANG: Grk, Sp; ♿ SA/SD 📷 🚹 🏥 $ Mcr WC NFI   2-
4 Weeks **VISA** 💳

Mallin, Jeffrey (MD)   N
Long Island Jewish Med Ctr

3003 New Hyde Park Rd 200; New Hyde Park, NY
11042; (516) 488-1888; **BDCERT:** Psyc 89; **MS:**
SUNY Stony Brook 82; **RES:** Med, Long Island
Jewish Med Ctr, New Hyde Park, NY 83-84; Albert
Einstein Med Ctr, Bronx, NY 84-87; **HOSP:** N Shore
Univ Hosp-Forest Hills; **SI:** *Peripheral Nerve Injuries;
Stroke Dementia Neuropathy;* **HMO:** Oxford Vytra
Magnacare PHS GHI +

LANG: Sp, Fr, Itl; ♿ 📞 📷 🏥 $ Mcr WC NFI
A Few Days 💳 **VISA** 💳

Mauser, Donald (MD)   N
South Nassau Comm Hosp

Donald I Masuser, MD PC, 294 W Merrick Rd;
Freeport, NY 11520; (516) 868-4500; **BDCERT:** N
69; **MS:** SUNY Hlth Sci Ctr 61; **RES:** IM,
Maimonides Med Ctr, Brooklyn, NY 62-64; N,
Mount Sinai Med Ctr, New York, NY 66-67; **FEL:** N,
Nat Inst Health, Bethesda, MD 64-66; **HOSP:**
Franklin Hosp Med Ctr; **SI:** *Epilepsy; Parkinson's
Disease*

♿ 📷 🚹 🏥 $ Mcr NFI   Immediately

Newman, Stephen (MD)   N
N Shore Univ Hosp-Plainview

Island Neurological Associates, PC, 824 Old
Country Rd; Plainview, NY 11803; (516) 822-
2230; **BDCERT:** N 78; **MS:** SUNY Buffalo 72; **RES:**
N, Nassau County Med Ctr, East Meadow, NY 73-
76; **FAP:** Clin Instr NYU Sch Med; **HOSP:** Mid-
Island Hosp; **SI:** *Headaches; Seizures;* **HMO:** Oxford
US Hlthcre United Healthcare PHS Magnacare +

♿ 📷 🚹 🏥 $ Mcr WC NFI   1 Week **VISA** 💳 💳

Ragone, Philip (MD)   N
N Shore Univ Hosp-Manhasset

1010 Northern Blvd Ste 136; Great Neck, NY
11021; **BDCERT:** IM 85; N 89; **MS:** NY Med Coll
82; **RES:** IM, Lenox Hill Hosp, New York, NY 82-85;
N, Albert Einstein Med Ctr, Bronx, NY 85-88; **FEL:**
EM, Albert Einstein Med Ctr, Bronx, NY 88-89;
FAP: Clin Instr Cornell U; **HOSP:** St Francis Hosp-
Roslyn

LANG: Itl, Sp; ♿ 📷 🚹 🏥 $ Mcr WC NFI
A Few Days

Schlesinger, Irwin (MD)   N
N Shore Univ Hosp-Manhasset

East Shore Neurological Associates, 333 E Shore Rd
204; Manhasset, NY 11030; (516) 482-2919;
BDCERT: N 94; **MS:** SUNY Hlth Sci Ctr 61; **RES:**
Bellevue Hosp Ctr, New York, NY 61-63; N, Jacobi
Med Ctr, Bronx, NY 65-68; **FAP:** Assoc Clin Prof;
HOSP: Long Island Jewish Med Ctr; **SI:** *Headache;
Peripheral Neuropathy;* **HMO:** Oxford Aetna Hlth
Plan CIGNA PHS PHCS +

LANG: Rom, Heb, Sp; ♿ 📞 📷 🚹 🏥 $ Mcr WC NFI
Immediately **VISA** 💳

Turner, Ira (MD) N
N Shore Univ Hosp-Plainview
Island Neurological Associates, 824 Old Country
Rd; Plainview, NY 11803; (516) 822-2230;
BDCERT: N 78; **MS:** SUNY Downstate 72; **RES:**
Nassau County Med Ctr, East Meadow, NY 76;
HOSP: Mid-Island Hosp; **SI:** *Headache; Epilepsy;*
HMO: Aetna Hlth Plan Blue Choice Metlife Prucare
⬚ ⬚ ⬚ ⬚ ⬚ Immediately **VISA** ⬚ ⬚

NUCLEAR MEDICINE

Margouleff, Donald (MD) NuM
N Shore Univ Hosp-Manhasset
300 Community Dr; Manhasset, NY 11030; (516)
562-4400; **BDCERT:** IM 65; NuM 72; **MS:**
Switzerland 56; **RES:** IM, VA Med Ctr-Brooklyn,
Brooklyn, NY 54-59; IM, VA Med Ctr, Houston, TX
61-62; **FEL:** NuM, Long Island Jewish Med Ctr, New
Hyde Park, NY 63-64; **FAP:** Prof NYU Sch Med; **SI:**
Thyroid Disease; Thyroid Cancer; **HMO:** Aetna Hlth
Plan GHI Blue Choice US Hlthcre United Healthcare
+

LANG: Sp, Fr, Itl, Ger; ⬚ ⬚ ⬚ ⬚ ⬚ ⬚ ⬚ ⬚ ⬚
Immediately **VISA** ⬚

Zanzi, Italo (MD) NuM
N Shore Univ Hosp-Manhasset
PO Box 586; Manhasset, NY 11030; (516) 562-
4400; **BDCERT:** NuM 75; **MS:** Chile 57; **RES:**
Nassau County Med Ctr, East Meadow, NY; U Clin
Hosp, Santiago, Chile; **FEL:** Hammersmith Hosp,
London, England; **HMO:** Aetna Hlth Plan Blue
Choice Blue Cross & Blue Shield

OBSTETRICS & GYNECOLOGY

Barbaccia, Ann (MD) ObG
Mercy Med Ctr
2000 N Village Ave; Rockville Centre, NY 11570;
(516) 678-4222; **BDCERT:** ObG 80; **MS:** NY Med
Coll 72; **RES:** Hartford Hosp, Hartford, CT 72-73;
Nassau County Med Ctr, East Meadow, NY 74-78;
HOSP: Nassau County Med Ctr; **SI:** *Gynecologic
Surgery; Abnormal Uterine Bleeding*
⬚ ⬚ ⬚ ⬚ ⬚ ⬚ 2-4 Weeks **VISA** ⬚

Bednoff, Stuart (MD) ObG
N Shore Univ Hosp-Manhasset
Schwartz & Garfinkel, 560 Northern Blvd 103;
Great Neck, NY 11021; (516) 482-8741; **BDCERT:**
ObG 68; **MS:** SUNY Downstate 61; **RES:** ObG, N
Shore Univ Hosp-Manhasset, Manhasset, NY 62-
66; **HOSP:** Long Island Jewish Med Ctr; **HMO:**
Aetna Hlth Plan PHS HealthNet Sel Pro
⬚ ⬚ ⬚ ⬚ ⬚ ⬚ Immediately ⬚ **VISA** ⬚

Benjamin, Fred (MD) ObG **PCP**
Long Island Jewish Med Ctr
3003 New Hyde Park Rd Ste 301; New Hyde Park,
NY 11042; (516) 437-2500; **MS:** England 60; **RES:**
ObG, England 67-71; **FEL:** EDM, England; **FAP:** Prof
ObG Albert Einstein Coll Med; **HOSP:** Mount Sinai
Med Ctr; **SI:** *Menopause; Gynecologic Endocrinology;*
HMO: Oxford Empire Blue Choice Magnacare MDLI
+

⬚ ⬚ ⬚ ⬚ ⬚ ⬚ ⬚ ⬚ ⬚ A Few Days ⬚ **VISA**
⬚

Bernstein, Robert (MD) ObG
N Shore Univ Hosp-Manhasset
Northern Obstetrical/Gynecology, 2110 Northern
Blvd 207; Manhasset, NY 11030; (516) 365-6100;
BDCERT: ObG 97; **MS:** Mexico 79; **RES:** ObG, N
Shore Univ Hosp-Manhasset, Manhasset, NY 80-
84; **FAP:** Assoc Clin Prof NYU Sch Med; **SI:**
Abnormal Pap Smears; High Risk Pregnancy; **HMO:**
Oxford

LANG: Sp; ⬚ ⬚ ⬚ ⬚ ⬚ ⬚ 2-4 Weeks **VISA** ⬚

Bialkin, Robert (MD)   ObG   PCP
Mercy Med Ctr
2000 N Village Ave 411; Rockville Ctr, NY 11570;
(516) 764-1344; **BDCERT:** ObG 68; **MS:** Univ Penn
60; **RES:** Bellevue Hosp Ctr, New York, NY 61-66;
HOSP: Franklin Hosp Med Ctr; **HMO:** Oxford US
Hlthcre Aetna Hlth Plan CIGNA GHI +
♿ ☽ ⌂ ★ ⊞ Mcr Immediately ■ VISA 💳

Brenner, Steven (MD)   ObG
Long Island Jewish Med Ctr
LI FertilityEndocrinology Assoc, 2001 Marcus Ave
SN213; Lake Success, NY 11042; (516) 358-6363;
BDCERT: ObG 85; RE 87; **MS:** SUNY Downstate 78;
RES: ObG, Beth Israel Med Ctr, New York, NY 79-
82; **FEL:** RE, New York University Med Ctr, New
York, NY 82-84; **FAP:** Asst Clin Prof ObG Albert
Einstein Coll Med; **HOSP:** JT Mather Mem Hosp Pt
Jfrson; **SI:** *Infertility*; **HMO:** US Hlthcre Oxford
United Healthcare Prucare Vytra +
♿ ★ ⌂ $ VISA

Divack, Daniel (MD)   ObG
Long Island Jewish Med Ctr
14 Glen Cove Rd; East Hills, NY 11577; (516) 484-
4300; **BDCERT:** ObG 67; ObG 78; **MS:** Washington
U, St Louis 56; **RES:** ObG, Bronx Muncipal Hosp Ctr,
Bronx, NY 59-63; **FAP:** Asst Clin Prof Albert
Einstein Coll Med; **HMO:** Oxford Aetna-US
Healthcare Blue Choice Magnacare GHI +
♿ SI ☽ ⌂ $ Mcr 2-4 Weeks ■ VISA 💳 💳

Dottino, Joseph (MD)   ObG
Mid-Island Hosp
79 Grand Ave; Massapequa, NY 11758; (516)
798-3376; **BDCERT:** ObG 88; **MS:** Georgetown U
51; **RES:** NY Hosp-Cornell Med Ctr, New York, NY
51-52; ObG, NY Hosp-Cornell Med Ctr, New York,
NY 52-53; **HOSP:** N Shore Univ Hosp-Plainview;
HMO: Blue Choice Independent Health Plan
♿ ☽ ⌂ ★ ⊞ Mcr Immediately VISA 💳 💳

Fleischer, Adiel (MD)   ObG
Long Island Jewish Med Ctr
NY Gottlieb Women's Comprehensive Health Ctr,
1554 Northern Blvd 5th Fl; Manhasset, NY 11030;
(718) 470-7636; **BDCERT:** ObG 82; MF 84; **MS:**
Romania 72; **FEL:** Albert Einstein Med Ctr, Bronx,
NY
♿ ⌂ ⊞ $ 1 Week

Garfinkel, Burton (MD)   ObG
N Shore Univ Hosp-Manhasset
560 Northern Blvd 103; Great Neck, NY 11021;
(516) 482-8741; **BDCERT:** ObG 65; **MS:** U Hlth
Sci/Chicago Med Sch 56; **RES:** Long Island Jewish
Med Ctr, New Hyde Park, NY 60; **FAP:** Asst Prof
NYU Sch Med; **HOSP:** Long Island Jewish Med Ctr;
HMO: PHS Aetna-US Healthcare Cost Care Sel Pro
♿ ☽ ⌂ ★ ⊞ $ 1 Week

Goldstein, Irwin (MD)   ObG
Mid-Island Hosp
79 Grand Ave; Massapequa, NY 11758; (516)
798-3376; **BDCERT:** ObG 92; **MS:** NY Med Coll 86;
RES: ObG, Maimonides Med Ctr, Brooklyn, NY 87-
90; **SI:** *Pap Smears*; **HMO:** Aetna-US Healthcare
Empire Magnacare Multiplan Oxford +
LANG: Heb; ♿ ☽ ⌂ ★ ⊞ $ Mcr Immediately
VISA 💳 💳

Greco, Helen (MD)   ObG
Long Island Jewish Med Ctr
1554 Northern Blvd 5th Fl; Manhasset, NY 11030;
(516) 390-9242; **BDCERT:** ObG 92; **MS:** NY Med
Coll 88; **RES:** Long Island Jewish Med Ctr, New
Hyde Park, NY 86-90; **HMO:** Oxford US Hlthcre
Magnacare
♿ ⌂ ★ ⊞ $ Mcr Immediately

Haselkorn, Joan (MD) ObG `PCP`
South Nassau Comm Hosp
Long Island Women's Health Care, MD,PC, 2260
Merrick Rd; Cedarhurst, NY 11516; (516) 295-
1313; **BDCERT:** ObG 90; **MS:** Israel 82; **RES:** ObG,
New York University Med Ctr, New York, NY 82-
86; **HOSP:** N Shore Univ Hosp-Manhasset; *SI:
Uterine Bleeding; Laparoscopic Surgery*; **HMO:** Oxford
Blue Choice GHI US Hlthcre NYLCare +

LANG: Heb; 🦽 🌙 🔒 🔧 🎂 $ Mcr 2-4 Weeks **VISA**
●

Hipps, Linda (MD) ObG
Winthrop Univ Hosp
601 Franklin Ave 215; Garden City, NY 11530;
(516) 742-4050; **BDCERT:** ObG 90; **MS:** Belgium
83; **RES:** Winthrop Univ Hosp, Mineola, NY 83-87;
HOSP: South Nassau Comm Hosp; *SI: Menopause;
Osteoporosis*; **HMO:** Oxford Empire Blue Choice
Magnacare Multiplan +

LANG: Fr; 🦽 🌙 🔒 🔧 🎂 $ Mcr

Jacob, Jessica (MD) ObG
N Shore Univ Hosp-Manhasset
3003 New Hyde Park Rd; New Hyde Park, NY
11042; (516) 488-8145; **BDCERT:** ObG 89; **MS:**
NYU Sch Med 83; **RES:** ObG, N Shore Univ Hosp-
Manhasset, Manhasset, NY 79-83; *SI: High Risk
Pregnancies*; **HMO:** PHCS Oxford Magnacare Aetna
Hlth Plan CIGNA +

🦽 🌙 🔒 🔧 🎂 $ Mcr 1 Week **VISA** ●

Khulpateea, Taru (MD) ObG
Winthrop Univ Hosp
4200 Sunrise Hwy; Massapequa, NY 11758; (516)
541-2100; **BDCERT:** ObG 82; **MS:** India 68; **RES:**
ObG, BYL NAIR Hosp, Bombay, India 70-72; ObG,
New York Methodist Hosp, Brooklyn, NY 74-78;
HOSP: Mid-Island Hosp; **HMO:** Vytra Blue Choice
Empire GHI Oxford +

LANG: Hin, Guj, Grk, Sp, Heb; 🦽 🌙 $

Krim, Eileen (MD) ObG
N Shore Univ Hosp-Manhasset
Northern ObsGyn, 2110 Northern Blvd 207;
Manhasset, NY 11030; (516) 365-6100; **BDCERT:**
ObG 82; **MS:** NY Med Coll 75; **RES:** ObG, Beth Israel
Med Ctr, New York, NY 75-79; **FEL:** MF, N Shore
Univ Hosp-Manhasset, Manhasset, NY 79-81; **FAP:**
Asst Clin Prof NYU Sch Med; *SI: Menopause;
Adolescent Gynecology*; **HMO:** Oxford PHCS
Independent Health Plan HIP Network

🦽 🌙 🔒 🔧 🎂 $ Mcr 4+ Weeks **VISA** ●

Krumholz, Burton (MD) ObG
Long Island Jewish Med Ctr
1554 Northern Blvd 5th Fl; Manhasset, NY 11030;
(516) 390-9242; **BDCERT:** ObG 61; **MS:** NY Med
Coll 53; **RES:** ObG, Metropolitan Hosp Ctr, New
York, NY 54-55; **RES:** Naval Med Ctr, Portsmouth, VA
55-57; **FAP:** Prof Albert Einstein Coll Med; **HOSP:**
Nassau County Med Ctr; *SI: Abnormal Pap Smears;
Vulvovaginal Disorders*; **HMO:** Blue Choice PHS US
Hlthcre CIGNA

🦽 🔒 🔧 🎂 $ Mcr 2-4 Weeks **VISA** ●

Kuncham, Sudha (MD) ObG
Mid-Island Hosp
Wantagh Ob Gyn, 1228 Wantagh Ave 201;
Wantagh, NY 11793; (516) 221-6500; **BDCERT:**
ObG 90; **MS:** India 77; **RES:** ObG, Beth Israel, New
York, NY; **HOSP:** Winthrop Univ Hosp; *SI:
Colposcopy with Biopsy*; **HMO:** Aetna-US Healthcare
CIGNA Prucare United Healthcare GHI +

🦽 🌙 🔒 🔧 🎂 $ Mcr A Few Days

Maulik, Dev (MD) ObG
Winthrop Univ Hosp
Winthrop University Hospital Obstetrics Dept, 259
1st St; Mineola, NY 11501; (516) 663-2264;
BDCERT: ObG 79; MF 87; **MS:** India 62; **RES:** ObG,
Calcutta, India 62-65; Affiliated Hospitals, London,
England 65-69; **FAP:** Prof SUNY Stony Brook
Mcr Mcd

Nimaroff, Michael (MD) ObG `PCP`
N Shore Univ Hosp-Manhasset

900 Northern Blvd Suite 220; Great Neck, NY 11021; (516) 466-0778; **BDCERT:** ObG 93; **MS:** UMDNJ-NJ Med Sch, Newark 87; **RES:** ObG, N Shore Univ Hosp-Manhasset, Manhasset, NY 88-91; **FAP:** Clin Prof Cornell U; **SI:** *Laparoscopic Surgery; Alternatives to Hysterectomy;* **HMO:** Oxford Aetna Hlth Plan US Hlthcre

🚻 🌙 📷 🎗 🏨 💲 Mcr WC NFI 2-4 Weeks

Pagnani, Daniel J (MD) ObG
N Shore Univ Hosp-Glen Cove

10 Medical Plaza; Glen Cove, NY 11542; (516) 671-3989; **BDCERT:** ObG 85; **MS:** Mexico 77; **RES:** S, Univ Hosp SUNY Stony Brook, Stony Brook, NY 78-80; ObG, Nassau County Med Ctr, East Meadow, NY 80-83; **SI:** *Laparoscopy; Laser Surgery;* **HMO:** Oxford Blue Choice Vytra Magnacare

LANG: Sp, Itl; 🚻 SI 🌙 📷 🎗 🏨 💲 NFI Immediately

Rabin, Jill (MD) ObG `PCP`
Long Island Jewish Med Ctr

1554 Northern Blvd 5th Fl; Manhasset, NY 11030; (718) 470-7690; **BDCERT:** ObG 97; **MS:** SUNY Downstate 81; **RES:** Albert Einstein Med Ctr, Bronx, NY; **FAP:** Assoc Prof ObG Albert Einstein Coll Med; **SI:** *Urogynecology*

LANG: Sp, Fr, Yd; 🚻 🏨 💲 Mcr 2-4 Weeks 🔳

Rebold, Bruce (MD) ObG
N Shore Univ Hosp-Plainview

87 Cold Spring Rd; Syosset, NY 11791; (516) 921-3168; **BDCERT:** ObG 84; **MS:** Mexico 77; **RES:** ObG, Nassau County Med Ctr, East Meadow, NY 78-82; **HOSP:** N Shore Univ Hosp-Glen Cove; **HMO:** Aetna Hlth Plan Choicecare Oxford Blue Choice PHCS +

LANG: Sp; 🚻 🌙 📷 🏨 💲 Mcr 4+ Weeks **VISA** 💳

Reinhardt, Henry (MD) ObG
N Shore Univ Hosp-Glen Cove

10 Medical Plaza 208; Glen Cove, NY 11542; (516) 676-7479; **BDCERT:** ObG 62; **MS:** NY Med Coll 49; **RES:** St Vincents Hosp & Med Ctr NY, New York, NY 49-50; ObG, St Vincents Hosp & Med Ctr NY, New York, NY 52-56; **HMO:** GHI Oxford United Healthcare Choicecare Prucare +

🚻 🌙 📷 🎗 🏨 💲 Mcr Immediately

Rifkin, Terry (MD) ObG `PCP`
N Shore Univ Hosp-Manhasset

Great Neck Obstetrics & Gynecology,PC, 900 Northern Blvd 220; Great Neck, NY 11021; (516) 466-0778; **BDCERT:** ObG 87; **MS:** Columbia P&S 81; **RES:** N Shore Univ Hosp-Manhasset, Manhasset, NY 81-85; **FAP:** Asst Clin Prof NYU Sch Med; **SI:** *Laparoscopic Surgery;* **HMO:** Oxford Aetna-US Healthcare

🚻 🌙 📷 🎗 🏨 💲 Mcr 2-4 Weeks

Rothbaum, David (MD) ObG `PCP`
N Shore Univ Hosp-Manhasset

East Shore Obstetrics & Gyn, 233 E Shore Rd 109; Great Neck, NY 11023; (516) 487-3450; **BDCERT:** ObG 88; **MS:** Boston U 82; **RES:** ObG, N Shore Univ Hosp-Manhasset, Manhasset, NY 82-86; ObG, N Shore Univ Hosp-Manhasset, Manhasset, NY 86; **FAP:** Clin Instr NYU Sch Med; **SI:** *Menopause, Osteoporosis; Fibroids;* **HMO:** HIP Network Oxford HIP Network Chubb NYLCare +

🚻 SI 📷 🎗 🏨 💲 Immediately 🔳 **VISA** 💳

Spector, Ira (MD) ObG
N Shore Univ Hosp-Manhasset

300 Old Country Rd # 201; Mineola, NY 11501; (516) 747-4404; **BDCERT:** ObG 74; **MS:** SUNY Hlth Sci Ctr 68; **RES:** Long Island Jewish Med Ctr, New Hyde Park, NY 69-72; **FEL:** Long Island Jewish Med Ctr, New Hyde Park, NY 74-75; **FAP:** Asst Prof SUNY Stony Brook; **HOSP:** Winthrop Univ Hosp; **SI:** *Reproductive Endo-Infertility; Menopause;* **HMO:** Oxford PHS Aetna Hlth Plan

🚻 SI 🌙 📷 🎗 🏨 💲 Immediately **VISA** 💳

Taubman, Richard (MD)   ObG
N Shore Univ Hosp-Glen Cove

900 Northern Blvd Ste 240; Great Neck, NY 11021; (516) 482-4343; **BDCERT:** ObG 98; **MS:** SUNY Downstate 80; **RES:** ObG, Long Island Jewish Med Ctr, New Hyde Park, NY 80-84; **FAP:** Clin Instr Albert Einstein Coll Med; **HOSP:** Long Island Jewish Med Ctr; *SI: Laparoscopic/Hysteroscopic; Hysterectomy Prevention;* **HMO:** Oxford Aetna-US Healthcare Vytra Multiplan GHI +

LANG: Sp; ♿ 🏥 🅲 🔯 ⚕ 🏧 Ⓢ Mcr NfI Immediately ▦ **VISA** 💳

Tydings, Lawrence (MD)   ObG   PCP
N Shore Univ Hosp-Plainview

700 Old Country Rd 205; Plainview, NY 11803; (516) 931-4800; **BDCERT:** ObG 75; **MS:** SUNY Downstate 69; **RES:** ObG, Long Island Jewish Med Ctr, New Hyde Park, NY 70-73; **FAP:** Asst Clin Prof SUNY Stony Brook; *SI: OB/GYN; Laparoscopy;* **HMO:** Aetna-US Healthcare Vytra Oxford GHI Empire +

LANG: Fr; ♿ 🏥 🅲 🔯 ⚕ 🏧 Ⓢ Mcr A Few Days ▦ **VISA** 💳

Vasudeva, Kusum (MD)   ObG
N Shore Univ Hosp-Manhasset

Long Island ObstetricsGyn, 1 Hollow Ln 107; New Hyde Park, NY 11042; (516) 365-9660; **BDCERT:** ObG 75; **MS:** India 68; **RES:** ObG, N Shore Univ Hosp-Manhasset, Manhasset, NY 69-73; **FEL:** MF, N Shore Univ Hosp-Manhasset, Manhasset, NY 73-75; **HMO:** Oxford Aetna-US Healthcare Blue Choice PHS Magnacare +

♿ 🔯 ⚕ 🏧 Ⓢ Mcr 2-4 Weeks

Veloso, Manuel (MD)   ObG
Long Beach Med Ctr

303 E Park Ave B; Long Beach, NY 11561; (516) 431-2828; **BDCERT:** ObG 74; **MS:** Philippines 66; **RES:** Kings County Hosp Ctr, Brooklyn, NY 68-72; **HOSP:** South Nassau Comm Hosp; **HMO:** Oxford Magnacare Sel Pro PHCS

♿ 🅲 🔯 ⚕ 🏧 Ⓢ Mcr 2-4 Weeks **VISA**

Weiss, Karen (MD)   ObG
Long Island Jewish Med Ctr

900 Northern Blvd 240; Great Neck, NY 11021; (516) 482-4343; **BDCERT:** ObG 90; **MS:** U Colo Sch Med 84; **RES:** ObG, Long Island Jewish Med Ctr, New Hyde Park, NY 85-88; **HMO:** Oxford US Hlthcre United Healthcare Vytra Sel Pro +

♿ 🅲 🔯 Ⓢ Mcr 4+ Weeks **VISA** 💳

OPHTHALMOLOGY

Burke, Stanley J (MD)   Oph
Mercy Med Ctr

200 Hempstead Ave; Lynbrook, NY 11563; (516) 593-7709; **BDCERT:** Oph 87; **MS:** SUNY Buffalo 81; **RES:** Univ Hosp SUNY Stony Brook, Stony Brook 85; **FEL:** Oph, Mass Eye & Ear Infirmary, Boston, MA; **HOSP:** Franklin Hosp Med Ctr

Cook, Jack (MD)   Oph
Winthrop Univ Hosp

199 Jericho Tpke 307; Floral Park, NY 11001; (516) 747-4011; **BDCERT:** Oph 80; **MS:** Albert Einstein Coll Med 75; **RES:** Oph, Long Island Jewish Med Ctr, New Hyde Park, NY 76-79; **FAP:** Asst Clin Prof Albert Einstein Coll Med

♿ 🏥 🅲 🔯 ⚕ 🏧 WC NfI 1 Week

Donnenfeld, Eric D (MD)   Oph
Mercy Med Ctr

Ophthalmic Consultants, 2000 N Village Ave 302; Rockville Centre, NY 11570; (516) 766-2519; **BDCERT:** Oph 85; **MS:** Dartmouth Med Sch 80; **RES:** Oph, Manhattan Eye, Ear & Throat Hosp, New York, NY 81-84; **FEL:** Refractive/Cornea, Wills Eye Hosp, Philadelphia, PA 84-85; **FAP:** Asst Prof Cornell U; *SI: Laser Vision Correction;* **HMO:** Oxford Aetna-US Healthcare MDNY Guardian US Hlthcre +

LANG: Sp; ♿ 🏥 🅲 🔯 ⚕ Ⓢ Mcr Mcd WC 2-4 Weeks **VISA** 💳

Garber, Perry (MD)　　　Oph
Long Island Jewish Med Ctr
1380 Northern Blvd F; Manhasset, NY 11030;
(516) 627-6630; **BDCERT:** Oph 76; **MS:** SUNY
Downstate 68; **RES:** S, Montefiore Med Ctr, Bronx,
NY 69-70; Oph, Bellevue Hosp Ctr, New York, NY
72-75; **FEL:** Oph PIS, New York Eye & Ear
Infirmary, New York, NY 75-76; Oph PIS,
Manhattan Eye, Ear & Throat Hosp, New York, NY
75-76; **FAP:** Assoc Clin Prof Oph Albert Einstein
Coll Med; **HOSP:** N Shore Univ Hosp-Manhasset; **SI:**
Eyelid Cosmetic; Reconstructive Surgery; **HMO:**
Oxford Aetna Hlth Plan Blue Choice CIGNA

🦽 🌗 📷 👤 🏨 💲 Mcr WC NFl　1 Week

Girardi, Anthony (MD)　　　Oph
N Shore Univ Hosp-Glen Cove
8 Med Plz; Glen Cove, NY 11542; (516) 676-4596;
BDCERT: Oph 85; **MS:** SUNY Hlth Sci Ctr 80; **RES:**
Oph, Kings County Hosp Ctr, Brooklyn, NY 81-84;
SI: *Cataract; Glaucoma*; **HMO:** Oxford Aetna-US
Healthcare United Healthcare Vytra

LANG: Itl, Sp; 🦽 🌗 📷 👤 🏨 💲 Mcr WC NFl　1 Week
VISA 💳 💳

Gold, Arthur (MD)　　　Oph
Franklin Hosp Med Ctr
1175 W Broadway # 21; Hewlett, NY 11557;
(516) 374-4199; **BDCERT:** Oph 66; **MS:** SUNY
Downstate 60; **RES:** Med, Long Island Jewish Med
Ctr, New Hyde Park, NY 60-61; Oph, Bellevue Hosp
Ctr, New York, NY 61-64; **FEL:** Oph, New York
University Med Ctr, New York, NY 61-64; **FAP:**
Assoc Clin Prof Albert Einstein Coll Med; **HOSP:**
Long Island Jewish Med Ctr; **SI:** *Cataract; Glaucoma*;
HMO: Oxford Empire GHI 1199 PHS +

LANG: Sp, Fr; 🌗 🌗 📷 👤 🏨 Mcr NFl　1 Week ***VISA***
💳

Goldberg, Leslie (MD)　　　Oph
N Shore Univ Hosp-Manhasset
Long Island Eye Surgeons, 2110 Northern Blvd
208; Manhasset, NY 11030; (516) 627-5113;
BDCERT: Oph 77; **MS:** U Hlth Sci/Chicago Med Sch
70; **RES:** Oph, New York University Med Ctr, New
York, NY 73-76; **FAP:** Asst Clin Prof Oph Cornell U;
HMO: Oxford Blue Cross Blue Choice Aetna-US
Healthcare Magnacare +

🦽 📷 👤 🏨 💲 Mcr　A Few Days ***VISA*** 💳 💳

Hatsis, Alexander (MD)　　　Oph
South Nassau Comm Hosp
2 Lincoln Ave 401; Rockville Centre, NY 11570;
(516) 763-4106; **BDCERT:** Oph 92; **MS:** Italy 78;
RES: Oph, Nassau County Med Ctr, East Meadow,
NY 80-81; **HOSP:** Mercy Med Ctr; **SI:** *Refractive
Surgery*; **HMO:** Aetna-US Healthcare Oxford Blue
Choice United Healthcare Empire +

LANG: Sp, Itl, Grk; 🦽 🌗 📷 👤 🏨 💲 Mcr Mod WC
A Few Days ***VISA*** 💳

Kasper, William (MD)　　　Oph
Winthrop Univ Hosp
Mineola Ophthalmology, 330 Old Country Rd 100;
Mineola, NY 11501; (516) 248-5773; **BDCERT:**
Oph 74; **MS:** Belgium 67; **RES:** Nassau County Med
Ctr, East Meadow, NY 69-71; **HOSP:** Mercy Med
Ctr; **SI:** *Cataract; Glaucoma*; **HMO:** Vytra Empire
Oxford GHI

LANG: Fr, Sp, Prt; 🦽 🌗 📷 👤 🏨 💲 Mcr WC NFl
Immediately 💳

Klein, Robert (MD)　　　Oph
Long Beach Med Ctr
Ophthalmology of Long Beach, 202 W Park Ave;
Long Beach, NY 11561; (516) 431-1101;
BDCERT: Oph 87; **MS:** SUNY Downstate 81; **RES:**
Long Island Coll Hosp, Brooklyn, NY 81-82; Univ
Hosp SUNY Bklyn, Brooklyn, NY 82-85; **HOSP:**
Long Island Coll Hosp; **HMO:** GHI Blue Choice Blue
Cross & Blue Shield Choicecare HealthNet +

🦽 🌗 📷 👤 🏨 💲 Mcr　Immediately

Lopez, Robert (MD)　　　Oph
Columbia-Presbyterian Med Ctr
230 Hilton Ave 118; Hempstead, NY 11550; (516)
481-1570; **BDCERT:** Oph 87; **MS:** Harvard Med
Sch 82; **RES:** Med, Winthrop Univ Hosp, Mineola,
NY 83-86; Oph, Columbia-Presbyterian Med Ctr,
New York, NY 83-86; **FEL:** Vitreoretinal S, NY
Hosp-Cornell Med Ctr, New York, NY 86-87; **FAP:**
Assoc Prof Columbia P&S; **HOSP:** Mercy Med Ctr;
SI: *Diabetic Retinopathy; Pediatric Retinal surgery*;
HMO: Oxford Aetna-US Healthcare Blue Cross &
Blue Shield United Healthcare Multiplan +

🦽 📷 👤 🏨 💲 Mcr Mod WC NFl　Immediately

Maisel, James (MD)   Oph
Winthrop Univ Hosp

400 S Oyster Bay Rd 305; Hicksville, NY 11801;
(516) 939-6100; **BDCERT:** Oph 83; **MS:** NY Med
Coll 78; **RES:** Oph, Nassau County Med Ctr, East
Meadow, NY 79-82; **FEL:** Retina, NY Hosp-Cornell
Med Ctr, New York, NY 82-83; **FAP:** Clin Instr NYU
Sch Med; **HOSP:** St Charles Hosp & Rehab Ctr; *SI:
Diabetic Retinopathy; Macular Degeneration;* **HMO:**
Aetna Hlth Plan Oxford PHS United Healthcare
Blue Cross & Blue Shield +

LANG: Itl, Chi; ⬤ ⬤ ⬤ ⬤ ⬤ ⬤ ⬤   Immediately
VISA ⬤

Marks, Alan (MD)   Oph
N Shore Univ Hosp-Manhasset

Long Island Eye Surgery, PC, 2110 Northern Blvd
208; Manhasset, NY 11030; (516) 627-5113;
BDCERT: Oph 83; **MS:** NY Med Coll 78; **RES:** Oph,
N Shore Univ Hosp-Manhasset, Manhasset, NY 79-
82; **HOSP:** St Francis Hosp-Roslyn; *SI: Cataract
Surgery; Laser Surgery;* **HMO:** Aetna Hlth Plan
Oxford Magnacare PHS PHCS +

⬤ ⬤ ⬤ ⬤ ⬤ ⬤ ⬤ ⬤ ⬤   1 Week **VISA** ⬤ ⬤

Nelson, David (MD)   Oph
Mercy Med Ctr

2000 N Village Ave 302; Rockville Centre, NY
11570; (516) 766-2519; **BDCERT:** Oph 77; **MS:**
SUNY Hlth Sci Ctr 72; **RES:** New York Eye & Ear
Infirmary, New York, NY 73-76; **HOSP:** South
Nassau Comm Hosp; *SI: Cataract; Glaucoma;* **HMO:**
Choicecare Oxford CIGNA Sanus-NYLCare Prucare
+

LANG: Ger, Grk, Sp; ⬤ ⬤ ⬤ ⬤ ⬤ ⬤ ⬤ ⬤ ⬤
⬤   2-4 Weeks

Packer, Samuel (MD)   Oph
N Shore Univ Hosp-Manhasset

North Shore Univ Hosp, 600 Northern Blvd Ste
220; Great Neck, NY 11021; (516) 465-8400;
BDCERT: Oph 73; **MS:** SUNY Hlth Sci Ctr 66; **RES:**
Yale-New Haven Hosp, New Haven, CT 67-71; **FEL:**
Yale-New Haven Hosp, New Haven, CT 67-68;
FAP: Clin Prof NYU Sch Med; **HOSP:** Long Island
Jewish Med Ctr; **HMO:** Aetna Hlth Plan PHS HIP
Network Oxford Chubb +

⬤ ⬤ ⬤ ⬤ ⬤ ⬤   A Few Days

Perry, Henry (MD)   Oph
Mercy Med Ctr

Ophthalmic Consultants of Long Island, 2000 N
Village Ave 302; Rockville Centre, NY 11570;
(516) 766-2519; **BDCERT:** Oph 77; **MS:** U
Cincinnati 71; **RES:** Nassau County Med Ctr, East
Meadow, NY 72; Hosp of U Penn, Philadelphia, PA
72-73; **FEL:** Pathology, Armed Forces Inst Path,
Washington, DC 75-76; Cornea, Mass Eye & Ear
Infirmary, Boston, MA 76-77; **FAP:** Assoc Clin Prof
Cornell U; **HOSP:** N Shore Univ Hosp-Syosset; *SI:
Keratoconus; Cataracts;* **HMO:** Empire Sanus-
NYLCare Oxford Blue Choice Aetna Hlth Plan +

LANG: Sp, Fr; ⬤ ⬤ ⬤ ⬤ ⬤ ⬤ ⬤ ⬤ ⬤ ⬤   1 Week
VISA ⬤

Prywes, Arnold (MD)   Oph
N Shore Univ Hosp-Plainview

Eye Care Assoc-Glaucoma Consultants of Long
Island, 4212 Hempstead Tpke; Bethpage, NY
11714; (516) 731-4800; **BDCERT:** Oph 78; **MS:**
Mt Sinai Sch Med 72; **RES:** Oph, Mount Sinai Med
Ctr, New York, NY 74-77; **FEL:** Oph, Mount Sinai
Med Ctr, New York, NY 73-74; **FAP:** Asst Clin Prof
Albert Einstein Coll Med; **HOSP:** Mid-Island Hosp;
SI: Glaucoma Surgery; Cataract Surgery & Implants;
HMO: CIGNA Oxford Prudential US Hlthcre
Prucare +

LANG: Fr, Sp, Rus; ⬤ ⬤ ⬤ ⬤ ⬤ ⬤ ⬤ ⬤ ⬤   2-
4 Weeks ⬤ **VISA** ⬤

Rubin, Laurence (MD)   Oph
Mid-Island Hosp

Mid Island Eye Physicians & Surgeons PC, 4277
Hempstead Tpke 109; Bethpage, NY 11714; (516)
796-4030; **BDCERT:** Oph 87; **MS:** NY Med Coll 80;
RES: New York Eye & Ear Infirmary, New York, NY
81-84; **HOSP:** N Shore Univ Hosp-Manhasset; *SI:
Cataract Surgery; Diabetic Retinopathy;* **HMO:** CIGNA
Aetna Hlth Plan Prucare Oxford +

LANG: Sp; ⬤ ⬤ ⬤ ⬤ ⬤ ⬤ ⬤ ⬤ ⬤ ⬤
A Few Days ⬤ **VISA** ⬤ ⬤

Rubin, Steven (MD)   Oph
N Shore Univ Hosp-Manhasset
600 Northern Blvd 220; Great Neck, NY 11021;
(516) 465-8444; **BDCERT:** Oph 83; **MS:** SUNY
Hlth Sci Ctr 78; **RES:** Jackson Mem Hosp, Miami, FL
78-79; Scheie Eye Inst, Philadelphia, PA 79-82;
FEL: Ped Oph, Wills Eye Hosp, Philadelphia, PA 82-
83; **FAP:** Assoc Prof NYU Sch Med; **HOSP:** Long
Island Jewish Med Ctr; *SI: Vision Problems Pediatric;
Strabismus;* **HMO:** Oxford Aetna Hlth Plan US
Hlthcre CIGNA Empire +
LANG: Itl; 🦽 🅲 🔓 🚼 🎦 Ⓢ Mcr 1 Week *VISA* 💳

Schwartz, Peter (MD)   Oph
N Shore Univ Hosp-Syosset
600 Northern Blvd 216; Great Neck, NY 11021;
(516) 466-0390; **BDCERT:** Oph 76; **MS:** SUNY
Hlth Sci Ctr 70; **RES:** Long Island Jewish Med Ctr,
New Hyde Park, NY 72-75; **FEL:** Mass Eye & Ear
Infirmary, Boston, MA 75-77; **HOSP:** Long Island
Jewish Med Ctr; **HMO:** Aetna Hlth Plan Blue Cross
& Blue Shield Blue Choice
🦽 SA/SU 🔓 🚼 🎦 Ⓢ Mcr A Few Days *VISA* 💳

Sturm, Richard (MD)   Oph
Mercy Med Ctr
Ophthalmic Consultants of Long Island, 200
Hempstead Ave; Lynbrook, NY 11563; (516) 593-
7709; **BDCERT:** Oph 89; **MS:** NY Med Coll 83; **RES:**
St Luke's Roosevelt Hosp Ctr, New York, NY 84-87;
FEL: Mass Eye & Ear Infirmary, Boston, MA 87-88;
HOSP: Long Island Jewish Med Ctr; *SI: Glaucoma;
Cataract;* **HMO:** Oxford US Hlthcre Prucare Empire
MDNY +
🦽 SA/SU 🅲 🔓 🚼 🎦 Ⓢ Mcr Mod WC A Few Days *VISA*
💳

Svitra, Paul (MD)   Oph
N Shore Univ Hosp-Manhasset
3003 New Hyde Park Rd 201; New Hyde Park, NY
11042; (516) 327-0505; **BDCERT:** Oph 90; **MS:**
Cornell U 84; **RES:** Oph, Mass Eye & Ear Infirmary,
Boston, MA 85-89; **FEL:** Retina Vitreous, Duke Eye
Ctr, Durham, NC 89-90; **FAP:** Asst Prof Cornell U;
SI: Macular Degeneration; Diabetic Retinopathy;
HMO: HIP Network Oxford Aetna-US Healthcare
GHI
🦽 SA/SU 🅲 🔓 🚼 🎦 Ⓢ Mcr Mod WC NFI Immediately

Udell, Ira (MD)   Oph
Long Island Jewish Med Ctr
Long Island Jewish Medical Center, 600 Northern
Blvd Ste 214; Great Neck, NY 11021; (516) 470-
2020; **BDCERT:** Oph 80; **MS:** Tulane U 74; **RES:**
Long Island Jewish Med Ctr, New Hyde Park, NY
76-79; **FEL:** Mass Eye & Ear Infirmary, Boston, MA
79-81; **FAP:** Prof Oph Albert Einstein Coll Med;
HOSP: Queens Hosp Ctr; *SI: Corneal Diseases;
Corneal Transplantation;* **HMO:** US Hlthcre CIGNA
Oxford Blue Choice
🦽 🔓 🎦 Ⓢ Mcr 2-4 Weeks *VISA* 💳

Weinstein, Joseph (MD)   Oph
Mid-Island Hosp
Eye Care Assoc, 4212 Hempstead Tpke; Bethpage,
NY 11714; (516) 731-4800; **BDCERT:** Oph 82;
MS: Albert Einstein Coll Med 77; **RES:** Long Island
Jewish Med Ctr, New Hyde Park, NY 78-81; **HOSP:**
Long Island Jewish Med Ctr; **HMO:** US Hlthcre
Oxford Multiplan
LANG: Sp, Rus; 🦽 SA/SU 🅲 🔓 🚼 🎦 Ⓢ Mcr WC NFI
A Few Days 💳 *VISA* 💳

Younger, Joseph (MD)   Oph
Winthrop Univ Hosp
520 Franklin Ave 101; Garden City, NY 11530;
(516) 741-4488; **BDCERT:** Oph 82; **MS:** Mexico
76; **RES:** Oph, U Louisville Hosp, Louisville, KY 77-
80; **FEL:** Retina, Joslin Diabetic Clinic, Boston, MA
80-81; *SI: Diabetic Eye Disease; Ocular Surgery;*
HMO: Aetna-US Healthcare Blue Cross & Blue
Shield GHI Oxford
LANG: Sp; 🦽 🅲 🔓 🚼 🎦 Ⓢ Mcr Mod WC NFI

ORTHOPAEDIC SURGERY

Asnis, Stanley (MD)   OrS
N Shore Univ Hosp-Manhasset
Orthopedic Associates, 800 Community Dr Fl 2;
Manhasset, NY 11030; (516) 627-8717; **BDCERT:**
OrS 76; **MS:** Washington U, St Louis 68; **RES:** OrS,
NY Hosp-Cornell Med Ctr, New York, NY 68-71;
FEL: OrS, Hosp For Special Surgery, New York, NY
72-75; **HOSP:** Hosp For Special Surgery; **SI:** *Hip
Replacement; Knee Replacement;* **HMO:** Oxford
Empire MDNY Health Source

🦽 📷 🔧 🛏 Mcr WC NFI   1 Week

Carroll, Michael (MD)   OrS
Brunswick Hosp Ctr
Island Orthopedic & SportsThrpy, 660 Broadway
100; Massapequa, NY 11758; (516) 798-0111;
BDCERT: OrS 83; **MS:** Georgetown U 76; **RES:**
Nassau County Med Ctr, East Meadow, NY 77-81;
Univ Hosp SUNY Stony Brook, Stony Brook, NY 77-
81; **FAP:** Asst Clin Instr SUNY Stony Brook; **SI:** *Hip
Replacement; Knee Replacement*

LANG: Sp; 🦽 📞 📷 🔧 🛏 $ Mcr WC NFI
Immediately 💳 **VISA** 💳 💳

Cataletto, Mauro (MD)   OrS
Winthrop Univ Hosp
200 Old Country Rd Ste 470; Mineola, NY 11501;
(516) 248-4488; **BDCERT:** OrS 89; **MS:** Mexico 78;
RES: Maimonides Med Ctr, Brooklyn, NY 84; **FEL:**
Hosp For Special Surgery, New York, NY 85; **FAP:**
Clin Instr S Cornell U; **HOSP:** Long Island Jewish
Med Ctr; **SI:** *Spine Surgery; Osteoporosis*

🦽 📞 📷 🛏 $ Mcr WC NFI   Immediately

Corso, Salvatore (MD)   OrS
N Shore Univ Hosp-Manhasset
205 Froehlich Farm Blvd; Woodbury, NY 11797;
(516) 364-0070; **BDCERT:** 95; **MS:** SUNY Hlth Sci
Ctr 87; **RES:** Long Island Jewish Med Ctr, New Hyde
Park, NY 87-92; **FEL:** Orthopaedic Research of VA,
Richmond, VA; **HOSP:** Winthrop Univ Hosp

🦽 📞 📷 🔧 🛏 Mcr WC NFI   Immediately 💳 **VISA**
💳

Dines, David (MD)   OrS
Long Island Jewish Med Ctr
935 Northern Blvd Ste 303; Great Neck, NY
11021; (516) 482-1037; **BDCERT:** OrS 80; **MS:**
UMDNJ-NJ Med Sch, Newark 74; **RES:** S, Hosp For
Special Surgery, New York, NY 75-76; OrS, Hosp
For Special Surgery, New York, NY 76-79; **FAP:**
Assoc Clin Prof Albert Einstein Coll Med; **HOSP:**
Hosp For Special Surgery; **SI:** *Shoulder Surgery;
Sports Medicine;* **HMO:** Health Source Sel Pro Beech
Street

🦽 🛏 $ Mcr WC NFI   1 Week 💳 **VISA** 💳

Garroway, Robert (MD)   OrS
South Nassau Comm Hosp
Long Island Orthopaedic Group PC, 125 Franklin
Ave; Valley Stream, NY 11580; (516) 825-7000;
BDCERT: OrS 85; **MS:** U Hlth Sci/Chicago Med Sch
77; **RES:** OrS, Univ Hosp SUNY Stony Brook, Stony
Brook, NY; Franklin Hosp Med Ctr, Valley Stream,
NY; **FEL:** HS, U of VA Health Sci Ctr, Charlottesville,
VA 83; Univ Hosp SUNY Stony Brook, Stony Brook,
NY 82; **HOSP:** Franklin Hosp Med Ctr; **SI:** *Knee
Arthroscopy Surgery;* **HMO:** Oxford GHI Magnacare
Empire

🦽 📷 🔧 🛏 $ Mcr WC NFI   A Few Days 💳 **VISA**

Illman, Arnold (MD)   OrS
Brunswick Hosp Ctr
NassauSuffolk Orthopedic Associates, PC, 4180
Sunrise Hwy; Massapequa, NY 11758; (516) 541-
7500; **BDCERT:** OrS 70; **MS:** Boston U 60; **RES:** S,
Mass Gen Hosp, Boston, MA 61-63; OrS, Lahey
Clinic, Burlington, MA 63-64; **FAP:** Assoc Prof OrS
SUNY Stony Brook; **HOSP:** N Shore Univ Hosp-
Plainview; **SI:** *Orthopedic Surgery; Sports Medicine;*
HMO: Oxford Empire CIGNA Multiplan United
Healthcare +

🦽 📷 🔧 🛏 $ Mcr WC NFI   A Few Days 💳 **VISA**
💳 💳

Leppard, John (MD)   OrS
N Shore Univ Hosp-Plainview
205 Froehlich Farm Blvd; Woodbury, NY 11797;
(516) 364-0070; **BDCERT:** OrS 86; **MS:** Bowman
Gray 76; **RES:** Columbia-Presbyterian Med Ctr,
New York, NY; **FEL:** Indiana Hand Ctr,
Indianapolis, IN; **HOSP:** Winthrop Univ Hosp;
HMO: Most

♿ 🅐 📷 💅 🏨 Mor WC NFI   Immediately **VISA** ●

Lesniewski, Peter (MD)   OrS
Winthrop Univ Hosp
100 Manetto Hill Rd 105; Plainview, NY 11803;
(516) 433-5757; **BDCERT:** OrS 85; **MS:** Cornell U
77; **RES:** S, N Shore Univ Hosp-Manhasset,
Manhasset, NY 77-80; OrS, Bellevue Hosp Ctr, New
York, NY 80-83; **HOSP:** N Shore Univ Hosp-
Plainview; **HMO:** United Healthcare Empire Blue
Choice Multiplan Chubb Anthem Health +

♿ 🅐 📷 🏨 💲 Mor WC NFI   A Few Days ▤ **VISA** ●

Marcus, Stephen (MD)   OrS
South Nassau Comm Hosp
South Island Orthopaedic Group, PC, 657 Central
Ave; Cedarhurst, NY 11516; (516) 295-0111;
BDCERT: OrS 73; **MS:** NY Med Coll 67; **RES:** Albert
Einstein Med Ctr, Bronx, NY 68-72; **HOSP:** St
John's Epis Hosp-S Shore; **HMO:** Sanus Oxford
United Healthcare 1199 Blue Choice +

LANG: Sp, Fr, Heb; ♿ 📷 💅 🏨 💲 Mor WC   1 Week
▤ **VISA**

Match, Ronald M (MD)   OrS
N Shore Univ Hosp-Glen Cove
3 School St 303A; Glen Cove, NY 11542; (516)
671-8779; **BDCERT:** OrS 67; **MS:** Jefferson Med
Coll 57; **RES:** Bellevue Hosp Ctr, New York, NY 57-
60; Hosp For Special Surgery, New York, NY 60-
64; **FEL:** HS, Columbia-Presbyterian Med Ctr, New
York, NY 68; **HMO:** None

Meinhard, Bruce (MD)   OrS
Nassau County Med Ctr
2201 Hempstead Tpke Rm 672; East Meadow, NY
11554; (516) 572-0123; **BDCERT:** OrS 81; **MS:**
Jefferson Med Coll 74; **RES:** S, Emory U Hosp,
Atlanta, GA; **FEL:** Switzerland; **FAP:** Clin Prof SUNY
Stony Brook; **HOSP:** N Shore Univ Hosp-Syosset; **SI:**
Fractures; **HMO:** GHI Aetna Hlth Plan Chubb
Prudential Empire +

♿ 📷 💅 🏨 💲 Mor WC NFI   2-4 Weeks ▤ **VISA** ●

Montero, Carlos (MD)   OrS
Mid-Island Hosp
Nassau Orthopedic Surgeons, 2920 Hempstead
Tpke; Levittown, NY 11756; (516) 735-4048;
BDCERT: OrS 74; **MS:** Argentina 68; **RES:** OrS,
Nassau County Med Ctr, East Meadow, NY 70-73;
FEL: HS, Nassau County Med Ctr, East Meadow, NY
73-74; **FAP:** Asst Clin Prof SUNY Stony Brook;
HOSP: N Shore Univ Hosp-Plainview; **HMO:** Aetna
Hlth Plan Blue Cross & Blue Shield CIGNA Metlife
Prucare +

LANG: Sp, Itl, Prt; ♿ 🅐 📷 🏨 💲 Mor WC NFI
Immediately **VISA**

Paul, Seth (MD)   OrS
South Nassau Comm Hosp
657 Central Ave; Cedarhurst, NY 11516; (516)
295-0111; **BDCERT:** OrS 90; HS 92; **MS:** Jefferson
Med Coll 81; **RES:** S, Mount Sinai Med Ctr, New
York, NY 81-82; OrS, Univ Hosp SUNY Stony
Brook, Stony Brook, NY 82-86; **FEL:** Hand & Upper
Extremity S, Columbia-Presbyterian Med Ctr, New
York, NY; **HOSP:** Peninsula Hosp Ctr; **HMO:**
Multiplan Oxford GHI 1199 US Hlthcre +

LANG: Sp, Fr, Heb; ♿ 📷 💅 🏨 💲 Mor WC NFI
Immediately ▤ **VISA** ● ▤

Rich, Daniel (MD)   OrS
N Shore Univ Hosp-Manhasset
Shelter Rock Orthopedic Group, 585 Plandome Rd
103; Manhasset, NY 11030; (516) 627-1525;
BDCERT: OrS 84; **MS:** Harvard Med Sch 77; **RES:**
SM, St Luke's Roosevelt Hosp Ctr, New York, NY
78-79; OrS, Hosp For Special Surgery, New York,
NY 79-82; **FAP:** Clin Instr Cornell U; **HOSP:** Hosp
For Special Surgery; **SI:** *Joint Replacement;* **HMO:** US
Hlthcre United Healthcare Prudential Oxford

♿ 🆔 🏨 💲 Mor WC   Immediately ▤ **VISA** ● ▤

Ross, Bruce (MD) OrS
Winthrop Univ Hosp
161 Willis Ave; Mineola, NY 11501; (516) 742-0034; **MS:** Mexico 76; **RES:** Long Island Jewish Med Ctr, New Hyde Park, NY 78-81; **FEL:** Nassau County Med Ctr, East Meadow, NY 81-82; **HOSP:** Mercy Med Ctr; *SI: Sports Injury; Total Joints*; **HMO:** Oxford Guardian Empire Blue Choice Vytra +

LANG: Sp; 🚹 📷 👤 🏨 Mcr WC NFI Immediately
VISA 💳

Shebairo, Raymond (MD) OrS
Long Island Jewish Med Ctr
1575 Hillside Ave 303; New Hyde Park, NY 11040; (516) 437-5500; **BDCERT:** OrS 82; **MS:** Med Coll Wisc 73; **RES:** OrS, Long Island Jewish Med Ctr, New Hyde Park, NY 74-77; **HOSP:** Mercy Med Ctr

🚹 📷 👤 🏨 💲 Mcr WC NFI Immediately ▦ *VISA* 💳

Simonson, Barry G (MD) OrS
N Shore Univ Hosp-Manhasset
825 Northern Blvd; Great Neck, NY 11021; (516) 627-0303; **BDCERT:** OrS 93; **MS:** Mt Sinai Sch Med 84; **RES:** Long Island Jewish Med Ctr, New Hyde Park, NY 86-90; **FEL:** New York University Med Ctr, New York, NY 90-91; **HOSP:** Long Island Jewish Med Ctr; *SI: Sports Medicine; Arthroscopic Surgery*; **HMO:** Magnacare Aetna Hlth Plan Oxford Blue Choice PHCS +

LANG: Fr, Sp, Heb; 🚹 🌙 📷 🏨 💲 Mcr WC NFI
Immediately ▦ 💳 🪪

Spinner, Morton (MD) OrS
Franklin Hosp Med Ctr
557 Central Ave; Cedarhurst, NY 11516; (516) 569-6323; **BDCERT:** OrS 60; **MS:** NYU Sch Med 51; **RES:** Bellevue Hosp Ctr, New York, NY 51-52; Hosp For Joint Diseases, New York, NY 55-57; **HMO:** None

📷 👤 🏨 💲 WC A Few Days

Watnik, Neil (MD) OrS
Long Island Jewish Med Ctr
Dept Orthopedic SurgeryLong Island Jewish Medical Center, 1554 Northern Blvd; Manhasset, NY 11030; (516) 627-9007; **BDCERT:** OrS 84; **MS:** NY Med Coll 86; **RES:** Univ Hosp SUNY Bklyn, Brooklyn, NY 86-91; **FEL:** SM, Hosp For Joint Diseases, New York, NY 91-92; **FAP:** Asst Prof OrS Albert Einstein Coll Med; **HOSP:** N Shore Univ Hosp-Manhasset; *SI: Sports Medicine; Dislocations*; **HMO:** Oxford US Hlthcre Magnacare Empire CIGNA +

🚹 ▦ 📷 👤 🏨 Mcr WC NFI Immediately

Weiss, Carl (MD) OrS
Mid-Island Hosp
Nassau Orthopedic Surgeons, 2920 Hempstead Tpke; Levittown, NY 11756; (516) 735-4048; **BDCERT:** OrS 93; **HS** 96; **MS:** SUNY Downstate 84; **RES:** OrS, Univ Hosp SUNY Stony Brook, Stony Brook, NY 85-89; **FEL:** HS, Orthopaedic Hosp, Los Angeles, CA 89-90; **HOSP:** Winthrop Univ Hosp; *SI: Hand/Wrist Problems; Knee Injuries*; **HMO:** Empire GHI Oxford Vytra US Hlthcre +

LANG: Sp; 🚹 🌙 📷 👤 🏨 💲 Mcr WC NFI
A Few Days *VISA*

Weiss, Leonard (MD) OrS
Winthrop Univ Hosp
2920 Hempstead Tpke; Levittown, NY 11756; (516) 735-4048; **BDCERT:** OrS 68; **MS:** Washington U, St Louis 57; **RES:** Univ Hosp SUNY Syracuse, Syracuse, NY 57-59; Case Western Reserve U Hosp, Cleveland, OH 62-65; **HOSP:** Mid-Island Hosp; **HMO:** Metlife Prucare Aetna Hlth Plan

🚹 🌙 📷 👤 🏨 💲 Mcr WC NFI Immediately *VISA* 💳

Zimmerman, Alan (MD) OrS
Long Beach Med Ctr

Park Avenue Orthopedic Assoc, 340 W Park Ave;
Long Beach, NY 11561; (516) 431-5000;
BDCERT: OrS 67; **MS:** NYU Sch Med 58; **RES:** S,
Lenox Hill Hosp, New York, NY 59-60; OrS,
Bellevue Hosp Ctr, New York, NY 60-63; **FAP:**
Adjct Clin Prof Coll Of Osteo Med-Pacific; **HOSP:**
South Nassau Comm Hosp; **SI:** *Hip & Knee Surgery;
Arthritis and Spine Rehab;* **HMO:** Oxford PHS Empire
Blue Cross & Shield Multiplan CIGNA +

LANG: Sp, Rus; ⬚ ⬚ ⬚ ⬚ ⬚ ⬚ ⬚ ⬚
A Few Days **VISA** ⬚

OTOLARYNGOLOGY

Abramson, Allan (MD) Oto
Long Island Jewish Med Ctr

L I Jewish Med Ctr Dept Oto, 27005 76th Ave; New
Hyde Park, NY 11042; (516) 470-7555; **BDCERT:**
Oto 72; **MS:** SUNY Downstate 67; **RES:** S, Long
Island Jewish Med Ctr, New Hyde Park, NY 67-68;
Oto, Mount Sinai Med Ctr, New York, NY 69-72;
FAP: Prof Oto Albert Einstein Coll Med; **SI:**
Laryngology; Photodynamic Therapy; **HMO:** Oxford
US Hlthcre CIGNA Chubb Multiplan +

LANG: Sp; ⬚ ⬚ ⬚ ⬚ ⬚ ⬚ ⬚ ⬚ 2-4 Weeks ⬚
VISA ⬚

Durante, Anthony (MD) Oto
Winthrop Univ Hosp

134 Mineola Blvd 301; Mineola, NY 11501; (516)
294-9363; **BDCERT:** Oto 75; **MS:** Italy 67; **RES:**
Albert Einstein Med Ctr, Bronx, NY 72-75; **HMO:**
Oxford Blue Cross & Blue Shield Choicecare CIGNA
Metlife +

⬚ ⬚ ⬚ ⬚ ⬚ ⬚ ⬚ ⬚ ⬚ Immediately ⬚
VISA ⬚

Glass, Walter (MD) Oto
N Shore Univ Hosp-Manhasset

333 E Shore Rd 102; Manhasset, NY 11030; (516)
482-8778; **BDCERT:** Oto 49; **MS:** Univ Vt Coll Med
43; **RES:** Columbia-Presbyterian Med Ctr, New
York, NY 47-49; **HOSP:** St Francis Hosp-Roslyn;
HMO: Oxford Magnacare CIGNA Aetna Hlth Plan

⬚ ⬚ ⬚ ⬚ ⬚ ⬚ ⬚ ⬚ Immediately ⬚ **VISA**
⬚

Goldofsky, Elliot (MD) Oto
Long Island Jewish Med Ctr

2001 Marcus Ave 125; Lake Success, NY 11042;
(516) 775-3377; **BDCERT:** Oto 90; **MS:** Mt Sinai
Sch Med 84; **RES:** Oto, Long Island Jewish Med Ctr,
New Hyde Park, NY 84-89; **FEL:** New York
University Med Ctr, New York, NY 89-90; **FAP:**
Assoc Clin Prof Oto Albert Einstein Coll Med; **HOSP:**
Winthrop Univ Hosp; **SI:** *Pediatrics Hearing Loss; Ear
Disorders;* **HMO:** Oxford Aetna Hlth Plan Blue
Choice PHCS

LANG: Heb, Itl, Sp; ⬚ ⬚ ⬚ ⬚ ⬚ ⬚ ⬚ ⬚
Immediately ⬚ **VISA** ⬚ ⬚ ⬚

Goldstein, Mark (MD) Oto
Long Island Jewish Med Ctr

The Otolaryngology and Facial Plastics Center, LLP,
600 Northern Blvd Ste 100; Great Neck, NY
11021; (516) 466-6888; **BDCERT:** Oto 79; **MS:**
Boston U 74; **RES:** S, Kaiser Hosp, Oakland, CA 74-
75; Oto, Boston U Med Ctr, Boston, MA 76-79;
FAP: Asst Clin Prof Oto NYU Sch Med; **HOSP:** N
Shore Univ Hosp-Forest Hills; **SI:** *Pediatric
Otolaryngology; Otology;* **HMO:** Oxford Aetna Hlth
Plan Magnacare PHS Prucare +

LANG: Sp; ⬚ ⬚ ⬚ ⬚ ⬚ ⬚ ⬚ A Few Days ⬚
VISA ⬚

Gordon, Michael A (MD) Oto
Long Island Jewish Med Ctr
Hearing & Speech Center, LI Jewish Med Ctr at 76th Ave; New Hyde Park, NY 11040; (718) 470-8922; **BDCERT:** Oto 93; **MS:** Albert Einstein Coll Med 86; **RES:** S, Albert Einstein Med Ctr, Bronx, NY 86-87; Oto, Montefiore Med Ctr, Bronx, NY 88-92; **FEL:** Oto N, Ear Research Foundation, Sarasota, FL 92-93; **FAP:** Asst Prof Albert Einstein Coll Med; *SI: Laser Stapes Surgery; Chronic Ear Infections*; **HMO:** Oxford Magnacare US Hlthcre Multiplan Blue Choice +

LANG: Heb; 🚻 🌙 🔒 👥 🎫 💲 Mcr 1 Week

Grosso, John (MD) Oto
N Shore Univ Hosp-Plainview
Long Island Ent Assoc, 875 Old Country Rd 100; Plainview, NY 11803; (516) 931-5552; **BDCERT:** Oto 93; **MS:** SUNY Syracuse 86; **RES:** U Hosp, Cincinnati, OH 88-92

🚻 SA 🌙 🔒 👥 🎫 💲 Mcr WC NFI A Few Days ▨ **VISA** 💳 💳

Mattucci, Kenneth (MD) Oto
N Shore Univ Hosp-Manhasset
North Shore Otolaryngology, 333 E Shore Rd 102; Manhasset, NY 11030; (516) 482-8778; **BDCERT:** Oto 70; **MS:** Bowman Gray 64; **RES:** NY Hosp-Cornell Med Ctr, New York, NY 64-66; New York Eye & Ear Infirmary, New York, NY 66-69; **FEL:** N, NY Hosp-Cornell Med Ctr, New York, NY 69-70; **FAP:** Clin Prof NY Med Coll; **HOSP:** St Francis Hosp-Roslyn; *SI: Otology; Neurotology*

LANG: Itl, Sp; 🚻 👥 🎫 💲 Mcr A Few Days ▨ **VISA** 💳

Modlin, Saul (MD) Oto
Winthrop Univ Hosp
975 Franklin Ave; Garden City, NY 11530; (516) 739-3999; **BDCERT:** Oto 95; **MS:** U Md Sch Med 88; **RES:** S, Montefiore Med Ctr, Bronx, NY 88-89; Oto, Albert Einstein Med Ctr, Bronx, NY 90-94; **FEL:** Montefiore Med Ctr, Bronx, NY 89-90; Ped Oto, Childrens Mem Med Ctr, Chicago, IL 94-95; **HOSP:** South Nassau Comm Hosp; *SI: ENT Problems Pediatric; Ear Sinus and Airway Problems*; **HMO:** Vytra Oxford Prucare GHI Empire +

LANG: Sp; 🚻 SA 🌙 🔒 👥 🎫 💲 Mcr WC NFI
Immediately

Rosner, Louis (MD) Oto
Mercy Med Ctr
South Shore Otolaryngology, 176 N Village Ave 1A; Rockville Centre, NY 11570; (516) 678-0303; **BDCERT:** Oto 82; **MS:** U Hlth Sci/Chicago Med Sch 78; **RES:** S, Loyola U Med Ctr, Chicago, IL; New York Eye & Ear Infirmary, New York, NY; **HOSP:** South Nassau Comm Hosp; *SI: Snoring*; **HMO:** Aetna Hlth Plan Blue Choice

🚻 🌙 👥 🎫 💲 Mcr NFI A Few Days **VISA** 💳

Setzen, Michael (MD) Oto
N Shore Univ Hosp-Manhasset
North Shore Otolaryngology, 333 E Shore Rd; Manhasset, NY 11030; (516) 482-8778; **BDCERT:** Oto 82; **MS:** South Africa 74; **RES:** Barnes Hosp, St Louis, MO 78-82; Cleveland Clinic Hosp, Cleveland, OH 77-78; *SI: Nasal & Sinus Surgery; Pediatric Otolaryngology*; **HMO:** NSHIP

🔒 👥 Mcr A Few Days ▨ **VISA** 💳

Tawfik, Bernard (MD) Oto
N Shore Univ Hosp-Glen Cove
3 School St Ste 304; Glen Cove, NY 11542; (516) 671-0085; **BDCERT:** Oto 77; **MS:** Johns Hopkins U 71; **RES:** Manhattan Eye, Ear & Throat Hosp, New York, NY 74-77; **HOSP:** Winthrop Univ Hosp; *SI: Endoscopic Sinus Surgery; Thyroid Surgery*; **HMO:** Blue Choice Vytra Sel Pro Magnacare Multiplan +

LANG: Fr, Sp; 🚻 🌙 🔒 👥 🎫 💲 Mcr NFI
Immediately

Youngerman, Jay (MD) Oto
Long Island Jewish Med Ctr
875 Old Country Rd 100; Plainview, NY 11803; (516) 931-5552; **BDCERT:** Oto 84; **MS:** Med Coll Va 79; **RES:** Oto, Long Island Jewish Med Ctr, New Hyde Park, NY 79-83; **HOSP:** N Shore Univ Hosp-Plainview; *SI: Pediatric Otolaryngology; Head, Neck & Sinus Surgery*; **HMO:** Empire JJ Newman MDLI Oxford

LANG: Sp; 🚻 SA 🌙 🔒 👥 🎫 💲 Mcr WC NFI
Immediately ▨ **VISA** 💳 💳

Zelman, Warren (MD)　　　Oto
Winthrop Univ Hosp
700 Stewart Ave; Garden City, NY 11530; (516)
739-3999; **BDCERT:** Oto 87; **MS:** U Hlth
Sci/Chicago Med Sch 82; **RES:** Univ Hosp SUNY
Stony Brook, Stony Brook, NY 82-84; **FEL:** Oto,
Manhattan Eye, Ear & Throat Hosp, New York, NY;
HOSP: Massapequa Gen Hosp; **SI:** *Head & Neck
Surgery;* **HMO:** Choicecare CIGNA Metlife PHS
Prucare +

⬥ ⬥ ⬥ ⬥ ⬥ ⬥ ⬥ ⬥ ⬥　Immediately

PAIN MANAGEMENT

Bluth, Mordecai (MD)　　　PM
Long Beach Med Ctr
Advanced Pain Management Services, 246 Long
Beach Rd PO Box 370; Island Park, NY 11558;
(516) 431-3113; **BDCERT:** Anes 78; PM 92; **MS:** U
Hlth Sci/Chicago Med Sch 65; **RES:** Anes, Univ
Hosp SUNY Bklyn, Brooklyn, NY 66-69; **FAP:** Aso
Clin Prof NY Coll Osteo Med; **SI:** *Disc Disease;
Sciatica;* **HMO:** Aetna Hlth Plan Oxford Blue Cross &
Blue Shield US Hlthcre

⬥ ⬥ ⬥ ⬥ ⬥ ⬥　A Few Days

Hanania, Michael (MD)　　　PM
Long Island Jewish Med Ctr
1554 Northern Blvd 4th Fl; Manhasset, NY 11030;
(516) 719-7246; **BDCERT:** Anes 93; PM 94; **MS:**
Mt Sinai Sch Med 88; **RES:** Anes, Mount Sinai Med
Ctr, New York, NY 89-92; **FAP:** Asst Prof Albert
Einstein Coll Med; **SI:** *Sciatica/Back Pain; Post
Herpetic Neuralgia;* **HMO:** Oxford GHI Magnacare
Aetna Hlth Plan PHS

⬥ ⬥ ⬥ ⬥ ⬥ ⬥ ⬥ ⬥　A Few Days **VISA** ⬤

Sinha, K (MD)　　　PM
Long Beach Med Ctr
Advanced Pain Management Svc, 455 Long Beach
Memorial Hospital; Long Beach, NY 11561; (516)
897-1265; **BDCERT:** Anes 83; PM 94; **MS:** India
74; **RES:** Anes, New York University Med Ctr, New
York, NY 80-81; **IM,** New York Methodist Hosp,
Brooklyn, NY 77-80; **SI:** *Pain Management; Cancer
Pain;* **HMO:** Oxford US Hlthcre

LANG: Hin; ⬥ ⬥ ⬥ ⬥ ⬥ ⬥ ⬥　A Few Days

PEDIATRIC ALLERGY & IMMUNOLOGY

Fagin, James (MD)　　　PA&I　　`PCP`
N Shore Univ Hosp-Manhasset
Division of General Pediatrics, N Shore Univ Hosp,
865 Northern Blvd 101; Great Neck, NY 11021;
(516) 622-5050; **BDCERT:** A&I 83; Ped 80; **MS:**
Belgium 76; **RES:** Ped, N Shore Univ Hosp-
Manhasset, Manhasset, NY 76-79; **FEL:** A&I,
Children's Hosp of Pittsburgh, Pittsburgh, PA 79-
81; **SI:** *Asthma; Allergic Disease;* **HMO:** Aetna Hlth
Plan Choicecare CIGNA Prucare Travelers +

LANG: Fr, Sp; ⬥ ⬥ ⬥ ⬥ ⬥ ⬥ ⬥　1 Week **VISA**
⬤

Pahwa, Savita (MD)　　　PA&I
N Shore Univ Hosp-Manhasset
North Shore University Hospital, 350 Community
Dr; Manhasset, NY 11030; (516) 562-4641;
BDCERT: Ped 76; A&I 77; **MS:** India 70; **RES:** Ped,
Univ Hosp SUNY Bklyn, Brooklyn, NY 72-73; Ped,
Mem Sloan Kettering Cancer Ctr, New York, NY
73-76; **FEL:** Ped A&I, Mem Sloan Kettering Cancer
Ctr, New York, NY 73-76; **FAP:** Prof Ped NYU Sch
Med; **SI:** *Immunology—Pediatrics; Pediatric HIV;*
HMO: +

⬥

PEDIATRIC CARDIOLOGY

Boxer, Robert A (MD)　　　PCd
N Shore Univ Hosp-Manhasset
300 Community Dr; Manhasset, NY 11030; (516)
562-3078; **BDCERT:** PCCM 96; PCd 79; **MS:**
Columbia P&S 72; **RES:** Columbia-Presbyterian
Med Ctr, New York, NY 72-74; Children's Hosp of
Buffalo, Buffalo, NY 75; **FEL:** Cv, Columbia-
Presbyterian Med Ctr, New York, NY 75-78; **FAP:**
Prof of Clin Ped NYU Sch Med; **SI:** *Marfan's and
Down's Syndrome; Congenital Heart Defects/Adult;*
HMO: Most

LANG: Sp, Fr; ⬥ ⬥ ⬥ ⬥ ⬥ ⬥ ⬥　Immediately
⬥ **VISA** ⬤

Cooper, Rubin (MD) **PCd**
N Shore Univ Hosp-Manhasset
North Shore Pediatric Cardiology Group, 300 Community Dr; Manhasset, NY 11030; (516) 562-3078; **BDCERT:** Ped 76; PCd 79; **MS:** NY Med Coll 71; **RES:** Ped, Strong Mem Hosp, Rochester, NY 71-73; Ped, Strong Mem Hosp, Rochester, NY 73; **FEL:** PCd, Strong Mem Hosp, Rochester, NY 73-75; **FAP:** Prof NYU Sch Med; **HOSP:** N Shore Univ Hosp-Forest Hills; ***SI:*** *Congenital Heart Disease; Rheumatic Fever, Sports Med*
LANG: Rus, Heb, Fr, Itl, Hin; Mcr Mcd WC NFI A Few Days VISA

Levchuck, Sean G (MD) **PCd**
St Francis Hosp-Roslyn
Pediatric Cardiology of Long Island, 100 Port Washington Blvd; Roslyn, NY 11576; (516) 365-3340; **BDCERT:** Ped 93; PCd 96; **MS:** West Indies 89; **RES:** Winthrop Univ Hosp, Mineola, NY 90-92; **FEL:** PCd, St Christopher's Hosp for Children, Philadelphia, PA 92-95; **HOSP:** Capital Health Sys-Mercer; ***SI:*** *Interventional Cardiology; Congenital Heart Disease*; **HMO:** Aetna Hlth Plan Oxford US Hlthcre Blue Choice
Mcd NFI Immediately VISA

Schiff, Russell (MD) **PCd**
N Shore Univ Hosp-Manhasset
2nd Office500 Montauk HighwayAtrium BuildingSuiteV West Islip New York, 300 Community Dr; Manhasset, NY 11795; (516) 562-3078; **BDCERT:** Ped 86; **MS:** SUNY Stony Brook 81; **RES:** Ped, Schneider Children's Hosp, New Hyde Park, NY 81-84; **FEL:** PCd, Schneider Children's Hosp, New Hyde Park, NY 84-86; **FAP:** Asst Prof Ped NYU Sch Med; ***SI:*** *Transesophageal Echocardiography; Fetal Echocardiography*; **HMO:** Aetna Hlth Plan Blue Choice Blue Cross & Blue Shield
LANG: Sp, Rus, Heb; Mcd 2-4 Weeks
VISA

Vallone, Ambrose (MD) **PCd**
St Francis Hosp-Roslyn
Pediatric Cardiology at Long Island, PC, 100 Port Washington Blvd Ste 107; Roslyn, NY 11576; (516) 365-3340; **BDCERT:** PCd 88; PCCM 90; **MS:** Johns Hopkins U 77; **RES:** Ped, Johns Hopkins Hosp, Baltimore, MD 77-78; Ped, Johns Hopkins Hosp, Baltimore, MD 78-80; **FEL:** PCd, Yale-New Haven Hosp, New Haven, CT 80-83; PCCM, Yale-New Haven Hosp, New Haven, CT 80-83; **FAP:** Asst Prof Ped U North Tx Hlth Sci Ctr, Coll Osteo Med; ***SI:*** *Pediatric Cardiology; Fetal Echocardiography*; **HMO:** Aetna-US Healthcare Vytra United Healthcare Oxford Blue Cross & Blue Shield +
LANG: Sp; Mcr Mcd NFI A Few Days
VISA

PEDIATRIC ENDOCRINOLOGY

Agdere, Levon (MD) **PEn**
New York Methodist Hosp
22 High Farms Rd; Glen Head, NY 11545; (718) 250-6911; **BDCERT:** Ped 89; PEn 91; **MS:** Turkey 81; **RES:** Ped, Lutheran Med Ctr, Brooklyn, NY 86; **FEL:** PEn, NY Hosp Cornell Med Ctr, New York, NY; ***SI:*** *Diabetes; Short Stature in Children*; **HMO:** Aetna-US Healthcare HealthNet Prucare HIP Network Oxford
LANG: Sp, Trk, Arm; Mcd 1 Week

Blumberg, Denise (MD) **PEn**
Nassau County Med Ctr
2201 Hempstead Tpke; East Meadow, NY 11554; (516) 572-6398; **BDCERT:** Ped 86; PEn 91; **MS:** Israel 82; **RES:** Ped, Brookdale Univ Hosp Med Ctr, Brooklyn, NY 82-85; **FEL:** PEn, New York University Med Ctr, New York, NY 85-88; **FAP:** Prof Ped SUNY Stony Brook; **HMO:** Multiplan Sanus Health First South Shore
Mcr Mcd 2-4 Weeks

Castro-Magana, Mariano (MD)PEn
Winthrop Univ Hosp
Winthrop University Hospital, Dept of
Endocrinology, Diabetes & Metabolism, 259 1st St;
Mineola, NY 11501; (516) 663-3069; **BDCERT:**
Ped 83; PEn 83; **MS:** El Salvador 74; **RES:** Ped,
Nassau County Med Ctr, East Meadow, NY 77-80;
FEL: PEn, Nassau County Med Ctr, East Meadow,
NY 80-82; **FAP:** Clin Prof NYU Sch Med; **SI:** *Puberty
Development-Growth; Sexual Development*
🔲 🔲 🔲 🔲 🔲 🔲 🔲 2-4 Weeks **VISA** 💳

Fort, Pavel (MD)   PEn
N Shore Univ Hosp-Manhasset
60 Argle Rd; Albertson, NY 11507; (516) 562-
4635; **BDCERT:** Ped 76; PEn 78; **MS:**
Czechoslovakia 69; **RES:** N Shore Univ Hosp-
Manhasset, Manhasset, NY 71-74; **FEL:** N Shore
Univ Hosp-Manhasset, Manhasset, NY; **FAP:** Assoc
Clin Prof Ped NYU Sch Med; **SI:** *Hormonal Disorders;
Diabetes Mellitus*; **HMO:** Oxford Empire Blue Cross &
Shield Aetna Hlth Plan Travelers CIGNA +
LANG: Sp, Fr, Heb, Czc; 🔲 🔲 🔲 🔲 🔲 🔲
4+ Weeks **VISA** 💳

Speiser, Phyllis W (MD)   PEn
N Shore Univ Hosp-Manhasset
300 Community Dr; Manhasset, NY 11030; (516)
562-4635; **BDCERT:** Ped 84; PEn 86; **MS:**
Columbia P&S 79; **RES:** Ped, Jacobi Med Ctr, Bronx,
NY 79-80; Albert Einstein Med Ctr, Bronx, NY 80-
82; **FEL:** PEn, NY Hosp-Cornell Med Ctr, New York,
NY 82-84; **FAP:** Assoc Prof Ped Cornell U; **SI:**
Puberty; Growth; **HMO:** Aetna Hlth Plan Oxford HIP
Network Blue Cross PPO Prudential +
LANG: Heb, Sp; 🔲 🔲 🔲 🔲 🔲 🔲 🔲 2-
4 Weeks 🔲 **VISA** 💳 💳 💳

PEDIATRIC GASTROENTEROLOGY

Aiges, Harvey (MD)   PGe
N Shore Univ Hosp-Manhasset
North Shore University Hosp, 300 Community Dr;
Manhasset, NY 11030; (516) 562-4640; **BDCERT:**
Ped 76; PGe 97; **MS:** NYU Sch Med 71; **RES:** Ped,
Jacobi Med Ctr, Bronx, NY 71-75; Ped, Jacobi Med
Ctr, Bronx, NY 74-75; **FEL:** Ge, NY Hosp-Cornell
Med Ctr, New York, NY 77-79; **FAP:** Prof NYU Sch
Med; **SI:** *Crohn's Disease; Liver Disease in Children*
LANG: Sp; 🔲 🔲 🔲 🔲 🔲 🔲 A Few Days 🔲
VISA 💳 💳

Daum, Fredric (MD)   PGe
N Shore Univ Hosp-Manhasset
North Shore University Hosp, 300 Community Dr;
Manhasset, NY 11030; (516) 562-0100; **BDCERT:**
Ped 72; PGe 90; **MS:** Tufts U 67; **RES:** Ped, Jacobi
Med Ctr, Bronx, NY 67-69; **FEL:** AM, Montefiore
Med Ctr, Bronx, NY 71-72; **FAP:** Prof Ped NYU Sch
Med; **SI:** *Pediatric and Adolescent Colitis; Liver Disease*
🔲 🔲 🔲 🔲 🔲 🔲 🔲 🔲 Immediately 🔲 **VISA**
💳 💳

Gold, David (MD)   PGe
Long Island Jewish Med Ctr
Schneider - Div of Ped Gastro and Nutrition, 269-
01 76th Ave; New Hyde Park, NY 11040; (516)
470-3430; **BDCERT:** Ped 90; PGe 95; **MS:** Albert
Einstein Coll Med 87; **RES:** Ped, Long Island Jewish
Med Ctr, New Hyde Park, NY 88-90; **FEL:** PGe,
Long Island Jewish Med Ctr, New Hyde Park, NY
90; **FAP:** Asst Prof Ped Albert Einstein Coll Med; **SI:**
Constipation; Gastroesophageal Reflux; **HMO:** Oxford
US Hlthcre CIGNA Guardian Prudential +
🔲 🔲 🔲 🔲 🔲 🔲 🔲 A Few Days **VISA** 💳

Sockolow, Robbyn (MD) PGe
Winthrop Univ Hosp
Winthrop University Hospital, Dept of
Gastroenterology, 222 Station Plaza North Ste 406;
Mineola, NY 11501; (516) 663-8534; **BDCERT:**
PGe 95; Ped 89; **MS:** NY Med Coll 86; **RES:** Ped,
Albert Einstein Med Ctr, Bronx, NY 86-89; **FEL:** PGe,
Mount Sinai Med Ctr, New York, NY 89-90; PGe,
Albert Einstein Med Ctr, Bronx, NY 90-92; **FAP:**
Asst Prof SUNY Stony Brook; **SI:** *Gastroesophageal
Reflux Disease;* **HMO:** Oxford Aetna-US Healthcare
Vytra Prucare Blue Cross PPO +
🔲 🔲 🔲 🔲 🔲 🔲 A Few Days 🔲 **VISA** 🔲

Weinstein, Toba (MD) PGe
Schneider Children's Hosp
269-01 76th Ave; New Hyde Park, NY 11040;
(718) 470-3430; **BDCERT:** PGe 92; **MS:** Columbia
P&S 86; **RES:** Ped, Children's Hosp Nat Med Ctr,
Washington, DC 87-89; **FEL:** PGe, Schneider
Children's Hosp, New Hyde Park, NY 89-91; **FAP:**
Asst Prof Albert Einstein Coll Med

PEDIATRIC HEMATOLOGY-ONCOLOGY

Lanzkowsky, Philip (MD) PHO
Schneider Children's Hosp
Schneider Children's Hospital,; New Hyde Park, NY
11040; (718) 470-3201; **BDCERT:** Ped 66; **MS:**
South Africa 54; **RES:** Red Cross War Mem
Children's Hosp, Cape Town, South Africa 59-60; St
Mary's Med Ctr, London, England 60-61; **FEL:** PHO,
Duke U Med Ctr, Durham, NC 61-62; PHO, U UT
Hosp, Salt Lake City, UT 62-63; **FAP:** Prof Albert
Einstein Coll Med; **SI:** *Leukemia; Childhood
Malignancies;* **HMO:** Oxford Aetna Hlth Plan United
Healthcare Empire Blue Cross & Shield Blue Shield +
🔲 🔲 🔲 🔲 🔲 🔲 Immediately 🔲 **VISA** 🔲

Paley, Carole (MD) PHO
Schneider Children's Hosp
Schneider Children's Hospital, 269-01 76th Ave; New
Hyde Park, NY 11040; (718) 470-3460; **BDCERT:**
Ped 89; PHO 92; **MS:** France 84; **RES:** Ped, St Luke's
Roosevelt Hosp Ctr, New York, NY 85-87; **FEL:** PHO,
Mem Sloan Kettering Cancer Ctr, New York, NY 87-
90; **FAP:** Asst Prof Albert Einstein Coll Med; **HMO:**
Oxford GHI Magnacare US Hlthcre CIGNA +
🔲 🔲 🔲 🔲 🔲 🔲

Weinblatt, Mark (MD) PHO
N Shore Univ Hosp-Manhasset
300 Community Dr; Manhasset, NY 11030; (516)
562-4634; **BDCERT:** Ped 80; **MS:** Albert Einstein
Coll Med 76; **RES:** Ped, Jacobi Med Ctr, Bronx, NY
76-79; **FEL:** PHO, Children's Hosp of Los Angeles,
Los Angeles, CA 79-81; **FAP:** Assoc Prof NYU Sch
Med; **SI:** *Pediatric Cancer; Bleeding Disorders;* **HMO:**
Aetna Hlth Plan Blue Cross & Blue Shield CIGNA
Oxford GHI +
LANG: Sp, Heb; 🔲 🔲 🔲 🔲 🔲 Immediately

PEDIATRIC INFECTIOUS DISEASE

Sood, Sunil (MD) Ped Inf
Schneider Children's Hosp
269-01 76th Ave; New Hyde Park, NY 11040;
(718) 470-3480; **BDCERT:** Ped 87; Ped Inf 94; **MS:**
India 76; **RES:** Ped, Brown Mem Hosp, Punjab,
India 78-81; Ped, Baltimore City Hosp, Baltimore,
MD 83; **FEL:** Ped, Tulane U Med Ctr, New Orleans,
LA 85-88; Inf, Georgetown U Hosp, Washington,
DC 83-85; **FAP:** Assoc Prof Albert Einstein Coll
Med; **SI:** *Lyme Disease;* **HMO:** Blue Choice Blue Cross
& Blue Shield Choicecare Magnacare
LANG: Hin, Ur, Pun; 🔲 🔲 🔲 🔲 🔲 🔲 🔲
Immediately 🔲 **VISA** 🔲

PEDIATRIC PULMONOLOGY

Narula, Pramod (MD) PPul
Winthrop Univ Hosp
12 Sterling Plaza; Roslyn, NY 11576; (516) 536-
5656; **BDCERT:** Ped 97; Pul 94; **MS:** India 77; **RES:**
Ped, Winthrop Univ Hosp, Mineola, NY 87-89; **FEL:**
PPul, Columbia-Presbyterian Med Ctr, New York,
NY; **FAP:** Asst Prof Columbia P&S; **SI:** *Asthma;
Muscular Dystrophy;* **HMO:** Oxford Aetna Hlth Plan
Vytra Blue Cross CIGNA +
LANG: Hin, Rom, Ur; 🔲 🔲 🔲 🔲 🔲 🔲 🔲 🔲
A Few Days

Schaeffer, Janis (MD)   PPul
Long Island Jewish Med Ctr

3003 New Hyde Park Rd 204; New Hyde Park, NY
11042; (516) 488-7575; **BDCERT:** Ped 84; PPul
96; **MS:** SUNY Hlth Sci Ctr 79; **RES:** Ped, Long
Island Jewish Med Ctr, New Hyde Park, NY 80-83;
FEL: PPul, Columbia-Presbyterian Med Ctr, New
York, NY 83-86; **FAP:** Albert Einstein Coll Med;
HOSP: N Shore Univ Hosp-Manhasset; **SI:** *Asthma*;
HMO: Magnacare Oxford

🚹 🔟 🚹 🏧 💲   A Few Days

PEDIATRIC
RHEUMATOLOGY

Ilowite, Norman Todd (MD)Ped Rhu
Schneider Children's Hosp

269th St & 76th Ave; New Hyde Park, NY 11042;
(718) 470-3530; **BDCERT:** Ped 85; Rhu 92; **MS:**
SUNY Downstate 79; **RES:** Ped, Children's Hosp Nat
Med Ctr, Washington, DC 79-82; **FEL:** Ped Rhu, U
WA Med Ctr, Seattle, WA 82-84; **FAP:** Assoc Prof
Ped Albert Einstein Coll Med; **SI:** *Juvenile Rheumatoid
Arthritis; Lyme Disease*; **HMO:** Oxford US Hlthcre
Aetna Hlth Plan GHI Vytra +

LANG: Sp, Can, Heb; 🚹 🔟 🚹 🏧 💲 🔟
A Few Days 📧 **VISA** 💳 🔟

PEDIATRIC SURGERY

Abrams, Martin (MD)   PS
Long Island Jewish Med Ctr

195 N Village Ave; Rockville Centre, NY 11570;
(516) 678-4900; **BDCERT:** PS 75; PS 85; **MS:** U
Hlth Sci/Chicago Med Sch 54; **RES:** S, Albert
Einstein Med Ctr, Bronx, NY 55-58; S, Bronx
Muncipal Hosp Ctr, Bronx, NY 58-59; **FEL:** PdS,
Children's Hosp of Philadelphia, Philadelphia, PA
59-60; **HOSP:** New York Methodist Hosp; **SI:**
General Pediatric Surgery; **HMO:** Aetna-US
Healthcare GHI Prudential HealthNet CIGNA +

LANG: Fr, Ger, Jpn; 🔟 🔟 🚹 🏧 🔟 🔟 🔟
Immediately

Becker, Jerrold (MD)   PS
Long Island Jewish Med Ctr

BSK Pediatrics Surgical Associates, 1300 Union
Tpke 107; New Hyde Park, NY 11040; (516) 352-
5750; **BDCERT:** S 55; PS 82; **MS:** NYU Sch Med 48;
RES: S, Montefiore Med Ctr, Bronx, NY 49-50; PdS,
Children's Hosp, Boston, MA 51-52; **FEL:** PdS,
Children's Hosp of Philadelphia, Philadelphia, PA
51-52; **FAP:** Clin Prof S NYU Sch Med; **SI:**
Inflammatory Bowel Disease; Pectus Excavatum;
HMO: Oxford Unicare Primary Plus Metlife
Magnacare +

🚹 🔟 🚹 🏧 💲 🔟 🔟   A Few Days

Bohrer, Stuart (MD)   PS
N Shore Univ Hosp-Manhasset

Children's Surgical Group, 2000 N Village Ave
311; Rockville Centre, NY 11570; (516) 766-
6606; **BDCERT:** S 95; PS 95; **MS:** Baylor 77; **RES:** S,
Johns Hopkins Hosp, Baltimore, MD 78-84; PdS,
Johns Hopkins Hosp, Baltimore, MD 84-86

LANG: Sp; 🚹 🔟 🏧 💲 🔟   2-4 Weeks **VISA**

Bronsther, Burton (MD)   PS
Long Island Jewish Med Ctr

195 N Village Ave; Rockville Centre, NY 11570;
(516) 678-4900; **BDCERT:** S 56; PS 82; **MS:** SUNY
Downstate 48; **RES:** Path, Montefiore Hosp, Bronx,
NY 50-51; S, Beth Israel Hosp, Boston, MA 51-56;
FEL: PdS, Chldns Meml Hosp, Chicago, IL 56-57;
FAP: Assoc Clin Prof PS Albert Einstein Coll Med;
HOSP: Brooklyn Hosp Ctr-Downtown; **SI:** *Second
Opinion Pediatric Surgery*

🚹 🔟 🚹 🏧 💲 🔟 🔟 🔟   A Few Days **VISA** 💳

Coren, Charles (MD)   PS
N Shore Univ Hosp-Manhasset

Children's Surgical Group, 320 Post Ave;
Westbury, NY 11590; (516) 997-1199; **BDCERT:**
PS 93; SCC 88; **MS:** U Cincinnati 78; **RES:** S, New
York University Med Ctr, New York, NY 79-83;
FEL: PdS, Univ Hosp SUNY Bklyn, Brooklyn, NY
83-85; **FAP:** Asst Prof S SUNY Hlth Sci Ctr; **HOSP:**
Winthrop Univ Hosp

Coryllos, Elizabeth (MD)　　　PS
Winthrop Univ Hosp

975 Franklin Ave 101; Garden City, NY 11530; (516) 671-6816; **BDCERT:** S 59; PS 53; **MS:** Cornell U 53; **RES:** S, Bellevue Hosp Ctr, New York, NY 54-57; **FEL:** S, Bellevue Hosp Ctr, New York, NY; PdS, Hosp For Sick Children, Toronto, Canada; **HOSP:** South Nassau Comm Hosp; *SI: Birth Defects In Newborns; Trauma/Sports Medicine*; **HMO:** Oxford GHI US Hlthcre Aetna Hlth Plan Empire Blue Cross +

♿ 🌙 📷 ⚕ 🏥 Mcd WC NFI A Few Days

Hong, Andrew (MD)　　　PS
Long Island Jewish Med Ctr

Schneider Childrens HospLI Jewish Med Ctr, 269-01 76th Ave; New Hyde Park, NY 11040; (718) 470-3574; **BDCERT:** PS 96; S 91; **MS:** U Wisc Med Sch 85; **RES:** S, Med Ctr Hosp of VT, Burlington, VT 85-90; **FEL:** PdS, Montreal Children's Hosp, Montreal, Canada 90-92; **FAP:** Asst Prof Albert Einstein Coll Med; **HOSP:** Schneider Children's Hosp; *SI: Minimal Access Laparoscopic; Neonatal Surgery*; **HMO:** Oxford US Hlthcre Magnacare Empire CIGNA +

LANG: Fr, Sp; ♿ 📷 ⚕ 🏥 Mcr Mcd WC NFI
Immediately 💬

Kessler, Edmund (MD)　　　PS
Long Island Jewish Med Ctr

1000 Northern Blvd Ste 250; Great Neck, NY 11570; (516) 498-9000; **BDCERT:** PS 83; **MS:** South Africa 68; **RES:** S, U Witwatersand, Johannesburg, South Africa 68-69; **FEL:** S, U Witwatersand, Johannesburg, South Africa 71-76; PdS, U Witwatersand, Johannesberg, South Africa 77-78; **FAP:** Clin Asst Prof S Cornell U; **HOSP:** New York Methodist Hosp; *SI: Tumors Pediatric; Adolescent Breast Problems*; **HMO:** HealthNet Blue Choice US Hlthcre Prucare United Healthcare +

♿ 🌙 📷 🏥 Mcr Mcd NFI

Kutin, Neil (MD)　　　PS
N Shore Univ Hosp-Manhasset

BSK Pediatric Surgical Associates, PC, 1300 Union Tpke 107; New Hyde Park, NY 11040; (516) 352-5750; **BDCERT:** S 80; PS 97; **MS:** NYU Sch Med 70; **RES:** S, New York University Med Ctr, New York, NY 71-74; S, New York University Med Ctr, New York, NY 74-75; **FEL:** PdS, Children's Hosp of Buffalo, Buffalo, NY 77-79; **FAP:** Asst Prof S NYU Sch Med; **HOSP:** Long Island Jewish Med Ctr; *SI: Hernia Repair; Intestinal Surgery*; **HMO:** Oxford GHI Aetna-US Healthcare Multiplan Empire +

LANG: Chi; ♿ 📷 🏥 💲 Immediately

PEDIATRICS

Adesman, Andrew (MD)　　　Ped
Schneider Children's Hosp

269-01 76th Ave SCH139; New Hyde Park, NY 11040; (718) 470-3540; **BDCERT:** Ped 87; **MS:** Univ Penn 81; **RES:** Ped, Children's Hosp Nat Med Ctr, Washington, DC 81-84; **FEL:** Child Development & Rehab, Children's Hosp of Philadelphia, Philadelphia, PA 84-86; **FAP:** Assoc Prof Albert Einstein Coll Med; *SI: Attention Deficit Disorders; Autism/Developmental Delay*; **HMO:** Oxford Aetna Hlth Plan

♿ 📷 ⚕ 🏥 💲 Mcd 2-4 Weeks 🩹 *VISA* 💬

Agulnek, Milton (MD)　　　Ped　 PCP
Long Island Jewish Med Ctr

1021 Old Country Rd; Plainview, NY 11803; (516) 935-4343; **BDCERT:** Ped 62; **MS:** NYU Sch Med 56; **RES:** Kings County Hosp Ctr, Brooklyn, NY 56-57; **HOSP:** N Shore Univ Hosp-Plainview; **HMO:** Chubb Champus Empire

LANG: Sp; SA/SO 🌙 📷 ⚕ 🏥 💲 NFI 2-4 Weeks

Ceron-Canas, L Carolina (MD)Ped `PCP`
Winthrop Univ Hosp

University Plaza Pediatrics, 877 Stewart Ave Ste 33; Garden City, NY; (516) 745-5621; **BDCERT:** Ped 93; **MS:** Dominica 86; **RES:** Ped, Nassau County Med Ctr, East Meadow, NY 90-92; Ped, Nassau County Med Ctr, East Meadow, NY 92-93; **HOSP:** N Shore Univ Hosp-Manhasset; *SI: Adolescent; Endocrinology;* **HMO:** Vytra Oxford NYLCare Aetna-US Healthcare CIGNA +

LANG: Sp, Frs, Fil, Fr; 🦽 🏥 📞 🔒 🚼 🛏 💲 🚾 NFI Immediately

Chianese, Maurice (MD) Ped `PCP`
N Shore Univ Hosp-Manhasset

ProHealth Care Associates, LLP, 2800 Marcus Ave Ste 207; Lake Success, NY 11021; (516) 466-1480; **BDCERT:** Ped 97; **MS:** NY Med Coll 86; **RES:** Ped, N Shore Univ Hosp-Manhasset, Manhasset, NY 86-89; Ped, N Shore Univ Hosp-Manhasset, Manhasset, NY 89-90; **FAP:** Asst Clin Prof Ped NYU Sch Med; **HOSP:** Schneider Children's Hosp; *SI: General Pediatrics; Pediatric Sports Medicine;* **HMO:** Aetna-US Healthcare Blue Choice HIP Network Oxford United Healthcare +

LANG: Sp; 🦽 🏥 📞 🔒 🚼 🛏 💲 Immediately **VISA** 💳

Copperman, Stuart (MD) Ped `PCP`
Long Island Jewish Med Ctr

3137 Hewlett Ave S; Merrick, NY 11566; (516) 378-3223; **BDCERT:** Ped 66; **MS:** SUNY Hlth Sci Ctr 60; **RES:** Long Island Jewish Med Ctr, New Hyde Park, NY 60-63; **FAP:** Assoc Prof Ped SUNY Stony Brook; **HOSP:** Winthrop Univ Hosp; *SI: Adolescent Medicine;* **HMO:** Aetna Hlth Plan Blue Cross & Blue Shield CIGNA

🦽 🏥 🔒 🚼 🛏 💲 Med NFI Immediately **VISA** 💳

Diamond, William (MD) Ped `PCP`
Winthrop Univ Hosp

1400 Wantagh Ave 102; Wantagh, NY 11793; (516) 221-6111; **BDCERT:** Ped 63; **MS:** NYU Sch Med 57; **RES:** New York University Med Ctr, New York, NY 57-58; Jacobi Med Ctr, Bronx, NY 58-60; **FEL:** Ped, Lincoln Med & Mental Hlth Ctr, Bronx, NY 60-61; **HOSP:** Long Island Jewish Med Ctr; **HMO:** Oxford CIGNA Vytra United Healthcare GHI +

LANG: Itl, Heb; 🦽 🏥 🔒 🚼 🛏 💲 Med NFI Immediately 🔳 **VISA** 💳 💳

Ente, Gerald (MD) Ped `PCP`
Winthrop Univ Hosp

530 Old Country Rd 1A; Westbury, NY 11590; (516) 333-2277; **BDCERT:** Ped 62; **MS:** NYU Sch Med 55; **RES:** Kings County Hosp Ctr, Brooklyn, NY 56-59; Jacobi Med Ctr, Bronx, NY 60; **HOSP:** Long Island Jewish Med Ctr; **HMO:** US Hlthcre Aetna Hlth Plan NYLCare Oxford GHI +

🦽 🏥 🔒 🚼 🛏 💲 Med NFI A Few Days 🔳 **VISA** 💳

Friedman, Eugene (MD) Ped
Long Island Jewish Med Ctr

271 Jericho Tpke; Floral Park, NY 11001; (516) 354-7575; **BDCERT:** Ped 73; **MS:** NY Med Coll 68; **RES:** Ped, Metropolitan Hosp Ctr, New York, NY; **FAP:** Asst Clin Prof Albert Einstein Coll Med; **HOSP:** Winthrop Univ Hosp; **HMO:** Oxford GHI United Healthcare Aetna-US Healthcare Multiplan +

LANG: Sp; 🦽 🏥 📞 🔒 🚼 🛏 💲 Immediately **VISA** 💳

Frogel, Michael (MD) Ped
Schneider Children's Hosp

Schneider Chldns Hosp, 269-01 76th Ave 173; New Hyde Park, NY 11040; (718) 470-3280; **BDCERT:** Ped 79; **MS:** Albert Einstein Coll Med 75; **RES:** Ped, Long Island Jewish Med Ctr, New Hyde Park, NY 77-78; Ped, Long Island Jewish Med Ctr, New Hyde Park, NY 76-77; **FAP:** Assoc Prof Ped Albert Einstein Coll Med

LANG: Sp; 🦽 4+ Weeks

Giannattasio, Thomas (MD) Ped `PCP`
Mid-Island Hosp
1130 Park Blvd; Massapequa Park, NY 11762;
(516) 541-6584; **BDCERT:** Ped 84; **MS:** Mexico 77;
RES: Ped, Nassau County Med Ctr, East Meadow,
NY 79-82; **HOSP:** Winthrop Univ Hosp; **HMO:**
Vytra Oxford GHI Multiplan Empire +
▨ ▣ ▤ A Few Days

Glatt, Hershel (MD) Ped `PCP`
South Nassau Comm Hosp
3051 Long Beach Rd; Oceanside, NY 11572; (516)
536-2000; **BDCERT:** Ped 77; **MS:** Belgium 69; **RES:**
Maimonides Med Ctr, Brooklyn, NY 69-72; **FAP:**
Asst Clin Prof SUNY Stony Brook; **HOSP:** Winthrop
Univ Hosp; **SI:** *Pediatric Cardiology;* **HMO:** Oxford
GHI Empire Blue Cross & Shield Chubb CIGNA +
♿ ▨ ▣ ▣ ▣ ▦ ▤ ▥ A Few Days **VISA** ⬤

Goldman, Arnold (MD) Ped `PCP`
Schneider Children's Hosp
332 Willis Ave; Roslyn Heights, NY 11577; (516)
621-4333; **BDCERT:** Ped 79; **MS:** NY Med Coll 73;
RES: Long Island Jewish Med Ctr, New Hyde Park,
NY 73-76; **FEL:** PHO, Long Island Jewish Med Ctr,
New Hyde Park, NY 77-78; **FAP:** Asst Clin Prof
Albert Einstein Coll Med; **HOSP:** N Shore Univ
Hosp-Manhasset; **HMO:** Oxford NSHIP Blue Choice
PHCS
▣ ▣ ▦ ▤ A Few Days

Good, Leonard (MD) Ped `PCP`
N Shore Univ Hosp-Manhasset
1380 Northern Blvd H; Manhasset, NY 11030;
(516) 365-5500; **BDCERT:** Ped 85; **MS:** Albert
Einstein Coll Med 79; **RES:** Ped, Jacobi Med Ctr,
Bronx, NY 79-82; **HOSP:** Long Island Jewish Med
Ctr; **HMO:** Oxford Blue Choice
♿ ▨ ▣ ▣ ▦ ▤ 1 Week

Gould, Eric (MD) Ped `PCP`
Long Island Jewish Med Ctr
15 Barstow Rd; Great Neck, NY 11021; (516) 829-
9409; **BDCERT:** Ped 76; **MS:** NYU Sch Med 70;
RES: Long Island Jewish Med Ctr, New Hyde Park,
NY 70-71; New York University Med Ctr, New
York, NY 73-74; **FEL:** ChAP, Albert Einstein Med
Ctr, Bronx, NY 74-76; **FAP:** Asst Prof NY Med Coll;
HOSP: N Shore Univ Hosp-Manhasset; *SI:*
Developmental Problems; Asthma; **HMO:** HIP
Network Oxford
♿ ▨ ▣ ▣ ▣ ▦ ▤ Immediately **VISA** ⬤

Green, Abraham (MD) Ped `PCP`
Long Island Jewish Med Ctr
Five Towns Pediatrics, 115 Franklin Ave;
Woodmere, NY 11598; (516) 295-1200; **BDCERT:**
Ped 84; **MS:** Albert Einstein Coll Med 79; **RES:** Ped,
Jacobi Med Ctr, Bronx, NY 79-80; Ped, Albert
Einstein Med Ctr, Bronx, NY 80-83; **HOSP:** N Shore
Univ Hosp-Syosset; **HMO:** MDNY Oxford Blue Cross
& Blue Shield PHS GHI +
LANG: Sp, Heb; ♿ ▨ ▣ ▣ ▣ ▦ ▤ ▥
Immediately ▩ **VISA** ⬤

Greensher, Joseph (MD) Ped
Winthrop Univ Hosp
Winthrop Pediatric Assoc, 222 Station Plaza North;
Mineola, NY 11501; (516) 663-2532; **BDCERT:**
Ped 65; **MS:** Switzerland 58; **RES:** Ped, Nassau
County Med Ctr, East Meadow, NY 60-62; **FAP:**
Prof Ped SUNY Stony Brook; **SI:** *Toxicology Poison*
Prevention; Injury Prevention; **HMO:** Blue Cross &
Blue Shield Choicecare Prucare Vytra Oxford +
LANG: Sp, Ger; ♿ ▨ ▣ ▣ ▣ ▦ ▦ ▦ ▦ ▥
Immediately

Heitler, Michael (MD) Ped **PCP**
N Shore Univ Hosp-Manhasset

Childrens Med Group, 1171 Old Country Rd 2A; Plainview, NY 11803; (516) 931-4343; **BDCERT:** Ped 66; **MS:** Albert Einstein Coll Med 59; **RES:** Ped, Long Island Jewish Med Ctr, New Hyde Park, NY 59-61; **FEL:** Ped, Queens Hosp Ctr, Jamaica, NY 62-64; **FAP:** Assoc Clin Prof Med NYU Sch Med; **HOSP:** Long Island Jewish Med Ctr; **SI:** *School and Learning Problems*; **HMO:** Oxford HealthNet Prucare Aetna Hlth Plan Vytra +

LANG: Sp, Grk, Itl, Sgn; 🔾 🆂 🅰 ⏰ 💲 🆖 Immediately ▮ **VISA** ●

Horowitz, Roy (MD) Ped
Winthrop Univ Hosp

Pediatric Associates Of LI, 173 Mineola Blvd Ste 100; Mineola, NY 11501; (516) 746-2299; **BDCERT:** Ped 73; **MS:** Belgium 68; **RES:** Ped, Montefiore Med Ctr, Bronx, NY 68-70; **FEL:** Ped, City Hospital of Montreal, Montreal, Canada 67; **FAP:** Asst Chrmn ChAP SUNY Stony Brook; **HMO:** Most

LANG: Bul;

Krilov, Leonard (MD) Ped
N Shore Univ Hosp-Manhasset

North Shore Hospital, 865 Northern Blvd 104; Great Neck, NY 11021; (516) 622-5094; **BDCERT:** Ped 83; Ped 94; **MS:** Columbia P&S 78; **RES:** Ped, Johns Hopkins Hosp, Baltimore, MD 78-81; **FEL:** Ped Inf, Children's Hosp, Boston, MA 81-84; **FAP:** Assoc Prof Ped NYU Sch Med; **HMO:** Aetna Hlth Plan Empire Magnacare HIP Network Oxford +

🔾 🆂 🅰 ⏰ 💲 A Few Days **VISA** ●

Levine, Harold (MD) Ped **PCP**
N Shore Univ Hosp-Manhasset

Oyster Bay Pediatrics, 229 South St; Oyster Bay, NY 11771; (516) 922-3131; **BDCERT:** Ped 66; **MS:** SUNY Downstate 60; **RES:** Mount Sinai Med Ctr, New York, NY 64-65; **HOSP:** Winthrop Univ Hosp

LANG: Sp; 🆂 🅰 🅈 ⏰ 💲 🅼 🆖 Immediately ▮ **VISA** ●

Levine, Jeremiah (MD) Ped
Schneider Children's Hosp

269-01 76th Ave; New Hyde Park, NY 11040; (718) 470-3430; **BDCERT:** Ped 85; Ge 97; **MS:** Harvard Med Sch 80; **RES:** Ped, Albert Einstein Med Ctr, Bronx, NY 80-83; **FEL:** PGe, Children's Hosp, Boston, MA 83-85; **FAP:** Assoc Prof Albert Einstein Coll Med; **SI:** *Crohn's Disease; Liver Disease*; **HMO:** Oxford US Hlthcre Vytra

LANG: Heb; 🔾 🅰 ⏰ 💲 🅼 A Few Days ▮ **VISA**

Levy, Morton (MD) Ped **PCP**
N Shore Univ Hosp-Manhasset

Roslyn Pediatric Associates LLP, 73 Garden St; Roslyn Heights, NY 11577; (516) 621-9360; **BDCERT:** Ped 66; **MS:** SUNY Downstate 61; **RES:** Kings County Hosp Ctr, Brooklyn, NY 61; Mount Sinai Med Ctr, New York, NY 63; **HOSP:** Schneider Children's Hosp; **HMO:** Oxford Blue Cross & Blue Shield Multiplan

LANG: Sp; 🔾 🆂 🅰 🅈 ⏰ 💲 Immediately ▮ **VISA** ● ◈

Marino, Ronald (DO)   Ped   **PCP**
Winthrop Univ Hosp
Winthrop Pediatric Assoc, 222 Station Plaza North
611; Mineola, NY 11501; (516) 663-2532;
BDCERT: Ped 83; **MS:** Mich St U 78; **RES:** Ped,
Doctors Hosp, Columbus, OH 81; **FEL:** Behavioral
Ped, U MD Hosp, Baltimore, MD 84-85; **FAP:** Assoc
Prof SUNY Stony Brook; **SI:** *Attention Deficit
Disorders; Enuresis (Bed Wetting)*; **HMO:** NYLCare
Oxford

⬥ 🈺 🌙 📷 👥 🎰 💲   Immediately *VISA* 💳

Markowitz, James (MD)   Ped
N Shore Univ Hosp-Manhasset
North Shore University Hosp, 300 Community Dr;
Manhasset, NY 11030; (516) 562-4642; **BDCERT:**
PGe 97; **MS:** Cornell U 77; **RES:** Ped, NY Hosp-
Cornell Med Ctr, New York, NY 77-80; **FEL:** PGe, N
Shore Univ Hosp-Manhasset, Manhasset, NY 80-
83; **FAP:** Assoc Prof NYU Sch Med; **SI:** *Inflammatory
Bowel Disease; Gastroesophageal Reflux*; **HMO:**
Oxford Vytra Aetna Hlth Plan CIGNA Prucare +

⬥ 📷 👥 🎰 💲 Mcr Mcd   Immediately ▦ *VISA* 💳
💳

Rabinowicz, Morris (MD)   Ped   **PCP**
N Shore Univ Hosp-Plainview
995 Old Country Rd; Plainview, NY 11803; (516)
935-7333; **BDCERT:** Ped 85; **MS:** SUNY Hlth Sci
Ctr 78; **RES:** Ped, Long Island Jewish Med Ctr, New
Hyde Park, NY 78-80; Ped, Brookdale Univ Hosp
Med Ctr, Brooklyn, NY 82-83; **HOSP:** Long Island
Jewish Med Ctr

⬥ 🈺 🌙 📷 👥 🎰 💲   A Few Days ▦ *VISA* 💳

St Louis, Yolaine (MD)   Ped   **PCP**
Bronx Lebanon Hosp Ctr
905 Uniondale Ave; Uniondale, NY 11553; (516)
485-4630; **BDCERT:** Ped 86; **MS:** Hahnemann U
81; **FEL:** PEn, Montefiore Med Ctr, Bronx, NY 84-
87; **FAP:** Assoc Albert Einstein Coll Med; **HOSP:**
Mercy Med Ctr; **SI:** *Diabetes; Short Stature*; **HMO:** US
Hlthcre Oxford Blue Cross & Blue Shield Vytra GHI
+

LANG: Fr, Cre; ⬥ 🈺 🌙 📷 🎰 💲 Mcd   A Few Days

Yadoo, Moshe (MD)   Ped   **PCP**
N Shore Univ Hosp-Glen Cove
Glen Harbor Pediatrics, 997 Glen Cove Ave; Glen
Head, NY 11545; (516) 759-1223; **BDCERT:** Ped
87; **MS:** SUNY Hlth Sci Ctr 83; **RES:** Ped, Brookdale
Univ Hosp Med Ctr, Brooklyn, NY 83-86; **FEL:** NP,
Long Island Jewish Med Ctr, New Hyde Park, NY
86-88; **HOSP:** N Shore Univ Hosp-Manhasset;
HMO: Oxford Aetna Hlth Plan Vytra US Hlthcre
NYLCare +

LANG: Heb, Itl, Sp; ⬥ 🈺 📷 👥 🎰 💲 Mcd
Immediately ▦ *VISA* 💳 💳

PHYSICAL MEDICINE & REHABILITATION

Cassvan, Arminius (MD)   PMR
Franklin Hosp Med Ctr
900 Franklin Ave; Valley Stream, NY 11582; (516)
256-6550; **BDCERT:** PMR 72; **MS:** Romania 52;
RES: PMR, New York Med Coll, New York, NY 67;
PMR, Mount Sinai Med Ctr, New York, NY 69; **FEL:**
PMR, Elmhurst City Hosp, New York, NY 68; **FAP:**
Assoc Clin Prof Med SUNY Stony Brook; **SI:**
*Electromyography-Evoked PO; Nerve Conduction
Studies*

LANG: Rom, Fr, Itl, Ger; ⬥ 📷 🎰 Mcr Mcd WC NFI
A Few Days

Root, Barry (MD)   PMR
N Shore Univ Hosp-Glen Cove
140 Jackson Ave; Syosset, NY 11791; (516) 921-
4812; **BDCERT:** PMR 88; **MS:** Ohio State U 84;
RES: Nassau County Med Ctr, East Meadow, NY 84-
87; **HOSP:** N Shore Univ Hosp-Syosset

Guide to symbols and abbreviations can be found on pages 110-113.

683

PLASTIC SURGERY

Acker, Gerald (MD)   PlS
Southside Hosp

1 Expressway Plaza 203; Roslyn Heights, NY
11577; (516) 484-8886; **BDCERT:** S 71; **MS:** Johns
Hopkins U 64; **RES:** PlS, Hosp of U Penn,
Philadelphia, PA 69-71; S, Mount Sinai Med Ctr,
New York, NY 65-69; **FEL:** Johns Hopkins Hosp,
Baltimore, MD 64-65; *SI: Cosmetic Surgery; Facial
Surgery*

🔲 🔲 🔲 🔲 🔲 *VISA*

Deane, Leland M (MD)   PlS
Winthrop Univ Hosp

999 Franklin Ave; Garden City, NY 11530; (516)
742-3404; **BDCERT:** PlS 90; **MS:** SUNY Hlth Sci Ctr
78; **RES:** S, New England Med Ctr, Boston, MA 78-
83; E VA Sch of Med, Norfolk, VA 83-85; **FEL:** HS,
Thomas Jefferson U Hosp, Philadelphia, PA 86;
FAP: Instr S; **HOSP:** N Shore Univ Hosp-Manhasset;
SI: Abdominoplasty; Liposuction; **HMO:** Oxford Vytra

🔲 🔲 🔲 🔲 🔲 🔲 🔲 🔲 Immediately▨
VISA 🔲

Di Gregorio, Vincent (MD)   PlS
Winthrop Univ Hosp

Long Island Plastic Surgical, 999 Franklin Ave;
Garden City, NY 11530; (516) 742-3404;
BDCERT: PlS 78; **MS:** Albany Med Coll 68; **RES:**
Boston Hosp, Boston, MA 69-70; Nassau County
Med Ctr, E Meadow, NY 74-76

LANG: Fr, Itl; 🔲 🔲 🔲 🔲 🔲 🔲 🔲 🔲 🔲
A Few Days ▨ *VISA* 🔲

Doctor, Naishad (MD)   PlS
Mercy Med Ctr

2000 N Village Ave 103; Rockville Centre, NY
11570; (516) 678-2517; **BDCERT:** PlS 93; S 91;
MS: India 74; **RES:** S, Univ Hosp SUNY Stony
Brook, Stony Brook, NY 83-87; PlS, U UT Hosp, Salt
Lake City, UT 88-90; **FEL:** Burns, Univ Hosp SUNY
Stony Brook, Stony Brook, NY 87-88; **HOSP:**
Winthrop Univ Hosp; **HMO:** United Healthcare
Multiplan Oxford Vytra

LANG: Hin; 🔲 🔲 🔲 🔲 🔲 🔲 🔲 🔲 1 Week

Duboys, Elliot (MD)   PlS
N Shore Univ Hosp-Plainview

Associated Plastic Surgeons, 800 Woodbury Rd;
Woodbury, NY 11797; (516) 822-8181; **BDCERT:**
PlS 85; **MS:** Belgium 77; **RES:** S, Univ Hosp SUNY
Stony Brook, Stony Brook, NY 77-82; PlS, Nassau
County Med Ctr, East Meadow, NY 82-84; **FAP:**
SUNY Stony Brook; **HOSP:** Univ Hosp SUNY Stony
Brook; *SI: Cosmetic and Reconstructive Surgery;
Congenital Deformities;* **HMO:** Oxford Magnacare
Vytra Blue Choice +

LANG: Fr; 🔲 🔲 🔲 🔲 🔲 🔲 🔲 🔲 🔲 A Few Days
VISA 🔲

Dubuoys, Elliot (MD)   PlS
N Shore Univ Hosp-Plainview

800 Woodbury Rd; Woodbury, NY 11797; (516)
921-2244; **BDCERT:** PlS 85; **MS:** Belgium 77; **RES:**
S, Univ Hosp SUNY Stony Brook, Stony Brook, NY
77-82; **FEL:** PlS, Nassau County Med Ctr, East
Meadow, NY 82-84; **FAP:** Assoc Clin Prof SUNY
Stony Brook; *SI: Reconstructive, Cosmetic; Pediatric;*
HMO: Oxford Vytra United Healthcare

LANG: Fr; 🔲 🔲 🔲 🔲 🔲 🔲 🔲 A Few Days *VISA*
🔲

Feinberg, Joseph (MD)   PlS
N Shore Univ Hosp-Manhasset

New York Plastic Surgical, 1201 Northern Blvd
202; Manhasset, NY 11030; (516) 869-8282;
BDCERT: PlS 80; **MS:** Cornell U 73; **RES:** S, NY
Hosp-Cornell Med Ctr, New York, NY 73-76; NY
Hosp-Cornell Med Ctr, New York, NY 76-78; **FEL:**
Mem Sloan Kettering Cancer Ctr, New York, NY
78; **FAP:** Asst Clin Prof S Cornell U; **HOSP:** NY
Hosp-Cornell Med Ctr; *SI: Cosmetic Surgery; Face
Lifts*

🔲 🔲 🔲 🔲 🔲 🔲 🔲 🔲 🔲 2-4 Weeks ▨ *VISA*

Freedman, Alan (MD)   PlS
Winthrop Univ Hosp

1575 Hillside Ave 100; New Hyde Park, NY 11040; (516) 488-8900; **BDCERT:** PlS 93; **MS:** Univ Mass Sch Med 81; **RES:** S, Hosp of U Penn, Philadelphia, PA 81-83; S, U KY Hosp, Lexington, KY 83-86; **FEL:** PlS, Mayo Clinic, Rochester, MN 87-89; PlS, Mem Sloan Kettering Cancer Ctr, New York, NY 89-90; **FAP:** Asst Prof S Albert Einstein Coll Med; **HOSP:** N Shore Univ Hosp-Manhasset; *SI: Reconstructive Microsurgery; Cosmetic Surgery;* **HMO:** GHI Magnacare PHS US Hlthcre Aetna Hlth Plan +

🔲 🔲 🔲 🔲 🔲 🔲 🔲 🔲 1 Week 🔲 **VISA** 🔲 🔲

Funt, David (MD)   PlS
South Nassau Comm Hosp

19 Irving Pl; Woodmere, NY 11598; (516) 295-0404; **BDCERT:** PlS 87; **MS:** Geo Wash U Sch Med 79; **RES:** PlS, Montefiore Med Ctr, Bronx, NY 83-85; S, Montefiore Med Ctr, Bronx, NY 79-83; **FAP:** Asst Clin Prof Albert Einstein Coll Med; **HOSP:** Winthrop Univ Hosp; *SI: Cosmetic Surgery; Liposuction;* **HMO:** GHI Oxford Magnacare CIGNA

🔲 🔲 🔲 🔲 🔲 🔲 🔲 🔲 🔲 1 Week **VISA** 🔲 🔲

Gallagher, Pamela (MD)   PlS
Winthrop Univ Hosp

Long Island Plastic Surgical, 999 Franklin Ave; Garden City, NY 11530; (516) 742-3404; **BDCERT:** PlS 80; **MS:** U Chicago-Pritzker Sch Med 74; **RES:** S, NY Hosp-Cornell Med Ctr, New York, NY 74-77; PlS, NY Hosp-Cornell Med Ctr, New York, NY 77-79; **FAP:** Clin Instr Cornell U; **HOSP:** N Shore Univ Hosp-Forest Hills; *SI: Cleft Lip and Palate Surgery; Breast Surgery;* **HMO:** Vytra Oxford MDLI Blue Cross Guardian +

🔲 🔲 🔲 🔲 🔲 🔲 🔲 🔲 🔲 2-4 Weeks 🔲 **VISA**

Gold, Alan (MD)   PlS
N Shore Univ Hosp-Manhasset

999 Franklin Ave; Garden City, NY 11530; (516) 742-3404; **BDCERT:** PlS 79; **MS:** SUNY Hlth Sci Ctr 71; **RES:** S, N Shore Univ Hosp-Manhasset, Manhasset, NY 71-75; PlS, Univ Hosp SUNY Bklyn, Brooklyn, NY 76-78; **FEL:** HS, Nassau County Med Ctr, East Meadow, NY 75-76; **FAP:** Assoc Clin Prof S Cornell U; **HOSP:** N Shore Univ Hosp-Glen Cove; *SI: Cosmetic Surgery*

LANG: Fr, Sp; 🔲 🔲 🔲 🔲 🔲 🔲 🔲 🔲 🔲 1 Week 🔲 **VISA** 🔲

Gotkin, Robert (MD)   PlS
Mercy Med Ctr

Cosmetique Dermatology, Laser & Plastic Surgery, LLP, 31 Northern Blvd; Greenvale, NY 11548; (516) 484-9000; **BDCERT:** PlS 90; **MS:** Howard U 80; **RES:** S, Univ Hosp SUNY Stony Brook, Stony Brook, NY 81-85; Georgetown U Hosp, Washington, DC 86-88; **FEL:** PlS, Georgetown U Hosp, Washington, DC 86-88; Burn Care, Univ Hosp SUNY Stony Brook, Stony Brook, NY 85-86; **HOSP:** Winthrop Univ Hosp; *SI: Facial Cosmetic Surgery; Breast & Body Contouring*

🔲 🔲 🔲 🔲 🔲 🔲 🔲 🔲 **VISA** 🔲

Grant, Robert (MD)   PlS
N Shore Univ Hosp-Manhasset

N Shore Univ Hosp Division of Plastic Surgery, 825 Northern Blvd; Great Neck, NY 11021; (516) 465-8770; **BDCERT:** S 91; PlS 93; **MS:** Albany Med Coll 83; **RES:** S, NY Hosp-Cornell Med Ctr, New York, NY 83-88; PlS, NY Hosp-Cornell Med Ctr, New York, NY 88-90; **FEL:** GVS, New York University Med Ctr, New York, NY 90-91; SHd, Bellevue Hosp Ctr, New York, NY 90-91; **FAP:** Asst Clin Prof NYU Sch Med; **HOSP:** NY Hosp-Cornell Med Ctr; *SI: Reconstructive Surgery; Cosmetic Surgery;* **HMO:** Oxford United Healthcare Aetna Hlth Plan HIP Network CIGNA +

🔲 🔲 🔲 🔲 🔲 🔲 🔲 🔲 🔲 🔲

Groeger, William (MD) PlS
Long Beach Med Ctr
1800 Rockaway Ave 210; Hewlett, NY 11557; (516) 887-5502; **BDCERT:** PlS 82; **MS:** SUNY Downstate 72; **RES:** S, Beth Israel Med Ctr, New York, NY 72-77; PlS, Univ Hosp SUNY Bklyn, Brooklyn, NY 77-79; **HOSP:** South Nassau Comm Hosp; **HMO:** GHI US Hlthcre Oxford United Healthcare Prucare +

♿ 📷 📷 📷 **S** Mcr NFl   A Few Days

Harris, Alvin H (MD) PlS
Long Island Jewish Med Ctr
1129 Northern Blvd 403; Manhasset, NY 11030; (516) 365-1041; **BDCERT:** PlS 66; S 63; **MS:** Harvard Med Sch 55; **RES:** PlS, U Hosp of Cleveland, Cleveland, OH 61-63; S, U Hosp of Cleveland, Cleveland, OH 55-61; **FEL:** Head & Neck S, Roswell Park Cancer Inst, Buffalo, NY 63; Nat Cancer Inst, Bethesda, MD 57-59; **FAP:** Asst Clin Prof PlS Cornell U; **HOSP:** N Shore Univ Hosp-Manhasset; *SI: Breast Surgery-Cosmetic Reconstruction; Cosmetic Surgery;* **HMO:** PHS Multiplan Aetna-US Healthcare CIGNA Oxford +

♿ 📷 📷 📷 📷 **S** Mcr Mcd WC NFl 2-4 Weeks
VISA

Karen, Joel (MD) PlS
N Shore Univ Hosp-Syosset
25 Central Park Rd; Plainview, NY 11803; (516) 822-3232; **BDCERT:** PlS 80; **MS:** U Hlth Sci/Chicago Med Sch 63; **RES:** S, New England Med Ctr, Boston, MA 63-69; PlS, U TX Med Branch Hosp, Galveston, TX 68-72; **FEL:** S, Malmo General Hospital, Lund, Sweden 66-67; **HOSP:** Mid-Island Hosp; *SI: Breast Surgery; Cosmetic Facial Surgery;* **HMO:** Oxford Aetna-US Healthcare Multiplan Magnacare GHI +

LANG: Swd; ♿ 📷 📷 📷 📷 **S** Mcr WC NFl 1 Week
VISA

Kaufman, Seth (MD) PlS
Long Beach Med Ctr
South Shore Plastic Surgical Group, PC, 1175 W Broadway; Hewlett, NY 11557; (516) 295-0085; **BDCERT:** PlS 80; **MS:** SUNY Hlth Sci Ctr 69; **RES:** S, Kings County Hosp Ctr, Brooklyn, NY 69-74; PlS, Kings County Hosp Ctr, Brooklyn, NY 74-76; **HOSP:** South Nassau Comm Hosp; *SI: Cosmetic Surgery; Ultrasonic Liposuction;* **HMO:** Oxford PHCS

LANG: Itl; ♿ 📷 📷 📷 **S** Mcr WC NFl *VISA*

Keller, Alex (MD) PlS
Long Island Jewish Med Ctr
900 Northern Blvd 130; Great Neck, NY 11021; (516) 482-1100; **BDCERT:** PlS 84; S 81; **MS:** NYU Sch Med 75; **RES:** S, Long Island Jewish Med Ctr, New Hyde Park, NY 78-80; PlS, New York University Med Ctr, New York, NY 80-82; **FEL:** Microsurgery, New York University Med Ctr, New York, NY 82-83; **FAP:** Asst Clin Prof PlS NYU Sch Med; **HOSP:** N Shore Univ Hosp-Forest Hills; *SI: Breast Reconstruction; Cosmetic Surgery;* **HMO:** Aetna Hlth Plan Blue Choice Choicecare

LANG: Fr, Sp, Heb; ♿ 📷 📷 📷 📷 **S** Mcr WC NFl
VISA

Kessler, Martin E (MD) PlS
South Nassau Comm Hosp
242 Merrick Rd Ste 302; Rockville Center, NY 11570; (516) 352-3533; **BDCERT:** PlS 87; HS 95; **MS:** Cornell U 80; **RES:** NY Hosp-Cornell Med Ctr, New York, NY 83-85; NY Hosp-Cornell Med Ctr, New York, NY 81-83; **FEL:** Microsurgery, Cleveland Clinic Hosp, Cleveland, OH 85-86; **HOSP:** Winthrop Univ Hosp; *SI: Aesthetic Surgery; Reconstructive Surgery;* **HMO:** Aetna Hlth Plan Choicecare US Hlthcre

LANG: Sp; ♿ 📷 📷 **S** Mcr WC NFl A Few Days
VISA

Leipziger, Lyle S (MD)   PlS
Long Island Jewish Med Ctr
900 Northern Blvd Ste 240; Great Neck, NY
11021; (516) 829-4588; **BDCERT:** PlS 94; **MS:**
Cornell U 85; **RES:** PlS, NY Hosp-Cornell Med Ctr,
New York, NY 88-90; **FEL:** Craniofacial S, Johns
Hopkins Hosp, Baltimore, MD; **FAP:** Asst Prof
Albert Einstein Coll Med; *SI: Cosmetic Surgery;
Breast Enhancement*; **HMO:** Oxford Blue Cross
Magnacare +

 ⛭ 📞 📷 📋 🏥 💲 Mcr NFI 2-4 Weeks **VISA** 💳

Lukash, Frederick (MD)   PlS
Long Island Jewish Med Ctr
1129 Northern Blvd; Manhasset, NY 11030; (516)
365-0194; **BDCERT:** PlS 82; **MS:** Tulane U 73;
RES: S, Emory U Hosp, Atlanta, GA 73-75; Univ
Hosp SUNY Stony Brook, Stony Brook, NY 75-80;
FEL: PlS, Mass Gen Hosp, Boston, MA 80-81; **FAP:**
Asst Prof S Albert Einstein Coll Med; **HOSP:**
Schneider Children's Hosp; *SI: Cosmetic Surgery;
Pediatric Plastic Surgery*

 ⛭ 📞 📷 📋 🏥 💲 WC NFI A Few Days 🏧 **VISA**
💳 💳

Silberman, Mark (MD)   PlS
N Shore Univ Hosp-Glen Cove
Plastic Surgery Group, 2001 Marcus Ave W98;
New Hyde Park, NY 11042; (516) 352-3533;
BDCERT: PlS 88; **MS:** SUNY Downstate 80; **RES:** S,
Mount Sinai Med Ctr, New York, NY 80; PlS, Univ
Hosp SUNY Bklyn, Brooklyn, NY 83-85; **HOSP:**
Winthrop Univ Hosp; *SI: Aesthetic Breast Surgery;
Liposuction*; **HMO:** Oxford Vytra

LANG: Sp; ⛭ 📞 📷 📋 🏥 Mcr WC NFI A Few Days
🏧 **VISA** 💳

Simpson, Roger (MD)   PlS
Nassau County Med Ctr
Long Island Plastic Surgical, 999 Franklin Ave;
Garden City, NY 11530; (516) 742-3404;
BDCERT: PlS 81; HS 89; **MS:** Belgium 74; **RES:** S,
Nassau Co Med Ctr, E Meadow, NY 74-78; PlS,
Nassau Co Med Ctr, E Meadow, NY 78-80; **FEL:** HS,
Roosevelt Hosp, New York, NY 80-81; **FAP:** Asst
Clin Prof S SUNY Stony Brook; **HOSP:** Winthrop
Univ Hosp; *SI: Hand Surgery; Breast Reconstruction*;
HMO: Choicecare CIGNA

 ⛭ 📞 📷 🏥 💲 Mcr Mcd WC NFI 2-4 Weeks 🏧 **VISA**

Sklansky, B Donald (MD)   PlS
N Shore Univ Hosp-Manhasset
1201 Northern Blvd 202; Manhasset, NY 11030;
(516) 869-8282; **BDCERT:** PlS 79; Oto 76; **MS:**
SUNY Downstate 69; **RES:** Hosp of U Penn,
Philadelphia, PA 69-70; Mass Gen Hosp, Boston,
MA 73-76; **FEL:** Mem Sloan Kettering Cancer Ctr,
New York, NY 77; Nat Cancer Inst, Bethesda, MD
71-73; **FAP:** Asst Clin Prof Cornell U; **HOSP:** NY
Hosp-Cornell Med Ctr; *SI: Cosmetic Surgery;
Liposuction*; **HMO:** Oxford Multiplan PHCS Aetna
Hlth Plan PHS +

 ⛭ 📞 📷 📋 🏥 💲 Mcr WC NFI 2-4 Weeks **VISA**

PSYCHIATRY

Bailine, Samuel (MD)   Psyc
Long Island Jewish Med Ctr
5 Ridgeway Rd; Port Washington, NY 11050;
(516) 883-3304; **BDCERT:** Psyc 70; **MS:** NYU Sch
Med 64; **RES:** Tulane U Med Ctr, New Orleans, LA
65-68; **FAP:** Asst Prof Psyc Albert Einstein Coll
Med; **HMO:** Travelers Blue Cross & Blue Shield GHI
Blue Choice HealthNet +

 📞 📷 📋 🏥 Mcr WC NFI 1 Week

Behr, Raymond (MD)   Psyc
Long Island Jewish Med Ctr
81 Arleigh Rd A; Great Neck, NY 11021; (516)
482-1980; **BDCERT:** Psyc 81; ChAP 82; **MS:** South
Africa 73; **RES:** Psyc, Long Island Jewish Med Ctr,
New Hyde Park, NY 76-78; **FEL:** ChAP, Long Island
Jewish Med Ctr, New Hyde Park, NY 78-80; **FAP:**
Asst Clin Prof Albert Einstein Coll Med; *SI:
Depression; Manic Depressive Illness*; **HMO:** None

 SA/SU 📷 📋 🏥 💲 1 Week

Benjamin, John (MD)   Psyc
Mercy Med Ctr
20 Canterbury Rd; Great Neck, NY 11021; (516)
482-7797; **BDCERT:** Psyc 83; GerPsy 92; **MS:**
India 69; **RES:** Psyc, N Shore Univ Hosp-Manhasset,
Manhasset, NY; **FEL:** Psyc, N Shore Univ Hosp-
Manhasset, Manhasset, NY; *SI: Depression; Anxiety
Disorders*; **HMO:** Oxford Empire Blue Cross & Shield
PHS United Healthcare

LANG: Pol; ⛭ 📷 📋 🏥 💲 A Few Days

Bhatt, Ashok (MD)   Psyc
Long Beach Med Ctr

Long Island Psychiatric Associates, PC, 871 E Park Ave; Long Beach, NY 11561; (516) 889-8844; **BDCERT:** Psyc 85; **MS:** India 76; **RES:** Psyc, Long Island Jewish Med Ctr, New Hyde Park, NY 77-81; *SI: Depression; Psychopharmacology;* **HMO:** Blue Cross VBH

LANG: Hin, Rom; ⚑ 🄲 🅰 🄼 🎞 🅂 Mcr
A Few Days

Budman, Cathy L (MD)   Psyc
N Shore Univ Hosp-Manhasset

Dept Psychiatry & Neurology N Shore Univ Hosp, 50 Murray Ave; Manhasset, NY 11030; (516) 562-3994; **BDCERT:** Psyc 91; **MS:** SUNY Buffalo 84; **RES:** Psyc, Langley Porter Psych Inst, San Francisco, CA 84-86; **FEL:** N Shore Univ Hosp-Manhasset, Manhasset, NY 88-90; N Shore Univ Hosp-Manhasset, Manhasset, NY 90-91; **FAP:** Asst Prof Psyc NYU Sch Med; *SI: Tourette's Syndrome; Neuropsychiatry-Child & Adult;* **HMO:** Oxford Blue Choice

⚑ 🄲 🅰 🄼 🎞 🅂 Mcr   A Few Days ▨ **VISA**

Carone, Patrick F (MD)   Psyc
Mercy Med Ctr

2000 N Village Ave #305; Rockville Centre, NY 11570; (516) 766-2871; **BDCERT:** Psyc 77; **MS:** Johns Hopkins U 70; **RES:** Yale-New Haven Hosp, New Haven, CT 74-76; **FEL:** Yale-New Haven Hosp, New Haven, CT 76; *SI: Geriatric Psychiatry; Depression;* **HMO:** Blue Cross & Blue Shield Oxford VBH Uniformed Services

⚑ 🅰 🄼 🎞 🅂 Mcr Mcd WC NfI   4+ Weeks

Fink, Max (MD)   Psyc
Univ Hosp SUNY Stony Brook

PO Box 457; St James, NY 11780; (718) 470-8366; **BDCERT:** Psyc 54; N 52; **MS:** NYU Sch Med 45; **RES:** N, Montefiore Med Ctr, Bronx, NY 48; N, Bellevue Hosp Ctr, New York, NY 49-51; **FEL:** Psyc, Hillside Hosp, Glen Oaks, NY 52-53; **FAP:** Prof Psyc SUNY Stony Brook; **HOSP:** Long Island Jewish Med Ctr; *SI: Electroshock and Depression; Psychopharmacology;* **HMO:** None

🅰 Mcr   A Few Days

Fleishman, Stewart (MD)   Psyc
Long Island Jewish Med Ctr

107 Northern Blvd; Great Neck, NY 11021; (516) 829-1958; **BDCERT:** Psyc 85; **MS:** Mexico 79; **RES:** Long Island Jewish Med Ctr, New Hyde Park, NY 80-84; **FEL:** Psyc Onc, Mem Sloan Kettering Cancer Ctr, New York, NY 84-86; **FAP:** Asst Clin Prof Albert Einstein Coll Med; *SI: Cancer Symptom Management; Cancer Survivors;* **HMO:** Oxford Empire Blue Cross & Shield

⚑ 🅂   1 Week

Glenn, Jules (MD)   Psyc

8 Preston Rd; Great Neck, NY 11023; (516) 482-6302; **BDCERT:** Psyc 57; **MS:** NYU Sch Med 46; **RES:** N, Bellevue Hosp Ctr, New York, NY 47-48; Psyc, USPHS Hosp, Fort Worth, TX 49-50; **FEL:** ChAP, NYS Psychiatric Institute, New York, NY 50-57; Child Psychoanalysis, NYS Psychiatric Institute, New York, NY 53-62; **FAP:** Clin Prof NYU Sch Med; *SI: Anxiety; Depression*

🅰 🄼 🎞 Mcr   A Few Days

Gross, Lillian (MD)   Psyc
N Shore Univ Hosp-Manhasset

55 Blue Bird; Great Neck, NY 11023; (516) 466-6360; **BDCERT:** Psyc 73; ChAP 74; **MS:** Duke U 59; **RES:** Ped, Kingsbrook Jewish Med Ctr, Brooklyn, NY 60-62; Psyc, Kings County Hosp Ctr, Brooklyn, NY 67-70; **FEL:** ChAP, Brooklyn Jewish Hosp, Brooklyn, NY; ChAP, Kings County Hosp Ctr, Brooklyn, NY; **FAP:** Assoc Clin Prof SUNY Downstate; *SI: Dissociative Disorders; Trauma;* **HMO:** NSHIP

⚑ 🄲 🅰 🄼 🎞 🅂 WC NfI   A Few Days

Katus, Eli (MD)   Psyc
N Shore Univ Hosp-Manhasset

1035 Route 106; East Norwich, NY 11732; (516) 922-5607; **BDCERT:** Psyc 90; ChAP 91; **MS:** Germany 82; **RES:** Psyc, N Shore Univ Hosp-Manhasset, Manhasset, NY 84; **FEL:** ChAP, N Shore Univ Hosp-Manhasset, Manhasset, NY 88; **HOSP:** Winthrop Univ Hosp; *SI: Psychopharmacology; Psychotherapy;* **HMO:** VBH CIGNA Aetna Hlth Plan Oxford

LANG: Nwg, Ger, Fr; ⚑ 🄲 🅰 🄼 🎞 🅂
A Few Days

Katz, Jack (MD) Psyc
N Shore Univ Hosp-Manhasset

400 Community Drive 81; Manhasset, NY 11030;
(516) 562-3065; **BDCERT:** Psyc 68; **MS:** Albert
Einstein Coll Med 60; **RES:** Med, Jackson Mem Hosp,
Miami, FL 60-61; Psyc, Montefiore Med Ctr, Bronx,
NY 64-66; **FEL:** Psyc, Albert Einstein Med Ctr,
Bronx, NY 66-68; **FAP:** Prof of Clin Psyc NYU Sch
Med; **SI:** *Eating Disorders; Anxiety & Depression;*
HMO: Aetna Hlth Plan HIP Network Oxford Merit
Behavioral Health Plans Multiplan +

🔧 🅲 📷 🔧 Mcr 1 Week

Martin, Robert (MD) Psyc
Long Island Jewish Med Ctr

14 Buckingham Ave; Great Neck, NY 11021;
(516) 482-6424; **BDCERT:** Psyc 72; **MS:** Med Coll
Ga 64; **RES:** Psyc, Mount Sinai Med Ctr, New York,
NY 65-68; **FAP:** Asst Clin Prof Albert Einstein Coll
Med; **HOSP:** N Shore Univ Hosp-Manhasset; **SI:**
Psychosomatics; Sleep/Insomnia; **HMO:** CIGNA
Travelers VBH

🔧 🅲 📷 🔧 🎬 Mcr A Few Days

Mendelsohn, Irwin (MD) Psyc
Nassau County Med Ctr

85 Orange Dr; Jericho, NY 11753; (516) 433-
5744; **BDCERT:** Psyc 69; **MS:** SUNY Hlth Sci Ctr
56; **RES:** IM, Jewish Hosp, Brooklyn, NY 57-59;
Psyc, Creedmoor State Hosp, 62-65; **FEL:** Cv, SUNY
Hlth Scie Ctr, Brooklyn, NY 59-60; Psyc, NY Sch
Psychiatry, 62-67; **FAP:** Asst Clin Prof Psyc SUNY
Stony Brook; **SI:** *Psychosomatic;* **HMO:** Blue Cross &
Blue Shield Independent Health Plan Metlife

🔧 📷 🔧 Mcr WC Immediately

Reddy, Stanley (MD) Psyc
Hempstead Gen Hosp Med Ctr

871 E Park Ave; Long Beach, NY 11561; (516)
889-8844; **BDCERT:** Psyc 81; **MS:** India 71; **RES:**
Elmhurst Hosp Ctr, Elmhurst, NY 74-78; **HOSP:**
Long Beach Med Ctr; **HMO:** Blue Cross

🔧 🅲 📷 🔧 Mcr

Sabot, Lawrence M (MD) Psyc
New York University Med Ctr

Lawrence M Sabot, MD PC, 38 Woodland Rd;
Roslyn, NY 11576; (516) 365-8924; **BDCERT:**
Psyc 70; ChAP 70; **MS:** SUNY Downstate 58; **RES:**
Psyc, Kings Co Hosp, Brooklyn, NY 59-62; **FEL:**
ChAP, Montefiore Med Ctr, Bronx, NY 62-64; **FAP:**
Assoc Clin Prof NYU Sch Med

🅲 🔧 🎬 Immediately

Sami, Sherif (MD) Psyc
N Shore Univ Hosp-Manhasset

7 Bond St; Great Neck, NY 11021; (516) 487-
9191; **BDCERT:** Psyc 73; GerPsy 95; **MS:** Egypt 61;
RES: Cairo Univ Hosp, Cairo, Egypt 64-66;
Elmhurst Hosp Ctr, Elmhurst, NY 67-69; **FEL:**
Albert Einstein Med Ctr, Bronx, NY 70; **HOSP:** Long
Island Jewish Med Ctr; **SI:** *Depression and Mood
Disorders; Panic Disorders/Geriatrics;* **HMO:** None

LANG: Ar; 🔧 🅲 📷 🔧 🎬 💲 Immediately

Wolfman, Cyrus (MD) Psyc
Brookdale Univ Hosp Med Ctr

973 Benton St; Woodmere, NY 11598; (516) 569-
5490; **BDCERT:** Psyc 70; **MS:** Univ Penn 54; **RES:**
Psyc, Philadelphia Gen Hosp, Philadelphia, PA 61-
64; **SI:** *Psychiatry; Psychotherapy;* **HMO:**
Independent Health Plan

🔧 🆂🅄 🅲 📷 🔧 🎬 Mcr Immediately

PULMONARY DISEASE

Blum, Alan (MD) Pul
South Nassau Comm Hosp

Pulmonary & Critical Care, 1800 Rockaway Ave
204; Hewlett, NY 11557; (516) 593-9500;
BDCERT: IM 81; Pul 97; **MS:** Mexico 77; **RES:** IM,
Elmhurst Hosp Ctr, Elmhurst, NY 78-81; **FEL:** Pul,
Elmhurst Hosp Ctr, Elmhurst, NY 81-83; **HOSP:**
Franklin Hosp Med Ctr; **SI:** *Chronic Obstructive Lung
Disease; Asthma*

LANG: Sp, Itl, Heb, Yd; 🔧 🅲 📷 🔧 🎬 💲 Mcr WC NFI
A Few Days

Guide to symbols and abbreviations can be found on pages 110-113.

689

Cohen, David (MD) Pul PCP
N Shore Univ Hosp-Manhasset
560 Northern Blvd Ste203; Great Neck, NY 11021; (516) 482-0600; **BDCERT:** IM 69; **MS:** SUNY Downstate 62; **RES:** IM, Jewish Hosp Med Ctr, Brooklyn, NY 62-64; U CO Hospital, Denver, CO 64-66; **FEL:** Pul, Albert Einstein Med Ctr, Bronx, NY 68-69; **SI:** *Primary Care; Respiratory Disease;* **HMO:** Oxford Blue Cross Chubb PHS

⬇ 🏥 🄲 🔳 🔳 🏧 🅂 Mcr   Immediately **VISA** 💳

Cohen, Michael (MD) Pul PCP
N Shore Univ Hosp-Manhasset
North Shore Internal Medicine Associates, PC, 560 Northern Blvd 203; Great Neck, NY 11021; (516) 482-0600; **BDCERT:** IM 72; **MS:** SUNY Syracuse 67; **RES:** IM/Pul, Montefiore Med Ctr, Bronx, NY 68-71; **FEL:** Pul, Long Island Jewish Med Ctr, New Hyde Park, NY 73-74; **FAP:** Asst Clin Prof Med Cornell U; **SI:** *Asthma*

⬇ 🏥 🄲 🔳 🔳 🏧 🅂 Mcr NfI A Few Days **VISA** 💳

Fein, Alan (MD) Pul
N Shore Univ Hosp-Manhasset
Director, Pulmonary & Critical Care Medicine, North Shore Hospital, 300 Community Dr 4 Levitt; Manhasset, NY 11030; (516) 562-4850; **BDCERT:** IM 76; Pul 78; **MS:** SUNY Downstate 73; **RES:** Albert Einstein Med Ctr, Bronx, NY 73-76; **FEL:** Pul, UC San Francisco Med Ctr, San Francisco, CA 76-78; **SI:** *Chronic Obstructive Lung Disease; Asthma*

⬇ 🄲 🔳 🔳 🏧 Mcr Mod WC NfI Immediately

Karp, Jason (MD) Pul
North Shore Pulm Assocs PC, 3003 New Hyde Park Rd; New Hyde Park, NY 11042; (516) 328-8700; **BDCERT:** IM 91; Pul 94; **MS:** SUNY Downstate 88; **RES:** IM, Montefiore Med Ctr, Bronx, NY 89-91; **FEL:** Pul, New York University Med Ctr, New York, NY 91

Marcus, Philip (MD) Pul
N Shore Univ Hosp-Manhasset
Nassau Chest Physicians, PC, 233 E Shore Rd 112; Great Neck, NY 11023; (516) 482-7810; **BDCERT:** Pul 78; CCM 89; **MS:** SUNY Downstate 73; **RES:** Long Island Jewish Med Ctr, New Hyde Park, NY 73-76; **FEL:** Pul, Queens Hosp Ctr, Jamaica, NY 76-77; VA Med Ctr-Northport, Northport, NY 77-78; **FAP:** Chrmn Med NY Coll Osteo Med; **HOSP:** St Francis Hosp-Roslyn; **SI:** *Asthma; Sarcoidosis;* **HMO:** Aetna Hlth Plan Vytra GHI United Healthcare Oxford +

LANG: Sp, Ger; ⬇ 🄲 🔳 🔳 🏧 🅂 Mcr Mod WC NfI Immediately 🔲 **VISA** 💳

Mermelstein, Steve (MD) Pul
Franklin Hosp Med Ctr
1800 Rockaway Ave 204; Hewlett, NY 11557; (516) 593-9500; **BDCERT:** IM 80; Pul 82; **MS:** Albert Einstein Coll Med 77; **RES:** Metropolitan Hosp Ctr, New York, NY 77-80; **FEL:** Pul, St Luke's Roosevelt Hosp Ctr, New York, NY 80-82; **HOSP:** South Nassau Comm Hosp

LANG: Heb; ⬇ 🄲 🏧 🅂 Mcr WC NfI A Few Days **VISA** 💳

Newmark, Ian (MD) Pul
N Shore Univ Hosp-Plainview
175 Jericho Tpke 320; Syosset, NY 11791; (516) 496-7900; **BDCERT:** Pul 86; CCM 89; **MS:** SUNY Hlth Sci Ctr 79; **RES:** IM, Nassau County Med Ctr, East Meadow, NY 79-82; **FEL:** Pul, Nassau County Med Ctr, East Meadow, NY 82-84; **FAP:** Asst Clin Prof SUNY Stony Brook; **HOSP:** N Shore Univ Hosp-Syosset; **SI:** *Asthma; Lung Cancer;* **HMO:** Oxford United Healthcare Vytra Blue Cross Aetna Hlth Plan +

⬇ 🄲 🔳 🔳 🏧 🅂 Mcr Mod WC NfI A Few Days

Niederman, Michael (MD) Pul
Winthrop Univ Hosp

Winthrop Pulmonary Assoc, 222 Station Plaza
North 400; Mineola, NY 11501; (516) 663-2834;
BDCERT: IM 80; Pul 83; **MS:** Boston U 77; **RES:** IM,
Northwestern Mem Hosp, Chicago, IL 77-80; **FEL:**
Pul, Yale-New Haven Hosp, New Haven, CT 80-83;
FAP: Prof Med SUNY Stony Brook; **SI:** *Chronic
Obstructive Lung Disease; Pneumonia;* **HMO:** Vytra
US Hlthcre Oxford United Healthcare NYLCare +

LANG: Sp; ⅏ ⓒ ⓐ ⊞ Mcr Mcd WC NFI 1 Week **VISA**
⬤

Rabinowitz, Stanley (MD) Pul
Mid-Island Hosp

4271 Hempstead Tpke 1; Bethpage, NY 11714;
(516) 796-3700; **BDCERT:** IM 79; Pul 82; **MS:** NY
Med Coll 76; **HOSP:** Brunswick Hosp Ctr
⅏ ⓒ ⓐ ⊞ ⓢ Mcr Mcd WC NFI Immediately

Rothman, Nathan (MD) Pul
St John's Epis Hosp-S Shore

360 Central Ave; Lawrence, NY 11559; (516)
569-6966; **BDCERT:** IM 77; Pul 82; **MS:** Albert
Einstein Coll Med 74; **RES:** Montefiore Med Ctr,
Bronx, NY 75-77; Montefiore Med Ctr, Bronx, NY;
FEL: Pul.; **HOSP:** South Nassau Comm Hosp; **SI:**
Chronic Obstructive Lung Disease; Asthma

LANG: Heb; ⅏ ⓐ ⅏ ⊞ ⓢ Mcr WC NFI A Few Days

Rubenstein, Roy (MD) Pul
Franklin Hosp Med Ctr

505 Hempstead Ave; Rockville Centre, NY 11570;
(516) 766-3343; **BDCERT:** IM 82; Pul 86; **MS:**
NYU Sch Med 78; **RES:** IM, Jacobi Med Ctr, Bronx,
NY 78-79; Jacobi Med Ctr, Bronx, NY 78-81; **FEL:**
Pul, Albert Einstein Med Ctr, Bronx, NY 81-82;
Albert Einstein Med Ctr, Bronx, NY 82-83; **HOSP:**
Mercy Med Ctr; **SI:** *Asthma*

⅏ ⓒ ⓐ ⅏ ⊞ ⓢ Mcr 1 Week

Schulster, Rita B (MD) Pul
Long Beach Med Ctr

442 E Waukena Ave; Oceanside, NY 11572; (516)
599-8234; **BDCERT:** IM 77; Pul 78; **MS:** Albert
Einstein Coll Med 70; **RES:** IM, Beth Israel Med Ctr,
New York, NY 71-73; IM, Beth Israel Med Ctr, New
York, NY 73-74; **FEL:** Pul, Long Island Jewish Med
Ctr, New Hyde Park, NY 74-75; Pul, Beth Israel
Med Ctr, New York, NY 75-76; **HOSP:** South
Nassau Comm Hosp; **SI:** *Asthma; Chronic Bronchitis;*
HMO: Blue Choice Oxford US Hlthcre PHS Aetna
Hlth Plan +

⅏ ⓐ ⅏ ⊞ ⓢ Mcr Mcd A Few Days

Wyner, Perry A (MD) Pul **PCP**
Mercy Med Ctr

Long Island Internal Med Assocs, 2 Lincoln Ave
201; Rockville Centre, NY 11570; (516) 536-
0600; **BDCERT:** IM 80; Pul 82; **MS:** Cornell U 77;
RES: Med Coll VA Hosp, Richmond, VA 77-80; **FEL:**
Pul, Bellevue Hosp Ctr, New York, NY; **HOSP:**
South Nassau Comm Hosp; **SI:** *Asthma; Smoking
Cessation;* **HMO:** Oxford Vytra United Healthcare
Blue Choice Multiplan +

LANG: Fr, Sp; ⅏ ⓒ ⓐ ⅏ ⊞ Mcr Immediately
VISA ⬤

Yang, Chin-tsun (MD) Pul
Franklin Hosp Med Ctr

505 Hempstead Ave; Rockville Centre, NY 11570;
(516) 766-3343; **BDCERT:** Pul 76; CCM 87; **MS:**
Taiwan 67; **RES:** IM, Taiwan 68-71; IM, Mount
Sinai Med Ctr, New York, NY 71-72; **FEL:** Pul,
Mount Sinai Med Ctr, New York, NY 74-76; **HOSP:**
Mercy Med Ctr; **SI:** *Chronic Lung Disease; Asthma,
Emphysema;* **HMO:** Chubb CIGNA Empire GHI
LANG: Chi; ⅏ SA ⓒ ⓐ ⅏ ⊞ ⓢ Mcr 1 Week

RADIATION ONCOLOGY

Bosworth, Jay (MD) RadRO
N Shore Univ Hosp-Manhasset
Long Island Radiation Therapy, 1129 Northern Blvd; Manhasset, NY 11030; (516) 365-6544; **BDCERT:** Rad 74; **MS:** Albert Einstein Coll Med 70; **RES:** Jacobi Med Ctr, Bronx, NY 71-74; **FAP:** Assoc Prof Rad NYU Sch Med; ***SI:*** *Prostate Seed Implants; Breast Cancer*; **HMO:** Blue Choice Empire US Hlthcre Vytra US Hlthcre +
LANG: Itl, Sp, Grk; ♿ ☎ 👤 📅 [Mcr] [Mcd] [WC] [NFI] A Few Days [AmEx] VISA [MasterCard]

Diamond, Ezriel (MD) RadRO
N Shore Univ Hosp-Plainview
688 Old Country Rd; Plainview, NY 11803; (516) 932-6007; **BDCERT:** Rad 82; **MS:** NYU Sch Med 78; **RES:** New York University Med Ctr, New York, NY 81; **FEL:** New York Methodist Hosp, Brooklyn, NY; **HOSP:** Mid-Island Hosp; **HMO:** Aetna Hlth Plan Oxford Prucare NYLCare Sel Pro +
♿ ☎ 📅 [Mcr] Immediately

Marin, Lorraine A (MD) RadRO
Long Island Jewish Med Ctr
Long Island Jewish Medical Center, 270-05 76th Ave; New Hyde Park, NY 11040; (718) 470-7194; **BDCERT:** Rad 86; Onc 83; **MS:** UC Davis 77; **RES:** IM, UC Davis Med Ctr, Sacramento, CA 78-80; **FEL:** Onc, Nat Cancer Inst, Bethesda, MD 81-83; RadRO, Nat Cancer Inst, Bethesda, MD 82-85; ***SI:*** *Cancer*; **HMO:** Most
LANG: Fr, Sp; ♿ [Mcr] [Mcd] A Few Days

Pollack, Jed (MD) RadRO
Long Island Jewish Med Ctr
Dept of Radiation Oncology, 270-05 76th Ave; New Hyde Park, NY 11040; (718) 470-7190; **BDCERT:** Rad 85; **MS:** U New Mexico 81; **RES:** RadRO, Mem Sloan Kettering Cancer Ctr, New York, NY 85; ***SI:*** *Head and Neck Cancer; Brain Tumors*; **HMO:** Oxford US Hlthcre 1199 CIGNA +
LANG: Sp, Heb, Chi, Fr, Yd; ♿ ☾ ☎ 📅 [Mcr] [Mcd] A Few Days VISA [MasterCard]

Rush, Stephen (MD) RadRO
St Francis Hosp-Roslyn
Long Island Radiation Therapy Ctr, 1129 Northern Blvd 101; Manhasset, NY 11030; (516) 365-6544; **BDCERT:** RadRO 90; **MS:** Howard U 83; **RES:** New York University Med Ctr, New York, NY 86-89; ***SI:*** *Brain, Head and Neck Tumors; Gynecological Cancer*
LANG: Sp, Grk, Itl; ♿ ☎ 👤 📅 [Mcr] Immediately

Saxe, Bruce (MD) RadRO
Winthrop Univ Hosp
700 Stewart Ave; Garden City, NY 11530; (516) 222-2020; **BDCERT:** Rad 66; NuM 72; **MS:** SUNY Hlth Sci Ctr 59; **RES:** Bellevue Hosp Ctr, New York, NY 59-63; Rad, Columbia-Presbyterian Med Ctr, New York, NY 63-66; **FAP:** Asst Clin Prof SUNY Stony Brook; ***SI:*** *Breast Cancer; Prostate Cancer*; **HMO:** Oxford US Hlthcre Vytra GHI
LANG: Chi, Chi; ♿ ☎ 📅 $ [Mcr] [Mcd] Immediately [AmEx] VISA [MasterCard] [Discover]

RADIOLOGY

Gold, Burton (MD) Rad
Winthrop Univ Hosp
Winthrop Radiology Associates, PC, 259 1st St; Mineola, NY 11501; (516) 663-2374; **BDCERT:** Rad 78; **MS:** Cornell U 74; **RES:** DR, NY Hosp-Cornell Med Ctr, New York, NY 75-78; **FAP:** Prof/ClinRad SUNY Stony Brook; ***SI:*** *Gastrointestinal Radiology; Breast Imaging*
♿ ☎ 📅 [Mcr] [Mcd] [WC] [NFI] Immediately

Goodman, Ken J (MD) Rad
St Francis Hosp-Roslyn
Physician's Diagnostic Imaging, 100 Port Washington Blvd; Roslyn, NY 11576; (516) 562-6511; **BDCERT:** Rad 77; **MS:** U Tex San Antonio 72; **RES:** N Shr Univ Hosp-Manhasset, Manhasset 73; NY Hosp-Cornell Med Ctr, New York, NY 74-77; **FEL:** NY Hosp-Cornell Med Ctr, New York, NY 77-78; ***SI:*** *Computer Tomography; Ultrasonography*; **HMO:** Oxford Magnacare MDNY PHS Sel Pro +
LANG: Fr, Sp; ♿ [SA SD] ☾ ☎ 👤 📅 [Mcr] [Mcd] [WC] [NFI]

Guide to symbols and abbreviations can be found on pages 110-113.

Hammel, Jay (MD)   Rad
Mid-Island Hosp

Bethpage MRI, 4273 Hempstead Tpke; Bethpage, NY 11714; (516) 579-5800; **BDCERT:** Rad 89; **MS:** SUNY Syracuse 84; **RES:** St Vincent's Med Ctr-Bridgeport, Bridgeport, CT 85-89; *SI: MRI; CT Scanning;* **HMO:** Oxford GHI Empire Multiplan Prucare +

[♿] [SA] [📞] [🏠] [🏨] [$] [Mcr] [Mcd] [WC] [NFI]   Immediately 🔲 *VISA* 💳

Khan, Arfa (MD)   Rad
Long Island Jewish Med Ctr

270-05 76th Ave C204; New Hyde Park, NY 11040; (718) 470-7177; **BDCERT:** Rad 71; **MS:** India 64; **RES:** Rad, Queens Hosp Ctr, Jamaica, NY 67-70; **FEL:** Rad, Long Island Jewish Med Ctr, New Hyde Park, NY 70-71; **FAP:** Assoc Prof Rad Albert Einstein Coll Med; *SI: Chest Radiology; Chest CT;* **HMO:** Oxford US Hlthcre Aetna-US Healthcare GHI

[♿] [SA] [🏠] [🏨] [Mcr] [Mcd]   Immediately 🔲 *VISA* 💳 🔲

Lefkowitz, Harvey (MD)   Rad
Hempstead Gen Hosp Med Ctr

Diagnostic Imaging Group, 750 Hicksville Rd; Seaford, NY 11783; (516) 520-3271; **BDCERT:** Rad 69; **MS:** SUNY Downstate 69; **RES:** Univ Hosp SUNY Bklyn, Brooklyn, NY 72-75; **HOSP:** Massapequa Gen Hosp; *SI: Breast Stereotactic Biopsy;* **HMO:** Oxford Empire GHI CIGNA Vytra +

LANG: Sp, Fr, Rus, Heb; [♿] [SA] [📞] [🏠] [🚹] [🏨] [$] [Mcr] [Mcd] [WC] [NFI]   Immediately

Rossi, Dennis (MD)   Rad
Long Beach Med Ctr

Long Island MRI, 1575 Hillside Ave 301; New Hyde Park, NY 11040; (516) 354-4200; **BDCERT:** Rad 73; **MS:** SUNY Downstate 68; **RES:** Rad, Montefiore Med Ctr, Bronx, NY 69-72; **FAP:** Assoc Clin Prof Rad SUNY Stony Brook

[♿] [SA] [📞] [🏠] [🏨] [$] [Mcr] [Mcd] [WC] [NFI]   Immediately

Sherman, Scott J (MD)   Rad
St Francis Hosp-Roslyn

100 Port Washington Blvd; Roslyn, NY 11576; (516) 562-6000; **BDCERT:** Rad 83; NuM 84; **MS:** Northwestern U 79; **RES:** Rad, NY Hosp-Cornell Med Ctr, New York, NY 80-83; NuM, NY Hosp-Cornell Med Ctr, New York, NY 84; **FEL:** Rad, NY Hosp-Cornell Med Ctr, New York, NY; *SI: CAT Scanning; Ultrasound*

LANG: Fr, Sp; [♿] [SA] [🏠] [🏨] [$] [Mcr] [Mcd] [WC] [NFI]   Immediately 🔲 *VISA* 💳

Weck, Steven (MD)   Rad
N Shore Univ Hosp-Glen Cove

North Shore Univ Hosp, Radiology; Glen Cove, NY 11542; (516) 674-7540; **BDCERT:** Rad 77; **MS:** NYU Sch Med 73; **RES:** Rad, New York University Med Ctr, New York, NY 73-77; *SI: Interventional Radiology;* **HMO:** Aetna Hlth Plan Oxford Empire Blue Cross & Shield Prudential Metlife +

[♿] [SA] [🏠] [🚹] [🏨] [$] [Mcr] [Mcd] [WC] [NFI]   A Few Days

Zito, Joseph (MD)   Rad

315 E Shore Rd; Manhasset, NY 11030; (516) 773-6611; **BDCERT:** Rad 78; **MS:** Georgetown U 74; **RES:** S, Montefiore Med Ctr, Bronx, NY 74-75; Rad, Georgetown U Hosp, Washington, DC 75-78; **FEL:** NR, Mass Gen Hosp, Boston, MA 78-79; **HMO:** Blue Choice CIGNA

[♿] [SA] [📞] [🏠] [🏨] [Mcr] [WC] [NFI] 🔲 *VISA* 💳

REPRODUCTIVE ENDOCRINOLOGY

Rosenfeld, David (MD)   RE
N Shore Univ Hosp-Manhasset

North Shore Univ Hospital, 300 Community Dr; Manhasset, NY 11030; (516) 562-4470; **BDCERT:** ObG 76; RE 80; **MS:** Univ Penn 70; **RES:** Hosp of U Penn, Philadelphia, PA 71-74; **FEL:** RE, Hosp of U Penn, Philadelphia, PA 74-76

[♿] [📞] [🏠] [🚹] [🏨] [$] [Mcr]

RHEUMATOLOGY

Blau, Sheldon P (MD)　　　Rhu
Winthrop Univ Hosp
566 Broadway; Massapequa, NY 11758; (516) 541-6262; **BDCERT:** IM 69; Rhu 72; **MS:** Albert Einstein Coll Med 61; **RES:** Montefiore Med Ctr, Bronx, NY 62-64; **FEL:** Rhu, Albert Einstein Med Ctr, Bronx, NY 64-65; *SI: Lupus; Rheumatoid Arthritis;* **HMO:** Blue Cross HealthNet

LANG: Yd; ⬛ ⬛ ⬛ ⬛ ⬛ ⬛ ⬛ Immediately ⬛
VISA ⬛

Carsons, Steven (MD)　　　Rhu
Winthrop Univ Hosp
222 Station Plaza North 430; Mineola, NY 11501; (516) 663-2097; **BDCERT:** IM 78; Rhu 80; **MS:** NY Med Coll 75; **RES:** IM, Maimonides Med Ctr, Brooklyn, NY 75-78; **FEL:** Rhu, Univ Hosp SUNY Bklyn, Brooklyn, NY 78-80; **FAP:** Assoc Prof Med SUNY Hlth Sci Ctr; *SI: Rheumatoid Arthritis; Sjogren's Syndrome;* **HMO:** Oxford Vytra Blue Choice Prucare United Healthcare +

⬛ ⬛ ⬛ ⬛ ⬛ ⬛ ⬛ 2-4 Weeks

Cohen, Daniel H (MD)　　　Rhu
St John's Epis Hosp-S Shore
Chief Rhu St Jhns Epis & Lg Bch Meml Hosps, 1157 Broadway; Hewlett, NY 11557; (516) 295-4481; **BDCERT:** Rhu 84; IM 81; **MS:** NYU Sch Med 78; **RES:** Columbia-Presbyterian Med Ctr, New York, NY 80-81; **FEL:** New York University Med Ctr, New York, NY 81-83; **FAP:** Clin Instr Med Columbia P&S; **HOSP:** Long Beach Med Ctr; *SI: Osteoporosis; Polymyalgia Rheumatica;* **HMO:** GHI Magnacare Multiplan

LANG: Sp; ⬛ ⬛ ⬛ ⬛ ⬛ ⬛ ⬛ ⬛ ⬛ 4+ Weeks

Meredith, Gary (MD)　　　Rhu
Mercy Med Ctr
242 Merrick Rd 303; Rockville Centre, NY 11570; (516) 536-9424; **BDCERT:** IM 84; Rhu 86; **MS:** NYU Sch Med 81; **RES:** Bellevue Hosp Ctr, New York, NY 81-84; **FEL:** Rhu, New York University Med Ctr, New York, NY 84-86; **FAP:** Clin Instr Med NYU Sch Med; **HOSP:** Franklin Hosp Med Ctr; *SI: Lupus; Gout;* **HMO:** Oxford MDNY Aetna Hlth Plan Empire GHI +

⬛ ⬛ ⬛ ⬛ ⬛ ⬛ 1 Week

Pellman, Elliot (MD)　　　Rhu　　PCP
Long Island Jewish Med Ctr
ProHealth Care Associates, 2800 Marcus Ave; Lake Success, NY 11042; (516) 622-6020; **BDCERT:** IM 83; **MS:** Mexico 79; **RES:** Long Island Jewish Med Ctr, New Hyde Park, NY 80-83; **FEL:** Rhu, Long Island Jewish Med Ctr, New Hyde Park, NY 83-85; **FAP:** Assoc Prof Albert Einstein Coll Med; **HOSP:** N Shore Univ Hosp-Forest Hills; *SI: Sports Medicine;* **HMO:** Blue Choice Oxford

⬛ ⬛ ⬛ ⬛ ⬛ 2-4 Weeks ⬛ *VISA* ⬛

Porges, Andrew (MD)　　　Rhu
NY Hosp Med Ctr of Queens
1157 Broadway; Hewlett, NY 11557; (516) 295-4481; **BDCERT:** IM 89; **MS:** Cornell U 86; **RES:** IM, NY Hosp-Cornell Med Ctr, New York, NY 86-89; **FEL:** Rhu, Hosp For Special Surgery, New York, NY 89-92; **FAP:** Asst Prof Cornell U; *SI: Rheumatology; Osteoporosis;* **HMO:** United Healthcare GHI Prudential

LANG: Sp, Itl; ⬛ ⬛ ⬛ ⬛ ⬛ ⬛ ⬛ A Few Days

Schorn, Karen (MD)　　　Rhu
N Shore Univ Hosp-Plainview
100 Manetto Hill Rd 306; Plainview, NY 11803; (516) 433-9026; **BDCERT:** IM 86; Rhu 92; **MS:** Mexico 82; **RES:** IM, Maimonides Med Ctr, Brooklyn, NY; **FEL:** Rhu, Univ Hosp SUNY Bklyn, Brooklyn, NY; **HOSP:** Mid-Island Hosp; *SI: Lupus; Osteoporosis;* **HMO:** Oxford ABC Health MDNY PHS Multiplan +

⬛ ⬛ ⬛ ⬛ ⬛ ⬛ ⬛ A Few Days

Sullivan, James (MD)   Rhu **PCP**
Winthrop Univ Hosp

566 Broadway; Massapequa, NY 11758; (516) 541-6262; **BDCERT:** IM 71; Rhu 80; **MS:** SUNY Hlth Sci Ctr 74; **RES:** U Mich Med Ctr, Ann Arbor, MI 74-77; **FEL:** U Mich Med Ctr, Ann Arbor, MI 77-79; **HMO:** Blue Cross Blue Choice

🔳 🔳 🔳 🔳 🔳 🔳 🔳 🔳 Immediately *VISA* 💳

Tiger, Louis H (MD)   Rhu
Winthrop Univ Hosp

566 Broadway; Massapequa, NY 11758; (516) 541-6262; **BDCERT:** IM 75; Rhu 76; **MS:** KY Med Sch, Louisville 67; **RES:** Maimonides Med Ctr, Brooklyn, NY 67-70; **FEL:** Rhu, Albert Einstein Med Ctr, Philadelphia, PA 72-74; **FAP:** Asst Clin Prof Med SUNY Stony Brook; **HOSP:** Mercy Med Ctr; *SI: Rheumatoid Arthritis; Connective Tissue Disorder;* **HMO:** Blue Choice Prucare Oxford Vytra CIGNA +

LANG: Sp, Yd, Heb; 🔳 🔳 🔳 🔳 🔳 🔳 🔳 Immediately *VISA* 💳

SPORTS MEDICINE

Hershon, Stuart (MD)   SM
N Shore Univ Hosp-Manhasset

Long Island Sports Medicine, 333 E Shore Rd Ste 101; Manhasset, NY 11030; (516) 466-3351; **BDCERT:** OrS 73; **MS:** NY Med Coll 63; **RES:** S, Georgetown U Hosp, Washington, DC 66-67; OrS, St Luke's Roosevelt Hosp Ctr, New York, NY 67-70; **FAP:** Asst Prof OrS Cornell U; **HMO:** Aetna Hlth Plan

Orlin, Harvey (MD)   SM
South Nassau Comm Hosp

36 Lincoln Ave Fl 3; Rockville Centre, NY 11570; (516) 536-2800; **BDCERT:** OrS 68; **MS:** SUNY Hlth Sci Ctr 61; **RES:** OrS, Bellevue Hosp Ctr, New York, NY 62-63; Columbia-Presbyterian Med Ctr, New York, NY 63-66; **HOSP:** Mercy Med Ctr; *SI: Arthroscopy; Total Joint Reconstruction;* **HMO:** Aetna-US Healthcare Blue Cross & Blue Shield United Healthcare Empire Vytra +

LANG: Itl, Sp, Prt; 🔳 🔳 🔳 🔳 🔳 🔳 🔳 🔳 🔳 Immediately 🔳 *VISA* 💳

Putterman, Eric A (MD)   SM
N Shore Univ Hosp-Manhasset

801 Merrick Ave; East Meadow, NY 11554; (516) 393-8800; **BDCERT:** OrS 88; **MS:** Mt Sinai Sch Med 80; **RES:** OrS, Bellevue Hosp Ctr, New York, NY 81-85; **FEL:** SM, Bellevue Hosp Ctr, New York, NY 85; **HOSP:** Winthrop Univ Hosp; *SI: Sports Injuries;* **HMO:** Aetna Hlth Plan Oxford Empire PHCS Magnacare +

🔳 🔳 🔳 🔳 🔳 🔳 🔳 🔳 🔳 Immediately 🔳 *VISA* 💳

Yerys, Paul (MD)   SM
Winthrop Univ Hosp

Island Sports Medicine, 30 Merrick Ave 100; East Meadow, NY 11554; (516) 794-7010; **BDCERT:** OrS 72; **MS:** SUNY Hlth Sci Ctr 61; **RES:** Meadowbrook Hosp, East Meadow, NY 65-70; **FAP:** Clin Prof SUNY Stony Brook; **HOSP:** Mercy Med Ctr

LANG: Hun, Sp; 🔳 🔳 🔳 🔳 🔳 🔳 🔳 🔳 1 Week 🔳

SURGERY

Auguste, Louis T (MD)   S
Long Island Jewish Med Ctr
410 Lakeville Rd 100; New Hyde Park, NY 11042;
(516) 775-2070; **BDCERT:** S 90; **MS:** Haiti 73;
RES: S, Long Island Jewish Med Ctr, New Hyde
Park, NY 75-80; **FEL:** S Onc, Roswell Park Cancer
Inst, Buffalo, NY 80-82; **FAP:** Assoc Clin Prof Albert
Einstein Coll Med; **HOSP:** N Shore Univ Hosp-
Manhasset; **SI:** *Breast Tumors; Thyroid/Parathyroid
Surgery;* **HMO:** Oxford Aetna-US Healthcare United
Healthcare 1199 Vytra +

LANG: Fr, Sp, Cre; A Few Days

Chanin, Irving (MD)   S
N Shore Univ Hosp-Glen Cove
1181 Old Country Rd; Plainview, NY 11803; (516)
681-6886; **BDCERT:** S 64; **MS:** SUNY Downstate
56; **RES:** Nassau County Med Ctr, East Meadow, NY
57-63; **FEL:** S, Nassau County Med Ctr, East
Meadow, NY 63-65; **HOSP:** Mid-Island Hosp;
HMO: US Hlthcre Oxford Blue Choice

 Immediately

Colantonio, Anthony (MD)   S
Winthrop Univ Hosp
General & Vascular Surgery of Long Island, 520
Franklin Ave; Garden City, NY 11530; (516) 746-
3310; **BDCERT:** S 90; **MS:** SUNY Hlth Sci Ctr 84;
RES: S, Montefiore Med Ctr, Bronx, NY 84-89; **FEL:**
GVS, UCLA Med Ctr, Los Angeles, CA 89-90; **HOSP:**
Mercy Med Ctr; **SI:** *Laparoscopic Surgery; Breast
Surgery;* **HMO:** Vytra Aetna Hlth Plan CIGNA GHI

LANG: Itl, Sp; Immediately

Conte, Charles (MD)   S
N Shore Univ Hosp-Manhasset
Northshore Surgical Oncology, 600 Northern Blvd
111; Great Neck, NY 11021; (516) 487-9454;
BDCERT: S 87; **MS:** Dartmouth Med Sch 81; **RES:**
Hartford Hosp, Hartford, CT 81-86; **FEL:** S Onc,
Roswell Park Cancer Inst, Buffalo, NY 86-88;
HOSP: Flushing Hosp Med Ctr; **SI:** *Breast Cancer;
Colon Cancer;* **HMO:** Oxford Aetna-US Healthcare
Magnacare PHCS

LANG: Sp; A Few Days *VISA*

De Risi, Dwight (MD)   S
N Shore Univ Hosp-Manhasset
North Shore Surgical Oncology Assoc, 600
Northern Blvd; Great Neck, NY 11021; (516) 487-
9454; **BDCERT:** S 79; **MS:** Georgetown U 73; **RES:**
S, N Shore Univ Hosp-Manhasset, Manhasset, NY
74-79; **FEL:** Path, N Shore Univ Hosp-Manhasset,
Manhasset, NY 78-79; **FAP:** Adjct Prof Cornell U;
HOSP: St Francis Hosp-Roslyn; **SI:** *Breast Disease;
Melanoma;* **HMO:** Aetna Hlth Plan Oxford

LANG: Sp, Itl; 1 Week
VISA

Forlenza, Ronald (MD)   S
N Shore Univ Hosp-Syosset
175 Jericho Tpke; Syosset, NY 11791; (516) 921-
2121; **BDCERT:** S 88; **MS:** Case West Res U 68;
RES: U WA Med Ctr, Seattle, WA 72-74; UCLA Med
Ctr, Los Angeles, CA 74-77; **HOSP:** Mid-Island
Hosp; **HMO:** Aetna Hlth Plan Travelers US Hlthcre
Choicecare

 Immediately

Friedman, Steven I (MD)   S
South Nassau Comm Hosp
77 N Centre Ave 207; Rockville Centre, NY 11570;
(516) 764-6206; **BDCERT:** S 82; **MS:** NY Med Coll
76; **RES:** Jacobi Med Ctr, Bronx, NY 76-78; Nassau
County Med Ctr, East Meadow, NY 78-81; **FAP:**
Clin Instr SUNY Stony Brook; **SI:** *Breast Surgery;
Laparoscopic Surgery;* **HMO:** Oxford Aetna Hlth Plan
GHI Vytra Empire +

 Immediately

Geiss, Alan (MD)   S
N Shore Univ Hosp-Manhasset
N Shore Univ Hosp, Director Laparoscopy Ctr, 221
Jericho Tpke; Syosset, NY 11791; (516) 496-2752;
BDCERT: S 96; **MS:** U Hlth Sci/Chicago Med Sch
70; **RES:** Albert Einstein Med Ctr, Bronx, NY 70-71;
Cleveland Clinic Hosp, Cleveland, OH 73-77; **FAP:**
Assoc Prof of Clin S Cornell U; **SI:** *Laparoscopic
Surgery; Abdominal Surgery;* **HMO:** Vytra Oxford
Blue Cross & Blue Shield Empire CIGNA +

 1 Week *VISA*

Goldberg, Max (MD) S
N Shore Univ Hosp-Manhasset

759 Lincoln Blvd; Long Beach, NY 11561; (516) 889-1600; **BDCERT:** S 70; **MS:** Ireland 59; **RES:** England 60-61; Central Middlesex Hosp, Middlesex, NJ 61-64; **SI:** *Laparoscopic Surgery; Breast Cancer; Colorectal;* **HMO:** Chubb Oxford Blue Choice Multiplan GHI +

LANG: Fr; ♿ 🅿 🏨 💲 Mcr WC NFI   A Few Days

Goldstein, Jonathon (MD) S
Mercy Med Ctr

G/S Surgical Associates, 30 Hempstead Ave Ste 144; Rockville Centre, NY 11570; (516) 764-5900; **BDCERT:** S 71; **MS:** Cornell U 63; **RES:** S, Bronx Muncipal Hosp Ctr, Bronx, NY 64-69; **FAP:** Asst Prof of Clin S SUNY Stony Brook; **HOSP:** South Nassau Comm Hosp; **SI:** *Breast Disease;* **HMO:** Most

♿ 🅂🄾 🅿 🚹 🏨 💲 Mcr WC NFI   Immediately **VISA** 💳

Gordon, Lawrence A (MD) S
Long Island Jewish Med Ctr

1300 Union Tpke 108; New Hyde Park, NY 11040; (516) 488-2743; **BDCERT:** S 71; **MS:** SUNY Downstate 64; **RES:** Long Island Jewish Med Ctr, New Hyde Park, NY 64-69; **HMO:** Oxford Multiplan Aetna Hlth Plan Magnacare US Hlthcre +

🅿 🚹 🏨 💲 Mcr WC NFI   Immediately

Grieco, Michael B (MD) S
N Shore Univ Hosp-Glen Cove

4 Med Plaza; Glen Cove, NY 11542; (516) 676-1060; **BDCERT:** S 80; CRS 82; **MS:** Albany Med Coll 74; **RES:** N Shore Univ Hosp-Manhasset, Manhasset, NY 74-79; **FEL:** S, Lahey Clinic, Burlington, MA 79-80; CRS, Baltimore City Hosp, Baltimore, MD 80-81; **FAP:** Asst Clin Prof S SUNY Stony Brook; **HOSP:** N Shore Univ Hosp-Manhasset; **SI:** *Breast Surgery; Abdominal Surgery;* **HMO:** Oxford Vytra Empire Aetna-US Healthcare MDNY +

♿ 📞 🅿 🚹 🏨 💲 Mcr WC NFI   Immediately

Held, Douglas (MD) S
Long Island Jewish Med Ctr

1300 Union Tpke 108; New Hyde Park, NY 11040; (516) 488-2743; **BDCERT:** CRS 87; S 87; **MS:** SUNY Downstate 86; **RES:** S, Long Island Jewish Med Ctr, New Hyde Park, NY 80-85; **FEL:** CRS, Lehigh Valley Hosp, Allentown, PA 85-86; **FAP:** Clin Instr S NYU Sch Med; **HOSP:** N Shore Univ Hosp-Manhasset; **SI:** *Abdominal Surgery; Breast Surgery;* **HMO:** Oxford Chubb Multiplan Magnacare US Hlthcre +

♿ 🅿 🏨 💲 Mcr WC   Immediately ▓ **VISA** 💳

Heller, Keith (MD) S
Long Island Jewish Med Ctr

200 Middle Neck Rd; Great Neck, NY 11021; (516) 487-0083; **BDCERT:** S 97; **MS:** NYU Sch Med 71; **RES:** S, Bellevue Hosp Ctr, New York, NY 71-76; **FEL:** S Onc, Mem Sloan Kettering Cancer Ctr, New York, NY 76-78; **FAP:** Clin Prof Albert Einstein Coll Med; **HOSP:** N Shore Univ Hosp-Manhasset; **SI:** *Head & Neck Tumors; Breast Tumors;* **HMO:** Oxford Aetna Hlth Plan GHI Blue Choice Most +

♿ 📞 🅿 🏨 💲 Mcr   A Few Days **VISA** 💳

Kantounis, Stratos (MD) S
South Nassau Comm Hosp

2 Lincoln Ave 400; Rockville Centre, NY 11570; (516) 763-6060; **BDCERT:** S 67; **MS:** SUNY Hlth Sci Ctr 58; **RES:** Bellevue Hosp Ctr, New York, NY 59-61; VA Med Ctr-Manh, New York, NY 62-64; **HOSP:** Long Beach Med Ctr; **HMO:** Blue Choice Metlife Chubb PHCS Oxford +

♿ 🅿 🚹 🏨 💲 Mcr Mcd WC NFI   Immediately

Katz, Paul (MD) S
Long Island Jewish Med Ctr

Metropolitan Surgical Group, 3003 New Hyde Park Rd 309; New Hyde Park, NY 11042; (516) 352-9682; **BDCERT:** S 78; **MS:** Hahnemann U 66; **RES:** S, Long Island Jewish Med Ctr, New Hyde Park, NY 70; **FAP:** Asst Clin Prof Albert Einstein Coll Med; **HOSP:** N Shore Univ Hosp-Glen Cove; **SI:** *Laparoscopic Surgery; Hernia Surgery;* **HMO:** GHI Oxford

LANG: Sp; ♿ 🅿 🏨 💲 Mcr WC NFI   Immediately

Guide to symbols and abbreviations can be found on pages 110-113.

697

Khalife, Michael (MD) S
Winthrop Univ Hosp

Nassau Surgical Associates, PC, 173 Mineola Blvd; Mineola, NY 11501; (516) 741-4131; **BDCERT:** S 95; **MS:** Lebanon 78; **RES:** S, Univ Hosp SUNY Stony Brook, Stony Brook, NY 78-79; **FAP:** Asst Clin Prof S SUNY Stony Brook; **HOSP:** N Shore Univ Hosp-Glen Cove; **SI:** *Laparoscopic Surgery; Breast Surgery*; **HMO:** Empire Oxford GHI Blue Choice Vytra +

LANG: Fr; 🚻 📞 🏠 👪 🏥 💲 Mcr WC NFI A Few Days
🟦 **VISA** 💳

Kim, Dong (MD) S
Winthrop Univ Hosp

877 Stewart Ave 10; Garden City, NY 11530; (516) 222-0502; **BDCERT:** S 73; **MS:** South Korea 66; **RES:** S, St Peter's Med Ctr, New Brunswick, NJ 67-68; S, Springfield Med Ctr, Springfield, MA 68-71; **FEL:** S Onc, Mem Sloan Kettering Cancer Ctr, New York, NY 71-74; **FAP:** Asst Lecturer S SUNY Stony Brook; **HOSP:** N Shore Univ Hosp-Plainview; **SI:** *Liver; Pancreas*; **HMO:** Vytra Oxford US Hlthcre GHI

🚻 📞 🏠 👪 🏥 Mcr Mod WC NFI Immediately

Kostroff, Karen (MD) S
Long Island Jewish Med Ctr

2001 Marcus Ave W270; Lake Success, NY 11042; (516) 775-7676; **BDCERT:** S 85; **MS:** Boston U 79; **RES:** S, NY Hosp-Cornell Med Ctr, New York, NY 79-83; NY Hosp-Cornell Med Ctr, New York, NY 83-84; **FEL:** S Onc, Brigham & Women's Hosp, Boston, MA 84-85; **FAP:** Asst Clin Prof Albert Einstein Coll Med; **HOSP:** N Shore Univ Hosp-Manhasset; **SI:** *Breast Cancer*; **HMO:** None

🚻 🏠 👪 🏥 💲 Immediately **VISA** 💳

Kurtz, Lewis (MD) S
Long Island Jewish Med Ctr

Metropolitan Surgical Group, 3003 New Hyde Park Rd 309; New Hyde Park, NY 11042; (516) 352-9682; **BDCERT:** S 90; **MS:** Italy 72; **RES:** S, Long Island Jewish Med Ctr, New Hyde Park, NY 73-77; **FEL:** S, Long Island Jewish Med Ctr, New Hyde Park, NY 77-78; **HOSP:** St Francis Med Ctr; **SI:** *Breast Surgery; Laparoscopic Surgery*; **HMO:** Oxford Aetna Hlth Plan Blue Choice GHI United Healthcare +

LANG: Sp, Itl; 🚻 📞 🏠 🏥 💲 Mcr WC A Few Days

Lanter, Bernard (MD) S
Peninsula Hosp Ctr

461 Golf Ct; N Woodmere, NY 11581; (516) 374-1619; **BDCERT:** S 67; **MS:** NYU Sch Med 55; **RES:** Albert Einstein Med Ctr, Bronx, NY 56-58; Brookdale Univ Hosp Med Ctr, Brooklyn, NY 58-60; **FEL:** CRS, Cleveland Clinic Hosp, Cleveland, OH 61; **HOSP:** St John's Epis Hosp-S Shore; **SI:** *Rectal Carcinoma; Rectal Prolapse*; **HMO:** Blue Choice Blue Cross Oxford US Hlthcre Multiplan +

🚻 SU 🏠 👪 🏥 💲 Mcr Mod WC NFI Immediately

Levin, Leroy (MD) S
Long Island Jewish Med Ctr

1000 Northern Blvd Ste 130; Great Neck, NY 11021; (516) 466-5260; **BDCERT:** S 70; CRS 70; **MS:** SUNY Downstate 62; **RES:** Long Island Jewish Med Ctr, New Hyde Park, NY 62-64; Long Island Jewish Med Ctr, New Hyde Park, NY 66-68; **FEL:** CRS, Cleveland Clinic Hosp, Cleveland, OH 68-69; **FAP:** Asst Prof S Cornell U; **HOSP:** N Shore Univ Hosp-Manhasset; **SI:** *Colon and Rectal Cancer Surgery; Inflammatory Bowel Disease*; **HMO:** Most

🚻 🏠 👪 🏥 💲 Mcr Mod WC Immediately **VISA** 💳

Mansouri, Hormoz (MD) S
Mid-Island Hosp

4277 Hempstead Tpke 108; Bethpage, NY 11714; (516) 735-7899; **BDCERT:** S 80; **MS:** Iran 64; **RES:** Nassau County Med Ctr, East Meadow, NY 69-71; Henry Ford Hosp, Detroit, MI 67-69; **FAP:** Asst Prof SUNY Stony Brook; **HOSP:** N Shore Univ Hosp-Plainview; **HMO:** Most

LANG: Per; 🚻 📞 🏠 🏥 💲 Mcr Mod WC NFI A Few Days

Mansouri, Mehran (MD) S
Mid-Island Hosp

4277 Hempstead Tpke Ste 108; Bethpage, NY 11714; (516) 735-7899; **BDCERT:** S 88; **MS:** Iran 78; **RES:** S, Nassau County Med Ctr, East Meadow, NY 82-87; **FEL:** GVS, Winthrop Univ Hosp, Mineola, NY 87-88; **HOSP:** N Shore Univ Hosp-Plainview; **HMO:** Most

LANG: Per; 🚻 📞 🏠 🏥 💲 Mcr Mod WC NFI A Few Days

Guide to symbols and abbreviations can be found on pages 110-113.

Maurer, Virginia (MD)   **S**
Winthrop Univ Hosp

243 Willis Ave; Mineola, NY 11501; (516) 742-1730; **BDCERT:** S 79; **MS:** Canada 71; **RES:** S, U Toronto Gen Hosp, Toronto, Canada 73-76; **FEL:** Lahey Clinic, Burlington, MA 77; *SI: Breast Surgery*; **HMO:** Oxford

LANG: Prt, Sp; ♿ 🕐 📷 👥 🏥 💲   Immediately

Monteleone, Frank (MD)   **S**
Winthrop Univ Hosp

Nassau Surgical Associates PC, 173 Mineola Blvd 302; Mineola, NY 11501; (516) 741-4131; **BDCERT:** S 96; **MS:** Italy 71; **RES:** Winthrop Univ Hosp, Mineola, NY 73-76; **FAP:** Asst Clin Prof S SUNY Stony Brook; *SI: Breast Surgery; Laparoscopic Surgery*; **HMO:** Vytra Oxford US Hlthcre GHI

LANG: Itl, Sp, Fr; ♿ 📷 🏥 💲 👥 📺 📱   1 Week 💳 **VISA** ⬤ 💳

Pesiri, Vincent (MD)   **S**
N Shore Univ Hosp-Glen Cove

3 School St 204; Glen Cove, NY 11542; (516) 759-2681; **BDCERT:** S 84; 93; **MS:** SUNY Downstate 78; **RES:** Kings County Hosp Ctr, Brooklyn, NY 78-83; **FEL:** GVS, Univ Hosp SUNY Bklyn, Brooklyn, NY 83-84; **HMO:** Vytra Oxford Blue Cross & Blue Shield Magnacare Empire +

LANG: Sp, Itl; ♿ 🕐 📷 👥 🏥 📺 📱 📱
A Few Days

Pomeranz, Lee (MD)   **S**
N Shore Univ Hosp-Plainview

100 Manetto Hill Rd 306; Plainview, NY 11803; (516) 822-1433; **BDCERT:** S 85; **MS:** SUNY Hlth Sci Ctr 79; **RES:** Albert Einstein Med Ctr, Bronx, NY 79-84; **HOSP:** Brunswick Hosp Ctr; *SI: Breast Cancer; Colon Cancer*; **HMO:** Oxford Aetna Hlth Plan CIGNA GHI United Healthcare +

♿ 🕐 📷 👥 🏥 📺 📱 📱 📱   Immediately

Procaccino, Angelo (MD)   **S**
N Shore Univ Hosp-Manhasset

North Shore Surgical Specialists, 310 E Shore Rd 203; Great Neck, NY 11023; (516) 482-8657; **BDCERT:** S 86; **MS:** NY Med Coll 79; **RES:** S, N Shore Univ Hosp-Manhasset, Manhasset, NY 79-84; **HOSP:** St Francis Med Ctr; *SI: Laparoscopic Surgery; Hernia Surgery*; **HMO:** Oxford Vytra Blue Choice CIGNA PHS +

♿ 📷 👥 🏥 💲 📺 📱 📱

Ramsey Jr, Walter S (MD)   **S**
Mid-Island Hosp

700 Old Country Rd; Plainview, NY 11803; (516) 681-1414; **BDCERT:** S 77; **MS:** Howard U 70; **RES:** Kings County Hosp Ctr, Brooklyn, NY 71-75; **FEL:** GVS, Univ Hosp SUNY Brooklyn, Brooklyn, NY 72-73; **HOSP:** N Shore Univ Hosp-Plainview

Rochman, Andrew (MD)   **S**
N Shore Univ Hosp-Plainview

100 Manetto Hill Rd 306; Plainview, NY 11803; (516) 822-1433; **BDCERT:** S 89; **MS:** Dominican Republic 80; **RES:** S, Long Island Coll Hosp, Brooklyn, NY 81-82; S, Maimonides Med Ctr, Brooklyn, NY 82-87; **FEL:** S, Maimonides Med Ctr, Brooklyn, NY 82-86; **HOSP:** Mid-Island Hosp; **HMO:** Aetna Hlth Plan Blue Choice Blue Cross & Blue Shield Choicecare CIGNA +

LANG: Sp; ♿ 🕐 📷 👥 🏥 📺 📱 📱   Immediately

Romero, Carlos (MD)   **S**
Winthrop Univ Hosp

Long Island Surgical Assoc, 297 Mineola Blvd; Mineola, NY 11501; (516) 741-6464; **BDCERT:** S 97; **MS:** Argentina 69; **RES:** Nassau County Med Ctr, East Meadow, NY 70-75; **FEL:** S, Med Coll VA Hosp, Richmond, VA; **HOSP:** Mercy Med Ctr; *SI: Laparoscopic Surgery; Head and Neck*; **HMO:** Blue Cross & Blue Shield Oxford Aetna Hlth Plan

♿ 📷 🏥 💲 📺 📱 📱   A Few Days **VISA**

Salzer, Peter (MD)   S
Mid-Island Hosp

4277 Hempstead Tpke 108; Bethpage, NY 11714;
(516) 735-7899; **BDCERT:** S 97; **MS:** Tufts U 70;
RES: S, Nassau County Med Ctr, East Meadow, NY
71-75; **FAP:** Asst Clin Prof S SUNY Stony Brook; **SI:**
Laparoscopic Cholecystectomy; Breast Cancer; **HMO:**
Magnacare MDNY Prudential Oxford US Hlthcre +

♿ 📷 📷 📺 **$** **WC** **NFI** Immediately

Stone, Alex (MD)   S
N Shore Univ Hosp-Manhasset

3003 New Hyde Park Rd 309; New Hyde Park, NY
11042; (516) 352-9682; **BDCERT:** S 72; **MS:** NYU
Sch Med 66; **RES:** S, Bellevue Hosp Ctr, New York,
NY 66-71; **FAP:** Clin Prof S Albert Einstein Coll
Med; **HOSP:** St Francis Hosp-Roslyn; **SI:**
Laparoscopic Surgery; Hernia Surgery; **HMO:** Oxford
Magnacare GHI

LANG: Sp; ♿ 📷 📺 **$** **Mcr** **WC** **NFI** Immediately

Vitale, Gerard (MD)   S
N Shore Univ Hosp-Glen Cove

10 Medical Plaza; Glen Cove, NY 11542; (516)
739-5224; **BDCERT:** S 89; **MS:** SUNY Buffalo 82;
RES: N Shore Univ Hosp-Manhasset, Manhasset,
NY; NY Hosp-Cornell Med Ctr, New York, NY; **FEL:**
GVS, St Vincent Hosp, Portland, OR; **HMO:**
Choicecare Blue Choice US Hlthcre Aetna Hlth Plan

♿ 📞 📷 📷 📺 **$** **WC** **NFI** A Few Days

Ward, Robert J (MD)   S
N Shore Univ Hosp-Syosset

Pro Health Care Assoc, 2800 Marcus Ave; Lake
Success, NY 11042; (516) 622-6120; **BDCERT:** S
84; **MS:** Columbia P&S 78; **RES:** St Vincents Hosp &
Med Ctr NY, New York, NY 78-79; St Vincents
Hosp & Med Ctr NY, New York, NY 79-83

♿ 📞 📷 📺 **Mcr** **Mcd** **WC** **NFI** 1 Week *VISA* ◉

THORACIC SURGERY

Beil, Arthur (MD)   TS
N Shore Univ Hosp-Manhasset

1380 Northern Blvd A; Manhasset, NY 11030;
(516) 627-1887; **BDCERT:** TS 67; S 66; **MS:**
Cornell U 59; **RES:** NY Hosp-Cornell Med Ctr, New
York, NY 60-65; **FEL:** NY Hosp-Cornell Med Ctr,
New York, NY 59-60; **FAP:** Chf CRS Cornell U

♿ 📺 1 Week

Bercow, Neil R (MD)   TS
St Francis Hosp-Roslyn

100 Port Washington Blvd; Roslyn, NY 11576;
(516) 365-8372; **BDCERT:** S 91; TS 94; **MS:** West
Indies 85; **RES:** S, Brooklyn Hosp Ctr, Brooklyn, NY
85-90; TS, Univ Hosp SUNY Bklyn, Brooklyn, NY
90-93; **SI:** *Arterial Bypass, Minimally Invasive;*
Acquired Cardiac Surgery; **HMO:** Oxford Aetna Hlth
Plan Empire Metlife

♿ 📞 📷 📷 📺 **Mcr** **Mcd** A Few Days

Damus, Paul S (MD)   TS
St Francis Hosp-Roslyn

100 Port Washington Blvd; Roslyn, NY 11576;
(516) 365-8372; **BDCERT:** S 75; TS 89; **MS:** UCLA
68; **RES:** S, UCLA, Los Angeles, CA 68-75; S,
Columbia Presby Med Ctr, New York, NY 77-79;
FEL: S, Harvard Med Sch, Cambridge, MA 70-72; S,
Hosp for Sick Children, Canada 79-80; **SI:** *Cardiac*
Surgery, Pacemaker; Thoracic & Vascular Surgery

Durban, Lawrence (MD)   TS
St Francis Hosp-Roslyn

Cardiothoracic Surgery PC, 100 Port Washington
Blvd; Roslyn, NY 11576; (516) 627-2173;
BDCERT: TS 90; S 88; **MS:** Cornell U 82; **RES:** NY-
Cornell Med Ctr, New York, NY 83-89; **HOSP:**
Nassau County Med Ctr; **HMO:** Choicecare Metlife

♿ 📷 📺 **Mcr** 1 Week ■ *VISA* ◉

Fox, Stewart (MD)   **TS**
South Nassau Comm Hosp

Long Island Thoracic Assoc, 77 N Centre Ave 215; Rockville Centre, NY 11570; (516) 594-9700; **BDCERT:** TS 89; S 79; **MS:** Med Coll Va 72; **RES:** S, Yale-New Haven Hosp, New Haven, CT 72-77; **FEL:** TS, MS Hershey Med Ctr, Hershey, PA; **HOSP:** Mercy Med Ctr; **SI:** *Thoracoscopy; Pacemakers*; **HMO:** Oxford Aetna Hlth Plan GHI PHS Empire Blue Cross & Shield +

🔲 🔲 🔲 🔲 🔲 🔲 A Few Days **VISA**

Hartman, Alan (MD)   **TS**
Winthrop Univ Hosp

Winthrop Cardiovascular & Thoracic Surgery PC, 120 Mineola Blvd Ste 300; Mineola, NY 11501; (516) 663-4400; **BDCERT:** TS 87; **MS:** Mt Sinai Sch Med 79; **RES:** New York University Med Ctr, New York, NY 79-83; Bellevue Hosp Ctr, New York, NY 83-84; **FEL:** New York University Med Ctr, New York, NY 84-86; Bellevue Hosp Ctr, New York, NY; **FAP:** Assoc Clin Prof SUNY Stony Brook; **HOSP:** Huntington Hosp; **HMO:** Aetna Hlth Plan Oxford Vytra United Healthcare CIGNA +

🔲 🔲 🔲 🔲 🔲 🔲 🔲 Immediately **VISA**

Hines, George L (MD)   **TS**
Winthrop Univ Hosp

Winthrop Cardiovascular & Thoracic Surgery, 120 Mineola Blvd Ste 300; Mineola, NY 11501; (516) 663-4400; **BDCERT:** TS 79; GVS 87; **MS:** Boston U 69; **RES:** Sinai Hosp, Detroit, MI 70-71; Long Island Jewish Med Ctr, New Hyde Park, NY 71-74; **FEL:** TS, New York University Med Ctr, New York, NY 74-76; **FAP:** Assoc Prof SUNY Stony Brook; **SI:** *Carotid Endarterectomy; Aortic Aneurysms*; **HMO:** Vytra Oxford Aetna Hlth Plan US Hlthcre

🔲 🔲 🔲 🔲 🔲 🔲 🔲 1 Week

Kline, Gary (MD)   **TS**
Long Island Jewish Med Ctr

LI Jewish Med CtrDept CTS, 27005 76th Ave; New Hyde Park, NY 11040; (718) 470-7460; **BDCERT:** TS 96; S 95; **MS:** Wayne State U Sch Med 86; **RES:** S, Detroit Med Ctr, Detroit, MI 86-91; Wayne Cnty Gen Hosp, Detroit, MI; **FEL:** TS, Hosp of U Penn, Philadelphia, PA; **SI:** *Coronary Bypass; Lung Resections*; **HMO:** Blue Cross & Blue Shield Oxford

LANG: Sp, Rus; 🔲 🔲 🔲 🔲 🔲 🔲 🔲

Mohtashemi, Manucher (MD)TS
Winthrop Univ Hosp

Winthrop Cardivascular & Thoracic Surgery PC, 120 Mineola Blvd Ste 300; Mineola, NY 11501; (516) 663-4400; **BDCERT:** TS 67; **MS:** Switzerland 58; **RES:** Cv, U of Alabama Hosp, Birmingham, AL 65-66; TS, Winthrop Univ Hosp, Mineola, NY 66-67; **FEL:** Cv, Montefiore Med Ctr, Bronx, NY 67-68; **FAP:** Assoc Clin Prof S SUNY Stony Brook; **SI:** *Open Heart Surgery; Vascular Surgery*; **HMO:** Blue Choice Vytra US Hlthcre Oxford

LANG: Per, Fr; 🔲 🔲 🔲 🔲 🔲 🔲 🔲 A Few Days **VISA** 🔲 🔲

Parnell, Vincent (MD)   **TS**
N Shore Univ Hosp-Manhasset

North Shore University Hosp, 300 Community Dr; Manhasset, NY 11030; (516) 562-4970; **BDCERT:** TS 84; **MS:** SUNY Downstate 76; **RES:** S, N Shore Univ Hosp-Manhasset, Manhasset, NY 81; TS, Harper Hosp, Detroit, MI 83; **FEL:** Cv, Children's Hosp of MI, Detroit, MI 84; **HOSP:** Univ Hosp SUNY Stony Brook; **SI:** *Congenital Heart Disease*

🔲 🔲 🔲 🔲 🔲 A Few Days

Robinson, Newell B (MD)   **TS**
St Francis Hosp-Roslyn

100 Port Washington Blvd; Roslyn, NY 11576; (516) 627-2173; **BDCERT:** S 85; TS 87; **MS:** U Miss Sch Med 77; **RES:** S, NY Hosp-Cornell Med Ctr, New York, NY 81-84; Mem Sloan Kettering Cancer Ctr, New York, NY 84; **FEL:** Trauma, U Washington, Seattle, WA; **SI:** *Cardiac Surgery, Pacemaker; Thoracic & Vascular Surgery*

🔲 🔲 🔲 🔲 1 Week 🔲 **VISA** 🔲

Saha, Chanchal (MD)   **TS**
N Shore Univ Hosp-Plainview

754 Old Country Rd; Plainview, NY 11803; (516) 931-0182; **BDCERT:** TS 90; S 77; **MS:** India 64; **RES:** Hosp For Joint Diseases, New York, NY 70-73; Huron Road Hosp, Cleveland, OH 65-70; **FEL:** Mount Sinai Med Ctr, New York, NY 73-76; **FAP:** Assoc Prof S Cornell U; **HOSP:** Mid-Island Hosp; **HMO:** Aetna Hlth Plan Blue Choice Vytra Empire PHS +

LANG: Hin, Bng; 🔲 🔲 🔲 🔲 🔲 🔲 🔲 🔲 A Few Days

Scott, William C (MD)   TS
Winthrop Univ Hosp

120 Mineola Blvd 300; Mineola, NY 11501; (516) 663-4400; **BDCERT:** TS 85; **MS:** Harvard Med Sch 74; **RES:** Mass Gen Hosp, Boston, MA 74-81; Stanford Med Ctr, Stanford, CA 81-84; **FEL:** SCC, Nat Inst Health, Bethesda, MD; **FAP:** Assoc Prof SUNY Stony Brook; **SI:** *Cardiac Surgery; Thoracic Surgery;* **HMO:** GHI HealthNet Choicecare

LANG: Sp; [symbols] Immediately **VISA** [symbol]

Slovin, Alvin (MD)   TS
Peninsula Hosp Ctr

South Shore Thoracic & Cardiovascular Surgical Group PC, 29 Piermont Ave; Hewlett, NY 11557; (516) 374-2351; **BDCERT:** S 70; TS 71; **MS:** SUNY Downstate 73; **RES:** S, Kings County Hosp Ctr, Brooklyn, NY 64-68; TS,; **SI:** *Carotid Endarterectomy; Lung Cancer Surgery*

LANG: Yd; [symbols]

Sutaria, Maganlal (MD)   TS
Winthrop Univ Hosp

120 Mineola Blvd 300; Mineola, NY 11501; (516) 663-4400; **BDCERT:** TS 71; S 70; **MS:** India 61; **RES:** S, Wilson Mem Med Ctr, Johnson City, NY 64-67; TS, St Francis Hosp-Roslyn, Roslyn, NY 67-68; **FEL:** TS, St Francis Hosp-Roslyn, Roslyn, NY 67-69; **FAP:** Asst Prof S SUNY Stony Brook; **SI:** *Esophageal Surgery;* **HMO:** Aetna Hlth Plan Blue Cross & Blue Shield Oxford CIGNA Metlife +

LANG: Hin, Guj; [symbols] A Few Days

Taylor, James R (MD)   TS
St Francis Hosp-Roslyn

100 Port Washington Blvd; Roslyn, NY 11576; (516) 627-2173; **BDCERT:** S 90; TS 93; **MS:** Med U SC, Charleston 84; **RES:** NY Hosp-Cornell Med Ctr, New York, NY 85-89; **FEL:** TS, NY Hosp-Cornell Med Ctr, New York, NY 89-91

Tirschwell, Perry (MD)   TS
South Nassau Comm Hosp

Long Island Thoracic Associates, 77 N Centre Ave 215; Rockville Centre, NY 11570; (516) 594-9700; **BDCERT:** TS 66; S 65; **MS:** Cornell U 58; **RES:** Jacobi Med Ctr, Bronx, NY 58; Albert Einstein Med Ctr, Bronx, NY 65; **FAP:** Asst Clin Prof SUNY Stony Brook; **HOSP:** Mercy Med Ctr; **SI:** *Pulmonary Surgery; Pacemakers;* **HMO:** Aetna Hlth Plan US Hlthcre Blue Cross & Blue Shield Prudential Oxford +

[symbols] Immediately **VISA** [symbol]

Tyras, Denis (MD)   TS
St Vincents Hosp & Med Ctr NY

27 Hemlock Dr; Great Neck, NY 11024; (516) 829-5580; **BDCERT:** S 73; TS 75; **MS:** Johns Hopkins U 68; **RES:** S, Johns Hopkins Hosp, Baltimore, MD 68-69; S, Emory U Hosp, Atlanta, GA 69-72; **FEL:** Cv, Emory U Hosp, Atlanta, GA 70-71; **FAP:** Prof S NY Med Coll; **SI:** *Cardiac Surgery;* **HMO:** HIP Network

[symbols] A Few Days **VISA** [symbol]

Weisz, Daniel (MD)   TS
St Francis Hosp-Roslyn

100 Port Washington Blvd; Roslyn, NY 11576; (516) 627-6213; **BDCERT:** S 73; TS 74; **MS:** Johns Hopkins U 67; **RES:** Johns Hopkins Hosp, Baltimore, MD 68-69; **FEL:** Barnes & Allied Hosp, 69-73

[symbols] 1 Week [symbol] **VISA** [symbol]

UROLOGY

Barbaris, Harry (MD)   U
St Francis Hosp-Roslyn

Urology Associates, 535 Plandome Rd 3; Manhasset, NY 11030; (516) 627-6188; **BDCERT:** U 77; **MS:** Georgetown U 69; **RES:** N Shore Univ Hosp-Manhasset, Manhasset, NY 70-71; Georgetown U Hosp, Washington, DC 71-75; **HOSP:** N Shore Univ Hosp-Manhasset; **SI:** *Prostate Disease; Bladder Cancer*

[symbols] Immediately [symbol] **VISA** [symbol]

Brock, William (MD)   U
Long Island Jewish Med Ctr

833 Northern Blvd; Great Neck, NY 11021; (516) 466-6953; **BDCERT:** U 80; **MS:** Emory U Sch Med 71; **RES:** NY Hosp-Cornell Med Ctr, New York, NY 71-73; UC San Diego Med Ctr, San Diego, CA 75-78; **FEL:** UC San Diego Med Ctr, San Diego, CA 78-79; U of Liverpool, Liverpool, England 79; **FAP:** Prof U Albert Einstein Coll Med; **HOSP:** N Shore Univ Hosp-Forest Hills; **HMO:** Oxford Multiplan Empire Blue Choice GHI +

LANG: Sp; ⬚ ⬚ ⬚ ⬚ ⬚ 2-4 Weeks ⬚ *VISA* ⬚

Bruno, Anthony (MD)   U
Winthrop Univ Hosp

230 Hilton Ave 206; Hempstead, NY 11550; (516) 565-3300; **BDCERT:** U 77; **MS:** Italy 68; **RES:** U, Bellevue Hosp Ctr, New York, NY 72-75; Winthrop Univ Hosp, Mineola, NY 72-75; **HOSP:** Franklin Hosp Med Ctr; **SI:** *Urinary Tract Problems; Sexual Dysfunction-Males*; **HMO:** Empire GHI Vytra Prucare Aetna Hlth Plan +

LANG: Itl, Sp; ⬚ ⬚ ⬚ ⬚ ⬚ ⬚ ⬚ ⬚

Buchbinder, Mitchell (MD)   U
Long Island Jewish Med Ctr

Lake Success Urological Assoc, 1300 Union Tpke 206; New Hyde Park, NY 11040; (516) 437-4228; **BDCERT:** U 76; **MS:** SUNY Downstate 69; **RES:** S, Long Island Jewish Med Ctr, New Hyde Park, NY 70-71; U, Long Island Jewish Med Ctr, New Hyde Park, NY 71-74; **FAP:** Asst Clin Prof Albert Einstein Coll Med; **HOSP:** N Shore Univ Hosp-Syosset; **SI:** *Prostate Disease; Kidney Stones*; **HMO:** Oxford Aetna-US Healthcare GHI PHCS

⬚ ⬚ ⬚ ⬚ ⬚ ⬚ 2-4 Weeks *VISA* ⬚

Fortunoff, Stephen (MD)   U
N Shore Univ Hosp-Glen Cove

North Nassau Urolgical Associates, 10 Medical Plaza 206; Glen Cove, NY 11542; (516) 676-2270; **BDCERT:** U 66; **MS:** Tulane U 58; **RES:** U, Columbia-Presbyterian Med Ctr, New York, NY 60-63; S, VA Med Ctr-Bronx, Bronx, NY 59-60; **FEL:** U, VA Med Ctr-Bronx, Bronx, NY 60-63; **FAP:** Asst Prof U Cornell U; **HOSP:** N Shore Univ Hosp-Manhasset; **SI:** *Prostate Bladder Kidney Disease; Cancer Kidney Stone/Laser*; **HMO:** Oxford CIGNA Prucare US Hlthcre

LANG: Sp, Itl; ⬚ ⬚ ⬚ ⬚ ⬚ ⬚ ⬚ ⬚ ⬚ A Few Days *VISA* ⬚

Hanna, Moneer (MD)   U
NY Hosp-Cornell Med Ctr

935 Northern Blvd 303; Great Neck, NY 11021; (516) 466-6950; **BDCERT:** U 78; **MS:** Egypt 63; **RES:** U Western Ontario, Ottawa, Canada 72-76; U London, London, England 70-72; **FEL:** Ped U, Hosp For Sick Children, Toronto, Canada 74-75; **HOSP:** Schneider Children's Hosp; **SI:** *Pediatric Urology; Reconstructive Surgery*; **HMO:** Oxford Magnacare Vytra Prucare CIGNA +

⬚ ⬚ ⬚ ⬚ ⬚ ⬚ ⬚ ⬚ 1 Week *VISA*

Harris, Steven (MD)   U
Long Beach Med Ctr

325 W Park Ave; Long Beach, NY 11561; (516) 431-9800; **BDCERT:** U 84; **MS:** Albert Einstein Coll Med 76; **RES:** S, Mount Sinai Med Ctr, New York, NY 76-77; U,; **FAP:** Asst Prof NY Coll Osteo Med; **HOSP:** South Nassau Comm Hosp; **SI:** *Impotence; Prostate Problems*; **HMO:** Aetna Hlth Plan Blue Choice Blue Cross & Blue Shield

LANG: Sp, Itl; ⬚ ⬚ ⬚ ⬚ ⬚ ⬚ ⬚

Kapoor, Deepak A (MD)   U
Mid-Island Hosp

Long Island Urological Associates, 4230 Hempstead Tpke Ste 200; Bethpage, NY 11714; (516) 796-2222; **BDCERT:** U 92; **MS:** Jefferson Med Coll 84; **RES:** Geisinger Med Ctr, Danville, PA 84-89; **HOSP:** N Shore Univ Hosp-Plainview; **HMO:** Most

LANG: Flm, Ger, Itl, Slv, Hin; ⬚ ⬚ ⬚ ⬚ ⬚ ⬚ ⬚ ⬚ ⬚ 1 Week *VISA* ⬚

Layne, Jeffrey (MD)   U
N Shore Univ Hosp-Plainview

1181 Old Country Rd; Plainview, NY 11803; (516) 993-6060; **BDCERT:** U 97; **MS:** SUNY Stony Brook 89; **RES:** S, New England Med Ctr, Boston, MA 89-91; U, New England Med Ctr, Boston, MA 91-95; **HOSP:** N Shore Univ Hosp-Syosset; **SI:** *Incontinence; Impotence;* **HMO:** Oxford Empire VBH GHI NYLCare +

🌙 🔒 🅿️ 🏥 💲 Mcr Mod WC NFI   Immediately

Leventhal, Arnold (MD)   U
Franklin Hosp Med Ctr

Five Towns Urology, 1800 Rockaway Ave 212; Hewlett, NY 11557; (516) 593-1838; **BDCERT:** U 92; **MS:** NYU Sch Med 84; **RES:** S, Bellevue Hosp Ctr, New York, NY 84-85; U, Bellevue Hosp Ctr, New York, NY 85-90; **FAP:** Instr NYU Sch Med; **SI:** *Stones, Urinary; Prostate;* **HMO:** Oxford US Hlthcre GHI Empire

♿ 🌙 🏥 💲 Mcr   1 Week

Lieberman, Elliott (MD)   U
N Shore Univ Hosp-Plainview

875 Old Country Rd 301; Plainview, NY 11803; (516) 931-1710; **BDCERT:** U 83; **MS:** SUNY Hlth Sci Ctr 76; **RES:** S, Mount Sinai Med Ctr, New York, NY 76-78; U, Univ Hosp SUNY Bklyn, Brooklyn, NY 78-81; **HOSP:** N Shore Univ Hosp-Manhasset; **SI:** *Urological Cancers; Interstitial Cystitis;* **HMO:** GHI Aetna Hlth Plan Vytra Oxford +

♿ 🆘 🌙 🔒 🅿️ 🏥 💲 Mcr WC NFI   A Few Days

Mellinger, Brett (MD)   U
Winthrop Univ Hosp

Winthrop Urology, 120 Mineola Blvd 320; Mineola, NY 11501; (516) 739-6300; **BDCERT:** U 90; **MS:** Ind U Sch Med 81; **RES:** S, St Vincents Hosp & Med Ctr NY, New York, NY 81-82; U, Univ Hosp SUNY Bklyn, Brooklyn, NY 82; **FEL:** U, NY Hosp-Cornell Med Ctr, New York, NY 85; **FAP:** Assoc Prof SUNY Stony Brook; **HOSP:** JT Mather Mem Hosp Pt Jfrson; **SI:** *Male Infertility; Impotence;* **HMO:** Vytra Oxford Aetna-US Healthcare Multiplan Prucare +

♿ 🅿️ 🏥 💲 Mcr   2-4 Weeks

Santoro, Michael (MD)   U
Mercy Med Ctr

30 Merrick Ave; East Meadow, NY 11554; (516) 794-4488; **BDCERT:** U 82; **MS:** SUNY Downstate 75; **RES:** S, Nassau County Med Ctr, East Meadow, NY 75-77; U, Nassau County Med Ctr, East Meadow, NY 77-80; **HOSP:** Winthrop Univ Hosp; **SI:** *Kidney Stones; Prostate Problems-Cancer;* **HMO:** Aetna Hlth Plan Oxford United Healthcare Vytra +

🔒 🅿️ 🏥 💲 Mcr NFI   Immediately

Shepard, Barry (MD)   U
Mercy Med Ctr

601 Franklin Ave 300; Garden City, NY 11530; (516) 742-3200; **BDCERT:** U 86; **MS:** SUNY Downstate 79; **RES:** Columbia-Presbyterian Med Ctr, New York, NY; **HOSP:** Winthrop Univ Hosp; **SI:** *Stones, Urinary; Urological Cancer;* **HMO:** GHI Empire Oxford Blue Cross

♿ 🌙 🔒 🅿️ 🏥 💲 Mcr WC NFI   1 Week **VISA** 💳

Smith, Arthur (MD)   U
Long Island Jewish Med Ctr

Dept of Urology at Long Island Jewish Medical Center, 27005 76th Ave; New Hyde Park, NY 11040; (718) 470-7221; **BDCERT:** U 80; **MS:** South Africa 62; **RES:** S, Baragwananath Hosp, Johannesburg, So Africa 66; Genl Hospital, Johannesburg, So Africa; **FEL:** Johannesburg Hospital, Johannesburg, So Africa; **HOSP:** N Shore Univ Hosp-Manhasset; **SI:** *Kidney Stones; Prostate Enlarged & Cancer;* **HMO:** Oxford US Hlthcre GHI Magnacare Multiplan +

LANG: Sp, Itl, Hin, Yd; ♿ 🔒 🅿️ 🏥 💲 Mcr WC Immediately 💳 **VISA** 💳

Sunshine, Robert (MD)   U
Mid-Island Hosp

4230 Hempstead Tpke 200; Bethpage, NY 11714; (516) 796-2222; **BDCERT:** U 87; **MS:** Mexico 77; **RES:** Long Island Jewish Med Ctr, New Hyde Park, NY 79-81; Mount Sinai Med Ctr, New York, NY 81-85; **HOSP:** N Shore Univ Hosp-Manhasset; **SI:** *Prostate Diseases; Male Sexual Dysfunction;* **HMO:** Aetna Hlth Plan Blue Choice Blue Cross & Blue Shield Independent Health Plan Prucare +

LANG: Sp, Grk; ♿ 🌙 🔒 🅿️ 🏥 💲 Mcr   A Few Days **VISA** 💳

Waldbaum, Robert (MD)   U
N Shore Univ Hosp-Manhasset
Urology Associates, 535 Plandome Rd # 3;
Manhasset, NY 11030; (516) 627-6188; **BDCERT:**
U 73; **MS:** Columbia P&S 62; **RES:** S, Columbia-
Presbyterian Med Ctr, New York, NY 65-66; U, NY
Hosp-Cornell Med Ctr, New York, NY 66-70; **FAP:**
Clin Prof Cornell U; **HOSP:** NY Hosp-Cornell Med
Ctr; *SI: Prostate Benign Hyperplasia; Prostate Cancer;*
HMO: Most

⚅ 🈳 🅒 🔂 🔧 🛏 🅢 Mcr WC NFI   1 Week **VISA** 💳

Ziegelbaum, Michael M (MD)   U
Long Island Jewish Med Ctr
Lake Success Urology Associates, 1300 Union Tpke
206; New Hyde Park, NY 11040; (516) 437-4228;
BDCERT: U 91; **MS:** Cornell U 82; **RES:** U, Cleveland
Clinic Hosp, Cleveland, OH 83-88; **FEL:** Stone
Disease, Univ Hosp SUNY Stony Brook, Stony
Brook, NY 88-89; **FAP:** Asst Prof Albert Einstein
Coll Med; **HOSP:** N Shore Univ Hosp-Glen Cove; *SI:*
Prostate Cancer; Female Urological Problems; **HMO:**
Aetna Hlth Plan GHI Oxford United Healthcare PHS
+

LANG: Fr, Ger; ⚅ 🔂 🔧 🛏 🅢 Mcr   Immediately
VISA 💳

VASCULAR SURGERY (GENERAL)

Berroya, Renato (MD)   GVS
St Francis Hosp-Roslyn
Long Island Surgical Specialists, PC, 639 Port
Washington Blvd; Port Washington, NY 11050;
(516) 883-2212; **BDCERT:** S 69; TS 74; **MS:**
Philippines 61; **RES:** Winthrop Univ Hosp, Mineola,
NY 64-68; St Francis Hosp-Roslyn, Roslyn, NY 68-
70; **FAP:** Asst Clin Instr Cornell U; **HOSP:** N Shore
Univ Hosp-Manhasset; *SI: Aneurysms; Carotid*
Artery; **HMO:** Oxford Blue Cross PPO Magnacare
Independent Health Plan Blue Choice PPO +

⚅ 🅒 🔂 🔧 🛏 🅢 Mcr WC NFI   Immediately **VISA** 💳

Chang, John (MD)   GVS
Long Island Jewish Med Ctr
Long Island Vascular Ctr, 1050 Northern Blvd;
Roslyn, NY 11576; (516) 484-3430; **BDCERT:** S
76; GVS 95; **MS:** South Korea 62; **RES:** S, Long
Island Jewish Med Ctr, New Hyde Park, NY 68-71;
GVS, Long Island Jewish Med Ctr, New Hyde Park,
NY 71-73; **FAP:** Assoc Prof S Albert Einstein Coll
Med; **HOSP:** St Francis Hosp-Roslyn; *SI: Circulation*
Problems of Legs; Chronic Artery Disease; **HMO:**
Magnacare Blue Cross PPO Oxford PHS Sel Pro +

⚅ 🔂 🛏 🅢 Mcr Mcd   2-4 Weeks

Faust, Glenn (MD)   GVS
Long Island Jewish Med Ctr
LIJMC - Dept of Surgery, 270-05 76th Ave; New
Hyde Park, NY 11040; (718) 470-7299; **BDCERT:**
S 93; GVS 95; **MS:** Yale U Sch Med 86; **RES:** S, Long
Island Jewish Med Ctr, New Hyde Park, NY 86-91;
FEL: GVS,; **FAP:** Asst Prof Albert Einstein Coll Med;
SI: Carotid Artery Surgery; Foot Surgery Diabetes;
HMO: Oxford GHI Blue Choice United Healthcare

⚅ 🛏 🅢 Mcr Mcd WC   A Few Days

Garvey, Julius W (MD)   GVS
Long Island Jewish Med Ctr
3003 New Hyde Park Rd 410; New Hyde Park, NY
11042; (516) 326-3255; **BDCERT:** GVS 70; TS 70;
MS: McGill U 61; **RES:** Harlem Hosp Ctr, New York,
NY 65-68; U MD Hosp, Baltimore, MD 68-70; **FAP:**
Assoc Prof S Albert Einstein Coll Med; **HOSP:**
Massapequa Gen Hosp; *SI: Laser Therapy for Spider*
Veins; Diabetic Foot; **HMO:** Oxford CIGNA US
Hlthcre United Healthcare GHI +

⚅ 🅒 🔂 🛏 🅢 Mcr Mcd   Immediately

Li Calzi, Luke (MD)   GVS
South Nassau Comm Hosp
77 N Centre Ave 208; Rockville Centre, NY 11570;
(516) 764-5455; **BDCERT:** S 81; **MS:** Albany Med
Coll 75; **RES:** S, Yale-New Haven Hosp, New Haven,
CT 75-80; **FEL:** GVS, New York University Med Ctr,
New York, NY 81-82; **FAP:** Asst Clin Prof SUNY
Stony Brook; *SI: Carotid Artery Surgery; Diabetic*
Wound Care; **HMO:** Oxford Aetna Hlth Plan CIGNA
Empire PHCS +

⚅ 🔂 🔧 🛏 Mcr WC NFI   A Few Days

Smirnov, Viktor (MD)   GVS
Winthrop Univ Hosp
30 Merrick Ave 109; East Meadow, NY 11554;
(516) 794-0444; **BDCERT:** S 87; GVS 93; **MS:**
Russia 72; **RES:** S, Univ Hosp SUNY Stony Brook,
Stony Brook, NY 80-85; **FEL:** GVS, Univ Hosp
SUNY Stony Brook, Stony Brook, NY 85-87; **HOSP:**
Mercy Med Ctr; *SI: Circulation Problems; Vein Disease*
of legs

LANG: Rus; ♿ 🕐 🔌 ⚕ 🛏 🆂 Mcr WC NFI
Immediately

SUFFOLK
COUNTY

GOOD SAMARITAN HOSPITAL MEDICAL CENTER

1000 MONTAUK HIGHWAY
WEST ISLIP, NEW YORK 11795
PHONE (516) 376-3000

Sponsorship	Voluntary Not-for-Profit
Beds	425 acute, 100 nursing home
Accreditation	Joint Commission on Accreditation of Health Care Organizations (JCAHO)

Good Samaritan Hospital Medical Center, "Suffolk's South Shore Health Care System," is affiliated with Catholic Health Services of Long Island and the New York College of Osteopathic Medicine. With over 600 attending physicians on the medical staff and residency programs in Emergency Medicine, Family Practice and Ob/Gyn as well as a traditional rotating internship, Good Samaritan is one of Long Island's leading health care systems.

SATELLITES OF GOOD SAMARITAN HOSPITAL MEDICAL CENTER

Good Samaritan Certified Home Health Care Agency-Founded in 1984, our home health agency provides a wide variety of comprehensive health care services to patients in the comfort of their own homes, including skilled nursing care as well as services provided by physical, occupational and speech therapists, medical social workers and home health aides, 7 days a week, 24 hours a day. *Accredited by the JCAHO.*

Good Samaritan Hospice-Founded in 1989 and one of the first hospital-based hospice programs on Long Island created to ease the pain of terminally ill patients and their families while offering professional care for the patient's final days. Hospice services are coordinated by an interdisciplinary team who insure continuity of patient and family care. *Accredited by the JCAHO.*

Good Samaritan Nursing Home-Founded in 1979, our 100-bed skilled nursing facility located in beautiful Sayville one block from the Great South Bay allows for personal attention to the needs of loved ones while emphasizing an interdisciplinary approach to meet the needs of each resident.

Good Samaritan Chronic Dialysis Center-Founded in 1976, our 25 station dialysis facility was the first Chronic Dialysis Center in Suffolk County. It provides free-standing dialysis services for patients with chronic kidney disease 20 hours a day, 6 days a week from 5:00 a.m. to 1:00 a.m. with ongoing support groups for patients and their families.

HomeCare America Superstore-The area's largest health care products source. Its mission is to be an after care patient education resource center complemented by a professional staff ranging from RNs to Orthotists who fit braces.

"INSTITUTES OF EXCELLENCE"

The Cancer Care Institute is a complete compendium of cancer care. The latest in diagnostic as well as surgical and nonsurgical treatment procedures create an unparalleled care center for those with breast, prostate and other cancers.

The Women's Health Institute has recognized that women have special health care needs and, as the "customary" care giver in their families, their needs often extend to other family members. Programs for moms and their babies are part and parcel of this institute.

The Vascular Care Institute with its minimally invasive radiological procedures as well as surgery and cutting edge techniques in angiography and stenting have been bringing about extraordinary results for patients with circulatory problems which previously restricted their abilities to ambulate.

The Prevention/Wellness Institute has been both a starting and focal point for the hospital in its patient care platform through our Chronic Pain Management Center, Pediatric Ambulatory Care Center/Family Asthma and Allergy Center, Nutrition and Food Service programs as well as community based forums.

The Cardiac Diagnostic Institute includes the latest approaches for detecting heart disease and susceptibility as well as damage. The most advanced imaging, mapping, and stress testing capabilities enables the cardiac care physician and professionals to clearly determine the extent of heart disease and help them to advise the patient and family.

Physician Referral	If you have any questions regarding the above organizations or Institutes, please call our *Physician & Health Referral Line at (516) 376-4444.*

ST. CHARLES HOSPITAL AND REHABILITATION CENTER

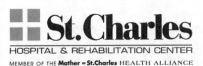

St. Charles
HOSPITAL & REHABILITATION CENTER
MEMBER OF THE **Mather ≈ St.Charles** HEALTH ALLIANCE

200 BELLE TERRE ROAD
PORT JEFFERSON, NEW YORK 11777
PHONE (516) 474-6000
FAX (516) 474-6270

Sponsorship	Voluntary Not-for-Profit
Beds	291 Total - 152 Acute Care, 105 Physical Medicine & Rehabilitation (Adult and Pediatric), 10 Traumatic Brain Injury, 24 Alcohol Rehabilitation
Accreditation	Joint Commission on Accreditation of Healthcare Organizations (JCAHO).

As Long Island's rehabilitation center, St. Charles Hospital and Rehabilitation Center has the largest and most diverse rehabilitation and related programs available in Nassau, Suffolk, Queens and Brooklyn region. Integrated with sophisticated orthopedic, spine and neurological services, St. Charles offers a seamless continuum of care through its inpatient, outpatient and subacute programs.

St. Charles is affiliated with John T. Mather Memorial Hospital through the Mather-St. Charles Health Alliance; and Good Samaritan Hospital, Mercy Medical Center and St. Francis Hospital as part of Catholic Health Services of Long Island.

St. Charles has over 600 attending medical staff and offers residency training of its own or in cooperation with SUNY Stony Brook in dentistry, orthopedics, pediatrics, family practice and physical medicine and rehabilitation (PM&R) and fellowship training in geriatric rehabilitation and neuro-rehabilitation.

INPATIENT PROGRAMS AND SERVICES

Adult Rehabilitation	In addition to such specialized programs as post cardiac surgery and pulmonary rehabilitation, St. Charles provides rehabilitation to individuals recovering from joint replacement surgery, stroke, neurological disorders, and many other conditions. Subacute rehabilitation is offered in conjunction with the Smithtown Healthcare Facility.
Pediatrics/TBI	In addition to providing acute care services, St. Charles has the first and only New York state designated pediatric traumatic brain injury (TBI) unit and pediatric rehabilitation unit on Long Island. Besides the finest physicians in orthopedics, rheumatology, neurology and pediatrics, full time staff includes a pediatric physiatrist, pediatric neuropsychologist, rehabilitation nurses, special educator, and physical, occupational and recreation therapists.
Maternity Services	With six birthing suites, two delivery/operating rooms, 36-bassinette nursery, 28 bed post-partum unit and a neo-natal intensive care unit, St. Charles has the newest, state-of-the-art maternity facilities on Long Island.

OUTPATIENT PROGRAMS AND SERVICES

Rehabilitation Network	With sites currently in Albertson, Melville, Port Jefferson Station, Smithtown, Riverhead and Patchogue, the St. Charles Rehabilitation Network provides quality therapeutic services for adults and children throughout Long Island. Additional sites will be opening in Manhattan, Brooklyn and Queens by the end of 1998.
Arthritis Institute of NY	A multi-disciplinary, multi-physician approach to the treatment of arthritis.
Diabetes Care Center	Program components include nutritional counseling, educational classes and consults with registered nurses working toward the ultimate goal of self management of diabetes. Medicare approved.
Physician Referral	Program information and physician referrals for over 600 physicians can be obtained at (516) 474-6030.

SPECIALTY & SUBSPECIALTY	ABBREVIATION	PAGE(S)
Addiction Psychiatry	AdP	711
Allergy & Immunology	A&I	711
Cardiology (Cardiovascular Disease)	Cv	712-713
Child & Adolescent Psychiatry	ChAP	713
Child Neurology	ChiN	713
Dermatology	D	713-715
Diagnostic Radiology	DR	715
Emergency Medicine	EM	715
Endocrinology, Diabetes & Metabolism	EDM	715-716
FAMILY PRACTICE	FP	716-718
Gastroenterology	Ge	718-719
Geriatric Medicine	Ger	719
Geriatric Psychiatry	GerPsy	720
Hand Surgery	HS	720
Hematology	Hem	720
Infectious Disease	Inf	720-721
INTERNAL MEDICINE	IM	721-723
Medical Genetics	MG	724
Medical Oncology*	Onc	724--725
Neonatal-Perinatal Medicine	NP	725
Nephrology	Nep	725-726
Neurological Surgery	NS	726
Neurology	N	726-727
OBSTETRICS & GYNECOLOGY	ObG	728-730
Occupational Medicine	OM	730
Ophthalmology	Oph	730-733
Orthopaedic Surgery	OrS	733-735
Otolaryngology	Oto	735-736
Pain Management	PM	736

SPECIALTY & SUBSPECIALTY	ABBREVIATION	PAGE(S)
Pediatric Cardiology	PCd	737
Pediatric Gastroenterology	PGe	737
Pediatric Hematology–Oncology*	PHO	737
Pediatric Nephrology	PNep	737
Pediatric Surgery	PS	738
PEDIATRICS (GENERAL)	Ped	738-740
Plastic Surgery	PlS	740-741
Psychiatry	Psyc	741-742
Pulmonary Disease	Pul	743-744
Radiation Oncology*	RadRO	744
Radiology	Rad	745
Reproductive Endocrinology	RE	745
Rheumatology	Rhu	745-746
Surgery	S	746-748
Thoracic Surgery (includes open heart surgery)	TS	748
Urology	U	749
Vascular Surgery (General)	GVS	749-750

Specialties in capital letters indicate Primary Care Specialties. However, many doctors will be certified in a subspecialty, but will practice predominantly primary care medicine. In our lists this will be indicated.

*Oncologists deal with Cancer

ADDICTION PSYCHIATRY

Blume, Sheila (MD)   AdP
South Oaks Hosp

South Oaks Hospital, 284 Green Ave; Sayville, NY 11782; (516) 589-7853; **BDCERT:** Psyc 68; **MS:** Harvard Med Sch 58; **RES:** Psyc, Central Islip Psych Ctr, Central Islip, NY 62-65; **FEL:** Psyc Biochemistry, Japan; **FAP:** Clin Prof Psyc SUNY Stony Brook; *SI: Addiction; Problem Gambling*

ALLERGY & IMMUNOLOGY

Cancellieri, Russell (MD)   A&I
Southampton Hosp

PO Box 5027; Southampton, NY 11968; (516) 283-3300; **BDCERT:** Ped 79; A&I 81; **MS:** Georgetown U 74; **RES:** Ped, Georgetown U Hosp, Washington, DC 75-77; A&I, St Luke's Roosevelt Hosp Ctr, New York, NY 77-79; **HMO:** Oxford Aetna Hlth Plan CIGNA

🅰 📷 🚻 🏥 $ Mcr WC   A Few Days **VISA** 💳

Chiaramonte, Joseph (MD)   A&I
Good Samaritan Hosp Med Ctr

Bay Shore Allergy Group, 649 Montauk Hwy; Bay Shore, NY 11706; (516) 665-2700; **BDCERT:** A&I 74; Ped 72; **MS:** Italy 65; **RES:** Brookdale Univ Hosp Med Ctr, Brooklyn, NY 67-68; **FEL:** A&I, Long Island Coll Hosp, Brooklyn, NY 71-72; **FAP:** Adjct Clin Prof NY Coll Osteo Med; **HOSP:** Long Island Jewish Med Ctr; *SI: Asthma Related Diseases*; **HMO:** Oxford Magnacare JJ Newman

LANG: Itl; 🅰 📞 📷 🏥 $ Mcr Mcd   2-4 Weeks **VISA** 💳

Lusman, Paul (MD)   A&I
JT Mather Mem Hosp Pt Jfrson

120 N Country Rd; Port Jefferson, NY 11777; (516) 928-4990; **BDCERT:** A&I 74; Ped 71; **MS:** Albert Einstein Coll Med 65; **RES:** Strong Mem Hosp, Rochester, NY 65-66; Bellevue Hosp Ctr, New York, NY 66-68; **FEL:** A&I, Duke U Med Ctr, Durham, NC 70-72; **FAP:** Asst Clin Prof SUNY Stony Brook; **HOSP:** Univ Hosp SUNY Stony Brook; *SI: Asthma; Hay Fever/Rose Fever*; **HMO:** Aetna Hlth Plan Blue Choice Oxford Vytra US Hlthcre +

🅰 📞 📷 🚻 🏥 $ Mcr Mcd WC   Immediately

Mayer, Daniel (MD)   A&I
Univ Hosp SUNY Stony Brook

University Medical Ctr; Stony Brook, NY 11790; (516) 444-1151; **BDCERT:** A&I 89; **MS:** Italy 78; **RES:** Albany Med Ctr, Albany, NY 81; **FEL:** A&I, Long Island Coll Hosp, Brooklyn, NY 87; **HOSP:** St John's Epis Hosp-Smithtown

Satnick, Steven (MD)   A&I
Univ Hosp SUNY Stony Brook

Allergy & Asthma Care, 233 Union Ave 206; Holbrook, NY 11741; (516) 588-4486; **BDCERT:** A&I 87; **MS:** SUNY Downstate 80; **RES:** IM, Univ Hosp SUNY Bklyn, Brooklyn, NY 80-84; **FEL:** A&I, Univ Hosp SUNY Bklyn, Brooklyn, NY 87; **HOSP:** Brookhaven Mem Hosp; *SI: Asthma; Allergic Rhinitis*; **HMO:** Most

LANG: Sp; 🅰 SA/SD 📞 📷 🚻 🏥 $ Mcr NFI
A Few Days

Young, Rosemarie (MD)   A&I
Nassau County Med Ctr

554 Larkfield Rd 10C; E Northport, NY 11731; (516) 368-4702; **BDCERT:** A&I 87; Ped 87; **MS:** Albert Einstein Coll Med 80; **RES:** IM, Albany Med Ctr, Albany, NY 80-84; **FEL:** A&I, Nat Jewish Med Ctr, Denver, CO 84-87; **FAP:** Asst Prof Ped SUNY Stony Brook; **HOSP:** Huntington Hosp; *SI: Asthma; Food Allergies*; **HMO:** Aetna-US Healthcare CIGNA Vytra Oxford Blue Choice +

🅰 SA/SD 📞 📷 🚻 🏥 $ Mcr   A Few Days

CARDIOLOGY (CARDIOVASCULAR DISEASE)

Altschul, Larry (MD)   Cv
Good Samaritan Hosp Med Ctr
1111 Montauk Hwy; West Islip, NY 11795; (516) 422-6565; **BDCERT:** Cv 83; IM 80; **MS:** SUNY Buffalo 77; **RES:** Nassau County Med Ctr, East Meadow, NY 77-80; **FEL:** Cv, Nassau County Med Ctr, East Meadow, NY 80-82; **HOSP:** Southside Hosp; **SI:** *Coronary Artery Disease; Congestive Heart Failure;* **HMO:** Oxford US Hlthcre Vytra Prucare
LANG: Sp, Grk; 🔲 🔲 🔲 🔲 🔲 🔲 🔲 🔲 🔲 🔲 A Few Days 🔲 **VISA** 🔵 🔲

Borek, Mark (MD)   Cv
St John's Epis Hosp-Smithtown
Island Cardiovascular Assoc, 496 Smithtown Byp 101; Smithtown, NY 11787; (516) 979-8880; **BDCERT:** IM 85; Cv 87; **MS:** SUNY Hlth Sci Ctr 81; **RES:** Nassau County Med Ctr, East Meadow, NY 81-84; **FEL:** Cv, Long Island Coll Hosp, Brooklyn, NY 85-87; **HOSP:** JT Mather Mem Hosp Pt Jfrson; **HMO:** Oxford US Hlthcre Vytra CIGNA
🔲 🔲 🔲 🔲 🔲 🔲 🔲 🔲 2-4 Weeks **VISA** 🔵

Chengot, Mathew (MD)   Cv
Brunswick Hosp Ctr
Amityville Heart Center, 129 Broadway; Amityville, NY 11701; (516) 598-3434; **BDCERT:** Cv 85; IM 83; **MS:** India 76; **RES:** Lincoln Med & Mental Hlth Ctr, Bronx, NY 80-82; **FEL:** Cv, Mt Sinai Med Ctr, Miami Beach, FL 82-84; **FAP:** Asst Clin Instr Cornell U; **HOSP:** Good Samaritan Hosp Med Ctr; **SI:** *Nuclear Cardiology; Lipid Management;* **HMO:** Aetna-US Healthcare Oxford Vytra PHS MDNY +
LANG: Sp, Hin, Itl; 🔲 🔲 🔲 🔲 🔲 🔲 🔲 🔲 🔲 🔲 Immediately

De Carlo, Alan (MD)   Cv
Southampton Hosp
365 County Rd 39A 9; Southampton, NY 11968; (516) 283-8888; **BDCERT:** IM 76; Cv 79; **MS:** Tufts U 73; **RES:** St Luke's Roosevelt Hosp Ctr, New York, NY; **HMO:** Blue Cross & Blue Shield Choicecare Travelers
🔲 🔲 🔲 🔲 4+ Weeks **VISA** 🔵

Dervan, John (MD)   Cv
Univ Hosp SUNY Stony Brook
North Suffolk Cardiology Associates, PC, 2500-1 Nesconset Hwy; Stony Brook, NY; (516) 689-7700; **BDCERT:** IM 79; Cv 85; **MS:** St Louis U 76; **RES:** IM, Faulkner Hosp, Boston, MA 76-77; **FEL:** Cv, Beth Israel Med Ctr, Boston, MA 80-82; Beth Israel Med Ctr, Boston, MA 82-83; **FAP:** Assoc Clin Prof SUNY Stony Brook; **HOSP:** St John's Epis Hosp-Smithtown; **SI:** *Interventional Cardiology;* **HMO:** Empire Oxford Vytra United Healthcare US Hlthcre +
LANG: Sp; 🔲 🔲 🔲 🔲 🔲 🔲 🔲 🔲 🔲 2-4 Weeks 🔲 **VISA** 🔵 🔲

Falco, Thomas (MD)   Cv
Central Suffolk Hosp
East End Cardiology, PC, 1333 E Main St; Riverhead, NY 11901; (516) 727-2100; **BDCERT:** IM 85; Cv 87; **MS:** Mexico 80; **RES:** IM, Winthrop Univ Hosp, Mineola, NY 82-84; Winthrop Univ Hosp, Mineola, NY 84-85; **FEL:** Cv, Albany Med Ctr, Albany, NY 85-87; **HOSP:** Eastern Long Island Hosp; **SI:** *Cardiology;* **HMO:** Vytra Oxford GHI Aetna-US Healthcare
🔲 🔲 🔲 🔲 🔲 🔲 1 Week **VISA** 🔵

Lense, Lloyd (MD)   Cv
JT Mather Mem Hosp Pt Jfrson
3400 Nesconset Hwy 105; E Setauket, NY 11733; (516) 689-1400; **BDCERT:** IM 80; Cv 83; **MS:** NYU Sch Med 77; **RES:** IM, Mount Sinai Med Ctr, New York, NY 77-80; **FEL:** Cv, Montefiore Med Ctr, Bronx, NY 80-83; **FAP:** SUNY Stony Brook; **HOSP:** St Charles Hosp & Rehab Ctr; **SI:** *Congestive Heart Failure; Hyperlipirdemia;* **HMO:** Oxford United Healthcare Aetna Hlth Plan Empire +
LANG: Sp; 🔲 🔲 🔲 🔲 🔲 🔲 🔲 Immediately 🔲 **VISA** 🔵

Masciello, Michael (MD)   Cv
Southside Hosp
2011 Union Blvd; Bay Shore, NY 11706; (516)
665-5517; **BDCERT:** IM 83; Cv 85; **MS:** U Miami
Sch Med 80; **RES:** Nassau County Med Ctr, East
Meadow, NY 82-85; **HOSP:** Good Samaritan Hosp
Med Ctr

🦽 🌙 🔒 🚹 🛏 Mcr Mcd WC NFI

Matilsky, Michael (MD)   Cv
Univ Hosp SUNY Stony Brook
Three Village Cardiology, 3400 Nesconset Hwy
105; East Setauket, NY 11733; (516) 689-1400;
BDCERT: IM 85; Cv 87; **MS:** SUNY Stony Brook 82;
RES: IM, Mount Sinai Med Ctr, New York, NY 82-
85; **FEL:** Cv, NY Hosp-Cornell Med Ctr, New York,
NY 85-88; **FAP:** Asst Prof of Clin Med SUNY Stony
Brook; **HOSP:** JT Mather Mem Hosp Pt Jfrson; *SI:*
Heart Failure; Angina Coronary Disease; **HMO:** Vytra
Oxford MDNY Aetna Hlth Plan US Hlthcre +

🦽 🔒 🚹 🛏 💲 Mcr 1 Week 📇 **VISA** 💳 💳 📇

Vlay, Stephen C (MD)   Cv
Univ Hosp SUNY Stony Brook
Suny Health Sciences Center, 100 Nicholls Rd
T17200; Stony Brook, NY 11794; (516) 444-
1060; **BDCERT:** IM 78; Cv 81; **MS:** Yale U Sch Med
75; **RES:** IM, Bellevue Hosp Ctr, New York, NY 75-
76; IM, Bellevue Hosp Ctr, New York, NY 76-78;
FEL: Cv, Bellevue Hosp Ctr, New York, NY 76-78;
Johns Hopkins Hosp, Baltimore, MD 78-81; *SI:*
Cardiac Arrhythmias; Pacemakers, Defibrillators;
HMO: Aetna Hlth Plan Blue Choice Blue Cross &
Blue Shield Choicecare HealthNet +

🦽 🔒 🚹 🛏 Mcr Mcd A Few Days

Yen, Owen (MD)   Cv
Univ Hosp SUNY Stony Brook
Shoreham Medical Svc, PO Box 879; Shoreham,
NY 11786; (516) 744-3303; **BDCERT:** IM 83; Cv
85; **MS:** SUNY Hlth Sci Ctr 80; **RES:** Univ Hosp
SUNY Stony Brook, Stony Brook, NY 80-83; **FEL:**
Univ Hosp SUNY Stony Brook, Stony Brook, NY;
FAP: Asst Clin Prof SUNY Stony Brook; **HOSP:** JT
Mather Mem Hosp Pt Jfrson; *SI: Heart Failure;*
Atypical Chest Pains

🦽 🌙 🔒 🛏 💲 Mcr Mcd NFI 2-4 Weeks **VISA** 💳

CHILD & ADOLESCENT PSYCHIATRY

Pomeroy, John (MD)   ChAP
Univ Hosp SUNY Stony Brook
Division of Developmental Disability, 100 Nicholls
Rd; Stony Brook, NY 11794; (516) 632-8983;
BDCERT: Psyc 84; **MS:** England 73; **RES:** U IA
Hosp, Iowa City, IA; **FAP:** Asst Lecturer Psyc SUNY
Stony Brook

🦽 🔒 🛏 💲 Mcr Mcd WC

CHILD NEUROLOGY

Andriola, Mary (MD)   ChiN
Univ Hosp SUNY Stony Brook
Dept of NeurologySUNY Stony Brook, 101 Nicholls
Rd T12020; Stony Brook, NY 11794; (516) 444-
2599; **BDCERT:** N 72; **MS:** Duke U 65; **RES:** Duke U
Med Ctr, Durham, NC 65-66; Ped, U FL Shands
Hosp, Gainesville, FL 66-67; **FEL:** N, U FL Shands
Hosp, Gainesville, FL 67-70; **FAP:** Assoc Prof SUNY
Stony Brook; *SI: Epilepsy; Attention Deficit Disorder;*
HMO: US Hlthcre Metlife Vytra Beech Street GHI +

🦽 🔒 🚹 🛏 Mcr Mcd NFI A Few Days 📇 💳 📇

DERMATOLOGY

Basuk, Pamela (MD)   D
Good Samaritan Hosp Med Ctr
260 Main St; Islip, NY 11751; (516) 277-8004;
BDCERT: D 88; **MS:** NYU Sch Med 84; **RES:** D,
Brown U Hosp, Providence, RI; **HMO:** Oxford
Prudential PHS Empire Blue Choice

🦽 🌙 🚹 🛏 💲 Mcr

Berger, Bernard (MD)   D
Southampton Hosp
319 Hampton Rd; Southampton, NY 11968; (516)
283-7722; **BDCERT:** D 75; **MS:** UC Irvine 63; **RES:**
Mount Sinai Med Ctr, New York, NY 68-71; Good
Samaritan Hosp, Los Angeles, CA 63-64; **FAP:** Asst
Clin Prof SUNY Stony Brook; *SI: Lyme Disease;*
HMO: None

🦽 🔒 🚹 🛏 💲 Mcr Mcd 1 Week

Clark, Richard (MD)   D
Univ Hosp SUNY Stony Brook
181 N Belle Meade Rd 5; E Setauket, NY 11733;
(516) 444-4200; **BDCERT:** D 80; **MS:** U Rochester
71; **RES:** Strong Mem Hosp, Rochester, NY 71-73;
FEL: A&I, Nat Inst Health, Bethesda, MD 73-76; D,
Mass Gen Hosp, Boston, MA 76-80; **FAP:**
Prof/Chrmn D SUNY Stony Brook; **HMO:** US
Hlthcre Aetna Hlth Plan Metlife Vytra Oxford +

LANG: Sp; ♿ ▣ ▥ ⏱ Ⓢ Ⓜ Ⓜ 4+ Weeks **VISA**
●

Miller, Richard L (MD)   D
JT Mather Mem Hosp Pt Jfrson
200 Main St; Setauket, NY 11733; (516) 751-
7070; **BDCERT:** D 75; **MS:** Duke U 68; **RES:** D,
Naval Med Ctr, San Diego, CA 91-94; **FAP:** Assoc
Prof D SUNY Stony Brook; **HOSP:** St Charles Hosp &
Rehab Ctr; **SI:** *Diseases of the Skin*; **HMO:** Magnacare
Oxford Blue Choice Multiplan PHS +

♿ Ⓒ ▣ ▥ ⏱ Ⓢ Ⓜ 2-4 Weeks

Moynihan, Gavan (MD)   D
Southside Hosp
332 E Main St; Bay Shore, NY 11706; (516) 666-
0500; **BDCERT:** D 77; **MS:** Howard U 73; **RES:**
USPHS Hosp, Baltimore, MD 74-76; **FEL:** D,
Columbia-Presbyterian Med Ctr, New York, NY;
FAP: Asst Prof SUNY Stony Brook; **HOSP:** Good
Samaritan Hosp Med Ctr; **SI:** *Melanoma; Skin Cancer*;
HMO: Empire Blue Cross & Shield Oxford MDNY
Blue Choice

LANG: Sp; ♿ Ⓢⓤ Ⓒ ▥ Ⓢ Ⓜ Ⓜ Ⓦ 1 Week ▦
VISA ●

Notaro, Antoinette (MD)   D
Eastern Long Island Hosp
PO Box 93, 13405 Main Rd; Mattituck, NY 11952;
(516) 298-1122; **BDCERT:** D 82; **MS:** SUNY Hlth
Sci Ctr 78; **RES:** St Vincents Hosp & Med Ctr NY,
New York, NY 78-79; Albert Einstein Med Ctr,
Bronx, NY 79-82; **FAP:** Asst Clin Prof SUNY Stony
Brook; **SI:** *Melanoma; Skin Cancer*; **HMO:** Vytra
Oxford United Healthcare Blue Shield

♿ ▣ ▥ ⏱ Ⓢ Ⓜ 2-4 Weeks ▦ **VISA** ●

Prestia, Alan (MD)   D
Huntington Hosp
180 E Pulaski Rd; Huntington Station, NY 11746;
(516) 425-3820; **BDCERT:** D 72; **MS:** SUNY Hlth
Sci Ctr 67; **RES:** VA Med Ctr-Brooklyn, Brooklyn,
NY 68-69; New York University Med Ctr, New
York, NY 69-71; **SI:** *Atopic Dermatitis; Melanoma*;
HMO: Aetna-US Healthcare Vytra Oxford United
Healthcare Blue Cross & Blue Shield +

LANG: Itl, Sp; ♿ ▣ ▥ ⏱ Ⓢ Ⓜ Ⓦ Ⓝ 2-4 Weeks
VISA ●

Puritz, Elliot (MD)   D
St John's Epis Hosp-Smithtown
327 E Middle Country Rd; Smithtown, NY 11787;
(516) 979-0909; **BDCERT:** D 72; **MS:** NY Med Coll
65; **RES:** NY Med Coll, Valhalla, NY 66-67; U NC
Hosp, Chapel Hill, NC 69-72; **HOSP:** South Oaks
Hosp; **SI:** *Acne; Eczema & Psoriasis*; **HMO:** Aetna
Hlth Plan JJ Newman Magnacare Oxford +

♿ Ⓒ ▥ ⏱ Ⓢ Ⓜ A Few Days

Skrokov, Robert (MD)   D
Good Samaritan Hosp Med Ctr
332 E Main St; Bay Shore, NY 11706; (516) 666-
0500; **BDCERT:** D 86; **MS:** SUNY Hlth Sci Ctr 82;
RES: Jacobi Med Ctr, Bronx, NY 82-83; Univ Hosp
SUNY Bklyn, Brooklyn, NY 83-86; **FAP:** Asst Clin
Prof D SUNY Stony Brook; **HOSP:** Southside Hosp;
SI: *Laser Surgery; Skin Signs of Systemic Disease*;
HMO: Empire Vytra GHI Blue Choice Prucare +

♿ Ⓢⓤ Ⓒ ▣ ▥ ⏱ Ⓢ Ⓜ Ⓦ 2-4 Weeks **VISA** ●

Tom, Jack (MD)   D
Mount Sinai Med Ctr
207 Hallock Rd Ste 211; Stony Brook, NY 11790;
(516) 444-0004; **BDCERT:** D 86; **MS:** NYU Sch
Med 82; **RES:** IM, New York University Med Ctr,
New York, NY 82-83; D, Mount Sinai Med Ctr, New
York, NY 83-86; **FAP:** Clin Instr Mt Sinai Sch Med;
HOSP: St John's Epis Hosp-Smithtown; **SI:** *Spider
Vein Sclerotherapy; Acne*; **HMO:** Aetna Hlth Plan
Blue Choice JJ Newman Oxford United Healthcare +

♿ Ⓒ ▣ ▥ ⏱ Ⓢ Ⓜ A Few Days

Tonnesen, Marcia (MD)   **D**
Univ Hosp SUNY Stony Brook
Stony Brook Dermatology Associates, PC, 181 N
Belle Meade Rd Ste 5; East Setauket, NY 11733;
(516) 444-4200; **BDCERT:** D 80; **MS:** U Utah 73;
RES: Harvard Med Sch, Cambridge, MA 76-79; **FEL:**
D, Harvard Med Sch, Cambridge, MA 79-81; **FAP:**
Assoc Prof SUNY Stony Brook; **HOSP:** VA Med Ctr-
Northport; **HMO:** Oxford Vytra United Healthcare
Blue Choice JJ Newman +

🚹 📠 🔧 🏥 💲 🖤 2-4 Weeks **VISA** 💳 🖃

Winston, Marvin (MD)   **D**
St Charles Hosp & Rehab Ctr
2 Medical Dr; Port Jefferson Station, NY 11776;
(516) 928-1555; **BDCERT:** D 65; **MS:** U Hlth
Sci/Chicago Med Sch 60; **RES:** D, Kings County
Hosp Ctr, Brooklyn, NY 61-64; **FAP:** Asst Clin Prof
SUNY Stony Brook; **HOSP:** JT Mather Mem Hosp Pt
Jfrson; **SI:** *Acne; General Dermatology;* **HMO:** United
Healthcare Blue Cross & Blue Shield Vytra Empire
Blue Cross & Shield GHI +

🚹 🆘 🎧 🔧 🏥 💲 🖤 A Few Days

DIAGNOSTIC
RADIOLOGY

Brancaccio, William (MD)   **DR**
Southampton Hosp
Radiological Health Services PC/South Hampton
Radiology, 1333 Roanoke Ave; Riverhead, NY
11901; (516) 727-2755; **BDCERT:** DR 81; **MS:**
Geo Wash U Sch Med 75; **RES:** Univ Hosp SUNY
Bklyn, Brooklyn, NY 76-79; **FEL:** New York
University Med Ctr, New York, NY 79-80; **HOSP:**
Central Suffolk Hosp; **SI:** *Abdominal Radiology;*
Mammography; **HMO:** MDNY Vytra Empire GHI US
Hlthcre +

LANG: Itl, Sp; 🚹 📠 🏥 🖤 🆖 Immediately
VISA 💳

Citron, Charles (MD)   **DR**
St Clare's Hosp & Health Ctr
St Charles Hosp - Dept of Radiology, 200 Belltaire
Rd; Port Jefferson, NY 11777; (516) 474-6163;
BDCERT: DR 74; **MS:** SUNY Downstate 70; **RES:**
DR, USPHS Hosp, Staten Island, NY 71-73; DR, Geo
Wash U Med Ctr, Washington, DC 73-74; **FEL:** NR,
Geo Wash U Med Ctr, Washington, DC 74; **HOSP:**
JT Mather Mem Hosp Pt Jfrson

🚹 🏥 🖤 🆖 1 Week

EMERGENCY
MEDICINE

Schiavone, Frederick M (MD)   **EM**
Univ Hosp SUNY Stony Brook
31 Pagnotta Dr; Port Jefferson Station, NY 11776;
(516) 444-2499; **BDCERT:** EM 90; IM 86; **MS:** Italy
83; **RES:** EM, Lincoln Med & Mental Hlth Ctr,
Bronx, NY 86-88; IM, Kings County Hosp Ctr,
Brooklyn, NY 84-86; **FAP:** Assoc Clin Prof SUNY
Stony Brook; **SI:** *Domestic Violence;* **HMO:** Vytra
Oxford Prucare Aetna Hlth Plan Blue Cross +

🚹 🆘 🎧 📠 🔧 🏥 🖤 🆖 Immediately 🔲
VISA 💳 🖃

ENDOCRINOLOGY,
DIABETES &
METABOLISM

Brand, Howard (MD)   **EDM**
St Charles Hosp & Rehab Ctr
323 Middle Country Rd; Smithtown, NY 11787;
(516) 360-7761; **BDCERT:** IM 87; EDM 91; **MS:**
UMDNJ-RW Johnson Med Sch 84; **RES:** IM, Mount
Sinai Med Ctr, New York, NY 84-87; VA Med Ctr-
Bronx, Bronx, NY 87-88; **FEL:** EDM, New York
University Med Ctr, New York, NY 88-90; **HOSP:** JT
Mather Mem Hosp Pt Jfrson; **SI:** *Thyroid Diseases;*
Pituitary Diseases

🚹 🎧 📠 🔧 🏥 💲 🖤 2-4 Weeks **VISA** 💳

Chowdhury, Fazlur R (MD) EDM
Good Samaritan Hosp Med Ctr
722 Montauk Hwy; West Islip, NY 11795; (516) 587-3340; **BDCERT:** IM 82; **MS:** India 67; **HOSP:** Southside Hosp; **HMO:** MDNY

🈯 🄰 🄷 Mcr A Few Days *VISA* 💳

Chown, Judith (MD) EDM
St John's Epis Hosp-Smithtown
12 Medical Dr; Port Jeffrsn Sta, NY 11776; (516) 331-9414; **BDCERT:** IM 72; **MS:** Canada 68; **RES:** IM, NY Hosp-Cornell Med Ctr, New York, NY 68-70; **FEL:** EDM, Univ CO Med Ctr, Denver, CO 71-72

♿ 🄰 🄼 🄷 💲 Mcr 4+ Weeks *VISA* 💳

Gioia, Leonard (MD) EDM
Southside Hosp
200 Howells Rd; Bay Shore, NY 11706; (516) 666-6275; **BDCERT:** IM 79; EDM 81; **MS:** SUNY Downstate 76; **RES:** St Vincents Hosp & Med Ctr NY, New York, NY 76-79; **FEL:** EDM, Boston U Med Ctr, Boston, MA 79-81; **HOSP:** Good Samaritan Hosp; **SI:** *Diabetes; Thyroid Disease;* **HMO:** Oxford CIGNA HealthNet Travelers

♿ 🆂🆄 🄰 🄼 🄷 💲 Mcr 1 Week ▦ *VISA* 💳

Kugler, David (DO) EDM
JT Mather Mem Hosp Pt Jfrson
JT Mather Meml Hosp of Pt Jeff - Dept of E, D, & M, 299 Ronkonkoma Ave; Lake Ronkonkoma, NY 11779; (516) 585-8100; **BDCERT:** EDM 95; IM 88; **MS:** NY Coll Osteo Med 82; **RES:** IM, Baptist Med Ctr, Brooklyn, NY 82-83; IM, Southeastern Med Ctr, North Miami Beach, FL 83-84; **FEL:** EDM, Univ Hosp SUNY Stony Brook, Stony Brook, NY 85-87; **FAP:** Assoc Prof IM SUNY Stony Brook; **HOSP:** St Charles Hosp & Rehab Ctr; **SI:** *Diabetes Mellitus; Thyroid;* **HMO:** Vytra Oxford Empire PHCS Prucare +

♿ 🄼 🄷 💲 Mcr 4+ Weeks

Wexler, Craig Barry (DO) EDM
Brookhaven Mem Hosp
286 Sills Rd 6; East Patchogue, NY 11772; (516) 758-5858; **BDCERT:** IM 81; EDM 89; **MS:** Chicago Coll Osteo Med 78; **RES:** IM, Long Island Jewish Med Ctr, New Hyde Park, NY 78-81; **FEL:** EDM, Long Island Jewish Med Ctr, New Hyde Park, NY 87-89; **SI:** *Diabetes; Thyroid Disorders;* **HMO:** Vytra US Hlthcre Oxford Empire Aetna Hlth Plan +

♿ 🆂🆄 🈯 🄰 🄼 🄷 💲 Mcr 2-4 Weeks

Wu, Ching-hui (MD) EDM
JT Mather Mem Hosp Pt Jfrson
2500-44 Route 347; Stony Brook, NY 11790; (516) 751-2185; **BDCERT:** IM 70; EDM 77; **MS:** Taiwan 59; **RES:** IM, Metropolitan Hosp Ctr, New York, NY 61-64; **FEL:** EDM, NY Med Coll, New York, NY 64-66; **FAP:** Asst Prof of Clin Med SUNY Stony Brook; **HOSP:** St Charles Hosp & Rehab Ctr; **SI:** *Thyroid Disease or Growth; Uncontrolled Diabetes;* **HMO:** Anthem Health Magnacare Blue Choice Oxford MDNY +

LANG: Man; ♿ 🈯 🄰 🄼 🄷 💲 Mcr WC A Few Days

FAMILY PRACTICE

Becker, Kenneth (MD) FP 🅿🅲🅿
JT Mather Mem Hosp Pt Jfrson
Northshore Family Practice, 12 Brewster Ln 12; East Setauket, NY 11733; (516) 941-4480; **BDCERT:** FP 87; **MS:** Dominica 84; **RES:** FP, St Joseph's Hosp-Paterson, Paterson, NJ 84-87; **FAP:** Asst Clin Prof FP SUNY Stony Brook; **HMO:** Aetna Hlth Plan Blue Choice Choicecare

LANG: Sp; 🆂🆄 🈯 🄰 🄼 🄷 Mcr Mcd NFI Immediately

Bilmes, Ernest (MD) FP 🅿🅲🅿
Brookhaven Mem Hosp
South Brookhaven Assoc, 258 S Ocean Ave; Patchogue, NY 11772; (516) 475-4280; **BDCERT:** FP 96; **MS:** U Hlth Sci/Chicago Med Sch 59; **RES:** Kings County Hosp Ctr, Brooklyn, NY 59-60

♿ 🆂🆄 🈯 🄰 🄷 Mcr WC 1 Week

Blyskal, Stanley (MD)   FP   `PCP`
Southside Hosp

126 E Main St; E Islip, NY 11730; (516) 581-0090;
BDCERT: FP 77; **MS:** Albany Med Coll 74; **RES:** FP,
Southside Hosp, Bay Shore, NY 77; **SI:** *Diabetes;
Women's Health*; **HMO:** Blue Choice Blue Cross &
Blue Shield Choicecare US Hlthcre Oxford +
LANG: Pol; ♿ 🈂 🅲 🔯 ♿ 🏠 🆂 Mcr WC NFI
Immediately

D'Esposito, Michael (MD)   FP   `PCP`
St John's Epis Hosp-Smithtown

120 E Northport Rd; Kings Park, NY 11754; (516)
269-1148; **BDCERT:** FP 89; **MS:** West Indies 84;
RES: FP, St Mary's Hosp, Hoboken, NJ

Ebarb, Raymond (MD)   FP   `PCP`
Good Samaritan Hosp Med Ctr

213 Montauk Hwy; W Sayville, NY 11796; (516)
563-6205; **BDCERT:** FP 87; **MS:** Mexico 82; **RES:**
Southside Hosp, Bay Shore, NY 84-87

Fishkin, Michael (DO)   FP   `PCP`
JT Mather Mem Hosp Pt Jfrson

2500 Nesconset Hwy 7; Stony Brook, NY 11790;
(516) 751-3322; **BDCERT:** FP 76; **MS:** Univ Osteo
Med & Hlth Sci 73; **RES:** FP, Nassau County Med
Ctr, East Meadow, NY 73-76; **FAP:** Assoc Prof
SUNY Stony Brook
♿ 🈂 🅲 🔯 ♿ 🆂 Mcr WC NFI   Immediately

Franco, John (MD)   FP   `PCP`
St John's Epis Hosp-Smithtown

9 Brooksite Dr; Smithtown, NY 11787; (516) 724-
1331; **BDCERT:** FP 78; Ger 95; **MS:** Mexico 74;
RES: Nassau County Med Ctr, East Meadow, NY 75-
78; **HMO:** Oxford MDNY Blue Cross & Blue Shield
♿ 🈂 🔯 ♿ 🏠 🆂 Mcr WC NFI ▨ *VISA* ●

Greenberg, Maury (MD)   FP   `PCP`
Univ Hosp SUNY Stony Brook

2500 Nesconset Hwy 24; Stony Brook, NY 11790;
(516) 751-5550; **BDCERT:** FP 85; **MS:** Albert
Einstein Coll Med 82; **RES:** Southside Hosp, Bay
Shore, NY 82-85; **FAP:** Prof SUNY Stony Brook; **SI:**
Obstetrics; Travel Medicine; **HMO:** United Healthcare
Empire GHI
♿ 🈂 🅲 🔯 ♿ 🏠 🆂   A Few Days

Greenblatt, Louis (DO)   FP   `PCP`
St John's Epis Hosp-Smithtown

Smithtown Family Medicine, 363 Rte 111;
Smithtown, NY 11787; (516) 366-1788; **BDCERT:**
FP 86; Ger 96; **MS:** NY Coll Osteo Med 83; **RES:** FP,
Univ Hosp SUNY Stony Brook, Stony Brook, NY 83-
86; **FAP:** Asst Clin Prof Med SUNY Stony Brook;
HOSP: Univ Hosp SUNY Stony Brook; **SI:** *Skin
Surgery; Pediatrics*; **HMO:** Empire Vytra Oxford GHI
CIGNA +
♿ 🈂 🅲 🔯 ♿ 🏠 🆂 Mcr WC NFI   Immediately

Guida, Anthony (MD)   FP   `PCP`
Good Samaritan Hosp

373 Sunrise Hwy; West Babylon, NY 11704; (516)
422-3377; **BDCERT:** FP 94; **MS:** SUNY Syracuse
79; **RES:** Univ Hosp SUNY Stony Brook, Stony
Brook, NY 79-82; **FAP:** Clin Instr SUNY Stony
Brook

Klein, Steven (MD)   FP   `PCP`
Southside Hosp

375 E Main St 11; Bay Shore, NY 11706; (516)
665-0760; **BDCERT:** FP 86; **MS:** Univ Vt Coll Med
83; **RES:** FP, Southside Hosp, Bay Shore, NY 83-86;
SI: *Diabetes Mellitus; Asthma*; **HMO:** Empire Vytra
Blue Choice Oxford PHS +
♿ 🈂 🅲 🔯 ♿ 🏠 🆂 Mcr WC NFI   Immediately ▨
VISA ● ▨

Korman, Elise (MD)   FP   `PCP`
Southampton Hosp
86 Old Town Rd; Southampton, NY 11968; (516)
283-0776; **BDCERT:** FP 71; **MS:** Temple U 61; **RES:**
Doctors Hosp, Seattle, WA 61-62; **HMO:**
Independent Health Plan JJ Newman
[SA/SU] [🔲] [👤] [🏠] [Mcd] [WC] [NFI]   A Few Days

Levites, Kenneth (MD)   FP   `PCP`
Southside Hosp
Great South Bay Family Medical Practice, 7
Montauk Hwy; W Sayville, NY 11796; (516) 567-
0770; **BDCERT:** FP 97; **MS:** Albany Med Coll 74;
RES: FP, Southside Hosp, Bay Shore, NY 74-77;
FAP: Asst Clin Prof FP SUNY Stony Brook; **HOSP:**
Good Samaritan Hosp Med Ctr; **SI:** *Pulmonary
Medicine; Occupational Medicine*; **HMO:** Aetna-US
Healthcare Oxford Vytra Blue Cross & Blue Shield
Unicare Primary Plus +
[♿] [SA/SU] [📞] [🔲] [👤] [🏠] [S] [Mcr] [WC]   A Few Days

Roth, Ronald (MD)   FP   `PCP`
St John's Epis Hosp-Smithtown
100 Maple Ave; Smithtown, NY 11787; (516)
265-7671; **BDCERT:** FP 91; **MS:** NY Med Coll 73;
RES: FP, Southside Hosp, Bay Shore, NY 76-78;
FAP: Assoc Prof SUNY Stony Brook; **HOSP:** Univ
Hosp SUNY Stony Brook; **HMO:** Vytra United
Healthcare Oxford Blue Choice
LANG: Sp; [♿] [SA/SU] [📞] [🔲] [👤] [🏠] [S] [Mcr] [WC] [NFI]
Immediately [====] **VISA** [💳] [💳]

Schwinn, Hans Diete (MD)   FP   `PCP`
Southampton Hosp
80 Old Riverhead Rd; Westhampton Bch, NY
11978; (516) 288-4004; **BDCERT:** FP 81; **MS:**
Germany 78; **RES:** Community Hosp, Glen Cove,
NY
LANG: Ger; [♿] [SA/SU] [📞] [🔲] [🏠] [S] [Mcr] [Mcd] [WC] [NFI]
Immediately

GASTROENTEROLOGY

Cohn, William (MD)   Ge
JT Mather Mem Hosp Pt Jfrson
LI Digestive Disease Consultants, 3400 Nesconset
Hwy 101; Setauket, NY 11733; (516) 751-8700;
BDCERT: IM 75; Ge 79; **MS:** Med Coll Va 72; **RES:**
IM, Med Coll VA Hosp, Richmond, VA 72-75; **FEL:**
Med Coll VA Hosp, Richmond, VA 75; Ge, Albert
Einstein Med Ctr, Bronx, NY 76; **FAP:** Asst Clin Prof
Med SUNY Stony Brook; **HOSP:** St Charles Hosp &
Rehab Ctr; **SI:** *Gastrointestinal Diseases; Liver
Diseases*; **HMO:** Blue Choice MDNY Aetna Hlth Plan
Lawrence Healthcare Oxford +
LANG: Sp; [♿] [🔲] [👤] [🏠] [S] [Mcr] [Mcd]   2-4 Weeks **VISA**
[💳]

Duva, Joseph (MD)   Ge
Central Suffolk Hosp
887 Old Country Rd A; Riverhead, NY 11901;
(516) 727-6122; **BDCERT:** IM 81; **MS:** Mt Sinai
Sch Med 78; **RES:** Nassau County Med Ctr, East
Meadow, NY 78-80; **FEL:** Ge, Nassau County Med
Ctr, East Meadow, NY 81-83; **SI:** *Intestinal
Disorders; Endoscopic Procedures*; **HMO:** Aetna Hlth
Plan Blue Cross & Blue Shield Metlife PHS Travelers
+
[♿] [🔲] [👤] [🏠] [S] [Mcr] [Mcd]   A Few Days **VISA** [💳]

Gecelter, Gary (MD)   Ge
Univ Hosp SUNY Stony Brook
Dept of Surgery T19 - HSC; Stony Brook, NY
11794; (516) 444-1793; **BDCERT:** S 90; Ge 92;
MS: South Africa 81; **RES:** S, Johannesburg
Hospital, Johannesburg, South Africa 85-90; **FEL:**
Ge, Johannesburg Hospital, Johannesburg, South
Africa 91-92; **FAP:** Asst Prof S SUNY Stony Brook;
HOSP: JT Mather Mem Hosp Pt Jfrson; **SI:** *Bile Duct
and Pancreas Cancer; Esophageal Diseases*; **HMO:**
Vytra US Hlthcre Oxford Blue Cross & Blue Shield
Empire +
LANG: Afr; [♿] [🔲] [👤] [🏠] [S] [Mcr] [Mcd] [WC] [NFI]
A Few Days **VISA** [💳] [💳]

Giorgini Jr, Gino (MD) Ge
Good Samaritan Hosp

375 E Main St Ste 21; Bay Shore, NY 11706; (516) 968-8288; **BDCERT:** IM 72; Ge 73; **MS:** UMDNJ-NJ Med Sch, Newark 66; **RES:** IM, Milwaukee Cty Gen Hosp, Milwaukee, WI 67-69; **FEL:** Ge, Rhode Island Hosp, Providence, RI 69-71; **HOSP:** Southside Hosp; **HMO:** Oxford US Hlthcre Empire MDNY Vytra +

⚙ 📷 ⊞ 💲 Mcr Mcd WC NFI A Few Days **VISA** ⬤

Harris, Alan I (MD) Ge
Huntington Hosp

Huntington Gastroenterology Associates, 152 E Main St Ste C; Huntington, NY 11743; (516) 421-2185; **BDCERT:** Ge 75; **MS:** Mt Sinai Sch Med 72; **RES:** Mount Sinai Med Ctr, New York, NY 72-75; **FEL:** Mount Sinai Med Ctr, New York, NY 75-77; **FAP:** Instr Med SUNY Stony Brook; *SI: Inflammatory Bowel Disease; Liver Disease;* **HMO:** Aetna Hlth Plan CIGNA Prucare Metro Empire Blue Choice +

⚙ 📷 👤 ⊞ 💲 Mcr A Few Days ▦ **VISA** ⬤

Harrison, Aaron R (MD) Ge
Southside Hosp

375 E Main St Ste 21; Bay Shore, NY 11706; (516) 968-8288; **BDCERT:** IM 77; Ge 79; **MS:** Albert Einstein Coll Med 74; **RES:** IM, Jacobi Med Ctr, Bronx, NY 74-77; **FEL:** Ge, UCLA Med Ctr, Los Angeles, CA 77-79; **FAP:** Asst Clin Prof Med SUNY Stony Brook; **HOSP:** Good Samaritan Hosp Med Ctr; *SI: Peptic Ulcer; Esophageal Reflux Disease;* **HMO:** Aetna Hlth Plan Vytra Oxford Empire MONY +

⚙ 📷 ⊞ 💲 Mcr Mcd WC NFI A Few Days **VISA** ⬤

Naso, Kristin (DO) Ge
Southampton Hosp

Second Office Southampton, 222 Manor Pl; Greenport, NY 11944; (516) 477-2500; **BDCERT:** IM 89; Ge 91; **MS:** NY Coll Osteo Med 85; **RES:** Long Island Coll Hosp, Brooklyn, NY 87-89; **FEL:** Ge, Long Island Coll Hosp, Brooklyn, NY; **HOSP:** Eastern Long Island Hosp

⚙ 📷 👤 ⊞ 💲 Mcr 1 Week

Pastrich, Howard Jay (MD) Ge
Brookhaven Mem Hosp

260 Patchogue-Yaphank Rd; Patchogue, NY 11772; (516) 289-0300; **BDCERT:** IM 83; Ge 87; **MS:** SUNY Hlth Sci Ctr 80; **RES:** IM, Nassau County Med Ctr, East Meadow, NY; **FEL:** Ge, Montefiore Med Ctr, Bronx, NY; Albert Einstein Med Ctr, Bronx, NY; **HMO:** Empire US Hlthcre Empire Blue Choice Sanus CIGNA +

LANG: Sp; ⚙ ⊞ 💲 Mcr Mcd 2-4 Weeks

Spielberg, Alan (MD) Ge
St John's Epis Hosp-Smithtown

St John's Medical Building, 48 Route 25A 203; Smithtown, NY 11787; (516) 724-1178; **BDCERT:** IM 77; Ge 79; **MS:** Belgium 74; **RES:** IM, Albany Med Ctr, Albany, NY 75-77; **FEL:** Ge, Albany Med Ctr, Albany, NY 77-79; *SI: Inflammatory Bowel Disease; Ulcer Disease;* **HMO:** Oxford Blue Choice GHI JJ Newman CIGNA +

LANG: Fr, Dut; ⚙ 📷 👤 ⊞ 💲 Mcr Mcd A Few Days

GERIATRIC MEDICINE

Fox, Elaine E (MD) Ger PCP
Southampton Hosp

61 Hill St; Southampton, NY 11968; (516) 287-1951; **BDCERT:** IM 79; Ger 88; **MS:** NY Med Coll 75; **RES:** St Luke's Roosevelt Hosp Ctr, New York, NY 75; IM, Stamford Hosp, Stamford, CT 77-78

⚙ 👤 ⊞ 💲 4+ Weeks

Guide to symbols and abbreviations can be found on pages 110-113.

719

GERIATRIC PSYCHIATRY

Steinberg, Alan (MD)   GerPsy
St John's Epis Hosp-Smithtown
East End Neuropsychiatric Associates, 2539 Middle
Country Rd; Centereach, NY 11720; (516) 737-
6434; **BDCERT:** Psyc 89; GerPsy 91; **MS:** Mt Sinai
Sch Med 83; **RES:** Med, Univ Hosp SUNY Stony
Brook, Stony Brook, NY 83-84; Psyc, Johns
Hopkins Hosp, Baltimore, MD 84-86; **FEL:** GerPsy,
NY Hosp-Cornell-Westchester, White Plains, NY
86-87; **FAP:** Asst Prof Med SUNY Stony Brook; **SI:**
Alzheimer's Disease; Depression; **HMO:** MDLI Empire
Oxford VBH

LANG: Sp; ⌖ ☎ 🖬 🖬 💲 Mcr Mcd WC NFI 2-4 Weeks

HAND SURGERY

Hurst, Lawrence (MD)   HS
Univ Hosp SUNY Stony Brook
181 Bellemeade Rd 2; E Setauket, NY 11733; (516)
444-3145; **BDCERT:** OrS 80; **MS:** Univ Vt Coll Med
73; **RES:** U NC Hosp, Chapel Hill, NC 74-78; **FEL:**
HS, Columbia-Presbyterian Med Ctr, New York, NY
78-79; **FAP:** Prof SUNY Stony Brook; **HOSP:** St
Charles Hosp & Rehab Ctr; **SI:** *Nerve Problems;
Dupuytren's;* **HMO:** CIGNA GHI Vytra Empire
Oxford +

⌖ ☎ 🖬 🖬 💲 Mcr Mcd WC NFI A Few Days **VISA** 💳

Mirza, M Ather (MD)   HS
St John's Epis Hosp-Smithtown
290 E Main St; Smithtown, NY 11787; (516) 361-
5302; **BDCERT:** OrS 78; HS 89; **MS:** India 66; **RES:**
Nassau County Med Ctr, East Meadow, NY 68-69;
FEL: HS, Cook Cty Hosp, Chicago, IL 72-73; **HOSP:**
Univ Hosp SUNY Stony Brook

⌖ 🄲 ☎ 🖬 💲 Mcr WC NFI 2-4 Weeks ▦ **VISA** 💳

HEMATOLOGY

Avvento, Louis (MD)   Hem
Central Suffolk Hosp
East End Hematology/Oncology, 1333 E Main St;
Riverhead, NY 11901; (516) 727-1214; **BDCERT:**
IM 85; **MS:** Italy 81; **RES:** Jamaica Med Ctr,
Jamaica, NY 83-85; **HOSP:** Southampton Hosp; **SI:**
Oncology

⌖ ☎ 🖬 💲 Mcr Mcd 2-4 Weeks ▦ **VISA** 💳 🏷

Gold, Kenneth (MD)   Hem
Good Samaritan Hosp Med Ctr
Oncology Associates, 370 E Main St 2; Bay Shore,
NY 11706; (516) 666-6752; **BDCERT:** Onc 83;
Hem 87; **MS:** Baylor 77; **RES:** Geo Wash U Med Ctr,
Washington, DC 78-81; **FEL:** Columbia-
Presbyterian Med Ctr, New York, NY 81-83; **HOSP:**
Southside Hosp; **HMO:** MDLI Aetna Hlth Plan Blue
Choice Chubb Cost Care +

LANG: Sp; ⌖ ☎ 🖬 💲 Mcr Mcd A Few Days **VISA**
💳

INFECTIOUS DISEASE

Collins, Adriane (DO)   Inf
Good Samaritan Hosp
786 Montauk Hwy; West Islip, NY 11730; (516)
376-6075; **BDCERT:** IM 95; **MS:** Cornell U 90; **RES:**
New York University Med Ctr, New York, NY 92-
93; **HMO:** Magnacare GHI US Hlthcre

⌖ ☎ 🖬 💲 Mcr Mcd WC NFI Immediately

Greenspan, Joel (MD)   Inf
N Shore Univ Hosp-Manhasset
44 S Bayles Ave; Pt Wash, NY 11050; (516) 767-
7771; **BDCERT:** IM 76; 79; **MS:** SUNY Syracuse 69;
RES: Med, Bellevue Hosp Ctr, New York, NY 70-72;
Ge, Bellevue Hosp Ctr, New York, NY 75-77; **FAP:**
Asst Clin Prof NYU Sch Med; **HMO:** Oxford US
Hlthcre

⌖ Mcr Mcd WC NFI

Klein, Arthur (DO)   Inf
St John's Epis Hosp-Smithtown
3400 Nesconset Hwy 108; E Setauket, NY 11733;
(516) 689-5400; **BDCERT:** IM 86; Inf 88; **MS:**
SUNY Hlth Sci Ctr 83; **RES:** Univ Hosp SUNY Stony
Brook, Stony Brook, NY 83; **FEL:** Inf, Univ Hosp
SUNY Stony Brook, Stony Brook, NY; **HMO:** None

🦽 🗝 📷 🛏 $ Mcr Mcd WC NFI 2-4 Weeks

Sacks-Berg, Anne (MD)   Inf
Huntington Hosp
Anne SacksBerg, MD, 21 Southdown Rd;
Huntington, NY 11743; (516) 423-9809;
BDCERT: IM 86; Inf 88; **MS:** SUNY Hlth Sci Ctr 82;
RES: IM, Winthrop Univ Hosp, Mineola, NY 83-86;
FEL: Inf, Winthrop Univ Hosp, Mineola, NY 86-88;
HMO: PHS

🦽 📷 🛏 $ Mcr WC NFI A Few Days

Samuels, Steven (MD)   Inf PCP
Good Samaritan Hosp Med Ctr
Suffolk Internal Medicine, 500 Montauk Hwy S; W
Islip, NY 11795; (516) 587-7733; **BDCERT:** IM 77;
Inf 82; **MS:** NY Med Coll 74; **RES:** IM, Nassau
County Med Ctr, East Meadow, NY 74-77; **FEL:** IP,
UC Irvine Med Ctr, Orange, CA 77-79; **HOSP:**
Southside Hosp; **SI:** *Lyme Disease; AIDS;* **HMO:**
Oxford Prucare PHS Vytra

🦽 🌙 📷 🛏 $ Mcr WC NFI 1 Week **VISA** 💳

Shah, Vijay (MD)   Inf
Mid-Island Hosp
129 Broadway; Amityville, NY; (516) 939-0149;
BDCERT: IM 91; Inf 96; **MS:** Other Foreign Country
84; **RES:** IM, Wyckoff Heights Med Ctr, Brooklyn,
NY 88-91; **FEL:** Inf, Nassau County Med Ctr, East
Meadow, NY 91; **HOSP:** N Shore Univ Hosp-
Plainview; **SI:** *HIV/AIDS Infection; Lyme Disease;*
HMO: Oxford Aetna-US Healthcare United
Healthcare CIGNA HIP Network +

LANG: Hin, Itl, Sp, Guj; 🦽 📷 🛏 $ Mcr Mcd WC
A Few Days

INTERNAL MEDICINE

Balot, Barry (DO)   IM
Good Samaritan Hosp Med Ctr
609 Route 109 # 1B; W Babylon, NY 11704;
(516) 669-8100; **BDCERT:** IM 89; Ger 94; **MS:** NY
Coll Osteo Med 85; **RES:** Univ Hosp SUNY Brooklyn,
Brooklyn, NY 86-87; Overlook Hosp, Summit, NJ
87-89; **HOSP:** Brunswick Hosp Ctr

Bernard, Robert (MD)   IM PCP
Central Suffolk Hosp
Family Care Medical Center, 6144 Rte 25A;
Wading River, NY 11792; (516) 929-5900;
BDCERT: IM 89; **MS:** Grenada 86; **RES:** IM, St
Joseph's Hosp-Paterson, Paterson, NJ 86-89; **SI:**
Heart Disease; Skin Disease; **HMO:** Vytra Oxford
MDNY Empire

🦽 🆘 🌙 📷 🛏 🛏 Mcr WC NFI Immediately 💳
VISA 💳

Biasetti, John (MD)   IM
JT Mather Mem Hosp Pt Jfrson
116 Terryville Rd; Port Jefferson Station, NY
11776; (516) 928-2002; **BDCERT:** IM 72; **MS:** NY
Med Coll 63; **RES:** IM, Nassau Cty Med Ctr, East
Meadow, NY 67-70

Chernaik, Robert (MD)   IM PCP
Brookhaven Mem Hosp
285 Sills Rd; Patchogue, NY 11772; (516) 654-
1800; **BDCERT:** IM 68; **MS:** UMDNJ-NJ Med Sch,
Newark 61; **RES:** Beth Israel Med Ctr, New York,
NY 62-63; Montefiore Med Ctr, Bronx, NY 63-64;
FEL: Path, U CO Hosp, Denver, CO 64-65; **FAP:** Asst
Clin Prof SUNY Downstate; **HMO:** Oxford JJ
Newman MDNY Empire Blue Shield

🦽 📷 🌙 🛏 $ Mcr WC NFI 4+ Weeks

Delman, Michael (MD) IM `PCP`
Southside Hosp

45 E Main St; E Islip, NY 11730; (516) 581-0737;
BDCERT: IM 72; Ge 75; **MS:** NY Med Coll 68; **RES:**
IM, Metropolitan Hosp Ctr, New York, NY 68-70;
Ge,; **FEL:** Ge, Metropolitan Hosp Ctr, New York, NY
72-73; Metropolitan Hosp Ctr, New York, NY; **FAP:**
Asst Clin Prof Med SUNY Stony Brook; **HOSP:** Good
Samaritan Hosp Med Ctr; *SI: Addiction Medicine*;
HMO: Aetna-US Healthcare CIGNA MDNY United
Healthcare Oxford +

[symbols] 2-4 Weeks **VISA**

Ells, Peter F (MD) IM
Univ Hosp SUNY Stony Brook

SUNY at Stony Brook, HSC T17 060; Stony Brook,
NY 11790; (516) 444-0580; **BDCERT:** IM 77; **MS:**
Tufts U 74; **RES:** IM, U of VA Health Sci Ctr,
Charlottesville, VA 74-77; **FEL:** Hem, UC San
Francisco Med Ctr, San Francisco, CA 77-81; **FAP:**
Asst Prof SUNY Stony Brook; *SI: Liver Disease;
Hepatitis*; **HMO:** Empire Vytra Oxford GHI US
Hlthcre +

[symbols] 1 Week **VISA**

Fleishman, Philip (MD) IM `PCP`
Southside Hosp

45 E Main St; E Islip, NY 11730; (516) 581-0737;
BDCERT: IM 69; **MS:** SUNY Hlth Sci Ctr 61; **RES:**
Kingsbrook Jewish Med Ctr, Brooklyn, NY 62-65;
FAP: Asst Clin Prof SUNY Stony Brook; **HOSP:**
Good Samaritan Hosp Med Ctr; *SI: Diabetes*; **HMO:**
Aetna Hlth Plan CIGNA

[symbols] A Few Days **VISA**

Frank, William (MD) IM
Good Samaritan Hosp Med Ctr

1308 Pine Dr; Bay Shore, NY 11706; (516) 666-
2808; **BDCERT:** IM 75; Nep 78; **MS:** U Iowa Coll
Med 72; **RES:** Long Island Jewish Med Ctr, New
Hyde Park, NY 72-73; **FEL:** Nep, Univ Hosp SUNY
Bklyn, Brooklyn, NY 75-77; **HOSP:** Southside
Hosp; **HMO:** Aetna Hlth Plan Choicecare HIP
Network

[symbols] A Few Days

Friedling, Steven (MD) IM `PCP`
St John's Epis Hosp-Smithtown

Branch Medical Assoc, 267 E Main St Bldg A;
Smithtown, NY 11787; (516) 724-2000; **BDCERT:**
IM 73; **MS:** SUNY Downstate 68; **RES:** IM, Barnes
Hosp, St Louis, MO 71-73; Onc, Nat Cancer Inst,
Bethesda, MD 69-71; **FEL:** Inf, Barnes Hosp, St
Louis, MO 73-74; **FAP:** Asst Clin Prof Med SUNY
Stony Brook; **HOSP:** Univ Hosp SUNY Stony Brook;
SI: Preventive Care; Managing Chronic Diseases;
HMO: Oxford Empire Blue Cross United Healthcare
PHS Vytra +

LANG: Vn, Heb, Swd; [symbols] 4+ Weeks

Goldfarb, Steven (MD) IM
Southampton Hosp

365 County Rd 39A Ste 5&6; Southampton, NY
11968; (516) 283-4048; **BDCERT:** IM 89; **MS:**
Italy 83; **RES:** IM, Berkshire Med Ctr, Pittsfield, MA
83-86; *SI: Medical Ethics; Lyme Disease*
LANG: Itl, Sp; [symbols] 4+ Weeks

Hallal, Edward (MD) IM `PCP`
Southside Hosp

180 E Main St; Bay Shore, NY 11706; (516) 665-
0027; **BDCERT:** IM 87; **MS:** Grenada 84; **RES:** New
York Methodist Hosp, Brooklyn, NY 84-87; **HOSP:**
Good Samaritan Hosp Med Ctr; **HMO:** Oxford
MDNY CIGNA Chubb

[symbols] 4+ Weeks **VISA**

Hertz, Howard M (MD) IM `PCP`
Good Samaritan Hosp Med Ctr

350 W Main St; Babylon, NY 11702; (516) 661-
2277; **MS:** Mexico 78; **RES:** Winthrop Univ Hosp,
Mineola, NY; **HMO:** Oxford Aetna-US Healthcare
GHI United Healthcare Prucare +

LANG: Sp, Ger, Grk, Pol, Itl; [symbols] A Few Days

Israel, Michael (MD) IM **PCP**
Southampton Hosp
94 Pantigo Rd; East Hampton, NY 11937; (516)
324-7700; **BDCERT:** IM 81; **MS:** Boston U 77; **RES:**
IM, Jackson Mem Hosp, Miami, FL 77-81; **HMO:**
Oxford MDNY Chubb JJ Newman
⟨symbols⟩ Immediately *VISA* ⬤

LaBarbera, Philip (MD) IM **PCP**
Brookhaven Mem Hosp
430 Montauk Hwy; Sayville, NY 11782; (516)
589-9303; **BDCERT:** FP 93; **MS:** Italy 75; **RES:** IM,
Brooklyn Hosp Ctr, Brooklyn, NY 75-78; **SI:**
Hypertension; Diabetes; **HMO:** CIGNA United
Healthcare MDNY Magnacare Mayan +
LANG: Itl; ⟨symbols⟩ A Few Days

Lalli, Corradino (MD) IM
St John's Epis Hosp-Smithtown
359 Route 111; Smithtown, NY 11787; (516)
366-0404; **BDCERT:** 79; Ger 88; **MS:** Albert
Einstein Coll Med 76; **RES:** IM, Nassau County Med
Ctr, East Meadow, NY 76-79; **FEL:** Pul, Nassau
County Med Ctr, East Meadow, NY 79-80; **FAP:**
Clin Instr SUNY Stony Brook; **SI:** *Preventive
Medicine; Dementia;* **HMO:** Vytra Oxford Blue Choice
United Healthcare PHS +
⟨symbols⟩ 2-4 Weeks

Lerner, Harvey (MD) IM **PCP**
St John's Epis Hosp-Smithtown
Smithtown Medical Specialists, 215 E Main St;
Smithtown, NY 11787; (516) 265-5858; **BDCERT:**
IM 74; **MS:** U Chicago-Pritzker Sch Med 57; **RES:**
Montefiore Med Ctr, Bronx, NY 58-59; Kings
County Hosp Ctr, Brooklyn, NY 59-61; **FAP:** Asst
Clin Prof SUNY Stony Brook; **HOSP:** Univ Hosp
SUNY Stony Brook; **SI:** *Risk Factor Management;
Chronic Fatigue;* **HMO:** Oxford Aetna Hlth Plan
Metlife Empire Prucare +
⟨symbols⟩ 2-4 Weeks *VISA*
⬤

Matkovic, Christopher (MD) IM
St John's Epis Hosp-Smithtown
80 Maple Ave 204; Smithtown, NY 11787; (516)
265-0075; **BDCERT:** IM 77; Inf 80; **MS:** Columbia
P&S 74; **RES:** Presbyterian U Hosp, Pittsburgh, PA
74-77; **FEL:** Presbyterian U Hosp, Pittsburgh, PA
77-79; **FAP:** Asst Clin Prof SUNY Stony Brook;
HMO: Oxford PHCS JJ Newman Lawrence
Healthcare
⟨symbols⟩ 1 Week

Nash, Bernard (MD) IM **PCP**
Good Samaritan Hosp Med Ctr
Suffolk Internal Medicine, 500 Montauk Hwy Suite
S; W Islip, NY 11795; (516) 587-7733; **BDCERT:**
Inf 82; IM 78; **MS:** Georgetown U 75; **RES:** IM, St
Elizabeth's Med Ctr, Boston, MA 76-78; **FEL:** Inf,
Boston U Med Ctr, Boston, MA 79-81; **HOSP:**
Southside Hosp; **SI:** *Lyme Disease; AIDS;* **HMO:**
Oxford Prucare Empire Vytra
⟨symbols⟩ 1 Week *VISA* ⬤

Romano, Rosario (MD) IM **PCP**
JT Mather Mem Hosp Pt Jfrson
Port Jefferson Internal Med Associates, 5225
Nesconset Hwy Ste 15; Port Jefferson Station, NY
11776; (516) 331-1000; **BDCERT:** IM 77; **MS:** NY
Med Coll 73; **RES:** IM, Lenox Hill Hosp, New York,
NY 74-77; **HOSP:** St Charles Hosp & Rehab Ctr;
HMO: Most
⟨symbols⟩ 2-4 Weeks

Simon, Lloyd (MD) IM **PCP**
Eastern Long Island Hosp
44210 C County Rd 48; Southold, NY 11971;
(516) 765-4150; **BDCERT:** IM 83; **MS:** SUNY
Buffalo 80; **RES:** IM, U Mass Med Ctr, Worcester,
MA 80-83; **SI:** *Addiction Medicine;* **HMO:** Vytra
Oxford US Hlthcre Blue Choice
⟨symbols⟩ A Few Days

Guide to symbols and abbreviations can be found on pages 110-113.

723

MEDICAL GENETICS

Hyman, David (MD)   **MG**
Univ Hosp SUNY Stony Brook
The Genetics Center,Inc, 48 Route 25A Ste 205;
Smithtown, NY 11787; (516) 862-3620; **BDCERT:**
MG 84; 83; **MS:** Univ IL Coll Med 78; **RES:** Yale-
New Haven Hosp, New Haven, CT 78-80; **FEL:**
Yale-New Haven Hosp, New Haven, CT 80-83;
HOSP: St John's Epis Hosp-Smithtown; **SI:** *Prenatal
Diagnosis; Cancer Susceptibility;* **HMO:** Oxford United
Healthcare Metlife Vytra Multiplan +

LANG: Ger, Ar, Fr; ♿ 🅢🅢 📞 📷 🎬 💲 Mcr Mcd
Immediately **VISA** 💳

MEDICAL ONCOLOGY

Berger, E Roy (MD)   **Onc**
JT Mather Mem Hosp Pt Jfrson
North Shore Hematology Oncology Associates, 235
N Belle Meade Rd; East Setauket, NY 11733; (516)
751-3000; **BDCERT:** Onc 77; Hem 76; **MS:** SUNY
Downstate 70; **RES:** Med, St Luke's Roosevelt Hosp
Ctr, New York, NY 71-73; **FEL:** Hem, St Luke's
Roosevelt Hosp Ctr, New York, NY 73-74; Onc,
Mem Sloan Kettering Cancer Ctr, New York, NY
74-75; **FAP:** Asst Clin Prof Med NY Med Coll;
HOSP: St John's Epis Hosp-Smithtown; **SI:** *Prostate
Cancer*

♿ 🅢🅢 📷 🧑 🎬 💲 Mcr Mcd WC NFl Immediately 📠
VISA 💳

Caruso, Rocco (MD)   **Onc**
Univ Hosp SUNY Stony Brook
2500 Nesconset Hwy 63; Stoney Brook, NY
11790; (516) 751-8305; **BDCERT:** Onc 95; IM 82;
MS: Univ Penn 79; **RES:** St Luke's Roosevelt Hosp
Ctr, New York, NY 80-82; **FEL:** Hem, New York
University Med Ctr, New York, NY 82-85; **FAP:**
Asst Prof of Clin Med SUNY Stony Brook; **HOSP:** JT
Mather Mem Hosp Pt Jfrson; **HMO:** Aetna Hlth Plan
Blue Choice Choicecare

♿ 📞 📷 🧑 🎬 Mcr Mcd Immediately

Dobbs, Joan (MD)   **Onc**
St John's Epis Hosp-Smithtown
North Shore Hematology Oncology Associates, 235
N Belle Meade Rd; East Setauket, NY 11733; (516)
751-3000; **BDCERT:** IM 71; Hem 77; **MS:** SUNY
Hlth Sci Ctr 60; **RES:** Med, Montefiore Med Ctr,
Bronx, NY 62-64; Path, Stanford Med Ctr, Stanford,
CA 61-62; **FEL:** Hem, Mount Sinai Med Ctr, New
York, NY 64-65; Hem, Maimonides Med Ctr,
Brooklyn, NY 65-66; **FAP:** SUNY Downstate;
HOSP: JT Mather Mem Hosp Pt Jfrson; **SI:** *Breast
Cancer; Ovarian Cancer;* **HMO:** Vytra Aetna Hlth
Plan CIGNA Oxford

LANG: Grk, Hin, Fr, Heb; ♿ 🎬 💲 Mcr Mcd
A Few Days 💳 **VISA**

Dosik, Michael (MD)   **Onc**
St Charles Hosp & Rehab Ctr
North Shore Hematology/Oncology Assoc, PC, 235
N Belle Meade Rd; East Setauket, NY 11733; (516)
751-3000; **BDCERT:** Onc 73; Hem 82; **MS:** Cornell
U 66; **RES:** UCLA Med Ctr, Los Angeles, CA 67-68;
FEL: Onc, Mem Sloan Kettering Cancer Ctr, New
York, NY; **HOSP:** JT Mather Mem Hosp Pt Jfrson; **SI:**
Breast Cancer; **HMO:** Vytra Oxford US Hlthcre
CIGNA

LANG: Grk, Flm, Sp; ♿ 🎬 💲 Mcr Mcd A Few Days
💳 **VISA** 💳

Fiore, John J (MD)   **Onc**
Univ Hosp SUNY Stony Brook
Health Science Center T17 80; Stony Brook, NY
11794; (516) 444-1727; **BDCERT:** Onc 82; Hem
82; **MS:** Tufts U 75; **RES:** IM, Boston VA Med Ctr,
Boston, MA 75-76; Boston VA Med Ctr, Boston, MA
76-79; **FEL:** Onc, Boston VA Med Ctr, Boston, MA
80-81; Mem Sloan Kettering Cancer Ctr, New York,
NY 81-84; **FAP:** Assoc Prof SUNY Stony Brook; **SI:**
Lung Cancer; **HMO:** US Hlthcre Oxford Aetna-US
Healthcare Travelers Metlife +

♿ 📷 🧑 🎬 💲 Mcr Mcd A Few Days

Lipshutz, Mark (MD)   Onc   `PCP`
Good Samaritan Hosp Med Ctr
HematologyOncology Assoc of W Suffolk, PC, 370 E
Main St 2; Bay Shore, NY 11706; (516) 666-6752;
BDCERT: Hem 78; Onc 79; **MS:** Penn State U-
Hershey Med Ctr 73; **RES:** IM, Cedars-Sinai Med Ctr,
Los Angeles, CA 73-75; **FEL:** Hem, Long Island
Jewish Med Ctr, New Hyde Park, NY 75-77; Long
Island Jewish Med Ctr, New Hyde Park, NY 77-78;
HOSP: Southside Hosp; **SI:** *Peripheral Stem Cell
Transplantation;* **HMO:** Aetna Hlth Plan Blue Choice
Blue Cross & Blue Shield Choicecare Prucare +
♿ 📷 🏦 $ Mcr Mod   1 Week **VISA** ●

Ostrow, Stanley (MD)   Onc
JT Mather Mem Hosp Pt Jfrson
All Island Hematology & Oncology, 2500
Nesconset Hwy Bld 8; Stony Brook, NY 11790;
(516) 751-5151; **BDCERT:** IM 78; **MS:** SUNY
Downstate 74; **RES:** Med, Jewish Mem Hosp, New
York, NY 75-76; **FEL:** Hem Onc, Nat Cancer Inst,
Bethesda, MD 76-80; **FAP:** Asst Prof SUNY Stony
Brook; **HOSP:** Brookhaven Mem Hosp
♿ 📷 🏦 🚹 🏦 Mcr Mod WC NFI   A Few Days

Samuel, Edward (MD)   Onc
JT Mather Mem Hosp Pt Jfrson
North Shore Hematology/Onc Assoc, 235
Bellemead Rd; East Setauket, NY 11733; (516)
751-3000; **BDCERT:** Onc 81; Hem 82; **MS:** Duke U
73; **RES:** IM, Duke U Med Ctr, Durham, NC 73-75;
Hem, Duke U Med Ctr, Durham, NC 75-76; **FEL:**
Hem, New York University Med Ctr, New York, NY
75-77; Onc, Mem Sloan Kettering Cancer Ctr, New
York, NY 77-78; **FAP:** Asst Clin Prof NYU Sch Med;
HOSP: St John's Epis Hosp-Smithtown; **SI:** *Cancer
Pain Management; Multiple Myeloma*
LANG: Sp; ♿ 📷 🏦 🏦 $ Mcr Mod   1 Week

Strauss, Barry (MD)   Onc
Southampton Hosp
353 Meeting House Ln; Southampton, NY 11968;
(516) 283-6611; **BDCERT:** Onc 75; IM 75; **MS:**
Geo Wash U Sch Med 71; **RES:** IM, Beth Israel Med
Ctr, New York, NY 71-72; IM, Beth Israel Med Ctr,
New York, NY 72-73; **FEL:** Onc, Nat Cancer Inst,
Bethesda, MD 73-74; Onc, Nat Cancer Inst,
Bethesda, MD 74-75; **SI:** *Lung Cancer; Ovarian
Cancer;* **HMO:** Vytra Oxford United Healthcare
Island Group
♿ Ⓕ 🏦 🚹 🏦 Mcr WC   A Few Days

NEONATAL-PERINATAL MEDICINE

De Cristofaro, Joseph D (MD) NP
Univ Hosp SUNY Stony Brook
Univ Hosp SUNY Stony Brook—Dept of Pediatrics,;
Stony Brook, NY 11794; (516) 444-3085;
BDCERT: Ped 86; **MS:** NYU Sch Med 81; **RES:** Ped,
Children's Hosp Med Ctr, Cincinnati, OH 81-84;
FEL: NP, NY Hosp-Cornell Med Ctr, New York, NY
84-86; **FAP:** Asst Prof SUNY Stony Brook; **SI:** *Apnea
of Infancy; SIDS;* **HMO:** Blue Choice Blue Cross &
Blue Shield Choicecare Vytra Oxford +
LANG: Sp; ♿ 🏦 🏦 $ Mcr Mod WC NFI   Immediately
■ **VISA** ●

NEPHROLOGY

Asad, Syed (MD)   Nep
Huntington Hosp
256 Broadway; Huntington Station, NY 11746;
(516) 423-4320; **BDCERT:** IM 73; Nep 78; **MS:**
Turkey 68; **RES:** IM, Nassau County Med Ctr, East
Meadow, NY 70-72; **FEL:** Nep, Nassau County Med
Ctr, East Meadow, NY 72-74; **FAP:** Assoc Clin Instr
Med SUNY Hlth Sci Ctr; **SI:** *Hemodialysis;
Hypertension*
♿ 🏦 🏦 Mcr Mod WC

Ilamathi, Ekambaram M (MD)Nep
St John's Epis Hosp-Smithtown

Suffolk Nephrology Consultants, PC, 2500 Route 347 Bldg14; Stony Brook, NY 11790; (516) 689-7800; **BDCERT:** Nep 78; **MS:** India 71; **RES:** Mount Sinai Med Ctr, New York, NY 73-74; Mount Sinai Med Ctr, New York, NY 74-76; **FEL:** Renal Disease, Nassau County Med Ctr, East Meadow, NY; **FAP:** Nep SUNY Stony Brook; **HOSP:** JT Mather Mem Hosp Pt Jfrson; **SI:** *Hypertension; Diabetes Mellitus*

♿ ☎ 🖼 📅 $ Mcr Mcd   A Few Days **VISA** 💳

Kirsch, Mitchell (MD)   Nep
St John's Epis Hosp-Smithtown

Suffolk Nephrology Consultants, 250026 Rte 347; Stony Brook, NY 11790; (516) 689-7800; **BDCERT:** IM 84; Nep 86; **MS:** NY Med Coll 81; **RES:** Nassau County Med Ctr, East Meadow, NY 81-84; **FEL:** Mount Sinai Med Ctr, New York, NY 84-86; **HOSP:** JT Mather Mem Hosp Pt Jfrson; **SI:** *Nephrology; Hypertension;* **HMO:** Empire Blue Choice US Hlthcre Aetna Hlth Plan Prucare Metlife +

♿ ☎ 🖼 📅 $ Mcr Mcd

NEUROLOGICAL SURGERY

Davis, Raphael (MD)   NS
Univ Hosp SUNY Stony Brook

Neurosurgery—SUNY Stony Brook Hosp, SUNY HSC T12 Rm 080; Stony Brook, NY 11794; (516) 444-1210; **BDCERT:** NS 90; **MS:** Mt Sinai Sch Med 81; **RES:** Mount Sinai Med Ctr, New York, NY 81-82; **HOSP:** JT Mather Mem Hosp Pt Jfrson; **HMO:** Aetna Hlth Plan Chubb

♿ ☎ 🖼 📅 Mcr Mcd WC NFI   Immediately **VISA** 💳 📧

Keuskamp, P Arjen (MD)   NS
St John's Epis Hosp-Smithtown

Midsuffolk Neurosurgical Assoc, 309 E Middle Country Rd 201; Smithtown, NY 11787; (516) 265-2020; **BDCERT:** NS 82; **MS:** Holland 71; **RES:** Montefiore Med Ctr, Bronx, NY 71-79; **FEL:** NS, Albert Einstein Med Ctr, Bronx, NY 75-77; **HOSP:** St Charles Hosp & Rehab Ctr; **SI:** *Neuro-Oncology; Spine Surgery;* **HMO:** Aetna Hlth Plan Oxford Vytra

LANG: Dut; ♿ ☎ 🖼 📅 $ Mcr Mcd WC NFI   A Few Days **VISA** 💳

NEUROLOGY

Anto, Cecily (MD)   N
Nassau County Med Ctr

521 Route 111 # 200; Hauppauge, NY 11788; (516) 724-4455; **BDCERT:** N 89; C/Nph 94; **MS:** India 76; **RES:** Lncln Med Ctr, Bronx, NY 78-79; Nassau Cty Med Ctr, East Meadow, NY 79-82; **FEL:** Nassau Cty Med, East Meadow, NY

Chernik, Norman (MD)   N
Brookhaven Mem Hosp

South Shore Neurological Associates, 280 E Main St; Bay Shore, NY 11706; (516) 666-3939; **BDCERT:** N 74; **MS:** St Louis U 65; **RES:** Mount Sinai Med Ctr, New York, NY 66-68; Kings County Hosp Ctr, Brooklyn, NY 68-69; **HOSP:** Central Suffolk Hosp; **SI:** *Acupuncture*

♿ 🖼 📅 $ Mcr Mcd WC NFI   1 Week ■ **VISA** 💳

Cohen, Daniel (MD)   N
Good Samaritan Hosp

Long Island Neurology, 370 E Main St Ste 1; Bay Shore, NY 11706; (516) 666-4767; **BDCERT:** N 86; **MS:** U Miami Sch Med 80; **RES:** N, Jackson Mem Hosp, Miami, FL 81-84; **HOSP:** Southside Hosp; **SI:** *Muscle and Nerve Problems; Stroke Treatment, Prevention;* **HMO:** Aetna-US Healthcare Oxford Empire Magnacare

♿ 🖼 📅 $ Mcr Mcd WC NFI   1 Week **VISA** 💳

Gudesblatt, Mark (MD) N
Southside Hosp

280 E Main St; Bay Shore, NY 11706; (516) 666-3939; **BDCERT:** N 86; **MS:** Cornell U 80; **RES:** Mount Sinai Med Ctr, New York, NY 81-84; **FEL:** N, Nat Inst Health, Bethesda, MD 84-85; Mount Sinai Med Ctr, New York, NY; **HOSP:** Good Samaritan Hosp Med Ctr; **HMO:** Choicecare Travelers

[symbols] Immediately [symbol]
VISA [symbols]

Kershaw, Paul (MD) N
Southampton Hosp

349 Meeting House Ln; Southampton, NY 11968; (516) 287-2500; **BDCERT:** N 90; **MS:** Tufts U 81; **RES:** IM, Faulkner Hosp, Boston, MA 81-84; N, Boston Med Ctr, Boston, MA 84-87; **HMO:** Aetna Hlth Plan Chubb MDLI

[symbols]

Mendelsohn, Frederic (MD) N
Univ Hosp SUNY Stony Brook

500 Portion Rd Ste 6; Ronkonkoma, NY 11779; (516) 737-0055; **BDCERT:** N 77; **MS:** KY Med Sch, Louisville 71; **RES:** N, Nassau County Med Ctr, East Meadow, NY; **FEL:** N, Nassau County Med Ctr, East Meadow, NY; **HMO:** Empire Choicecare Metlife US Hlthcre Aetna Hlth Plan +

[symbols] 1 Week

Moreta, Henry (MD) N
Southside Hosp

South Shore Neurologic Associates, 280 E Main St; Bay Shore, NY 11706; (516) 666-3939; **BDCERT:** N 87; **MS:** Harvard Med Sch 77; **RES:** NY Hosp-Cornell Med Ctr, New York, NY 78-79; **HOSP:** Good Samaritan Hosp Med Ctr

[symbols] Immediately [symbol]
VISA [symbols]

Newman, George (MD & PhD) N
Univ Hosp SUNY Stony Brook

Neurology Associates—SUNYat Stony Brook HSC, T12020; Stony Brook, NY 11794; (516) 444-2599; **BDCERT:** N 82; **MS:** U Va Sch Med 76; **RES:** IM, Roger Williams Med Ctr, Providence, RI 76-78; **FEL:** N, U of VA Health Sci Ctr, Charlottesville, VA 78-81; **FAP:** Assoc Prof SUNY Stony Brook; **HOSP:** VA Med Ctr-Northport; **SI:** *Stroke; Stroke Prevention*; **HMO:** Empire Oxford Vytra US Hlthcre Aetna Hlth Plan +

LANG: Sp; [symbols] Immediately
VISA [symbols]

Vaillancourt, Phillippe (MD) N
Univ Hosp SUNY Stony Brook

Neurology AssociatesStony Brk, 101 Nicholls Rd T12020; Stony Brook, NY 11794; (516) 444-2599; **BDCERT:** N 86; **MS:** McGill U 78; **RES:** N, Mount Sinai Med Ctr, New York, NY 80-83; **FAP:** Asst Prof SUNY Stony Brook; **SI:** *Headache; Chronic Pain/General Neurology*; **HMO:** GHI Oxford Vytra Aetna Hlth Plan CIGNA +

[symbols] **VISA** [symbols]

Zippin, Allen (MD) N
St John's Epis Hosp-Smithtown

Mid Suffolk NeuroSurgical Associates, 309 E Middle Country Rd 201; Smithtown, NY 11787; (516) 265-2020; **BDCERT:** N 73; **MS:** Canada 55; **RES:** Med, New Mt Sinai Med Ctr, Montreal, Canada 63-64; S, Jewish Gen Hosp, Montreal, Canada 64-65; **FEL:** NS, Albert Einstein Med Ctr, Bronx, NY 65-69; **HOSP:** St Charles Hosp & Rehab Ctr; **SI:** *Pain Management; Lower Back Problems*; **HMO:** Aetna Hlth Plan Oxford HealthNet Prucare Travelers +

[symbols] Immediately **VISA** [symbols]

OBSTETRICS & GYNECOLOGY

Baker, David (MD) ObG
Univ Hosp SUNY Stony Brook
100 Nicholls Rd; Stony Brook, NY 11794; (516) 444-2775; **BDCERT:** ObG 79; MF 81; **MS:** SUNY Hlth Sci Ctr 73; **RES:** Hosp of U Penn, Philadelphia, PA 74; **FEL:** MF, Med Ctr Hosp of VT, Burlington, VT 77-79; **HOSP:** Bridgeport Hosp; **SI:** *Sexually Transmitted Diseases; Infection in Pregnancy*
🦽 📷 🎖 🛏 S Mcr Mcd WC NFi A Few Days 📠 *VISA* 💳 💳

Chalas, Eva (MD) ObG
Univ Hosp SUNY Stony Brook
Long Island Gynecologic Oncologists PC, 994 Jericho Tpke; Smithtown, NY 11787; (516) 864-5440; **BDCERT:** ObG 88; GO 90; **MS:** SUNY Stony Brook 81; **RES:** Univ Hosp SUNY Stony Brook, Stony Brook, NY 81-85; **FEL:** GO, Mem Sloan Kettering Cancer Ctr, New York, NY 85-87; **FAP:** Assoc Clin Prof GO SUNY Stony Brook; **HOSP:** St John's Epis Hosp-Smithtown; **SI:** *Gynecologic Cancers; Breast Diseases*; **HMO:** Oxford Vytra Aetna Hlth Plan Blue Cross & Blue Shield CIGNA +
LANG: Sp, Fr, Czc; 🦽 📷 🎖 🛏 S Mcr Mcd
A Few Days

Davenport, Deborah M (MD)ObG
Univ Hosp SUNY Stony Brook
Three Village ObGYN, 100 S Jersey Ave Ste 16; East Setauket, NY 11733; (516) 689-6400; **BDCERT:** ObG 86; **MS:** Univ Penn 75; **RES:** ObG, Hosp of U Penn, Philadelphia, PA 75-76; ObG, Univ Hosp SUNY Stony Brook, Stony Brook, NY 80-83; **FAP:** Asst Clin Prof SUNY Stony Brook; **HOSP:** JT Mather Mem Hosp Pt Jfrson; **SI:** *Menopause*; **HMO:** Empire Blue Choice Oxford Vytra United Healthcare JJ Newman +
🦽 📷 🎖 🛏 S Mcr Mcd 4+ Weeks *VISA* 💳 💳

Gentilesco, Michael (MD) ObG PCP
St John's Epis Hosp-Smithtown
OB/OGN Specialities, PC, 48 Route 25A 207; Smithtown, NY 11787; (516) 862-3800; **BDCERT:** ObG 87; **MS:** Albert Einstein Coll Med 80; **RES:** ObG, Columbia-Presbyterian Med Ctr, New York, NY 80-84; **HOSP:** Univ Hosp SUNY Stony Brook; **HMO:** Aetna Hlth Plan Vytra Oxford PHS Sel Pro +
🦽 📷 🎖 🛏 S 2-4 Weeks *VISA* 💳

Giammarino, Anthony (MD)ObG
St Charles Hosp & Rehab Ctr
Suffolk OBGYN LLP, 118 N Country Rd; Port Jefferson, NY 11777; (516) 473-7171; **BDCERT:** ObG 69; **MS:** Italy 60; **RES:** Univ Hosp SUNY Stony Brook, Stony Brook, NY; **HOSP:** JT Mather Mem Hosp Pt Jfrson; **SI:** *Menopause; Menstrual Disorders*; **HMO:** Choicecare Aetna Hlth Plan Prucare Travelers
LANG: Itl, Sp; 🦽 📷 🎖 🛏 S Mcr Mcd
A Few Days 📠 *VISA*

Goldman, Mitchell (MD) ObG
Southside Hosp
971 Montauk Hwy; Oakdale, NY 11769; (516) 589-4344; **BDCERT:** ObG 63; **MS:** U Hlth Sci/Chicago Med Sch 55; **RES:** ObG, Kings County Hosp Ctr, Brooklyn, NY 55-60; **HOSP:** Good Samaritan Hosp Med Ctr; **SI:** *Laparoscopic Surgery; Sonograms*; **HMO:** US Hlthcre Vytra Oxford Empire Magnacare +
LANG: Hin, Sp; 🦽 📷 🎖 🛏 S Mcr A Few Days *VISA* 💳

Hirt, Paula (MD) ObG
Good Samaritan Hosp Med Ctr
83 W Main St; E Islip, NY 11730; (516) 277-5800; **BDCERT:** ObG 85; **MS:** NYU Sch Med 79; **RES:** New York University Med Ctr, New York, NY 79-83; **HMO:** Aetna Hlth Plan Blue Choice Choicecare HealthNet Independent Health Plan +
🦽 📷 🎖 🛏 S Mcr 2-4 Weeks *VISA* 💳 💳

Judge, Peter (MD) ObG
Good Samaritan Hosp
ObGyn Southbay, 320 Montauk Hwy; West Islip,
NY 11718; (516) 587-2500; **BDCERT:** ObG 93;
MS: Georgetown U 85; **RES:** St Vincents Hosp &
Med Ctr NY, New York, NY 85-91; **HMO:** Aetna
Hlth Plan Blue Choice Blue Cross & Blue Shield

Kaplan, Robert (MD) ObG **PCP**
St John's Epis Hosp-Smithtown
363 Route 111 100; Smithtown, NY 11787; (516)
265-5550; **BDCERT:** ObG 66; **MS:** SUNY Hlth Sci
Ctr 57; **RES:** ObG, Nassau County Med Ctr, East
Meadow, NY 63; **HMO:** Prudential Oxford MDNY
🖮 🕻 🗖 🗷 🎟 💲 🗠 A Few Days

Kramer, Robert (DO) ObG
JT Mather Mem Hosp Pt Jfrson
North Harbor Ob/Gyn Assoc, 16 Roosevelt Ave;
Port Jeffrsn Station, NY 11776; (516) 331-1919;
BDCERT: ObG 95; **MS:** Coll Of Osteo Med-Pacific
80; **RES:** ObG, Maimonides Med Ctr, Brooklyn, NY
81-85; **HOSP:** St Charles Hosp & Rehab Ctr; **HMO:**
Aetna-US Healthcare Vytra Oxford Blue Choice
Prucare +
🖮 🕻 🗖 🗷 🎟 💲 A Few Days **VISA** 🖸

Mann, Charles (MD) ObG
St John's Epis Hosp-Smithtown
48 Route 25A 207; Smithtown, NY 11787; (516)
862-3800; **BDCERT:** ObG 79; **MS:** Creighton U 74;
RES: Barnes Hosp, St Louis, MO 74-77; **HOSP:** Univ
Hosp SUNY Stony Brook

Matalon, Martin (MD) ObG
Southside Hosp
Medical Arts Obstetrics & Gyn, 375 E Main St 4;
Bay Shore, NY 11706; (516) 665-8226; **BDCERT:**
ObG 73; **MS:** U Cincinnati 66; **RES:** ObG, Brookdale
Univ Hosp Med Ctr, Brooklyn, NY 67-71; **HMO:**
Aetna Hlth Plan Choicecare HIP Network US
Hlthcre
🖮 🕻 🗖 🗷 🎟 💲 🗠 🗷 🗷 2-4 Weeks 🖸 **VISA**
🖸

Ott, Allen (MD) ObG
Southampton Hosp
Hamptons Gynecology Obstetrics, 235 Osborne
Ave; Riverhead, NY 11901; (516) 727-3422;
BDCERT: ObG 79; **MS:** Boston U 72; **RES:** ObG,
Hosp of U Penn, Philadelphia, PA 73-76; Hosp of U
Penn, Philadelphia, PA 73-76; **HMO:** Aetna Hlth
Plan Choicecare
🖮 🗷

Pallotta, John (MD) ObG
Good Samaritan Hosp
ObGyn Southbay, 320 Montauk Hwy; West Islip,
NY 11795; (516) 587-5033; **BDCERT:** ObG 65;
MS: NY Med Coll 55; **RES:** ObG, NY Med Coll, New
York, NY 58-62; **FAP:** Assoc Clin Prof NY Coll
Osteo Med; **SI:** *High Risk Obstetrics; Vaginal Surgery;*
HMO: Oxford CIGNA Aetna-US Healthcare Empire
MDNY +
LANG: Itl, Sp; 🖮 🗷 🕻 🗖 🗷 🎟 💲 🗠 🗷 1 Week
🖸 **VISA** 🖸

Rochelson, Burton (MD) ObG **PCP**
Univ Hosp SUNY Stony Brook
Three Village ObGyn, 100 S Jersey Ave Ste 16;
Setauket, NY 11733; (516) 689-6400; **BDCERT:**
ObG 84; MF 88; **MS:** U Mich Med Sch 78; **RES:** Long
Island Jewish Med Ctr, New Hyde Park, NY 82; **FEL:**
MF, Univ Hosp SUNY Stony Brook, Stony Brook,
NY; **FAP:** Assoc Clin Prof SUNY Stony Brook; **SI:**
High Risk Pregnancy; Ultrasound; **HMO:** Vytra
Oxford Multiplan Empire MDNY +
🖮 🕻 🗖 🗷 🎟 🗠 🗷 2-4 Weeks **VISA** 🖸

San Roman, Gerardo (MD) ObG **PCP**
St Charles Hosp & Rehab Ctr
118 N Country Rd; Port Jefferson, NY 11777;
(516) 473-7171; **BDCERT:** ObG 89; **MS:** Johns
Hopkins U 81; **RES:** ObG, NY Hosp-Cornell Med Ctr,
New York, NY 81-85; **HOSP:** JT Mather Mem Hosp
Pt Jfrson; **SI:** *Infertility; Osteoporosis;* **HMO:** Vytra
Choicecare Empire Aetna Hlth Plan GHI +
LANG: Sp, Itl; 🖮 🗷 🕻 🗖 🗷 🎟 💲 🗠 🗷
A Few Days 🖸 **VISA** 🖸 🖸

Schwarz, Richard (MD) ObG
Univ Hosp SUNY Stony Brook

101 Nicholls Rd; Stony Brook, NY 11794; (516) 444-1608; **BDCERT:** ObG 63; MF 74; **MS:** Jefferson Med Coll 55; **RES:** Los Angeles Cty Hosp, Los Angeles, CA 80-81; Kaiser Fdn Hosp, Los Angeles, CA 81-82; **HOSP:** New York Methodist Hosp

Tesauro, William (MD) ObG `PCP`
Good Samaritan Hosp Med Ctr

750 Montauk Hwy; W Islip, NY 11795; (516) 669-5900; **BDCERT:** ObG 69; **MS:** NY Med Coll 62; **RES:** ObG, New York Methodist Hosp, Brooklyn, NY 63-67; **HOSP:** Southside Hosp; **SI:** *Female Infertility; Gynecological Surgery;* **HMO:** Aetna Hlth Plan Oxford Metlife Metlife PHCS +

LANG: Itl; 🖥 🌙 🔒 📺 🏧 💲 Immediately

OCCUPATIONAL MEDICINE

Hailoo, Wajdy (MD) OM
Univ Hosp SUNY Stony Brook

Center for Occupational & Environmental Medicine, SUNY Stony Brook Sch Med HSC, 3L086; Stony Brook, NY 11794; (516) 444-2196; **BDCERT:** OM 88; PrM 89; **MS:** Iraq 69; **RES:** Med, Port General Hospital, Basra, Iraq 71-74; OM, Mount Sinai Med Ctr, New York, NY 84-87; **FEL:** OM, U London, London, England 75-77; Pul, Mount Sinai Med Ctr, New York, NY 85-87; **FAP:** Assoc Prof SUNY Stony Brook; **SI:** *Asbestos, Dust Lung Disease; Toxicology;* **HMO:** Vytra JJ Newman Chubb Blue Cross & Blue Shield Magnacare +

LANG: Sp, Ar; ♿ 🖥 🌙 🔒 📺 🏧 💲 Mcr Mcd WC NFI 1 Week ▦ **VISA** 💳 📷

Mendelsohn, Sara L (MD) OM
Univ Hosp SUNY Bklyn

SUNY Stony Brook Level 3 Rm 086; Stony Brook, NY 11794; (516) 444-2167; **BDCERT:** OM 93; **MS:** Boston U 88; **RES:** U of Illinois, Chicago, IL 89-91; **FEL:** Illinois Masonic Med Ctr, Chicago, IL 88-89

OPHTHALMOLOGY

Apisson, John (MD) Oph
JT Mather Mem Hosp Pt Jfrson

640 Belleterre Rd G; Port Jefferson, NY 11777; (516) 331-1414; **BDCERT:** Oph 69; **MS:** Emory U Sch Med 61; **RES:** Oph, New York Eye & Ear Infirmary, New York, NY 65-68; Oph, New York Eye & Ear Infirmary, New York, NY 68-69; **HOSP:** St Charles Hosp & Rehab Ctr; **SI:** *Cataract Microsurgery; Glaucoma;* **HMO:** Oxford Aetna-US Healthcare MDNY Multiplan Blue Choice +

LANG: Arm, Fr; ♿ 🖥 🌙 🔒 📺 🏧 💲 Mcr WC NFI A Few Days

Aries, Philip (MD) Oph
Southside Hosp

Suffolk Opthalmology Associates, 375 E Main St 24; Bay Shore, NY 11706; (516) 665-1330; **BDCERT:** Oph 75; **MS:** NY Med Coll 67; **RES:** Oph, Nassau County Med Ctr, East Meadow, NY 70-73; **HOSP:** Good Samaritan Hosp Med Ctr; **SI:** *Cataracts; Glaucoma;* **HMO:** CIGNA Oxford Empire Blue Cross & Blue Shield US Hlthcre +

LANG: Sp; ♿ 🖥 🌙 🔒 📺 🏧 💲 Mcr Mcd WC NFI 2-4 Weeks ▦ 💳

Beyrer, Charles R (MD) Oph
Southside Hosp

Suffolk Ophthalmology Associates, PC, 375 E Main St 24; Bay Shore, NY 11706; (516) 665-1330; **BDCERT:** Oph 68; **MS:** Switzerland 62; **RES:** New York Eye & Ear Infirmary, New York, NY 63-66; **FEL:** Retina, New York Eye & Ear Infirmary, New York, NY 65-67; **FAP:** Clin Prof SUNY Stony Brook; **HOSP:** Good Samaritan Hosp Med Ctr; **SI:** *Diabetic Retinopathy; Macula Degeneration;* **HMO:** Oxford Vytra US Hlthcre JJ Newman

LANG: Sp, Ger; ♿ 🔒 📺 🏧 💲 Mcr Mcd WC NFI A Few Days ▦ **VISA** 💳

Bogaty, Stanley (MD) Oph
JT Mather Mem Hosp Pt Jfrson
Long Island Eye Physicians, 251 E Oakland Ave;
Port Jefferson, NY 11777; (516) 473-5329;
BDCERT: Oph 74; MS: U Hlth Sci/Chicago Med Sch
66; RES: Oph, Beth Israel Med Ctr, New York, NY
69-72; FAP: Asst Clin Prof Oph SUNY Stony Brook;
HOSP: St Charles Hosp & Rehab Ctr; SI: Cataracts;
Glaucoma; HMO: Vytra Oxford MDNY US Hlthcre
Blue Choice +

🔳 🔳 🔳 🔳 🔳 🔳 🔳 🔳 A Few Days **VISA** 💳

Cossari, Alfred (MD) Oph
JT Mather Mem Hosp Pt Jfrson
Children's Eye Care of LI, 311 Barnum Ave; Port
Jefferson, NY 11777; (516) 928-6400; BDCERT:
Oph 76; MS: Italy 69; RES: Nassau County Med Ctr,
East Meadow, NY 71-74; FEL: Johns Hopkins Hosp,
Baltimore, MD 74; Children's Hosp Nat Med Ctr,
Washington, DC 75; HOSP: St Charles Hosp &
Rehab Ctr; SI: Pediatric Ophthalmology; Adult
Strabismus; HMO: Aetna Hlth Plan Oxford

LANG: Itl, Sp, Grk; 🔳 🔳 🔳 🔳 🔳 🔳 🔳 🔳 🔳 2-
4 Weeks 🔳 **VISA** 💳

Di Leo, Frank (MD) Oph
Southampton Hosp
137 Hampton Rd; Southampton, NY 11968; (516)
283-5152; BDCERT: Oph 87; MS: Albert Einstein
Coll Med 81; RES: Oph, St Luke's Roosevelt Hosp
Ctr, New York, NY 82-85; SI: Small Incision
Cataract; Surgery; HMO: Oxford Empire US Hlthcre
Vytra MDNY +

LANG: Sp; 🔳 🔳 🔳 🔳 🔳 🔳 A Few Days 🔳
VISA 💳

Martin, Sidney A (MD) Oph
St John's Epis Hosp-Smithtown
91 Maple Ave; Smithtown, NY 11787; (516) 265-
8780; BDCERT: Oph 63; MS: SUNY Hlth Sci Ctr 55;
RES: Baltimore Eye & Ear Hosp, Baltimore, MD 58-
61; FAP: Clin Instr SUNY Stony Brook; HOSP:
Nassau County Med Ctr; SI: Cataract Surgery;
Refractive Surgery; HMO: Aetna Hlth Plan Blue
Choice Blue Cross & Blue Shield Choicecare
HealthNet +

🔳 🔳 🔳 🔳 🔳 🔳 🔳 🔳 🔳 Immediately

Michalos, Peter (MD) Oph
Southampton Hosp
Benton Plaza, Southhampton Eye Associates, PC,
365 County Rd 39A Ste 11; Southampton, NY
11968; (516) 283-8604; BDCERT: Oph 91; MS:
SUNY Downstate 86; RES: S, NY Hosp-Cornell Med
Ctr, New York, NY 86-87; Oph, St Luke's Roosevelt
Hosp Ctr, New York, NY 87-90; FEL: Oph Plastic
and Reconstructive S, Columbia-Presbyterian Med
Ctr, New York, NY 90-91; FAP: Asst Clin Prof Oph
Columbia P&S; HOSP: Columbia-Presbyterian Med
Ctr; SI: Cataract Surgery, Small Incision; Lid Tumor
Tearing Disorder; HMO: Oxford GHI Empire Aetna-
US Healthcare

LANG: Grk, Sp; 🔳 🔳 🔳 🔳 🔳 🔳 🔳 Immediately
VISA 💳

Morabito, Carmine D (MD) Oph
Good Samaritan Hosp Med Ctr
375 E Main St; Bay Shore, NY 11706; (516) 655-
1330; BDCERT: Oph 71; MS: Switzerland 62; RES:
Oph, Hosp of U Penn, Philadelphia, PA 66-69;
HOSP: Southside Hosp

Morris, Robert (MD) Oph
St John's Epis Hosp-Smithtown
222 E Main St 330; Smithtown, NY 11787; (516)
724-4488; BDCERT: Oph 74; MS: SUNY Syracuse
66; RES: Univ Hosp SUNY Bklyn, Brooklyn, NY 69-
72; HMO: Aetna Hlth Plan Blue Choice Blue Cross
& Blue Shield Choicecare CIGNA +

🔳 🔳 🔳 🔳 🔳 🔳 🔳 🔳 🔳 2-4 Weeks

Nattis, Richard (MD) Oph
Good Samaritan Hosp Med Ctr
Eye Physcians and Surgeons, 786 Montauk Hwy FL
2; West Islip, NY 11795; (516) 661-5400;
BDCERT: Oph 85; MS: NY Med Coll 80; RES: St
Vincents Hosp & Med Ctr NY, New York, NY 81-84;
FAP: Asst Clin Prof NY Coll Osteo Med; HOSP:
Brunswick Hosp Ctr; SI: Cataract Surgery;
Nearsightedness; HMO: Oxford Aetna Hlth Plan
Prucare MDNY

LANG: Sp; 🔳 🔳 🔳 🔳 🔳 🔳 🔳 🔳 🔳 🔳
Immediately **VISA** 💳

Nudelman, Jeffrey Stuart (MD)Oph
Good Samaritan Hosp
Lindenhurst Eye Physicians & Surgerons,PC, 150 E
Sunrise Hwy FL2; West Islip, NY 11795; (516)
661-5400; **BDCERT:** Oph 89; **MS:** U Cincinnati 84;
RES: Mount Sinai Hosp, Cleveland, OH 84-85; Oph,
Mount Sinai Hosp, Cleveland, OH 85-88; **FEL:** Oph,
Manhattan Eye, Ear & Throat Hosp, New York, NY
88-89; **HOSP:** Brunswick Hosp Ctr; *SI: Crossed Eyes;
Lazy Eye;* **HMO:** Aetna Hlth Plan Oxford United
Healthcare Magnacare Multiplan +
LANG: Sp; 🔲 🔲 🔲 🔲 🔲 🔲 🔲 🔲 🔲 🔲 🔲 2-
4 Weeks **VISA** 💳

O'Brien, John D (MD)   Oph
Southside Hosp
Suffolk Opthalmology Assoc, 375 E Main St 24;
Bayshore, NY 11706; (516) 665-1330; **BDCERT:**
Oph 67; **MS:** NY Med Coll 60; **RES:** St Vincents
Hosp & Med Ctr NY, New York, NY 60-64; **HOSP:**
Good Samaritan Hosp Med Ctr
LANG: Sp; 🔲 🔲 🔲 🔲 🔲 🔲 🔲 🔲 🔲 🔲 🔲 1 Week
💳 **VISA** 💳

O'Malley, Grace M (MD)   Oph
Southampton Hosp
186 Old Towne Rd; Southampton, NY 11968;
(516) 283-3533; **BDCERT:** Oph 89; **MS:** NY Med
Coll 81; **RES:** Oph, NY Med Coll, Vallhalla, NY 85;
HOSP: Univ Hosp SUNY Stony Brook

Pizzarello, Louis (MD)   Oph
Southampton Hosp
1228 Roanoke Ave; Riverhead, NY 11901; (516)
727-6555; **BDCERT:** Oph 80; **MS:** U Va Sch Med
75; **RES:** Oph, Columbia-Presbyterian Med Ctr, New
York, NY 76-79; **FAP:** Instr Oph Columbia P&S; *SI:
Diabetic Laser Therapy*
LANG: Itl, Fr, Sp; 🔲 🔲 🔲 🔲 🔲 🔲 🔲 🔲 🔲 2-
4 Weeks **VISA**

Romanelli, John (MD)   Oph
St John's Epis Hosp-Smithtown
222 E Main St 331; Smithtown, NY 11787; (516)
724-4488; **BDCERT:** Oph 92; **MS:** Harvard Med
Sch 87; **RES:** Oph, Manhattan Eye, Ear & Throat
Hosp, New York, NY 88-91; **HOSP:** South Oaks
Hosp; **HMO:** Oxford GHI Aetna-US Healthcare
🔲 🔲 🔲 🔲 🔲 🔲 🔲 🔲 🔲 🔲 🔲 Immediately

Rothberg, Charles (MD)   Oph
Brookhaven Mem Hosp
1641 Route 112 C; Medford, NY 11763; (516)
758-5300; **BDCERT:** Oph 89; **MS:** SUNY Hlth Sci
Ctr 83; **RES:** Oph, Univ Hosp SUNY Bklyn,
Brooklyn, NY 84-87; *SI: Cataract Surgery; Refractive
Surgery;* **HMO:** Oxford Vytra Aetna-US Healthcare
Blue Choice PPO
🔲 🔲 🔲 🔲 🔲 🔲 🔲 🔲 🔲 🔲 2-4 Weeks

Schneck, Gideon (MD)   Oph
Univ Hosp SUNY Stony Brook
Building 17 - Suite 65, 2500 Route 347; Stony
Brook, NY 11790; (516) 246-9140; **BDCERT:** Oph
91; **MS:** Boston U 86; **RES:** Northwestern Mem
Hosp, Chicago, IL 87-90; **FEL:** Oculoplastic &
Reconstructive S, IL Eye & Ear Infirmary, Chicago,
IL 90-91; **FAP:** Asst Clin Prof Oph SUNY Stony
Brook; **HOSP:** St John's Epis Hosp-S Shore; *SI:
Diseases and Surgery of the Eyelids; Thyroid Eye
Disease;* **HMO:** Aetna Hlth Plan Blue Cross GHI HIP
Network Blue Choice +
🔲 🔲 🔲 🔲 🔲 🔲 🔲 🔲 🔲 1 Week

Sibony, Patrick (MD)   Oph
Univ Hosp SUNY Stony Brook
33 Research Way; Setauket, NY 11733; (516)
444-4090; **BDCERT:** Oph 87; **MS:** Boston U 81;
RES: Boston U Med Ctr, Boston, MA 78-81; **FEL:** Eye
& Ear Hosp, Pittsburgh, PA 81-82; **FAP:** Prof Oph
SUNY Stony Brook; **HMO:** Oxford US Hlthcre US
Hlthcre CIGNA Aetna Hlth Plan +
🔲 🔲 🔲 🔲 🔲 🔲 🔲 2-4 Weeks **VISA** 💳 💳

Stoller, Gerald (MD)   Oph
St Charles Hosp & Rehab Ctr

Long Island Eye Physicians & Surgeons, PC, 251 E
Oakland Ave; Port Jefferson, NY 11777; (516) 473-
5329; **BDCERT:** Oph 73; **MS:** Temple U 66; **RES:**
Oph, Bronx Muncipal Hosp Ctr, Bronx, NY 68-71;
FAP: Asst Clin Prof Oph SUNY Stony Brook; **HOSP:**
JT Mather Mem Hosp Pt Jfrson; **SI:** *Retina; Cataracts;*
HMO: Vytra Oxford MDNY US Hlthcre Blue Choice
+

♿ 📷 🏧 $ Mcr Mcd WC **VISA** 💳

Wasserman, Robert L (MD) Oph
Eastern Long Island Hosp

303 Griffing Ave; Riverhead, NY 11901; (516)
727-8353; **BDCERT:** Oph 71; **MS:** Albert Einstein
Coll Med 62; **RES:** Thomas Jefferson U Hosp,
Philadelphia, PA 66-69; N, Bronx Muncipal Hosp
Ctr, Bronx, NY 65-66; **HOSP:** Southampton Hosp

♿ SA/SU 📷 🏧 $ Mcr WC NFI 1 Week

Weber, Pamela (MD)   Oph
Univ Hosp SUNY Stony Brook

Eastern Long Island Retina Associates, 1500
William Floyd Pkwy; Shirley, NY 11967; (516)
924-4300; **BDCERT:** Oph 89; **MS:** Columbia P&S
84; **RES:** Oph, New York Eye & Ear Infirmary, New
York, NY 87-89; **FEL:** Retina, Mass Eye & Ear
Infirmary, Boston, MA 89-90; **FAP:** Asst Prof SUNY
Stony Brook; **HOSP:** St Charles Hosp & Rehab Ctr;
SI: *Diabetic Retinopathy; Macular Degeneration;*
HMO: Vytra Prudential Oxford US Hlthcre Empire
+

♿ 📷 🏧 $ Mcr Mcd WC NFI Immediately

Zweibel, Lawrence (MD)   Oph
St John's Epis Hosp-Smithtown

91 Maple Ave; Smithtown, NY 11787; (516) 265-
8780; **BDCERT:** Oph 77; **MS:** Albany Med Coll 72;
RES: French Hosp, New York, NY 76; **FAP:** Clin
Instr SUNY Stony Brook; **HOSP:** Univ Hosp SUNY
Stony Brook; **SI:** *Refractive Surgery; Cataract Surgery;*
HMO: Oxford US Hlthcre MDNY Blue Cross & Blue
Shield Magnacare +

♿ SA/SU ☎ 📷 🚹 🏧 $ Mcr Mcd WC NFI Immediately

ORTHOPAEDIC SURGERY

Bleifeld, Charles (MD)   OrS
St John's Epis Hosp-Smithtown

48 Route 25A Suite 106; Smithtown, NY 11787;
(516) 862-3660; **BDCERT:** OrS 75; **MS:** Geo Wash
U Sch Med 68; **RES:** St Luke's Rsvlt Ctr, New York,
NY 69-70; Hosp For Special Surgery, New York, NY
70-73

Boccio, Richard (MD)   OrS
St John's Epis Hosp-Smithtown

290 E Main St 700; Smithtown, NY 11787; (516)
265-6991; **BDCERT:** OrS 93; **MS:** Wayne State U
Sch Med 86; **RES:** OrS, Univ Hosp SUNY Stony
Brook, Stony Brook, NY 87-91; **HOSP:** Univ Hosp
SUNY Stony Brook; **SI:** *Foot & Ankle Surgery;* **HMO:**
Empire Vytra

♿ ☎ 📷 🚹 🏧 $ Mcr WC NFI 2-4 Weeks **VISA** 💳

Dowling, Thomas (MD)   OrS
St John's Epis Hosp-Smithtown

Long Island Spine Specialists, PC, 2171 Jericho
Tpke 304; Commack, NY 11725; (516) 462-2225;
BDCERT: OrS 90; **MS:** Boston U 81; **RES:** N Shore
Univ Hosp-Manhasset, Manhasset, NY 81-83; Univ
Hosp SUNY Stony Brook, Stony Brook, NY 83-87;
FEL: Spine S, U Toronto Gen Hosp, Toronto,
Canada; **HOSP:** Huntington Hosp; **SI:** *Scoliosis
Surgery; Disc Surgery*

LANG: Fr, Sp; ♿ 📷 🚹 🏧 $ Mcr WC NFI 1 Week
VISA 💳

Dubrow, Eric N (MD)   OrS
St Charles Hosp & Rehab Ctr

6 Medical Dr; Port Jefferson Station, NY 11776;
(516) 928-5112; **BDCERT:** OrS 86; **MS:** Belgium
79; **RES:** Nassau County Med Ctr, East Meadow, NY
79-80; Univ Hosp SUNY Stony Brook, Stony Brook,
NY 80-84; **FAP:** Asst Clin Prof SUNY Stony Brook;
HOSP: JT Mather Mem Hosp Pt Jfrson; **SI:** *Total Joint
Replacement; Sports Medicine;* **HMO:** Aetna Hlth
Plan Vytra Oxford Magnacare Empire +

LANG: Fr; ♿ SA/SU ☎ 📷 🚹 🏧 $ Mcr WC NFI A Few Days
VISA 💳

Guide to symbols and abbreviations can be found on pages 110-113.

733

Ellstein, Jerry (MD) OrS
Huntington Hosp

Hand Surgery Assoc Long Island, 166 E Main St; Huntington, NY 11743; (516) 427-4263; **BDCERT:** OrS 86; HS 89; **MS:** Mexico 77; **RES:** Mount Sinai Med Ctr, New York, NY 78-83; **FEL:** Indiana Hand Ctr, Indianapolis, IN 83-84; **FAP:** Asst Clin Prof OrS SUNY Stony Brook; **HOSP:** Long Island Jewish Med Ctr; *SI: Pediatric Congenital Defects;* **HMO:** Oxford United Healthcare Multiplan Magnacare Blue Choice +

LANG: Pol, Sp; ⌖ ▣ ⌗ ▦ � ⎕ ▦ ▦ ▦ 1 Week **VISA** ●

Healy Jr, William (MD) OrS
Huntington Hosp

196 E Main St; Huntington, NY 11743; (516) 271-8300; **BDCERT:** OrS 70; **MS:** NY Med Coll 61; **RES:** St Vincents Hosp & Med Ctr NY, New York, NY 61-62; St Vincents Hosp & Med Ctr NY, New York, NY 62-63; **FEL:** New York University Med Ctr, New York, NY 65-68; **FAP:** Assoc Clin Prof OrS SUNY Stony Brook; **HOSP:** Univ Hosp SUNY Stony Brook; *SI: Medical Legal Orthopaedics*

⌖ ▣ ▦ ▦ ▦ ▦ ▦ A Few Days

Kurtz, Neil J (MD) OrS
St Charles Hosp & Rehab Ctr

6 Medical Dr; Port Jefferson Station, NY 11776; (516) 331-9313; **BDCERT:** OrS 77; **MS:** NYU Sch Med 71; **RES:** OrS, U of Pittsburgh Med Ctr, Pittsburgh, PA 73-76; **FEL:** PMR, New York University Med Ctr, New York, NY 72-73; **FAP:** Assoc Clin Prof OrS SUNY Stony Brook; **HOSP:** JT Mather Mem Hosp Pt Jfrson; *SI: Joint Replacement Surgery; Arthroscopic Surgery;* **HMO:** Most

⌖ ▣ ▦ ▦ ⎕ ▦ ▦ ▦ 1 Week **VISA** ●

Levin, Paul Edward (MD) OrS
St Charles Hosp & Rehab Ctr

625 Belle Terre Rd 202; Port Jefferson, NY 11777; (516) 476-1600; **BDCERT:** OrS 88; **MS:** SUNY Downstate 80; **RES:** OrS, Montefiore Med Ctr, Bronx, NY 80-85; **FEL:** OrS Trauma, Hermann Hosp, Houston, TX 85-86; Fracture Care, Kentospital, Kentospital, Switzerland 86; **FAP:** Asst Prof SUNY Stony Brook; **HOSP:** JT Mather Mem Hosp Pt Jfrson; *SI: Orthopaedic Trauma; Fractures;* **HMO:** Vytra Magnacare US Hlthcre Anthem Health

⌖ ◖ ▣ ▦ ▦ ⎕ ▦ ▦ ▦ A Few Days **VISA** ●

Mango, Enrico S (MD) OrS
St John's Epis Hosp-Smithtown

290 E Main St 700; Smithtown, NY 11787; (516) 361-4802; **BDCERT:** OrS 83; **MS:** Creighton U 76; **RES:** OrS, Univ Hosp SUNY Stony Brook, Stony Brook, NY 77-81; **FAP:** Asst Clin Prof OrS SUNY Stony Brook; *SI: Sports Medicine; Knee & Shoulder Surgery;* **HMO:** Vytra Oxford MDNY Magnacare PHS +

⌖ ▥ ◖ ▣ ▦ ▦ ⎕ ▦ ▦ ▦ Immediately ▦ **VISA** ●

Ratzan, Sanford (MD) OrS
Good Samaritan Hosp Med Ctr

375 E Main St 1; Bay Shore, NY 11706; (516) 665-8790; **BDCERT:** OrS 73; **MS:** Columbia P&S 65; **RES:** S, St Luke's Roosevelt Hosp Ctr, New York, NY 66-67; OrS, St Luke's Roosevelt Hosp Ctr, New York, NY 69; **HOSP:** Southside Hosp; *SI: Arthroscopic Surgery; Sports Medicine*

⌖ ▥ ◖ ▣ ▦ ▦ ▦ ▦ ▦ ▦ **VISA** ●

Skilbred, Arne (MD) OrS
Southampton Hosp

Southampton Orthopedic Group, 315 Meeting House Ln; Southampton, NY 11968; (516) 283-0355; **BDCERT:** OrS 66; **MS:** Columbia P&S 56; **RES:** S, St Luke's Roosevelt Hosp Ctr, New York, NY 56-58; OrS, Columbia-Presbyterian Med Ctr, New York, NY 60-62; **FEL:** OrS, Columbia-Presbyterian Med Ctr, New York, NY 63-64; **SI:** *Total Joint Replacements; Arthroscopies;* **HMO:** Blue Cross & Blue Shield Oxford Aetna Hlth Plan Anthem Health Vytra +

LANG: Nwg; ♿ 📷 ⚕ 🏥 💲 Mcr WC NFI 1 Week
VISA 💳

Stillwell, William (MD) OrS
St John's Epis Hosp-Smithtown

48 Route 25a 7; Smithtown, NY 11787; (516) 862-3007; **BDCERT:** OrS 80; **MS:** NY Med Coll 73; **RES:** S, Med Coll VA Hosp, Richmond, VA 74-75; OrS, St Luke's Roosevelt Hosp Ctr, New York, NY 75-78; **FEL:** New England Baptist Hosp, Boston, MA 78-79; **FAP:** Clin Instr OrS Columbia P&S; **SI:** *Hips; Knees;* **HMO:** PHCS Sel Pro

♿ 💲 WC 🖼 **VISA** 💳

Tabershaw, Richard (MD) OrS
Good Samaritan Hosp Med Ctr

Suffolk Orthopedic Assoc, 375 E Main St 1; Bay Shore, NY 11706; (516) 665-8790; **BDCERT:** OrS 97; **MS:** Georgetown U 80; **RES:** St Vincents Hosp & Med Ctr NY, New York, NY 80-83; Columbia-Presbyterian Med Ctr, New York, NY 83-86; **HOSP:** Southside Hosp; **SI:** *Shoulder Problems; Knee & Sports Injuries*

LANG: Sp; ♿ 📷 ⚕ 🏥 💲 Mcr WC NFI 2-4 Weeks
VISA 💳 🖼

Weissberg, David (MD) OrS
Huntington Hosp

180 E Pulaski Rd; Huntington Station, NY 11746; (516) 425-2140; **BDCERT:** OrS 87; **MS:** SUNY Downstate 80; **RES:** OrS, Univ Hosp SUNY Stony Brook, Stony Brook, NY

OTOLARYNGOLOGY

Caruso, Anthony (MD) Oto
Southampton Hosp

580 County Rd 39A; Southampton, NY 11968; (516) 283-4412; **BDCERT:** Oto 79; **MS:** Jefferson Med Coll 75; **RES:** S, Mercy Fitzgerald Hosp, Darby, PA 75-76; Oto, Thomas Jefferson U Hosp, Philadelphia, PA 76-79; **HOSP:** Central Suffolk Hosp; **SI:** *Sinus Endoscopic Surgery; Head and Neck Surgery;* **HMO:** Oxford Vytra CIGNA Aetna-US Healthcare

♿ 📷 ⚕ 🏥 💲 Mcl WC NFI Immediately **VISA** 💳

Chitkara, Dev (MD) Oto
St John's Epis Hosp-Smithtown

29 Manor Rd; Smithtown, NY 11787; (516) 979-0311; **BDCERT:** Oto 67; **MS:** India 61; **RES:** Long Island Coll Hosp, Brooklyn, NY 63-64; Boston Med Ctr, Boston, MA 66-67; **FEL:** Georgetown U Hosp, Washington, DC 67-70; **SI:** *Pediatric Otolaryngology; Salivary Glands & Sinuses;* **HMO:** Oxford Vytra Aetna Hlth Plan Empire Blue Cross & Shield GHI +

♿ 🌙 📷 ⚕ 🏥 💲 Mcr Mcl WC NFI A Few Days

Dash, Greg (MD) Oto
Good Samaritan Hosp Med Ctr

1111 Montauk Hwy Fl 2; West Islip, NY 11795; (516) 422-2700; **BDCERT:** Oto 87; **MS:** Columbia P&S 82; **RES:** St Luke's Rsvlt Ctr-St Luke's Div, New York, NY 82-83; NY Eye & Ear Infirm, New York, NY 83-87; **HOSP:** Southside Hosp

DeBlasi, Henry (MD) Oto
Mid-Island Hosp

42 Bluegrass Ln; Levittown, NY 11756; (516) 731-6644; **BDCERT:** Oto 96; **MS:** NY Med Coll 89; **RES:** Oto, New York Eye & Ear Infirmary, New York, NY 97-95; Oto, St Vincents Hosp & Med Ctr NY, New York, NY 90-91; **HOSP:** Winthrop Univ Hosp; **SI:** *Facial Plastic Surgery*

♿ 🅿 🌙 📷 ⚕ 🏥 💲 Mcr WC NFI A Few Days 🖼
VISA 💳 🖼

Guide to symbols and abbreviations can be found on pages 110-113.

735

Katz, Arnold (MD)   Oto
Univ Hosp SUNY Stony Brook

Department of Otolaryngology, 33 Research Way; Setauket, NY 11733; (516) 444-4122; **BDCERT:** Oto 76; **MS:** Washington U, St Louis 67; **RES:** U IA Hosp, Iowa City, IA 72-76; **FAP:** Chf Oto SUNY Stony Brook; **SI:** *Facial Skin Cancer Repair*; **HMO:** Oxford Vytra Empire Magnacare US Hlthcre +

LANG: Sp; 🔲 🔲 🔲 🔲 🔲 🔲 🔲 🔲 🔲 2-4 Weeks 🔲 **VISA** 🔲 🔲

Lipinsky, Edward John (MD)   Oto
St John's Epis Hosp-Smithtown

300 E Main St 1; Smithtown, NY 11787; (516) 265-3727; **BDCERT:** Oto 76; **MS:** NYU Sch Med 72; **RES:** Oto, Washington Hosp Ctr, Washington, DC 72-76; **HOSP:** Univ Hosp SUNY Stony Brook; **HMO:** Aetna Hlth Plan US Hlthcre Vytra Oxford

🔲 🔲 🔲 🔲 🔲 🔲 🔲 🔲 🔲 2-4 Weeks

Litman, Richard (MD)   Oto
JT Mather Mem Hosp Pt Jfrson

Lithan, Sher, Shangold, MDPC, 251 E Oakland Ave; Port Jefferson, NY 11777; (516) 928-0188; **BDCERT:** Oto 76; **MS:** Bowman Gray 71; **RES:** Jacobi Med Ctr, Bronx, NY 71-72; S, Long Island Jewish Med Ctr, New Hyde Park, NY 72-73; **FEL:** Oto, Albert Einstein Med Ctr, Bronx, NY 73-76; **FAP:** Asst Prof SUNY Stony Brook; **HOSP:** St Charles Hosp & Rehab Ctr; **SI:** *Pediatric Otolaryngology; Head & Neck Surgery*; **HMO:** Aetna-US Healthcare Oxford Magnacare United Healthcare Vytra +

🔲 🔲 🔲 🔲 🔲 🔲 🔲 🔲 2-4 Weeks **VISA** 🔲

Sampogna, Dominick (MD)   Oto
Southside Hosp

375 E Main St 17; Bay Shore, NY 11706; (516) 665-2430; **BDCERT:** Oto 71; **MS:** Boston U 65; **RES:** Boston U Med Ctr, Boston, MA 65-67; **HOSP:** Good Samaritan Hosp Med Ctr

LANG: Itl; 🔲 🔲 🔲 🔲 🔲 🔲 🔲 A Few Days

Smouha, Eric (MD)   Oto
Univ Hosp SUNY Stony Brook

Department Of Otolaryngology-SUNY Hosp Stony Brook, 37 Research Way; Setauket, NY 11733; (516) 444-4121; **BDCERT:** Oto 86; **MS:** McGill U 81; **RES:** S, St Vincents Hosp & Med Ctr NY, New York, NY 82-83; Oto, Manhattan Eye, Ear & Throat Hosp, New York, NY 83-86; **FEL:** Oto N, Ear Research Foundation, Sarasota, FL 86-87; **FAP:** Asst Prof SUNY Stony Brook

🔲 🔲 🔲 🔲 🔲 🔲 🔲 🔲 2-4 Weeks 🔲 **VISA** 🔲 🔲

Staro, Frank (MD)   Oto
Southside Hosp

Otolaryngology Head & Neck Surgery, 375 E Main St 17; Bay Shore, NY 11730; (516) 665-2430; **BDCERT:** Oto 76; S 85; **MS:** Boston U 70; **RES:** S, Boston U Med Ctr, Boston, MA 70-72; Boston U Med Ctr, Boston, MA 72-75; **HOSP:** Good Samaritan Hosp Med Ctr; **SI:** *Pediatric Ear Problems; Sinus Disease*; **HMO:** Aetna-US Healthcare Empire Anthem Health Vytra +

LANG: Sp, Itl; 🔲 🔲 🔲 🔲 🔲 🔲 🔲 🔲 A Few Days

PAIN MANAGEMENT

Gargiulo, Juan (MD)   PM
Southampton Hosp

East End Anesthesiologists/East End Pain Mgmt, 240 Meeting House Ln; Southampton, NY 11968; (516) 726-8350; **BDCERT:** Anes 93; PM 97; **MS:** Uruguay 84; **RES:** Lincoln Hosp, Bronx, NY 87-88; Westchester County Med Ctr, Valhalla, NY 89-91; **HMO:** MDNY Oxford US Hlthcre JJ Newman

LANG: Sp; 🔲 🔲 🔲 🔲 🔲 🔲 🔲 🔲 Immediately

PEDIATRIC CARDIOLOGY

Biancaniello, Thomas (MD) PCd
Univ Hosp SUNY Stony Brook
100 Nicholls Rd P; Stony Brook, NY 11794; (516) 444-2585; **BDCERT:** Ped 79; PCd 81; **MS:** NY Med Coll 75; **RES:** Ped, N Shore Univ Hosp-Manhasset, Manhasset, NY 75-77; **FEL:** PCd, Cincinnati Gen Hosp, Cincinnati, OH 77-80; **FAP:** Prof SUNY Stony Brook; *SI: Cardiac Catheterization*; **HMO:** Empire Blue Cross & Blue Shield Aetna Hlth Plan CIGNA Oxford +

⬥ 🄲 🄰 🄺 🄼 🄎 Mcr Mcd WC 2-4 Weeks **VISA** 💳

Reitman, Milton (MD) PCd
St Francis Hosp-Roslyn
Pediatric CardiologyLong Isld, 631 Montauk Hwy 4; West Islip, NY 11795; (516) 669-9624; **BDCERT:** Ped 74; **MS:** NY Med Coll 69; **RES:** Flower Fifth Ave Hosp, New York, NY 69-71; **FEL:** PCd, Texas Children's Hosp, Houston, TX; **HMO:** Oxford United Healthcare Aetna Hlth Plan GHI

⬥ 🄰 🄺 🄎 🄎 Mcd NFl A Few Days **VISA** 💳

PEDIATRIC GASTROENTEROLOGY

Lowenheim, Mark Saul (MD)PGe
Univ Hosp SUNY Stony Brook
Univ Hosp SUNY Stony Brook,; Stony Brook, NY 11794; (516) 444-8115; **BDCERT:** Ped 88; PGe 95; **MS:** Dominican Republic 84; **RES:** Elmhurst Hosp Ctr, Elmhurst, NY 85-86; **FEL:** PGe, Mount Sinai Med Ctr, New York, NY 87-89

⬥ 🄰 🄺 🄎 Mcd

PEDIATRIC HEMATOLOGY-ONCOLOGY

Parker, Robert (MD) PHO
Univ Hosp SUNY Stony Brook
Pediatrics, HSC T11 Rm 029; Stony Brook, NY 11794; (516) 444-7720; **BDCERT:** Ped 83; PHO 84; **MS:** Brown U 76; **RES:** Med, Roger Williams Med Ctr, Providence, RI 76-77; Ped, Rhode Island Hosp, Providence, RI 77-79; **FEL:** PHO, Nat Cancer Inst, Bethesda, MD 79-81; Hem, Nat Cancer Inst, Bethesda, MD 81-84; **FAP:** Assoc Prof Ped SUNY Stony Brook; *SI: Pediatric Cancer; Bleeding Disorders*; **HMO:** Vytra Aetna-US Healthcare Oxford Metlife CIGNA +

LANG: Sp, Hin; ⬥ 🄰 🄺 🄎 🄎 Mcr Mcd WC NFl
Immediately 📋 **VISA** 💳

PEDIATRIC NEPHROLOGY

Fine, Richard (MD) PNep
Univ Hosp SUNY Stony Brook
SUNY Stony Brook Sch Med; Stony Brook, NY 11794; (516) 444-2716; **BDCERT:** Ped 67; PNep 74; **MS:** Temple U 62; **RES:** Boston Med Ctr, Boston, MA 62-63; Children's Hosp of Los Angeles, Los Angeles, CA 64-66; **FAP:** Prof Ped SUNY Stony Brook; **HOSP:** St Charles Hosp & Rehab Ctr; *SI: Transplants; Nephrology*; **HMO:** Blue Choice Blue Cross & Blue Shield Choicecare CIGNA HealthNet +

⬥ 🄎 🄲 🄰 🄺 Mcr Mcd 1 Week

Stewart, Charles (MD) PNep
Univ Hosp SUNY Stony Brook
SUNYat Stony Brook Children's Svc, PC-Dept of Ped, 100 Nicholls Rd; Stony Brook, NY 11794; (516) 444-2585; **BDCERT:** Ped 96; PNep 96; **MS:** Georgetown U 79; **RES:** Childrens Hosp, Washington, DC 80-82; **FEL:** PNep, Georgetown U Med Ctr, Washington, DC 83-86; **FAP:** Assoc Prof Ped SUNY Stony Brook; *SI: Hypertension - Pediatric; Renal Failure - Pediatric*; **HMO:** Most

⬥ 🄲 🄰 🄎 Mcr Mcd NFl 1 Week **VISA** 💳

Guide to symbols and abbreviations can be found on pages 110-113.

737

PEDIATRIC SURGERY

Kugaczewski, Jane T (MD)   PS
Univ Hosp SUNY Stony Brook
Stony Brook Surgical AssociatesSUNY at Stony Brook, 34 Harbor Rd HSC T19; Stony Brook, NY 11794; (516) 444-2045; **BDCERT:** S 97; PS 92; **MS:** 81; **RES:** S, Hosp of U Penn, Philadelphia, PA 81-86; **FEL:** PdS, Univ Hosp SUNY Bklyn, Brooklyn, NY 87-89; **FAP:** Asst Prof S SUNY Stony Brook; *SI: Neonatal Surgery; Anorectal Malformations*
LANG: Sp, Pol; ▣ ▣ ▣ ▣ ▣ ▣ ▣ ▣ ▣
A Few Days

Priebe, Cedric J (MD)   PS
Univ Hosp SUNY Stony Brook
Stony Brook Surgical Associates, PC SUNY Stony Brook, 101 Nicholls Rd T19020; Stony Brook, NY 11794; (516) 444-2045; **BDCERT:** S 61; PS 93; **MS:** Cornell U 55; **RES:** S, St Luke's Roosevelt Hosp Ctr, New York, NY 55-60; PdS, Ohio State U Hosp, Columbus, OH 65-67; **FAP:** Prof SUNY Stony Brook; **HOSP:** St Charles Hosp & Rehab Ctr; *SI: Hernia & Testicular Surgery; Gastrointestinal Surgery;* **HMO:** Empire Aetna Hlth Plan Oxford US Hlthcre JJ Newman +
LANG: Sp; ▣ ▣ ▣ ▣ ▣ ▣ ▣ ▣ 1 Week ▨ *VISA* ▣

Winick, Martin (MD)   PS
St John's Epis Hosp-Smithtown
2500 Route 347 Bldg 10; Stony Brook, NY 11790; (516) 427-1300; **BDCERT:** S 66; PS 75; **MS:** SUNY Downstate 60; **RES:** S, Jewish Hosp Med Ctr, Brooklyn, NY 61-66; PS, St Christopher's Hosp for Children, Philadelphia, PA 65-66; **FAP:** Assoc Clin Prof SUNY Stony Brook; **HOSP:** St Charles Hosp & Rehab Ctr; *SI: Hernia Surgery; Undescended Testicles*
▣ ▣ ▣ ▣ ▣ ▣ A Few Days

PEDIATRICS

Adler, Albert (MD)   Ped   PCP
St John's Epis Hosp-Smithtown
1 Teapot Ln; Smithtown, NY 11787; (516) 265-7272; **BDCERT:** Ped 63; **MS:** Switzerland 58; **RES:** Ped, Queens Hosp Ctr, Jamaica, NY 58-61; **FEL:** Ped, Queens Hosp Ctr, Jamaica, NY; **HOSP:** Univ Hosp SUNY Stony Brook; **HMO:** Vytra Oxford Blue Cross & Blue Shield PHCS GHI +
▣ ▣ ▣ ▣ ▣ ▣ ▣ ▣ ▣ Immediately

Ancona, Richard (MD)   Ped   PCP
St John's Epis Hosp-Smithtown
Branch Pediatric & Adolescent Group, 300 E Middle Country Rd; Smithtown, NY 11787; (516) 979-6466; **BDCERT:** Ped 81; **MS:** Germany 75; **RES:** Long Island Coll Hosp, Brooklyn, NY 75-78; **FEL:** PHO, Long Island Coll Hosp, Brooklyn, NY; **HMO:** Aetna Hlth Plan Blue Choice Blue Cross & Blue Shield Choicecare HealthNet +
▣ ▣ ▣ ▣ ▣ ▣ ▣ Immediately

Augustine, V M (MD)   Ped   PCP
Southside Hosp
160 Middle Rd; Sayville, NY 11782; (516) 589-5533; **BDCERT:** Ped 79; **MS:** India 70; **RES:** Harlem Hosp Ctr, New York, NY 74-76; **FEL:** NP, Harlem Hosp Ctr, New York, NY 76-78; *SI: Asthma; Gastroenteritis;* **HMO:** Blue Cross & Blue Shield Oxford Vytra JJ Newman CIGNA +
LANG: Mly; ▣ ▣ ▣ ▣ ▣ ▣ ▣ Immediately

Cusumano, Barbara (MD)   Ped   PCP
Southampton Hosp
Southampton Pediatric Associates, 325 Meeting House Ln; Southampton, NY 11968; (516) 283-7733; **BDCERT:** Ped 96; **MS:** U Hlth Sci/Chicago Med Sch 84; **RES:** Ped, NY Hosp-Cornell Med Ctr, New York, NY 84-87; **HMO:** Aetna Hlth Plan Oxford US Hlthcre CIGNA Vytra +
▣ ▣ ▣ ▣ ▣ ▣ ▣ ▣ 2-4 Weeks ▨ ▣

Festa, Robert (MD) Ped PCP
Univ Hosp SUNY Stony Brook

635 Belleterre Rd; Port Jefferson, NY 11777; (516)
331-6200; **BDCERT:** Ped 78; **MS:** SUNY Downstate
72; **RES:** Ped, Montefiore Med Ctr, Bronx, NY 73-75

♿ 🆘 🌙 📷 🚹 🏨 💲 Med WC NFI Immediately 🔲
VISA ● 💳

Gottlieb, Robert (MD) Ped PCP
Southampton Hosp

Southampton Pediatric Assoc, 325 Meeting House
Ln C; Southampton, NY 11968; (516) 283-7733;
BDCERT: Ped 84; **MS:** NYU Sch Med 78; **RES:** Ped,
Bellevue Hosp Ctr, New York, NY 78-81; **FEL:** Ped,
Bellevue Hosp Ctr, New York, NY 81-83; **SI:** *Well
Baby Care; Colic;* **HMO:** Vytra MDNY Oxford US
Hlthcre

♿ 🆘 🌙 📷 🚹 🏨 💲 Med Immediately 🔲 **VISA**
●

Grello, Fred W (MD) Ped PCP
Good Samaritan Hosp Med Ctr

390 Montauk Hwy; West Islip, NY 11795; (516)
422-0700; **BDCERT:** Ped 62; **MS:** Georgetown U
55; **RES:** Nat Naval Med Ctr, Bethesda, MD 56-60;
HOSP: Southside Hosp

♿ 🆘 📷 🚹 Med NFI A Few Days

Hauptman, Martin (MD) Ped
St John's Epis Hosp-Smithtown

363 Route 111; Smithtown, NY 11787; (516)
979-7222; **BDCERT:** Ped 68; **MS:** Univ Penn 63;
RES: NY Hosp-Cornell Med Ctr, New York, NY 64-
67; **HOSP:** Univ Hosp SUNY Stony Brook

Kaplan, Martin (MD) Ped PCP
St Charles Hosp & Rehab Ctr

12 Med Dr B; Port Jefferson Station, NY 11776;
(516) 331-1710; **BDCERT:** Ped 77; **MS:** NYU Sch
Med 72; **RES:** Bellevue Hosp Ctr, New York, NY 72-
74; Duke U Med Ctr, Durham, NC 74-75; **HOSP:**
Univ Hosp SUNY Stony Brook; **SI:** *Asthma;
Developmental Problems;* **HMO:** Oxford Empire Blue
Cross & Blue Shield

LANG: Sp, Fr, Ger; ♿ 🌙 📷 🚹 🏨 💲 Med WC NFI
1 Week 🔲 **VISA** ●

Kolker, Harvey (MD) Ped PCP
St Charles Hosp & Rehab Ctr

111 Sylvan Ave; Miller Place, NY 11764; (516)
928-4888; **BDCERT:** Ped 71; **MS:** SUNY Downstate
66; **RES:** Washington, DC 67-69; **FAP:** Assoc Clin
Prof SUNY Stony Brook; **HOSP:** JT Mather Mem
Hosp Pt Jfrson; **HMO:** Aetna Hlth Plan Prucare
Oxford

🆘 📷 🚹 🏨 💲 NFI A Few Days **VISA** ●

Lifshitz, Miriam (MD) Ped PCP
St Charles Hosp & Rehab Ctr

St Charles Hospital, 200 Belle Terre Rd; Port
Jefferson, NY 11777; (516) 474-6000; **BDCERT:**
Ped 89; **MS:** Laval U, Quebec 60; **RES:** Ped,
Cumberland Med Ctr, Brooklyn, NY 78-80; **FEL:**
NP, Cumberland Med Ctr, Brooklyn, NY 80-82; **SI:**
Newborn Intensive Care; Newborn Regular Care;
HMO: Vytra Magnacare US Hlthcre

LANG: Rus; ♿ 🆘 🌙 📷 🚹 🏨 💲 Med Immediately
🔲 **VISA** ● 💳

Manners, Richard (MD) Ped
St John's Epis Hosp-Smithtown

1770 Motor Pkwy; Hauppauge, NY 11788; (516)
434-1770; **BDCERT:** Ped 80; **MS:** Albert Einstein
Coll Med 75; **RES:** U MN Med Ctr, Minneapolis, MN
75-78; **FEL:** Ped, U MN Med Ctr, Minneapolis, MN;
HOSP: Univ Hosp SUNY Stony Brook; **HMO:** Aetna
Hlth Plan Choicecare Vytra Oxford Blue Cross &
Blue Shield +

♿ 🆘 🌙 📷 🚹 🏨 💲 NFI **VISA** ● 💳

Musiker, Seymour (MD) Ped PCP
Univ Hosp SUNY Stony Brook

2233 Nesconset Hwy; Lake Grove, NY 11755;
(516) 585-4440; **BDCERT:** Ped 66; **MS:** U Hlth
Sci/Chicago Med Sch 61; **RES:** Ped, Jacobi Med Ctr,
Bronx, NY; Albert Einstein Med Ctr, Bronx, NY 61-
64; **HOSP:** St Charles Hosp & Rehab Ctr; **HMO:**
Aetna Hlth Plan United Healthcare JJ Newman
Oxford Multiplan +

♿ 🆘 📷 🚹 🏨 Med NFI A Few Days **VISA** ●

Guide to symbols and abbreviations can be found on pages 110-113.

739

Parker, Margaret (DO)   Ped
Univ Hosp SUNY Stony Brook

Dept of Pediatrics, Stony Brook Children's Services,
Univ Hosp at Stony Brook 40; Stony Brook, NY
11794; (516) 444-7720; **BDCERT:** Ped 95; CCM
97; **MS:** Brown U 77; **RES:** IM, Roger Williams Med
Ctr, Providence, RI 77-80; **FEL:** CCM, Nat Inst
Health, Bethesda, MD 80-82; **FAP:** Assoc Clin Prof
Med SUNY Stony Brook; *SI: Severe Infections;
Asthma;* **HMO:** CIGNA Vytra Blue Cross & Blue
Shield Oxford US Hlthcre +

[♿] [SA/SU] [☎] [📷] [🔍] [🛏] [Mcr] [NFI] Immediately

Quinn, Joseph (MD)   Ped   PCP
Southampton Hosp

Southhampton Pediatric Assoicates, 325 Meeting
House Ln C; Southampton, NY 11968; (516) 283-
7733; **BDCERT:** Ped 87; **MS:** Univ Vt Coll Med 81;
RES: Ped, NY Hosp-Cornell Med Ctr, New York, NY
82-84; **FEL:** Ped, U MD Hosp, Baltimore, MD 81-82;
HMO: Oxford Vytra MDNY HealthNet Blue Choice
+

[♿] [SA/SU] [☎] [📷] [🔍] [🛏] [$] [Mcr] A Few Days ▒▒ **VISA** ●

Rehman, Hafiz (MD)   Ped   PCP
Good Samaritan Hosp Med Ctr

375 E Main St Ste 7; Bay Shore, NY 11706; (516)
666-6780; **BDCERT:** Ped 79; **MS:** Pakistan 72;
RES: Ped, Good Samaritan Hosp Med Ctr, West Islip,
NY 75-77; **HOSP:** Southside Hosp; **HMO:** Most

LANG: Pak; [♿] [SA/SU] [📷] [🔍] [🛏] [$] [Mcr] [WC] [NFI]
A Few Days

Wilson, Thomas (MD)   Ped
Univ Hosp SUNY Stony Brook

SUNY HSC T11SUNY Stony Brook; Stony Brook,
NY 11794; (516) 444-3429; **BDCERT:** Ped 83;
MS: Univ Penn 73; **RES:** Children's Hosp Med Ctr,
Oakland, CA 74-76; **FEL:** PEn, U VA,
Charlottesville, VA 77-82

[♿] [📷] [🛏] [Mcr]

PLASTIC SURGERY

Adler, Hilton C (MD)   PlS
JT Mather Mem Hosp Pt Jfrson

Suffolk Plastic Surgeons, PC, 181 Belle Meade Rd
Ste 6; E Setauket, NY 11733; (516) 751-4400;
BDCERT: PlS 94; HS 87; **MS:** SUNY Downstate 79;
RES: S, U Miami Hosp, Miami, FL 79-80; PlS,
Albany Med Ctr, Albany, NY 83-85; **FEL:** Head &
Neck S, Beth Israel Med Ctr, New York, NY 81;
Burn S, Albany Med Ctr, Albany, NY 83; **FAP:** Clin
Instr SUNY Stony Brook; **HOSP:** St Charles Hosp &
Rehab Ctr; *SI: Plastic/Reconstructive/Surgery; Hand
Surgery;* **HMO:** Vytra Empire Blue Choice PPO
MDNY Multiplan +

LANG: Sp, Itl; [♿] [📷] [🔍] [🛏] [$] [Mcr] [Mcd] [WC] [NFI] 2-
4 Weeks ▒▒ **VISA** ●

Anton, John (MD)   PlS
Southampton Hosp

138 Old Town Rd; Southampton, NY 11968; (516)
283-9100; **BDCERT:** PlS 92; **MS:** Univ Vt Coll Med
81; **RES:** S, Deaconess Hosp, Boston, MA 81-84;
FEL: S, Mass Gen Hosp, Boston, MA 84-86; **HOSP:**
Central Suffolk Hosp; *SI: Face Lifts;* **HMO:** MDNY

[🔍] [🛏] [$] [Mcr] [NFI] 1 Week ▒▒ **VISA** ●

De Bellis, Joseph L (MD)   PlS
Southampton Hosp

80 Sanford Pl; Southampton, NY 11968; (516)
287-1234; **BDCERT:** PlS 84; **MS:** Georgetown U
86; **RES:** S, St Vincents Hosp & Med Ctr NY, New
York, NY 86-91; PlS, NY Hosp-Cornell Med Ctr,
New York, NY 91-93; **FEL:** Craniofacial S, Necker-
Enfant-Malade, Paris, France 93-94; PlS, Clinic
Belvedore, Clinic Belvedore 93-94; **HOSP:** Univ
Hosp SUNY Stony Brook; *SI: Hand Surgery; Face
Lifts;* **HMO:** None

LANG: Fr; [♿] [☎] [📷] [🛏] [$] [Mcr] [WC] [NFI] 2-4 Weeks ▒▒
VISA ●

Garcia, Ariel (MD) PlS
Good Samaritan Hosp Med Ctr

800 Montauk Hwy; West Islip, NY 11795; (516) 665-7946; **BDCERT:** PlS 80; **MS:** Philippines 61; **RES:** S, Bronx Lebanon Hosp Ctr, Bronx, NY 61-67; PlS, Montefiore Med Ctr, Bronx, NY 68-69; **HOSP:** Southside Hosp; *SI: Liposuction; Breast Reduction*

♿ 🌙 🔒 🚹 🏧 Mcr WC NFI A Few Days

Klindt, Joyce (MD) PlS
Good Samaritan Hosp Med Ctr

375 E Main St # 28; Bay Shore, NY 11706; (516) 665-2486; **BDCERT:** PlS 84; **MS:** Mt Sinai Sch Med 76; **RES:** Mount Sinai Med Ctr, New York, NY 76-80; Columbia Presbyterian Med Ctr, New York, NY 80-82; **FEL:** Manhattan Eye, Ear & Throat Hosp, New York, NY 81; NY Hosp-Cornell Med Ctr, New York, NY 80; **HOSP:** Southside Hosp

PSYCHIATRY

Carlson, Gabrielle A (MD) Psyc
Univ Hosp SUNY Stony Brook

SUNY Stony Brook, Putnam Hall, South Campus, 101 Nicholls Rd; Stony Brook, NY 11794; (516) 632-8840; **BDCERT:** Psyc 75; ChAP 78; **MS:** Cornell U 68; **RES:** Psyc, Barnes Hosp, St Louis, MO 68-70; Nat Inst Mental Health, Bethesda, MD 70-72; **FEL:** ChAP, UCLA Med Ctr, Los Angeles, CA 74-78; **FAP:** Lecturer SUNY Stony Brook

♿ 🔒 🚹 💲 Mcr Md 4+ Weeks 🈺 **VISA** 💳

Castroll, Robert (MD) Psyc
St John's Epis Hosp-Smithtown

222 Middle Country Rd Suite 210; Smithtown, NY 11787; (516) 265-6868; **BDCERT:** Psyc 85; **MS:** Univ Kans Sch Med 80; **RES:** Univ Hosp SUNY Stony Brook, Stony Brook, NY 81-84

Crasta, Jovita (MD) Psyc
Brunswick Hall Psych Hosp

80 Louden Ave; Amityville, NY 11701; (516) 789-3183; **BDCERT:** Psyc 81; **MS:** Meml U-St Johns, Newfoundland 81; **RES:** Psyc, Nassau County Med Ctr, East Meadow, NY 83-87; *SI: Depression, Panic; Stress Management;* **HMO:** Prucare GHI

♿ 🌙 🔒 🏧 Mcr WC NFI

Crovello, James (MD) Psyc
JT Mather Mem Hosp Pt Jfrson

625 Belle Terre Rd 203; Port Jefferson, NY 11777; (516) 928-8330; **BDCERT:** Psyc 70; **MS:** SUNY Hlth Sci Ctr 63; **RES:** Long Island Jewish Med Ctr, New Hyde Park, NY 64-67; **HOSP:** St Charles Hosp & Rehab Ctr; *SI: Depression; Anxiety Disorders;* **HMO:** MDNY

♿ 🔒 🏧 💲 2-4 Weeks

Derman, Robert (MD) Psyc
JT Mather Mem Hosp Pt Jfrson

33 Landing Ln; Port Jefferson, NY 11777; (516) 928-5773; **BDCERT:** Psyc 69; **MS:** Northwestern U 60; **RES:** Menninger Clinic, Topeka, KS 63-66; *SI: Depression; Panic Disorder;* **HMO:** Empire Blue Cross & Shield United Healthcare Mental Behavioral Care Sanus-NYLCare

♿ 🌙 🔒 🏧 💲 Mcr WC 1 Week

Eltan, Noam (MD) Psyc
Eastern Long Island Hosp

Eastern Long Island Hospital, 201 Manor Pl; Greenport, NY 11944; (516) 477-4975; **BDCERT:** Psyc 98; **MS:** Israel 86; **RES:** Psyc, Shalvata Hospital, Tel Aviv, Israel 86-91; **FEL:** Psyc, Sackler School of Med, Tel Aviv, Israel 88-95; **FAP:** Asst Clin Prof SUNY Stony Brook; **HOSP:** Univ Hosp SUNY Stony Brook; *SI: Anxiety Disorders; Depression;* **HMO:** First Choice Multiplan 1199 Health Choice American Health Plan +

LANG: Heb, Fr, Itl; ♿ 🌙 🚹 Mcr Md 1 Week

Hauben, Robert (MD)   Psyc
Southampton Hosp

351 Meeting House Ln; Riverhead, NY 11901;
(516) 283-9191; **MS:** Georgetown U 59; **RES:** Psyc,
Menninger Clinic, Topeka, KS 64; **FAP:** Asst Clin
Prof; *SI: Psychopharmacology; Psychotherapy;* **HMO:**
NYS Empire Plan

LANG: Dut, Fr; 🔲 🔲 🔲 🔲 🔲 🔲 🔲 1 Week

Lee, Kwang Soo (MD)   Psyc
Brunswick Hosp Ctr

80 Louden Ave; Amityville, NY 11701; (516) 789-
7448; **BDCERT:** Psyc 79; **MS:** South Korea 65; **RES:**
Booth Mem Hosp, Flushing, NY 66-67; Bellevue
Hosp Ctr, New York, NY 67-70; **FEL:** Amer Inst
Psychoanalysis, New York, NY 69; **HMO:** MDNY
NYNEX VBH Vytra

🔲 🔲 🔲 🔲 🔲 🔲 🔲 1 Week

Nass, Jack (MD)   Psyc
South Oaks Hosp

350 W Main St; Babylon, NY 11702; (516) 321-
7697; **BDCERT:** Psyc 80; GerPsy 90; **MS:** Belgium
75; **RES:** Psyc, Long Island Jewish Med Ctr, New
Hyde Park, NY 75-79; **FAP:** Adjct Prof SUNY Stony
Brook; *SI: Geriatrics; Mood Disorders*

🔲 🔲 🔲 🔲 🔲 🔲 🔲 A Few Days 🔲 *VISA*
🔲 🔲

Oxenhorn, Sanford (MD)   Psyc
Southampton Hosp

186A Old Town Rd Box 1550; Southampton, NY
11969; (516) 283-5585; **BDCERT:** Psyc 66; **MS:**
SUNY Hlth Sci Ctr 51; **RES:** IM, Montefiore Med Ctr,
Bronx, NY 52-53; **FEL:** Psyc, Albert Einstein Med
Ctr, Bronx, NY 60-62

🔲 🔲 🔲 🔲 🔲

Packard, William (MD)   Psyc

887 Old Country Rd; Riverhead, NY 11901; (516)
727-3596; **BDCERT:** Psyc 81; **MS:** Cornell U 76;
RES: St Luke's Roosevelt Hosp Ctr, New York, NY
77-80; **FEL:** FPsy, New York University Med Ctr,
New York, NY 83-84; **FAP:** Asst Prof SUNY Stony
Brook; *SI: Psychopharmacology; Depressive Disorders;*
HMO: VBH MBS Suffolk EmHC

🔲 🔲 🔲 🔲 🔲 🔲 🔲 🔲 1 Week

Pott, Nicholas (DO)   Psyc
Eastern Long Island Hosp

Windsway Prof Ctr PO Box 170, 44210 F Rte 48;
Southold, NY 11971; (516) 765-5191; **BDCERT:**
Psyc 78; **MS:** Univ N E Coll Osteo Med Biddeford 63

Rosen, Bruce (MD)   Psyc
St John's Epis Hosp-Smithtown

North Shore Psychiatric Consultants, PC, 222 E
Middle Country Rd 210; Smithtown, NY 11787;
(516) 265-6868; **BDCERT:** Psyc 76; GerPsy 96;
MS: Loyola U-Stritch Sch Med, Maywood 71; **RES:**
Psyc, Long Island Jewish Med Ctr, New Hyde Park,
NY 71-74; **FEL:** Psychotherapy, Long Island Jewish
Med Ctr, New Hyde Park, NY 74-75; **FAP:** Asst Clin
Prof Psyc SUNY Stony Brook; *SI: Depression and
Anxiety;* **HMO:** Empire Vytra United Healthcare

LANG: Sp; 🔲 🔲 🔲 🔲 🔲 🔲 2-4 Weeks *VISA* 🔲

Schwartz, Michael (MD)   Psyc
Huntington Hosp

33 E Carver St; Huntington, NY 11743; (516) 385-
3313; **BDCERT:** Psyc 84; **MS:** U Miami Sch Med 77;
RES: Psyc, Mount Sinai Med Ctr, New York, NY 81;
FEL: Nat Inst Health, Bethesda, MD; **FAP:** Assoc
Prof SUNY Stony Brook; **HOSP:** Univ Hosp SUNY
Stony Brook; *SI: Mood Disorders; Personality
Disorders*

🔲 🔲 🔲 2-4 Weeks 🔲

Solomon, Randall (MD)   Psyc

3771 Nesconset Hwy 103; Centereach, NY 11720;
(516) 751-3199; **BDCERT:** Psyc 90; **MS:** SUNY
Buffalo 84; **RES:** U of Pittsburgh Med Ctr,
Pittsburgh, PA 84-85; Psych Inst, Pittsburgh, PA
85-88; **HMO:** Anthem Health MDNY CIGNA

🔲 🔲 🔲 🔲 🔲 🔲 🔲 🔲 🔲 1 Week

Guide to symbols and abbreviations can be found on pages 110-113.

PULMONARY DISEASE

Bergman, Marion (MD)   Pul
Brookhaven Mem Hosp
Suffolk Chest Physicians, 73 S Ocean Ave;
Patchogue, NY 11772; (516) 654-4577; **BDCERT:**
IM 79; Pul 82; **MS:** U Va Sch Med 74; **RES:** IM, Univ
Hosp SUNY Bklyn, Brooklyn, NY 77-79; **FEL:** Pul,
Univ Hosp SUNY Stony Brook, Stony Brook, NY 79-
81

  🔵 🔲 📶 🏧 💲 Mcr Mcd WC   1 Week

Bernardini, Dennis (MD)   Pul
Huntington Hosp
175 E Main St; Huntington, NY 11743; (516) 424-
3787; **BDCERT:** Pul 87; Ger 96; **MS:** Johns Hopkins
U 80; **RES:** IM, St Luke's Roosevelt Hosp, New York,
NY 81-83; **FEL:** Pul, Univ Hosp SUNY Stony Brook,
Stony Brook, NY 83-85; **FAP:** Clin Instr SUNY
Stony Brook

Enden, Jay B (MD)   Pul
Southside Hosp
370 E Main St Ste 27; Bay Shore, NY 11706; (516)
666-5864; **BDCERT:** IM 87; Pul 90; **MS:** SUNY
Hlth Sci Ctr 84; **RES:** IM, Long Island Jewish Med
Ctr, New Hyde Park, NY 84-87; **FEL:** CCM, Albert
Einstein Med Ctr, Bronx, NY; Albert Einstein Med
Ctr, Bronx, NY; **HOSP:** Good Samaritan Hosp Med
Ctr

  🔲 📶 🏧 Mcr Mcd WC NFl   Immediately **VISA** 💳

Glaser, Morton (MD)   Pul
JT Mather Mem Hosp Pt Jfrson
60 N Country Rd 203; Port Jefferson, NY 11777;
(516) 928-3444; **BDCERT:** IM 80; Pul 84; **MS:** Med
Coll Wisc 76; **RES:** IM, Roger Williams Med Ctr,
Providence, RI 76-79; **FEL:** Pul, Univ Hosp SUNY
Stony Brook, Stony Brook, NY 79-81; **FAP:** Asst
Clin Instr SUNY Stony Brook; **HOSP:** St Charles
Hosp & Rehab Ctr; **HMO:** None

  🔵 🏧 💲 Mcr Mcd WC NFl   1 Week

Scheuch, Robert (MD)   Pul
Southampton Hosp
Southampton Pulmonary Medicine, PC, 50 N Main
St; South Hampton, NY 11968; (516) 283-8008;
BDCERT: IM 85; Pul 90; **MS:** Univ Mass Sch Med
82; **RES:** IM, St Vincent Hosp, Worcester, MA 82-
84; IM, Westchester County Med Ctr, Valhalla, NY
84-85; **FEL:** Pul, NY Med Coll, New York, NY 85-
87; **SI:** Asthma; Emphysema; **HMO:** MDNY Vytra
Oxford Health Plus Aetna-US Healthcare +

  🔵 🔲 📶 💲 Mcr   2-4 Weeks

Schneyer, Barton (MD)   Pul
St John's Epis Hosp-Smithtown
267 E Main St Bldg C; Smithtown, NY 11787;
(516) 361-7444; **BDCERT:** IM 75; Pul 80; **MS:**
Jefferson Med Coll 72; **RES:** Thomas Jefferson U
Hosp, Philadelphia, PA 72-73; Montefiore Med Ctr,
Bronx, NY 73-75; **FEL:** Pul, Montefiore Med Ctr,
Bronx, NY; **SI:** Asthma; Emphysema; **HMO:** Vytra
Oxford Empire Magnacare US Hlthcre +

  🔵 🔵 🔲 🏧 📶 💲 Mcr NFl   A Few Days **VISA** 💳

Sklarek, Howard (MD)   Pul
Southampton Hosp
Southampton Pulmonary Medicine, PC, 50 N Main
St; Southampton, NY 11968; (516) 283-8008;
BDCERT: IM 84; Pul 86; **MS:** SUNY Buffalo 81;
RES: IM, Nassau County Med Ctr, East Meadow, NY
81-84; **FEL:** Pul/CCM, Winthrop Univ Hosp,
Mineola, NY 84-86; **SI:** Asthma and Shortness of
Breath; Chronic Lung Disease; **HMO:** MDNY US
Hlthcre Oxford Vytra Health Source +

  🔵 🔲 🏧 📶 Mcr Mcd NFl   1 Week

Tow, Tony (MD)   Pul
Southside Hosp
Long Island Lung Center, 370 E Main St Suite 5;
Bay Shore, NY 11706; (516) 666-5800; **BDCERT:**
IM 82; Pul 84; **MS:** Cornell U 79; **RES:** IM, NY
Hosp-Cornell Med Ctr, New York, NY 79-82; **FEL:**
Pul, Mount Sinai Med Ctr, New York, NY 82-84;
HOSP: Good Samaritan Hosp Med Ctr; **SI:** Asthma;
Chronic Lung Disease; **HMO:** HIP Network Aetna
Hlth Plan Oxford CIGNA Prucare +

  LANG: Chi, Sp; 🔵 🔲 🏧 💲 Mcr Mcd WC NFl
Immediately **VISA** 💳

Walser, Lawrence (MD)   Pul
Central Suffolk Hosp

1333 Roanoke Ave; Riverhead, NY 11901; (516) 727-2523; **BDCERT:** IM 82; **MS:** SUNY Downstate 79; **RES:** Berkshire Med Ctr, Pittsfield, MA 80-82; **FEL:** Pul, Univ Hosp SUNY Stony Brook, Stony Brook, NY 82-84; **HOSP:** Eastern Long Island Hosp

🦽 🏥 📶 Mcr Mcd WC

Weiner, Jerome (MD)   Pul
Good Samaritan Hosp

LI Lung Center, 370 E Main St Ste 5; Bay Shore, NY 11706; (516) 666-5800; **BDCERT:** IM 80; CCM 87; **MS:** Mt Sinai Sch Med 77; **RES:** Med, Mount Sinai Med Ctr, New York, NY 78-80; **FEL:** Pul, Montefiore Med Ctr, Bronx, NY 80; **HOSP:** Southside Hosp

Wohlberg, Gary (MD)   Pul
Southside Hosp

370 E Main St Suite 5; Bay Shore, NY 11706; (516) 666-5800; **BDCERT:** IM 85; Pul 86; **MS:** SUNY Hlth Sci Ctr 81; **RES:** Long Island Jewish Med Ctr, New Hyde Park, NY 81-84; **FEL:** Montefiore Med Ctr, Bronx, NY 84-86; **HOSP:** Good Samaritan Hosp Med Ctr

LANG: Sp; 🦽 📶 🏥 📶 Mcr WC NFl 1 Week **VISA** 💳

RADIATION ONCOLOGY

Benninghoff, David (MD) RadRO
Huntington Hosp

3 Broad Path West; Huntington, NY 11743; (516) 864-5600; **BDCERT:** Rad 56; **MS:** Columbia P&S 52; **RES:** Temple U Hosp, Philadelphia, PA 56; **FEL:** Case Western Reserve U Hosp, Cleveland, OH; **HOSP:** St John's Epis Hosp-Smithtown; **HMO:** Blue Choice Blue Cross & Blue Shield Choicecare CIGNA HealthNet +

🦽 📶 🏥 Mcr Mcd WC NFl Immediately

Fiore, Americo S (MD)   RadRO
Southampton Hosp

Southampton Hosp, Herricks Ln; Southampton, NY 11968; (516) 727-2755; **BDCERT:** RadRO 65; **MS:** Italy 58; **RES:** RadRO, Metropolitan Hosp Ctr, New York, NY 60-63; Rad, Columbia-Presbyterian Med Ctr, New York, NY 63-65; **FEL:** RadRO, Columbia-Presbyterian Med Ctr, New York, NY 65-67; **FAP:** Instr Columbia P&S; **HOSP:** Central Suffolk Hosp; **SI:** *Breast; Prostate;* **HMO:** Vytra Oxford Empire Aetna Hlth Plan MDLI +

LANG: Sp, Itl; 🦽 📶 📶 🏥 📶 🏥 📶 WC NFl Immediately **VISA**

Meek, Allen (MD)   RadRO
Univ Hosp SUNY Stony Brook

University Hospital Dept of Radiation Oncology, 100 Nicholls Rd 643; Stony Brook, NY 11794; (516) 444-2200; **BDCERT:** RadRO 83; IM 79; **MS:** Johns Hopkins U 74; **RES:** IM, Johns Hopkins Hosp, Baltimore, MD 74-79; Rad, Johns Hopkins Hosp, Baltimore, MD 80-82; **FEL:** Onc, Johns Hopkins Hosp, Baltimore, MD 79-80; **FAP:** Chrmn SUNY Stony Brook; **SI:** *Breast Cancer; Prostate Cancer;* **HMO:** Oxford US Hlthcre Empire Blue Choice Vytra

🦽 📶 🏥 📶 Mcr Mcd WC NFl Immediately **VISA** 💳 📶

Mullen, Edward (MD)   RadRO
Good Samaritan Hosp Med Ctr

1000 Montauk Hwy; W Islip, NY 11795; (516) 669-1103; **BDCERT:** RadRO 91; **MS:** U Va Sch Med 86; **RES:** Columbia-Presbyterian Med Ctr, New York, NY 86-90; **SI:** *Prostate Seed Implantation;* **HMO:** Oxford GHI Aetna Hlth Plan US Hlthcre Choicecare +

🦽 📶 🏥 📶 Mcr Mcd Immediately

RADIOLOGY

Mack, Walter J (MD)   Rad
Southampton Hosp
265 Herrick Rd; Southampton, NY 11978; (516) 726-8410; **BDCERT:** Rad 61; **MS:** NY Med Coll 56; **RES:** Rad, Nat Naval Med Ctr, Bethesda, MD; Rad, U Chicago Hosp, Chicago, IL; **HOSP:** Central Suffolk Hosp

McIvor, John (MD)   Rad
Good Samaritan Hosp Med Ctr
South Shore Radiologists, PC, 759 Montauk Hwy; W Islip, NY 11795; (516) 669-1103; **BDCERT:** Rad 72; **MS:** Cornell U 63; **RES:** S, Bellevue Hosp Ctr, New York, NY 64-66; Rad, Montefiore Med Ctr, Bronx, NY 68-71; **SI:** *Angioplasty; Stenting;* **HMO:** MDNY Aetna Hlth Plan US Hlthcre Oxford Blue Cross +

LANG: Sp; [symbols] Immediately [symbols] **VISA** [symbol]

Trachtenberg, Albert (MD)   Rad
St Charles Hosp & Rehab Ctr
Radiological Health Services, P C, 80 Maple Ave; Smithtown, NY 11787; (516) 265-5777; **BDCERT:** Rad 62; **MS:** Switzerland 57; **RES:** Rad, VA Med Ctr-Manh, New York, NY 58-59; Rad, VA Med Ctr-Bronx, Bronx, NY 59-61; **FAP:** Asst Clin Prof FP SUNY Stony Brook; **HOSP:** JT Mather Mem Hosp Pt Jfrson; **SI:** *Cat Scanning; Mammography;* **HMO:** Vytra MDNY GHI Blue Cross Oxford +

LANG: Fr, Ger, Sp, Itl; [symbols] Immediately **VISA**

REPRODUCTIVE ENDOCRINOLOGY

Kenigsberg, Daniel (MD)   RE
JT Mather Mem Hosp Pt Jfrson
Long Island Fertility & Endocrinology/IVF Assoc PC, 625 Belle Terre Rd 200; Port Jefferson, NY 11777; (516) 331-7575; **BDCERT:** ObG 85; RE 87; **MS:** NY Med Coll 78; **RES:** ObG, Johns Hopkins Hosp, Baltimore, MD 78-82; **FEL:** RE, Nat Inst Health, Bethesda, MD 82-84; **FAP:** Assoc Prof SUNY Stony Brook; **HOSP:** St Charles Hosp & Rehab Ctr; **SI:** *In Vitro Fertilization; Infertility;* **HMO:** US Hlthcre Prucare Oxford Vytra United Healthcare +

LANG: Sp; [symbols] 1 Week **VISA** [symbol]

RHEUMATOLOGY

Bennett, Ronald (MD)   Rhu
St Charles Hosp & Rehab Ctr
Rheumatology Associates of Long Island, 315 E Middle Country Rd; Smithtown, NY 11787; (516) 360-7778; **BDCERT:** IM 75; Rhu 80; **MS:** SUNY Hlth Sci Ctr 72; **RES:** IM, Nassau County Med Ctr, East Meadow, NY 72-75; **FEL:** Rhu, Kings County Hosp Ctr, Brooklyn, NY 75-77; **FAP:** Asst Clin Prof Med SUNY Stony Brook; **HOSP:** JT Mather Mem Hosp Pt Jfrson; **SI:** *Rheumatoid Arthritis; Systemic Lupus;* **HMO:** Elderplan JJ Newman United Healthcare Vytra US Hlthcre +

[symbols] 2-4 Weeks

Bulanowski, Michael (MD)   Rhu
Southampton Hosp
365 County Rd 39A Ste 10; Southampton, NY 11968; (516) 287-2425; **MS:** SUNY Downstate 81; **RES:** IM, Nassau County Med Ctr, East Meadow, NY; **FEL:** Rhu, UC Irvine Med Ctr, Orange, CA; **SI:** *Rheumatoid Arthritis; Lyme Disease;* **HMO:** Island Group

[symbols] A Few Days

Hamburger, Max (MD)   Rhu
St John's Epis Hosp-Smithtown

Rheumatology Associates of Long Island, 315 E
Middle Country Rd; Smithtown, NY 11787; (516)
360-7778; **BDCERT:** IM 77; Rhu 80; **MS:** Albert
Einstein Coll Med 73; **RES:** IM, Bellevue Hosp Ctr,
New York, NY 73-76; **FEL:** A&I, Nat Inst Health,
Bethesda, MD 76-79; **FAP:** Asst Clin Prof Med
SUNY Stony Brook; **HOSP:** JT Mather Mem Hosp Pt
Jfrson; *SI: Lupus; Osteoporosis;* **HMO:** Oxford Vytra
Empire Aetna-US Healthcare MDNY +

▨ ⊞ S Mcr Mcd NFI 1 Week

Kaell, Alan (MD)   Rhu
St Charles Hosp & Rehab Ctr

Arthritis Care & Rehab Assoc, 315 E Middle
Country Rd; Smithtown, NY 11787; (516) 360-
7778; **BDCERT:** IM 81; Rhu 84; **MS:** Brown U 78;
RES: Strong Mem Hosp, Rochester, NY 78-79;
Strong Mem Hosp, Rochester, NY 79-81; **FEL:** Rhu,
Hosp For Special Surgery, New York, NY 81-83; NY
Hosp-Cornell Med Ctr, New York, NY; **FAP:** Clin
Prof SUNY Stony Brook; **HOSP:** JT Mather Mem
Hosp Pt Jfrson; *SI: Geriatrics; Osteoporosis*

♿ ℂ ▨ ⊞ S 1 Week

Repice, Michael (MD)   Rhu
Huntington Hosp

5 E Main St; Huntington, NY 11743; (516) 271-
1640; **BDCERT:** IM 76; **MS:** Georgetown U 73; **RES:**
Rhu, Univ of Mass Med Ctr, Worcester, MA 74-77;
HOSP: Good Samaritan Hosp

Tan, Mark (MD)   Rhu
JT Mather Mem Hosp Pt Jfrson

315 Middle Country Rd; Smithtown, NY 11787;
(516) 360-7778; **BDCERT:** IM 89; Rhu 94; **MS:**
SUNY Buffalo 83; **RES:** Univ Hosp SUNY Stony
Brook, Stony Brook, NY 84-86; **FEL:** Rhu, Johns
Hopkins Hosp, Baltimore, MD 87-89; **FAP:** SUNY
Stony Brook

LANG: Sp; ♿ ℂ ▨ ▨ ⊞ S Mcr WC NFI 4+ Weeks

SURGERY

Capizzi, Anthony (MD)   S
Good Samaritan Hosp Med Ctr

786 Montauk Hwy; W Islip, NY 11795; (516) 669-
3700; **BDCERT:** S 89; **MS:** NY Med Coll 83; **RES:**
Montefiore Med Ctr, Bronx, NY 83-88; **HOSP:**
Brunswick Hosp Ctr; *SI: Laparoscopic Surgery; Breast
Diseases;* **HMO:** Aetna Hlth Plan Oxford Prucare

♿ ℂ ▨ ▨ ⊞ S Mcr Mcd WC NFI A Few Days▨
VISA

Cohen, Bradley (MD)   S
Good Samaritan Hosp Med Ctr

Island Surgical & Vascular Grp, 111 Carleton Ave
2; Islip Terrace, NY 11752; (516) 581-4400;
BDCERT: S 89; **MS:** Mt Sinai Sch Med 83; **RES:**
Lenox Hill Hosp, New York, NY 83-88; **FEL:** Mem
Sloan Kettering Cancer Ctr, New York, NY 88-89;
HOSP: Southside Hosp; *SI: Breast Diseases;
Abdominal Problems;* **HMO:** US Hlthcre Oxford
Choicecare NYLCare Blue Cross +

LANG: Sp, Rus, Itl; ♿ ℂ ▨ ▨ ⊞ Mcr WC NFI
A Few Days▨ **VISA** ▨ ▨

Craig, Nicholas (MD)   S
JT Mather Mem Hosp Pt Jfrson

North Country Surgery PC, 41 N Country Rd; Port
Jefferson, NY 11777; (516) 928-8300; **BDCERT:** S
93; **MS:** Italy 82; **RES:** S, Hosp of St Raphael, New
Haven, CT 84-88; **HOSP:** St Charles Hosp & Rehab
Ctr; **HMO:** Aetna Hlth Plan Choicecare Metlife

LANG: Sp, Grk; ♿ ▨ ⊞ S Mcr WC NFI 1 Week

De Angelis, Vincent (MD)   S
Good Samaritan Hosp Med Ctr

786 Montauk Hwy; W Islip, NY 11795; (516) 669-
3700; **BDCERT:** S 64; **MS:** NY Med Coll 58; **RES:** St
Vincents Hosp & Med Ctr NY, New York, NY 58-59;
NY Med Coll, New York, NY 59-63; *SI: Breast
Cancer Surgery; Surgical Oncology;* **HMO:** Oxford
Aetna Hlth Plan US Hlthcre Prucare PHS +

LANG: Itl, Sp; ♿ ℂ ▨ ▨ ⊞ Mcr Mcd WC NFI
Immediately

Eghrari, Massoud (MD)   **S**
St John's Epis Hosp-Smithtown

Breast Surgery Office, 50 Karl Ave; Smithtown, NY 11787; (516) 724-3399; **BDCERT:** S 68; **MS:** France 56; **RES:** Baptist Med Ctr, Kansas City, MO 58; Med Ctr Hosp of VT, Burlington, VT 60-61; **FEL:** St Clare's Hosp & Health Ctr, New York, NY; St Clare's Hosp & Health Ctr, New York, NY; **FAP:** Asst Clin Prof S SUNY Stony Brook; **HOSP:** Univ Hosp SUNY Stony Brook; *SI: Breast Surgery; Diseases of Breast;* **HMO:** Oxford US Hlthcre Blue Choice MDNY

LANG: Fr, Frs; 🔲 🔲 🔲 🔲 🔲 🔲 🔲 🔲 🔲 🔲 Immediately

Gallagher, John F (MD)   **S**
Southside Hosp

375 E Main St; Bay Shore, NY 11706; (516) 665-5000; **BDCERT:** S 93; **MS:** U Chicago-Pritzker Sch Med 74; **RES:** S, NY Hosp-Cornell Med Ctr, New York, NY 74-76; S, NY Hosp-Cornell Med Ctr, New York, NY 76-79; **FEL:** GVS, Newark Beth Israel Med Ctr, Newark, NJ 81-82

Martinez, Alfred (MD)   **S**
St John's Epis Hosp-Smithtown

20 Manor Rd; Smithtown, NY 11787; (516) 360-3399; **BDCERT:** S 66; **MS:** Italy 58; **RES:** St John's Epis Hosp-Smithtown, Smithtown, NY 58-63; **FEL:** Kings County Hosp Ctr, Brooklyn, NY; Meadowbrook Hosp, East Meadow, NY; **HOSP:** South Nassau Comm Hosp; **HMO:** Aetna Hlth Plan Vytra Oxford MDNY

LANG: Sp, Itl; 🔲 🔲 🔲 🔲 🔲 🔲 🔲 🔲 Immediately 🔲 **VISA** 🔲 🔲

O'Hea, Brian (MD)   **S**
Univ Hosp SUNY Stony Brook

University Hospital and Medical Center at Stony Brook, Dept of Surgery, SUNY HSC Stony Brook, Nicholls Road; Stony Brook, NY 11794; (516) 444-1793; **BDCERT:** S 92; **MS:** Georgetown U 86; **RES:** S, St Vincent's, New York, NY 86-91; **FEL:** S, Memorial Sloan Kettering, New York, NY 95-96; **FAP:** Asst Prof SUNY Stony Brook; *SI: Breast Cancer*

🔲 🔲 🔲 🔲 🔲 🔲 1 Week **VISA** 🔲

Pastewski, Andrew (MD)   **S**
Univ Hosp SUNY Stony Brook

4 Phyllis Dr B3; Patchogue, NY 11772; (516) 289-4700; **BDCERT:** S 72; **MS:** Argentina 60; **RES:** S, Rhode Island Hosp, Providence, RI 66-70; **TS,** Rhode Island Hosp, Providence, RI 71-72

Petrillo, Anthony (MD)   **S**
Southampton Hosp

238 Old Town Rd; Southampton, NY 11968; (516) 283-2100; **BDCERT:** S 79; **MS:** UMDNJ-NJ Med Sch, Newark 69; **RES:** Kings County Hosp Ctr, Brooklyn, NY 70-76; *SI: Breast Disease;* **HMO:** Vytra Heritage Aetna Hlth Plan MDNY Oxford +

🔲 🔲 🔲 🔲 🔲 🔲 🔲 🔲 A Few Days 🔲 **VISA** 🔲

Ricca, Richard (MD)   **S**
Southampton Hosp

335A Meeting House Ln; Southampton, NY 11968; (516) 287-6570; **BDCERT:** S 86; **MS:** NY Med Coll 79; **RES:** Med, U Miami Hosp, Miami, FL 79-80; S, Univ Hosp SUNY Stony Brook, Stony Brook, NY 80-81; **FEL:** S, Boston U Med Ctr, Boston, MA 81-82; S, Univ Hosp SUNY Stony Brook, Stony Brook, NY 82-85; *SI: Hernias; Breast;* **HMO:** Vytra Oxford Aetna-US Healthcare MDNY

🔲 🔲 🔲 🔲 🔲 🔲 🔲

Robinson, John (MD)   **S**
St John's Epis Hosp-Smithtown

222 E Main St 102; Smithtown, NY 11787; (516) 360-1720; **BDCERT:** S 80; **MS:** Washington U, St Louis 70; **RES:** Jewish Hosp of St Louis, St Louis, MO 70-76; **FEL:** Cancer Immunology, Mass Gen Hosp, Boston, MA; *SI: Breast and Colon; Hernia Surgery;* **HMO:** Blue Choice Blue Cross & Blue Shield Choicecare CIGNA HealthNet +

🔲 🔲 🔲 🔲 🔲 🔲 🔲 🔲 🔲 🔲 🔲 Immediately

Schoenwald, Robert (MD)   **S**
Good Samaritan Hosp Med Ctr

375 E Main St; Bay Shore, NY 11706; (516) 665-5000; **BDCERT:** S 85; **MS:** Univ IL Coll Med 74; **RES:** Cook Cty Hosp, Chicago, IL 74-75; **FEL:** Cv, U IL Med Ctr, Chicago, IL; **HOSP:** Southside Hosp

🔲 🔲 🔲 🔲 🔲 🔲 🔲 Immediately

Sconzo, Frank (MD)   S
Brookhaven Mem Hosp

286 Sills Rd 5; East Patchogue, NY 11772; (516)
654-3100; **BDCERT:** S 67; **MS:** NY Med Coll 51;
RES: Brooklyn Meth Hosp, Brooklyn, NY 55-58;
Brooklyn Meth Hosp, Brooklyn, NY 52-53

⬆ 🏥 🏢 🅂 Mcr Mcd WC NFI   Immediately

Simon, John (MD)   S
Southside Hosp

375 E Main St 26; Bay Shore, NY 11706; (516)
665-5000; **BDCERT:** S 92; **MS:** India 81; **RES:** S,
SIA, India 82-85; **HOSP:** Good Samaritan Hosp
Med Ctr; **SI:** *Laparoscopic Surgery*

⬆ 🄲 🄰 🏥 🏢 🅂 Mcr WC NFI   A Few Days

Warm, Hillard (MD)   S
JT Mather Mem Hosp Pt Jfrson

Cosmetic Surgery of New York,PC, 4616 Nesconset
Hwy; Port Jeffrsn Sta, NY 11776; (516) 473-5800;
BDCERT: PlS 90; **MS:** Mexico 79; **RES:** S, Millard
Fillmore Health Sys, Buffalo, NY 81-85; PlS, Med U
of SC Med Ctr, Charleston, SC 86-88; **SI:** *Face &
Eyelid Lifts; Breast Enlargements*

LANG: Sp; ⬆ 🆂🅰 🄲 🄰 🏥 🏢 🅂 Mcr WC NFI
Immediately 💳 **VISA** 💳 💳

Ziviello, Alfred (MD)   S
JT Mather Mem Hosp Pt Jfrson

251 E Oakland Ave 202; Port Jefferson, NY 11777;
(516) 928-3332; **BDCERT:** S 63; **MS:** U Ottawa 57;
RES: Med Coll VA Hosp, Richmond, VA 58-62;
FAP: Asst Prof S SUNY Stony Brook; **HOSP:** St
Charles Hosp & Rehab Ctr; **SI:** *Breast Surgery;
Gallbladder Surgery*; **HMO:** US Hlthcre Aetna Hlth
Plan Prucare Blue Cross & Blue Shield

🄰 🏥 🅂 Mcr WC   A Few Days

THORACIC SURGERY

Bilfinger, Thomas (MD)   TS
Univ Hosp SUNY Stony Brook

101 Nicholls Rd FL 19; Stony Brook, NY 11794;
(516) 444-1820; **BDCERT:** TS 90; SCC 90; **MS:**
Switzerland 78; **RES:** U Chicago Hosp, Chicago, IL
80-82; U TX Med Branch Hosp, Galveston, TX 82-
86; **FEL:** TS, U TX Med Branch Hosp, Galveston, TX
86-88; **FAP:** Assoc Prof SUNY Stony Brook; **HOSP:**
JT Mather Mem Hosp Pt Jfrson; **HMO:** Vytra HIP
Network US Hlthcre CIGNA Aetna-US Healthcare +

LANG: Ger, Itl, Fr; ⬆ 🄲 🄰 🏥 Mcr Mcd WC
A Few Days 💳 **VISA** 💳 💳

Dranitzke, Richard (MD)   TS
St Charles Hosp & Rehab Ctr

Richard J Dranitxke, MD, PC, 635 Belle Terre Rd
201; Port Jefferson, NY 11777; (516) 473-1602;
BDCERT: TS 76; S 74; **MS:** Columbia P&S 66; **RES:**
S, Bellevue Hosp Ctr, New York, NY 69-73; TS,
Albany Med Ctr, Albany, NY 73-75; **HOSP:** JT
Mather Mem Hosp Pt Jfrson; **SI:** *General Vascular
Surgery; Thoracic Surgery*; **HMO:** Vytra US Hlthcre
Oxford GHI Empire +

⬆ 🄰 🏥 🅂 Mcr Mcd WC NFI   Immediately

Palatt, Terry (MD)   TS
Good Samaritan Hosp Med Ctr

Island Surgical & Vascular Grp, 111 Carleton Ave
2; Islip Terrace, NY 11752; (516) 581-4400;
BDCERT: TS 89; S 87; **MS:** Grenada 81; **RES:** TS,
Maimonides Med Ctr, Brooklyn, NY 86;
Maimonides Med Ctr, Brooklyn, NY 82; **FEL:** Cv,
Univ Hosp SUNY Bklyn, Brooklyn, NY 88

⬆ 🏥 🅂 Mcr Mcd NFI   A Few Days 💳 **VISA** 💳
💳

Rubenstein, Richard (MD)   TS
Brookhaven Mem Hosp

250 Yaphank Rd; E Patchogue, NY 11772; (516)
475-1013; **BDCERT:** TS 82; S 79; **MS:** SUNY
Downstate 72; **RES:** Beth Israel Med Ctr, New York,
NY 72-77; Charlotte Mem Hosp, Charlotte, NC 77-
79; **FEL:** Mayo Clinic, Rochester, MN; **HMO:** Oxford
Choicecare Aetna Hlth Plan Prucare

UROLOGY

Beccia, David (MD) U
Southside Hosp
332 E Main St; Bay Shore, NY 11706; (516) 665-3737; **BDCERT:** U 79; **MS:** NY Med Coll 70; **RES:** S, Hartford Hosp, Hartford, CT 70-73; U, Boston U Med Ctr, Boston, MA 74-77; **HOSP:** Good Samaritan Hosp Med Ctr; **SI:** *Prostate Cancer; Erectile Dysfunction*; **HMO:** Oxford United Healthcare Vytra Aetna-US Healthcare

LANG: Sp, Grk; ⬢ 🌓 🔒 🏢 $ Mcr Mcd WC NFI 1 Week 🎫 **VISA** 😊 🔲

Cruickshank, David (MD) U
Southampton Hosp
315 Meeting House Ln; Southampton, NY 11968; (516) 283-0323; **BDCERT:** U 78; **MS:** SUNY Downstate 70; **RES:** St Vincents Hosp & Med Ctr NY, New York, NY 70-72; Univ Hosp SUNY Bklyn, Brooklyn, NY 73-76; **HOSP:** Eastern Long Island Hosp; **SI:** *Prostate; Vasectomy—No Scalpel*; **HMO:** Aetna Hlth Plan US Hlthcre Vytra Blue Choice MDNY +

⬢ 🔒 🏢 $ Mcr WC NFI 2-4 Weeks **VISA** 😊

Frischer, Zelik (MD) U
Univ Hosp SUNY Stony Brook
Department Of Urology, 2500 Nesconset Hwy 9D; Stony Brook, NY 11790; (516) 444-6270; **BDCERT:** U 90; **MS:** Russia 60; **RES:** U, Tel Aviv, Israel 73-78; U, Leningrad, USSR 65-69; **FEL:** U, Beth Israel Med Ctr, New York, NY 84-86; **FAP:** Prof U SUNY Stony Brook

Pastore, Louis (MD) U
Brookhaven Mem Hosp
250 Yaphank Rd 15; East Patchogue, NY 11772; (516) 475-5051; **BDCERT:** U 74; **MS:** Canada 65; **RES:** Kings County Hosp Ctr, Brooklyn, NY 66-67; **HOSP:** JT Mather Mem Hosp Pt Jfrson; **HMO:** Aetna Hlth Plan Blue Choice Choicecare

Waltzer, Wayne (MD) U
Univ Hosp SUNY Stony Brook
Dept of Urology, 2500 Nesconset Hwy 9D; Stony Brook, NY 11790; (516) 689-6210; **BDCERT:** U 80; **MS:** Univ Pittsburgh 73; **RES:** Presbyterian U Hosp, Pittsburgh, PA; **FEL:** Renal Transplantation, Mayo Clinic, Rochester, MN; **HOSP:** St John's Epis Hosp-Smithtown; **SI:** *Urologic Cancer; Reconstructive Urology Surgery*; **HMO:** Empire GHI Aetna Hlth Plan CIGNA

LANG: Heb, Rus, Kor, Ur; ⬢ 🔒 🏢 🏢 $ Mcr Mcd WC NFI 1 Week 🎫 **VISA** 😊 🔲

Wasnick, Robert (MD) U
Univ Hosp SUNY Stony Brook
2500 Nesconset Hwy 9D; Stony Brook, NY 11790; (516) 444-6270; **BDCERT:** U 82; **MS:** Jefferson Med Coll 74; **RES:** St Vincents Hosp & Med Ctr NY, New York, NY 74-77; Univ Hosp SUNY Bklyn, Brooklyn, NY 77-80; **FEL:** England; **HOSP:** St Charles Hosp & Rehab Ctr; **SI:** *Hypospadias; Undescended Testes*; **HMO:** Oxford Magnacare Vytra Oxford GHI +

⬢ 🌓 🔒 🏢 🏢 $ Mcr Mcd WC NFI A Few Days **VISA** 😊

VASCULAR SURGERY (GENERAL)

Anker, Eli (MD) GVS
Good Samaritan Hosp Med Ctr
111 Carleton Ave 2; Islip Terrace, NY 11752; (516) 581-4400; **BDCERT:** S 80; **MS:** Albert Einstein Coll Med 72; **RES:** Montefiore Med Ctr, Bronx, NY 72-76; **FEL:** GVS, Newark Beth Israel Med Ctr, Newark, NJ 76-77; **HOSP:** Southside Hosp; **SI:** *Angioplasty and Stents; Sclerotherapy*; **HMO:** Aetna Hlth Plan CIGNA NYLCare Blue Choice GHI +

⬢ 🌓 🔒 🏢 🏢 $ Mcr WC NFI 1 Week **VISA** 😊

Guide to symbols and abbreviations can be found on pages 110-113.

749

Arnold, Thomas E (MD) GVS
JT Mather Mem Hosp Pt Jfrson
Suffolk Vascular Associates, 5225 Route 347 60;
Port Jefferson, NY 11776; (516) 476-9100; **MS:**
SUNY Downstate 85; **RES:** S, Medical College of PA,
Philadelphia, PA 87-91; S, Presbeterian Univ of PA,
Philadelphia, PA 86-87; **HOSP:** St Charles Hosp &
Rehab Ctr

♿ 🅲 🔲 🛏 🅂 Mcr Mcd WC NFI 1 Week **VISA** 💳

Francfort, John (MD) GVS
Good Samaritan Hosp Med Ctr
Great South Bay Surgical Associates, 375 E Main St
Ste 26; Bay Shore, NY 11706; (516) 665-5000;
BDCERT: S 87; GVS 89; **MS:** UMDNJ-NJ Med Sch,
Newark 80; **RES:** S, Hosp of U Penn, Philadelphia,
PA 80-86; **FEL:** GVS, Northwestern Mem Hosp,
Chicago, IL 86-87; **HOSP:** Southside Hosp; *SI:
Vascular Surgery; Breast Surgery;* **HMO:** Oxford
Aetna Hlth Plan Vytra Blue Cross

♿ 🅲 🔲 🛏 🅂 Mcr Mcd WC NFI A Few Days

Giron, Fabio (MD) GVS
Univ Hosp SUNY Stony Brook
Stony Brook Surgical Associates, PC, SUNY Stony
Brook Sch Med Dept of Surg; Stony Brook, NY
11794; (516) 444-2040; **BDCERT:** GVS 91; **MS:**
Spain 54; **RES:** S, Univ Hosp of Madrid, Madrid,
Spain 56-60; **FEL:** Mount Sinai Med Ctr, New York,
NY 66-67; Mount Sinai Med Ctr, New York, NY 67-
68; **FAP:** Prof SUNY Stony Brook; *SI: Abdominal
Aortic Aneurysm; Carotid Endarterectomy;* **HMO:**
Empire Vytra Oxford CIGNA GHI +

♿ 🔲 🧍 🛏 🅂 Mcr Mcd WC NFI 2-4 Weeks

Gredysa, Leslaw (MD) GVS
Southampton Hosp
234 Hampton Rd; Southampton, NY 11968; (516)
287-1433; **BDCERT:** S 95; **MS:** Poland 82; **RES:**
Poland 82-83; Wyckoff Heights Med Ctr, Brooklyn,
NY 88-90; **FEL:** GVS, Nassau County Med Ctr, East
Meadow, NY; St Francis Hosp-Roslyn, Roslyn, NY;
HOSP: Central Suffolk Hosp

♿ 🔲 🧍 🛏 🅂 Mcr Mcd WC NFI Immediately

Pollina, Robert M (MD) GVS
JT Mather Mem Hosp Pt Jfrson
Suffolk Vascular Associates, 522560 Rte 347; Port
Jefferson, NY 11772; (516) 654-0585; **BDCERT:**
TS 94; **MS:** SUNY Hlth Sci Ctr 88; **RES:** S, Kings
County Hosp Ctr, Brooklyn, NY 89-92; **FEL:** GVS,
Maimonides Med Ctr, Brooklyn, NY 93-94; **HOSP:**
St Charles Hosp & Rehab Ctr; *SI: Varicose Veins; All
Circulatory Disorders;* **HMO:** Oxford Vytra Blue
Cross & Blue Shield US Hlthcre

♿ 🔲 🛏 🅂 Mcr Mcd WC NFI Immediately 💳 **VISA** 💳

Ricotta, John (MD) GVS
Univ Hosp SUNY Stony Brook
Dept of Surgery-SUNY at Stony Brook, Nicholls Rd;
Stony Brook, NY 11794; (516) 444-7875;
BDCERT: GVS 80; **MS:** Johns Hopkins U 73; **RES:**
Johns Hopkins Hosp, Baltimore, MD 73-76; Johns
Hopkins Hosp, Baltimore, MD 77-79; **FEL:** Johns
Hopkins Hosp, Baltimore, MD 76-77; **FAP:** Prof
SUNY Stony Brook; *SI: Aneurysms; Carotid Surgery;*
HMO: Vytra Empire Oxford Sel Pro US Hlthcre +
LANG: Itl, Sp; 🅲 🔲 🧍 🛏 🅂 Mcr Mcd NFI 1 Week

WESTCHESTER COUNTY

SAINT AGNES HOSPITAL

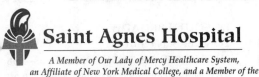

Saint Agnes Hospital

*A Member of Our Lady of Mercy Healthcare System,
an Affiliate of New York Medical College, and a Member of the
Catholic Health Care Network.*

**SAINT AGNES HOSPITAL
305 NORTH STREET
WHITE PLAINS, NY 10605
(914) 681-4500
FAX (914) 681-4948**

Sponsorship	Not-for-Profit; Sponsored by the Archdiocese of New York
Beds	189
Accreditation	Joint Commission on Accreditation of Healthcare Organizations, Association of American Medical Colleges, New York State Department of Health

A MEMBER OF OUR LADY OF MERCY HEALTHCARE SYSTEM

Serving Westchester, Rockland, and Putnam counties from its location in White Plains, Saint Agnes Hospital is a member of Our Lady of Mercy Healthcare System. The system is comprised of three hospitals (Our Lady of Mercy Medical Center, the Florence D'Urso Pavilion and Saint Agnes Hospital), an ambulatory care pavilion, six Medical Villages (physician office sites), senior citizen housing, a physician-hospital organization, a residence for unwed mothers, and a home health agency.

Saint Agnes Hospital provides a full range of medical and surgical services, comprehensive outpatient services, same-day surgery services and 24-hour emergency care for adults and children. Saint Agnes Hospital is a teaching affiliate of New York Medical College, which sponsors most of the hospital's residency programs.

THE THOMAS AND AGNES CARVEL FOUNDATION CHILDREN'S REHABILITATION CENTER

For children with developmental disabilities, Saint Agnes Hospital offers The Thomas and Agnes Carvel Foundation Children's Rehabilitation Center. Saint Agnes is renowned for its Children's Rehabilitation Center, which offers the only comprehensive, year-round outpatient program in the Westchester area for children with cerebral palsy, spina bifida and other developmentally disabling conditions. Using a unique blend of medical, therapeutic and educational services, the Center treats more than 2,000 children each year. The children range in age from birth through age 21, and represent every race and creed. With an extensive staff of experts, brand new facilities, and a wealth of resources, staff members are able to help each child learn and work to his or her greatest potential. In addition, a satellite facility in Carmel serves Putnam County residents.

CENTERS OF EXCELLENCE

Saint Agnes Hospital has designated ten Centers of Excellence which reflect the hospital's commitment to quality care and services. These include:

Maternity Services, The Center for Breast Diseases, The Center for Geriatrics, Multiple Sclerosis Center,

The Cancer Institute, The Institute for Minimally Invasive Surgery, The Diabetes Treatment Center,

The Hyperbaric Chamber Center, The Balance Function Center and The Dialysis Center

Saint Agnes Hospital operates a toll-free, 7 days a week, 24 hours a day physician referral service (1-800-628-1008). Multilingual operators are available, with computerized access to more than 600 staff and affiliated physicians. More than 80 percent of the physicians are board certified in their fields.

SAINT JOSEPH'S MEDICAL CENTER

127 SOUTH BROADWAY
YONKERS, NY 10701
PHONE (914) 378-7535 FAX (914) 965-4838
www.saintjosephs.org e-mail: sjmcgen@chcn.org

Sponsorship	Voluntary, Not-for-Profit, sponsored by Sisters of Charity of St. Vincent de Paul
Beds	194 acute (29 Psych, 37 dedicated Geriatric, 9 Pediatric), 200 nursing home (40 Alzheimer's)
Accreditation	Joint Commission on Accreditation of Health Care Organizations (JCAHO), NYS Department of Health

GENERAL DESCRIPTION

A progressive health care facility offering comprehensive inpatient and outpatient programs and services in all medical specialties, except Obstetrics.

PHILOSOPHY

Committed to medical excellence, providing the latest technology, and treating every patient with dignity, respect and concern.

TEACHING PROGRAMS/AFFILIATIONS

The only Family Practice Residency Program in Westchester County and a surgical residency with Lincoln Hospital in the Bronx. Affiliated with New York Medical College and a member of the Catholic Health Care Network, Excel Care and Pinnacle Health System.

CENTERS OF EXCELLENCE

Geriatrics	A full continuum of care, including a nursing home, acute inpatient unit, long-term home health care, medical and social day care programs and speech and hearing center.
Primary Care	Modern Family Health Center for affordable primary and preventive care and Urgent Care Centers for minor emergencies.
Oncology	Bone Marrow Transplant program, ABBI breast biopsy system, accredited mammography unit, prostate seed implantation, chemotherapy and spiral CAT scan. (Radiation therapy located across the street.)
Surgery	Holmium laser, endo-urology, micro-neurosurgery and state-of-the-art ophthalmology surgery.

SPECIAL PROGRAMS

Mental Health	A secure 29-bed inpatient psychiatric unit, outpatient clinic, emergency psychiatric services, continuing day treatment, supportive case management and substance abuse programs.
Pediatrics	Children's Evaluation and Rehabilitation Center for children with physical and developmental disabilities, numerous physician Pediatric subspecialists and school-based programs.
Renal Dialysis	Inpatient renal dialysis unit, continuous ambulatory (CAPD) and continuous cycling (CCPD) peritoneal dialysis programs.
Emergency Medicine	Emergency Medical Control Hospital for the City of Yonkers, Chest Pain Center, Stroke Team, Asthma Treatment Center and Fast Track service.
Physician Referral	Please call our free telephone referral at (914) 378-7830 (weekdays from 8 a.m. to 5 p.m.) for access to more than 250 qualified and respected physicians on the Medical Staff, a majority of whom are Board Certified, many frequently published leaders in their fields.

UNITED HOSPITAL MEDICAL CENTER

406 BOSTON POST ROAD
PORT CHESTER, NY 10573
PHONE: (914) 934-3000
FAX: (914) 934-3411
WEBSITE: WWW.UHMC.COM

ponsorship	Voluntary Not-for-Profit
eds	311 licensed (including 40 nursing home beds)
ccreditation	Joint Commission on Accreditation of Healthcare Organizations (JCAHO)

OMMUNITY HOSPITAL AND MEMBER OF A LARGE HEALTHCARE SYSTEM

nited has served the communities of Harrison, Larchmont, Mamaroneck, Port Chester, Purchase, Rye
nd Rye Brook, NY since 1889 and is a member of The New York and Presbyterian Healthcare Network,
ne of the largest health care systems in the world.

nited's staff of 300 physicians represents 50 specialties. 95% are either Board Certified (83%) or Board Eligible.

EDICAL PROGRAMS AND COMMUNITY SERVICES

der Care:	*Center for Geriatric Health:* addresses health problems associated with aging. *Health Outreach:* for ages 65+, provides health screenings and education for maintaining health. *Senior Day Care Center:* provides safe environment for seniors who aren't as independent as they once were or have decreased physical or mental functioning. *Skilled Nursing Pavilion:* A nursing residence for older adults requiring ongoing medical care, offers therapeutic and social enrichment opportunities
he Center for Holistic Medicine:	Certified practitioners treat patients with acupuncture, Alexander Technique, herbology, massage, nutrition, reflexology, biofeedback and/or imagery.
evel II Nursery:	Directed by a Neonatologist, provides care for premature babies.
Iew Rochelle lcoholism Clinic:	Serves those whose lives, and the lives of their families, co-dependents and significant others, have been disrupted by addiction.
ain Management enter:	Treats and rehabilitates patients suffering from chronic pain due to arthritis, cancer, migraine, back injury, etc.
nited Hospital Iospice:	Offers comfort and support for terminally ill patients and their families. Care is given primarily in the home, enabling families to remain together.
nited Walk-In:	Open 11:00 a.m. -11:00 p.m., 7 days a week, provides treatment for minor emergencies.
ECP. Enhanced xternal ounterpulsation:	A noninvasive therapy for angina pectoris, decreases chest pain. United is the only hospital in NY offering EECP commercially.
hysician Referral:	United offers a free telephone and internet physician referral service.

PHONE # (914)934-3414

SPECIALTY & SUBSPECIALTY	ABBREVIATION	PAGE(S)
Allergy & Immunology	A&I	757-758
Anesthesiology	Anes	758
Cardiology (Cardiovascular Disease)	Cv	758-763
Child & Adolescent Psychiatry	ChAP	763-764
Child Neurology	ChiN	764
Colon & Rectal Surgery	CRS	765
Dermatology	D	765-768
Diagnostic Radiology	DR	768-769
Emergency Medicine	EM	769
Endocrinology, Diabetes & Metabolism	EDM	769-771
FAMILY PRACTICE	FP	771-773
Gastroenterology	Ge	773-776
Geriatric Medicine	Ger	777
Gynecologic Oncology*	GO	777
Hand Surgery	HS	777
Hematology	Hem	777-778
Infectious Disease	Inf	778-779
INTERNAL MEDICINE	IM	779-787
Maternal & Fetal Medicine	MF	787
Medical Genetics	MG	787
Medical Oncology*	Onc	787-789
Neonatal-Perinatal Medicine	NP	789
Nephrology	Nep	789-790
Neurological Surgery	NS	791
Neurology	N	791-793
Neuroradiology	NRad	793
Nuclear Medicine	NuM	793
Nuclear Radiology	NR	793
OBSTETRICS & GYNECOLOGY	ObG	794-799
Ophthalmology	Oph	799-804
Orthopaedic Surgery	OrS	804-807
Otolaryngology	Oto	808-810
Pain Management	PM	810

SPECIALTY & SUBSPECIALTY	ABBREVIATION	PAGE(S)
Pediatric Cardiology	PCd	810-811
Pediatric Endocrinology	PEn	811-812
Pediatric Gastroenterology	PGe	812
Pediatric Hematology–Oncology*	PHO	812-813
Pediatric Nephrology	PNep	813
Pediatric Pulmonology	PPul	813
Pediatric Surgery	PS	813-814
PEDIATRICS (GENERAL)	Ped	814-819
Physical Medicine & Rehabilitation	PMR	819
Plastic Surgery	PlS	819-821
Preventive Medicine	PrM	821
Psychiatry	Psyc	821-826
Pulmonary Disease	Pul	826-828
Radiation Oncology*	RadRO	828
Radiology	Rad	829
Rheumatology	Rhu	829-830
Sports Medicine	SM	830-831
Surgery	S	831-835
Surgical Critical Care	SCC	835
Thoracic Surgery (includes open heart surgery)	TS	835-836
Urology	U	836-839
Vascular Surgery (General)	GVS	839-840

Specialties in capital letters indicate Primary Care Specialties. However, many doctors will be certified in a subspecialty, but will practice predominantly primary care medicine. In our lists this will be indicated.

*Oncologists deal with Cancer

ALLERGY & IMMUNOLOGY

Baum, Carol (MD) A&I
White Plains Hosp Ctr
210 Westchester Ave; White Plains, NY 10604;
(914) 682-6479; **BDCERT:** IM 86; A&I 89; **MS:**
NYU Sch Med 83; **RES:** IM, St Luke's Roosevelt
Hosp Ctr, New York, NY 83-86; **FEL:** A&I, NY Hosp-
Cornell Med Ctr, New York, NY 86-88; **FAP:** Clin
Instr Cornell U; **HOSP:** NY Hosp-Cornell Med Ctr;
SI: Asthma; Hay Fever; **HMO:** Kaiser Permanente
LANG: Sp; ♿ 🅲 🔂 🔊 🛏 🆂 Mcr Mcd A Few Days
📧

Fusillo, Christine (MD) A&I
Phelps Mem Hosp Ctr
1600 Harrison Ave 104; Mamaroneck, NY 10543;
(914) 381-2285; **BDCERT:** A&I 87; **MS:** NYU Sch
Med 80; **RES:** Bellevue Hosp Ctr, New York, NY 81-
83; **FEL:** A&I, St Luke's Roosevelt Hosp Ctr, New
York, NY 85; **HOSP:** Westchester Med Ctr; *SI:*
Asthma; Food Allergy

Geraci, Kira (MD) A&I
United Hosp Med Ctr
10 Rye Ridge Plaza 215; Rye Brook, NY 10573;
(914) 251-1245; **BDCERT:** A&I 85; Ped 84; **MS:**
Columbia P&S 80; **RES:** Ped, NY Hosp-Cornell Med
Ctr, New York, NY 80-83; **FEL:** A&I, NY Hosp-
Cornell Med Ctr, New York, NY 83-85; **FAP:** Clin
Instr Cornell U; **HOSP:** St Agnes Hosp; *SI:* Asthma;
Sinusitis; **HMO:** Blue Cross & Blue Shield Oxford
Pomco
LANG: Itl; ♿ 🔂 🔊 🛏 🆂 1 Week **VISA** 💳

Gerardi, Anthony (MD) A&I
St John's Riverside Hosp
984 N Broadway 307; Yonkers, NY 10701; (914)
476-8877; **BDCERT:** IM 72; **MS:** SUNY Hlth Sci Ctr
58; **RES:** IM, St Luke's Roosevelt Hosp Ctr, New
York, NY 58; A&I, St Luke's Roosevelt Hosp Ctr,
New York, NY 61-62; **HOSP:** Yonkers Gen Hosp; *SI:*
Asthma; Hay Fever; **HMO:** Oxford Blue Choice
United Healthcare Pomco PHS +
LANG: Itl; ♿ 🅲 🔂 🔊 🛏 Mcr A Few Days

Goldman, Neil C (MD) A&I
Hudson Valley Hosp Ctr
Hudson Valley Asthma and Allergy Assoc, PC, 35 S
Riverside Ave Ste 106; Croton On Hudson, NY
10520; (914) 271-0001; **BDCERT:** A&I 77; **MS:**
NY Med Coll 66; **RES:** IM, Beth Israel Med Ctr, New
York, NY 67-68; IM, Metropolitan Hosp Ctr, New
York, NY 68-69; **FEL:** A&I, Jewish Hosp Med Ctr,
Brooklyn, NY 69-70; **HOSP:** Phelps Mem Hosp Ctr;
SI: Allergies; Asthma; **HMO:** Blue Choice PHS Oxford
US Hlthcre Multiplan +
♿ 🆂🄰 🅲 🔂 🔊 🛏 🆂 Mcr 1 Week **VISA** 💳 📧

Golub, James (MD) A&I
Sound Shore Med Ctr-Westchester
150 Lockwood Ave 36; New Rochelle, NY 10801;
(914) 235-1888; **BDCERT:** A&I 72; **MS:** Columbia
P&S 53; **RES:** Mount Sinai Med Ctr, New York, NY
58-59; Bellevue Hosp Ctr, New York, NY 57-58;
FEL: Cv, Columbia-Presbyterian Med Ctr, New
York, NY 56-57; **HOSP:** Westchester Med Ctr
LANG: Sp; ♿ 🆂🄰 🔂 🔊 🛏 🆂 Mcr Mcd WC
Immediately **VISA** 💳

Hermance, William (MD) A&I
St Agnes Hosp
333 W Post Rd; White Plains, NY 10606; (914)
997-1688; **BDCERT:** A&I 74; **MS:** U Rochester 60;
RES: St Luke's Roosevelt Hosp Ctr, New York, NY
60-67; **HOSP:** Lenox Hill Hosp; **HMO:** Aetna Hlth
Plan CIGNA Metlife Magnacare
♿ 🔂 🔊 🛏 Mcr WC NFI Immediately

Josephson, Barry (MD) A&I
St Joseph's Med Ctr-Yonkers
50 Riverdale Ave; Yonkers, NY 10701; (914) 965-
8866; **BDCERT:** A&I 77; PA&I 62; **MS:** NYU Sch
Med 55; **RES:** Ped, NY Hosp-Cornell Med Ctr, New
York, NY 56-58; **FEL:** A&I, Strong Mem Hosp,
Rochester, NY 60-62; **FAP:** Clin Instr NY Med Coll;
SI: Asthma; Food Allergy; **HMO:** Oxford Pomco Blue
Cross & Blue Shield Metlife PHS +
LANG: Sp; ♿ 🆂🄰 🅲 🔂 🔊 🛏 🆂 Mcr NFI
A Few Days

Guide to symbols and abbreviations can be found on pages 110-113.

757

Larkin, Aimee (MD)   A&I
White Plains Hosp Ctr
170 Maple Ave 508; White Plains, NY 10601;
(914) 946-7187; **BDCERT:** A&I 74; **MS:** Columbia
P&S 50; **RES:** Kings County Hosp Ctr, Brooklyn, NY
52-53; **HOSP:** St Agnes Hosp; **SI:** *Asthma; Hay
Fever;* **HMO:** Oxford Pomco SWCHP Aetna Hlth
Plan

♿ 📷 🚾 🏛 Mcr   A Few Days **VISA** ●

Mendelsohn, Lois (MD)   A&I
Northern Westchester Hosp Ctr
Allergy Associates of Westchester, 86 Smith Ave;
Mt Kisco, NY 10549; (914) 666-7171; **BDCERT:**
IM 89; A&I 91; **MS:** NY Med Coll 86; **RES:** IM,
Lenox Hill Hosp, New York, NY 86-89; **FEL:** A&I,
Mount Sinai Med Ctr, New York, NY 89-91; **SI:**
Asthma; Hay Fever; **HMO:** Oxford Aetna Hlth Plan
Pomco Empire Prucare +

🌑 📷 🚾 🏛 Ⓢ Mcr   Immediately ■ **VISA** ● ■

Rivenson, Melanie (MD)   A&I
Westchester Med Ctr
105 Stevens Ave 608; Mt Vernon, NY 10550;
(914) 667-5310; **BDCERT:** A&I 79; **MS:** Romania
55; **RES:** Ped, St Luke's Roosevelt Hosp Ctr, New
York, NY 71-72; A&I, St Luke's Roosevelt Hosp Ctr,
New York, NY 72-79; **HOSP:** Mount Vernon Hosp;
SI: *Asthma; Sinusitis;* **HMO:** Blue Cross & Blue Shield
Empire GHI Multiplan Oxford +

♿ Ⓢ 🌑 📷 🚾 🏛 Ⓢ Mcr Mcd   Immediately

ANESTHESIOLOGY

Altman, Jill (MD)   Anes
Sound Shore Med Ctr-Westchester
16 Guion Pl; New Rochelle, NY 10802; (914) 725-
2430; **BDCERT:** Anes 87; **MS:** U Conn Sch Med 81;
RES: Hartford Hosp, Hartford, CT 81-84; **FEL:** ObG,
Hartford Hosp, Hartford, CT 84-85; **HMO:** Oxford
SWCHP US Hlthcre Aetna-US Healthcare Pomco +

Frost, Elizabeth (MD)   Anes
Westchester Med Ctr
9 Heathcote Rd; Scarsdale, NY 10583; (914) 594-
7693; **BDCERT:** Anes 66; **MS:** Scotland 61; **RES:**
IM, Englewood Hosp, Englewood, NJ 63-64; Anes,
NY Hosp-Cornell Med Ctr, New York, NY 64-66;
FAP: Prof NY Med Coll; **SI:** *Anesthesia For
Neurosurgery;* **HMO:** Aetna Hlth Plan Blue Choice
Blue Cross & Blue Shield Oxford Magnacare +
LANG: Sp, Jpn, Kor, Hin, Fr;

O'Leary, John (MD)   Anes
Cabrini Med Ctr
Premium Point, Rd; New Rochelle, NY 10801;
(914) 636-8441; **BDCERT:** Anes 66; **MS:**
Georgetown U 60; **RES:** Anes, Columbia-
Presbyterian Med Ctr, New York, NY 61-62; Anes,
Columbia-Presbyterian Med Ctr, New York, NY 63-
65

📷 🚾 🏛 Mcr Mcd WC NFI

CARDIOLOGY (CARDIOVASCULAR DISEASE)

Becker, Richard (MD)   Cv
Hudson Valley Hosp Ctr
1985 Crompond Rd D; Peekskill, NY 10566; (914)
736-0703; **BDCERT:** IM 82; Cv 87; **MS:** NY Med
Coll 79; **RES:** Lenox Hill Hosp, New York, NY 80-
82; **FEL:** Cv, Westchester County Med Ctr, Valhalla,
NY 82-84; **HOSP:** Westchester Med Ctr; **HMO:** Blue
Choice Blue Cross & Blue Shield CIGNA HealthNet
Independent Health Plan +

LANG: Sp, Itl; ♿ Ⓢ 🌑 📷 🚾 🏛 Ⓢ Mcr Mcd WC NFI
Immediately

Bleiberg, Melvyn (MD)   Cv
St Joseph's Med Ctr-Yonkers
127 S Broadway; Yonkers, NY 10701; (914) 965-
6060; **BDCERT:** IM 78; Cv 81; **MS:** Albert Einstein
Coll Med 74; **RES:** Brookdale Univ Hosp Med Ctr,
Brooklyn, NY 75-77; **FEL:** Cv, Brookdale Univ Hosp
Med Ctr, Brooklyn, NY 77-79; **FAP:** Asst Clin Prof
NY Med Coll

♿ 📷 🚾 🏛 Ⓢ Mcr Mcd WC NFI   A Few Days

Cohen, Martin (MD)   Cv
Westchester Med Ctr
Cardiology Consultants of Westchester, 19 Bradhurst Ave; Hawthorne, NY 10532; (914) 593-7800; **BDCERT:** IM 83; Cv 85; **MS:** SUNY Hlth Sci Ctr 80; **RES:** Univ Hosp SUNY Bklyn, Brooklyn, NY 80-83; **FEL:** Cv, Univ Hosp SUNY Bklyn, Brooklyn, NY 83-85; Westchester County Med Ctr, Valhalla, NY 85-86; **FAP:** Assoc Prof of Clin Med NY Med Coll; **SI:** *Cardiac Catheterization; Cardiac Electrophysiology*; **HMO:** Oxford Aetna Hlth Plan GHI Prucare

⌨ ⬛ ▦ ▦ $ Mcr Mcd WC   A Few Days ▦ **VISA** ⬤ ◨

Cooper, Jerome (MD)   Cv
Sound Shore Med Ctr-Westchester
Westchester Heart Specialists, 150 Lockwood Ave 28; New Rochelle, NY 10801; (914) 633-7870; **BDCERT:** IM 68; Cv 73; **MS:** SUNY Hlth Sci Ctr 61; **RES:** IM, Baltimore City Hosp, Baltimore, MD 61-63; CV, Montefiore Med Ctr, Bronx, NY 63-64; **FEL:** Med, Johns Hopkins Hosp, Baltimore, MD 65-66; Cv, Johns Hopkins Hosp, Baltimore, MD 66-67; **FAP:** Assoc Clin Prof Albert Einstein Coll Med; **HOSP:** Montefiore Med Ctr; **SI:** *Clinical Cardiology; Drug Trials*; **HMO:** PHS Empire Blue Choice United Healthcare Oxford GHI +

⌨ ⬛ ▦ ▦ $ Mcr Mcd NFI   2-4 Weeks **VISA** ⬤

DeLuca, Albert (MD)   Cv
Westchester Med Ctr
Cardiology Consultants of Westchester, 311 North St Ste .403; White Plains, NY 106055; (914) 428-2600; **BDCERT:** Cv 93; IM 89; **MS:** SUNY Downstate 86; **RES:** IM, Mount Sinai Med Ctr, New York, NY 86-87; IM, Mount Sinai Med Ctr, New York, NY 87-89; **FEL:** Cv, Westchester County Med Ctr, Valhalla, NY 89-91; Cv, Westchester County Med Ctr, Valhalla, NY 91-92; **FAP:** Asst Prof Med NY Med Coll; **HOSP:** St Agnes Hosp; **SI:** *Cardiac Diseases*

⌨ ⬛ ▦ ▦ $ Mcr Mcd WC NFI   A Few Days ▦ **VISA** ⬤

Epstein, Stanley (MD)   Cv
Columbia-Presbyterian Med Ctr
Westchester Cardiology Assoc, One Elm St 1B; Tuckahoe, NY 10707; (914) 337-7600; **BDCERT:** IM 67; Cv 75; **MS:** U Hlth Sci/Chicago Med Sch 58; **RES:** IM, Jewish Hosp Med Ctr, Brooklyn, NY 58-60; IM, San Francisco Gen Hosp, San Francisco, CA 60-61; **FEL:** Cv, Montefiore Med Ctr, Bronx, NY 62-67; **FAP:** Clin Prof Med Columbia P&S; **HOSP:** Lawrence Hosp; **SI:** *Stress Testing; Echocardiography*; **HMO:** Oxford Empire Blue Cross & Shield Aetna Hlth Plan Prucare Columbia-Cornell Care +

⌨ ⬛ ▦ Mcr Mcd   A Few Days ▦ **VISA** ⬤ ◨

Fass, Arthur (MD)   Cv
Phelps Mem Hosp Ctr
465 N State Rd; Briarcliff Manor, NY 10510; (914) 762-5810; **BDCERT:** IM 79; Cv 81; **MS:** NY Med Coll 76; **RES:** Metropolitan Hosp Ctr, New York, NY 77-79; **FEL:** Cv, Westchester County Med Ctr, Valhalla, NY 79-81; **FAP:** Asst Clin Prof Med NY Med Coll; **HOSP:** Westchester Med Ctr; **SI:** *Coronary Artery Disease; Mitral Valve Prolapse*; **HMO:** Oxford US Hlthcre Prucare Blue Choice CIGNA +

⌨ ⬛ ▦ $ Mcr WC NFI   2-4 Weeks

Feld, Michael (MD)   Cv
Phelps Mem Hosp Ctr
200 S Broadway E; Tarrytown, NY 10591; (914) 631-2895; **BDCERT:** IM 80; Cv 83; **MS:** Penn State U-Hershey Med Ctr 77; **RES:** Montefiore Med Ctr, Bronx, NY 77-80; IM, Montefiore Med Ctr, Bronx, NY 81; **FEL:** Cv, Montefiore Med Ctr, Bronx, NY; **FAP:** Asst Clin Prof Albert Einstein Coll Med; **HOSP:** Community Hosp At Dobbs Ferry; **SI:** *Pacemaker Therapy*; **HMO:** Oxford PHS CIGNA Independent Health Plan Empire Blue Cross & Shield +

⌨ ⬛ ▦ ▦ $ Mcr   A Few Days **VISA** ⬤ ◨

Feldman, Richard (MD)   Cv
Montefiore Med Ctr
Riverside Cardiology Assoc, 955 Yonkers Ave Ste 200; Yonkers, NY 10704; (914) 237-1332; **BDCERT:** IM 84; Cv 87; **MS:** Tulane U 81; **RES:** Lenox Hill Hosp, New York, NY; **FEL:** Cv, Temple U Hosp, Philadelphia, PA; **FAP:** Asst Prof IM Albert Einstein Coll Med; **SI:** *Catheterizations*; **HMO:** Oxford Blue Cross Aetna Hlth Plan US Hlthcre

⌨ ⬛ ▦ ▦ $ Mcr   A Few Days ▦ **VISA** ⬤

Fishbach, Mitchell (MD)   Cv
Lawrence Hosp

Westchester Cardiology Associates, 1 Elm St; Tuckahoe, NY 10707; (914) 337-7600; **BDCERT:** IM 80; Cv 83; **MS:** Albert Einstein Coll Med 77; **RES:** IM, Montefiore Med Ctr, Bronx, NY 77-78; IM, Montefiore Med Ctr, Bronx, NY 78-80; **FEL:** Cv, Montefiore Med Ctr, Bronx, NY 80-82; **FAP:** Asst Prof Columbia P&S; **HOSP:** Montefiore Med Ctr; **SI:** *Noninvasive Cardiology; Sports Medicine/ Cardiology;* **HMO:** US Hlthcre Blue Choice Oxford NYLCare CIGNA +

♿ 📞 🔒 👤 🏠 $ Mcr Immediately **VISA** 💳

Frishman, William (MD)   Cv
Westchester Med Ctr

Westchester Medical Center Med Rsrch Assoc, Munger Pavillion; Valhalla, NY 10595; (914) 594-4383; **BDCERT:** IM 72; Cv 75; **MS:** Boston U 69; **RES:** Montefiore Med Ctr, Bronx, NY 69-71; Jacobi Med Ctr, Bronx, NY 71-72; **FEL:** Cv, NY Hosp-Cornell Med Ctr, New York, NY 72-74; **FAP:** Chrmn Med NY Med Coll; **SI:** *Cardiac Drugs; Cardiac Disease Prevention;* **HMO:** Blue Choice Pomco GHI

LANG: Sp; ♿ 🔒 👤 🏠 1 Week

Gabelman, Gary (MD)   Cv
Montefiore Med Ctr

1 Elm St 1B; Tuckahoe, NY 10707; (914) 337-7600; **BDCERT:** IM 88; Cv 91; **MS:** Mt Sinai Sch Med 85; **RES:** Montefiore Med Ctr, Bronx, NY 85-89; Montefiore Med Ctr, Bronx, NY 88-89; **FEL:** Cv, Montefiore Med Ctr, Bronx, NY; **HOSP:** Columbia-Presbyterian Med Ctr; **SI:** *Non-Invasive Cardiology;* **HMO:** Aetna Hlth Plan Blue Choice Prucare Metlife Oxford +

♿ 📞 🔒 👤 🏠 $ Mcr Immediately **VISA** 💳

Gitler, Bernard (MD)   Cv
Sound Shore Med Ctr-Westchester

Westchester Heart Specialists, 150 Lockwood Ave 28; New Rochelle, NY 10801; (914) 633-7870; **BDCERT:** IM 79; Cv 81; **MS:** Cornell U 76; **RES:** IM, Jacobi Med Ctr, Bronx, NY 76-79; **FEL:** Cv, Montefiore Med Ctr, Bronx, NY 79-81; **FAP:** Assoc Clin Prof Med Albert Einstein Coll Med; **HOSP:** Montefiore Med Ctr; **SI:** *Non-Invasive and Invasive Cardiology; Sports Cardiology Medicine;* **HMO:** United Healthcare PHS Empire Blue Choice Oxford GHI +

♿ 🔒 👤 🏠 $ Mcr Mcd WC NFl 2-4 Weeks ▦ **VISA** 💳

Golier, Francis (MD)   Cv
Phelps Mem Hosp Ctr

200 S Broadway SteE; Tarrytown, NY 10591; (914) 631-2895; **BDCERT:** IM 72; Cv 78; **MS:** Med Coll Wisc 69; **RES:** IM, Lenox Hill Hosp, New York, NY 69-72; **FEL:** Cv, Montefiore Med Ctr, Bronx, NY 72-74; **FAP:** Asst Prof Albert Einstein Coll Med; **HOSP:** Montefiore Med Ctr; **SI:** *Transesophageal Echo; Stress Echoes;* **HMO:** PHS Oxford Multiplan Magnacare

LANG: Pol; ♿ 🔒 👤 🏠 $ Mcr WC NFl 1 Week **VISA** 💳 ✉

Greif, Richard H (MD)   Cv
St Joseph's Med Ctr-Yonkers

127 S Broadway; Yonkers, NY 10701; (914) 378-7584; **BDCERT:** Cv 81; **MS:** NY Med Coll 75; **RES:** Metropolitan Hosp Ctr, New York, NY 75-78; **FEL:** St Vincents Hosp & Med Ctr NY, New York, NY 79-81; **FAP:** Asst Prof of Clin Med NY Med Coll; **HMO:** Oxford Prucare Aetna-US Healthcare Empire Blue Cross

♿ 🔒 🏠 $ Mcr Mcd WC 2-4 Weeks

Heidenberg, William (MD)　　Cv　**PCP**
White Plains Hosp Ctr

85 Old Mamaroneck Rd; White Plains, NY 10605; (914) 948-2650; **BDCERT:** IM 67; Cv 75; **MS:** Univ Pittsburgh 60; **RES:** Montefiore Med Ctr, Bronx, NY 60-62; VA Med Ctr-Bronx, Bronx, NY 62-63; **FEL:** Cv, Montefiore Med Ctr, Bronx, NY 63-64; Cv, Yale-New Haven Hosp, New Haven, CT 66-67; **FAP:** Asst Clin Prof Columbia P&S; **HOSP:** Columbia-Presbyterian Med Ctr; **SI:** *Echocardiography; Nuclear Cardiology;* **HMO:** PHS Oxford Blue Choice Pomco +

🚻 📷 ♿ 🏧 $ Mcr WC NFI　Immediately

Kay, Richard (MD)　　Cv
Westchester Med Ctr

19 Bradhurst Ave Ste 16; Hawthorne, NY 10532; (914) 593-7800; **BDCERT:** IM 79; **MS:** Johns Hopkins U 76; **RES:** IM, Columbia-Presbyterian Med Ctr, New York, NY 76-79; **FEL:** Cv, Mount Sinai Med Ctr, New York, NY 79-81; **FAP:** Assoc Prof NY Med Coll; **HOSP:** St Agnes Hosp; **SI:** *Preventive Cardiology; Congestive Heart Failure*

🚻 🌙 📷 ♿ 🏧 $ Mcr Mcd WC　Immediately **VISA** 💳

Keltz, Theodore (MD)　　Cv
Montefiore Med Ctr

150 Lockwood Ave 28; New Rochelle, NY 10801; (914) 633-7870; **BDCERT:** IM 83; Cv 85; **MS:** Albany Med Coll 80; **RES:** Mount Sinai Med Ctr, New York, NY 81-83; **FEL:** Cv, Montefiore Med Ctr, Bronx, NY 83-85; **FAP:** Clin Prof Albert Einstein Coll Med; **SI:** *Coronary Disease; Valvular Heart Disease;* **HMO:** PHS Blue Choice United Healthcare Oxford

🚻 📷 ♿ 🏧 $ Mcr WC NFI　Immediately **VISA** 💳

Levine, Evan (MD)　　Cv
Montefiore Med Ctr

Riverside Cardiology, 955 Yonkers Ave Ste 200; Yonkers, NY 10704; (914) 237-1332; **BDCERT:** IM 88; **MS:** Mt Sinai Sch Med 85; **RES:** IM, Montefiore Med Ctr, Bronx, NY 85-88; **FEL:** Cv, Montefiore Med Ctr, Bronx, NY 88-90; **HOSP:** St John's Riverside Hosp; **HMO:** Most

🚻 📷 ♿ 🏧 $ Mcr WC　Immediately 💳 **VISA** 💳 💳

Levy, James (MD)　　Cv
United Hosp Med Ctr

Cardiology Associates, 32 Rye Ridge Plaza; Port Chester, NY 10573; (914) 251-1070; **BDCERT:** IM 66; Cv 73; **MS:** NYU Sch Med 58; **RES:** Bellevue Hosp Ctr, New York, NY 59-60; Westchester County Med Ctr, Valhalla, NY 61-62; **FEL:** Cv, New York University Med Ctr, New York, NY 60-61; **FAP:** Assoc Clin Prof Med NY Med Coll; **HOSP:** Westchester Med Ctr; **HMO:** Independent Health Plan Pomco CIGNA US Hlthcre Oxford +

🚻 💳 📷 ♿ 🏧 $ Mcr Mcd WC NFI　A Few Days

Marano, Anthony (MD)　　Cv　**PCP**
White Plains Hosp Ctr

20 Old Mamaroneck Rd; White Plains, NY 10605; (914) 948-8838; **BDCERT:** IM 67; Cv 77; **MS:** Cornell U 60; **RES:** IM, St Luke's Roosevelt Hosp Ctr, New York, NY 61; **FEL:** Cv, Mount Sinai Med Ctr, New York, NY 63-64; **HOSP:** St Agnes Hosp; **HMO:** Oxford Aetna Hlth Plan PHS Chubb Pomco +

🚻 📷 ♿ 🏧 Mcr　1 Week

Matos, Marshall (MD)　　Cv
Montefiore Med Ctr-Weiler/Einstein Div

140 Lockwood Ave 310; New Rochelle, NY 10801; (914) 576-7171; **BDCERT:** Cv 85; **MS:** Albert Einstein Coll Med 77; **RES:** Bronx Muncipal Hosp Ctr, Bronx, NY 78-81; **FAP:** Asst Prof Med Albert Einstein Coll Med; **HOSP:** Sound Shore Med Ctr-Westchester; **SI:** *Coronary Artery Disease; Heart Rhythm Disorders;* **HMO:** Aetna Hlth Plan Oxford US Hlthcre PHS GHI +

🚻 📷 🏧 $　A Few Days **VISA** 💳

McClung, John A (MD)　　Cv
Westchester Med Ctr

Cardiology Consulting of Westchester PC, 19 Bradhurst Ave; Hawthorne, NY 10532; (914) 593-7800; **BDCERT:** IM 80; Cv 83; **MS:** NY Med Coll 75; **RES:** IM, Lincoln Med & Mental Hlth Ctr, Bronx, NY 75-79; IM, Our Lady of Mercy Med Ctr, Bronx, NY 75-79; **FEL:** Cv, Westchester County Med Ctr, Valhalla, NY 80-82; **FAP:** Assoc Prof Med NY Med Coll; **SI:** *Valvular Heart Disease; Peripheral Vascular Disease;* **HMO:** Aetna-US Healthcare Oxford Prudential Empire Blue Cross & Shield CIGNA +

🚻 📷 ♿ 🏧 $ Mcr WC NFI　A Few Days 💳 **VISA** 💳 💳

Medina, Emma (MD)   Cv
Sound Shore Med Ctr-Westchester

140 Lockwood Ave 310; New Rochelle, NY 10801; (914) 632-1600; **BDCERT:** IM 82; Cv 85; **MS:** NYU Sch Med 79; **RES:** Jacobi Med Ctr, Bronx, NY; **FEL:** Jacobi Med Ctr, Bronx, NY; **FAP:** Asst Clin Prof Albert Einstein Coll Med; **HOSP:** Montefiore Med Ctr-Weiler/Einstein Div; **HMO:** Blue Cross & Blue Shield Oxford Aetna Hlth Plan

[symbols] A Few Days

Mercando, Anthony (MD)   Cv
Lawrence Hosp

1 Elm St 1B; Tuckahoe, NY 10707; (914) 337-7600; **BDCERT:** IM 83; Cv 87; **MS:** Harvard Med Sch 80; **RES:** IM, Montefiore Med Ctr, Bronx, NY 80-84; **FEL:** Cv, Montefiore Med Ctr, Bronx, NY 84-86; **FAP:** Assoc Clin Prof Med Columbia P&S; **HOSP:** Columbia-Presbyterian Med Ctr; **SI:** *Arrhythmias; Cholesterol Abnormalities;* **HMO:** Oxford Empire Aetna Hlth Plan Independent Health Plan +

[symbols] A Few Days *VISA* ⬤ ▣

Mercurio, Peter (MD)   Cv
Northern Westchester Hosp Ctr

1888 Commerce St; Yorktown Heights, NY 10598; (914) 962-4000; **BDCERT:** IM 78; Cv 83; **MS:** NYU Sch Med 75; **RES:** IM, Bellevue Hosp Ctr, New York, NY 75-79; **FEL:** Cv, Bellevue Hosp Ctr, New York, NY 79-81; **HOSP:** Westchester Med Ctr; **SI:** *Echocardiography; Stress Echoes;* **HMO:** Oxford Pomco Aetna-US Healthcare CIGNA

[symbols] 1 Week

Monteferrante, Judith (MD)   Cv
White Plains Hosp Ctr

Primary Care & Cardiovascular Associates, 222 Westchester Ave 405; White Plains, NY 10604; (914) 946-3135; **BDCERT:** IM 81; Cv 85; **MS:** Mt Sinai Sch Med 78; **RES:** IM, St Vincents Hosp & Med Ctr NY, New York, NY 78-81; **FEL:** Cv, Westchester County Med Ctr, Valhalla, NY 81-83; **FAP:** Asst Clin Prof Columbia P&S; **HOSP:** St Agnes Hosp; **SI:** *Nuclear Cardiology; Women's Heart Disease*

[symbols] 1 Week ▦ *VISA* ⬤

Moser, Stuart (MD)   Cv
Montefiore Med Ctr

955 Yonkers Ave; Yonkers, NY 10704; (914) 237-1332; **BDCERT:** Cv 91; IM 88; **MS:** NY Med Coll 85; **RES:** Montefiore Med Ctr, Bronx, NY 85-88; **FEL:** Cv, Montefiore Med Ctr, Bronx, NY 88-90; **HOSP:** St John's Riverside Hosp; **HMO:** US Hlthcre Prucare GHI Aetna Hlth Plan Oxford +

[symbols] Immediately ▦ *VISA* ⬤ ▣

Ozick, Hershel (MD)   Cv
Sound Shore Med Ctr-Westchester

Sound Shore Cardiology PC, 175 Memorial Hwy 11; New Rochelle, NY 10801; (914) 235-3535; **BDCERT:** IM 80; CCM 89; **MS:** NYU Sch Med 77; **RES:** IM, Univ Hosp SUNY Bklyn, Brooklyn, NY 77-80; **FEL:** Cv, New York University, New York, NY 80-81; Cv, Maimonides Med Ctr, Brooklyn, NY 81-83; **FAP:** Asst Clin Prof Med NY Med Coll; **HOSP:** Westchester Med Ctr; **SI:** *Preventive Cardiology; Nutrition;* **HMO:** CIGNA Aetna Hlth Plan Prucare GHI US Hlthcre +

LANG: Sp; [symbols] Immediately

Pucillo, Anthony (MD)   Cv
Westchester Med Ctr

19 Broadhurst Ave; Hawthorne, NY 10532; (914) 593-7800; **BDCERT:** IM 81; Cv 83; **MS:** Mt Sinai Sch Med 78; **RES:** Columbia-Presbyterian Med Ctr, New York, NY 79-80; Columbia-Presbyterian Med Ctr, New York, NY 80-81; **FEL:** Columbia-Presbyterian Med Ctr, New York, NY; Columbia-Presbyterian Med Ctr, New York, NY; **HOSP:** St Agnes Hosp; **SI:** *Cardiology;* **HMO:** Aetna Hlth Plan Blue Choice CIGNA Oxford Prucare +

[symbols] A Few Days

Rubin, David (MD)   Cv
Columbia-Presbyterian Med Ctr

222 Westchester Ave; White Plains, NY 10604; (914) 428-3888; **BDCERT:** Cv 81; CE 92; **MS:** Columbia P&S 75; **RES:** Columbia-Presbyterian Med Ctr, New York, NY 75-78; **FEL:** Cv, Mount Sinai Med Ctr, New York, NY 78-80; **FAP:** Assoc Prof of Clin Med Columbia P&S; **HOSP:** Westchester Med Ctr; **SI:** *Radio Frequency Ablation;* **HMO:** Oxford PHS Prucare Independent Health Plan Aetna-US Healthcare +

[symbols] 1 Week

Stampfer, Morris (MD)   Cv
Sound Shore Med Ctr-Westchester

175 Memorial Hwy 2; New Rochelle, NY 10801; (914) 576-2828; **BDCERT:** IM 70; Cv 75; **MS:** Albert Einstein Coll Med 63; **RES:** IM, Jacobi Med Ctr, Bronx, NY 63-65; **FEL:** Cv, Nat Inst Health, Bethesda, MD 65-68; *SI: Stress Testing; Echocardiography;* **HMO:** Oxford Blue Choice GHI PHS

♿ ■ **S** **Mcr** **NFI**

Tartaglia, Joseph J (MD)   Cv
St Agnes Hosp

311 North St 301; White Plains, NY 10605; (914) 946-3388; **BDCERT:** IM 88; Cv 91; **MS:** Italy 84; **RES:** Path, N Shore Univ Hosp-Plainview, Plainview, NY 84-86; Med, Our Lady of Mercy Med Ctr, Bronx, NY 85-88; **FEL:** Cv, N Shore Univ Hosp-Manhasset, Manhasser, NY 88-90; **FAP:** Assoc Clin Prof; **HOSP:** United Hosp Med Ctr; *SI: Noninvasive Cardiology; Angina Pectoris;* **HMO:** CIGNA Independent Health Plan Oxford Prucare US Hlthcre +

LANG: Itl; ♿ ☎ ■ ♀ 🏥 **S** **Mcr** **Mcd** **WC** **NFI**
A Few Days

Weiss, Melvin (MD)   Cv
Westchester Med Ctr

Cardiology Consultants of Westchester, 19 Bradhurst Ave; Hawthorne, NY 10532; (914) 593-7800; **BDCERT:** IM 72; **MS:** SUNY Hlth Sci Ctr 67; **RES:** Kings County Hosp Ctr, Brooklyn, NY 67-68; NY Hosp-Cornell Med Ctr, New York, NY 70-71; **FEL:** Columbia-Presbyterian Med Ctr, New York, NY 71-72; **FAP:** Prof Med NY Med Coll; *SI: Coronary Artery Disease; Heart Failure;* **HMO:** Most

♿ ☎ ☎ 🏥 **S** **Mcr** **Mcd** **WC** **NFI** A Few Days

Weissman, Ronald (MD)   Cv
White Plains Hosp Ctr

311 North St 403; White Plains, NY 10605; (914) 684-0204; **BDCERT:** IM 80; Cv 83; **MS:** NY Med Coll 77; **RES:** Long Island Jewish Med Ctr, New Hyde Park, NY 77-80; **FEL:** Cv, Long Island Jewish Med Ctr, New Hyde Park, NY 80-82; **FAP:** Asst Clin Prof Med NY Med Coll; **HOSP:** St Agnes Hosp; *SI: Heart Failure; Coronary Artery Disease;* **HMO:** Oxford SWCHP PHS CIGNA Pomco +

LANG: Prt; ♿ ☎ ♀ 🏥 **S** **Mcr** **WC** **NFI** A Few Days

Zevon, Sanford (MD)   Cv
White Plains Hosp Ctr

33 Davis Ave; White Plains, NY 10605; (914) 948-3630; **BDCERT:** IM 65; Cv 74; **MS:** SUNY Syracuse 58; **RES:** Jewish Hosp of Bklyn, Brooklyn, NY 59-60; Mt Zion Hosp, San Francisco, CA 60-61; **FEL:** Cv, Montefiore Med Ctr, Bronx, NY

Zimmerman, Franklin (MD)   Cv
Phelps Mem Hosp Ctr

465 N State Rd; Briarcliff Manor, NY 10510; (914) 762-5810; **BDCERT:** IM 83; Cv 87; **MS:** Brown U 80; **RES:** St Luke's Roosevelt Hosp Ctr, New York, NY 80-83; **FEL:** Cv, St Luke's Roosevelt Hosp Ctr, New York, NY 84-88; **FAP:** Asst Clin Prof Columbia P&S; **HOSP:** Westchester Med Ctr; *SI: Preventive Cardiology;* **HMO:** Oxford US Hlthcre Empire PHS Prucare +

♿ ☎ ♀ 🏥 **S** **Mcr** **WC** **NFI** 1 Week

CHILD & ADOLESCENT PSYCHIATRY

Cohen, Lee (MD)   ChAP
Columbia-Presbyterian Med Ctr

623 Warburton Ave; Hastings On Hudson, NY 10706; (914) 478-1330; **BDCERT:** Psyc 87; ChAP 88; **MS:** SUNY Stony Brook 82; **RES:** Ped, Mount Sinai Med Ctr, New York, NY 82-83; Psyc, Mount Sinai Med Ctr, New York, NY 83-85; **FEL:** ChAP, Columbia-Presbyterian Med Ctr, New York, NY 83-87; **FAP:** Asst Prof of Clin Psyc Columbia P&S; *SI: Psychopharmacology; Depression*

☎ ☎ ♀ 🏥 **S** 2-4 Weeks

Greenhill, Laurence (MD)   ChAP
Columbia-Presbyterian Med Ctr

9 Country Rd; Mamaroneck, NY 10343; (914) 381-2436; **BDCERT:** Psyc 76; **MS:** Albert Einstein Coll Med 67; **RES:** Psyc, Bronx Muncipal Hosp Ctr, Bronx, NY 68-71; Psyc, Bronx Muncipal Hosp Ctr, Bronx, NY 72-74; **FAP:** Assoc Prof Columbia P&S; **HOSP:** Columbia-Presbyterian Med Ctr; *SI: Attention Deficit Disorders; Adolescent Depression*

SA/SD ☎ ☎ ♀ **S** 4+ Weeks

Guide to symbols and abbreviations can be found on pages 110-113.

763

Hyler, Irene (MD)　　　ChAP
NY Hosp-Cornell-Westchester

2A Berkeley Rd; Scarsdale, NY 10583; (914) 472-8447; **BDCERT:** Psyc 84; ChAP 86; **MS:** Albert Einstein Coll Med 79; **RES:** Psyc, Albert Einstein Med Ctr, Bronx, NY 79-82; **FEL:** ChAP, Albert Einstein Med Ctr, Bronx, NY 82-84; **FAP:** Asst Clin Prof ChAP Cornell U; **SI:** *Psychotherapy; Psychoanalysis;* **HMO:** Oxford PHS Empire CIGNA +

🦽 📷 🔳 🏥 💲 Mcr NFi　1 Week

Kernberg, Paulina (MD)　　ChAP
NY Hosp-Cornell Med Ctr

21 Bloomingdale Rd; White Plains, NY 10605; (914) 997-5951; **BDCERT:** ChAP 71; **MS:** Chile 59; **RES:** Psyc, Menninger Clinic, Topeka, KS 63-65; **FAP:** Dir ChAP Cornell U

LANG: Sp, Ger, Fr; 🦽 🈂 🔳 📷 💲　1 Week

Rubinstein, Boris (MD)　　ChAP
Columbia-Presbyterian Med Ctr

623 Warburton Ave; Hastings On Hudson, NY 10706; (914) 478-1330; **BDCERT:** ChAP 81; Psyc 79; **MS:** Mexico 70; **RES:** Ped, Children's Hosp, Boston, MA 71-74; Psyc, Albert Einstein Med Ctr, Bronx, NY 74-76; **FEL:** ChAP, Albert Einstein Med Ctr, Bronx, NY 76-78; **FAP:** Asst Clin Prof Columbia P&S; **SI:** *Psychopharmacology*

LANG: Sp, Heb; 🔳 📷 🔳 🏥 💲　2-4 Weeks

Seaver, Robert (MD)　　　ChAP
Blythedale Children's Hosp

39 Smith Ave; Mt Kisco, NY 10549; (914) 241-8979; **BDCERT:** Psyc 84; ChAP 86; **MS:** Mt Sinai Sch Med 73; **RES:** Ped, Mount Sinai Med Ctr, New York, NY 73-75; Psyc, NY Hosp-Cornell-Westchester, White Plains, NY; **FEL:** Ambulatory Ped, St Luke's Roosevelt Hosp Ctr, New York, NY 75-76; ChAP, Jacobi Med Ctr, Bronx, NY 84-85; **HMO:** None

🔳 📷 🔳 🏥 💲　2-4 Weeks

Slater, Jonathan (MD)　　ChAP
Columbia-Presbyterian Med Ctr

1 Bridge St Ste 24; Irvington, NY 10533; (914) 591-4040; **BDCERT:** Psyc 91; ChAP 93; **MS:** Columbia P&S 85; **RES:** Psyc, Columbia-Presbyterian Med Ctr, New York, NY 87-90; **FEL:** Columbia-Presbyterian Med Ctr, New York, NY 90-92; NYS Psychiatric Institute, New York, NY 85-86; **FAP:** Asst Clin Prof Columbia P&S; **SI:** *Psychopharmacology; Medical Illness*

🔳 📷 🏥 💲 Mcr　A Few Days

CHILD NEUROLOGY

Jacobson, Ronald (MD)　　ChiN
Westchester Med Ctr

125 S Broadway; White Plains, NY 10605; (914) 997-1692; **BDCERT:** N 84; **MS:** Albert Einstein Coll Med 75; **RES:** Yale-New Haven Hosp, New Haven, CT 75-79; **FEL:** U MN Med Ctr, Minneapolis, MN 79-82; **HOSP:** White Plains Hosp Ctr; **HMO:** Oxford Well Care

🦽 🈂 🔳 📷 📷 🏥 💲 Mcd　1 Week

Kutscher, Martin (MD)　　ChiN
Westchester Med Ctr

Pediatric Neurological Associates, 125 S Broadway; White Plains, NY 10605; (914) 997-1692; **BDCERT:** N 88; Ped 85; **MS:** Columbia P&S 81; **RES:** Ped, St Christopher's Hosp for Children, Philadelphia, PA 82; N, Albert Einstein Med Ctr, Bronx, NY 84; **FEL:** ChiN, Albert Einstein Med Ctr, Bronx, NY 87; **HOSP:** White Plains Hosp Ctr; **SI:** *Seizures; Attention Deficit Disorder;* **HMO:** Aetna-US Healthcare Well Care Oxford Child Health Plus Kaiser Permanente +

🦽 📷 🏥 💲　Immediately

COLON & RECTAL SURGERY

Burg, Richard (MD)   CRS
White Plains Hosp Ctr
12 Greenridge Ave 201; White Plains, NY 10605; (914) 949-0760; **BDCERT:** CRS 77; S 71; **MS:** Tulane U 65; **RES:** S, U WI Sch Med, Milwaukee, WI 65-70; **FEL:** CRS, St Vincents Hosp & Med Ctr NY, New York, NY 76-77; **HOSP:** Sound Shore Med Ctr-Westchester; **HMO:** Aetna Hlth Plan Blue Cross & Blue Shield HealthNet PHS Oxford +

🆘 💳 🔒 👪 🏥 Mcr   Immediately

Cohen, Martin (MD)   CRS
Northern Westchester Hosp Ctr
666 Lexington Ave Ste 101; Mt Kisco, NY 10549; (914) 666-2778; **BDCERT:** CRS 86; **MS:** Hahnemann U 79; **RES:** S, Long Island Jewish Med Ctr, New Hyde Park, NY 80; **HOSP:** Hudson Valley Hosp Ctr; **HMO:** Oxford Pomco SWCHP Empire

🔒 🏥 👪 📅 💲 WC **VISA** 💳

Krakovitz, Evan (MD)   CRS
Hudson Valley Hosp Ctr
1985 Crompond Rd; Peekskill, NY 10566; (914) 736-0050; **BDCERT:** S 95; CRS 97; **MS:** Hahnemann U 89; **RES:** S, Hosp of U Penn, Philadelphia, PA 89-94; **FEL:** CRS, RWJ Univ Hosp-New Brunswick, New Brunswick, NJ 94-95; *SI: Colon Cancer; Hemorrhoid Treatment;* **HMO:** Oxford Prucare PHS US Hlthcre Empire Blue Cross & Shield +

🔒 🏥 👪 📅 💲 Mcr Mcd WC NFI   A Few Days 💳 **VISA** 💳 💳

DERMATOLOGY

Bank, David (MD)   D
Columbia-Presbyterian Med Ctr
The Center of Dermatology, Cosmetic and Laser Sugery, 359 E Main St 4G/E; Mt Kisco, NY 10549; (914) 241-3003; **BDCERT:** D 89; **MS:** Columbia P&S 85; **RES:** IM, Montefiore Med Ctr, Bronx, NY 85-86; D, Columbia-Presbyterian Med Ctr, New York, NY 86-89; **FAP:** Columbia P&S; **HOSP:** Northern Westchester Hosp Ctr; *SI: Liposuction; Laser Surgery;* **HMO:** Oxford SWCHP Pomco First Health

🔒 🆘 💳 🔒 👪 🏥 💲 Mcr   A Few Days 💳 **VISA** 💳 💳

Berkowitz, Rhonda (MD)   D
Phelps Mem Hosp Ctr
124 S Highland Ave; Ossining, NY 10562; (914) 941-5769; **BDCERT:** D 86; **MS:** NYU Sch Med 82; **RES:** N Shore Univ Hosp-Manhasset, Manhasset, NY 82-83; Columbia-Presbyterian Med Ctr, New York, NY 83-86

💳 🔒 👪 🏥 Mcr   Immediately **VISA** 💳

Bronin, Andrew (MD)   D
United Hosp Med Ctr
4 Rye Ridge Plaza; Port Chester, NY 10573; (914) 253-8080; **BDCERT:** D 81; **MS:** NY Med Coll 75; **RES:** NY Hosp-Cornell Med Ctr, New York, NY 76-79; **FAP:** Assoc Clin Prof Yale U Sch Med; **HOSP:** Greenwich Hosp; *SI: Malignant Melanoma; Pediatric Dermatology;* **HMO:** None

🔒 💳 🔒 👪 🏥 💲   Immediately 💳 **VISA** 💳

Di Pietro, Joseph (MD)   D
Sound Shore Med Ctr-Westchester
12 Studio Arcade; Bronxville, NY 10708; (914) 779-6666; **MS:** Loyola U-Stritch Sch Med, Maywood 73; **RES:** D, NY Hosp-Cornell Med Ctr, New York, NY 75-78; **HOSP:** Lawrence Hosp; *SI: Skin Cancer Treatment; Pediatric Dermatology;* **HMO:** GHI Pomco Oxford US Hlthcre Empire +

LANG: Itl, Sp, Prt; 🔒 🆘 🔒 👪 🏥 💲 Mcr
Immediately

Eisenstat, Barrett (MD)   D
Westchester Med Ctr

Pleasantville Dermatology Assoc, 427 Bedford Rd Ste 310; Pleasantville, NY 10570; (914) 769-3253; **BDCERT:** D 80; **MS:** NYU Sch Med 75; **RES:** IM, Lenox Hill Hosp, New York, NY 75-76; Path, New York University Med Ctr, New York, NY 76-77; **FEL:** D, New York University Med Ctr, New York, NY 77-80; **FAP:** Asst Clin Prof NY Med Coll; **HMO:** Blue Choice PPO GHI Metlife Pomco

♿ 🆂 🄲 🔒 🔧 🛏 🅂 ᴹᶜ A Few Days

Eisert, Jack (MD)   D
Phelps Mem Hosp Ctr

Dermatology Group of Westchester, 200 S Broadway; Tarrytown, NY 10591; (914) 631-4666; **BDCERT:** D 61; **MS:** SUNY Hlth Sci Ctr 56; **RES:** D, Columbia-Presbyterian Med Ctr, New York, NY 57-60; **HOSP:** Columbia-Presbyterian Med Ctr; **HMO:** Prucare Oxford Aetna Hlth Plan CIGNA

LANG: Sp; ♿ 🆂 🄲 🔒 🔧 🛏 🅂 ᴹᶜ ᵂᶜ Immediately *VISA* ●

Felsenstein, Jerome M (MD)   D
Phelps Mem Hosp Ctr

100 S Highland Ave; Ossining, NY 10562; (914) 941-5770; **BDCERT:** D 76; **MS:** NYU Sch Med 71; **RES:** D, Kings County Hosp Ctr, Brooklyn, NY 72-75; **HOSP:** New York University Med Ctr; **HMO:** Oxford Blue Choice PHS GHI

♿ 🆂 🄲 🔒 🔧 🛏 🅂 ᴹᶜ Immediately

Goldberg, Neil (MD)   D
Westchester Med Ctr

222 Westchester Ave; White Plains, NY 10604; (914) 761-8140; **BDCERT:** D 86; **MS:** Northwestern U 82; **RES:** Lenox Hill Hosp, New York, NY 82-83; D, Northwestern U, Chicago, IL 83-86; **HOSP:** Lawrence Hosp; **HMO:** GHI Oxford CIGNA US Hlthcre

♿ 🆂 🄲 🔒 🔧 🛏 🅂 ᴹᶜ Immediately ▨ *VISA* ●

Grossman, Marc (MD)   D
Columbia-Presbyterian Med Ctr

12 Greenridge Ave; White Plains, NY 10605; (914) 946-1101; **BDCERT:** D 77; IM 77; **MS:** Univ Penn 74; **RES:** IM, Hosp of U Penn, Philadelphia, PA 74-76; **FEL:** D, Columbia-Presbyterian Med Ctr, New York, NY 76-79; **FAP:** Clin Prof D; **HOSP:** White Plains Hosp Ctr; **SI:** *Psoriasis; Infection*

LANG: Sp; ♿ 🄲 🔒 🔧 🛏 Immediately

Halperin, Alan (MD)   D
Montefiore Med Ctr-Weiler/Einstein Div

91 Weyman Ave; New Rochelle, NY 10805; (914) 636-0136; **BDCERT:** D 75; **MS:** NYU Sch Med 70; **RES:** D, Albert Einstein Med Ctr, Bronx, NY 71-73; **FAP:** Assoc Clin Prof Med Albert Einstein Coll Med; **HOSP:** Montefiore Med Ctr

Kaplan, Sherri (MD)   D
Community Hosp At Dobbs Ferry

547 Saw Mill River Rd 2B; Ardsley, NY 10502; (914) 693-7191; **BDCERT:** D 87; **MS:** NY Med Coll 83; **RES:** IM, Lenox Hill Hosp, New York, NY 83-84; D, NY Med Coll, New York, NY 84-87; **FAP:** Asst Clin Prof D NY Med Coll; **HOSP:** Sound Shore Med Ctr-Westchester; **SI:** *Pediatric Dermatology*; **HMO:** Most

LANG: Sp; ♿ 🆂 🄲 🔒 🔧 🛏 ᴹᶜ

Klar, Tobi (MD)   D
Sound Shore Med Ctr-Westchester

150 Lockwood Ave 20; New Rochelle, NY 10801; (914) 636-2039; **BDCERT:** D 89; **MS:** SUNY Hlth Sci Ctr 81; **RES:** Univ Hosp SUNY Bklyn, Brooklyn, NY 81-86; **HOSP:** Montefiore Med Ctr-Weiler/Einstein Div; **HMO:** Oxford PHS Blue Choice Magnacare

♿ 🄲 🔒 🛏 🅂 ᴹᶜ ᴹᵈ Immediately

Guide to symbols and abbreviations can be found on pages 110-113.

Klein, Lester (MD)   **D**
St John's Riverside Hosp

Westchester Dermatology, PC, 984 N Broadway 315; Yonkers, NY 10701; (914) 963-0010; **BDCERT:** D 55; **MS:** U Hlth Sci/Chicago Med Sch 48; **RES:** D, NY Polyclinic Hosp, New York, NY 49-52; **HOSP:** St Joseph's Med Ctr-Yonkers; *SI: Skin Cancer; Psoriasis;* **HMO:** Blue Shield GHI Oxford US Hlthcre

LANG: Itl, Sp; 🚻 🆘 🔒 👪 🏨 💲 Mcr WC NFI A Few Days ▨ *VISA* ⬤

Lerman, Jay (MD)   **D**
St Agnes Hosp

280 Dobbs Ferry Rd 205; White Plains, NY 10607; (914) 949-9196; **BDCERT:** D 74; **MS:** SUNY Downstate 69; **RES:** D, Jacobi Med Ctr, Bronx, NY 70-73; **FAP:** Asst Clin Prof Albert Einstein Coll Med; **HOSP:** White Plains Hosp Ctr; *SI: Acne; Eczema;* **HMO:** Aetna Hlth Plan Oxford Empire Blue Choice

🚻 🌙 🔒 👪 🏨 💲 Mcr A Few Days

Levy, Ross (MD)   **D**
Montefiore Med Ctr

90 S Bedford Rd; Mt Kisco, NY 10549; (914) 242-1355; **BDCERT:** D 81; **MS:** Albert Einstein Med Sch 76; **RES:** IM, Montefiore Med Ctr, Bronx, NY 76-78; **FEL:** D, Albert Einstein Med Ctr, Bronx, NY 78-81; **FAP:** Assoc Clin Prof Med Albert Einstein Coll Med; **HOSP:** Northern Westchester Hosp Ctr; *SI: Laser Surgery; Skin Cancer Surgery;* **HMO:** Oxford Aetna Hlth Plan Physician's Health Plan Independent Health Plan

LANG: Sp; 🚻 🌙 🔒 👪 🏨 💲 Mcr WC NFI A Few Days ▨ *VISA* ⬤

Lukash, Barbara (MD)   **D**
St Joseph's Med Ctr-Yonkers

824 Bronx River Rd 1A; Yonkers, NY 10708; (914) 237-2400; **BDCERT:** D 80; **MS:** Tulane U 76; **RES:** D, U Chicago Hosp, Chicago, IL 77-80; **HOSP:** Columbia-Presbyterian Med Ctr; *SI: Skin Cancer;* **HMO:** Oxford Aetna-US Healthcare Prudential GHI Pomco +

🌙 👪 💲 Mcr 1 Week *VISA*

Mackler, Karen (MD)   **D**
Sound Shore Med Ctr-Westchester

150 Lockwood Ave 34; New Rochelle, NY 10801; (914) 576-7070; **BDCERT:** D 83; Ped 78; **MS:** NYU Sch Med 73; **RES:** Ped, NY Hosp-Cornell Med Ctr, New York, NY 73-76; D, Montefiore Med Ctr, Bronx, NY 80-83; **FAP:** Asst Prof D Albert Einstein Coll Med; *SI: Pediatric Dermatology;* **HMO:** Oxford United Healthcare Aetna Hlth Plan GHI Pomco +

🚻 🆘 🔒 👪 🏨 💲 Mcr A Few Days

Mattison, Timothy (MD)   **D**
Northern Westchester Hosp Ctr

90 S Bedford Rd; Mt Kisco, NY 10549; (914) 241-1050; **BDCERT:** D 80; **MS:** Dartmouth Med Sch 76; **RES:** D, New York University Med Ctr, New York, NY 77-80; **HMO:** Oxford Aetna Hlth Plan PHS

🚻 💲 Mcr Mcd Immediately *VISA* ⬤

Narins, Rhoda (MD)   **D**
White Plains Hosp Ctr

Derm Surgery and Laser Ctr2nd ofc on Park Av,NYC, 222 Westchester Ave 300; White Plains, NY 10604; (914) 684-1000; **BDCERT:** D 70; **MS:** NYU Sch Med 65; **RES:** D, New York University Med Ctr, New York, NY 66-69; **HOSP:** Bellevue Hosp Ctr; *SI: Liposuction; Laser-Resurfacing;* **HMO:** None

🚻 🌙 👪 🏨 2-4 Weeks *VISA* ⬤

Rosenthal, Elizabeth (MD)   **D**
United Hosp Med Ctr

1600 Harrison Ave 303; Mamaroneck, NY 10543; (914) 698-2190; **BDCERT:** D 75; **MS:** NYU Sch Med 67; **RES:** Henry Ford Hosp, Detroit, MI 68-69; St Luke's Roosevelt Hosp Ctr, New York, NY 69-70; **FAP:** Asst Clin Prof Albert Einstein Coll Med; *SI: Acne; Pediatric Dermatology;* **HMO:** Oxford CIGNA Empire Aetna-US Healthcare PHS +

LANG: Fr; 🚻 🆘 🌙 🔒 👪 🏨 💲 Mcr WC A Few Days ▨ *VISA* ⬤ 🎴

Safai, Bijan (MD)　　　　**D**
Westchester Med Ctr

Vosburgh Pavillion, New York Medical College;
Valhalla, NY 10595; (914) 594-4566; **BDCERT:** D
74; **MS:** Iran 65; **RES:** Med, VA Med Ctr-Manh,
New York, NY; D, New York University Med Ctr,
New York, NY; **FEL:** Immunology, Mem Sloan
Kettering Cancer Ctr, New York, NY; **FAP:** Prof NY
Med Coll; **HOSP:** Our Lady of Mercy Med Ctr; **HMO:**
Blue Choice Aetna Hlth Plan Pomco

♿ 🅂🄰 📞 🔒 📋 🏥 💲 Mcr ▦ **VISA** 💳

Schliftman, Alan (MD)　　　　**D**
White Plains Hosp Ctr

222 Westchester Ave; White Plains, NY 10604;
(914) 761-1400; **BDCERT:** D 81; **MS:** Geo Wash U
Sch Med 77; **RES:** D, Albert Einstein Med Ctr,
Bronx, NY 78-80; **HOSP:** St Agnes Hosp; **SI:** *Laser
Surgery; Diseases of Skin, Nail, Hair;* **HMO:** Oxford
Aetna Hlth Plan GHI PHS US Hlthcre +

♿ 🅂🄰 📞 🔒 📋 🏥 💲 Mcr Immediately ▦ **VISA**
💳

Soriano, Dale (MD)　　　　**D**
Sound Shore Med Ctr-Westchester

Abadir Associates, 90 S Ridge St LL3; Rye Brook,
NY 10573; (914) 937-5500; **BDCERT:** D 74; **MS:**
Australia 67; **RES:** D, Bellevue Hosp Ctr, New York,
NY; **FEL:** PlS, England/Australia; **SI:** *Cosmetic
Surgery and Dermatology; Skin Cancer;* **HMO:** Oxford
Blue Choice PHS Magnacare PHCS +

LANG: Fr; ♿ 📞 🔒 📋 🏥 💲 Mcr A Few Days **VISA**
💳

Stillman, Michael (MD)　　　　**D**
Northern Westchester Hosp Ctr

39 Smith Ave; Mt Kisco, NY 10549; (914) 241-
3330; **BDCERT:** D 73; **MS:** SUNY Hlth Sci Ctr 67;
RES: D, New York University Med Ctr, New York,
NY 70-73; **SI:** *Skin Cancer-Moles-Melanoma; Acne-
Warts-Eczema;* **HMO:** Aetna-US Healthcare Oxford
Pomco PHS CIGNA +

♿ 🔒 📋 🏥 Mcr Immediately

Sturza, Jeffrey (MD)　　　　**D**
Phelps Mem Hosp Ctr

200 S Broadway; Tarrytown, NY 10591; (914)
631-4666; **BDCERT:** D 88; **MS:** SUNY Hlth Sci Ctr
84; **RES:** D, Cook Cty Hosp, Chicago, IL 85-88;
HOSP: Community Hosp At Dobbs Ferry; **SI:**
Psoriasis Phototherapy; Laser Surgery; **HMO:** Oxford
US Hlthcre United Healthcare GHI

♿ 🅂🄰 📞 🔒 📋 🏥 💲 Mcr A Few Days **VISA** 💳

Treiber, Ruth Kaplan (MD)　　**D**
United Hosp Med Ctr

175 Purchase St; Rye, NY 10580; (914) 967-
2153; **BDCERT:** D 83; **MS:** Cornell U 78; **RES:** IM,
NY Hosp-Cornell Med Ctr, New York, NY 78-80; D,
Columbia-Presbyterian Med Ctr, New York, NY 80-
83; **FAP:** Assoc Clin Prof D Columbia P&S; **HOSP:**
Columbia-Presbyterian Med Ctr; **SI:** *Acne; Botox
Laser Skin Cancer Rx;* **HMO:** Oxford

LANG: Sp; 🔒 📋 🏥 💲 2-4 Weeks **VISA** 💳

Zweibel, Stuart M (MD)　　　　**D**
Northern Westchester Hosp Ctr

83 S Bedford Rd; Mt Kisco, NY 10549; (914) 242-
2020; **BDCERT:** D 89; **MS:** Mt Sinai Sch Med 85;
RES: D, Rhode Island Hosp, Providence, RI 86-89;
FEL: Mohs S, U of WI Hosp, Madison, WI 90-91;
FAP: Asst Clin Prof NYU Sch Med; **HOSP:** New York
University Med Ctr; **SI:** *Mohs Micrographic Surgery;
Laser Surgery;* **HMO:** Oxford Aetna-US Healthcare
United Healthcare Prucare GHI +

LANG: Fr; ♿ 🅂🄰 📞 🔒 📋 🏥 💲 Mcr **VISA** 💳

DIAGNOSTIC RADIOLOGY

Berliner, Stewart R (MD)　　　**DR**
Our Lady of Mercy Med Ctr

Bronx- Westchester Radiology, PC, 14 Stratford Rd;
New Rochelle, NY 10804; (718) 920-9188;
BDCERT: DR 93; NR 96; **MS:** NY Med Coll 88; **RES:**
DR, Univ Hosp SUNY Bklyn, Brooklyn, NY 89-93;
FEL: NR, Thomas Jefferson U Hosp, Philadelphia,
PA 93-94; ChiN, Children's Hosp of Philadelphia,
Philadelphia, PA 94-95; **SI:** *Neurology*

♿ 🅂🄰 📞 🔒 🏥 💲 Mcr Mcd WC NFl Immediately **VISA**
💳

Freeman, Susan (MD)   **DR**
Westchester Med Ctr
University Imaging Medical Associates,
Westchester Med Center, Macy Pavilion; Valhalla,
NY 10595; (914) 493-7552; **BDCERT:** Rad 83;
NuM 84; **MS:** NY Med Coll 79; **RES:** IM,
Maimonides Med Ctr, Brooklyn, NY 79-80; DR,
Mount Sinai Med Ctr, New York, NY 80-81; **FEL:**
NuM, Westchester County Med Ctr, Valhalla, NY
83-84; **FAP:** Asst Prof NY Med Coll; **SI:** *Pediatric
Urology; Thyroid Cancer;* **HMO:** Oxford Well Care
Pomco US Hlthcre Independent Health Plan +

LANG: Fr, Sp; 🚻 🔄 🛏 Mcr Mcd WC NFI Immediately
▨ **VISA** 💳 💳

Miller, Karen (MD)   **DR**
Phelps Mem Hosp Ctr
Phelps Radiology, PC Phelps Memorial Hosp, 701 N
Broadway; Sleepy Hollow, NY 10591; (914) 366-
3450; **BDCERT:** DR 90; **MS:** NY Med Coll 81; **RES:**
DR, NY Med Coll, Valhalla, NY 86-90; **FEL:** Cross
Sectional Imaging, NY Med Coll, Valhalla, NY 90-
91; **SI:** *Cross Section Imaging*

LANG: Sp, Fr, Ar, Prt, Itl; 🚻 🔄 🛏 🅂 Mcr Mcd WC
NFI A Few Days

Swirsky, Michael (MD)   **DR**
Westchester Med Ctr
University Imaging & Medical Assoc PC/NY Med
College, Westchester Med Center; Valhalla, NY
10595; (914) 493-8759; **BDCERT:** DR 79; **MS:**
Case West Res U 75; **RES:** DR, Strong Mem Hosp,
Rochester, NY 75-79; **FAP:** Assoc Clin Prof Rad NY
Med Coll; **SI:** *Digestive & Urinary Problems; Breast
Imaging;* **HMO:** Pomco Oxford CIGNA Well Care

LANG: Sp, Rus; 🚻 🔄 🛏 Mcr Mcd WC NFI Immediately
VISA 💳 💳

EMERGENCY
MEDICINE

Kyi, Michael (MD)   **EM**
Phelps Mem Hosp Ctr
701 N Broadway; Tarrytown, NY 10591; (914)
366-3590; **BDCERT:** EM 91; **MS:** Burma 73; **RES:**
Mount Vernon Hosp, Mt Vernon, NY 80-81; St
Francis Hosp, Jersey City, NJ 81-83; **HOSP:**
Northern Westchester Hosp Ctr; **HMO:** Most
🚻 🄲 🔄 🛏 🛏 Mcr Mcd WC NFI Immediately

Nigro, Emil (MD)   **EM**
Phelps Mem Hosp Ctr
Raymond Rd; N Salem, NY 10560; (914) 366-
3598; **BDCERT:** EM 84; **MS:** Mexico 75; **RES:**
Westchester County Med Ctr, Valhalla, NY 76-79
🚻 🄢 🄲 🔄 🛏 🛏 Mcr Mcd WC NFI

ENDOCRINOLOGY,
DIABETES &
METABOLISM

Albin, Joan (MD)   **EDM**
Sound Shore Med Ctr-Westchester
140 Lockwood Ave 212; New Rochelle, NY 10801;
(914) 235-8503; **BDCERT:** EDM 72; **MS:** NY Med
Coll 67; **RES:** Montefiore Med Ctr, Bronx, NY 69-
70; **FEL:** EDM, Mount Sinai Med Ctr, New York, NY
70-72; **FAP:** Assoc Clin Prof Med Albert Einstein
Coll Med; **HOSP:** Montefiore Med Ctr; **SI:** *Diabetes;
Thyroid Disease;* **HMO:** Blue Cross & Blue Shield
Oxford Pomco
🚻 🄲 🔄 🛏 🛏 🅂 WC 1 Week

Becker, Carolyn (MD)   **EDM**
Northern Westchester Hosp Ctr
Mt Kisco Medical Group, 90 S Bedford Rd; Mt Kisco,
NY 10549; (914) 241-1050; **BDCERT:** IM 85; EDM
89; **MS:** Howard U 82; **RES:** IM, Michael Reese
Hosp Med Ctr, Chicago, IL 83-85; **FEL:** EDM, Mass
Gen Hosp, Boston, MA 85-86; **SI:** *Osteoporosis;
Thyroid Disease;* **HMO:** Oxford Aetna Hlth Plan PHS
Prucare +
🚻 🛏 🅂 Mcr 4+ Weeks

Bloomgarden, David (MD) EDM
White Plains Hosp Ctr
Endocrinology & Diabetes Associates, 222
Westchester Ave 306; White Plains, NY 10604;
(914) 684-0202; **BDCERT:** IM 80; EDM 83; **MS:**
NYU Sch Med 77; **RES:** Jacobi Medical Center,
Bronx, NY 77-80; **FEL:** EDM, Albert Einstein Med
Ctr, Bronx, NY 80-82; *SI: Diabetes; Osteoporosis;*
HMO: Oxford PHS Independent Health Plan Pomco
SWCHP +

♿ 🅲 🗂 🎏 🛏 🅂 Mcr 1 Week ▒ *VISA* 💳

Blum, David (MD)   EDM   PCP
Sound Shore Med Ctr-Westchester
175 Memorial Hwy 17; New Rochelle, NY 10801;
(914) 633-8680; **BDCERT:** IM 77; **MS:**
Northwestern U 74; **RES:** Mount Sinai Med Ctr,
New York, NY 74-77; **FEL:** Mount Sinai Med Ctr,
New York, NY 77-79

♿ SA/SU 🅲 🗂 🎏 🛏 🅂 Immediately *VISA* 💳

Eufemio, Michael (MD)   EDM
Sound Shore Med Ctr-Westchester
140 Lockwood Ave 308; New Rochelle, NY 10801;
(914) 636-5700; **BDCERT:** IM 68; EDM 72; **MS:**
Geo Wash U Sch Med 60; **RES:** IM, DC Gen Hosp,
Washington, DC 61-62; IM, VA Med Ctr-Bronx,
Bronx, NY 64-66; **FEL:** EDM, VA Med Ctr-Bronx,
Bronx, NY 66-67; **FAP:** Assoc Clin Prof Med NY
Med Coll; **HOSP:** Calvary Hosp; *SI: Osteoporosis;*
Thyroid; **HMO:** Oxford PHS Empire Blue Cross &
Shield Pomco Aetna Hlth Plan +

LANG: Itl; ♿ 🅲 🗂 🛏 Mcr 1 Week

Hellerman, James (MD)   EDM
Phelps Mem Hosp Ctr
200 S Broadway 100; Tarrytown, NY 10591;
(914) 631-9300; **BDCERT:** EDM 79; **MS:** U
Rochester 76; **RES:** IM, Montefiore Med Ctr, Bronx,
NY 80; **FEL:** EDM, Mass Gen Hosp, Boston, MA 84;
HOSP: Hudson Valley Hosp Ctr

♿ SA/SU 🅲 🛏 🅂 Mcr Immediately

Kantor, Alan (MD)   EDM   PCP
Northern Westchester Hosp Ctr
1940 Commerce St; Yorktown Heights, NY 10598;
(914) 245-1111; **BDCERT:** IM 81; EDM 83; **MS:**
South Africa 75; **RES:** Groote Schuur Hosp, Cape
Town, South Africa 76-77; Long Island Jewish Med
Ctr, New Hyde Park, NY 79-81; **FEL:** Mem Sloan
Kettering Cancer Ctr, New York, NY 81-83; *SI:*
Thyroid/Endocrine Tumors; Insulin Pumps,
Osteoporosis; **HMO:** Oxford Pomco WHSN Blue
Cross & Blue Shield

♿ 🗂 🎏 🛏 🅂 Mcr WC NFI A Few Days

Kleinbaum, Jerry (MD)   EDM   PCP
Hudson Valley Hosp Ctr
1985 Crompond Rd; Peekskill, NY 10566; (914)
736-1100; **BDCERT:** IM 79; **MS:** Tufts U 76; **RES:**
Bronx Muncipal Hosp Ctr, Bronx, NY 77-80; **FEL:**
EDM, Albert Einstein Med Ctr, Bronx, NY 80; *SI:*
Geriatric Medicine; Diabetes; **HMO:** Most

♿ SA/SU 🅲 🗂 🛏 🅂 Mcr NFI 4+ Weeks

Marshall, Merville (MD)   EDM
Westchester Med Ctr
New York Medical College,; Valhalla, NY 10595;
(914) 594-4429; **BDCERT:** IM 77; EDM 81; **MS:**
Columbia P&S 74; **RES:** St Luke's Roosevelt Hosp
Ctr, New York, NY 74-76; **FEL:** EDM, Nat Inst
Health, Bethesda, MD 76-79; **FAP:** Assoc Prof NY
Med Coll; *SI: Thyroid; Diabetes;* **HMO:** Prucare US
Hlthcre Aetna Hlth Plan Oxford Well Care +

♿ 🛏 🅂 Mcr 4+ Weeks

Ross, Herbert (MD)   EDM
White Plains Hosp Ctr
33 Davis Ave; White Plains, NY 10605; (914) 946-
5354; **BDCERT:** IM 64; EDM 72; **MS:** Switzerland
55; **RES:** VA Med Ctr-Brooklyn, Brooklyn, NY 57-
59; Montefiore Med Ctr, Bronx, NY 61-62; **FEL:**
EDM, Flower Fifth Ave Hosp, New York, NY 62-63;
FAP: Assoc Prof Med Albany Med Coll; *SI: Diabetes;*
Thyroid and Osteoporosis; **HMO:** Oxford Aetna Hlth
Plan PHS Blue Cross & Blue Shield Pomco +

LANG: Tag, Ger, Sp, Itl; ♿ SA/SU 🗂 🎏 🛏 🅂 Mcr WC NFI
A Few Days *VISA* 💳

Segal, Nancy (MD) EDM
United Hosp Med Ctr

14 Rye Ridge Plaza 141; Rye Brook, NY 10573; (914) 253-6940; **BDCERT:** IM 80; EDM 83; **MS:** NY Med Coll 77; **RES:** IM, St Vincents Hosp & Med Ctr NY, New York, NY 77-80; **FEL:** EDM, St Luke's Roosevelt Hosp Ctr, New York, NY 81-83; **FAP:** Asst Clin Prof NY Med Coll; **HOSP:** Westchester Med Ctr; *SI: Thyroid Disorders; Pituitary Disorders;* **HMO:** Blue Cross Oxford Magnacare CIGNA Pomco +

⬡ ⬡ ⬡ ⬡ ⬡ ⬡ 2-4 Weeks

Socolow, Edward (MD) EDM
Northern Westchester Hosp Ctr

359 E Main St 4A; Mt Kisco, NY 10549; (914) 666-5200; **BDCERT:** IM 65; EDM 73; **MS:** Yale U Sch Med 58; **RES:** Med, UCLA Med Ctr, Los Angeles, CA 59-60; New England Med Ctr, Boston, MA 63-64; **FEL:** Thyroid, Mass Gen Hosp, Boston, MA 60-63; EDM, Boston Med Ctr, Boston, MA 64-68; **FAP:** Assoc Clin Prof Med Albert Einstein Coll Med; *SI: Thyroid Nodules/Tumors; Diabetes;* **HMO:** Oxford Aetna Hlth Plan United Healthcare Blue Cross & Blue Shield Pomco +

⬡ ⬡ ⬡ ⬡ ⬡ ⬡ A Few Days 🔲 *VISA* 🔲 🔲

Southren, A Louis (MD) EDM
Westchester Med Ctr

Route 100 Munger Pavilion; Valhalla, NY 10595; (914) 493-7578; **BDCERT:** IM 63; EDM 72; **MS:** U Hlth Sci/Chicago Med Sch 55; **RES:** Mount Sinai Med Ctr, New York, NY 55-56; VA Med Ctr-Brooklyn, Brooklyn, NY 56-57; **FEL:** EDM, Mount Sinai Med Ctr, New York, NY 58-59; Jewish Hosp Med Ctr, Brooklyn, NY 59-61; **FAP:** Prof Med NY Med Coll; *SI: Cushing's Disease; Adrenogenital Syndromes;* **HMO:** GHI Empire Blue Cross & Shield Metlife Well Care

⬡ ⬡ ⬡ ⬡ ⬡ ⬡ A Few Days

Stangel, John (MD) EDM
United Hosp Med Ctr

70 Maple Ave; Rye, NY 10580; (914) 967-6800; **BDCERT:** EDM 76; **MS:** NY Med Coll 69; **RES:** Mount Sinai Med Ctr, New York, NY 70-74; **FEL:** RE, Metropolitan Hosp Ctr, New York, NY 74-76; **HOSP:** Northern Westchester Hosp Ctr; *SI: Infertility; Pregnancy Loss;* **HMO:** Pomco Oxford Independent Health Plan PHS United Healthcare +

LANG: Fr, Sp; ⬡ ⬡ ⬡ ⬡ ⬡ ⬡ 1 Week 🔲 *VISA* 🔲

FAMILY PRACTICE

Apuzzo, Thomas (MD) FP **PCP**
St Joseph's Med Ctr-Yonkers

955 Yonkers Ave; Yonkers, NY 10704; (914) 237-0994; **BDCERT:** FP 89; **MS:** Italy 85; **RES:** St Joseph's Med Ctr, Yonkers, NY; **FEL:** Brooklyn Hosp Ctr-Caledonian, Brooklyn, NY; **HOSP:** St John's Riverside Hosp

Coloka-Kump, Rodika (DO) FP **PCP**
St Joseph's Med Ctr-Yonkers

Kump and Sayegh Family Medical Services PC, 461 Riverdale Ave; Yonkers, NY 10705; (914) 965-0117; **BDCERT:** FP 92; **MS:** NY Coll Osteo Med 88; **RES:** New York Methodist Hosp, Brooklyn, NY 88-89; St Joseph's Med Ctr-Yonkers, Yonkers, NY 89-91; **HOSP:** St John's Riverside Hosp; **HMO:** United Healthcare Blue Choice Oxford CIGNA Magnacare +

LANG: Sp, Rus, Ar; ⬡ ⬡ ⬡ ⬡ ⬡ ⬡ ⬡ A Few Days

DeAlleaume, Lauren (MD) FP **PCP**
St Joseph's Med Ctr-Yonkers

St Josephs Family Hlth Ctr, 81 S Broadway; Yonkers, NY 10701; (914) 375-3200; **BDCERT:** FP 95; FP 89; **MS:** Columbia P&S 86; **RES:** FP, Overlook Hosp, Summit, NJ 86-89; **FEL:** NY Med Coll, New York, NY 76-77; **FAP:** Asst Prof NY Med Coll; *SI: Women's Health;* **HMO:** Oxford Aetna-US Healthcare Health Source Community Choice

⬡ ⬡ ⬡ ⬡ ⬡ ⬡ ⬡ 4+ Weeks

Guide to symbols and abbreviations can be found on pages 110-113.

771

Donovan, Denis (MD)　　FP　　PCP
United Hosp Med Ctr

125 Milton Rd; Rye, NY 10580; (914) 967-7902;
BDCERT: FP 86; MS: Georgetown U 60; RES: St
Vincents Hosp & Med Ctr NY, New York, NY 61-63;
HOSP: NY Hosp-Cornell Med Ctr

Goldstein, Lawrence (MD)　　FP　　PCP
Community Hosp At Dobbs Ferry

200 S Broadway Ste 106; Tarrytown, NY 10591;
(914) 366-0633; MS: Mt Sinai Sch Med 89; RES:
FP, North Shore Univ Hosp, , NY 90-93; HOSP:
Phelps Mem Hosp Ctr; HMO: Oxford US Hlthcre
Blue Cross & Blue Shield United Healthcare

LANG: Sp, Prt; 🚻 📶 🌙 📷 🚼 🏧 📠 Mcr Mcd WC NFI
Immediately VISA ●

Gottesfeld, Peter (MD)　　FP　　PCP
Northern Westchester Hosp Ctr

49 Smith Ave; Mt Kisco, NY 10549; (914) 241-
7800; BDCERT: FP 88; MS: UMDNJ-RW Johnson
Med Sch 85; RES: FP, Thomas Jefferson U Hosp,
Philadelphia, PA 85-88; HMO: Pomco US Hlthcre
Aetna Hlth Plan Blue Choice

LANG: Sp, Ger, Fr, Itl; 🚻 🌙 📷 🚼 🏧 📠 Mcr WC NFI
Immediately 📇 VISA ●

Griffith, Barbara (MD)　　FP　　PCP
St Joseph's Med Ctr-Yonkers

296 Kimball Ave; Yonkers, NY 10704; (914) 776-
7758; BDCERT: FP 85; MS: Dominican Republic
82; RES: St Joseph's Med Ctr-Yonkers, Yonkers, NY;
SI: Correctional Healthcare; HMO: US Hlthcre
Genesis Blue Cross & Blue Shield Oxford

LANG: Sp; 📶 🌙 🏧 📠 Mcr Mcd WC NFI　1 Week

Halbach, Joseph (MD)　　FP　　PCP
St Joseph's Med Ctr-Yonkers

St Josephs/Thomas and Agnes Carvel FdnFam Hlth
Ctr, 127 S Broadway; Yonkers, NY 10701; (914)
375-3200; BDCERT: FP 94; MS: Univ IL Coll Med
78; RES: Montefiore Med Ctr, Bronx, NY 78-81;
FAP: Asst Clin Prof NY Med Coll; SI: HIV Infection;
HMO: US Hlthcre Oxford

LANG: Sp; 🚻 📷 🚼 🏧 📠 Mcr Mcd　2-4 Weeks

Heinegg, Philip (MD)　　FP　　PCP
Sound Shore Med Ctr-Westchester

Larchmont Family Practice, 1890 Palmer Ave 305;
Larchmont, NY 10538; (914) 834-9606; BDCERT:
FP 83; MS: France 80; RES: Univ Hosp SUNY Stony
Brook, Stony Brook, NY 80-83; FAP: Asst Clin Prof
FP SUNY Stony Brook; HMO: Aetna Hlth Plan Blue
Choice Pomco Oxford PHS +

🚻 📶 📷 🚼 🏧 📠 Mcr VISA ●

Kelly, Stephen P (MD)　　FP　　PCP
Community Hosp At Dobbs Ferry

18 Ashford Ave MW; Dobbs Ferry, NY 10522;
(914) 693-1660; BDCERT: FP 78; MS: U
Cincinnati 75; RES: Ventura Cty Med Ctr, Ventura,
CA 76; FP, Rutgers Univ, , NJ 76-78; FEL: Tropical
Medicine, Harvard Med Sch, Cambridge, MA 78-
79; HOSP: St John's Riverside Hosp; SI: Tropical
Medicine; Weight Management; HMO: Oxford United
Healthcare CIGNA Aetna-US Healthcare Prucare +

LANG: Sp, Rus; 🚻 📶 🌙 📷 🚼 🏧 📠 Mcr WC NFI
Immediately

Merker, Edward (MD)　　FP　　PCP
Phelps Mem Hosp Ctr

Family Medical Care, PC, 180 Marble Ave;
Pleasantville, NY 10570; (914) 769-7300;
BDCERT: FP 81; MS: Albert Einstein Coll Med 81;
RES: Overlook Hosp, Summit, NJ 81-84; HMO:
Prucare Blue Choice Oxford PHS

LANG: Itl, Sp; 🚻 📶 🌙 📷 🚼 🏧 📠 Mcr Mcd WC NFI
Immediately 📇 VISA ● 📇

Miller, Daniel (MD)　　FP　　PCP
St Joseph's Med Ctr-Yonkers

St Joseph'sThomas & Agnes Foundation Family
Hlth Ctr, 81 S Broadway; Yonkers, NY 10701;
(914) 375-3200; BDCERT: FP 88; MS: U
Cincinnati 84; RES: FP, Montefiore Med Ctr, Bronx,
NY 84-87; FAP: Asst Prof NY Med Coll; SI:
Comprehensive Family Care; Parenting; HMO: Aetna-
US Healthcare Oxford Genesis Health Source Child
Health Plus +

LANG: Sp; 🚻 📶 🌙 📷 🚼 📠 Mcr Mcd　1 Week

Miller, Ellen G (MD) FP **PCP**
St Joseph's Med Ctr-Yonkers

St Joseph's Med Ctr—Family Health Ctr, 81 S Broadway; Yonkers, NY 10701; (914) 375-3200; **BDCERT:** FP 80; **MS:** U Rochester 77; **RES:** FP, Montefiore, Bronx, NY 77-80; **FAP:** Asst Prof Med NY Med Coll; **SI:** *Women's Healthcare*; **HMO:** Aetna-US Healthcare Oxford Community Choice Health Source

LANG: Sp, Ar; 🔲 🔲 🔲 🔲 🔲 🔲 2-4 Weeks

Piccirilli, Dora (MD) FP **PCP**
Phelps Mem Hosp Ctr

180 Marble Ave; Pleasantville, NY 10570; (914) 769-7300; **BDCERT:** FP 91; **MS:** SUNY Hlth Sci Ctr 88; **RES:** Overlook Hosp, Summit, NJ 89-91; **HMO:** Pomco Metlife Oxford Blue Choice US Hlthcre +

🔲 🔲 🔲 🔲 🔲 🔲 🔲 🔲 🔲 🔲 Immediately **VISA** 💳 💳

Sincero, Domenico (MD) FP **PCP**
Phelps Mem Hosp Ctr

200 S Broadway; Tarrytown, NY 10591; (914) 631-3727; **BDCERT:** FP 71; **MS:** Italy 50; **RES:** U, Wilkes Barre Gen Hosp, Wilkes Barre, PA 55-56; **HOSP:** Community Hosp At Dobbs Ferry; **HMO:** Oxford CIGNA Metlife PHS Travelers +

🔲 🔲 🔲 🔲 🔲 🔲 🔲 Immediately

Strongwater, Richard (MD) FP **PCP**
Phelps Mem Hosp Ctr

180 Marble Ave; Pleasantville, NY 10570; (914) 769-7300; **BDCERT:** FP 84; **MS:** SUNY Syracuse 81; **RES:** FP, Overlook Hosp, Summit, NJ 81-84

🔲 🔲 🔲 🔲 🔲 🔲 🔲 🔲 🔲 🔲 Immediately 💳 **VISA** 💳 💳

Sutton, Ira (MD) FP **PCP**
Sound Shore Med Ctr-Westchester

77 Quaker Ridge Rd 101; New Rochelle, NY 10804; (914) 636-0077; **BDCERT:** FP 83; **MS:** Albert Einstein Coll Med 80; **RES:** Rhode Island Hosp, Providence, RI 80-83; **FAP:** Clin Instr Albert Einstein Coll Med; **HOSP:** Sound Shore Med Ctr-Westchester; **SI:** *Preventive Medicine*; **HMO:** PHS Blue Cross United Healthcare Oxford Health Source +

🔲 🔲 🔲 🔲 🔲 🔲 🔲 🔲 A Few Days **VISA** 💳

Yudin, Howard (MD) FP **PCP**
United Hosp Med Ctr

10 Rye Ridge Plaza 207; Rye Brook, NY 10573; (914) 251-1261; **BDCERT:** FP 84; **MS:** Canada 74; **RES:** Jewish Gen Hosp, Montreal, Canada 74-76; **HOSP:** Sound Shore Med Ctr-Westchester; **HMO:** Blue Choice Pomco GHI SWCHP NY Hosp Hlth +

LANG: Fr, Sp; 🔲 🔲 🔲 🔲 🔲 🔲 Immediately **VISA** 💳

GASTROENTEROLOGY

Abemayor, Elie (MD) Ge
Northern Westchester Hosp Ctr

91 Smith Ave; Mt Kisco, NY 10549; (914) 241-9026; **BDCERT:** IM 88; Ge 95; **MS:** SUNY Hlth Sci Ctr 85; **RES:** IM, Washington Hosp Ctr, Washington, DC 85; IM, Bellevue Hosp Ctr, New York, NY 86-88; **FEL:** Ge, VA Med Ctr-Manh, New York, NY 88-90; **FAP:** Clin Instr NYU Sch Med; **HOSP:** New York University Med Ctr; **SI:** *Inflammatory Bowel Disease; Hepatobiliary Disease*; **HMO:** Oxford Aetna Hlth Plan Pomco CIGNA SWCHP +

LANG: Fr; 🔲 🔲 🔲 🔲 🔲 🔲 1 Week **VISA** 💳

Antonelle, Michael (MD) Ge
St Agnes Hosp

311 North St Ste 301; White Plains, NY 10605; (914) 949-7171; **MS:** NY Med Coll 62; **RES:** N, NY Med Coll, Valhalla, NY; **FEL:** IM, Metropolitan Hosp Ctr, New York, NY; **HOSP:** White Plains Hosp Ctr

🔲 🔲 🔲 🔲 🔲 🔲 🔲

Antonelle, Robert (MD)   Ge   PCP
St Agnes Hosp
Gastroenterologysts Consultants of Westchester, 311 North St Ste 302; White Plains, NY 10605; (914) 949-7171; **BDCERT:** IM 92; **MS:** NY Med Coll 89; **RES:** IM, Westchester County Med Ctr, Valhalla, NY 92-94; **HOSP:** White Plains Hosp Ctr; **HMO:** Aetna Hlth Plan Oxford CIGNA Empire Blue Cross & Shield US Hlthcre +

LANG: Sp; ⚕ 📷 🎥 📅 $ Mcr   1 Week

Auerbach, Mitchell E (MD)   Ge
St Joseph's Med Ctr-Yonkers
Westchester Digestive Disease Group, 1 Apple Hill Lane; Chappaqua, NY 10514; (914) 969-1115; **BDCERT:** IM 94; Ge 98; **MS:** Tufts U 91; **RES:** Mount Sinai Med Ctr, New York, NY 92-94; **HOSP:** St John's Riverside Hosp; **SI:** *Ulcerative Colitis and Crohn's Disease*; **HMO:** Oxford Aetna Hlth Plan Blue Cross & Blue Shield GHI

LANG: Sp; ⚕ 📷 🎥 📅 $ Mcr Mcd   Immediately

Chinitz, Marvin (MD)   Ge
Northern Westchester Hosp Ctr
90 S Bedford Rd; Mt Kisco, NY 10549; (914) 241-1050; **BDCERT:** IM 81; Ge 85; **MS:** Boston U 78; **RES:** IM, Boston Med Ctr, Boston, MA 78-81; **FEL:** Montefiore Hosp, Bronx, NY 82-84; **FAP:** Clin Instr Med Albert Einstein Coll Med; **SI:** *Gastroenterology; Liver Diseases*

⚕ 📷 🎥 📅 $ Mcr   A Few Days

Dworkin, Brad (MD)   Ge
Westchester Med Ctr
Route 100 Munger Pavilion 206; Valhalla, NY 10595; (914) 594-7337; **BDCERT:** IM 79; **MS:** Jefferson Med Coll 76; **RES:** IM, NY Hosp-Cornell Med Ctr, New York, NY 76-79; **FEL:** Ge, Mem Sloan Kettering Cancer Ctr, New York, NY 79-81; Nutrition, Mem Sloan Kettering Cancer Ctr, New York, NY 81-82; **FAP:** Assoc Prof Med NY Med Coll; **HMO:** Prucare Oxford Independent Health Plan US Hlthcre CIGNA +

⚕ 📷 🎥 📅 $ Mcr Mcd NFI   1 Week

Field, Barry (MD)   Ge
Phelps Mem Hosp Ctr
Westchester Gastroenterology, 777 N Broadway 305; North Tarrytown, NY 10591; (914) 366-6120; **BDCERT:** IM 76; Ge 79; **MS:** Albert Einstein Coll Med 72; **RES:** Montefiore Med Ctr, Bronx, NY 72-73; Metropolitan Hosp Ctr, New York, NY 73-76; **FEL:** Ge, Harbor Gen Hosp, Los Angeles, CA 76-78; **SI:** *Inflammatory Bowel Disease; Colorectal Cancer Detection*; **HMO:** Blue Choice PHS CIGNA Blue Choice Magnacare +

⚕ 📷 🎥 📅 $ Mcr Mcd   Immediately **VISA** ⬤

Genn, David (MD)   Ge
Hudson Valley Hosp Ctr
MidHudson Gastroenterology Associates, 1985 Crompond Rd; Peekskill, NY 10566; (914) 739-2400; **BDCERT:** IM 92; Ge 93; **MS:** Boston U 88; **RES:** IM, Montefiore Med Ctr, Bronx, NY 88-91; **FEL:** Ge, Westchester County Med Ctr, Valhalla, NY 91-93; **HOSP:** Phelps Mem Hosp Ctr; **SI:** *Liver Disease; Colon Cancer Screening*; **HMO:** Oxford Aetna-US Healthcare PM Care Prucare Pomco +

LANG: Sp; ⚕ 📷 🎥 📅 $ Mcr Mcd   A Few Days

Goldblatt, Robert (MD)   Ge
United Hosp Med Ctr
25 S Regent St; Port Chester, NY 10573; (914) 937-4646; **BDCERT:** IM 78; Ge 79; **MS:** Geo Wash U Sch Med 74; **RES:** IM, U FL Shands Hosp, Gainesville, FL 75-77; **FEL:** Ge, Yale-New Haven Hosp, New Haven, CT 77-79; **FAP:** Asst Clin Prof Cornell U; **HOSP:** NY Hosp-Cornell Med Ctr; **SI:** *Endoscopy; Biliary Tract Diseases*; **HMO:** Oxford Prucare PHS Pomco Aetna Hlth Plan +

⚕ ☾ 📷 🎥 📅 $ Mcr Mcd WC   A Few Days **VISA** ⬤ ⬛

Halata, Michael (MD)   Ge
Westchester Med Ctr
Wchstr Hosp CtrDept/Ped/Div Ped Gas, Munger Pavilion; Valhalla, NY 10595; (914) 594-4610; **BDCERT:** Ped 80; PGe 90; **MS:** UMDNJ-NJ Med Sch, Newark 74; **HOSP:** St Agnes Hosp

Heier, Stephen (MD) Ge
Westchester Med Ctr

Gastroenterology Consultants of Westchester, Munger Pavilion Rm 408; Valhalla, NY 10595; (914) 493-8699; **BDCERT:** IM 79; Ge 81; **MS:** Albany Med Coll 76; **RES:** Flower Fifth Ave Hosp, New York, NY 76-79; Metropolitan Hosp Ctr, New York, NY 76-79; **FEL:** Tufts U, Boston, MA 79-81; Lemuel Shattuck Hosp, Boston, MA; **SI:** *Esophageal Cancer; Stone Removal-ERCP*; **HMO:** Oxford Well Care Independent Health Plan Prucare CIGNA +

🕭 🖸 🐜 🛗 🚭 🖾 🖾 2-4 Weeks **VISA** ⬤

Katz, Henry (MD) Ge
Montefiore Med Ctr

1234 Central Park Ave; Yonkers, NY 10704; (914) 793-1600; **BDCERT:** IM 83; Ge 85; **MS:** Albany Med Coll 80; **RES:** Bellevue Hosp Ctr, New York, NY 80-83; **FEL:** Ge, Montefiore Med Ctr, Bronx, NY 83-85; **FAP:** Clin Instr Med Albert Einstein Coll Med; **HOSP:** Community Hosp At Dobbs Ferry; **HMO:** Blue Choice Blue Cross & Blue Shield CIGNA GHI

🕭 🖸 🐜 🛗 🖾 A Few Days

Kozicky, Orest (MD) Ge
St John's Riverside Hosp

Westchester Digestinve Deisease Group, LLP, 469 N Broadway; Yonkers, NY 10701; (914) 969-1115; **BDCERT:** Ge 87; IM 85; **MS:** NY Med Coll 81; **RES:** IM, Jacobi Med Ctr, Bronx, NY 81-85; **FEL:** Ge, Montefiore Med Ctr, Bronx, NY 85-87; **FAP:** Asst Clin Instr Albert Einstein Coll Med; **HOSP:** St Joseph's Med Ctr-Yonkers; **SI:** *Colitis; Peptic Ulcer Disease*; **HMO:** Oxford US Hlthcre Blue Choice CIGNA GHI +

LANG: Ukr, Sp; 🕭 🖸 🛗 🖾 🖾 2-4 Weeks

Kressner, Michael (MD) Ge
Sound Shore Med Ctr-Westchester

120 E Prospect Ave 102; Mt Vernon, NY 10550; (914) 664-4466; **BDCERT:** IM 80; Ge 83; **MS:** SUNY Buffalo 77; **RES:** IM, Albert Einstein Med Ctr, Bronx, NY 77-80; **FEL:** Ge, Albert Einstein Med Ctr, Bronx, NY 80-82; **FAP:** Asst Clin Prof NY Med Coll; **HOSP:** Mount Vernon Hosp; **SI:** *Reflex Diseases; Colonic Polyps*; **HMO:** Aetna Hlth Plan PHS Blue Cross & Blue Shield GHI Oxford +

LANG: Sp; 🕭 🖸 🐜 🛗 🚭 🖾 🖾 🖾 🖾 Immediately

Landau, Steven (MD) Ge `PCP`
White Plains Hosp Ctr

30 Greenridge Ave 2K; White Plains, NY 10605; (914) 328-8555; **BDCERT:** IM 87; **MS:** NYU Sch Med 81; **RES:** Jacobi Med Ctr, Bronx, NY 81-84; **FEL:** Mount Sinai Med Ctr, New York, NY 84-86; **SI:** *Inflammatory Bowel Disease; Ulcer Disease*; **HMO:** PHS Aetna Hlth Plan Oxford SWCHP Pomco +

LANG: Sp, Fr, Ger, Heb, Yd; 🕭 🖸 🐜 🛗 🚭 🖾 🖾 A Few Days

Lebovics, Edward (MD) Ge
Westchester Med Ctr

Munger Pavilion 206; Valhalla, NY 10595; (914) 493-7337; **BDCERT:** IM 83; Ge 85; **MS:** NYU Sch Med 80; **RES:** Jewish Hosp of St Louis, St Louis, MO 80-83; **FEL:** Ge, Mount Sinai Med Ctr, New York, NY 83-84; NY Med Coll, Valhalla, NY 84-86; **SI:** *Therapeutic Endoscopy; Chronic Viral Hepatitis*; **HMO:** Aetna Hlth Plan Oxford Pomco Prucare GHI +

LANG: Sp; 🕭 🖸 🐜 🛗 🚭 🖾 1 Week **VISA**

Liss, Mark (MD) Ge
Sound Shore Med Ctr-Westchester

140 Lockwood Ave 318; New Rochelle, NY 10801; (914) 633-0888; **BDCERT:** IM 80; Ge 83; **MS:** Mt Sinai Sch Med 77; **RES:** IM, Mount Sinai Med Ctr, New York, NY 77-80; **FEL:** Ge, Montefiore Med Ctr, Bronx, NY 80-82; **HOSP:** Montefiore Med Ctr; **HMO:** CIGNA Sanus-NYLCare HealthNet Blue Choice Oxford +

🕭 🔘 🖸 🐜 🛗 🚭 1 Week

Mehta, Rekha (MD) Ge
Sound Shore Med Ctr-Westchester

140 Lockwood Ave; New Rochelle, NY 10801; (914) 632-9455; **BDCERT:** IM 84; Ge 87; **MS:** India 72; **RES:** New Rochelle Hosp Med Ctr, New Rochelle, NY; **FEL:** Med U of SC Med Ctr, Charleston, SC; Clinical Nutrition, U of Pittsburgh Med Ctr, Pittsburgh, PA; **HOSP:** Calvary Hosp; **HMO:** Aetna Hlth Plan Blue Cross & Blue Shield Oxford Empire Pomco +

🕭 🖸 🛗 🖾 🖾 🖾 A Few Days

Guide to symbols and abbreviations can be found on pages 110-113.

775

Neschis, Martin (MD) **Ge**
United Hosp Med Ctr
25 S Regent St; Port Chester, NY 10573; (914) 937-4646; **BDCERT:** IM 66; Ge 72; **MS:** SUNY Hlth Sci Ctr 58; **RES:** VA Med Ctr-Bronx, Bronx, NY 59-60; IM, Maimonides Med Ctr, Brooklyn, NY 62-64; **FEL:** Ge, Wadsworth VA Hosp, Los Angeles, CA 64-65; ***SI:*** *Gastroesophageal Reflux; Peptic Ulcer Disease;* **HMO:** SWCHP Oxford PHS Pomco Blue Cross +
LANG: Yd, Itl; ♿ ☎ 🚹 📅 $ [Mcr] [Mcd] A Few Days
American Express VISA MasterCard

Rosemarin, Jack (MD) **Ge**
White Plains Hosp Ctr
222 Westchester Ave 308; White Plains, NY 10604; (914) 683-1555; **BDCERT:** IM 82; Ge 83; **MS:** NY Med Coll 72; **RES:** NY Med Coll, Valhalla, NY 78-81; **FEL:** Ge, Yale-New Haven Hosp, New Haven, CT; **HOSP:** St Agnes Hosp; ***SI:*** *Nutrition; Colon Cancer*
♿ ☎ 🚹 📅 [Mcr] [NFI] Immediately American Express VISA MasterCard Discover

Rosenthal, William (MD) **Ge**
Westchester Med Ctr
Route 100 Munger Pavilion Rm 206; Valhalla, NY 10595; (914) 594-4418; **BDCERT:** Ge 64; **MS:** SUNY Hlth Sci Ctr 50; **RES:** VA Med Ctr-Brooklyn, Brooklyn, NY 51-52

Salama, Meir (MD) **Ge**
St John's Riverside Hosp
955 Yonkers Ave 200; Yonkers, NY 10704; (914) 237-0011; **BDCERT:** IM 90; Ge 93; **MS:** NY Med Coll 87; **RES:** IM, Montefiore Medical Ctr, Bronx, NY 87-90; **FEL:** Ge, NY Medical School, Valhalla, NY 90-92; **HOSP:** St Joseph's Med Ctr-Yonkers; ***SI:*** *Colonoscopy; Endoscopy;* **HMO:** Aetna Hlth Plan Oxford US Hlthcre 1199 Empire +
LANG: Sp; ♿ ☎ 📅 [Mcr] 1 Week

Shapiro, Neil (MD) **Ge** [PCP]
United Hosp Med Ctr
1600 Harrison Ave 305; Mamaroneck, NY 10543; (914) 698-0448; **BDCERT:** IM 78; Ge 87; **MS:** Wayne State U Sch Med 75; **RES:** Beth Israel Med Ctr, New York, NY 75-78; **FEL:** Ge, Montefiore Med Ctr, Bronx, NY 78-80; **HMO:** Blue Cross & Blue Shield Prucare PHS Oxford US Hlthcre +
♿ ☎ 🚹 📅 [Mcr] [Mcd] A Few Days

Taffet, Sanford (MD) **Ge**
Sound Shore Med Ctr-Westchester
140 Lockwood Ave 110; New Rochelle, NY 10801; (914) 636-5222; **BDCERT:** IM 80; Ge 81; **MS:** NY Med Coll 76; **RES:** IM, Maimonides Med Ctr, Brooklyn, NY 76-79; **FEL:** Ge, Albert Einstein Med Ctr, Bronx, NY 79-81; **FAP:** Assoc Clin Prof Med NY Med Coll; **HOSP:** Mount Vernon Hosp; ***SI:*** *Inflammatory Bowel Disease; Liver Disease;* **HMO:** Aetna Hlth Plan Blue Choice Oxford PHS US Hlthcre +
♿ ☎ 🚹 📅 [Mcr] [Mcd] [WC] [NFI] Immediately

Torman, Julie (MD) **Ge**
Phelps Mem Hosp Ctr
11 Dove Ct; Croton-on-Hudson, NY 10520; (914) 271-4212; **BDCERT:** IM 83; Ge 89; **MS:** U Nevada 80; **RES:** IM, Brigham & Women's Hosp, Boston, MA 80-81; IM, Harvard Med Sch, Cambridge, MA 81-83; **FEL:** GO, Stanford Med Ctr, Stanford, CA 83-85; **HOSP:** Hudson Valley Hosp Ctr; ***SI:*** *Colon Cancer Screening; Swallowing Difficulty;* **HMO:** PHS Oxford US Hlthcre Independent Health Plan Blue Choice +
LANG: Sp; ♿ ☾ ☎ 🚹 📅 $ [Mcr] [Mcd] Immediately

Wayne, Peter (MD) **Ge**
St Joseph's Med Ctr-Yonkers
469 N Broadway; Yonkers, NY 10701; (914) 969-1115; **BDCERT:** IM 79; Ge 81; **MS:** Albert Einstein Coll Med 76; **RES:** Montefiore Med Ctr, Bronx, NY 76-79; **FEL:** Ge, Mount Sinai Med Ctr, New York, NY 79-81; **HOSP:** St John's Riverside Hosp; ***SI:*** *Hepatitis & Liver Disease; Pancreatic Disease;* **HMO:** Oxford GHI Aetna Hlth Plan CIGNA PHS +
LANG: Sp; ♿ ☎ 📅 $ [Mcr] 2-4 Weeks

Guide to symbols and abbreviations can be found on pages 110-113.

GERIATRIC MEDICINE

Juthani, Virendra (MD)   Ger   **PCP**
Bronx Lebanon Hosp Ctr
17 Pheasant Run; Scarsdale, NY 10583; (914)
723-4575; **BDCERT:** IM 77; Ger 88; **MS:** India 69;
RES: Med, Jewish Meml Hospital, New York, NY 71-
72; Cv, Jewish Meml Hospital, New York, NY 72-
73; **FEL:** Albert Einstein Med Ctr, Bronx, NY 73-74;
FAP: Asst Prof Med Albert Einstein Coll Med; *SI:*
Dementia
LANG: Hin, Rom; 🚹 ☷ ☰

Pousada, Lidia (MD)   Ger   **PCP**
Sound Shore Med Ctr-Westchester
Sound Shore Med CtrGeriatrics Assoc of
Westchester, 16 Guion Pl; New Rochelle, NY
10802; (914) 637-1646; **BDCERT:** IM 87; Ger 90;
MS: NY Med Coll 80; **RES:** IM, Montefiore Med Ctr,
Bronx, NY 80-83; **FEL:** Ger, New York University
Med Ctr, New York, NY 78-79; **FAP:** Assoc Prof NY
Med Coll; *SI: Urinary Incontinence; Memory Loss;*
HMO: Oxford Aetna Hlth Plan GHI Blue Cross &
Blue Shield
LANG: Sp, Chi, Itl, Fr; 🚹 ☷ 👪 ☰ ☷ ☷
Immediately ▨ *VISA* ● ▨

GYNECOLOGIC ONCOLOGY

Chuang, Linus (MD)   GO
Westchester Med Ctr
NY Med Coll Dept Ob Gynec, Macy Pavilion 2nd Fl;
Valhalla, NY 11021; (914) 493-8846; **BDCERT:**
ObG 95; GO 97; **MS:** Taiwan 81; **RES:** ObG,
Flushing Hosp Med Ctr, Flushing, NY 86-90; **FEL:**
GO, MD Anderson Cancer Ctr, Houston, TX 90-94;
FAP: Asst Prof NY Med Coll; **HOSP:** Sound Shore
Med Ctr-Westchester
LANG: Sp; 🚹 👪 ☰ ☷ ☷ 2-4 Weeks ▨ *VISA*
● ▨

Kwon, Tae (MD)   GO
Our Lady of Mercy Med Ctr
305 North St; White Plains, NY 10605; (914) 681-
7171; **BDCERT:** ObG 78; GO 81; **MS:** South Korea
65; **RES:** GO, Lenox Hill Hosp, New York, NY 74-
76; **FEL:** Lenox Hill Hosp, New York, NY 74-76; U
Miss Med Ctr, Jackson, MS 76-78; **HOSP:** St Agnes
Hosp; **HMO:** Oxford Independent Health Plan
Magnacare
LANG: Kor; 🚹 ☷ ☰ ☷ 1 Week

HAND SURGERY

Purcell, Ralph (MD)   HS
Phelps Mem Hosp Ctr
200 S Broadway 104; Tarrytown, NY 10591;
(914) 631-1142; **BDCERT:** OrS 89; **MS:** Columbia
P&S 80; **RES:** IM, Baylor Coll Med, Houston, TX 79-
80; S, Beth Israel Med Ctr, Boston, MA 80-82; **FEL:**
HS, New York University Med Ctr, New York, NY;
HOSP: White Plains Hosp Ctr; *SI: Orthopedic*
Surgery; Plastic Surgery; **HMO:** Aetna Hlth Plan
PHCS US Hlthcre Lawrence Healthcare Well Care +
🚹 ☾ ☷ 👪 ☰ ☷ ☷ ☷ ☷ ☷ 2-4 Weeks

HEMATOLOGY

Biers, Martin (MD)   Hem   **PCP**
White Plains Hosp Ctr
15 Chester Ave; White Plains, NY 10601; (914)
946-3553; **BDCERT:** IM 70; Hem 72; **MS:** SUNY
Hlth Sci Ctr 55; **RES:** Kings County Hosp Ctr,
Brooklyn, NY 55-56; VA Med Ctr-Brooklyn,
Brooklyn, NY 56-57; **FEL:** Mount Sinai Med Ctr,
New York, NY 57-58; Mount Sinai Med Ctr, New
York, NY 58-59; **HMO:** Aetna Hlth Plan Pomco
PHS Oxford Vytra +
🚹 ☷ 👪 ☰ ☷ A Few Days

Fass, Richard (MD) Hem PCP
St John's Riverside Hosp

Advanced Oncology Associates, 385 Palisades Ave; Yonkers, NY 10703; (914) 476-7600; **BDCERT:** IM 73; Hem 74; **MS:** U Hlth Sci/Chicago Med Sch 66; **RES:** Lenox Hill Hosp, New York, NY 67-71; **FEL:** Hem, Albert Einstein Med Ctr, Bronx, NY 73-75; **SI:** *Breast Cancer; Iron Storage Diseases;* **HMO:** PHS Empire Blue Choice Oxford

[symbols] A Few Days

Schwartz, Simeon (MD) Hem
United Hosp Med Ctr

The Westchester Medical Group PC, 14 Rye Ridge Plaza 229; Port Chester, NY 10573; (914) 253-8200; **BDCERT:** IM 80; Hem 84; **MS:** Yale U Sch Med 77; **RES:** Med, NY Hosp-Cornell Med Ctr, New York, NY 77-80; NY Hosp-Cornell Med Ctr, New York, NY 79-80; **FEL:** Hem, Mem Sloan Kettering Cancer Ctr, New York, NY 80-83; **FAP:** Asst Clin Prof Med NY Med Coll; **HOSP:** White Plains Hosp Ctr; **HMO:** Aetna-US Healthcare Blue Choice Oxford PHS Pomco +

LANG: Sp; [symbols] A Few Days *VISA*

INFECTIOUS DISEASE

Berkey, Peter (MD) Inf
St Joseph's Med Ctr-Yonkers

Southern Westchester Infectious Disease Med Grp, 970 N Broadway 212; Yonkers, NY 10701; (914) 376-1543; **BDCERT:** Inf 85; IM 88; **MS:** U Puerto Rico 80; **RES:** IM, Westchester County Med Ctr, Valhalla, NY 80-84; **FEL:** Inf, MD Anderson Cancer Ctr, Houston, TX 86-88; **HOSP:** St John's Riverside Hosp; **HMO:** Blue Cross & Blue Shield Oxford Metlife Aetna-US Healthcare

[symbols] 1 Week

Haber, Stuart (MD) Inf PCP
St Agnes Hosp

Oncology Hematology Associates, 707 Westchester Ave Suite 110; White Plains, NY 10604; (914) 328-9696; **BDCERT:** IM 86; **MS:** NYU Sch Med 83; **RES:** Emory U Hosp, Atlanta, GA; **FEL:** Emory U Hosp, Atlanta, GA; **HOSP:** United Hosp Med Ctr; **SI:** *HIV Infection;* **HMO:** Aetna Hlth Plan Blue Cross & Blue Shield Oxford US Hlthcre

[symbols] A Few Days *VISA*

Hewlett, Dial (MD) Inf
Lincoln Med & Mental Hlth Ctr

955 Yonkers Ave 17; Yonkers, NY 10704; (914) 237-7090; **BDCERT:** IM 80; Inf 84; **MS:** U Wisc Med Sch 76; **RES:** IM, Harlem Hosp Ctr, New York, NY 76-80; **FEL:** Inf, Montefiore Med Ctr, Bronx, NY; Albert Einstein Med Ctr, Bronx, NY; **FAP:** Assoc Prof Med NY Med Coll; **HOSP:** Lawrence Hosp; **HMO:** Oxford Excelcare CIGNA Aetna-US Healthcare Blue Cross & Blue Shield +

[symbols] 2-4 Weeks

Horowitz, Harold (MD) Inf
Westchester Med Ctr

209 SE Macy Pavilion Southeast; Valhalla, NY 10595; (914) 493-8865; **BDCERT:** IM 83; Inf 88; **MS:** NYU Sch Med 79; **RES:** IM, U of WI Hosp, Madison, WI 81-83; **FEL:** Inf, New England Med Ctr, Boston, MA 84-86; **FAP:** Assoc Prof NY Med Coll; **SI:** *HIV-AIDS;* **HMO:** Oxford Pomco GHI US Hlthcre Well Care +

LANG: Sp; [symbols] 1 Week *VISA*

Moorjani, Harish (MD) Inf
Phelps Mem Hosp Ctr

Hudson Infectious Diseases Assoc, 540 N State Rd; Briarcliff Manor, NY 10510; (914) 762-2276; **BDCERT:** IM 92; Inf 94; **MS:** India 86; **RES:** IM, Univ of Med & Dent NJ Hosp, Newark, NJ 89-90; IM, Univ of Med & Dent NJ Hosp, Newark, NJ 90-92; **FEL:** Inf, Univ Hosp SUNY Stony Brook, Stony Brook, NY 92-94; **SI:** *Lyme Disease; HIV;* **HMO:** Oxford Blue Choice Aetna-US Healthcare Independent Health Plan CIGNA +

LANG: Fr, Sp, Hin; [symbols] Immediately

Nadelman, Robert (MD) **Inf**
Westchester Med Ctr
95 Grasslands Rd; Valhalla, NY 10595; (914) 493-8865; **BDCERT:** IM 83; Inf 88; **MS:** Albert Einstein Coll Med 80; **RES:** IM, Beth Israel Med Ctr, New York, NY 80-83; **FEL:** Inf, Beth Israel Med Ctr, New York, NY 83-85; **FAP:** Assoc Prof NY Med Coll
♿ $ A Few Days

Rush, Thomas (MD) **Inf**
Phelps Mem Hosp Ctr
540 N State Rd; Briarcliff Manor, NY 10510; (914) 762-2276; **BDCERT:** IM 81; Inf 84; **MS:** Rush Med Coll 78; **RES:** Med, Genesee Hosp, Rochester, NY 79-81; **FEL:** Inf, Strong Mem Hosp, Rochester, NY 81-83; **FAP:** Asst Clin Prof Med NY Med Coll; ***SI:*** *HIV Infection; Lyme Disease*; **HMO:** Aetna-US Healthcare CIGNA Independent Health Plan Physician's Health Plan +
♿ ☎ 👤 📅 $ [Mcr] [Mcd] [WC] A Few Days

Welch, Peter (MD) **Inf**
Northern Westchester Hosp Ctr
400 E Main St; Mt Kisco, NY 10549; (914) 666-1308; **BDCERT:** IM 77; Inf 80; **MS:** SUNY Buffalo 74; **RES:** NY Hosp-Cornell Med Ctr, New York, NY 74-77; **FEL:** Inf, NY Hosp-Cornell Med Ctr, New York, NY; ***SI:*** *Lyme Disease*; **HMO:** Oxford Blue Cross & Blue Shield Aetna-US Healthcare US Hlthcre
♿ ☎ 👤 📅 $ [Mcr] [Mcd] [NFI] A Few Days

Wormser, Gary (MD) **Inf**
Westchester Med Ctr
Route 100 Macy Pavilion 209SE; Valhalla, NY 10595; (914) 493-8865; **BDCERT:** IM 81; Inf 82; **MS:** Johns Hopkins U 72; **RES:** Mount Sinai Med Ctr, New York, NY 72-75; **FEL:** Inf, Mount Sinai Med Ctr, New York, NY 75-77; ***SI:*** *HIV; Lyme*
♿ ☎ 👤 📅 $ [Mcr] 2-4 Weeks

INTERNAL MEDICINE

Abenavoli, T J (MD) **IM** [PCP]
United Hosp Med Ctr
446 Westchester Ave; Port Chester, NY 10573; (914) 939-1573; **BDCERT:** IM 79; Cv 81; **MS:** NYU Sch Med 76; **RES:** VA Med Ctr-Manh, New York, NY; IM, Bellevue Hosp Ctr, New York, NY 76-79; **FEL:** Cv, VA Med Ctr-Manh, New York, NY; New York University Med Ctr, New York, NY 79-81; **HMO:** Blue Choice Oxford
♿ ☾ ☎ 👤 📅 $ [Mcr] Immediately

Alpert, Barbara (MD) **IM** [PCP]
Northern Westchester Hosp Ctr
Mount Kisco Medical Group, 90 S Bedford Rd; Mt Kisco, NY 10549; (914) 241-1050; **BDCERT:** IM 87; **MS:** Univ Penn 84; **RES:** NY Hosp-Cornell Med Ctr, New York, NY 84-87; ***SI:*** *Prevention of Osteoporosis*; **HMO:** PHS Aetna-US Healthcare Oxford
LANG: Sp; ♿ [SA SU] 👤 📅 $ [Mcr] 2-4 Weeks VISA MasterCard

Alter, Sheldon (MD) **IM** [PCP]
White Plains Hosp Ctr
33 Davis Ave; White Plains, NY 10605; (914) 946-5354; **BDCERT:** IM 67; **MS:** U Hlth Sci/Chicago Med Sch 61; **RES:** Montefiore Med Ctr, Bronx, NY 61-64; **FEL:** St Luke's Roosevelt Hosp Ctr, New York, NY 64-66; **HMO:** Blue Cross & Blue Shield PHS Oxford Aetna Hlth Plan
♿ [SA SU] ☎ 👤 📅 [Mcr] A Few Days American Express VISA

Altholz, Jeffrey (MD) **IM** [PCP]
Phelps Mem Hosp Ctr
160 S Central Ave; Elmsford, NY 10523; (914) 631-2099; **BDCERT:** IM 92; **MS:** Albert Einstein Coll Med 86; **RES:** Boston U Med Ctr, Boston, MA 86-87; St Vincents Hosp & Med Ctr NY, New York, NY 87-90; **HOSP:** Community Hosp At Dobbs Ferry; ***SI:*** *General Medicine; Addictions/Recovery*; **HMO:** Most
LANG: Prt, Heb, Sp; ♿ [SA SU] ☾ ☎ 👤 📅 $ [Mcr] [WC] [NFI] Immediately VISA MasterCard

Berk, Paul D (MD)   IM
Mount Sinai Med Ctr

East Mountain Rd South, RR 2 BO; Gold Spring, NY 10516; (212) 241-6479; **BDCERT:** IM 70; Hem 72; **MS:** Columbia P&S 64; **RES:** IM, Columbia-Presbyterian Med Ctr, New York, NY 65-66; Nat Inst Health, Bethesda, MD 66-69; **FEL:** Hem, Columbia-Presbyterian Med Ctr, New York, NY 69-70; **FAP:** Prof Med Mt Sinai Sch Med; **SI:** *Liver Diseases; Hematology/Myeloproliferative*; **HMO:** Oxford Health Source PHS Blue Cross PPO Preferred Care +

🔲 🔲 🔲 🔲 🔲 🔲 4+ Weeks 🔲 **VISA** 🔲

Boufford, Timothy (MD)   IM
Lawrence Hosp

1 Stone Pl; Bronxville, NY 10708; (914) 337-9004; **BDCERT:** IM 75; **MS:** U Mich Med Sch 71; **RES:** IM, Harlem Hosp Ctr, New York, NY 71-74; **FEL:** Nep,; **FAP:** Asst Clin Prof Med Columbia P&S; **HOSP:** St Joseph's Med Ctr-Yonkers; **SI:** *Hypertension; Kidney Diseases*; **HMO:** Blue Choice Oxford CIGNA

🔲 🔲 🔲 🔲 🔲 🔲

Chia, Gloria (MD)   IM
Phelps Mem Hosp Ctr

777 N Broadway; N Tarrytown, NY 10591; (914) 941-0453; **BDCERT:** IM 96; **MS:** Philippines 65; **RES:** IM, VA Med Ctr-Brooklyn, Brooklyn, NY 67-69; Hem, Long Island Coll Hosp, Brooklyn, NY 69-71; **FEL:** Onc, Albert Einstein Med Ctr, Bronx, NY 72-74; **FAP:** Asst Clin Attng; **SI:** *Breast; Lung*; **HMO:** PHS United Healthcare

🔲 🔲 🔲 🔲 🔲 2-4 Weeks

Colangelo, Daniel (MD)   IM   PCP
United Hosp Med Ctr

1600 Harrison Ave 102; Mamaroneck, NY 10543; (914) 698-4466; **BDCERT:** IM 94; **MS:** NYU Sch Med 80; **RES:** Lenox Hill Hosp, New York, NY 80-83; **HOSP:** White Plains Hosp Ctr; **HMO:** Oxford PHS Pomco CIGNA Empire Blue Choice +

🔲 🔲 🔲 🔲 🔲 🔲 🔲 🔲 4+ Weeks

Croen, Kenneth (MD)   IM   PCP
White Plains Hosp Ctr

259 Heathcote Rd; Scarsdale, NY 10583; (914) 723-8100; **BDCERT:** IM 84; Inf 89; **MS:** Albert Einstein Coll Med 80; **RES:** IM, Columbia-Presbyterian Med Ctr, New York, NY 80-84; **FEL:** Inf, Nat Inst Health, Bethesda, MD 84-89; **FAP:** Asst Clin Prof Med Columbia P&S; **SI:** *Infectious Diseases; Herpes Virus Infections*; **HMO:** Oxford United Healthcare Blue Choice PHS +

LANG: Sp; 🔲 🔲 🔲 🔲 🔲 🔲 🔲 🔲 A Few Days 🔲 🔲 🔲

De Angelis, Arthur (MD)   IM   PCP
United Hosp Med Ctr

Weschester MedicalGroup, 16 Rye Ridge Plaza; Rye Brook, NY 10573; (914) 253-6464; **BDCERT:** IM 75; Cv 77; **MS:** SUNY Buffalo 69; **RES:** Buffalo Gen Hosp, Buffalo, NY 69-70; Montefiore Med Ctr, Bronx, NY 70-71; **FEL:** Cv, Mount Sinai Med Ctr, New York, NY 73-75; **FAP:** Asst Clin Prof Med Cornell U; **SI:** *Elevated Cholesterol*; **HMO:** Aetna-US Healthcare Oxford CIGNA PHS Pomco +

LANG: Sp, Itl; 🔲 🔲 🔲 🔲 🔲 🔲 🔲 🔲 🔲 🔲 🔲 Immediately 🔲 **VISA** 🔲

De Matteo, Robert (MD)   IM   PCP
St John's Riverside Hosp

970 N Broadway 209; Yonkers, NY 10701; (914) 965-3366; **BDCERT:** IM 88; **MS:** Mexico 82; **RES:** Mount Sinai Med Ctr, New York, NY 82-85; **FEL:** Westchester County Med Ctr, Valhalla, NY 86-88; **HOSP:** St Joseph's Med Ctr-Yonkers; **HMO:** Oxford Aetna-US Healthcare Blue Choice CIGNA United Healthcare +

🔲 🔲 🔲 🔲 🔲 🔲 A Few Days

Dennett, Ronald (MD)   IM   PCP
Lawrence Hosp

1254 Central Park Ave; Yonkers, NY 10704; (914) 965-1771; **BDCERT:** IM 80; **MS:** Univ Vt Coll Med 77; **RES:** U CO Hosp, Denver, CO 77-80; **HOSP:** Montefiore Med Ctr; **HMO:** Oxford PHS Blue Choice Pomco

🔲 🔲 🔲 🔲 🔲 🔲 🔲 A Few Days

Dieck, Eileen (MD)   IM
Northern Westchester Hosp Ctr
83 S Bedford Rd; Mt Kisco, NY 10549; (914) 666-5077; **BDCERT:** IM 89; **MS:** NY Med Coll 86; **RES:** Westchester County Med Ctr, Valhalla, NY 86-89

Epstein, Carol (MD)   IM
United Hosp Med Ctr
Oxford Medical Group, 707 Westchester Ave 110; White Plains, NY 10604; (914) 328-0050; **BDCERT:** IM 87; Inf 92; **MS:** Mt Sinai Sch Med 83; **RES:** IM, Beth Israel Med Ctr, New York, NY 83-86; **FEL:** Inf, Beth Israel Med Ctr, New York, NY 86-88; **HOSP:** St Agnes Hosp; *SI: Lyme Disease; HIV Infection*
LANG: Sp, Itl; 🚻 🔾 🕍 🎛 🆂 🆆 🕥   A Few Days **VISA** 💳

Faber, Andrew (MD)   IM   **PCP**
Community Hosp At Dobbs Ferry
Irvington Medical Associates, 116 Main St; Irvington, NY 10533; (914) 591-7557; **BDCERT:** IM 87; Ger 90; **MS:** Mexico 82; **RES:** IM, Metropolitan Hosp Ctr, New York, NY 84-87; **FEL:** Ge, Ruth Taylor Inst, Hawthorne, NY 87-89; **FAP:** Asst Clin Prof Med NY Med Coll; **HOSP:** Phelps Mem Hosp Ctr; *SI: Alzheimer's Disease;* **HMO:** Oxford CIGNA Aetna-US Healthcare Empire Oxford +
LANG: Sp; 🕍 🔾 🕍 🎛 🆂 🕥   A Few Days **VISA** 💳

Fazio, Nelson M (MD)   IM   **PCP**
Lawrence Hosp
1 Pondfield Rd West Ste 1R; Bronxville, NY 10708; (914) 771-5750; **BDCERT:** IM 86; **MS:** NY Med Coll 81; **RES:** IM, Lincoln Med & Mental Hlth Ctr, Bronx, NY 81-82; Westchester County Med Ctr, Valhalla, NY 82-84; **FEL:** Inf, Montefiore Med Ctr, Bronx, NY 93-94; **FAP:** Asst Prof NY Med Coll; **HOSP:** Our Lady of Mercy Med Ctr; *SI: Hypertension; Obesity;* **HMO:** US Hlthcre Oxford CIGNA Amerihealth Blue Choice +
LANG: Sp; 🚻 🕍 🔾 🕍 🎛 🆂 🕥 🕥   A Few Days

Federman, Harold (MD)   IM   **PCP**
Northern Westchester Hosp Ctr
Katonah Medical Group, 111 Bedford Rd; Katonah, NY 10536; (914) 232-3135; **BDCERT:** IM 72; **MS:** NYU Sch Med 64; **RES:** Bellevue Hosp Ctr, New York, NY 68-71; Yale-New Haven Hosp, New Haven, CT 64-65; **FAP:** Asst Prof NYU Sch Med; **HMO:** CIGNA Oxford PHS Index Aetna Hlth Plan +
🚻 🕍 🔾 🕍 🎛 🆂 🕥 🆆 🕥   1 Week

Finkelstein, Michael (MD)   IM   **PCP**
Northern Westchester Hosp Ctr
175 King St; Chappaqua, NY 10514; (914) 238-4777; **BDCERT:** IM 89; **MS:** Univ Penn 86; **RES:** IM, Lenox Hill Hosp, New York, NY 86-89
🚻 🔾 🕍 🎛   Immediately 🔳 **VISA** 💳

Goldberg, Roy J (MD)   IM   **PCP**
Sound Shore Med Ctr-Westchester
Sickels Ave & May St; New Rochelle, NY 10801; (914) 632-1234; **BDCERT:** IM 85; Ger 92; **MS:** Albert Einstein Coll Med 82; **RES:** IM, Montefiore Med Ctr, Bronx, NY 82-85; **FAP:** Asst Clin Prof Med NY Med Coll; *SI: Geriatrics;* **HMO:** Oxford PHS Pomco
🚻 🕍 🔾 🕍 🎛 🆂 🕥 🕥 🆆 🕥   Immediately

Goldman, Jack S (MD)   IM   **PCP**
St Joseph's Med Ctr-Yonkers
32 Hyatt Ave; Yonkers, NY 10704; (914) 237-8686; **BDCERT:** IM 75; Ge 79; **MS:** Albert Einstein Coll Med 61; **RES:** IM, Bronx Lebanon Hosp Ctr, Bronx, NY 62-63; IM, VA Med Ctr-Bronx, Bronx, NY 63-66; **FEL:** Ge, VA Med Ctr-Bronx, Bronx, NY 64-65; **HOSP:** Montefiore Med Ctr; **HMO:** Aetna Hlth Plan GHI Blue Cross & Blue Shield Oxford United Healthcare +
LANG: Fr, Heb, Yd; 🚻 🔾 🕍 🎛 🆂 🕥 🕥 🆆
A Few Days

Gutstein, Sidney (MD)   IM   PCP
Northern Westchester Hosp Ctr

90 S Bedford Rd; Mt Kisco, NY 10549; (914) 241-1050; **BDCERT:** IM 66; Ge 72; **MS:** NYU Sch Med 58; **RES:** IM, Bronx Muncipal Hosp Ctr, Bronx, NY 62-63; **FEL:** Ge, Bronx Muncipal Hosp Ctr, Bronx, NY 63; **FAP:** Assoc Clin Prof Med Albert Einstein Coll Med; **SI:** *High Blood Pressure; High Cholesterol;* **HMO:** Aetna-US Healthcare Oxford Prudential PHS Independent Health Plan +

LANG: Sp, Yd, Ger; 👤 🈚 🌙 🔒 🚲 📷 💲 Mcr NFI A Few Days ▨ **VISA** 💳 💳

Healy, Elaine (MD)   IM   PCP
Westchester Med Ctr

Comprehensive Adult Med Svc, 311 North St 307; White Plains, NY 10605; (914) 684-6845; **BDCERT:** IM 86; Ger 90; **MS:** SUNY Buffalo 82; **RES:** IM, Westchester County Med Ctr, Valhalla, NY 83-85; **FAP:** Asst Clin Prof IM NY Med Coll; **HOSP:** St Agnes Hosp

👤 🈚 📷 📺 💲 Mcr WC NFI Immediately ▨ **VISA** 💳 ▨

Heckman, Bruce (MD)   IM   PCP
Phelps Mem Hosp Ctr

14 Dove CT; Croton On Hudson, NY 10520; (914) 941-1334; **BDCERT:** IM 72; **MS:** NY Med Coll 67; **RES:** NY Med Coll, Valhalla, NY 67-70; **FEL:** Hem, NY Med Coll, Valhalla, NY 70-71; **HOSP:** Westchester Med Ctr; **HMO:** Oxford US Hlthcre Pomco Prucare

👤 🈚 🌙 🈚 🚲 📷 💲 Mcr WC NFI Immediately **VISA** 💳

Herzog, David (MD)   IM   PCP
Sound Shore Med Ctr-Westchester

140 Lockwood Ave Annex; New Rochelle, NY 10801; (914) 235-3311; **BDCERT:** IM 84; **MS:** Mt Sinai Sch Med 81; **RES:** St Luke's Roosevelt Hosp Ctr, New York, NY 81-84; **SI:** *Cholesterol and Lipids; Preventative Care Medicine;* **HMO:** Oxford PHS Chubb PHCS Blue Choice +

👤 🈚 📷 🚲 📺 💲 2-4 Weeks

Higgins, William (MD)   IM
Hudson Valley Hosp Ctr

1985 Crompond Rd; Cortlandt Manor, NY 10566; (914) 739-3597; **BDCERT:** IM 91; **MS:** Geo Wash U Sch Med 86; **RES:** IM, Lenox Hill Hosp, New York, NY 86-89; **FEL:** Pul, Lenox Hill Hosp, New York, NY 89; **FAP:** Asst Clin Prof Med NY Med Coll; **SI:** *Asthma;* **HMO:** Oxford Pomco GHI CIGNA US Hlthcre +

👤 🈚 🌙 📷 📺 Mcr WC NFI Immediately ▨ **VISA** 💳 💳

Hopkins, Arthur (MD)   IM   PCP
Montefiore Med Ctr

6 Xavier Drve 610; Yonkers, NY 10704; (914) 376-5550; **BDCERT:** IM 86; **MS:** Univ Penn 83; **RES:** Hosp of U Penn, Philadelphia, PA 84-86; **HMO:** Oxford Blue Cross CIGNA Prucare NYLCare +

👤 🈚 🌙 📷 🚲 📺 💲 Mcr NFI Immediately ▨ **VISA** 💳 💳

Hurwitz, Harvey (MD)   IM   PCP
Phelps Mem Hosp Ctr

7 Morningside Ct; Ossining, NY 10562; (914) 762-3521; **BDCERT:** IM 71; **MS:** Boston U 62; **RES:** Yale-New Haven Hosp, New Haven, CT 65-68; **SI:** *Stress Management;* **HMO:** PHS Blue Choice Oxford Independent Health Plan Magnacare +

LANG: Fr; 👤 🈚 🚲 📺 💲 Mcr Mod WC NFI 1 Week

Isaacs, Ellen (MD)   IM   PCP
St Joseph's Med Ctr-Yonkers

385 Palisade Ave; Yonkers, NY 10703; (914) 963-9493; **BDCERT:** IM 72; Cv 81; **MS:** NYU Sch Med 69; **RES:** IM, Bellevue Hosp Ctr, New York, NY 69-72; **FEL:** Cv, St Vincents Hosp & Med Ctr NY, New York, NY 72-74; **FAP:** Asst Prof NY Med Coll; **SI:** *General Medicine; Heart Disease;* **HMO:** CIGNA GHI Independent Health Plan Magnacare Oxford +

LANG: Sp; 👤 🌙 📷 🚲 📺 Mcr Mod NFI Immediately

Jonas, Darrell (DO)   IM   **PCP**
Sound Shore Med Ctr-Westchester

New Rochelle Hosp Med Ctr, 3765 Riverdale Ave; Riverdale, NY 10463; (914) 632-5000; **BDCERT:** IM 91; **MS:** NY Coll Osteo Med 87; **RES:** IM, Long Island Jewish Med Ctr, New Hyde Park, NY 88-91; **FAP:** Clin Instr NY Med Coll; **HMO:** Oxford Aetna-US Healthcare WHSN Pomco PHCS +

♿ ☽ ▣ ♟ ▦ **S** Mcr Wc   Immediately ▨ **VISA** ◉

Kalchthaler, Thomas (DO)   IM   **PCP**
St Joseph's Med Ctr-Yonkers

Geriatric Services, 69 S Broadway; Yonkers, NY 10701; (914) 376-5555; **BDCERT:** IM 76; Ger 92; **MS:** Chicago Coll Osteo Med 71; **RES:** Michael Reese Hosp Med Ctr, Chicago, IL 71-72; IM, Elmhurst Hosp Ctr, Elmhurst, NY 72-75; **FEL:** Ger, Elmhurst Hosp Ctr, Elmhurst, NY 73-74; **FAP:** Asst Prof Med NY Med Coll; **HOSP:** Sound Shore Med Ctr-Westchester; **SI:** *Geriatrics*; **HMO:** Empire Blue Cross & Shield Oxford US Hlthcre CIGNA

LANG: Fr, Sp, Heb, Fil, Itl; ♿ ▣ ♟ ▦ **S** Mcr Mcd NFl 2-4 Weeks

Kaplan, Kenneth (MD)   IM   **PCP**
Phelps Mem Hosp Ctr

160 N State Rd; Briarcliff Manor, NY 10510; (914) 762-3821; **BDCERT:** IM 70; **MS:** NYU Sch Med 62; **RES:** Bellevue Hosp Ctr, New York, NY 60-66; **FEL:** Cv, New York University Med Ctr, New York, NY 68-69; **SI:** *Cardiology; Vascular Ultrasound*; **HMO:** PHS Oxford Empire Blue Cross Teamsters Prucare +

▣ ♟ ▦   A Few Days

Kapoor, Satish (MD)   IM   **PCP**
Phelps Mem Hosp Ctr

777 N Broadway 300; North Tarrytown, NY 10591; (914) 631-2070; **BDCERT:** IM 79; **MS:** India 72; **RES:** Kingsbrook Jewish Med Ctr, Brooklyn, NY; **FEL:** Pul, Queens Hosp Ctr, Jamaica, NY 79-80; **HOSP:** Community Hosp At Dobbs Ferry; **HMO:** Oxford PHS CIGNA Aetna Hlth Plan Independent Health Plan +

LANG: Hin, Sp, Itl; ♿ ♻ ☽ ▣ ♟ ▦ **S** Mcr Mcd Wc NFl A Few Days **VISA** ◉ ▨

Klecatsky, Lawrence (MD)   IM
Sound Shore Med Ctr-Westchester

16 Guion Pl; New Rochelle, NY 10801; (914) 637-1375; **BDCERT:** IM 74; **MS:** U Minn 67; **RES:** Philadelphia Gen Hosp, Philadelphia, PA 67-68; IM, New Rochelle Hosp Med Ctr, New Rochelle, NY 70-73; **FAP:** Asst Prof EM NY Med Coll; **SI:** *Emergency Medicine; Sports Medicine*

♿ ♻ ☽ ▣ ♟ ▦ ▦ Mcr Mcd Wc NFl   Immediately ▨ **VISA** ◉ ⚖

Lans, David (DO)   IM   **PCP**
Sound Shore Med Ctr-Westchester

838 Pelhamdale Ave; New Rochelle, NY 10801; (914) 235-5577; **BDCERT:** IM 84; Rhu 88; **MS:** Univ Osteo Med & Hlth Sci 81; **RES:** IM, Univ Hosp SUNY Bklyn, Brooklyn, NY 81-85; **FEL:** A&I, New England Med Ctr, Boston, MA 85-87; Rhu, Hosp For Special Surgery, New York, NY 87-89; **FAP:** Asst Clin Prof Med Albert Einstein Coll Med; **HOSP:** Montefiore Med Ctr; **SI:** *Preventive Health Care; Osteoporosis*; **HMO:** Oxford Empire United Healthcare PHS

☽ ▣ ♟ ▦ **S** Mcr   1 Week **VISA** ◉

Lebofsky, Martin (MD)   IM   **PCP**
Lawrence Hosp

1 Stone Pl; Bronxville, NY 10708; (914) 337-9004; **BDCERT:** IM 75; Nep 78; **MS:** Albert Einstein Coll Med 72; **RES:** IM, Harlem Hosp Ctr, New York, NY 73-75; **FEL:** Nep, Montefiore Med Ctr, Bronx, NY 76-78; **HOSP:** St Joseph's Med Ctr-Yonkers

♿ ▣ ♟ ▦ **S** Mcr Mcd

Lechner, Michael (MD)   IM   **PCP**
Phelps Mem Hosp Ctr

245 N Broadway; North Tarrytown, NY 10591; (914) 762-0722; **BDCERT:** IM 68; **MS:** Albert Einstein Coll Med 61; **RES:** Westchester County Med Ctr, Valhalla, NY 61-63; **FEL:** Long Island Jewish Med Ctr, New Hyde Park, NY 63-65; **SI:** *Nursing Home Medicine; Office Geriatrics*; **HMO:** Empire Blue Cross & Shield PHS Prucare Oxford US Hlthcre +

♿ ▣ ♟ ▦ Mcr NFl   A Few Days

Lester, Thomas (MD)   IM
Northern Westchester Hosp Ctr
Katonah Medical Group, 111 Bedford Rd; Katonah, NY 10536; (914) 232-3135; **BDCERT:** IM 82; Onc 87; **MS:** Rutgers U 79; **RES:** Mount Sinai Med Ctr, New York, NY 80-82; **FEL:** Hem, Mount Sinai Med Ctr, New York, NY 82-84; Onc, Mem Sloan Kettering Cancer Ctr, New York, NY 84-86; *SI: Oncology; Hematology*

[symbols]

Lipman, Marvin (MD)   IM
White Plains Hosp Ctr
Scarsdale Medical Group, 259 Heathcote Rd; Scarsdale, NY 10583; (914) 723-8100; **BDCERT:** IM 66; EDM 72; **MS:** Columbia P&S 54; **RES:** IM, Columbia-Presbyterian Med Ctr, New York, NY 54-56; IM, Mass Gen Hosp, Boston, MA 58-60; **FEL:** EDM, Columbia-Presbyterian Med Ctr, New York, NY 60-61; **FAP:** Clin Prof NY Med Coll; *SI: Diabetes Mellitus; Thyroid Diseases*

LANG: Sp; [symbols] 2-4 Weeks *VISA* ⬤

Matz, Robert (MD)   IM
Mount Sinai Med Ctr
32 Buena Vista Dr; Hastings On Hudson, NY 10706; (212) 241-0780; **BDCERT:** IM 63; **MS:** NYU Sch Med 56; **RES:** Jacobi Med Ctr, Bronx, NY 56-60; **FEL:** Albert Einstein Med Ctr, Bronx, NY 59-60; Albert Einstein Med Ctr, Bronx, NY 62-63; **FAP:** Prof Med Mt Sinai Sch Med; *SI: Diabetes Mellitus; Metabolic Disorders*

[symbols] 1 Week

Melman, Martin (MD)   IM   PCP
Phelps Mem Hosp Ctr
Croton Medical Assoc, 87 Grand St; Croton On Hudson, NY 10520; (914) 271-4845; **BDCERT:** IM 77; **MS:** NY Med Coll 74; **RES:** IM, Metropolitan Hosp Ctr, New York, NY 74-77; **FEL:** IM, Westchester County Med Ctr, Valhalla, NY 77-78; **HOSP:** Hudson Valley Hosp Ctr; *SI: Hypertension; Asthma*

[symbols] 1 Week *VISA* ⬤

Mettu, Sudhaker (MD)   IM   PCP
St John's Riverside Hosp
Riverside Medical Group, 1010 N Broadway; Yonkers, NY 10701; (914) 968-3535; **BDCERT:** IM 95; **MS:** India 73; **RES:** IM, Misericordia Hosp, Bronx, NY 79-82; **HOSP:** Community Hosp At Dobbs Ferry; *SI: Hypertension; Diabetes Mellitus*

[symbols] A Few Days [symbols] *VISA* ⬤

Morelli, Michael (MD)   IM   PCP
Lawrence Hosp
1 Pondfield Rd 205; Bronxville, NY 10708; (914) 337-1610; **BDCERT:** IM 84; Pul 86; **MS:** NYU Sch Med 81; **RES:** Bellevue Hosp Ctr, New York, NY 81-84; **FEL:** PMR, Bellevue Hosp Ctr, New York, NY 84-86; **HMO:** Blue Choice HealthNet Independent Health Plan CIGNA

LANG: Itl; [symbols] 2-4 Weeks

Noto, Rocco (MD)   IM   PCP
Northern Westchester Hosp Ctr
Yorktown Adult's Pediatric Medicine, 358 Downing Dr; Yorktown Heights, NY 10598; (914) 245-0256; **MS:** Mexico 84; **RES:** Ped, Westchester County Med Ctr, Valhalla, NY 84-87; IM, Maimonides Med Ctr, Brooklyn, NY 87-89; **HMO:** Oxford Pomco PHS Blue Choice +

LANG: Itl, Sp; [symbols] Immediately *VISA* ⬤

Pappas, Steven (MD)   IM   PCP
Sound Shore Med Ctr-Westchester
266 White Plains; Eastchester, NY 10707; (914) 793-1115; **BDCERT:** IM 82; EM 89; **MS:** Albert Einstein Coll Med 78; **RES:** St Luke's Roosevelt Hosp Ctr, New York, NY 81; **HOSP:** Phelps Mem Hosp Ctr; **HMO:** GHI Pomco

[symbols] A Few Days [symbols] *VISA* ⬤

Park, Tai (MD)　　　　IM　　PCP
Phelps Mem Hosp Ctr

1 S Lawn Ave; Elmsford, NY 10523; (914) 592-7400; **BDCERT:** IM 93; **MS:** South Korea 71; **RES:** Our Lady of Mercy Med Ctr, Bronx, NY 86; **HMO:** Aetna Hlth Plan Blue Choice Blue Cross & Blue Shield CIGNA Oxford +

🅂 ⬜ 🚹 🏨 💲 ⬜ ⬜ Immediately

Peterson, Stephen J (MD)　　IM　　PCP
Westchester Med Ctr

Westchester Medical Center, Ste 504; Valhalla, NY 10595; (914) 493-8370; **BDCERT:** IM 85; **MS:** 82; **RES:** IM, Metropolitan Hosp, Philadelphia, PA 82-86; **FAP:** Assoc Prof NY Med Coll; *SI: General Internal Medicine*; **HMO:** Oxford CIGNA US Hlthcre Independent Health Plan PHS +

LANG: Sp, Itl; ⬜ 🅂 ⬜ ⬜ 🚹 💲 ⬜ ⬜ ⬜

Pleasset, Maxwell (MD)　　IM
Northern Westchester Hosp Ctr

3630 Hill Blvd 101; Jefferson Valley, NY 10535; (914) 245-5525; **BDCERT:** IM 76; **MS:** Univ Pittsburgh 68; **RES:** IM, NY Hosp-Cornell Med Ctr, New York, NY 74-76; *SI: Geriatrics; Health Maintenance*; **HMO:** Aetna Hlth Plan Metlife Oxford PHS United Healthcare +

⬜ 🅂 ⬜ 🚹 🏨 💲 ⬜ ⬜

Ravikumar, Sunita (MD)　　IM　　PCP
Phelps Mem Hosp Ctr

777 N Broadway 300; N Tarrytown, NY 10591; (914) 366-7800; **BDCERT:** IM 83; **MS:** India 76; **RES:** IM, Westchester County Med Ctr, Valhalla, NY 79-82; **FEL:** EDM, Westchester County Med Ctr, Valhalla, NY 82-84; **HOSP:** Westchester Med Ctr; **HMO:** CIGNA Aetna Hlth Plan Independent Health Plan PHS Oxford +

⬜ ⬜ ⬜ 🚹 🏨 ⬜ ⬜ ⬜ ⬜ Immediately

Reda, Dominick (MD)　　IM
St Joseph's Med Ctr-Yonkers

461 Riverdale Ave; Yonkers, NY 10705; (914) 965-0621; **BDCERT:** IM 87; Nep 90; **MS:** Italy 83; **RES:** IM, Our Lady of Mercy Med Ctr, Bronx, NY 84-87; **FEL:** Nep, Lincoln Med & Mental Hlth Ctr, Bronx, NY 87-89; *SI: Nephrology*; **HMO:** Blue Cross & Blue Shield US Hlthcre Oxford

⬜ ⬜ 🚹 🏨 💲 ⬜ ⬜ 1 Week

Richards, Ernest (MD)　　IM　　PCP
United Hosp Med Ctr

The Rye Medical Group, 269 Purchase St; Rye, NY 10580; (914) 967-4444; **BDCERT:** IM 72; **MS:** Columbia P&S 60; **RES:** IM, St Luke's Roosevelt Hosp Ctr, New York, NY 61-62; IM, St Luke's Roosevelt Hosp Ctr, New York, NY 64-66; **FEL:** Columbia-Presbyterian Med Ctr, New York, NY 66-67; *SI: Respiratory Illnesses*; **HMO:** Aetna Hlth Plan Oxford Empire Blue Cross & Shield CIGNA US Hlthcre +

LANG: Sp; ⬜ 🅂 ⬜ 🚹 🏨 💲 ⬜ ⬜ ⬜ ⬜
A Few Days **VISA** 💳 💳

Ridge, Gerald (MD)　　IM　　PCP
Lawrence Hosp

14 Studio Arcade; Bronxville, NY 10708; (914) 779-9066; **BDCERT:** IM 83; Ger 97; **MS:** UC San Francisco 79; **RES:** IM, Albert Einstein Med Ctr, Bronx, NY 79-81; N, Columbia-Presbyterian Med Ctr, New York, NY 81-82; **FEL:** IM, NY Hosp-Cornell Med Ctr, New York, NY 82-83; **FAP:** Assoc Clin Prof Med Columbia P&S; **HOSP:** Columbia-Presbyterian Med Ctr; *SI: Geriatric Medicine*; **HMO:** Oxford Blue Choice PHS CIGNA

⬜ ⬜ 🚹 🏨 💲 A Few Days

Rosch, Elliott (MD)　　IM　　PCP
St John's Riverside Hosp

Riverside Medical Group, 1010 N Broadway; Yonkers, NY 10701; (914) 965-4424; **BDCERT:** IM 81; **MS:** Univ Penn 78; **RES:** Pennsylvania Hosp, Philadelphia, PA 78-81; *SI: Hypertension; Osteoporosis*; **HMO:** PHS Blue Choice Empire Oxford

LANG: Prt, Hin; ⬜ 🚹 💲 ⬜ 4+ Weeks ▦ **VISA** 💳 💳

Rummo, Nicholas (MD)   **IM**
Northern Westchester Hosp Ctr
34 S Bedford Rd; Mt Kisco, NY 10549; (914) 241-
1050; **BDCERT:** IM 72; **MS:** Duke U 69; **RES:** St
Luke's Roosevelt Hosp Ctr, New York, NY 70-72;
FEL: Pul, Duke U Med Ctr, Durham, NC 73-75;
Columbia-Presbyterian Med Ctr, New York, NY 75-
76; *SI: Asthma*; **HMO:** Oxford Aetna Hlth Plan
United Healthcare Independent Health Plan
NYLCare +

⬤ 🔲 🔲 🔲 🔲 🔲 🔲 🔲 🔲 *VISA* ⬤

Sabba, Stephen (MD)   **IM**
Phelps Mem Hosp Ctr
55 Ryder Rd; Maryknoll, NY 10545; (914) 941-
7590; **BDCERT:** IM 88; Ge 91; **MS:** NYU Sch Med
85; **RES:** IM, New York University Med Ctr, New
York, NY 85-88; **FEL:** Ge, New York Universtiy Med
Ctr, New York, NY 88-89; **HOSP:** Community Hosp
At Dobbs Ferry

Seicol, Noel (MD)   **IM**   **PCP**
United Hosp Med Ctr
33 Cedar St; Rye, NY 10580; (914) 967-3483;
BDCERT: IM 84; A&I 84; **MS:** SUNY Hlth Sci Ctr
50; **RES:** IM, Montefiore Med Ctr, Bronx, NY 51-52;
IM, Beth Israel Med Ctr, New York, NY 52-53; **FEL:**
Cv, VA Med Ctr-Bronx, Bronx, NY 53-54; *SI:*
Asthma and Allergies; Menopause & Osteoporosis;
HMO: United Healthcare NYLCare Empire Blue
Cross & Shield Oxford PHS +

⬤ 🔲 🔲 🔲 🔲 🔲 🔲 🔲 🔲 A Few Days

Sheehy, Albert (MD)   **IM**   **PCP**
Phelps Mem Hosp Ctr
Heritage Medical Group, LLP, 777 N Broadway Ste
300; N Tarrytown, NY 10591; (914) 631-2070;
BDCERT: IM 82; **MS:** U Rochester 63; **RES:** St
Vincents Hosp & Med Ctr NY, New York, NY 63-67;
Kings County Hosp Ctr, Brooklyn, NY 67-68; **FEL:**
Pul, Kings County Hosp Ctr, Brooklyn, NY 68-69;
HMO: PHS Oxford CIGNA US Hlthcre HealthNet +

LANG: Itl; ⬤ 🔲 🔲 🔲 🔲 🔲 🔲

Soltren, Rafael (MD)   **IM**   **PCP**
Phelps Mem Hosp Ctr
100 S Highland Ave; Ossining, NY 10562; (914)
941-1277; **BDCERT:** IM 85; **MS:** Cornell U 81; **RES:**
Montefiore Med Ctr, Bronx, NY 81-84

⬤ 🔲 🔲 🔲 🔲 🔲 🔲 🔲 A Few Days

Starke, Charles (MD)   **IM**   **PCP**
Phelps Mem Hosp Ctr
516 N State Rd; Briarcliff Manor, NY 10510; (914)
762-4460; **BDCERT:** IM 78; **MS:** Albert Einstein
Coll Med 75; **RES:** Georgetown U Hosp,
Washington, DC 75-78; **FAP:** Instr Mt Sinai Sch
Med; **HOSP:** Westchester Med Ctr; **HMO:**
Independent Health Plan Pomco PHS Oxford Blue
Choice +

⬤ 🔲 🔲 🔲 🔲 🔲 🔲 🔲 Immediately

Sullivan, Brenda (MD)   **IM**   **PCP**
St John's Riverside Hosp
955 Yonkers Ave; Yonkers, NY 10704; (914) 237-
1260; **BDCERT:** IM 92; **MS:** SUNY Hlth Sci Ctr 85;
RES: IM, Bronx Muncipal Hosp Ctr, Bronx, NY 85-
88; **HMO:** CIGNA Oxford

Weinberg, Harlan (MD)   **IM**
Northern Westchester Hosp Ctr
225 Veterans Rd Ste 201; Yorktown Heights, NY
10598; (914) 962-8430; **BDCERT:** IM 84; Pul 86;
MS: U Conn Sch Med 81; **RES:** Northwestern Mem
Hosp, Chicago, IL 81-84; **FEL:** Cedars-Sinai Med
Ctr, Los Angeles, CA 84-86; **HOSP:** Hudson Valley
Hosp Ctr; *SI: Pulmonary Critical Care*

⬤ 🔲 🔲 🔲 🔲 🔲 🔲 🔲 🔲 Immediately *VISA* ⬤
🔲

Wolfe, Mary (MD)   **IM**   **PCP**
Phelps Mem Hosp Ctr
14 Church St 208; Ossining, NY 10562; (914)
941-1334; **BDCERT:** IM 80; EM 86; **MS:** Penn State
U-Hershey Med Ctr 76; **RES:** IM, Rochester Gen
Hosp, Rochester, NY 76-77; IM, Westchester
County Med Ctr, Valhalla, NY 77-79; *SI: Women's*
Health; **HMO:** Oxford Pomco US Hlthcre
Independent Health Plan PHS +

⬤ 🔲 🔲 🔲 🔲 🔲 🔲 🔲 🔲 A Few Days *VISA* ⬤

Zarlengo, Marco (MD)   IM   `PCP`
Phelps Mem Hosp Ctr

115 Maple St; Croton On Hudson, NY 10520;
(914) 271-3583; **BDCERT:** IM 72; Nep 75; **MS:**
Creighton U 69; **RES:** Med, Harlem Hosp Ctr, New
York, NY 71-72; Med, Harlem Hosp Ctr, New York,
NY 73; **FEL:** Nep, Peter Bent Brigham Hosp, Boston,
MA 73-75; Nep, Peter Bent Brigham Hosp, Boston,
MA 75; *SI: Hypertension; Renal Failure;* **HMO:**
CIGNA PHS Oxford Pomco Excelcare +

🔣 🔣 🔣 🔣 🔣 🔣 🔣 🔣   Immediately ***VISA*** 💳

Zarowitz, William (MD)   IM   `PCP`
White Plains Hosp Ctr

210 Westchester Ave; White Plains, NY 10604;
(914) 682-0700; **BDCERT:** IM 81; **MS:** NY Med
Coll 78; **RES:** IM, Montefiore Med Ctr, Bronx, NY
78-81; **FAP:** Adjct Prof Med NY Med Coll; *SI:*
Occupational Health; **HMO:** Kaiser Permanente
LANG: Sp, Prt; 🔣 🔣 🔣 🔣 🔣 🔣 🔣 🔣 🔣
Immediately ***VISA*** 💳 💳

MATERNAL & FETAL MEDICINE

Brustman, Lois (MD)   MF
Our Lady of Mercy Med Ctr

700 Mc Lean Ave; Yonkers, NY 10704; (718) 920-
9647; **BDCERT:** ObG 86; MF 90; **MS:** NY Med Coll
79; **RES:** ObG, Albert Einstein Med Ctr, Bronx, NY
80-84; **FEL:** MF, Albert Einstein Med Ctr, Bronx, NY
86-88; **FAP:** Assoc Prof NY Med Coll; **HOSP:**
Montefiore Med Ctr-Weiler/Einstein Div; *SI: Diabetes*
in Pregnancy; Fetal Assessment; **HMO:** US Hlthcre
Oxford Blue Choice GHI

LANG: Sp; 🔣 🔣 🔣 🔣 🔣 🔣 🔣 🔣 🔣
A Few Days 🔣 ***VISA*** 💳

MEDICAL GENETICS

Brenholz, Pauline (MD)   MG
Phelps Mem Hosp Ctr

280 Mamaroneck Ave 203; White Plains, NY
10605; (914) 997-6535; **BDCERT:** MG 82; Ped 82;
MS: Albert Einstein Coll Med 73; **RES:** Ped,
Montefiore Med Ctr, Bronx, NY 74-75; Ped,
Montefiore Med Ctr, Bronx, NY 75-76; **FEL:** MG,
Albert Einstein Med Ctr, Bronx, NY 76-79; *SI:*
Prenatal Diagnosis; Inherited Diseases; **HMO:** Oxford
CIGNA United Healthcare Aetna Hlth Plan Blue
Cross & Blue Shield +

LANG: Pol; 🔣 🔣 🔣 🔣 🔣 ***VISA*** 💳 💳

Shapiro, Lawrence R (MD)   MG
Westchester Med Ctr

Westchester Medical Center,; Valhalla, NY 10595;
(914) 347-3010; **BDCERT:** Ped 67; CG 82; **MS:**
NYU Sch Med 62; **RES:** Los Angeles Children's
Hosp, Los Angeles, CA 62-64; Bellevue Hosp Ctr,
New York, NY 64-65; **FEL:** Genetics, New York
University Med Ctr, New York, NY 63; Genetics,
Mount Sinai Med Ctr, New York, NY 67-68

MEDICAL ONCOLOGY

Ahmed, Tauseef (MD)   Onc
Westchester Med Ctr

Route 250 Munger Pavillon; Valhalla, NY 10595;
(914) 493-8374; **BDCERT:** Onc 80; Hem 83; **MS:**
Pakistan 76; **RES:** Sinai Hosp, Detroit, MI 77-80;
FEL: Onc, Mem Sloan Kettering Cancer Ctr, New
York, NY; Hem,; **FAP:** Prof NY Med Coll; **HOSP:** St
Agnes Hosp; *SI: Breast Cancer; Lymphomas Hodgkin's*
Disease; **HMO:** Oxford Aetna Hlth Plan Prudential
Magnacare

LANG: Sp, Heb, Kor, Pun, Ur; 🔣 🔣 🔣 🔣 🔣 🔣 🔣
A Few Days

Bernhardt, Bernard (MD)   Onc
Sound Shore Med Ctr-Westchester
Advanced Oncology Associates, 50 Guion Pl; New Rochelle, NY 10801; (914) 632-5397; **BDCERT:** Onc 73; Hem 72; **MS:** Northwestern U 61; **RES:** IM, DC Gen Hosp, Washington, DC 61-63; IM, NY Med Coll, Valhalla, NY 65-66; **FEL:** Hem, Montefiore Med Ctr, Bronx, NY 67-68; **FAP:** Clin Prof Med NY Med Coll; **HOSP:** United Hosp Med Ctr; **HMO:** Oxford Aetna Hlth Plan PHS Blue Choice Pomco +

🚫 🚗 📷 💲 ☎ Mcr Mcd   A Few Days ▓ **VISA** 💳 ☎ 📷

Feldman, Stuart (MD)   Onc
White Plains Hosp Ctr
14 Rye Ridge Plaza 229; Port Chester, NY 10573; (914) 253-8200; **BDCERT:** IM 80; Onc 85; **MS:** Geo Wash U Sch Med 77; **RES:** NY Hosp-Cornell Med Ctr, New York, NY 77-80; **FEL:** Hem Onc, Mem Sloan Kettering Med Ctr, New York, NY 80-83; **HOSP:** Mem Sloan Kettering Cancer Ctr

Friedman, Eliot (MD)   Onc
Hudson Valley Hosp Ctr
707 Westchester Ave Suite 110; White Plains, NY 10604; (914) 328-9696; **BDCERT:** IM 84; Onc 87; **MS:** U Chicago-Pritzker Sch Med 81; **RES:** U Chicago Hosp, Chicago, IL 81-84; **FEL:** Onc, Harvard Med Sch, Cambridge, MA 84-87; **HMO:** US Hlthcre PHS Oxford

LANG: Sp, Itl; 🚫 📷 👤 🏠 💲 Mcr Mcd WC Immediately

Mills, Nancy Ellyn (MD)   Onc
Phelps Mem Hosp Ctr
Mem Sloan Kettering Canc Ctr at Phelps Hosp Ctr, 777 N Broadway Ste 102; Sleepy Hollow, NY 10591; (914) 366-0664; **BDCERT:** IM 90; Onc 93; **MS:** Mt Sinai Sch Med 87; **RES:** IM, Mount Sinai Med Ctr, New York, NY 87-90; **FEL:** Hem, New York University Med Ctr, New York, NY 90-93; Onc, New York University Med Ctr, New York, NY 90-93; **FAP:** Asst Clin Prof Med NYU Sch Med; **SI:** Breast Cancer; Lymphoma; **HMO:** PHS Oxford Blue Cross & Blue Shield

🚫 📷 👤 🏠 Mcr 2-4 Weeks

Mittelman, Abraham (MD) Onc
Westchester Med Ctr
Westchester Oncology Group, Munger Pavilion Rm250; Valhalla, NY 10595; (914) 285-8374; **BDCERT:** IM 80; **MS:** Mexico 77; **RES:** Kings County Hosp Ctr, Brooklyn, NY; **FEL:** Mem Sloan Kettering Cancer Ctr, New York, NY; **HOSP:** St Agnes Hosp; **SI:** Breast Cancer; Melanoma; **HMO:** Blue Choice Oxford GHI Aetna-US Healthcare Pomco +

LANG: Sp, Ur, Mly, Pun; 🚫 🚗 📷 👤 🏠 Mcr Mcd **VISA** 💳

Nelson, John C (MD)   Onc
Westchester Med Ctr
Westchester County Med Ctr, Munger Pavillion; Valhalla, NY 10595; (914) 493-8353; **BDCERT:** IM 74; Hem 76; **MS:** Harvard Med Sch 71; **RES:** IM, Mount Sinai Med Ctr, New York, NY 72-74; **FEL:** Hem, NY Med Coll, Valhalla, NY 74-76; **HOSP:** United Hosp Med Ctr

🚫 🚗 📷 🏠 Mcr WC NFI Immediately

Phillips, Elizabeth (MD)   Onc
Sound Shore Med Ctr-Westchester
Advanced Oncology Associates, 50 Guion Place Pl 32; New Rochelle, NY 10801; (914) 632-5397; **BDCERT:** IM 74; Onc 77; **MS:** U Wash, Seattle 69; **RES:** Med, Harlem Hosp Ctr, New York, NY 70-72; Hem, Montefiore Med Ctr, Bronx, NY 72-73; **FEL:** Mem Sloan Kettering Cancer Ctr, New York, NY 73-75; **FAP:** Assoc Clin Prof NY Med Coll; **HOSP:** United Hosp Med Ctr; **SI:** Breast Cancer; Complementary Medicine; **HMO:** Oxford PHS Aetna-US Healthcare Blue Cross & Blue Shield Magnacare +

LANG: Fr, Sp; 🚫 📷 👤 🏠 💲 Mcr Mcd **VISA** 💳

Puccio, Carmelo (MD)   Onc
Westchester Med Ctr
New York Medical College, Munger Pavillion 250; Valhalla, NY 10595; (914) 493-8374; **BDCERT:** IM 84; Onc 89; **MS:** Mexico 79; **RES:** Maimonides Med Ctr, Brooklyn, NY 81-84; **FEL:** NY Med Coll, Valhalla, NY; **HOSP:** St Agnes Hosp; **SI:** Solid Tumor; **HMO:** Aetna Hlth Plan GHI Well Care US Hlthcre Oxford +

LANG: Sp; 🚫 🚗 📷 👤 🏠 Mcr Mcd WC A Few Days

Rosen, Norman (MD)   Onc
Montefiore Med Ctr

984 N Broadway 502; Yonkers, NY 10701; (718)
549-2755; **BDCERT:** Onc 77; **MS:** Tufts U 72; **RES:**
Med, Montefiore Med Ctr, Bronx, NY 73-75; **FEL:**
Onc, Montefiore Med Ctr, Bronx, NY 75-76;
Montefiore Med Ctr, Bronx, NY 76-77; **FAP:** Asst
Clin Prof Albert Einstein Coll Med; **HOSP:** St John's
Riverside Hosp; **HMO:** Oxford Blue Cross Aetna
Hlth Plan Prucare US Hlthcre +

LANG: Sp; ☒ ☎ ⊞ Ⓜ Immediately

Sadan, Sara (MD)   Onc
White Plains Hosp Ctr

12 Greenridge Ave 401; White Plains, NY 10605;
(914) 948-6600; **BDCERT:** IM 92; Onc 95; **MS:**
Israel 84; **RES:** IM, St Luke's Roosevelt Hosp Ctr,
New York, NY 89-91; **FEL:** Onc, Mem Sloan
Kettering Cancer Ctr, New York, NY 91-94; Hem,
Mem Sloan Kettering Cancer Ctr, New York, NY
91-94; **HMO:** Oxford PHS Blue Cross Aetna Hlth
Plan

LANG: Heb, Sp; ☒ ☎ ⚑ ⊞ Ⓢ Ⓜ A Few Days

Saponara, Eduardo (MD)   Onc
Lawrence Hosp

Eduardo Sapanara MD PC, 77 Pondfield Rd;
Bronxville, NY 10708; (914) 793-1500; **BDCERT:**
IM 77; Onc 79; **MS:** Peru 73; **RES:** IM, Flower Fifth
Ave Hosp, New York, NY 73-74; IM, NY Med Coll,
Valhalla, NY 77-76; **FEL:** Hem Onc, NY Med Coll,
New York, NY 77-78; Neoplastic Dis, Mount Sinai
Med Ctr, New York, NY; **FAP:** Sr Clin Instr Onc Mt
Sinai Sch Med; **HOSP:** Mount Sinai Med Ctr; **SI:**
Breast, Colon, Prostate Cancers; Preventive Medicine;
HMO: Empire Oxford CIGNA PHS Pomco +

LANG: Sp, Itl; ☒ Ⓒ ☎ ⚑ ⊞ Ⓢ Ⓜ A Few Days

Schneider, Robert (MD)   Onc
Northern Westchester Hosp Ctr

439 E Main St; Mt Kisco, NY 10549; (914) 666-
8976; **BDCERT:** IM 79; Onc 85; **MS:** Albert Einstein
Coll Med 75; **RES:** Jacobi Med Ctr, Bronx, NY 75-
78; **FEL:** Mem Sloan Kettering Cancer Ctr, New
York, NY 78-80; **HOSP:** Westchester Med Ctr;
HMO: None

☒ Ⓒ ☎ ⚑ ⊞ Ⓜ Ⓜ A Few Days

NEONATAL-PERINATAL MEDICINE

Reale, Mario (MD)   NP
Westchester Med Ctr

192 Valley Rd; Katonah, NY 10536; (914) 493-
8487; **BDCERT:** Ped 82; **MS:** Argentina 69; **RES:**
Maimonides Med Ctr, Brooklyn, NY 72-74; **FEL:**
SUNY Downstate, Brooklyn, NY 76-77

2-4 Weeks

NEPHROLOGY

Buzzeo, Louis (MD)   Nep
Phelps Mem Hosp Ctr

777 N Broadway St Suite 203; Sleepy Hollow, NY
10591; (914) 332-9100; **BDCERT:** IM 75; Nep 78;
MS: Tufts U 72; **RES:** St Vincents Hosp & Med Ctr
NY, New York, NY 72-75; St Vincents Hosp & Med
Ctr NY, New York, NY 73-75; **FEL:** Nep, New York
University Med Ctr, New York, NY 75-77; **FAP:**
Asst Prof NY Med Coll; **HMO:** Oxford PHS Metlife

Ⓒ ☎ ⚑ ⊞ Ⓢ Ⓜ 4+ Weeks

Das Gupta, Manash K (MD)   Nep
St Joseph's Med Ctr-Yonkers

9A Central Park Ave; Yonkers, NY 10705; (914)
376-3330; **BDCERT:** IM 80; Nep 90; **MS:** India 66;
RES: IM, Methodits Hosp, Brooklyn, NY 71-72;
Nep, Montefiore Med Ctr, Bronx, NY 72-74; **FAP:**
Assoc Clin Prof Albert Einstein Coll Med; **SI:** *Kidney
Diseases; Dialysis;* **HMO:** Oxford US Hlthcre

LANG: Bng, Hin; ☎ ⊞ Ⓜ 1 Week

Garrick, Renee (MD)   Nep   **PCP**
Westchester Med Ctr

Westchester Medical Center,; Valhalla, NY 10595;
(914) 493-7701; **BDCERT:** IM 81; Nep 84; **MS:**
Rush Med Coll 78; **RES:** IM, Jacobi Med Ctr, Bronx,
NY 78-81; IM, Albert Einstein Med Ctr, Bronx, NY
78-81; **FEL:** Nep, Hosp of U Penn, Philadelphia, PA
81-85; **HOSP:** St Agnes Hosp

☒ ☎ ⚑ ⊞ Ⓜ Ⓜ NFI A Few Days **VISA** 💳

Guide to symbols and abbreviations can be found on pages 110-113.

789

Goldstein, Barry (MD) Nep
Sound Shore Med Ctr-Westchester
120 Pelham Rd; New Rochelle, NY 10805; (914)
636-2611; **BDCERT:** IM 76; **MS:** NY Med Coll 73;
RES: Metropolitan Hosp Ctr, New York, NY 74-76;
FEL: Renal Disease, Metropolitan Hosp, New York,
NY 76-77; **HMO:** Aetna Hlth Plan

Goodman, Alvin (MD) Nep
Westchester Med Ctr
Westchester Co Hosp — Dept of Nephrology, Route
100; Valhalla, NY 10595; (914) 285-7701;
BDCERT: IM 65; Nep 72; **MS:** Switzerland 55; **RES:**
IM, Kingsbrook Jewish Med Ctr, Brooklyn, NY 56-
57; IM, Yale-New Haven Hosp, New Haven, CT 62-
63; **FEL:** Nep, Yale-New Haven Hosp, New Haven,
CT 60-62; **FAP:** Prof NY Med Coll; *SI: Kidney
Disease; Dialysis, Artificial Kidney;* **HMO:** Aetna Hlth
Plan Blue Choice Blue Cross & Blue Shield CIGNA
LANG: Fr; ▣ ▣ ▥ ▥ ▥ ▥ ▥ A Few Days ▥
VISA ▣

Meggs, Leonard (MD) Nep
Westchester Med Ctr
95 Grasslands Rd; Valhalla, NY 10595; (914) 285-
7701; **BDCERT:** IM 79; Nep 81; **MS:** Yale U Sch
Med 75; **RES:** Columbia-Presbyterian Med Ctr, New
York, NY 75-78; **FEL:** Nep, Brigham & Women's
Hosp, Boston, MA; **FAP:** Prof NY Med Coll; *SI:
Hypertension; Diabetic Renal Disease*
▣ ▣ ▣ ▣ ▥ ▥ ▥ ▥ Immediately

Natarajan, Sam (MD) Nep
United Hosp Med Ctr
Renal Associates, 222 Westchester Ave 201; White
Plains, NY 10604; (914) 683-6474; **BDCERT:** IM
77; **MS:** India 66; **RES:** IM, Mercy Fitzgerald Hosp,
Darby, PA 71; IM, Cumberland Med Ctr, Brooklyn,
NY 72; **FEL:** St Luke's Roosevelt Hosp Ctr, New
York, NY 73; St Luke's Roosevelt Hosp Ctr, New
York, NY 75; **HOSP:** White Plains Hosp Ctr; *SI:
Kidney Failure, Chronic; Dialysis;* **HMO:** Kaiser
Permanente Oxford US Hlthcre
LANG: Pun, Rus; ▣ ▣ ▣ ▥ ▥ ▣ ▥ ▥
A Few Days

Rie, Jonathan (MD) Nep **PCP**
White Plains Hosp Ctr
33 Davis Ave; White Plains, NY 10605; (914) 946-
5354; **BDCERT:** IM 88; Nep 90; **MS:** NY Med Coll
85; **RES:** Montefiore Med Ctr, Bronx, NY 85-86;
Montefiore Med Ctr, Bronx, NY 86-88; **FEL:**
Montefiore Med Ctr, Bronx, NY 88-89; Montefiore
Med Ctr, Bronx, NY 89-90; **HMO:** Oxford PHS
Anthem Health Blue Choice NYLCare +
▣ ▣ ▣ ▥ ▥ ▣ ▥ ▥ A Few Days *VISA* ▣

Saltzman, Martin (MD) Nep
Northern Westchester Hosp Ctr
41 S Bedford Rd; Mt Kisco, NY 10549; (914) 666-
5588; **BDCERT:** IM 77; Nep 78; **MS:** SUNY Hlth Sci
Ctr 72; **RES:** IM, Kings County Hosp Ctr, Brooklyn,
NY 72-73; Harlem Hosp Ctr, New York, NY 73-74;
FEL: Nep, Univ Hosp SUNY Bklyn, Brooklyn, NY
74-76; *SI: Renal Disease, Acute and Chronic;
Hypertension & Nephritis;* **HMO:** Blue Choice Pomco
PHS Oxford
▣ ▥ ▣ ▥ ▥ A Few Days

Stein, Martin F (MD) Nep
St Joseph's Med Ctr-Yonkers
127 S Broadway; Yonkers, NY 10701; (914) 378-
7581; **BDCERT:** IM 77; **MS:** Albany Med Coll 62;
RES: Med, St Luke's Roosevelt Hosp Ctr, New York,
NY 63-65; Med, VA Med Ctr-Bronx, Bronx, NY 65-
66; **FAP:** Assoc Clin Prof Med NY Med Coll; **HMO:**
Oxford Prudential Empire Blue Cross & Shield
CIGNA +
LANG: Ger; ▣ ▣ ▥ ▥ Immediately

NEUROLOGICAL SURGERY

Benzil, Deborah (MD)   NS
Westchester Med Ctr
Neurological & Spine Surgery Associates, Route 100 Munger Pavilion; Valhalla, NY 10595; (914) 403-8302; **BDCERT:** NS 97; **MS:** U Md Sch Med 85; **RES:** NS, Rhode Island Hosp, Providence, RI 87-94; **FEL:** NS, Nat Inst Health, Bethesda, MD; **FAP:** Assoc Prof NY Med Coll; **SI:** *Peripheral Nerve Repair; Stereotactic Radiosurgery;* **HMO:** Oxford GHI Empire Blue Cross & Blue Shield US Hlthcre +

LANG: Sp; ♿ 🅰 🏠 💲 Mcr Mcd WC NFI   1 Week

Duffy, Kent (MD)   NS
Westchester Med Ctr
22 Westchester Ave 202; White Plains, NY 10604; (914) 948-2288; **BDCERT:** NS 93; **MS:** Temple U 80; **RES:** NS, UCLA Med Ctr, Los Angeles, CA 82-88

Kasoff, Samuel (MD)   NS
Westchester Med Ctr
3141 Route 9 W; New Windsor, NY 12553; (914) 562-9200; **BDCERT:** NS 76; **MS:** Univ Pittsburgh 63; **RES:** Albert Einstein Coll Med,, Bronx, NY 73; **HOSP:** United Hosp Med Ctr

Lansen, Thomas (MD)   NS
Lawrence Hosp
Neurosurgeons of New York, 222 Westchester Ave 202; White Plains, NY 10604; (914) 948-8448; **BDCERT:** NS 83; **MS:** Med Coll Wisc 73; **RES:** New York University Med Ctr, New York, NY 73-74; U FL Shands Hosp, Gainesville, FL 75-80; **HOSP:** Northern Westchester Hosp Ctr; **HMO:** Oxford Aetna-US Healthcare US Hlthcre GHI Anthem Health +

♿ 🅰 🏠 💲 Mcr Mcd WC NFI   1 Week

Oestreich, Herbert (MD)   NS
White Plains Hosp Ctr
New York Medical College; Valhalla, NY 10595; (914) 493-8392; **BDCERT:** NS 66; **MS:** Cornell U 57; **RES:** Montefiore Med Ctr, Bronx, NY 58; **HOSP:** Westchester Med Ctr; **SI:** *Radiosurgery*

♿ 🅰 🚼 🏠 Mcr Mcd WC NFI   A Few Days

Rosner, Saran (MD)   NS
Phelps Mem Hosp Ctr
245 Saw Mill River Rd; Hawthorne, NY 10532; (914) 741-2666; **BDCERT:** NS 86; **MS:** Columbia P&S 76; **RES:** NS, Columbia-Presbyterian Med Ctr, New York, NY 78-72; S, Johns Hopkins Hosp, Baltimore, MD 76-78; **FEL:** Microneurosurgery, U FL Shands Hosp, Gainesville, FL 82; **FAP:** Instr Columbia P&S; **HOSP:** Hudson Valley Hosp Ctr; **SI:** *Spinal Surgery; Tumors of the Brain & Spine;* **HMO:** Oxford US Hlthcre Pomco GHI +

LANG: Itl; ♿ 🅰 🚼 🏠 💲 Mcr WC NFI   A Few Days

Stern, Jack (MD)   NS
White Plains Hosp Ctr
Neurosurgical Group, 222 Westchester Ave 202; White Plains, NY 10604; (914) 948-6688; **BDCERT:** NS 82; **MS:** Albert Einstein Coll Med 71; **RES:** N, Bellevue Hosp Ctr, New York, NY 74-76; N, Columbia-Presbyterian Med Ctr, New York, NY 76-80; **HOSP:** Lenox Hill Hosp

LANG: Sp, Fr, Heb; ♿ 🅲 🅰 🏠 💲 Mcr Mcd WC NFI
A Few Days 🔲

NEUROLOGY

Ahluwalia, Brij Mohan Singh (MD)   N
Westchester Med Ctr
Route 100 Munger Pavilion 4th Fl; Valhalla, NY 10595; (914) 594-4293; **BDCERT:** N 74; **MS:** India 61; **RES:** Rajindra Hosp Patiala India, Patiala, India 62-63; Beekman Downtown Hosp, New York, NY 68; **HMO:** Prucare Pomco Oxford

Brown, Alan Joseph (MD)   N
St John's Riverside Hosp

984 N Broadway 417; Yonkers, NY 10701; (914) 968-2322; **BDCERT:** N 68; **MS:** Vanderbilt U Sch Med 60; **RES:** N, Jacobi Med Ctr, Bronx, NY 62-65; VA Med Ctr-Bronx, Bronx, NY 61-62; *SI: Neck & Back Pain; Dementia;* **HMO:** Oxford US Hlthcre Aetna-US Healthcare CIGNA SWCHP +

LANG: Sp, Ger, Fr; 🔲 🔲 🔲 🔲 Mcr WC NFI

Dickoff, David (MD)   N
St John's Riverside Hosp

984 N Broadway 509; Yonkers, NY 10701; (914) 968-0620; **BDCERT:** N 87; **MS:** Albany Med Coll 82; **RES:** IM, Mount Sinai Med Ctr, New York, NY 82-83; N, Mount Sinai Med Ctr, New York, NY 83-86; **FEL:** Columbia-Presbyterian Med Ctr, New York, NY 86-87; **HOSP:** St Joseph's Med Ctr-Yonkers; *SI: Parkinson's Disease; Peripheral Neuropathy;* **HMO:** Oxford CIGNA Aetna Hlth Plan Prucare

LANG: Fr, Sp; 🔲 🔲 🔲 🔲 🔲 Mcr WC NFI A Few Days ▪▪▪ **VISA** ●

Green, Mark (MD)   N
Northern Westchester Hosp Ctr

Mount Kisco Med Group, 90 S Bedford Rd; Mt Kisco, NY 10549; (914) 241-1050; **BDCERT:** N 78; **MS:** Albert Einstein Coll Med 74; **RES:** N, Albert Einstein Med Ctr, Bronx, NY 75-79; Montefiore Med Ctr, Bronx, NY; **FAP:** Assoc Clin Prof N NY Med Coll; *SI: Headache;* **HMO:** Aetna Hlth Plan Prucare Oxford US Hlthcre

🔲 🔲 🔲 🔲 🔲 Mcr 4+ Weeks **VISA**

Gross, Elliott (MD)   N
United Hosp Med Ctr

32 Rye Ridge Plaza; Rye Brook, NY 10573; (914) 251-1010; **BDCERT:** N 69; **MS:** Albert Einstein Coll Med 62; **RES:** N, Albert Einstein Med Ctr, Bronx, NY 63-66; **FEL:** N, Albert Einstein Med Ctr, Bronx, NY 68-70; **FAP:** Asst Prof of Clin Albert Einstein Coll Med; *SI: Headache; Alzheimer;* **HMO:** Aetna Hlth Plan Prucare CIGNA Pomco Oxford +

LANG: Sp, Heb, Fr; 🔲 🔲 🔲 🔲 Mcr Mod WC NFI Immediately

Koppel, Barbara (MD)   N
Westchester Med Ctr

Route 100 Munger Pavilion 401; Valhalla, NY 10595; (914) 594-4293; **BDCERT:** N 83; **MS:** Columbia P&S 78; **RES:** Med, Montefiore U Hosp, Pittsburgh, PA 78-79; N, Columbia-Presbyterian Med Ctr, New York, NY 79-82; **FAP:** Prof NY Med Coll; **HOSP:** Metropolitan Hosp Ctr; *SI: Neurological Complications AIDS; Seizures;* **HMO:** Magnacare Empire Blue Cross Aetna-US Healthcare Oxford

LANG: Sp; 🔲 🔲 🔲 🔲 🔲 Mcr NFI A Few Days **VISA** ●

Kranzler, L Stephan (MD)   N
White Plains Hosp Ctr

30 Davis Ave; White Plains, NY 10605; (914) 946-9444; **BDCERT:** N 90; **MS:** Univ Penn 85; **RES:** Hosp of U Penn, Philadelphia, PA 86; N, Columbia-Presbyterian Med Ctr, New York, NY 89; **HMO:** Oxford Aetna-US Healthcare Pomco Blue Choice

LANG: Sp, Itl, Fr; 🔲 🔲 🔲 🔲 Mcr Mod WC NFI 1 Week **VISA** ●

Marks, Stephen (MD)   N
Westchester Med Ctr

10 Stewart Pl; White Plains, NY 10603; (914) 594-4296; **BDCERT:** N 85; **MS:** NY Med Coll 80; **RES:** N, Mount Sinai Med Ctr, New York, NY 81-84; **FEL:** Cv, Duke U Med Ctr, Durham, NC 84-85; **FAP:** Asst Prof NY Med Coll; *SI: Cerebrovascular Disease; Dementia;* **HMO:** Blue Choice Lawrence Healthcare Aetna Hlth Plan Oxford CIGNA +

🔲 🔲 🔲 🔲 🔲 Mcr WC 4+ Weeks **VISA** ●

Robbins, John (MD)   N
Phelps Mem Hosp Ctr

Sarah S Rosner MC & John B Robins, MD, PC, 245 Saw Mill River Rd; Hawthorne, NY 10532; (914) 741-2666; **BDCERT:** NS 91; **MS:** Brown U 78; **RES:** S, Montefiore Med Ctr, Bronx, NY 81-82; NS, NY Hosp-Cornell Med Ctr, New York, NY 86-88; **HOSP:** Northern Westchester Hosp Ctr; *SI: Spinal Surgery; Brain Tumors;* **HMO:** Most

🔲 🔲 🔲 🔲 🔲 Mcr WC NFI A Few Days

Rothman, Allan (MD) N
Phelps Mem Hosp Ctr

325 S Highland Ave; Briarcliff Manor, NY 10510; (914) 941-0788; **BDCERT:** N 84; **MS:** SUNY Hlth Sci Ctr 77; **RES:** Mount Sinai Med Ctr, New York, NY 77-78; N, Mount Sinai Med Ctr, New York, NY 78-81; *SI: Parkinson's Disease; Migraine*

🛆 📷 🚗 🏥 💲 Mcr WC NFI Immediately **VISA** 💳

Selman, Jay E (MD) N
Northern Westchester Hosp Ctr

117 Smith Ave; Mt Kisco, NY 10549; (914) 241-1616; **BDCERT:** N 80; **MS:** U Tex SW, Dallas 73; **RES:** Ped, Jacobi Med Ctr, Bronx, NY 73-75; NS, Jacobi Med Ctr, Bronx, NY 75-78; **FAP:** Asst Prof NS Columbia P&S; **HMO:** Oxford PHS Chubb

LANG: Sp, Fr, Dan, Ger, Itl; 🛆 📷 🚗 🏥 💲 Mcr WC NFI A Few Days **VISA** 💳

Singh, Avtar (MD) N
White Plains Hosp Ctr

303 North St 202; White Plains, NY 10605; (914) 946-2552; **BDCERT:** N 78; **MS:** India 67; **RES:** N, Metropolitan Hosp Ctr, New York, NY 73-76; **HOSP:** St Agnes Hosp; *SI: Stroke Management; Epilepsy;* **HMO:** Aetna Hlth Plan Blue Choice Aetna-US Healthcare Independent Health Plan Oxford +

LANG: Sp, Hin, Ur, Pun; 🛆 SA/SU 💳 📷 🚗 🏥 💲 Mcr WC NFI 1 Week **VISA** 💳

Weintraub, Michael (MD) N
Phelps Mem Hosp Ctr

325 S Highland Ave; Briarcliff Manor, NY 10510; (914) 941-0788; **BDCERT:** N 72; **MS:** SUNY Buffalo 66; **RES:** N, EJ Meyer Mem Hosp, Buffalo, NY 67-68; **FEL:** N, Yale-New Haven Hosp, New Haven, CT 68-70; **FAP:** Clin Prof NY Med Coll; **HOSP:** Putnam Hosp Ctr; *SI: Pain Management; Carpal Tunnel Syndrome*

LANG: Sp; 🛆 📷 🚗 🏥 💲 Mcr Mcd WC NFI A Few Days **VISA** 💳

NEURORADIOLOGY

Tenner, Michael (MD) NRad
Westchester Med Ctr

Route 100 Munger Pavilion; Valhalla, NY 10595; (914) 347-2010; **BDCERT:** Rad 67; **MS:** U Md Sch Med 60; **RES:** U MD Hosp, Baltimore, MD 61-62; US Army Med Corp, 62-64; **FEL:** NR, Columbia-Presbyterian Med Ctr, New York, NY 66-67; **HMO:** Well Care Oxford GHI Pomco Prudential +

LANG: Sp; 🛆 📷 💳 🚗 🏥 💲 Mcr Mcd WC NFI A Few Days **VISA** 💳

NUCLEAR MEDICINE

Patel, Kamini (MD) NuM
Bronx Lebanon Hosp Ctr

27 Maole Ave; Dobbs Ferry, NY 10522; (914) 562-1661; **BDCERT:** NuM 85; **MS:** India 71; **RES:** IM, United Hosp Med Ctr, Port Chester, NY 80-83; NuM, Montefiore Med Ctr, Bronx, NY 83-85; **FAP:** Instr NuM Albert Einstein Coll Med

NUCLEAR RADIOLOGY

Perez, Louis A (MD) NR
Lawrence Hosp

55 Palmer Ave; Bronxville, NY 10708; (914) 237-4902; **BDCERT:** NR 74; **MS:** SUNY Hlth Sci Ctr 66; **RES:** Rad, Bronx Muncipal Hosp Ctr, Bronx, NY 67-70

Guide to symbols and abbreviations can be found on pages 110-113.

793

OBSTETRICS & GYNECOLOGY

Adachi, Akinori (MD)   ObG   **PCP**
Montefiore Med Ctr
30 Lockwood Rd; Scarsdale, NY 10583; (718) 519-3879; **BDCERT:** ObG 73; **MS:** Japan 63; **RES:** Jewish Mem Hosp, New York, NY 65-68; **FEL:** GO, NY Med Coll, Valhalla, NY 68-69; Gynecologic EDM, Metropolitan Hosp Ctr, New York, NY 70-71; **FAP:** Assoc Prof Albert Einstein Coll Med; *SI: GYN Checkup, Cancer Therapy; Pelvic Reconstruction*; **HMO:** Aetna Hlth Plan Blue Choice CIGNA Oxford Bronx Health +

LANG: Jpn; [icons] A Few Days **VISA** 💳

Armbruster, Robert (MD)   ObG
Lawrence Hosp
77 Pondfield Rd; Bronxville, NY 10708; (914) 337-3227; **BDCERT:** ObG 84; **MS:** Washington U, St Louis 77; **RES:** UCLA Med Ctr, Los Angeles, CA 77-79; NY Hosp-Cornell Med Ctr, New York, NY 79-81; **HMO:** Oxford Prucare CIGNA US Hlthcre Pomco +

LANG: Sp, Grk, Fr; [icons] 2-4 Weeks

Barad, David (MD)   ObG
Montefiore Med Ctr-Weiler/Einstein Div
20 Beacon Hill Dr; Dobbs Ferry, NY 10522; (914) 693-8820; **BDCERT:** ObG 85; GO 94; **MS:** UMDNJ-RW Johnson Med Sch 78; **RES:** ObG, Columbia-Presbyterian Med Ctr, New York, NY 79-82; **FEL:** ObG, Brigham & Women's Hosp, Boston, MA 82-84; **HOSP:** Community Hosp At Dobbs Ferry; *SI: Infertility; Fibroids; Endometriosis Laparoscopy*

[icons] **VISA** 💳

Burns, Elisa (MD)   ObG
Northern Westchester Hosp Ctr
90 S Bedford Rd; Mt Kisco, NY 10549; (914) 241-1050; **BDCERT:** ObG 88; ObG 98; **MS:** Columbia P&S 82; **RES:** Columbia-Presbyterian Med Ctr, New York, NY 82-86; *SI: Menopause; Colposcopy*; **HMO:** United Healthcare Oxford Aetna Hlth Plan PHS Independent Health Plan +

[icons] 2-4 Weeks

Carolan, Stephen (MD)   ObG   **PCP**
United Hosp Med Ctr
14 Rye Ridge Plaza 244; Rye Brook, NY 10573; (914) 253-4912; **BDCERT:** ObG 90; **MS:** NY Med Coll 84; **RES:** U Conn Hlth Ctr, Farmington, CT 84-88; *SI: Minimally Invasive Surgery; Fibroids*; **HMO:** Oxford Aetna Hlth Plan US Hlthcre NYLCare CIGNA +

LANG: Sp; [icons] 1 Week **VISA** 💳 [icon]

D'Amico, Vincent M (MD)   ObG
White Plains Hosp Ctr
30 Greenridge Ave; White Plains, NY 10605; (914) 428-4400; **BDCERT:** ObG 75; **MS:** NY Med Coll 68; **RES:** Metropolitan Hosp Ctr, New York, NY; **HOSP:** Westchester Med Ctr; *SI: Laparoscopic Surgery*; **HMO:** Aetna Hlth Plan Independent Health Plan

LANG: Sp; [icons] Immediately [icon] **VISA** 💳 💳

Du Vigneaud, Vincent (MD) ObG
St Agnes Hosp
50 Popham Rd; Scarsdale, NY 10583; (914) 472-6555; **BDCERT:** ObG 68; **MS:** Cornell U 59; **RES:** ObG, Columbia-Presbyterian Med Ctr, New York, NY 60-63; ObG, St Luke's Roosevelt Hosp Ctr, New York, NY 63-65; **FAP:** Asst Clin Prof ObG Cornell U; **HOSP:** United Hosp Med Ctr; **HMO:** Aetna Hlth Plan CIGNA Oxford Metlife Oxford +

LANG: Itl, Sp; [icons] A Few Days

Eilen, Bonnie (MD) ObG
White Plains Hosp Ctr

30 Davis Ave; White Plains, NY 10605; (914) 946-7274; **BDCERT:** ObG 83; **MS:** Albert Einstein Coll Med 77; **RES:** ObG, Bronx Municipal Hosp, Bronx, NY

Florio, Philip (MD) ObG **PCP**
St John's Riverside Hosp

1022 N Broadway; Yonkers, NY 10701; (914) 963-0284; **BDCERT:** ObG 81; **MS:** SUNY Syracuse 74; **RES:** ObG, St Barnabas Med Ctr, Livingston, NJ 74-78; **SI:** *High Risk Obstetric; Hormone Therapy;* **HMO:** Oxford Blue Choice Aetna Hlth Plan PHS

LANG: Itl, Sp; [symbols] Immediately
VISA [symbols]

Friedman, Norman (MD) ObG
St John's Riverside Hosp

984 N Broadway LL04; Yonkers, NY 10701; (914) 965-2900; **BDCERT:** ObG 67; **MS:** SUNY Hlth Sci Ctr 55; **RES:** Long Island Coll Hosp, Brooklyn, NY 59-62; **HMO:** Aetna-US Healthcare Blue Choice Oxford United Healthcare Independent Health Plan +

LANG: Sp, Itl; [symbols] A Few Days

Giuffrida, Regina (MD) ObG **PCP**
Northern Westchester Hosp Ctr

Mt Kisco Medical Group, 90 S Bedford Rd; Mt Kisco, NY 10549; (914) 241-1050; **BDCERT:** ObG 96; **MS:** NY Med Coll 80; **RES:** ObG, UC San Diego Med Ctr, San Diego, CA 80-84; **SI:** *Menopause;* **HMO:** Aetna-US Healthcare Oxford PHS

LANG: Sp; [symbols] 2-4 Weeks **VISA** [symbols]

Grano, Vanessa (MD) ObG
United Hosp Med Ctr

14 Rye Ridge Plaza 244; Rye Brook, NY 10573; (914) 253-4912; **BDCERT:** ObG 95; **MS:** SUNY Downstate 88; **RES:** ObG, Columbia-Presbyterian Med Ctr, New York, NY; **SI:** *Colposcopy of Cervical Problems; Breast Feeding;* **HMO:** Aetna-US Healthcare CIGNA PHS Prucare Oxford +

[symbols] 1 Week **VISA** [symbols]

Greenlee, Robert (MD) ObG
Sound Shore Med Ctr-Westchester

838 Pelhamdale Ave; New Rochelle, NY 10801; (914) 235-2900; **BDCERT:** ObG 82; **MS:** Mexico 75; **RES:** ObG, St Lukes Hosp, New York, NY 77-80

LANG: Sp; [symbols] 1 Week [symbols] **VISA** [symbols]

Hayworth, Scott (MD) ObG **PCP**
Northern Westchester Hosp Ctr

Mt Kisco Medical Group, 90 S Bedford Rd; Mt Kisco, NY 10549; (914) 241-1050; **BDCERT:** ObG 90; **MS:** Cornell U 84; **RES:** ObG, Mount Sinai Med Ctr, New York, NY 84-88; **SI:** *Laser Surgery; Laparoscopic Surgery;* **HMO:** Oxford PHS United Healthcare Aetna-US Healthcare Prudential +

[symbols] 1 Week [symbols] **VISA** [symbols]

Henderson, Cassandra (MD) ObG
Montefiore Med Ctr-Weiler/Einstein Div

1 Madison Ave; Larchmont, NY 10538; (718) 405-8200; **BDCERT:** ObG 87; **MS:** Loyola U-Stritch Sch Med, Maywood 80; **RES:** ObG, U Chicago Hosp, Chicago, IL 84-88; **HOSP:** Montefiore Med Ctr; **HMO:** Aetna Hlth Plan Blue Choice Blue Cross & Blue Shield CIGNA HIP Network +

Howard, James (MD) ObG **PCP**
White Plains Hosp Ctr

170 Maple Ave Ste 309; White Plains, NY 10601; (914) 949-8338; **BDCERT:** ObG 66; **MS:** Jefferson Med Coll 59; **RES:** Pennsylvania Hosp, Philadelphia, PA 63; **SI:** *Infertility;* **HMO:** PHS Oxford

LANG: Sp; [symbols] Immediately [symbols] **VISA** [symbols]

Kalinsky, Jay (MD) ObG `PCP`
Hudson Valley Hosp Ctr
Hudson Valley OB-GYN Assoiciates, 1985
Crompond Rd Ste B; Peekskill, NY 10566; (914)
739-1697; **BDCERT:** ObG 80; **MS:** U Miami Sch
Med 73; **RES:** ObG, Bronx Muncipal Hosp Ctr,
Bronx, NY 74-77; *SI: Midwifery; High Risk
Pregnancies*; **HMO:** Aetna-US Healthcare CIGNA
PPO United Healthcare Oxford Magnacare +
♿ 🅂🅄 🌙 📷 👤 🎦 💲 Mcr 4+ Weeks 💳 *VISA* 💳
💳

Klugman, Susan (MD) ObG `PCP`
Montefiore Med Ctr-Weiler/Einstein Div
1 Madison Ave; Larchmont, NY 10583; (914) 834-
4422; **BDCERT:** ObG 95; **MS:** NYU Sch Med 88;
RES: ObG, Albert Einstein Med Ctr, Bronx, NY 88-
92; **FAP:** Asst Prof ObG Albert Einstein Coll Med; *SI:
High Risk Pregnancy; Laparoscopy—Adolescents*;
HMO: Most
LANG: Itl, Sp; ♿ 📷 👤 🎦 💲 Mcr 1 Week *VISA* 💳

Loiacono, Anthony F (MD) ObG
White Plains Hosp Ctr
280 Mamaroneck Ave; White Plains, NY 10605;
(914) 949-0108; **BDCERT:** ObG 66; **MS:** SUNY
Downstate 59; **RES:** ObG, St John's Epis Hosp-S
Shore, Far Rockaway, NY 59-63; **FAP:** Asst Clin
Prof NY Med Coll; **HOSP:** St Agnes Hosp; *SI:
Laparoscopic Surgery; Endometrial Ablation*; **HMO:**
CIGNA Blue Choice Oxford PHS Pomco +
LANG: Itl; ♿ 📷 👤 🎦 💲 Mcr WC NFI A Few Days

Mastrantonio, John (MD) ObG
Montefiore Med Ctr-Weiler/Einstein Div
191525 Central Ave; Yonkers, NY 10710; (914)
961-0201; **BDCERT:** ObG 74; **MS:** SUNY Hlth Sci
Ctr 67; **RES:** Bronx Muncipal Hosp Ctr, Bronx, NY
68-72; **FAP:** Asst Clin Prof Albert Einstein Coll Med;
HOSP: Montefiore Med Ctr; **HMO:** Oxford Aetna-US
Healthcare United Healthcare PHS GHI +
LANG: Itl; ♿ 🅂🅄 🌙 📷 👤 🎦 Mcr A Few Days

Meacham, Kevin (MD) ObG
Sound Shore Med Ctr-Westchester
2071 Boston Post Rd; Larchmont, NY 10538;
(914) 833-1000; **BDCERT:** ObG 93; **MS:** NY Med
Coll 86; **RES:** ObG, Long Island Jewish Med Ctr,
New Hyde Park, NY 87-90; *SI: Laparoscopic Surgery;
Infertility*; **HMO:** Oxford Pomco Aetna Hlth Plan US
Hlthcre +
LANG: Sp; ♿ 🅂🅄 🌙 📷 👤 🎦 💲 Mcr NFI 2-4 Weeks
💳 *VISA* 💳 💳

Mendelowitz, Lawrence (MD)ObG `PCP`
Phelps Mem Hosp Ctr
Sleepy Hollow Medical Group, 99 N Broadway;
Tarrytown, NY 10591; (914) 631-0337; **BDCERT:**
ObG 82; **MS:** NYU Sch Med 76; **RES:** ObG, Bellevue
Hosp Ctr, New York, NY 76-80; **FAP:** Clin Instr NY
Med Coll; **HOSP:** Westchester Med Ctr; *SI: Pelvic
Reconstructive Surgery*; **HMO:** PHS CIGNA Oxford
Independent Health Plan Prucare +
LANG: Sp; ♿ 🌙 📷 👤 🎦 💲 Mcr Mcd WC NFI
Immediately *VISA* 💳

Mendelowitz, Mark (MD) ObG
Phelps Mem Hosp Ctr
Sleepyhollow Medical Group, 99 N Broadway;
Tarrytown, NY 10591; (914) 631-0337; **BDCERT:**
ObG 88; **MS:** NYU Sch Med 82; **RES:** ObG, U Hosp,
Cincinnati, OH; **HOSP:** Westchester Med Ctr; **HMO:**
US Hlthcre PHS GHI Lawrence Healthcare
Independent Health Plan +
LANG: Sp; ♿ 📷 👤 🎦 💲 Mcr WC NFI 4+ Weeks
VISA 💳

Mootabar, Hamid (MD) ObG
Lawrence Hospital
Amniocentesis & Genetics Ctr, 1990 Central Park
Ave; Yonkers, NY 10710; (914) 337-2102;
BDCERT: ObG 75; **MS:** Iran 66; **RES:** Lawrence
Hosp, Bronxville, NY 68-69; ObG, St Luke's
Roosevelt Hosp Ctr, New York, NY 74; **FEL:** MF, St
Luke's Roosevelt Hosp Ctr, New York, NY 74-78;
FAP: Assoc Clin Prof ObG SUNY Buffalo; **HOSP:**
Staten Island Univ Hosp-North

Nelson, William (MD)   ObG
Montefiore Med Ctr-Weiler/Einstein Div
Rye Brook Ob/Gyn, 14 Rye Ridge Plaza 244; Rye Brook, NY 10573; (914) 253-4912; **BDCERT:** ObG 81; **MS:** Albert Einstein Coll Med 60; **RES:** ObG, Maimonides Med Ctr, Brooklyn, NY 61-65; **FAP:** Asst Clin Prof Albert Einstein Coll Med; *SI: Menopause; Perimenopause;* **HMO:** Oxford Aetna-US Healthcare PHS Pomco SWCHP +

⟨symbols⟩ 2-4 Weeks ▨ *VISA* ⬤ ⬤

Neubardt, Selig (MD)   ObG   PCP
Sound Shore Med Ctr-Westchester
2071 Boston Post Rd; Larchmont, NY 10538; (914) 833-1000; **BDCERT:** ObG 56; **MS:** SUNY Hlth Sci Ctr 52; **RES:** Maimonides Med Ctr, Brooklyn, NY 52-53; Maimonides Med Ctr, Brooklyn, NY 53-55; **FEL:** ObG, Albert Einstein Med Ctr, Bronx, NY 55-58; **FAP:** Asst Clin Prof Albert Einstein Coll Med; *SI: Office Gynecology; Menopause;* **HMO:** Oxford

⟨symbols⟩ Immediately *VISA*

Nigro, Antoinette (MD)   ObG   PCP
Northern Westchester Hosp Ctr
1825 Commerce St; Yorktown Heights, NY 10598; (914) 962-5060; **BDCERT:** ObG 93; **MS:** NY Med Coll 86; **RES:** ObG, Flushing Hosp/Queens Hosp, Queens, NY 87-90

⟨symbols⟩ 4+ Weeks ▨ *VISA* ⬤ ▨

Novendstern, Joel (MD)   ObG
Northern Westchester Hosp Ctr
666 Lexington Ave; Mt Kisco, NY 10549; (914) 666-0019; **BDCERT:** ObG 82; **MS:** Georgetown U 75; **RES:** ObG, NY Med Coll, New York, NY 75-79; **HOSP:** United Hosp Med Ctr; *SI: Infertility; Reproductive Surgery;* **HMO:** Oxford Aetna Hlth Plan United Healthcare CIGNA GHI +

LANG: Sp; ⟨symbols⟩ A Few Days *VISA* ⬤

Oberlander, Samuel (MD)   ObG
Montefiore Med Ctr-Weiler/Einstein Div
1254 Central Park Ave; Yonkers, NY 10704; (914) 423-4111; **BDCERT:** ObG 74; **MS:** Harvard Med Sch 65; **RES:** ObG, Bronx Muncipal Hosp Ctr, Bronx, NY 66-67; **HOSP:** Lawrence Hosp; **HMO:** Aetna Hlth Plan Blue Cross & Blue Shield CIGNA HealthNet Montefiore IPA +

⟨symbols⟩ 1 Week

Orofino, Michael (MD)   ObG
Lawrence Hosp
45 Mill Rd; Eastchester, NY 10709; (914) 793-2070; **BDCERT:** ObG 95; **MS:** Mexico 79; **RES:** NY Med Coll, Valhalla, NY 79-84; Lincoln Med & Mental Hlth Ctr, Bronx, NY; **HOSP:** Mount Vernon Hosp

⟨symbols⟩ Immediately

Parker, Albert (MD)   ObG
United Hosp Med Ctr
Ryebrook OBGYN, 14 Rye Ridge Plaza; Port Chester, NY 10573; (914) 253-4912; **BDCERT:** ObG 67; **MS:** Harvard Med Sch 58; **RES:** Boston Med Ctr, Boston, MA; **HOSP:** NY Hosp-Cornell Med Ctr; **HMO:** CIGNA Prucare Oxford Aetna Hlth Plan

⟨symbols⟩ A Few Days

Pawl, Nancy (MD)   ObG
Sound Shore Med Ctr-Westchester
110 Lockwood Ave 300; New Rochelle, NY 10801; (914) 632-8164; **BDCERT:** ObG 91; **MS:** Harvard Med Sch 80; **RES:** Columbia-Presbyterian Med Ctr, New York, NY 80-84; **HMO:** Aetna Hlth Plan Blue Choice Travelers HealthNet

⟨symbols⟩ 4+ Weeks ▨ *VISA* ⬤

Razmzan, Shahram (MD)   ObG
St John's Riverside Hosp
Southern Westchester OB/GYN Associates, LLP, 656 Yonkers Ave; Yonkers, NY 10704; (914) 963-3366; **BDCERT:** ObG 89; **MS:** Grenada 82; **RES:** ObG, NY Med Coll, Valhalla, NY 83-87; **HOSP:** St Joseph's Med Ctr-Yonkers; *SI: Laparoscopic Surgery; High Risk Pregnancy;* **HMO:** Oxford US Hlthcre United Healthcare Magnacare Prudential +

LANG: Sp, Itl; ⟨symbols⟩ A Few Days

Reilly, Kevin B (MD) ObG PCP
Northern Westchester Hosp Ctr
90 S Bedford Rd; Mt Kisco, NY 10549; (914) 241-1050; **BDCERT:** ObG 79; **MS:** SUNY Hlth Sci Ctr 70; **RES:** ObG, Columbia-Presbyterian Med Ctr, New York, NY 73-77; **HOSP:** Westchester Med Ctr; *SI: Ultrasound; Genetic Screening and Testing;* **HMO:** Oxford Aetna Hlth Plan PHS

♿ 🔲 🔲 🔲 🔲 🔲 🔲 🔲 A Few Days

Schneider, Ronald (MD) ObG
Sound Shore Med Ctr-Westchester
Obstetric & Gynecological Assoc of Westchester, PC, 110 Lockwood Ave 300; New Rochelle, NY 10801; (914) 632-8164; **BDCERT:** ObG 81; **MS:** NY Med Coll 75; **RES:** Long Island Jewish Med Ctr, New Hyde Park, NY 75-79; **HOSP:** Sound Shore Med Ctr-Westchester; *SI: Surgery*

LANG: Sp; ♿ 🔲 🔲 🔲 🔲 🔲 🔲 2-4 Weeks
VISA 💳

Semple, Sandra (MD) ObG
Phelps Mem Hosp Ctr
280 Dobbs Ferry Rd 308; White Plains, NY 10607; (914) 946-5202; **BDCERT:** ObG 88; **MS:** Temple U 80; **RES:** Harlem Hosp Ctr, New York, NY 81; **HOSP:** St Agnes Hosp; **HMO:** US Hlthcre PHS Oxford Metlife

♿ 🔲 🔲 🔲 🔲 🔲 🔲 A Few Days

Shojai, E Mohajer (MD) ObG
St John's Riverside Hosp
944 N Broadway Ste 207; Yonkers, NY 10701; (914) 969-6677; **BDCERT:** ObG 76; **MS:** Iran 64; **RES:** ObG, Harlem Hosp Ctr, New York, NY 68-69; ObG, St Luke's Roosevelt Hosp Ctr, New York, NY 69-72; **FEL:** Family Planning, Harlem Hosp Ctr, New York, NY 72-74; **HOSP:** St Joseph's Med Ctr-Yonkers; **HMO:** Oxford US Hlthcre CIGNA PHS United Healthcare +

LANG: Per; ♿ 🔲 🔲 🔲 🔲 🔲 🔲 A Few Days

Silverman, Barney (MD) ObG PCP
White Plains Hosp Ctr
Westchester Gynecologists, 170 Maple Ave 309; White Plains, NY 10601; (914) 949-8338; **BDCERT:** ObG 73; **MS:** KY Med Sch, Louisville 64; **RES:** Hosp U Penn, Philadelphia, PA 67-71; **FAP:** Assoc Clin Prof Yale U Sch Med; **HMO:** PHS

LANG: Sp; ♿ 🔲 🔲 🔲 🔲 🔲 🔲 🔲 A Few Days
VISA 💳

Suvannavejh, Chaisurat (MD)ObG
Mount Vernon Hosp
559 Gramatan Ave; Mt Vernon, NY 10552; (914) 668-8601; **BDCERT:** ObG 76; **MS:** Thailand 68; **RES:** Mount Vernon Hosp, Mt Vernon, NY 70-73; **HOSP:** Lawrence Hosp; **HMO:** Oxford Blue Choice Sanus-NYLCare CIGNA Magnacare +

Tejani, Nergesh (MD) ObG PCP
Westchester Square Med Ctr
Route 100 Macy Pavilion; Valhalla, NY 10595; (914) 493-1575; **BDCERT:** ObG 75; **MF** 79; **MS:** India 56; **RES:** ObG, New York Methodist Hosp, Brooklyn, NY 71-73; *SI: Maternal Fetal Medicine;* **HMO:** Aetna Hlth Plan Oxford GHI Prucare US Hlthcre +

♿ 🔲 🔲 🔲 🔲 🔲 **VISA** 💳

Ullman, Joel (MD) ObG
Sound Shore Med Ctr-Westchester
Gynecology & Obstetric Assoc, 2071 Boston Post Rd; Larchmont, NY 10538; (914) 833-1000; **BDCERT:** ObG 71; **MS:** NY Med Coll 63; **RES:** ObG, Beth Israel Med Ctr, New York, NY 64-69; **FAP:** Asst Clin Prof Albert Einstein Coll Med; *SI: Laparoscopic Surgery; Hysteroscopic Surgery;* **HMO:** Oxford Blue Shield Metlife CIGNA Aetna Hlth Plan +

LANG: Sp; ♿ 🔲 🔲 🔲 🔲 🔲 🔲 1 Week **VISA** 💳

Witt, Barry (MD)   ObG
Montefiore Med Ctr

Montefiore Fertility & Hormone Center, 20 Beacon Hill Dr; Dobbs Ferry, NY 10522; (914) 693-8820; **BDCERT:** ObG 91; RE 92; **MS:** NY Med Coll 84; **RES:** ObG, Albert Einstein Med Ctr, Bronx, NY 84-88; **FEL:** RE, Tulane U Med Ctr, New Orleans, LA 88-90; **FAP:** Asst Prof Albert Einstein Coll Med; **HOSP:** Community Hosp At Dobbs Ferry; **SI:** *Infertility; In Vitro Fertilization;* **HMO:** Oxford US Hlthcre PHS

♿ 🔳 **C** 📷 🚹 📆 **S**   2-4 Weeks 💳 ***VISA*** 💳

Young, Constance (MD)   ObG
Phelps Mem Hosp Ctr

Scarboro Ob/Gyn, 100 S Highland Ave; Ossining, NY 10562; (914) 762-5540; **BDCERT:** ObG 90; **MS:** Cornell U 83; **RES:** N Shore Univ Hosp-Manhasset, Manhasset, NY 83-87; **HOSP:** Westchester Med Ctr; **HMO:** Oxford Aetna Hlth Plan PHS Blue Choice

♿ 📷 🚹 📆 **S** Mcr   2-4 Weeks ***VISA*** 💳

Young, Zenaida (MD)   ObG
Sound Shore Med Ctr-Westchester

345 Gramatan Ave; Mt Vernon, NY 10552; (914) 699-2525; **BDCERT:** ObG 83; **MS:** Philippines 72; **RES:** ObG, Newark Beth Israel Med Ctr, Newark, NJ 76-80; **HMO:** HealthNet Metlife PHS

LANG: Fil; **C** 📷 📆 **S** Mcr   1 Week ***VISA*** 💳

OPHTHALMOLOGY

Barest, Herman (MD)   Oph
Northern Westchester Hosp Ctr

344 E Main St 103; Mt Kisco, NY 10549; (914) 666-3477; **BDCERT:** Oph 59; **MS:** Middlesex U Sch Med 46; **RES:** Montefiore Med Ctr, Bronx, NY 56-58; **HOSP:** Montefiore Med Ctr; **SI:** *Neuro-Ophthalmology;* **HMO:** Oxford Aetna-US Healthcare CIGNA PHS Pomco +

LANG: Itl, Fr; ♿ 🔳 📷 🚹 📆 **S** Mcr WC NFI   Immediately

Bauer, Robert (MD)   Oph
Phelps Mem Hosp Ctr

Hudson Valley Eye Associates, 55 S Broadway; Tarrytown, NY 10591; (914) 631-9191; **BDCERT:** Oph 70; **MS:** SUNY Downstate 70; **RES:** Montefiore Med Ctr, Bronx, NY 71-72; Oph, New York University Med Ctr, New York, NY 72-75; **HMO:** Aetna Hlth Plan Oxford Metlife PHS GHI +

♿ 🔳 📷 📆 **S** Mcr WC   2-4 Weeks ***VISA*** 💳

Beckerman, Barry (MD)   Oph
Northern Westchester Hosp Ctr

344 E Main St 406; Mt Kisco, NY 10549; (914) 666-3764; **BDCERT:** Oph 73; Med 65; **MS:** NYU Sch Med 65; **RES:** S, New England Med Ctr, Boston, MA 65-67; Oph, New York University Med Ctr, New York, NY 68-70; **FEL:** Med, New York University Med Ctr, New York, NY 71-72; **FAP:** Asst Clin Prof Albert Einstein Coll Med; **HOSP:** Montefiore Med Ctr; **HMO:** Pomco Oxford

♿ 📷 🚹 📆 **S**   2-4 Weeks

Bocian, Franklin (MD)   Oph
Sound Shore Med Ctr-Westchester

Eye Specialist of Westchester, 140 Lockwood Ave 220; New Rochelle, NY 10801; (914) 235-9500; **BDCERT:** Oph 70; **MS:** SUNY Hlth Sci Ctr 64; **RES:** Oph, Kings County Hosp Ctr, Brooklyn, NY 65-69; **HMO:** Oxford Aetna Hlth Plan United Healthcare PHS Pomco +

LANG: Sp, Itl, Fr, Heb; ♿ 🔳 **C** 📷 🚹 📆 **S** Mcr Mcd WC NFI   A Few Days 💳 ***VISA*** 💳

Brustein, Harris (MD)   Oph
Sound Shore Med Ctr-Westchester

77 Quaker Ridge Rd 203; New Rochelle, NY 10804; (914) 235-0022; **BDCERT:** Oph 76; **MS:** Albert Einstein Coll Med 70; **RES:** Montefiore Med Ctr, Bronx, NY 71-74; **FEL:** Children's Hosp, Boston, MA 74-75; **HMO:** Oxford PHS United Healthcare GHI PHCS +

LANG: Sp; ♿ 🔳 **C** 📷 🚹 📆 **S** Mcr WC NFI   1 Week

Guide to symbols and abbreviations can be found on pages 110-113.

799

Burris, James (MD) Oph
White Plains Hosp Ctr

170 Maple Ave 208; White Plains, NY 10601;
(914) 949-4414; **BDCERT:** Oph 64; **MS:** Boston U
56; **RES:** New York Eye & Ear Infirmary, New York,
NY 60-63; **HOSP:** St Agnes Hosp; *SI: Cataract;
Glaucoma;* **HMO:** Oxford PHS CIGNA Empire Aetna
Hlth Plan +

LANG: Sp; 🚹 🌙 📷 🚼 🎬 💲 Mcr WC NFI 1 Week
VISA 💮

Casper, Daniel (MD) Oph
Columbia-Presbyterian Med Ctr

66 Milton Rd; Rye, NY 10580; (914) 967-4400;
BDCERT: Oph 91; **MS:** Albany Med Coll 85; **RES:**
Oph, Columbia-Presbyterian Med Ctr, New York,
NY 86-89; **FEL:** Oculoplastic & Orbital S, Columbia-
Presbyterian Med Ctr, New York, NY 89-90; **FAP:**
Asst Clin Prof Oph Columbia P&S; **HOSP:** Phelps
Mem Hosp Ctr; **HMO:** +

LANG: Sp; 🚹 ⬛ 📷 🚼 🎬 💲 Mcr WC Immediately

Chess, Jeremy (MD) Oph
Yonkers Gen Hosp

6 Xavier Dr 710; Yonkers, NY 10704; (914) 376-
2273; **BDCERT:** Oph 77; **MS:** Boston U 70; **RES:**
Boston U Med Ctr, Boston, MA 74; **FEL:** Harvard
Med Sch, Cambridge, MA; *SI: Retina;* **HMO:** Oxford
US Hlthcre HealthNet Aetna Hlth Plan GHI +

LANG: Heb, Ger, Sp; 🚹 📷 🎬 💲 Mcr Mod WC NFI
A Few Days **VISA**

Dieck, William (MD) Oph
Northern Westchester Hosp Ctr

359 E Main St 3H; Mt Kisco, NY 10549; (914)
666-4939; **BDCERT:** Oph 90; **MS:** NY Med Coll 83;
RES: NY Med Coll, Valhalla, NY 85-88; **HOSP:**
Westchester Med Ctr

LANG: Rus; 🚹 🌙 📷 🚼 🎬 💲 Mcr WC NFI 2-
4 Weeks **VISA** 💮

Forman, Scott (MD) Oph
Westchester Med Ctr

Westchester Medical Center,; Valhalla, NY 10595;
(914) 493-7666; **BDCERT:** Oph 89; **MS:** UMDNJ-
RW Johnson Med Sch 81; **RES:** NY Med Coll, New
York, NY 83-86; **FEL:** Oph, Columbia-Presbyterian
Med Ctr, New York, NY 86-87; **FAP:** Assoc Clin
Prof NY Med Coll; **HOSP:** St Agnes Hosp; *SI: Botox
Treatment; Eye Muscle Surgery;* **HMO:** PHS Blue
Choice US Hlthcre Prucare Oxford +

🚹 📷 🚼 🎬 💲 Mcr Mod WC NFI 2-4 Weeks ▨▨ **VISA**
💮

Glassman, Morris (MD) Oph
Northern Westchester Hosp Ctr

1940 Commerce St 301; Yorktown Heights, NY
10598; (914) 962-5506; **BDCERT:** Oph 75; **MS:**
NYU Sch Med 68; **RES:** Albert Einstein Med Ctr,
Bronx, NY 71-74; Montefiore Med Ctr, Bronx, NY
71-74; *SI: Cataract; Glaucoma;* **HMO:** Oxford Aetna
Hlth Plan US Hlthcre PHS United Healthcare +

LANG: Sp, Yd, Heb, Fr; 🚹 🌙 📷 🚼 🎬 💲 Mcr Mod WC
NFI A Few Days **VISA** 💮

Greenbaum, Allen (MD) Oph
White Plains Hosp Ctr

Westchester Eye Associates, 170 Maple Ave 402;
White Plains, NY 10601; (914) 949-9200;
BDCERT: Oph 85; **MS:** Mt Sinai Sch Med 79; **RES:**
Oph, Beth Israel Med Ctr, New York, NY 79-80;
Mount Sinai Med Ctr, New York, NY 80-83; **FAP:**
Instr Mt Sinai Sch Med; **HOSP:** St Agnes Hosp; *SI:
Cataract; Refractive Surgery;* **HMO:** Oxford PHS
Pomco United Healthcare Blue Cross +

LANG: Sp; 🚹 ⬛ 🌙 📷 🚼 🎬 💲 Mcr WC NFI 1 Week
VISA 💮

Greenberg, Steven (MD) Oph
United Hosp Med Ctr

282 Harrison Ave; Harrison, NY 10528; (914)
835-1031; **BDCERT:** Oph 87; **MS:** U Conn Sch Med
82; **RES:** New York University Med Ctr, New York,
NY 83-86; **FEL:** Strabismus, Manhattan Eye, Ear &
Throat Hosp, New York, NY 86-87; **HOSP:**
Manhattan Eye, Ear & Throat Hosp; *SI: Strabismus;
Pediatric Ophthalmology;* **HMO:** PHS Aetna-US
Healthcare Oxford United Healthcare CIGNA +

🚹 ⬛ 📷 🚼 🎬 💲 Mcr Mod WC NFI 1 Week **VISA** 💮

Hayworth, Nan (MD)   Oph
Northern Westchester Hosp Ctr
Mount Kisco Medical Group, 90 S Bedford Rd 304B;
Mt Kisco, NY 10549; (914) 242-1408; **BDCERT:**
Oph 92; **MS:** Cornell U 85; **RES:** Oph, Mount Sinai
Med Ctr, New York, NY 86-89; **FAP:** Clin Instr Oph
Mt Sinai Sch Med; **SI:** *Cataract Surgery; Glaucoma;*
HMO: Aetna-US Healthcare Oxford PHS United
Healthcare Prudential +

🦽 ⬛ 📷 📧 🎬 💲 Mc WC 4+ Weeks ▓▓ **VISA** 💳

Horowitz, Marc (MD)   Oph
Westchester Med Ctr
209 Harwood Bldg; Scarsdale, NY 10583; (914)
723-5511; **BDCERT:** Oph 83; **MS:** Mt Sinai Sch
Med 78; **RES:** IM, St Luke's Roosevelt Hosp Ctr, New
York, NY 79; Oph, St Luke's Roosevelt Hosp Ctr,
New York, NY 82; **FEL:** Ped Oph, Children's Hosp of
Philadelphia, Philadelphia, PA 83; **FAP:** Clin Prof
NY Med Coll; **HOSP:** White Plains Hosp Ctr; **SI:**
Retinopathy of Prematurity; Pediatric Cataracts;
HMO: Pomco Guardian

🦽 📷 🎬 💲 Mc 2-4 Weeks

Kelly, Nancy (MD)   Oph
St Joseph's Med Ctr-Yonkers
632 Palmer Rd; Yonkers, NY 10701; (914) 337-
3600; **BDCERT:** Oph 87; **MS:** NY Med Coll 78; **RES:**
Oph, Lincoln Med & Mental Hlth Ctr, Bronx, NY 78-
79; Our Lady of Mercy Med Ctr, Bronx, NY 78-82;
HMO: Blue Choice Oxford Prudential US Hlthcre
GHI +

LANG: Sp; 🦽 📷 🎬 🎬 Mc Md WC Immediately ▓▓

Lateiner, Lloyd (MD)   Oph
Sound Shore Med Ctr-Westchester
110 Lockwood Ave; New Rochelle, NY 10801;
(914) 235-8886; **MS:** NY Med Coll 73; **RES:** Santa
Barbara Gen, 73-74; Beth Israel, 74-77

Lederman, Martin (MD)   Oph
White Plains Hosp Ctr
Ophthalmology Consultants, 10 Chester Ave;
White Plains, NY 10601; (914) 684-6888;
BDCERT: Oph 71; **MS:** Albert Einstein Coll Med 64;
RES: Oph, Jacobi Med Ctr, Bronx, NY 65-68; **FEL:**
Ped Oph, Children's Hosp Nat Med Ctr,
Washington, DC 68-69; **FAP:** Asst Clin Prof
Columbia P&S; **HOSP:** Columbia-Presbyterian Med
Ctr; **SI:** *Pediatric Eye and Ear;* **HMO:** Oxford United
Healthcare Pomco PHS Aetna Hlth Plan +

🦽 ⬛ 📧 📷 🎬 🎬 💲 Mc Md WC Immediately ▓▓
VISA 💳

Levin, Henry (MD)   Oph
Sound Shore Med Ctr-Westchester
421 Huguenot St 24; New Rochelle, NY 10801;
(914) 632-7882; **BDCERT:** Oph 87; **MS:** Mt Sinai
Sch Med 80; **RES:** Oph, Metropolitan Hosp Ctr, New
York, NY 82-85; **SI:** *No Stitch Cataract Surgery;*
Glaucoma Care; **HMO:** Oxford Aetna Hlth Plan GHI
PHS Blue Choice +

🦽 📷 🎬 🎬 💲 Mc Md WC NFI A Few Days

Magaro, Joseph (MD)   Oph
Lawrence Hosp
77 Pondfield Rd; Bronxville, NY 10708; (914) 337-
8844; **BDCERT:** Oph 67; **MS:** Boston U 61; **RES:**
Manhattan Eye, Ear & Throat Hosp, New York, NY
65; **HOSP:** Manhattan Eye, Ear & Throat Hosp;
HMO: Aetna Hlth Plan Blue Choice Blue Cross &
Blue Shield CIGNA Metlife +

LANG: Fr, Itl; 🦽 ⬛ 📷 📧 🎬 Mc WC NFI
Immediately

Mardirossian, Jonathan (MD)Oph
White Plains Hosp Ctr
33 Davis Ave; White Plains, NY 10605; (914) 684-
0020; **BDCERT:** Oph 78; **MS:** Cornell U 72; **RES:**
Manhattan Eye, Ear & Throat Hosp, New York, NY;
FEL: NY Hosp-Cornell Med Ctr, New York, NY; St
John's Eye Hosp, New York, NY; **HOSP:** St Agnes
Hosp; **SI:** *Retinal Detachment; Diabetic Retinopathy;*
HMO: Oxford Aetna Hlth Plan First Option Pomco

LANG: Fr, Ger, Itl; 🦽 📧 🎬 Immediately **VISA** 💳

Markowitz, Allan (MD)   Oph
Northern Westchester Hosp Ctr
3505 Hill Blvd # K; Yorktown Heights, NY 10598;
(914) 245-3303; **BDCERT:** Oph 79; **MS:** Albert
Einstein Coll Med 74; **RES:** Oph, Albert Einstein Med
Ctr, Bronx, NY 75-78; **FAP:** Assoc Clin Prof Albert
Einstein Coll Med; *SI: Cataract*; **HMO:** Independent
Health Plan PHS

 ⬛ ⬛ ⬛ ⬛ A Few Days

McKee, Heather (MD)   Oph
St Agnes Hosp
200 S Broadway 202; Tarrytown, NY 10591;
(914) 631-7300; **BDCERT:** Oph 81; **MS:** Duke U
76; **RES:** U Mich Med Ctr, Ann Arbor, MI 76-77;
Strong Mem Hosp, Rochester, NY 77-80; **FAP:**
Assoc Clin Prof NY Med Coll; **HOSP:** Community
Hosp At Dobbs Ferry

 ⬛ ⬛ ⬛ ⬛ ⬛ ⬛ ⬛ ⬛ ⬛ ⬛ A Few Days

Mennin, Gerald (MD)   Oph
Yonkers Gen Hosp
45 Ludlow St 618; Yonkers, NY 10705; (914) 969-
6995; **BDCERT:** Oph 64; **MS:** SUNY Hlth Sci Ctr 58;
RES: Jacobi Med Ctr, Bronx, NY; **FAP:** Clin Prof
Albert Einstein Coll Med; **HOSP:** Montefiore Med
Ctr-Weiler/Einstein Div; **HMO:** Aetna Hlth Plan
Blue Choice PHS Pomco Oxford +

LANG: Sp; ⬛ ⬛ ⬛ ⬛ ⬛ ⬛ ⬛ ⬛ ⬛
Immediately ⬛

Mickatavage, Robert (MD)   Oph
United Hosp Med Ctr
66 Nutton Rd; Rye, NY 10580; (914) 967-4400;
BDCERT: Oph 66; **MS:** Temple U 58; **RES:** Oph,
Bascom Palmer Eye Inst, Miami, FL 61-64

Mignone, Biagio (MD)   Oph
Mount Vernon Hosp
148 Stevens Ave; Mt Vernon, NY 10550; (914)
664-6001; **BDCERT:** Oph 80; **MS:** NY Med Coll 75;
RES: Oph, Univ of Med & Dent NJ Hosp, Newark, NJ
75-79; **FAP:** Asst Clin Prof NYU Sch Med; **HOSP:**
Our Lady of Mercy Med Ctr; *SI: Cataract Surgery;
Glaucoma*; **HMO:** Aetna Hlth Plan PHS Pomco
Oxford Blue Cross & Blue Shield +

LANG: Arm, Sp, Prt; ⬛ ⬛ ⬛ ⬛ ⬛ ⬛ ⬛ ⬛ ⬛
⬛ Immediately ⬛ *VISA* ⬛

Miller, Brian (MD)   Oph
United Hosp Med Ctr
1600 Harrison Ave; Mamaroneck, NY 10543;
(914) 698-0670; **BDCERT:** Oph 75; **MS:** Temple U
71; **RES:** Oto, Temple U Hosp, Philadelphia, PA 72-
75; **FAP:** Asst Clin Prof Albert Einstein Coll Med

 ⬛ ⬛ ⬛ ⬛ ⬛ ⬛ ⬛ 2-4 Weeks *VISA* ⬛

Mooney, Robert (MD)   Oph
Northern Westchester Hosp Ctr
359 E Main St; Mt Kisco, NY 10549; (914) 666-
4939; **BDCERT:** Oph 82; **MS:** Italy 72; **RES:**
Westchester County Med Ctr, Valhalla, NY 74-77

Morello, Robert (MD)   Oph
Sound Shore Med Ctr-Westchester
120 Warren St; New Rochelle, NY 10801; (914)
633-7214; **BDCERT:** Oph 85; **MS:** Mexico 76; **RES:**
IM, Bronx Lebanon Hosp Ctr, Bronx, NY 77-78;
Oph, Bronx Lebanon Hosp Ctr, Bronx, NY 78-81;
HOSP: Calvary Hosp; *SI: Geriatric Ophthalmology*;
HMO: Blue Choice PHS Oxford Aetna Hlth Plan US
Hlthcre +

LANG: Sp, Fr, Itl; ⬛ ⬛ ⬛ ⬛ ⬛ ⬛ ⬛ ⬛
4+ Weeks ⬛ *VISA* ⬛

Most, Richard W (MD) Oph
Northern Westchester Hosp Ctr
101 S Bedford Rd 401; Mt Kisco, NY 10549; (914) 241-9288; **BDCERT:** Oph 77; **MS:** Italy 71; **RES:** Path, Maimonides Med Ctr, Brooklyn, NY 72-73; Oph, Lenox Hill Hosp, New York, NY 73-76; **FEL:** Ped Oph, Bellevue Hosp Ctr, New York, NY 76-77; Ped Oph, Children's Hosp Nat Med Ctr, Washington, DC 78; **HOSP:** St Agnes Hosp; *SI: Strabismus/Amblyopia; Tear Duct Problems*; **HMO:** Aetna Hlth Plan CIGNA Oxford Pomco PHS +

LANG: Itl, Sp; [symbols] 1 Week [symbols] *VISA* [symbols]

O'Rourke, James (MD) Oph
Westchester Med Ctr
Dept of Ophthalmology, Route 100 Macy Pavilion; Valhalla, NY 10595; (914) 493-7865; **BDCERT:** Oph 51; **MS:** Georgetown U 43; **RES:** Columbia-Presbyterian Med Ctr, New York, NY 49-51; **FAP:** Assoc Chrmn&Prof NY Coll Osteo Med; **HMO:** Magnacare Oxford Aetna-US Healthcare Pomco

[symbols] 1 Week

Palumbo, John (MD) Oph
St Joseph's Med Ctr-Yonkers
984 N Broadway 407; Yonkers, NY 10701; (914) 965-8100; **BDCERT:** Oph 82; **MS:** Mt Sinai Sch Med 73; **RES:** Mount Sinai Med Ctr, New York, NY 75-78; **FEL:** Mount Sinai Med Ctr, New York, NY 75; **HOSP:** Yonkers Gen Hosp; **HMO:** Oxford Blue Choice CIGNA US Hlthcre

LANG: Sp; [symbols] 1 Week

Phillips, Howard (MD) Oph
Phelps Mem Hosp Ctr
Hudson Valley Eye Associates, 55 S Broadway; Tarrytown, NY 10591; (914) 631-9191; **BDCERT:** Oph 82; **MS:** NYU Sch Med 77; **RES:** New York University Med Ctr, New York, NY 78-81; **FEL:** Med Retina, New York University Med Ctr, New York, NY 81-82; *SI: Refractive Surgery; Corneal Problems*; **HMO:** Oxford PHS US Hlthcre CIGNA Well Care +

[symbols] 1 Week *VISA* [symbols]

Ray, Audell (MD) Oph
Lawrence Hosp
Bronxville Eye Care Assoc, 77 Pondfield Rd; Bronxville, NY 10708; (914) 337-8844; **BDCERT:** Oph 79; **MS:** Columbia P&S 74; **RES:** Oph, Manhattan Eye, Ear & Throat Hosp, New York, NY 75-78; **FAP:** Dir Oph Unknown/other New York Sch ool; **HOSP:** Manhattan Eye, Ear & Throat Hosp; *SI: Cataracts*; **HMO:** US Hlthcre Oxford Blue Choice Pomco United Healthcare +

LANG: Sp; [symbols] Immediately

Salzman, Jacqueline (MD) Oph
Phelps Mem Hosp Ctr
200 S Broadway 211; Tarrytown, NY 10591; (914) 332-5394; **BDCERT:** Oph 85; **MS:** NYU Sch Med 79; **RES:** Bellevue Hosp Ctr, New York, NY 80-83; **FEL:** Oph, Bellevue Hosp Ctr, New York, NY 83-84; **HOSP:** Westchester Med Ctr; *SI: Cataract Surgery; Laser Surgery*; **HMO:** Oxford PHS Aetna Hlth Plan CIGNA

[symbols] A Few Days *VISA* [symbols]

Solomon, Ira (MD) Oph
Lawrence Hosp
Bronxville Eye Care Associates, 77 Pondfield Rd; Bronxville, NY 10708; (914) 337-8844; **BDCERT:** Oph 89; **MS:** Jefferson Med Coll 82; **RES:** Oph, Montefiore Med Ctr, Bronx, NY; **FEL:** Glaucoma, New York Eye & Ear Infirmary, New York, NY 86-87; **FAP:** Asst Clin Prof Albert Einstein Coll Med; **HOSP:** Lenox Hill Hosp; *SI: Glaucoma; Medical Laser Surgery*; **HMO:** Aetna Hlth Plan Blue Choice Blue Cross & Blue Shield Pomco

[symbols] A Few Days

Guide to symbols and abbreviations can be found on pages 110-113.

803

Solomon, Sherry (MD)   Oph
Lawrence Hosp

Retina Consultations, 915 Palmer Rd; Bronxville, NY 10708; (914) 793-6900; **BDCERT:** Oph 91; **MS:** Albert Einstein Coll Med 86; **RES:** Lenox Hill Hosp, New York, NY 87; Montefiore Med Ctr, Bronx, NY 87-90; **FEL:** New York University Med Ctr, New York, NY 90-91; **FAP:** Clin Instr Albert Einstein Coll Med; **HOSP:** Sound Shore Med Ctr-Westchester; **SI:** *Macular Degeneration; Diabetic Retinopathy;* **HMO:** US Hlthcre Blue Cross & Blue Shield GHI Oxford

LANG: Sp; 🚻 🏧 🄲 📷 🛏 Mcr Mcl WC NFI Immediately

Stein, Mitchell (MD)   Oph
Northern Westchester Hosp Ctr

69 S Moger Ave; Mount Kisco, NY 10549; (914) 666-2961; **BDCERT:** Oph 87; IM 82; **MS:** Albert Einstein Coll Med 79; **RES:** IM, St Francis Hosp Med Ctr, Hartford, CT 79-80; IM, Jacobi Med Ctr, Bronx, NY 80-82; **FEL:** Oph, Mount Sinai Med Ctr, New York, NY 86-87; **FAP:** Asst Clin Prof Albert Einstein Coll Med; **SI:** *Cataract; Corneal Disease;* **HMO:** Oxford Aetna Hlth Plan Pomco CIGNA

LANG: Sp; 🚻 📷 🎿 🛏 💲 Mcr WC NFI 1 Week **VISA** 💳

Sussman, John (MD)   Oph
Phelps Mem Hosp Ctr

200 S Broadway 204; Tarrytown, NY 10591; (914) 631-6844; **BDCERT:** Oph 65; **MS:** NYU Sch Med 59; **RES:** Oph, Montefiore Med Ctr, Bronx, NY 60-63; **SI:** *Glaucoma; Cataract Surgery;* **HMO:** Oxford PHS Aetna-US Healthcare Prucare Pomco +

🚻 🏧 📷 🎿 🛏 💲 Mcr Mcl WC NFI Immediately

Taffet, Simeon (MD)   Oph
Mount Vernon Hosp

40 E Sidney Ave; Mt Vernon, NY 10550; (914) 668-0110; **BDCERT:** Oph 62; **MS:** Switzerland 55; **RES:** Jacobi/Bronx Muni Hosp Ctr, Bronx, NY 57-60; **FAP:** Assoc Clin Prof Oph Albert Einstein Coll Med; **HOSP:** Manhattan Eye, Ear & Throat Hosp; **SI:** *Glaucoma; Low Vision;* **HMO:** None

LANG: Fr, Dut, Ger; 🚻 📷 🎿 🛏 💲 Mcr Mcl WC NFI

Zaidman, Gerald (MD)   Oph
Westchester Med Ctr

Route 100 Macy Pavilion; Valhalla, NY 10595; (914) 493-1599; **BDCERT:** Oph 81; **MS:** Albert Einstein Coll Med 75; **RES:** Ger, Beth Abraham Hosp, Bronx, NY 76-77; Oph, Lenox Hill Hosp, New York, NY 77-80; **FEL:** Cornea & External Disease, U of Pittsburgh Med Ctr, Pittsburgh, PA 80-82; **FAP:** Assoc Prof Oph NY Med Coll; **HOSP:** Our Lady of Mercy Med Ctr; **SI:** *Corneal Transplants; Refractive Surgery (Myopia);* **HMO:** Aetna-US Healthcare Oxford Independent Health Plan Blue Choice GHI +

LANG: Sp; 🚻 📷 🛏 💲 Mcr Mcl WC NFI Immediately

ORTHOPAEDIC SURGERY

Brown, Charles (MD)   OrS
Northern Westchester Hosp Ctr

Mt Kisco Medical Group, 90 S Bedford Rd; Mt Kisco, NY 10549; (914) 241-1050; **BDCERT:** OrS 77; **MS:** Columbia P&S 69; **RES:** S, Columbia-Presbyterian Med Ctr, New York, NY 70-71; OrS, Columbia-Presbyterian Med Ctr, New York, NY 71-75; **FEL:** OrS, Columbia-Presbyterian Med Ctr, New York, NY 75-76; **SI:** *Arthroscopic Surgery; Joint Replacement Surgery;* **HMO:** Oxford Aetna Hlth Plan PHS NYLCare

🚻 🛏 💲 Mcr WC NFI Immediately **VISA** 💳

Burak, George (MD)   OrS
Phelps Mem Hosp Ctr

239 N Broadway; N Tarrytown, NY 10591; (914) 631-7777; **BDCERT:** OrS 71; **MS:** SUNY Syracuse 64; **RES:** OrS, Kings County Hosp Ctr, Brooklyn, NY 66-69; S, Kings County Hosp Ctr, Brooklyn, NY 65-66; **FAP:** Asst Instr OrS SUNY Downstate; **SI:** *Sports Injuries; Arthritis*

LANG: Sp, Itl; 🚻 📷 🎿 🛏 💲 Mcr WC NFI A Few Days 💳

Cristofaro, Robert (MD)   OrS
United Hosp Med Ctr
Blind Brook Lane & Purchase St; Rye, NY 10580; (914) 967-8708; **BDCERT:** OrS 78; **MS:** SUNY Hlth Sci Ctr 71; **RES:** Montefiore Med Ctr, Bronx, NY 73; Montefiore Med Ctr, Bronx, NY 76; **FEL:** Rancho Los Amigos Med Ctr, Downey, CA; **HOSP:** Sound Shore Med Ctr-Westchester; *SI: Pediatric Orthopedics*; **HMO:** Most

LANG: Sp; ♿ 📷 🧍 🏥 **S** Mcr WC NFI   2-4 Weeks ▨ **VISA** ●

Dobson, Chauncey (MD)   OrS
Phelps Mem Hosp Ctr
200 S Broadway 104; Tarrytown, NY 10591; (914) 631-1142; **BDCERT:** OrS 62; **MS:** USC Sch Med 54; **RES:** S, Los Angeles Hosp, Los Angeles, CA 54-59; Columbia Presbyterian Med Ctr, New York, NY 58-59; **HOSP:** Community Hosp At Dobbs Ferry

Edelson, Charles (MD)   OrS
St Joseph's Med Ctr-Yonkers
970 N Broadway 204; Yonkers, NY 10701; (914) 476-4343; **BDCERT:** OrS 79; **MS:** NY Med Coll 73; **RES:** OrS, Montefiore Med Ctr, Bronx, NY 75-78; S, Montefiore Med Ctr, Bronx, NY 74-75

Elfenbein, Joseph (MD)   OrS
United Hosp Med Ctr
875 Mamaroneck Ave; Mamaroneck, NY 10543; (914) 698-4180; **BDCERT:** OrS 74; **MS:** Albert Einstein Coll Med 63; **RES:** S, Hosp For Joint Diseases, New York, NY 68; OrS, Hosp For Joint Diseases, New York, NY 66-69; **HOSP:** Sound Shore Med Ctr-Westchester; *SI: Endoscopic Carpal Tunnel Surgery*

Galeno, John (MD)   OrS
St Agnes Hosp
222 Westchester Ave 204; White Plains, NY 10604; (914) 288-0030; **BDCERT:** OrS 87; **MS:** Italy 79; **RES:** Westchester County Med Ctr, Valhalla, NY 79-84; **FEL:** Toronto Gen Hosp, Toronto, Canada; **HOSP:** Westchester Med Ctr; *SI: Spine Surgery; Sports Medicine*; **HMO:** Oxford CIGNA Aetna-US Healthcare US Hlthcre Independent Health Plan +

LANG: Sp, Itl; ♿ **C** 📷 🧍 **S** Mcr WC NFI Immediately **VISA** ●

Gundy, Edward (MD)   OrS
United Hosp Med Ctr
2 Rye Ridge Plaza; Rye Brook, NY 10573; (914) 253-9199; **BDCERT:** OrS 83; **MS:** Cornell U 76; **RES:** St Luke's Roosevelt Hosp Ctr, New York, NY 76-78; Hosp For Special Surgery, New York, NY 78-81; *SI: Joint Replacement; Sport Medicine*; **HMO:** Oxford Prucare CIGNA US Hlthcre +

♿ 🧍 📷 **S** Mcr WC NFI 1 Week ▨ **VISA** ● ▨

Holder, Jonathan (MD)   OrS
St Agnes Hosp
311 North St Ste 406; White Plains, NY 10605; (914) 428-5666; **BDCERT:** OrS 92; **MS:** NY Med Coll 85; **RES:** Metropolitan Hosp Ctr, New York, NY 85-90; **HOSP:** White Plains Hosp Ctr; **HMO:** Aetna Hlth Plan US Hlthcre Oxford Empire Blue Choice GHI +

♿ 🧍 📷 **S** Mcr WC Immediately ▨ **VISA** ● ▨

Krishnamurthy, Shanker (MD)OrS
Hudson Valley Hosp Ctr
Community Orthopedic Assoc, 1985 Crompond Rd; Peekskill, NY 10566; (914) 739-2121; **BDCERT:** OrS 84; **MS:** India 70; **RES:** NY Med Coll, Valhalla, NY 79-82; **HMO:** Oxford Aetna-US Healthcare PHS Independent Health Plan SWCHP +

LANG: Hin, Tam, Kan; ♿ 📷 🧍 🏥 **S** Mcr Mcd WC NFI A Few Days **VISA** ●

Levin, Howard (MD)   OrS
Northern Westchester Hosp Ctr
1888 Commerce St; Yorktown Heights, NY 10598;
(914) 962-7712; **BDCERT:** OrS 79; **MS:** SUNY Hlth
Sci Ctr 73; **RES:** OrS, Hosp For Joint Diseases, New
York, NY 74-78; **SI:** *Knee Surgery; Shoulder Surgery;*
HMO: SWCHP Amerihealth Empire Blue Cross &
Shield Oxford Pomco +

♿ 📷 🚹 🏩 $ Mcr WC NFI   Immediately

Maddalo, Anthony (MD)   OrS
Phelps Mem Hosp Ctr
239 N Broadway; N Tarrytown, NY 10591; (914)
631-7777; **BDCERT:** OrS 88; **MS:** NY Med Coll 81;
RES: Lenox Hill Hosp, New York, NY 81-86; **HOSP:**
Community Hosp At Dobbs Ferry; **SI:** *Sports Injuries;*
Arthroscopic Surgery; **HMO:** Blue Choice Oxford
Multiplan

LANG: Itl, Sp, Prt; ♿ 📷 🏩 $ Mcr WC NFI
Immediately **VISA** 💳 💳

Mann, Ronald (MD)   OrS
Northern Westchester Hosp Ctr
Northern Westchester Orthopedic Associates, 1888
Commerce St; Yorktown Heights, NY 10598; (914)
962-7712; **BDCERT:** OrS 97; **MS:** Univ Penn 80;
RES: S, Mount Sinai Med Ctr, New York, NY 80-82;
OrS, Mount Sinai Med Ctr, New York, NY 82-85;
FEL: Ped OrS, Hosp For Special Surgery, New York,
NY 85-86; **SI:** *Pediatric Orthopedics;* **HMO:** Oxford
PHS Aetna Hlth Plan Empire

♿ 📷 🚹 🏩 $ Mcr WC NFI   A Few Days

Mazella, John S (MD)   OrS
Northern Westchester Hosp Ctr
39 Smith Ave; Mt Kisco, NY 10549; (914) 241-
1808; **BDCERT:** OrS 69; **MS:** Cornell U 59; **RES:** S,
Geo Wash U Med Ctr, Washington, DC 59-61; OrS,
Bellevue Hosp Ctr, New York, NY 64-66; **FAP:** Asst
Clin Prof OrS NYU Sch Med; **SI:** *Sports Medicine;*
Knee Surgery; **HMO:** Oxford Aetna Hlth Plan United
Healthcare Blue Choice Magnacare +

♿ 🏦 📷 🏩 $ Mcr WC NFI   A Few Days **VISA** 💳

Nelson Jr, John M (MD)   OrS
United Hosp Med Ctr
Cristofro Nelson Delbello, Blind Brook Lane &
Purchase St; Rye, NY 10580; (914) 967-8708;
BDCERT: OrS 87; OrS 98; **MS:** Mt Sinai Sch Med
79; **RES:** S, Mount Sinai Med Ctr, New York, NY 79-
80; OrS, Hosp For Joint Diseases, New York, NY 80-
84; **FEL:** Ped OrS, Scottish Rite Children's Hosp,
Atlanta, GA 84-85; **FAP:** Instr NY Med Coll; **HOSP:**
Sound Shore Med Ctr-Westchester; **SI:** *Pediatric*
Orthopedics/ Sports Medicine; Joint Replacement
Surgery; **HMO:** Aetna Hlth Plan Independent
Health Plan CIGNA Pomco Oxford +

LANG: Sp; ♿ 📷 $ Mcr WC NFI   A Few Days 💳
VISA 💳

Peress, Richard (MD)   OrS
Phelps Mem Hosp Ctr
Park Professional Building, Suite 1, 100 S Highland
Ave; Ossining, NY 10562; (914) 762-9300;
BDCERT: OrS 89; **MS:** Columbia P&S 81; **RES:**
Columbia-Presbyterian Med Ctr, New York, NY 83-
86; St Luke's Roosevelt Hosp Ctr, New York, NY
81-83; **FEL:** Scoliosis & Spine S, Kosair Hosp,
Louisville, KY; **HOSP:** St Agnes Hosp; **HMO:** PHS

♿ 📷 🚹 🏩 $ Mcr WC NFI   A Few Days **VISA** 💳

Ricciardelli, Charles (MD)   OrS
Westchester Med Ctr
19 Broadhurst Ave 4; Hawthorne, NY 10538;
(914) 347-5822; **BDCERT:** OrS 77; **MS:** Italy 70;
RES: S, NY Med Coll, New York, NY 73; OrS, NY
Med Coll, New York, NY 76; **SI:** *Sports Medicine;*
Arthritis Surgery; **HMO:** Oxford Pomco Magnacare
Anthem Health Medichoice +

LANG: Itl; ♿ 📳 🚹 🏩 $ Mcr WC NFI   1 Week

Rizzo, Thomas (MD)   OrS
Lawrence Hosp
77 Pondfield Rd; Bronxville, NY 10708; (914) 337-
1118; **BDCERT:** OrS 65; **MS:** Georgetown U 56;
RES: S, St Vincents Hosp & Med Ctr NY, New York,
NY 57-58; Hosp For Special Surgery, New York, NY
58-59; **FEL:** OrS, Newington Children's Hosp,
Newington, CT 61-62; **FAP:** Clin Instr Cornell U;
HOSP: Hosp For Special Surgery; **SI:** *Foot & Ankle;*
General Orthopedics; **HMO:** Aetna Hlth Plan Chubb
Empire

♿ 📷 🚹 🏩 Mcr WC NFI   2-4 Weeks **VISA**

Schulman, Lawrence (MD)   OrS
St John's Riverside Hosp
984 N Broadway LLO3; Yonkers, NY 10701; (914)
969-8150; **BDCERT:** OrS 72; **MS:** SUNY Downstate
63; **RES:** Hosp For Joint Diseases, New York, NY 66-
70; **HOSP:** Community Hosp At Dobbs Ferry; *SI:*
Total Joint Replacement; Sports Injuries; **HMO:** Oxford
PHS Magnacare Aetna Hlth Plan Empire Blue Cross
& Shield +

⬦ 🔲 🔲 🔲 🔲 Mcr Mcd WC NFI   A Few Days

Seebacher, J Robert (MD)   OrS
Phelps Mem Hosp Ctr
239 N Broadway; Sleepy Hollow, NY 10591; (914)
631-7777; **BDCERT:** OrS 84; **MS:** Georgetown U
76; **RES:** S, Mount Sinai Med Ctr, New York, NY;
FEL: Ped Oto, Hosp For Sick Children, Toronto,
Canada; **HOSP:** Westchester Med Ctr; *SI: Hips and*
Knees; Pediatric Orthopaedic Surgery; **HMO:** PHS
Oxford HealthNet Blue Choice Magnacare +

⬦ 🔲 🔲 Mcr Mcd WC NFI   4+ Weeks ▨ *VISA* 💳 💳

Small, Steven (MD)   OrS
Hudson Valley Hosp Ctr
Community Orthopadics, 1985 Crompond Rd Bldg
E; Peekskill, NY 10566; (914) 739-2121; **BDCERT:**
OrS 86; **MS:** NY Med Coll 79; **RES:** NY Med Coll,
Valhalla, NY 80-84; **HMO:** Most

⬦ 🔲 🔲 🔲 Mcr WC NFI   1 Week *VISA* 💳

Taddonio, Rudolph (MD)   OrS
Westchester Med Ctr
Scoliosis & Spinal Surgery, 19 Bradhurst Ave;
Hawthorne, NY 10532; (914) 347-3884;
BDCERT: OrS 77; **MS:** NY Med Coll 71; **RES:**
Metropolitan Hosp Ctr, New York, NY 72-75; **FEL:**
S, Rush Presbyterian-St Lukes Med Ctr, Chicago, IL
75-76; **HOSP:** Stamford Hosp; *SI: Scoliosis Surgery;*
Spine Surgery Reconstruction; **HMO:** Oxford Prucare
Aetna Hlth Plan US Hlthcre

⬦ 🔲 🔲 🔲 Mcr WC NFI   A Few Days

Walsh, William (MD)   OrS
St Agnes Hosp
311 North St 406; White Plains, NY 10605; (914)
428-5666; **BDCERT:** OrS 72; **MS:** NY Med Coll 64;
RES: St Vincents Hosp & Med Ctr NY, New York, NY
64-66; Bellevue Hosp Ctr, New York, NY 68-71;
FAP: Assoc Prof NY Med Coll; **HOSP:** White Plains
Hosp Ctr; *SI: Reconstructive Knee Surgery; Sports*
Medicine-Running; **HMO:** Oxford Genesis Prucare
CIGNA Aetna-US Healthcare +

LANG: Ger, Itl, Sp; ⬦ 🔲 🔲 🔲 🔲 Mcr WC NFI
Immediately *VISA* 💳

Zelicof, Steven (MD & PhD)   OrS
Westchester Med Ctr
311 North St 206; White Plains, NY 10605; (914)
686-0111; **BDCERT:** OrS 92; **MS:** Univ Penn 83;
RES: S, Lenox Hill Hosp, New York, NY 84-85; OrS,
Hosp For Special Surgery, New York, NY 85-89;
FEL: PlS, Brigham & Women's Hosp, Boston, MA
89-90; **FAP:** Assoc Clin Prof OrS NY Med Coll;
HOSP: Hosp For Special Surgery; *SI: Joint—*
Replacement; Sports Medicine; **HMO:** Oxford Prucare
Aetna-US Healthcare Pomco CIGNA +

LANG: Itl, Rom; ⬦ 🔲 🔲 🔲 🔲 🔲 Mcr WC NFI
Immediately ▨ *VISA*

Zitzmann, Eric (MD)   OrS
White Plains Hosp Ctr
Westchester Orthopaedic Assoc, 222 Westchester
Ave; White Plains, NY 10604; (914) 946-1010;
BDCERT: OrS 70; **MS:** Cornell U 61; **RES:** S, NY
Hosp-Cornell Med Ctr, New York, NY 62-63; OrS,
Columbia-Presbyterian Med Ctr, New York, NY 65-
68; **FAP:** Assoc Clin Prof OrS NY Med Coll; **HOSP:**
St Agnes Hosp; *SI: Hip & Knee Replacement; Foot*
Surgery; **HMO:** Oxford PHS Prudential Pomco
Aetna Hlth Plan +

LANG: Sp, Ger, Itl; ⬦ 🔲 🔲 🔲 🔲 Mcr WC NFI
A Few Days ▨ *VISA* 💳

OTOLARYNGOLOGY

Bergstein, Michael (MD)   Oto
Phelps Mem Hosp Ctr

Ear, Nose and Associates, PC, 200 S Broadway Rd
201; Tarrytown, NY 10591; (914) 631-3053;
BDCERT: Oto 90; **PlS** 94; **MS:** Mt Sinai Sch Med 85;
RES: Oto, Mount Sinai Med Ctr, New York, NY 85-
90; **FEL:** PlS, UC San Francisco Med Ctr, San
Francisco, CA 90-91; **FAP:** Asst Clin Prof Mt Sinai
Sch Med; **HOSP:** Hudson Valley Hosp Ctr; *SI:*
Endoscopic Sinus Surgery; Facial Plastic Surgery;
HMO: Oxford PHS US Hlthcre Empire Blue Cross &
Shield CIGNA +

LANG: Sp, Fr, Heb; 🔲 🔲 🔲 🔲 🔲 🔲 🔲 🔲 🔲
Immediately 🔲 **VISA** 🔲 🔲

Brown-Wagner, Marie (MD) Oto
Westchester Med Ctr

Route 100 Macy Pavilion 1042B; Valhalla, NY
10595; (914) 285-7891; **BDCERT:** Oto 82; S 82;
MS: Tufts U 76; **RES:** Montefiore Med Ctr, Bronx,
NY 76-78; Jacobi Med Ctr, Bronx, NY 78-80; **FEL:**
Albert Einstein Med Ctr, Bronx, NY 81; **HOSP:** St
Agnes Hosp; **HMO:** Aetna Hlth Plan Blue Choice
Independent Health Plan Lawrence Healthcare

🔲 🔲 🔲 🔲 🔲 🔲 🔲 🔲 1 Week 🔲 **VISA** 🔲

Flynn, William (MD)   Oto
Sound Shore Med Ctr-Westchester

150 Lockwood Ave 38; New Rochelle, NY 10801;
(914) 636-0104; **BDCERT:** Oto 70; **MS:** NY Med
Coll 60; **RES:** NY Med Coll, New York, NY 64-66;
NY Hosp-Cornell Med Ctr, New York, NY 66-69;
HOSP: Lawrence Hosp; **HMO:** Blue Choice
HealthNet Independent Health Plan PHS Oxford +

🔲 🔲 🔲 🔲 🔲 🔲 Immediately **VISA** 🔲

Fox, Mark (MD)   Oto
Lawrence Hosp

700 White Plains Rd 30; Scarsdale, NY 10583;
(914) 725-4266; **BDCERT:** Oto 79; **MS:** NY Med
Coll 73; **RES:** S, Metropolitan Hosp Ctr, New York,
NY 73-74; Manhattan Eye, Ear & Throat Hosp,
New York, NY 76-79; **FAP:** Clin Instr Columbia
P&S; **HOSP:** Sound Shore Med Ctr-Westchester; *SI:*
Sinus & Nasal Surgery; Head/Neck Tumor Surgery;
HMO: Aetna-US Healthcare United Healthcare GHI
Pomco Oxford +

🔲 🔲 🔲 🔲 🔲 🔲 🔲 🔲 🔲 A Few Days **VISA** 🔲

Jamal, Habib (MD)   Oto
United Hosp Med Ctr

14 Rye Ridge Plaza Ste 231; Rye Brook, NY 10573;
(914) 253-2985; **BDCERT:** Oto 79; **MS:** Pakistan
74; **RES:** S, Baylor Coll Med, Houston, TX 74-76;
Oto, Albert Einstein Med Ctr, Bronx, NY 76-79;
HMO: Prucare US Hlthcre PHS Oxford CIGNA +

🔲 🔲 🔲 🔲 🔲 🔲 🔲 🔲 🔲 🔲 Immediately **VISA**
🔲

Jay, Judith (MD)   Oto
Phelps Mem Hosp Ctr

425 N State Rd; Briarcliff Manor, NY 10510; (914)
945-0505; **BDCERT:** Oto 84; **MS:** Hahnemann U
79; **RES:** S, Abington Mem Hosp, Abington, PA 79-
80; Oto, Mount Sinai Med Ctr, New York, NY 81-
84; **HOSP:** Mount Sinai Med Ctr; *SI: Endoscopic*
Sinus Surgery; Tinnitus; **HMO:** PHS Oxford Blue
Choice Multiplan Magnacare +

🔲 🔲 🔲 🔲 🔲 🔲 🔲 🔲 🔲 A Few Days 🔲 **VISA**
🔲

Kase, Steven (MD)   Oto
White Plains Hosp Ctr

1 Old Mamaroneck Rd 1B; White Plains, NY
10605; (914) 681-0300; **BDCERT:** Oto 81; **MS:**
Loyola U-Stritch Sch Med, Maywood 76; **RES:** S, St
Francis Hosp, Evanston, IL 76-77; Oto, New York
Eye & Ear Infirmary, New York, NY 77-80; **HOSP:**
St Agnes Hosp; *SI: Sinus Disease; Pediatric E.N.T.;*
HMO: Oxford PHS Pomco Aetna Hlth Plan United
Healthcare +

LANG: Sp; 🔲 🔲 🔲 🔲 🔲 🔲 🔲 🔲 🔲
Immediately **VISA** 🔲

Kates, Matthew (MD) Oto
Sound Shore Med Ctr-Westchester
Ear Nose & Throat, 150 Lockwood Ave 38; New Rochelle, NY 10801; (914) 636-0104; **BDCERT:** Oto 92; **MS:** Cornell U 86; **RES:** Oto, Manhattan Eye, Ear & Throat Hosp, New York, NY 88-91; **HOSP:** Lawrence Hosp; *SI: Sinus Disease & Surgery; Thyroid Surgery;* **HMO:** Blue Choice Blue Choice PHS Aetna Hlth Plan CIGNA +

LANG: Sp; 🔣 🔣 🔣 🔣 🔣 🔣 🔣 🔣 🔣 Immediately **VISA** 💳

Lawrence, David (MD) Oto
United Hosp Med Ctr
1600 Harrison Ave G104; Mamaroneck, NY 10543; (914) 381-2274; **BDCERT:** Oto 74; **MS:** Albany Med Coll 69; **RES:** Lenox Hill Hosp, New York, NY 70-71; New York Eye & Ear Infirmary, New York, NY 71-74; **HOSP:** New York Eye & Ear Infirmary; *SI: Pediatric ENT Problems; Sinusitis;* **HMO:** Oxford Aetna Hlth Plan Pomco PHS SWCHP +

LANG: Fr; 🔣 🔣 🔣 🔣 🔣 🔣 🔣 🔣 Immediately **VISA** 💳

Lewis, Lawrence (MD) Oto
Northern Westchester Hosp Ctr
495 Main St; Mt Kisco, NY 10549; (914) 241-0516; **BDCERT:** Oto 76; **MS:** SUNY Buffalo 69; **RES:** S, Montefiore Med Ctr, Bronx, NY 69-71; **FEL:** Oto, U Conn Hlth Ctr, Farmington, CT 73-76; *SI: Sinus Surgery; Facial Plastic Surgery;* **HMO:** Oxford PHS Aetna Hlth Plan Pomco Blue Cross & Blue Shield +

🔣 🔣 🔣 🔣 🔣 🔣 🔣 🔣 🔣 Immediately

Meiteles, Lawrence (MD) Oto
Westchester Med Ctr
Cedarwood Hall 4th Fl; Valhalla, NY 10595; (914) 493-7891; **BDCERT:** Oto 92; **MS:** Albert Einstein Coll Med 86; **RES:** S, Montefiore Med Ctr, Bronx, NY 87; Oto, New York Eye & Ear Infirmary, New York, NY 91; **FEL:** Ont N S, U Mich Med Ctr, Ann Arbor, MI; Wayne Cnty Gen Hosp, Detroit, MI; **HOSP:** St Agnes Hosp; *SI: Middle Ear Imbalance; Neurotology;* **HMO:** Most

LANG: Sp; 🔣 🔣 🔣 🔣 🔣 2-4 Weeks 🔣 **VISA** 💳 🔣

Moscatello, Augustine (MD) Oto
Westchester Med Ctr
Cedarwood Hall, 1042B; Valhalla, NY 10595; (914) 493-7891; **BDCERT:** Oto 87; **MS:** Mt Sinai Sch Med 82; **RES:** Mount Sinai Med Ctr, New York, NY 82-87; **FAP:** Assoc Prof NY Med Coll; **HOSP:** St Agnes Hosp; *SI: Pediatric Otolaryngology; Sinus & Nasal Disease;* **HMO:** Pomco GHI CIGNA US Hlthcre Oxford +

LANG: Sp, Itl; 🔣 🔣 🔣 🔣 🔣 🔣 🔣 2-4 Weeks **VISA** 💳 🔣

Murray, Joseph P (MD) Oto
St John's Riverside Hosp
Ear, Nose & Throat Associates, 984 N Broadway Ste 400; Yonkers, NY 10701; (914) 963-8588; **BDCERT:** Oto 73; **MS:** SUNY Downstate 68; **RES:** Oto, Nat Naval Med Ctr, Bethesda, MD 70-73; **HMO:** Most GHI Empire Blue Cross & Blue Shield

🔣 🔣 🔣 🔣 🔣 🔣 🔣 🔣 🔣 1 Week 🔣 **VISA** 💳 🔣

Nevins, Stuart (MD) Oto
White Plains Hosp Ctr
Ear, Nose & Throat Associates, 170 Maple Ave Ste 101; White Plains, NY 10601; (914) 949-4242; **BDCERT:** Oto 68; **MS:** Albany Med Coll 60; **RES:** S, Albany Med Ctr, Albany, NY 62; Oto, Manhattan Eye, Ear & Throat Hosp, New York, NY 64-67; **HMO:** Aetna Hlth Plan Blue Cross & Blue Shield HealthNet Most

🔣 🔣 🔣 🔣 🔣 🔣 🔣 Immediately **VISA** 💳

Rock, Erwin (MD) Oto
St John's Riverside Hosp
970 N Broadway 110; Yonkers, NY 10701; (914) 963-1488; **BDCERT:** Oto 53; **MS:** U Hlth Sci/Chicago Med Sch 48; **RES:** Oto, Harlem Hosp Ctr, New York, NY 49-51; **FEL:** Oto, Harlem Hosp Ctr, New York, NY; *SI: Otology; Neurotology;* **HMO:** Blue Cross & Blue Shield Independent Health Plan PHS Pomco Oxford +

🔣 🔣 🔣 🔣 🔣 🔣 🔣 🔣

Ryback, Hyman (MD)   Oto
White Plains Hosp Ctr
79 East Post Rd Fl 3; White Plains, NY 10601;
(914) 949-3888; **BDCERT:** Oto 77; **MS:** Canada
70; **RES:** Mount Sinai Med Ctr, New York, NY 77;
HOSP: St Agnes Hosp; **SI:** *Endoscopic Sinus Surgery;*
Laryngeal Head & Neck Surgery; **HMO:** Most Aetna-
US Healthcare CIGNA Blue Choice
LANG: Fr, Itl, Heb, Jpn, Sp; 🔳 🔳 🔳 🔳 🔳 🔳 🔳 🔳
🔳 Immediately 🔳 **VISA** 🔳

Schaffer, Dean (MD)   Oto
Northern Westchester Hosp Ctr
51 Bedford Rd; Katonah, NY 10536; (914) 232-
3112; **BDCERT:** Oto 80; **MS:** Albert Einstein Coll
Med 76; **RES:** Montefiore Med Ctr, Bronx, NY 76-
77; Johns Hopkins Hosp, Baltimore, MD 77-80; **SI:**
Nasal & Sinus Symptoms; **HMO:** Prucare Oxford
CIGNA Pomco SWCHP +
LANG: Fr; 🔳 🔳 🔳 🔳 🔳 🔳 🔳 🔳 Immediately
🔳 **VISA** 🔳

Shapiro, Barry (MD)   Oto
Phelps Mem Hosp Ctr
Hudson Ent & Sinus Assoc, 425 N State Rd;
Briarcliff Manor, NY 10510; (914) 945-0505;
BDCERT: Oto 83; **MS:** Mt Sinai Sch Med 78; **RES:** S,
Mount Sinai Med Ctr, New York, NY 78-79; Oto,
Mount Sinai Med Ctr, New York, NY 79-82; **FAP:**
Asst Clin Prof Oto Mt Sinai Sch Med; **SI:** *Endoscopic*
Sinus Surgery; Head/Neck Oncology; **HMO:** Oxford
Pomco PHS Prucare United Healthcare +
🔳 🔳 🔳 🔳 🔳 🔳 🔳 🔳 A Few Days 🔳 **VISA**
🔳

Siglock, Timothy (MD)   Oto
Hudson Valley Hosp Ctr
Valley Ear, Nose & Throat Medicine & Surgery, PC,
3630 Hill Blvd Ste 202; Jefferson Valley, NY
10535; (914) 245-7700; **BDCERT:** Oto 86; **MS:**
Belgium 81; **RES:** New York Eye & Ear Infirmary,
New York, NY 82-86; **FEL:** Oto, House Ear Inst, Los
Angeles, CA 86-87; **SI:** *Care of the Voice;*
Microsurgery of the Ear; **HMO:** Oxford GHI Pomco
United Healthcare Magnacare +
LANG: Fr, Sp; 🔳 🔳 🔳 🔳 🔳 🔳 🔳 🔳 🔳
A Few Days **VISA** 🔳

Vecchiotti, Arthur (MD)   Oto
Phelps Mem Hosp Ctr
245 N Broadway 101; Sleepy Hollow, NY 10591;
(914) 631-6161; **BDCERT:** Oto 78; **MS:** Italy 71;
RES: Metropolitan Hosp Ctr, New York, NY 75;
Manhattan Eye, Ear & Throat Hosp, New York, NY
76-78; **HOSP:** Westchester Med Ctr; **SI:** *Pediatric*
Otolaryngology; Allergy; **HMO:** Oxford PHS United
Healthcare Pomco Excelcare +
LANG: Itl, Sp; 🔳 🔳 🔳 🔳 🔳 🔳 🔳 A Few Days

PAIN MANAGEMENT

Lu, Gabriel (MD)   PM
Montefiore Med Ctr
112 Penn Rd; Scarsdale, NY 10583; (914) 725-
4240; **BDCERT:** Anes 84; **MS:** Taiwan 68; **RES:** S,
St Louis U Hosp, St Louis, MO 74-76; Anes, Albert
Einstein Med Ctr, Bronx, NY 76-77; **FAP:** Assoc
Prof Albert Einstein Coll Med; **HOSP:** Jacobi Med
Ctr; **SI:** *Lower Back Pain & Neck Pain; Acupuncture;*
HMO: Empire Blue Cross & Shield Oxford GHI HIP
Network HMO Blue +
LANG: Chi, Sp; 🔳 🔳 🔳 🔳 🔳 🔳 🔳 🔳
A Few Days

PEDIATRIC CARDIOLOGY

Fish, Bernard (MD)   PCd
Westchester Med Ctr
Munger Pavilion, Rte 100 601; Valhalla, NY
10595; (914) 594-4370; **BDCERT:** Ped 74; PCd
75; **MS:** U Chicago-Pritzker Sch Med 69; **RES:** Ped,
Montefiore Med Ctr, Bronx, NY 70-71; PCd,
Montefiore Med Ctr, Bronx, NY 71-73; **FEL:** PCd,
Yale-New Haven Hosp, New Haven, CT 73-75;
FAP: Asst Prof Ped NY Med Coll; **HOSP:** St John's
Riverside Hosp; **SI:** *Noninvasive Testing; Fetal*
Echocardiography; **HMO:** PHS Blue Choice Oxford
United Healthcare US Hlthcre +
🔳 🔳 🔳 🔳 🔳 🔳 🔳 Immediately **VISA** 🔳

Gewitz, Michael (MD) PCd
Westchester Med Ctr

Route 100 Munger Pavilion 618; Valhalla, NY 10595; (914) 594-4370; **BDCERT:** Ped 79; PCd 81; **MS:** Hahnemann U 74; **RES:** Ped, Children's Hosp of Philadelphia, Philadelphia, PA 74-76; Ped, Hosp For Sick Children, England 76-77; **FEL:** PCd, Yale-New Haven Hosp, New Haven, CT 77-79; **FAP:** Chf PCd NY Med Coll; **HOSP:** Our Lady of Mercy Med Ctr; **SI:** *Congenital Heart Disease; Pediatric Heart Disease*; **HMO:** Oxford Aetna Hlth Plan Prucare CIGNA Anthem Health +

♿ 🅿 🏧 💲 Ⓜ �Ⓦ A Few Days 💳 **VISA** ●

Levin, Aaron (MD) PCd
Westchester Med Ctr

NY Medical College, Rte100 Munger Pavilion 618; Valhalla, NY 10595; (914) 594-4370; **BDCERT:** PCd 66; **MS:** South Africa 53; **RES:** Coronation Hosp, Johannesberg, South Africa 55-60; Charing Cross Hosp, London, England 62; **FEL:** PCd, Duke U Med Ctr, Durham, NC 64-66; **FAP:** Prof NY Med Coll; **SI:** *Congenital Heart Disease; Pediatric Heart Disease*; **HMO:** Aetna-US Healthcare Kaiser Permanente Oxford United Healthcare Magnacare +

LANG: Afk; ♿ 🅿 🚹 🏧 💲 Ⓜ Immediately 💳 **VISA** ●

Snyder, Michael (MD) PCd
Westchester Med Ctr

Faculty Practice Associates, Munger Pavilion; Valhalla, NY 10595; (914) 594-4370; **BDCERT:** Ped 84; Cv 85; **MS:** Cornell U 79; **RES:** Ped, NY Hosp-Cornell Med Ctr, New York, NY 79-82; **FEL:** PCd, NY Hosp-Cornell Med Ctr, New York, NY 82-84; **FAP:** Asst Prof NY Med Coll; **SI:** *Pediatric Heart Murmurs*; **HMO:** Oxford PHS Aetna Hlth Plan Empire Blue Cross United Healthcare +

♿ 🅿 🚹 🏧 💲 Ⓜ Ⓜ A Few Days **VISA** ●

Woolf, Paul (MD) PCd
Westchester Med Ctr

Pediatric Cardiology, Munger Pavilion; Valhalla, NY 10595; (914) 594-4370; **BDCERT:** Ped 82; PCd 83; **MS:** Columbia P&S 77; **FEL:** Cv, Children's Hosp of Philadelphia, Philadelphia, PA; **SI:** *Rhythm Disorders*; **HMO:** Aetna Hlth Plan HealthNet Travelers Oxford

LANG: Sp; ♿ 🅿 🏧 💲 Ⓜ Ⓜ Ⓦ Ⓝ Immediately **VISA** ●

PEDIATRIC ENDOCRINOLOGY

Breidbart, Scott (MD) PEn
Westchester Med Ctr

Route 100 Munger Pavilion 140; Valhalla, NY 10595; (914) 493-7584; **BDCERT:** Ped 87; PEn 97; **MS:** Columbia P&S 83; **RES:** Ped, Columbia-Presbyterian Med Ctr, New York, NY 83-85; Ped, Westchester County Med Ctr, Valhalla, NY 85-86; **FEL:** PEn, Montefiore Med Ctr, Bronx, NY 86-88; **FAP:** Asst Prof NY Med Coll; **HMO:** Most

♿ 🅿 🚹 🏧 💲 Ⓜ Ⓜ Immediately **VISA** ●

Handelsman, Dan (MD) PEn PCP
Phelps Mem Hosp Ctr

325 S Highland Ave; Briarcliff Manor, NY 10510; (914) 762-0015; **BDCERT:** Ped 73; **MS:** Albert Einstein Coll Med 68; **RES:** Ped, Montefiore Med Ctr, Bronx, NY 69-71; **FEL:** Metabolism & Genetics, Albert Einstein Med Ctr, Bronx, NY; **FAP:** Assoc Clin Instr Ped NYU Sch Med; **HOSP:** Westchester Med Ctr

♿ ⓈⒶ Ⓒ 🅿 🚹 🏧 💲 Ⓜ Ⓝ A Few Days **VISA** ●

Lebinger, Tessa (MD) PEn
White Plains Hosp Ctr

811 N Broadway 204; White Plains, NY 10603; (914) 682-8756; **BDCERT:** Ped 82; PEn 83; **MS:** Albert Einstein Coll Med 76; **RES:** Ped, Jacobi Med Ctr, Bronx, NY 76-78; **FEL:** PEn, Montefiore Med Ctr, Bronx, NY; Albert Einstein Med Ctr, Bronx, NY 79-81; **FAP:** Asst Clin Prof Ped Albert Einstein Coll Med; **HOSP:** Montefiore Med Ctr; **SI:** *Diabetes; Growth Problems In Children*

♿ Ⓒ 🅿 🚹 🏧 💲 Ⓜ Immediately

Romano, Alicia (MD) PEn
Westchester Med Ctr
Route 100 Munger Pavilion; Valhalla, NY 10595;
(914) 493-7584; **BDCERT:** PEn 89; **MS:** SUNY
Hlth Sci Ctr 85; **RES:** Schneider Children's Hosp,
New Hyde Park, NY 85-88; **FEL:** PEn, Schneider
Children's Hosp, New Hyde Park, NY; **HOSP:** Our
Lady of Mercy Med Ctr; **HMO:** US Hlthcre Oxford
Champus CIGNA

♿ 📷 🏨 Ⓢ 🄪 4+ Weeks **VISA** 💳

PEDIATRIC GASTROENTEROLOGY

Benkov, Keith (MD) PGe
Mount Sinai Med Ctr
Pediatric Gastroenterology, 147 Underhill Ave Fl 1;
White Plains, NY 10604; (914) 681-0333;
BDCERT: PGe 84; **MS:** Mt Sinai Sch Med 79; **RES:**
Ped, Mount Sinai Med Ctr, New York, NY 79-82;
FEL: Ped GI, Mount Sinai Med Ctr, New York, NY
82-84; **FAP:** Asst Lecturer Mt Sinai Sch Med;
HOSP: Englewood Hosp & Med Ctr; **SI:** *Inflammatory
Bowel Disease; Liver Disease;* **HMO:** Oxford US
Hlthcre Prucare

LANG: Sp; ♿ 📷 👨 🏨 Ⓢ 2-4 Weeks 💳 **VISA**
💳

Glassman, Mark (MD) PGe
Sound Shore Med Ctr-Westchester
16 Guion Pl; New Rochelle, NY 10801; (914) 637-
1122; **BDCERT:** Ped 83; PGe 90; **MS:** SUNY Buffalo
78; **RES:** Yale-New Haven Hosp, New Haven, CT
78-81; **FEL:** Ge, Children's Hosp of Philadelphia,
Philadelphia, PA 81-83; **FAP:** Prof Ped NY Med
Coll; **HOSP:** Greenwich Hosp; **SI:** *Inflammatory
Bowel Disease; Gastroenterological Reflux;* **HMO:**
Aetna Hlth Plan CIGNA PHS United Healthcare
Blue Cross +

♿ 📷 👨 🏨 Ⓢ 🄪 Immediately

Newman, Leonard (MD) PGe
Westchester Med Ctr
Route 100 Munger Pavilion 123; Valhalla, NY
10595; (914) 594-4280; **BDCERT:** Ped 75; PGe
90; **MS:** NY Med Coll 70; **RES:** NY Med Coll, New
York, NY 71-72; NY Med Coll, New York, NY 72-
73; **FEL:** Ge, Albert Einstein Med Ctr, Bronx, NY 73-
74; **FAP:** Prof NY Med Coll; **SI:** *Pediatric Colitis;
Ileitis—Crohn's Disease;* **HMO:** Oxford US Hlthcre
Well Care Independent Health Plan

♿ 📷 🏨 Ⓢ 🄪 A Few Days **VISA** 💳

PEDIATRIC HEMATOLOGY-ONCOLOGY

Bonilla, Mary Ann (MD) PHO
Mem Sloan Kettering Cancer Ctr
United Medical Center, 15 S 9th St; Newark, NJ
07107; (973) 972-4300; **BDCERT:** Ped 90; PHO
90; **MS:** Loyola U-Stritch Sch Med, Maywood 81;
RES: Brookdale Univ Hosp Med Ctr, Brooklyn, NY
82-83; Brookdale Univ Hosp Med Ctr, Brooklyn, NY
83-84; **FEL:** Hem, Mem Sloan Kettering Cancer Ctr,
New York, NY 84-88; **HOSP:** St Barnabas Med Ctr-
Livingston

Jayabose, Somasundaram (MD)PHO
Westchester Med Ctr
Route 100 Munger Pavilion RM110; Valhalla, NY
10595; (914) 493-7997; **BDCERT:** Ped 75; PHO
76; **MS:** India 69; **RES:** Ped, Metropolitan Hosp Ctr,
New York, NY 71-73; **FEL:** PHO, Long Island
Jewish Med Ctr, New Hyde Park, NY; **FAP:** Assoc
Prof Ped NY Med Coll; **HOSP:** Good Samaritan
Hosp; **SI:** *Sickle Cell Disease; Bone Marrow
Transplantation;* **HMO:** Aetna Hlth Plan Empire
Oxford CIGNA GHI +

LANG: Sp, Trk; ♿ 📷 🏨 Ⓢ 🄪 Ⓦ 🄵 Immediately

Guide to symbols and abbreviations can be found on pages 110-113.

Tugal, Oya (MD)   PHO
Westchester Med Ctr

Rt 100 Munger Pav-Westchester Med Ctr 110; Valhalla, NY 10595; (914) 493-7997; **BDCERT:** Ped 86; **MS:** Turkey 74; **RES:** Ped, Hacettepe Med Ctr, Turkey 74-77; Ped, Westchester County Med Ctr, Valhalla, NY 83-85; **FEL:** A&I, Hacettepe Med Ctr, Turkey 77-78; **PHO**, Mount Sinai Med Ctr, New York, NY 85-87; **FAP:** Assoc Prof NY Med Coll; **HOSP:** Good Samaritan Hosp; *SI: Leukemia & Lymphomas; Histiocytosis;* **HMO:** Aetna Hlth Plan Pomco GHI Oxford CIGNA +

LANG: Sp, Trk; 👤 📷 🔧 🏥 $ Mcd WC NFI Immediately **VISA** 💳

PEDIATRIC
NEPHROLOGY

Weiss, Robert Allen (MD)   PNep
Westchester Med Ctr

Munger Pavilion, Munger Pav-Westchester Med Ctr; Valhalla, NY 10595; (914) 493-7583; **BDCERT:** Ped 76; Nep 79; **MS:** Georgetown U 71; **RES:** Ped, Bellevue Hosp Ctr, New York, NY 72-74; **FEL:** PNep, Albert Einstein Med Ctr, Bronx, NY; **FAP:** Sr Prof Ped NY Med Coll; *SI: Nephritic Syndrome; Kidney Transplantation*

👤 📷 🏥 $ Mcd

Zuckerman, Andrea (MD)   PNep
Westchester Med Ctr

Dept of Pediatrics, New York Medical College; Valhalla, NY 10595; (914) 493-7583; **BDCERT:** Ped 85; PNep 88; **MS:** Harvard Med Sch 80; **RES:** Ped, Johns Hopkins Hosp, Baltimore, MD 80-83; PNep, Mount Sinai Med Ctr, New York, NY 86-87; **FEL:** PNep, Children's Hosp Med Ctr, Cincinnati, OH 83-84; PNep, NY Hosp-Cornell Med Ctr, New York, NY 84-86; **FAP:** Asst Prof NY Med Coll; **HOSP:** Metropolitan Hosp Ctr; *SI: Lupus;* **HMO:** Oxford Kaiser Permanente US Hlthcre CIGNA Pomco +

LANG: Sp, Fr, Ger, Swd; 👤 📷 🔧 🏥 $ Mcd Mcd 1 Week **VISA** 💳

PEDIATRIC
PULMONOLOGY

Dozor, Allen (MD)   PPul
Westchester Med Ctr

95 Grassland Rd; Valhalla, NY 10595; (914) 493-7585; **BDCERT:** Ped 81; **MS:** Penn State U-Hershey Med Ctr 77; **RES:** Ped, St Vincents Hosp & Med Ctr NY, New York, NY 77-80; **FEL:** PPul, Children's Hosp, Boston, MA 80-82; **FAP:** Assoc Prof Ped NY Med Coll; *SI: Asthma; Cystic Fibrosis;* **HMO:** Oxford Aetna Hlth Plan Independent Health Plan Prucare Metlife +

👤 📷 🔧 🏥 $ Mcd A Few Days 🏧 **VISA** 💳 💳

PEDIATRIC SURGERY

Holgersen, Leif (MD)   PS
St Luke's Roosevelt Hosp Ctr

1 Elm St 1A; Tuckahoe, NY 10707; (914) 337-2455; **BDCERT:** S 71; PS 75; **MS:** UMDNJ-NJ Med Sch, Newark 65; **RES:** St Luke's Roosevelt Hosp Ctr, New York, NY 66-70; Children's Hosp of Philadelphia, Philadelphia, PA 72-74; **FAP:** Asst Prof Columbia P&S; **HOSP:** St John's Riverside Hosp; **HMO:** Aetna Hlth Plan Oxford Pomco United Healthcare Empire Blue Choice +

👤 🌙 📷 🏥 $ Mcd NFI A Few Days

Liebert, Peter (MD)   PS
White Plains Hosp Ctr

270 White Plains Rd; Eastchester, NY 10707; (914) 337-5678; **BDCERT:** S 68; Ped 95; **MS:** Harvard Med Sch 61; **RES:** Peter Bent Brigham Hosp, Boston, MA 61-64; Montefiore Med Ctr, Bronx, NY 64-66; **FEL:** Ped, Children's Hosp of Philadelphia, Philadelphia, PA 66-68; **FAP:** Assoc Prof S Columbia P&S; **HOSP:** Columbia-Presbyterian Med Ctr; *SI: Pediatric Hernias All Types; Intestinal Abnormalities;* **HMO:** Oxford CIGNA Kaiser Permanente Prucare PHS +

👤 📷 🔧 🏥 $ Mcd NFI A Few Days

San Filippo, J Anthony (MD)   PS
St Agnes Hosp
Westchester Co Med Ctr/St Agnes Hosp, 311 North
St; Valhalla, NY 10595; (914) 761-5437;
BDCERT: S 73; **PS** 75; **MS:** Georgetown U 65; **RES:**
S, Bellevue Hosp Ctr, New York, NY 66-67; N Shore
Univ Hosp-Manhasset, Manhasset, NY; **FEL:** Ped,
Children's Hosp of Buffalo, Buffalo, NY; **HOSP:**
Westchester Med Ctr; *SI: Congenital Newborn
Surgery; Tumors in Childhood;* **HMO:** Oxford Blue
Cross & Blue Shield US Hlthcre GHI Servitas +
⟨symbols⟩   A Few Days

Slim, Michel (MD)   PS
Westchester Med Ctr
Munger Pavillion/Westchester Med Ctr, Ped Surg,
New York Medical College 321; Valhalla, NY
10595; (914) 493-7620; **BDCERT:** TS 62; **PS** 91;
MS: Lebanon 54; **RES:** American U Med Ctr, Beirut,
Lebanon 54-58; Cleveland Metro Gen Hosp,
Cleveland, OH 58-59; **FEL:** Children's Hosp of
Pittsburgh, Pittsburgh, PA 60-62; TS, Hosp For
Sick Children, Toronto, Canada 70; **FAP:** Prof NY
Med Coll; *SI: Pediatric Trauma; Neonatal Surgery*
LANG: Fr, Ar; ⟨symbols⟩
Immediately

Zitsman, Jeffrey (MD)   PS
Our Lady of Mercy Med Ctr
BronxWestchester Pediatric Surgery, 688 White
Plains Rd 223; Scarsdale, NY 10583; (914) 722-
6737; **BDCERT:** PS 95; Ped 93; **MS:** Tufts U 76;
RES: S, New England Med Ctr, Boston, MA 76-81;
FEL: PdS, Babies Hosp, New York, NY 83-85; **FAP:**
Asst Clin Prof Columbia P&S; **HOSP:** Columbia-
Presbyterian Med Ctr; *SI: Pediatric Laparoscopy;
Chestwall Repair;* **HMO:** Oxford Aetna-US
Healthcare GHI Magnacare Prucare +
LANG: Sp; ⟨symbols⟩   A Few Days

PEDIATRICS

Amler, David (MD)   Ped   PCP
White Plains Hosp Ctr
15 Chester Ave; White Plains, NY 10601; (914)
948-4422; **BDCERT:** Ped 74; **MS:** SUNY Buffalo 69;
RES: Bellevue Hosp Ctr, New York, NY 69-70; New
York University Med Ctr, New York, NY 70-72;
FAP: Clin Instr NYU Sch Med; **HOSP:** St Agnes
Hosp; **HMO:** Oxford PHS Pomco Pomco
⟨symbols⟩   Immediately ▦ *VISA* ●

Baskind, Larry (MD)   Ped   PCP
Hudson Valley Hosp Ctr
Riverside Pediatrics, 35 S Riverside Ave 5; Croton-
On-Hudson, NY 10520; (914) 271-2424;
BDCERT: Ped 96; **MS:** UMDNJ-NJ Med Sch, Newark
83; **RES:** Children's Hosp of NJ, Newark, NJ 83-87;
HOSP: Westchester Med Ctr; *SI: Homeopathy;* **HMO:**
Oxford Aetna Hlth Plan Blue Choice Independent
Health Plan Multiplan +
LANG: Sp, Itl; ⟨symbols⟩   Immediately
VISA ●

Berger, Leonard (MD)   Ped   PCP
St Agnes Hosp
731 Saw Mill River Rd; Ardsley, NY 10502; (914)
693-2133; **BDCERT:** Ped 64; **MS:** Geo Wash U Sch
Med 57; **RES:** Kings County Hosp Ctr, Brooklyn, NY
60-62; **HOSP:** White Plains Hosp Ctr; *SI:
Developmental Disabilities; Mental Retardation;* **HMO:**
Oxford Aetna Hlth Plan United Healthcare PHCS
Independent Health Plan +
⟨symbols⟩   Immediately

Berkowitz, Norman (MD)   Ped   PCP
United Hosp Med Ctr
Pediatric Associates, 12 Rye Ridge Plaza; Rye
Brook, NY 10573; (914) 251-1100; **BDCERT:** Ped
72; **MS:** SUNY Buffalo 67; **RES:** Ped, Mount Sinai
Med Ctr, New York, NY 68-70; **FEL:** Ped, St
Christopher's Hosp for Children, Philadelphia, PA
72-73; **FAP:** Clin Instr Psyc Cornell U; **HOSP:**
Greenwich Hosp; **HMO:** Oxford
LANG: Sp; ⟨symbols⟩   A Few Days *VISA*
●

814

Berman, Morton (MD) Ped **PCP**
White Plains Hosp Ctr

14 Soundview Ave; White Plains, NY 10606;
(914) 948-7016; **BDCERT:** Ped 72; **MS:** NYU Sch
Med 66; **RES:** Ped, Bellevue Hosp Ctr, New York,
NY 66-68; Ped, Univ Hosp SUNY Bklyn, Brooklyn,
NY 66-68; **FEL:** Ped, Bellevue Hosp Ctr, New York,
NY 69-70; Univ Hosp SUNY Bklyn, Brooklyn, NY
69-70; **FAP:** NYU Sch Med; **HOSP:** Blythedale
Children's Hosp; **HMO:** Oxford Chubb PHS Pomco
Blue Cross & Blue Shield +

LANG: Sp; 🔳 🔳 🔳 🔳 🔳 🔳 Immediately **VISA** 💳

Blumencranz, Harriet (MD) Ped
Northern Westchester Hosp Ctr

PO Box 488; Goldens Bridge, NY 10526; (914)
232-2600; **BDCERT:** Ped 82; **MS:** U Tenn Ctr Hlth
Sci, Memphis 76; **RES:** Ped, U FL Shands Hosp,
Gainesville, FL 71-77; Ped, Mount Sinai Med Ctr,
New York, NY 79-80; **FEL:** PGe, Mount Sinai Med
Ctr, New York, NY 80-82; **FAP:** Lecturer Mt Sinai
Sch Med; **SI:** *Pediatric Nutrition; Pediatric Preventive
Medicine;* **HMO:** Oxford Pomco Blue Choice CIGNA
United Healthcare +

🔳 🔳 🔳 🔳 🔳 🔳 🔳 🔳 1 Week **VISA** 💳

Bomback, Fredric (MD) Ped **PCP**
White Plains Hosp Ctr

Westchester Pediatrics, 99 Fieldstone Dr; Hartsdale,
NY 10530; (914) 428-2120; **BDCERT:** Ped 72;
MS: NYU Sch Med 69; **RES:** Ped, Albert Einstein
Med Ctr, Bronx, NY 69-70; Ped, Albert Einstein
Med Ctr, Bronx, NY 70-72; **FEL:**
Genetics/Metabolism, Albert Einstein Med Ctr,
Bronx, NY 74-76; **FAP:** Clin Prof Ped Columbia
P&S; **HOSP:** Columbia-Presbyterian Med Ctr; **SI:**
Infectious Disease; Complicated Diagnoses; **HMO:**
Oxford PHS Pomco Aetna Hlth Plan

LANG: Sp; 🔳 🔳 🔳 🔳 🔳 🔳 🔳 🔳 🔳
Immediately

Brittis, Robert (MD) Ped **PCP**
St John's Riverside Hosp

984 N Broadway Ste 506; Yonkers, NY 10701;
(914) 963-7668; **MS:** Italy 63; **RES:** Ped,
Hackensack U Med Ctr, Hackensack, NJ 64-65; Ped,
Kings County Hosp Ctr, Brooklyn, NY 69-71; **HMO:**
Oxford United Healthcare Pomco Blue Cross PHS +

LANG: Itl; 🔳 🔳 🔳 🔳 🔳 🔳 🔳 Immediately **VISA**
💳

Brown, Jeffrey (MD) Ped **PCP**
United Hosp Med Ctr

12 Rye Ridge Plaza; Rye Brook, NY 10573; (914)
251-1100; **BDCERT:** Ped 72; **MS:** U Md Sch Med
65; **RES:** Mount Sinai Med Ctr, New York, NY 68-
70; **FEL:** NY Hosp-Cornell Med Ctr, New York, NY
70-71; **FAP:** Assoc Clin Prof Psyc Cornell U; **HOSP:**
NY Hosp-Cornell Med Ctr; **HMO:** Oxford

🔳 🔳 🔳 🔳 🔳 🔳 🔳 🔳 **VISA** 💳

Conway Jr, Edward E (MD) Ped
Beth Israel Med Ctr

17 Whittier St; Hartsdale, NY 10530; (212) 870-
9692; **BDCERT:** PCCM 96; Ped 96; **MS:** SUNY Hlth
Sci Ctr 84; **RES:** Ped, Albert Einstein Med Ctr,
Bronx, NY 84-85; Ped, Albert Einstein Med Ctr,
Bronx, NY 85-87; **FEL:** PCCM, Albert Einstein Med
Ctr, Bronx, NY 88-90; **FAP:** Assoc Ped Albert
Einstein Coll Med; **SI:** *Head Injury; Child Abuse;*
HMO: Chubb Prucare Oxford Aetna Hlth Plan US
Hlthcre +

LANG: Sp, Arm; 🔳 🔳 🔳 🔳 🔳 🔳 🔳 🔳
Immediately

Costa, John (MD) Ped **PCP**
Northern Westchester Hosp Ctr

Mount Kisco Medical Group, 1825 Commerce St;
Yorktown Heights, NY 10598; (914) 962-8989;
BDCERT: Ped 72; **MS:** St Louis U 66; **RES:**
Columbia-Presbyterian Med Ctr, New York, NY 67-
68; **FEL:** NP, Columbia-Presbyterian Med Ctr, New
York, NY 71-72; **SI:** *Neonatology; General Pediatrics;*
HMO: Oxford Aetna Hlth Plan US Hlthcre PHS
NYLCare +

🔳 🔳 🔳 🔳 🔳 🔳 🔳 🔳 Immediately 🔳 **VISA**
💳

Guide to symbols and abbreviations can be found on pages 110-113.

815

Coven, Barbara (MD)　　　Ped　PCP
White Plains Hosp Ctr
210 Westchester Ave; White Plains, NY 10604;
(914) 682-0700; **BDCERT:** Ped 86; **MS:** Boston U
80; **RES:** Boston Med Ctr, Boston, MA 80-82; **FEL:**
ChiN, Children's Hosp, Boston, MA 83; *SI:*
Psychosomatic Childhood Illness; **HMO:** Kaiser
Permanente
LANG: Sp; ⬥ 🆘 🔲 🔲 🔲 🔲 $ Med WC NFI
A Few Days ▦ *VISA* 💳 🔲

Dreyfus, Norma (MD)　　　Ped　PCP
Sound Shore Med Ctr-Westchester
2345 Boston Post Rd; Larchmont, NY 10538;
(914) 833-7540; **BDCERT:** Ped 71; **MS:** Columbia
P&S 66; **RES:** Jacobi Med Ctr, Bronx, NY 67-69;
Albert Einstein Med Ctr, Bronx, NY 67-69; **FAP:**
Asst Clin Prof Albert Einstein Coll Med; **HOSP:**
Montefiore Med Ctr
⬥ 🆘 🔲 🔲 🔲 $ Immediately *VISA* 💳

Edis, Gloria (MD)　　　Ped　PCP
Lawrence Hosp
Scarsdale Pediatric Assoc, 2 Overhill Rd 200;
Scarsdale, NY 10583; (914) 725-0800; **BDCERT:**
Ped 70; **MS:** NYU Sch Med 63; **RES:** Montefiore Med
Ctr, Bronx, NY 63-64; Columbia-Presbyterian Med
Ctr, New York, NY 66-68; **FAP:** Asst Clin Prof
Cornell U; **HOSP:** White Plains Hosp Ctr; **HMO:**
Oxford Independent Health Plan PHS United
Healthcare Multiplan +
LANG: Sp; ⬥ 🆘 🔲 🔲 🔲 🔲 $ NFI Immediately
VISA 💳 🔲

Hartz, Cindi (MD)　　　Ped
United Hosp Med Ctr
1415 Boston Post Rd; Larchmont, NY 10538;
(914) 833-1502; **BDCERT:** Ped 89; **MS:** Mt Sinai
Sch Med 83; **RES:** Mount Sinai Med Ctr, New York,
NY 83-86; **FEL:** Hem & Onc, Mount Sinai Med Ctr,
New York, NY 86-87

Hetzler, Theresa (MD)　　　Ped　PCP
Westchester Med Ctr
Children's Physicians of Westchester, LLP, 19
Bradhurst Ave; Hawthorne, NY 10532; (914) 493-
7897; **BDCERT:** Ped 91; **MS:** Albany Med Coll 88;
RES: Ped, Westchester County Med Ctr, Valhalla,
NY 88-91; **FEL:** Ped, Westchester County Med Ctr,
Valhalla, NY; **FAP:** Asst Prof NY Med Coll; **HMO:**
Oxford Aetna Hlth Plan Empire Prucare US Hlthcre
+
⬥ 🆘 🔲 🔲 🔲 $ Med A Few Days *VISA* 💳

Inch, Eugene (MD)　　　Ped　PCP
St John's Riverside Hosp
984 N Broadway LL10; Yonkers, NY 10701; (914)
965-3670; **BDCERT:** Ped 78; **MS:** SUNY Hlth Sci
Ctr 68; **RES:** U Hosp, Cincinnati, OH 69; Children's
Hosp Med Ctr, Cincinnati, OH 71-73; **FAP:** Asst
Clin Prof Albert Einstein Coll Med; **HOSP:**
Westchester Med Ctr; *SI: Behavioral*
Problems/Attention Deficit Hyperactivity Disorder;
Asthma; **HMO:** Aetna Hlth Plan Oxford United
Healthcare Health Source PHS +
LANG: Sp; ⬥ 🆘 🔲 🔲 🔲 $ WC NFI *VISA* 💳 🔲

Katz, Kenneth (MD)　　　Ped　PCP
White Plains Hosp Ctr
99 Fieldstone Dr; Hartsdale, NY 10530; (914) 428-
2120; **BDCERT:** Ped 78; **MS:** NY Med Coll 73; **RES:**
Ped, Bronx Muncipal Hosp Ctr, Bronx, NY 73-76;
FEL: Ped, Albert Einstein Med Ctr, Bronx, NY 76-
78; **FAP:** Clin Prof Columbia P&S; **HOSP:** Columbia-
Presbyterian Med Ctr; **HMO:** Oxford PHS
⬥ 🔲 🔲 🔲 $ Med 2-4 Weeks

Levine, Steven (MD)　　　Ped　PCP
Northern Westchester Hosp Ctr
Pediatric Associates of Northern Westchester, 666
Lexington Ave 107; Mt Kisco, NY 10549; (914)
666-4742; **BDCERT:** Ped 85; Ped EM 92; **MS:**
Albert Einstein Coll Med 81; **RES:** Ped, Jacobi Med
Ctr, Bronx, NY 81-85; **FAP:** Asst Clin Prof NY Med
Coll
⬥ 🔲 $ ▦ *VISA* 💳 🔲

Levitt, Miriam (MD)   Ped   **PCP**
Lawrence Hosp

1 Pondfield Rd; Bronxville, NY 10708; (914) 961-3604; **BDCERT:** Ped 75; **MS:** Albert Einstein Coll Med 71; **RES:** Montefiore Med Ctr, Bronx, NY 72-73; **FAP:** Asst Clin Prof Ped Albert Einstein Coll Med; **HOSP:** Montefiore Med Ctr; **HMO:** CIGNA Oxford

🔲 🔲 🔲 🔲 🔲 🔲 Immediately

Lubell, David (MD)   Ped   **PCP**
Phelps Mem Hosp Ctr

Briarcliff Pediatrics Associates, PC, 325 S Highland Ave; Briarcliff Manor, NY 10510; (914) 762-0015; **BDCERT:** Ped 68; **MS:** NYU Sch Med 62; **RES:** Children's Hosp of Pittsburgh, Pittsburgh, PA 62-64; Boston Med Ctr, Boston, MA 64-65; **FEL:** Behavioral Ped, Children's Hosp, Boston, MA 65-66; **HMO:** Aetna Hlth Plan Blue Choice Blue Cross & Blue Shield HIP Network HealthNet +

🔲 🔲 🔲 🔲 🔲 🔲 🔲 Immediately **VISA** 🔲

Lubell, Harry R (MD)   Ped   **PCP**
Phelps Mem Hosp Ctr

Pediatrics of Sleepy Hollow, LLP, 245 N Broadway 201; North Tarrytown, NY 10591; (914) 332-4141; **BDCERT:** Ped 69; **MS:** U Hlth Sci/Chicago Med Sch 64; **RES:** Ped, Montefiore Med Ctr, Bronx, NY 65-67; **FEL:** PHO, Babies Hosp, New York, NY 69-70; **FAP:** Asst Clin Prof Ped NY Med Coll; **HOSP:** Westchester Med Ctr; **HMO:** Aetna Hlth Plan CIGNA PHS Oxford Prucare +

🔲 🔲 🔲 🔲 🔲 🔲 🔲 1 Week

Marcus, Judith (MD)   Ped
Columbia-Presbyterian Med Ctr

147 Underhill Ave; White Plains, NY 10604; (914) 684-0220; **BDCERT:** Ped 76; **MS:** NYU Sch Med 71; **RES:** Ped, Albert Einstein Med Ctr, Bronx, NY 72-74; **FEL:** PHO, NY Hosp-Cornell Med Ctr, New York, NY; PHO, Mem Sloan Kettering Cancer Ctr, New York, NY 78-79; **FAP:** Clin Prof Ped Columbia P&S; **HOSP:** White Plains Hosp Ctr; **HMO:** Blue Cross & Blue Shield Anthem Health GHI Oxford PHS +

LANG: Sp, Heb; 🔲 🔲 🔲 🔲 🔲 🔲 🔲 Immediately

Noto, Richard (MD)   Ped
Westchester Med Ctr

Westchester County Med Ctr—Pediatrics, Route 100 Munger Pavilion 103; Valhalla, NY 10595; (914) 285-7584; **BDCERT:** Ped 81; **MS:** Mt Sinai Sch Med 76; **RES:** Beth Israel Med Ctr, New York, NY 78; **FEL:** NY Hosp-Cornell Med Ctr, New York, NY 79; N Shore Univ Hosp-Plainview, Plainview, NY 81; **HMO:** Aetna Hlth Plan Blue Choice Blue Cross & Blue Shield HealthNet Independent Health Plan +

🔲 🔲 🔲 🔲 🔲 🔲 🔲 Immediately **VISA** 🔲

Richel, Peter (MD)   Ped   **PCP**
Northern Westchester Hosp Ctr

14 Smith Ave; Mt Kisco, NY 10549; (914) 666-6655; **BDCERT:** Ped 90; **MS:** Dominican Republic 83; **RES:** Albany Med Ctr, Albany, NY 83-86; **FEL:** PM, St Luke's Roosevelt Hosp Ctr, New York, NY 87-88; **FAP:** Asst Clin Prof Albert Einstein Coll Med; **HMO:** Oxford Pomco SWCHP

LANG: Sp, Fr, Grk; 🔲 🔲 🔲 🔲 🔲 Immediately 🔲 **VISA** 🔲

Rifkinson-Mann, Stephanie (MD)   Ped
St Agnes Hosp

503 Grasslands Rd 108; Valhalla, NY 10595; (914) 345-2111; **MS:** U Puerto Rico 81; **RES:** S, Mount Sinai Med Ctr, New York, NY 81-82; NS, Mount Sinai Med Ctr, New York, NY 82-87; **FEL:** Nat Hosp For Nervous Diseases, London, England 83; Ped NS, New York University Med Ctr, New York, NY 87-88; **HOSP:** Westchester Med Ctr; **HMO:** Empire Blue Cross & Shield Oxford US Hlthcre Independent Health Plan

🔲 🔲 🔲 🔲 🔲 🔲 🔲 🔲 A Few Days

Sidoti, Eugene (MD)   Ped   **PCP**
Lawrence Hosp

1254 Central Park Ave; Yonkers, NY 10704; (914) 423-7700; **BDCERT:** Ped 63; **MS:** SUNY Downstate 57; **RES:** Jacobi Med Ctr, Bronx, NY 57-61; **FAP:** Assoc Clin Prof Ped Albert Einstein Coll Med; **HOSP:** Montefiore Med Ctr; *SI: Cleft Lip and Palate; Craniofacial Abnormalities;* **HMO:** Oxford Blue Choice CIGNA United Healthcare Magnacare +

LANG: Itl; 🔲 🔲 🔲 🔲 🔲 🔲 🔲 🔲 2-4 Weeks **VISA** 🔲

Guide to symbols and abbreviations can be found on pages 110-113.

817

Silverman, Jason (MD)　　Ped　PCP
Sound Shore Med Ctr-Westchester
140 Lockwood Ave; New Rochelle, NY 10801; (914) 235-3800; **BDCERT:** Ped 65; **MS:** Boston U 60; **RES:** Rhode Island Hosp, Providence, RI 60-61; Yale-New Haven Hosp, New Haven, CT 61-63; **HMO:** Most

⌖ 🅂🄾 🅲 🄰 🅈 🎟 🅂 🄼 Immediately **VISA** ⊜

Stillman, Margaret (MD)　　Ped　PCP
Phelps Mem Hosp Ctr
245 N Broadway 201; N Tarrytown, NY 10591; (914) 332-4141; **BDCERT:** Ped 83; **MS:** Columbia P&S 77; **RES:** Babies Hosp, New York, NY 77-80; **FEL:** Behavioral Ped, U MD Hosp, Baltimore, MD 80-82; *SI: Behavioral Pediatric Problems*; **HMO:** Aetna Hlth Plan CIGNA PHS Prucare

⌖ 🅂🄾 🄰 🎟 🅂 2-4 Weeks

Versfelt, Mary (MD)　　Ped　PCP
United Hosp Med Ctr
Pediatric Associates, 12 Rye Ridge Plaza; Rye Brook, NY 10573; (914) 251-1100; **BDCERT:** Ped 83; **MS:** Columbia P&S 78; **RES:** Babies Hosp, New York, NY 78-81; **FAP:** Assoc Clin Prof Ped Columbia P&S; **HOSP:** Greenwich Hosp; **HMO:** Oxford

⌖ 🅂🄾 🅲 🄰 🅈 🎟 🅂 2-4 Weeks **VISA** ⊜

Wager, Marc (MD)　　Ped　PCP
Sound Shore Med Ctr-Westchester
Pediatric GroupNew Rochelle, 140 Lockwood Ave 115; New Rochelle, NY 10801; (914) 235-3800; **BDCERT:** Ped 86; **MS:** Albert Einstein Coll Med 81; **RES:** Ped, Jacobi Med Ctr, Bronx, NY 81-84; **FEL:** AM, Montefiore Med Ctr, Bronx, NY 84-86; **FAP:** Clin Instr Albert Einstein Coll Med; *SI: Adolescent Medicine*; **HMO:** Aetna Hlth Plan Oxford Chubb PHS

⌖ 🅂🄾 🅲 🄰 🅈 🎟 🅂 🄼 A Few Days **VISA** ⊜

Wasserman, Eugene (MD)　　Ped　PCP
United Hosp Med Ctr
1600 Harrison Ave 307; Mamaroneck, NY 10543; (914) 698-0564; **BDCERT:** Ped 61; **MS:** U Hlth Sci/Chicago Med Sch 56; **RES:** Ped, Mount Sinai Med Ctr, New York, NY 57-59; **FAP:** Clin Prof Ped NY Med Coll; **HOSP:** St Agnes Hosp; **HMO:** Prucare Oxford US Hlthcre Pomco PHS +

LANG: Sp, Heb; ⌖ 🄰 🅈 🎟 🅂 🄽🄵 Immediately

Weiss-Harrison, Adrienne (MD)Ped
Sound Shore Med Ctr-Westchester
School Physician, Distr Of New Rochelle, 515 North Ave; New Rochelle, NY 10801; (914) 576-4264; **BDCERT:** Ped 84; **MS:** Cornell U 79; **RES:** NY Hosp-Cornell Med Ctr, New York, NY 80-82; **FEL:** Ambulatory Ped, NY Hosp-Cornell Med Ctr, New York, NY 82-83; **FAP:** Clin Instr Ped Cornell U; **HOSP:** NY Hosp-Cornell-Westchester; *SI: Asthma; AD HD & LD*

🅂🄾 🅲 🅈 🎟 🅂 🄼🄲🅆🄲 🄽🄵 2-4 Weeks

Weissman, Michael H (MD)　Ped
Northern Westchester Hosp Ctr
90 S Bedford Rd; Mt Kisco, NY 10590; (914) 241-1050; **BDCERT:** Ped 76; **MS:** Washington U, St Louis 76; **RES:** Ped, Jacobi Med Ctr, Bronx, NY 76-80; **HMO:** Oxford Metlife

⌖ 🅂🄾 🅲 🄰 🅈 🎟 🅂 🄼 🄽🄵 Immediately

Wenick, Gary (MD)　　Ped　PCP
Danbury Hosp
Paterson Park Medical Center, Old Route 22 Paterson Park Med Ctr Ste107; Brewster, NY 10509; (914) 279-2323; **BDCERT:** Ped 87; **PEn** 89; **MS:** NY Med Coll 82; **RES:** Ped, U Conn Hlth Ctr, Farmington, CT 82-83; Ped, Schneider Children's Hosp, New Hyde Park, NY 83-85; **FEL:** PEn, Schneider Children's Hosp, New Hyde Park, NY 85-87; *SI: Pediatric Endocrinology*; **HMO:** CIGNA PHS Prucare Oxford

⌖ 🅂🄾 🅲 🄰 🅈 🎟 🅂 🄲🅆 🄽🄵 1 Week

Zimmerman, Lester (MD) Ped
Sound Shore Med Ctr-Westchester
Soundshore Pediatrics, 110 Lockwood Ave 200;
New Rochelle, NY 10801; (914) 235-1400;
BDCERT: Ped 83; **MS:** Holland 55; **RES:** Ped, Bronx
Muncipal Hosp Ctr, Bronx, NY 58-60; **FEL:** Child
Development, Bronx Muncipal Hosp Ctr, Bronx, NY
60-62; **FAP:** Assoc Clin Prof Albert Einstein Coll
Med; **HOSP:** Montefiore Med Ctr-Weiler/Einstein
Div; **SI:** *Adolescents*

🔲 🔲 🔲 🔲 🔲 Immediately **VISA** 💳

PHYSICAL MEDICINE & REHABILITATION

Gristina, Jerome (MD) PMR
Sound Shore Med Ctr-Westchester
150 Lockwood Ave 10; New Rochelle, NY 10801;
(914) 636-4466; **BDCERT:** PMR 66; **MS:** Italy 59

Hinterbuchner, Catherine (MD)PMR
Metropolitan Hosp Ctr
Route 100 Munger Pavilion; Valhalla, NY 10595;
(914) 594-4275; **BDCERT:** PMR 62; **MS:** Greece
51; **RES:** French Hosp, New York, NY 54-55;
Kingsbrook Jewish Med Ctr, Brooklyn, NY 55-56;
FEL: Kingsbrook Jewish Med Ctr, Brooklyn, NY 56-
57; Metropolitan Hosp, New York, NY 59-60;
HOSP: Westchester Med Ctr

Randolph, Audrey (MD) PMR
St Agnes Hosp
311 North St; White Plains, NY 10595; (914) 428-
6838; **BDCERT:** PMR 70; **MS:** Med Coll PA 64; **RES:**
New York University Med Ctr, New York, NY 65-
68; **FAP:** Prof NY Med Coll; **HMO:** Pomco Oxford
Prucare

🔲 🔲 🔲 🔲 🔲 🔲 🔲 🔲 Immediately

Salzano, Anthony (MD) PMR
Westchester Square Med Ctr
Physical Medicine & Rehabilitation, 815 Mc Lean
Ave; Yonkers, NY 10704; (914) 237-4555;
BDCERT: PMR 89; **MS:** Italy 82; **RES:** PMR,
Montefiore Med Ctr, Bronx, NY 85-88; **FAP:** Asst
Clin Prof Albert Einstein Coll Med; **HOSP:** Our Lady
of Mercy Med Ctr; **SI:** *Pain Control; Braces and
Artificial Limbs*; **HMO:** GHI Blue Choice Oxford
Prucare PHS +

LANG: Itl, Sp, Kor, Chi, Tag; 🔲 🔲 🔲 🔲 🔲 🔲 🔲
🔲 1 Week

Stern, Peter (MD) PMR
Burke Rehabilitation Hosp
Burke Rehab Hosp, 785 Mamaroneck Ave Apt D;
White Plains, NY 10605; (914) 597-2332;
BDCERT: PMR 63; **MS:** Austria 45; **RES:** IM,
Nuremberg City Hosp, Nuremberg, Germany 45-
50; Ottowa Univ Hosp, Ottawa, Canada 58-59;
FEL: PMR, New York University Med Ctr, New
York, NY 58-61; **FAP:** Clin Prof Cornell U; **HOSP:**
United Hosp Med Ctr; **SI:** *Spinal Injury; Amputation
Rehab*; **HMO:** PHS Oxford Empire Blue Choice
🔲 🔲 🔲 🔲 🔲 🔲 🔲 🔲 1 Week

PLASTIC SURGERY

Bernard, Robert (MD) PlS
White Plains Hosp Ctr
10 Chester Ave; White Plains, NY 10601; (914)
241-1911; **BDCERT:** PlS 75; S 73; **MS:** Univ Vt Coll
Med 67; **RES:** S, New York University Med Ctr, New
York, NY; PlS, New York University Med Ctr, New
York, NY; **HOSP:** Northern Westchester Hosp Ctr;
SI: *Cosmetic Surgery; Breast Reconstruction*; **HMO:**
Oxford Pomco
🔲 🔲 🔲 🔲 🔲 🔲 🔲 1 Week **VISA** 💳

Bonanno, Philip C (MD)   PlS
Northern Westchester Hosp Ctr

Plastic & Reconstructive Surgery, PC, 400 E Main
St 2 N; Mt Kisco, NY 10549; (914) 241-0265;
BDCERT: S 69; PlS 72; **MS:** Albany Med Coll 63;
RES: S, Univ Hosp SUNY Bklyn, Brooklyn, NY 64-
68; PlS, New York University Med Ctr, New York,
NY 68-70; **FAP:** Assoc Clin Prof PlS NYU Sch Med;
SI: Facial Cosmetic Surgery; Head & Neck Surgery;
HMO: Oxford Pomco Aetna-US Healthcare First
Health Amerihealth +

♿ 📷 🏩 $ 🆁 🆐   2-4 Weeks ■■■ **VISA** ●

Goldstein, Steven (MD)   PlS
Montefiore Med Ctr-Weiler/Einstein Div

955 Yonkers Ave; Yonkers, NY 10704; (914) 237-
0050; **BDCERT:** Oto 87; **MS:** SUNY Buffalo 82; **RES:**
S, Bellevue Hosp Ctr, New York, NY 82-87; **FEL:**
Facial PlS, Mount Sinai Med Ctr, New York, NY;
FAP: Clin Instr NYU Sch Med; **HOSP:** Westchester
Square Med Ctr; *SI: Facial Plastic Surgery; Endoscopic
Sinus Surgery;* **HMO:** Oxford GHI

♿ ☽ 📷 📷 🏩 $ Immediately ■■■ **VISA** ●

Khoury, F Frederic (MD)   PlS
White Plains Hosp Ctr

22 Rye Ridge Plaza; Rye Brook, NY 10573; (914)
253-9300; **BDCERT:** PlS 82; **MS:** Lebanon 71; **RES:**
S, St Luke's Roosevelt Hosp Ctr, New York, NY 72-
77; PlS, St Luke's Roosevelt Hosp Ctr, New York,
NY 77; **FEL:** S, St Louis Hosp, Paris, France 77;
FAP: Clin Instr Columbia P&S; **HOSP:** United Hosp
Med Ctr; *SI: Facial Cosmetic Surgery; Liposuction;*
HMO: Oxford

LANG: Fr, Itl, Sp; ♿ 📷 📷 🏩 $ 🆐 🆐
Immediately

Kleinman, Andrew (MD)   PlS
Sound Shore Med Ctr-Westchester

175 Memorial Hwy LL17; New Rochelle, NY
10801; (914) 632-8500; **BDCERT:** PlS 89; **MS:** U
Rochester 79; **RES:** S, Geo Wash U Med Ctr,
Washington, DC 79-81; S, Harvard Surgical
Service, Boston, MA 81-83; **FEL:** PlS, Baylor Med
Ctr, Dallas, TX 83-85; **HOSP:** United Hosp Med Ctr;
SI: Cosmetic Surgery; Laser Surgery; **HMO:** Oxford
Pomco Aetna Hlth Plan

♿ 📷 📷 🏩 🆐 🆐 🆐   Immediately ■■■ **VISA** ●

Miclat Jr, Marciano (MD)   PlS
Sound Shore Med Ctr-Westchester

175 Memorial Hwy 24; New Rochelle, NY 10801;
(914) 636-8657; **BDCERT:** PlS 78; **MS:** Philippines
69; **RES:** S, Albert Einstein Med Ctr, Bronx, NY 71-
74; PlS, Albert Einstein Med Ctr, Bronx, NY 74-77;
SI: Cosmetic Surgery; Hand Surgery; **HMO:** First
Health SWCHP

♿ 📷 🏩 $ 🆐   Immediately **VISA** ●

Petro, Jane (MD)   PlS
Westchester Med Ctr

Route 100 Macy Pavilion; Valhalla, NY 10595;
(914) 493-8660; **BDCERT:** PlS 82; **MS:** Penn State
U-Hershey Med Ctr 72; **RES:** St Joseph Infirmary,
Louisville, KY 72-73; Harrisburg Hosp, Harrisburg,
PA 74-76; **FEL:** Montefiore Med Ctr, Bronx, NY 79-
80; **HOSP:** St Agnes Hosp; **HMO:** Aetna Hlth Plan
Blue Choice PHS Prucare Pomco +

LANG: Sp; ♿ ☽ 📷 🏩 $ 🆐 🆐 🆐 🆐   1 Week
VISA ●

Reiffel, Robert (MD)   PlS
White Plains Hosp Ctr

12 Greenridge Ave 203; White Plains, NY 10605;
(914) 683-1400; **BDCERT:** PlS 81; **MS:** Columbia
P&S 72; **RES:** St Luke's Roosevelt Hosp Ctr, New
York, NY 72-77; S, New York University Med Ctr,
New York, NY 77-79; **FEL:** HS, New York
University Med Ctr, New York, NY 79-80; **HOSP:** St
Agnes Hosp; *SI: Cosmetic and Reconstructive Surgery;
Hand Surgery;* **HMO:** Aetna Hlth Plan Blue Cross &
Blue Shield

♿ 🗄 📷 📷 🏩 $ 🆐 🆐 🆐   2-4 Weeks ■■■ **VISA**
● 💳

Salzberg, C Andrew (MD)   PlS
Westchester Med Ctr

New York GroupPlastic Surgery, Grasslands Rd;
Valhalla, NY 10595; (914) 493-8660; **BDCERT:**
PlS 89; **MS:** U Fla Coll Med 81; **RES:** Mount Sinai
Med Ctr, New York, NY 84-87; **HOSP:** St Agnes
Hosp; *SI: Cosmetic Surgery; Breast Reconstruction;*
HMO: Most

LANG: Sp; ♿ 🗄 ☽ 📷 📷 🏩 $ 🆐 🆐 🆐 🆐
A Few Days **VISA** ●

Soley, Robert (MD) PlS
White Plains Hosp Ctr
Associated Plastic Surgeons, 170 Maple Ave 211;
White Plains, NY 10601; (914) 997-9600;
BDCERT: PlS 72; S 70; **MS:** NYU Sch Med 59; **RES:**
S, Mount Sinai Med Ctr, New York, NY 60-65; PlS,
Hosp of U Penn, Philadelphia, PA 67-69; **FAP:** Asst
Clin Prof NY Med Coll; **HOSP:** St Agnes Hosp; *SI:*
Aging Face and Eyes; **HMO:** Oxford Blue Choice
CIGNA

🔲 🔲 🔲 🔲 🔲 🔲 A Few Days

PREVENTIVE MEDICINE

Cimino, Joseph (MD) PrM
Westchester Med Ctr
Route 100 Munger Pavilion; Valhalla, NY 10595;
(914) 594-4253; **BDCERT:** PrM OM 69; **MS:** SUNY
Buffalo 62; **RES:** Westchester County Med Ctr,
Valhalla, NY 62-63; Harvard Med Sch, Cambridge,
MA 63-65; **FEL:** PrM, NYC Dept Hlth, New York,
NY 65-66; **FAP:** Prof NY Med Coll; **HOSP:** Our Lady
of Mercy Med Ctr; *SI: Nutrition; Environmental*
Medicine

🔲 🔲 🔲 🔲 🔲 🔲 🔲 1 Week

Mamtani, Ravinder (MD) PrM
Westchester Med Ctr
Route 100 Munger Pavilion; Valhalla, NY 10595;
(914) 896-0492; **BDCERT:** PrM 89; **MS:** India 75;
RES: Derby Health Auth, England 78-81; Our Lady
of Mercy Med Ctr, Bronx, NY 86-87; **HOSP:** Our
Lady of Mercy Med Ctr

Williams, Christine (MD) PrM
Nyack Hosp
Child Health Center AHF, 1 Dana Rd; Valhalla, NY
10595; (914) 789-7239; **BDCERT:** Ped 84; PrM
84; **MS:** Univ Pittsburgh 67; **RES:** Ped, Mass Gen
Hosp, Boston, MA 67-68; Ped, Hosp Med College of
PA, Philadelphia, PA 72-73; **FEL:** Ped, Johns
Hopkins Hosp, Baltimore, MD 69-71; Karolinska
Inst, Stockholm, Sweden 71-72; **FAP:** Clin Prof
Path NY Med Coll; *SI: Cholesterol; Preventive*
Cardiology; **HMO:** Oxford Prucare GHI Aetna-US
Healthcare

🔲 🔲 🔲 🔲 🔲 🔲 🔲 2-4 Weeks

PSYCHIATRY

Addonizio, Gerard (MD) Psyc
NY Hosp-Cornell-Westchester
21 Bloomingdale Rd; White Plains, NY 10605;
(914) 997-5864; **BDCERT:** Psyc 83; **MS:** Columbia
P&S 78; **RES:** Yale-New Haven Hosp, New Haven,
CT 79-82; **FAP:** Assoc Prof Cornell U; *SI: Depression;*
Combining Med & Therapy; **HMO:** Empire

🔲 🔲 🔲 🔲 🔲 🔲 🔲 A Few Days

Alexopoulos, George (MD) Psyc
NY Hosp-Cornell Med Ctr
21 Bloomingdale Rd; White Plains, NY 10605;
(914) 997-5767; **BDCERT:** Psyc 78; GerPsy 92;
MS: Greece 80; **RES:** Psyc, UMDNJ-Camden,
Camden, NJ 77; **FEL:** Psyc, Cornell U Med Coll,
Ithaca, NY 78; *SI: Depression; Psychopharmacology*
LANG: Grk; 🔲 🔲 🔲 🔲 2-4 Weeks

Badikian, Arthur (MD) Psyc
St Agnes Hosp
303 North St 204; White Plains, NY 10605; (914)
948-4277; **BDCERT:** Psyc 81; **MS:** U Fla Coll Med
76; **RES:** NY Med Coll, Valhalla, NY 80; **HOSP:** St
Vincent's Med Ctr-Westchester; **HMO:** Aetna Hlth
Plan Blue Choice CIGNA HealthNet Independent
Health Plan +

Blumenfield, Michael (MD) Psyc
Westchester Med Ctr

16 Donellan Rd; Scarsdale, NY 10583; (914) 472-5035; **BDCERT:** Psyc 70; **MS:** SUNY Downstate 64; **RES:** Psyc, Kings County Hospital Center, Brooklyn, NY 65-68; **FEL:** Psyc, Univ Hosp SUNY Bklyn, Brooklyn, NY 70; **FAP:** Prof Psyc NY Med Coll; **HOSP:** White Plains Hosp Ctr; **SI:** *Psychopharmacology*; **HMO:** Blue Choice Oxford PHS

♿ 💠 📱 📷 📹 📺 Mcr WC NFI   A Few Days

Brancucci, Marion (MD) Psyc
Westchester Med Ctr

10 Old Mamaroneck Rd; White Plains, NY 10605; (914) 428-0681; **BDCERT:** Psyc 82; **MS:** NY Med Coll 57; **RES:** Westchester County Med Ctr, Valhalla, NY 78-81; **SI:** *Depression; Panic Disorders*; **HMO:** Aetna-US Healthcare Oxford GHI

♿ 💠 📱 📷 📹 Mcr Mod   A Few Days

Brescia, Robert (MD) Psyc
Calvary Hosp

303 Wolves Ln; Pelham, NY 10803; (914) 738-8537; **BDCERT:** Psyc 83; **MS:** SUNY Hlth Sci Ctr 77; **RES:** NY Hosp-Cornell Med Ctr-Westchester, White Plains, NY

Docherty, John P (MD) Psyc
NY Hosp-Cornell-Westchester

21 Bloomingdale Rd; White Plains, NY 10605; (914) 997-5796; **BDCERT:** Psyc 77; **MS:** Univ Penn 70; **RES:** Psyc, Yale-New Haven Hosp, New Haven, CT 71-74; Bio Psyc, NIMH, 74-76

Dolan, Anna (MD) Psyc
Yonkers Gen Hosp

984 N Broadway; Yonkers, NY 10701; (914) 476-1208; **BDCERT:** Psyc 76; **MS:** St Louis U 60; **RES:** Philadelphia Gen Hosp, Philadelphia, PA 66-68; St Louis U Hosp, St Louis, MO 61-62; **HOSP:** St John's Riverside Hosp; **SI:** *Depression; Anxiety States*

♿ 💠 📷 📹 📺 💵   2-4 Weeks

Dulit, Everett P (MD) Psyc
Four Winds Hosp

16 Sage Terr; Scarsdale, NY 10583; (914) 725-2673; **BDCERT:** Psyc 79; **MS:** U Minn 58; **RES:** Psyc, Jacobi Med Ctr, Bronx, NY 59-62; **FEL:** ChAP, Jacobi Med Ctr, Bronx, NY 62-66; **FAP:** Assoc Clin Prof Psyc Albert Einstein Coll Med; **HOSP:** NY Hosp-Cornell-Westchester; **SI:** *Adolescents; Family*; **HMO:** Empire

💠 📷 📹 📺 Mcr Mod NFI   Immediately

Gabel, Richard (MD) Psyc
White Plains Hosp Ctr

12 Green Ridge Ave; White Plains, NY 10605; (914) 681-0202; **BDCERT:** Psyc 82; **MS:** NYU Sch Med 76; **RES:** Mass Gen Hosp, Boston, MA 76-80; **SI:** *Anxiety Disorders; Mood Disorders*; **HMO:** Oxford

♿ 📷 📺 💵 Mcr Mod   2-4 Weeks

Halmi, Katherine (MD) Psyc
NY Hosp-Cornell-Westchester

21 Bloomingdale Rd; White Plains, NY 10605; (914) 997-5875; **BDCERT:** Psyc 77; **MS:** U Iowa Coll Med 65; **RES:** Ped, U IA Hosp, Iowa City, IA 70; Psyc, U IA Hosp, Iowa City, IA 72

📷 📹 📺 💵 Mcr Mod   Immediately 💳 *VISA* 💳

Halpern, Abraham L (MD) Psyc
Westchester Med Ctr

720 The Parkway; Mamaroneck, NY 10543; (914) 698-2136; **BDCERT:** Psyc 61; FPsy 94; **MS:** Canada 52; **RES:** Warren State Hosp, Warren, PA 57-60; Toronto Western Hosp, Toronto, Canada 52-53; **FAP:** Prof Psyc NY Med Coll; **HOSP:** Rye Hosp Ctr; **SI:** *Forensic Psychiatry*

💠 📷 💵 WC

Kaitz, Ronald (MD) Psyc
White Plains Hosp Ctr

Prefered Psychiatrics of Westchester, 250 E Hartsdale Ave Ste 15; Hartsdale, NY 10530; (914) 725-5959; **BDCERT:** Psyc 86; **MS:** NY Med Coll 78; **RES:** Psyc, NY Med Coll, Valhalla, NY 78-82; **HOSP:** St Vincent's Med Ctr-Westchester

♿ 💠 📷 📹 📺 Mcr NFI   A Few Days

Kernberg, Otto (MD)   Psyc
NY Hosp-Cornell Med Ctr

21 Bloomingdale Rd; White Plains, NY 10605;
(914) 997-5714; **BDCERT:** Psyc 70; **MS:** Chile 53;
RES: Psyc, Psychiatric Clinic, Santiago, Chile 54-
57; **FEL:** Psyc, Johns Hopkins Hospital, Baltimore,
MD 59-60; **FAP:** Prof Psyc Cornell U

LANG: Ger, Fr, Sp; 🏥 📞 👤

Klagsbrun, Samuel C (MD) Psyc
Four Winds Hosp

Four Winds Hosp; Katonah, NY 10536; (914) 763-
8151; **BDCERT:** Psyc 77; **MS:** U Hlth Sci/Chicago
Med Sch 62; **RES:** Psyc, Yale-New Haven Hosp,
New Haven, CT; **FAP:** Clin Prof Albert Einstein Coll
Med; **SI:** *Death and Dying; Emotions & Cancer*

LANG: Flm, Heb, Yd; 👤 📞 👤 🏥 NFI 1 Week

Levin, Andrew Paul (MD)   Psyc
St Vincent's Med Ctr-Westchester

St Vincents Hosp, 275 North St; Harrison, NY
10528; (914) 967-6500; **BDCERT:** Psyc 85; **MS:**
Univ Penn 80; **RES:** Psyc, NYS Psychiatric Institute,
New York, NY 81-84; **FEL:** Psyc, NYS Psychiatric
Institute, New York, NY 84-86; **FAP:** Asst Prof Psyc
NY Med Coll; **SI:** *Trauma and Dissociation; Forensic
Psychiatry;* **HMO:** Oxford VBH

LANG: Sp; 👤 📞 👤 🏥 💲 Mcr Mcd NFI 1 Week

Lew, Arthur (MD)   Psyc
Sound Shore Med Ctr-Westchester

225 Lyncroft Rd; New Rochelle, NY 10804; (914)
632-9679; **BDCERT:** Psyc 74; **MS:** SUNY
Downstate 68; **RES:** Psyc, Univ Hosp SUNY Bklyn,
Brooklyn, NY; **SI:** *Child Psychiatry; Adult & Child
Analysis*

📞 📞 👤 🏥 NFI

Lituchy, Stanley (MD)   Psyc
NY Hosp-Cornell Med Ctr

250 Garth Rd; Scarsdale, NY 10583; (914) 725-
2055; **BDCERT:** Psyc 66; **MS:** NYU Sch Med 55;
RES: VA Med Ctr-Bronx, Bronx, NY 60-61; NYS
Psychiatric Institute, New York, NY 59-60; **FEL:**
Psychoanalytic Med, NYS Psychiatric Institute,
New York, NY; **FAP:** Asst Prof Cornell U; **HOSP:**
Long Island Jewish Med Ctr; **SI:** *Personality
Problems; Psychoanalysis*

👤 🏥 📞 📞 👤 🏥 Mcr A Few Days

Loeb, Laurence (MD)   Psyc
NY Hosp-Cornell-Westchester

180 E Hartsdale Ave 1C; Hartsdale, NY 10530;
(914) 723-1446; **BDCERT:** Psyc 59; **MS:** SUNY
Downstate 53; **RES:** Psyc, NY Hosp-Cornell-
Westchester, White Plains, NY 54-55; ChAP, NY
Hosp-Cornell-Westchester, White Plains, NY 57;
FEL: ChAP, Albert Einstein Med Ctr, Bronx, NY 53-
60; **FAP:** Assoc Clin Prof; **SI:** *Forensic Psychiatry*

LANG: Fr; 📞 🏥 Immediately

Mendelson, Harold (MD)   Psyc

70 Salem Rd; Pound Rigde, NY 10516; (914) 545-
0374; **BDCERT:** Psyc 67; **MS:** SUNY Hlth Sci Ctr
60; **RES:** Kings County Hosp Ctr, Brooklyn, NY 61-
64; **FEL:** ChAP, Long Island Jewish Med Ctr, New
Hyde Park, NY 67-69; **SI:** *General Psychiatry;
Psychopharmacology;* **HMO:** None

📞 📞 👤 🏥 💲 Mcr A Few Days

Meyers, Barnett (MD)   Psyc
NY Hosp-Cornell-Westchester

21 Bloomingdale Rd; White Plains, NY 10605;
(914) 997-5721; **BDCERT:** Psyc 75; GerPsy 91;
MS: NYU Sch Med 66; **RES:** Jacobi Med Ctr, Bronx,
NY 69-72; **FAP:** Prof Cornell U; **SI:** *Depression;
Geriatrics*

👤 📞 👤 🏥 Mcr 2-4 Weeks

Milone, Richard (MD)   Psyc
St Vincent's Med Ctr-Westchester
120 Forest Ave; Rye, NY 10580; (914) 967-0220;
BDCERT: Psyc 70; **MS:** Creighton U 63; **RES:** St
Vincents Hosp & Med Ctr NY, New York, NY 64-67;
HOSP: United Hosp Med Ctr; **HMO:** Oxford US
Hlthcre Empire Blue Cross & Shield

♿ 🖳 📺 Mcr   1 Week

Neschis, Ronald (MD)   Psyc
St Joseph's Med Ctr-Yonkers
18 Linden Ave; Larchmont, NY 10538; (914) 834-
3470; **BDCERT:** Psyc 72; **MS:** SUNY Downstate 63;
RES: Psyc, Montefiore Med Ctr, Bronx, NY 66-69;
FAP: Adjct Clin Prof Cornell U; **HOSP:** Rye Hosp Ctr;
HMO: Blue Choice Blue Cross & Blue Shield
Independent Health Plan

♿ SA/SU ☾ 🖳 🚹 📺 Mcr   A Few Days

O'Connell, Barbara E (MD)   Psyc
NY Hosp-Cornell-Westchester
240 Brevoort Ln; Rye, NY 10580; (914) 698-
5387; **BDCERT:** Psyc 78; **MS:** Columbia P&S 51;
RES: Jacobi Med Ctr, Bronx, NY 59-60; **FEL:** ChAP,
Jacobi Med Ctr, Bronx, NY 61; *SI: Forensic
Psychiatry; Geriatric Psychiatry;* **HMO:** None

♿ SA/SU 🖳 🚹 📺 Mcr   Immediately

O'Connell, Ralph (MD)   Psyc
St Vincents Hosp & Med Ctr NY
New York Medical College; Valhalla, NY 10595;
(914) 594-4900; **BDCERT:** Psyc 71; **MS:** Cornell U
63; **RES:** Psyc, St Vincents Hosp & Med Ctr NY, New
York, NY 67-69; **FAP:** NY Med Coll

Pagliaro, Salvatore (MD)   Psyc
Rye Hosp Ctr
510 N Broadway; White Plains, NY 10603; (914)
946-0583; **BDCERT:** Psyc 71; **MS:** Columbia P&S
92; **RES:** Psyc, Colum Presb Med Ctr, New York, NY
92-93; NY Hosp-Cornell Med Ctr/Westch, White
Plains, New York, NY

Perlman, Barry Bruce (MD) Psyc
St Joseph's Med Ctr-Yonkers
St Joseph's Med Ctr-Dept of Psychiatry, 127 S
Broadway; Yonkers, NY 10701; (914) 378-7342;
BDCERT: Psyc 77; **MS:** Yale U Sch Med 71; **RES:**
Psyc, Mount Sinai Med Ctr, New York, NY 72-75;
HMO: Oxford Excelcare MBC VBH

♿ ☾ 🖳 🚹 📺 S Mcr WC   1 Week

Perry, Bradford (MD)   Psyc
NY Hosp-Cornell-Westchester
455 S Central Park Ave Ste 214; Scarsdale, NY
10583; (914) 472-2167; **BDCERT:** Psyc 89; **MS:** U
Miami Sch Med 84; **RES:** NY Hosp-Cornell-
Westchester, White Plains, NY; Public Psyc,
Columbia-Presbyterian Med Ctr, New York, NY;
FAP: Asst Prof Cornell U; **HOSP:** White Plains Hosp
Ctr; *SI: Anxiety; Mood Disorders;* **HMO:** Empire Blue
Cross & Shield Aetna Hlth Plan US Hlthcre

♿ ☾ 🖳 🚹 📺 S Mcr NFI   A Few Days

Roff, George (MD)   Psyc
Rye Hosp Ctr
1600 Harrison Ave; Mamaroneck, NY 10543;
(914) 698-8755; **BDCERT:** Psyc 76; **MS:** Albany
Med Coll 65; **RES:** Psyc, NY Hosp-Cornell-
Westchester, White Plains, NY 66-69

Rowntree, Ellen (MD)   Psyc
NY Hosp-Cornell-Westchester
1 Macy Ave; White Plains, NY 10605; (914) 328-
5616; **BDCERT:** Psyc 77; **MS:** Columbia P&S 68;
RES: Jacobi Med Ctr, Bronx, NY 75; **FEL:**
Psychoanalysis, Columbia-Presbyterian Med Ctr,
New York, NY 84; **FAP:** Assoc Clin Prof Psyc
Cornell U; *SI: Individual Psychotherapy;
Psychoanalysis;* **HMO:** None

☾ 🚹 📺   1 Week

Russakoff, L Mark (MD)   Psyc
Phelps Mem Hosp Ctr
701 N Broadway; Sleepy Hollow, NY 10591; (914) 366-3600; **BDCERT:** Psyc 76; **MS:** SUNY Downstate 71; **RES:** Yale-New Haven Hosp, New Haven, CT 72-75; **SI:** *Psychopharmacology; Affective Disorders;* **HMO:** Oxford

🦽 🈺 🈯 🏧 🅂 Mcr   2-4 Weeks

Scharfman, Edward (MD)   Psyc
St Vincents Hosp & Med Ctr NY
111 N Central Ave 421; Hartsdale, NY 10530; (914) 632-6646; **BDCERT:** Psyc 83; **MS:** SUNY Hlth Sci Ctr 78; **RES:** Psyc, Univ Hosp SUNY Bklyn, Brooklyn, NY 78-81; Kings County Hosp Ctr, Brooklyn, NY 81-82; **FEL:** Psychopharmacology, New England Med Ctr, Boston, MA 82-84; New England Med Ctr, Boston, MA 82-83; **FAP:** Asst Clin Prof NY Med Coll; **HOSP:** Sound Shore Med Ctr-Westchester; **SI:** *Mood Disorders; Panic Phobic Anxiety Disorders*

LANG: Heb; 🦽 🈺 🈯 🏧 🅂 Mcr   A Few Days

Seaman, Cheryl (MD)   Psyc
721 Long Hill Rd West; Briarcliff Manor, NY 10510; (914) 762-4712; **BDCERT:** Psyc 86; **MS:** Columbia P&S 79; **RES:** NY Hosp-Cornell Med Ctr, New York, NY 79-83; **SI:** *Depression; Anxiety*

LANG: Fr; 🦽 🈺 🈯 🏧 🏧   1 Week

Singer, Elliot (MD)   Psyc
Rye Hosp Ctr
754 Boston Post Rd; Rye, NY 10580; (914) 967-4567; **BDCERT:** Psyc 77; **MS:** Univ Vt Coll Med 65; **RES:** NY Hosp-Cornell Med Ctr, New York, NY 68-71; **FAP:** Asst Clin Prof NY Med Coll; **SI:** *Psychopharmacology; Individual Psychotherapy;* **HMO:** GHI Mental Behavioral Care Independent Health Plan Oxford

🦽 🈴 🈯 🏧 Mcr NFI   A Few Days

Stock, Howard (MD)   Psyc
White Plains Hosp Ctr
260 Garth Rd; Scarsdale, NY 10583; (914) 723-0180; **BDCERT:** Psyc 73; **MS:** Albert Einstein Coll Med 63; **RES:** Psyc, Kings County Hosp Ctr, Brooklyn, NY 67-68; Psyc, Brookdale Univ Hosp Med Ctr, Brooklyn, NY 68-69; **HMO:** None

🦽 🈯 🈯 🏧   A Few Days

Sullivan, Timothy (MD)   Psyc
St Vincent's Med Ctr-Westchester
StVincent's Hosp & Med Center Westchester, 275 North St; Harrison, NY 10528; (914) 925-5485; **BDCERT:** Psyc 86; IM 81; **MS:** Dartmouth Med Sch 77; **RES:** IM, St Vincents Hosp & Med Ctr NY, New York, NY 77-80; Psyc, NY Hosp-Cornell-Westchester, White Plains, NY 81-84; **FEL:** Hem Onc, St Vincents Hosp & Med Ctr NY, New York, NY 80-81; Psyc, NY Hosp-Cornell-Westchester, White Plains, NY 84-85; **FAP:** Asst Clin Prof Psyc NY Med Coll; **SI:** *Mental Illness-Severe; Psychotherapy & Medication;* **HMO:** Oxford VBH MBC

🦽 🈺 🈯 🏧 Mcr Mcd   A Few Days

Sussman, Robert (MD)   Psyc
United Hosp Med Ctr
167 Purchase St; Rye, NY 10580; (914) 967-1363; **BDCERT:** Psyc 64; AdP 93; **MS:** SUNY Buffalo 57; **RES:** Stanford Med Ctr, Stanford, CA 58-60; Hillside Hosp, Glen Oaks, NY 62-63; **FEL:** Psyc, Columbia-Presbyterian Med Ctr, New York, NY 65-67; **FAP:** Asst Clin Prof Psyc Cornell U; **SI:** *Substance Abuse; Psychopharmacology;* **HMO:** Prucare Oxford VBH Blue Cross GHI +

🈺 🈯 🈯 🏧 🅂 Mcr   A Few Days

Terkelsen, Kenneth (MD)   Psyc
NY Hosp-Cornell Med Ctr
21 Bloomingdale Rd; White Plains, NY 10605; (914) 997-5896; **BDCERT:** Psyc 77; **MS:** Jefferson Med Coll 69; **RES:** Albert Einstein Med Ctr, Bronx, NY 70-73; **FEL:** Albert Einstein Med Ctr, Bronx, NY 73-75; **FAP:** Assoc Prof of Clin Psyc Cornell U

🦽 🈺 🈯 Mcr Mcd   1 Week

Tischler, Gary L (MD)   Psyc
NY Hosp-Cornell-Westchester
21 Bloomingdale Rd; White Plains, NY 10605;
(914) 997-8690; **MS:** Univ Penn 61; **RES:** Yale-
New Haven Hosp, New Haven, CT 62-65

Travin, Sheldon (MD)   Psyc
Bronx Lebanon Hosp Ctr
901 N Broadway 19; White Plains, NY 10603;
(914) 428-2454; **BDCERT:** Psyc 72; **MS:** NY Med
Coll 64; **RES:** Jewish Hosp Med Ctr, Brooklyn, NY
64-65; Metropolitan Hosp Ctr, New York, NY 65-
68; **FAP:** Prof Albert Einstein Coll Med; **SI:** *Deviant
Sexual Disorders; Alcohol Substance Abuse;* **HMO:**
Blue Cross & Blue Shield

🔲 🔳 🔲 🔲 🔲 🔲 Immediately

Turato, Mariann (MD)   Psyc
Phelps Mem Hosp Ctr
17 Maple Ave; N Tarrytown, NY 10591; (914)
524-7266; **BDCERT:** Psyc 92; **MS:** Albert Einstein
Coll Med 86; **RES:** NY Hosp-Cornell-Westchester,
White Plains, NY 87-90; **SI:** *Anxiety Disorders;
Women's Issues*

🔲 🔲 🔲 🔲 🔲 🔲 🔲 A Few Days

Zolkind, Neil (MD)   Psyc
Westchester Med Ctr
280 Dobbs Ferry Rd; White Plains, NY 10607;
(914) 332-5162; **BDCERT:** Psyc 81; **MS:** Geo Wash
U Sch Med 76; **RES:** Psyc, UCLA Neuropsychiatric
Hosp, Los Angeles, CA 77-80; **FAP:** Asst Prof NY
Med Coll; **SI:** *Depression; Anxiety;* **HMO:** Oxford
Prudential Aetna Hlth Plan GHI Empire Blue Cross
& Shield +

🔲 🔲 🔲 🔲 🔲 🔲 🔲 🔲

Zucker, Arnold (MD)   Psyc
Mount Vernon Hosp
120 E Prospect Ave; Mt Vernon, NY 10550; (914)
668-2332; **BDCERT:** Psyc 63; **MS:** SUNY Hlth Sci
Ctr 54; **RES:** Psyc, Kings County Hosp Ctr,
Brooklyn, NY 55-56; Psyc, Albert Einstein Med Ctr,
Bronx, NY 59-60; **SI:** *Psychoanalysis; Religion-
Psychiatry*
LANG: Yd; 🔲 🔲 🔲 🔲 🔲 🔲 🔲 🔲 A Few Days

PULMONARY DISEASE

Brill, Joseph (MD)   Pul
St John's Riverside Hosp
547 Saw Mill River Rd 1E; Ardsley, NY 10502;
(914) 674-0140; **BDCERT:** IM 88; Pul 92; **MS:**
Mexico 81; **RES:** Elmhurst Hosp Ctr, Elmhurst, NY
85-86; **FEL:** Pul, Elmhurst Hosp Ctr, Elmhurst, NY
86-88; **HOSP:** St Joseph's Med Ctr-Yonkers; **HMO:**
Aetna Hlth Plan Oxford US Hlthcre GHI PHS +

🔲 🔲 🔲 🔲 🔲 🔲 🔲 🔲 A Few Days

Casino, Joseph (MD)   Pul
Sound Shore Med Ctr-Westchester
77 Quaker Ridge Rd Ste 200a; New Rochelle, NY
10801; (914) 636-7936; **BDCERT:** Pul 90; CCM
91; **MS:** Italy 84; **RES:** St Michael's Med Ctr,
Newark, NJ 84-85; New Rochelle Hosp Med Ctr,
New Rochelle, NY 85-88; **FEL:** CCM, RWJ Univ
Hosp-New Brunswick, New Brunswick, NJ 88-91;
FAP: Asst Clin Prof Med NY Med Coll; **SI:** *Asthma;
Sleep Disorders;* **HMO:** Aetna Hlth Plan Oxford
CIGNA GHI PHS +

LANG: Itl; 🔲 🔲 🔲 🔲 🔲 🔲 Immediately

Chodosh, Ronald (MD)   Pul   **PCP**
Phelps Mem Hosp Ctr
14 Church St; Ossining, NY 10562; (914) 762-
4141; **BDCERT:** IM 71; Pul 78; **MS:** Switzerland
65; **RES:** IM, Maimonides Med Ctr, Brooklyn, NY
68-70; **FEL:** Pul, Albert Einstein/Bronx Muni Hosp,
Bronx, NY 70-71; **FAP:** Asst Prof Med Albert
Einstein Coll Med; **HOSP:** Northern Westchester
Hosp Ctr; **HMO:** Oxford Aetna-US Healthcare PHS
CIGNA Well Care +

LANG: Ger, Sp; 🔲 🔲 🔲 🔲 🔲 🔲 Immediately

Guide to symbols and abbreviations can be found on pages 110-113.

Delorenzo, Lawrence (MD)   Pul
Westchester Med Ctr
Pulmonary Area Westchester Med Center 2G; Valhalla, NY 10595; (914) 493-7518; **BDCERT:** IM 79; Pul 82; **MS:** NY Med Coll 76; **RES:** Metropolitan Hosp Ctr, New York, NY 79; **FEL:** Pul, Metropolitan Hosp Ctr, New York, NY; **HOSP:** St Agnes Hosp; *SI: Critical Care Medicine*; **HMO:** Aetna Hlth Plan Blue Cross & Blue Shield Independent Health Plan Prucare Travelers +

LANG: Itl, Sp; 🦽 🔂 🚗 🏥 Mcr WC NFI Immediately
VISA 💳

DiCosmo, Bruno F (MD)   Pul
United Hosp Med Ctr
745 E Boston Post Rd; Mamaroneck, NY 10543; (914) 698-6900; **BDCERT:** Pul 91; CCM 92; **MS:** U Conn Sch Med 88; **RES:** IM, U Conn Hlth Ctr, Farmington, CT 88-91; **FEL:** Pul, Yale-New Haven Hosp, New Haven, CT 91-94; CCM, Yale-New Haven Hosp, New Haven, CT 91-94; **FAP:** Clin Instr Yale U Sch Med; **HOSP:** St Agnes Hosp; *SI: Chronic Obstructive Pulmonary Disease; Asthma*; **HMO:** Oxford PHS Aetna-US Healthcare Blue Cross & Blue Shield Prucare +

LANG: Itl, Sp; 🦽 SD 🌙 🔂 🚗 🏥 S Mcr Mcd WC NFI
A Few Days 🛏 **VISA** 💳

Frimer, Richard (MD)   Pul
New York University Med Ctr
170 Maple Ave 1; White Plains, NY 10601; (914) 328-0932; **BDCERT:** IM 83; **MS:** SUNY Buffalo 80; **RES:** IM, Montefiore Med Ctr, Bronx, NY 83; IM, Montefiore Med Ctr, Bronx, NY 82; **FEL:** PM, New York University Med Ctr, New York, NY 84-85

Lehrman, Gary (MD)   Pul
Phelps Mem Hosp Ctr
160 N State Rd; Briarcliff Manor, NY 10510; (914) 762-8383; **BDCERT:** IM 82; Pul 86; **MS:** NYU Sch Med 79; **RES:** Long Island Jewish Med Ctr, New Hyde Park, NY

🦽 🔂 🚗 🏥 S Mcr Immediately

Lehrman, Stuart (MD)   Pul
Westchester Med Ctr
Westchester Med Center; Valhalla, NY 10595; (914) 493-7518; **BDCERT:** Pul 84; CCM 87; **MS:** SUNY Hlth Sci Ctr 78; **RES:** Cedars-Sinai Med Ctr, Los Angeles, CA 78-81; **FEL:** Pul, Cedars-Sinai Med Ctr, Los Angeles, CA 81-83; **FAP:** Assoc Clin Prof Med NY Med Coll; **HOSP:** St Agnes Hosp; *SI: Lung Cancer; Pulmonary Hypertension*; **HMO:** Blue Choice Champus CIGNA GHI

🦽 🔂 🚗 🏥 S Mcr WC NFI Immediately

Maguire, George (MD)   Pul
Westchester Med Ctr
Route 100 Macy Pavilion; Valhalla, NY 10595; (914) 285-7518; **BDCERT:** IM 75; **MS:** SUNY Hlth Sci Ctr 72; **RES:** Univ Hosp SUNY Downstate, Brooklyn, NY; **FEL:** Univ Hosp SUNY Downstate, Brooklyn, NY

Meixler, Steven (MD)   Pul
White Plains Hosp Ctr
170 Maple Ave 1; White Plains, NY 10601; (914) 328-0932; **BDCERT:** IM 87; Pul 90; **MS:** Boston U 84; **RES:** VA Med Ctr-Manh, New York, NY 84-88; **FEL:** Pul, Bellevue Hosp Ctr, New York, NY 88-90; *SI: Asthma; Chronic Cough*; **HMO:** PHS Blue Choice Oxford Chubb Aetna Hlth Plan +

LANG: Sp; 🦽 🔂 🚗 🏥 S WC NFI Immediately
VISA

Schreiber, Michael (MD)   Pul
St John's Riverside Hosp
970 N Broadway 304; Yonkers, NY 10701; (914) 423-8517; **BDCERT:** IM 76; Pul 78; **MS:** U Ariz Coll Med 73; **RES:** IM, Montefiore Med Ctr, Bronx, NY 73-76; **FEL:** Pul, New York University Med Ctr, New York, NY 76-78; **FAP:** Asst Clin Prof NY Med Coll; *SI: Asthma; Emphysema*; **HMO:** Blue Cross Oxford PHS United Healthcare CIGNA +

🦽 🔂 🚗 🏥 S Mcr A Few Days

Sherling, Bruce E (MD)   Pul
United Hosp Med Ctr

745 E Boston Post Rd; Mamaroneck, NY 10543;
(914) 698-6900; **BDCERT:** IM 76; Pul 78; **MS:** NY
Med Coll 73; **RES:** Med, Metropolitan Hosp, New
York, NY 73-76; **FEL:** Pul, NY Med Coll, Valhalla,
NY 77; Pul, Lenox Hill Hosp, New York, NY 77-78;
FAP: Instr Med NY Med Coll

Volcovici, Guido (MD)   Pul   PCP
St Joseph's Med Ctr-Yonkers

984 N Broadway Ste 419; Yonkers, NY 10701;
(914) 968-5446; **BDCERT:** IM 85; Pul 88; **MS:**
Romania 62; **RES:** IM, Jewish Hosp Med Ctr,
Brooklyn, NY 71-74; **FEL:** Pul, VA Med Center
Manhattan, New York, NY 74-76; *SI: Asthma;
Emphysema;* **HMO:** Blue Cross US Hlthcre GHI
Oxford +

LANG: Fr, Rom, Rus, Sp; ♿ 🆘 🅲 📷 🧑 🛏 Mcr Mcd
WC NFI Immediately

RADIATION
ONCOLOGY

Brimberg, Arthur (MD)   RadRO
St John's Riverside Hosp

Riverhill Radiation Oncology, 970 N Broadway
101; Yonkers, NY 10701; (914) 969-1600;
BDCERT: Rad 68; **MS:** U Hlth Sci/Chicago Med Sch
61; **RES:** RadRO, Bronx Muncipal Hosp Ctr, Bronx,
NY 64-67; **FEL:** Rad, Albert Einstein Med Ctr,
Bronx, NY 67-69; **HOSP:** Lawrence Hosp; *SI:
Prostate Therapy; Breast and Lung Cancer;* **HMO:**
Oxford Blue Cross & Blue Shield PHS United
Healthcare Pomco +

LANG: Sp; ♿ 📷 🛏 Mcr Mcd WC NFI Immediately

Lehrman, David B (MD)   RadRO
Sound Shore Med Ctr-Westchester

The Center for Radiation Oncology, 175 Memorial
Hwy LL5; New Rochelle, NY 10801; (914) 633-
3525; **BDCERT:** RadRO 80; **MS:** Dalhousie U 74;
RES: RadRO, New York University Med Ctr, New
York, NY 80; S, Univ Hosp SUNY Bklyn, Brooklyn,
NY 75-77; **FAP:** Visiting Prof Albert Einstein Coll
Med; *SI: Breast Cancer; Prostate Seed Implants;* **HMO:**
Oxford GHI Chubb Blue Cross & Blue Shield

LANG: Sp; ♿ 📷 🧑 🛏 🅂 Mcr Mcd Immediately 🅰
VISA 💳

Moorthy, Chitti (MD)   RadRO
Westchester Med Ctr

Westchester Med Ctr - Dept of Radiation Medicine -
MACY Pavillion, Route 100 RM 1297; Valhalla,
NY 10595; (914) 493-1408; **BDCERT:** RadRO 79;
MS: India 74; **RES:** S, Michael Reese Hosp Med Ctr,
Chicago, IL 75-76; RadRO, Michael Reese Hosp
Med Ctr, Chicago, IL 76-79; **FEL:** Brachytherapy,
Mem Sloan Kettering Cancer Ctr, New York, NY
79-80; **FAP:** Prof of Clin Rad NY Med Coll; **HOSP:**
Lincoln Med & Mental Hlth Ctr; *SI: Radiation
Medicine; Oncology;* **HMO:** Aetna-US Healthcare
Magnacare Oxford GHI

LANG: Itl, Chi, Sp; ♿ 🆘 🅲 📷 🧑 🛏 Mcr Mcd
Immediately 🅰 VISA 💳 📇

Usas, Craig (MD)   RadRO
Northern Westchester Hosp Ctr

449 North State Road BriarCliff Manor NY, 400
Main St; Mt Kisco, NY 10510; (914) 945-0346;
BDCERT: RadRO 79; **MS:** Mexico 74; **RES:**
Columbia-Presbyterian Med Ctr, New York, NY 75-
78; **HMO:** PHS Oxford Prudential Aetna Hlth Plan

LANG: Sp; ♿ 📷 🛏 Mcr Mcd WC Immediately 🅰
VISA 💳

RADIOLOGY

Botet, Jose (MD)   Rad
St Agnes Hosp

305 North St; White Plains, NY 10605; (914) 681-4500; **BDCERT:** DR 82; **MS:** Mexico 73; **RES:** St Luke's Roosevelt Hosp Ctr, New York, NY 74-78; **FEL:** Mem Sloan Kettering Cancer Ctr, New York, NY 78-79

♿

Chisolm, Alvin (MD)   Rad
Sound Shore Med Ctr-Westchester

16 Guion Pl; New Rochelle, NY 10801; (914) 632-5000; **BDCERT:** Rad 73; **MS:** NY Med Coll 68; **RES:** Montefiore Med Ctr, Bronx, NY 69-72; **SI:** *Body Imaging; Mammography*; **HMO:** Oxford PHS Blue Cross & Blue Choice

LANG: Sp, Heb; ♿ ▣ ▣ ▣ ▣ ▣ ▣ ▣ ▣
Immediately ▣ **VISA** ▣

Khoury, Paul (MD)   Rad
White Plains Hosp Ctr

White Plains Radiology Assoc, 122 Maple Ave; White Plains, NY 10577; (914) 681-1260; **MS:** Lebanon 73; **RES:** Hotel Dieu de France Hosp, Beirut, Lebanon 73-75; St Luke's Roosevelt Hosp Ctr, New York, NY 76-78; **HOSP:** St Agnes Hosp; **HMO:** US Hlthcre Aetna Hlth Plan Oxford CIGNA +

LANG: Fr, Sp, Itl; ♿ ▣ ▣ ▣ ▣ ▣ ▣ ▣ ▣
Immediately ▣ **VISA** ▣ ▣

Klein, Robert M (MD)   Rad
Westchester Med Ctr

Westchester Med Center; Valhalla, NY 10595; (914) 493-8056; **BDCERT:** Rad 71; NuM 75; **MS:** SUNY Hlth Sci Ctr 63; **RES:** Rad, Kings County Hosp Ctr, Brooklyn, NY 66-69; **FAP:** Prof of Clin Rad NY Med Coll; **SI:** *Musculoskeletal Radiology; Bone Densitometry*; **HMO:** Well Care Oxford Aetna-US Healthcare Pomco Independent Health Plan +

LANG: Sp; ♿ ▣ ▣ ▣ ▣ ▣ ▣ ▣ A Few Days
VISA ▣

Kutcher, Rosalyn (MD)   Rad
White Plains Hosp Ctr

White Plains Radiology Associates, Davis Ave and East Post Rd Rd; White Plains, NY 10601; (914) 681-1260; **BDCERT:** Rad 75; **MS:** SUNY Hlth Sci Ctr 70; **RES:** DR, Montefiore Med Ctr, Bronx, NY 71-74; **SI:** *Mammography; Ultrasound*; **HMO:** Blue Cross & Blue Shield Aetna Hlth Plan Oxford HIP Network +

♿ ▣ ▣ ▣ ▣ ▣   A Few Days

McCarthy, Joseph (MD)   Rad
Westchester Med Ctr

Ardsley Radiology, 933 Saw Mill River Rd; Ardsley, NY 10502; (914) 693-4900; **BDCERT:** Rad 75; NuM 75; **MS:** SUNY Buffalo 70; **RES:** Rad, Columbia-Presbyterian Med Ctr, New York, NY 72-73; Rad, New York University Med Ctr, New York, NY 73-75; **FEL:** NuM, Univ Hosp SUNY Bklyn, Brooklyn, NY 75-76; **SI:** *Open MRI Osteoporosis; Contour Mammography*; **HMO:** Oxford Aetna Hlth Plan SWCHP Blue Choice NYLCare +

LANG: Sp, Prt, Lth; ♿ ▣ ▣ ▣ ▣ ▣ ▣ ▣ ▣ ▣
1 Week ▣ **VISA** ▣ ▣

RHEUMATOLOGY

Barone, Richard (MD)   Rhu
Sound Shore Med Ctr-Westchester

421 Huguenot St Ste 53; New Rochelle, NY; (914) 235-3065; **MS:** Ind U Sch Med 71; **RES:** Med, Brooklyn Jewish Hosp, Brooklyn, NY 71-74; **FEL:** Rhu, Jewish Hosp Med Ctr, Brooklyn, NY 74-76; **FAP:** Assoc Clin Prof NY Med Coll; **SI:** *Rheumatoid Arthritis; Psoriatic Arthritis*; **HMO:** Pomco US Hlthcre Blue Choice Physician's Health Plan Aetna Hlth Plan +

LANG: Itl; ♿ ▣ ▣ ▣ ▣   1 Week

Berger, Jack (MD)   Rhu
White Plains Hosp Ctr

15 Chester Ave; White Plains, NY 10601; (914) 946-3553; **BDCERT:** IM 79; Rhu 82; **MS:** Albert Einstein Coll Med 76; **RES:** Bellevue Hosp Ctr, New York, NY 77-79; **FEL:** Bellevue Hosp Ctr, New York, NY 79-81

Burns, Mark (MD)   Rhu
Sound Shore Med Ctr-Westchester

421 Huguenot St 53; New Rochelle, NY 10801; (914) 235-3065; **BDCERT:** Rhu 80; **MS:** UC San Francisco 77; **RES:** IM, Montefiore Med Ctr, Bronx, NY 77-80; **FEL:** Rhu, Montefiore Med Ctr, Bronx, NY 81-83; **FAP:** Asst Clin Prof Med Albert Einstein Coll Med; **HOSP:** Montefiore Med Ctr; **SI:** *Lupus; Rheumatoid Arthritis*; **HMO:** Aetna Hlth Plan Blue Cross PHS Pomco Oxford +

🔲 🔲 🔲 🔲 🔲 🔲 A Few Days

Chodock, Allen (MD)   Rhu   PCP
United Hosp Med Ctr

1600 Harrison Ave G107; Mamaroneck, NY 10543; (914) 698-2902; **BDCERT:** IM 71; **MS:** Univ Pittsburgh 63; **RES:** IM, Montefiore Med Ctr, Bronx, NY 64-69; **FEL:** Rhu, Montefiore Med Ctr, Bronx, NY 68-69; **HOSP:** Montefiore Med Ctr; **HMO:** Oxford

LANG: Sp; 🔲 🔲 🔲 🔲 🔲 🔲 🔲 Immediately
VISA 🔲 🔲 🔲

Faltz, Lawrence L (MD)   Rhu
Phelps Mem Hosp Ctr

701 N Broadway; Sleepy Hollow, NY 10591; (914) 366-1005; **BDCERT:** IM 79; Rhu 82; **MS:** NYU Sch Med 72; **RES:** NC Mem Hosp, Chapel Hill, NC 72-74; Bellevue Hosp Ctr, New York, NY 78-79; **FEL:** Rhu, Bellevue Hosp Ctr, New York, NY 79-80; **FAP:** Assoc Prof of Clin Med Mt Sinai Sch Med; **HMO:** Oxford NYLCare Multicare Empire Blue Cross & Shield

🔲 🔲 🔲 🔲 🔲 🔲 🔲 🔲 Immediately

Futran-Sheinberg, Jacobo (MD)Rhu
St John's Riverside Hosp

944 N Broadway Suite 201; Yonkers, NY 10701; (914) 968-4695; **BDCERT:** IM 95; Rhu 96; **MS:** Mexico 80; **RES:** Nat Med Center, Mexico City, Mexico 80-81; IM, Nat Med Center, Mexico City, Mexico 81-84; **FEL:** Rhu, U Toronto Gen Hosp, Toronto, Canada 84-86; IM, U IA Hosp, Iowa City, IA 86-88; **HOSP:** Hosp For Special Surgery; **SI:** *Arthritis; Lupus*; **HMO:** Oxford PHS PHCS Pomco +

LANG: Sp, Heb; 🔲 🔲 🔲 🔲 🔲 🔲 🔲 A Few Days

Reinitz, Elizabeth (MD)   Rhu   PCP
White Plains Hosp Ctr

259 Heathcote Rd; Scarsdale, NY 10583; (914) 723-8100; **BDCERT:** Rhu 79; **MS:** Albert Einstein Coll Med 76; **RES:** IM, Boston Med Ctr, Boston, MA 77-79; **FEL:** Rhu, Montefiore Med Ctr, Bronx, NY 79-81

🔲 🔲 🔲 🔲 🔲 🔲 🔲 🔲 A Few Days *VISA* 🔲

Sloane, Lori (MD)   Rhu
Northern Westchester Hosp Ctr

Northern Metropolitan Medical, 206 Veterans Rd; Yorktown Heights, NY 10598; (914) 962-5501; **BDCERT:** IM 89; Rhu 91; **MS:** SUNY Hlth Sci Ctr 86; **RES:** IM, Jacobi Med Ctr, Bronx, NY 86-89; **FEL:** Rhu, Montefiore Med Ctr, Bronx, NY 89-91; **FAP:** Asst Clin Instr Albert Einstein Coll Med; **SI:** *Lupus; Rheumatoid Arthritis*; **HMO:** Aetna Hlth Plan Oxford Blue Cross & Blue Choice

🔲 🔲 🔲 🔲 🔲 🔲 2-4 Weeks 🔲 *VISA* 🔲 🔲

Weinstein, Arthur (MD)   Rhu
Westchester Med Ctr

N Y Medical College-Lyme Disease Research, Munger Pavilion G52; Valhalla, NY 10595; (914) 594-4311; **BDCERT:** Rhu 76; DLI 86; **MS:** Canada 67; **RES:** Toronto Gen Hosp, Toronto, Canada 67-68; Toronto Wellesley Hosp, Toronto, Canada 68-69; **FEL:** Rhu, Hammersmith Hosp, London, England 69-71; Toronto Wellesley Hosp, Toronto, Canada 71-72; **FAP:** Adjct Prof Med NY Med Coll; **SI:** *Lyme Disease Research; Lupus*; **HMO:** +

🔲 🔲

SPORTS MEDICINE

Cavaliere, Gregg (MD)   SM
Phelps Mem Hosp Ctr

239 N Broadway; N Tarrytown, NY 10591; (914) 631-7777; **BDCERT:** OrS 95; **MS:** NY Med Coll 87; **RES:** Lenox Hill Hosp, New York, NY 87-92; **FEL:** Ped OrS, Children's Hosp, Boston, MA 90-91; SM, New York University Med Ctr, New York, NY 92-93; **HOSP:** Community Hosp At Dobbs Ferry; **HMO:** Oxford PHS Independent Health Plan

🔲 🔲 🔲 🔲 🔲 🔲 🔲 🔲 Immediately *VISA* 🔲
🔲

Luks, Howard J (MD)   **SM**
Westchester Med Ctr
New York Medical College, Department of
Orthopedics, Mercy Pavillion; Valhalla, NY 10595;
(917) 493-8737; **MS:** NY Med Coll 91; **RES:** OrS,
Long Island Jewish Med Ctr, New Hyde Park, NY
92-96; **FEL:** SM, Hosp for Joint Diseases, New York,
NY 96-97; **HOSP:** St Agnes Hosp; **HMO:** Oxford
PHS Independent Health Plan Aetna Hlth Plan
Pomco

LANG: Sp, Fr, Sgn; [symbols]
A Few Days [symbols] **VISA** [symbols]

SURGERY

Ashikari, Roy (MD)   **S**
St Agnes Hosp
St Agnes Hosp, 305 North St; White Plains, NY
10605; (914) 681-9478; **BDCERT:** S 67; **MS:**
Japan 58; **RES:** S, Mount Sinai Med Ctr, New York,
NY 61-64; S, Mem Sloan Kettering Cancer Ctr, New
York, NY 66-68; **FEL:** Mount Sinai Med Ctr, New
York, NY 64-65; **FAP:** Prof S NY Med Coll; **HOSP:**
Beth Israel Med Ctr; **SI:** *Breast Surgery;* **HMO:**
Oxford Aetna-US Healthcare Empire Blue Cross
Pomco

LANG: Jpn; [symbols] Immediately

Bentivegna, Saverio (MD)   **S**
Westchester Med Ctr
Dept of Surgery NY Medical College, Munger
Pavilion; Valhalla, NY 10595; (914) 493-7619;
BDCERT: S 58; **MS:** NY Med Coll 50; **RES:** IM,
Fordham Hosp, Bronx, NY 51-52; S, Metropolitan
Hosp Ctr, New York, NY 52-57; **SI:** *Breast Surgery;*
HMO: Aetna Hlth Plan Blue Shield Oxford Pomco
Independent Health Plan +

LANG: Itl, Sp; [symbols] A Few Days

Cehelsky, John Ihor (MD)   **S**
Northern Westchester Hosp Ctr
Mt Kisco Medical Group, 34 S Bedford Rd; Mt Kisco,
NY 10549; (914) 242-1360; **BDCERT:** S 83; **MS:**
Ohio State U 77; **RES:** St Luke's Roosevelt Hosp Ctr,
New York, NY 77-82; **FEL:** CCM, Bayley Seton
Hosp, Staten Island, NY; **SI:** *Laparoscopic Surgery;*
Breast; **HMO:** Oxford Aetna Hlth Plan Prucare US
Hlthcre

LANG: Ukr; [symbols]
A Few Days **VISA** [symbols]

Chafizadeh, Mohsen (MD)   **S**
St John's Riverside Hosp
984 N Broadway L5; Yonkers, NY 10701; (914)
964-1774; **BDCERT:** S 69; **MS:** France 57; **RES:** S,
Jersey City Med Ctr, Jersey City, NJ 57-63; **FAP:**
Asst Prof S NY Med Coll; **HOSP:** Community Hosp
At Dobbs Ferry; **SI:** *Breast Surgery; Abdominal
Surgery;* **HMO:** Blue Cross & Blue Shield Oxford
Aetna-US Healthcare United Healthcare

[symbols] Immediately

Cooperman, Avram M (MD)   **S**
Community Hosp At Dobbs Ferry
128 Ashford Ave; Dobbs Ferry, NY 10522; (914)
693-0055; **BDCERT:** S 72; **MS:** Howard U 65; **RES:**
S, Mayo Clinic, Rochester, MN 66-71; **FEL:** Liver
Trans, Mayo Clinic, Rochester, MN 66-71; **HOSP:**
Beth Israel Med Ctr; **SI:** *Pancreaticobiliary Surgery;
Laparoscopic Surgery;* **HMO:** HealthNet Empire Blue
Choice

[symbols] Immediately [symbols] **VISA** [symbols]

De Angelis, Roger (MD)   **S**
St John's Riverside Hosp
17 Greenvale Ave; Yonkers, NY 10703; (914) 965-
2026; **BDCERT:** S 76; **MS:** Columbia P&S 68; **RES:**
S, St Luke's Roosevelt Hosp Ctr, New York, NY 68-
72; **SI:** *Breast Gallbladder Colon; Minimally Invasive
Surgery;* **HMO:** Oxford PHS Blue Choice Aetna Hlth
Plan

LANG: Tag; [symbols] Immediately
VISA [symbols]

De Caprio, Vincent (MD)   S
United Hosp Med Ctr
478 Westchester Ave; Port Chester, NY 10573;
(914) 937-0707; **BDCERT:** S 67; **MS:** SUNY
Downstate 57; **RES:** S, Grasslands Hosp, Valhalla,
NY 61-65; *SI: Breast Surgery; Laparoscopic
Cholecystectomy;* **HMO:** Prudential Aetna Hlth Plan
Oxford Pomco Magnacare +
LANG: Itl; ⬚ ⬚ ⬚ ⬚ ⬚ ⬚ ⬚ ⬚   A Few Days

Elwyn, Katherine (MD)   S
Community Hosp At Dobbs Ferry
98 Grand St; Croton On Hudson, NY 10520; (914)
271-6649; **BDCERT:** S 83; **MS:** SUNY Hlth Sci Ctr
76; **RES:** S, Univ Hosp SUNY Bklyn, Brooklyn, NY
77-81; **HOSP:** Hudson Valley Hosp Ctr; *SI: Breast
Surgery;* **HMO:** Oxford Blue Choice CIGNA GHI
⬚ ⬚ ⬚ ⬚ ⬚ ⬚   1 Week **VISA** ⬤

Finkelstein, Jacob (MD)   S
United Hosp Med Ctr
33 Cedar St; Rye, NY 10580; (914) 967-7979;
BDCERT: S 70; **MS:** NYU Sch Med 63; **RES:** Mount
Sinai Med Ctr, New York, NY 64-69
⬚ ⬚ ⬚ ⬚ ⬚ ⬚   4+ Weeks

Finley, David (MD)   S
White Plains Hosp Ctr
311 North St 308; White Plains, NY 10605; (914)
684-5884; **BDCERT:** S 79; **MS:** Columbia P&S 73;
RES: S, U of VA Health Sci Ctr, Charlottesville, VA
74-75; Med Ctr Hosp of VT, Burlington, VT 75-78;
FEL: GVS, Bellevue Hosp Ctr, New York, NY 78-79;
NY Hosp-Cornell Med Ctr, New York, NY 78-79;
HOSP: St Agnes Hosp; *SI: Gallbladder & Hernia;
Laparoscopic Surgery;* **HMO:** Oxford PHS Empire
Blue Cross & Shield Aetna Hlth Plan Prucare +
⬚ ⬚ ⬚ ⬚ ⬚ ⬚ ⬚   A Few Days ⬚ **VISA**

Garcia Jr, Jose G (MD)   S
Hudson Valley Hosp Ctr
325 Nelson Ave; Peekskill, NY 10566; (914) 737-
1311; **BDCERT:** S 82; **MS:** Philippines 63; **RES:** S,
Our Lady of Mercy Med Ctr, Bronx, NY 65-69; **FEL:**
S, Our Lady of Mercy Med Ctr, Bronx, NY 69-70;
Mem Sloan Kettering Cancer Ctr, New York, NY
70-71; *SI: Laparoscopic Surgery*
LANG: Sp; ⬚ ⬚ ⬚ ⬚ ⬚ ⬚ ⬚ ⬚   Immediately

Genovese, Matthew L (MD)   S
St Joseph's Med Ctr-Yonkers
127 S Broadway 4A; Yonkers, NY 10701; (914)
378-7800; **BDCERT:** S 69; **MS:** Italy 63; **RES:** S,
Misericordia Hosp, Bronx, NY 64-68; **FAP:** Asst
Prof NY Med Coll; *SI: Gallbladder; Hernia;* **HMO:** Blue
Shield GHI Oxford US Hlthcre
LANG: Itl; ⬚ ⬚ ⬚ ⬚ ⬚ ⬚ ⬚   Immediately

Gomez, Rolando (MD)   S
Lawrence Hosp
77 Pondfield Rd Fl 2; Bronxville, NY 10708; (914)
793-2212; **BDCERT:** S 76; **MS:** Peru 57; **RES:**
Springfield Med Ctr, Springfield, MA 58-60;
Metropolitan Hosp Ctr, New York, NY 71; **FEL:**
Peter Bent Brigham Hosp, Boston, MA 60-63; GVS,
Texas Heart Inst, Houston, TX 67; *SI: Vascular
Surgery; Varicose Veins*
⬚ ⬚ ⬚ ⬚ ⬚ ⬚   A Few Days

Gordon, Mark (MD)   S
White Plains Hosp Ctr
311 North St 308; White Plains, NY 10605; (914)
684-5884; **BDCERT:** S 88; **MS:** Northwestern U 82;
RES: S, NY Hosp-Cornell Med Ctr, New York, NY
82-87; **FEL:** S Onc, Mem Sloan Kettering Cancer
Ctr, New York, NY 87-89; **HOSP:** St Agnes Hosp;
HMO: Aetna Hlth Plan Blue Choice CIGNA
HealthNet Travelers +
⬚ ⬚ ⬚ ⬚ ⬚ ⬚ ⬚ ⬚   A Few Days

Josephson, Lynn (MD)   S
White Plains Hosp Ctr
170 Maple Ave 502; White Plains, NY 10601;
(914) 949-4609; **BDCERT:** S 92; **MS:** Mt Sinai Sch
Med 77; **RES:** Columbia-Presbyterian Med Ctr, New
York, NY 77-81; *SI: Breast Surgery; Laparoscopic
Gallbladders;* **HMO:** Oxford Blue Choice PHS Oxford
SWCHP +
⬚ ⬚ ⬚ ⬚ ⬚ ⬚ ⬚ ⬚ ⬚   A Few Days **VISA** ⬤

Kaplan, Sidney (MD)   S
Mount Vernon Hosp
504 Gramatan Ave; Mt Vernon, NY 10552; (914)
664-7323; **BDCERT:** S 65; **MS:** SUNY Buffalo 55;
RES: VA Med Ctr-Bronx, Bronx, NY 59-63

Kassel, Barry (MD) S
Northern Westchester Hosp Ctr
41 S Bedford Rd; Mount Kisco, NY 10549; (914) 666-6727; **BDCERT:** S 80; **MS:** SUNY Buffalo 73; **RES:** Albert Einstein Med Ctr, Bronx, NY 75-77; New York University Med Ctr, New York, NY 77-79; **SI:** *Breast Surgery; Laparoscopic Surgery;* **HMO:** Oxford Aetna Hlth Plan Prudential NYLCare PHS +

 ♿ 🌙 🔲 👥 🏥 $ Mcr Mcd WC NFl 1 Week

Kim, Zung Wan (MD) S
United Hosp Med Ctr
265 Purchase St; Rye, NY 10580; (914) 967-2588; **BDCERT:** S 73; **MS:** South Korea 64; **RES:** Hosp For Joint Diseases, New York, NY 66; New York Methodist Hosp, Brooklyn, NY 67-70; **HMO:** Oxford CIGNA Aetna Hlth Plan US Hlthcre PHS +

 ♿ 🔲 👥 🏥 Mcr Mcd WC NFl Immediately

Lee, Chong Sung (MD) S
United Hosp Med Ctr
18 Rye Ridge Plaza; Rye Brook, NY 10573; (914) 251-1614; **BDCERT:** S 81; **MS:** South Korea 70; **RES:** Bronx Lebanon Hosp Ctr, Bronx, NY 73-78; **SI:** *Laparoscopic Surgery; Colorectal Surgery;* **HMO:** Oxford CIGNA Metlife Prucare Sanus-NYLCare +

LANG: Sp, Kor; ♿ SU 🔲 👥 🏥 Mcr Mcd WC NFl Immediately

Marrero, Vito A (MD) S
St Agnes Hosp
Mid-Westcheste Surgical Associates, 311 North St Ste 204; White Plains, NY 10605; (914) 949-3988; **BDCERT:** S 79; **MS:** Switzerland 71; **RES:** S, Beth Israel Med Ctr, New York, NY 72-74; S, Univ Hosp SUNY Stony Brook, Stony Brook, NY 74-78; **FAP:** Assoc Prof of Clin S NY Med Coll; **HOSP:** White Plains Hosp Ctr; **SI:** *Laparoscopic Surgery; Breast Surgery;* **HMO:** CIGNA US Hlthcre Oxford GHI Aetna Hlth Plan +

 ♿ 🔲 👥 🏥 $ Mcr Mcd WC NFl Immediately

Molt, Patrick (MD) S
St Agnes Hosp
303 North St 207; White Plains, NY 10605; (914) 949-6716; **BDCERT:** S 84; **MS:** Mt Sinai Sch Med 78; **RES:** S, Mount Sinai Med Ctr, New York, NY 78-83; **FEL:** S Onc, Mem Sloan Kettering Cancer Ctr, New York, NY; **FAP:** Asst Prof S NY Med Coll; **HOSP:** White Plains Hosp Ctr; **SI:** *Surgical Oncology; Breast Cancer;* **HMO:** Oxford Prucare Blue Shield US Hlthcre +

 ♿ 🔲 👥 🏥 Mcr Mcd WC NFl 1 Week **VISA** 💳

Piper, James (MD) S
Westchester Med Ctr
Route 100 Macy Pavilion; Valhalla, NY 10595; (914) 285-7000; **BDCERT:** S 90; **MS:** U Iowa Coll Med 84; **RES:** U Iowa Coll Med, Iowa City, IA 84-89; **FEL:** Transplant S, U Iowa Coll Med, Iowa City, IA 89-91; Liver Transplant & Hepatobiliary S, U Chicago, Chicago, IL 90-91

Policastro, Anthony (MD) S
Westchester Med Ctr
Route 100 Macy Pavilion 220; Valhalla, NY 10595; (914) 594-4887; **BDCERT:** S 91; **MS:** Creighton U 85; **RES:** Westchester County Med Ctr, Valhalla, NY 85-90; **FEL:** Westchester County Med Ctr, Valhalla, NY 90-91

Rajdeo, Heena (MD) S
Westchester Med Ctr
Westchester Surgical Consultants, Munger Pavilion 551; Valhalla, NY 10595; (914) 493-7378; **BDCERT:** S 82; **MS:** India 69; **RES:** Westchester County Med Ctr, Valhalla, NY 77-82; Kem Hosp, Bombay, India 69-72; **FEL:** GI Endoscopy, Lincoln Med & Mental Hlth Ctr, Bronx, NY 82; **FAP:** Asst Prof S NY Med Coll; **SI:** *Laparoscopy/Heartburn/Hernia; Surgery in Dialysis Patients;* **HMO:** Oxford Aetna Hlth Plan CIGNA Pomco Multiplan +

LANG: Sp, Hin; ♿ 🔲 👥 🏥 $ Mcr Mcd WC NFl Immediately **VISA** 💳

Rangraj, Madhu S (MD) S
Sound Shore Med Ctr-Westchester
Soundshore, 140 Lockwood Ave; New Rochelle, NY 10801; (914) 632-9650; **BDCERT:** S 88; **MS:** India 72; **RES:** S, New Rochelle Hosp Med Ctr, New Rochelle, NY 73-78; S, VA Med Ctr, Castle Point, NY 78-80

Raniolo, Robert (MD) S
Phelps Mem Hosp Ctr
777 N Broadway 204; Sleepyhollow, NY 10591; (914) 631-3660; **BDCERT:** S 89; **MS:** Mexico 81; **RES:** Lincoln Med & Mental Hlth Ctr, Bronx, NY 87-88; Lincoln Med & Mental Hlth Ctr, Bronx, NY 83-87; **HMO:** Well Care Sanus-NYLCare Travelers Premier Pomco +

LANG: Sp; 🦽 ☎ 🚻 🛏 Mcr WC NFI 1 Week

Roeder, Werner (MD) S
Lawrence Hosp
77 Pondfield Rd; Bronxville, NY 10708; (914) 793-0996; **BDCERT:** S 71; **MS:** NY Med Coll 70; **RES:** NY Med Coll, New York, NY 70; **FAP:** Asst Clin Prof S Columbia P&S; **HOSP:** Columbia-Presbyterian Med Ctr; *SI: Breast Diseases; Laparoscopic Surgery;* **HMO:** Oxford Blue Cross & Blue Shield PHS Independent Health Plan Magnacare +

🦽 ☎ 🚻 🛏 Mcr WC NFI A Few Days

Savino, John (MD) S
Westchester Med Ctr
NY Med Coll, Dept of Surg, Westchester Med Ctr, Munger Pavillion; Valhalla, NY 10595; (914) 594-4352; **BDCERT:** S 75; **SCC** 87; **MS:** Italy 68; **RES:** Metropolitan Hosp Ctr, New York, NY 69-74; **FAP:** Prof S NY Med Coll; *SI: Pancreas; Colorectal Surgery;* **HMO:** Most

🦽 ☎ 🚻 🛏 Mcr Mcd WC NFI Immediately

Sayegh, Naseem E (MD) S
St Joseph's Med Ctr-Yonkers
Southern Westchester Surgical Associates, PC, 127 S Broadway Ste 4A; Yonkers, NY 10701; (914) 378-7800; **BDCERT:** S 97; **MS:** Mexico 82; **RES:** S, Lincoln Med & Mental Hlth Ctr, Bronx, NY 83; S, NY Med Coll, New York, NY 87; **FEL:** CCM, Lincoln Med & Mental Hlth Ctr, Bronx, NY 88; **FAP:** Assoc Clin Prof S NY Med Coll; **HOSP:** St John's Riverside Hosp; *SI: Breast Surgery; Gastrointestinal Surgery;* **HMO:** Empire Blue Cross & Shield US Hlthcre Oxford CIGNA Prudential +

LANG: Ar, Sp, Itl; 🦽 ☎ 🚻 🛏 $ Mcr Mcd WC NFI 1 Week

Tomasula, John (MD) S
Westchester Med Ctr
Grasslands Rd; Valhalla, NY 10595; (914) 285-1990; **BDCERT:** S 88; **MS:** NYU Sch Med 81; **RES:** S, Univ Hosp SUNY Buffalo, Buffalo, NY 81-86; **FEL:** Transplantation, Univ Hosp SUNY Buffalo, Buffalo, NY 86-87

Voges, Peter (MD) S
Lawrence Hosp
77 Pondfield Rd; Bronxville, NY 10708; (914) 793-0922; **BDCERT:** S 73; **MS:** Germany 62; **RES:** NY Med Coll, New York, NY 65-70; **HMO:** Blue Choice Blue Cross & Blue Shield HealthNet

LANG: Ger; 🦽 ☎ 🚻 🛏 $ Mcr WC NFI Immediately

Walsh, Bruce (MD) S
Sound Shore Med Ctr-Westchester
140 Lockwood Ave 103; New Rochelle, NY 10801; (914) 636-3373; **BDCERT:** S 87; **SCC** 92; **MS:** Mexico 79; **RES:** S, New Rochelle Hosp Med Ctr, New Rochelle, NY 81-86; **FEL:** S, Westchester County Med Ctr, Valhalla, NY 86-87; **HMO:** Blue Choice Oxford Chubb US Hlthcre

🦽 ☎ 🚻 $ Mcr WC NFI Immediately

Wertkin, Martin (MD)   **S**
Phelps Mem Hosp Ctr
200 S Broadway 100; Tarrytown, NY 10591;
(914) 631-5533; **BDCERT:** S 80; **MS:** SUNY Hlth
Sci Ctr 72; **RES:** S, Mount Sinai Med Ctr, New York,
NY 72-78; **HOSP:** Community Hosp At Dobbs
Ferry; **SI:** *Breast Surgery; Breast Disease;* **HMO:**
Aetna Hlth Plan Blue Choice Oxford PHS United
Healthcare +

🦽 🔂 🔆 🎢 Mcr Mcd WC NFI   Immediately

SURGICAL CRITICAL CARE

Cerabona, Thomas D (MD)   **SCC**
Westchester Med Ctr
Route 100 Munger Pavilion; Valhalla, NY 10595;
(914) 493-7221; **BDCERT:** S 88; **SCC** 89; **MS:** NY
Med Coll 82; **RES:** NY Med Coll, Valhalla, NY 82-
87; **FEL:** Trauma & CCM, NY Med Coll, Valhalla, NY
87-88

THORACIC SURGERY

DelGuercio, Louis (MD)   **TS**
Westchester Med Ctr
14 Pryer Ln; Larchmont, NY 10538; (914) 493-
7621; **BDCERT:** S 59; TS 61; **MS:** Yale U Sch Med
53; **RES:** Columbia-Presbyterian Med Ctr, New
York, NY 53-54; St Vincents Hosp & Med Ctr NY,
New York, NY 54-58; **FEL:** TS, Cleveland Metro
Gen Hosp, Cleveland, OH 58-60

🦽 🔂 🔆 🎢 Mcr Mcd WC NFI   Immediately

Gayola, George (MD)   **TS**
Sound Shore Med Ctr-Westchester
150 Lockwood Ave; New Rochelle, NY 10801;
(914) 235-5335; **BDCERT:** TS 63; S 62; **MS:** Italy
51; **RES:** S, Columbia-Presbyterian Med Ctr, New
York, NY 53-55; New Rochelle Hosp Med Ctr, New
Rochelle, NY 55-60; **FEL:** TS, New York University
Med Ctr, New York, NY; Albert Einstein Med Ctr,
Bronx, NY; **HOSP:** Lawrence Hosp

🦽 🔂 🎢 Mcr Mcd WC NFI   Immediately

Kim, Shihan (MD)   **TS**
Bronx Lebanon Hosp Ctr
5 Shoreview Cir; New Rochelle, NY 10803; (914)
738-0889; **BDCERT:** S 71; TS 76; **MS:** South Korea
58; **RES:** TS, Brooklyn Hosp Ctr-Downtown,
Brooklyn, NY 61-63; TS, Univ Hosp SUNY Bklyn,
Brooklyn, NY 63-65; **FEL:** Bronx Lebanon Hosp Ctr,
Bronx, NY 85; **FAP:** Asst Clin Prof S Albert Einstein
Coll Med; **HOSP:** Our Lady of Mercy Med Ctr; **SI:**
Surgery; Thoracic Surgery; **HMO:** US Hlthcre
LANG: Kor; 🅂 Mcr Mcd   1 Week

Miller, Hyman (MD)   **TS**
Westchester Square Med Ctr
970 N Broadway 209; Yonkers, NY 10701; (914)
963-1553; **BDCERT:** TS 78; S 76; **MS:** NYU Sch
Med 66; **RES:** Albert Einstein Med Ctr, Bronx, NY;
TS, U UT Hosp, Salt Lake City, UT; **HOSP:**
Greenwich Hosp; **SI:** *Lung Surgery; Vascular Surgery;*
HMO: Oxford US Hlthcre Prucare PHS NYLCare +
LANG: Fr, Itl; 🦽 🔂 🔆 🎢 🅂 Mcr   A Few Days

Moggio, Richard (MD)   **TS**
Westchester Med Ctr
Route 100 Macy Pavilion E203; Valhalla, NY
10595; (914) 285-7676; **BDCERT:** TS 79; **MS:**
Yale U Sch Med 71; **RES:** Yale-New Haven Hosp,
New Haven, CT 71-76; **FEL:** New York University
Med Ctr, New York, NY 76-78

🆂🅂🅄 🅲 🔂 🔆 🎢 Mcr Mcd WC NFI   Immediately

Pooley, Richard (MD)   **TS**
Westchester Med Ctr
PO Box 434; Elmsford, NY 10523; (914) 493-
7676; **BDCERT:** TS 77; **MS:** Tufts U 65; **RES:** Mary
Hitchcock Mem Hosp, Hanover, NH; Metropolitan
Hosp Ctr, New York, NY 70-73; **FEL:** Columbia-
Presbyterian Med Ctr, New York, NY 73-75; **HMO:**
Aetna Hlth Plan Blue Choice Blue Cross & Blue
Shield HealthNet Independent Health Plan +

🦽 🔂 🔆 🎢 Mcr Mcd WC NFI   A Few Days

Guide to symbols and abbreviations can be found on pages 110-113.

835

Reed, George (MD)   **TS**
Westchester Med Ctr

Westchester Medical Ctr, PO Box 434; Elmsford, NY 10523; (914) 493-7676; **BDCERT:** TS 52; **MS:** NYU Sch Med 51; **RES:** Bellevue Hosp Ctr, New York, NY 51-56; **FEL:** Bellevue Hosp Ctr, New York, NY 56-59; **FAP:** Prof S NY Med Coll; **SI:** *Cardiothoracic Surgery*; **HMO:** Aetna Hlth Plan Blue Choice Blue Cross & Blue Shield CIGNA Independent Health Plan +

♿ 📷 📷 Mcr Mcd WC NFI   1 Week

Sarabu, Mohan (MD)   **TS**
Westchester Med Ctr

Cardiac Surgery Group, 61 Hirst Rd; Briarcliff Manor, NY 10510; (914) 493-7676; **BDCERT:** S 81; TS 83; **MS:** India 73; **RES:** S, Union Mem Hosp, Baltimore, MD 76-78; S, New Rochelle Hosp Med Ctr, New Rochelle, NY 78-80; **FEL:** TS, Univ Hosp SUNY Syracuse, Syracuse, NY 80-82; **FAP:** Assoc Prof S NY Med Coll; **SI:** *Minimally Invasive Cardiovascular Surgery*; **HMO:** CIGNA Aetna Hlth Plan Blue Cross & Blue Shield Independent Health Plan Metlife +

LANG: Tel, Hin; ♿ 📷 📷 📷 S Mcr Mcd   1 Week

Streisand, Robert (MD)   **TS**
White Plains Hosp Ctr

10 Chester Ave; White Plains, NY 10601; (914) 948-6633; **BDCERT:** TS 75; S 73; **MS:** SUNY Downstate 66; **RES:** Kings County Hosp Ctr, Brooklyn, NY 68-73; **FEL:** Baylor Coll Med, Houston, TX 67-68; **HOSP:** St John's Riverside Hosp; **SI:** *Thoracostomies-Video Assisted*; **HMO:** Aetna Hlth Plan Independent Health Plan Blue Cross & Blue Shield Pomco

♿ 📷 📷 📷 Mcr Mcd WC NFI   1 Week

UROLOGY

Alexander, Martin (MD)   **U**
United Hosp Med Ctr

33 Cedar St; Rye, NY 10580; (914) 967-8719; **BDCERT:** U 73; **MS:** NYU Sch Med 64; **RES:** Greenwich Hosp, Greenwich, CT 66; U, New York University Med Ctr, New York, NY 67-70; **HOSP:** Greenwich Hosp; **HMO:** Most

♿ ☎ 📷 📷 📷 S Mcr   Immediately

Bromberg, Warren (MD)   **U**
Northern Westchester Hosp Ctr

Mt Kisco Medical Group, 34 S Bedford Rd; Mt Kisco, NY 10549; (914) 242-1520; **BDCERT:** U 93; **MS:** Johns Hopkins U 85; **RES:** U, Northwestern Mem Hosp, Chicago, IL 87-91; Northwestern Mem Hosp, Chicago, IL 87-91; **SI:** *Prostate Cancer; Incontinence*; **HMO:** Oxford Aetna Hlth Plan United Healthcare PHS Pomco +

♿ ☎ 📷 📷 📷 S Mcr WC NFI   Immediately ■ **VISA** ●

Choudhury, Muhammad (MD) U
Westchester Med Ctr

Munger Pavilion; Valhalla, NY 10595; (914) 594-4305; **BDCERT:** U 82; **MS:** Bangladesh 72; **RES:** Columbia-Presbyterian Med Ctr, New York, NY 77-78; NY Med Coll, New York, NY 78-80; **FEL:** U, Roswell Park Cancer Inst, Buffalo, NY 80-81; **FAP:** Prof U NY Med Coll; **HOSP:** St Agnes Hosp; **SI:** *Urologic Cancer*; **HMO:** Oxford Independent Health Plan CIGNA Well Care

♿ 📷 📷 📷 Mcr Mcd WC NFI   A Few Days **VISA** ●

Eshghi, Majid (MD)   **U**
Our Lady of Mercy Med Ctr

4170 Bronx Blvd; Bronx, NY 10466; (718) 920-9695; **BDCERT:** U 87; **MS:** Iran 76; **RES:** S, St Barnabas Med Ctr, Livingston, NJ 80-81; U, Long Island Jewish, New Hyde Park, NY 81-85; **FEL:** New York Medical College, New York, NY 87; **HMO:** Oxford Blue Choice Well Care

Fagin, Bernard (MD)   U
Hudson Valley Hosp Ctr

East Hudson Urology Group, 3505 Hill Blvd G;
Yorktown Heights, NY 10598; (914) 245-2622;
BDCERT: U 77; **MS:** NY Med Coll 67; **RES:** S,
Brookdale Univ Hosp Med Ctr, Brooklyn, NY 68-69;
Albert Einstein Med Ctr, Bronx, NY 69-73; *SI: Laser
Prostatectomy; Prostate Cancer;* **HMO:** Aetna-US
Healthcare Blue Choice Oxford Pomco

🔵 ⬛ 🔲 🔳 🔲 🔲 Mcr WC NFI   1 Week

Glassman, Charles (MD)   U
White Plains Hosp Ctr

170 Maple Ave 104; White Plains, NY 10601;
(914) 949-7556; **BDCERT:** U 80; **MS:** Tufts U 73;
RES: S, UC San Francisco Med Ctr, San Francisco,
CA 74-75; U, UC San Francisco Med Ctr, San
Francisco, CA 75-78; **FEL:** Ped U, Mayo Clinic,
Rochester, MN 78-79; **FAP:** Asst Clin Prof NY Med
Coll; **HOSP:** St Agnes Hosp; *SI: Prostate Cancer;
Impotence;* **HMO:** PHS Aetna Hlth Plan Chubb
Oxford Empire Blue Choice +

LANG: Sp; 🔲 ⬛ 🔲 🔲 🔲 🔲 Mcr Mcd WC NFI
Immediately *VISA* 💳

Gursel, Erol (MD)   U
St Joseph's Med Ctr-Yonkers

944 N Broadway 202; Yonkers, NY 10701; (914)
969-5577; **BDCERT:** U 76; **MS:** Turkey 54; **RES:**
Cerrahpasa Hosp, Istanbul, Turkey; Sinai Hosp,
Detroit, MI; **FEL:** Columbia-Presbyterian Med Ctr,
New York, NY; **HOSP:** St John's Riverside Hosp;
HMO: Aetna Hlth Plan Blue Choice Blue Cross &
Blue Shield CIGNA HealthNet +

🔲 🔲 🔲 Mcr Mcd WC NFI   Immediately

Hershman, Jack (MD)   U
Phelps Mem Hosp Ctr

777 N Broadway 309; Sleepy Hollow, NY 10591;
(914) 631-3331; **BDCERT:** U 88; **MS:** Mt Sinai Sch
Med 81; **RES:** S, Lenox Hill Hosp, New York, NY 81-
83; U, Montefiore Med Ctr, Bronx, NY 83-86; **FAP:**
Clin Instr U Cornell U; **HOSP:** Westchester Med Ctr;
SI: Prostate Cancer; Kidney Stones; **HMO:** Oxford PHS
US Hlthcre GHI +

LANG: Sp; 🔲 ⬛ 🔲 🔲 🔲 🔲 Mcr   A Few Days

Housman, Arno (MD)   U
Phelps Mem Hosp Ctr

325 S Highland Ave; Briarcliff Manor, NY 10510;
(914) 941-0617; **BDCERT:** U 89; **MS:** SUNY
Downstate 80; **RES:** TS, Univ Hosp SUNY Bklyn,
Brooklyn, NY 80-83; U, Yale-New Haven Hosp,
New Haven, CT 83-86; **FAP:** Asst NY Med Coll; *SI:
Renal Stones-Laser; Urologic Cancer Specialist;* **HMO:**
Oxford Pomco PHS US Hlthcre

LANG: Sp, Fr; 🔲 ⬛ 🔲 🔲 🔲 🔲 Mcr WC NFI
A Few Days

Kogan, Stanley J (MD)   U
Westchester Med Ctr

311 North St 310; White Plains, NY 10605; (914)
948-8765; **BDCERT:** U 76; **MS:** SUNY Hlth Sci Ctr
66; **RES:** S, Montefiore Med Ctr, Bronx, NY 67-68;
U, Montefiore Med Ctr, Bronx, NY 70-73; **FEL:** Ped
U, Montefiore Med Ctr, Bronx, NY; Alder Hey
Children's Hosp, Liverpool, England 73-74; **FAP:**
Clin Prof U NY Med Coll; **HOSP:** NY Hosp-Cornell
Med Ctr; *SI: Pediatric Genital Surgery; Kidney-
Urinary Problems;* **HMO:** Child Health Plus Aetna-
US Healthcare Oxford Well Care

LANG: Sp; 🔲 🔲 🔲 🔲 🔲 Mcr Mcd WC NFI
A Few Days *VISA* 💳

Levitt, Selwyn (MD)   U
Westchester Med Ctr

Route 100 Macy Pavilion; Valhalla, NY 10595;
(914) 285-8628; **BDCERT:** U 72; **MS:** South Africa
61; **RES:** U, Bronx Muncipal Hosp Ctr, Bronx, NY
63-67; **FEL:** Ped, Babies Hosp, New York, NY 67-
68; Ped, Hosp For Sick Children, Toronto, Canada
68-69; **FAP:** Clin Prof U NY Med Coll; **HOSP:**
Montefiore Med Ctr-Weiler/Einstein Div; *SI: Urinary
Tract Reflux (Infection); Hypospadias & Genital
Surgery;* **HMO:** Prucare Blue Choice CIGNA Chubb
Oxford +

🔲 🔲 🔲 🔲 🔲 Mcd   Immediately ▦ *VISA* 💳

Mallouh, Camille (MD)   U
Metropolitan Hosp Ctr

Route 100 Munger Pavilion 460; Valhalla, NY
10595; (914) 594-4300; **BDCERT:** U 68; **MS:**
Lebanon 57; **RES:** U, Metropolitan Hosp Ctr, New
York, NY 59-62; **HOSP:** Westchester Med Ctr

LANG: Fr; Mcr Mcd   2-4 Weeks

Matthews, Gerald J (MD) U
Westchester Med Ctr

Urological Faculty Associates, New York Medical College; Valhalla, NY 10595; (914) 594-4305; **MS:** NY Med Coll 86; **RES:** U, Lenox Hill Hosp, New York, NY 89-93; **FEL:** Inf, Rockefeller Univ Hosp, New York, NY 93-95; **FAP:** Asst Prof NY Med Coll; **HOSP:** St Agnes Hosp; **SI:** *Infertility; Impotence*; **HMO:** Oxford Aetna-US Healthcare Prucare GHI CIGNA +

🔲 🔲 🔲 🔲 🔲 🔲 🔲 🔲 🔲 🔲 A Few Days 🔲 **VISA** 🔲

Megalli, Maguid (MD) U
St Joseph's Med Ctr-Yonkers

StJoseph's Medical Center, 127 S Broadway; Yonkers, NY 10701; (914) 378-7499; **BDCERT:** U 75; **MS:** Egypt 64; **RES:** St Mary Abbotts Hosp, London, England 68-69; Columbia-Presbyterian Med Ctr, New York, NY 70-73; **FEL:** Columbia-Presbyterian Med Ctr, New York, NY 73-74

Motola, Jay Alan (MD) U
Hudson Valley Hosp Ctr

East Hudson Urology Group, 1985 Crompond Rd; Peekskill, NY 10519; (914) 739-1219; **BDCERT:** U 95; **MS:** SUNY Stony Brook 86; **RES:** S, Long Island Jewish Med Ctr, New Hyde Park, NY 87-88; U, Long Island Jewish Med Ctr, New Hyde Park, NY 88-92; **SI:** *Stone Disease; Male Infertility*

LANG: Sp; 🔲 🔲 🔲 🔲 🔲 🔲 🔲 🔲 🔲 2-4 Weeks 🔲 **VISA** 🔲

Owens, George (MD) U
St Agnes Hosp

311 North St; White Plains, NY 10605; (914) 946-1406; **BDCERT:** U 86; **MS:** NY Med Coll 79; **RES:** S, Montefiore Med Ctr, Bronx, NY 79-80; U, Albert Einstein Med Ctr, Bronx, NY 81-84; **HOSP:** Westchester Med Ctr; **SI:** *Impotence; Prostate Disease*; **HMO:** Blue Choice Oxford CIGNA Blue Cross

LANG: Sp, Prt; 🔲 🔲 🔲 🔲 🔲 🔲 🔲 1 Week

Putignano, Joseph (MD) U
Lawrence Hosp

26 Pondfield Rd W; Bronxville, NY 10708; (914) 793-1200; **BDCERT:** U 75; **MS:** Canada 65; **RES:** St Luke's Roosevelt Hosp Ctr, New York, NY 65-71; **HOSP:** Westchester Med Ctr; **HMO:** Aetna Hlth Plan Blue Choice Blue Cross & Blue Shield CIGNA HealthNet +

🔲 🔲 🔲 🔲 🔲 🔲 🔲 🔲 Immediately 🔲 **VISA** 🔲 🔲

Riechers, Roger (MD) U
Northern Westchester Hosp Ctr

34 S Bedford Rd; Mt Kisco, NY 10549; (914) 242-1520; **BDCERT:** U 76; **MS:** NYU Sch Med 68; **RES:** Mount Sinai Med Ctr, New York, NY 69-73; **SI:** *Pediatric Urology/Incontinence; Prostate Cancer*; **HMO:** Oxford Aetna Hlth Plan United Healthcare PHS Prucare +

LANG: Fr; 🔲 🔲 🔲 🔲 🔲 🔲 🔲 1 Week **VISA** 🔲

Roberts, Larry P (MD) U
Sound Shore Med Ctr-Westchester

175 Memorial Hwy 32; New Rochelle, NY 10801; (914) 235-2929; **BDCERT:** U 81; **MS:** U Miami Sch Med 74; **RES:** U, Albert Einstein Med Ctr, Bronx, NY 76-79; S, U Miami Hosp, Miami, FL 75-76; **HOSP:** Westchester Med Ctr; **SI:** *Male Infertility; Erectile Dysfunction*; **HMO:** Oxford GHI PHS Blue Choice

LANG: Sp, Itl, Fr; 🔲 🔲 🔲 🔲 🔲 🔲 🔲 Immediately

Sayegh, Neil (MD) U
Yonkers Gen Hosp

Southern Westchester Urology Group, PC, 944 N Broadway 202; Yonkers, NY 10701; (914) 969-5577; **BDCERT:** U 84; **MS:** NY Med Coll 82; **RES:** U, NY Med Coll, Valhalla, NY 79-81; U, NY Med Coll, Valhalla, NY 81-82; **FAP:** Asst Lecturer U NY Med Coll; **HOSP:** St Joseph's Med Ctr-Yonkers; **SI:** *Prostate Cancer; Sexual Dysfunction*; **HMO:** US Hlthcre Oxford PHS Aetna Hlth Plan NYLCare +

LANG: Sp; 🔲 🔲 🔲 🔲 🔲 🔲 🔲 🔲 🔲 A Few Days

Schrager, Alan (MD)   U
United Hosp Med Ctr

1600 Harrison Ave G102; Mamaroneck, NY
10543; (914) 698-8106; **BDCERT:** U 75; **MS:** U
Hlth Sci/Chicago Med Sch 66; **RES:** S, Maimonides
Med Ctr, Brooklyn, NY 69-70; U, Univ Hosp SUNY
Bklyn, Brooklyn, NY 70-73; **HOSP:** Sound Shore
Med Ctr-Westchester; **SI:** *Diseases of the Prostate;
Sexual Dysfunction;* **HMO:** Blue Cross GHI Blue
Choice Oxford US Hlthcre +

LANG: Sp, Itl; 🅰 🔲 📷 👤 🎫 NFI   A Few Days

Shalit, Shimon (MD)   U
White Plains Hosp Ctr

12 Greenridge Ave; White Plains, NY 10605; (914)
949-0608; **BDCERT:** U 79; **MS:** Israel 57; **RES:**
Beilinson Hosp, Tel Aviv, Israel 59-62; U, Bellevue
Hosp Ctr, New York, NY 62-65; **FAP:** Assoc Prof
NYU Sch Med; **HOSP:** St Agnes Hosp; **SI:** *Prostate
Diseases; Incontinence and Stones;* **HMO:** Blue Cross &
Blue Shield Oxford PHS Aetna-US Healthcare PHCS
+

LANG: Ger, Heb, Rus; 🅰 🌙 🔲 📷 👤 🎫 Mcr WC NFI
A Few Days **VISA** 💳

Tozzo, Pellegrino (MD)   U
Sound Shore Med Ctr-Westchester

Sound Shore Urology, 120 Warren St; New
Rochelle, NY 10801; (914) 636-2121; **BDCERT:** U
71; **MS:** Switzerland 60; **RES:** S, Westchester
County Med Ctr, Valhalla, NY 60-63; U, St Luke's
Roosevelt Hosp Ctr, New York, NY 63-67; **FAP:**
Assoc Prof U NY Med Coll; **HOSP:** Westchester Med
Ctr; **SI:** *Sexual Dysfunction(Impotence)-Male;
Infertility-Male;* **HMO:** Oxford Blue Cross & Blue
Shield CIGNA Aetna Hlth Plan

LANG: Itl, Fr, Ger, Sp; 🅰 🔲 📷 🎫 💲 Mcr Mcd WC NFI
Immediately 🔲 **VISA** 💳

Tucci, Paul (MD)   U
Our Lady of Mercy Med Ctr

955 Yonkers Ave 102; Yonkers, NY 10704; (914)
668-2682; **BDCERT:** U 60; **MS:** NY Med Coll 51;
RES: S, Flower Fifth Ave Hosp, New York, NY 52-
53; U, Metropolitan Hosp Ctr, New York, NY 53-
55; **HOSP:** Lawrence Hosp; **HMO:** Oxford Prucare
Aetna-US Healthcare US Hlthcre Chubb +

LANG: Itl; 🅰 🌙 🔲 🎫 💲 Mcr WC NFI   A Few Days

VASCULAR SURGERY (GENERAL)

Babu, Sateesh (MD)   GVS
Westchester Med Ctr

Vascular Associates of Westchester, LLP, 777 N
Broadway Ste 310; Tarrytown, NY 10595; (914)
366-4270; **BDCERT:** S 76; GVS 83; **MS:** India 69;
RES: Jewish Memorial Hosp, New York, NY 72-75;
S, Metropolitan Hosp Ctr, New York, NY 72-75;
FEL: GVS, Metropolitan Hosp Ctr, New York, NY
76-77; **FAP:** Assoc Prof S NY Med Coll; **HOSP:** St
Agnes Hosp; **SI:** *Carotid Artery Disease; Aortic
Aneurysms;* **HMO:** Oxford Pomco Independent
Health Plan Blue Cross & Blue Choice Aetna-US
Healthcare +

🅰 🔲 📷 👤 🎫 💲 Mcr Mcd NFI

Butt, Khalid (MD)   GVS
Westchester Med Ctr

Route 100 Macy Pavilion 1048; Valhalla, NY
10595; (914) 493-1990; **BDCERT:** S 72; TS 72;
MS: Pakistan 62; **RES:** Queens Hosp Ctr, Jamaica,
NY 64-65; Kings County Hosp Ctr, Brooklyn, NY
65-70; **FEL:** TS, Kings County Hosp Ctr, Brooklyn,
NY 70-71

🅰 SA/SU 🔲 👤 🎫 Mcr Mcd   Immediately

Karanfilian, Richard (MD)   GVS
Sound Shore Med Ctr-Westchester

150 Lockwood Ave 14; New Rochelle, NY 10801;
(914) 636-1700; **BDCERT:** S 84; GVS 89; **MS:** Italy
77; **RES:** S, Univ of Med & Dent NJ Hosp, Newark,
NJ 78-83; **FEL:** GVS, Univ of Med & Dent NJ Hosp,
Newark, NJ 83-85; **FAP:** Assoc Clin Prof NY Med
Coll; **HOSP:** St Agnes Hosp; **SI:** *Carotid Artery
Surgery; Treatment of Varicose Vein;* **HMO:** Oxford
Aetna Hlth Plan PHS Blue Choice CIGNA +

LANG: Itl, Sp, Kor; 🅰 🔲 📷 👤 🎫 💲 Mcr WC NFI
A Few Days

Majlessi, Heshmat (MD)   GVS
United Hosp Med Ctr

233 Purchase St; Rye, NY 10580; (914) 967-
0400; **BDCERT:** S 81; **MS:** Iran 67; **RES:** NY Med
Coll, Valhalla, NY 74-80; **SI:** *Vein Treatments;* **HMO:**
Oxford Prucare Aetna Hlth Plan

🅰 🔲 👤 🎫 Mcr   1 Week

Schwartz, Kenneth (MD)   GVS
White Plains Hosp Ctr
Vascular Surgical Associates, 14 Harwood Ct Ste
326; Scarsdale, NY 10583; (914) 723-7737;
BDCERT: S 91; **MS:** Albert Einstein Coll Med 77;
RES: S, Montefiore Med Ctr, Bronx, NY 77-81; **FEL:**
GVS, USC Med Ctr, Los Angeles, CA 81-82; **FAP:**
Assoc Clin Prof NY Coll Osteo Med; **HMO:** Oxford
Aetna-US Healthcare CIGNA Pomco Metropolitan
+

🔲 🌙 📷 📺 🛏 Mcr Mcd WC NFI A Few Days

Shah, Pravin (MD)   GVS
Westchester Med Ctr
216 E Macy Pavilion E; Valhalla, NY 10595; (914)
493-8800; **BDCERT:** S 74; GVS 84; **MS:** India 67;
RES: Misericordia Hosp, Bronx, NY 69-73; **FEL:** Ellis
Hosp, Schenectady, NY 74-75; **HOSP:** Phelps Mem
Hosp Ctr; **HMO:** Independent Health Plan Blue
Choice Oxford Well Care PHS +

📷 📺 🛏 Mcr Immediately **VISA** 💳

Tannenbaum, Gary (MD)   GVS
St John's Riverside Hosp
984 N Broadway 501; Yonkers, NY 10701; (914)
965-2606; **BDCERT:** GVS 94; S 90; **MS:** Columbia
P&S 83; **RES:** S, Columbia-Presbyterian Med Ctr,
New York, NY 83-90; **FEL:** GVS, New England
Deaconess Hosp, Boston, MA 90-92; **HOSP:** St
Joseph's Med Ctr-Stamford; *SI: Diabetic Vascular
Disease; Wound Care*; **HMO:** Oxford PHS Aetna Hlth
Plan GHI +

🔲 📅 📷 📺 🛏 $ Mcr WC 4+ Weeks

Weintraub, Neil (MD)   GVS
White Plains Hosp Ctr
14 Harwood Ct 326; Scarsdale, NY 10583; (914)
723-7737; **BDCERT:** S 85; **MS:** U Hlth Sci/Chicago
Med Sch 79; **RES:** S, New York University Med Ctr,
New York, NY 79-84; **FEL:** GVS, New York
University Med Ctr, New York, NY 84-85; **FAP:**
Asst Clin Instr NY Med Coll; **HOSP:** St Joseph's Med
Ctr-Yonkers; *SI: Carotid Artery Disease; Abdominal
Aortic Aneurysm*; **HMO:** Oxford CIGNA Kaiser
Permanente Aetna Hlth Plan US Hlthcre +

🔲 📷 📺 🛏 $ Mcr 1 Week 💳 **VISA** 💳

ROCKLAND COUNTY

THE VALLEY HOSPITAL

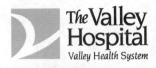

223 NORTH VAN DIEN AVENUE
RIDGEWOOD, NEW JERSEY 07450
(201) 447-8000

Sponsorship:	Voluntary Not-for Profit
Beds:	412 Acute Care Beds
Accreditation:	Accreditation with Commendation, Joint Commission on Accreditation of Healthcare Organizations

PROFILE

Serving more than 350,000 people in Bergen County and adjoining communities, The Valley Hospital is affiliated with Columbia-Presbyterian Medical Center in New York and is part of Valley Health System, a four-county healthcare system.

MEDICAL STAFF

The Valley Hospital has 600 members on its Active Medical Staff, and approximately 90.5% of the Active Staff are Board Certified.

Cardiology	Valley Hospital's cardiology service includes a full range of diagnostic and interventional cardiac treatments, including cardiac surgery, coronary angioplasty and electrophysiology studies. Valley was the first hospital in northern New Jersey to perform the MIDCAB, or Minimally Invasive Direct Coronary Artery Bypass, procedure.
Oncology	Certified by the American College of Surgeons as a *Community Hospital Comprehensive Cancer Program*, Valley provides more radiation therapy treatments than any other hospital in New Jersey, and is widely known for its prostate seed implant program. Additional innovative treatments include Peripheral Stem Cell Transplantation and Intensity Modulated Radiation Therapy. Plans are underway for a free-standing, full-service Cancer Center, designed to bring clinical and social services to patients and their families in one easily-accessible location.
Obstetrics	The hospital offers a full range of maternity services, including Perinatology Services, a newly renovated and enhanced Neonatal Intensive Care Unit directed by two full-time neonatologists, a Maternal & Child Health home care program, and a full-service *Center for Child Development & Wellness*. The completion of new Labor/Delivery/Recovery/Post-Partum Suites in 1998 will offer expectant mothers additional birthing options.
Orthopedics	One of the hospital's newest innovations is its Total Joint Replacement Center offering comprehensive care surrounding hip, knee and shoulder replacements.
Pediatrics	Valley has a comprehensive Pediatric program that includes a Neonatal Intensive Care Unit, overseen by two, full time Board Certified neonatologists, a *Center for Child Development & Wellness*, which is directed by a Board Certified Neonatologist and offers a wide variety of therapeutic services including developmental pediatrics and genetic counseling, and a Center specializing in the diagnosis and treatment of Pediatric Epilepsy and other seizure disorders. In addition, through its affiliation with Columbia-Presbyterian Medical Center, Valley can offer the services of a wide variety of subspecialists so patients can be evaluated and treated in a convenient and local setting.
Physician and Program Referral Service	Valley Connection - A free, seven-day, 24 hour telephone referral service providing callers with information on programs the hospital offers and the more than 600 Active Medical Staff physicians affiliated with The Valley Hospital. Call 1-800-VALLEY 1.

Specialties in capital letters indicate Primary Care Specialties. However, many doctors will be certified in a subspecialty, but will practice predominantly primary care medicine. In our lists this will be indicated.

*Oncologists deal with Cancer

ALLERGY & IMMUNOLOGY

Bosso, John (MD)   A&I
Nyack Hosp
Orangetown Allergy & Asthma, 2 Crossfield Ave
406; West Nyack, NY 10994; (914) 353-9600;
BDCERT: IM 88; A&I 91; **MS:** SUNY Buffalo 85;
RES: IM, Staten Island Univ Hosp, Staten Island,
NY; **FEL:** A&I, Scripps Clinical Research
Foundation, La Jolla, CA 88-90; **FAP:** Asst Clin Prof
Med NY Med Coll; *SI: Asthma;* **HMO:** Independent
Health Plan Metlife Prucare
[symbols] 2-4 Weeks *VISA*

CARDIOLOGY (CARDIOVASCULAR DISEASE)

Roth, Richard (MD)   Cv
Good Samaritan Hosp
7 Medical Park Dr C; Pomona, NY 10970; (914)
362-1365; **BDCERT:** IM 78; Cv 81; **MS:** Yale U Sch
Med 75; **RES:** IM, Boston Med Ctr, Boston, MA 76-
78; **FEL:** Cv, Boston U Med Ctr, Boston, MA 78-80;
HOSP: Nyack Hosp
[symbols] A Few Days

DERMATOLOGY

Waldorf, Donald (MD)   D
Good Samaritan Hosp Med Ctr
57 N Middletown Rd; Nanuet, NY 10954; (914)
623-7077; **BDCERT:** D 65; **MS:** Univ Penn 62;
HOSP: Nyack Hosp; **HMO:** Independent Health
Plan Oxford
[symbols] 1 Week *VISA*

DIAGNOSTIC RADIOLOGY

Weingarten, Marvin J (MD)   DR
Good Samaritan Hosp
Orange Radiology, 505 Route 208; Monroe, NY
10950; (914) 783-3444; **BDCERT:** Rad 83; **MS:**
NY Med Coll 79; **RES:** Rad, Maimonides Med Ctr,
Brooklyn, NY 79-80; Rad, NY Med Coll, Valhalla,
NY 80-83; **HOSP:** Helen Hayes Hosp
[symbols] Immediately *VISA*

ENDOCRINOLOGY, DIABETES & METABOLISM

Josef, Minna (MD)   EDM
Nyack Hosp
Diabetes & Endocrin Consultants, PC, 2 Crosfield
Ave Ste 204; West Nyack, NY 10994; (914) 358-
6266; **BDCERT:** IM 88; EDM 91; **MS:** NYU Sch Med
85; **RES:** Med, Columbia-Presbyterian Med Ctr,
New York, NY 85-88; **FEL:** EDM, Columbia-
Presbyterian Med Ctr, New York, NY 88-91; **HOSP:**
Good Samaritan Hosp; *SI: General Endocrinology;
Osteoporosis;* **HMO:** Oxford US Hlthcre CIGNA
Independent Health Plan Prucare +
[symbols] 2-4 Weeks *VISA*

INTERNAL MEDICINE

Friedman, Sam (MD)   IM   PCP
Good Samaritan Hosp Med Ctr
1 Medical Park Dr; Pomona, NY 10970; (914)
354-9500; **BDCERT:** IM 66; Ge 69; **MS:** SUNY
Downstate 59; **RES:** IM, Montefiore Med Ctr, Bronx,
NY 60-61; IM, Philadelphia Gen Hosp,
Philadelphia, PA 61-62; **FEL:** Ge, Montefiore Med
Ctr, Bronx, NY 64-65; **HOSP:** Nyack Hosp; *SI:
Gastroenterology;* **HMO:** Oxford United Healthcare
Blue Choice CIGNA
LANG: Yd; [symbols] 1 Week

King, Thomas (MD)   **IM**   `PCP`
Good Samaritan Hosp Med Ctr

16 Stony Ridge; Stony Point, NY 10980; (914) 429-8080; **BDCERT:** IM 89; **MS:** Mexico 84; **RES:** IM, Harlem Hosp/Columbia U, New York, NY 87-89; **FAP:** Clin Instr NY Med Coll; **HMO:** US Hlthcre CIGNA Empire Oxford Chubb +

LANG: Sp; 🔲 🔲 🔲 🔲 🔲 🔲 🔲   A Few Days

Leahy, Mary (MD)   **IM**   `PCP`
Nyack Hosp

2 Crossfield Ave 421; West Nyack, NY 10994; (914) 353-1161; **BDCERT:** IM 88; **MS:** Italy 83; **RES:** IM, Misericordia Hosp, Bronx, NY 84-86; **FEL:** Nep, West County Med, Valhalla, NY 86-88

LANG: Itl; 🔲 🔲 🔲 🔲 🔲 🔲 🔲   4+ Weeks

Pomerantz, Barry (MD)   **IM**
Good Samaritan Hosp Med Ctr

Ramapo Cardiology Assoc, 56 S Main St; Spring Valley, NY 10977; (914) 356-0292; **BDCERT:** IM 71; **MS:** NY Med Coll 63; **RES:** IM, St Vincents Hosp & Med Ctr NY, New York, NY 64-65; IM, Michael Reese Hosp Med Ctr, Chicago, IL 67-68; **FEL:** Cv, Colorado Med Ctr, Denver, CO 68-70; *SI: Lipid Abnormality; Hypertension*

🔲 🔲 🔲 🔲 🔲 🔲 🔲 🔲   A Few Days 🔲 **VISA** 💳

NEONATAL-PERINATAL MEDICINE

Mendoza, Glenn (MD)   **NP**
Good Samaritan Hosp

255 Lafayette Ave; Suffern, NY 10901; (914) 368-5104; **BDCERT:** NP 85; Ped 83; **MS:** Philippines 76; **RES:** FP, Elyria Mem Hosp, Elyria, OH 79; Ped, Brooklyn Jewish Hosp, Brooklyn, NY 80-83; **FEL:** NP, Mount Sinai Med Ctr, New York, NY 85-86; **FAP:** Asst Prof Ped Columbia P&S; **HOSP:** Valley Hosp; *SI: Hyperbilirubinemia; Oxygen Transport*; **HMO:** Oxford US Hlthcre Aetna Hlth Plan Well Care Blue Cross & Blue Shield +

NEPHROLOGY

Kozin, Arthur (MD)   **Nep**
Nyack Hosp

Rockland Renal Assoc, 2 Crossfield Ave 312; West Nyack, NY 10994; (914) 358-2400; **BDCERT:** IM 85; Nep 88; **MS:** Albert Einstein Coll Med 82; **RES:** IM, Montefiore Med Ctr, Bronx, NY 82-85; **FEL:** Nep, Bellevue Hosp Ctr, New York, NY 85-87; **HOSP:** Good Samaritan Hosp; *SI: Hypertension; Diabetes Mellitus*; **HMO:** Oxford US Hlthcre Well Care PHS CIGNA +

🔲 🔲 🔲 🔲 🔲 🔲 🔲 🔲 🔲   A Few Days **VISA** 💳

Shapiro, Kenneth (MD)   **Nep**
Good Samaritan Hosp

Rockland Renal Assoc, 2 Crossfield Ave 312; West Nyack, NY 10994; (914) 358-2400; **BDCERT:** IM 78; Nep 80; **MS:** Rush Med Coll 75; **RES:** IM, Albany Med Ctr, Albany, NY 75-78; **FEL:** Nep, New England Med Ctr, Boston, MA 78-80; **FAP:** Asst Clin Prof NY Med Coll; **HOSP:** Nyack Hosp; *SI: High Blood Pressure; Lupus*; **HMO:** Oxford Aetna Hlth Plan

LANG: Fr; 🔲 🔲 🔲 🔲 🔲 🔲   A Few Days **VISA** 💳

NEUROLOGICAL SURGERY

Oppenheim, Jeffery (MD)   **NS**
Nyack Hosp

Hudson Valley Neurosurgical Associates, 222 Route 59 205; Suffern, NY 10901; (914) 368-0286; **BDCERT:** NS 96; **MS:** Cornell U 88; **RES:** NS, Mount Sinai Med Ctr, New York, NY 88-94; **FAP:** Instr Columbia P&S; **HOSP:** Good Samaritan Hosp; *SI: Herniated Disks; Brain Tumors*; **HMO:** Oxford Well Care PHCS Genesis

🔲 🔲 🔲 🔲 🔲 🔲   Immediately 🔲 **VISA** 💳

Spitzer, Daniel (MD)　　　　NS
Nyack Hosp

Hudson Valley Neurosurgical Associates, 222 Route 59 205; Suffern, NY 10901; (914) 368-0286; **BDCERT:** NS 92; **MS:** NYU Sch Med 83; **RES:** N, Montefiore Med Ctr, Bronx, NY 83-89; **FAP:** Asst Clin Prof N Columbia P&S; **HOSP:** Good Samaritan Hosp; *SI: Brain Tumors; Spinal Surgery*

LANG: Fr; 🔲 🌙 📷 📋 🏥 💲 Mcr WC NFl　A Few Days **VISA** 💳

OTOLARYNGOLOGY

Levine, Marc Joel (MD)　　　　Oto
Nyack Hosp

Otolaryngology of Rockland, 11 Medical Park Dr Ste 206; Pomona, NY 10970; (914) 362-3333; **BDCERT:** Oto 92; **MS:** SUNY Stony Brook 80; **RES:** S, Montefiore Med Ctr, Bronx, NY 80-82; Oto, Mount Sinai Med Ctr, New York, NY 82-85; *SI: Thyroid; Parathyroid*; **HMO:** US Hlthcre Oxford Empire

🔲 🌙 📷 📋 🏥 💲 Mcr WC NFl　A Few Days 🔲 **VISA** 💳 💳

Plotkin, Roger (MD)　　　　Oto
Nyack Hosp

603 Route 304; New City, NY 10956; (914) 634-4005; **BDCERT:** Oto 71; **MS:** U Wisc Med Sch 62; **RES:** S, Beth Israel Med Ctr, New York, NY 65-66; Oto, New York Eye & Ear Infirmary, New York, NY 67-70; **FAP:** Asst Clin Prof NY Med Coll; **HOSP:** Good Samaritan Hosp; *SI: Hearing Loss; Thyroid & Parotid Surgery*; **HMO:** Oxford United Healthcare Empire PHCS

🔲 📷 📋 🏥 💲 Mcr WC NFl　1 Week **VISA** 💳

PAIN MANAGEMENT

Burns, Paul (MD)　　　　PM
Good Samaritan Hosp

Ramapo Anesthesiologists—Pain Management, 133 Lafayette Ave; Suffern, NY 10901; (914) 357-5745; **BDCERT:** Anes 84; PM 96; **MS:** SUNY Buffalo 78; **RES:** Anes, NY Hosp-Cornell Med Ctr, New York, NY 79-81; *SI: Pain Management*

🔲 📷 🏥 💲 Mcr Mcd WC NFl　1 Week 🔲 **VISA** 💳

PEDIATRICS

Puder, Douglas (MD)　　　Ped　PCP
Nyack Hosp

Clarkstown Pediatric Assoc, 160 N Midland Ave; Nyack, NY 10960; (914) 353-2600; **BDCERT:** Ped 87; **MS:** NYU Sch Med 82; **RES:** NYU/Bellevue Hosp, New York, NY; **FEL:** Ambulatory Ped, New York University Med Ctr, New York, NY 85-87; **HMO:** Aetna Hlth Plan Oxford HIP Network US Hlthcre +

🔲 SA/SU 🌙 📷 📋 🏥 💲 Mcd　Immediately 🔲 **VISA** 💳 💳

Siegal, Elliot (MD)　　　Ped　PCP
Nyack Hosp

Clarkstown Pediatric Assoc, 200 E Eckerson Rd; New City, NY 10956; (914) 352-5511; **BDCERT:** Ped 75; PEn 78; **MS:** Univ Penn 68; **RES:** Ped, NY Hosp-Cornell Med Ctr, New York, NY 69-71; **FEL:** PEn, NY Hosp-Cornell Med Ctr, New York, NY 71-72; *SI: Thyroid Diseases; Short Stature*; **HMO:** Aetna Hlth Plan GHI Oxford US Hlthcre United Healthcare +

🔲 SA/SU 🌙 📷 📋 🏥 💲 Mcd NFl　Immediately 🔲 **VISA** 💳 💳

PSYCHIATRY

Esser, Aristide (MD)   Psyc
Rye Hosp Ctr
Psychiatry PC, 337 N Main St Ste 2; New City, NY
10956; (914) 639-6723; **BDCERT:** Psyc 70; **MS:**
Holland 55; **RES:** Psyc, Univ of Leyden Med Sch,
Netherlands 57-61; **FEL:** Psyc, Yale-New Haven
Hosp, New Haven, CT 61-62; **FAP:** Prof NYU Sch
Med; **HOSP:** Good Samaritan Hosp Med Ctr; *SI:
Attention Deficit Disorders; Obsessive Compulsive
Disorders;* **HMO:** PHS Oxford Well Care VBH Merit
Behavioral Health Plans +

LANG: Dut, Ger, Fr, Ilo; ⬛ ⬛ ⬛ ⬛ ⬛ ⬛ ⬛ ⬛
⬛ Immediately

PULMONARY DISEASE

Hodes, David (MD)   Pul   PCP
Good Samaritan Hosp
2 Crosfield Ave 318; West Nyack, NY 10994; (914)
353-5600; **BDCERT:** IM 76; Pul 78; **MS:** NYU Sch
Med 73; **RES:** Med, St Luke's Roosevelt Hosp Ctr,
New York, NY 74-76; **FEL:** Pul, NYU-Bellevue Hosp
Ctr, New York, NY 76-78

⬛ ⬛ ⬛ ⬛ ⬛ ⬛ ⬛ ⬛ ⬛ ⬛ 2-4 Weeks ⬛
VISA ⬛

Osei, Clement (MD)   Pul
Good Samaritan Hosp Med Ctr
Rockland Pulmonary Assoc, 2 Crosfield Ave 318;
West Nyack, NY 10994; (914) 353-5600;
BDCERT: IM 75; Pul 78; **MS:** Germany 70; **RES:** IM,
Mount Sinai Med Ctr, New York, NY 72-73; IM,
Mount Sinai Med Ctr, New York, NY 73-75; **FEL:**
Pul, Mount Sinai Med Ctr, New York, NY 75-77; *SI:
Asthma; Emphysema;* **HMO:** Oxford Aetna-US
Healthcare
LANG: Ger; ⬛ ⬛ ⬛ ⬛ ⬛ 1 Week ⬛ **VISA** ⬛

RADIOLOGY

Bobroff, Lewis (MD)   Rad
Good Samaritan Hosp Med Ctr
Rockland Diagnostics Inc, 11 N Airmont Rd;
Suffern, NY 10901; (914) 368-5000; **BDCERT:**
Rad 74; **MS:** Harvard Med Sch 69; **RES:** Rad,
Montefiore Med Ctr, Bronx, NY 70-73; **FEL:** Rad,
Montefiore Med Ctr, Bronx, NY 72-73; *SI:
Interventional Radiology; Mammography;* **HMO:**
Aetna Hlth Plan Blue Choice Blue Cross & Blue
Shield

⬛ ⬛ ⬛ ⬛ ⬛ ⬛ ⬛ ⬛ ⬛ ⬛ Immediately **VISA**
⬛

Boltin, Harry (MD)   Rad
Good Samaritan Hosp Med Ctr
Rockland Diagnostics Inc, 11 N Airmont Rd;
Suffern, NY 10901; (914) 368-5196; **BDCERT:**
Rad 68; **MS:** UMDNJ-RW Johnson Med Sch 63;
RES: Montefiore Med Ctr, Bronx, NY 64-67; **HMO:**
Blue Choice Blue Cross & Blue Shield CIGNA

A Few Days

Geller, Mark (MD)   Rad
Nyack Hosp
Rockland Radiology Group, 18 Squadron Blvd;
New City, NY 10956; (914) 634-9729; **BDCERT:**
Rad 89; **MS:** SUNY Downstate 85; **RES:** DR, NY
Med Coll, Valhalla, NY 85-89; **FAP:** Asst Clin Prof
Rad NY Med Coll; *SI: MRI; CT Scan; Ultrasound;*
HMO: US Hlthcre Oxford GHI Blue Cross & Blue
Choice

LANG: Sp, Rus, Itl; ⬛ ⬛ ⬛ ⬛ ⬛ ⬛ ⬛ ⬛ ⬛ ⬛
Immediately ⬛ **VISA** ⬛ ⬛

Peck, Harvey (MD)   Rad
Good Samaritan Hosp
Ramapo Radiology Assoc, 972 Route 45; Pomona,
NY 10970; (914) 354-7700; **BDCERT:** Rad 60;
MS: Yale U Sch Med 53; **RES:** Mount Sinai Med Ctr,
New York, NY 53-54; Rad, Mount Sinai Med Ctr,
New York, NY 57-60; **FEL:** Path, Mount Sinai Med
Ctr, New York, NY 54-55; **HMO:** Oxford
Metropolitan Aetna-US Healthcare Prucare GHI +

⬛ ⬛ ⬛ ⬛ ⬛ ⬛ ⬛ ⬛ ⬛ ⬛ Immediately **VISA**
⬛ ⬛

Schwartz, Joel (MD) Rad
Nyack Hosp
Mid Rockland Imaging Assoc, 18 Squadron Blvd;
New City, NY 10956; (914) 634-9729; **BDCERT:**
DR 90; **MS:** SUNY Syracuse 85; **RES:** DR, New York
University Med Ctr, New York, NY 88-90; **FEL:** NR,
New York University Med Ctr, New York, NY 89-
91; **FAP:** Clin Instr NYU Sch Med; *SI:*
Neuroradiology

LANG: Sp; 🦽 🔊 🌙 📷 🎬 📶 📶 📶 *VISA* 💳 💳

Tash, Robert R (MD) Rad
Good Samaritan Hosp Med Ctr
11 N Airmont Rd; Suffern, NY 10901; (914) 357-
7245; **BDCERT:** Rad 87; **MS:** NY Med Coll 83; **RES:**
Rad, Westchester County Med Ctr, Valhalla, NY
83-87; **FEL:** NR, Yale-New Haven Hosp, New
Haven, CT 87-89; *SI: Neuroradiology*; **HMO:** Most

🦽 📶 🎬 📶 📶 📶 📶 A Few Days

RHEUMATOLOGY

Becker, Alfred (MD) Rhu
Good Samaritan Hosp Med Ctr
Arthritis AssociatesRockland, 222 Route 59 204;
Suffern, NY 10901; (914) 357-6464; **BDCERT:** IM
69; Rhu 72; **MS:** Albert Einstein Coll Med 62; **RES:**
IM, Pittsburgh Med Ctr, Pittsburgh, PA 65-67; **FEL:**
Rhu, Albert Einstein Med Ctr, Bronx, NY 67-68;
FAP: Clin Prof Med Columbia P&S; **HMO:**
HealthNet US Hlthcre Blue Choice Oxford Prucare
+

LANG: Yd; 🦽 🌙 📷 📶 🎬 📶 📶 📶 📶 2-4 Weeks

SURGERY

Facelle, Thomas (MD) S
Good Samaritan Hosp Med Ctr
Ramapo Valley Surgical Assoc, 100 Route 59 101;
Suffern, NY 10901; (914) 357-8800; **BDCERT:** S
85; S 93; **MS:** NY Med Coll 79; **RES:** S, NY Hosp-
Cornell Med Ctr, New York, NY 79-84; **FAP:** Clin
Instr S NY Med Coll; **HOSP:** Nyack Hosp; *SI:*
Laparoscopic Surgery; Cancer Surgery

🦽 📷 📶 🎬 📶 📶 📶 📶 📶 Immediately *VISA* 💳

Gorenstein, Lyall (MD) S
Columbia-Presbyterian Med Ctr
Rockland Thoracic Assoc, 5 Medical Park Dr A;
Pomona, NY 10970; (914) 362-0075; **BDCERT:**
TS 93; **MS:** Canada 83; **RES:** S, U Toronto Gen
Hosp, Canada 84-88; U Toronto Gen Hosp, Canada
90; **FEL:** TS, MD Anderson Cancer Ctr, Houston, TX
89-90; **HMO:** Oxford US Hlthcre

Rella, Anthony (MD) S
Good Samaritan Hosp Med Ctr
Suffern Surgical Associates, 134 Route 59; Suffern,
NY 10901; (914) 357-7377; **BDCERT:** S 64; **MS:**
NY Med Coll 59; **RES:** S, St Vincents Hosp, New
York, NY 60-64; *SI: Colon and Rectal; Vascular;*
HMO: US Hlthcre Oxford PHS Independent Health
Plan

🦽 📷 📶 🎬 📶 📶 📶 📶 A Few Days

Simon, Lawrence (MD) S
Nyack Hosp
Phillips Hill Surgical Assoc, PC, 11 Medical Park Dr
Ste 203; Pomona, NY 10970; (914) 354-2241;
BDCERT: S 71; **MS:** SUNY Syracuse 65; **RES:** S, St
Luke's Roosevelt Hosp Ctr, New York, NY 66-70;
FEL: American Cancer Society,; **HOSP:** Good
Samaritan Hosp; *SI: Minimally Invasive Surgery;*
Breast Surgery; **HMO:** Oxford US Hlthcre Empire
GHI Independent Health Plan +

🦽 📷 📶 📶 📶 📶 📶 A Few Days

Vladeck, Bob (MD) S
Good Samaritan Hosp Med Ctr
Ramapo Valley Surgical Assoc, 100 Route 59 101;
Suffern, NY 10901; (914) 357-8800; **BDCERT:** S
74; **MS:** Albert Einstein Coll Med 67; **RES:** S, Mount
Sinai Med Ctr, New York, NY 67-73; *SI: Breast*
Disease; **HMO:** Aetna-US Healthcare Oxford PHS
CIGNA GHI +

LANG: Sp; 🦽 📷 📶 📶 📶 📶 📶 📶 A Few Days
VISA 💳

UROLOGY

Kroll, Richard (MD)   **U**
Good Samaritan Hosp Med Ctr
Rockland Urology Assoc, PC, 6 Medical Park Dr
BLDG 6; Pomona, NY 10970; (914) 354-5000;
BDCERT: U 80; **MS:** Albany Med Coll 72; **RES:** S, St
Vincents Hosp & Med Ctr NY, New York, NY 72-74;
U, Columbia-Presbyterian Med Ctr, New York, NY
74-78; **FAP:** Clin Instr U Columbia P&S; **HOSP:**
Nyack Hosp; *SI: Prostate Disorders; Urinary Stones;*
HMO: Aetna Hlth Plan US Hlthcre Oxford Empire
CIGNA +

♿ 🖼 ⚕ 🏥 **S** Mc Md Wc NFl   2-4 Weeks *VISA*

Rudin, Leonard (MD)   **U**
Good Samaritan Hosp Med Ctr
Rockland Urology Assoc, 6 Medical Park Dr BLDG
6; Pomona, NY 10970; (914) 354-5000; **BDCERT:**
U 76; **MS:** SUNY Syracuse 66; **RES:** U, Columbia-
Presbyterian Med Ctr, New York, NY 70-74; S, St
Luke's Roosevelt Hosp Ctr, New York, NY 67-68;
FAP: Instr U Columbia P&S

850

THE STATE OF NEW JERSEY

SAINT BARNABAS HEALTH CARE SYSTEM

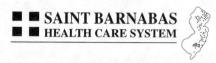

95 OLD SHORT HILLS ROAD
WEST ORANGE, NEW JERSEY 07052
(973) 322-5000
WWW.SAINTBARNABAS.COM

Sponsorship:	Not-for-Profit
Beds:	3,866 acute care beds; 1,487 nursing home beds
Accreditation:	Joint Commission on Accreditation of Healthcare Organizations; American Osteopathic Association; Accreditation Council for Graduate Medical Education.

SYSTEM AFFILIATES

New Jersey's largest integrated healthcare delivery system includes 465-bed Clara Maass Medical Center in Belleville; 596-bed Community Medical Center in Toms River; 157-bed Irvington General Hospital; 350-bed Kimball Medical Center in Lakewood; 527-bed Monmouth Medical Center in Long Branch; 607-bed Newark Beth Israel Medical Center; 620-bed Saint Barnabas Medical Center in Livingston; 201-bed Union Hospital; 231-bed Wayne General Hospital; and 217-bed West Hudson Hospital in Kearny. Also includes 10 nursing homes, 40 ambulatory care facilities, three geriatric centers, an inpatient psychiatric facility, a state-wide behavioral health network, and comprehensive home care and hospice care.

The Saint Barnabas Health Care System and Mount Sinai Health System in New York have a comprehensive strategic alliance and academic affiliation. Saint Barnabas Medical Center and Newark Beth Israel Medical Center are major teaching affiliates of the Mount Sinai School of Medicine. Monmouth Medical Center is a major teaching affiliate of MCP - Hahnemann Medical School in Philadelphia. The Saint Barnabas System is a major clinical campus for the New York College of Osteopathic Medicine.

PATIENTS, EMPLOYEES, PHYSICIANS

The system provides treatment and services for more than 183,300 inpatients and same day surgery patients, 342,000 Emergency Department patients and 1.32 million outpatient visits, and delivers more than 16,000 babies annually. Includes 22,300 employees (third largest private employer in N.J.), 4,620 physicians, 443 residents with 40 programs in virtually all specialties and subspecialties.

SPECIAL PROGRAMS AND SERVICES

Ambulatory Care	New Saint Barnabas Ambulatory Care Center in Livingston, one of only a few in U.S., sets new standard, offering broad array of programs and services for patients in one location with highest quality medical care, technology, patient satisfaction, comfort and convenience.
Burn Services	The Burn Center at Saint Barnabas is New Jersey's only certified burn treatment facility equipped to treat pediatric through geriatric burn patients with a full range of specialized services.
Cardiac Services	Newark Beth Israel Medical Center, with The Heart Hospital of New Jersey and Children's Hospital of New Jersey, is state's only center for heart and lung transplants and is NJ's most comprehensive cardiac program for adult and pediatric cardiac surgery, cardiac transplantation, interventional cardiology services, and clinical and diagnostic cardiology.

Diabetes	Joslin Center for Diabetes at Saint Barnabas, an affiliate of world-renowned Boston center, the leader in diabetes treatment, education and research, offers comprehensive care for adults and children with diabetes and their families. The System has six Joslin Divisions.
Neuroscience and Neurosurgery	The team of dedicated neurosurgeons, specially trained nurses, anesthesiologists and radiologists at Saint Barnabas diagnose and treat the most complicated neurological conditions, including skull-base surgery and complex spine surgery. The Neurosciences Center has sophisticated monitoring systems for diagnosis and management of difficult epilepsy cases.
Obstetrics and Gynecology	More than 16,000 babies delivered annually. Saint Barnabas Medical Center, with 6,143 deliveries, is one of only 22 hospitals (3.5%) in the U.S. performing more than 6,000 deliveries a year. Exceptional services for high-risk or complicated pregnancies. The world-class Institute for Reproductive Medicine and Science at Saint Barnabas, reporting one of the highest pregnancy rates in the nation, is at the forefront of research into improved clinical embryology procedures, pioneering many of the assisted reproductive techniques in use today. Extensive women's health education offered. Saint Barnabas Gynecologic Oncology Division one of five largest and most recognized in northeast. Respected Osteoporosis and Mammography programs.
Oncology	Comprehensive cancer programs provide state-of-the-art treatment for adults and children for all types of cancer and offer patients access to wide variety of clinical trials investigating promising new treatments. Widely recognized facilities for gynecologic cancers. Includes the nationally recognized Jacqueline M. Wilentz Comprehensive Breast Center and new Breast Center of Ambulatory Care Center. Three Valerie Fund Children's Centers for Cancer and Blood Disorders which treat more infants, children, and adolescents with cancer and blood disorders than other facilities in New Jersey. The well respected Center for Hospice Care, a Saint Barnabas System affiliate, provides services for a variety of end-stage diseases including cancer, heart, Parkinson's, kidney and Alzheimer's.
Pediatrics	Widely recognized facilities and programs throughout state, including Children's Hospital of New Jersey at Newark Beth Israel Medical Center with outstanding pediatric specialists to provide comprehensive preventive, diagnostic, therapeutic and rehabilitative health care services. Three hospitals are state-designated Regional Perinatal Centers with Level III, (the highest level), Neonatal Intensive Care Units (NICU), caring for 2,100 premature and sick infants annually. Saint Barnabas Medical Center is one of only 16 hospitals (3.3%) in the U.S. to treat more than 1,000 infants each year in the NICU.
The Refractive Surgery Center	Offers a comprehensive array of laser refractive surgical procedures to reduce dependence on contact lenses and glasses for nearsighted, farsighted or astigmatic patients.
Renal Transplant	The Renal Transplant Centers at Newark Beth Israel Medical Center and Saint Barnabas Medical Center are among the 10 most active of 240 programs in the U.S. With 30 years of experience, our transplant teams are the most experienced in NJ in adult kidney/pancreas transplants and pediatric and adult kidney procedures. Both short-term and long-term graft survivals exceed national averages.
Physician Referral	The Saint Barnabas Physician Referral Service provides a free, seven-day, 24-hour telephone service connecting to a network of over 4,600 primary care physicians and specialists in every field. 1-888-SBHS-123.

BERGEN COUNTY

ENGLEWOOD HOSPITAL AND MEDICAL CENTER

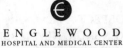

ENGLEWOOD
HOSPITAL AND MEDICAL CENTER
AN AFFILIATE OF MOUNT SINAI SCHOOL OF MEDICINE

We treat you with world-class medicine. And we treat you with respect.

350 Engle Street
Englewood, New Jersey 07631
(201) 894-3000
(201) 569-6126

Sponsorship	Acute Care Teaching Hospital Not-for-Profit
Beds	520
Accreditation	Joint Commission on Accreditation of Healthcare Organizations (JCAHO)
	American College of Radiology, American College of Pathology
	Intersocietal Commission for the Accreditation of Vascular Laboratories
	American College of Graduate Medical Education
	American Association of Colleges of Podiatric Medicine
	Medical Society of New Jersey, Committee on Medical Education

GENERAL DESCRIPTION

Englewood Hospital and Medical Center provides primary, secondary and tertiary care and is a leader in innovative services and state-of-the-art clinical programs.

AFFILIATIONS AND TEACHING PROGRAMS

Englewood Hospital and Medical Center is a member of The Mount Sinai Health System. Through its affiliation with the Mount Sinai School of Medicine, residents in surgery, pediatrics and pathology, as well as critical care medicine fellows rotate through Englewood Hospital and Medical Center. The institution also maintains a free-standing residency program in medicine and a fellowship in vascular surgery.

SPECIAL PROGRAMS

Bloodless Care	The New Jersey Institute for the Advancement of Bloodless Medicine and Surgery recognized by TIME Magazine as a "Hero of Medicine," is a national and international research, education and referral center for care without the use of blood transfusions.
Breast Care	The Cytodiagnosis and Breast Care Center, recognized by the federal government as a national model for breast cancer diagnosis and management, minimizes the anxiety of invasive procedures and hospitalization by providing a unique approach to breast cancer detection that reduces to one day the average diagnosis time of three to six weeks.
Wound Care	With an over 80 percent successful healing rate for chronic wounds, ranking our results among the best in the United States, The Wound Care Center involves a team of physicians, nurses, podiatrists, physical therapists and orthotists with special training and experience in wound management and has the only Hyperbaric Oxygen Chamber in Northern New Jersey.
Post-Polio	The Post-Polio Institute offers polio survivors a comprehensive treatment program addressing the effects aging and 'overuse abuse' have on the polio survivor's function.
Radiology	In addition to the latest Magnetic Resonance Imaging and CT-Scan capabilities in the region, the only hospital-based superconducting Open MRI ideal for larger patients, children and adults with claustrophobia is available at the Medical Center.
Pediatrics	In addition to over 60 world class pediatricians, the Pediatric Specialty Center offers specialized care in cardiology, urology, infectious disease, pulmonology, gastroenterology, allergy/immunology, neurology, anesthesiology, endocrinology, hematology, neonatology, ophthalmology, orthopedics, otolaryngology, and surgery.
Obesity	The Surgical Weight Reduction and Support Center provides a surgical alternative to the severely overweight under the medical direction of a nationally known board certified Gastrointestinal Surgeon with special certification in Surgical Critical Care.
Neonatology	The Neonatal Intensive Care Nursery (Level III) cares for infants born as early as three months prematurely and weighing as little as 2.2 pounds.
Physician Referral	Please call The Medical Connection toll free at 1-877-EHMCMDS.

HACKENSACK UNIVERSITY MEDICAL CENTER

30 PROSPECT AVE.
HACKENSACK, NEW JERSEY 07601
PHONE (201) 996-2000
FAX (201) 996-3452

Sponsorship:	A not-for-profit, teaching hospital affiliated with the University of Medicine and Dentistry of New Jersey–New Jersey Medical School and a member of the University Health System of New Jersey.
Beds:	A 629 bed, tertiary-care hospital that serves as the center of healthcare for Northern New Jersey.
Accreditation:	Joint Commission on the Accreditation of Healthcare Organizations.

BACKGROUND

Founded in 1888 as Bergen County's first hospital, Hackensack University Medical Center has demonstrated more than a century of growth and progress in response to the needs of the communities it serves. The medical center continues to be the largest provider of inpatient and outpatient services in New Jersey.

MEDICAL/DENTAL STAFF

There are more than 800 members on the medical/dental staff. These physicians and dentists represent a full spectrum of medical and dental specialties and subspecialties.

NURSING EXCELLENCE

Honored since 1995 as the first hospital in New Jersey–one of nine in the nation–to receive the Magnet Award for Nursing Excellence from the American Nurses Credentialing Center.

ACCOMPLISHMENTS

Six National Rankings	The medical center, in 1996, received six national rankings from U.S. News and World Report's "America's Best Hospitals," in Cardiology, Geriatrics, Gastroenterology, Otolaryngology, Orthopedics, and Rheumatology.
Quality Leader Award	For the last two years in a row, the medical center was the recipient of the Quality Leader Award in Bergen and Passaic counties.
Highest Risk-Adjusted Survival Rates for Cardiac Surgery	In 1997, the New Jersey State Department of Health and Human Services announced that the medical center's Coronary Artery Bypass Program has the highest patient survival rates in the state.
Kidney Transplant Center Designation	In 1998, the New Jersey Department of Health designated the medical center as a Kidney Transplant Center.

SPECIALTIES

Oncology	The medical center's Northern New Jersey Cancer Center is one of the state's most comprehensive outpatient treatment centers for adults, offering state-of-the-art diagnosis, treatment, and management of all cancers.
Pediatric Oncology	The medical center's DON IMUS-WFAN Pediatric Center for Tomorrow's Children is home to the Tomorrow's Children's Institute for Cancer and Blood Disorders, the largest program of its kind in the state.
Trauma Center	Hackensack University Medical Center is the state-designated trauma center for Bergen County.
Physician Referral	Physician Referral Service representatives offer information on more than 800 doctors representing more than 50 specialties. Call (201) 996-2020

THE VALLEY HOSPITAL

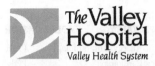

223 NORTH VAN DIEN AVENUE
RIDGEWOOD, NEW JERSEY 07450
(201) 447-8000

Sponsorship:	Voluntary Not-for Profit
Beds:	412 Acute Care Beds
Accreditation:	Accreditation with Commendation, Joint Commission on Accreditation of Healthcare Organizations

PROFILE

Serving more than 350,000 people in Bergen County and adjoining communities, The Valley Hospital is affiliated with Columbia-Presbyterian Medical Center in New York and is part of Valley Health System, a four-county healthcare system.

MEDICAL STAFF

The Valley Hospital has 600 members on its Active Medical Staff, and approximately 90.5% of the Active Staff are Board Certified.

Cardiology	Valley Hospital's cardiology service includes a full range of diagnostic and interventional cardiac treatments, including cardiac surgery, coronary angioplasty and electrophysiology studies. Valley was the first hospital in northern New Jersey to perform the MIDCAB, or Minimally Invasive Direct Coronary Artery Bypass, procedure.
Oncology	Certified by the American College of Surgeons as a *Community Hospital Comprehensive Cancer Program*, Valley provides more radiation therapy treatments than any other hospital in New Jersey, and is widely known for its prostate seed implant program. Additional innovative treatments include Peripheral Stem Cell Transplantation and Intensity Modulated Radiation Therapy. Plans are underway for a free-standing, full-service Cancer Center, designed to bring clinical and social services to patients and their families in one easily-accessible location.
Obstetrics	The hospital offers a full range of maternity services, including Perinatology Services, a newly renovated and enhanced Neonatal Intensive Care Unit directed by two full-time neonatologists, a Maternal & Child Health home care program, and a full-service *Center for Child Development & Wellness*. The completion of new Labor/Delivery/Recovery/Post-Partum Suites in 1998 will offer expectant mothers additional birthing options.
Orthopedics	One of the hospital's newest innovations is its Total Joint Replacement Center offering comprehensive care surrounding hip, knee and shoulder replacements.
Pediatrics	Valley has a comprehensive Pediatric program that includes a Neonatal Intensive Care Unit, overseen by two, full time Board Certified neonatologists, a *Center for Child Development & Wellness*, which is directed by a Board Certified Neonatologist and offers a wide variety of therapeutic services including developmental pediatrics and genetic counseling, and a Center specializing in the diagnosis and treatment of Pediatric Epilepsy and other seizure disorders. In addition, through its affiliation with Columbia-Presbyterian Medical Center, Valley can offer the services of a wide variety of subspecialists so patients can be evaluated and treated in a convenient and local setting.

Physician and Program Referral Service	Valley Connection - A free, seven-day, 24 hour telephone referral service providing callers with information on programs the hospital offers and the more than 600 Active Medical Staff physicians affiliated with The Valley Hospital. Call 1-800-VALLEY 1.

Specialties in capital letters indicate Primary Care Specialties. However, many doctors will be certified in a subspecialty, but will practice predominantly primary care medicine. In our lists this will be indicated.

*Oncologists deal with Cancer

ALLERGY & IMMUNOLOGY

Falk, Theodore (MD)   A&I
Holy Name Hosp
Teaneck Allergy, PA, 63 Grand Ave; River Edge, NJ 07661; (201) 487-2900; **BDCERT:** A&I 82; **MS:** Belgium 77; **RES:** Ped, Long Island Jewish Med Ctr, New Hyde Park, NY 78-79; **HOSP:** Englewood Hosp & Med Ctr; **SI:** *Asthma and Allergies; Chronic Fatigue;* **HMO:** Blue Cross & Blue Shield PHS PHCS CIGNA

🛆 🖩 🕻 🖻 🔳 🛗 🅂   A Few Days **VISA** 💳

Goodstein, Carolyn E (MD)   A&I
Englewood Hosp & Med Ctr
180 N Dean St; Englewood, NJ 07631; (201) 871-4755; **BDCERT:** IM 74; A&I 74; **MS:** SUNY Downstate 64; **RES:** IM, Montefiore Med Ctr, Bronx, NY 65-67; **FEL:** A&I, St Luke's Roosevelt Hosp Ctr, New York, NY 69-71; **FAP:** Assoc Clin Prof Med Columbia P&S; **HOSP:** Hackensack Univ Med Ctr; **SI:** *Allergic Rhinitis; Asthma;* **HMO:** Oxford CIGNA Aetna Hlth Plan Prudential Blue Cross & Blue Shield +

🛆 🕻 🖻 🛗 🅂 🖭   Immediately

Harish, Ziv (MD)   A&I
Englewood Hosp & Med Ctr
200 Engle St Ste 18; Englewood, NJ 07631; (201) 871-7475; **BDCERT:** Ped 89; **MS:** Israel 83; **RES:** Albert Einstein Med Ctr, Bronx, NY 88; **FEL:** A&I, Albert Einstein Med Ctr, Bronx, NY 91; **FAP:** Asst Prof Albert Einstein Coll Med; **HOSP:** Bronx Lebanon Hosp Ctr; **SI:** *Asthma; Food Allergy;* **HMO:** US Hlthcre PHS First Option Aetna Hlth Plan Blue Cross & Blue Shield +

🛆 🖩 🕻 🖻 🛗 🖭   Immediately **VISA** 💳 💳

Michelis, Mary Ann (MD)   A&I
Hackensack Univ Med Ctr
30 Prospect Ave; Hackensack, NJ 07601; (201) 996-2065; **BDCERT:** A&I 81; **MS:** Univ Pittsburgh 75; **RES:** Lenox Hill Hosp, New York, NY 76-78; NY Hosp-Cornell Med Ctr, New York, NY 76-78; **FEL:** Rockefeller Univ Hosp, New York, NY 80-81; **FAP:** Assoc Clin Prof UMDNJ New Jersey Sch Osteo Med; **SI:** *Atopic Allergies; Immune Disorders;* **HMO:** Oxford QualCare

🛆 🖩 🕻 🖻 🔳 🛗 🅂 🅆   A Few Days **VISA** 💳

ANESTHESIOLOGY

Raggi, Robert (MD)   Anes
Holy Name Hosp
33 Hillside Ave; Cresskill, NJ 07626; (201) 568-1994; **BDCERT:** Anes 85; **MS:** Georgetown U 78

CARDIOLOGY (CARDIOVASCULAR DISEASE)

Berkowitz, Robert (MD) Cv
Valley Hosp

Cardiology Associates of Bergen/Passaic, PA, 31-00 Broadway; Fair Lawn, NJ 07410; (201) 796-2255; **BDCERT:** IM 88; Cv 91; **MS:** Yale U Sch Med 84; **RES:** IM, Bronx Muncipal Hosp Ctr, Bronx, NY 84-87; **FEL:** Cv, Albert Einstein Med Ctr, Bronx, NY 87-89; **HOSP:** Hackensack Univ Med Ctr; **SI:** *Congestive Heart Failure; Hypertension;* **HMO:** Oxford HMO Blue First Option CIGNA PHCS +

LANG: Sp, Rus; ⬛ ⬛ ⬛ ⬛ ⬛ ⬛ ⬛ ⬛ ⬛ ⬛ A Few Days ⬛ **VISA** ⬛ ⬛

Blood, David (MD) Cv
Englewood Hosp & Med Ctr

163 Engle St; Englewood, NJ 07631; (201) 569-3313; **BDCERT:** IM 72; Cv 75; **MS:** Columbia P&S 66; **RES:** IM, Bellevue Hosp Ctr, New York, NY 66; IM, Harlem Hosp Ctr, New York, NY 71-72; **FEL:** Cv, Columbia-Presbyterian Med Ctr, New York, NY 72-74; **FAP:** Assoc Clin Instr Columbia P&S; **HOSP:** Columbia-Presbyterian Med Ctr; **SI:** *Nuclear Cardiology; Heart Transplantation;* **HMO:** NYLCare Oxford Aetna Hlth Plan

⬛ ⬛ ⬛ ⬛ ⬛ ⬛ ⬛ A Few Days ⬛ **VISA** ⬛ ⬛

Eisenberg, Sheldon (MD) Cv
Pascack Valley Hosp

Westwood Cardiology Assoc, 333 Old Hook Rd 200; Westwood, NJ 07675; (201) 664-0201; **BDCERT:** IM 79; Cv 81; **MS:** Cornell U 76; **RES:** IM, N Shore Univ Hosp-Manhasset, Manhasset, NY 76-77; **FEL:** Cv, N Shore Univ Hosp-Manhasset, Manhasset, NY 79-81; **HOSP:** Hackensack Univ Med Ctr; **SI:** *Non-Invasive Cardiac Tests; Preventive Cardiology;* **HMO:** Oxford US Hlthcre First Option Blue Cross & Blue Shield

⬛ ⬛ ⬛ ⬛ ⬛ ⬛ ⬛ ⬛ ⬛ 1 Week **VISA** ⬛

Goldberg, Theodore H (MD) Cv
Pascack Valley Hosp

Westwood Cardiology Associates, 333 Old Hook Rd Ste 200; Westwood, NJ 07675; (201) 664-0201; **BDCERT:** IM 63; **MS:** Univ Vt Coll Med 52; **RES:** IM, Montefiore Med Ctr, Bronx, NY 53-54; IM, Jersey City Med Ctr, Jersey City, NJ 57-59; **HOSP:** Hackensack Univ Med Ctr; **SI:** *Preventive Cardiology; Heart Failure;* **HMO:** Oxford US Hlthcre Empire Blue Cross CIGNA First Option +

⬛ ⬛ ⬛ ⬛ ⬛ ⬛ ⬛ ⬛ ⬛ 1 Week **VISA** ⬛

Goldfischer, Jerome D (MD) Cv
Englewood Hosp & Med Ctr

1555 Center Ave; Fort Lee, NJ 07024; (201) 945-1144; **BDCERT:** IM 62; Cv 75; **MS:** NYU Sch Med 55; **RES:** IM, Montefiore Med Ctr, Bronx, NY 59-60; Cv, Montefiore Med Ctr, Bronx, NY 60-61; **FEL:** Cv, Montefiore Med Ctr, Bronx, NY 61-63; **FAP:** Asst Prof Albert Einstein Coll Med; **HOSP:** Montefiore Med Ctr; **SI:** *Heart Disease*

⬛ ⬛ ⬛ ⬛ ⬛ 1 Week ⬛ **VISA** ⬛

Landers, David (MD) Cv
Holy Name Hosp

Bergan Cardiology, 222 Cedar Lane; Teaneck, NJ 07666; (201) 907-0442; **BDCERT:** IM 83; Cv 87; **MS:** Georgetown U 79; **RES:** St Vincents, New York, NY 80-82; **FEL:** Cv, Westchester Co Med, Valhalla, NY 84-85

⬛ ⬛ ⬛ ⬛ ⬛ ⬛ Immediately

Lauricella, Joseph (MD) Cv
Holy Name Hosp

Bergen Cardiology, 292 Columbia Ave; Fort Lee, NJ 07024; (201) 224-0050; **BDCERT:** IM 85; **MS:** Mexico 78; **RES:** IM, Rutgers U Med Ctr, New Brunswick, NJ

⬛ ⬛ ⬛ ⬛ ⬛ ⬛ ⬛ 4+ Weeks

Livelli, Frank (MD)　　　Cv
Columbia-Presbyterian Med Ctr

311 Oakdene Ave; Leonia, NJ 07605; (201) 461-5959; **BDCERT:** IM 79; Cv 81; **MS:** Harvard Med Sch 76; **RES:** IM, Columbia-Presbyterian Med Ctr, New York, NY 76-79; Cv, Columbia-Presbyterian Med Ctr, New York, NY 79-82; **FAP:** Assoc Clin Prof Cv Columbia P&S; *SI: Coronary Disease—Myopathy; Arrhythmias/Defibrillators*; **HMO:** Oxford

♿ 🅒 🔟 👤 🎫 💲　2-4 Weeks *VISA* 💳

Rothman, Howard (MD)　　　Cv
Englewood Hosp & Med Ctr

2200 Fletcher Ave; Fort Lee, NJ 07024; (201) 461-6200; **BDCERT:** IM 75; Cv 79; **MS:** U Cincinnati 70; **RES:** IM, NY Hosp-Cornell Med Ctr, New York, NY 73-75; **FEL:** Cv, NY Hosp-Cornell Med Ctr, New York, NY 74-76; **FAP:** Asst Clin Prof Cv Columbia P&S; **HOSP:** Columbia-Presbyterian Med Ctr; *SI: Cholesterol Control; Coronary Disease*; **HMO:** Oxford Aetna Hlth Plan PHS PHCS

♿ 🔟 🔟 👤 🎫 💲 🅼　A Few Days *VISA* 💳

Sotsky, Gerald (MD)　　　Cv
Valley Hosp

Valley Heart Group, PA, 75 N Maple Ave; Ridgewood, NJ 07450; (201) 670-8660; **BDCERT:** IM 84; Cv 89; **MS:** Mt Sinai Sch Med 81; **RES:** IM, Mount Sinai Med Ctr, New York, NY 81-84; **FEL:** Cv, Mount Sinai Med Ctr, New York, NY 84-86; **HMO:** Blue Cross & Blue Shield

♿ 🅒 🔟 👤 🎫 🅼　A Few Days

Strobeck, John (MD)　　　Cv
Valley Hosp

Heart Lung Center, 297 Lafayette Ave; Hawthorne, NJ 07506; (201) 652-0088; **BDCERT:** IM 79; Cv 83; **MS:** U Cincinnati 74; **RES:** Med, Harvard Med Sch, Cambridge, MA 75-76; **FEL:** Cv, Albert Einstein Med Ctr, Bronx, NY 76-78; **FAP:** Asst Clin Prof Med Albert Einstein Coll Med

♿ 🔟 👤 🎫 💲 🅼 🆆 🆕　A Few Days *VISA* 💳

Weinstock, Murray (MD)　　　Cv
Hackensack Univ Med Ctr

150 Overlook Ave; Hackensack, NJ 07601; (201) 489-5999; **BDCERT:** Cv 75; **MS:** Boston U 65; **RES:** Cv, VA Hosp-Bronx, Bronx, NY 69-70

CHILD & ADOLESCENT PSYCHIATRY

Levine, Allwyn (MD)　　　ChAP
Valley Hosp

Psychiatry Associates of Ridgewood, 179 S Maple Ave; Ridgewood, NJ 07450; (201) 652-4335; **BDCERT:** Psyc 77; ChAP 81; **MS:** SUNY Buffalo 67; **RES:** Psyc, U Mich Med Ctr, Ann Arbor, MI 71-73; **FEL:** ChAP, U Mich Med Ctr, Ann Arbor, MI 73-75; *SI: Forensic Psychiatry*; **HMO:** None

LANG: Heb; 🅒 🔟 👤 🎫 🆕　A Few Days

COLON & RECTAL SURGERY

Helbraun, Mark (MD)　　　CRS
Hackensack Univ Med Ctr

101 Prospect Ave 1J; Hackensack, NJ 07601; (201) 666-7007; **BDCERT:** CRS 78; **MS:** Wayne State U Sch Med 72; **RES:** S, NY Hosp-Cornell Med Ctr, New York, NY 73-77; **FEL:** CRS, Lahey Clinic, Burlington, MA 77-78; **HOSP:** Pascack Valley Hosp; **HMO:** Aetna Hlth Plan Blue Choice Blue Cross & Blue Shield CIGNA Sanus +

♿ 🅒 🔟 👤 🎫 🅼 🆕　Immediately

McConnell, John (MD)　　CRS
Valley Hosp

North Jersey Colon & Rectal Surgery Associates, 414 Saddle River Rd; Fair Lawn, NJ 07410; (201) 791-4002; **BDCERT:** CRS 80; S 80; **MS:** Columbia P&S 74; **RES:** S, St Luke's Roosevelt Hosp Ctr, New York, NY 75-79; **FEL:** CRS, Lehigh Valley Hosp, Allentown, PA 79-80; **HOSP:** Chilton Mem Hosp; **HMO:** Aetna Hlth Plan Blue Cross & Blue Shield CIGNA Prudential United Healthcare +

🦽 🔲 🔳 🏠 💲 Mcr Mcd WC NFI 1 Week ▓ **VISA** ● ▣

Nizin, Joel (MD)　　CRS
Valley Hosp

North Jersey Colon & Rectal, 414 Saddle River Rd; Fair Lawn, NJ 07410; (201) 791-4002; **BDCERT:** CRS 87; **MS:** Howard U 78; **RES:** S, St Luke's Roosevelt Hosp Ctr, New York, NY 78-83; **FEL:** CRS, U MN Med Ctr, Minneapolis, MN 83-84

🦽

Waxenbaum, Steven (MD)　CRS
Valley Hosp

127 Union St; Ridgewood, NJ 07450; (201) 447-4466; **BDCERT:** S 94; CRS 95; **MS:** UMDNJ-RW Johnson Med Sch 88; **RES:** S, Westchester County Med Ctr, Valhalla, NY 88-93; **FEL:** CRS, Lehigh Valley Hosp, Allentown, PA 93-94; **HOSP:** Englewood Hosp & Med Ctr; **SI:** *Laparoscopic Colon Surgery; Hemorrhoids;* **HMO:** HMO Blue Prudential Oxford Aetna Hlth Plan United Healthcare +

🦽 🔲 🏠 🏠 Mcr WC NFI A Few Days **VISA** ●

White, Ronald (MD)　　CRS
Englewood Hosp & Med Ctr

127 Union St; Ridgewood, NJ 07450; (201) 447-4466; **BDCERT:** S 87; CRS 88; **MS:** Boston U 81; **RES:** S, Montefiore Med Ctr, Bronx, NY 81-86; **FEL:** CRS, Univ of Med & Dent NJ Hosp, Newark, NJ 86-87; **HOSP:** Valley Hosp; **SI:** *Hemorrhoids; Laparoscopic Surgery;* **HMO:** Aetna Hlth Plan CIGNA Prucare Oxford PHS +

LANG: Sp; 🦽 🔲 🏠 🏠 💲 Mcr WC NFI A Few Days **VISA** ●

CRITICAL CARE MEDICINE

Cornell, James (MD & PhD) CCM
Valley Hosp

New Jersey Associates in Medicine, PA, 31-00 Fair Lawn Ave; Fair Lawn, NJ 07410; (201) 796-2255; **BDCERT:** IM 92; **MS:** Cornell U 88; **RES:** IM, NY Hosp-Cornell Med Ctr, New York, NY 88-91; Mem Sloan Kettering Cancer Ctr, New York, NY 90-91; **FEL:** CCM, NY Hosp-Cornell Med Ctr, New York, NY 91-94; Pul, NY Hosp-Cornell Med Ctr, New York, NY 91-94; **HOSP:** Barnert Hosp; **SI:** *Breathing Disorders;* **HMO:** Oxford Aetna-US Healthcare CIGNA HMO Blue United Healthcare +

LANG: Sp; 🦽 🔳 🔲 🏠 🏠 💲 Mcr WC NFI A Few Days **VISA** ● ▣

DERMATOLOGY

Baxt, Saida (MD)　　　D
Valley Hosp

Cosmedical NJ, 351 Evelyn St; Paramus, NJ 07652; (201) 265-1300; **BDCERT:** D 71; **MS:** NYU Sch Med 66; **RES:** D, Kings County Hosp Ctr, Brooklyn, NY 66-67; D, Kings County Hosp Ctr, Brooklyn, NY 67-70; **FEL:** D, Kings County Hosp Ctr, Brooklyn, NY 69-70; **SI:** *Acne; Rosacea*

LANG: Itl; 🦽 🔳 🔲 🏠 🏠 💲 1 Week ▓ **VISA** ●

Fine, Herbert (MD)　　　D
Pascack Valley Hosp

390 Old Hook Rd; Westwood, NJ 07675; (201) 666-9550; **BDCERT:** D 69; **MS:** U Hlth Sci/Chicago Med Sch 61; **RES:** D, Bellevue Hosp Ctr, New York, NY 64-67

Fishman, Miriam (MD) **D**
Englewood Hosp & Med Ctr
216 Engle St 104; Englewood, NJ 07631; (201) 569-5678; **BDCERT:** D 84; **MS:** NYU Sch Med 78; **RES:** Ped, Montefiore Med Ctr, Bronx, NY 79-81; D, Albert Einstein Med Ctr, Bronx, NY 81-84; ***SI:** Pediatric Dermatology*; **HMO:** Oxford First Option
LANG: Sp, Yd, Fr, Heb; ♿ ☎ 📅 $ 2-4 Weeks

Fried, Sharon (MD) **D**
Englewood Hosp & Med Ctr
180 N Dean St; Englewood, NJ 07631; (201) 568-1120; **BDCERT:** IM 83; D 87; **MS:** NYU Sch Med 80; **RES:** IM, NY Hosp-Cornell Med Ctr, New York, NY 80-83; D, Univ Hosp SUNY Bklyn, Brooklyn, NY 83-85; ***SI:** Skin Cancer; Acne*; **HMO:** Oxford CIGNA PPO United Healthcare Blue Cross & Blue Shield Premier +
LANG: Sp, Heb; ♿ ☾ ☎ 👤 📅 $ [Mcr] 2-4 Weeks
VISA MasterCard

Heldman, Jay (MD) **D**
Valley Hosp
2300 Route 208 S; Fair Lawn, NJ 07410; (201) 797-7770; **BDCERT:** D 81; **MS:** Columbia P&S 77; **RES:** Columbia-Presbyterian Med Ctr, New York, NY 77-78; D, Mount Sinai Med Ctr, New York, NY 78-81; ***SI:** General Dermatology; Dermatological Surgery*; **HMO:** Blue Cross & Blue Shield PHCS United Healthcare Oxford
♿ [SA SU] ☾ ☎ 👤 📅 $ [Mcr]

Janniger, Camila (MD) **D**
Univ of Med & Dent NJ Hosp
42 Locust Ave; Wallington, NJ 07057; (973) 472-5044; **BDCERT:** D 90; **MS:** Poland 87; **RES:** D, Univ of Med & Dent NJ Hosp, Newark, NJ 87-90; **FAP:** Asst Prof D

Pellicci, Virginia (MD) **D**
Valley Hosp
Dermatology Associates, 348 S Maple Ave; Glen Rock, NJ 07452; (201) 652-6060; **BDCERT:** D 79; **MS:** Cornell U 75; **RES:** D, New York University Med Ctr, New York, NY 76-79
♿ ☾

Scherl, Sharon (MD) **D**
Englewood Hosp & Med Ctr
180 N Dean St; Englewood, NJ 07631; (201) 568-8400; **BDCERT:** D 92; **MS:** NY Med Coll 88; **RES:** D, Metropolitan Hosp Ctr, New York, NY 89-92; ***SI:** General & Pediatric Dermatology; Skin Cancer Surgery*; **HMO:** Oxford Blue Choice Blue Cross & Blue Shield First Option PHS +
LANG: Heb, Sp; ♿ [SA SU] ☾ 👤 📅 $ [Mcr] 2-4 Weeks
VISA

Sweeney, Eugene (MD) **D**
Holy Name Hosp
773 Teaneck Rd; Teaneck, NJ 07666; (201) 837-3939; **BDCERT:** D 67; **MS:** NYU Sch Med 60; **RES:** D, Columbia-Presbyterian Med Ctr, New York, NY 63-66; **FAP:** Asst Prof Columbia P&S; ***SI:** Skin Cancer; Pediatric Dermatology*; **HMO:** Blue Choice Blue Cross & Blue Shield Oxford Blue Cross
LANG: Sp; ☾ ☎ 👤 📅 [Mcr] [NFI] A Few Days

DIAGNOSTIC RADIOLOGY

Adler, Jonathan (MD) **DR**
Englewood Hosp & Med Ctr
309 Engle St 1; Englewood, NJ 07631; (201) 894-3417; **BDCERT:** Rad 73; **MS:** UMDNJ-NJ Med Sch, Newark 66; **RES:** DR, Albert Einstein Med Ctr, Bronx, NY 67-68; DR, Albert Einstein Med Ctr, Bronx, NY 71-73; **FAP:** Asst Clin Prof Albert Einstein Coll Med; ***SI:** CT Scan*
♿ [SA SU] ☾ ☎ 📅 [Mcr] [Mcd] [WC] Immediately

Baldassare, Jack L (MD) **DR**
Westchester Square Med Ctr
Englewood Imaging Ctr, 177 N Dean St Fl P2; Englewood, NJ 07631; (201) 871-1950; **BDCERT:** DR 79; **MS:** SUNY Hlth Sci Ctr 74; **RES:** DR, Bronx Muncipal Hosp Ctr, Bronx, NY 76-79; ***SI:** Magnetic Resonance Imaging*; **HMO:** Oxford US Hlthcre Aetna Hlth Plan Guardian Travelers +
LANG: Sp, Hin, Itl, Kor; ♿ [SA SU] ☾ ☎ 📅 $ [Mcr] [Mcd] [WC] [NFI] Immediately American Express VISA MasterCard

Budin, Joel A (MD)   DR
Hackensack Univ Med Ctr
Hackensack Radiology Group, 30 S Newman St;
Hackensack, NJ 07601; (201) 488-1188; **BDCERT:**
DR 75; **MS:** Columbia P&S 69; **RES:** DR, Columbia-
Presbyterian Med Ctr, New York, NY 72-75; *SI:*
Neuroradiology; **HMO:** Blue Cross & Blue Shield
CIGNA Travelers US Hlthcre

LANG: Sp; 🚪 🅂🅄 🌙 🗄 🎴 Mcr Mod WC   1 Week **VISA**
⬤

Leichter, Jair (MD)   DR
Chilton Mem Hosp
Fair Lawn Diag Imaging, 1904 Fair Lawn Ave; Fair
Lawn, NJ 07410; (973) 835-4981; **BDCERT:** DR
72; **MS:** Austria 63; **RES:** Bronx Muncipal Hosp Ctr,
Bronx, NY 65-68; **FEL:** Angiography, Bronx
Muncipal Hosp Ctr, Bronx, NY 69-70; **FAP:** Asst
Clin Prof Rad Albert Einstein Coll Med

🚪 🌙 🗄 Mcr WC NFI   A Few Days

Rambler, Louis (MD)   DR
Valley Hosp
20 Franklin Tpke; Waldin, NJ 07463; (201) 445-
8822; **BDCERT:** DR 77; **MS:** Cornell U 71; **RES:** DR,
Columbia-Presbyterian Med Ctr, New York, NY 74-
77; *SI: Ultrasound*

🚪 🅂🅄 🌙 🗄 🎴 🎴 Mcr Mod WC NFI   2-4 Weeks **VISA**
⬤

EMERGENCY
MEDICINE

Baddoura, Rashid (MD)   EM
Valley Hosp
Valley Hospital, 223 N Van Dien Ave; Ridgewood,
NJ 07450; (201) 447-8737; **BDCERT:** EM 82; **IM**
80; **MS:** Lebanon 74; **RES:** IM, St Joseph's Hosp-
Paterson, Paterson, NJ 74-76; **FEL:** Pul, Duke U
Med Ctr, Durham, NC 76-79; *SI: Myocardial*
Infarction; Respiratory Distress; **HMO:** Blue Cross &
Blue Shield First Option

🚪 🅂🅄 🌙 🗄 🎴 🎴 Mcr Mod WC NFI   4+ Weeks

Schreibman, Barbara (MD)   EM
Englewood Hosp & Med Ctr
350 Engle St; Englewood, NJ 07631; (201) 894-
3450; **BDCERT:** EM 94; **MS:** Mexico 83; **RES:** S,
Maimonides Med Ctr, Brooklyn, NY 84-86; EM,
Elmhurst Hosp Ctr, Elmhurst, NY 89-92; **FEL:** Med,
Maimonides Med Ctr, Brooklyn, NY 88-89; S,
Maimonides Med Ctr, Brooklyn, NY 86-88

Schwab, Richard (MD)   EM
Holy Name Hosp
718 Teaneck Rd; Teaneck, NJ 07666; (201) 833-
3229; **BDCERT:** EM 83; **MS:** USC Sch Med 77; **RES:**
EM, UCLA Med Ctr, Los Angeles, CA 78-80; **HMO:**
Blue Choice

🚪 🅂🅄 🌙 🗄 🎴 🎴 Mcr Mod WC NFI   Immediately

ENDOCRINOLOGY,
DIABETES &
METABOLISM

Goldman, Michael (MD)   EDM   **PCP**
Englewood Hosp & Med Ctr
600 E Palisade Ave; Englewood Cliffs, NJ 07632;
(201) 568-1108; **BDCERT:** IM 80; EDM 81; **MS:**
NY Med Coll 73; **RES:** Englewood Hosp, Englewood,
NJ 76-78; **FEL:** Columbia-Presbyterian Med Ctr,
New York, NY; *SI: Thyroid Diseases; Diabetes;* **HMO:**
Oxford United Healthcare PHCS CIGNA PHS +

LANG: Sp; 🚪 🅂🅄 🌙 🗄 🎴 💲   4+ Weeks **VISA** ⬤

Kirschner-Levy, Stacy (MD) EDM   **PCP**
Pascack Valley Hosp
228 Rivervale Rd; Rivervale, NJ 07675; (201) 666-
4040; **BDCERT:** IM 89; **MS:** NY Med Coll 85; **RES:**
IM, Long Island Jewish Med Ctr, New Hyde Park,
NY 85-88; **FEL:** EDM, Nassau County Med Ctr, East
Meadow, NY 88-90; **HOSP:** Valley Hosp; *SI: Thyroid*
Disease; Diabetes; **HMO:** CIGNA Sanus-NYLCare US
Hlthcre Aetna Hlth Plan First Option +

LANG: Sp, Heb; 🚪 🅂🅄 🌙 🗄 🎴 🎴 💲 WC
A Few Days 🏧 **VISA** ⬤

Litvin, Yair (MD) EDM
Englewood Hosp & Med Ctr

245 Engle St FL1; Englewood, NJ 07631; (201) 569-5242; **MS:** Israel 73; **RES:** Hassadah Hosp, Jerusalem, Israel 74-79; **FEL:** Hassadah Hosp, Jerusalem, Israel 79-82; Albert Einstein Med Ctr, Bronx, NY 82-84; **HOSP:** Newark Beth Israel Med Ctr; **HMO:** Oxford Blue Cross & Blue Shield CIGNA Chubb

🦽 📷 🅿 🏨 💲 Mcr A Few Days 📧

Tohme, Jack (MD) EDM
Valley Hosp

265 Ackerman Ave Ste 101; Ridgewood, NJ 07450; (201) 444-4363; **BDCERT:** IM 78; EDM 79; **MS:** Lebanon 74; **RES:** IM, Johns Hopkins Hosp, Baltimore, MD 73; IM, American U Med Ctr, Beirut, Lebanon 74-76; **FEL:** EDM, Columbia-Presbyterian Med Ctr, New York, NY 76-77; EDM, Barnes Hosp, St Louis, MO 77-78; **FAP:** Asst Clin Prof Columbia P&S; **HOSP:** Columbia-Presbyterian Med Ctr; **SI:** Osteoporosis; Thyroid Disorders; **HMO:** Oxford Blue Cross & Blue Shield First Option United Healthcare Aetna Hlth Plan +

LANG: Fr, Ar; 🦽 📷 🏨 💲 Mcr Mcd 2-4 Weeks **VISA** 💳

Wehmann, Robert (MD & PhD)EDM
Pascack Valley Hosp

99 Kinderkamack Rd 202; Westwood, NJ 07675; (201) 666-1400; **BDCERT:** IM 77; EM 79; **MS:** Albany Med Coll 74; **RES:** IM, VA Med Ctr, Washington, DC 74-76; **FEL:** EM, Nat Inst Health, Bethesda, MD 76-79; **HOSP:** Hackensack Univ Med Ctr; **SI:** Thyroid Fine Needle Biopsy; Diabetes; **HMO:** US Hlthcre First Option CIGNA PHCS PHS +

🦽 📷 🅿 🏨 💲 Mcr 1 Week **VISA** 💳

Wiesen, Mark (MD) EDM **PCP**
Hackensack Univ Med Ctr

870 Palisade Ave 203; Teaneck, NJ 07666; (201) 836-5655; **BDCERT:** EDM 78; IM 75; **MS:** Columbia P&S 75; **RES:** IM, Brookdale Univ Hosp Med Ctr, Brooklyn, NY 75-78; **FEL:** EDM, Mount Sinai Med Ctr, New York, NY 78-81; **FAP:** Asst Clin Prof UMDNJ New Jersey Sch Osteo Med; **HOSP:** Holy Name Hosp; **HMO:** Blue Cross & Blue Shield Oxford Magnacare CIGNA Aetna Hlth Plan +

🦽 🌙 📷 🏨 💲 Mcr 1 Week **VISA** 💳

FAMILY PRACTICE

Bello, Mary (MD) FP **PCP**
Valley Hosp

400 Franklin Tpke 106; Mahwah, NJ 07430; (201) 327-3333; **BDCERT:** FP 89; **MS:** West Indies 84; **RES:** FP, St Joseph's Hosp-Paterson, Paterson, NJ 84-87; **FAP:** Asst Clin Prof UMDNJ-NJ Med Sch, Newark; **HMO:** CIGNA Prucare First Option PHS PHCS +

🦽 📷 🅿 🏨 💲 Mcr

Gross, Harvey (MD) FP **PCP**
Englewood Hosp & Med Ctr

370 Grand Ave; Englewood, NJ 07631; (201) 569-8786; **BDCERT:** FP 82; **MS:** Boston U 70; **RES:** Montefiore Med Ctr, New York, NY 70-73; **HOSP:** Holy Name Hosp; **SI:** Geriatric Medicine; **HMO:** Most

🦽 🌙 📷 🅿 🏨 💲 Mcr WC 2-4 Weeks

Karatoprak, Ohan (MD) FP **PCP**
Holy Name Hosp

420 Deerwood Rd; Fort Lee, NJ 07024; (201) 886-8877; **BDCERT:** FP 86; Ger 94; **MS:** Turkey 77; **RES:** S, Brookdale Univ Hosp Med Ctr, Brooklyn, NY 82-83; FP, Southside Hosp, Bay Shore, NY 83-86; **FAP:** Clin Instr UMDNJ New Jersey Sch Osteo Med

Nickles, Steven (DO) FP **PCP**
Valley Hosp

50 S Franklin Tpke; Ramsey, NJ 07446; (201) 327-0500; **BDCERT:** FP 90; **MS:** Univ Osteo Med & Hlth Sci 87; **RES:** FP, Montefiore Med Ctr, New York, NY; **HMO:** Blue Cross & Blue Shield CIGNA

🌙 🅿 🏨 Mcr WC NFI 2-4 Weeks 📧 **VISA** 💳

Perkel, David (DO) FP **PCP**
Valley Hosp

6 Brandywine Pl; Oakland, NJ 07436; (201) 337-6662; **BDCERT:** FP 76; **MS:** Kirksville Coll Osteo Med 63; **RES:** FP, Memorial Osteopathic, York, PA 63-64

Guide to symbols and abbreviations can be found on pages 110-113.

867

GASTROENTEROLOGY

Feit, David (MD)   Ge
Hackensack Univ Med Ctr

Hackensack Digestive Disease Associates, PA, 385 Prospect Ave; Hackensack, NJ 07601; (201) 488-3003; **BDCERT:** IM 84; Ge 89; **MS:** Columbia P&S 81; **RES:** IM, Columbia-Presbyterian Med Ctr, New York, NY 81-84; **FEL:** Ge, Columbia-Presbyterian Med Ctr, New York, NY 86-87; **FAP:** Asst Clin Instr Columbia P&S; **HOSP:** Holy Name Hosp; *SI: Chronic Hepatitis;* **HMO:** Oxford Prudential Aetna-US Healthcare Magnacare CIGNA +

♿ ⬛ 🔧 ⏟ S WC NFI A Few Days 💳 **VISA** 💳

Friedrich, Ivan (MD)   Ge
Englewood Hosp & Med Ctr

420 Grand Ave; Englewood, NJ 07631; (201) 569-7044; **BDCERT:** IM 81; **MS:** Albany Med Coll 76; **RES:** Med, Montefiore Med Ctr, Bronx, NY 77-79; **FEL:** GO, Mount Sinai Med Ctr, New York, NY 79-82; *SI: Endoscopy; Endoscopic Biliary Therapy;* **HMO:** Aetna Hlth Plan Blue Choice Blue Cross & Blue Shield CIGNA United Healthcare +

♿ ⬛ ⏟ S Mcr NFI **VISA** 💳

Georgsson, Maria (MD)   Ge
Englewood Hosp & Med Ctr

663 Palisade Ave; Fort Lee, NJ 07010; (201) 945-0491; **BDCERT:** IM 95; **MS:** Columbia P&S 90; **RES:** IM, Columbia Presbyterian Med Ct, New York, NY 91-93; **FEL:** Ge, Univ Hosp SUNY Stony Brook, Stony Brook, NY 93-96

Goldfarb, Joel (MD)   Ge   PCP
Holy Name Hosp

1600 Parker Ave; Fort Lee, NJ 07024; (201) 461-2507; **BDCERT:** IM 78; Ge 81; **MS:** NYU Sch Med 75; **RES:** IM, Bellevue Hosp Ctr, New York, NY 75-78; **FEL:** Hepatology, Yale-New Haven Hosp, New Haven, CT 78-79; Ge, Columbia-Presbyterian Med Ctr, New York, NY 79-81; **FAP:** Asst Clin Prof Med Mt Sinai Sch Med; **HOSP:** Englewood Hosp & Med Ctr; *SI: Liver and Biliary Disease; Colon Cancer*

LANG: Sp, Itl; ♿ ⬛ 🔧 ⏟ S Mcr A Few Days **VISA** 💳

Margulis, Stephen (MD)   Ge
Pascack Valley Hosp

Bergen Gastrology, 466 Old Hook Rd 1; Emerson, NJ 07630; (201) 967-8221; **BDCERT:** IM 84; Ge 87; **MS:** Brown U 81; **RES:** IM, NY Hosp-Cornell Med Ctr, New York, NY 81-84; **FEL:** GO, NY Hosp-Cornell Med Ctr, New York, NY 84-87; **FAP:** Asst Clin Prof Cornell U; **HOSP:** Valley Hosp; *SI: Hepatitis-Liver Diseases; Endoscopy;* **HMO:** Blue Choice Blue Cross & Blue Shield Sanus-NYLCare HMO Blue

LANG: Sp, Itl, Heb; ♿ ⬛ ⬛ 🔧 ⏟ S Mcr Mcd WC NFI **VISA** 💳

Panella, Vincent (MD)   Ge
Englewood Hosp & Med Ctr

420 Grand Ave; Englewood, NJ 07631; (201) 569-7044; **BDCERT:** IM 85; Ge 87; **MS:** NY Med Coll 82; **RES:** IM, N Shore Univ Hosp-Manhasset, Manhasset, NY 83-85; **FEL:** Ge, Mem Sloan Kettering Cancer Ctr, New York, NY 86-87; **FAP:** Asst Clin Prof Mt Sinai Sch Med; **HOSP:** Holy Name Hosp; *SI: Colon Cancer; Liver Disease;* **HMO:** Oxford CIGNA Prudential PHS Aetna-US Healthcare +

LANG: Slv, Itl; ♿ ⬛ 🔧 ⏟ S Mcr A Few Days **VISA** 💳

Rubin, Kenneth (DO)   Ge
Englewood Hosp & Med Ctr

420 Grand Ave; Englewood, NJ 07631; (201) 569-7044; **BDCERT:** IM 78; Ge 81; **MS:** UMDNJ New Jersey Sch Osteo Med 75; **RES:** Med, Bronx Muncipal Hosp Ctr, Bronx, NY 75-76; IM, Bronx Muncipal Hosp Ctr, Bronx, NY 76-79; **FEL:** Ge, Mount Sinai Med Ctr, New York, NY 79-81; **FAP:** Asst Clin Prof Med Mt Sinai Sch Med; **HOSP:** Mount Sinai Med Ctr; *SI: Colon Cancer; Inflammatory Bowel Disease;* **HMO:** Oxford CIGNA Aetna-US Healthcare Prudential PHS +

LANG: Sp, Itl; ♿ ⬛ ⬛ 🔧 ⏟ S Mcr A Few Days **VISA** 💳

Rubinoff, Mitchell (MD)   Ge
Valley Hosp

Gastrointestinal Associates, 140 Chestnut St 300; Ridgewood, NJ 07450; (201) 444-2600; **BDCERT:** IM 82; Ge 85; **MS:** Mt Sinai Sch Med 79; **RES:** IM, Columbia-Presbyterian Med Ctr, New York, NY 79-82; **FEL:** Ge, Columbia-Presbyterian Med Ctr, New York, NY 82-85; **HMO:** Oxford First Option HMO Blue CIGNA

🔲 🔲 🔲 🔲 🔲 Mcr Mcd WC NFI A Few Days **VISA** 💳

Scherl, Newton (MD)   Ge
Englewood Hosp & Med Ctr

1555 Center Ave; Fort Lee, NJ 07024; (201) 945-6564; **BDCERT:** IM 62; Ge 65; **MS:** Med Coll Wisc 55; **RES:** Mount Sinai Med Ctr, New York, NY 55-56; VA Med Ctr-Bronx, Bronx, NY 56-57; **FEL:** Montefiore Med Ctr, Bronx, NY 59-60; Ge, VA Med Ctr-Manh, New York, NY 60-61; **FAP:** Asst Clin Prof Mt Sinai Sch Med; **HOSP:** Holy Name Hosp; *SI: Colonoscopy; Gastroscopy;* **HMO:** Oxford First Option Aetna Hlth Plan Prucare

🔲 🔲 🔲 🔲 Mcr Immediately **VISA** 💳

Zingler, Barry (MD)   Ge
Englewood Hosp & Med Ctr

Scherl Chessler, 1555 Center Ave; Fort Lee, NJ 07024; (201) 945-6564; **BDCERT:** IM 88; Ge 91; **MS:** Rutgers U 85; **RES:** IM, New York University Med Ctr, New York, NY 85-88; **FEL:** Ge, New York University Med Ctr, New York, NY 88-90; **HMO:** Oxford GHI Guardian

LANG: Sp; 🔲 🔲 🔲 🔲 🔲 🔲 Mcr Immediately **VISA** 💳

Zucker, Ira (MD)   Ge
Pascack Valley Hosp

Pascack Gastroenterology Assoc, 400 Old Hook Rd 21; Westwood, NJ 07675; (201) 664-0011; **BDCERT:** IM 84; Ge 87; **MS:** U Hlth Sci/Chicago Med Sch 81; **RES:** IM, St Vincents Hosp & Med Ctr NY, New York, NY 82-84; **FEL:** Ge, St Vincents Hosp & Med Ctr NY, New York, NY 84

GYNECOLOGIC ONCOLOGY

Gafori, Iraj (MD)   GO PCP
Hackensack Univ Med Ctr

140 Prospect Ave 3; Hackensack, NJ 07601; (201) 489-1808; **BDCERT:** ObG 79; **MS:** Iran 91; **RES:** ObG, WV U Hosp, Morgantown, WV 74-77; S, Albert Einstein Med Ctr, Bronx, NY; **FEL:** ObG, Philadelphia, PA; **FAP:** Assoc Clin Prof ObG UMDNJ New Jersey Sch Osteo Med; **HOSP:** Newark Beth Israel Med Ctr; **HMO:** Most

🔲 🔲 🔲 🔲 🔲 🔲 Mcr Mcd 1 Week

HAND SURGERY

Fakharzadeh, Frederick (MD) HS
Hackensack Univ Med Ctr

312 Forest Ave Fl 2; Paramus, NJ 07652; (201) 967-5950; **BDCERT:** OrS 96; **MS:** Columbia P&S 80; **RES:** S, St Luke's Roosevelt Hosp Ctr, New York, NY 80-82; OrS, Columbia-Presbyterian Med Ctr, New York, NY 82-85; **FEL:** HS, Thomas Jefferson U Hosp, Philadelphia, PA 85-86; **FAP:** Asst Clin Prof UMDNJ New Jersey Sch Osteo Med; **HOSP:** Valley Hosp; **HMO:** Oxford CIGNA First Option United Healthcare

🔲 🔲 🔲 🔲 WC NFI 2-4 Weeks **VISA** 💳 💳

Miller, Anne (MD)   HS
Holy Name Hosp

Englewood Orthopedic Associates, 97 Engle St; Englewood, NJ 07631; (201) 569-2770; **BDCERT:** OrS 91; HS 92; **MS:** Harvard Med Sch 83; **RES:** Montefiore Med Ctr, Bronx, NY 88; **FEL:** HS, New England Med Ctr, Boston, MA 88-89; **HOSP:** Englewood Hosp & Med Ctr; *SI: Arthritis Reconstruction; Wrist Injuries*

LANG: Sp; 🔲 🔲 🔲 🔲 🔲 Mcr WC NFI 2-4 Weeks **VISA** 💳

Rosenstein, Roger (MD)   HS
Hackensack Univ Med Ctr

312 Forest Ave; Paramus, NJ 07652; (201) 967-
5950; **BDCERT:** OrS 84; HS 89; **MS:** Columbia P&S
75; **RES:** S, St Luke's Roosevelt Hosp Ctr, New York,
NY 75-77; OrS, Columbia-Presbyterian Med Ctr,
New York, NY 77-80; **FEL:** HS, Thomas Jefferson U
Hosp, Philadelphia, PA 80-81; **FAP:** Asst Clin Prof
UMDNJ-NJ Med Sch, Newark; **HOSP:** Valley Hosp;
SI: Arthritis; Nerve Problems; **HMO:** Oxford First
Option Blue Cross CIGNA

🔲 🔲 🔲 🔲 🔲 🔲   Immediately **VISA** 💳

HEMATOLOGY

Fernbach, Barry (MD)   Hem
Valley Hosp

Hematology Associates Of NJ, 174 Union St;
Ridgewood, NJ 07450; (201) 444-2528; **BDCERT:**
IM 74; Onc 77; **MS:** Harvard Med Sch 71; **RES:** IM,
Mount Sinai Med Ctr, New York, NY 72-73; Hem,
Mount Sinai Med Ctr, New York, NY 75-76; **FEL:**
Neoplastic Disease, Mount Sinai Med Ctr, New
York, NY 76-77; *SI: Oncology*

🔲 🔲 🔲 🔲 🔲 🔲 🔲   Immediately

Forte, Francis (MD)   Hem
Englewood Hosp & Med Ctr

25 Rockwood Pl; Englewood, NJ 07631; (201)
568-5250; **BDCERT:** Hem 72; Onc 73; **MS:** Albert
Einstein Coll Med 64; **RES:** Med, Mount Sinai Med
Ctr, New York, NY 64-68; Med, Mount Sinai Med
Ctr, New York, NY 67-68; **FEL:** Hem, Mount Sinai
Med Ctr, New York, NY 68-69; **FAP:** Asst Prof Med
Mt Sinai Sch Med; **HOSP:** Holy Name Hosp; *SI:
Breast Cancer; Hematologic Disorders;* **HMO:** Oxford
US Hlthcre Blue Cross & Blue Shield Empire Blue
Choice QualCare +

LANG: Sp, Itl, Heb; 🔲 🔲 🔲 🔲 🔲 🔲   1 Week
VISA 💳

Frank, Martin (MD)   Hem
Chilton Mem Hosp

Hematology/Oncology Associates–Collins Pavillion,
97 W Pkwy; Pompton Plains, NJ 07444; (973)
831-5451; **BDCERT:** IM 85; Hem 90; **MS:** Geo
Wash U Sch Med 82; **RES:** Montefiore Med Ctr,
Bronx, NY

🔲 🔲 🔲 🔲 🔲 🔲 🔲   1 Week

Harper, Harry (MD)   Hem
Holy Name Hosp

Northern Nj Cancer Assoc, 5 Summit Ave FL2;
Hackensack, NJ 07601; (201) 996-5900; **BDCERT:**
IM 80; Hem 82; **MS:** Baylor 77; **RES:** IM, NY Hosp-
Cornell Med Ctr, New York, NY 80; **FEL:** Hem Onc,
Mem Sloan Kettering Cancer Ctr, New York, NY
80-83

Israel, Alan (MD)   Hem
Pascack Valley Hosp

261 Old Hook Rd; Westwood, NJ 07675; (201)
666-4949; **BDCERT:** IM 82; **MS:** NYU Sch Med 79;
RES: IM, Mount Sinai Med Ctr, New York, NY 79-
82; **FEL:** Hem, Mem Sloan Kettering Cancer Ctr,
New York, NY 82-84; Long Island Jewish Med Ctr,
New Hyde Park, NY 84; **HOSP:** Valley Hosp; **HMO:**
Sanus CIGNA Empire Blue Choice First Option
Chubb +

🔲 🔲 🔲 🔲 🔲 🔲   Immediately

Spielvogel, Arthur (MD)   Hem
Valley Hosp

Hematology Associates Of Nj, 174 Union St;
Ridgewood, NJ 07450; (201) 444-2528; **BDCERT:**
IM 74; **MS:** Hahnemann U 59; **RES:** Med, Seton
Hall Coll Med, South Orange, NJ; **FEL:** Hem, New
England Med Ctr, Boston, MA; Hem, Montefiore
Med Ctr, Bronx, NY; **FAP:** Prof; *SI: Coagulation
Disorder; Lymphomas;* **HMO:** Aetna Hlth Plan Blue
Choice Blue Cross & Blue Shield

LANG: Sp; 🔲 🔲 🔲 🔲 🔲 🔲 🔲   Immediately

INFECTIOUS DISEASE

Birch, Thomas (MD)   Inf
Englewood Hosp & Med Ctr

Leonia Medical Assoc, 25 Rockwood Pl; Englewood, NJ 07631; (201) 568-3335; **BDCERT:** IM 86; Inf 94; **MS:** U Wisc Med Sch 83; **RES:** IM, Montefiore Med Ctr, Bronx, NY 84-86; **FEL:** Inf, Montefiore Med Ctr, Bronx, NY; **FAP:** Asst Prof NY Med Coll; **HOSP:** Holy Name Hosp; **SI:** *HIV Infections/AIDS; Lyme Disease;* **HMO:** CIGNA Oxford Aetna Hlth Plan Blue Cross & Blue Shield First Option +

⚅ 🄲 📷 🚹 🎬 🅂 Mcr WC NFi   A Few Days

Gross, Peter (MD)   Inf
Hackensack Univ Med Ctr

30 Prospect Ave; Hackensack, NJ 07601; (201) 487-4088; **BDCERT:** IM 71; Inf 76; **MS:** Yale U Sch Med 64; **RES:** Yale-New Haven Hosp, New Haven, CT 65-66; Med, Peter Bent Brigham Hosp, Boston, MA 68-69; **FEL:** Inf, Yale-New Haven Hosp, New Haven, CT 69-71; **FAP:** Prof Med UMDNJ New Jersey Sch Osteo Med; **HMO:** Aetna Hlth Plan Blue Cross & Blue Shield CIGNA Metlife

⚅ 📷 🚹 🎬 🅂 Mcr WC NFi   Immediately 🟫 **VISA** 💮 ▱

Kocher, Jeffrey (MD)   Inf
Englewood Hosp & Med Ctr

25 Rockwood Pl; Englewood, NJ 07631; (201) 568-3335; **BDCERT:** IM 83; Inf 86; **MS:** Cornell U 80; **RES:** NY Hosp-Cornell Med Ctr, New York, NY 80-83; **FEL:** Inf, NY Hosp-Cornell Med Ctr, New York, NY; **HOSP:** Pascack Valley Hosp

⚅ 🄲 📷 🚹 🎬 🅂 Mcr   Immediately

Levine, Jerome (MD)   Inf
Hackensack Univ Med Ctr

Center for Infectious Disease, 385 Prospect Ave; Hackensack, NJ 07601; (201) 487-4088; **BDCERT:** IM 79; **MS:** NYU Sch Med 76; **RES:** IM, VA Med Ctr-Manh, New York, NY 76-80; IM, VA Med Ctr-Manh, New York, NY 77-79; **FEL:** Inf, VA Med Ctr-Manh, New York, NY 80-82; **FAP:** Assoc Prof Med UMDNJ New Jersey Sch Osteo Med; **SI:** *AIDS;* **HMO:** Oxford CIGNA Prudential Magnacare Blue Cross & Blue Shield of NJ +

⚅ 📷 🎬 🅂 Mcr Mcd NFi   Immediately **VISA** 💮

INTERNAL MEDICINE

Andron, Richard (MD)   IM   **PCP**
Englewood Hosp & Med Ctr

154 Engle St; Englewood, NJ 07631; (201) 871-1515; **BDCERT:** IM 77; Rhu 80; **MS:** Temple U 74; **RES:** IM, Temple U Hosp, Philadelphia, PA 74-77; **FEL:** Rhu, New York University Med Ctr, New York, NY 77-79; **FAP:** Clin Instr Med NY Med Coll; **HOSP:** Holy Name Hosp; **SI:** *Rheumatoid Arthritis; Osteoporosis;* **HMO:** Oxford

LANG: Heb; ⚅ 🄲 📷 🚹 🎬 🅂 Mcr Mcd WC NFi
A Few Days 🟫 **VISA** 💮

Angeli, Stephen (MD)   IM
Holy Name Hosp

222 Cedar Lane; Teaneck, NJ 07666; (201) 836-1788; **BDCERT:** IM 84; **MS:** SUNY Downstate 81; **RES:** IM, Univ Hosp SUNY Bklyn, Brooklyn, NY 81-84; **FEL:** Cv, St Michael's Med Ctr, Newark, NJ 84-86; **HOSP:** Hackensack Univ Med Ctr; **SI:** *Cardiac Catheterization; Angioplasty & Stents;* **HMO:** Oxford Aetna Hlth Plan Mastercare First Option

LANG: Itl, Sp; ⚅ 🄲 📷 🚹 🎬 🅂 Mcr   1 Week

Bromberg, Assia (MD)   IM
Valley Hosp

Internal Medicine & Cardiology of Bergen Passaic, 3100 Broadway; Fairlawn, NJ 07410; (201) 796-2255; **BDCERT:** IM 89; Pul 92; **MS:** Israel 74; **RES:** Chaim Sheba Med Ctr, Tel Aviv, Israel 77-81; Englewood Hosp, Englewood, NJ 86-89; **FEL:** Pul, New York University Med Ctr, New York, NY 89-92; **SI:** *Women's Wellness; Asthma;* **HMO:** CIGNA Oxford HMO Blue Magnacare Guardian +

LANG: Heb, Sp; ⚅ 🄲 📷 🎬 🅂 Mcr 🟫 **VISA** 💮

Brunnquell, Stephen (MD)   IM   **PCP**
Englewood Hosp & Med Ctr

274 County Rd; Tenafly, NJ 07670; (201) 568-0493; **BDCERT:** IM 92; **MS:** UMDNJ-NJ Med Sch, Newark 89; **RES:** Montefiore Med Ctr, Bronx, NY 90-92; **HOSP:** Pascack Valley Hosp

⚅ 🆂🆄 🄲 📷 🚹 🎬 🅂 Mcr WC NFi   1 Week **VISA** 💮

Cohen, Sally (MD)   IM   PCP
Valley Hosp
Prospect Medical, 301 Godwin Ave; Midland Park, NJ 07432; (201) 444-4526; **BDCERT:** IM 87; **MS:** Columbia P&S 84; **RES:** St Luke's Roosevelt Hosp, New York, NY 84-85; IM, St Luke's Roosevelt Hosp, New York, NY 85-87; **HMO:** Aetna Hlth Plan Blue Cross & Blue Shield CIGNA

🔣 1 Week

Di Pasquale, Laurene (MD)   IM
Pascack Valley Hosp
99 Kinderkamack Rd; Westwood, NJ 07675; (201) 664-8663; **BDCERT:** IM 93; **MS:** U Puerto Rico 82; **RES:** Mountainside Hosp, Montclair, NJ 85-88; **FEL:** Pul, Bronx Lebanon Hosp Ctr, Bronx, NY 88-90; **HOSP:** Hackensack Univ Med Ctr; *SI: Asthma; Sleep Disorders*; **HMO:** Oxford First Option HIP Network PHCS CIGNA +

LANG: Sp, Rus, Ar; 🔣 Immediately *VISA* 💳

Engler, Mitchell (MD)   IM
Holy Name Hosp
Bergen Medical Alliance, 180 N Dean St; Englewood, NJ 07631; (201) 568-8010; **BDCERT:** IM 81; CCM 93; **MS:** Boston U 78; **RES:** IM, St Luke's Roosevelt Hosp Ctr, New York, NY 78-81; **FEL:** Pul, St Luke's Roosevelt Hosp Ctr, New York, NY 81-83; *SI: Pulmonary & Critical Care*

LANG: Sp; 🔣 1 Week ▆ *VISA* 💳 💳

Fields, Sheila (MD)   IM   PCP
Pascack Valley Hosp
261 Old Hook Rd; Westwood, NJ 07675; (201) 666-4949; **BDCERT:** IM 73; **MS:** SUNY Hlth Sci Ctr 68; **RES:** Mount Sinai Med Ctr, New York, NY 71-73; **HOSP:** Valley Hosp; **HMO:** US Hlthcre

🔣 2-4 Weeks *VISA* 💳

Jarrett, Adam (MD)   IM
Valley Hosp
Medical Office, 301 Godwin Ave; Midland Park, NJ 07432; (201) 444-4526; **BDCERT:** IM 92; **MS:** Geo Wash U Sch Med 89; **RES:** IM, NY Hosp-Cornell Med Ctr, New York, NY 89-92; **HMO:** Oxford CIGNA Prudential First Option United Healthcare +

Knackmuhs, Gary (MD)   IM
Valley Hosp
141 Dayton St; Ridgewood, NJ 07450; (201) 447-6468; **BDCERT:** IM 79; Inf 82; **MS:** NY Med Coll 76; **RES:** Med, Mt Sinai, New York, NY 77-79; **FEL:** Inf, Montefiore, Bronx, NY 79-81

Lau, Henry (MD)   IM
Hackensack Univ Med Ctr
211 Essex St Ste 403; Hackensack, NJ 07601; (201) 646-0044; **BDCERT:** IM 77; Cv 80; **MS:** Taiwan 73; **RES:** Hackensack U Med Ctr, Hackensack, NJ 73-78; **FEL:** Hackensack U Med Ctr, Hackensack, NJ 79-80; **HMO:** Oxford Physician's Health Plan Mastercare

LANG: Man, Can; 🔣 2-4 Weeks

Leifer, Bennett (MD)   IM   PCP
Valley Hosp
Medical Offices, 301 Godwin Ave; Midland Park, NJ 07432; (201) 444-4526; **BDCERT:** IM 90; Ger 92; **MS:** SUNY Syracuse 86; **RES:** IM, Hartford Hosp, Hartford, CT 86-89; **FEL:** Ger, Mount Sinai Med Ctr, New York, NY 89-91; **FAP:** Clin Instr Ger Mt Sinai Sch Med; *SI: Geriatrics/Internal Medicine; Dementia/Alzheimzers Disease*

🔣 A Few Days *VISA* 💳

Melamed, Marc (MD)   IM
Valley Hosp
43 Yawpo Ave 5; Oakland, NJ 07436; (201) 337-1122; **BDCERT:** IM 80; CCM 97; **MS:** NYU Sch Med 77; **RES:** IM, Montefiore Med Ctr, Bronx, NY 77-80; **FEL:** CCM, Montefiore Med Ctr, Bronx, NY 80-81; *SI: Asthma; Hypertension*

🔣 4+ Weeks

Miguel, Eduardo (MD)   IM   `PCP`
Englewood Hosp & Med Ctr

154 Engle St; Englewood, NJ 07631; (201) 871-3280; **BDCERT:** IM 82; **MS:** Uruguay 66; **RES:** IM, VA Med Ctr-Manh, New York, NY 68-69; IM, NY Polyclinic Hosp, New York, NY 70-72; **FEL:** Rhu, Albert Einstein Med Ctr, Bronx, NY 72-73; **FAP:** Clin Instr Mt Sinai Sch Med

LANG: Sp; 🔲 🔲 🔲 🔲 🔲 🔲 🔲 🔲

Nevins, Michael (MD)   IM   `PCP`
Pascack Valley Hosp

354 Old Hook Rd 203; Westwood, NJ 07675; (201) 666-3030; **BDCERT:** IM 69; **MS:** Tufts U 62; **RES:** Kingsbrook Jewish Med Ctr, Brooklyn, NY 62-64; Mount Sinai Med Ctr, New York, NY 66-67; **FEL:** Cv, Mount Sinai Med Ctr, New York, NY; **SI:** Geriatrics; **HMO:** Oxford First Option Blue Cross & Blue Shield

🔲 🔲 🔲 🔲 🔲 Immediately

Pelavin, Martin (MD)   IM   `PCP`
Pascack Valley Hosp

Old Tappan Medical Group, 215 Old Tappan Rd; Old Tappan, NJ 07675; (201) 666-1000; **BDCERT:** IM 76; **MS:** NYU Sch Med 73; **RES:** Montefiore Med Ctr, Bronx, NY 73-76; **HMO:** Oxford US Hlthcre First Option Empire Blue Cross & Shield Prucare +

🔲 🔲 🔲 🔲 🔲 🔲 🔲 🔲 🔲 🔲 A Few Days

Rosner, Steven (MD)   IM   `PCP`
Pascack Valley Hosp

Old Hook Medical Associates LLC, 333 Old Hook Rd 201; Westwood, NJ 07675; (201) 666-7887; **BDCERT:** IM 79; Rhu 94; **MS:** NY Med Coll 76; **RES:** Albert Einstein Med Ctr, Bronx, NY 76-77; Metropolitan Hosp Ctr, New York, NY 77-79; **FEL:** Univ Hosp SUNY Bklyn, Brooklyn, NY 79-81; **FAP:** Asst Clin Prof Med UMDNJ-NJ Med Sch, Newark; **HOSP:** Valley Hosp; **SI:** Rheumatoid Arthritis; Fibromyalgia; **HMO:** Oxford US Hlthcre CIGNA Blue Cross & Blue Shield Prucare +

🔲 🔲 🔲 🔲 🔲 🔲 🔲 🔲 🔲 1 Week 🔲 **VISA** 🔲 🔲

Roth, Joseph (MD)   IM
Gen Hosp Ctr At Passaic

71 Union Ave; Rutherford, NJ 07070; (201) 842-0020; **BDCERT:** IM 84; **MS:** Univ Pittsburgh 81; **RES:** Lenox Hill Hosp, New York, NY 84; **FEL:** Ge, U Conn Hlth Ctr, Farmington, CT; **HOSP:** Passaic Beth Israel Hosp

Schuster, Joseph (MD)   IM
Holy Name Hosp

175 Cedar Ln; Teaneck, NJ 07666; (201) 692-7766; **BDCERT:** IM 84; **MS:** Albany Med Coll 81; **RES:** IM, St Luke's Roosevelt Hosp Ctr, New York, NY 81-82; IM, Univ Hosp SUNY Bklyn, Brooklyn, NY 82-84; **HOSP:** Hackensack Univ Med Ctr

🔲 🔲 🔲 🔲 🔲 🔲 🔲 🔲 Immediately

Scibetta, Maria (MD)   IM   `PCP`
Valley Hosp

Doctor's Park of Ramsey, 42 N Franklin Tpke; Ramsey, NJ 07446; (201) 327-8765; **BDCERT:** IM 93; **MS:** UMDNJ-RW Johnson Med Sch 90; **RES:** IM, Mount Sinai Med Ctr, New York, NY 90-93

LANG: Fr, Sp; 🔲 🔲 🔲 🔲 🔲 🔲 🔲 2-4 Weeks

Volpe, Anthony Peter (MD)   IM   `PCP`
Pascack Valley Hosp

466 Old Hook Rd Ste 14; Emerson, NJ 07630; (201) 262-6485; **BDCERT:** IM 95; **MS:** Mexico 81; **RES:** IM, Huron Road Hosp, Cleveland, OH 83-84; IM, Texas Tech U School of Med, Galveston, TX 84-86; **HMO:** Oxford Unicare Primary Plus First Option Prudential Aetna-US Healthcare +

LANG: Sp; 🔲 🔲 🔲 🔲 🔲 🔲 🔲 1 Week

Wasserman, Kenneth (MD)   IM   `PCP`
Englewood Hosp & Med Ctr

401 S Van Brunt St Ste 402; Englewood, NJ 07631; (201) 567-1140; **BDCERT:** IM 82; **MS:** Albert Einstein Coll Med 79; **RES:** IM, Lenox Hill Hosp, New York, NY 79-82; **HOSP:** Holy Name Hosp; **HMO:** Oxford Blue Cross CIGNA Prudential First Option +

LANG: Sp; 🔲 🔲 🔲 🔲 🔲 🔲 🔲 A Few Days 🔲 **VISA** 🔲 🔲

Weisholtz, Steven (MD)   IM   **PCP**
Englewood Hosp & Med Ctr

Leonia Medical Assoc, 25 Rockwood Pl; Englewood,
NJ 07631; (201) 568-3335; **BDCERT:** IM 81; Inf
83; **MS:** Univ Penn 78; **RES:** NY Hosp-Cornell Med
Ctr, New York, NY 79-81; **FEL:** Inf, NY Hosp-
Cornell Med Ctr, New York, NY 81-83; **HOSP:** Holy
Name Hosp; **HMO:** Oxford Aetna Hlth Plan CIGNA
Guardian First Option +

🚻 🌙 🔄 🗄 🛏 💲 Mcr WC NFI   1 Week

Weizman, Howard (MD)   IM
Valley Hosp

Bergen Hypertension & Renal, 44 Godwin Ave;
Midland Park, NJ 07432; (201) 447-0013;
BDCERT: IM 85; Nep 85; **MS:** Albert Einstein Coll
Med 82; **RES:** IM, Bronx Muncipal Hosp Ctr, Bronx,
NY 82-85; **FEL:** Nep, Mount Sinai Med Ctr, New
York, NY 85-87

🚻 SA/SU 🌙 🔄 🗄 🛏 💲 Mcr Mcd   A Few Days **VISA** 💳

Wierum, Carl (MD)   IM   **PCP**
Englewood Hosp & Med Ctr

245 Engle St; Englewood, NJ 07631; (201) 871-
3680; **BDCERT:** IM 58; **MS:** Cornell U 51; **RES:** NY
Hosp-Cornell Med Ctr, New York, NY 51-54; **FEL:**
Arthritis & Metabolic Disease, NY Hosp-Cornell Med
Ctr, New York, NY 54; **FAP:** Asst Prof Med Mt Sinai
Sch Med; **SI:** *Endocrinology*

🚻 🔄 🛏 🗄 Mcr   A Few Days

MATERNAL & FETAL MEDICINE

Frieden, Faith (MD)   MF
Englewood Hosp & Med Ctr

350 Engle St; Englewood, NJ 07631; (201) 894-
3573; **BDCERT:** ObG 91; MF 92; **MS:** Mt Sinai Sch
Med 84; **RES:** ObG, Beth Israel Med Ctr, New York,
NY 84-88; **FEL:** MF, Bellevue Hosp Ctr, New York,
NY 88-90; **FAP:** Asst Prof Mt Sinai Sch Med; **SI:**
Fetal Ultrasound; Prenatal Diagnosis; **HMO:** Oxford
AARP Blue Cross & Blue Shield Multiplan

🚻 🔄 🛏 🗄 💲 Mcr Mcd   A Few Days **VISA** 💳

MEDICAL ONCOLOGY

Attas, Lewis (MD)   Onc
Englewood Hosp & Med Ctr

25 Rockwood Pl; Englewood, NJ 07631; (201)
568-5250; **BDCERT:** Onc 87; Hem 88; **MS:** Mt
Sinai Sch Med 82; **RES:** IM, Montefiore Med Ctr,
Bronx, NY 83-85; **FEL:** Onc, N Shore Univ Hosp-
Manhasset, Manhasset, NY 85-88; **FAP:** Assoc Prof
Mt Sinai Sch Med; **HOSP:** Holy Name Hosp; *SI:
Breast Cancer; Lymphoma*; **HMO:** Oxford Chubb
Empire

LANG: Sp, Heb; 🚻 🔄 🛏 💲 Mcr Mcd   A Few Days
VISA 💳

Pascal, Mark (MD)   Onc
Hackensack Univ Med Ctr

5 Summit Ave; Hackensack, NJ 07601; (201) 996-
5900; **BDCERT:** Onc 77; **MS:** Jefferson Med Coll 73;
RES: IM, NY Hosp-Cornell Med Ctr, New York, NY
73-77; **FEL:** Hem Onc, Mem Sloan Kettering Cancer
Ctr, New York, NY 77-79; **HOSP:** Holy Name Hosp;
SI: Lung Cancer; **HMO:** Prucare CIGNA Guardian
Blue Cross & Blue Shield Oxford +

LANG: Sp, Rus; 🚻 🛏 🛏 💲 Mcr Mcd   A Few Days
VISA 💳

Schleider, Michael (MD)   Onc
Englewood Hosp & Med Ctr

25 Rockwood Pl; Englewood, NJ 07631; (201)
568-5250; **BDCERT:** Onc 77; Hem 76; **MS:** Univ
Penn 69; **RES:** Med, NY Hosp-Cornell Med Ctr, New
York, NY 72-74; **FEL:** Hem Onc, NY Hosp-Cornell
Med Ctr, New York, NY 74-77; **FAP:** Asst Prof Mt
Sinai Sch Med; **HOSP:** Holy Name Hosp; *SI: Breast
Cancer; Bloodless Surgery*; **HMO:** Oxford Aetna-US
Healthcare First Option Blue Shield PHS +

LANG: Heb, Sp, Itl; 🚻 🔄 🛏 💲 Mcr Mcd   1 Week
VISA 💳

Waintraub, Stanley (MD)   Onc
Hackensack Univ Med Ctr

Northern NJ Cancer Associates, 5 Summit Ave;
Hackensack, NJ 07601; (201) 996-5900; **BDCERT:**
Onc 80; Hem 82; **MS:** NY Med Coll 77; **RES:**
Metropolitan Hosp Ctr, New York, NY 78-80; **FEL:**
Montefiore Med Ctr, Bronx, NY 80-81; Mem Sloan
Kettering Cancer Ctr, New York, NY 82-83; **HOSP:**
Holy Name Hosp; *SI: Breast Cancer; Bleeding
Disorders*; **HMO:** US Hlthcre CIGNA Empire Blue
Cross & Shield Prucare QualCare +

LANG: Yd, Rus, Sp; ⬚ ⬚ ⬚ ⬚ ⬚ ⬚ ⬚
A Few Days **VISA** ⬚

NEONATAL-PERINATAL MEDICINE

Manginello, Frank (MD)   NP
Valley Hosp

The Valley Hospital, 223 N Van Dien Ave 3N;
Ridgewood, NJ 07450; (201) 447-8388; **BDCERT:**
Ped 78; NP 79; **MS:** Georgetown U 73; **RES:** Ped,
Georgetown U Hosp, Washington, DC 73-74; Ped,
Georgetown U Hosp, Washington, DC 74-75; **FEL:**
Perinatal Pul, NY Hosp-Cornell Med Ctr, New York,
NY 75-77

Pane, Carmella (MD)   NP
Valley Hosp

223 N Van Dien Ave; Ridgewood, NJ 07450; (201)
447-8288; **BDCERT:** Ped 88; NP 89; **MS:** Geo
Wash U Sch Med 84; **RES:** Ped, Children's Hosp of
Philadelphia, Philadelphia, PA 84-87; **FEL:** NP,
Children's Hosp of Philadelphia, Philadelphia, PA
87-89; **HOSP:** Good Samaritan Hosp Med Ctr; *SI:
Prematurity; Multiple Births*

⬚ ⬚ ⬚ ⬚ ⬚

Perl, Harold (MD)   NP   **PCP**
Hackensack Univ Med Ctr

30 Prospect Ave; Hackensack, NJ 07601; (201)
996-5304; **BDCERT:** Ped 80; NP 83; **MS:** Albert
Einstein Coll Med 75; **RES:** Montefiore Med Ctr,
Bronx, NY 75-78; **FEL:** Albert Einstein Med Ctr,
Bronx, NY 78-80

⬚ ⬚ ⬚ ⬚ Immediately

Sison, Joseph (MD)   NP
Englewood Hosp & Med Ctr

Englewood Hospital & Medical Center, Dept of
NeonatalPerinatal Medicine, 350 Engle St;
Englewood, NJ 07631; (201) 894-3321; **BDCERT:**
Ped 92; **MS:** Philippines 84; **RES:** Ped, Jersey Shore
Med Ctr, Neptune, NJ 89; **FEL:** NP, NY Hosp-Cornell
Med Ctr, New York, NY 93-95; **FAP:** Clin Prof Mt
Sinai Sch Med; *SI: Diseases of Newborn*; **HMO:** Blue
Cross & Blue Shield Oxford Prudential First Option
United Healthcare +

LANG: Sp, Tag; ⬚ ⬚ **VISA** ⬚ ⬚

NEPHROLOGY

Grodstein, Gerald (MD)   Nep   **PCP**
Englewood Hosp & Med Ctr

177 N Dean St 207; Englewood, NJ 07631; (201)
567-0446; **BDCERT:** IM 80; Nep 80; **MS:** SUNY
Downstate 74; **RES:** Med, Kings County Hosp Ctr,
Brooklyn, NY 75-77; **FEL:** Nep, UCLA Med Ctr, Los
Angeles, CA 76-78; *SI: Hypertension*

LANG: Sp; ⬚ ⬚ ⬚ ⬚ ⬚ Immediately ⬚ **VISA**
⬚ ⬚

Kozlowski, Jeffrey (MD)   Nep   **PCP**
Valley Hosp

Bergen Hypertension and Renal Associates, 44
Godwin Ave; Midland Park, NJ 07432; (201) 447-
0013; **BDCERT:** IM 81; **MS:** NYU Sch Med 78; **RES:**
VA Med Ctr-Manh, New York, NY 78; New York
University Med Ctr, New York, NY 82; **FEL:** Nep,
New York University Med Ctr, New York, NY 82-
84; **HOSP:** Hackensack Univ Med Ctr; *SI: Dialysis*

⬚ ⬚ ⬚ ⬚ ⬚ ⬚ ⬚ ⬚ 2-4 Weeks **VISA** ⬚

Levin, David (MD)   Nep
Holy Name Hosp

870 Palisade Ave 202; Teaneck, NJ 07666; (201)
836-0897; **BDCERT:** IM 79; Nep 81; **MS:** UMDNJ-
NJ Med Sch, Newark 76; **RES:** IM, Jacobi Med Ctr,
Bronx, NY 76-79; **FEL:** Nep, Albert Einstein Med
Ctr, Bronx, NY 79-81; **HOSP:** Hackensack Univ
Med Ctr; *SI: Hypertension; Dialysis*; **HMO:** Oxford
Aetna Hlth Plan CIGNA Prucare US Hlthcre +

LANG: Sp, Itl, Heb; ⬚ ⬚ ⬚ ⬚ ⬚ ⬚ Immediately

Guide to symbols and abbreviations can be found on pages 110-113.

875

Needle, Mark (MD)　　　Nep
St Joseph's Hosp-Patterson

North Jersey Nephrology Assoc, 1715 Maple Ave; Fair Lawn, NJ 07410; (201) 796-1200; **BDCERT:** IM 66; Nep 76; **MS:** Tufts U 59; **RES:** IM, U Chicago Hosp, Chicago, IL 59-61; IM, New England Med Ctr, Boston, MA 63-64; **FEL:** Nep, New England Med Ctr, Boston, MA 61-63; **FAP:** Assoc Clin Prof UMDNJ New Jersey Sch Osteo Med; **SI:** *Renal Diseases; Lupus;* **HMO:** Aetna Hlth Plan Blue Choice Blue Cross & Blue Shield Oxford US Hlthcre +

[⅄] [◎] [⊞] [S] [Mcr] [Mod]　A Few Days

NEUROLOGICAL SURGERY

Bruce, Jeffrey (MD)　　　NS
Columbia-Presbyterian Med Ctr

Neurological Assocs of NJ, 82 E Allendale Rd Ste 2A; Saddle River, NJ 07458; (201) 327-8600; **BDCERT:** NS 93; **MS:** UMDNJ-RW Johnson Med Sch 83; **RES:** Columbia-Presbyterian Med Ctr, New York, NY 83-90; **FEL:** NS, Nat Inst Health, Bethesda, MD 84-85; **FAP:** Assoc Prof Columbia P&S; **SI:** *Brain Tumors; Skull Base Tumors;* **HMO:** Oxford PHS Blue Cross & Blue Shield Independent Health Plan Chubb +

LANG: Sp; [⅄] [◎] [⅋] [⊞] [Mcr] [Mod] [NFI]　Immediately [▩] **VISA** [●] [▥]

Carpenter, Duncan (MD)　　　NS
Valley Hosp

225 Dayton St; Ridgewood, NJ 07450; (201) 612-0020; **BDCERT:** NS 87; **MS:** Columbia P&S 78; **RES:** NS, Columbia-Presbyterian Med Ctr, New York, NY 80-85; **SI:** *Brain Tumors; Spine*
1 Week

Goulart, Hamilton (MD)　　　NS
Valley Hosp

225 Dayton St; Ridgewood, NJ 07450; (201) 612-0020; **BDCERT:** NS 85; **MS:** Brazil 75; **RES:** NS, Mount Sinai Med Ctr, New York, NY 77-82; **SI:** *Spine Surgery; Microsurgery;* **HMO:** +

LANG: Sp; [⅄] [◎] [⅋] [⊞] [Mcr] [WC] [NFI]　1 Week

Pelosi, Richard (MD)　　　NS
St Joseph's Hosp-Patterson

BergenPassaic Neurosurgical, 617 Paramus Rd; Paramus, NJ 07652; (201) 445-8666; **BDCERT:** NS 71; **MS:** UMDNJ-NJ Med Sch, Newark 61; **RES:** S, VA Med Ctr-Bronx, Bronx, NY 62-63; N, Columbia-Presbyterian Med Ctr, New York, NY 63-67; **FAP:** Asst Clin Prof N UMDNJ-NJ Med Sch, Newark; **SI:** *Spinal Disorders; Brain Tumors;* **HMO:** Blue Shield CIGNA Oxford Prucare

[⅄] [◎] [⊞] [S] [Mcr] [Mod] [WC] [NFI]　1 Week

Quest, Donald (MD)　　　NS
Columbia-Presbyterian Med Ctr

82 E Allendale Rd; Saddle River, NJ 07458; (201) 327-8600; **BDCERT:** NS 79; **MS:** Columbia P&S 70; **RES:** S, Mass Gen Hosp, Boston, MA 70-71; Columbia-Presbyterian Med Ctr, New York, NY 71-76; **FAP:** Prof Columbia P&S; **HOSP:** Valley Hosp; **SI:** *Carotid Artery Disease;* **HMO:** Blue Choice Oxford PHS

LANG: Sp; [⅄] [◎] [⅋] [⊞] [S] [Mcr] [Mod] [WC] [NFI]
A Few Days [▩] **VISA** [●] [▥]

NEUROLOGY

Alweiss, Gary (MD)　　　N
Englewood Hosp & Med Ctr

Willner and Alweis, 200 Grand Ave 101; Englewood, NJ 07631; (201) 894-5805; **BDCERT:** N 93; **MS:** Mt Sinai Sch Med 88; **RES:** Mount Sinai Med Ctr, New York, NY 89-92; **FEL:** Columbia-Presbyterian Med Ctr, New York, NY 92-93; **FAP:** Asst Clin Prof Columbia P&S; **SI:** *Headaches; Nerve Injuries;* **HMO:** HMO Blue First Option Aetna Hlth Plan Guardian Oxford +

[⅄] [◎] [⅋] [⊞] [S] [Mcr] [WC] [NFI]　Immediately **VISA** [●]

Jotkowitz, Seymour (MD)   N
Hackensack Univ Med Ctr

272 Atlantic St; Hackensack, NJ 07601; (201)
488-3765; **BDCERT:** N 69; **MS:** Albert Einstein Coll
Med 62; **RES:** Barnes Hosp, St Louis, MO 63; Albert
Einstein Med Ctr, Bronx, NY 63-66; **FAP:** Clin Prof
UMDNJ-NJ Med Sch, Newark; **HOSP:** Univ of Med &
Dent NJ Hosp; *SI: Parkinson's Disease;*
Botox/Neuropathy; **HMO:** Oxford

LANG: Sp, Heb, Yd; 🅖 📞 🔓 🚼 🛏 $ Mcr WC NFI
A Few Days **VISA** 💳

Klein, Patricia (MD)   N
Pascack Valley Hosp

10 Fairview Ave; Westwood, NJ 07675; (201) 261-
3600; **BDCERT:** N 80; **MS:** UMDNJ-NJ Med Sch,
Newark 76; **RES:** Univ of Med & Dent NJ Hosp,
Newark, NJ 76-79; **HOSP:** Holy Name Hosp; *SI:*
Parkinson's Disease; Seizures; **HMO:** Most

🅖 📞 🔓 🛏 $ Mcr WC NFI 1 Week **VISA** 💳 💳

Perron, Reed (MD)   N
Valley Hosp

Neurology Group Of Bergen Cnty, 106 Prospect St;
Ridgewood, NJ 07450; (201) 444-0868; **BDCERT:**
N 74; **MS:** U Rochester 66; **RES:** Cleveland Clinic
Hosp, Cleveland, OH 69-70; Albert Einstein Med
Ctr, Bronx, NY 70-73

Rabin, Aaron (MD & PhD)   N
Englewood Hosp & Med Ctr

177 N Dean St; Englewood, NJ 07631; (201) 568-
3412; **BDCERT:** N 81; **MS:** Albert Einstein Coll Med
76; **RES:** N, Albert Einstein Coll Med, Bronx, NY 77-
80; **FEL:** CE, Neur Inst-Columbia Presby, New York,
NY 80-81; **FAP:** Asst Clin Prof N Columbia P&S;
HOSP: Holy Name Hosp

Van Engel, Daniel (MD)   N
Valley Hosp

Neurology Group Of Bergen County, 1200 E
Ridgewood Ave; Ridgewood, NJ 07450; (201) 444-
0868; **BDCERT:** N 80; **MS:** SUNY Syracuse 73;
RES: N, Albert Einstein Med Ctr, Bronx, NY 75-78;
IM, NY Hosp-Cornell Med Ctr, New York, NY 74-
75; **HMO:** US Hlthcre CIGNA Oxford Aetna Hlth
Plan First Option +

WC

Willner, Joseph (MD)   N
Englewood Hosp & Med Ctr

200 Grand Ave 101; Englewood, NJ 07631; (201)
894-5805; **BDCERT:** N 78; **MS:** NYU Sch Med 70;
RES: NR, Columbia-Presbyterian Med Ctr, New
York, NY 74-77; **FAP:** Assoc Prof of Clin N
Columbia P&S; **HMO:** Aetna Hlth Plan Blue Cross &
Blue Shield Empire Chubb Oxford +

🅖 🔓 🚼 🛏 $ Mcr WC NFI 2-4 Weeks

OBSTETRICS & GYNECOLOGY

Alvarez, Manuel (MD)   ObG
Hackensack Univ Med Ctr

Hackensack U Med CtrDept OB/GYN Chairman, 30
Prospect Ave; Hackensack, NJ 07601; (201) 996-
2439; **BDCERT:** ObG 90; MF 91; **MS:** Dominican
Republic 81; **RES:** ObG, St Joseph's Hosp-Paterson,
Paterson, NJ 83-87; **FEL:** MF, Mount Sinai Med Ctr,
New York, NY 87-89; CCM (ObG), Mount Sinai
Med Ctr, New York, NY 89-90; **FAP:** Adjct Prof
ObG NYU Sch Med; **HOSP:** New York University
Med Ctr; *SI: Multiple Births; High Risk Pregnancy;*
HMO: Oxford Blue Cross Prudential Aetna-US
Healthcare

LANG: Frs, Sp; 🅖 📞 🔓 🛏 $ Mcr WC NFI
Immediately **VISA** 💳

Banzon, Manuel (MD)   ObG
Meadowlands Hosp Med Ctr

1 W Ridgewood Ave; Paramus, NJ 07652; (201) 251-8750; **BDCERT:** ObG 79; **MS:** Philippines 62; **RES:** Jersey City Med Ctr, Jersey City, NJ 64-69; **HOSP:** Valley Hosp; **SI:** *Infertility Treatment*; **HMO:** Blue Cross CIGNA Oxford PHS Prucare +

LANG: Fil; ♿ ☾ 🔒 🏥 🎬 S Mcr NFl   A Few Days 🟦 **VISA**

Berkman, Steven (MD)   ObG
Pascack Valley Hosp

Pinnacle Medical Group, PA, 1 Sears Dr; Paramus, NJ 07652; (201) 599-4921; **BDCERT:** ObG 77; **MS:** SUNY Downstate 71; **RES:** ObG, Kings County Hosp Ctr, Brooklyn, NY 71-75; **SI:** *High Risk Obstetrics; Menopause*; **HMO:** HIP Network

♿ ☾ 🔒 🎬 S   A Few Days **VISA** 💳

Butler, David (MD)   ObG   **PCP**
Holy Name Hosp

420 Grand Ave 201; Englewood, NJ 07631; (201) 871-4040; **BDCERT:** ObG 72; **MS:** SUNY Hlth Sci Ctr 65; **RES:** St Vincents Hosp & Med Ctr NY, New York, NY 65-70; **HOSP:** Englewood Hosp & Med Ctr; **HMO:** Blue Cross & Blue Shield Oxford PHCS Travelers Prucare +

LANG: Itl; ♿ 🅢 ☾ 🔒 🏥 🎬 S Mcr Mcd
Immediately 🟦 **VISA** 💳 🔳

Coven, Roger (MD)   ObG   **PCP**
Valley Hosp

Valley Center for Women's Health, 1 W Ridgewood Ave 208; Paramus, NJ 07652; (201) 447-2200; **BDCERT:** ObG 86; **MS:** UMDNJ-NJ Med Sch, Newark 80; **RES:** ObG, Thomas Jefferson U Hosp, Philadelphia, PA 80-84; **HOSP:** Hackensack Univ Med Ctr; **SI:** *High Risk Obstetrics; General Gynecology*; **HMO:** Oxford CIGNA Prucare Metlife Aetna-US Healthcare +

♿ 🅢 ☾ 🔒 🏥 🎬 S   A Few Days **VISA** 💳

Dotto, Myles (MD)   ObG
Pascack Valley Hosp

595 Chestnut Ridge Rd; Woodcliff Lane, NJ 07675; (201) 391-5443; **BDCERT:** ObG 84; **MS:** UMDNJ-NJ Med Sch, Newark 76; **RES:** Women & Infants Hosp, Providence, RI 79-82; **HOSP:** Valley Hosp; **SI:** *Laparoscopic Surgery; Infertility*; **HMO:** US Hlthcre Oxford NYLCare

♿ 🅢 ☾ 🔒 🏥 🎬 S Mcr   A Few Days **VISA** 💳

Faust, Michael (MD)   ObG
Valley Hosp

1 W Ridgewood Ave 208; Paramus, NJ 07652; (201) 447-2200; **BDCERT:** ObG 89; **MS:** Univ Pittsburgh 83; **RES:** ObG, Thomas Jefferson U Hosp, Philadelphia, PA 83-87; **HOSP:** Hackensack Univ Med Ctr; **HMO:** Aetna Hlth Plan United Healthcare CIGNA Oxford Blue Cross & Blue Shield +

LANG: Ar, Fr, Sp; ♿ 🅢 ☾ 🔒 🏥 🎬 S   2-4 Weeks **VISA** 💳

Friedman, Harvey Y (MD)   ObG
Englewood Hosp & Med Ctr

180 N Dean St; Englewood, NJ 07631; (201) 871-4346; **BDCERT:** ObG 87; **MS:** NYU Sch Med 81; **RES:** ObG, New York University Med Ctr, New York, NY 81-85; **HOSP:** Hackensack Univ Med Ctr; **SI:** *High Risk Pregnancy; Operative Gynecology*; **HMO:** Blue Cross & Blue Shield Oxford CIGNA PHCS Prucare +

LANG: Sp, Yd, Heb; ♿ ☾ 🔒 🏥 🎬 S Mcr   1 Week 🟦 **VISA** 💳 🔳

Ginsburg, Eugene (MD)   ObG
Valley Hosp

Valley ObGYN Associates, 140 Chestnut St 305; Ridgewood, NJ 07450; (201) 447-5757; **BDCERT:** ObG 77; **MS:** KY Med Sch, Louisville 65; **RES:** U CO Hosp, Denver, CO 69-70; Mount Sinai Med Ctr, New York, NY 71-75; **SI:** *Hysteroscopy/Laparoscopy; Urinary Incontinence*; **HMO:** Blue Cross & Blue Shield Oxford CIGNA First Option Metlife +

♿ ☾ 🔒 🏥 🎬 S Mcr WC   A Few Days **VISA** 💳

Gross, Arthur H (MD)　　ObG
Englewood Hosp & Med Ctr
Comprehensive Health Care, 450 Lewis St; Fort Lee,
NJ 07024; (201) 894-9599; **MS:** Brown U 92; **RES:**
ObG, Albert Einstein Med Ctr, Bronx, NY 92-96;
FAP: Asst Clin Instr Mt Sinai Sch Med; **SI:**
Laparoscopic Surgery; Vaginal Birth After Cesarean;
HMO: Oxford US Hlthcre Chubb United Healthcare
Blue Cross & Blue Shield +

LANG: Sp, Heb; 🔲 🆂 🆈 🔲 🔲 🔲 🆖 Mcr WC NFI
Immediately ▦ *VISA* ● 🔲

Hurst, Wendy (MD)　　ObG
Englewood Hosp & Med Ctr
370 Grand Ave; Englewood, NJ 07631; (201) 894-
9599; **BDCERT:** ObG 92; **MS:** Tufts U 86; **RES:**
Pennsylvania Hosp, Philadelphia, PA 86-90;
HOSP: Holy Name Hosp; **SI:** *Laparoscopic Surgery;*
Preconception Planning; **HMO:** Oxford US Hlthcre
CIGNA Prucare PHCS +

LANG: Sp; 🔲 🔲 🔲 🔲 🔲 🆂 4+ Weeks ▦ *VISA*
●

McCormack, Barbara (MD) ObG
Englewood Hosp & Med Ctr
Mc Cormack & Suarez, 2 Dean Dr FL2; Tenafly, NJ
07670; (201) 569-5151; **BDCERT:** ObG 89; **MS:**
Albert Einstein Coll Med 71; **RES:** ObG, Bronx
Muncipal Hosp Ctr, Bronx, NY 71-75; **FAP:** Clin
Instr Albert Einstein Coll Med

LANG: Sp; 🔲 🔲 🔲 🆂 2-4 Weeks *VISA* ●

Schulze, Ruth (MD)　　ObG
Valley Hosp
Obstetrics & Gynecology, 43 Yawpo Ave 4;
Oakland, NJ 07436; (201) 337-5500; **BDCERT:**
ObG 89; **MS:** SUNY Stony Brook 83; **RES:** ObG,
Baystate Med Ctr, Springfield 84-87

Tobias, Theodore (MD)　　ObG　**PCP**
Englewood Hosp & Med Ctr
Engle Street ObGyn Assoc, 286 Engle St;
Englewood, NJ 07631; (201) 569-6190; **BDCERT:**
ObG 71; **MS:** SUNY Hlth Sci Ctr 62; **RES:** ObG, St
Luke's Roosevelt Hosp Ctr, New York, NY 65-68;
FAP: Sr Clin Instr Mt Sinai Sch Med; **HMO:** Aetna
Hlth Plan Chubb Oxford CIGNA Premier +

LANG: Ger, Itl, Sp; 🔲 🔲 🔲 🔲 🔲 🆂 Mcr 2-
4 Weeks ▦ *VISA* ● 🔲

Viscardi, Anthony (MD)　　ObG　**PCP**
Pascack Valley Hosp
577 Chestnut Ridge Rd; Wood Clifflake, NJ 07675;
(201) 307-9050; **BDCERT:** ObG 77; **MS:** UMDNJ-
NJ Med Sch, Newark 68; **RES:** ObG, Maimonides
Med Ctr, Brooklyn, NY 69-70; **HOSP:** Valley Hosp;
HMO: Oxford United Healthcare Aetna Hlth Plan
Prudential

🔲 🔲 🔲 🔲 🆂 Mcr 1 Week *VISA*

OPHTHALMOLOGY

Burke, Patricia (MD)　　Oph
Holy Name Hosp
751 Teaneck Rd; Teaneck, NJ 07666; (201) 833-
0006; **BDCERT:** Oph 91; **MS:** UMDNJ-NJ Med Sch,
Newark 86; **RES:** Oph, Columbia-Presbyterian Med
Ctr, New York, NY 87-90; **FEL:** Oph, Manhattan
Eye, Ear & Throat Hosp, New York, NY 90-91; **SI:**
Cornea; Cataracts; **HMO:** Oxford First Option
Prudential QualCare

🆂 🔲 🔲 🔲 🔲 🆂 WC NFI 1 Week

Kaiden, Jeffrey (MD)　　Oph
Pascack Valley Hosp
Westwood Ophthalmology Assoc, 300 Fairview
Ave; Westwood, NJ 07675; (201) 666-4014;
BDCERT: Oph 78; **MS:** U Fla Coll Med 73; **RES:**
Oph., Mount Sinai Med Ctr, New York, NY 74-77;
FAP: Clin Instr Mt Sinai Sch Med; **SI:** *Glaucoma;*
Cataracts; **HMO:** Oxford Aetna-US Healthcare First
Option CIGNA CHN +

LANG: Sp, Fr, Rus, Chi; 🔲 🆂 🔲 🔲 🔲 🔲 🆂 Mcr Mcd
WC NFI *VISA* ●

Kaiden, Richard (MD)   Oph
Pascack Valley Hosp

Westwood Ophthalmology Associates, PA, 300 Fariview Ave; Westwood, NJ 07675; (201) 666-4014; **BDCERT:** Oph 73; **MS:** Albert Einstein Coll Med 66; **RES:** Montefiore Med Ctr, Bronx, NY 68-71; **SI:** *Cataract and Refractive Surgery*; **HMO:** Aetna-US Healthcare Oxford First Option Guardian

LANG: Sp, Itl; ⬛ 🆂 🄲 🄶 🄼 🄷 🆂 Mcr Mcd WC NFI 2-4 Weeks **VISA** 💳

Silbert, Glenn (MD)   Oph
Hackensack Univ Med Ctr

316 State St; Hackensack, NJ 07601; (201) 342-8115; **BDCERT:** Oph 85; **MS:** Columbia P&S 79; **RES:** Oph, New York University Med Ctr, New York, NY 80-83; **SI:** *Cataract Surgery*; **HMO:** PHCS Aetna-US Healthcare CIGNA United Healthcare Magnacare +

🄲 🄶 🄼 🄷 🆂 Mcr WC NFI Immediately

Solomon, Edward (MD)   Oph
Valley Hosp

85 S Maple Ave 3; Ridgewood, NJ 07450; (201) 444-3010; **BDCERT:** Oph 76; **MS:** Tufts U 68; **RES:** Oph, New York University Med Ctr, New York, NY 71-74; **HMO:** CIGNA Metlife

⬛ 🄲 🄶 🄼 🄷 🆂 WC 2-4 Weeks

Stabile, John (MD)   Oph
Englewood Hosp & Med Ctr

Tenafly Eye Associates, 1111 Dean Dr; Tenafly, NJ 07670; (201) 567-5995; **BDCERT:** Oph 81; **MS:** NY Med Coll 76; **RES:** IM, Lincoln Med & Mental Hlth Ctr, Bronx, NY 76-77; Oph, St Luke's Roosevelt Hosp Ctr, New York, NY 77-80; **FEL:** Oculoplastic S, Columbia-Presbyterian Med Ctr, New York, NY 80-81; **FAP:** Clin Instr Columbia P&S; **HOSP:** Holy Name Hosp; **SI:** *Cataracts; Oculoplastics*; **HMO:** Oxford CIGNA Blue Cross & Blue Shield First Option +

LANG: Sp; ⬛ 🆂 🄲 🄶 🄼 🄷 🆂 Mcr Mcd WC NFI Immediately ▦ **VISA** 💳 ▦

Weinberg, Martin (MD)   Oph
Englewood Hosp & Med Ctr

405 Cedar Ln; Teaneck, NJ 07666; (201) 836-8333; **BDCERT:** Oph 89; **MS:** Eastern VA Med Sch, Norfolk 79; **RES:** Oph, Kings County Hosp Ctr, Brooklyn, NY 83-86; Manhattan Eye, Ear & Throat Hosp, New York, NY 86-87; **FEL:** Oph, Hosp of U Penn, Philadelphia, PA 81-83; Oph, Manhattan Eye, Ear & Throat Hosp, New York, NY 86-88; **HOSP:** Hackensack Univ Med Ctr; **HMO:** CIGNA First Option Oxford United Healthcare

🄲 🄶 🄼 🄷 🆂 Mcr Mcd WC NFI 2-4 Weeks

ORTHOPAEDIC SURGERY

Altman, Wayne (MD)   OrS
Mountainside Hosp

85 Orient Way Fl 3; Rutherford, NJ 07070; (201) 438-5888; **BDCERT:** OrS 88; **HS** 92; **MS:** UMDNJ-NJ Med Sch, Newark 77; **RES:** Univ of Med & Dent NJ Hosp, Newark, NJ 82; **FEL:** HS, Thomas Jefferson U Hosp, Philadelphia, PA 82-83; **HOSP:** Meadowlands Hosp Med Ctr; **HMO:** Oxford Aetna Hlth Plan US Hlthcre NYLCare Prucare +

LANG: Sp; ⬛ 🄷 🆂 Mcr WC A Few Days ▦ **VISA** 💳

Andronaco, John (MD)   OrS
Hackensack Univ Med Ctr

385 Prospect Ave; Hackensack, NJ 07601; (201) 489-3933; **BDCERT:** OrS 79; **MS:** Mexico 72; **RES:** OrS, Univ of Med & Dent NJ Hosp, Newark, NJ 73-74; S, Univ of Med & Dent NJ Hosp, Newark, NJ 74-78; **HMO:** Aetna Hlth Plan Blue Cross & Blue Shield CIGNA

LANG: Sp; ⬛ 🄶 🄷 🆂 Mcr WC 1 Week ▦ **VISA** 💳 ▦

Berman, Mark (MD)   OrS
Hackensack Univ Med Ctr
306 Atlantic St; Hackensack, NJ 07601; (201) 489-8250; **BDCERT:** OrS 89; **MS:** Mt Sinai Sch Med 81; **RES:** Mount Sinai Med Ctr, New York, NY 81-83; Univ Hosp SUNY Bklyn, Brooklyn, NY 83-86; **FEL:** SM, Lenox Hill Hosp, New York, NY 86-87; **HOSP:** St Vincent's Med Ctr-Bridgeport; **SI:** *Sports Medicine; Knee Injuries;* **HMO:** CIGNA Oxford
🔲 🔲 🔲 🔲 🔲 🔲 🔲 🔲 2-4 Weeks *VISA* 🔲 🔲

Brenner, Stephen (MD)   OrS
Pascack Valley Hosp
440 Old Hook Rd Fl 2; Emerson, NJ 07630; (201) 261-3333; **BDCERT:** OrS 85; **MS:** Mexico 74; **RES:** Hosp For Joint Diseases, New York, NY 76-80; **FAP:** OrS; **HOSP:** Hosp For Joint Diseases; **SI:** *Sports Medicine;* **HMO:** Aetna-US Healthcare Blue Cross & Blue Shield Magnacare US Hlthcre Mastercare +
LANG: Sp; 🔲 🔲 🔲 🔲 🔲 🔲 🔲 🔲 🔲
Immediately 🔲 *VISA* 🔲 🔲

Doidge, Robert (DO)   OrS
Englewood Hosp & Med Ctr
Englewood Knee & sports Medicine, PC, 370 Grand Ave Ste 100; Englewood, NJ 07631; (201) 567-5700; **MS:** Philadelphia Coll Osteo Med 86; **RES:** Oakland Gen Hosp, Madison Hts, MI 87-91; **FEL:** SM, Michigan St U, East Lansing, MI 91-92; **HOSP:** Pascack Valley Hosp; **SI:** *Knees Surgery; Shoulders Surgery;* **HMO:** CIGNA PHCS Prucare Chubb
LANG: Sp; 🔲 🔲 🔲 🔲 🔲 🔲 🔲 🔲 A Few Days
VISA 🔲

Gurland, Mark (MD)   OrS
Hackensack Univ Med Ctr
216 Engle St; Englewood, NJ 07631; (201) 568-4066; **BDCERT:** HS 80; **MS:** NYU Sch Med 79; **RES:** S, Hosp of U Penn, Philadelphia, PA 79-80; OrS, Hosp For Joint Diseases, New York, NY 80-84; **FEL:** HS, Thomas Jefferson U Hosp, Philadelphia, PA 84; **HOSP:** Englewood Hosp & Med Ctr; **SI:** *Carpal Tunnel Syndrome; Wrist Problems/Arthritis;* **HMO:** Oxford Health Source United Healthcare First Option QualCare +
LANG: Sp; 🔲 🔲 🔲 🔲 🔲 🔲 🔲 🔲 1 Week *VISA* 🔲

Hartzband, Mark (MD)   OrS
Hackensack Univ Med Ctr
2 Forest Ave; Paramus, NJ 07652; (201) 587-1111; **BDCERT:** OrS 86; **MS:** Canada 78; **RES:** S, Montefiore Med Ctr, Bronx, NY 78-84; OrS, Montefiore Med Ctr, Bronx, NY 82; **SI:** *Total Knee Replacement; Total Hip Replacement;* **HMO:** Blue Cross & Blue Shield CIGNA Oxford Chubb Travelers +
🔲 🔲 🔲 🔲 🔲 🔲 🔲 🔲 A Few Days 🔲 *VISA* 🔲 🔲

Livingston, Lawrence (MD)   OrS
Pascack Valley Hosp
595 Chestnut Ridge Rd 5; Woodcliff Lake, NJ 07675; (201) 573-1202; **BDCERT:** OrS 81; **MS:** Med Coll Wisc 75; **RES:** OrS, Hosp For Joint Diseases, New York, NY 76-80; **SI:** *Arthroscopic Knee and Shoulder Surgery; Knee & Hip Replacement Surgery;* **HMO:** Aetna-US Healthcare First Option PHCS Prudential
🔲 🔲 🔲 🔲 🔲 🔲 🔲 🔲 🔲 *VISA* 🔲

Lloyd, J Mervyn (MD)   OrS
Pascack Valley Hosp
223 Old Hook Rd; Westwood, NJ 07675; (201) 666-0013; **BDCERT:** OrS 86; **MS:** England 71; **RES:** St George's Hosp, London, England 78; Mt Carmel Hosp, Detroit, MI 81; **SI:** *Knee Problems; Hip Arthritis;* **HMO:** Oxford Aetna Hlth Plan QualCare Multicare PHS +
🔲 🔲 🔲 🔲 🔲 🔲 🔲 🔲 A Few Days *VISA* 🔲

Longobardi, Raphael (MD)   OrS
Holy Name Hosp
870 Pallisade Ave 205; Teaneck, NJ 07666; (201) 836-1663; **MS:** NYU Sch Med 90; **RES:** OrS, NYU Med Ctr, New York, NY 91-95; **FEL:** SM, Knoxville Orthopaedic /U of Tenessee, Knoxville, TN 95-96; **SI:** *Shoulder Injuries;* **HMO:** Most
🔲 🔲 🔲 🔲 🔲 🔲 🔲 🔲 🔲 1 Week 🔲 *VISA* 🔲 🔲

Pizzurro, Joe (MD)   OrS
Valley Hosp
Vly Ridge Orth, 85 S Maple Ave; Ridgewood, NJ
07450; (201) 445-2830; **BDCERT:** OrS 72; **MS:** St
Louis U 63; **RES:** OrS, Bellevue Hosp Ctr, New York,
NY 68-71; **SI:** *Joint Replacement*; **HMO:** Oxford First
Option Blue Cross & Blue Shield PHS Magnacare +
♿ 🌙 📷 🕐 🎬 💲 ♿ 🆕 A Few Days **VISA** 💳

Salzer, Richard (MD)   OrS
Englewood Hosp & Med Ctr
97 Engle St; Englewood, NJ 07631; (201) 569-
2770; **BDCERT:** OrS 79; **MS:** Tufts U 73; **RES:**
Parkland Mem Hosp, Dallas, TX 73-74; Hosp For
Special Surgery, New York, NY 75-78; **FAP:** Clin
Instr Cornell U; **HOSP:** Holy Name Hosp; **HMO:**
Guardian CIGNA Magnacare Blue Cross & Blue
Shield Oxford +
LANG: Sp; ♿ 📶 📞 🎬 🕐 💲 ⓜ ♿ 🆕
A Few Days

Self, Edward (MD)   OrS
Valley Hosp
385 S Maple Ave 101; Glen Rock, NJ 07452; (201)
447-1188; **BDCERT:** OrS 80; **MS:** Columbia P&S
70; **RES:** S, St Luke's Roosevelt Hosp Ctr, New York,
NY 71-72; OrS, Columbia-Presbyterian Med Ctr,
New York, NY 74-77; **FAP:** NY Coll Osteo Med; **SI:**
Shoulder Disorders; **HMO:** Travelers Mastercare
♿ 📷 🎬 🕐 💲 ♿ 🆕 **VISA** 💳

Weinstein, Joel (MD)   OrS
Englewood Hosp & Med Ctr
Englewood Orth Assocs PA 2nd Ofc in Ft Lee, 97
Engle St; Englewood, NJ 07631; (201) 569-2770;
BDCERT: OrS 71; **MS:** Columbia P&S 62; **RES:**
Bellevue Hosp Ctr, New York, NY 65-66; Columbia-
Presbyterian Med Ctr, New York, NY 66-69; **FEL:**
Columbia-Presbyterian Med Ctr, New York, NY 69-
70; **FAP:** Assoc Prof Columbia P&S; **HOSP:** Holy
Name Hosp; **SI:** *Joint Reconstruction; Sports Injuries*;
HMO: Oxford First Option CIGNA Prucare
Magnacare +
♿ 🎬 🕐 💲 ⓜ ♿ 🆕 A Few Days 💳 **VISA** 💳

OTOLARYNGOLOGY

Eisenberg, Lee (MD)   Oto
Englewood Hosp & Med Ctr
Chestnut ENT Associates, 177 N Dean St;
Englewood, NJ 07631; (201) 567-2771; **BDCERT:**
Oto 77; **MS:** SUNY Hlth Sci Ctr 71; **RES:** S, Valley
Med Ctr, Fresno, CA 73-74; UC San Francisco Med
Ctr, San Francisco, CA 74-77; **FAP:** Assoc Clin Prof
Columbia P&S; **HOSP:** Hackensack Univ Med Ctr;
SI: *Pediatric ENT; Thyroid Surgery*; **HMO:** Oxford
First Option Aetna Hlth Plan American Health Plan
Guardian +
♿ 📶 📞 📷 🎬 🕐 💲 ⓜ Immediately 💳 **VISA**
💳 💳

Katz, Harry (MD)   Oto
Valley Hosp
Ridgewood Ear Nose & Throat, 44 Godwin Ave FL2;
Midland Park, NJ 07432; (201) 445-2900;
BDCERT: Oto 82; **MS:** NYU Sch Med 77; **RES:** Oto,
New York University Med Ctr, New York, NY 78-81

Lehrer, Joel (MD)   Oto
Holy Name Hosp
Northern Jersey ENT Associates PA, 315 Cedar
Lane; Teaneck, NJ 07666; (201) 837-2174;
BDCERT: Oto 64; **MS:** SUNY Syracuse 56; **RES:** S,
Kings County Hosp Ctr, Brooklyn, NY 59-60; Oto,
Mount Sinai Med Ctr, New York, NY 61-63; **FEL:**
Oto, Mount Sinai Med Ctr, New York, NY 63-64;
FAP: Assoc Clin Prof UMDNJ New Jersey Sch Osteo
Med; **SI:** *Dizziness and Imbalance; Ear Infections /
Hearing Loss*; **HMO:** Aetna-US Healthcare Oxford
CIGNA Blue Shield PHS +
LANG: Sp, Ur, Kor; ♿ 📞 📷 🎬 🕐 💲 ⓜ ♿ 🆕
1 Week **VISA** 💳 💳

Low, Ronald (MD) Oto
Hackensack Univ Med Ctr
Bergen Ear Nose & Throat, 920 Main St; Hackensack, NJ 07601; (201) 489-6520; **BDCERT:** Oto 74; **MS:** U Hlth Sci/Chicago Med Sch 69; **RES:** Oto, New York University Med Ctr, New York, NY 71-74; **S**, Montefiore Med Ctr, Bronx, NY 70-71; **HOSP:** Pascack Valley Hosp; **HMO:** Aetna Hlth Plan CIGNA Sanus-NYLCare Most

♿ ▣ 👤 🏢 💲 Mcr NFI 2-4 Weeks

Scherl, Michael (MD) Oto
Englewood Hosp & Med Ctr
219 Old Hook Rd; Westwood, NJ 07675; (201) 666-8787; **BDCERT:** Oto 87; **MS:** Albany Med Coll 82; **RES:** S, Mount Sinai Med Ctr, New York, NY 82-84; Oto, Mount Sinai Med Ctr, New York, NY 84-87; **FAP:** Clin Instr Mt Sinai Sch Med; **HOSP:** Pascack Valley Hosp; **SI:** *Head & Neck Surgery; Nasal & Sinus Treatment;* **HMO:** Oxford Prudential Aetna-US Healthcare PHS First Option +

LANG: Sp, Fr; ♿ 🆘 🌙 ▣ 👤 🏢 💲 Mcr WC NFI
A Few Days 🎫 **VISA** 💳 💳

Steckowych, Jayde (MD) Oto
Englewood Hosp & Med Ctr
177 N Dean St; Englewood, NJ 07631; (201) 567-2771; **BDCERT:** Oto 93; **MS:** Philippines 81; **RES:** S, Harlem Hosp Ctr, New York, NY 81-83; IM, Harlem Hosp Ctr, New York, NY 86-88; **FEL:** Oto, St Luke's Roosevelt Hosp Ctr, New York, NY 83; Columbia-Presbyterian Med Ctr, New York, NY 88-92; **FAP:** Clin Instr Columbia P&S; **HOSP:** Hackensack Univ Med Ctr; **SI:** *Sinusitis; Voice Problems;* **HMO:** Oxford Magnacare PHCS Aetna-US Healthcare

♿ 🆘 🌙 ▣ 👤 🏢 💲 Mcr Immediately 🎫 **VISA**
💳 💳

Surow, Jason (MD) Oto
Valley Hosp
Ridgewood Ear Nose & Throat, 44 Godwin Ave FL2; Midland Park, NJ 07432; (201) 445-2900; **BDCERT:** Oto 87; **MS:** Univ Penn 82; **RES:** Oto, Hosp of U Penn, Philadelphia, PA 86-87; **SI:** *Sinusitis & Nasal Disorders; Voice Disorders;* **HMO:** CIGNA Oxford First Option Prudential Aetna-US Healthcare +

♿ 🌙 ▣ 👤 🏢 💲 Mcr NFI A Few Days **VISA** 💳

PEDIATRIC ALLERGY & IMMUNOLOGY

Colenda, Maryann (MD) PA&I
Englewood Hosp & Med Ctr
810 Abbott Blvd 2nd FL; Fort Lee, NJ 07024; (201) 224-2256; **BDCERT:** Ped 76; A&I 79; **MS:** NYU Sch Med 71

🌙 ▣ 🏢 💲 Mcr A Few Days

Hicks, Patricia (MD) PA&I
Valley Hosp
119 1st St; Ho Ho Kus, NJ 07423; (201) 444-5277; **BDCERT:** A&I 81; Ped 78; **MS:** Hahnemann U 73; **RES:** Ped, Babies Hosp, New York, NY 73-76; **FEL:** A&I, Columbia-Presbyterian Med Ctr, New York, NY 79-81; **SI:** *Asthma Management; Chronic Sinusitis Cough*

♿ 🌙 ▣ 👤 🏢 💲 A Few Days 🎫 **VISA** 💳 💳

PEDIATRIC CARDIOLOGY

Marans, Zvi (MD) PCd
Valley Hosp
Valley Hosp, Dept of Cardio Cardiovasc, 223 N Van Dien Ave; Ridgewood, NJ 07450; (201) 599-0026; **BDCERT:** Ped 88; PCd 91; **MS:** Penn State U-Hershey Med Ctr 84; **RES:** Ped, Montefiore Med Ctr, Bronx, NY 84-87; **FEL:** PCd, Columbia-Presbyterian Med Ctr, New York, NY 87-90; **FAP:** Asst Clin Prof Ped Columbia P&S

Guide to symbols and abbreviations can be found on pages 110-113.

883

Messina, John (MD) PCd
St Joseph's Hosp-Patterson

Pediatric Cardiology Associates, 57 Willowbrook Blvd Fl 4; Wayne, NJ 07470; (973) 754-2529; **BDCERT:** Ped 89; **MS:** West Indies 86; **RES:** Ped, St Joseph's Hosp-Patterson, Paterson, NJ 86-88; **FEL:** PCd, NY Hosp-Cornell Med Ctr, New York, NY 89-92; **FAP:** Chf PCd; **HOSP:** Valley Hosp; **SI:** *Congenital Heart Disease; Interventional Cardiology*; **HMO:** Oxford CIGNA First Option Blue Cross HMO Blue +

LANG: Sp, Grk, Itl; 🦽 🏧 ☎ 🅿 🎦 Mcr Mcd WC NFI Immediately ▦ **VISA** 💳 ◪

Tozzi, Robert (MD) PCd
Hackensack Univ Med Ctr

30 Prospect Ave; Hackensack, NJ 07601; (201) 487-7617; **BDCERT:** Ped 87; PCd 91; **MS:** UMDNJ-NJ Med Sch, Newark 83; **RES:** Ped, Univ of Med & Dent NJ Hosp, Newark, NJ; **FEL:** PCd, New York University Med Ctr, New York, NY; **HOSP:** Valley Hosp; **SI:** *Fetal Echocardiography; Sports Readiness Evaluation*; **HMO:** Aetna-US Healthcare United Healthcare CIGNA Oxford Prucare +

LANG: Sp; 🦽 🌙 ☎ 🅿 🎦 Mcr Mcd A Few Days **VISA** 💳

PEDIATRIC HEMATOLOGY-ONCOLOGY

Diamond, Steven (MD) PHO
Hackensack Univ Med Ctr

Tomorrows Children Institute, 30 Prospect Ave; Hackensack, NJ 07901; (201) 996-5435; **BDCERT:** Ped 79; PHO 80; **MS:** Univ Penn 74; **RES:** Ped, Mount Sinai Med Ctr, New York, NY 74-77; **FEL:** PHO, Beth Israel Med Ctr, New York, NY 77-79; **FAP:** Asst Clin Prof Columbia P&S; **SI:** *Pediatric Cancer; Sickle Cell Disease*

🦽 🎦 💲 Mcd Immediately

Halpern, Steven (MD) PHO
Hackensack Univ Med Ctr

30 prospect Ave; Hackensack, NJ 07601; (201) 996-5653; **BDCERT:** PHO 82; **MS:** U Hlth Sci/Chicago Med Sch 76; **RES:** St Christopher's Hosp for Children, Philadelphia, PA 76; **FEL:** Children's Hosp of Philadelphia, Philadelphia, PA 79-82

LANG: Sp, Heb; 🦽 ☎ 🅿 🎦 Mcd NFI Immediately **VISA** 💳

Harris, Michael (MD) PHO
Hackensack Univ Med Ctr

Tomorrows Children's Institute, 30 Prospect Ave; Hackensack, NJ 07601; (201) 996-5437; **BDCERT:** Ped 74; PHO 74; **MS:** Albert Einstein Coll Med 69; **RES:** Ped, Children's Hosp of Philadelphia, Philadelphia, PA 69-71; **FEL:** PHO, Children's Hosp of Philadelphia, Philadelphia, PA 71-74; **FAP:** Prof Ped UMDNJ New Jersey Sch Osteo Med; **HMO:** Oxford US Hlthcre HMO Blue Blue Select Prucare +

LANG: Sp, Heb, Itl; 🦽 ☎ 🅿 🎦 💲 Mcd Immediately **VISA** 💳

PEDIATRIC INFECTIOUS DISEASE

Boscamp, Jeffrey (MD) Ped Inf
Hackensack Univ Med Ctr

30 Prospect Ave; Hackensack, NJ 07601; (201) 996-5308; **BDCERT:** Ped 94; **MS:** NY Med Coll 81; **RES:** Ped, Columbia-Presbyterian Med Ctr, New York, NY 81-84; IM, Greenwich Hosp, Greenwich, CT 84-85; **FEL:** Inf, Albert Einstein Med Ctr, Bronx, NY 85-87; **FAP:** Asst Prof Ped UMDNJ New Jersey Sch Osteo Med; **HOSP:** Morristown Mem Hosp; **SI:** *Lupus*; **HMO:** Oxford HIP Network Blue Cross & Blue Shield First Option QualCare +

🦽 ☎ 🎦 💲 Mcr Mcd Immediately **VISA** 💳

PEDIATRIC RHEUMATOLOGY

Kimura, Yukiko (MD)   Ped Rhu
Hackensack Univ Med Ctr
Hackensack Medical Ctr, 30 Prospect Ave;
Hackensack, NJ 07601; (201) 996-9815; **BDCERT:**
Ped 87; Ped Rhu 92; **MS:** Albert Einstein Coll Med
82; **RES:** Ped, Babies Hosp, New York, NY 82-85;
FEL: Ped Rhu, Columbia-Presbyterian Med Ctr,
New York, NY 87-90; **FAP:** Asst Prof Ped UMDNJ-
NJ Med Sch, Newark; **SI:** *Juvenile Arthritis; Lupus;*
HMO: Blue Cross & Blue Shield Oxford Aetna Hlth
Plan CIGNA US Hlthcre +

🦽 🅿 ♿ 💲 Mcr Mcd NFI **VISA** 💳

PEDIATRIC SURGERY

Friedman, David (MD)   PS
Englewood Hosp & Med Ctr
Pediatric Surgical Associates, PA, 1501 Broadway
Ste 38; Fairlawn, NJ 07410; (201) 794-8010;
BDCERT: S 77; PS 82; **MS:** SUNY Downstate 71;
RES: S, Univ Hosp SUNY Bklyn, Brooklyn, NY 76;
FEL: PdS, Univ Hosp SUNY Bklyn, Brooklyn, NY;
HOSP: Valley Hosp; **HMO:** Oxford Aetna-US
Healthcare Blue Shield CIGNA NYLCare +

LANG: Sp, Hin, Brm; 🦽 🌙 🅿 ♿ 💲 Mcr Mcd NFI
A Few Days **VISA** 💳

Gandhi, Rajinder (MD)   PS
Valley Hosp
1501 Broadway 38; Fairlawn, NJ 07410; (201)
794-8010; **BDCERT:** S 75; PS 97; **MS:** Burma 66;
RES: S, Albert Einstein Med Ctr, Bronx, NY 75-77;
Ge, Columbia-Presbyterian Med Ctr, New York, NY
74-75; **FEL:** PdS, Columbia-Presbyterian Med Ctr,
New York, NY 75-77; **FAP:** Asst Clin Prof S
Columbia P&S; **HOSP:** Englewood Hosp & Med Ctr;
SI: *Pediatric Laparoscopy; Pediatric Flexible
Laparoscopy*

LANG: Hin, Pun, Brm; 🦽 🌙 🅿 ♿ ♿ 💲 Mcd
A Few Days **VISA** 💳

Valda, Victor (MD)   PS
St Joseph's Hosp-Patterson
5 Summit Ave 6; Hackensack, NJ 07601; (201)
343-6885; **BDCERT:** S 74; PS 95; **MS:** Bolivia 62;
RES: Mt Zion Hosp, San Francisco, CA 68; Maricopa
Med Ctr, Phoenix, AZ 68-72; **FEL:** St Christopher's
Hosp for Children, Philadelphia, PA 72-74; **HMO:**
Oxford QualCare Blue Cross & Blue Shield Prucare

LANG: Sp; 🦽 🅿 ♿ ♿ 💲 Mcr Mcd   1 Week

PEDIATRICS

Asnes, Russell (MD)   Ped   PCP
Englewood Hosp & Med Ctr
Tenafly Pediatrics, 32 Franklin St; Tenafly, NJ
07670; (201) 569-2400; **BDCERT:** Ped 69; **MS:**
Tufts U 63; **RES:** Boston Med Ctr, Boston, MA 63-
64; Johns Hopkins Hosp, Baltimore, MD 64; **FAP:**
Clin Prof Ped Columbia P&S; **HOSP:** Hackensack
Univ Med Ctr; **HMO:** Aetna Hlth Plan

🦽 🏧 🅿 ♿ ♿ 💲   Immediately **VISA** 💳 💳

Buchalter, Maury (MD)   Ped   PCP
Hackensack Univ Med Ctr
Tenafly Pediatrics, 32 Franklin St; Tenafly, NJ
07670; (201) 569-2400; **BDCERT:** Ped 88; **MS:** Mt
Sinai Sch Med 84; **RES:** Mount Sinai Med Ctr, New
York, NY 84-87; **FEL:** Inf, Children's Hosp of Los
Angeles, Los Angeles, CA 88; **HOSP:** Englewood
Hosp & Med Ctr; **HMO:** Aetna Hlth Plan CIGNA
Oxford US Hlthcre United Healthcare +

LANG: Sp; 🦽 🏧 🌙 🅿 ♿ ♿ 💲 WC NFI
Immediately **VISA** 💳 💳

Connor, Thomas (MD)   Ped
St Barnabas Hosp-Bronx
414 Saddle River Rd; Fair Lawn, NJ 07410; (201)
794-1366; **BDCERT:** Ped 73; PCd 77; **MS:** Italy 66;
RES: Ped, Grasslands Hosp, Valhalla, NY 68-70; NY
Hosp-Cornell Med Ctr, New York, NY 69; **FEL:** PCd,
Yale-New Haven Hosp, New Haven, CT 70-72;
FAP: Asst Prof Columbia P&S; **HMO:** Aetna Hlth
Plan Blue Choice Blue Cross & Blue Shield

De Maria, Frank (MD) Ped **PCP**
Valley Hosp

Valley Pediatric Assoc, 357 Forest Rd; Mahwah, NJ 07430; (201) 891-7272; **BDCERT:** Ped 66; **MS:** UMDNJ-NJ Med Sch, Newark 61; **RES:** Jersey City Med Ctr, Jersey City, NJ 62-64; **FAP:** Asst Clin Prof Nova SE Univ, Coll Osteo Med; **SI:** *Learning Disorders; Handicapped Children;* **HMO:** Oxford Blue Choice CIGNA Prucare Empire Blue Shield +

LANG: Itl, Sp; 🔲 🔲 🔲 🔲 🔲 🔲 🔲 *VISA* ⬤

Hages, Harry (MD) Ped **PCP**
Pascack Valley Hosp

215 Old Tappan Rd; Old Tappan, NJ 07675; (201) 666-1000; **BDCERT:** Ped 73; **MS:** Univ Pittsburgh 66; **RES:** Ped, Children's Hosp of Pittsburgh, Pittsburgh, PA 67-68; Ped, NY Hosp-Cornell Med Ctr, New York, NY 68-69; **HMO:** Oxford US Hlthcre Aetna Hlth Plan PHCS First Option +

LANG: Itl, Grk, Sp; 🔲 🔲 🔲 🔲 🔲 🔲 🔲 🔲 🔲 🔲 🔲 Immediately

Harlow, Paul (MD) Ped **PCP**
Hackensack Univ Med Ctr

90 Prospect Ave; Hackensack, NJ 07601; (201) 342-4001; **BDCERT:** Ped 79; **MS:** SUNY Hlth Sci Ctr 74; **RES:** Jacobi Med Ctr, Bronx, NY 74-77; **FEL:** PHO, Children's Hosp of Los Angeles, Los Angeles, CA; **HOSP:** Holy Name Hosp; **HMO:** Chubb Prucare US Hlthcre CIGNA Cost Care +

🔲 🔲 🔲 🔲 🔲 🔲 🔲 A Few Days *VISA* ⬤

Hyatt, Alexander (MD) Ped
Englewood Hosp & Med Ctr

350 Engle St; Englewood, NJ 07631; (201) 894-3158; **BDCERT:** Ped 81; Inf 94; **MS:** Mt Sinai Sch Med 75; **RES:** Johns Hopkins Hosp, Baltimore, MD 75-78; **FEL:** Inf, Mount Sinai Med Ctr, New York, NY 78-79; Johns Hopkins Hosp, Baltimore, MD 79-80; **FAP:** Assoc Prof Mt Sinai Sch Med; **HOSP:** Mount Sinai Med Ctr; **SI:** *Pediatric Infectious Disease*

LANG: Sp; 🔲 🔲 🔲 🔲 🔲 1 Week 🔲 *VISA* ⬤ 🔲

Kanter, Alan (MD) Ped **PCP**
Englewood Hosp & Med Ctr

Metropolitan Pediatric Group, 704 Palisade Ave; Teaneck, NJ 07666; (201) 836-4301; **BDCERT:** Ped 77; **MS:** Albert Einstein Coll Med 70; **RES:** Ped, St Christopher's Hosp for Children, Philadelphia, PA 70-71; Ped, Montefiore Med Ctr, Bronx, NY 74-75; **FAP:** Assoc Clin Instr Columbia P&S; **HOSP:** Columbia-Presbyterian Med Ctr; **SI:** *Attention Deficit Disorders; Autistic Spectrum Disorder;* **HMO:** Oxford GHI First Option Blue Cross & Blue Shield PHS +

LANG: Yd, Heb, Sp; 🔲 🔲 🔲 🔲 🔲 🔲 🔲 🔲 Immediately *VISA* ⬤

Kolsky, Neil (MD) Ped **PCP**
Holy Name Hosp

Pedimedica, 870 Palisade Ave; Teaneck, NJ 07666; (201) 692-1661; **BDCERT:** Ped 72; **MS:** UMDNJ-NJ Med Sch, Newark 66; **RES:** Ped, Johns Hopkins, Baltimore, MD 67-69

LANG: Heb, Sp, Rus; 🔲 🔲 🔲 🔲 🔲 🔲 🔲 Immediately 🔲 *VISA* ⬤

Namerow, David (MD) Ped **PCP**
Valley Hosp

Pediatri Care Assoc, 2020 Fair Lawn Ave; Fair Lawn, NJ 07410; (201) 791-4545; **BDCERT:** Ped 77; **MS:** KY Med Sch, Louisville 72; **RES:** Ped, Children's Hosp Med Ctr, Cincinnati, OH 72-75; U MD Hosp, Baltimore, MD 75-77; **FAP:** Adjct Prof Cornell U; **SI:** *Adolescent Medicine; Behavioral Disorders;* **HMO:** Aetna-US Healthcare Oxford CIGNA/CoMed HMO Blue

LANG: Per, Flm, Sp; 🔲 🔲 🔲 🔲 🔲 🔲 🔲 Immediately *VISA* ⬤ 🔲

Novogroder, Michael (MD) Ped **PCP**
Englewood Hosp & Med Ctr

704 Palisade Ave; Teaneck, NJ 07666; (201) 836-4301; **BDCERT:** Ped 74; **MS:** SUNY Hlth Sci Ctr 69; **RES:** Ped, Jacobi Med Ctr, Bronx, NY 69-73; **FEL:** PEn, NY Hosp-Cornell Med Ctr, New York, NY; **FAP:** Assoc Prof Ped Columbia P&S; **SI:** *Endocrinology/Growth; Puberty Disorders;* **HMO:** Most

🔲 🔲 🔲 🔲 🔲 🔲 🔲 4+ Weeks *VISA*

Rozdeba, Christopha (MD)   Ped
St Joseph's Hosp-Patterson
42 Locust Ave; Wallington, NJ 07057; (201) 777-
0090; **BDCERT:** Ped 86; **MS:** Poland 78; **RES:**
UMDNJ, Newark, NJ 80-83

Rubin, Mitchell H (MD)   Ped
Valley Hosp
23-00 Route 208; Fair Lawn, NJ 07410; (212)
423-6262; **BDCERT:** Ped 85; **MS:** UMDNJ-NJ Med
Sch, Newark 78; **RES:** Ped, St Luke's Roosevelt
Hosp Ctr, New York, NY 79-80; Ped, Newark Beth
Israel Med Ctr, Newark, NJ 81-82; **FEL:** ChiN, New
York University Med Ctr, New York, NY 80-81

Schuss, Steven (MD)   Ped   [PCP]
Englewood Hosp & Med Ctr
Teanick Pediatrics, 197 Cedar Ln; Teaneck, NJ
07666; (201) 836-7171; **BDCERT:** Ped 86; **MS:**
Albert Einstein Coll Med 79; **RES:** Montefiore Med
Ctr, Bronx, NY 79-82; **FEL:** Ped, Montefiore Med
Ctr, Bronx, NY; **FAP:** Asst Clin Prof Ped Albert
Einstein Coll Med; **HOSP:** Holy Name Hosp; **HMO:**
Oxford PHS PHCS First Option QualCare +

🔣 🔣 🔣 🔣 🔣 🔣 2-4 Weeks **VISA** 💳

Wolmer, Donald (MD)   Ped   [PCP]
Pascack Valley Hosp
Chestnut Ridge Pediatrics, 595 Chestnut Ridge Rd
4; Woodcliff Lake, NJ 07675; (201) 391-2020;
BDCERT: Ped 65; **MS:** Albert Einstein Coll Med 60;
RES: Ped, Jacobi Med Ctr, Bronx, NY 60-63; **FAP:**
Asst Clin Prof Albert Einstein Coll Med; **HOSP:**
Valley Hosp; **HMO:** CIGNA US Hlthcre Oxford
Prucare

🔣 🔣 🔣 🔣 🔣 🔣 🔣 Immediately

PHYSICAL MEDICINE & REHABILITATION

Liss, Donald (MD)   PMR
Englewood Hosp & Med Ctr
Physical Medicine & Rehab Ctr, 15 Engle St 205;
Englewood, NJ 07631; (201) 567-2277; **BDCERT:**
PMR 84; **MS:** Wayne State U Sch Med 79; **RES:**
Med, Columbia-Presbyterian Med Ctr, New York,
NY 80-82; Med, Columbia-Presbyterian Med Ctr,
New York, NY 80-82; **SI:** *Sports Medicine; Low Back
Pain-Arthritis;* **HMO:** Oxford NYLCare Aetna-US
Healthcare CIGNA United Healthcare +

LANG: Sp, Rus; 🔣 🔣 🔣 🔣 🔣 🔣 🔣 🔣 🔣 🔣
1 Week **VISA** 💳

Zimmerman, Jerald (MD)   PMR
Englewood Hosp & Med Ctr
350 Engle St; Englewood, NJ 07631; (201) 894-
3288; **BDCERT:** PMR 89; **MS:** Univ IL Coll Med 82;
RES: OrS, U MN Med Ctr, Minneapolis, MN 83-85;
FEL: PMR, Columbia-Presbyterian Med Ctr, New
York, NY 85-88; **FAP:** Asst Prof PMR UMDNJ New
Jersey Sch Osteo Med; **SI:** *Post Polio Syndrome/Joint
Replacement; Muscular Skeletal Med*

LANG: Sp; 🔣 🔣 🔣 🔣 🔣 🔣 🔣 2-4 Weeks 🔣
VISA 💳 💳

PLASTIC SURGERY

Bloomenstein, Richard (MD) PlS
Englewood Hosp & Med Ctr
177 N Dean St 201; Englewood, NJ 07631; (201)
569-2244; **BDCERT:** PlS 70; **MS:** SUNY Downstate
59; **RES:** S, Kings County Hosp Ctr, Brooklyn, NY
64-65; PlS, Montefiore Med Ctr, Bronx, NY 65-67;
HOSP: Valley Hosp; **SI:** *Cosmetic Surgery; Face &
Body Reconstruction;* **HMO:** CIGNA Guardian
Oxford Aetna Hlth Plan

🔣 🔣 🔣 🔣 🔣 🔣 🔣 🔣 1 Week **VISA** 💳

Guide to symbols and abbreviations can be found on pages 110-113.

887

D'Amico, Richard (MD) PlS
Englewood Hosp & Med Ctr

180 N Dean St 3NE; Englewood, NJ 07631; (201) 567-9595; **BDCERT:** PlS 86; **MS:** NYU Sch Med 76; **RES:** IM, Georgetown U Hosp, Washington, DC 76-77; S, Strong Mem Hosp, Rochester, NY 81; **FEL:** PlS, Columbia-Presbyterian Med Ctr, New York, NY 83; **HOSP:** Holy Name Hosp; **HMO:** Aetna Hlth Plan Multiplan Empire Blue Choice

[symbols] 2-4 Weeks **VISA** [symbol]

DiPirro, Earl (MD) PlS
Englewood Hosp & Med Ctr

Teaneck Prof Ctr, 185 Cedar Ln; Teaneck, NJ 07666; (201) 692-1122; **BDCERT:** PlS 69; **MS:** NY Med Coll 61; **RES:** PlS, NY Hosp-Cornell Med Ctr, New York, NY 64-65; PlS, NY Hosp-Cornell Med Ctr, New York, NY 65-67; **FEL:** NY Hosp-Cornell Med Ctr, New York, NY 67; **FAP:** Instr UMDNJ New Jersey Sch Osteo Med; **HOSP:** Pascack Valley Hosp; **SI:** *Laser Surgery; Cosmetic Surgery*; **HMO:** Beech Street Premier

LANG: Itl; [symbols] 1 Week

Hall, Craig (MD) PlS
Hackensack Univ Med Ctr

Metropolitan Plastic Surgery, 140 Prospect Ave 20; Hackensack, NJ 07601; (201) 488-2101; **BDCERT:** PlS 90; **MS:** U Chicago-Pritzker Sch Med 81; **RES:** S, Montefiore Med Ctr, Bronx, NY 81-85; PlS, Montefiore Med Ctr, Bronx, NY 85-87; **FEL:** S, Humana Intl Craniofacial Inst, 87-88; **FAP:** Assoc Prof PlS UMDNJ New Jersey Sch Osteo Med; **SI:** *Craniofacial*

LANG: Ger, Sp, Heb; [symbols] 1 Week [symbol] **VISA** [symbol]

Rauscher, Gregory (MD) PlS
Hackensack Univ Med Ctr

Metropolitan Plastic Surgery, 321 Essex St; Hackensack, NJ 07601; (201) 488-1034; **BDCERT:** PlS 79; HS 90; **MS:** SUNY Downstate 72; **RES:** S, Kings County Hosp Ctr, Brooklyn, NY 72-76; PlS, Kings County Hosp Ctr, Brooklyn, NY 76-78; **FEL:** Microsurgery, Kings County Hosp Ctr, Brooklyn, NY 74-75; **FAP:** Prof UMDNJ New Jersey Sch Osteo Med; **HMO:** Aetna Hlth Plan Blue Cross & Blue Shield CIGNA

[symbols] 4+ Weeks **VISA** [symbol]

Sperling, Richard (MD) PlS
Pascack Valley Hosp

43 Yawpo Ave 6; Oakland, NJ 07436; (201) 337-3434; **BDCERT:** PlS 85; **MS:** Cornell U 70; **RES:** S, St Luke's Roosevelt Hosp Ctr, New York, NY 70-72; PlS, Univ Hosp SUNY Stony Brook, Stony Brook, NY 77-79; **FEL:** HS, St Luke's Roosevelt Hosp Ctr, New York, NY 76; **HOSP:** Valley Hosp; **SI:** *Cosmetic Surgery; Hand Surgery*

[symbols] A Few Days **VISA** [symbol]

PSYCHIATRY

Blackinton, Charles (MD) Psyc
Englewood Hosp & Med Ctr

111 Dean Dr; Tenafly, NJ 07670; (201) 568-8288; **BDCERT:** Psyc 79; **MS:** Columbia P&S 73; **RES:** Mary Imogene Bassett Hosp, Cooperstown, NY 73-74; Columbia-Presbyterian Med Ctr, New York, NY 74-76; **SI:** *Depression; Adjustment to Life Changes*; **HMO:** First Option PHS Aetna Hlth Plan

[symbols] A Few Days

Brenner, Ronald (MD) Psyc
St John's Epis Hosp-Smithtown

67 Walnut Ct; Englewood, NJ 07631; (718) 869-7248; **BDCERT:** Psyc 79; Psyc 73; **MS:** Spain 78; **RES:** Psyc, St Luke's Roosevelt Hosp Ctr, New York, NY 75-78; **FEL:** Psyc, New York University Med Ctr, New York, NY 78-79; **FAP:** Prof Psyc SUNY Hlth Sci Ctr; **HOSP:** Long Island Jewish Med Ctr; **SI:** *Depression and Dementia; Panic Attacks*; **HMO:** Oxford Health First Merit Behavioral Health Plans Empire Blue Cross & Shield

LANG: Sp, Ger; [symbols] A Few Days

Chertoff, Harvey (MD) Psyc
Englewood Hosp & Med Ctr

205 Engle St; Englewood, NJ 07631; (201) 567-4970; **BDCERT:** Psyc 78; **MS:** Albert Einstein Coll Med 66; **RES:** Columbia-Presbyterian Med Ctr, New York, NY 67-70; **FAP:** Asst Clin Prof Psyc Columbia P&S; **HOSP:** Columbia-Presbyterian Med Ctr; **SI:** *Mood Disorders; Anxiety Disorders*; **HMO:** Oxford Aetna Hlth Plan

[symbols] 1 Week

Farkas, Edward (MD)   Psyc
Holy Name Hosp

175 Cedar Ln A; Teaneck, NJ 07666; (201) 692-8354; **BDCERT:** Psyc 88; GerPsy 91; **MS:** Italy 79; **RES:** Psyc, Bronx Lebanon Hosp Ctr, Bronx, NY 79-81; Psyc, St Luke's Roosevelt Hosp Ctr, New York, NY 81-83; **FEL:** Psyc, William A White Inst, New York, NY 82-83; **SI:** *Geriatric Psychiatry; Depression*; **HMO:** CIGNA GHI Oxford

LANG: Itl; 🚹 🏧 🌙 📷 🚼 🏨 💲 Mcr Mcd

Gardner, Richard A (MD)   Psyc
Columbia-Presbyterian Med Ctr

155 County Rd; Cresskill, NJ 07626; (201) 567-8989; **BDCERT:** Psyc 63; ChAP 66; **MS:** SUNY Hlth Sci Ctr 56; **RES:** Psyc, Columbia-Presbyterian Med Ctr, New York, NY 57-59; ChAP, Columbia-Presbyterian Med Ctr, New York, NY 59-62; **FAP:** Clin Prof ChAP Columbia P&S; **SI:** *Child Custody Litigation; Sex Abuse*; **HMO:** None

📷 🚼 🏨 💲   A Few Days 🔲 *VISA* 💳

Gurland, Frances (MD)   Psyc
Hackensack Univ Med Ctr

216 Engle St; Englewood, NJ 07631; (201) 568-4066; **BDCERT:** Psyc 91; **MS:** SUNY Hlth Sci Ctr 89; **RES:** Psyc, St Luke's Roosevelt Hosp Ctr, New York, NY 89-91; **FEL:** ChAP, Mount Sinai Med Ctr, New York, NY 92-94; **FAP:** Asst Clin Instr ChAP Mt Sinai Sch Med; **SI:** *Eating Disorders-Post Partum Depression; Attention Deficit Disorder*; **HMO:** None

🚹 🌙 📷 🚼 🏨 💲 WC   1 Week *VISA* 💳

Narula, Amarjot (MD)   Psyc
Valley Hosp

65 N Maple Ave; Ridgewood, NJ 07450; (201) 670-4423; **BDCERT:** Psyc 92; **MS:** India 79; **RES:** Metropolitan Hosp Ctr, New York, NY 88-89; Psyc, Middletown Psyc Ctr, Middletown, NY 84-88; **HOSP:** Barnert Hosp; **SI:** *Geriatric Psychiatry*

LANG: Pun, Hin, Ur; 🌙 📷 🚼 🏨 💲 Mcd

Rosenfeld, David (MD)   Psyc
Valley Hosp

265 Ackerman Ave; Ridgewood, NJ 07450; (201) 447-5630; **MS:** UMDNJ-RW Johnson Med Sch 88; **RES:** Psyc, Mount Sinai Med Ctr, New York, NY; Psyc, Bergen Pines Hosp, Paramus, NJ; **SI:** *Mood Disorders; Geriatric Psychiatry*

LANG: Rom; 🚹 🌙 📷 🚼 🏨 💲 Mcr *VISA* 💳

Videtti, Nicholas (MD)   Psyc
Valley Hosp

127 Union St; Ridgewood, NJ 07450; (201) 444-4103; **BDCERT:** Psyc 79; **MS:** Italy 61; **RES:** Psyc, VA Hosp, Lyons, NJ 63-66; **SI:** *Psychopharmacology; Electroconvulsive Therapy*; **HMO:** None

🚹 🌙 📷 🚼 🏨 💲 Mcr   1 Week

Wagle, Sharad (MD)   Psyc
Pascack Valley Hosp

Pascack Valley Psychiatric, 270 Old Hook Rd FL2; Westwood, NJ 07675; (201) 358-2323; **BDCERT:** Psyc 96; **MS:** India 71; **RES:** Hackensack Univ Med Ctr, Hackensack, NJ 73-76; Psychoanaltic Inst, Brooklyn, NY 75-78; **FEL:** ChAP, Albert Einstein Hosp, Bronx, NY 76-78; **HOSP:** Holy Name Hosp

🚹 🌙 📷 🏨 Mcr   A Few Days *VISA* 💳

PULMONARY DISEASE

Amoruso, Robert (MD)   Pul
St Joseph's Hosp-Patterson

Associates for Respiratory Help, 2308 Maple Ave; Fairlawn, NJ 07410; (201) 796-8477; **BDCERT:** IM 79; Pul 81; **MS:** Italy 75; **RES:** St Joseph's Hosp, Chicago, IL 75-79; **FEL:** Univ of Med & Dent NJ Hosp, Newark, NJ 79-81; **HOSP:** Wayne Gen Hosp; **SI:** *Critical Care Medicine; Sleep Disorders*; **HMO:** First Option CIGNA Prucare Oxford QualCare +

🚹 📷 🚼 🏨 Mcr   1 Week *VISA* 💳

Guide to symbols and abbreviations can be found on pages 110-113.

889

Birns, Robert (MD)   Pul
Holy Name Hosp

Pulmonary Associates of NJ, 200 Grand Ave 102; Englewood, NJ 07631; (201) 871-3636; **BDCERT:** IM 74; Pul 76; **MS:** Washington U, St Louis 70; **RES:** IM, Boston Med Ctr, Boston, MA 71-72; **FEL:** Chest Disease, Boston Med Ctr, Boston, MA 72-73

🔽 🆂🆂 🅲 🔁 🎟 Mcr Mcd WC Immediately ▨ **VISA** 💳 💳

Brauntuch, Glenn (MD)   Pul   PCP
Englewood Hosp & Med Ctr

Englewood Bergen Medical, 180 Engle St; Englewood, NJ 07631; (201) 567-2050; **BDCERT:** IM 81; Pul 84; **MS:** Columbia P&S 78; **RES:** Pul, Columbia-Presbyterian Med Ctr, New York, NY 78-84; **HMO:** CIGNA Metlife

🔽 🅲 🎟 🆂 Mcr WC NFl A Few Days ▨ **VISA** 💳 💳

Grizzanti, Joseph (DO)   Pul
Valley Hosp

Bergen Health Affiliates, 1501 Broadway 4; Fairlawn, NJ 07410; (201) 794-6505; **BDCERT:** IM 79; Pul 82; **MS:** Philadelphia Coll Osteo Med 79; **RES:** Univ of Med & Dent NJ Hosp, Newark, NJ 76-79; **FEL:** Pul, Albert Einstein Med Ctr, Bronx, NY 79-81; **HMO:** Oxford First Option CIGNA Blue Cross PHCS +

🔽 🅲 🔁 🔣 🎟 🆂 Mcr WC NFl 1 Week ▨ **VISA** 💳

Malovany, Robert (MD)   Pul   PCP
Englewood Hosp & Med Ctr

Bergen Medical Alliance, 180 Dean St; Englewood, NJ 07631; (201) 568-8010; **BDCERT:** IM 73; Pul 76; **MS:** Jefferson Med Coll 70; **RES:** IM, Montefiore Med Ctr, Bronx, NY 70-73; **FEL:** Pul, Montefiore Med Ctr, Bronx, NY 73-75; **FAP:** Asst Prof Mt Sinai Sch Med; **HOSP:** Holy Name Hosp; **SI:** *Asthma; Emphysema;* **HMO:** Oxford CIGNA US Hlthcre Chubb Blue Cross & Blue Shield +

LANG: Sp; 🔽 🅲 🔁 🔣 🎟 🆂 Mcr WC NFl 1 Week ▨ **VISA** 💳 💳

Polkow, Melvin (MD)   Pul
Hackensack Univ Med Ctr

211 Essex St 302; Hackensack, NJ 07601; (201) 498-1311; **BDCERT:** IM 80; Pul 82; **MS:** SUNY Downstate 77; **RES:** Lenox Hill Hosp, New York, NY 77-80; **FEL:** Pul, Univ Hosp SUNY Stony Brook, Stony Brook, NY 80-82; **FAP:** Asst Clin Prof UMDNJ New Jersey Sch Osteo Med; **SI:** *Asthma; Sarcoidosis;* **HMO:** Oxford US Hlthcre Prucare Blue Choice QualCare +

🔽 🅲 🔁 🎟 🆂 Mcr 1 Week

Rose, Henry (MD)   Pul
Passaic Beth Israel Hosp

639 Ridge Rd; Lyndhurst, NJ 07071; (201) 939-8741; **BDCERT:** IM 82; **MS:** UMDNJ-NJ Med Sch, Newark 79; **RES:** Med, Univ of Med & Dent NJ Hosp, Newark, NJ 80-82; **FEL:** Pul, Bronx Muncipal Hosp Ctr, Bronx, NY 82-84; **FAP:** Clin Instr UMDNJ New Jersey Sch Osteo Med; **SI:** *Asthma; Emphysema;* **HMO:** Aetna Hlth Plan Oxford PHS Travelers United Healthcare +

🔽 🅲 🔁 🔣 🎟 🆂 Mcr A Few Days

Simon, Clifford J (MD)   Pul   PCP
Englewood Hosp & Med Ctr

Englewood Medical & Pulmonary Assoc, 180 Engle St; Englewood, NJ 07631; (201) 567-2050; **BDCERT:** IM 76; Pul 80; **MS:** Cornell U 73; **RES:** Dartmouth Hitchcock Med Ctr, Lebanon, NH 73-75; **FEL:** Pul, Bellevue Hosp Ctr, New York, NY 75-77; **HOSP:** Holy Name Hosp; **SI:** *Asthma/Chronic Obstructive Pulmonary Disease; Emphysema;* **HMO:** Oxford United Healthcare Chubb CIGNA First Option +

🔽 🔁 🔣 🎟 🆂 Mcr NFl Immediately ▨ **VISA** 💳

RADIATION ONCOLOGY

Dubin, David (MD)   RadRO
Englewood Hosp & Med Ctr
350 Engle St; Englewood, NJ 07631; (201) 894-3125; **BDCERT:** Rad 91; **MS:** Albert Einstein Coll Med 86; **RES:** RadRO, St Barnabas Med Ctr, Livingston, NJ 86-90; *SI: Breast Cancer; Prostate Cancer;* **HMO:** Oxford First Option HMO Blue CIGNA PHCS +

LANG: Sp, Fr, Heb, Yd, Hin; 🔲 📞 🛏 Mcr Mcd NFi Immediately ▨ **VISA** 💳 💳

Greenblatt, David (MD)   RadRO
Valley Hosp
130 Beech Rd; Englewood, NJ 07631; (201) 447-8000; **BDCERT:** Rad 86; **MS:** SUNY Syracuse 80; **RES:** DR, Westchester County Med Ctr, Valhalla, NY 81-83; **FEL:** Brachytherapy, Mem Sloan Kettering Cancer Ctr, New York, NY 86

Jones, Harold (MD)   RadRO
Englewood Hosp & Med Ctr
350 Engle St; Englewood, NJ 07631; (201) 894-3125; **BDCERT:** Rad 63; **MS:** SUNY Downstate 58; **RES:** VA Med Ctr-Bronx, Bronx, NY 58-61; **FEL:** Royal Marsden Hosp, London, England 65-67
LANG: Sp; 🔲 📞 🛏 A Few Days

RADIOLOGY

Kaufman, Stephen (MD)   Rad
Pascack Valley Hosp
Sharlin Radiological Assocs, PO BOX 694; Westwood, NJ 07675; (201) 342-7558; **BDCERT:** NuM 76; **MS:** NY Med Coll 65; **RES:** Maimonides Med Ctr, Brooklyn, NY 65-67; Mount Sinai Med Ctr, New York, NY 69-72

🔲 📞 🚹 🛏 Mcr WC NFi Immediately **VISA** 💳

Lubat, Edward (MD)   Rad
Valley Hosp
20 N Franklin Tpke; Waldick, NJ 07463; (201) 445-8822; **BDCERT:** Rad 89; NuM 89; **MS:** Jefferson Med Coll 82; **RES:** Rad, New York University Med Ctr, New York, NY 85-88; **FEL:** NuM, New York University Med Ctr, New York, NY 84-85; **FAP:** Asst Clin Prof Rad NYU Sch Med; *SI: Abdomen and Chest Imaging; Bone and Joint Imaging*
🔲 🆘 🌙 🛏 Mcr Mcd WC Immediately **VISA** 💳

Myers, Dale (MD)   Rad
Englewood Hosp & Med Ctr
Englewood Radiologic Group, PA, 309 Engle St 1; Englewood, NJ 07631; (201) 871-1230; **BDCERT:** Rad 63; **MS:** Ohio State U 57; **RES:** Cincinnati Gen Hosp, Cincinnati, OH 61-63
LANG: Sp, Itl, Ger, Fr; 🔲 🆘 🌙 📞 🛏 Mcr Mcd WC A Few Days

Sorabella, Philip (MD)   Rad
Valley Hosp
Radiology Associates of Ridgewood, PA, 20 Franklin Tpke; Waldwick, NJ 07463; (201) 447-8210; **BDCERT:** DR 74; **MS:** Columbia P&S 68; **RES:** DR/NuM, Columbia-Presbyterian Med Ctr, New York, NY; **HMO:** Oxford HMO Blue CIGNA First Option Prucare +

🔲 🆘 🌙 📞 🛏 Mcr Mcd WC NFi A Few Days **VISA** 💳

REPRODUCTIVE ENDOCRINOLOGY

Navot, Daniel (MD)   RE
Pascack Valley Hosp
400 Old Hook Rd; Westwood, NJ 07675; (201) 666-4200; **BDCERT:** ObG 92; RE 94; **MS:** Israel 78; **RES:** Hassadah Hosp, Jerusalem, Israel 77-78; **FEL:** Jones Inst For Reproductive Med, Norfolk, VA; **HMO:** First Option Empire Blue Choice US Hlthcre QualCare

RHEUMATOLOGY

Kopelman, Rima (MD)   Rhu
Valley Hosp

Prospect Medical Offices, 301 Godwin Ave; Midland Park, NJ 07432; (201) 444-4526; **BDCERT:** IM 80; Rhu 84; **MS:** Columbia P&S 77; **RES:** Columbia-Presbyterian Med Ctr, New York, NY 77-81; **FEL:** Rhu, Columbia-Presbyterian Med Ctr, New York, NY 81-83; **FAP:** Asst Prof Med Columbia P&S; **HOSP:** Columbia-Presbyterian Med Ctr; *SI: Rheumatoid Arthritis; Lupus;* **HMO:** Aetna Hlth Plan Blue Cross & Blue Shield Chubb CIGNA Oxford +

🦽 🔦 🏥 🛏 💲 Mcr Mcd WC   A Few Days **VISA** 💳

Marcus, Ralph (MD)   Rhu
Hackensack Univ Med Ctr

870 Palisade Ave 204; Teaneck, NJ 07666; (201) 692-0203; **BDCERT:** IM 75; Rhu 76; **MS:** Albert Einstein Coll Med 69; **RES:** Maimonides Med Ctr, Brooklyn, NY 69-70; Mount Sinai Med Ctr, New York, NY 73-74; **FEL:** Hosp For Special Surgery, New York, NY 74-76; Nat Inst Health, Bethesda, MD 70-72; **FAP:** Asst Clin Prof UMDNJ-NJ Med Sch, Newark; **HOSP:** Holy Name Hosp; *SI: Osteoporosis; Rheumatoid Arthritis;* **HMO:** Oxford First Option HMO Blue United Healthcare QualCare +

🦽 📞 🔦 🏥 🛏 💲 WC   2-4 Weeks **VISA** 💳

Salem, Noel (MD)   Rhu
Englewood Hosp & Med Ctr

285 Engle St; Englewood, NJ 07631; (201) 871-0223; **BDCERT:** IM 76; Rhu 78; **MS:** SUNY Buffalo 72; **RES:** IM, USPHS Hosp, Baltimore, MD 72-74; **FEL:** Rhu, Columbia-Presbyterian Med Ctr, New York, NY 74-76; **FAP:** Asst Prof Mt Sinai Sch Med; **HMO:** Aetna Hlth Plan Blue Cross & Blue Shield Metlife Oxford US Hlthcre +

🦽 🔦 Mcr WC   A Few Days

Zalkowitz, Alan (MD)   Rhu   PCP
Valley Hosp

New Jersey Associates in Medicine, PA, 31-00 Broadway; Fair Lawn, NJ 07410; (201) 796-2255; **BDCERT:** IM 77; Rhu 91; **MS:** Belgium 70; **RES:** Med, Yale-New Haven Hosp, New Haven, CT 70-71; **FEL:** Rhu, Mount Sinai Med Ctr, New York, NY 72-74; **HOSP:** Barnert Hosp; *SI: Lupus;* **HMO:** CIGNA First Option HMO Blue PHS United Healthcare +

LANG: Sp; 🦽 📞 🔦 🏥 🛏 💲 Mcr WC NFI
A Few Days 📠 **VISA** 💳 📷

SPORTS MEDICINE

Savatsky, Gary (MD)   SM
Hackensack Univ Med Ctr

Orthopaedic Spine and Sports Medicine Center, 2 Forest Ave; Paramus, NJ 07652; (201) 587-1111; **BDCERT:** OrS 86; OrS 97; **MS:** Columbia P&S 75; **RES:** S, St Luke's Roosevelt Hosp Ctr, New York, NY 76-78; OrS, Hosp For Special Surgery, New York, NY 80-83; **FEL:** OrS, Hosp For Special Surgery, New York, NY 78-79; **HOSP:** Meadowlands Hosp Med Ctr; *SI: Sports Medicine; Shoulder and Knee Problems;* **HMO:** Oxford CIGNA Aetna-US Healthcare HMO Blue QualCare +

LANG: Sp, Grk, Ger; 🦽 📞 🔦 🏥 🛏 💲 Mcr WC NFI   2-4 Weeks 📠 **VISA** 💳

SURGERY

Ahlborn, Thomas (MD)   S
Valley Hosp

385 S Maple Ave; Ridgewood, NJ 07452; (201) 444-5757; **BDCERT:** S 86; **MS:** Columbia P&S 80; **RES:** S, Columbia-Presbyterian Med Ctr, New York, NY 80-85; **FEL:** GVS, Columbia-Presbyterian Med Ctr, New York, NY 85-86; **HOSP:** Pascack Valley Hosp; **HMO:** Oxford First Option

🦽 📞 🔦 🏥 🛏 💲 Mcr WC NFI   A Few Days **VISA** 💳

Benson, Douglas (MD) S
Hackensack Univ Med Ctr

DeGroote,Manno PA, 83 Summit Ave; Hackensack, NJ 07601; (201) 996-1022; **BDCERT:** S 77; **MS:** UMDNJ-NJ Med Sch, Newark 71; **RES:** UMDNJ Mental Health Ctr, Piscataway, NJ 71-75; **FAP:** Asst Clin Prof UMDNJ-NJ Med Sch, Newark; **HOSP:** Holy Name Hosp; **SI:** *Laparoscopic Surgery; Breast Cancer*

LANG: Sp, Itl; 🔣 Immediately **VISA**

Bruck, Harold (MD) S
Valley Hosp

385 S Maple Ave 204; Ridgewood, NJ 07452; (201) 652-2800; **BDCERT:** S 69; **MS:** Columbia P&S 62; **RES:** S, Bellevue Hosp Ctr, New York, NY 62-68; S, Columbia-Presbyterian Med Ctr, New York, NY 67-68; **SI:** *Breast Diagnosis and Surgery; Melanoma & Surgery/Oncology;* **HMO:** Oxford Blue Cross & Blue Shield United Healthcare Prudential First Option +

🔣 A Few Days

Bufalini, Bruno (MD) S
Englewood Hosp & Med Ctr

200 Grand Ave; Englewood, NJ 07631; (201) 871-0303; **MS:** Italy 71; **RES:** Englewood Hosp, Englewood, NJ 76; **SI:** *Laparoscopic Surgery; Cryoablation;* **HMO:** First Option CIGNA Premier

LANG: Itl; 🔣 Immediately **VISA**

Elias, Steven (MD) S
Holy Name Hosp

180 N Dean St FL2; Englewood, NJ 07631; (201) 568-8666; **BDCERT:** S 87; **MS:** SUNY Buffalo 79; **RES:** S, Millard Fillmore Hosp, Buffalo, NY 79-81; **FEL:** GVS, Englewood Hosp, Englewood, NJ 84-85; **FAP:** Asst Prof S Mt Sinai Sch Med; **HOSP:** Englewood Hosp & Med Ctr

Fried, Kenneth (MD) S
Englewood Hosp & Med Ctr

180 N Dean St; Englewood, NJ 07631; (201) 568-1120; **BDCERT:** S 94; 78; **MS:** NYU Sch Med 78; **RES:** New York University Med Ctr, New York, NY 83; **FEL:** Peripheral VS, New York University Med Ctr, New York, NY; **FAP:** Asst Clin Instr Mt Sinai Sch Med; **HOSP:** Holy Name Hosp; **SI:** *Carotid Artery Surgery; Breast Diseases;* **HMO:** Oxford Aetna-US Healthcare Blue Cross & Blue Shield Prucare United Healthcare +

LANG: Sp, Heb, Fr; 🔣 A Few Days

Geuder, James (MD) S
Hackensack Univ Med Ctr

466 Old Hook Rd 5; Emerson, NJ 07630; (201) 599-2005; **BDCERT:** S 87; GVS 90; **MS:** Med Coll Wisc 81; **RES:** S, Univ of Med & Dent NJ Hosp, Newark, NJ 81-86; **FEL:** GVS, New York University Med Ctr, New York, NY 87-88; **HOSP:** Passaic Beth Israel Hosp; **SI:** *Vascular Surgery*

🔣 1 Week

Ibrahim, Ibrahim (MD) S
Englewood Hosp & Med Ctr

375 Engle St; Englewood, NJ 07631; (201) 894-0400; **BDCERT:** S 74; **MS:** NYU Sch Med 66; **RES:** S, New York University Med Ctr, New York, NY 67-73; **FEL:** GVS, New York University Med Ctr, New York, NY; **HOSP:** Meadowlands Hosp Med Ctr; **SI:** *Laparoscopic Surgery; Gastric Bypass Surgery;* **HMO:** Aetna Hlth Plan Blue Cross & Blue Shield Metlife Oxford

🔣 Immediately **VISA** 💳

Joseph, Patricia (MD) S
Holy Name Hosp

401 S Van Brunt St 404; Englewood, NJ 07631; (201) 567-5111; **BDCERT:** S 85; **MS:** U Fla Coll Med 79; **RES:** S, Montefiore Med Ctr, Bronx, NY 80-84; **FAP:** Clin Instr Mt Sinai Sch Med; **HOSP:** Englewood Hosp & Med Ctr; **SI:** *Breast Cancer;* **HMO:** Oxford CIGNA First Option United Healthcare GHI +

LANG: Sp; 🔣 1 Week **VISA** 💳

Guide to symbols and abbreviations can be found on pages 110-113.

893

Kagan, Andrew (MD)   S
Hackensack Univ Med Ctr

101 Prospect Ave 1D; Hackensack, NJ 07601; (201) 342-7979; **BDCERT:** S 73; **MS:** NY Med Coll 622; **RES:** S, Lenox Hill Hosp, New York, NY 68-72; S, VA Hosp-Bronx, Bronx, NY 69-70; **HMO:** Oxford, Qualcare, MagnaCare, PHCS, Blue Cross & Blue Shield

Manno, Joseph (MD)   S
Holy Name Hosp

83 Summit Ave; Hackensack, NJ 07601; (201) 646-0010; **BDCERT:** S 88; **MS:** Oral Roberts Sch Med 82; **RES:** S, Univ of Med & Dent NJ Hosp, Newark, NJ 82-83; S, Univ of Med & Dent NJ Hosp, Newark, NJ 83-87; **FEL:** GVS, Univ of Med & Dent NJ Hosp, Newark, NJ 87-89; **SI:** *Gallbladder Disease; Arterial Disease;* **HMO:** Aetna Hlth Plan US Hlthcre Oxford First Option Blue Cross +

LANG: Itl; ♿ ⌂ 👫 🕐 💲 Mcr Mcd WC NFI 2-4 Weeks

Tsoukas, Elias (MD)   S
Valley Hosp

245 E Main St; Ramsey, NJ 07446; (201) 327-0220; **BDCERT:** S 64; **MS:** St Louis U 58; **RES:** Philadelphia Gen Hosp, Philadelphia, PA 59-63; Thomas Jefferson U Hosp, Philadelphia, PA 59-63; **HMO:** Aetna Hlth Plan Travelers Oxford First Option +

⌂ 👫 🕐 💲 Mcr Mcd WC NFI A Few Days

Walsky, Robert (MD)   S
Pascack Valley Hosp

466 Old Hook Rd 10; Emerson, NJ 07630; (201) 967-1105; **BDCERT:** S 76; **MS:** KY Med Sch, Louisville 69; **RES:** Mount Sinai Med Ctr, New York, NY 70-75

♿ ⌂ 🕐 💲 Mcd WC NFI Immediately

Yiengpruksawan, Anusak (MD)S
Valley Hosp

Valley Hosp—Surgery, 223 N Van Dien Ave; Ridgewood, NJ 07450; (201) 567-9728; **BDCERT:** S 90; **MS:** Japan 78; **RES:** S, Harlem Hosp Ctr, New York, NY 84-89; **FEL:** Mem Sloan Kettering Cancer Ctr, New York, NY 89

♿ 👫 🕐 Mcd NFI A Few Days

THORACIC SURGERY

Hutchinson, John (MD)   TS
Hackensack Univ Med Ctr

30 Prospect Ave; Hackensack, NJ 07601; (201) 488-8440; **BDCERT:** TS 64; S 63; **MS:** Meharry Med Coll 57; **RES:** U IA Hosp, Iowa City, IA 57-64; **FEL:** TS, U IA Hosp, Iowa City, IA 62-64; **FAP:** Assoc Clin Prof TS Columbia P&S; **SI:** *Cardiac Surgery;* **HMO:** Oxford United Healthcare Aetna-US Healthcare Blue Cross & Blue Shield

LANG: Fr, Sp, Heb; ♿ ⌂ 🕐 Mcr Mcd NFI A Few Days 🔲

Lee, Youngick (MD)   TS
Valley Hosp

145 Prospect St; Ridgewood, NJ 07450; (201) 652-3641; **BDCERT:** TS 76; **MS:** South Korea 63; **RES:** S, St Clare's Hosp & Health Ctr, New York, NY 64-68; TS, Metropolitan Hosp Ctr, New York, NY 68-70; **FEL:** Cv, St Vincents Hosp & Med Ctr NY, New York, NY 81-82; **FAP:** Asst Clin Prof S NY Med Coll; **HOSP:** Englewood Hosp & Med Ctr; **SI:** *Lung Surgery;* **HMO:** Aetna-US Healthcare Magnacare CIGNA Oxford NYLCare +

LANG: Chi, Kor, Ger; ♿ 🕐 💲 Mcr Mcd WC A Few Days

Nichols, Francis (MD)   TS
Hackensack Univ Med Ctr

Hackensack Univ Med Ctr—Surgery Dept, 90 Prospect Ave; Hackensack, NJ 07601; (201) 343-3433; **BDCERT:** TS 94; S 90; **MS:** U Va Sch Med 84; **RES:** S, Mayo Grad Sch, Rochester, MN 84-89; **FEL:** TS, Mayo Grad Sch, Rochester, MN 89-92; **FAP:** Asst Clin Prof TS UMDNJ-NJ Med Sch, Newark; **HMO:** Aetna Hlth Plan Blue Cross & Blue Shield

♿ ⌂ 👫 🕐 WC NFI Immediately

UROLOGY

Berdini, Jeffrey (MD)　　　U
Pascack Valley Hosp
92 Kinderkamack Rd; Woodcliff Lake, NJ 07675; (201) 391-1515; **BDCERT:** U 80; **MS:** UMDNJ-NJ Med Sch, Newark 73; **RES:** Univ of Med & Dent NJ Hosp, Newark, NJ 73-78; **HOSP:** Valley Hosp; **HMO:** Oxford CIGNA Aetna-US Healthcare Blue Shield United Healthcare +

  ♿ 🌙 📷 🗝 🎟 💲 　A Few Days

Cohen, Stephen (MD)　　　U
Valley Hosp
North Jersey Urological, 2515 Fair Lawn Ave; Fair Lawn, NJ 07410; (201) 791-9100; **BDCERT:** U 73; **MS:** Bowman Gray 63; **RES:** S, Montefiore Med Ctr, Bronx, NY 65-66; U, Mount Sinai Med Ctr, New York, NY 67-69; **SI:** *Prostate Cancer*; **HMO:** Oxford HMO Blue Blue Cross Prudential CIGNA +

  ♿ 🌙 🗝 WC 　1 Week 🔲 **VISA** 💳

Frey, Howard (MD)　　　U
Valley Hosp
4 Godwin Ave; Midland Park, NJ 07432; (201) 444-7070; **BDCERT:** U 85; **MS:** Johns Hopkins U 77; **RES:** Johns Hopkins Hosp, Baltimore, MD 77-79; UCLA Med Ctr, Los Angeles, CA 79-83; **SI:** *Urologic Cancer; Prostate*; **HMO:** Blue Choice Blue Cross & Blue Shield CIGNA Sanus

  LANG: Tag, Sp; ♿ 🏧 🌙 📷 🗝 🎟 💲 　Immediately
🔲 **VISA** 💳 💳

Katz, Steven (MD)　　　U
Englewood Hosp & Med Ctr
The Urology Center of Englewood, 75 S Dean St; Englewood, NJ 07631; (201) 816-1900; **BDCERT:** U 78; **MS:** SUNY Buffalo 69; **RES:** U, Metropolitan Hosp Ctr, New York, NY 72-76; **HOSP:** Holy Name Hosp; **SI:** *Vasectomy-No Scalpel; Prostatectomy*; **HMO:** Oxford Guardian Travelers Blue Cross & Blue Shield US Hlthcre +

  LANG: Sp; ♿ 🏧 📷 🗝 🎟 💲 Mcr Mcd WC
A Few Days **VISA** 💳

Vitenson, Jack (MD)　　　U
Hackensack Univ Med Ctr
Urologic InstituteNew Jersey, 331 Summit Ave; Hackensack, NJ 07601; (201) 489-8900; **BDCERT:** U 74; **MS:** NY Med Coll 65; **RES:** S, VA Med Ctr-Manh, New York, NY 66-67; U, Metropolitan Hosp Ctr, New York, NY 67-70; **FAP:** Asst Clin Prof UMDNJ New Jersey Sch Osteo Med; **SI:** *Prostate Disease; Erectile Function*; **HMO:** Oxford Blue Cross & Blue Shield US Hlthcre Aetna Hlth Plan Prucare +

  LANG: Fr; ♿ 🗝 🎟 💲 Mcr NFI 　A Few Days **VISA** 💳

Wasserman, Gary (MD)　　　U
Englewood Hosp & Med Ctr
106 Grand Ave; Englewood, NJ 07631; (201) 569-7777; **BDCERT:** U 93; **MS:** Tulane U 85; **RES:** Geo Wash U Med Ctr, Washington, DC 85-87; Tulane U Med Ctr, New Orleans, LA 87-91; **HOSP:** Holy Name Hosp; **HMO:** Aetna Hlth Plan Blue Choice Blue Cross & Blue Shield PHS

  LANG: Sp; ♿ 🌙 📷 🗝 🎟 💲 Mcr Mcd 　Immediately
VISA 💳

VASCULAR SURGERY (GENERAL)

Dardik, Herbert (MD)　　　GVS
Englewood Hosp & Med Ctr
Englewood Surgical Associates, PA, 375 Engle St; Englewood, NJ 07631; (201) 894-0400; **BDCERT:** S 66; **MS:** NYU Sch Med 60; **RES:** S, Montefiore Med Ctr, Bronx, NY 60-65; **SI:** *Leg By-Pass Surgery; Aortic-Aneurysm Surgery*; **HMO:** Oxford US Hlthcre Aetna Hlth Plan Blue Cross & Blue Shield Prudential +

  LANG: Sp, Yd, Ar; ♿ 📷 🗝 🎟 💲 Mcr Mcd WC NFI
A Few Days **VISA** 💳

De Groote, Robert (MD)   GVS
Hackensack Univ Med Ctr

DeGroote/Manno/Napolitano/Benson/Poole, 83
Summit Ave; Hackensack, NJ 07601; (201) 646-
0010; **BDCERT:** S 85; GVS 88; **MS:** Mexico 79; **RES:**
S, Univ of Med & Dent NJ Hosp, Newark, NJ 80-84;
FEL: CCM, Univ of Med & Dent NJ Hosp, Newark,
NJ; GVS, Hackensack U Med Ctr, Hackensack, NJ;
HOSP: Holy Name Hosp; *SI: Hernia; Carotid Artery*;
HMO: US Hlthcre Oxford First Option CIGNA
Metropolitan +

  ♿ 🅲 🔲 🎟 🆂 Mcr Mcd WC NFi Immediately

Sussman, Barry (MD)   GVS
Englewood Hosp & Med Ctr

Englewood Surgical Associates, PA, 375 Engle St;
Englewood, NJ 07631; (201) 894-0400; **BDCERT:**
S 80; GVS 88; **MS:** NYU Sch Med 73; **RES:** New
York University Med Ctr, New York, NY 73-78;
FEL: GVS, Englewood Hosp, Englewood, NJ 78-79;
HOSP: Holy Name Hosp; *SI: Breast Surgery;
Vascular Surgeries-all*; **HMO:** Aetna Hlth Plan Blue
Cross & Blue Shield Oxford Travelers US Hlthcre +

LANG: Heb; ♿ 🔲 🅟 🎟 🆂 Mcr Mcd WC 2-4 Weeks
▭ *VISA* 💳 📇

Wengerter, Kurt (MD)   GVS
Montefiore Med Ctr-Weiler/Einstein Div

381 Grant Ave; Cresskill, NJ 07626; (201) 871-
7085; **BDCERT:** S 88; GVS 91; **MS:** SUNY
Downstate 80; **RES:** S, Montefiore Med Ctr, Bronx,
NY 81-85; **FEL:** GVS, Montefiore Med Ctr, Bronx,
NY 85-87; **HMO:** HIP Network US Hlthcre PHS
Blue Choice Travelers +

  ♿ 🔲 🎟 Mcr Mcd WC Immediately

Wolodiger, Fred (MD)   GVS
Englewood Hosp & Med Ctr

Englewood Surgical Associates, 375 Engle St;
Englewood, NJ 07631; (201) 894-0400; **BDCERT:**
S 86; GVS 90; **MS:** SUNY Hlth Sci Ctr 80; **RES:** UC
San Diego Med Ctr, San Diego, CA 80-81; N Shore
Univ Hosp-Manhasset, Manhasset, NY 81-85; **FEL:**
GVS, Englewood Hosp, Englewood, NJ 85-87;
HOSP: Holy Name Hosp; *SI: Laparascopic Surgery*;
HMO: US Hlthcre Aetna Hlth Plan Blue Shield
Oxford Prudential +

  ♿ 🔲 🅟 🎟 🆂 Mcr Mcd WC NFi Immediately *VISA* 💳

ESSEX
COUNTY

Specialties in capital letters indicate Primary Care Specialties. However, many doctors will be certified in subspecialty, but will practice predominantly primary care medicine. In our lists this will be indicated.

*Oncologists deal with Cancer

ADDICTION PSYCHIATRY

Patel, Pankaj (MD)   AdP
St Vincent's Med Ctr-Richmond
603 Village Dr; Avenel, NJ 07001; (732) 634-0020; **BDCERT:** Psyc 94; **MS:** India 81; **RES:** Psyc, St Vincent's Med Ctr-Richmond, Staten Island, NY 81-84; **HOSP:** Bayley Seton Hosp

ALLERGY & IMMUNOLOGY

Bielory, Leonard (MD)   A&I   PCP
Univ of Med & Dent NJ Hosp
UMDNJ—Allergy & Ummunology Dept, 90 Bergen St 4700; Newark, NJ 07103; (973) 972-2762; **BDCERT:** A&I 85; IM 84; **MS:** UMDNJ-NJ Med Sch, Newark 80; **RES:** U MD Hosp, Baltimore, MD 80-82; **FEL:** A&I, Nat Inst Health, Bethesda, MD 82-85; **FAP:** Dir A&I UMDNJ New Jersey Sch Osteo Med; **HMO:** CIGNA US Hlthcre

🚹 🅲 🄰 🅈 🎬 🆂 Mcr Mcd WC 2-4 Weeks *VISA* ⬛ ⬛

Weiss, Steven (MD)   A&I
St Barnabas Med Ctr-Livingston
Allergy Asthma & Immunology, 209 S Livingston Ave 6; Livingston, NJ 07039; (973) 992-4171; **BDCERT:** A&I 87; IM 85; **MS:** U Hlth Sci/Chicago Med Sch 82; **RES:** IM, St Luke's Roosevelt Hosp Ctr, New York, NY 82-85; **FEL:** A&I, St Luke's Roosevelt Hosp Ctr, New York, NY 85-87; **FAP:** Clin Instr Columbia P&S; **SI:** *Asthma; Chronic Sinusitis;* **HMO:** Prucare Oxford CIGNA Blue Cross First Option +

🚹 🆂🄳 🅲 🄰 🅈 🎬 🆂 WC

CARDIAC ELECTROPHYSIOLOGY

Correia, Joaquim (MD)   CE
Univ of Med & Dent NJ Hosp
183 Adams St; Newark, NJ 07105; (201) 589-8668; **BDCERT:** Cv 91; CE 94; **MS:** NYU Sch Med 86; **RES:** Columbia-Presbyterian Med Ctr, New York, NY 86-89; **FEL:** Columbia-Presbyterian Med Ctr, New York, NY 89-92; Columbia-Presbyterian Med Ctr, New York, NY 92-93; **FAP:** Asst Prof UMDNJ-NJ Med Sch, Newark; **HOSP:** St Elizabeth Hosp; **SI:** *Arrhythmias; Pacemakers;* **HMO:** Oxford US Hlthcre Empire Blue Cross & Shield First Option

LANG: Prt, Sp, Chi; 🚹 🆂🄳 🅲 🄰 🅈 🎬 🆂 Mcr Mcd
A Few Days

CARDIOLOGY (CARDIOVASCULAR DISEASE)

Ciccone, John (MD)   Cv
St Barnabas Med Ctr-Livingston
374 Millburn Ave; Millburn, NJ 07041; (973) 467-1544; **BDCERT:** Cv 82; **MS:** UMDNJ-NJ Med Sch, Newark 79; **RES:** Univ of Med & Dent NJ Hosp, Newark, NJ 81-82; Newark Beth Israel Med Ctr, Newark, NJ 80-81; **FEL:** Newark Beth Israel Med Ctr, Newark, NJ 82-84; **FAP:** Clin Prof UMDNJ-NJ Med Sch, Newark; **HOSP:** Morristown Mem Hosp; **HMO:** Aetna-US Healthcare HMO Blue CIGNA Blue Cross & Blue Shield

LANG: Sp, Prt; 🚹 🄰 🅈 🎬 🆂 Mcr Mcd 2-4 Weeks

Dwyer, Edward (MD)   Cv
Univ of Med & Dent NJ Hosp
MSB 1536, 185 S Orange Ave; Newark, NJ 07103; (973) 972-2574; **BDCERT:** IM 68; Cv 70; **MS:** Columbia P&S 61; **RES:** IM, St Luke's Roosevelt Hosp Ctr, New York, NY 64-66; Cv, St Luke's Roosevelt Hosp Ctr, New York, NY 63-64; **FEL:** Cv, Columbia-Presbyterian Med Ctr, New York, NY 64-65; **FAP:** Prof Med UMDNJ-NJ Med Sch, Newark

🚹 🄰 🎬 Mcr Mcd 1 Week

Klapholz, Marc (MD)   Cv
Univ of Med & Dent NJ Hosp

NJ Med Sch - Medical Science Bldg, 185 S Orange Ave Ste I-574; Newark, NJ 07103; (973) 972-2297; **BDCERT:** IM 89; Cv 91; **MS:** Albert Einstein Coll Med 86; **RES:** IM, Bronx Muncipal Hosp Ctr, Bronx, NY 86-89; **FEL:** Cv, Bronx Muncipal Hosp Ctr, Bronx, NY 89-92; **FAP:** Dir Cv UMDNJ New Jersey Sch Osteo Med; **SI:** *Interventional Cardiology; Congestive Heart Failure;* **HMO:** US Hlthcre CIGNA

LANG: Heb, Sp; 1 Week **VISA**

Rogal, Gary J (MD)   Cv
St Barnabas Med Ctr-Livingston

769 Northfield Ave 220; W Orange, NJ 07052; (201) 731-9442; **BDCERT:** IM 81; Cv 83; **MS:** Geo Wash U Sch Med 78; **RES:** IM, Long Island Jewish Med Ctr, New Hyde Park, NY 78-81; **FEL:** Cv, Strong Mem Hosp, Rochester, NY 81-84; **HOSP:** Beth Israel Med Ctr; **SI:** *Angioplasty; Heart Failure;* **HMO:** CIGNA Oxford Blue Cross & Blue Shield First Option Prudential +

LANG: Sp; 2-4 Weeks

Rothbart, Stephen (DO)   Cv
Newark Beth Israel Med Ctr

Newark Beth Israel Medical Center, 201 Lyons Ave G4; Newark, NJ 07112; (973) 926-8590; **BDCERT:** IM 81; Cv 83; **MS:** UMDNJ New Jersey Sch Osteo Med 77; **RES:** IM, Univ of Med & Dent NJ Hosp, Newark, NJ 77-78; Cv, Univ of Med & Dent NJ Hosp, Newark, NJ; **FEL:** Cv, Newark Beth Israel Med Ctr, Newark, NJ 80-82; CE, Beth Israel Med Ctr, Boston, MA 82-83; **FAP:** UMDNJ New Jersey Sch Osteo Med; **HOSP:** St Barnabas Med Ctr-Livingston; **SI:** *Heart Palpitations; Dizziness or Fainting;* **HMO:** Prucare United Healthcare Oxford CIGNA First Option +

LANG: Sp; Immediately **VISA**

Werres, Roland (MD)   Cv
Newark Beth Israel Med Ctr

The Heart Specialist PA, 2130 Millburn Ave A4; Millburn, NJ 07041; (973) 275-9300; **BDCERT:** IM 74; Cv 77; **MS:** Germany 67; **RES:** IM, Newark Beth Israel Med Ctr, Newark, NJ 72-74; **FEL:** Cv, Newark Beth Israel Med Ctr, Newark, NJ 74-76; **HOSP:** St Barnabas Med Ctr-Livingston; **SI:** *Interventional Cardiology; Congestive Heart Failure;* **HMO:** Aetna Hlth Plan Blue Choice Blue Cross & Blue Shield Choicecare CIGNA +

LANG: Sp, Ger, Pol; Immediately **VISA**

CHILD & ADOLESCENT PSYCHIATRY

Bartlett, Jacqueline (MD)   ChAP
Univ of Med & Dent NJ Hosp

University Psychiatric Associates, 185 S Orange Ave 501; Newark, NJ 07103; (973) 972-2727; **BDCERT:** Psyc 83; **MS:** U Cincinnati 71; **RES:** Ped, Montefiore/Einstein Hosp, Bronx, NY 74-76; Psyc, Columbia-Presbyterian Med Ctr, New York, NY 79-81; **FEL:** ChAP, Columbia-Presbyterian Med Ctr, New York, NY 77-79; **FAP:** Assoc Prof UMDNJ New Jersey Sch Osteo Med; **SI:** *Stress Related Problems; Behavior/School Problems;* **HMO:** Greenspring

A Few Days

Clemente, Jack (MD)   ChAP
Mountainside Hosp

326 Park St; Upper Montclair, NJ 07043; (973) 783-4669; **BDCERT:** Psyc 72; ChAP 73; **MS:** NY Med Coll 63; **RES:** Psyc, Metropolitan Hosp Ctr, New York, NY 64-66; ChAP, Metropolitan Hosp Ctr, New York, NY 66-68; **FAP:** Asst Clin Prof UMDNJ New Jersey Sch Osteo Med; **HOSP:** Newark Beth Israel Med Ctr; **SI:** *Attention Deficit Disorders; Depression & Anxiety;* **HMO:** None

A Few Days

DERMATOLOGY

Abbey, Albert (MD)   D
St Barnabas Med Ctr-Livingston
Center for Dermatology, PA, 101 Old Short Hills Rd
401; W Orange, NJ 07052; (973) 736-9535;
BDCERT: D 72; **MS:** Tufts U 64; **RES:** IM, Boston
Med Ctr, Boston, MA 64-66; D, NY Hosp-Cornell
Med Ctr, New York, NY 68-72; **FAP:** Asst Clin Prof
Med UMDNJ-NJ Med Sch, Newark

Brodkin, Roger (MD)   D
St Barnabas Med Ctr-Livingston
101 Old Short Hills Rd 401; W Orange, NJ 07052;
(973) 736-9535; **BDCERT:** D 64; **MS:** Jefferson Med
Coll 58; **RES:** Bellevue Hosp Ctr, New York, NY 59-
62; New York University Med Ctr, New York, NY
60-62; **FAP:** Clin Prof D UMDNJ New Jersey Sch
Osteo Med; **HOSP:** Univ of Med & Dent NJ Hosp; *SI:
Benign and Malignant Tumors; Pediatric/Adolescent
Allergy*; **HMO:** First Option Blue Cross & Blue Shield
Magnacare Health Source

LANG: Fr, Sp; 🅰 📞 📷 🔧 🛏 💲 Mc WC
A Few Days **VISA** 💳

Connolly, Adrian L (MD)   D
St Barnabas Med Ctr-Livingston
Dermatology & Cutaneous Surgery Ctr, 101 Old
Short Hills Rd; W Orange, NJ 07052; (201) 731-
9600; **BDCERT:** D 79; **MS:** UMDNJ-NJ Med Sch,
Newark 75; **RES:** D, New York University Med Ctr,
New York, NY 76-79; **FEL:** Mohs S, New York
University Med Ctr, New York, NY 79-81; **FAP:**
Asst Clin Prof UMDNJ New Jersey Sch Osteo Med;
SI: Skin Cancer; **HMO:** First Option Oxford Prucare
Blue Cross & Blue Shield

LANG: Sp, Rus; 🅰 📞 📷 🔧 🛏 Mc 2-4 Weeks 💳
VISA 💳 💳

Gottlieb, Alice (MD)   D
RWJ Univ Hosp-New Brnsw
RWJ Hosp, 1 Robert Wood Johnson Pl; New
Brunswick, NJ 08903; (732) 235-7098; **BDCERT:**
IM 93; D 93; **MS:** Cornell U 80; **RES:** D, NY Hosp-
Cornell Med Ctr, New York, NY; IM, NY Hosp-
Cornell Med Ctr, New York, NY; **FEL:** Rhu, Hosp For
Special Surgery, New York, NY; **FAP:** Dir D UMDNJ
New Jersey Sch Osteo Med; **HOSP:** Rockefeller Univ
Hosp; *SI: Psoriasis*

LANG: Sp, Tag; 🅰 🛏 Mc Mc WC 2-4 Weeks **VISA**
💳

Schwartz, Robert A (MD)   D
185 S Orange Ave; Newark, NJ 07103; (973) 982-
6255; **BDCERT:** D 78; **MS:** NY Med Coll 74; **RES:** D,
U Hosp, Cincinnati, OH 75-77; D, Roswell Park
Cancer Inst, Buffalo, NY 77-78; **FEL:** D, RWJ Univ
Hosp-New Brunswick, New Brunswick, NJ; **FAP:**
Prof D; **HMO:** United Healthcare

Seibt, R Stephen (MD)   D
St Luke's Roosevelt Hosp Ctr
92 Old Northfield Rd; W Orange, NJ 07052; (973)
736-0885; **MS:** U Minn 76; **RES:** USPHS Hosp,
Baltimore, MD 77-80; **FAP:** Assoc Prof D Columbia
P&S; **HOSP:** Columbia-Presbyterian Med Ctr; *SI:
Skin Malignancies; Aging Skin*; **HMO:** Blue Shield
Multiplan Chubb Amerihealth GHI +

🅰 📞 📷 🔧 🛏 💲 Mc WC   A Few Days

EMERGENCY MEDICINE

Almeida, Victor (DO)   EM
Union Hosp-New Jersey
19 J Nob Hill; Roseland, NJ 07068; (908) 687-
1900; **BDCERT:** EM 95; **MS:** UMDNJ, Sch Osteo
Med 90; **RES:** EM, Thomas Jefferson, Philadelphia,
PA

ENDOCRINOLOGY, DIABETES & METABOLISM

Schneider, George (MD)   EDM
Newark Beth Israel Med Ctr
204 Eagle Rock Ave; Roseland, NJ 07068; (973)
228-2047; **BDCERT:** IM 71; EDM 73; **MS:** Tufts U
65; **RES:** Bellevue Hosp Ctr, New York, NY 65-67;
Strong Mem Hosp, Rochester, NY 69-70; **FEL:** EDM,
Yale-New Haven Hosp, New Haven, CT 70-72;
FAP: Assoc Clin Prof Med UMDNJ-NJ Med Sch,
Newark; **HOSP:** St Barnabas Med Ctr-Livingston;
SI: Thyroid Diseases; Diabetes Mellitus; **HMO:** First
Option Blue Cross & Blue Shield Prucare CIGNA
QualCare +

🔲 🔲 🔲 🔲 🔲 2-4 Weeks

FAMILY PRACTICE

Giuliano, Michael (DO)   FP   PCP
Mountainside Hosp
622 Franklin Ave; Nutley, NJ 07110; (973) 667-
8493; **BDCERT:** FP 89; **MS:** Philadelphia Coll Osteo
Med 81; *SI: Geriatric;* **HMO:** Aetna Hlth Plan Blue
Choice Blue Cross & Blue Shield

🔲 🔲 🔲 🔲 🔲 🔲 2-4 Weeks

Johnson, Mark (MD)   FP   PCP
Univ of Med & Dent NJ Hosp
New Jersey Family Practice Ctr, 90 Bergen St Ste
300; Newark, NJ 07103; (973) 972-2111;
BDCERT: FP 82; **MS:** UMDNJ-NJ Med Sch, Newark
79; **RES:** U of S AL Med Ctr, Mobile, AL 79-82; **FEL:**
RWJ Univ Hosp-New Brunswick, New Brunswick,
NJ 82-84; Onc, NC Mem Hosp, Chapel Hill, NC;
FAP: Chrmn FP UMDNJ New Jersey Sch Osteo Med;
HOSP: Clara Maass Med Ctr; *SI: Mitral Valve
Prolapse; Hypertension;* **HMO:** US Hlthcre First
Option HMO Blue United Healthcare

LANG: Sp; 🔲 🔲 🔲 🔲 🔲 🔲 🔲 🔲 🔲
A Few Days **VISA** 🔲 🔲

McCampbell, Edwin (MD)   FP   PCP
East Orange Gen Hosp
85 S Harrison St 104; E Orange, NJ 07018; (201)
672-3829; **BDCERT:** FP 74; **MS:** Howard U 68;
RES: Kaiser Hosp, Oakland, CA; **FEL:** FP, Howard U
Hosp, Washington, DC; Howard U Hosp,
Washington, DC; **FAP:** Assoc Prof UMDNJ New
Jersey Sch Osteo Med; **HOSP:** St Barnabas Med Ctr-
Livingston; *SI: Stress Management; Personal
Counseling;* **HMO:** HMO Blue Aetna-US Healthcare
CIGNA Oxford United Healthcare +

🔲 🔲 🔲 🔲 🔲 🔲 🔲 🔲 🔲 🔲 2-4 Weeks

GASTROENTEROLOGY

De Pasquale, Joseph (MD)   Ge
St Barnabas Med Ctr-Livingston
North Jersey Gastroenterology, 741 Northfield Ave
101; West Orange, NJ 07052; (973) 736-1991;
BDCERT: IM 86; Ge 89; **MS:** Italy 83; **RES:** IM, St
Michael's Med Ctr, New York, NY 86-88; **FEL:** Ge,
St Michael's Med Ctr, New York, NY 83-86; **HOSP:**
St Michael's Med Ctr; **HMO:** 1199 Aetna Hlth Plan
Empire Blue Cross & Shield First Health Oxford +

LANG: Sp, Itl; 🔲 🔲 🔲 🔲 🔲 🔲 Immediately

Leevy, C M (MD)   Ge
Univ of Med & Dent NJ Hosp
New Jersey Medical School Liver Center and
Sammy Davis Jr Liver Institute, 150 Bergen St;
Newark, NJ 07103; (973) 972-4534; **BDCERT:** IM
51; Ge 90; **MS:** U Mich Med Sch 44; **RES:** IM, Jersey
City Med Ctr, Jersey City, NJ 44-45; PHO, Jersey
City Med Ctr, Jersey City, NJ 45-48; **FEL:**
Hepatology, U Toronto Gen Hosp, Totonto, Canada
51; Hepatology, Boston Med Ctr, Boston, MA 58-
59; **FAP:** Prof UMDNJ New Jersey Sch Osteo Med;
SI: Hepatitis; Cirrhosis, Liver Cancer; **HMO:** US
Hlthcre Blue Cross & Blue Shield CIGNA Prudential
+

LANG: Sp, Itl, Prt, Fr, Pol; 🔲 🔲 🔲 🔲 🔲 🔲 🔲 🔲
2-4 Weeks 🔲 **VISA** 🔲

Mogan, Glen (MD)   Ge
St Barnabas Med Ctr-Livingston
Advanced Gastroenterology, 741 N Field Ave 204;
West Orange, NJ 07052; (973) 731-8686;
BDCERT: IM 78; Ge 81; **MS:** SUNY Syracuse 75;
RES: IM, Mount Sinai Med Ctr, New York, NY 75-
76; IM, Mount Sinai Med Ctr, New York, NY 76-78;
FEL: Ge, Mount Sinai Med Ctr, New York, NY 78-
79; Ge, Mount Sinai Med Ctr, New York, NY 79-80;
FAP: Assoc Clin UMDNJ New Jersey Sch Osteo Med;
SI: *Colitis; Ulcers;* **HMO:** Aetna-US Healthcare
Oxford Prucare

LANG: Ger; 🚫 🔟 🏧 💲 Mcr Mcd A Few Days ▦
VISA 💳 💳

Schrader, Zalman (MD)   Ge
St Barnabas Med Ctr-Livingston
Affliates In Gastrenterology, 101 Old Short Hills Rd
217; W Orange, NJ 07052; (973) 731-4600;
BDCERT: Ge 68; **MS:** Albert Einstein Coll Med 61;
RES: Jacobi Med Ctr, Bronx, NY 61-62; **FEL:** NY
Hosp-Cornell Med Ctr, New York, NY 67-69; *SI:*
Inflammatory Bowel Disease; **HMO:** Blue Cross &
Blue Shield CIGNA Oxford Aetna Hlth Plan US
Hlthcre +

🚫 🔟 🏧 🔟 💲 Mcr Mcd 1 Week **VISA** 💳

Sloan, William (MD)   Ge
St Barnabas Med Ctr-Livingston
101 Old Short Hills Rd 217; W Orange, NJ 07052;
(973) 731-4600; **BDCERT:** IM 72; Ge 72; **MS:** Univ
Penn 65; **RES:** Mount Sinai Med Ctr, New York, NY
66-67; Mount Sinai Med Ctr, New York, NY 69-70;
FEL: Ge, Mount Sinai Med Ctr, New York, NY;
HOSP: Morristown Mem Hosp; *SI: Liver Disease;*
Inflammatory Bowel Disease; **HMO:** HMO Blue
CIGNA US Hlthcre Prucare First Option +
LANG: Sp; 🚫 🔟 🏧 🔟 💲 Mcr Mcd WC NFI
A Few Days ▦ **VISA** 💳 💳

Trotman, Bruce W (MD)   Ge
Univ of Med & Dent NJ Hosp
185 S Orange Ave msbH538; Newark, NJ 07103;
(973) 972-5252; **BDCERT:** IM 71; Ge 73; **MS:** Univ
Penn 69; **RES:** IM, Hosp of U Penn, Philadelphia,
PA 69-71; **FEL:** Ge, Hosp of U Penn, Philadelphia,
PA 71-73; **FAP:** Prof UMDNJ New Jersey Sch Osteo
Med; *SI: Gallbladder Disease; Hepatitis;* **HMO:** HMO
Blue US Hlthcre Empire Blue Cross & Shield Prucare

🚫 🔟 🏧 🔟 💲 Mcr Mcd NFI 1 Week **VISA** 💳

GERIATRIC MEDICINE

Gambert, Steven R (MD)   Ger
Univ of Med & Dent NJ Hosp
UMDNJ Hosp Newark, 150 Bergen St Level I, Rm
248; Newark, NJ 07103; (973) 972-0412;
BDCERT: IM 78; Ger 88; **MS:** Columbia P&S 75;
RES: IM, Dartmouth Hitchcock Med Ctr, Lebanon,
NH 75-77; **FEL:** EDM & Ger, Beth Israel Med Ctr,
Boston, MA 77-79; **FAP:** Prof Med UMDNJ New
Jersey Sch Osteo Med; *SI: Thyroid; Aging*
🚫 🔟 💲 Mcr Mcd 4+ Weeks **VISA** 💳

GYNECOLOGIC ONCOLOGY

Denehy, Thad (MD)   GO
St Barnabas Med Ctr-Livingston
St Barnabas Med Ctr, Old Short Hills Rd; Livingston,
NJ 07039; (973) 322-5280; **BDCERT:** ObG 91; **MS:**
Bowman Gray 84; **RES:** ObG, St Barnabas Med Ctr,
Livingston, NJ 85-88; **FEL:** GO, Strong Mem Hosp,
Rochester, NY 88-90; *SI: Gynecologic Cancers;*
Reconstructive Pelvic Surgery; **HMO:** United
Healthcare Oxford First Option Cost Care US
Hlthcre +
LANG: Itl; 🚫 🌙 🔟 🏧 🔟 Mcr Mcd WC 1 Week ▦
VISA 💳

Gregori, Caterina (MD) GO
St Barnabas Med Ctr-Livingston

St Barnabas Med Ctr, Old Short Hill Rd; Livingston, NJ 07039; (973) 322-5280; **BDCERT:** ObG 69; GO 74; **MS:** Italy 57; **RES:** ObG, Newark City Hosp, Newark, NJ 63-66; **FEL:** GO, Newark City Hosp, Newark, NJ 66-68; **SI:** *Gynecologic Cancers; Reconstructive Pelvic Surgery;* **HMO:** Oxford Blue Cross & Blue Shield PHCS Aetna Hlth Plan United Healthcare +

🚗 📷 ♿ Mcr Mcd WC 1 Week 💳 *VISA* 💳

HEMATOLOGY

Zauber, N Peter (MD) Hem
St Barnabas Med Ctr-Livingston

22 Old Short Hills Rd # 108; Livingston, NJ 07039; (973) 533-9299; **BDCERT:** IM 76; Hem 78; **MS:** Johns Hopkins U 71; **RES:** Baltimore City Hosp, Baltimore, MD 75-76; **FEL:** Hem & Onc, Presbyterian U Hosp, Pittsburgh, PA 76-78

INFECTIOUS DISEASE

Johnson, Edward (MD) Inf
St Michael's Med Ctr

5 Franklin Ave Ste 110; Belleville, NJ 07109; (201) 751-3399; **BDCERT:** IM 80; Inf 84; **MS:** Italy 75; **RES:** St Michael's Med Ctr, Newark, NJ 75-78; **FEL:** St Michael's Med Ctr, Newark, NJ 78-80; **HOSP:** Clara Maass Med Ctr; **SI:** *Fungal Infections; Travel & Tropical Diseases;* **HMO:** Prucare US Hlthcre Chubb Blue Select Multiplan +

LANG: Itl; 🚗 🌙 ♿ ♿ S Mcr Mcd WC 1 Week

Kapila, Rajendra (MD) Inf
Hosp Ctr at Orange

185 Central Ave Ste 409; East Orange, NJ 07018; (973) 675-8545; **BDCERT:** IM 77; Inf 78; **MS:** India 64; **RES:** Newark City Hosp, Newark, NJ 68-69; **FEL:** Newark City Hosp, Newark, NJ 71-73; **HOSP:** Univ of Med & Dent NJ Hosp; **SI:** *HIV;* **HMO:** Most

LANG: Hin; 🚗 📷 ♿ ♿ S Mcr Mcd 1 Week

INTERNAL MEDICINE

Amin, Jashvantkumar S (MD) IM
Hosp Ctr at Orange

JS Ajmin MD PA, 181 Franklin Ave 302; Nutley, NJ 07110; (973) 235-1300; **BDCERT:** IM 76; Ger 76; **MS:** India 68; **RES:** IM, Shadyside Hosp, Pittsburgh, PA 70-71; IM, Univ of Med & Dent NJ Hosp, Newark, NJ 71-72; **FEL:** Hem Onc, Univ of Med & Dent NJ Hosp, Newark, NJ 72-74; **FAP:** Clin Instr UMDNJ New Jersey Sch Osteo Med; **HOSP:** Clara Maass Med Ctr; **SI:** *Anemia, Leukemia, Lymphoma; Cancer Treatment;* **HMO:** CIGNA Aetna-US Healthcare Blue Cross & Blue Shield Prudential Oxford +

LANG: Hin, Guj; 🚗 🌙 📷 ♿ ♿ S A Few Days

Chrisanderson, Donna (MD) IM
Hosp Ctr at Orange

Metabolic Associates, 2040 Milburn Ave; Maplewood, NJ; (973) 378-9070; **BDCERT:** IM 94; **MS:** Med Coll Ga 88; **RES:** Greenwich Hosp, Greenwich, CT 89-91; **FEL:** U of Alabama Hosp, Birmingham, AL 91-93

Decosimo, Diana R (MD) IM PCP
Univ of Med & Dent NJ Hosp

Women's Wellness Center, 90 Bergen St; Newark, NJ 07103; (973) 972-2777; **BDCERT:** IM 79; Ger 92; **MS:** Boston U 74; **RES:** St Vincents Hosp & Med Ctr NY, New York, NY 74-75; Worcester City Hosp, Worcester, MA 75-77; **FEL:** U Mass Med Ctr, Worcester, MA 77-79; **FAP:** Assoc Prof UMDNJ New Jersey Sch Osteo Med; **SI:** *Women's Health; Prevention;* **HMO:** Blue Cross & Blue Shield Aetna-US Healthcare Mercy Health Plans QualCare Prudential +

LANG: Sp; 🚗 ♿ 🌙 📷 ♿ ♿ Mcr Mcd WC
A Few Days 💳 *VISA* 💳 💳

Di Giacomo, William (MD) IM PCP
St Michael's Med Ctr

1072 S Orange Ave; Newark, NJ 07106; (201) 623-5309; **BDCERT:** IM 78; **MS:** Mexico 74; **RES:** St Michael's Med Ctr, Newark, NJ 75-78; **HOSP:** Overlook Hosp

LANG: Sp; ♿ 🌙 📷 ♿ ♿ S Immediately

Dower, Samuel (MD)　　IM
St Barnabas Hosp-Bronx

Josyln Center For Diabetes, 200 S Orange Ave; Livingston, NJ 07039; (973) 322-7200; **BDCERT:** IM 84; EDM 87; **MS:** NYU Sch Med 81; **RES:** IM, Albert Einstein Med Ctr, Bronx, NY 82-84; **FEL:** EDM, Mount Sinai Med Ctr, New York, NY 84-85

Gewirtz, George (MD)　　IM
St Barnabas Med Ctr-Livingston

Joselyn Center, 200 S Orange Ave; Livingston, NJ 07039; (973) 322-7200; **BDCERT:** IM 72; **MS:** Harvard Med Sch 65; **RES:** Columbia-Presbyterian Med Ctr, New York, NY 70-71; **HMO:** Most

⬆ 🅂🄰 📷 🄺 🎬 🅂 Mcr Mcd　4+ Weeks ▦ **VISA** ●

Haggerty, Mary (MD)　　IM　　PCP
Newark Beth Israel Med Ctr

201 Lyons Ave; Newark, NJ 07112; (201) 926-7472; **BDCERT:** IM 83; Ger 90; **MS:** UMDNJ-NJ Med Sch, Newark 79; **RES:** IM, Univ of Med & Dent NJ Hosp, Newark, NJ 79; **FAP:** Assoc Clin Prof UMDNJ-NJ Med Sch, Newark; **HOSP:** Univ of Med & Dent NJ Hosp; *SI: Preventive Medicine; Hypertension*; **HMO:** Aetna-US Healthcare HMO Blue CIGNA Oxford First Option +

⬆ 🅲 📷 🄺 🎬 🅂 Mcr Mcd　2-4 Weeks

Kramer, Neil (MD)　　IM
St Barnabas Med Ctr-Livingston

200 S Orange Ave; Livingston, NJ 07039; (201) 322-7400; **BDCERT:** IM 77; Rhu 80; **MS:** Univ Penn 74; **RES:** VA Med Ctr-Manh, New York, NY 75-78; **FEL:** Rhu, New York University Med Ctr, New York, NY 78-80

⬆ 📷 🄺 🎬 Mcr Mcd NFI　4+ Weeks ▦ **VISA** ●

Labissiere, Jean-Claude (MD)　IM
Hosp Ctr at Orange

280 Henry St; Orange, NJ 07050; (201) 676-6661; **BDCERT:** IM 88; **MS:** Haiti 77; **RES:** IM, Lincoln Med & Mental Hlth Ctr, Bronx, NY 81-84; **FEL:** Pul, Univ of Med & Dent NJ Hosp, Newark, NJ 84-86; **HOSP:** St Barnabas Med Ctr-Livingston; **HMO:** HMO Blue GHI Oxford Magnacare

LANG: Fr, Sp; ⬆ 🅲 📷 🎬 🅂 Mcr　A Few Days

Peyser, Donald (MD)　　IM
St Barnabas Med Ctr-Livingston

225 Millburn Ave 104A; Millburn, NJ 07041; (201) 467-5800; **BDCERT:** IM 68; **MS:** U Rochester 58; **RES:** IM, Boston VA Med Ctr, Boston, MA 61-63; **FEL:** Cv, Peter Bent Brigham Hosp, Boston, MA 63-64; *SI: Heart Disease*

⬆ 📷 🄺 🎬 🅂 Mcr　1 Week

Reichman, Lee (MD)　　IM
Univ of Med & Dent NJ Hosp

New Jersey Medical School National Tuberculosis Center, 65 Bergen St GB1; Newark, NJ 07107; (973) 972-3270; **BDCERT:** IM 72; Pul 72; **MS:** NYU Sch Med 64; **RES:** Bellevue Hosp Ctr, New York, NY 67-68; Harlem Hosp Ctr, New York, NY 68-70; **FEL:** Pul, Harlem Hosp Ctr, New York, NY; **HOSP:** Union Hosp-New Jersey

LANG: Sp; ⬆ 📷 🎬 Mcr Mcd WC　Immediately

Smith, Leon G (MD)　　IM
St Michael's Med Ctr

189 Eagle Rock Ave; Roseland, NJ 07068; (973) 877-5482; **BDCERT:** IM 63; Inf 74; **MS:** Georgetown U 56; **RES:** Georgetown U Hosp, Washington, DC 56-57; IM, Yale-New Haven Hosp, New Haven, CT 60-62; **FEL:** Inf, Yale University, New Haven, CT 59-60; **HOSP:** Univ of Med & Dent NJ Hosp; *SI: Infectious Disease*

⬆ 📷 🄺 🎬 🅂 Mcr Mcd　4+ Weeks

Soroko, Theresa (MD)　　IM
Clara Maass Med Ctr

Infectious Disease Group, 199 Broad St 2A; Bloomfield, NJ 07003; (973) 748-4583; **BDCERT:** IM 88; Inf 92; **MS:** Grenada 85; **RES:** IM, St Michael's Med Ctr, New York, NY 86-88; **FEL:** Inf, St Michael's Med Ctr, Newark, NJ 88; **HOSP:** Mountainside Hosp

LANG: Itl; ⬆ 📷 🄺 🎬 🅂 Mcr WC　A Few Days

Guide to symbols and abbreviations can be found on pages 110-113.

905

Wangenheim, Paul (MD)   IM
St Barnabas Med Ctr-Livingston

Consultants In Cardiology, 374 Millburn Ave 402;
Millburn, NJ 07041; (201) 467-1544; **BDCERT:** IM
87; Cv 87; **MS:** UMDNJ-NJ Med Sch, Newark 82;
RES: VA Med Ctr, Orange, NJ 82-85; Univ of Med &
Dent NJ Hosp, Newark, NJ 85; **FEL:** Cv, Newark
Beth Israel Med Ctr, Newark, NJ 85-87; **HOSP:**
Morristown Mem Hosp; **SI:** *Invasive Cardiology;*
Echocardiology; **HMO:** First Option Guardian
🔲 🔲 🔲 🔲 🔲 Mcr Mcd WC NFi Immediately

Wu, Chia (MD)   IM   PCP
Hosp Ctr at Orange

35 Park Ave; West Orange, NJ 07052; (973) 325-
3445; **BDCERT:** IM 72; **MS:** Taiwan 69; **RES:** Med,
Martland Hosp, Newark, NJ 70-72; **FEL:** Cv,
Martland Hosp, Newark, NJ 72-74; **FAP:** Asst Clin
Prof Med UMDNJ New Jersey Sch Osteo Med; **HOSP:**
JT Mather Mem Hosp Pt Jfrson; **SI:** *Cardiology;*
HMO: Aetna Hlth Plan Blue Choice Prucare
LANG: Chi; 🔲 🔲 🔲 🔲 🔲 Mcr WC 2-4 Weeks

Zucker, Mark (MD)   IM
Newark Beth Israel Med Ctr

Heart Failure Treatment & Transplant Program,
201 Lyons Ave ACC4; Newark, NJ 07112; (973)
926-7205; **BDCERT:** IM 84; **MS:** Northwestern U
81; **RES:** IM, Northwestern Mem Hosp, Chicago, IL
81-84; **FEL:** Cv, Northwestern Mem Hosp, Chicago,
IL 84-87; **FAP:** Asst Prof UMDNJ New Jersey Sch
Osteo Med; **SI:** *Heart Transplantation; Heart Failure;*
HMO: Aetna-US Healthcare Oxford First Option
Blue Choice CIGNA +
LANG: Sp; 🔲 🔲 🔲 🔲 Mcr Mcd WC NFi A Few Days

MEDICAL GENETICS

Desposito, Franklin (MD)   MG
Univ of Med & Dent NJ Hosp

UMDNJ Hosp, 150 Bergen St; Newark, NJ 07103;
(973) 972-5276; **BDCERT:** CG 82; Ped 86; **MS:** U
Hlth Sci/Chicago Med Sch 57; **RES:** Ped, Long
Island Jewish Med Ctr, New Hyde Park, NY 58-61;
FEL: Hem, U WI Sch Med, Milwaukee, WI 61-63;
FAP: Prof Ped UMDNJ-NJ Med Sch, Newark; **SI:**
Birth Defects; Family Genetic Disorders; **HMO:** HMO
Blue Mercy Health Plans Aetna-US Healthcare
Prucare Prudential +
LANG: Sp, Prt, Fr; 🔲 🔲 🔲 🔲 🔲 🔲 Mcr Mcd WC 2-
4 Weeks

MEDICAL ONCOLOGY

Decter, Julian A (MD)   Onc
St Barnabas Med Ctr-Livingston

101 Old Short Hills Rd 405; W Orange, NJ 07052;
(201) 926-7140; **BDCERT:** Hem 74; Onc 75; **MS:**
NYU Sch Med 66; **RES:** Ohio State U Hosp,
Columbus, OH; **FEL:** New York University Med Ctr,
New York, NY; Nat Cancer Inst, Bethesda, MD;
FAP: Assoc Prof UMDNJ New Jersey Sch Osteo Med;
HOSP: Newark Beth Israel Med Ctr; **SI:**
Lymphoma/Leukemia/Myeloma; Breast/Lung Cancer;
HMO: Prucare HMO Blue Aetna Hlth Plan Oxford
US Hlthcre +
LANG: Sp, Itl, Fr, Rus; 🔲 🔲 🔲 🔲 🔲 🔲 Mcr Mcd
Immediately

Lowenthal, Dennis (MD)   Onc
Overlook Hosp

150 Morris Ave; Springfield, NJ 07081; (973) 376-
5777; **BDCERT:** Hem 96; Onc 95; **MS:** Boston U 79;
RES: IM, Montefiore Med Ctr, Bronx, NY 80-82;
FEL: Hem, Montefiore Med Ctr, Bronx, NY 82-83;
Onc, Mem Sloan Kettering Cancer Ctr, New York,
NY 84-86; **FAP:** Clin Instr Med Columbia P&S; **SI:**
Lymphoma Leukemia; Breast Cancer; **HMO:** HIP
Network CIGNA Blue Cross & Blue Shield Oxford
Aetna Hlth Plan +
🔲 🔲 🔲 🔲 Mcr A Few Days **VISA** 💳

Michaelson, Richard (MD)   Onc
St Barnabas Med Ctr-Livingston

St Barnabas, 92 Old Short Hills Rd; Livingston, NJ 07021; (973) 322-5362; **BDCERT:** IM 81; Onc 81; **MS:** Univ Penn 76; **RES:** IM, Hosp of U Penn, Philadelphia, PA 77-79; **FEL:** Onc, Mem Sloan Kettering Cancer Ctr, New York, NY 79-81; **SI:** *Breast Cancer;* **HMO:** Aetna-US Healthcare Blue Select First Option CIGNA Prucare +

🚻 📞 🔒 🏥 🛏 Mcr Mcd 2-4 Weeks ▨ **VISA** 📇

Weiss, Stanley H (MD)   Onc
Univ of Med & Dent NJ Hosp

42 Ridge Dr; Livingston, NJ 07039; (201) 982-4623; **BDCERT:** IM 81; Onc 85; **MS:** Harvard Med Sch 78; **RES:** IM, Montefiore Med Ctr, Bronx, NY 78-81; **FEL:** Nat Cancer Inst, Bethesda, MD 82-85; Epidemiology, Nat Cancer Inst, Bethesda, MD 83-87; **FAP:** Assoc Prof UMDNJ-NJ Med Sch, Newark; **SI:** *Breast Diseases; HIV*

🚻 📞 🔒 🏥 🛏 Mcr Mcd A Few Days

NEPHROLOGY

Byrd, Lawrence H (MD)   Nep
St Barnabas Hosp-Bronx

Hypertension & Renal Group, 22 Old Short Hills Rd 212; Livingston, NJ 07039; (201) 994-4550; **BDCERT:** Nep 78; **MS:** Penn State U-Hershey Med Ctr 73; **RES:** Med, Univ of Med & Dent NJ Hosp, Newark, NJ 74-76; **FEL:** Nep, NY Hosp-Cornell Med Ctr, New York, NY 76-78; **HOSP:** Bayonne Hosp; **SI:** *Hypertension*

🚻 📞 🔒 🏥 🛏 $ A Few Days **VISA** 📇

Grasso, Michael (MD)   Nep
Newark Beth Israel Med Ctr

Nephrology Group, 111 Northfield Ave 311; West Orange, NJ 07052; (973) 325-2103; **BDCERT:** IM 74; Nep 76; **MS:** U Md Sch Med 70; **RES:** U MD Hosp, Baltimore, MD 71-74; **FEL:** Nep, Newark Beth Israel Med Ctr, Newark, NJ 74-76; **HOSP:** Hosp Ctr at Orange

🚻 🔒 🛏 $ Mcr Mcd 1 Week

Lyman, Neil (MD)   Nep
St Barnabas Med Ctr-Livingston

769 Northfield Ave 200; W Orange, NJ 07052; (973) 736-2212; **BDCERT:** IM 76; Nep 80; **MS:** Albert Einstein Coll Med 73; **RES:** Mount Sinai Med Ctr, New York, NY 73-76; **FEL:** Boston Med Ctr, Boston, MA 76-77; Mount Sinai Med Ctr, New York, NY 77-79; **FAP:** Asst Prof Nep UMDNJ-NJ Med Sch, Newark; **HOSP:** Clara Maass Med Ctr; **SI:** *Hemodialysis; Peritoneal Dialysis;* **HMO:** Prucare CIGNA Oxford

LANG: Sp, Heb, Itl; 🚻 🔒 🛏 Mcr Mcd A Few Days **VISA** 📇

Thomsen, Stephen (MD)   Nep   `PCP`
Christ Hosp

123 Highland Ave; Glen Ridge, NJ 07028; (973) 429-1881; **BDCERT:** IM 81; **MS:** Italy 77; **RES:** IM, Mountainside Hosp, Montclair, NJ 77-80; **FEL:** Nep, Univ of Med & Dent NJ Hosp, Newark, NJ 80-82; **HOSP:** Mountainside Hosp; **SI:** *Diabetes; Hypertension;* **HMO:** Oxford First Option Aetna Hlth Plan Blue Cross & Blue Shield Empire Blue Cross & Shield +

LANG: Itl, Sp; 🚻 🔒 🏥 🛏 $ Mcr Mcd A Few Days

NEUROLOGICAL SURGERY

Carmel, Peter (MD)   NS
Univ of Med & Dent NJ Hosp

90 Bergen St 7300; Newark, NJ 07103; (973) 972-2323; **BDCERT:** NS 68; **MS:** NYU Sch Med 60; **RES:** Columbia-Presbyterian Med Ctr, New York, NY 66; **FEL:** Neuroanatomy, Nat Inst Health, Bethesda, MD; **HOSP:** Hackensack Univ Med Ctr

🚻 🔒 🛏 $ Mcr Mcd WC A Few Days

Hubschmann, Otakar (MD)   NS
St Barnabas Med Ctr-Livingston

101 Old Short Hills Rd #409; W Orange, NJ
07052; (973) 325-6732; **BDCERT:** NS 78; **MS:**
Czechoslovakia 67; **RES:** Albert Einstein Coll Med,
Bronx, NY; **FEL:** C/NPh, U Texas,, Texas, TX;
C/NPh, Albert Einstein Coll Med,, Bronx, NY;
HOSP: Newark Beth Israel Med Ctr; **HMO:**
Prudential Oxford US Hlthcre HMO Blue First
Option +

LANG: Czc, Pol, Sp; 🚹 📷 🏠 💲 Mcr Mcd WC NFI
A Few Days

Schulder, Michael (MD)   NS
Univ of Med & Dent NJ Hosp

Neurological Surgery, 90 Bergen St 7300; Newark,
NJ 07103; (973) 972-2907; **BDCERT:** NS 91; **MS:**
Columbia P&S 82; **RES:** NS, Montefiore Med Ctr,
Bronx, NY 82-88; **FAP:** Assoc Prof UMDNJ New
Jersey Sch Osteo Med; **HOSP:** Hackensack Univ Med
Ctr; *SI: Brain Tumors; Sterotactic Radiosurgery;*
HMO: Aetna Hlth Plan CIGNA NYLCare Prucare
Blue Cross & Blue Shield +

LANG: Sp, Fr, Heb, Rus; 🚹 📷 🏠 💲 Mcr Mcd WC NFI
A Few Days **VISA** 💳

NEUROLOGY

Cook, Stuart (MD)   N
St Barnabas Med Ctr-Livingston

185 S Orange Ave H506; Newark, NJ 07103;
(973) 972-5208; **BDCERT:** N 70; **MS:** Univ Vt Coll
Med 62; **RES:** Univ Hosp SUNY Syracuse, Syracuse,
NY 62-63; Albert Einstein Med Ctr, Bronx, NY 65-
68; **HOSP:** Univ of Med & Dent NJ Hosp; *SI: Multiple
Sclerosis; Peripheral Neuropathy;* **HMO:** CIGNA

🚹 📷 👥 🏠 💲   4+ Weeks ▦ **VISA** 💳

Frankel, Jeffrey (MD)   N
St Barnabas Med Ctr-Livingston

Essex Neurological Assoc, 340 E Northfield Rd 2A;
Livingston, NJ 07039; (973) 994-3322; **BDCERT:**
N 72; **MS:** U Chicago-Pritzker Sch Med 66; **RES:** N,
Albert Einstein Med Ctr, Bronx, NY 67-70; **FAP:**
Assoc Clin Prof N UMDNJ New Jersey Sch Osteo
Med; **HMO:** Prucare CIGNA Prucare Magnacare
Cost Care +

🚹 📷 🏠 💲 Mcd WC NFI

Koenigsberger, M Richard (MD)   N
Univ of Med & Dent NJ Hosp

185 S Orange Ave; Newark, NJ 07103; (973) 972-
5204; **BDCERT:** Ped 66; ChiN 72; **MS:** U Chicago-
Pritzker Sch Med 59; **RES:** Ped, Columbia-
Presbyterian Med Ctr, New York, NY 60-62; **FEL:**
ChiN, Columbia-Presbyterian Med Ctr, New York,
NY 65-68; **FAP:** Assoc Prof ChiN UMDNJ New
Jersey Sch Osteo Med; **HOSP:** Hackensack Univ Med
Ctr; *SI: Neonatal Care;* **HMO:** CIGNA Beech Street
Blue Choice HMO Blue Magnacare +

LANG: Sp, Chi, Kor, Fr; 🚹 📷 👥 🏠 💲 Mcd NFI   2-
4 Weeks **VISA** 💳 🏧

Marks, David A (MD)   N
Univ of Med & Dent NJ Hosp

150 Bergen St Ste 4100; Newark, NJ 07103; (973)
972-2550; **BDCERT:** N 89; **MS:** South Africa 83;
RES: N, Boston Med Ctr, Boston, MA 85-88; **FEL:**
Neurophysiology, New England Med Ctr, Boston,
MA 88-89; Epilepsy, Yale-New Haven Hosp, New
Haven, CT 89-91; **FAP:** Assoc Prof Med UMDNJ-NJ
Med Sch, Newark; *SI: Epilepsy—Seizure; Headache—
Migraine*

LANG: Sp, Rus; 🚹 📷 👥 🏠 💲 Mcr Mcd WC NFI
A Few Days ▦ **VISA** 💳 🏧

Ruderman, Marvin (MD) N
St Barnabas Med Ctr-Livingston
Neurology Associates, 33 Clinton Rd 109; West Caldwell, NJ 07006; (973) 227-3344; **BDCERT:** N 81; **MS:** Columbia P&S 76; **RES:** Med, St Luke's Roosevelt Hosp Ctr, New York, NY 76-77; N, Barnes Hosp, St Louis, MO 77-80; **FEL:** Neuromuscular, Columbia-Presbyterian Med Ctr, New York, NY 80-81; **FAP:** Asst Clin Prof N UMDNJ New Jersey Sch Osteo Med; **HOSP:** Mountainside Hosp; ***SI:*** *Neuromuscular Disorders*; **HMO:** Blue Cross & Blue Shield United Healthcare Aetna-US Healthcare First Option
♿ ☾ ☎ 👤 📅 $ [Mcr] [WC] [NFI] 1 Week

OBSTETRICS & GYNECOLOGY

Apuzzio, Joseph (MD) ObG
Univ of Med & Dent NJ Hosp
185 S Orange Ave E506; Newark, NJ 07103; (973) 972-5557; **BDCERT:** ObG 78; MF 84; **MS:** UMDNJ-NJ Med Sch, Newark 73; **RES:** Univ of Med & Dent NJ Hosp, Newark, NJ 73-76; **FEL:** MF, Univ of Med & Dent NJ Hosp, Newark, NJ 80-82; **FAP:** Prof ObG; **HOSP:** St Elizabeth Hosp; ***SI:*** *High Risk Obstetrics; Prenatal Diagnosis*; **HMO:** Aetna Hlth Plan Blue Cross & Blue Shield CIGNA
LANG: Sp; ♿ [SA SU] ☎ 👤 📅 [Mcr] [Mcd] A Few Days VISA

Bardeguez, Arlene (MD) ObG
Univ of Med & Dent NJ Hosp
University OBGYN Associates, 90 Bergen St 50100; Newark, NJ 07103; (973) 972-2700; **BDCERT:** ObG 88; MF 89; **MS:** U Puerto Rico 81; **RES:** Catholic Med Ctr Bklyn & Qns, Jamaica, NY 85; **FEL:** MF, Nassau County Med Ctr, East Meadow, NY 85-87; **HMO:** Aetna Hlth Plan Empire
♿ ☎ 👤 📅 $ [Mcr] [Mcd] A Few Days VISA [MasterCard]

Breen, James (MD) ObG
St Barnabas Med Ctr-Livingston
Old Short Hills Rd Ste 401; Livingston, NJ 07039; (973) 533-5280; **BDCERT:** ObG 61; **MS:** Northwestern U 52; **RES:** ObG, Walter Reed Army Med Ctr, Washington, DC 54-57; **FEL:** GO, Walter Reed Army Med Ctr, Washington, DC 57-58; Path, Armed Forces Inst, Washington, DC 60-61; **HMO:** Cost Care First Option HMO Blue Oxford
♿ ☎ 📅 $ [Mcr] [Mcd] 2-4 Weeks [MasterCard]

Cooperman, Alan (MD) ObG [PCP]
Overlook Hosp
235 Millburn Ave; Millburn, NJ 07041; (201) 467-9440; **BDCERT:** ObG 79; **MS:** Italy 68; **RES:** ObG, Newark Beth Israel Med Ctr, Newark, NJ 70-73; **FAP:** Asst Clin Prof UMDNJ New Jersey Sch Osteo Med; **HOSP:** St Barnabas Med Ctr-Livingston; **HMO:** Oxford CIGNA US Hlthcre Chubb
♿ ☾ ☎ 👤 📅 $ [Mcr] [WC] Immediately [American Express] VISA [MasterCard] [Discover]

Luciani, R L (MD) ObG
Overlook Hosp
Associates Of Female Hlth Care, PA, 235 Millburn Ave; Millburn, NJ 07901; (973) 467-9440; **BDCERT:** ObG 82; **MS:** UMDNJ-NJ Med Sch, Newark 76; **RES:** ObG, St Barnabas Med Ctr, Livingston, NJ 76-80; **HOSP:** St Barnabas Med Ctr-Livingston; ***SI:*** *Laparoscopic Surgery; High risk Obstetrics*; **HMO:** US Hlthcre Prucare CIGNA Oxford Blue Cross & Blue Shield +
♿ [SA SU] ☾ ☎ 👤 📅 $ [Mcr] 2-4 Weeks VISA [MasterCard]

Sama, Jahir (MD) ObG
Univ of Med & Dent NJ Hosp
366 S Orange Ave; South Orange, NJ 07079; (973) 763-8303; **BDCERT:** ObG 72; **MS:** India 59; **RES:** ObG, Sir J J Group of Teach Hosp/Grant Med Coll, Bombay, India 60-63; ObG, Martland Hosp, Newark, NJ 67-69; **FEL:** GO, Newark City Hosp, Newark, NJ 65-67; **FAP:** Assoc Prof UMDNJ New Jersey Sch Osteo Med; **HOSP:** Clara Maass Med Ctr; ***SI:*** *Gynecologic Cancer; Gynecologic Incontinence*; **HMO:** HMO Blue Prucare First Option Oxford CIGNA +
LANG: Sp, Guj, Hin; [SA SU] ☾ ☎ 📅 $ [Mcr] A Few Days VISA [MasterCard]

Sladowski, Catherine (MD) ObG
St Barnabas Med Ctr-Livingston
West Essex OB/GYN, PC, 207 Pompton Ave;
Verona, NJ 07044; (973) 239-0052; **BDCERT:** ObG
76; **MS:** Med Coll PA 70; **RES:** St Barnabas Med Ctr,
Livingston, NJ 71-74

C 🔲 ⊞ Mcr 4+ Weeks **VISA** ●

Weiss, Gerson (MD)   ObG
Hackensack Univ Med Ctr
Center For Fertility Medicine, 90 Bergen St;
Newark, NJ 071007103; (201) 393-7444;
BDCERT: ObG 71; **MS:** NYU Sch Med 64; **RES:** IM,
Baltimore City Hosp, Baltimore, MD 64-65; ObG,
New York University Med Ctr, New York, NY 65-
69; **FEL:** RE, U of Pittsburgh Med Ctr, Pittsburgh,
PA 71-73; **FAP:** Prof UMDNJ-NJ Med Sch, Newark;
SI: *Infertility; Menopause;* **HMO:** US Hlthcre Metlife
Blue Cross

LANG: Sp; 🔲 🔲 🔲 ⊞ Mcr 1 Week

OPHTHALMOLOGY

Ball, Charles (MD)   Oph
St Barnabas Med Ctr-Livingston
Short Hills Opthalmology Group, 551 Millburn
Ave; Short Hills, NJ 07078; (973) 379-2544;
BDCERT: Oph 69; **MS:** NYU Sch Med 62; **RES:** Oph,
Bellevue Hosp Ctr, New York, NY 63-67; **HOSP:**
Newark Beth Israel Med Ctr; **SI:** *Cataract Surgery;*
Glaucoma; **HMO:** Blue Cross & Blue Choice HMO
Blue US Hlthcre CIGNA First Option +

LANG: Sp, Ger; 🔲 SA 🔲 🔲 ⊞ Mcr Mod WC 1 Week
VISA ●

Caputo, Anthony (MD)   Oph
Columbus Hosp
556 Eagle Rock Ave 203; Roseland, NJ 07068;
(973) 228-3111; **BDCERT:** Oph 76; **MS:** Italy 69;
RES: Oph, Univ of Med & Dent NJ Hosp, Newark, NJ
71-74; **FEL:** Ped Oph, Wills Eye Hosp, Philadelphia,
PA 74-75; **FAP:** Clin Prof Oph UMDNJ-NJ Med Sch,
Newark; **SI:** *Strabismus;* **HMO:** Oxford Aetna-US
Healthcare CIGNA First Option Blue Cross & Blue
Shield +

LANG: Sp, Itl, Ger; 🔲 ⊞ Mcr Mod WC NFI 1 Week **VISA**
●

Frohman, Larry (MD)   Oph
Univ of Med & Dent NJ Hosp
University Ophthalmology Associates, 90 Bergen St
6100; Newark, NJ 07103; (973) 972-2025;
BDCERT: Oph 85; **MS:** Univ Penn 80; **RES:** Oph,
Bellevue Hosp Ctr, New York, NY 81-84; **FEL:** Oph,
Bellevue Hosp Ctr, New York, NY 84-85; **FAP:**
Assoc Prof Oph UMDNJ New Jersey Sch Osteo Med;
HOSP: St Barnabas Med Ctr-Livingston; **SI:**
Unexplained Visual Loss; Systematic Disease (Eye);
HMO: Oxford CIGNA Prucare US Hlthcre HMO
Blue +

LANG: Fr, Sp, Prt, Chi, Itl; 🔲 🔲 ⊞ S Mcr Mod NFI 2-
4 Weeks **VISA**

Hersh, Peter (MD)   Oph
Univ of Med & Dent NJ Hosp
University Eye Assoc of NJ, 90 Bergen St 6100;
Newark, NJ 07103; (201) 982-2020; **BDCERT:**
Oph 87; **MS:** Johns Hopkins U 82; **RES:** Mass Eye &
Ear Infirmary, Boston, MA; Harvard Med Sch,
Cambridge, MA 86; **FEL:** Cornea, Mass Eye & Ear
Infirmary, Boston, MA; Harvard Med Sch,
Cambridge, MA; **HOSP:** Hackensack Univ Med Ctr;
SI: *Corneal Transplantation*

🔲 SA C 🔲 ⊞ S Mcr WC 1 Week ▦ **VISA** ●

Norris, John (MD)   Oph
Hosp Ctr at Orange
Northern New Jersey Eye Institute, 71 2nd St;
South Orange, NJ 07079; (973) 763-2203;
BDCERT: Oph 73; **MS:** NYU Sch Med 65; **RES:** Oph,
UMDNJ Mental Health Ctr, Piscataway, NJ 68-71;
Misericordia Hosp, Bronx, NY 66; **FAP:** Assoc Clin
Prof UMDNJ New Jersey Sch Osteo Med; **HOSP:**
Univ of Med & Dent NJ Hosp; **SI:** *Cataracts*

LANG: Sp, Fr; 🔲 SA 🔲 🔲 ⊞ S Mcr Mod WC NFI
1 Week

Wagner, Rudolph (MD) Oph
St Barnabas Med Ctr-Livingston

Children's Eye Care Ctr at Columbus Hospital, 495 N 13th St; Newark, NJ 07107; (973) 485-3186; **BDCERT:** Oph 83; **MS:** UMDNJ-NJ Med Sch, Newark 78; **RES:** Univ of Med & Dent NJ Hosp, Newark, NJ 79-82; **FEL:** Ped Oph, Wills Eye Hosp, Philadelphia, PA; **FAP:** Assoc Clin Prof Oph UMDNJ New Jersey Sch Osteo Med; **HOSP:** Univ of Med & Dent NJ Hosp; **SI:** *Strabismus Surgery; Botox Injections*; **HMO:** US Hlthcre Oxford First Option United Healthcare Prucare +

LANG: Sp; ⓩ ⬡ ⬛ ⏰ ⬛ ⬛ ⬛ ⬛ ⬛
A Few Days

Zarbin, Marco (MD) Oph
Univ of Med & Dent NJ Hosp

Univ of Med & Dent NJ Hosp—Oph Dept, 90 Bergen St 6100; Newark, NJ 07103; (973) 972-2038; **BDCERT:** Oph 89; **MS:** Johns Hopkins U 84; **RES:** Johns Hopkins Hosp, Baltimore, MD 85-88; **FEL:** Retina Vitreous Disease, Johns Hopkins Hosp, Baltimore, MD 88-90; **HMO:** First Option Magnacare

ⓩ ⬡ ⏰ ⬛ ⬛ ⬛ ⬛ ⬛ A Few Days *VISA* ⬤ ⬛

ORTHOPAEDIC SURGERY

Behrens, Fred (MD) OrS
Univ of Med & Dent NJ Hosp

University Orthopaedic Specialists, 90 Bergen St Ste 1200; Newark, NJ 07103; (973) 972-5350; **BDCERT:** OrS 83; **MS:** Switzerland 68; **RES:** McGill Teaching Hosp, Montreal, Canada 70-76; **FEL:** McGill Teaching Hosp, Montreal, Canada 76-77; U of VA Health Sci Ctr, Charlottesville, VA; **FAP:** Prof UMDNJ New Jersey Sch Osteo Med; **HOSP:** Overlook Hosp; **SI:** *Problem Fractures & Complications.; Limb Deformities*; **HMO:** Oxford Multiplan US Hlthcre CIGNA QualCare +

LANG: Sp, Prt, Itl, Fr, Ger; ⓩ ⬡ ⏰ ⬛ ⬛ ⬛ ⬛ ⬛
A Few Days ⬛ *VISA* ⬤ ⬛

Benvenia, Joseph (MD) OrS
Univ of Med & Dent NJ Hosp

90 Bergen St #1200; Newark, NJ 07103; (973) 972-2153; **BDCERT:** OrS 92; **MS:** UMDNJ-NJ Med Sch, Newark 84; **RES:** Univ of Med & Dent NJ Hosp, Newark, NJ 84-89; **FEL:** Case Western Reserve U Hosp, Cleveland, OH 90-91; **SI:** *Muscular Skeletal Oncology*

ⓩ ⬡ ⏰ ⬛ ⬛ ⬛ ⬛ 1 Week ⬛ *VISA* ⬤ ⬛

Decter, Edward (MD) OrS
St Barnabas Med Ctr-Livingston

315 E Northfield Rd; Livingston, NJ 07039; (973) 535-9000; **BDCERT:** OrS 82; **MS:** Creighton U 75; **RES:** Hosp For Joint Diseases, New York, NY 76-80; Temple U, Philadelphia, PA 75-76; **HMO:** Prucare Metlife US Hlthcre Magnacare First Option +

ⓩ ⬡ ⬛ ⏰ ⬛ ⬛ ⬛ ⬛ Immediately *VISA* ⬤

Gennace, Ronald (MD) OrS
West Hudson Hosp

629 Belgrove Drive; Kearny, NJ 07032; (201) 997-8777; **BDCERT:** OrS 82; **MS:** UMDNJ-NJ Med Sch, Newark 76; **RES:** St Joseph's Hosp, Paterson, NJ 76-80

Schob, Clifford (MD) OrS
Overlook Hosp

159 Millburn Ave; Millburn, NJ 07041; (973) 258-1177; **BDCERT:** OrS 92; **MS:** UMDNJ New Jersey Sch Osteo Med 82; **RES:** S, Long Island Jewish Med Ctr, New Hyde Park, NY 82-84; OrS, Long Island Jewish Med Ctr, New Hyde Park, NY 84-88; **FEL:** SM, American Sports Med Inst, Birmingham, AL 89; **SI:** *Sports Injury; Arthroscopic Surgery*; **HMO:** PHS HMO Blue Blue Cross & Blue Shield CIGNA Oxford +

ⓩ ⬛ ⬡ ⏰ ⬛ ⬛ ⬛ ⬛ A Few Days *VISA* ⬤

Guide to symbols and abbreviations can be found on pages 110-113.

911

OTOLARYNGOLOGY

Baredes, Soly (MD)   Oto
Univ of Med & Dent NJ Hosp
90 Bergen St 7200; Newark, NJ 07103; (973) 226-
3444; **BDCERT:** Oto 81; **MS:** Columbia P&S 76;
RES: S, St Luke's Roosevelt Hosp Ctr, New York, NY
76-77; Oto, Columbia-Presbyterian Med Ctr, New
York, NY 77-80; **FEL:** Head & Neck S, Beth Israel
Med Ctr, New York, NY 80-81; **FAP:** Assoc Clin
Prof Oto UMDNJ New Jersey Sch Osteo Med; **HOSP:**
St Barnabas Med Ctr-Livingston; **SI:** *Head and Neck
Tumors; Voice and Swallowing Disorders*; **HMO:**
QualCare Blue Cross & Blue Shield First Option
Magnacare US Hlthcre +

🚻 🔲 🔣 🏧 $ Mcr Mcd WC NFI   1 Week **VISA** 💳

Chandrasekhar, Sujana (MD) Oto
Univ of Med & Dent NJ Hosp
NJMS Doctors Office Center, 90 Bergen St Ste 7200;
Newark, NJ 07103; (973) 972-2537; **BDCERT:** Oto
93; **MS:** Mt Sinai Sch Med 86; **RES:** Oto, New York
University Med Ctr, New York, NY 86-92; **FEL:**
Neurotology, House Ear Inst, Los Angeles, CA 93;
FAP: Asst Prof UMDNJ New Jersey Sch Osteo Med;
HOSP: St Barnabas Med Ctr-Livingston; **SI:** *Hearing
& Balance Disorder; Facial Nerve, Acoustic Tumors*;
HMO: First Option Aetna Hlth Plan US Hlthcre UHP
+

LANG: Sp, Kan, Grk, Pol; 🚻 🔲 🔣 🏧 $ Mcr Mcd WC
NFI   1 Week **VISA** 💳

Fieldman, Robert (MD)   Oto
St Barnabas Med Ctr-Livingston
Associates In Otolaryngology of NJ, 741 Northfield
Ave 104; W Orange, NJ 07052; (201) 243-0600;
BDCERT: Oto 86; **MS:** Tulane U 81; **RES:** Oto, NY
Hosp-Cornell Med Ctr, New York, NY; **HOSP:**
Newark Beth Israel Med Ctr; **SI:** *Chronic Sinusitis;
Pediatric Otolaryngology*; **HMO:** Aetna-US
Healthcare CIGNA Oxford Blue Cross & Blue Shield
Guardian +

LANG: Sp; 🚻 🔲 🔣 🏧 $ Mcr WC NFI   Immediately
▦ **VISA** 💳 ▬

Jahn, Anthony (MD)   Oto
St Barnabas Med Ctr-Livingston
556 Eagle Rock Ave 201; Roseland, NJ 07068;
(973) 226-2262; **BDCERT:** Oto 79; **MS:** Canada
74; **RES:** Oto, U Toronto Gen Hosp, Totonto,
Canada 74; **FAP:** Prof Oto Columbia P&S; **HOSP:** St
Luke's Roosevelt Hosp Ctr; **SI:** *Ear Diseases, Hearing
Loss, Vertigo; Disorders of the Voice*; **HMO:** First
Option Blue Cross & Blue Shield Prucare
Physician's Health Plan

LANG: Sp, Hun; 🚻 🔲 🔣 🏧 🏨 $ WC NFI   1 Week
VISA 💳

Levey, Mark (MD)   Oto
St Barnabas Med Ctr-Livingston
Assoc In Otolaryngology, 741 Northfield Ave 104;
West Orange, NJ 07052; (973) 243-0600;
BDCERT: Oto 70; **MS:** NY Med Coll 62; **RES:** Oto,
Mount Sinai Med Ctr, New York, NY 65-69; **FAP:**
Assoc UMDNJ-RW Johnson Med Sch; **SI:** *Nose/Sinus
Disease; Tumors of the Head /Neck*; **HMO:** Oxford Blue
Cross Magnacare First Option Prudential +

LANG: Sp; 🚻 🔲 🔣 🏧 🏨 $ Mcr WC NFI
Immediately **VISA** 💳

PEDIATRIC ALLERGY & IMMUNOLOGY

Fost, Arthur (MD)   PA&I
Clara Maass Med Ctr
Allergy, Asthma Finer Center of NJ, 5 Franklin Ave
102; Belleville, NJ 07109; (973) 759-2029;
BDCERT: A&I 72; Ped 68; **MS:** Jefferson Med Coll
63; **RES:** Children's Hosp of Philadelphia,
Philadelphia, PA 65-66; St Vincents Hosp & Med
Ctr NY, New York, NY 66-68; **HMO:** Aetna Hlth
Plan Blue Cross & Blue Shield CIGNA

🚻 🔲 🔣 🏧 🏨 Mcr Mcd WC   A Few Days ▦ **VISA**

PEDIATRIC CARDIOLOGY

Langsner, Alan (MD)   **PCd**
St Vincents Hosp & Med Ctr NY
405 Northfield Ave Ste 204; West Orange, NJ
07052; (973) 736-8883; **BDCERT:** Ped 83; **MS:**
Mexico 77; **RES:** Ped, Metropolitan Hosp Ctr, New
York, NY 78-80; **FEL:** PCd, New York University
Med Ctr, New York, NY 81-83; **FAP:** Asst Clin Prof
Ped NYU Sch Med; **HOSP:** New York University
Med Ctr; **SI:** *Pediatric Cardiology; Fetal
Echocardiology;* **HMO:** Aetna Hlth Plan CIGNA GHI
US Hlthcre Empire +

LANG: Sp; 🔲 🔲 🔲 🔲 🔲 🔲 🔲 Immediately

PEDIATRIC ENDOCRINOLOGY

Skuza, Kathryn (MD)   **PEn**
United Hosp Med Ctr
UMDNJ/NJ Medical School185 SO Orange Ave,
185 S Orange Ave; Newark, NJ 07103; (973) 972-
2100; **BDCERT:** Ped 87; PEn 89; **MS:** Poland 82;
RES: Ped, Univ of Med & Dent NJ Hosp, Newark, NJ
82-85; **FEL:** EDM, Univ of Med & Dent NJ Hosp,
Newark, NJ 85-88; **FAP:** Asst Prof UMDNJ New
Jersey Sch Osteo Med; **HOSP:** St Barnabas Med Ctr-
Livingston; **SI:** *Pediatric Diabetes; Thyroid Disorders;*
HMO: Prudential Oxford US Hlthcre QualCare
American Health Plan +

LANG: Pol, Ukr, Ar; 🔲 🔲 🔲 🔲 🔲 🔲 🔲 🔲 🔲
A Few Days **VISA** 💳

PEDIATRIC GASTROENTEROLOGY

Sunaryo, Francis (MD)   **PGe**
Children's Hosp of New Jersey
400 Osborne Terr; Newark, NJ 07112; (973) 926-
7328; **BDCERT:** Ped 97; PGe 90; **MS:** Indonesia 73;
RES: Ped, Misericordia Hosp, Bronx, NY 77-78;
Ped, N Shore Univ Hosp-Manhasset, Manhasset,
NY 78-79; **FEL:** PGe, Children's Hosp of
Philadelphia, Philadelphia, PA 79-82; **FAP:** Asst
Prof UMDNJ New Jersey Sch Osteo Med; **SI:**
Inflammatory Bowel Disease; Pediatric Liver Disease;
HMO: Blue Cross & Blue Shield Aetna Hlth Plan
Prucare US Hlthcre Oxford +

LANG: Sp, Rus; 🔲 🔲 🔲 🔲 🔲 🔲 2-4 Weeks

PEDIATRIC HEMATOLOGY-ONCOLOGY

Kamalakar, Peri (MD)   **PHO**
Newark Beth Israel Med Ctr
Valerie Fund Childrens Ct;Childrens Hospital of
New Jersey, 7 Nicholas Ct; Edison, NJ 07112; (973)
926-7161; **BDCERT:** Ped 75; **MS:** India 67; **RES:**
Newark Beth Israel Med Ctr, Newark, NJ 70-73;
FEL: PHO, Children's Hosp of Buffalo, Buffalo, NY;
HOSP: Monmouth Med Ctr; **SI:** *Leukemia & Solid
Tumors; Sickle Cell;* **HMO:** Prucare Blue Cross First
Option US Hlthcre Oxford +

LANG: Sp, Hin; 🔲 🔲 🔲 🔲 🔲 🔲 Immediately

PEDIATRIC INFECTIOUS DISEASE

Minnefor, Anthony (MD) Ped Inf
St Barnabas Med Ctr-Livingston
Director of Pediatric - St Barnabas Med Ctr, 12
Bahama Rd; Morris Plains, NJ 07950; (973) 533-
5690; **BDCERT:** Ped 70; Ped Inf 94; **MS:** UMDNJ-NJ
Med Sch, Newark 63; **RES:** Ped A&I, Yale-New
Haven Hosp, New Haven, CT 64-66; **FEL:** Inf, Johns
Hopkins Hosp, Baltimore, MD 68-70; **FAP:** Assoc
Clin Prof UMDNJ New Jersey Sch Osteo Med; *SI:*
Fever of Unknown Origin; Recurrent Infections; **HMO:**
Oxford HMO Blue CIGNA Aetna Hlth Plan
Amerihealth +

🔊 📷 🏠 💲 🏥 2-4 Weeks

PEDIATRIC NEPHROLOGY

Salcedo, Jose (MD)   PNep
St Joseph's Hosp-Patterson
703 Main St; Patersn, NJ 07053; (973) 928-2547;
BDCERT: Ped 76; PNep 76; **MS:** Mexico 70; **RES:**
Ped, Martland Hosp, Newark, NJ 71-74; **FEL:** Nep,
Children's Hosp Nat Med Ctr, Washington, DC 74-
76; Nep, Armed Forces Inst Path, Washington, DC
76-77; **HOSP:** Univ of Med & Dent NJ Hosp; *SI:*
Pediatric Dialysis; Kidney Biopsies; **HMO:** CIGNA US
Hlthcre Aetna Hlth Plan HIP Network NYLCare +

LANG: Sp; 🔊 📞 📷 🏠 🏥 💲 🏥 🏥 🏥
A Few Days

PEDIATRIC PULMONOLOGY

Aguila, Helen (MD)   PPul
Univ of Med & Dent NJ Hosp
150 Bergen St G-102; Newark, NJ 07103; (973)
972-0380; **BDCERT:** PPul 89; Ped 83; **MS:**
Philippines 74; **RES:** PPul, Univ Hosp SUNY Bklyn,
Brooklyn, NY 77-80; PM, Kings County Hosp Ctr,
Brooklyn, NY 79-80; **FEL:** PPul, Wayne Cnty Gen
Hosp, Detroit, MI 80-83; **FAP:** Asst Prof PPul
UMDNJ New Jersey Sch Osteo Med

LANG: Fil, Sp; 🔊 📷 🏥 🏥 4+ Weeks

Bisberg, Dorothy Stein (MD)PPul
Children's Hosp of New Jersey
Children's Hosp NJ/Newark Beth Israel Med Ctr,
201 Lyons Ave; South Oange, NJ 07079; (973)
926-7328; **BDCERT:** Ped 77; PPul 92; **MS:** Cornell
U 72; **RES:** Ped, Montefiore Med Ctr, Bronx, NY 72-
74; Ped, Bronx Lebanon Hosp Ctr, Bronx, NY 74-
75; **FAP:** Asst Prof of Clin Ped UMDNJ New Jersey
Sch Osteo Med; *SI: Asthma; Cystic Fibrosis;* **HMO:**
Blue Cross First Option Aetna-US Healthcare Oxford
NYLCare +

🔊 📷 👥 🏥 💲 🏥 🏥 1 Week

Kottler, William (MD)   PPul
Union Hosp-New Jersey
200 S Orange Ave 107; Livingston, NJ 07039;
(973) 322-7300; **BDCERT:** Ped 90; PPul 94; **MS:**
France 87; **RES:** Ped, Overlook Hosp, Summit, NJ
87-90; **FEL:** Pul, U FL Shands Hosp, Gainesville, FL
91-93; **FAP:** Asst Prof UMDNJ New Jersey Sch
Osteo Med; **HOSP:** St Barnabas Med Ctr-Livingston;
SI: Pediatric Asthma; Pediatric Lung Disease; **HMO:**
Prucare Aetna Hlth Plan Blue Cross Pinnacle

LANG: Fr; 🔊 📷 👥 🏥 💲 🏥 Immediately

Turcios, Nelson (MD)   PPul
Univ of Med & Dent NJ Hosp

Doctors Office Ctr NJ Med School, 90 Bergen St;
Newark, NJ 07103; (973) 972-4815; **BDCERT:** Ped
82; PPul 92; **MS:** El Salvador 73; **RES:** U Miss Med
Ctr, Jackson, MS 77-78; U MD Hosp, Baltimore, MD
78-80; **FEL:** Pul, Children's Hosp Nat Med Ctr,
Washington, DC; **HOSP:** Somerset Med Ctr

LANG: Sp; ⬧ ⬧ ⬧ ⬧ ⬧ ⬧ Immediately **VISA**
⬧

PEDIATRIC SURGERY

Bethal, Colin (MD)   PS
Univ of Med & Dent NJ Hosp

185 S Orange Ave; Newark, NJ 07103; (973) 972-
2404; **BDCERT:** PS 96; **MS:** Columbia P&S 87; **RES:**
S, Yale University, New Haven, CT 93-95; S, Yale
University, New Haven, CT 87-90; **FEL:** PdS,
Children's Hospital, Columbus, OH 96-97

PEDIATRICS

Boodish, Wesley (MD)   Ped   **PCP**
St Barnabas Med Ctr-Livingston

159 Milburn Ave; Millburn, NJ 07401; (973) 912-
0155; **BDCERT:** Ped 65; **MS:** England 60; **RES:** Ped,
US Naval Hosp, Philadelphia, PA 62-64; **HOSP:**
Overlook Hosp; **HMO:** Prucare Oxford CIGNA PHS
PHCS +

⬧ ⬧ ⬧ ⬧ ⬧ ⬧ ⬧ ⬧ **VISA** ⬧

Gruenwald, Laurence D (MD)   Ped
St Barnabas Med Ctr-Livingston

173 S Orange Ave 1B; South Orange, NJ 07079;
(973) 762-0400; **BDCERT:** Ped 81; **MS:** UMDNJ-NJ
Med Sch, Newark 75; **RES:** Ped, Children's Hosp
Nat Med Ctr, Washington, DC 75-78; **HOSP:**
Overlook Hosp

⬧ ⬧ ⬧ ⬧ ⬧ ⬧ ⬧ Immediately ⬧

Johnson, Robert (MD)   Ped
Univ of Med & Dent NJ Hosp

185 S Orange Ave; Newark, NJ 07103; (973) 972-
5377; **BDCERT:** Ped 77; **MS:** UMDNJ-NJ Med Sch,
Newark 72; **RES:** Martland Hosp, Newark, NJ 68-
72; **FEL:** New York University Med Ctr, New York,
NY 74-76; **FAP:** Prof Ped UMDNJ-NJ Med Sch,
Newark; **SI:** *Adolescent Medicine (ages 12-25);*
HIV/AIDS; **HMO:** Aetna Hlth Plan

⬧ ⬧ ⬧ ⬧ ⬧ ⬧ ⬧ ⬧ A Few Days ⬧ **VISA**
⬧

Khanna, Yash (MD)   Ped
Hosp Ctr at Orange

Family Medicine/Pediatrics, 280 Henry St; Orange,
NJ 07050; (973) 678-2900; **BDCERT:** Ped 78; **MS:**
64; **RES:** Ped, St Michael's Med Ctr, New York, NY
71-72; Ped, St Michael's Med Ctr, New York, NY
72-73; **HOSP:** Montclair Comm Hosp; **SI:** *Bronchial
Asthma; Preventive Medicine;* **HMO:** US Hlthcre
United Healthcare CIGNA PPO NYLCare Amer Pref
Prov +

LANG: Hin, Pun, Guj; ⬧ ⬧ ⬧ ⬧ ⬧ ⬧ ⬧ ⬧ ⬧
⬧ ⬧ Immediately

Marcus, Richard (MD)   Ped   **PCP**
Clara Maass Med Ctr

242 Washington Ave Ste A; Nutley, NJ 07110;
(201) 667-6676; **BDCERT:** Ped 88; **MS:** UMDNJ-NJ
Med Sch, Newark 82; **RES:** Univ of Med & Dent NJ
Hosp, Newark, NJ 82-85; **FAP:** Asst Prof UMDNJ
New Jersey Sch Osteo Med; **HOSP:** Mountainside
Hosp; **HMO:** HMO Blue Oxford HIP Network
CIGNA Aetna-US Healthcare +

⬧ ⬧ ⬧ ⬧ ⬧ ⬧ A Few Days **VISA** ⬧ ⬧

Oleske, James (MD)   Ped   **PCP**
Univ of Med & Dent NJ Hosp

UMDNJNJ Med Sch, 185 S Orange Ave; Newark, NJ
07103; (201) 982-5066; **BDCERT:** Ped 76; A&I
77; **MS:** UMDNJ-NJ Med Sch, Newark 71; **RES:** Ped,
Martland Hosp, Newark, NJ 72-73; **FEL:** MPH,
Columbia-Presbyterian Med Ctr, New York, NY 74;
FAP: Prof UMDNJ New Jersey Sch Osteo Med; **SI:**
Infectious Diseases; Allergy

⬧ ⬧ ⬧ ⬧ ⬧ ⬧ ⬧ ⬧ ⬧ A Few Days ⬧ **VISA**
⬧ ⬧

Pak, Jayoung (MD)   Ped
Univ of Med & Dent NJ Hosp

185 S Orange Ave; Newark, NJ 07103; (973) 972-5204; **BDCERT:** Ped 91; ChiN 93; **MS:** South Korea 78; **RES:** EWHA Womans U, South Korea 79-83; Univ of Med & Dent NJ Hosp, Newark, NJ 86; **FEL:** Univ of Med & Dent NJ Hosp, Newark, NJ 88; Columbia-Presbyterian Med Ctr, New York, NY 91; *SI: Neurology;* **HMO:** Blue Choice CIGNA Cost Care First Option Multiplan +

LANG: Chi, Kor, Fr, Sp, Prt; ♿ ⌂ 🏥 $ Mcd A Few Days 💳 *VISA* 💳 💳

Prystowsky, Barry (MD)   Ped
Clara Maass Med Ctr

562 Kingsland St; Nutley, NJ 07110; (201) 667-0003; **BDCERT:** Ped 86; **MS:** UMDNJ-NJ Med Sch, Newark 81; **RES:** Ped, Univ of Med & Dent NJ Hosp, Newark, NJ 84; *SI: Cardiac Diseases Pediatric;* **HMO:** Aetna Hlth Plan Prucare HMO Blue CIGNA United Healthcare +

SA/SU ⌂ 🅿 🏥 $ Mcd NFI

Prystowsky, Milton (MD)   Ped   PCP
Clara Maass Med Ctr

562 Kingsland St; Nutley, NJ 07110; (201) 667-0003; **BDCERT:** Ped 51; S 72; **MS:** Med U SC, Charleston 44; **RES:** PCd, Johns Hopkins Hosp, Baltimore, MD 48-51; Ped, Kings County Hosp Ctr, Brooklyn, NY 44-46; **FAP:** Clin Prof Ped UMDNJ, Sch Osteo Med; *SI: Cardiac Diseases;* **HMO:** Aetna Hlth Plan Blue Choice Blue Cross & Blue Shield CIGNA Metlife +

SA/SU ⌂ 🅿 🏥 $ Mcd NFI 2-4 Weeks

Rich, Andrea (MD)   Ped
Montefiore Med Ctr

59 Club Rd; Montclair, NJ 07043; (718) 920-4321; **BDCERT:** Ped 85; **MS:** Boston U 79; **RES:** Ped, Montefiore Med Ctr, Bronx, NY 80-82; **FAP:** Asst Prof Albert Einstein Coll Med

Shaw, Jennifer (MD)   Ped   PCP
Overlook Hosp

Summit Medical Group, 85 Woodland Rd; Short Hills, NJ 07078; (201) 379-2488; **MS:** U Conn Sch Med 89; **RES:** Long Island Jewish Med Ctr, New Hyde Park, NY 89-94; **FEL:** Ped, Long Island Jewish Med Ctr, New Hyde Park, NY 94; **HOSP:** St Barnabas Med Ctr-Livingston; *SI: ADHD; Behavioral Pediatrics;* **HMO:** US Hlthcre Oxford ABC Health Blue Cross & Blue Choice CIGNA +

LANG: Sp; ♿ SA/SU 🌙 ⌂ 🅿 🏥 $ NFI 2-4 Weeks 💳 *VISA* 💳

Torre, Arthur (MD)   Ped
St Joseph's Hosp-Patterson

25 Hollywood Ave; Fairfield, NJ 07004; (973) 882-0880; **BDCERT:** Ped 75; **MS:** UMDNJ-NJ Med Sch, Newark 70; **RES:** Ped, Martland Hosp, Newark, NJ 71-72; **FEL:** Ped A&I, Martland Hosp, Newark, NJ 72-73; **FAP:** Assoc Clin Prof UMDNJ-NJ Med Sch, Newark; *SI: Pediatric Asthma; Dive Medicine;* **HMO:** Blue Cross & Blue Shield QualCare John Hancock Oxford Health Choice +

SA/SU ⌂ 🅿 🏥 $ Mcd A Few Days

PHYSICAL MEDICINE & REHABILITATION

Delisa, Joel (MD)   PMR
Kessler Inst For Rehab

1199 Pleasant Valley Way; W Orange, NJ 07052; (973) 243-6805; **BDCERT:** PMR 77; **MS:** U Wash, Seattle 68; **RES:** U WA Med Ctr, Seattle, WA 75; **HOSP:** Univ of Med & Dent NJ Hosp

♿ ⌂ 🅿 🏥 Mcr Mcd WC NFI Immediately

Flanagan, Steven Robert (MD)PMR
VA Med Ctr, E Orange

77 Stanford Ave; West Orange, NJ 07052; (800) 226-0926; **BDCERT:** PMR 93; **MS:** UMDNJ-NJ Med Sch, Newark 88

Kirshblum, Steven C (MD) PMR
Kessler Inst For Rehab

1199 Pleasant Valley Way; West Orange, NJ
07052; (973) 731-3600; **BDCERT:** PMR 91; **MS:** U
Hlth Sci/Chicago Med Sch 86; **RES:** PMR, Mount
Sinai Med Ctr, New York, NY 87-90; *SI: Spinal Cord
Injury*

LANG: Sp, Heb, Pol; ♿ 🄲 🄰 🄵 🎫 Mcr Mcd WC NFI
A Few Days *VISA* 💳

Nadler, Scott (DO)   PMR
Univ of Med & Dent NJ Hosp

Univ Rehab Assocs, 90 Bergern St Ste 3100;
Newark, NJ 07103; (973) 972-2802; **BDCERT:**
PMR 95; **MS:** UMDNJ New Jersey Sch Osteo Med
90; **RES:** PMR, Univ of Med & Dent NJ Hosp,
Newark, NJ 91-94; **FEL:** SM, Kessler Inst for
Rehabilitation, East Orange, NJ 94-95; **FAP:** Asst
Prof UMDNJ-NJ Med Sch, Newark; *SI: Sports
Medicine; Low Back Pain*; **HMO:** Blue Cross Oxford
First Option QualCare GHI +

LANG: Sp, Itl, Prt; ♿ 🄰 🄵 🎫 🅂 Mcr Mcd WC NFI
A Few Days *VISA* 💳 💳

PLASTIC SURGERY

Morrow, Todd (MD)   PlS
St Barnabas Med Ctr-Livingston

741 Northfield Ave 104; W Orange, NJ 07052;
(973) 243-0600; **BDCERT:** Oto 92; PlS 95; **MS:**
Jefferson Med Coll 86; **RES:** Univ of Med & Dent NJ
Hosp, Newark, NJ 86-91; **FEL:** Facial Plastic &
Reconstructive S, U Toronto Gen Hosp, Ontario,
Canada; **FAP:** Asst Prof UMDNJ-NJ Med Sch,
Newark; **HOSP:** Newark Beth Israel Med Ctr; *SI:
Nasal Recontouring; Facial Rejuvenation*; **HMO:** First
Option HMO Blue CIGNA Prucare Aetna Hlth Plan
+

LANG: Sp; ♿ 🅂🄳 🄲 🄰 🄵 🎫 🅂 Mcr WC NFI
Immediately 📧 *VISA* 💳 💳 💳

Tutela, Rocco (MD)   PlS
Columbus Hosp

405 Northfield Ave 100; West Orange, NJ 07052;
(973) 669-1240; **BDCERT:** PlS 82; **MS:** Italy 69;
RES: PlS, Univ of Med & Dent NJ Hosp, Newark, NJ
74-76; **S,** Univ of Med & Dent NJ Hosp, Newark, NJ
71-74; **HMO:** Aetna Hlth Plan Blue Choice Blue
Cross & Blue Shield

♿ 🄲 🄰 🄵 🎫 🅂 Mcr Mcd WC NFI 2-4 Weeks

PSYCHIATRY

Nucci, Annamaria (MD)   Psyc
NY Hosp-Cornell Med Ctr

5 Westview Ct; Cedar Grove, NJ 07009; (973) 857-
2609; **BDCERT:** Psyc 78; **MS:** Italy 71; **RES:** Psyc,
NY Hosp-Cornell Med Ctr, New York, NY 71-75;
FEL: ChAP, NY Hosp-Cornell Med Ctr, New York,
NY 75-78; **HOSP:** Mountainside Hosp; *SI:
Psychotherapy; Psychopharmacotherapy*

LANG: Itl; 🅂🄳 🄲 🄰 🄵 🎫 🅂 A Few Days

Schleifer, Steven (MD)   Psyc
Univ of Med & Dent NJ Hosp

185 S Orange Ave; Newark, NJ 07103; (973) 982-
7117; **BDCERT:** Psyc 80; **MS:** Mt Sinai Sch Med 75;
RES: Los Angeles Cty Hosp, Los Angeles, CA 75-76;
Mount Sinai Med Ctr, New York, NY 76-79; **HOSP:**
Hackensack Univ Med Ctr; *SI: Depression*

♿ 🄲 🄰 Mcr A Few Days

Silver, Bennett (MD)   Psyc
Overlook Hosp

206 Millburn Ave; Millburn, NJ 07041; (973) 376-
1020; **BDCERT:** Psyc 79; **MS:** SUNY Downstate 74;
RES: Psyc, Mount Sinai Med Ctr, New York, NY 75-
78; **FEL:** ChAP, Mount Sinai Med Ctr, New York,
NY 78-80; **HOSP:** St Mary's Hosp; *SI:
Psychopharmacology; Child & Adolescent Psych*;
HMO: CIGNA PHCS

♿ 🅂🄳 🄲 🄵 🎫 🅂 Mcr A Few Days

Squires, Sandra (MD)   Psyc
NW Covenant Med Ctr-Riverside

In Health Associates, 376 Route 15 101; Sparta, NJ
07871; (973) 579-6700; **BDCERT:** Psyc 93; ChAP
94; **MS:** NY Med Coll 88; **RES:** Psyc, St Vincents
Hosp & Med Ctr NY, New York, NY 88-91; ChAP,
St Vincents Hosp & Med Ctr NY, New York, NY 91-
93; *SI: Attention Deficit Disorders; Depression*

Templeton, Hilda (MD)   Psyc
St Barnabas Med Ctr-Livingston

22 Old Short Hills Rd 217; Livingston, NJ 07039;
(973) 535-3131; **BDCERT:** Psyc 89; **MS:** UMDNJ-
NJ Med Sch, Newark 78; **RES:** Univ of Med & Dent
NJ Hosp, Newark, NJ 78-79; Rutgers U Med Ctr,
New Brunswick, NJ 79-82; *SI: Depression; Anxiety
Disorders*

♿ 🅒 📷 👥 🏨 Mcr   1 Week

PULMONARY DISEASE

Johanson, Waldemar (MD)   Pul
Univ of Med & Dent NJ Hosp

UMDNJ—Dept Med, 185 S Orange Ave; Newark, NJ
7103; (973) 972-4595; **BDCERT:** IM 69; Pul 74;
MS: U Minn 62; **RES:** IM, U MN Med Ctr,
Minneapolis, MN 65-67; **FEL:** Pul, U Texas SW Med
Ctr, Dallas, TX 67-69; **FAP:** Chrmn UMDNJ-NJ Med
Sch, Newark; *SI: Environmental Injuries; Chronic
Lung Disease;* **HMO:** Aetna-US Healthcare UHP
HMO Blue Amerihealth QualCare +

LANG: Sp; ♿ 📷 👥 🏨 Mcr Mod WC NFI *VISA* 💳 📷

Karetzky, Monroe (MD)   Pul
Newark Beth Israel Med Ctr

Newark Beth Israel Med Center, Dept of Pul Disease,
201 Lyons Ave; Newark, NJ 07112; (973) 926-
7597; **BDCERT:** PM 74; CCM 89; **MS:** Cornell U 63;
RES: Mary Imogene Bassett Hosp, Cooperstown,
NY; IM, Mary Imogene Bassett Hosp, Cooperstown,
NY; **FEL:** CP, Mary Imogene Bassett Hosp,
Cooperstown, NY; **FAP:** Asst Clin Prof UMDNJ New
Jersey Sch Osteo Med; *SI: Asthma; Sleep Disorders*

LANG: Sp, Fil; ♿ 📷 👥 🏨 S Mcr Mod WC NFI
Immediately *VISA*

McDonough, Michael (MD) Pul
Newark Beth Israel Med Ctr

Comprehensive Pulmonary & Critical Care
Associates, 2040 Millburn Ave 401; Maplewood,
NJ 07040; (973) 736-6800; **BDCERT:** Pul 90; CCM
91; **MS:** UMDNJ-NJ Med Sch, Newark 82; **RES:** IM,
UMDNJ-Univ Hosp, Newark, NJ 82-85; **FEL:** Pul,
Univ of Med & Dent of NJ Univ Hosp, , NJ 85-87;
FAP: Assoc Prof UMDNJ New Jersey Sch Osteo Med;
HOSP: Bayonne Hosp; *SI: Lung Cancer; Lung
Transplantation;* **HMO:** Aetna-US Healthcare Oxford
Blue Cross & Blue Choice First Option Prucare +

LANG: Hin, Sp; ♿ 📷 👥 🏨 S Mcr Mod WC NFI
Immediately

Safirstein, Benjamin (MD)   Pul
Mountainside Hosp

Montclair Medical Group, 62 S Fullerton Street;
Montclair, NJ 07042; (973) 744-3900; **BDCERT:**
IM 70; **MS:** U Hlth Sci/Chicago Med Sch 65; **RES:**
Mount Sinai Med Ctr, New York, NY 65-69; **FEL:**
Inst Disease of Chest, London, England 71-72;
HOSP: St Michael's Med Ctr; *SI: Asthma; Sarcoidosis;*
HMO: Oxford Magnacare Blue Cross Multicare

LANG: Ger; ♿ 📷 👥 🏨 S Mcr Mod   1 Week *VISA*

RADIATION ONCOLOGY

Zablow, Andrew (MD)   RadRO
St Barnabas Med Ctr-Livingston

Physicians In Rad/Onc, 94 Old Short Hills Rd;
Livingston, NJ 07039; (973) 322-5630; **BDCERT:**
RadRO 86; **MS:** Mexico 81; **RES:** RadRO, St
Barnabas Med Ctr, Livingston, NJ 82-86; *SI:
Prostate Cancer; Breast Cancer;* **HMO:** Prucare Blue
Cross & Blue Shield US Hlthcre

LANG: Sp; ♿ 📷 👥 🏨 S Mcr Mod WC   Immediately

RADIOLOGY

Devereux, Corinne (MD) Rad
Clara Maass Med Ctr

Clara Maass Med Onc, 1 Clara Maass Dr; Belleville,
NJ 07109; (973) 450-2270; **BDCERT:** RadRO 77;
MS: Med Coll PA 71; **RES:** Rad, Bellevue Hosp Ctr,
New York, NY 72-74; **Hosp** of U Penn,
Philadelphia, PA 74-76; **FEL:** Mem Sloan Kettering
Cancer Ctr, New York, NY 79; *SI: Breast Cancer;
Prostate Cancer;* **HMO:** Aetna Hlth Plan Blue Choice
Blue Cross & Blue Shield

LANG: Fr, Sp; ♿ ☎ 🚗 🏥 Mcr Mcd NFI

REPRODUCTIVE ENDOCRINOLOGY

Bergh, Paul A (MD) RE
St Barnabas Med Ctr-Livingston

Institute for Reproductive Med & Science of St
Barnabas Hosp, 94 Old Short Hills Rd East Wing;
Livingston, NJ 07039; (973) 322-8286; **BDCERT:**
ObG 92; RE 94; **MS:** UMDNJ-RW Johnson Med Sch
83; **RES:** DR, Med Ctr Hosp of VT, Burlington, VT
84-85; ObG, St Barnabas Med Ctr, Livingston, NJ
85-89; **FEL:** RE, Mount Sinai Med Ctr, New York,
NY 89-91; *SI: Infertility; Implantation;* **HMO:** Blue
Cross & Blue Shield Prucare First Option Magnacare
NJ Plus +

LANG: Sp, Prt; ♿ 🚗 🏥 💲 2-4 Weeks
VISA ⊖

RHEUMATOLOGY

Paolino, James (MD) Rhu
St Barnabas Med Ctr-Livingston

2168 Millburn Ave 205; Maplewood, NJ 07040;
(973) 762-3738; **BDCERT:** IM 72; Rhu 73; **MS:**
Jefferson Med Coll 66; **RES:** IM, St Vincents Hosp &
Med Ctr NY, New York, NY 66-70; **FEL:** Rhu, Univ
Hosp SUNY Bklyn, Brooklyn, NY 70-71; **FAP:** Asst
Clin Prof UMDNJ New Jersey Sch Osteo Med; **HOSP:**
Hosp Ctr at Orange; *SI: Rheumatoid Arthritis; Lupus;*
HMO: Aetna-US Healthcare GHI Blue Choice First
Option

♿ SA/SO ⊙ ☎ 🚗 🏥 💲 Mcr WC NFI 1 Week

Rosenstein, Elliot D (MD) Rhu
St Barnabas Med Ctr-Livingston

Arthritis & Rheumatic Disease Center at St
Barnabas, 200 S Orange Ave; Livingston, NJ
07039; (973) 322-7400; **BDCERT:** IM 82; Rhu 84;
MS: Mt Sinai Sch Med 78; **RES:** Bellevue Hosp Ctr,
New York, NY 78-82; **FEL:** Bellevue Hosp Ctr, New
York, NY 82-84; **FAP:** Assoc Prof Rhu Mt Sinai Sch
Med; **HOSP:** Newark Beth Israel Med Ctr; *SI:
Rheumatoid Arthritis; Lupus;* **HMO:** Blue Choice
HMO Blue PHCS First Option Cost Care +

♿ ⊙ ☎ 🚗 🏥 💲 Mcr Mcd 4+ Weeks **VISA** ⊖

SURGERY

Brief, Donald (MD) S
Newark Beth Israel Med Ctr

225 Millburn Ave; Millburn, NJ 07041; (973) 379-
5888; **BDCERT:** S 65; **MS:** Harvard Med Sch 57;
RES: Peter Bent Brigham Hosp, Boston, MA 57-64;
FEL: Harvard Med Sch, Cambridge, MA 63-64;
FAP: Clin Prof S UMDNJ New Jersey Sch Osteo Med;
HOSP: St Barnabas Med Ctr-Livingston; *SI:
Parathyroid and Thyroid; Breast Cancer Surgery;*
HMO: US Hlthcre Blue Cross & Blue Shield Aetna
Hlth Plan Oxford US Hlthcre +

LANG: Fr, Sp; ♿ ☎ 🚗 🏥 Mcr Mcd WC NFI 2-4 Weeks
⊠ **VISA** ⊖

Guide to symbols and abbreviations can be found on pages 110-113.

919

Chang, Patrick (MD)   S
St Barnabas Med Ctr-Livingston

Northfield Surgical Assoc, 299 E Northfield Rd; Livingston, NJ 07039; (973) 992-3464; **BDCERT:** S 78; **MS:** Australia 70; **RES:** S, St Barnabas Med Ctr, Livingston, NJ 72-76; **FEL:** Onc, Mem Sloan Kettering Cancer Ctr, New York, NY 78-80; **FAP:** Assoc Clin Prof UMDNJ New Jersey Sch Osteo Med; **HOSP:** Union Hosp-New Jersey; *SI: Melanoma; Laparoscopic Surgery;* **HMO:** Aetna Hlth Plan HMO Blue CIGNA Prudential

LANG: Chi, Sp; 🚹 📷 🚹 🏥 🅢 Mcr Mcd WC NFI

Deitch, Edwin (MD)   S
Univ of Med & Dent NJ Hosp

UMDNJ/NJ, 185 S Orange Ave G506; Newark, NJ 07103; (973) 982-5045; **BDCERT:** S 79; **MS:** U Md Sch Med 73; **RES:** S, USPHS Hosp, Baltimore, MD 74-76; S, USPHS Hosp, Baltimore, MD 76-78; *SI: Burns; Critical Care;* **HMO:** Blue Cross & Blue Shield Mercy Health Plans Amerihealth Empire Aetna-US Healthcare +

🚹 📷 🚹 🏥 🅢 Mcr Mcd WC NFI Immediately **VISA** 💳

Filippone, Dennis (MD)   S
St Barnabas Med Ctr-Livingston

St Barnabas Medical Center-Livingston, Dept of Surgery, 94 Old Short Hills Rd; Livingston, NJ 07039; (973) 322-5195; **BDCERT:** S 65; **MS:** Albany Med Coll 56; **RES:** S, Albany Mem Hosp, Albany, NY 56-57; S, Med Coll VA Hosp, Richmond, VA 59-64; **FEL:** Research Transplantation, Med Coll VA Hosp, Richmond, VA 61-62; **FAP:** Assoc Clin Prof S UMDNJ-NJ Med Sch, Newark; *SI: Gallbladder Surgery; Cancer Surgery;* **HMO:** Aetna-US Healthcare Blue Cross & Blue Shield Prudential First Option Magnacare +

🚹 📷 🚹 🏥 🅢 Mcr Mcd WC NFI A Few Days

Fletcher, Stephen H (MD)   S
St Barnabas Med Ctr-Livingston

349 E Northfield Rd Ste 212; Livingston, NJ 07039; (201) 379-2424; **BDCERT:** S 73; **MS:** Geo Wash U Sch Med 67; **RES:** Geo Wash U Sch Med,, Washington, DC 68-72; Hartford Hosp, Hartford, CT 67-68; **HOSP:** Overlook Hosp

Gardner, Bernard (MD)   S
Univ of Med & Dent NJ Hosp

185 S Orange Ave; Newark, NJ 07103; (973) 972-5501; **BDCERT:** S 66; **MS:** NYU Sch Med 56; **RES:** S, Mount Sinai Med Ctr, New York, NY 57-58; S, UC San Francisco Med Ctr, San Francisco, CA 60-65; **FEL:** Onc, UC San Francisco Med Ctr, San Francisco, CA 60-61; **FAP:** Prof UMDNJ-NJ Med Sch, Newark; *SI: Breast Cancer; Pancreatic Biliary Cancer;* **HMO:** Blue Cross Aetna Hlth Plan United Healthcare Amerihealth

LANG: Sp; 🚹 📷 🚹 🏥 Mcr Mcd WC NFI **VISA** 💳

Huston, Jan A (MD)   S
Newark Beth Israel Med Ctr

Millburn Surgical Assoc, 225 Millburn Ave 104B; Millburn, NJ 07041; (973) 379-5888; **BDCERT:** S 88; GVS 88; **MS:** Mich St U 82; **RES:** S, St Barnabas Med Ctr, Livingston, NJ 82-87; GVS, Lehigh Valley Hosp, Allentown, PA 87-88; **FAP:** Asst Prof S UMDNJ New Jersey Sch Osteo Med; *SI: Breast Problems; Laparoscopic Surgery;* **HMO:** US Hlthcre Oxford Prudential Blue Cross & Blue Shield First Option +

🚹 📷 🏥 🅢 Mcr Mcd WC NFI 2-4 Weeks **VISA** 💳

Livingston, David (MD)   S
Univ of Med & Dent NJ Hosp

University Hospital NJ Trauma Center, 150 Bergen St; Newark, NJ 07103; (973) 972-4900; **BDCERT:** S 96; SCC 90; **MS:** Albany Med Coll 81; **RES:** S, Bellevue Hosp Ctr, New York, NY 81-86; **FEL:** Trauma, U Louisville Hosp, Louisville, KY 86-88; **FAP:** Assoc Prof UMDNJ-NJ Med Sch, Newark

🚹 🚹 🏥 🅢 Mcr Mcd WC NFI 1 Week **VISA** 💳

Munoz, Eric (MD)   S
Long Island Jewish Med Ctr

UMDNJ- Univ Hospital-, 150 Bergan St Rm D215; Newark, NJ 07103; (973) 972-4300; **BDCERT:** S 82; **MS:** Albert Einstein Coll Med 74; **RES:** S, Yale-New Haven Hosp, New Haven, CT 74-78; **FAP:** Asst Prof S SUNY Syracuse; **HOSP:** Queens Hosp Ctr; *SI: General Surgery; Breast Surgery;* **HMO:** Most

🚹 📷 🏥 Mcr Mcd WC NFI Immediately ▨ **VISA** 💳

Padberg, Frank (MD)   **S**
Univ of Med & Dent NJ Hosp

Center for Vascular Disease, 90 Bergen St Ste 2300;
East Orange, NJ 07018; (973) 972-9371; **BDCERT:**
S 86; GVS 95; **MS:** U Ark Sch Med 73; **RES:** S, New
England Deaconess Hosp, Boston, MA 73-80; S,
Aberdean Royal Infirmary, Aberdeen, Scotland 76-
77; **FEL:** GVS, Lahey Clinic, Burlington, MA 80-81;
Nutrition/Metabolism, New Eng Deaconess Hosp,
Boston, MA 77; **FAP:** Prof S UMDNJ New Jersey Sch
Osteo Med; **HOSP:** St Michael's Med Ctr; *SI: Surgery
for Venous Disease; Aneurysm*; **HMO:** Aetna-US
Healthcare Empire Amerihealth First Option

🔲 🔲 🔲 🔲 🔲 🔲 🔲 🔲 1 Week **VISA** 🔵

Santoro, Elissa (MD)   **S**
St Barnabas Med Ctr-Livingston

Breast Care & Treatment Center, 200 S Orange
Ave; Livingston, NJ 07039; (973) 533-0222;
BDCERT: S 71; **MS:** Med Coll PA 65; **RES:** S, Magee
Women's Hosp, Philadelphia, PA 66-67; S, St
Vincents Hosp & Med Ctr NY, New York, NY 67-70;
FEL: St Vincents Hosp & Med Ctr NY, New York, NY
68-69; S Onc, New York University Med Ctr, New
York, NY 70-71; *SI: Breast Diseases and Surgery*;
HMO: Prucare Oxford Magnacare QualCare
Multiplan +

LANG: Sp, Ukr, Ger; 🔲 🔲 🔲 🔲 🔲 🔲 🔲 🔲
A Few Days **VISA** 🔵

Seltzer, Murray (MD)   **S**
St Barnabas Med Ctr-Livingston

200 S Orange Ave 101; Livingston, NJ 07039;
(973) 992-8484; **BDCERT:** S 72; **MS:** Univ Penn
65; **RES:** Hosp of U Penn, Philadelphia, PA 66-71;
FEL: Bredso Cancer Researc, New York, NY; **FAP:**
Prof S; *SI: Breast Surgery; Breast Cancer*; **HMO:**
Prucare Oxford Magnacare First Option PHCS +

🔲 🔲 🔲 🔲 🔲 Immediately **VISA** 🔵

THORACIC SURGERY

Forman, Mark (MD)   **TS**
Columbus Hosp

Northfield Surgical Associates, 299 E Northfield Rd;
Livingston, NJ 07039; (973) 992-3464; **BDCERT:**
S 83; TS 87; **MS:** Tulane U 76; **RES:** S, Long Island
Jewish Med Ctr, New Hyde Park, NY 76-81; TS,
Montefiore Med Ctr, Bronx, NY 81-82; **FEL:** TS,
Montefiore Med Ctr, Bronx, NY 82-84; **HMO:** HMO
Blue Aetna Hlth Plan Prudential CIGNA

LANG: Chi, Sp; 🔲 🔲 🔲 🔲 🔲 🔲 🔲 🔲 1 Week
🔲 **VISA** 🔵

McCormick, John R (MD)   **TS**
Univ of Med & Dent NJ Hosp

Univ of Med & Dent NJ Hosp, 185 S Orange Ave
G595; Newark, NJ 07103; (973) 972-5678;
BDCERT: TS 75; **MS:** Boston U 65; **RES:** TS, U of
Alabama Hosp, Birmingham, AL 72-73; **FEL:**
Boston U Med Ctr, Boston, MA 64-71; **FAP:** Prof S
UMDNJ-NJ Med Sch, Newark; **HOSP:** St Elizabeth
Hosp; *SI: Cardiothoracic Surgery; Open Heart &
Cardiac Surgery*; **HMO:** Most

LANG: Sp; 🔲 🔲 🔲 🔲 🔲 🔲 🔲 Immediately

UROLOGY

Ciccone, Patrick (MD)   **U**
Columbus Hosp

Urology Consultants, 349 E Northfield Rd 201;
Livingston, NJ 07039; (973) 759-6180; **BDCERT:**
U 75; **MS:** Georgetown U 67; **RES:** S, VA Med Ctr-
East Orange, East Orange, NJ 68-69; U, VA Med
Ctr-East Orange, East Orange, NJ 69-72; **FAP:** Clin
Instr UMDNJ New Jersey Sch Osteo Med

Irwin, Robert (MD)   **U**
Univ of Med & Dent NJ Hosp

185 S Orange Ave G536; Newark, NJ 07103; (201)
982-4488; **BDCERT:** U 76; **MS:** Harvard Med Sch
67; **RES:** Mass Gen Hosp, Boston, MA 73; **HMO:** US
Hlthcre CIGNA

🔲 🔲 🔲 🔲 🔲 🔲 🔲 🔲 Immediately **VISA** 🔲

Katz, Jeffrey (MD)   U
St Barnabas Hosp-Bronx
741 Northfield Ave # 206; W Orange, NJ 07052;
(201) 325-6100; **BDCERT:** U 78; **MS:** Italy 70;
RES: S, Mt Sinai,, Miami Beach, FL 72-73; U, Albert
Einstein Coll Med, Bronx, NY 73-76

Strauss, Bernard (MD)   U
St Barnabas Med Ctr-Livingston
741 Northfield Ave 206; W Orange, NJ 07052;
(201) 325-6100; **BDCERT:** U 73; **MS:** Albert
Einstein Coll Med 64; **RES:** S, Marquette U,
Milwaukee, WI 65-66; **FEL:** U, Bronx Muncipal
Hosp Ctr, Bronx, NY 66-69; **FAP:** Asst Clin Prof
UMDNJ New Jersey Sch Osteo Med; *SI: Urinary
Stone Disease; Urologic Cancer Surgery;* **HMO:** HMO
Blue Prudential Aetna-US Healthcare CIGNA
Magnacare +

LANG: Sp, Itl, Heb, Grk; ♿ 🅿 ⛑ 🏨 Mcr Mcd WC NFI
A Few Days **VISA** 💳

VASCULAR SURGERY (GENERAL)

Brener, Bruce (MD)   GVS
Newark Beth Israel Med Ctr
Millburn Surgical Associates, 225 Millburn Ave
104B; Millburn, NJ 07041; (973) 379-5888;
BDCERT: GVS 83; **MS:** Harvard Med Sch 66; **RES:**
S, Peter Bent Brigham Hosp, Boston, MA 68-72;
HOSP: Union Hosp-New Jersey
♿ 🅿 🏨 💲 Mcr Mcd WC 1 Week **VISA** 💳

Hobson, Robert W, II (MD)   GVS
St Michael's Med Ctr
Medical Science Bldg, G532; NJ Medical School,
185 S Orange Ave; Newark, NJ 07103; (973) 972-
6633; **BDCERT:** S 72; GVS 83; **MS:** Geo Wash U
Sch Med 63; **RES:** S, Walter Reed Army Med Ctr,
Washington, DC 67-71; **FEL:** GVS, Walter Reed
Army Med Ctr, Washington, DC 72-73; **FAP:**
Dir/VasSurg UMDNJ-NJ Med Sch, Newark; **HOSP:**
Northwest Covenant Med Ctr; *SI: Stroke: Carotid
Disease; Aortic Aneurysm;* **HMO:** Oxford US Hlthcre
HIP Network HMO Blue Amerihealth +
LANG: Sp; ♿ 🅿 ⛑ 🏨 💲 Mcr Mcd NFI 2-4 Weeks

HUDSON
COUNTY

SPECIALTY & SUBSPECIALTY	ABBREVIATION	PAGE(S)
Cardiology (Cardiovascular Disease)	Cv	925
Dermatology	D	925-926
Endocrinology, Diabetes & Metabolism	EDM	926
FAMILY PRACTICE	FP	926
Gastroenterology	Ge	926-927
Geriatric Medicine	Ger	927
Gynecologic Oncology*	GO	927
Infectious Disease	Inf	927
INTERNAL MEDICINE	IM	928-929
Medical Oncology*	Onc	929
Neonatal-Perinatal Medicine	NP	929
Neurology	N	929
OBSTETRICS & GYNECOLOGY	ObG	930
Ophthalmology	Oph	930
Orthopaedic Surgery	OrS	931
Otolaryngology	Oto	931
Pediatric Surgery	PS	931
PEDIATRICS (GENERAL)	Ped	931
Physical Medicine & Rehabilitation	PMR	931
Psychiatry	Psyc	932
Pulmonary Disease	Pul	932
Rheumatology	Rhu	932
Surgery	S	933
Thoracic Surgery (includes open heart surgery)	TS	933
Urology	U	933-934
Vascular Surgery (General)	GVS	934

Specialties in capital letters indicate Primary Care Specialties. However, many doctors will be certified in a subspecialty, but will practice predominantly primary care medicine. In our lists this will be indicated.

*Oncologists deal with Cancer

CARDIOLOGY (CARDIOVASCULAR DISEASE)

Baruchin, Mitchell (MD)   Cv
Christ Hosp
Pavonia Medical Assoc, 600 Pavonia Ave CD; Jersey City, NJ 07306; (201) 216-3070; **BDCERT:** IM 87; Cv 91; **MS:** Mt Sinai Sch Med 84; **RES:** IM, Beth Israel Med Ctr, New York, NY 84-87; **FEL:** Cv, Beth Israel Med Ctr, New York, NY 89-92; **FAP:** Clin Instr Mt Sinai Sch Med; **HOSP:** Gen Hosp Ctr At Passaic; **SI:** *Preventive Cardiology/Lipids; Nuclear Cardiology;* **HMO:** HMO Blue Aetna Hlth Plan CIGNA Prucare

LANG: Sp, Pol, Hin, Fr, Tag; 🔲 📞 👤 🏢 💲 Mcr
VISA 🔲

Cruz, Merle Correa (MD)   Cv
St Francis Hosp-Jersey City
25 McWilliams Pl; Jersey City, NJ 07302; (201) 653-7533; **BDCERT:** Cv 85; **MS:** Philippines 76; **RES:** Jersey City Med Ctr, Jersey City, NJ 79-82; **FEL:** Brookdale Univ Hosp Med Ctr, Brooklyn, NY 82-84; **SI:** *Heart Disease;* **HMO:** United Healthcare Empire Blue Cross & Shield Multiplan Prudential

LANG: Tag, Sp; 🔲 📞 🏢 💲 Mcr Mcd   2-4 Weeks

Elkind, Barry M (MD)   Cv
Bayonne Hosp
The Heart Group, PA, 273 Avenue A; Bayonne, NJ 07002; (201) 858-0800; **BDCERT:** Cv 81; IM 79; **MS:** UMDNJ-NJ Med Sch, Newark 76; **RES:** IM, Boston Med Ctr, Boston, MA 76-79; **FEL:** New England Med Ctr, Boston, MA 79-82; **HOSP:** Newark Beth Israel Med Ctr; **SI:** *Coronary Artery Disease; Cardiac Testing*

📞 👤 🏢 💲 Mcr Mcd   Immediately 🔲

Moussa, Ghias (MD)   Cv   **PCP**
Greenville Hosp
1815 Kennedy Blvd; Jersey City, NJ 07305; (201) 333-3311; **BDCERT:** Cv 91; **MS:** Syria 79; **RES:** IM, Jersey City Med Ctr, Jersey City, NJ 86-89; **FEL:** Cv, Jersey City Med Ctr, Jersey City, NJ 89-91; **FAP:** Assoc Prof Cv; **SI:** *Valvular Heart Diseases; Congestive Heart Failure;* **HMO:** PHS American Health Plan US Hlthcre Amerihealth

LANG: Fr, Sp, Ar; 🔲 📶 📞 🔲 👤 🏢 Mcr Mcd WC
A Few Days

Sandhu, M Y (MD)   Cv
Bayonne Hosp
719 Avenue C; Bayonne, NJ 07002; (201) 339-3710; **MS:** India 77; **RES:** VA Med Ctr-Bronx, Bronx, NY 77; **FEL:** Cv, Jersey City Med Ctr, Jersey City, NJ 78

📞 🔲 👤 🏢 💲 Mcr Mcd   Immediately

DERMATOLOGY

Blank, Ellen (MD)   D
Mount Sinai Med Ctr
333 Avenue C; Bayonne, NJ 07002; (201) 858-4800; **BDCERT:** D 79; **MS:** Mt Sinai Sch Med 75; **RES:** Beth Israel Med Ctr, New York, NY 75-76; Mount Sinai Med Ctr, New York, NY 76-79; **HOSP:** Bayonne Hosp

📶 🔲 👤 🏢 💲   1 Week

Blank, Ellen (MD)   D
Mount Sinai Med Ctr
Hudson Richmond Dermatology, 333 Avenue C; Bayonne, NJ 07002; (201) 858-4800; **BDCERT:** D 79; **MS:** Mt Sinai Sch Med 75; **RES:** Beth Israel Med Ctr, New York, NY 75-76; Mt Sinai Med Ctr, New York, NY 76-79

Kopec, Anna V (MD)   D
Bayonne Hosp

730 Kennedy Blvd; Bayonne, NJ 07002; (201) 858-4300; **BDCERT:** D 80; **MS:** UMDNJ-NJ Med Sch, Newark 75; **RES:** Albert Einstein Med Ctr, Bronx, NY 76-79; Univ of Med & Dent NJ Hosp, Newark, NJ 75-76; **FAP:** Assoc Clin Prof Albert Einstein Coll Med; *SI: Skin Cancer; Aging Skin;* **HMO:** QualCare

▦ ▧ ▨ ▤ ▦   Immediately

ENDOCRINOLOGY, DIABETES & METABOLISM

Cam, Jenny (MD)   EDM
St Francis Hosp-Jersey City

25 Mc Williams Pl 303; Jersey City, NJ 07302; (201) 656-6003; **BDCERT:** IM 88; EDM 89; **MS:** Philippines 79; **RES:** IM, Interfaith Med Ctr, Brooklyn, NY 84-87; **FEL:** EDM, Univ of Med & Dent NJ Hosp, Newark, NJ 87-89; **HOSP:** Christ Hosp; *SI: Diabetes; Thyroid Disorders;* **HMO:** Blue Cross & Blue Shield Oxford Aetna Hlth Plan Prucare Guardian +

▤ ▦ ▤ ▦ ▦ ▦   2-4 Weeks

FAMILY PRACTICE

Castro, Zoila Yolanda (MD)   FP   PCP

2954 Kennedy Blvd; Jersey City, NJ 07306; (201) 653-6666; **BDCERT:** FP 94; **MS:** Mexico 87; **RES:** Hospital del Seguro Social, Mexico City, Mexico 87; **FEL:** FP, JFK Med Ctr, Edison, NJ 90-93

LANG: Sp; ▤ ▧ ▦ ▨ ▤ ▦ ▦ ▦
Immediately *VISA* 💳

Grapa, Octavian (MD)   FP   PCP
Palisades Med Ctr

6040 Boulevard East St; West New York, NJ 07093; (201) 868-4346; **MS:** Romania 1955; **RES:** Reddy Memorial Hospital, Montreal, Canada; **HOSP:** Meadowlands Hosp Med Ctr; **HMO:** Guardian CIGNA

▤ ▦ ▧ ▦ ▨ ▤ ▦ ▦   Immediately

Levine, Martin S (DO)   FP   PCP
Christ Hosp

789 Avenue C; Bayonne, NJ 07002; (201) 339-2620; **BDCERT:** FP 83; **MS:** Kirksville Coll Osteo Med 80; **RES:** FP, Kennedy Mem Hosp, Stratford, NJ 80-83; **FAP:** Asst Clin Prof UMDNJ, Sch Osteo Med; **HOSP:** Bayonne Hosp; *SI: Sports Medicine; Osteopathic Manipulation*

▦ ▧ ▤ ▦ ▦ ▦ ▦   Immediately

Sand, Jay P (MD)   FP   PCP
Jersey City Med Ctr

196 Jewett Ave; Jersey City, NJ 07304; (201) 332-3354; **MS:** Holland 56; **RES:** IM, Irvington General Hospital, Irvington, NJ 58-58; **HMO:** Most

LANG: Sp, Dut, Fr; ▦ ▨ ▤ ▦ ▦   A Few Days

Sklower, Jay A (DO)   FP   PCP
Christ Hosp

Pavonia Medical Associates, 600 Pavonia Ave Ste AB; Jersey City, NJ 07306; (201) 216-3040; **BDCERT:** FP 78; **MS:** U Hlth Sci/Chicago Med Sch 71; **RES:** Union Mem Hosp, Baltimore, MD 72; **HOSP:** Jersey City Med Ctr; **HMO:** Most

LANG: Sp; ▤ ▦ ▧ ▦ ▨ ▤ ▦ ▦ ▦ ▦ ▦
4+ Weeks *VISA* 💳

GASTROENTEROLOGY

Hahn, John Charles (MD)   Ge
Bayonne Hosp

183 Avenue B; Bayonne, NJ 07002; (201) 823-0450; **BDCERT:** IM 88; Ge 91; **MS:** UMDNJ-NJ Med Sch, Newark 85; *SI: Colon Polyps; Peptic Ulcer Disease*

▤ ▦ ▤ ▦ ▦   Immediately

Prakash, Anaka (MD)   Ge
Bayonne Hosp
132 W 39th St; Bayonne, NJ 07002; (201) 858-8444; **BDCERT:** Ge 77; Ger 92; **MS:** India 73; **RES:** St Joseph's Hosp-Paterson, Paterson, NJ 73-75; **FEL:** Univ of Med & Dent NJ Hosp, Newark, NJ 75-77; **HOSP:** Greenville Hosp; *SI: Gall Bladder & Liver; Endoscopy;* **HMO:** Aetna Hlth Plan QualCare CIGNA Corporate Care HIP Network +

LANG: Sp; 🔵 🔲 🔲 🔲 🔲 🔲 🔲 Immediately

Siebel, Wayne D (MD)   Ge
Christ Hosp
600 Pavonia Ave; Jersey City, NJ 07306; (201) 216-3065; **BDCERT:** IM 89; Ge 93; **MS:** SUNY Hlth Sci Ctr 86; **RES:** IM, RWJ Univ Hosp-New Brunswick, New Brunswick, NJ 86; **FEL:** Ge, Univ of Med & Dent NJ Hosp, Newark, NJ 89-91; **HOSP:** Meadowlands Hosp Med Ctr; **HMO:** Oxford Prucare CIGNA

🔲 🔲 🔵 🔲 🔲 🔲 🔲 🔲 🔲 🔲 Immediately 🔲
VISA 🔲

Siegel, Wayne (MD)   Ge
Christ Hosp
Pavonia Medical Assoc, 600 Pavonia Ave FG; Jersey City, NJ 07306; (201) 216-3065; **BDCERT:** Ge 93; IM 89; **MS:** SUNY Syracuse 86; **RES:** IM, RWJ Univ Hosp-New Brunswick, New Brunswick, NJ 86-89; **FEL:** Ge, Univ of Med & Dent NJ Hosp, Newark, NJ 89-91; **FAP:** Clin Instr UMDNJ New Jersey Sch Osteo Med; **HOSP:** Meadowlands Hosp Med Ctr; *SI: Liver Disease-Hepatitis; Digestive Diseases;* **HMO:** Oxford HMO Blue US Hlthcre Prucare CIGNA +

LANG: Sp; 🔲 🔵 🔲 🔲 🔲 🔲 🔲 A Few Days **VISA** 🔲 🔲

Spira, Robert S (MD)   Ge
St Michael's Med Ctr
655 Kearny Ave; Kearny, NJ 07032; (201) 736-1991; **BDCERT:** IM 78; Ge 81; **MS:** NYU Sch Med 75; **RES:** NYU Med Ctr, New York, NY 75-78; Bellevue Hosp Ctr, New York, NY 75-78; **FEL:** VA Med Ctr-Manhattan, New York, NY 79-81; **HOSP:** Clara Maass Med Ctr

GERIATRIC MEDICINE

Brown, Mitchell Lee (MD)   Ger   **PCP**
Bayonne Hosp
2 Joan Ree Terrace; Bayonne, NJ 07002; (201) 339-2220; **BDCERT:** IM 90; Ger 92; **MS:** West Indies 87; **RES:** IM, St Elizabeth Hosp, Elizabeth, NJ 87-90; **FEL:** Ger, St Vincents Hosp & Med Ctr NY, New York, NY 90-92; **HOSP:** Christ Hosp; *SI: Alzheimer's Disease;* **HMO:** Amerihealth Blue Cross & Blue Shield Prudential Oxford HMO Blue +

LANG: Sp; 🔲 🔲 🔲 🔲 🔲 🔲 Immediately

GYNECOLOGIC ONCOLOGY

Sommers, Gara M (MD)   GO
Christ Hosp
129 Washington St; Hoboken, NJ 07030; (201) 792-9011; **BDCERT:** ObG 90; **MS:** NYU Sch Med 81; **RES:** New York University Med Ctr, New York, NY 81-85; **FEL:** GO, Barnes Hosp, St Louis, MO 85-88; **HOSP:** Bayonne Hosp

INFECTIOUS DISEASE

Bellomo, Spartaco (MD)   Inf
Christ Hosp
142 Palisade Ave 209; Jersey City, NJ 07306; (201) 653-8336; **BDCERT:** IM 85; Inf 90; **MS:** Italy 78; **RES:** Inf, St Michael's Med Ctr, New York, NY 81-83; **FEL:** Inf, St Michael's Med Ctr, New York, NY 79-81

LANG: Itl, Grk; 🔲 🔲 🔵 🔲 🔲 🔲 A Few Days

INTERNAL MEDICINE

Bains, Yatinder (MD)   IM   PCP
Jersey City Med Ctr

One Robertson Drive, Bedminster Medical Plaza 1818; Bedminster, NJ 07921; (908) 781-1100; **BDCERT:** IM 91; Ge 93; **MS:** UMDNJ-NJ Med Sch, Newark 87; **RES:** Ge, Univ of Med & Dent NJ Hosp, Newark, NJ 90-92; IM, Univ of Med & Dent NJ Hosp, Newark, NJ 87-90; **FEL:** Ge, Univ of Med & Dent NJ Hosp, Newark, NJ 90-92; **FAP:** Assoc Prof Ge UMDNJ New Jersey Sch Osteo Med; **HOSP:** Somerset Med Ctr

LANG: Hin, Rom; ♿ 📞 🔲 📧 🏠 Mcr WC NFI Immediately

Cardiello, Gary P (MD)   IM
Christ Hosp

834 Avenue C; Bayonne, NJ 07002; (201) 436-8888; **BDCERT:** IM 83; **MS:** Italy 1983; **RES:** St Michaels Hospital, Newark, NJ 83-86; **HOSP:** St Michael's Med Ctr

Condo, Dominick (MD)   IM   PCP
Bayonne Hosp

209 Avenue B; Bayonne, NJ 07002; (201) 436-2800; **BDCERT:** IM 84; Ger 94; **MS:** Mexico 80; **RES:** IM, St Michael's Med Ctr, Newark, NJ 82-84; **FEL:** St Michael's Med Ctr, Newark, NJ 81-82; **HMO:** HMO Blue Oxford QualCare Aetna Hlth Plan CIGNA +

LANG: Itl, Sp; ♿ 📞 🔲 📧 🏠 $ Mcr 1 Week

Dedousis, John T (MD)   IM   PCP
Bayonne Hosp

1166 Kennedy Blvd; Bayonne, NJ 07002; (201) 339-1133; **BDCERT:** IM 93; **MS:** Dominica 85; **RES:** UMDNJ-Newark, Newark, NJ

📞 🔲 🏠 $ Mcr Mcd A Few Days

Douedi, Hani Ramses (MD)   IM
Jersey City Med Ctr

Jersey City Med Ctr — Internal Med Dept, 50 Baldwin Ave; Jersey City, NJ 07304; (201) 915-2448; **BDCERT:** IM 95; **MS:** Egypt 82; **RES:** Jersey City Med Ctr, Jersey City, NJ 92-95; **FEL:** Cv, Jersey City Med Ctr, Jersey City, NJ 95

LANG: Grk; ♿ 📧 📞

Hoffman, Mark Andrew (MD)IM   PCP
Bayonne Hosp

South Hudson Medical Associates, 19 E 27th St; Bayonne, NJ 07002; (201) 339-1414; **BDCERT:** IM 89; **MS:** Boston U 83; **RES:** IM, St Joseph's Hosp-Paterson, Paterson, NJ 83-86; **SI:** *Preventive Medicine*

LANG: Sp; ♿ 📧 📞 🔲 🏠 🏠 $ Mcr WC Immediately

Kozel, Joseph Martin (MD)   IM   PCP
St Mary's Hosp

330 Clinton St; Hoboken, NJ 07030; (201) 656-3519; **BDCERT:** IM 84; **MS:** Mexico 73; **RES:** FP, St Mary Hosp, Hoboken, NJ 76-79; IM, St Michael's Med Ctr, Newark, NJ 79-80; **FEL:** Pul, St Michael's Med Ctr, Newark, NJ 80-81; **HOSP:** St Francis Hosp-Jersey City; **SI:** *Asthma*; **HMO:** Oxford Pinnacle Blue Cross & Blue Shield HIP Network QualCare +

LANG: Sp, Itl; ♿ 📞 🔲 🏠 🏠 $ A Few Days

Mutterperl, Mitchell (MD)   IM
Bayonne Hosp

19 W 33rd St B2; Bayonne, NJ 07002; (201) 858-0090; **BDCERT:** IM 85; **MS:** Italy 81; **RES:** IM, Univ of Med & Dent NJ Hosp, Newark, NJ 82-85; **HMO:** Oxford United Healthcare Prudential Corporate Care Blue Cross +

📞 🔲 🏠 🏠 $ Mcr 2-4 Weeks

Perlmutter, Barbara (MD)   IM
St Mary's Hosp

330 Clinton Street; Hoboken, NJ 07030; (201) 963-5886; **BDCERT:** IM 79; Ger 90; **MS:** UMDNJ-NJ Med Sch, Newark 76; **RES:** IM, Overlook Hosp, Summit, NJ 76-79; **FAP:** Asst Clin Prof Med NY Med Coll; **HOSP:** Bayley Seton Hosp

Simone, Don (MD)   IM
Bayonne Hosp
Simone & Condo, MD, 209 Avenue B; Bayonne, NJ
07002; (201) 436-2800; **BDCERT:** IM 83; **MS:**
Rutgers U 80; **RES:** IM, St Michael's Med Ctr,
Newark, NJ 81-83; **HMO:** Blue Choice
LANG: Sp, Itl; 🔲 🔲 🔲 🔲 🔲 🔲 🔲 🔲
A Few Days

Wagner, Michael L (MD)   IM
Greenville Hosp
198 Stevens Ave; Jersey City, NJ 07305; (201)
434-7824; **BDCERT:** IM 73; **MS:** UMDNJ-NJ Med
Sch, Newark 61; **RES:** IM, Jersey City Med Ctr,
Jersey City, NJ 61-63; IM, Columbia-Presbyterian
Med Ctr, New York, NY 63-65; **FEL:** Columbia-
Presbyterian Med Ctr, New York, NY 64-65; **FAP:**
Asst Clin Prof Med UMDNJ-NJ Med Sch, Newark;
HOSP: St Francis Hosp-Jersey City

Wozniak, D (MD)   IM
Bayonne Hosp
19 E 27th; Bayonne, NJ 07002; (201) 823-1066;
BDCERT: IM 79; **MS:** UMDNJ-NJ Med Sch, Newark
76; **RES:** Med, St Joseph's Hosp-Paterson, Paterson,
NJ 77-79; Univ of Med & Dent NJ Hosp, Newark, NJ
76-77
LANG: Sp; 🔲 🔲 🔲 🔲 🔲 🔲 🔲 🔲 🔲
A Few Days

MEDICAL ONCOLOGY

Iyengar, Devarajan P (MD)   Onc
Bayonne Hosp
777 Avenue C; Bayonne, NJ 07002; (201) 858-
1211; **BDCERT:** IM 82; Onc 85; **MS:** India 77; **RES:**
IM, St Clare's Hosp & Health Ctr, New York, NY 77-
80; **FEL:** Hem Onc, Univ of Med & Dent NJ Hosp,
Newark, NJ 81-82; Newark Beth Israel Med Ctr,
Newark, NJ 82-83; *SI: Breast Cancer; Colon & Rectal
Cancer;* **HMO:** ABC Health HMO Blue Oxford
CIGNA Prucare +
LANG: Pol, Hin, Sp; 🔲 🔲 🔲 🔲 🔲 🔲 🔲
Immediately

NEONATAL-PERINATAL MEDICINE

Aly, Sayed (MD)   NP   **PCP**
Bayonne Hosp
770 Kennedy Blvd; Bayonne, NJ 07002; (201)
823-3769; **BDCERT:** Ped 94; **MS:** Egypt 77; **RES:**
Hahnemann U Hosp, Philadelphia, PA; **FEL:** NP,
Babies Hosp, New York, NY; Columbia-
Presbyterian Med Ctr, New York, NY; **FAP:** Asst
Clin Prof Ped Columbia P&S
LANG: Ar; 🔲 🔲 🔲 🔲   Immediately

NEUROLOGY

Anselmi, Gregory (MD)   N
Bayonne Hosp
Hudson Neurosciences, 1222 Kennedy Blvd;
Bayonne, NJ 07002; (201) 339-6531; **BDCERT:** N
94; **MS:** Italy 88; **RES:** IM, St Vincent's Med Ctr-
Richmond, Staten Island, NY 88-89; N, St Vincents
Hosp & Med Ctr NY, New York, NY 89-92; **FEL:**
Neuromuscular, Univ Hosp SUNY Bklyn, Brooklyn,
NY 92-93; **HOSP:** St Francis Hosp-Jersey City; *SI:
Migraine Headaches; Multiple Sclerosis;* **HMO:** Aetna-
US Healthcare CIGNA Prudential Blue Cross & Blue
Shield
LANG: Itl, Sp; 🔲 🔲 🔲 🔲 🔲 🔲 🔲 🔲 🔲 🔲
Immediately

Sadeghi, H (MD)   N
Bayonne Hosp
631 Broadway Fl 3; Bayonne, NJ 07002; (201)
823-2888; **BDCERT:** N 77; **MS:** Iran 67; **RES:**
Northern Westchester Hosp Ctr, Mt Kisco, NY 71-
72; Univ of Med & Dent NJ Hosp, Newark, NJ 72-
75; **FAP:** Asst Clin Prof UMDNJ New Jersey Sch
Osteo Med; **HOSP:** Christ Hosp; *SI: Headaches and
Epilepsy; Neck Pain and Low Back Pain;* **HMO:** Oxford
Aetna-US Healthcare Blue Cross & Blue Shield
CIGNA
🔲 🔲 🔲 🔲 🔲 🔲 🔲 🔲 🔲 🔲   Immediately

Guide to symbols and abbreviations can be found on pages 110-113.

929

OBSTETRICS & GYNECOLOGY

Masson, Lalitha (MD)   ObG
St Mary's Hosp
506 Washington St; Hoboken, NJ 07030; (201) 963-8554; **BDCERT:** ObG 73; **MS:** India 64; **RES:** Margaret Hague Hosp, Jersey City, NJ 67-69; St Clares Hosp, New York, NY 69-70; **FEL:** Infertility, NJ Sch Med, Newark, NJ 70-71

Pelosi, Marco A (MD)   ObG
Bayonne Hosp
350 Kennedy Blvd; Bayonne, NJ 07002; (201) 858-1800; **BDCERT:** ObG 74; **MS:** Peru 68; **RES:** ObG, Univ of Med & Dent NJ Hosp, Newark, NJ 68-72; **FEL:** Onc, Univ of Med & Dent NJ Hosp, Newark, NJ 72-74; **HOSP:** Meadowlands Hosp Med Ctr; *SI: Laparoscopy; Advanced Pelvic Surgery*; **HMO:** Aetna-US Healthcare Oxford Blue Cross & Blue Shield CIGNA NYLCare +
LANG: Sp, Itl, Fr, Prt; ⬛ ⬛ ⬛ ⬛ ⬛ ⬛ ⬛ ⬛ ⬛ A Few Days ⬛ **VISA** ⬛ ⬛

Uy, Vena (MD)   ObG   **PCP**
Christ Hosp
142 Palisades Ave Ste 102; Jersey City, NJ 07306; (201) 653-0506; **BDCERT:** ObG 77; **MS:** Philippines 68; **RES:** ObG, Jersey City Med Ctr, Jersey City, NJ 70-73; **FEL:** ObG Path, Magee Women's Hosp, Philadelphia, PA 73-74; **HOSP:** Meadowlands Hosp Med Ctr; **HMO:** Oxford Prucare Aetna-US Healthcare NYLCare TPA +
LANG: Chi, Fil; ⬛ ⬛ ⬛ ⬛ ⬛ ⬛ 1 Week

OPHTHALMOLOGY

Constad, William H (MD)   Oph
Jersey City Med Ctr
Hudson Eye Physician and Surgeons, 600 Pavonia Ave 6th Fl; Jersey City, NJ 07306; (201) 963-3937; **BDCERT:** Oph 85; **MS:** Med Coll PA 80; **RES:** Oph, Univ of Med & Dent NJ Hosp, Newark, NJ 80-84; **FEL:** Cornea & External Disease, New York Eye & Ear Infirmary, New York, NY 84-85; **FAP:** Assoc Clin Prof Oph UMDNJ New Jersey Sch Osteo Med; **HOSP:** Univ of Med & Dent NJ Hosp; *SI: Corneal Transplants; Cataract Surgery*; **HMO:** Oxford Aetna-US Healthcare Blue Cross & Blue Shield United Healthcare CIGNA +
LANG: Sp; ⬛ ⬛ ⬛ ⬛ ⬛ ⬛ ⬛ ⬛ ⬛ A Few Days ⬛ **VISA** ⬛ ⬛

Fasano, Carl (MD)   Oph
Palisades Med Ctr
229 60th St; West New York, NJ 07093; (201) 863-0665; **BDCERT:** Oph 64; **MS:** Temple U 56; **RES:** Northeastern Hosp, Philadelphia, PA 56-57; Oph, Manhattan Eye, Ear & Throat Hosp, New York, NY 57-59; **FEL:** Oph, Manhattan Eye, Ear & Throat Hosp, New York, NY 59-60

Lagoda, Boleslaw (MD)   Oph
Bayonne Hosp
813 Kennedy Blvd; Bayonne, NJ 07002; (201) 823-2473; **BDCERT:** Oph 75; FP 95; **MS:** Poland 65; **RES:** Christ Hosp, Jersey City, NJ 66-67; Univ of Med & Dent NJ Hosp, Newark, NJ 70-73; **HMO:** Magnacare Oxford CIGNA Blue Cross & Blue Shield Blue Cross & Blue Shield +
LANG: Pol; ⬛ ⬛ ⬛ ⬛ ⬛ ⬛ ⬛ ⬛ ⬛ Immediately

ORTHOPAEDIC SURGERY

Granadir, Charles (MD)   OrS
West Hudson Hosp
586 Kearny Avenue; Kearny, NJ; (201) 997-7667;
BDCERT: OrS 89; **MS:** Hahnemann U 79; **RES:**
Montefiore Med Ctr, Bronx, NY 79-84

Irving III, Henry C (MD)   OrS
Meadowlands Hosp Med Ctr
Tolentino & Irving, 600 Pavonia Ave; Jersey City,
NJ 07306; (201) 216-9300; **BDCERT:** OrS 80; **MS:**
Meharry Med Coll 72; **RES:** Univ of Med & Dent NJ
Hosp, Newark, NJ 72-77; **HOSP:** Jersey City Med
Ctr; *SI: Joint Replacement Surgery; Knee Surgery*
LANG: Sp; ♿ 🅲 🄖 🅗 🎟 🆂 Mcr Mcd WC NFI 1 Week
▥ VISA ●

OTOLARYNGOLOGY

Laskey, Richard S (MD)   Oto
Meadowlands Hosp Med Ctr
330 Clinton St Suite 305; Hoboken, NJ 07030;
(201) 795-5103; **BDCERT:** Oto 84; **MS:** Albert
Einstein Coll Med 79; **RES:** Oto, NYU Med Ctr, New
York, NY 80-83; PlS, Boston U Med Ctr, Boston,
MA 84-86

PEDIATRIC SURGERY

Garrow, Eugene (MD)   PS
Jersey City Med Ctr
Children's Surgery of NJ PA, 45 Gifford Ave; Jersey
City, NJ 07304; (201) 434-1208; **BDCERT:** PS 64;
MS: SUNY Hlth Sci Ctr 58; **RES:** Montefiore Med
Ctr, Bronx, NY 59-63; Children's Hosp of MI,
Detroit, MI 63-64; **FAP:** Assoc Clin Prof UMDNJ
New Jersey Sch Osteo Med; **HOSP:** Christ Hosp;
HMO: Prucare Aetna-US Healthcare Oxford United
Healthcare NYLCare +
🅲 🄖 🅗 🎟 🆂 Mcd NFI 2-4 Weeks

PEDIATRICS

Al-Salihi, Farouk (MD)   Ped   PCP
St Francis Med Ctr
1810 Kennedy Blvd; Jersey City, NJ 07304; (201)
451-9799; **BDCERT:** Ped 66; **MS:** Iraq 68; **RES:** U
KS Med Ctr, Kansas City, KS 64; St Luke's Roosevelt
Hosp Ctr, New York, NY 65; **FEL:** Bellevue Hosp Ctr,
New York, NY 65; **HMO:** Mercy Health Plans
American Health Plan GHI Sanus
♿ 🅲 🄖 🅗 🎟 🆂 Mcr Mcd Immediately

Rhee, Jung (MD)   Ped
Christ Hosp
142 Palisades Ave; Jersey City, NJ; (201) 798-
1333; **BDCERT:** Ped 80; **MS:** South Korea 65; **RES:**
Korea U Hosp, Seoul, South Korea 69-70; Nat Med
Ctr, Seoul, South Korea 70-74; **HMO:** Oxford Blue
Choice Blue Select CIGNA US Hlthcre +
LANG: Kor; 🆂🄐 🅲

Skirtkus, Aldonna (MD)   Ped
West Hudson Hosp
381 Kearny Avenue; Kearny, NJ; (201) 991-4824;
BDCERT: Ped 71; **MS:** Univ Penn 66; **RES:** U
Maryland, Baltimore, MD 66-67; Ped, Children's
Hosp Nat Med Ctr, Washington, DC 67-69

PHYSICAL MEDICINE & REHABILITATION

Fischberg, Juan (MD)   PMR
Palisades Med Ctr
321 60th St; West New York, NJ 07093; (201)
295-9003; **BDCERT:** PMR 88; **MS:** Argentina 71;
RES: North General Hosp, New York, NY 83-84;
Albert Einstein Med Ctr, Bronx, NY 84-87
LANG: Sp, Ger; ♿ 🄖 🎟 🆂 Mcr WC NFI A Few Days

PSYCHIATRY

Gewolb, Eric B (MD)   Psyc
Bayonne Hosp
830 Kennedy Blvd; Bayonne, NJ 07002; (201) 339-0200; **BDCERT:** Psyc 79; **MS:** Tulane U 74; **RES:** Psyc, Mount Sinai Med Ctr, New York, NY 75-78; **HMO:** Blue Cross QualCare Health Choice Oxford
📞 🏠 ♿ 🏥 💲   Immediately

Jacoby, Jacob (MD)   Psyc
654 Avenue C Suite 201; Bayonne, NJ 07002; (201) 339-0323; **BDCERT:** Psyc 93; **AM** 93; **MS:** SUNY Buffalo 80; **RES:** Psyc, U of Pittsburgh Med Ctr, Pittsburgh, PA 80-81; Psyc, Western Psyc Inst, Pittsburgh, PA 81-83; **FEL:** Alcoholism, Albert Einstein Med Ctr, Bronx, NY 83; **FAP:** Assoc Clin Prof Psyc UMDNJ New Jersey Sch Osteo Med; *SI: Psychopharmacology; Mood Disorders*; **HMO:** Blue Cross & Blue Shield Oxford United Healthcare QualCare IPA +
♿ 🏠 ♿ 🏥 💲   Immediately

Kurani, Devendra (MD)   Psyc
Christ Hosp
221 Palisade Ave Fl 2; Jersey City, NJ 07306; (201) 656-3116; **BDCERT:** Psyc 86; **MS:** Burma 75; **RES:** Psyc, Harlem Hosp Ctr, New York, NY 82-83; Psyc, Warley Hosp, Brentwood, England 78-81; **FEL:** DK Hosp, Raipurlindia, India 75-76; *SI: Depression; Anxiety Disorders*; **HMO:** CIGNA Blue Cross & Blue Shield Prudential Aetna Hlth Plan Oxford +
📞 🏠 ♿ 🏥 💲 Mcr WC NFI   A Few Days

Moraille, Pascale (MD)   Psyc   PCP
St Mary's Hosp
St Mary's Hospital; Hoboken, NJ 07030; (201) 792-8200; **BDCERT:** Psyc 93; **ChAP** 95; **MS:** U Puerto Rico 88; **RES:** Univ of Med & Dent NJ Hosp, Newark, NJ 88-90; **FEL:** Univ of Med & Dent NJ Hosp, Newark, NJ 90-92
LANG: Sp, Fr, Cre;

PULMONARY DISEASE

Elamir, Mazhar (MD)   Pul
Christ Hosp
Jersey City Breathing Ctr, 192 Harrison Ave; Jersey City, NJ 07304; (201) 333-5363; **MS:** Egypt 81; **RES:** IM, Jersey City Med Ctr, Jersey City, NJ 86; **FEL:** Pul, Brooklyn Hosp Ctr-Downtown, Brooklyn, NY 92; *SI: Sleep Disorders; Allergy Test*
LANG: Sp, Ar; ♿ 🏥 📞 🏠 🏥 💲 Mcr Mcd
Immediately

Scerbo, Joseph (MD)   Pul
St Mary's Hosp
330 Clinton Street; Hoboken, NJ 07030; (201) 656-3519; **BDCERT:** IM 74; Pul 76; **MS:** Italy 59; **RES:** IM, St Michael's Hosp, Newark, NJ 64-66; Pul, East Orange VA Hosp, East Orange, NJ 66-67

RHEUMATOLOGY

Scarpa, Nicholas P (DO)   Rhu
Univ of Med & Dent NJ Hosp
Pavonia Medical Assoc, 600 Pavonia Ave CD; Jersey City, NJ 07306; (201) 216-3050; **BDCERT:** Rhu 86; IM 83; **MS:** UMDNJ New Jersey Sch Osteo Med 80; **RES:** IM, Hackensack U Med Ctr, Hackensack, NJ 80-83; **FEL:** NY Hosp-Cornell Med Ctr, New York, NY 85; **FAP:** Asst Clin Prof Rhu UMDNJ-NJ Med Sch, Newark; **HOSP:** Christ Hosp; *SI: Lupus; Osteoporosis*; **HMO:** Prucare Oxford HMO Blue Guardian Blue Cross & Blue Shield +
LANG: Itl, Sp, Hin, Pol; ♿ 📞 ♿ 🏥 💲 Mcr WC
1 Week *VISA* 💳

SURGERY

Anfang, David (MD)   S
Bayonne Hosp
809 Kennedy Blvd; Bayonne, NJ 07002; (201) 858-3355; **BDCERT:** S 81; **MS:** SUNY Downstate 73; **RES:** New York University Med Ctr, New York, NY; New York University Med Ctr, New York, NY; *SI: Vascular Surgery;* **HMO:** None

🌙 📷 🧑 🏧 Mcr Mcd WC NFi   A Few Days

Gildengers, Jaime (MD)   S
Palisades Med Ctr
313 60th St; West New York, NJ; (201) 854-0406; **BDCERT:** S 76; **MS:** Argentina 65; **RES:** S, Mt Sinai Med Ctr, Miami Beach, FL 68-70; S, St Clare's Hosp & Health Ctr, New York, NY 70-74; **FAP:** Asst Clin Prof UMDNJ New Jersey Sch Osteo Med; *SI: Gallbladder-Colon; Breast, Hernia;* **HMO:** Oxford Prudential Magnacare CIGNA Blue Shield +

LANG: Itl, Sp, Heb; 🏧 🌙 🧑 🏧 S Mcr WC
A Few Days

McGovern Jr, Patrick Joseph (MD)   S
Bayonne Hosp
Hudson Surgical Group, 631 Broadway; Bayonne, NJ 07002; (201) 858-5705; **BDCERT:** S 93; **MS:** UMDNJ-NJ Med Sch, Newark 78; **RES:** S, Univ of Med & Dent NJ Hosp, Newark, NJ 78-79; S, Univ of Med & Dent NJ Hosp, Newark, NJ 79-83; **FEL:** GVS, RWJ Univ Hosp-New Brunswick, New Brunswick, NJ 83-84; **HOSP:** Christ Hosp; *SI: Varicose Veins Laser Surgery; Gallbladder Disease;* **HMO:** Prucare Oxford Aetna-US Healthcare NYLCare HMO Blue +

LANG: Itl, Sp; 🏧 🏧 📷 🏧 S Mcr Mcd WC
Immediately **VISA** 💳

Popovich, Joseph F (MD)   S
Christ Hosp
Hudson Surgical Group, 3284 John F Kennedy Blvd; Jersey City, NJ 07306; (201) 656-0646; **BDCERT:** S 94; **MS:** UMDNJ-RW Johnson Med Sch 87; **RES:** Med Ctr Hosp of VT, Burlington, VT 91-93; Univ of Med & Dent NJ Hosp, Newark, NJ 88-91; **FEL:** St Francis Med Ctr, Trenton, NJ 78-88; **HOSP:** Meadowlands Hosp Med Ctr; **HMO:** Oxford US Hlthcre Blue Choice 32BJ Aetna Hlth Plan +

🏧 📷 🏧 Mcr Mcd WC NFi

Sultan, Ronald H (MD)   S
Christ Hosp
2255 John F Kennedy Blvd; Jersey City, NJ 07304; (201) 434-3305; **BDCERT:** S 81; **MS:** NYU Sch Med 73; **RES:** S, Albert Einstein Med Ctr, Philadelphia, PA 77-80; S, Bronx Lebanon Hosp Ctr, Bronx, NY 74-77; **FEL:** Kings County Hosp Ctr, Brooklyn, NY 73-74; **HOSP:** Greenville Hosp; *SI: Hernia Repairs; Gallbladder-Laparascopic;* **HMO:** Aetna Hlth Plan CIGNA Blue Shield Oxford

LANG: Sp, Heb; 🏧 🌙 S Mcr WC   Immediately

THORACIC SURGERY

Demos, Nicholas (MD)   TS
Christ Hosp
142 Palisade Ave 100; Jersey City, NJ 07306; (201) 420-1486; **BDCERT:** TS 65; GVS 83; **MS:** Northwestern U 55; **RES:** TS, BS Pollak Hosp, Jersey City, NJ 63-65; SM, Northwestern Mem Hosp, Chicago, IL 56-63; **FEL:** Cv.; Passavant Pavillion, Chicago, IL 55-56; **FAP:** Assoc Prof S UMDNJ New Jersey Sch Osteo Med; **HOSP:** St Mary's Hosp; *SI: Diseases of Esophagus; Circulation Problems;* **HMO:** Aetna-US Healthcare Blue Cross & Blue Shield

LANG: Sp, Grk, Itl; 🏧 🏧 🌙 📷 🧑 🏧 Mcr Mcd WC
A Few Days 📠 **VISA** 💳 💳

UROLOGY

Katz, Herbert I (MD)   U
Bayonne Hosp
631 Broadway; Bayonne, NJ 07002; (201) 823-1303; **BDCERT:** U 81; **MS:** Temple U 74; **RES:** S, Abington Mem Hosp, Abington, PA 74-76; U, Albert Einstein Med Ctr, Bronx, NY 76-79; *SI: Urologic Cancer; Impotency;* **HMO:** Oxford Aetna-US Healthcare GHI HMO Blue

LANG: Sp; 🏧 🌙 📷 🧑 🏧 Mcr WC NFi   Immediately

Shulman, Yale (MD)   U
Christ Hosp

2255 Kennedy Blvd; Jersey City, NJ 07304; (201)
433-1057; **BDCERT:** U 84; **MS:** Albert Einstein Coll
Med 76; **RES:** S, Montefiore Med Ctr, Bronx, NY 76-
78; U, New York University Med Ctr, New York, NY
78-82; **FAP:** Asst Clin Prof U NYU Sch Med; **HOSP:**
Bayonne Hosp; *SI: Sexual Dysfunction; Prostate
Disease & Cancer;* **HMO:** Aetna Hlth Plan HMO Blue
Prucare Travelers

LANG: Sp, Heb; 🔲 🔲 🔲 🔲 🔲 🔲 🔲 🔲 🔲 🔲
Immediately

Steigman, Elliott G (MD)   U
Christ Hosp

142 Palisade Ave 211; Jersey City, NJ 07306; (201)
435-2244; **BDCERT:** U 82; **MS:** SUNY Downstate
75; **RES:** U, Univ Hosp SUNY Bklyn, Brooklyn, NY
77-80; SM, Brooklyn Hosp Ctr, Brooklyn, NY 75-
77; **HOSP:** St Francis Hosp-Jersey City; **HMO:** Blue
Cross & Blue Shield Aetna Hlth Plan Oxford Prucare
GHI +

LANG: Sp, Tag; 🔲 🔲 🔲 🔲 🔲 🔲 🔲   A Few Days

VASCULAR SURGERY (GENERAL)

Zitani Jr, Alfred M (MD)   GVS
St Mary's Hosp-Passaic

331 Grand St; Hoboken, NJ 07030; (201) 420-
7903; **BDCERT:** S 59; **MS:** Geo Wash U Sch Med
49; **RES:** Jersey City Med Ctr, Jersey City, NJ 50-51;
HOSP: Meadowlands Hosp Med Ctr; **HMO:** Oxford
Prucare

🔲 🔲 🔲 🔲 🔲 Immediately **VISA** 🔲

MERCER
COUNTY

SPECIALTY & SUBSPECIALTY	ABBREVIATION	PAGE(S)
Allergy & Immunology	A&I	937
Cardiology (Cardiovascular Disease)	Cv	937
Colon & Rectal Surgery	CRS	938
Dermatology	D	938
Diagnostic Radiology	DR	938
Emergency Medicine	EM	939
Endocrinology, Diabetes & Metabolism	EDM	939
FAMILY PRACTICE	FP	939
Gastroenterology	Ge	939
Infectious Disease	Inf	940
INTERNAL MEDICINE	IM	940-941
Medical Oncology*	Onc	941
Neonatal-Perinatal Medicine	NP	941
Nephrology	Nep	941-942
Neurological Surgery	NS	942
Neurology	N	942-943
OBSTETRICS & GYNECOLOGY	ObG	943
Ophthalmology	Oph	943
Orthopaedic Surgery	OrS	943-945
Otolaryngology	Oto	945
Pain Management	PM	945
Pediatric Allergy & Immunology	PA&I	946
Pediatric Endocrinology	PEn	946
PEDIATRICS (GENERAL)	Ped	946
Physical Medicine & Rehabilitation	PMR	946
Plastic Surgery	PlS	947
Psychiatry	Psyc	947
Pulmonary Disease	Pul	948
Radiation Oncology*	RadRO	948
Radiology	Rad	948-949
Rheumatology	Rhu	949
Surgery	S	949-950
Thoracic Surgery (includes open heart surgery)	TS	950
Urology	U	950-951
Vascular Surgery (General)	GVS	951

Specialties in capital letters indicate Primary Care Specialties. However, many doctors will be certified in a subspecialty, but will practice predominantly primary care medicine. In our lists this will be indicated.

*Oncologists deal with Cancer

ALLERGY & IMMUNOLOGY

Caucino, Julie (DO)   A&I
Somerset Med Ctr
Princeton Allergy & AsthmaBuilding #4, 414 Executive Dr; Princeton, NJ 08540; (609) 921-2202; **BDCERT:** A&I 93; IM 91; **MS:** Kirksville Coll Osteo Med 87; **RES:** RWJ Univ Hosp-New Brunswick, New Brunswick, NJ 88-91; **FEL:** Albert Einstein Med Ctr, Bronx, NY 91; **FAP:** Clin Instr UMDNJ-RW Johnson Med Sch; **SI:** *Asthma; Allergies;* **HMO:** CIGNA Blue Cross HMO Blue Aetna Hlth Plan Oxford +

⬧ 🔲 🔓 🔳 🔲 💲 A Few Days **VISA** 💳

Ricketti, Anthony (MD)   A&I
St Francis Med Ctr
Allergy & Pulmonary Assoc, 1542 Kuser Rd B7; Trenton, NJ 08619; (609) 581-1400; **BDCERT:** A&I 83; Pul 86; **MS:** Hahnemann U 78; **RES:** IM, Cleveland Clinic Hosp, Cleveland, OH 79-81; A&I, Northwestern Mem Hosp, Chicago, IL 81-83; **FEL:** Pul, Northwestern Mem Hosp, Chicago, IL 83-84; **FAP:** Asst Clin Prof UMDNJ-RW Johnson Med Sch; **HOSP:** RWJ Univ Hosp-New Brnsw; **SI:** *Asthma During Pregnancy;* **HMO:** Blue Cross US Hlthcre Prucare Oxford CIGNA +

⬧ 🔓 🔳 🔲 💲 🔲 🔲 🔲 1 Week

Southern, D Loren (MD)   A&I
Med Ctr At Princeton
414 Executive Dr; Princeton, NJ 08540; (609) 921-2202; **BDCERT:** Ped 76; **MS:** Columbia P&S 71; **RES:** Ped, Columbia-Presbyterian Med Ctr, New York, NY 72-74; **FEL:** A&I, Columbia-Presbyterian Med Ctr, New York, NY 74-76; **FAP:** Clin Instr Med UMDNJ-RW Johnson Med Sch; **SI:** *Asthma, Pediatric and;* **HMO:** Aetna Hlth Plan Blue Cross & Blue Shield Oxford CIGNA Prucare +

LANG: Itl, Rus; ⬧ 🔲 🔓 🔳 🔲 💲 A Few Days **VISA** 💳

CARDIOLOGY (CARDIOVASCULAR DISEASE)

Costin, Andrew (MD)   Cv
Med Ctr At Princeton
419 N Harrison St; Princeton, NJ 08540; (609) 924-9300; **BDCERT:** IM 89; Cv 93; **MS:** Yale U Sch Med 86; **RES:** IM, NY Hosp-Cornell Med Ctr, New York, NY; **FEL:** Cv, Hosp of U Penn, Philadelphia, PA; **HMO:** Oxford Aetna Hlth Plan

⬧ 🔲 🔓 🔳 🔲 💲 🔲 A Few Days **VISA** 💳

George, Abraham (MD)   Cv
Capital Health Sys-Mercer
416 Bellevue Ave # 301; Trenton, NJ 08618; (609) 695-6363; **BDCERT:** IM 81; Cv 83; **MS:** India 73; **RES:** S, French Hosp, New York, NY 76-77; IM, St Francis Med Ctr, Trenton, NY 77-80; **FEL:** Cv, Ky Sch Med, Louisville, KY 80-82

Mercuro, T John (MD)   Cv
Med Ctr At Princeton
Princeton Interventional Cardiology, 181 N Harrison St; Princeton, NJ 08540; (609) 921-2800; **BDCERT:** IM 88; Cv 91; **MS:** UMDNJ-RW Johnson Med Sch 85; **RES:** IM, RWJ Univ Hosp-New Brunswick, New Brunswick, NJ 85-88; **FEL:** Cv, Presbyterian Med Ctr, Philadelphia, PA 88-91; **FAP:** Clin Instr IM Univ Penn; **SI:** *Cardiac Catheterization; Coronary Angioplasty/Stent;* **HMO:** CIGNA First Option Oxford United Healthcare US Hlthcre +

LANG: Itl; ⬧ 🔓 🔲 💲 🔲 🔲 🔲 2-4 Weeks

COLON & RECTAL SURGERY

Hardy III, Howard (MD)   CRS
St Francis Med Ctr
3131 Princeton Pike 201 Bl 3C; Trenton, NJ 08648; (609) 896-1700; **BDCERT:** CRS 91; **MS:** Columbia P&S 80; **RES:** S, St Luke's Roosevelt Hosp Ctr, New York, NY 85-86; **FEL:** S, Texas Med Ctr, Houston, TX 85-86; **HOSP:** Capital Health Sys-Fuld
🛇 🞟 🛏 🛇 🞟 A Few Days

Proshan, Steven Gerald (MD)CRS
St Francis Med Ctr
1345 Kuser Rd; Trenton, NJ 08619; (609) 585-1400; **BDCERT:** CRS 96; S 95; **MS:** Columbia P&S 89; **RES:** S, Albert Einstein Med Ctr, Bronx, NY 90-94; **FEL:** CRS, UMDNJ-RW Johnson, Plainfield, NJ 94-95; **HOSP:** RWJ Univ Hosp-Hamilton; **SI:** *Colon and Rectal Cancer; Hemorrhoids*
🛇 🌙 🞟 🞟 🛏 🛇 🞟 🞟 🞟 🞟 Immediately **VISA** 🞟

DERMATOLOGY

Kazenoff, Steven (MD)   D
Med Ctr At Princeton
Princeton Medical Group PA, 419 N Harrison St; Princeton, NJ 08540; (609) 924-9300; **BDCERT:** D 85; IM 82; **MS:** Jefferson Med Coll 79; **RES:** IM, Univ Hosp SUNY Stony Brook, Stony Brook, NY 80-82; D, U Hosp of Cleveland, Cleveland, OH 82-85; **FAP:** Asst Clin Prof UMDNJ-RW Johnson Med Sch; **HMO:** Aetna-US Healthcare Oxford
🛇 🞟 🞟 🞟 🛏 🛇 🞟 2-4 Weeks **VISA** 🞟

Kessel, Daniel (MD)   D
St Francis Med Ctr
2063 Klockner Rd; Hamilton, NJ 08690; (609) 890-2600; **BDCERT:** D 87; **MS:** Temple U 83; **RES:** IM, Abington Mem Hosp, Abington, PA 83-84; **FEL:** D, New York Med Coll, New York, NY 84-87

Kostrzewa, Raymond (MD)   D
St Francis Med Ctr
1345 Kuser Rd 4; Trenton, NJ 08619; (609) 585-3311; **BDCERT:** D 71; **MS:** Jefferson Med Coll 56; **RES:** Skin & Cancer Hosp, Temple 67-70; **SI:** *Acne; Rashes*
🛇 🞟 🞟 🛏 🛇 🞟 2-4 Weeks

Rosenthal, Albert L (MD)   D
Capital Health Sys-Mercer
Lawernceville Dermatology Associates PC, 74 Franklin Corner Rd; Lawrenceville, NJ 08648; (609) 896-3232; **BDCERT:** D 60; **MS:** Tufts U 51; **RES:** D, Rhode Island Hosp, Providence, RI 52-53; D, Mass Gen Hosp, Boston, MA 55-56; **FEL:** D, New York University Med Ctr, New York, NY; **FAP:** Clin Prof D; **HMO:** Blue Choice Blue Cross & Blue Shield CIGNA Prucare Travelers +
🛇 🞟 🌙 🞟 🞟 🞟 🛏 🛇 🞟 🞟 Immediately

Sciallis, Gabriel F (MD)   D
Capital Health Sys-Fuld
2211 Whitehorse Mercerville Rd; Mercerville, NJ 08619; (609) 890-0500; **BDCERT:** D 75; **MS:** Geo Wash U Sch Med 70; **RES:** Mayo Clinic, Rochester, MN 74; **FAP:** Instr D; **HOSP:** RWJ Univ Hosp-Hamilton; **SI:** *Early Diagnosis of Cancer; Acne Treatment;* **HMO:** US Hlthcre NYLCare Prucare
🛇 🞟 🞟 🛏 🛇 🞟 🞟 2-4 Weeks **VISA** 🞟

DIAGNOSTIC RADIOLOGY

Namm, Joel (MD)   DR
St Francis Med Ctr
Radiology Affiliates of Central NJ, 1255 Whitehorse Mercerville; Hamilton Township, NJ 08619; (609) 585-8800; **BDCERT:** Rad 71; **MS:** SUNY Downstate 66; **RES:** Rad, Univ Hosp SUNY Bklyn, Brooklyn, NY 67-70; **FEL:** Rad, Yale-New Haven Hosp, New Haven, CT 70-71; **FAP:** Asst Prof Yale U Sch Med; **HMO:** HMO Blue Blue Cross & Blue Shield Pinnacle NJ Plus
🛇 🌙 🞟 🛏 🞟 🞟 🞟 🞟 Immediately

EMERGENCY MEDICINE

Sussman, Cindy (MD)   EM
RWJ Univ Hosp-Hamilton

R W Johnson Univ Hosp, Dept of Emerg Med, One
Hamilton Health Pl; Hamilton, NJ 08690; (609)
586-7900; **BDCERT:** EM 96; **MS:** Med Coll PA 82;
RES: EM, Hosp Med College of PA, Philadelphia, PA
82-85

[symbols] Immediately **VISA**

ENDOCRINOLOGY, DIABETES & METABOLISM

Willard, David (MD)   EDM
Med Ctr At Princeton

Montgomery Internal Medicine, 727 State Rd;
Princeton, NJ 08540; (609) 924-0115; **BDCERT:**
IM 70; EDM 73; **MS:** Tufts U 64; **RES:** Boston VA
Med Ctr, Boston, MA 66-68; Maine Med Ctr,
Portland, ME 65-66; **FEL:** EDM, Boston U Med Ctr,
Boston, MA 70-72

[symbols] Immediately **VISA**

FAMILY PRACTICE

Carty, Elyse (MD)   FP   PCP
Capital Health Sys-Mercer

Bordentown Family Medical Ctr, 1 3rd St;
Bordentown, NJ 08505; (609) 298-2005;
BDCERT: FP 92; **MS:** NY Med Coll 82; **RES:** FP,
Mountainside Hosp, Montclair, NJ 82-85; **HMO:**
Aetna-US Healthcare Corporate Care Oxford
NYLCare Blue Cross & Blue Shield +

[symbols] A Few Days

Carty, Robert (MD)   FP   PCP
Capital Health Sys-Mercer

Bordentown Family Medical Ctr, 1 3rd St;
Bordentown, NJ 08505; (609) 298-2005;
BDCERT: FP 97; **MS:** UMDNJ-RW Johnson Med Sch
81; **RES:** FP, Mountainside Hosp, Montclair, NJ 81-
84; **HMO:** Aetna-US Healthcare Corporate Care
Oxford NYLCare Blue Cross & Blue Shield +

[symbols] A Few Days

Rednor, Jeffrey (DO)   FP   PCP
RWJ Univ Hosp-Hamilton

1007 Washington Blvd; Robbinsville, NJ 08691;
(609) 448-4353; **BDCERT:** FP 92; **MS:** UMDNJ-NJ
Med Sch, Newark 89; **RES:** FP, UMDNJ-NJ- Newark,
Newark, NJ 90-92; Kennedy Memorial, Stratford,
NJ 90-92; **FEL:** Doctor's Hospital, Columbus, OH
89-90; **SI:** *Osteopathy;* **HMO:** Most

[symbols] A Few Days

GASTROENTEROLOGY

De Antonio, Joseph (MD)   Ge
Capital Health Sys-Fuld

2999 Princeton Pike; Lawrence, NJ 08648; (609)
882-2185; **BDCERT:** IM 89; Ge 91; **MS:** St Louis U
82; **SI:** *Liver Disease*

LANG: Sp; [symbols] 2-4 Weeks

Sachs, Jonathan (MD)   Ge
Med Ctr At Princeton

Princeton Gastroenterology, 281 Witherspoon St
230; Princeton, NJ 08540; (609) 924-1422;
BDCERT: IM 87; Ge 89; **MS:** Med Coll PA 84; **RES:**
IM, Temple U Hosp, Philadelphia, PA 84-87; **FEL:**
Ge, Hosp of U Penn, Philadelphia, PA 87-89; **SI:**
Digestive Problems; Colon Cancer Prevention; **HMO:**
Oxford Aetna-US Healthcare First Option Prucare
HMO Blue +

LANG: Fr; [symbols] A Few Days **VISA**

Guide to symbols and abbreviations can be found on pages 110-113.

939

INFECTIOUS DISEASE

Aufiero, Patrick (MD)   Inf
RWJ Univ Hosp-Hamilton

2085 Klockner Rd; Hamilton, NJ 08690; (609) 587-4122; **BDCERT:** Inf 96; IM 95; **MS:** West Indies 84; **RES:** IM, St Michael's Med Ctr, Newark, NJ 87-89; **FEL:** Inf, St Michael's Med Ctr, Newark, NJ 89-91; **HOSP:** Capital Health Sys-Mercer

♿ Ⓒ 🖺 🚗 🏥 Ⓢ Mcr Mcd WC NFI 1 Week

Nahass, Ronald (MD)   Inf
RWJ Univ Hosp-New Brnsw

11 State Rd 200; Princeton, NJ 08540; (609) 497-1068; **BDCERT:** IM 85; Inf 88; **MS:** UMDNJ-RW Johnson Med Sch 82; **RES:** IM, RWJ Univ Hosp-New Brunswick, New Brunswick, NJ 82-85; **FEL:** Inf, RWJ Univ Hosp-New Brunswick, New Brunswick, NJ 86-88; **FAP:** Asst Clin Prof UMDNJ-RW Johnson Med Sch; **HOSP:** RWJ Univ Hosp-New Brnsw; *SI: HIV Treatment-Clinical Trials; Lyme Disease;* **HMO:** Aetna-US Healthcare Prucare Blue Cross First Option CIGNA +

LANG: Sp; ♿ 🖺 🏥 Ⓢ Mcr WC NFI A Few Days ■ **VISA** 💳

Porwancher, Richard (MD)   Inf
St Francis Med Ctr

Infectious Disease Consultants, 601 Hamilton Ave; Trenton, NJ 08629; (609) 599-5150; **BDCERT:** IM 80; Inf 82; **MS:** Northwestern U 77; **RES:** IM, Med Coll WI, Milwaukee, WI 78-80; **FEL:** Inf, VA Med Ctr, Washington, DC 80-82; *SI: Lyme disease*

♿ 🖺 🏥 Ⓢ Mcr Mcd WC 2-4 Weeks

INTERNAL MEDICINE

Ackley Jr, Alexander (MD)   IM
Med Ctr At Princeton

Medical Center Dept—Medicine, 253 Witherspoon St; Princeton, NJ 08540; (609) 497-4310; **BDCERT:** IM 72; **MS:** Coll Physicians & Surgeons 67; **RES:** Inf, UC San Francisco Med Ctr, San Francisco, CA 71-74; Columbia-Presbyterian Med Ctr, New York, NY 67-69

♿

Deitz, Joel (MD)   IM   **PCP**
Med Ctr At Princeton

Princeton Medical Associates, 253 Witherspoon St; Princeton, NJ 08540; (609) 497-4301; **BDCERT:** Pul 84; CCM 87; **MS:** Tufts U 77; **RES:** IM, Med Coll VA Hosp, Richmond, VA 78-80; **FEL:** Pul, Duke U Med Ctr, Durham, NC 81-84; **FAP:** Asst Prof Med UMDNJ-RW Johnson Med Sch; **HMO:** Prudential CIGNA PHCS Oxford First Option +

♿ 🚗 🏥 Ⓢ Mcr Mcd WC A Few Days **VISA** 💳

Kropinicki, William (MD)   IM
Capital Health Sys-Mercer

160 Lawrenceville Rd; Lawrenceville, NJ 08648; (609) 989-5151; **BDCERT:** IM 87; **MS:** Poland 83; **RES:** IM, Perth Amboy Gen Hosp, Perth Amboy, NJ 84-87

Lancefield, Margaret (MD)   IM   **PCP**
Med Ctr At Princeton

Medical Center at Princeton, 253 Witherspoon St; Princeton, NJ 08540; (609) 497-4301; **BDCERT:** IM 87; **MS:** Yale U Sch Med 84; **RES:** IM, Hosp of U Penn, Philadelphia, PA 84-87; **FAP:** Assoc Clin Prof UMDNJ-RW Johnson Med Sch; **HMO:** Oxford CIGNA First Option Amerihealth

♿ 🖺 🏥 Ⓢ Mcr 2-4 Weeks **VISA** 💳

Laub, Edward (MD)   IM   **PCP**
Capital Health Sys-Fuld

2055 Klockner Rd; Trenton, NJ 08690; (609) 586-8060; **BDCERT:** IM 79; **MS:** UMDNJ-NJ Med Sch, Newark 76; **RES:** Univ Hosp SUNY Buffalo, Buffalo, NY 76; **HMO:** US Hlthcre Prucare Amerihealth CIGNA HMO Blue +

♿ 🖺 🚗 🏥 WC NFI Immediately

Murray, Simon (MD)   IM
Med Ctr At Princeton

Montgomery Internal Medicine Group, 727 State
Rd; Princeton, NJ 08540; (609) 921-6410;
BDCERT: IM 85; **MS:** Indonesia 80; **RES:** IM, RWJ
Univ Hosp-Hamilton, Hamilton, NJ 80-84; **FAP:**
Asst Clin Instr Med UMDNJ-RW Johnson Med Sch;
SI: Wellness and Nutrition; Hyperlipidemia; **HMO:**
CIGNA Aetna Hlth Plan Oxford Prudential

LANG: Chi, Sp; ⬚ ⬚ ⬚ ⬚ ⬚ ⬚ ⬚ ⬚ ⬚
A Few Days ⬚ **VISA** ⬚

Rothberg, Harvey (MD)   IM   **PCP**
Med Ctr At Princeton

419 N Harrison St; Princeton, NJ 08540; (609)
924-9300; **BDCERT:** IM 61; Hem 80; **MS:** Harvard
Med Sch 53; **RES:** Mass Gen Hosp, Boston, MA 53-
55; Mass Gen Hosp, Boston, MA 58-59; **FEL:** Hem,
Walter Reed Army Med Ctr, Washington, DC 55-
58; **FAP:** Clin Prof UMDNJ-RW Johnson Med Sch;
HMO: Oxford Aetna Hlth Plan Unicare Primary
Plus Physician's Health Plan Blue Choice +

⬚ ⬚ ⬚ ⬚ ⬚ ⬚ ⬚ A Few Days **VISA** ⬚ ⬚

MEDICAL ONCOLOGY

Grossman, Bernard (MD)   Onc
Capital Health Sys-Mercer

408 Bellevue Ave; Trenton, NJ 08618; (609) 396-
5800; **BDCERT:** Onc 79; Hem 80; **MS:** Temple U
74; **RES:** Albany Med Ctr, Albany, NY 74-77; **FEL:**
Fox Chase Cancer Ctr,; **HMO:** US Hlthcre Aetna
Hlth Plan Prucare Premier

⬚ ⬚ ⬚ ⬚ ⬚ Immediately

Kane, Michael J (MD)   Onc
RWJ Univ Hosp-Hamilton

5 Hamilton Health Pl Ste 12; Hamilton, NJ 08690;
(609) 631-6960; **BDCERT:** Onc 89; **MS:** UMDNJ-NJ
Med Sch, Newark 83; **RES:** Thomas Jefferson U
Hosp, Philadelphia, PA 83-86; **FEL:** Neoplastic
Disease, Mount Sinai Med Ctr, New York, NY 86-
88; **FAP:** Assoc Prof UMDNJ-RW Johnson Med Sch;
SI: Breast Cancer; Colon Cancer; **HMO:** Pinnacle
Prudential Aetna-US Healthcare Oxford

LANG: Fr; ⬚ ⬚ ⬚ ⬚ ⬚ ⬚ ⬚ A Few Days **VISA**
⬚

Yi, Peter (MD)   Onc
Med Ctr At Princeton

419 N Harrison St; Princeton, NJ 08540; (609)
924-9300; **BDCERT:** IM 87; Onc 89; **MS:** Cornell U
84; **RES:** Brigham & Women's Hosp, Boston, MA
84-87; **FEL:** NY Hosp-Cornell Med Ctr, New York,
NY 87-90; **HMO:** Oxford Aetna Hlth Plan

⬚ ⬚ ⬚ ⬚ ⬚ ⬚ ⬚ Immediately **VISA** ⬚

NEONATAL-PERINATAL
MEDICINE

Axelrod, Randi (MD)   NP
Capital Health Sys-Mercer

Pediatric Medical Group, 446 Bellevue Rd; Trenton,
NJ 08607; (609) 394-4000; **BDCERT:** Ped 90; **NP**
93; **MS:** Mt Sinai Sch Med 87; **RES:** Ped, St
Christopher's Hospital for Children, Philadelphia,
PA 88-90

LANG: Sp; ⬚ ⬚ ⬚ ⬚ A Few Days ⬚ **VISA** ⬚
⬚

NEPHROLOGY

Singh, Ajay (MD)   Nep
Med Ctr At Princeton

Medical Center At Princeton, 253 Witherspoon St;
Princeton, NJ 08540; (609) 497-4301; **BDCERT:**
IM 86; Nep 90; **MS:** Jefferson Med Coll 83; **RES:** IM,
RWJ Univ Hosp-Hamilton, Hamilton, NJ 83-86;
FEL: Nep, Case Western Reserve U Hosp, Cleveland,
OH 86-87; **FAP:** Assoc Prof of Clin Med UMDNJ-RW
Johnson Med Sch; *SI: Kidney Disease; Hypertension;*
HMO: Prudential First Option Amerihealth Blue
Cross PHCS +

LANG: Pun; ⬚ ⬚ ⬚ ⬚ ⬚ ⬚ A Few Days **VISA**
⬚

Somerstein, Michael (MD)   Nep
Capital Health Sys-Fuld
40 Fuld St 1A; Trenton, NJ 08638; (609) 599-
1004; **BDCERT:** IM 77; **MS:** U Cincinnati 66; **RES:**
Nep, Hahnemann U Hosp, Philadelphia, PA 69-70;
FEL: IM, Hahnemann U Hosp, Philadelphia, PA 67-
69; Philadelphia General Hosp, Philadelphia, PA
66-67; **HOSP:** St Francis Med Ctr; *SI: High Blood
Pressure; Diabetes*; **HMO:** Aetna Hlth Plan US
Hlthcre CIGNA Metlife HMO Blue +

⛑ 📷 🏥 🎫 Mcr Mcd   1 Week

Sudhakar, Telechery (MD)   Nep
Capital Health Sys-Fuld
40 Fuld St Ste 401; Trenton, NJ 08638; (609) 599-
1004; **BDCERT:** Nep 77; **MS:** India 71; **RES:** Helene
Fuld Med Ctr, Trenton, NJ 74-76; **HOSP:** Mercy
Med Ctr

⛑ 📷 🏥 🎫 S Mcr Mcd   2-4 Weeks

Wei, Fong (MD)   Nep
Med Ctr At Princeton
Princeton Medical Group, PC, 419 N Harrison St;
Princeton, NJ 08540; (609) 924-9300; **BDCERT:**
IM 76; Nep 76; **MS:** Tufts U 67; **RES:** IM, Boston
Med Ctr, Boston, MA 67-69; IM, Bronx Muncipal
Hosp Ctr, Bronx, NY 69-70; **FEL:** Nep, U NC Hosp,
Chapel Hill, NC 70; Nep, U NC Hosp, Chapel Hill,
NC 71; **FAP:** Assoc Clin Prof UMDNJ-RW Johnson
Med Sch; *SI: Hypertension; Nephritis*; **HMO:** Oxford
Beech Street

⛑ 🅂🄾 🎫 S Mcr   1 Week **VISA** 🔵 ▬

NEUROLOGICAL SURGERY

Abud, Ariel (MD)   NS
Capital Health Sys-Fuld
3100 Princeton Pike; Lawrenceville, NJ 08648;
(609) 771-9089; **BDCERT:** NS 76; **MS:** Mexico 66;
RES: Hackensack U Med Ctr, Hackensack, NJ 67;
NS, Univ Hosp, Saskatoon, Canada 68; **FEL:**
Neuroanatomy, Univ Hosp, Saskatoon, Canada 69;
HOSP: Capital Health Sys-Mercer; *SI: Tremor
Surgery; Implants for Pain Relief*; **HMO:** Aetna Hlth
Plan Blue Choice Blue Cross & Blue Shield CIGNA

⛑ 📷 🏥 🎫 S Mcr Mcd WC NFI   A Few Days 🔳 **VISA**
🔵

Pizzi, Francis (MD)   NS
St Francis Med Ctr
8 Quakerbridge Plz A; Trenton, NJ 08619; (609)
890-0345; **BDCERT:** NS 77; **MS:** NY Med Coll 69;
RES: Hosp of U Penn, Philadelphia, PA 70-75;
HOSP: Capital Health Sys-Mercer; *SI: Spinal Disc
Surgery Same Day*; **HMO:** Most

⛑ 📷 🎫 S Mcr Mcd WC NFI   Immediately **VISA** 🔵

NEUROLOGY

Livingstone, Ian (MD)   N
Med Ctr At Princeton
11 State Rd 300; Princeton, NJ 08540; (609) 683-
5404; **BDCERT:** N 83; Psyc 83; **MS:** South Africa
73; **RES:** N, Baragwanath Gen Hosp, Johannesberg,
South Africa 74-76; N, Harvard Longwood
Program, Boston, MA 80-82; **FEL:** MG, Regional
Neurological Centre, Newcastle-Upon-Tyne,
England 82-83; U of Newcastle-Upon-Tyne,
Newcastle-Upon-Tyne, England 82-83; **FAP:** Asst
Clin Prof N UMDNJ-RW Johnson Med Sch; *SI:
Headache Management*; **HMO:** Blue Cross & Blue
Shield CIGNA Prucare Travelers Oxford +

⛑ 📷 🏥 🎫 Mcr WC   4+ Weeks **VISA** 🔵

Witte, Arnold (MD)　　　N
Capital Health Sys-Mercer
433 Bellevue Ave 1st Fl; Trenton, NJ 08618; (609)
989-0055; **BDCERT:** IM 81; N 83; **MS:** Tufts U 77;
RES: Med, Univ Hosps Cleveland, Cleveland, OH 77-
79; N, Hosp of U Penn, Philadelphia, PA 79-82;
FEL: Hosp of U Penn, Philadelphia, PA 82-83

OBSTETRICS & GYNECOLOGY

Brickner, Gary (MD)　　　ObG
RWJ Univ Hosp-Hamilton
1 Hamilton Health Pl; Hamilton, NJ 08690; (609)
586-7900; **BDCERT:** ObG 81; **MS:** Univ Pittsburgh
75; **RES:** ObG, Pennsylvania Hosp, Philadelphia,
PA 75-79; **HOSP:** Capital Health Sys-Mercer

OPHTHALMOLOGY

Matossian, Cynthia (MD)　　Oph
Capital Health Sys-Fuld
1230 Pkwy Ave 103; Trenton, NJ 08628; (609)
882-8833; **BDCERT:** Oph 86; **MS:** Penn State U-
Hershey Med Ctr 81; **RES:** Geo Wash U Med Ctr,
Washington, DC 85; **HOSP:** Med Ctr At Princeton;
SI: Cataract Surgery and Implants; Glaucoma; **HMO:**
HMO Blue Aetna Hlth Plan American Health Plan
LANG: Fr; ♿ 🅂🄰 🌙 📷 👪 🛏 🅂 Mcr Mcd WC NFI
A Few Days **VISA** 💳 💳

Pica, Vincent (MD)　　　Oph
RWJ Univ Hosp-Hamilton
3105 Nottingham Way; Trenton, NJ 08619; (609)
587-4287; **BDCERT:** Oph 69; **MS:** Med Coll Wisc
56; **RES:** Oph, Hosp of U Penn, Philadelphia, PA 63-
64; Oph, Univ of Med & Dent NJ Hosp, Newark, NJ
64-66; **FAP:** Instr UMDNJ-NJ Med Sch, Newark;
HOSP: St Francis Med Ctr; *SI: Cataract; Glaucoma;*
HMO: Aetna-US Healthcare CIGNA NJ Plus Blue
Cross & Blue Shield
LANG: Itl; ♿ 📷 👪 🛏 🅂 Mcr Mcd WC NFI
Immediately **VISA** 💳

Wong, Michael (MD)　　　Oph
Med Ctr At Princeton
419 N Harrison St 104; Princeton, NJ 08540;
(609) 921-9437; **BDCERT:** Oph 83; **MS:** Albany
Med Coll 78; **RES:** IM, Albany Med Ctr, Albany, NY
78-79; Oph, Wills Eye Hosp, Philadelphia, PA 79-
82; **FAP:** Clin Instr UMDNJ-RW Johnson Med Sch;
SI: Laser Vision Correction; Cataract Surgery; **HMO:**
Oxford US Hlthcre Blue Cross & Blue Shield CIGNA
Prucare +
♿ 🅂🄰 📷 👪 🛏 🅂 Mcr WC NFI　2-4 Weeks **VISA** 💳

Wong, Richard (MD)　　　Oph
Med Ctr At Princeton
419 N Harrison St 104; Princeton, NJ 08540;
(609) 921-9437; **BDCERT:** Oph 87; IM 82; **MS:**
UMDNJ-NJ Med Sch, Newark 79; **RES:** Oph, Wills
Eye Hosp, Philadelphia, PA 82-85; IM, Thomas
Jefferson U Hosp, Philadelphia, PA 79-82; *SI:*
Cataract Surgery; Refractive Surgery; **HMO:** Aetna
Hlth Plan CIGNA Oxford United Healthcare
American Health Plan +
♿ 🅂🄰 🌙 📷 👪 🛏 🅂 Mcr Mcd　2-4 Weeks **VISA** 💳

ORTHOPAEDIC SURGERY

Abrams, Jeffrey (MD)　　　OrS
Med Ctr At Princeton
Princeton Orthopaedic Associates, 325 Princeton
Ave; Princeton, NJ 08540; (609) 924-8131;
BDCERT: OrS 88; **MS:** SUNY Syracuse 80; **RES:**
OrS, Thomas Jefferson U Hosp, Philadelphia, PA
81-85; **FEL:** Shoulder S, U Of Western Ontario,
London, Canada 85-86; SM, Hughston Sports Med
Hosp, Columbus, OH 86; *SI: Shoulder Surgery; Sports*
Medicine; **HMO:** Aetna Hlth Plan CIGNA Oxford
United Healthcare Blue Cross & Blue Shield +
LANG: Sp; ♿ 🅂🄰 🌙 📷 🛏 🅂 Mcr WC NFI　1 Week
VISA 💳

Costa, Leon (MD)   OrS
Med Ctr At Princeton

256 Bunn Dr; Princeton, NJ 08540; (609) 924-9229; **BDCERT:** OrS 88; **MS:** Geo Wash U Sch Med 80; **RES:** NY Orthopaedic Hosp, New York, NY; OrS, Helen Hayes Hosp, Rockland, NY 84; **SI:** *Sports Medicine;* **HMO:** Oxford First Option CIGNA Amerihealth CIGNA

♿ ☽ 📷 🏯 ⛶ ♻ Mcr WC NFI   Immediately **VISA** 💳

Eingorn, David (MD)   OrS
Capital Health Sys-Mercer

416 Bellevue Ave # 302; Trenton, NJ 08618; (609) 392-7106; **BDCERT:** OrS 86; **MS:** Temple U 79; **RES:** OrS, Thomas Jefferson U Hosp, Philadelphia, PA 80; **HOSP:** St Mary's Hosp-Passaic

Ford, Edward (MD)   OrS
Capital Health Sys-Mercer

Mercer Bucks Orthopaedics, 3120 Princeton Pike; Lawrenceville, NJ 08648; (609) 896-0444; **BDCERT:** OrS 88; **MS:** UMDNJ-NJ Med Sch, Newark 80; **RES:** St Joseph's Hosp-Paterson, Paterson, NJ 81-85

♿ ☽ 📷 ⛶ ♻ Mcr WC NFI   2-4 Weeks **VISA** 💳

Glick, Ronald (MD)   OrS
Capital Health Sys-Fuld

2320 Brunswick Pike; Lawrenceville, NJ 08648; (609) 394-3804; **BDCERT:** OrS 77; **MS:** U Md Sch Med 68; **RES:** OrS, Albert Einstein Med Ctr, Philadelphia 75

Gomez, William (MD)   OrS
St Francis Med Ctr

Trenton Orthopedic Group, 1675 Whitehorse Mercerville Rd; Trenton, NJ 08619; (609) 890-3200; **BDCERT:** OrS 90; **MS:** Columbia P&S 82; **RES:** S, St Vincents Hosp & Med Ctr NY, New York, NY 82-84; OrS, Columbia-Presbyterian Med Ctr, New York, NY 84-87; **FEL:** SM, U of Pittsburgh Med Ctr, Pittsburgh, PA 87-88; **HOSP:** RWJ Univ Hosp-Hamilton; **SI:** *Sports Medicine; Arthroscopic Surgery;* **HMO:** CIGNA Prudential Blue Cross Aetna Hlth Plan

LANG: Sp; ♿ ☽ 📷 🏯 ⛶ ♻ Mcr WC NFI
Immediately 💳 **VISA** 💳 💳

Grenis, Michael (MD)   OrS
Med Ctr At Princeton

256 Bunn Dr; Princeton, NJ 08540; (609) 924-9229; **BDCERT:** OrS 92; **MS:** NY Med Coll 84; **RES:** S, NYU-Bellevue Hosp Ctr, New York, NY 84-85; OrS, NYU-Bellevue Hosp Ctr, New York, NY 85-89; **FEL:** HS, NYU-Bellevue Hosp Ctr, New York, NY 89-90; **HOSP:** Capital Health Sys-Mercer; **HMO:** Blue Cross & Blue Shield Oxford CIGNA First Option

♿ ☽ 📷 🏯 ⛶ ♻ Mcr WC NFI   Immediately **VISA** 💳

Sporn, Aaron (MD)   OrS
RWJ Univ Hosp-Hamilton

Medical Arts Building, 8 Quakerbridge Plz; Mercerville, NJ 08619; (609) 587-4600; **BDCERT:** OrS 86; **MS:** Columbia P&S 78; **RES:** S, St Luke's Roosevelt Hosp Ctr, New York, NY 78-80; OrS, New York University Med Ctr, New York, NY 80-83; **FEL:** OrS, Midwest Inst for Orthopaedics, Cincinnati, OH 83-84; **FAP:** Clin Instr Hahnemann U; **HOSP:** St Francis Hosp-Jersey City; **SI:** *Knee Problems; Sports Medicine;* **HMO:** US Hlthcre Blue Select PHCS Ethix

♿ 📷 🏯 ⛶ ♻ Mcr Mcd WC NFI   Immediately **VISA** 💳 💳

Taitsman, James (MD)   OrS
Capital Health Sys-Mercer

Associated Orthopedics/Sports, 123 Franklin
Corner Rd # 114; Lawrenceville, NJ 08648; (609)
896-0707; **BDCERT:** OrS 77; S 79; **MS:** U
Rochester 71; **RES:** S, Yale-New Haven Hosp, New
Haven, CT 72-73; OrS, Yale-New Haven Hosp, New
Haven, CT 73-76; **FAP:** Instr Yale U Sch Med;
HOSP: RWJ Univ Hosp-Hamilton; *SI: Orthopaedic
Surgery; Sports Medicine;* **HMO:** ABC Health Blue
Cross & Blue Shield HMO Blue Prucare CIGNA +

LANG: Ger; 🔲 🔲 🔲 🔲 🔲 🔲 🔲 🔲
Immediately

OTOLARYNGOLOGY

Davidson, William (MD)   Oto
Capital Health Sys-Mercer

1230 Parkway Ave 300; Trenton, NJ 08628; (215)
504-9400; **BDCERT:** Oto 87; **MS:** U Va Sch Med
82; **RES:** Rutgers U Med Ctr, New Brunswick, NJ; S,
U of Texas Med Sch, Houston, TX; **FEL:** Oto,
Presbyterian Med Ctr, Philadelphia, PA; U of Texas
Med Sch, Houston, TX; **HMO:** US Hlthcre Oxford
Aetna Hlth Plan NYLCare

🔲 🔲 🔲 🔲 🔲 🔲 🔲 Immediately **VISA** 🔲 🔲

Farmer, H Stephen (MD)   Oto
Med Ctr At Princeton

Princeton Otolaryngology Assoc, 457 N Harrison
St 101; Princeton, NJ 08540; (609) 924-0518;
BDCERT: Oto 66; **MS:** Washington U, St Louis 59;
RES: S, Mount Sinai Med Ctr, New York, NY 60-61;
Oto, Barnes Hosp, St Louis, MO 64-66; **FAP:** Assoc
Clin Prof S UMDNJ-RW Johnson Med Sch; *SI: Ear
Surgery; Snoring and Sleep Apnea;* **HMO:** Aetna-US
Healthcare HIP Network CIGNA Prucare US
Hlthcre +

LANG: Sp, Grk; 🔲 🔲 🔲 🔲 🔲 🔲 🔲 1 Week **VISA**
🔲 🔲

Kay, Scott (MD)   Oto
Med Ctr At Princeton

Princeton Otolaryngology Assoc, 457 N Harrison
St 101; Princeton, NJ 08540; (609) 924-0518;
BDCERT: Oto 93; **MS:** Univ Penn 86; **RES:** Oto,
Columbia-Presbyterian Med Ctr, New York, NY 88-
92; S, Mount Sinai Med Ctr, New York, NY 87-88;
FEL: Facial PlS, Shadyside Hosp, Pittsburgh, PA 92-
93; **FAP:** Asst Prof Columbia P&S; *SI: Facial
Cosmetic Surgery; Facial Paralysis;* **HMO:** CIGNA
Prudential Amerihealth Aetna-US Healthcare First
Option +

LANG: Sp; 🔲 🔲 🔲 🔲 🔲 🔲 🔲 2-4 Weeks 🔲
VISA 🔲 🔲

Li, Ronald (MD)   Oto
Med Ctr At Princeton

812 Executive Dr; Princeton, NJ 08540; (609)
921-1000; **BDCERT:** Oto 90; **MS:** Mt Sinai Sch Med
84; **RES:** Montefiore Med Ctr, Bronx, NY 84-89;
Albert Einstein Med Ctr, Bronx, NY 84-89; **FAP:**
Clin Instr Oto UMDNJ-RW Johnson Med Sch; *SI:
Facial plastic surgery;* **HMO:** Aetna Hlth Plan CIGNA
Oxford First Option

🔲 🔲 🔲 🔲 🔲 🔲 🔲 Immediately **VISA** 🔲

PAIN MANAGEMENT

Loren, Gary Mark (MD)   PM
St Francis Med Ctr

1666 Hamilton Ave; Hamilton Township, NJ
08629; (609) 584-9080; **BDCERT:** Anes 88; **MS:**
Univ Pittsburgh 84; **RES:** Anes, Long Island Jewish
Med Ctr, New Hyde Park, NY 85-87; **FEL:** Ped, Long
Island Jewish Med Ctr, New Hyde Park, NY 87-88;
SI: Pain Management

🔲 🔲 🔲 🔲 🔲 🔲 🔲 🔲 🔲 🔲 A Few Days 🔲
VISA 🔲 🔲

PEDIATRIC ALLERGY & IMMUNOLOGY

Winant, John (MD) PA&I
Med Ctr At Princeton
8 Quakerbridge Plz; Mercerville, NJ 08619; (609) 890-8782; **BDCERT:** Ped 80; A&I 81; **MS:** U Cincinnati 75; **RES:** Ped, Children's Hosp Med Ctr, Cincinnati, OH 75-76; Ped, Children's Hosp Med Ctr, Cincinnati, OH 76-78; **FEL:** A&I, Children's Hosp Med Ctr, Cincinnati, OH 78-80; **SI:** *Asthma*; **HMO:** Amerihealth CIGNA Oxford First Option Prudential +

🦽 🏠 👥 🛏 💲 Med *VISA* 💳

PEDIATRIC ENDOCRINOLOGY

Boim, Marilynn (MD) PEn PCP
Capital Health Sys-Mercer
Hamilton Pediatric Assoc, 2400 Whitehorse Mercerville Rd; Mercerville, NJ 08619; (609) 587-4200; **BDCERT:** Ped 87; PEn 97; **MS:** Emory U Sch Med 82; **RES:** Ped, Mt Sinai Hosp, New York, NY; **FEL:** PEn, Mt Sinai Hosp, New York, NY; **SI:** *Endocrinology*

🦽 🆘 🌙 🏠 👥 🛏 💲 Med Immediately▓ *VISA* 💳 ✍

PEDIATRICS

Baiser, Dennis (MD) Ped PCP
RWJ Univ Hosp-Hamilton
Hamilton Pediatric Assoc, 2400 Whitehorse Mercerville Rd; Mercerville, NJ 08619; (609) 587-4200; **BDCERT:** Ped 83; **MS:** NY Med Coll 78; **RES:** Ped, Children's Hosp of Buffalo, Buffalo, NY 78-81; **FAP:** Instr Univ Penn; **SI:** *Developmental Evaluation; Asthma*; **HMO:** Aetna-US Healthcare Prucare HMO Blue Amerihealth Oxford +

🦽 🆘 🌙 🏠 👥 🛏 💲 Med NFI Immediately▓ *VISA* 💳 ✍

Mondestin, Harry (MD) Ped PCP
Capital Health Sys-Fuld
40 Fuld St 309; Trenton, NJ 08638; (609) 989-9125; **BDCERT:** Ped 85; NP 91; **MS:** Haiti 77; **RES:** Ped, Kingsbrook Jewish Med Ctr, Brooklyn, NY 80-83; **FEL:** Rutgers U Med Ctr, New Brunswick, NJ 83-85

LANG: Fr, Sp; 🦽 🌙 🏠 👥 🛏 💲 Med NFI 1 Week

PHYSICAL MEDICINE & REHABILITATION

Carabelli, Robert (MD) PMR
St Francis Hosp-Jersey City
The Back Rehab Institute, 1245 Whitehouse-Mercerville Rd Ste 424; Trenton, NJ 08619; (609) 581-2400; **BDCERT:** PMR 86; **MS:** West Indies 81; **RES:** Hosp of U Penn, Philadelphia, PA 82-84; **FAP:** Lecturer UMDNJ New Jersey Sch Osteo Med
🦽 🏠 🛏 💲 Med Med WC NFI 1 Week *VISA* 💳

Gribbin, Dorota (MD) PMR
RWJ Univ Hosp-Hamilton
Comprehensive Pain and Rehabilitation Center, 2333 WhitehorseMercerville 8; Hamilton, NJ 06819; (609) 588-0540; **BDCERT:** PMR 93; **MS:** Poland 84; **RES:** PMR, NY Hosp-Cornell Med Ctr, New York, NY 89-92; **FAP:** Asst Clin Prof Columbia P&S; **SI:** *Spine Problems & Sports Med; Pain Management*; **HMO:** Oxford CIGNA Amerihealth PHCS +

LANG: Fr, Czc, Rus; 🦽 🆘 🌙 🏠 👥 🛏 💲 Med WC NFI Immediately

Lutz, Gregory (MD) PMR
Hosp For Special Surgery
Hospital for Special Surgery - Bldg 4, 3131 Princeton Pike Ste 100; Lawrenceville, NJ 08648; (609) 896-9190; **BDCERT:** PMR 93; **MS:** Georgetown U 88; **RES:** Mayo Clinic, Rochester, MN 89-92; **FEL:** Hosp For Special Surgery, New York, NY 92-93; **FAP:** Asst Prof PMR Cornell U; **HOSP:** Med Ctr At Princeton; **SI:** *Muscular—Skeletal Disorders*; **HMO:** Amerihealth Blue Cross Oxford CIGNA First Option +

🦽 🏠 👥 🛏 💲 Med WC NFI A Few Days *VISA* 💳

PLASTIC SURGERY

Cimino, Ernest (MD)   PlS
Capital Health Sys-Mercer
Yardley Plastic Surgery, 416 Bellevue Ave 404;
Trenton, NJ 08618; (609) 396-5509; **BDCERT:** PlS
91; **MS:** NYU Sch Med 82; **RES:** S, St Vincents Hosp
& Med Ctr NY, New York, NY 82-86; PlS, Indiana U
Med Ctr, Indianapolis, IN 86-89; *SI: Cosmetic
Surgery; Breast Procedures*; **HMO:** United Healthcare
Carpenters Prucare

[symbols] 2-4 Weeks **VISA** [symbol]

Drimmer, Marc Alan (MD) PlS
Med Ctr At Princeton
Princeton Plastic Surgery, 842 State Rd; Princeton,
NJ 08540; (609) 924-1026; **BDCERT:** PlS 81; **MS:**
Belgium 74; **RES:** Beth Israel Med Ctr, New York,
NY 75-77; Univ Hosp SUNY Syracuse, Syracuse,
NY 77-79; **FAP:** Assoc Clin Prof UMDNJ-RW
Johnson Med Sch; *SI: Cosmetic Surgery; Hand
Surgery*

LANG: Fr; [symbols] 1 Week
VISA [symbol]

Smotrich, Gary (MD)   PlS
Capital Health Sys-Mercer
Lawrenceville Plastic Surgery, 3131 Princeton Pike
Ste 205; Lawrenceville, NJ 08648; (609) 896-
2525; **BDCERT:** PlS 91; **MS:** U Conn Sch Med 82;
RES: S, Boston U Med Ctr, Boston, MA 82-87; PlS, U
Louisville Hosp, Louisville, KY 87-89; **HMO:** Aetna
Hlth Plan Blue Choice Blue Cross & Blue Shield

PSYCHIATRY

Huberman, Roberta (MD) Psyc
Mount Sinai Med Ctr
245 Nassau St; Princeton, NJ 08540; (609) 252-
0660; **BDCERT:** Psyc 93; ChAP 94; **MS:** Harvard
Med Sch 66; **RES:** Georgetown U Hosp,
Washington, DC 66; UC San Francisco Med Ctr,
San Francisco, CA 73; **FEL:** ChAP, Mount Sinai Med
Ctr, New York, NY 87; *SI: Family Psychiatry; Child
& Adolescent Psych*

[symbols] 1 Week

Khouri, Phillippe John (MD) Psyc
Med Ctr At Princeton
Princeton House, 905 Herrontown Rd; Princeton,
NJ 08540; (609) 497-3300; **BDCERT:** Psyc 77;
GerPsy 94; **MS:** Lebanon 72; **RES:** IM, American U
Med Ctr, Beirut, Lebanon 71-72; Psyc, Strong Mem
Hosp, Rochester, NY 72-73; **FEL:** Psychopathology,
Nat Inst Mental Health, Bethesda, MD 95-97; **FAP:**
Prof Psyc UMDNJ-NJ Med Sch, Newark; **HOSP:** RWJ
Univ Hosp-New Brnsw; *SI: Manic Depressive Illness;
Alzheimer's Disease*

LANG: Fr, Ar; [symbols] 1 Week

Leifer, Marvin W (MD)   Psyc
Med Ctr At Princeton
243 Russell Rd; Princeton, NJ 08540; (609) 497-
1810; **BDCERT:** Psyc 77; AdP 77; **MS:** SUNY
Downstate 70; **RES:** Psyc, Albert Einstein Med Ctr,
Bronx, NY 71-74; **FEL:** Psyc, Albert Einstein Med
Ctr, Bronx, NY 74-76; **FAP:** Assoc Prof UMDNJ-RW
Johnson Med Sch; **HOSP:** Capital Health Sys-
Mercer; *SI: Depression; Attention Deficit Disorder*

[symbols] 1 Week

Schneider, Samuel (MD) Psyc
Med Ctr At Princeton
330 N Harrison St; Princeton, NJ 08540; (609)
924-3980; **BDCERT:** Psyc 84; IM 78; **MS:** Univ
Penn 75; **RES:** IM, Hershey Med Ctr, Hershey, PA
75-77; Psyc, UMDNJ-Rutgers Med Sch, Piscataway,
NJ 80-82

PULMONARY DISEASE

Goldblatt, Kenneth (MD)   Pul
Med Ctr At Princeton
Medical Center At Princeton, 253 Witherspoon St;
Princeton, NJ 08540; (609) 497-4301; **BDCERT:**
IM 75; Pul 78; **MS:** NY Med Coll 72; **RES:** IM, St
Luke's Roosevelt Hosp Ctr, New York, NY 72-73;
IM, Rutgers U Med Ctr, New Brunswick, NJ 73-75;
FEL: Pul, Rutgers U Med Ctr, New Brunswick, NJ
75-77; **FAP:** Assoc Clin Prof Med UMDNJ-RW
Johnson Med Sch; *SI: Chronic Obstructive Lung
Disease; Asthma;* **HMO:** Prudential CIGNA Oxford
Amerihealth First Option +

⑂ 🄰 🝆 🎬 🅂 Mcr Mcd WC   1 Week **VISA** ⬤

Harman, John (MD)   Pul   PCP
Capital Health Sys-Mercer
2480 Pennington Rd Ste 104; Trenton, NJ 08638;
(609) 737-7544; **BDCERT:** IM 72; **MS:** Univ Penn
69; **RES:** IM, Presbyterian Med Ctr, Philadelphia,
PA 70-72; **HMO:** Blue Choice Blue Cross & Blue
Shield Prucare Oxford First Option +

🄰 🝆 🎬 Mcr WC   2-4 Weeks

Seelagy, Marc (MD)   Pul
St Francis Med Ctr
Allergy & Pulmonary Assoc, 1542 Kuser Rd B7;
Trenton, NJ 08619; (609) 581-1400; **BDCERT:** Pul
92; **MS:** U Chicago-Pritzker Sch Med 86; **RES:** IM, U
CO Hosp, Denver, CO 86-89; **FEL:** Pul, Johns
Hopkins Hosp, Baltimore, MD 90-93; Sleep
Disorders, Johns Hopkins Hosp, Baltimore, MD 92-
93; **FAP:** Clin Instr UMDNJ-RW Johnson Med Sch;
HOSP: RWJ Univ Hosp-Hamilton; *SI: Sleep
Disorders; Complex Lung Disorders;* **HMO:** Oxford
Prucare US Hlthcre Multicare Blue Cross & Blue
Shield +

⑂ 🄲 🄰 🝆 🎬 Mcr WC NFI   A Few Days

RADIATION ONCOLOGY

Baumann, John (MD)   RadRO
Med Ctr At Princeton
Princeton Radiology Assoc, 253 Witherspoon St;
Princeton, NJ 08540; (609) 497-4304; **BDCERT:**
Rad 81; **MS:** Harvard Med Sch 77; **RES:** IM, Walter
Reed Army Med Ctr, Washington, DC 77-78; Rad,
Harvard Joint Ctr Radiation Therapy, Boston, MA
78-81; *SI: Breast Cancer; Prostate Cancer;* **HMO:** HIP
Network Prucare Blue Cross & Blue Shield Oxford
CIGNA +

⑂ 🄰 🝆 🎬 Mcr Mcd WC NFI   A Few Days **VISA** ⬤

Fram, Daniel K (MD)   RadRO
Capital Health Sys-Mercer
Capital Health at Mercer Med Ctr for Radiation, 446
Bellevue Ave; Trenton, NJ 08607; (609) 394-
4244; **BDCERT:** RadRO 91; **MS:** Univ Vt Coll Med
85; **RES:** Madigan Army Med Ctr, 85-86; Kenner
Army Com Hosp, Petersburg, VA 86-87; **FAP:** Prof
Penn State U-Hershey Med Ctr; **HMO:** Most

LANG: Fr; ⑂ 🄰 🝆 🎬 Mcr Mcd WC   1 Week

Soffen, Edward (MD)   RadRO
Med Ctr At Princeton
Princeton Radiology Associates, 185 Shadybrook
Ln; Princeton, NJ 08540; (609) 497-4304;
BDCERT: RadRO 91; **MS:** Temple U 86; **RES:** Med,
Cooper Hosp, Camden, NJ 87; RadRO, Hosp of U
Penn, Philadelphia, PA 88-90; **FAP:** Asst Prof
UMDNJ-RW Johnson Med Sch; **HOSP:** Centrastate
Med Ctr; *SI: Prostate Seed Implant; Conformal 3D
Radiation*

⑂ 🄰 🝆 🎬 Mcr Mcd   Immediately ▦ **VISA** ⬤

RADIOLOGY

Greenberg, Andrew (MD)   Rad
Med Ctr At Princeton
Princeton Radiology Assoc, 253 Witherspoon St;
Princeton, NJ 08540; (609) 497-4304; **BDCERT:**
RadRO 92; **MS:** UMDNJ-NJ Med Sch, Newark 87;
RES: RadRO, Hosp U Penn, Philadelphia, PA 88-91

Welt, H (MD) Rad
RWJ Univ Hosp-Hamilton

Radiology Affiliates Of NJ, 1255 Whitehorse Mercerville Rd 514; Mercerville, NJ 08619; (609) 585-8800; **BDCERT:** NuM 74; Rad 73; **MS:** NYU Sch Med 67; **RES:** Rad, New York University Med Ctr, New York, NY 72-73; Rad, New York University Med Ctr, New York, NY 68-70; **SI:** *Nuclear Medicine*

[symbols] Immediately

RHEUMATOLOGY

Carney, Alexander (MD) Rhu
Med Ctr At Princeton

8 Quakerbridge Plz H; Mercerville, NJ 08619; (609) 588-9044; **BDCERT:** IM 72; **MS:** Cornell U 66; **RES:** IM, U IA Hosp, Iowa City, IA 69-72; **FEL:** Rhu, U IA Hosp, Iowa City, IA 72-74; **SI:** *General Rheumatology*; **HMO:** Blue Cross & Blue Shield US Hlthcre First Option QualCare Prucare +

[symbols] 2-4 Weeks

Gordon, Richard (MD) Rhu
St Francis Med Ctr

2275 Whitehorse Mercerville Rd 8; Mercerville, NJ 08619; (609) 587-9898; **BDCERT:** IM 78; Rhu 80; **MS:** Jefferson Med Coll 75; **RES:** IM, Geo Wash U Med Ctr, Washington, DC 75-78; **FEL:** Rhu, Georgetown U Hosp, Washington, DC 78-79; St Vincent Hosp, Worcester, MA 79-80; **HOSP:** Capital Health Sys-Fuld; **SI:** *Osteoporosis; Rheumatoid Arthritis*; **HMO:** Prucare Blue Cross & Blue Shield CIGNA HMO Blue Aetna-US Healthcare +

[symbols] 1 Week

Pinals, Robert (MD) Rhu
Med Ctr At Princeton

253 Witherspoon St; Princeton, NJ 08540; (609) 497-4301; **BDCERT:** IM 63; Rhu 74; **MS:** U Rochester 56; **RES:** Strong Mem Hosp, Rochester, NY 56-57; Boston Med Ctr, Boston, MA 59-60; **FEL:** Rhu, Mass Gen Hosp, Boston, MA; **FAP:** Prof Med UMDNJ-RW Johnson Med Sch; **HOSP:** RWJ Univ Hosp-New Brnsw; **HMO:** First Option CIGNA PHCS

[symbols] 2-4 Weeks **VISA** ●

SURGERY

Abouchedid, Claude (MD) S
RWJ Univ Hosp-Hamilton

1542 Kuser Rd B3; Trenton, NJ 08619; (609) 585-2323; **BDCERT:** S 68; **MS:** Lebanon 63; **RES:** Mem Sloan Kettering Cancer Ctr, New York, NY 67; St Francis Med Ctr, Trenton, NJ 63-67; **FEL:** St Francis Med Ctr, Trenton, NJ 62; **HMO:** Aetna Hlth Plan Blue Choice Blue Cross & Blue Shield

LANG: Fr; [symbols] 2-4 Weeks

Chandler, James (MD) S
Med Ctr At Princeton

Princeton Surgical Assoc, 281 Witherspoon St 120; Princeton, NJ 08540; (609) 921-7223; **BDCERT:** S 65; SCC 89; **MS:** U Mich Med Sch 57; **RES:** S, Oregon Health Sci U Hosp, Portland, OR 61-64; S, Boston Med Ctr, Boston, MA 57-58; **FAP:** Clin Prof S UMDNJ-RW Johnson Med Sch; **SI:** *Breast Problems; Cancer; Thyroid Nodules; Cancer*; **HMO:** First Option Oxford HIP Network Aetna-US Healthcare United Healthcare +

[symbols] A Few Days **VISA** ●

Clay, Lucius (MD) S
Med Ctr At Princeton

Princeton Surgical Assoc, 281 Witherspoon St 120; Princeton, NJ 08540; (609) 921-7223; **BDCERT:** CRS 86; S 85; **MS:** U Va Sch Med 79; **RES:** S, St Luke's Roosevelt Hosp Ctr, New York, NY 80-84; **FEL:** CRS, Ochsner Fdn Hosp, New Orleans, LA 84-85; **FAP:** Asst Clin Prof S UMDNJ-NJ Med Sch, Newark; **SI:** *Colon Cancer; Endoscopy*; **HMO:** CIGNA Prucare Oxford HIP Network

[symbols] 1 Week **VISA** ●

Guide to symbols and abbreviations can be found on pages 110-113.

949

Fares II, Louis G (MD)   S
St Francis Med Ctr

Fares Surgical Associates, PC, 1345 Kuser Rd Ste 1; Trenton, NJ 08619; (609) 585-1400; **BDCERT:** S 86; **MS:** U Md Sch Med 78; **RES:** S, St Barnabas Med Ctr, Livingston, NJ 78-84; **FAP:** Asst Clin Prof S UMDNJ-RW Johnson Med Sch; **HOSP:** RWJ Univ Hosp-Hamilton; *SI: Breast Surgery; Minimally Invasive Surgery;* **HMO:** Aetna-US Healthcare Blue Cross & Blue Shield HMO Blue Oxford

LANG: Sp, Fr; 🚪 🔒 🏧 💲 Mcr Mcd WC NFI Immediately **VISA** 💳

Goldman, Kenneth Alan (MD)   S
Med Ctr At Princeton

Princeton Surgical Assocites, 281 Witherspoon St Ste 120; Princeton, NJ 08540; (609) 921-7223; **BDCERT:** S 94; GVS 96; **MS:** NYU Sch Med 88; **RES:** S, Bellevue Hospital, New York, NY 89-93; **FEL:** GVS, New York University Med Ctr, New York, NY 93-94; **FAP:** Asst Clin Prof S UMDNJ-RW Johnson Med Sch; *SI: Carotid Artery Surgery; Aortic Aneurysm Surgery;* **HMO:** Oxford Blue Cross Aetna Hlth Plan Amerihealth Prudential +

LANG: Sp; 🚪 SA/SD 🔒 💊 🏧 💲 Mcr Mcd WC NFI A Few Days 💳 **VISA** 💳

Jordan, Lawrence (MD)   S
Med Ctr At Princeton

Princeton Medical Group, 419 N Harrison St; Princeton, NJ 08540; (609) 924-9300; **BDCERT:** S 89; **MS:** Cornell U 83; **RES:** Columbia-Presbyterian Med Ctr, New York, NY 83-88; *SI: Laparoscopic Surgery;* **HMO:** Oxford US Hlthcre Prucare CIGNA

🚪 SA/SD 🔒 💊 🏧 💲 Mcr WC NFI Immediately 💳 **VISA** 💳

Kahn, Steven (MD)   S
Med Ctr At Princeton

419 N Harrison St; Princeton, NJ 08540; (609) 924-9300; **BDCERT:** S 75; GVS 75; **MS:** NY Med Coll 67; **RES:** U Mich Med Ctr, Ann Arbor, MI 67-73; **FAP:** Asst Clin Prof S UMDNJ-RW Johnson Med Sch; *SI: Vascular Problems; Cancer;* **HMO:** Aetna Hlth Plan Prucare CIGNA Oxford

LANG: Sp; 🚪 SA/SD 🔒 💊 🏧 💲 Mcr Mcd WC NFI Immediately 💳 **VISA** 💳 💳

Schell, Harold S (MD)   S
Capital Health Sys-Mercer

416 Bellevue Ave 406; Trenton, NJ 08618; (609) 392-8100; **BDCERT:** S 91; **MS:** Boston U 70; **RES:** SM, St Vincents Hosp & Med Ctr NY, New York, NY 71-75; *SI: Breast Diseases; Thyroid and Parathyroid;* **HMO:** US Hlthcre Aetna Hlth Plan Oxford HMO Blue

LANG: Itl; 🚪 🔒 🏧 💲 Mcr Mcd A Few Days

THORACIC SURGERY

Ahmad, Imtiaz (MD)   TS
RWJ Univ Hosp-Hamilton

1760 Whitehorse Hamilton 5; Trenton, NJ 08690; (609) 890-2966; **BDCERT:** TS 72; S 72; **MS:** Pakistan 61; **RES:** Northwestern Mem Hosp, Chicago, IL 67-68; S, Michael Reese Hosp Med Ctr, Chicago, IL 69-71; **FEL:** Peripheral VS, Northwestern Mem Hosp, Chicago, IL 67; **HOSP:** St Francis Med Ctr; **HMO:** Metlife

LANG: Ar, Fr, Pun; 🚪 🔒 💊 🏧 Mcr Mcd WC NFI 1 Week

UROLOGY

Orland, Steven (MD)   U
Capital Health Sys-Fuld

6 Colonial Lake Dr D; Lawrenceville, NJ 08648; (609) 882-5564; **BDCERT:** U 89; U 98; **MS:** Columbia P&S 81; **RES:** S, Hosp of U Penn, Philadelphia, PA 82-83; U, Hosp of U Penn, Philadelphia, PA 83-87; *SI: Urinary Incontinence; Prostate Diseases;* **HMO:** HIP Network CIGNA Aetna-US Healthcare Oxford HMO Blue +

LANG: Sp; 🚪 🔒 💊 🏧 💲 Mcr WC NFI Immediately

Rogers, Brad (MD)   U
Capital Health Sys-Mercer

Mercer Urology Assoc, 416 Bellevue Ave Ste 407; Trenton, NJ 08618; (609) 393-2045; **BDCERT:** U 84; **MS:** Jefferson Med Coll 77; **RES:** U, Jackson Mem Hosp, Miami, FL 79-82; S, Montefiore Med Ctr, Bronx, NY 78-79; **HMO:** Most

Rossman, Barry (MD)   U
Med Ctr At Princeton

Urology Group Of Princeton, 281 Witherspoon St
100; Princeton, NJ 08903; (609) 924-6487;
BDCERT: U 91; **MS:** Boston U 83; **RES:** S, Albert
Einstein Med Ctr, Bronx, NY 83-85; U, Montefiore
Med Ctr, Bronx, NY 85-89; **FAP:** Clin Prof UMDNJ
New Jersey Sch Osteo Med; **HOSP:** Univ of Med &
Dent NJ Hosp; *SI: Urinary Incontinence; Prostate
Cancer;* **HMO:** Aetna Hlth Plan CIGNA Blue Cross &
Blue Shield First Option NYLCare +

LANG: Sp, Fr; 🔲 🔲 🔲 🔲 🔲 🔲 🔲 🔲 🔲 2-
4 Weeks ▨ **VISA** 🔲

VASCULAR SURGERY (GENERAL)

Abud, Alfredo (MD)   GVS
Capital Health Sys-Fuld

123 Franklin Corner Rd; Lawrenceville, NJ 08648;
(609) 896-0242; **MS:** Mexico 66; **RES:** St Francis
Med Ctr, Trenton, NJ 75-79; **FEL:** Cleveland Clinic
Hosp, Cleveland, OH 79-80; **HOSP:** St Francis Med
Ctr; **HMO:** Aetna Hlth Plan Blue Cross & Blue Shield
CIGNA

🔲 🔲 🔲 🔲 🔲 🔲 🔲 🔲 Immediately

MIDDLESEX
COUNTY

SPECIALTY & SUBSPECIALTY	ABBREVIATION	PAGE(S)
Allergy & Immunology	A&I	955
Cardiology (Cardiovascular Disease)	Cv	955
Colon & Rectal Surgery	CRS	956
Diagnostic Radiology	DR	956
Endocrinology, Diabetes & Metabolism	EDM	956-957
FAMILY PRACTICE	FP	957
Gastroenterology	Ge	957
Gynecologic Oncology*	GO	958
Hand Surgery	HS	958
Infectious Disease	Inf	958
INTERNAL MEDICINE	IM	958-959
Maternal & Fetal Medicine	MF	960
Medical Oncology*	Onc	960
Nephrology	Nep	960
Neurological Surgery	NS	961
Neurology	N	961
Nuclear Medicine	NuM	962
OBSTETRICS & GYNECOLOGY	ObG	962
Occupational Medicine	OM	962
Ophthalmology	Oph	962
Orthopaedic Surgery	OrS	962-963
Otolaryngology	Oto	963
Pain Management	PM	963
Pediatric Cardiology	PCd	964
Pediatric Nephrology	PNep	964
Pediatric Surgery	PS	964
PEDIATRICS (GENERAL)	Ped	964-965
Plastic Surgery	PlS	965
Psychiatry	Psyc	966
Pulmonary Disease	Pul	966
Radiation Oncology*	RadRO	967
Radiology	Rad	967
Reproductive Endocrinology	RE	967
Rheumatology	Rhu	967-968
Surgery	S	968-969
Thoracic Surgery (includes open heart surgery)	TS	969
Urology	U	970
Vascular Surgery (General)	GVS	970

Specialties in capital letters indicate Primary Care Specialties. However, many doctors will be certified in a subspecialty, but will practice predominantly primary care medicine. In our lists this will be indicated.

*Oncologists deal with Cancer

ALLERGY & IMMUNOLOGY

Sullivan, Bessie (MD)　　A&I
Muhlenberg Regional Med Ctr

37 Progress St A2; Edison, NJ 08820; (908) 753-1133; **BDCERT:** A&I 75; **MS:** Med Coll PA 67; **RES:** IM, Roosevelt Hosp, Edison, NJ 68-70; **FEL:** Rhu, Roosevelt Hosp, Edison, NJ 70-72; Rhu, New York University Med Ctr, New York, NY 72-74; **HOSP:** JFK Med Ctr; *SI: Lupus; Osteoporosis;* **HMO:** Blue Cross & Blue Shield CIGNA Oxford PHS Sanus-NYLCare +

🚻 🅲 🅖 🔟 🛏 🅢 🆆 2-4 Weeks 🔲 **VISA** 💳 🔳

CARDIOLOGY (CARDIOVASCULAR DISEASE)

Burns, John J (MD)　　Cv
RWJ Univ Hosp-New Brnsw

Cardi Assocs New Brunswick, 31 River Rd; Highland Park, NJ 08904; (732) 545-0170; **BDCERT:** IM 78; Cv 81; **MS:** Hahnemann U 75; **RES:** Med, RWJ Univ Hosp-Hamilton, Hamilton, NJ 76-78; Med, UC Irvine Med Ctr, Orange, CA 75-76; **FEL:** Cv, Presbyterian Med Ctr, Philadelphia, PA 78-80; **FAP:** Asst Clin Prof UMDNJ-RW Johnson Med Sch; **HOSP:** St Peter's Med Ctr; *SI: Interventional Cardiology; Coronary Artery Disease;* **HMO:** Blue Shield Oxford First Option AARP

🅖 🔟 🛏 🅜 🆖

Kostis, John B (MD)　　Cv
RWJ Univ Hosp-New Brnsw

PO Box 19, 1 Robert Wood Johnson Pl 4th Fl; New Brunswick, NJ 08903; (732) 235-7208; **BDCERT:** Cv 73; IM 73; **MS:** Greece 60; **RES:** IM, Evangelismos Hosp, Athens, Greece 63-64; **FEL:** Cumberland Med Ctr, Brooklyn, NY 65-67; Philadelphia Gen Hosp, Philadelphia, PA 67-68; **FAP:** Prof Med UMDNJ-RW Johnson Med Sch; **HOSP:** St Peter's Med Ctr; *SI: Heart Diseases; Hypertension;* **HMO:** HIP Network Oxford CIGNA CoMed First Option +

🚻 🅖 🔟 🛏 🅜 🅟 🆖 A Few Days **VISA** 💳

Mermelstein, Erwin (MD)　　Cv
RWJ Univ Hosp-New Brnsw

Cardiology Assoc New Brunswick, 31 River Rd; Highland Park, NJ 08904; (732) 545-0170; **BDCERT:** IM 81; Cv 83; **MS:** Cornell U 78; **RES:** IM, NY Hosp-Cornell Med Ctr, New York, NY 79-81; **FEL:** Cv, Hosp of U Penn, Philadelphia, PA 81-83; **FAP:** Asst Clin Prof Med UMDNJ New Jersey Sch Osteo Med; *SI: Coronary Angioplasty; Cardiac Catheterization;* **HMO:** US Hlthcre Oxford CIGNA/CoMed

LANG: Prt, Heb; 🚻 🅖 🔟 🛏 🅢 🅜 🆆 🆖 2-4 Weeks

Spotnitz, Alan J (MD)　　Cv
RWJ Univ Hosp-New Brnsw

1 Robert Wood Johnson Pl; New Brunswick, NJ 08903; (732) 235-7805; **BDCERT:** Cv 81; **MS:** Columbia P&S 70; **RES:** S, Beth Israel Med Ctr, Boston, MA 71-75; **HMO:** US Hlthcre Pinnacle Americaid Blue Cross Banner +

🚻 🅖 🔟 🛏 🅢 🅜 🅟 🆆 🆖 A Few Days 🔲 **VISA** 💳

Stroh, Jack (MD)　　Cv
RWJ Univ Hosp-New Brnsw

New Brunswick Cardiology Group, 7 Wirt St; New Brunswick, NJ 08901; (732) 545-7874; **BDCERT:** IM 87; Cv 89; **MS:** Albert Einstein Coll Med 84; **RES:** IM, Boston U Med Ctr, Boston, MA 84-87; **FEL:** Cv, New York University Med Ctr, New York, NY 87-90; **FAP:** Asst Instr UMDNJ New Jersey Sch Osteo Med; *SI: Angioplasty; Hypertension;* **HMO:** Aetna Hlth Plan Blue Choice Blue Cross & Blue Shield

🚻 🅖 🔟 🛏 🅢 🅜 🅟

Wajnberg, Alexander (MD)　　Cv
Univ of Med & Dent NJ Hosp

3 Hospital Plz #417; Old Bridge, NJ 08857; (732) 360-1169; **BDCERT:** IM 84; Cv 87; **MS:** SUNY Hlth Sci Ctr 81; **RES:** Univ Hosp SUNY Bklyn, Brooklyn, NY 81-82; Rutgers U Med Ctr, New Brunswick, NJ 82-84; **FEL:** Cv, Rutgers U Med Ctr, New Brunswick, NJ 84-86; **HOSP:** Raritan Bay Med Ctr-Old Bridge; *SI: Coronary Artery Disease; Hypertension;* **HMO:** Prucare US Hlthcre QualCare First Option GHI +

LANG: Pol, Rus, Ger, Itl; 🚻 🅲 🅖 🔟 🛏 🅢 🅜 🅟 🆆 2-4 Weeks

COLON & RECTAL SURGERY

Salvati, Eugene (MD)   **CRS**
Muhlenberg Regional Med Ctr
98 James St 207; Edison, NJ 08820; (908) 756-6640; **BDCERT:** CRS 56; S 62; **MS:** U Md Sch Med 47; **RES:** S, St Vincent's Hosp, Indianapolis, IN 50-51; Veterans Hosp, Indianapolis, IN 51-52; **FEL:** CRS, Allentown Gen Hosp, Allentown, PA 54-56; **FAP:** Clin Prof S UMDNJ-RW Johnson Med Sch; **HOSP:** JFK Med Ctr; **HMO:** Aetna Hlth Plan CIGNA CoMed Connecticut Gen Cost Care +

🔲 🔲 🔲 🔲 🔲 1 Week **VISA** 🔲

Zinkin, Lewis (MD)   **CRS**
St Peter's Med Ctr
B3 Brier Hill Ct; East Brunswick, NJ 08816; (732) 238-2662; **BDCERT:** CRS 78; S 86; **MS:** UMDNJ-NJ Med Sch, Newark 70; **RES:** S, St Vincents Hosp & Med Ctr NY, New York, NY 73-77; CRS, Greater Baltimore Med Ctr, Baltimore, MD 77-78; **FAP:** Assoc Clin Prof S UMDNJ New Jersey Sch Osteo Med; **HOSP:** RWJ Univ Hosp-New Brnsw; **SI:** *Colon Cancer; Inflammatory Bowel Disease*; **HMO:** US Hlthcre Aetna-US Healthcare HMO Blue Prucare NYLCare +

🔲 🔲 🔲 🔲 🔲 🔲 🔲 🔲 2-4 Weeks

DIAGNOSTIC RADIOLOGY

Siegel, Randall (MD)   **DR**
RWJ Univ Hosp-New Brnsw
Radiology Group of New Brunswick, 800 Ryders Lane; East Brunswick, NJ 08816; (732) 937-8617; **BDCERT:** DR 91; 95; **MS:** Univ Penn 86; **RES:** DR, RWJ Univ Hosp-New Brunswick, New Brunswick, NJ 87-91; **FEL:** VIR, RWJ Univ Hosp-New Brunswick, New Brunswick, NJ 91-92; **FAP:** Instr UMDNJ-RW Johnson Med Sch; **HOSP:** St Peter's Med Ctr; **SI:** *Endovascular Therapy; Dialysis Grafts & Access*; **HMO:** HMO Blue CIGNA QualCare Oxford US Hlthcre +

LANG: Sp; 🔲 🔲 🔲 🔲 🔲 🔲 🔲 🔲 A Few Days 🔲 **VISA** 🔲

ENDOCRINOLOGY, DIABETES & METABOLISM

Amorosa, Louis (MD)   **EDM**
St Peter's Med Ctr
1 Robert Wood Johnson Pl CN19; New Brunswick, NJ 08903; (732) 235-7219; **BDCERT:** IM 72; **MS:** UMDNJ-NJ Med Sch, Newark 69; **RES:** Med, Bronx Muncipal Hosp Ctr, Bronx, NY 71-72; Med, Kings County Hosp Ctr, Brooklyn, NY 72-73; **FEL:** EDM, Mount Sinai Med Ctr, New York, NY 73-75; **FAP:** Prof of Clin Med UMDNJ-RW Johnson Med Sch; **HOSP:** RWJ Univ Hosp-New Brnsw; **SI:** *Diagnosis of Thyroid Disease; Treatment of Diabetes Mellitus*; **HMO:** Aetna Hlth Plan Blue Cross & Blue Shield CIGNA HIP Network

🔲 🔲 🔲 🔲 🔲 🔲 🔲 **VISA** 🔲 🔲

Bucholtz, Harvey K (MD)   **EDM**
Newark Beth Israel Med Ctr
1692 Oak Tree Rd; Edison, NJ 08820; (732) 549-7470; **BDCERT:** EDM 75; IM 73; **MS:** SUNY Hlth Sci Ctr 68; **RES:** IM, Montefiore Med Ctr, Bronx, NY 68-69; IM, U Mich Med Ctr, Ann Arbor, MI 69-71; **FEL:** EDM, Duke U Med Ctr, Durham, NC 73-75; **FAP:** Asst Clin Prof UMDNJ New Jersey Sch Osteo Med; **HOSP:** Rahway Hosp; **SI:** *Diabetes Complications Prevention; Thyroid Disorders*

🔲 🔲 🔲 🔲 🔲 🔲 A Few Days **VISA** 🔲

Salas, Max (MD)   **EDM**
St Peter's Med Ctr
St Peter's Med Ctr, 254 Easton Ave 4th Fl.; New Brunswick, NJ 08901; (732) 745-8574; **BDCERT:** Ped 69; PEn 86; **MS:** Mexico 63; **RES:** Ped, Children's Hosp, Boston, MA 65-67; Ped, Children's Hosp, Sheffield, England 67-68; **FEL:** Ped Oto, Children's Hosp of Pittsburgh, Pittsburgh, PA 77-79; Ped, N Shore Univ Hosp-Manhasset, Manhasset, NY 79-80; **FAP:** Assoc Prof Ped UMDNJ-RW Johnson Med Sch; **HOSP:** RWJ Univ Hosp-New Brnsw; **SI:** *Thyroid Growths; Puberty—Diabetes*

LANG: Sp; 🔲 🔲 🔲 🔲 🔲 🔲 2-4 Weeks 🔲 **VISA** 🔲 🔲

Spiler, Ira (MD) EDM
Raritan Bay Med Ctr-Perth Amboy

3 Hospital Plz Ste 307; Old Bridge, NJ 08857; (732) 360-1122; **BDCERT:** IM 76; EDM 79; **MS:** Albert Einstein Coll Med 71; **RES:** Bronx Muncipal Hosp Ctr, Bronx, NY 72-73; Med, Boston Med Ctr, Boston, MA 75-76; **FEL:** EDM, New England Med Ctr, Boston, MA 76-78; **FAP:** Assoc Clin Prof Med UMDNJ-RW Johnson Med Sch

♿ 🌙 📷 🏥 Mcr Mcd 4+ Weeks

FAMILY PRACTICE

Lansing, Martha (MD) FP PCP

Family Health Ctr, 666 Plainsboro Rd Ste 632; Plainsboro, NJ 08536; (609) 275-0487; **BDCERT:** FP 92; **MS:** U Okla Coll Med 82; **RES:** FP, Williamsport U, Williamsport, PA 84-85; *SI: Women's Health; Psychosomatic Illness;* **HMO:** Aetna-US Healthcare CIGNA Blue Cross & Blue Shield HMO Blue Amerihealth +

LANG: Sp; ♿ 🌙 📷 🏥 🏥 S Mcr Mcd WC NFI
A Few Days *VISA* 💳 💳

Sinha, Gopal Krishna (MD) FP PCP

606 Roosevelt Ave; Carteret, NJ 07008; (732) 541-6521; **BDCERT:** FP 77; IM 97; **MS:** India 65; **RES:** IM, Union Mem Hosp, Baltimore, MD 72-73; *SI: Primary Care Hypertension; Immunization, Diabetes;* **HMO:** Prucare Oxford Aetna-US Healthcare United Healthcare HMO Blue +

LANG: Hin, Sp; ♿ 🌙 📷 🏥 🏥 Mcr Mcd WC NFI
Immediately 📠 *VISA* 💳

Swee, David (MD) FP PCP
RWJ Univ Hosp-New Brnsw

1 Penn Plaza; New Brunswick, NJ 08901; (732) 828-5962; **BDCERT:** FP 77; **MS:** Canada 75; **RES:** Dalhousie U, Montreal, Canada 74-75; Somerset Med Ctr, Somerville, NJ 75-77; **HOSP:** St Peter's Med Ctr; **HMO:** Amerihealth CIGNA Prucare US Hlthcre HMO Blue +

♿ 🌙 📷 🏥 🏥 S Mcr Mcd WC NFI A Few Days

Tierney, Peter (MD) FP PCP
Med Ctr At Princeton

Plainsboro Family Physicians, 666 Plainsboro Rd 1316; Plainsboro, NJ 08536; (609) 275-8100; **BDCERT:** FP 86; **MS:** U Va Sch Med 83; **RES:** FP, Hunterdon Med Ctr, Flemington, NJ 83-86; **HMO:** Aetna Hlth Plan Blue Choice CIGNA US Hlthcre Prucare +

♿ 🌙 📷 🏥 🏥 S Mcr A Few Days *VISA*

GASTROENTEROLOGY

Hodes, Steven (MD) Ge
Raritan Bay Med Ctr-Perth Amboy

Gastroenterology Consultants, PA, 760 Amboy Ave; Edison, NJ 08837; (732) 225-9455; **BDCERT:** IM 77; **MS:** Albert Einstein Coll Med 74; **RES:** Montefiore Med Ctr, Bronx, NY 75-76; **FEL:** Ge, Mount Sinai Med Ctr, New York, NY 76-77; **HOSP:** JFK Med Ctr; **HMO:** Blue Cross Prudential United Healthcare Aetna Hlth Plan

♿ 🌙 📷 🏥 S Mcr Mcd A Few Days *VISA* 💳

Patel, Kamalesh (MD) Ge PCP
JFK Med Ctr

291 Amboy Ave; Woodbridge, NJ 07095; (732) 634-0020; **BDCERT:** Ge 83; IM 90; **MS:** Univ Penn 71; **RES:** IM, Thomas Jefferson U Hosp, Philadelphia, PA 87-90; **FEL:** Ge, Thomas Jefferson U Hosp, Philadelphia, PA 90-92; *SI: Prevention of Colon Cancer; Nutrition;* **HMO:** Blue Cross & Blue Shield US Hlthcre CIGNA Prudential Most +

LANG: Hin, Guj; ♿ 🌙 📷 🏥 🏥 S Mcr Mcd NFI *VISA*
💳

Rosenheck, David (MD) Ge
JFK Med Ctr

Gastroenterology Consultants, PA, 760 Amboy Ave; Edison, NJ 08837; (732) 225-9455; **BDCERT:** IM 86; **MS:** UMDNJ-NJ Med Sch, Newark 83; **RES:** Univ of Med & Dent NJ Hosp, Newark, NJ 84-86; **FEL:** Ge, Univ of Med & Dent NJ Hosp, Newark, NJ 86-88; **HOSP:** Raritan Bay Med Ctr-Old Bridge; **HMO:** Blue Cross Prudential United Healthcare Aetna Hlth Plan

♿ 🌙 📷 🏥 S Mcr Mcd *VISA* 💳

GYNECOLOGIC ONCOLOGY

Goldberg, Michael (MD) **GO**
RWJ Univ Hosp-New Brnsw
130 Easton Ave; New Brunswick, NJ 08901; (732) 828-3300; **BDCERT:** ObG 77; GO 80; **MS:** Italy 70; **RES:** ObG, Maimonides Med Ctr, Brooklyn, NY 72-75; **FEL:** GO, Jackson Mem Hosp, Miami, FL 75-77; **FAP:** Clin Prof GO UMDNJ-RW Johnson Med Sch; **HOSP:** St Peter's Med Ctr; **HMO:** Sanus-NYLCare HealthNet HIP Network CIGNA
☾ ☎ 📅 $ [Mcr] A Few Days VISA MasterCard

HAND SURGERY

Coyle, Michael (MD) **HS**
RWJ Univ Hosp-New Brnsw
University Orthopaedic Assoc, 215 Easton Ave; New Brunswick, NJ 08901; (732) 545-0400; **BDCERT:** OrS 78; HS 89; **MS:** Columbia P&S 68; **RES:** S, UC San Francisco Med Ctr, San Francisco, CA 68-70; OrS, Columbia-Presbyterian Med Ctr, New York, NY 73-76; **FEL:** HS (PlS), Columbia-Presbyterian Med Ctr, New York, NY 76-77; **FAP:** Clin Prof OrS; ***SI:*** *Hand Injuries—Sport; Hand—Arthritic*
LANG: Sp, Prt; ♿ ☎ 🏥 📅 $ [Mcr] [Mcd] [WC] [NFI] 1 Week VISA MasterCard

INFECTIOUS DISEASE

Gartenberg, Gary (MD) **Inf**
RWJ Univ Hosp-New Brnsw
Highland Park Medical Assoc, 205 N 2nd Ave; Highland Park, NJ 08904; (732) 545-7243; **BDCERT:** IM 76; **MS:** UMDNJ-NJ Med Sch, Newark 73; **RES:** IM, Mt Sinai, New York, NY 74-76; **FEL:** Inf, Mt Sinai, New York, NY 77-78; **FAP:** Assoc Clin Prof UMDNJ-RW Johnson Med Sch
🏥 📅 $ [Mcr] [WC] [NFI] 1 Week VISA MasterCard

John, Joseph (MD) **Inf**
RWJ Univ Hosp-New Brnsw
1 Robert Wood Johnson Pl CN19; New Brunswick, NJ 08901; (732) 235-7712; **BDCERT:** IM 73; Inf 78; **MS:** Case West Res U 70; **RES:** Rush Presbyterian-St Lukes Med Ctr, Chicago, IL 70-73; **FEL:** Strong Mem Hosp, Rochester, NY 73-74; Med, Med U of SC Med Ctr, Charleston, SC 76-77; **FAP:** Prof UMDNJ-RW Johnson Med Sch; ***SI:*** *HIV; Chronic Fatigue Syndrome*; **HMO:** US Hlthcre Blue Cross & Blue Shield Oxford
♿ ☎ 🏥 📅 [Mcr] [Mcd] [WC] 2-4 Weeks American Express VISA MasterCard Discover

Sensakovic, John (MD) **Inf**
St Michael's Med Ctr
111 James St; Edison, NJ 08820; (732) 549-3449; **BDCERT:** IM 82; Inf 84; **MS:** UMDNJ-NJ Med Sch, Newark 77; **RES:** IM, St Michael's Med Ctr, Newark, NJ 77-80; **FEL:** Inf, St Michael's Med Ctr, Newark, NJ 80-82; **HOSP:** JFK Med Ctr; ***SI:*** *Lyme Disease; HIV Infection*; **HMO:** First Option
♿ ☾ ☎ 🏥 📅 $ [Mcr] [WC] [NFI] 1 Week

Weinstein, Melvin (MD) **Inf**
RWJ Univ Hosp-New Brnsw
RW Johnson Med Sch, 1 Robert Wood Johnson Pl; New Brunswick, NJ 08901; (732) 235-7713; **BDCERT:** IM 75; Inf 78; **MS:** Geo Wash U Sch Med 70; **RES:** IM, Hartford Hosp, Hartford, CT 73-75; **FEL:** Inf, U CO Hosp, Denver, CO 75-77; **FAP:** Prof UMDNJ-RW Johnson Med Sch; ***SI:*** *Bloodstream Infections; Osteomyelitis*; **HMO:** Aetna-US Healthcare HIP Network HMO Blue First Option QualCare +
☾ 🏥 📅 $ [Mcr] [Mcd] [NFI] 1 Week VISA MasterCard

INTERNAL MEDICINE

Bullock, Richard (MD) **IM** [PCP]
JFK Med Ctr
1511 Park Ave Fl 3; S Plainfield, NJ 07080; (908) 755-6633; **BDCERT:** IM 84; **MS:** Mt Sinai Sch Med 81; **RES:** Mount Sinai Med Ctr, New York, NY 81-84; **HOSP:** Muhlenberg Regional Med Ctr; **HMO:** United Healthcare Oxford NYLCare PHCS
♿ ☾ ☎ 🏥 📅 $ [Mcr] 4+ Weeks American Express VISA MasterCard Discover

Guide to symbols and abbreviations can be found on pages 110-113.

Carson, Jeffrey (MD)   IM
RWJ Univ Hosp-New Brnsw
125 Paterson St 2302; New Brunswick, NJ 08903;
(732) 235-7122; **BDCERT:** IM 80; **MS:**
Hahnemann U 77; **RES:** Med, Hahnemann U Hosp,
Philadelphia, PA 78-80; **FEL:** IM, Hosp of U Penn,
Philadelphia, PA 80-82; **FAP:** Prof IM UMDNJ-RW
Johnson Med Sch; **SI:** *Blood Clot; Blood Transfusion;*
HMO: Blue Cross & Blue Shield First Option HIP
Network US Hlthcre

🔄 📷 👥 🏥 💲 Mcr Mcd WC NFI 2-4 Weeks

DeSilva Jr, Derrick M (MD)   IM
Raritan Bay Med Ctr-Perth Amboy
760 Amboy Avenue; Edison, NJ 08837; (732) 738-
8080; **MS:** Dominican Republic 82; **RES:** IM,
Raritan Bay Med Ctr, Perth Amboy, NJ 85-88;
HOSP: Raritan Bay Med Ctr-Old Bridge; **SI:**
Integrative Medicine; **HMO:** None
LANG: Sp; 🔄 ☾ A Few Days ●

Gil, Constante (MD)   IM   PCP
Raritan Bay Med Ctr-Perth Amboy
262 Kings St; Perth Amboy, NJ 08861; (732) 826-
1609; **BDCERT:** IM 90; **MS:** Dominican Republic
81; **RES:** IM, Raritan Bay Med Ctr, Perth Amboy, NJ
85-89; **FAP:** Asst Clin Prof Med UMDNJ-RW
Johnson Med Sch; **HMO:** US Hlthcre Prucare HIP
Network Oxford QualCare +
LANG: Sp; 🔄 📶 📷 👥 🏥 💲 Mcr A Few Days

Lenger, Ellis Steven (MD)   IM
RWJ Univ Hosp-New Brnsw
579 Cranbury Rd B; East Brunswick, NJ 08816;
(732) 390-1995; **BDCERT:** IM 82; Ge 87; **MS:**
SUNY Downstate 79; **RES:** NY Hosp-Cornell Med
Ctr, New York, NY 80-82; Ge, Beth Israel Med Ctr,
Boston, MA 82-84; **FAP:** Asst Clin Prof Med
UMDNJ-RW Johnson Med Sch; **SI:** *Diseases of the
Bile Duct; Ulcer Disease;* **HMO:** CIGNA US Hlthcre
HMO Blue HMO Blue Metlife +
LANG: Heb; 🔄 📷 👥 🏥 💲 Mcr Mcd A Few Days

Leventhal, Elaine (MD & PhD)IM
RWJ Univ Hosp-New Brnsw
125 Paterson St 2310; New Brunswick, NJ 08901;
(732) 235-7145; **BDCERT:** IM 79; Ger 88; **MS:** U
Wisc Med Sch 74; **RES:** U of WI Hosp, Madison, WI
74-77; U WI Sch Med, Milwaukee, WI 77-79; **FEL:**
Ger, William S Middleton Mem VA Hosp, Madison,
WI 79-81; **FAP:** Prof UMDNJ-RW Johnson Med
Sch; **SI:** *Geriatrics*
LANG: Fr, Sp; 🔄 📷 👥 🏥 💲 Mcr 2-4 Weeks▨
VISA ●

Middleton, John (DO)   IM
Raritan Bay Med Ctr-Perth Amboy
Raritan Bay Infectious Disease, 3 Hospital Plz 208;
Old Bridge, NJ 08857; (732) 360-2700; **BDCERT:**
IM 73; Inf 80; **MS:** UMDNJ-NJ Med Sch, Newark
70; **RES:** Med, Cornell Affil Hosps, New York, NY
71-72; NY Hosp, New York, NY 72-73; **FEL:** Inf,
RWJ Univ Hosp-New Brunswick, New Brunswick,
NJ 75-77; **FAP:** Assoc Clin Prof Med Rutgers U; **SI:**
HIV-AIDS; Osteomyelitis; **HMO:** US Hlthcre CIGNA
Oxford Blue Cross & Blue Shield QualCare +

🔄 ☾ 🏥 💲 Mcr Mcd WC 2-4 Weeks

Sherman, Richard (MD)   IM
RWJ Univ Hosp-New Brnsw
University Medical Group, 1 Robert Wood Johnson
Pl CN19; New Brunswick, NJ 08903; (732) 235-
7778; **BDCERT:** IM 78; Nep 80; **MS:** Albert Einstein
Coll Med 75; **RES:** IM, Metropolitan Hosp Ctr, New
York, NY 75-77; **FEL:** Nep, Albert Einstein Med Ctr,
Bronx, NY 77-79; **FAP:** Prof Med UMDNJ-RW
Johnson Med Sch; **SI:** *Hemodialysis; Peritoneal
Dialysis;* **HMO:** US Hlthcre First Option Oxford
QualCare Amerihealth +

🔄 📷 🏥 Mcr Mcd WC NFI 1 Week **VISA** ●

Guide to symbols and abbreviations can be found on pages 110-113.

959

MATERNAL & FETAL MEDICINE

Nochimson, David (MD)   MF
RWJ Univ Hosp-New Brnsw
254 Easton Ave; New Brunswick, NJ 08903; (732)
828-3000; **BDCERT:** ObG 71; MF 76; **MS:** NY Med
Coll 64; **RES:** Cedars Lebanon Hosp, Los Angeles,
CA 65-69; **FEL:** NP, USC Sch Med, Los Angeles, CA
71-72; **HOSP:** St Peter's Med Ctr

MEDICAL ONCOLOGY

Hait, William (MD & PhD)   Onc
Univ of Med & Dent NJ Hosp
195 Little Albany St; New Brunswick, NJ 08901;
(732) 235-8064; **BDCERT:** Onc 87; IM 82; **MS:**
Univ Penn 78; **RES:** Yale-New Haven Hosp, New
Haven, CT 82-83; **HOSP:** RWJ Univ Hosp-New
Brnsw; *SI: Breast Cancer*

[symbols] 1 Week [symbols] **VISA** [symbols]

Miskoff, A R (DO)   Onc
JFK Med Ctr
3 Hospital Plz; Old Bridge, NJ 08857; (732) 287-
2690; **BDCERT:** Hem 82; Onc 75; **MS:** Coll Of Osteo
Med-Pacific 68; **RES:** IM, Brooke Army Med Ctr,
San Antonio, TX 70-72; **FEL:** HS, Walter Reed
Army Med Ctr, Washington, DC 72-74; **HOSP:**
Raritan Bay Med Ctr-Old Bridge; *SI: Breast Cancer;*
Lung Cancer; **HMO:** Aetna Hlth Plan HIP Network
CIGNA First Option Blue Cross & Blue Shield +

[symbols] Immediately

Nissenblatt, Michael (MD)   Onc
RWJ Univ Hosp-New Brnsw
205 Easton Ave; New Brunswick, NJ 08901; (732)
828-9570; **BDCERT:** IM 76; Onc 79; **MS:** Columbia
P&S 73; **RES:** Johns Hopkins Hosp, Baltimore, MD
73-74; **FEL:** Johns Hopkins Hosp, Baltimore, MD
75-78; **FAP:** Prof; **HOSP:** St Peter's Med Ctr; *SI:*
Breast Cancer; Lung Cancer; **HMO:** CIGNA Oxford US
Hlthcre First Option HMO Blue +

[symbols] Immediately [symbols]

Shypula, Gregory (MD)   Onc
Raritan Bay Med Ctr-Perth Amboy
Oncocare, LLC, 1030 St Georges Ave Ste 307;
Avenel, NJ 07001; (732) 750-1200; **BDCERT:** IM
89; Onc 91; **MS:** Poland 81; **RES:** T Marciniak U,
Wroclaw, Poland 82-84; Raritan Bay Med Ctr,
Perth Amboy, NJ 86-89; **FEL:** St Luke's Roosevelt
Hosp Ctr, New York, NY 89-92; **FAP:** Assoc Clin
Prof Med Columbia P&S; **HOSP:** JFK Med Ctr; *SI:*
Breast Cancer; Cancers of the Blood; **HMO:** Aetna-US
Healthcare Prucare CIGNA Blue Cross & Blue
Shield United Healthcare +

LANG: Pol, Rus; [symbols] A Few Days
VISA [symbols]

NEPHROLOGY

Covit, Andrew (MD)   Nep
RWJ Univ Hosp-New Brnsw
NephrologyHypertension Assoc, 8 Old Bridge Tpke;
South River, NJ 08882; (732) 390-4888; **BDCERT:**
IM 82; Nep 86; **MS:** SUNY Downstate 79; **RES:** NY
Hosp-Cornell Med Ctr, New York, NY 80-82; **FEL:**
Nep, NY Hosp-Cornell Med Ctr, New York, NY 82-
84; **FAP:** Assoc Prof Med UMDNJ-RW Johnson Med
Sch; *SI: Hypertension;* **HMO:** Oxford US Hlthcre
Aetna Hlth Plan CIGNA

LANG: Kor; [symbols] 2-
4 Weeks **VISA** [symbols]

NEUROLOGICAL SURGERY

Nosko, Michael (MD & PhD) NS
RWJ Univ Hosp-New Brnsw
University Neurosurgical Associates, 125 Paterson
St Suite 1200; New Brunswick, NJ 08901; (732)
235-7757; **BDCERT:** NS 93; **MS:** Canada 82; **RES:**
Toronto Gen Hosp, Toronto, Canada 83; NS, Walter
Mackenzie Ctr, Edmonton, Canada 86-91; **FEL:**
Alberta Heritage Fnd Med Rsrch, Alberta, Canada
83-86; **FAP:** Assoc Prof UMDNJ-RW Johnson Med
Sch; **HOSP:** St Peter's Med Ctr; **SI:** *Cerebral*
Aneurysms; Brain Tumors; **HMO:** US Hlthcre HIP
Network CIGNA Prucare HMO Blue +

LANG: Sp; ⬤ ⬤ ⬤ ⬤ ⬤ ⬤ ⬤ ⬤ 1 Week ▨
VISA ⬤ ⬤

NEUROLOGY

Friedlander, Marvin (MD) N
St Peter's Med Ctr
Neurology Association of Central NJ, 754 Highway
18 North 110; East Brunswick, NJ 08816; (908)
688-8800; **BDCERT:** NS 94; **MS:** SUNY Hlth Sci Ctr
82; **RES:** N, Albert Einstein Med Ctr, Bronx, NY 90;
IM, RWJ Univ Hosp-New Brunswick, New
Brunswick, NJ 89; **FEL:** Lyons VA Med Ctr, East
Orange, NJ 93; **HOSP:** RWJ Univ Hosp-New Brnsw;
SI: *Stroke; Epilepsy;* **HMO:** CIGNA Oxford First
Option Blue Cross PPO

⬤ ⬤ ⬤ ⬤ ⬤ ⬤ ⬤ 1 Week **VISA** ⬤

Gainey, Patrick (MD) N
RWJ Univ Hosp-New Brnsw
Neurology Association of Central NJ, 754 Highway
18 North 110; East Brunswick, NJ 08816; (732)
613-1300; **BDCERT:** N 93; **MS:** UMDNJ-RW
Johnson Med Sch 88; **RES:** RWJ Univ Hosp-New
Brunswick, New Brunswick, NJ 88-89; N, Univ of
Med & Dent NJ Hosp, Newark, NJ 89-92; **FEL:** Univ
of Med & Dent NJ Hosp, Newark, NJ 92-93; **HOSP:**
St Peter's Med Ctr; **SI:** *Stroke; Epilepsy;* **HMO:** CIGNA
Oxford First Option Blue Cross PPO

LANG: Fil; ⬤ ⬤ ⬤ ⬤ ⬤ ⬤ ⬤ 1 Week **VISA** ⬤

Gizzi, Martin (MD & PhD) N
JFK Med Ctr
65 James St 107; Edison, NJ 08820; (732) 321-
7010; **BDCERT:** N 90; **MS:** U Miami Sch Med 85;
RES: Mount Sinai Med Ctr, New York, NY 85-89;
FEL: N/Oph, Mount Sinai Med Ctr, New York, NY;
SI: *Neuro-Ophthalmology;* **HMO:** HMO Blue First
Option Mastercare US Hlthcre Oxford +

⬤ ⬤ ⬤ ⬤ ⬤ ⬤ ⬤ 2-4 Weeks **VISA** ⬤

Golbe, Lawrence (MD) N
RWJ Univ Hosp-New Brnsw
RWJ Medical School/University Medical Grp/Dept
of Neurology, 97 Paterson St; New Brunswick, NJ
08901; (732) 235-7729; **BDCERT:** N 84; **MS:** NYU
Sch Med 78; **RES:** Bellevue Hosp Ctr, New York, NY
80-83; **FAP:** Prof N UMDNJ-RW Johnson Med Sch;
SI: *Parkinsonism; Movement Disorders*

⬤ ⬤ ⬤ ⬤ ⬤ 4+ Weeks **VISA** ⬤

Lepore, Frederick (MD) N
RWJ Univ Hosp-New Brnsw
Dept of Neurology, Robert Wood Johnson Medical
School, 97 Paterson St Rm 225; New Brunswick,
NJ 08901; (732) 235-7731; **BDCERT:** N 81; **MS:** U
Rochester 75; **RES:** IM, U Mich Med Ctr, Ann Arbor,
MI 75-76; N, U of VA Health Sci Ctr, Charlottesville,
VA 76-79; **FEL:** N/Oph, Bascom Palmer Eye Inst,
Miami, FL; **FAP:** Prof UMDNJ-RW Johnson Med
Sch; **SI:** *Blepharospasm; Optic Neuritis;* **HMO:** HIP
Network US Hlthcre Oxford Cost Care American
Health Plan +

⬤ ⬤ ⬤ ⬤ ⬤ ⬤ ⬤ 2-4 Weeks

Sage, Jacob (MD) N
RWJ Univ Hosp-New Brnsw
Dept Neurology, RW Johnson Med Sch CN19; New
Brunswick, NJ 08903; (732) 937-7733; **BDCERT:**
N 79; **MS:** Univ Pittsburgh 72; **RES:** NR, Pittsburgh
Med Ctr, Pittsburgh, PA 78; **FEL:** NR, NY Hosp-
Cornell Med Ctr, New York, NY 78-80; **FAP:** Prof
UMDNJ-RW Johnson Med Sch; **SI:** *Parkinson's*
Disease; Dystonia

⬤ ⬤ ⬤ ⬤ ⬤ ⬤ ⬤ ⬤ 4+ Weeks **VISA** ⬤

Guide to symbols and abbreviations can be found on pages 110-113.

961

NUCLEAR MEDICINE

Stahl, Theodore (MD) NuM
RWJ Univ Hosp-New Brnsw

303 George St; New Brunswick, NJ 08901; (732) 249-4410; **BDCERT:** NuM 72; **MS:** Hahnemann U 57; **RES:** Albert Einstein Med Ctr, Philadelphia, PA 58-59

OBSTETRICS & GYNECOLOGY

Bachmann, Gloria (MD) ObG
RWJ Univ Hosp-New Brnsw

University Medical Group, 125 Patterson St 4th Fl; New Brunswick, NJ 08901; (732) 235-7627; **BDCERT:** ObG 81; **MS:** Univ Penn 74; **RES:** Hosp of U Penn, Philadelphia, PA 78; **FAP:** Prof UMDNJ-RW Johnson Med Sch; **HOSP:** St Peter's Med Ctr; *SI: Menopause; Domestic Violence*; **HMO:** CIGNA First Option US Hlthcre HMO Blue Oxford +

LANG: Sp; 🚹 📞 🔲 🔳 🔲 🔲 🔲 🔲 Immediately

Knuppel, Robert A (MD) ObG
St Peter's Med Ctr

University Medical Group, 125 Robert Wood Johnson Pl 4th Fl; New Brunswick, NJ 08903; (732) 235-7643; **BDCERT:** ObG 80; MF 81; **MS:** UMDNJ-NJ Med Sch, Newark 73; **RES:** ObG, New England Med Ctr, Boston, MA 73-76; **FEL:** MF, New England Med Ctr, Boston, MA 76-78; **FAP:** Prof UMDNJ-RW Johnson Med Sch; *SI: High Risk Obstetrics; Office Gynecology*; **HMO:** CIGNA Aetna-US Healthcare Oxford Blue Cross & Blue Shield

🔲 📞 🔲 🔲 🔲 🔲 🔲 🔲 Immediately 🔲 **VISA** ●

OCCUPATIONAL MEDICINE

Kipen, Howard (MD) OM
RWJ Univ Hosp-New Brnsw

681 Frelinghuysem Rd; Piscataway, NJ 08855; (732) 445-0182; **BDCERT:** IM 82; OM 86; **MS:** UC San Francisco 79; **RES:** IM, Columbia Presbyterian Med Ctr, New York, NY 79-82; OM, Mount Sinai Med Ctr, New York, NY 83-84

OPHTHALMOLOGY

Santamaria II, Jaime (MD) Oph
Raritan Bay Med Ctr-Old Bridge

Santamaria Eye Institute, 104 Market St; Perth Amboy, NJ 08861; (732) 826-5159; **BDCERT:** Oph 79; **MS:** Columbia P&S 73; **RES:** Columbia-Presbyterian Med Ctr, New York, NY 75-78; **FEL:** Oph, Columbia-Presbyterian Med Ctr, New York, NY 74-75; **FAP:** Asst Prof Oph Columbia P&S; **HOSP:** JFK Med Ctr; *SI: Cataract Surgery; Corneal Surgeries*; **HMO:** Prudential Aetna-US Healthcare CIGNA Oxford HIP Network +

LANG: Chi, Sp; 🚹 🔲 📞 🔲 🔲 🔲 🔲 🔲 🔲 A Few Days **VISA** ● 🔲

ORTHOPAEDIC SURGERY

Garfinkel, Matthew (MD) OrS
JFK Med Ctr

EdisonMetuchen Orthopedic Grp, 10 Parsonage Rd 500; Edison, NJ 08837; (732) 494-6226; **BDCERT:** OrS 94; **MS:** Cornell U 86; **RES:** Montefiore Med Ctr, Bronx, NY 87-91; **FEL:** SM, Lankenau Hosp, Philadelphia, PA 91-92; **HOSP:** JFK Med Ctr; *SI: Knee Injuries; Shoulder Problems*; **HMO:** Oxford Blue Cross & Blue Shield CIGNA Aetna Hlth Plan +

LANG: Sp, Pol, Itl; 🚹 🔲 🔲 🔲 🔲 🔲 🔲 🔲 A Few Days 🔲 **VISA** ● 🔲

Leddy, Joseph (MD)   OrS
RWJ Univ Hosp-New Brnsw

University Orthopedic Assoc, 215 Easton Ave; New Brunswick, NJ 08901; (732) 545-0400; **BDCERT:** OrS 72; **MS:** Jefferson Med Coll 65; **RES:** S, NY Hosp-Cornell Med Ctr, New York, NY 65-67; OrS, Columbia-Presbyterian Med Ctr, New York, NY 67-70; **FEL:** HS, Los Angeles, CA; **FAP:** Prof UMDNJ-RW Johnson Med Sch; **HOSP:** St Peter's Med Ctr; *SI: Hand Surgery; Upper Extremity;* **HMO:** Aetna-US Healthcare First Option Oxford CIGNA

LANG: Sp; ♿ ⚲ ⏰ 🖼 🏧 $ Mcr Mcd WC NFI A Few Days **VISA**

Lombardi, Joseph (MD)   OrS
JFK Med Ctr

10 Parsonage Rd Ste 500; Edison, NJ 08837; (732) 494-6226; **BDCERT:** OrS 87; **MS:** UMDNJ-RW Johnson Med Sch 78; **RES:** St Vincents Hosp & Med Ctr NY, New York, NY 78-79; Univ of Med & Dent NJ Hosp, Newark, NJ 79-83; **FEL:** Long Beach Mem Med Ctr, Long Beach, CA 83-84; **HOSP:** Rahway Hosp; *SI: Laser Surgery;* **HMO:** Oxford United Healthcare Blue Choice US Hlthcre Blue Shield +

♿ ☾ ⚲ 🖼 🏧 $ Mcr WC NFI A Few Days **VISA** 💳

Zawadsky, Joseph (MD)   OrS
RWJ Univ Hosp-New Brnsw

215 Easton Ave; New Brunswick, NJ 08901; (732) 545-0400; **BDCERT:** OrS 67; **MS:** Columbia P&S 55; **RES:** Columbia-Presbyterian Med Ctr, New York, NY 56; Columbia-Presbyterian Med Ctr, New York, NY 63; **FEL:** Columbia-Presbyterian Med Ctr, New York, NY; Columbia-Presbyterian Med Ctr, New York, NY; **FAP:** Prof UMDNJ New Jersey Sch Osteo Med; **HOSP:** St Peter's Med Ctr; *SI: Knee & Joint Reconstruction; Sports Medicine;* **HMO:** Aetna Hlth Plan Blue Cross Oxford HIP Network US Hlthcre +

♿ ⚲ 🖼 🏧 $ Mcr Mcd WC NFI 2-4 Weeks 🔲 **VISA** 💳 📇

OTOLARYNGOLOGY

Aruna, Pasalai N (MD)   Oto
JFK Med Ctr

408 New Brunswick Ave; Fords, NJ 08863; (732) 738-9090; **BDCERT:** Oto 81; **MS:** India 72; **RES:** Univ of Med & Dent NJ Hosp, Newark, NJ 75-77; Oto, Univ of Med & Dent NJ Hosp, Newark, NJ 77-80; **FAP:** Clin Instr UMDNJ New Jersey Sch Osteo Med; **HOSP:** Rahway Hosp; **HMO:** Most

♿ 🏧 ☾ ⚲ 🖼 🏧 $ Mcr WC NFI A Few Days

Rosenbaum, Jeffrey (MD)   Oto
St Peter's Med Ctr

5 Cornwall Dr B3; East Brunswick, NJ 08816; (732) 238-0300; **BDCERT:** Oto 78; **MS:** Albany Med Coll 73; **RES:** S, Hartford Hosp, Hartford, CT 74-75; Oto, New York University Med Ctr, New York, NY 75-78; **FEL:** PlS, Wayne Cnty Gen Hosp, Detroit, MI 78-79; **FAP:** Assoc Prof NYU Sch Med; **HMO:** Blue Cross & Blue Shield Prucare Sanus-NYLCare

WC

PAIN MANAGEMENT

Choi, Young (MD)   PM
RWJ Univ Hosp-New Brnsw

New Jersey Institute, UMDNJRobert Wood Johnson Medical School, 125 Paterson St Suite 6100; New Brunswick, NJ 08901; (732) 235-6444; **BDCERT:** Anes 90; PM 93; **MS:** South Korea 73; **RES:** Anes, Yale-New Haven Hosp, New Haven, CT 83; **FEL:** PM, RWJ Univ Hosp-New Brunswick, New Brunswick, NJ 91; **FAP:** Asst Prof UMDNJ-RW Johnson Med Sch; *SI: Back Pain Syndrome; Reflex Sympathetic Dystrophy;* **HMO:** Blue Cross & Blue Shield Prudential First Option HIP Network Oxford +

LANG: Kor, Sp; ♿ ⚲ 🖼 $ Mcr Mcd WC NFI 2-4 Weeks **VISA** 💳

Guide to symbols and abbreviations can be found on pages 110-113.

963

PEDIATRIC CARDIOLOGY

Gaffney, Joseph (MD)   PCd
St Peter's Med Ctr

Pediatric Cardiology Assoc, 254 Easton Ave 312;
New Brunswick, NJ 08901; (732) 545-8882;
BDCERT: Ped 88; PCd 91; **MS:** NY Med Coll 81;
RES: Ped, Brookdale Univ Hosp Med Ctr, Brooklyn,
NY 81-84; **FEL:** PCd, Babies Hosp, New York, NY
84-87; **FAP:** Asst Clin Prof Ped Columbia P&S; **SI:**
Fetal Echocardiography; Cardiac Catheterization;
HMO: CIGNA US Hlthcre First Option Oxford

[symbols] 2-4 Weeks

PEDIATRIC NEPHROLOGY

Weiss, Lynne (MD)   PNep
RWJ Univ Hosp-New Brnsw

1 Robert Wood Johnson Pl; New Brunswick, NJ
08903; (732) 235-6230; **BDCERT:** Ped 79; PNep
82; **MS:** Hahnemann U 74; **RES:** Ped, Michael
Reese Hosp Med Ctr, Chicago, IL 74-77; **FEL:** PNep,
Michael Reese Hosp Med Ctr, Chicago, IL 77-79;
FAP: Clin Prof Ped UMDNJ-RW Johnson Med Sch;
HOSP: St Peter's Med Ctr

[symbols] A Few Days **VISA**

PEDIATRIC SURGERY

Krasna, Irwin (MD)   PS
RWJ Univ Hosp-New Brnsw

UMDNJRobert Wood Johnson Schl, PO Box 19, 1
Robert Wood Johnson Pl; New Brunswick, NJ
08901; (732) 235-7821; **BDCERT:** TS 64; PS 75;
MS: U Hlth Sci/Chicago Med Sch 55; **RES:** Mount
Sinai Med Ctr, New York, NY 55-62; **FEL:** PS,
Montreal Children's Hosp, Montreal, Canada 62;
FAP: Prof S UMDNJ-RW Johnson Med Sch; **HOSP:**
St Peter's Med Ctr; **SI:** *New Born Surgery; Childhood
Cancer;* **HMO:** US Hlthcre CIGNA First Option HMO
Blue Oxford +

[symbols] A Few Days **VISA**

Price, Mitchell (MD)   PS
RWJ Univ Hosp-New Brnsw

UMDNJ Robert Wood Johnson Medical School, 1
Robert Wood Johnson Pl CN19; New Brunswick, NJ
08903; (732) 235-7821; **BDCERT:** S 96; PS 98;
MS: U Chicago-Pritzker Sch Med 86; **RES:** New
York University Med Ctr, New York, NY 86-88;
New York University Med Ctr, New York, NY 91-
94; **FEL:** Children's Hosp, Denver, CO 94-96;
Columbia-Presbyterian Med Ctr, New York, NY 88-
91; **FAP:** Asst Prof S UMDNJ-RW Johnson Med Sch;
HOSP: St Peter's Med Ctr; **SI:** *Laparoscopic Surgery
Pediatric; Congenital Lesions;* **HMO:** First Option
Oxford US Hlthcre

LANG: Sp; [symbols] A Few Days
VISA

PEDIATRICS

Carver, David (MD)   Ped
RWJ Univ Hosp-New Brnsw

1 Robert Wood Johnson Pl; New Brunswick, NJ
08901; (732) 235-7900; **BDCERT:** Ped 62; **MS:**
Duke U 55; **RES:** Ped, Children's Hosp, Boston, MA
58-61; **FEL:** Inf, Case Western Reserve U Hosp,
Cleveland, OH 56-58; Harvard Med Sch,
Cambridge, MA 61-63; **FAP:** Chrmn UMDNJ-RW
Johnson Med Sch; **HOSP:** St Peter's Med Ctr; **SI:**
Infectious Disease; **HMO:** Aetna-US Healthcare
QualCare HIP Network

[symbols] A Few Days

Cohen, Richard (MD)   Ped   PCP
St Peter's Med Ctr

North Brunswick Pediatrics, 1598 US Highway
130; North Brunswick, NJ 08902; (732) 297-
0603; **BDCERT:** Ped 74; **MS:** Jefferson Med Coll 68;
RES: Ped, St Luke's Roosevelt Hosp Ctr, New York,
NY 68-69; Ped, St Luke's Roosevelt Hosp Ctr, New
York, NY 69-70; **FEL:** Ped, Thomas Jefferson U
Hosp, Philadelphia, PA 70-72; **FAP:** Asst Clin Prof
UMDNJ New Jersey Sch Osteo Med; **HOSP:** RWJ
Univ Hosp-New Brnsw; **HMO:** Aetna Hlth Plan
CIGNA First Option US Hlthcre CoMed +

[symbols] 2-4 Weeks **VISA**

Drachtman, Richard (MD)   Ped
RWJ Univ Hosp-New Brnsw

Cancer Institute of New Jersey, 195 Little Albany
St; New Brunswick, NJ 08903; (732) 235-7898;
BDCERT: Ped 88; **MS:** U Hlth Sci/Chicago Med Sch
84; **RES:** Ped, N Shore Univ Hosp-Manhasset,
Manhasset, NY 84-88; **FEL:** PHO, Mount Sinai Med
Ctr, New York, NY 89-91; **FAP:** Assoc Prof UMDNJ
New Jersey Sch Osteo Med; **HOSP:** St Peter's Med
Ctr; *SI: Pediatric Cancer; Sickle Cell Disease;* **HMO:**
Aetna Hlth Plan Blue Choice Blue Cross & Blue
Shield

⟨symbols⟩ A Few Days

Ettinger, Lawrence (MD)   Ped
RWJ Univ Hosp-New Brnsw

Cancer Inst NJ, 195 Little Albany St; New
Brunswick, NJ 08901; (732) 235-7898; **BDCERT:**
Ped 78; PHO 78; **MS:** Case West Res U 73; **RES:**
Ped, U MD Hosp, Baltimore, MD 74-75; Ped,
Children's Hosp of Buffalo, Buffalo, NY 75-76; **FEL:**
PHO, Roswell Park Cancer Inst, Buffalo, NY 76-78;
FAP: Assoc Prof Ped UMDNJ-RW Johnson Med Sch;
HOSP: St Peter's Med Ctr; *SI: Pediatric Cancer;
Childhood Blood Disorders;* **HMO:** Aetna Hlth Plan
CIGNA Blue Cross & Blue Shield CoMed Prucare +

⟨symbols⟩ Immediately **VISA** ⟨symbol⟩

Rhoads, Frances (MD)   Ped   PCP
St Peter's Med Ctr

Pediatric Faculty Group, 254 Easton Ave; New
Brunswick, NJ 08901; (732) 745-8600; **BDCERT:**
Ped 81; **MS:** England 65; **RES:** Ped, Philadelphia
Gen Hosp, Philadelphia, PA 66-68; Ped, Kapiolani
Children's Med Ctr, Honolulu, HI 73; **FEL:** ChDev,
Kapiolani Children's Med Ctr, Honolulu, HI 73-75;
FAP: Clin Prof Ped UMDNJ-RW Johnson Med Sch;
HMO: Aetna Hlth Plan Oxford Mercy Health Plans
First Option Americaid +

LANG: Sp; ⟨symbols⟩ A Few Days **VISA**
⟨symbols⟩

PLASTIC SURGERY

Borah, Gregory (MD)   PlS
RWJ Univ Hosp-New Brnsw

UMDNJ - Division of Plastic Surgery, 1 Robert Wood
Johnson Pl MEB 584; New Brunswick, NJ 08903;
(732) 235-7865; **BDCERT:** PlS 86; HS 96; **MS:**
Harvard Med Sch 78; **RES:** S, Mass Gen Hosp,
Boston, MA 78-83; PlS, Yale-New Haven Hosp,
New Haven, CT 83-85; **FAP:** Chf UMDNJ-RW
Johnson Med Sch; **HOSP:** Med Ctr At Princeton; *SI:
Hand Surgery;* **HMO:** HMO Blue First Option Oxford
Aetna-US Healthcare CIGNA +

⟨symbols⟩ 1 Week **VISA** ⟨symbol⟩

Choi, Mihye (MD)   PlS
RWJ Univ Hosp-New Brnsw

Medical Education Building, 1 Robert Wood
Johnson Pl MEB 584; New Brunswick, NJ 08901;
(732) 235-7865; **BDCERT:** PlS 98; **MS:** U
Rochester 87; **RES:** S, Beth Israel Med Ctr, Boston,
MA 87-90; PlS, Mount Sinai Med Ctr, New York,
NY 92-95; **FEL:** HS, New York University Med Ctr,
New York, NY 95-96; **FAP:** Asst Prof UMDNJ-RW
Johnson Med Sch; **HOSP:** St Peter's Med Ctr; *SI:
Hand Surgery;* **HMO:** HMO Blue First Option Oxford
CIGNA Aetna-US Healthcare +

⟨symbols⟩ 1 Week **VISA** ⟨symbol⟩

Nini, Kevin (MD)   PlS
St Peter's Med Ctr

Adult & Pediatric Surgery, 561 Cranbury Rd K;
East Brunswick, NJ 08816; (732) 390-1720;
BDCERT: S 90; PlS 94; **MS:** UMDNJ-RW Johnson
Med Sch 84; **RES:** S, Pennsylvania Hosp,
Philadelphia, PA 84-89; PlS, U FL Shands Hosp,
Gainesville, FL 89-90; **FEL:** Craniofacial S, U Miami
Hosp, Miami, FL 90-91; *SI: Cosmetic Surgery; Breast
Surgery*

⟨symbols⟩ 1 Week ⟨symbol⟩ **VISA** ⟨symbol⟩

Guide to symbols and abbreviations can be found on pages 110-113.

965

PSYCHIATRY

Escobar, Javier I (MD)   Psyc
RWJ Univ Hosp-New Brnsw
University Medical Group, 1 Robert Wood Johnson Pl; New Brunswick, NJ 08903; (732) 828-3000; **BDCERT:** Psyc 77; **MS:** Colombia 67; **RES:** St Vincent DePaul, Colombia 67-68; Psyc, Univ Hosp of Madrid, Madrid, Spain 68-69; **FEL:** Psyc, U MN Med Ctr, Minneapolis, MN 69-72; MG, U MN Med Ctr, Minneapolis, MN 72-73; **FAP:** Chrmn Psyc UMDNJ-RW Johnson Med Sch; **HOSP:** Med Ctr At Princeton; *SI: Depression; Psychopharmacology*
LANG: Sp; 🚫 🌙 🏠 🛏 Mcr Mcd WC **VISA** ⬤

Jones Jr, Frank (MD)   Psyc
RWJ Univ Hosp-Hamilton
671 Hoes Ln; Piscataway, NJ 08854; (732) 235-5611; **BDCERT:** Psyc 77; **MS:** Case West Res U 72; **RES:** Psyc, Boston Med Ctr, Boston, MA 72-73; Psyc, Worcester City Hosp, Worcester, MA 73-75; **FAP:** Prof of Clin Psyc UMDNJ-RW Johnson Med Sch

Schwartz, Arthur (MD)   Psyc
RWJ Univ Hosp-Hamilton
675 Hoes Ln; Piscataway, NJ 08854; (732) 235-4463; **BDCERT:** Psyc 67; **MS:** Harvard Med Sch 61; **RES:** Psyc, Yale-New Haven Hosp, New Haven, CT 62-65; *SI: Psychopharmacology; Psychotherapy*
🏠 🛏 🛏 S Mcr 1 Week **VISA** ⬤

PULMONARY DISEASE

Goldberg, Jory (MD)   Pul   PCP
Med Ctr at Princeton
9 Centre Dr 100A; Jamesburg, NJ 08831; (609) 655-1700; **BDCERT:** IM 81; Pul 84; **MS:** Mexico 76; **RES:** IM, City Hospital, Elmhurst, NY 78-79; IM, Monmouth Hospital, Long Ridge 79-80; **FEL:** Pul, Bergen County Hosp, Livingston 81-82; *SI: Chronic Obstructive Lung Disease; Asthma*; **HMO:** Amerihealth CIGNA Prudential First Option
LANG: Sp; 🚫 🌙 🏠 🛏 🛏 S Mcr 1 Week

Melillo, Nicholas (MD)   Pul
JFK Med Ctr
Middlesex Pulmonary Assoc, 106 James St; Edison, NJ 08820; (732) 906-0091; **BDCERT:** Pul 86; CCM 87; **MS:** UMDNJ-NJ Med Sch, Newark 79; **RES:** IM, St Michael's Med Ctr, Newark, NJ 80-83; **FEL:** Pul, St Michael's Med Ctr, Newark, NJ 83; CCM, St Michael's Med Ctr, New York, NY 85; *SI: Asthma; Lung Cancer*; **HMO:** CIGNA HMO Blue Oxford First Option PHS +
LANG: Sp; 🚫 🏠 🛏 🛏 S Mcr NFI

Riley, David (MD)   Pul
RWJ Univ Hosp-New Brnsw
RWJ Hosp, 1 Robert Wood Johnson Pl; New Burnswick, NJ 08901; (732) 235-7840; **BDCERT:** IM 80; Pul 74; **MS:** U Md Sch Med 68; **RES:** IM, Baltimore City Hosp, Baltimore, MD 68-70; IM, Johns Hopkins Hosp, Baltimore, MD 72-73; **FEL:** Pul, Hosp of U Penn, Philadelphia, PA 70-72; **FAP:** Prof UMDNJ-RW Johnson Med Sch; *SI: Lung Fibrosis (Scarring)*; **HMO:** First Option HIP Network PHCS QualCare US Hlthcre +
🚫 🏠 🛏 Mcr Mcd A Few Days ▦ **VISA** ⬤ ▦

Wolf, Barry (MD)   Pul
JFK Med Ctr
Pulmonary Internists, 2 Lincoln Hwy Ste 301; Edison, NJ 08820; (732) 549-7380; **BDCERT:** Pul 88; CCM 90; **MS:** NYU Sch Med 82; **RES:** IM, Bellevue Hosp Ctr, New York, NY 82-85; **FEL:** CCM, Bellevue Hosp Ctr, New York, NY 85-86; Bellevue Hosp Ctr, New York, NY 86-88; **HOSP:** RWJ Univ Hosp-New Brnsw; *SI: Asthma*; **HMO:** Oxford CIGNA United Healthcare PHS US Hlthcre +
LANG: Heb; 🚫 🌙 🏠 🛏 🛏 S Mcr WC NFI
A Few Days **VISA**

RADIATION ONCOLOGY

Haas, Alexander (MD)   RadRO
St Peter's Med Ctr
St Peters Med Ctr, 254 Easton Ave; New Brunswick, NJ 08901; (732) 745-8590; **BDCERT:** RadRO 72; **MS:** Yugoslavia 62; **RES:** DR, U WA Med Ctr, Seattle, WA 66-67; RadRO, U WA Med Ctr, Seattle, WA 70-72; **FEL:** Thomas Jefferson U Hosp, Philadelphia, PA 72-73; **FAP:** Assoc Clin Prof Rad UMDNJ-RW Johnson Med Sch; **HOSP:** RWJ Univ Hosp-Hamilton; **HMO:** Aetna Hlth Plan Blue Cross & Blue Shield CIGNA HMO Blue HIP Network +
LANG: Crt; ♿ 🏠 🏨 Mcr Mod

Macher, Mark (MD)   RadRO
JFK Med Ctr
MidState Radiation Oncology, 65 James St; Edison, NJ 08820; (732) 321-7167; **BDCERT:** RadRO 86; **MS:** Howard U 82; **RES:** Rad, New York University Med Ctr, New York, NY 82-85; **FEL:** Rad, Univ Hosp SUNY Bklyn, Brooklyn, NY 85-86; **FAP:** Clin Instr SUNY Downstate
♿ 🏨 Mcr Mod   A Few Days

RADIOLOGY

George, Louis (MD)   Rad
JFK Med Ctr
60 James St; Edison, NJ 08820; (732) 632-1650; **BDCERT:** Rad 87; **MS:** UMDNJ-NJ Med Sch, Newark 83; **RES:** Rad, Univ of Med & Dent NJ Hosp, Newark, NJ 84-88; **FEL:** Angiography & Interventional Radiology, Hosp of U Penn, Philadelphia, PA 88-89; **SI:** Angioplasty Stents; CT/US Guided Biopsies; **HMO:** US Hlthcre Blue Cross & Blue Shield First Option Beech Street PHS +
LANG: Chi, Sp, Hin; ♿ 🈂 🅲 🏠 🏨 💲 Mcr Mod WC NFI
A Few Days 🅰 VISA 💳 💳

Sweeney, William (MD)   Rad
St Peter's Med Ctr
Dept Radiation Oncology, St Peters Med Ctr; New Brunswick, NJ 08901; (732) 745-8590; **BDCERT:** Rad 66; **MS:** Univ Penn 59; **RES:** Rad, Columbia-Presbyterian Med Ctr, New York, NY 63-66; **FAP:** Assoc Clin Prof UMDNJ-RW Johnson Med Sch; **SI:** Radiation Oncology; **HMO:** Aetna Hlth Plan HIP Network Blue Cross & Blue Shield US Hlthcre QualCare +
♿ 🏠 🏨 Mcr Mod   1 Week

REPRODUCTIVE ENDOCRINOLOGY

Kemmann, Ekkehard (MD)   RE
RWJ Univ Hosp-New Brnsw
Umdnj Medical School, 303 George St 250; New Brunswick, NJ 08901; (732) 235-7630; **BDCERT:** ObG 75; **MS:** Germany 67; **RES:** ObG, Kings County Hosp Ctr, Brooklyn, NY 70-73; **FEL:** EDM, Univ Hosp SUNY Bklyn, Brooklyn, NY 74-76; **FAP:** Prof ObG UMDNJ-RW Johnson Med Sch; **HMO:** Aetna Hlth Plan Blue Cross & Blue Shield CIGNA

RHEUMATOLOGY

Seibold, James R (MD)   Rhu
RWJ Univ Hosp-New Brnsw
UMDNJ Scleroderma Program, 1 Robert Wood Johnson Pl MEB556; New Brunswick, NJ 08903; (732) 235-7520; **BDCERT:** IM 78; Rhu 80; **MS:** SUNY Downstate 75; **RES:** IM, Long Island Jewish Med Ctr, New Hyde Park, NY 75-78; **FEL:** Rhu, U of Pittsburgh Med Ctr, Pittsburgh, PA 78-80; **FAP:** Prof Med UMDNJ-RW Johnson Med Sch; **SI:** Scleroderma; Raynaud's Phenomenon; **HMO:** US Hlthcre Aetna Hlth Plan CIGNA First Option Blue Cross & Blue Shield +
LANG: Rus, Sp; ♿ 🏠 🏨 💲 Mcr Mod NFI   4+ Weeks
VISA 💳

Guide to symbols and abbreviations can be found on pages 110-113.

967

Sigal, Leonard (MD)   Rhu
RWJ Univ Hosp-New Brnsw

125 Paterson St 3100; New Brunswick, NJ 08901;
(732) 235-7210; **BDCERT:** Rhu 84; **MS:** Stanford U
76; **RES:** Mount Sinai Med Ctr, New York, NY 76-
79; **FEL:** Rhu, Yale-New Haven Hosp, New Haven,
CT 81-84; **A&I,** Yale-New Haven Hosp, New
Haven, CT 82-84; **SI:** *Lyme Disease; Rheumatoid
Arthritis*; **HMO:** CIGNA QualCare HMO Blue Oxford
First Option +

🚹 📷 🅿 🛏 🅂 Mcr Mcd WC NFI   2-4 Weeks ▦ **VISA**
⬤ 🈸

SURGERY

August, David (MD)   S
RWJ Univ Hosp-New Brnsw

Cancer Institute NJ, 195 Little Albany St; New
Brunswick, NJ 08901; (732) 235-7701; **BDCERT:**
S 87; SCC 91; **MS:** Yale U Sch Med 80; **RES:** S, Yale-
New Haven Hosp, New Haven, CT 80-86; **FEL:** S,
Nat Cancer Inst, Bethesda, MD 82-84; **FAP:** Assoc
Prof UMDNJ-RW Johnson Med Sch; **SI:**
Gastrointestinal Cancer; Breast Cancer; **HMO:** Aetna-
US Healthcare CIGNA First Option HMO Blue
Oxford +

🚹 📷 🅿 🛏 🅂 Mcr Mcd WC NFI   A Few Days

Boyarsky, Andrew (MD)   S
RWJ Univ Hosp-New Brnsw

UMDNJ—RW Johnson Med School, Dept Surgery,;
New Brunswick, NJ 08903; (732)235-7920;
BDCERT: S 86; **MS:** 80; **RES:** S, RWJ Univ Hosp-
New Brunswick, New Brunswick, NJ 80-85; **FEL:**
GVS, Maimonides Med Ctr, Brooklyn, NY 85-86;
FAP: Assoc Prof of Clin S UMDNJ-RW Johnson Med
Sch; **SI:** *General & Trauma Surgery; Advanced
Laparoscopy*

LANG: Sp; 🚹 📷 🅿 🛏 Mcr Mcd WC NFI   Immediately

Brolin, Robert E (MD)   S
RWJ Univ Hosp-New Brnsw

University Medical Group, 1 Robert Wood Johnson
Pl 512; New Brunswick, NJ 08903; (732) 235-
7762; **BDCERT:** S 81; **MS:** U Mich Med Sch 74;
RES: U of Pittsburgh Med Ctr, Pittsburgh, PA 74-
80; **FAP:** Prof UMDNJ-RW Johnson Med Sch; **SI:**
Morbid Obesity; Gastrointestinal Surgery; **HMO:** HMO
Blue PM Care CIGNA First Option Oxford +

🚹 📷 🛏 🅂 Mcr Mcd NFI   2-4 Weeks

Chung-Loy, Harold (MD)   S
JFK Med Ctr

Surgical Practices Associates, PA, 3436 Progress St
B1; Edison, NJ 08820; (908) 756-7755; **BDCERT:** S
95; **MS:** Howard U 80; **RES:** S, Mount Sinai Med
Ctr, New York, NY 80-85; **FEL:** Mount Sinai Med
Ctr, New York, NY 82-83; **HOSP:** Rahway Hosp; **SI:**
Renal Transplantation; **HMO:** Aetna Hlth Plan
CIGNA US Hlthcre Oxford Blue Shield +

🚹 🌙 📷 🅿 🛏 🅂 Mcr Mcd WC NFI

Dasmahapatra, Kumar (MD)   S
Raritan Bay Med Ctr-Perth Amboy

Comprehensive Surgical Associates, 473 Amboy
Ave; Perth Amboy, NJ 08861; (732) 442-1331;
BDCERT: S 80; **MS:** India 74; **RES:** Grace Hosp,
Detroit, MI 79; **FEL:** Roswell Park Cancer Inst,
Buffalo, NY 82; **HOSP:** JFK Med Ctr; **HMO:** Oxford
QualCare First Option US Hlthcre CIGNA +

🚹 📷 🅿 🛏 🅂 Mcr Mcd WC NFI   Immediately **VISA** ⬤

Greco, Ralph S (MD)   S
RWJ Univ Hosp-New Brnsw

Dept of Surgery, 1 Robert Wood Johnson Pl; New
Brunswick, NJ 08903; (732) 235-7765; **BDCERT:**
S 74; **MS:** Yale U Sch Med 68; **RES:** S, Yale-New
Haven Hosp, New Haven, CT 69-75; **FAP:** Prof S
UMDNJ-RW Johnson Med Sch; **SI:** *Endocrine &
Breast Surgery; Surgical Oncology*; **HMO:** CIGNA
CoMed First Option HMO Blue US Hlthcre +

🚹 📷 🅿 🛏 Mcr Mcd WC NFI   2-4 Weeks

Konigsberg, Stephen (MD)   S
RWJ Univ Hosp-New Brnsw

Highland Park Surgical Associates, 31 River Rd;
Highland Park, NJ 08904; (732) 846-9500;
BDCERT: S 70; **MS:** Harvard Med Sch 62; **RES:** S,
Peter Bent Brigham Hosp, Boston, MA 63-66; S,
Albert Einstein Med Ctr, Bronx, NY 66-68; **FEL:**
Harvard Med Sch, Cambridge, MA 65-66; **HOSP:** St
Peter's Med Ctr; **HMO:** Oxford First Option US
Hlthcre US Hlthcre US Hlthcre +

LANG: Sp; 🔲🔲🔲🔲🔲🔲🔲🔲🔲 2-4 Weeks

Lewis, Ralph (MD)   S
Univ of Med & Dent NJ Hosp

Cardio Thoracic Surgical Group, 185 Livingston
Ave; New Brunswick, NJ 08901; (908) 725-0555;
BDCERT: TS 88; S 66; **MS:** Cornell U 58; **RES:** NY
Hosp-Cornell Med Ctr, New York, NY 59-65; **FAP:**
Clin Prof S UMDNJ New Jersey Sch Osteo Med;
HOSP: St Peter's Med Ctr; **HMO:** HIP Network US
Hlthcre Aetna Hlth Plan

LANG: Sp; 🔲🔲🔲🔲🔲🔲 1 Week

Simpson, Alec (MD)   S
Muhlenberg Regional Med Ctr

Park Avenue Surgical Associates, PA, 1511 Park
Ave; S Plainfield, NJ 07080; (908) 561-9500;
BDCERT: S 78; GVS 87; **MS:** Panama 70; **RES:** S,
Beth Israel Med Ctr, New York, NY 72-77; **FEL:**
GVS, RWJ Univ Hosp-New Brunswick, New
Brunswick, NJ 77-78; **FAP:** Asst Clin Prof UMDNJ-
RW Johnson Med Sch; **HOSP:** JFK Med Ctr; **SI:**
Stroke Prevention; Diabetic Ulcers; **HMO:** Oxford
CIGNA Aetna-US Healthcare Blue Shield NYLCare
+

LANG: Sp; 🔲🔲🔲🔲🔲🔲🔲🔲🔲🔲
Immediately ▨ **VISA** 💳

Swaminathan, A P (MD)   S
Raritan Bay Med Ctr-Perth Amboy

Comprehensive Surgical Associates, 473 Amboy
Ave; Perth Amboy, NJ 08861; (732) 442-1331;
BDCERT: S 74; **MS:** India 68; **RES:** Univ of Med &
Dent NJ Hosp, Newark, NJ; **FEL:** Univ of Med & Dent
NJ Hosp, Newark, NJ; **HOSP:** JFK Med Ctr; **SI:**
Breast; Laparoscopic Surgery

🔲🔲🔲🔲🔲🔲🔲 A Few Days **VISA** 💳

Wapnir, Irene (MD)   S
RWJ Univ Hosp-New Brnsw

RWJ Hosp, 1 Robert Wood Johnson Pl; New
Brunswick, NJ 08903; (732) 235-7868; **BDCERT:**
S 86; **MS:** Mexico 80; **RES:** S, NY Med Coll, New
York, NY 80-85; RWJ Univ Hosp-Hamilton,
Hamilton, NJ 87-88; **FAP:** Assoc Prof UMDNJ-RW
Johnson Med Sch; **SI:** Breast Cancer Surgery; **HMO:**
CIGNA CoMed First Option HMO Blue US Hlthcre +

LANG: Sp, Heb; 🔲🔲🔲🔲🔲🔲🔲🔲🔲
A Few Days

Zullo, Joseph (MD)   S
St Peter's Med Ctr

7 Wirt St; New Brunswick, NJ 08901; (732) 249-
3020; **BDCERT:** S 65; **MS:** Georgetown U 56; **RES:**
Walter Reed Army Med Ctr, Washington, DC 60-
64; **HOSP:** RWJ Univ Hosp-New Brnsw

THORACIC SURGERY

Mackenzie, James (MD)   TS
RWJ Univ Hosp-New Brnsw

University Medical Group, 125 Patterson St; New
Brunswick, NJ 08903; (732) 235-7802; **BDCERT:**
TS 88; **MS:** Mich St U 51; **RES:** S, U Mich Med Ctr,
Ann Arbor, MI 52-58; TS, U Mich Med Ctr, Ann
Arbor, MI 58-60; **FAP:** Prof UMDNJ-RW Johnson
Med Sch; **HMO:** US Hlthcre CoMed First Option
Blue Cross & Blue Shield CIGNA +

LANG: Sp; 🔲🔲🔲🔲🔲🔲 1 Week **VISA** 💳

Sisler, Glenn (MD)   TS
St Peter's Med Ctr

Cardio Thoracic Surgical Group, 185 Livingston
Ave; New Brunswick, NJ 08901; (732) 725-0555;
BDCERT: TS 70; **MS:** NYU Sch Med 61; **RES:**
Bellevue Hospital Ctr-NYU, New York, NY 68-70;
FAP: Assoc Prof of Clin S UMDNJ New Jersey Sch
Osteo Med; **HOSP:** Somerset Med Ctr; **HMO:** HIP
Network US Hlthcre Aetna Hlth Plan

LANG: Sp; 🔲🔲🔲🔲🔲🔲🔲 1 Week

Guide to symbols and abbreviations can be found on pages 110-113.

969

UROLOGY

Grubman, Jerold (MD)   U
JFK Med Ctr

Urological Surgical Assoc, 10 Parsonage Rd Ste .
118; Edison, NJ 08837; (732) 494-9400; **BDCERT:**
U 76; **MS:** Albert Einstein Coll Med 66; **RES:** U,
Bronx Muncipal Hosp Ctr, Bronx, NY 70-73; **FAP:**
Instr Rutgers U; **HOSP:** Raritan Bay Med Ctr-Perth
Amboy; *SI: Prostate Cancer; Interstitial Cystitis;*
HMO: Aetna-US Healthcare Oxford First Option
United Healthcare CIGNA +

LANG: Sp, Ukr; ♿ 🆘 🔄 📷 ✆ 🏥 $ Mcr Mcd WC
Immediately *VISA* ● ▦

Solomon, Michael (MD)   U
St Peter's Med Ctr

Genito Urinary Surgeons of NJ, 585 Cranbury Rd;
East Brunswick, NJ 08816; (732) 390-8700;
BDCERT: U 81; **MS:** Univ Penn 73; **RES:** New
England Deaconess Hosp, Boston, MA 73-76; U,
Lahey Clinic, Burlington, MA 76-79; **FEL:** Ped U,
Mass Gen Hosp, Boston, MA 81; **FAP:** Assoc Clin
Prof UMDNJ-RW Johnson Med Sch; **HOSP:** RWJ
Univ Hosp-New Brnsw; *SI: Pediatric & Urology;*
Adult Urology

♿ ✆ 📷 🏥 $ Mcr Mcd WC NFI 2-4 Weeks ▦ *VISA*
● ▦

Weiss, Robert E (MD)   U
RWJ Univ Hosp-New Brnsw

Robert Wood Johnson Medical, 1 Robert Wood
Johnson Pl CN19; New Brunswick, NJ 08903;
(732) 235-7776; **BDCERT:** U 96; **MS:** NYU Sch
Med 85; **RES:** S, Mount Sinai Med Ctr, New York,
NY 85-87; U, Mount Sinai Med Ctr, New York, NY
87-91; **FEL:** U, Mem Sloan Kettering Cancer Ctr,
New York, NY 91-94; **FAP:** Asst Prof U UMDNJ-RW
Johnson Med Sch; **HOSP:** St Peter's Med Ctr; *SI:*
Prostate Disease; Bladder Cancer; **HMO:** HIP Network
Aetna Hlth Plan US Hlthcre Blue Cross & Blue
Shield Oxford +

♿ 🔄 📷 🏥 Mcr Mcd WC NFI A Few Days

VASCULAR SURGERY (GENERAL)

Graham, Alan (MD)   GVS
RWJ Univ Hosp-New Brnsw

1 Robert Wood Johnson Pl; New Brunswick, NJ
08901; (732) 235-7816; **BDCERT:** S 85; **MS:**
Queens U 79; **RES:** S, McGill Teaching Hosp,
Ontario, Canada 80-84; **FEL:** GVS, U Chicago Hosp,
Chicago, IL 85; **FAP:** Assoc Prof UMDNJ-RW
Johnson Med Sch; *SI: Carotid Artery; Aortic*
Aneurysm; **HMO:** Aetna Hlth Plan US Hlthcre
CIGNA Oxford First Option +

♿ 🏥 $ Mcr Mcd WC NFI 2-4 Weeks ▦ *VISA* ● ▦

MONMOUTH COUNTY

SPECIALTY & SUBSPECIALTY	ABBREVIATION	PAGE(S)
Allergy & Immunology	A&I	973
Anesthesiology	Anes	973
Cardiology (Cardiovascular Disease)	Cv	973
Colon & Rectal Surgery	CRS	973
Dermatology	D	974
Emergency Medicine	EM	974
Endocrinology, Diabetes & Metabolism	EDM	974
FAMILY PRACTICE	FP	974
Gastroenterology	Ge	975
Gynecologic Oncology*	GO	975
Hand Surgery	HS	975
Hematology	Hem	975
INTERNAL MEDICINE	IM	975-976
Medical Oncology*	Onc	976
Nephrology	Nep	977
Neurology	N	977
OBSTETRICS & GYNECOLOGY	ObG	977
Ophthalmology	Oph	978
Orthopaedic Surgery	OrS	978
Otolaryngology	Oto	978-979
Pain Management	PM	979
PEDIATRICS (GENERAL)	Ped	979
Plastic Surgery	PlS	979
Psychiatry	Psyc	980
Pulmonary Disease	Pul	980
Radiation Oncology*	RadRO	980
Radiology	Rad	980
Rheumatology	Rhu	980
Sports Medicine	SM	981
Surgery	S	981-982
Thoracic Surgery (includes open heart surgery)	TS	982
Urology	U	982-983

Specialties in capital letters indicate Primary Care Specialties. However, many doctors will be certified in a subspecialty, but will practice predominantly primary care medicine. In our lists this will be indicated.

*Oncologists deal with Cancer

ALLERGY & IMMUNOLOGY

Gross, Gary L (MD) A&I
Jersey Shore Med Ctr

Atlantic Allergy, Asthma & Immunology
Associates of NJ, LLC, 3200 Sunset Ave 208; Ocean
Township, NJ 07712; (732) 988-7880; **BDCERT:**
A&I 87; Ped 86; **MS:** NYU Sch Med 81; **RES:** Ped,
Children's Hosp Nat Med Ctr, Washington, DC 81-
84; **FEL:** A&I, Children's Hosp of Los Angeles, Los
Angeles, CA 84-86; **FAP:** Asst Clin Prof UMDNJ-
RW Johnson Med Sch; **HOSP:** Monmouth Med Ctr;
SI: *Asthma; Cough;* **HMO:** Prudential Blue Cross &
Blue Shield CIGNA Oxford

♿ 🌙 📷 🔧 🏧 💲 Mcr Mcd WC NFI 1 Week ▨ **VISA**
⬭ 🔷

Picone, Frank (MD)  A&I
Riverview Med Ctr

Allergy and Asthma Consultants, PA, 709
Sycamore Ave; Tinton Falls, NJ 07701; (732) 747-
8188; **BDCERT:** A&I 75; **MS:** UMDNJ-NJ Med Sch,
Newark 67; **RES:** Jackson Mem Hosp, Miami, FL 68-
69; **FEL:** A&I, Children's Hosp, Boston, MA 72-74;
FAP: Asst Clin Prof Hahnemann U; **HOSP:**
Monmouth Med Ctr; **SI:** *Asthma; Sinus;* **HMO:**
Oxford Blue Cross PPO USHE Prudential United
Healthcare +

♿ 🌙 📷 🔧 🏧 💲 Mcr Mcd A Few Days ▨ **VISA**
⬭ 🔷

ANESTHESIOLOGY

Handlin, David (MD) Anes
Bayshore Community Hosp

Bayshore Community HospitalGarden State
Anesthesia, 727 N Beers St; Holmdel, NJ 07733;
(732) 739-5853; **BDCERT:** Anes 86; **MS:** Columbia
P&S 80; **RES:** PM, Columbia-Presbyterian Med Ctr,
New York, NY 81-83; **FEL:** Chronic Pain,
Columbia-Presbyterian Med Ctr, New York, NY 83-
84; **SI:** *Chronic Pain; Back and Neck Pain*

♿ 📷 🔧 🏧 Mcr Mcd WC 1 Week

CARDIOLOGY (CARDIOVASCULAR DISEASE)

Checton, John (MD) Cv
Monmouth Med Ctr

Monmouth Cardiology Associates, LLC, 215
Brighton Ave; Long Branch, NJ 07740; (732) 222-
5143; **BDCERT:** IM 81; **MS:** UMDNJ-NJ Med Sch,
Newark 78; **RES:** IM, Monmouth Med Ctr, Long
Branch, NJ 78-81; **FEL:** Cv, U Louisville Hosp,
Louisville, KY 81-83; **FAP:** Asst Clin Instr; **HOSP:**
Jersey Shore Med Ctr

♿ 📷 🔧 🏧 💲 Mcr Mcd

Daniels, Jeff (MD) Cv
Monmouth Med Ctr

Monmouth Cardiology Associates, LLC, 215
Brighton Ave; Long Branch NJ, NJ 07740; (732)
222-5143; **BDCERT:** IM 83; Cv 85; **MS:** Albany
Med Coll 80; **RES:** IM, Mount Sinai Med Ctr, New
York, NY 80-83; **FEL:** Cv, Mount Sinai Med Ctr,
New York, NY 83-85; **FAP:** Asst Prof Med
Hahnemann U

♿ 📷 🔧 🏧 💲 Mcr Mcd 2-4 Weeks

COLON & RECTAL SURGERY

Arvanitis, Michael (MD) CRS
Monmouth Med Ctr

Wellington Medical Group, 1131 Broad St;
Shrewsbury, NJ 07702; (732) 542-1840; **BDCERT:**
CRS 91; **MS:** Hahnemann U 82; **RES:** Med, St
Vincents Hosp & Med Ctr NY, New York, NY 82-87;
FEL: CRS, Cleveland Clinic Hosp, Cleveland, OH 87-
88; **SI:** *Cancer; Inflammatory Bowel Disease*

♿ 🌙 📷 🏧 💲 Mcr Mcd WC NFI A Few Days ▨ **VISA**
⬭

Guide to symbols and abbreviations can be found on pages 110-113.

973

DERMATOLOGY

Grossman, Kenneth (MD)   **D**
Riverview Med Ctr

180 White Rd 103; Little Silver, NJ 07739; (732) 842-5222; **BDCERT:** D 83; IM 80; **MS:** SUNY Hlth Sci Ctr 77; **RES:** IM, Nassau County Med Ctr, East Meadow, NY 77-80; D, Albert Einstein Med Ctr, Bronx, NY 80-83; **HOSP:** Monmouth Med Ctr; *SI: Skin Cancer; Psoriasis;* **HMO:** First Option GHI United Healthcare PHCS HMO Blue +

[⛑] [SN] [🔊] [👤] [🏚] [S]   4+ Weeks

Hametz, Irwin (MD)   **D**
Centrastate Med Ctr

7755 Schanck Rd B3; Freehold, NJ 07728; (732) 462-9800; **BDCERT:** D 78; **MS:** NY Med Coll 73; **RES:** Long Island Jewish Med Ctr, New Hyde Park, NY 73-75; Rhode Island Hosp, Providence, RI 75-78; **FAP:** Asst Clin Prof UMDNJ-RW Johnson Med Sch; **HMO:** CIGNA Prucare Oxford Blue Cross First Option +

LANG: Itl; [⛑] [SN] [📞] [🔊] [👤] [🏚] [S] [Mcr] [WC] [NFl]   2-4 Weeks *VISA*

Orsini, William (MD)   **D**
Monmouth Med Ctr

223 Monmouth Rd; W Long Branch, NJ 07764; (732) 870-2992; **BDCERT:** D 77; **MS:** UMDNJ-NJ Med Sch, Newark 72; **RES:** Monmouth Med Ctr, Long Branch, NJ 73-75

[⛑] [S] [Mcr] *VISA* 💳

EMERGENCY MEDICINE

Kessler, Stuart (MD)   **EM**
Jersey Shore Med Ctr

30 Crossridge Cir; Marlboro, NJ 07746; (732) 776-4510; **BDCERT:** EM 92; IM 90; **MS:** U South Fla Coll Med 85; **RES:** EM, Boston Med Ctr, Boston, MA 88-91; IM, Long Island Jewish Med Ctr, New Hyde Park, NY 86-88

ENDOCRINOLOGY, DIABETES & METABOLISM

Luria, Martin (MD)   **EDM**
Monmouth Med Ctr

170 Morris Ave; Long Branch, NJ 07740; (732) 222-8874; **BDCERT:** IM 78; EDM 77; **MS:** NYU Sch Med 71; **RES:** IM, Univ Hosp SUNY Bklyn, Brooklyn, NY 79; **FEL:** EDM, Mount Sinai Med Ctr, New York, NY; **HOSP:** Riverview Med Ctr; *SI: Blood Sugar Problems; Thyroid Diseases;* **HMO:** First Option QualCare

[⛑] [📞] [👤] [🏚] [S] [Mcr] [WC]   A Few Days

Nassberg, B (MD)   **EDM**
Bayshore Community Hosp

Monmouth Endocrinology Associates, 723 N Beers St 2G; Holmdel, NJ 07733; (732) 739-0200; **BDCERT:** IM 82; EDM 84; **MS:** Belgium 79; **RES:** IM, Mountainside Hosp, Montclair, NJ 79-82; **FEL:** EDM, MS Hershey Med Ctr, Hershey, PA 82-84; *SI: Thyroid Disease; Diabetes;* **HMO:** First Option Empire Blue Cross

LANG: Fr; [⛑] [SN] [📞] [🔊] [👤] [🏚] [S] [Mcr]   2-4 Weeks

FAMILY PRACTICE

Haddad, A John (MD)   **FP**   **PCP**
Riverview Med Ctr

370 State Highway 35; Red Bank, NJ 07701; (732) 758-0048; **BDCERT:** FP 85; **MS:** Italy 82; **RES:** JFK Med Ctr, Edison, NJ 83-85

LANG: Itl; [⛑] [📞] [🔊] [S] [Mcr] [Mcd]   2-4 Weeks *VISA* 💳

Senz, Ronald (MD)   **FP**   **PCP**
Monmouth Med Ctr

37 E Washington Ave; Atlantic Highlands, NJ 07716; (732) 291-3430; **BDCERT:** FP 73; Ger 96; **MS:** Med Coll Wisc 67; **RES:** FP, Monmouth Med, Long Branch, NJ; **HMO:** Oxford First Option Blue Cross & Blue Shield

[🏚] [S] [Mcr] [WC] [NFl]   A Few Days *VISA* 💳

GASTROENTEROLOGY

Fiest, Thomas (DO)　　　**Ge**
Monmouth Med Ctr

Monmouth Gastroenterology, 279 3rd Ave 305;
Long Branch, NJ 07740; (732) 870-9100;
BDCERT: IM 89; Ge 95; **MS:** Philadelphia Coll Osteo
Med 85; **RES:** IM, Monmouth Med Ctr, Long
Branch, NJ 86-89; **FEL:** Ge, Jersey City Med Ctr,
Jersey City, NJ 90-93; **FAP:** Chf Med Hahnemann U;
HOSP: Jersey Shore Med Ctr; **SI:** *Colitis; Liver
Disorders*; **HMO:** Oxford US Hlthcre QualCare First
Option CIGNA +

🔲 🔲 🔲 🔲 🔲 🔲 🔲 🔲 🔲 A Few Days **VISA** 💳

Turtel, Penny (MD)　　　**Ge**
Monmouth Med Ctr

Shore Gastroenterology Assoc, 1907 Hwy 35 Ste 1;
Oakhurst, NJ 07755; (732) 517-0060; **BDCERT:**
IM 89; Ge 91; **MS:** Cornell U 86; **RES:** IM, Mount
Sinai Med Ctr, New York, NY 86-89; **FEL:** Ge,
Mount Sinai Med Ctr, New York, NY 89-91; **FAP:**
Instr UMDNJ New Jersey Sch Osteo Med; **HOSP:**
Jersey Shore Med Ctr; **SI:** *Inflammatory Bowel
Disease; Liver Diseases*; **HMO:** Amerihealth Oxford
Blue Cross & Blue Choice US Hlthcre QualCare +

LANG: Heb, Sp; 🔲 🔲 🔲 🔲 🔲 🔲 🔲 2-4 Weeks
🔲 💳

GYNECOLOGIC ONCOLOGY

Hackett, Thomas (DO)　　　**GO**
Monmouth Med Ctr

Atlantic Gynecologic Oncology, 1540 Highway
138 Ste 205; Wall, NJ 07719; (732) 280-5464;
BDCERT: ObG 89; GO 95; **MS:** UMDNJ New Jersey
Sch Osteo Med 83; **RES:** Naval Med Ctr, San Diego,
CA 84-87; **FEL:** MS Hershey Med Ctr, Hershey, PA
90-92; **FAP:** Asst Prof; **HOSP:** Jersey Shore Med Ctr;
SI: *Uterine Cancer; Cervical Cancer*; **HMO:** Guardian
Blue Cross & Blue Shield US Hlthcre HMO Blue
CIGNA +

🔲 🔲 🔲 🔲 🔲 🔲 🔲 🔲 1 Week **VISA** 💳 💳

HAND SURGERY

Chekofsky, Kenneth (MD)　　**HS**
Centrastate Med Ctr

2 Industrial Way West; Eatontown, NJ 07724;
(732) 542-4477; **BDCERT:** OrS 84; HS 89; **MS:** Mt
Sinai Sch Med 76; **RES:** Lenox Hill Hosp, New York,
NY 77-80; **FEL:** Hip Reconstructive S, Hosp For
Special Surgery, New York, NY 80-81; U Miami
Hosp, Miami, FL 82; **SI:** *Carpal Tunnel Syndrome*;
HMO: Blue Shield Oxford Prudential Affordable
Hlth Plan United Healthcare +

🔲 🔲 🔲 🔲 🔲 🔲 Immediately **VISA** 💳

HEMATOLOGY

Walsh, Christina (MD)　　**Hem**
Riverview Med Ctr

365 Broad St; Red Bank, NJ 07701; (732) 530-
8666; **BDCERT:** Hem 80; **MS:** Georgetown U 77;
RES: Georgetown U Hosp, Washington, DC 77-80

LANG: Sp; 🔲 🔲 🔲 🔲 🔲 🔲 1 Week 🔲 **VISA**
💳

INTERNAL MEDICINE

Burkett, Eric (MD)　　**IM**　　**PCP**
Monmouth Med Ctr

Monmouth Medical Group, 223 Monmouth Rd;
West Long Branch, NJ 07764; (732) 229-3838;
BDCERT: IM 76; Ger 92; **MS:** Hahnemann U 71;
RES: IM, Monmouth Med Ctr, Long Branch, NJ 71-
73; IM, Monmouth Med Ctr, Long Branch, NJ 75-
76; **SI:** *Hypertension; Diabetes Mellitus*; **HMO:** Aetna-
US Healthcare Blue Cross First Option Prudential
Oxford +

🔲 🔲 🔲 🔲 🔲 🔲 1 Week **VISA** 💳

Guide to symbols and abbreviations can be found on pages 110-113.

975

Courtney, Barbara (MD)   IM   PCP
Monmouth Med Ctr

Monmouth Medical Group, 223 Monmouth Rd;
West Long Branch, NJ 07764; (732) 229-3838;
BDCERT: IM 80; Ger 92; **MS:** Hahnemann U 77;
RES: IM, Monmouth Med Ctr, Long Branch, NJ 77-
80; **FAP:** Assoc Clin Prof Med Hahnemann U; *SI:*
Post Menopausal Health; **HMO:** HMO Blue
Prudential US Hlthcre First Option

🔲 🔲 🔲 🔲 🔲 🔲 🔲

Davis, George (MD)   IM
Monmouth Med Ctr

279 3rd Ave 510; Long Branch, NJ 07740; (732)
870-0650; **BDCERT:** IM 76; Pul 79; **MS:**
Hahnemann U 87; **RES:** IM, Monmouth Med Ctr,
Long Branch, NJ 73; IM, Monmouth Med Ctr, Long
Branch, NJ 74; **FEL:** Pul, Monmouth Med Ctr, Long
Branch, NJ 77; *SI: Asthma; Emphysema*; **HMO:**
Oxford Aetna-US Healthcare HMO Blue First Option
CIGNA +

🔲 🔲 🔲 🔲 🔲 🔲

Glowacki, Jan S (MD)   IM   PCP
Riverview Med Ctr

569 River Rd; Fair Haven, NJ 07701; (732) 530-
0100; **BDCERT:** IM 80; **MS:** Jefferson Med Coll 77;
RES: Monmouth Med Ctr, Long Branch, NJ 77-80;
HOSP: Monmouth Med Ctr; *SI: Preventive Medicine*;
HMO: Most

🔲 🔲 🔲 🔲 🔲 🔲 🔲 🔲 🔲 🔲 A Few Days **VISA**
🔲

Schwartz, Mitchell (MD)   IM
Monmouth Med Ctr

Shore Gastroenterology Associates, PC, 1907 Hwy
35 # 1; Oakhurst, NJ 07755; (732) 517-0060;
BDCERT: IM 86; Ge 89; **MS:** Albert Einstein Coll
Med 83; **RES:** IM, Bronx Muncipal Hosp Ctr, Bronx,
NY 83-84; IM, Bronx Muncipal Hosp Ctr, Bronx,
NY 84-86; **FEL:** Ge, Montefiore Med Ctr, Bronx, NY
87-89; **FAP:** Asst Clin Prof Med Hahnemann U;
HOSP: Jersey Shore Med Ctr; *SI: Biliary Disease*;
HMO: Empire Oxford US Hlthcre First Option

🔲 🔲 🔲 🔲 🔲 🔲 1 Week 🔲 **VISA** 🔲

MEDICAL ONCOLOGY

Fitzgerald, Denis (MD)   Onc
Riverview Med Ctr

Hematology Oncology of Central New Jersey, 365
Broad St; Red Bank, NJ 07701; (732) 530-8666;
BDCERT: Onc 85; Hem 86; **MS:** SUNY Hlth Sci Ctr
78; **RES:** St Vincents Hosp & Med Ctr NY, New
York, NY 78-82; **FEL:** Hem, Strong Mem Hosp,
Rochester, NY 84-85; Onc, Strong Mem Hosp,
Rochester, NY 82-84; *SI: Breast Cancer; Lung*
Cancer; **HMO:** PHCS Oxford US Hlthcre Magnacare
First Option +

LANG: Sp; 🔲 🔲 🔲 🔲 🔲 🔲 A Few Days 🔲
VISA 🔲

Greenberg, Susan (MD)   Onc
Monmouth Med Ctr

39 Sycamore Ave; Little Silver, NJ 07739; (732)
576-8610; **BDCERT:** IM 81; Onc 83; **MS:** Med Coll
PA 78; **RES:** IM, Hosp Med College of PA,
Philadelphia, PA 78-81; **FEL:** Hem Onc, Columbia-
Presbyterian Med Ctr, New York, NY 81-83; **HOSP:**
Jersey Shore Med Ctr; *SI: Breast Cancer; Lymphoma*;
HMO: Oxford Prudential Blue Cross & Blue Shield
First Option CIGNA +

🔲 🔲 🔲 🔲 🔲 🔲 🔲 A Few Days

Sharon, David (MD)   Onc
Monmouth Med Ctr

Monmouth Hematology Oncology, 279 3rd Ave
203; Long Branch, NJ 07740; (732) 222-1711;
BDCERT: IM 80; Onc 82; **MS:** NY Med Coll 77; **RES:**
IM, Beth Israel Med Ctr, New York, NY 77-80; **FEL:**
Neoplastic Disease, Mount Sinai Med Ctr, New
York, NY 80-82; *SI: Breast Cancer; General Medical*
Oncology

🔲 🔲 🔲 🔲 🔲 🔲 A Few Days

NEPHROLOGY

Arbes, Spiros (MD)   Nep
Monmouth Med Ctr
Hypertension & Nephrology Partners, 6 Industrial Way West Suite B; Eatontown, NJ 07724; (732) 460-1200; **BDCERT:** IM 86; **MS:** Philippines 82; **RES:** IM, Jersey Shore Med Ctr, Neptune, NJ 82-85; **FEL:** Nep, Mount Sinai Med Ctr, New York, NY 85-87; **HOSP:** Riverview Med Ctr; **SI:** *Hypertension; Kidney Disease;* **HMO:** Aetna Hlth Plan Blue Choice Oxford Blue Shield Blue Cross +

LANG: Sp; 🔲 🔲 🔲 🔲 🔲 🔲 1 Week

Flis, Raymond S (DO)   Nep
Monmouth Med Ctr
Hypertension & Nephrology Associates, 6 Industrial Way West Ste B; Eatontown, NJ 07724; (732) 460-1200; **BDCERT:** IM 74; Nep 76; **MS:** Kirksville Coll Osteo Med 71; **RES:** IM, Cooper Hosp, Camden, NJ 71-74; **FEL:** Nep, Thomas Jefferson U Hosp, Philadelphia, PA 74-75; Nep, Temple U Hosp, Philadelphia, PA 75-76; **FAP:** Asst Clin Prof Hahnemann U; **HOSP:** Riverview Med Ctr; **SI:** *Kidney Disease; Hypertension;* **HMO:** Aetna-US Healthcare First Option CIGNA Blue Cross Oxford +

LANG: Sp; 🔲 🔲 🔲 🔲 🔲 🔲 🔲 🔲 🔲 A Few Days **VISA** 🔲

NEUROLOGY

Gilson, Noah (MD)   N
Monmouth Med Ctr
107 Monmouth Rd; West Long Branch, NJ 07764; (732) 222-6238; **BDCERT:** N 87; **MS:** Loyola U-Stritch Sch Med, Maywood 82; **RES:** N, Mount Sinai Med Ctr, New York, NY 83-8; **HOSP:** Riverview Med Ctr; **SI:** *Multiple Sclerosis; Epilepsy;* **HMO:** First Option CIGNA US Hlthcre Aetna Hlth Plan Oxford +

LANG: Grk; 🔲 🔲 🔲 🔲 🔲 🔲 🔲 🔲 🔲 1 Week

Herman, Martin (MD)   N
Monmouth Med Ctr
107 Monmouth Rd; West Long Branch, NJ 07764; (732) 222-6238; **BDCERT:** Psyc 73; **MS:** Northwestern U 64; **RES:** N, U of VA Health Sci Ctr, Charlottesville, VA 67-70; **FEL:** CNph, Columbia-Presbyterian Med Ctr, New York, NY 70-71; **FAP:** Assoc Clin Prof Hahnemann U; **HOSP:** Riverview Med Ctr; **SI:** *Epilepsy; Migraines;* **HMO:** First Option Prucare CIGNA US Hlthcre Magnacare +

🔲 🔲 🔲 🔲 🔲 2-4 Weeks

OBSTETRICS & GYNECOLOGY

Goldstein, Steven (MD)   ObG
Centrastate Med Ctr
501 Iron Bridge Rd 4; Freehold, NJ 07728; (732) 431-1807; **BDCERT:** ObG 91; **MS:** SUNY Downstate 85; **RES:** Univ of Med & Dent NJ Hosp, Newark, NJ 85-89; **SI:** *Ultrasound; Abnormal Pap Smears;* **HMO:** United Healthcare Oxford HMO Blue Prudential First Option +

🔲 🔲 🔲 🔲 🔲 🔲 🔲 🔲 1 Week 🔲 **VISA**

Rothenberg, Eugene (MD)   ObG
Monmouth Med Ctr
59 Avenue At The Common #205; Shrewsbury, NJ 07702; (732) 542-0800; **BDCERT:** ObG 67; **MS:** Tufts U 57; **RES:** ObG, U of Illinois Med Ctr, Chicago, IL 61-64; **FAP:** Asst Clin Prof Hahnemann U; **SI:** *Gynecologic Surgery; Lapapascopic Surgery*

🔲 🔲 🔲 🔲 🔲 🔲 🔲 1 Week **VISA**

OPHTHALMOLOGY

Goldberg, Daniel (MD) **Oph**
Monmouth Med Ctr

Atlantic Eye Physicians, 279 3rd Ave 204; Long Branch, NJ 07740; (732) 222-7373; **BDCERT:** Oph 79; **MS:** SUNY Downstate 74; **RES:** Oph, Univ Hosp SUNY Bklyn, Brooklyn, NY 75-78; **FEL:** Cornea/Ant Segment, Eye & Ear Hosp, Pittsburgh, PA 78-79; **HOSP:** Jersey Shore Med Ctr; *SI: Laser Vision Correction; Corneal Transplants;* **HMO:** Blue Cross & Blue Shield Aetna-US Healthcare Oxford United Healthcare

LANG: Sp, Grk; 👓 🌙 📷 🐟 🏧 💲 Mcr Mcd WC NFi 2-4 Weeks ▨ *VISA* 💳 📇

Talansky, Marvin (MD) **Oph**
Jersey Shore Med Ctr

Eye Diagnostic Ctr, 3333 Fairmont Ave; Asbury Park, NJ 07712; (732) 988-4000; **BDCERT:** Oph 78; **MS:** Med U SC, Charleston 73; **RES:** Oph, Med U of SC Med Ctr, Charleston, SC 75-78; **FEL:** Retina, Med U of SC Med Ctr, Charleston, SC 85-86; **FAP:** Clin Instr Hahnemann U; *SI: Cataracts; Diabetic Eye Disease;* **HMO:** US Hlthcre QualCare CIGNA Blue Cross & Blue Shield Prucare +

👓 SA 🌙 📷 🐟 🏧 💲 Mcr Mcd WC NFi 1 Week *VISA* 💳

ORTHOPAEDIC SURGERY

Absatz, Michael (MD) **OrS**
Monmouth Med Ctr

Shore Orthopaedic Group, 35 Gilbert Street South; Tinton Falls, NJ 07701; (732) 530-1515; **BDCERT:** OrS 90; **MS:** Columbia P&S 82; **RES:** OrS, Bellevue Hosp Ctr, New York, NY; **FEL:** Kerlan-Jobe Ortho Clinic, Inglewood, CA; **HOSP:** Riverview Med Ctr; *SI: Total Joint Replacement; Arthritis;* **HMO:** Aetna-US Healthcare United Healthcare Prucare Oxford First Option +

👓 📷 🏧 💲 Mcr WC NFi ▨ *VISA* 💳 📇

Berkowitz, Steven (MD) **OrS**
Jersey Shore Med Ctr

Seaview Orthopaedic & Medical Associates, 2040 6th Ave; Neptune, NJ 07753; (732) 775-4802; **BDCERT:** OrS 81; **MS:** SUNY Hlth Sci Ctr 75; **RES:** Maimonides Med Ctr, Brooklyn, NY 75-77; Columbia-Presbyterian Med Ctr, New York, NY 77-80; **FEL:** OrS, Columbia-Presbyterian Med Ctr, New York, NY 79-80; **HOSP:** Med Ctr of Ocean County; *SI: Arthroscopic Surgery; Shoulder Surgery;* **HMO:** Blue Cross Aetna Hlth Plan Prucare NY Life GHI +

LANG: Sp; 👓 📷 🐟 🏧 💲 Mcr WC NFi 1 Week *VISA* 💳

Dennis, Robert (MD) **OrS**
Jersey Shore Med Ctr

Seaview Orthopaedics, 2040 6th Ave B; Neptune City, NJ 07753; (732) 775-4802; **BDCERT:** OrS 77; **MS:** Temple U 71; **RES:** OrS, Montefiore Med Ctr, Bronx, NY 72-75; **HMO:** Aetna Hlth Plan Blue Cross & Blue Shield US Hlthcre QualCare Options +

LANG: Sp; 👓 📷 🏧 💲 Mcr WC A Few Days ▨ *VISA* 💳

OTOLARYNGOLOGY

Rossos, Paul (MD) **Oto**
RWJ Univ Hosp-Hamilton

501 Iron Bridge Rd 11; Freehold, NJ 07728; (732) 409-2500; **BDCERT:** Oto 88; **MS:** Grenada 81; **RES:** Oto, Univ of Med & Dent NJ Hosp, Newark, NJ 83-86; UMDNJ Hospital, Newark, NJ 82-83; *SI: Pediatrics; Sinus Disease;* **HMO:** US Hlthcre Oxford American Health Plan QualCare Blue Cross & Blue Shield +

LANG: Grk; 📷 🐟 🏧 💲 Mcr A Few Days

Winarsky, Eric (MD)   Oto
Monmouth Med Ctr

Central Jersey Otolaryngolgoy, 1131 Broad St; Shrewsbury, NJ 07702; (732) 389-3388; **BDCERT:** Oto 82; **MS:** Belgium 76; **RES:** IM, Monmouth Med Ctr, Long Branch, NJ 76-77; S, Monmouth Med Ctr, Long Branch, NJ 77-78; **FEL:** Oto, Univ of Med & Dent NJ Hosp, Newark, NJ 78-81; **HOSP:** Riverview Med Ctr; *SI: Nasal & Sinus Disease; Sleep & Snoring Disorders*; **HMO:** HMO Blue US Hlthcre Oxford

LANG: Fr, Sp; 🔲 🔲 🔲 🔲 🔲 🔲 🔲 🔲
A Few Days **VISA** 🔲

PAIN MANAGEMENT

Bram, Harris (MD)   PM
Monmouth Med Ctr

Pain Management Associates, 200 White Rd 205; Little Silver, NJ 07739; (732) 345-1180; **BDCERT:** Anes 93; PM 96; **MS:** U Ark Sch Med 88; **RES:** Anes, Hahnemann U Hosp, Philadelphia, PA 89-92; **FEL:** PM, Thomas Jefferson U Hosp, Philadelphia, PA 92-93; **HOSP:** Community Hosp At Dobbs Ferry; *SI: Chronic Neck and Lower Back Pain; Pre and Post Surgical Pain*

🔲 🔲 🔲 🔲 🔲 🔲 🔲 🔲 A Few Days 🔲 **VISA** 🔲

PEDIATRICS

Lefrak, Steven (MD)   Ped   **PCP**
Riverview Med Ctr

272 Broad St; Red Bank, NJ 07701; (732) 741-0456; **BDCERT:** Ped 73; **MS:** Jefferson Med Coll 68; **RES:** Ped, Monmouth Med Ctr, Long Branch, NJ 69-71; **FAP:** Asst Prof Hahnemann U; **HOSP:** Monmouth Med Ctr; *SI: Medical Genetics*; **HMO:** HMO Blue Blue Cross & Blue Shield US Hlthcre CIGNA HIP Network +

🔲 🔲 🔲 🔲 🔲 🔲 🔲 Immediately 🔲 **VISA** 🔲 🔲

PLASTIC SURGERY

Dudick, Stephen T (MD)   PlS
Monmouth Med Ctr

70 E Front St; Red Bank, NJ 07701; (732) 741-1303; **BDCERT:** PlS 93; **MS:** Mexico 75; **RES:** S, St Vincents Hosp & Med Ctr NY, New York, NY 78-81; PlS, Indiana U Med Ctr, Indianapolis, IN 81; **FAP:** Sr Clin Instr S Hahnemann U; **HOSP:** Riverview Med Ctr; *SI: Mastectomy/Reconstructive; Trauma*; **HMO:** QualCare First Option CHN

🔲 🔲 🔲 🔲 🔲 🔲 🔲 🔲 A Few Days

Hetzler, Peter (MD)   PlS
Riverview Med Ctr

200 White Rd 211; Little Silver, NJ 07739; (732) 219-0447; **BDCERT:** PlS 91; S 89; **MS:** U Mich Med Sch 81; **RES:** S, MS Hershey Med Ctr, Hershey, PA 81-86; PlS, MS Hershey Med Ctr, Hershey, PA 86-88; **FEL:** Microsurgery, York Hosp, York, PA 88; S, Manhattan Eye, Ear & Throat Hosp, New York, NY 88-89; **HOSP:** Manhattan Eye, Ear & Throat Hosp; *SI: Breast Reconstruction; Melanoma*; **HMO:** Magnacare QualCare American Health Plan

🔲 🔲 🔲 🔲 🔲 🔲 🔲 🔲 2-4 Weeks **VISA** 🔲

Samra, Said (MD)   PlS
Bayshore Community Hosp

733 N Beers St U1; Holmdel, NJ 07733; (732) 739-2100; **BDCERT:** PlS 88; **MS:** Syria 73; **RES:** S, Univ of Med & Dent NJ Hosp, Newark, NJ 75-80; **FEL:** PlS, St Barnabas Med Ctr, Livingston, NJ 80-82; **HOSP:** Raritan Bay Med Ctr-Perth Amboy; *SI: Facial Rejuvenation; Breast Surgery*; **HMO:** QualCare First Option US Hlthcre Oxford Prucare +

LANG: Sp, Fr, Ar; 🔲 🔲 🔲 🔲 🔲 🔲 🔲 🔲 🔲 🔲 🔲 A Few Days **VISA** 🔲 🔲

PSYCHIATRY

Rubin, Kenneth (MD)   Psyc
Monmouth Med Ctr

170 Morris Ave D; Long Branch, NJ 07740; (732) 870-3535; **BDCERT:** Psyc 79; **MS:** SUNY Downstate 74; **RES:** Kings County Hosp Ctr, Brooklyn, NY 74-77; **FAP:** Assoc Clin Prof Med Coll PA; *SI: Depression; Anxiety;* **HMO:** Aetna Hlth Plan First Option Blue Cross US Hlthcre

♿ 💧 🍺 📷 📺 🍻 💵 🚽 A Few Days

PULMONARY DISEASE

Kosinski, Robert (MD)   Pul
Monmouth Med Ctr

Monmouth Pulmonary Consultants, 422 Morris Ave 7; Long Branch, NJ 07740; (732) 571-5151; **BDCERT:** IM 90; Pul 92; **MS:** MC Ohio, Toledo 87; **RES:** IM, Monmouth Med Ctr, Long Branch, NJ 87-90; **FEL:** Pul, Hahnemann U Hosp, Philadelphia, PA 90-92; Hosp Med College of PA, Philadelphia, PA 92-93; **HOSP:** Jersey Shore Med Ctr; *SI: Sleep Apnea;* **HMO:** Blue Cross Aetna-US Healthcare Prucare Magnacare United Healthcare +

♿ 💧 📷 📺 🍻 💵 Mcr WC A Few Days

RADIATION ONCOLOGY

Kornmehl, Carol (MD)   RadRO
Monmouth Med Ctr

Monmouth Medical Radiology, 300 2nd Ave; Long Branch, NJ 07740; (908) 870-5064; **BDCERT:** RadRO 88; **MS:** SUNY Downstate 84; **RES:** Univ Hosp SUNY Bklyn, Brooklyn, NY; **FAP:** Asst Clin Prof; *SI: Internal Radiation for GYN; Tumors as an outpatient;* **HMO:** CIGNA Oxford HIP Network First Option HMO Blue +

♿ 📷 📺 🍻 Mcr Mcd Immediately

RADIOLOGY

Schultz, Sidney (MD)   Rad
Monmouth Med Ctr

Monmouth Medical Center, 300 2nd Ave; Long Branch, NJ 07740; (732) 923-6806; **BDCERT:** Rad 63; **MS:** SUNY Downstate 58; **RES:** Med, Bellevue Hosp Ctr, New York, NY 58-59; Rad, Montefiore Med Ctr, Bronx, NY 59-62; **FAP:** Assoc Clin Prof Hahnemann U

RHEUMATOLOGY

Schwartzberg, Mori (MD)   Rhu
Jersey Shore Med Ctr

Shore Rheumatalogy, 10 Neptune Blvd 106; Neptune, NJ 07753; (732) 988-5030; **BDCERT:** IM 76; Rhu 78; **MS:** SUNY Syracuse 73; **RES:** IM, Nassau County Med Ctr, East Meadow, NY 73-76; **FEL:** Rhu, Albert Einstein Med Ctr, Philadelphia, PA 76-78; **FAP:** Asst Clin Prof Med UMDNJ-RW Johnson Med Sch; *SI: Rheumatoid Arthritis; Lyme Disease;* **HMO:** None

♿ 📷 📺 🍻 💵 4+ Weeks

Wasser, Kenneth (MD)   Rhu
Riverview Med Ctr

43 N Gilbert St No; Tinton Falls, NJ 07701; (732) 530-7999; **BDCERT:** IM 81; Rhu 82; **MS:** Case West Res U 77; **RES:** U Hosp of Cleveland, Cleveland, OH 77-80; Rhu, U Hosp of Cleveland, Cleveland, OH 80-82; **FAP:** Clin Instr Hahnemann U; **HOSP:** Monmouth Med Ctr; **HMO:** First Option HMO Blue Aetna-US Healthcare CIGNA Affordable Hlth Plan +

♿ 💧 💵 2-4 Weeks

SPORTS MEDICINE

Bade III, Harry A (MD)　　SM
Riverview Med Ctr
Professional Orthopedics Assoc, 776 Shrewsbury
Ave 201; Tinton Falls, NJ 07724; (732) 530-4949;
BDCERT: OrS 84; **MS:** Jefferson Med Coll 76; **RES:** S,
St Luke's Roosevelt Hosp Ctr, New York, NY 76-78;
OrS, Hosp For Special Surgery, New York, NY 78-
81; **FEL:** Shoulder-Cervical Spine, Hosp For Special
Surgery, New York, NY 81-82; Hand, St Luke's
Roosevelt Hosp Ctr, New York, NY 81-82; **HOSP:**
Monmouth Med Ctr; **HMO:** Blue Cross & Blue Shield
First Option Allied Health United Healthcare
Prudential +

🔲 🔲 🔲 🔲 🔲 🔲 🔲 🔲 🔲 A Few Days **VISA** 💳

Sclafani, Michael (MD)　　SM
Jersey Shore Med Ctr
Orthopedic Institute of Central Jersey, 2164 Route
35; Sea Girt, NJ 08750; (732) 974-0404; **BDCERT:**
OrS 96; **MS:** NYU Sch Med 88; **RES:** OrS, New York
University Med Ctr, New York, NY 88-93; **FEL:** SM,
American Sports Med Inst, Birmingham, AL 93-94;
SI: Anterior Cruciate Ligament; Shoulder Instability;
HMO: +

🔲 🔲 🔲 🔲 🔲 🔲 🔲 🔲 🔲 A Few Days 🔲
VISA 💳 💳

SURGERY

Arbour, Robert (MD)　　S
Bayshore Community Hosp
Matawan Medical Assoc, 213 Main St; Matawan,
NJ 07747; (732) 566-2363; **BDCERT:** S 72; **MS:**
UMDNJ-NJ Med Sch, Newark 65; **RES:** S,
Georgetown U Hosp, Washington, DC 66-71; IM,
Jersey City Med Ctr, Jersey City, NJ 66; **HOSP:**
Riverview Med Ctr; *SI: Vascular Surgery;* **HMO:** First
Option US Hlthcre Oxford Prucare Blue Choice +

🔲 🔲 🔲 🔲 🔲 🔲 🔲 🔲 🔲 1 Week 🔲 💳

Averbach, David (MD)　　S
Monmouth Med Ctr
157 Pavilion Ave; Long Branch, NJ 07740; (732)
229-7373; **BDCERT:** S 68; **MS:** Univ Penn 61; **RES:**
Monmouth Med Ctr, Long Branch, NJ 61-66; **FAP:**
Assoc Prof Hahnemann U; **HOSP:** Jersey Shore Med
Ctr; *SI: Breast Surgery; Laparoscopic Surgery;* **HMO:**
HMO Blue US Hlthcre Blue Shield HIP Network
Choicecare +

🔲 🔲 🔲 🔲 🔲 🔲 🔲

Goldfarb, Michael (MD)　　S
Monmouth Med Ctr
48 Pavilion Ave; Long Branch, NJ 07740; (732)
870-6060; **BDCERT:** S 73; **MS:** NYU Sch Med 67;
RES: Beth Israel Med Ctr, New York, NY 67-72;
FAP: Assoc Prof Hahnemann U; *SI: Breast Surgery;
Laparoscopy;* **HMO:** Blue Cross & Blue Shield First
Option Aetna Hlth Plan CIGNA Oxford +

🔲 🔲 🔲 🔲 🔲 🔲 🔲 🔲 A Few Days **VISA** 💳

Klein, Gerald (MD)　　S
Monmouth Med Ctr
Coastal Pediatric Surg Assoc, 1 Industrial Way
West A; Eatontown, NJ 07724; (732) 935-0480;
BDCERT: S 65; **MS:** Switzerland 60; **RES:** S,
Brookdale, Brooklyn, NY 60-65; Winnipeg, Canada
67-68; **FEL:** U Manitoba, Canada 65-67; **FAP:** Asst
Clin Prof Hahnemann U; **HMO:** Aetna Hlth Plan
Blue Choice Blue Cross & Blue Shield

Sarokhan, John (MD)　　S
Jersey Shore Med Ctr
608 Hwy 71; Brielle, NJ 08730; (732) 223-4848;
BDCERT: S 62; **MS:** Boston U 46; **RES:** Boston Med
Ctr, Boston, MA 48-50; Hartford Hosp, Hartford, CT
50-51; **FEL:** Mem Sloan Kettering Cancer Ctr, New
York, NY 52-54; **FAP:** Asst Prof S UMDNJ New
Jersey Sch Osteo Med; **HOSP:** Jersey Shore Med Ctr

🔲 🔲 🔲 🔲 🔲 🔲 Immediately

Schwartz, Mark (MD)   **S**
Monmouth Med Ctr

Atlantic Surgical Group, 157 Pavilion Ave; Long Branch, NJ 07740; (732) 229-7373; **BDCERT:** S 91; **MS:** Hahnemann U 83; **RES:** S, Monmouth Med Ctr, Long Branch, NJ 83-88; **HOSP:** Jersey Shore Med Ctr; **SI:** *Laparoscopic Surgery; Breast Surgery;* **HMO:** US Hlthcre Blue Select Prudential First Option CIGNA +

LANG: Sp, Fr, Heb; 🔲 🌙 🔲 🔲 🔲 🔲 🔲 🔲 🔲
A Few Days

THORACIC SURGERY

Heleotis, Thomas (MD)   **TS**
Jersey Shore Med Ctr

Jersey Shore Cardiothoracic, 239 W Sylvania Ave; Neptune City, NJ 07753; (732) 775-9077; **BDCERT:** S 87; **MS:** Italy 78; **RES:** S, Monmouth Med Ctr, Long Branch, NJ 78-83; TS, Boston U Med Ctr, Boston, MA 83-86; **HOSP:** Riverview Med Ctr; **SI:** *Pacemakers Defibrillators; Lung Cancer*

LANG: Grk, Itl, Sp; 🔲 🔲 🔲 🔲 🔲 🔲 🔲 🔲 🔲
A Few Days

Sills, Charles (MD)   **TS**
Monmouth Med Ctr

Chest & Cardiovascular Assoc, 255 3rd Ave; Long Branch, NJ 07740; (732) 571-4114; **BDCERT:** TS 70; **MS:** Rush Med Coll 61; **RES:** S, Albert Einstein Med Ctr, Bronx, NY 67; TS, Albert Einstein Med Ctr, Bronx, NY 67-68; **FAP:** Asst Clin Prof Hahnemann U; **SI:** *Lung Cancer; Pacemakers;* **HMO:** Blue Choice Blue Cross & Blue Shield Metlife Blue Cross & Blue Shield First Option +

🔲 🔲 🔲 🔲 🔲 🔲 A Few Days

UROLOGY

Ebani, Jack (MD)   **U**
Jersey Shore Med Ctr

1820 Corlies Ave; Neptune, NJ 07753; (732) 774-4551; **BDCERT:** U 87; **MS:** SUNY Hlth Sci Ctr 79; **RES:** S, N Shore Univ Hosp-Manhasset, Manhasset, NY 79-81; U, New York University Med Ctr, New York, NY 81-85; **HOSP:** Monmouth Med Ctr; **SI:** *Prostate Cancer; Incontinence;* **HMO:** PHCS PHS HMO Blue Magnacare Ethix +

LANG: Sp; 🔲 🔲 🔲 🔲 🔲 🔲 🔲   Immediately

Geltzeiler, Jules (MD)   **U**
Monmouth Med Ctr

Shore Urology, 279 3rd Ave Ste 101; Long Branch, NJ 07740; (732) 222-2111; **BDCERT:** U 86; U 94; **MS:** Hahnemann U 79; **RES:** S, Monmouth Med Ctr, Long Branch, NJ 79-81; U, Geo Wash U Med Ctr, Washington, DC 81-83; **HOSP:** Jersey Shore Med Ctr; **SI:** *Prostate Cancer; Incontinence;* **HMO:** Aetna Hlth Plan Guardian Blue Cross & Blue Shield US Hlthcre Oxford +

🔲 🔲 🔲 🔲 🔲 🔲 🔲 A Few Days **VISA** 🔲

Grebler, Arnold (MD)   **U**
Monmouth Med Ctr

Shore Urology, 279 3rd Ave 101; Long Branch, NJ 07740; (732) 732-2222; **BDCERT:** U 82; **MS:** Italy 74; **RES:** S, Maimonides Med Ctr, Brooklyn, NY 74-76; U, Maimonides Med Ctr, Brooklyn, NY 76-79; **FAP:** Assoc Clin Prof Hahnemann U; **HOSP:** Jersey Shore Med Ctr; **SI:** *Urologic Cancer Surgery; Stone Disease;* **HMO:** Aetna Hlth Plan Blue Cross & Blue Shield CIGNA Prucare Travelers +

LANG: Itl, Sp; 🔲 🔲 🔲 🔲 🔲 🔲 A Few Days **VISA** 🔲

Linn, Gary (MD)　　　　U
Jersey City Med Ctr

Coastal Urology Associates, 1915 6th Ave;
Neptune, NJ 07753; (732) 988-3313; **BDCERT:** U
80; **MS:** Cornell U 73; **RES:** S, NY Hosp-Cornell Med
Ctr, New York, NY 72-74; U, Mem Sloan Kettering
Cancer Ctr, New York, NY 74-78; **HOSP:** Jersey
Shore Med Ctr; *SI: Urologic Oncology; Pediatric
Urology;* **HMO:** US Hlthcre Oxford HMO Blue
Magnacare American Health Plan +

 ⌖ ☎ ♿ ▦ 🆂 Mcr Mcd WC NFI　A Few Days ***VISA*** ⬤

Litvin, Y Samuel (MD)　　　U
Monmouth Med Ctr

Shore Urology, 279 3rd Ave 101; Long Branch, NJ
07740; (732) 222-2111; **BDCERT:** U 94; **MS:**
UCLA 86; **RES:** S, Beth Israel Med Ctr, New York,
NY 86-88; U, Beth Israel Med Ctr, New York, NY
88-91; **HOSP:** Riverview Med Ctr; *SI: Prostate
Cancer; Male Infertility;* **HMO:** CIGNA Aetna-US
Healthcare Prucare HMO Blue

LANG: Sp; ♿ ☾ ☎ ♿ ▦ 🆂 Mcr WC　Immediately
▦ ***VISA*** ⬤

Rotolo, James (MD)　　　U
Jersey Shore Med Ctr

2130 Hwy 35 126; Sea Girt, NJ 08750; (732) 974-
2297; **BDCERT:** U 92; **MS:** Georgetown U 84; **RES:**
S, Georgetown U Hosp, Washington, DC 84-86; U,
Georgetown U Hosp, Washington, DC 86-90;
HOSP: Med Ctr of Ocean County; **HMO:** Oxford
Blue Cross & Blue Shield Prucare First Option US
Hlthcre +

 ♿ ☎ ♿ ▦ 🆂 Mcr WC　2-4 Weeks

MORRIS
COUNTY

MORRIS COUNTY

Specialties in capital letters indicate Primary Care Specialties. However, many doctors will be certified in a subspecialty, but will practice predominantly primary care medicine. In our lists this will be indicated.

*Oncologists deal with Cancer

ALLERGY & IMMUNOLOGY

Applebaum, Eric (MD)   **A&I**
Morristown Mem Hosp
Allergic & Asthmatic Comprehensive Care of NJ PA,
50 Cherry Hill Rd 301; Parsippany, NJ 07054;
(973) 335-1700; **BDCERT:** A&I 93; IM 90; **MS:**
Albert Einstein Coll Med 87; **RES:** IM, Long Island
Jewish Med Ctr, New Hyde Park, NY 88-90; **FEL:**
A&I, Long Island Jewish Med Ctr, New Hyde Park,
NY 90-92; **FAP:** Instr Med Albert Einstein Coll Med;
HOSP: NW Covenant Med Ctr-Riverside; *SI:
Asthma;* **HMO:** Blue Cross & Blue Shield CIGNA
PHCS

LANG: Heb; 🔧 🌙 🏠 🏨 💲 Med   A Few Days **VISA**
💳 💳

CARDIOLOGY (CARDIOVASCULAR DISEASE)

Casale Jr, Alfred Stanley (MD) Cv
Morristown Mem Hosp
Mid Atlantic Surg Assoc, 100 Madison Ave;
Morristown, NJ 07960; (973) 971-7300; **BDCERT:**
TS 98; S 95; **MS:** Johns Hopkins U 80; **RES:** TS,
Johns Hopkins Hosp, Baltimore, MD 85-88; **FEL:** TS,
Mem Sloan Kettering Cancer Ctr, New York, NY
87; *SI: Coronary Valve Repair and Replacement;
Coronary Artery Bypass*

🔧 🏠 🏥 🏨 Med Med WC NFI   A Few Days 🏨 **VISA**
💳 💳

Fisch, Arthur (MD)   **Cv**
Morristown Mem Hosp
Morristown Cardiology Assoc, 182 South St 5;
Morristown, NJ 07960; (973) 267-3944; **BDCERT:**
IM 72; Cv 75; **MS:** Boston U 69; **RES:** IM, UCLA
Med Ctr, Los Angeles, CA 70-72; **FEL:** Cv, Hosp of U
Penn, Philadelphia, PA 72-74; **FAP:** Clin Instr Med

CHILD NEUROLOGY

Grossman, Elliot (MD)   **ChiN**
St Barnabas Med Ctr-Livingston
205 Ridgedale; Florham Park, NJ 07932; (973)
966-6333; **BDCERT:** ChiN 90; Ped 87; **MS:**
Meharry Med Coll 80; **RES:** Ped, Bellevue Hosp Ctr,
New York, NY 80-82; Ped, Boston Med Ctr, Boston,
MA 82-83; **FEL:** Ped N, Boston Med Ctr, Boston, MA
83-86; **HOSP:** Morristown Mem Hosp; *SI:
Headaches; School Problems;* **HMO:** Prucare Blue
Cross & Blue Shield CIGNA HMO Blue Prucare +

🔧 🏠 🏨 💲 WC   1 Week 🏨 **VISA** 💳

COLON & RECTAL SURGERY

Moskowitz, Richard (MD)   CRS
Morristown Mem Hosp
Colon Surgery & Proctology, 130 Speedwell Ave;
Morris Plains, NJ 07950; (973) 267-1225;
BDCERT: CRS 85; S 91; **MS:** Penn State U-Hershey
Med Ctr 78; **RES:** S, Long Island Jewish Med Ctr,
New Hyde Park, NY; **HOSP:** Northwest Covenant
Med Ctr; *SI: Ulcerative Colitis; Rectal Cancer;* **HMO:**
Aetna-US Healthcare Oxford CIGNA HMO Blue
Prucare +

🔧 🌙 🏠 🏥 🏨 💲 Med   Immediately **VISA** 💳

DERMATOLOGY

Almeida, Laila (MD)   **D**
NW Covenant Med Ctr-Riverside
Dematology Associates of Morris, 199 Baldwin Rd
230; Parsippany, NJ 07054; (973) 335-2560;
BDCERT: IM 86; **MS:** U Mich Med Sch 83; **RES:**
Columbia-Presbyterian Med Ctr, New York, NY 83-
86; D, Columbia-Presbyterian Med Ctr, New York,
NY 86-89

LANG: Sp; 🔧 🌙 🏨 💲 Med Med   2-4 Weeks

Bisaccia, Emil (MD) D
Morristown Mem Hosp

Affiliated Dermatologists, 182 South St 1;
Morristown, NJ 07960; (973) 267-0300; **BDCERT:**
D 84; **MS:** MC Ohio, Toledo 79; **RES:** IM,
Morristown Mem Hosp, Morristown, NJ 79-80; D,
Ohio State U Hosp, Columbus, OH 80-82; **FEL:** IM,
Columbia-Presbyterian Med Ctr, New York, NY 82-
83; **FAP:** Assoc Clin Prof D Columbia P&S; **HOSP:**
Columbia-Presbyterian Med Ctr; **SI:** *Skin Cancer—
Cosmetic Surgery; Cutaneous T-Cell Lymphoma*;
HMO: Oxford CIGNA Prudential United Healthcare
PHCS +

[symbols] *VISA*

Weinberg, Harvey (MD) D
Columbia-Presbyterian Med Ctr

Dermatology Associates of Morris, 199 Baldwin Rd
230; Parsippany, NJ 07054; (973) 335-2560;
BDCERT: D 74; **MS:** SUNY Buffalo 69; **RES:** D,
USPHS, Staten Island, NY 70-72; D, Colum-Presby
Med Ctr, New York, NY 72-73; **FAP:** Asst Clin Prof
Columbia P&S; **HOSP:** NW Covenant Med Ctr-
Riverside; **SI:** *Psoriasis Phototherapy; Laser Surgery*;
HMO: Oxford CIGNA PHS HMO Blue Prudential +
LANG: Sp; [symbols] 2-4 Weeks

DIAGNOSTIC RADIOLOGY

Claps, Richard (MD) DR
Union Hosp-New Jersey

95 Madison Ave FL1; Morristown, NJ 07960; (973)
984-1111; **BDCERT:** NRad 78; NuM 75; **MS:** NY
Med Coll 68; **RES:** Rad, Metropolitan Hosp Ctr, New
York, NY 69-72; **SI:** *General Radiology CT- Scan;
Ultrasound Mammography*; **HMO:** GHI CIGNA
Oxford Blue Cross & Blue Shield United Healthcare
+
LANG: Sp; [symbols] Immediately

EMERGENCY MEDICINE

Gerardi, Michael (MD) EM
Morristown Mem Hosp

Morristown Memorial Hospital Emergency Medical
Associates, 100 Madison Ave; Livingston, NJ
07960; (973) 971-8919; **BDCERT:** EM 95; Ped 91;
MS: Georgetown U 85; **RES:** IM, Emory U Hosp,
Atlanta, GA 85-89; Ped, Emory U Hosp, Atlanta,
GA 85-89; **FAP:** Asst Clin Instr Med UMDNJ New
Jersey Sch Osteo Med; **SI:** *Pediatric Emergency
Medicine; Headaches*; **HMO:** Aetna Hlth Plan Blue
Choice Blue Cross & Blue Shield

[symbols] Immediately

ENDOCRINOLOGY, DIABETES & METABOLISM

Usiskin, Keith (MD) EDM
Morristown Mem Hosp

101 Madison Ave 305; Morristown, NJ 07960;
(973) 267-9099; **BDCERT:** EDM 89; IM 87; **MS:**
UMDNJ-RW Johnson Med Sch 84; **RES:** IM, Med
Coll VA Hosp, Richmond, VA 85-87; **FEL:** EDM,
Med Coll VA Hosp, Richmond, VA 87-89; **HMO:**
CIGNA
[symbol]

FAMILY PRACTICE

Holland Jr, Elbridge (MD) FP PCP
Overlook Hosp

Chatham Family Practice Assoc, 492 Main St;
Chatham, NJ 07928; (973) 635-2432; **BDCERT:**
FP 78; Ger 88; **MS:** U Chicago-Pritzker Sch Med 75;
RES: FP, Overlook Hosp, Summit, NJ 75-78; **FAP:**
Asst Prof of Clin Med Columbia P&S; **HMO:** Blue
Cross & Blue Shield CIGNA US Hlthcre

GASTROENTEROLOGY

Dalena, John (MD)　　　Ge
Morristown Mem Hosp

7 Prospeck St; Madison, NJ 07940; (973) 377-
5300; **BDCERT:** IM 88; Ge 91; **MS:** UMDNJ-NJ Med
Sch, Newark 85; **RES:** Mount Sinai Med Ctr, New
York, NY 85-88; **FEL:** Ge, Univ of Med & Dent NJ
Hosp, Newark, NJ 88-90

Freedman, Pamela (MD)　　　Ge
NW Covenant Med Ctr-Riverside

Gastroenterology Associates of North Jersey, 369
W Blackwell; Dover, NJ 07801; (973) 361-7660;
BDCERT: IM 83; **MS:** Albert Einstein Coll Med 80;
RES: IM, Montefiore Med Ctr, Bronx, NY 81-83;
FEL: Bellevue Hosp Ctr, New York, NY 83-85;
HMO: Aetna Hlth Plan Blue Choice Blue Cross &
Blue Shield

🦽 SA SO 🄲 📠 👥 🏥 Mcr WC　4+ Weeks

Rosh, Joel (MD)　　　Ge
Morristown Mem Hosp

Pediatric Gastroenterology & Nutrition, 100
Madison Ave; Morristown, NJ 07962; (973) 971-
5676; **BDCERT:** Ped 89; PGe 92; **MS:** Albert
Einstein Coll Med 86; **RES:** Ped, Columbia-
Presbyterian Med Ctr, New York, NY 87-89; **FEL:**
PGe, Mount Sinai Med Ctr, New York, NY 89-91;
FAP: Asst Prof of Clin Ped Columbia P&S; **HOSP:**
Overlook Hosp; **SI:** *Inflammatory Bowel Disease;
Pediatric Liver Disease;* **HMO:** Blue Cross & Blue
Shield CIGNA Oxford Prudential Aetna-US
Healthcare +

🦽 📠 👥 🏥 💲 Mcl NFI　Immediately 🟦AMERICAN EXPRESS **VISA** 💳

Samach, Michael (MD)　　　Ge
Morristown Mem Hosp

Affiliates In Gastroenterology, 101 Madison Ave
100; Morristown, NJ 07960; (973) 455-0404;
BDCERT: IM 74; Ge 79; **MS:** NYU Sch Med 71; **RES:**
IM, Montefiore Med Ctr, Bronx, NY 71-74; **FEL:** Ge,
Montefiore Med Ctr, Bronx, NY 76-78; **FAP:** Asst
Clin Prof Columbia P&S; **SI:** *Colonoscopy; Esophageal
Reflux;* **HMO:** United Payors CIGNA Oxford Prucare
Blue Cross & Blue Shield +

🦽 📠 👥 🏥 Mcr Mcl　Immediately **VISA** 💳 🟥

Soriano, John (MD)　　　Ge
Northwest Covenant Med Ctr

Morris County Gastroenterology, 16 Pocono Rd
310; Denville, NJ 07834; (973) 627-4430;
BDCERT: IM 86; Ge 93; **MS:** Mexico 81; **RES:** IM,
Morristown Mem Hosp, Morristown, NJ 83-87;
FEL: Ge, Long Island Coll Hosp, Brooklyn, NY 87-
89; **HOSP:** Morristown Mem Hosp; **SI:** *Colon and
Rectal Cancer Screening; Peptic Ulcer Disease;* **HMO:**
CIGNA Blue Cross & Blue Shield Prucare

🦽 📠 👥 🏥 💲 Mcr　1 Week **VISA** 💳

Stein, Lawrence (MD)　　　Ge
Morristown Mem Hosp

101 Madison Ave 100; Morristown, NJ 07960;
(973) 455-0404; **BDCERT:** IM 72; Ge 73; **MS:** U
Minn 65; **RES:** Albert Einstein Med Ctr, Bronx, NY
65-67; Albert Einstein Med Ctr, Bronx, NY 69-70;
FEL: Albert Einstein Med Ctr, Bronx, NY 70-72;
HOSP: St Barnabas Med Ctr-Livingston

🦽 📠 👥 🏥 💲 Mcr Mcl WC NFI　Immediately 🟦AMERICAN EXPRESS
VISA 💳 🟥

HAND SURGERY

Ende, Leigh (MD)　　　HS
Northwest Covenant Med Ctr

121 Center Grove Rd; Randolph, NJ 07869; (973)
366-5565; **BDCERT:** OrS 89; HS 90; **MS:** Tulane U
78; **RES:** OrS, Univ of Med & Dent NJ Hosp, Newark,
NJ 79-83; **FEL:** HS, Columbia Presbyterian Med Ctr,
New York, NY 83-84; **SI:** *Arthritis; Carpal Tunnel
Syndrome*

Guide to symbols and abbreviations can be found on pages 110-113.

989

Miller, Jeffrey (MD)   HS
Morristown Mem Hosp

North Jersey Hand Surgery, 300 Madison Ave Fl 2; Madison, NJ 07940; (973) 377-1456; **BDCERT:** OrS 89; HS 91; **MS:** Univ Pittsburgh 81; **RES:** S, Geo Wash U Med Ctr, Washington, DC 81; OrS, Boston U Med Ctr, Boston, MA 82-86; **FEL:** HS, Thomas Jefferson U Hosp, Philadelphia, PA 86-87; **FAP:** Instr UMDNJ New Jersey Sch Osteo Med; **HOSP:** Overlook Hosp; *SI: Carpal Tunnel Syndrome; Dupuytren's Disease;* **HMO:** Blue Choice Blue Cross & Blue Shield CIGNA Metlife Sanus-NYLCare +

LANG: Sp; 🔲 🔲 🔲 🔲 🔲 🔲 🔲 🔲 🔲
A Few Days **VISA** 💳

INFECTIOUS DISEASE

Allegra, Donald (MD)   Inf
Northwest Covenant Med Ctr

Infectious Disease Assoc, 765 Rte 10 East; Dover, NJ 07869; (973) 989-0068; **BDCERT:** IM 78; Inf 82; **MS:** Harvard Med Sch 74; **RES:** IM, U CO Hosp, Denver, CO 74-75; **FEL:** Inf, Emory U Hosp, Atlanta, GA 80-81; *SI: Tropical Medicine;* **HMO:** Most

🔲 🔲 🔲 🔲 🔲 🔲 🔲 🔲 A Few Days **VISA** 💳

McManus, Edward (MD)   Inf
Northwest Covenant Med Ctr

Infectious Diease Associates, 765 Route 10 East; Randolph, NJ 07869; (973) 989-0068; **BDCERT:** IM 85; Inf 88; **MS:** UMDNJ-NJ Med Sch, Newark 82; **RES:** IM, U of WI Hosp, Madison, WI 82-85; IM, U of WI Hosp, Madison, WI 85-86; **FEL:** Inf, Nat Inst Health, Bethesda, MD 86-89; **HOSP:** Morristown Mem Hosp; **HMO:** CIGNA Oxford Prucare Aetna-US Healthcare HMO Blue +

🔲 🔲 🔲 🔲 🔲 🔲 🔲 🔲 🔲 A Few Days **VISA** 💳

INTERNAL MEDICINE

Pond, William (MD)   IM **PCP**
Morristown Mem Hosp

95 Madison Ave; Morristown, NJ 07960; (973) 538-1388; **BDCERT:** IM 80; Ger 88; **MS:** Tufts U 77; **RES:** Overlook Hosp, Summit, NJ 77-80; **HMO:** CoMed CIGNA Aetna-US Healthcare NYLCare

🔲 🔲 🔲 🔲 🔲 🔲 2-4 Weeks **VISA** 💳

Scaduto, Phillip (MD)   IM **PCP**
Northwest Covenant Med Ctr

223 W Main St; Boonton, NJ 07005; (973) 335-7900; **BDCERT:** IM 86; Ge 90; **MS:** UMDNJ-NJ Med Sch, Newark 83; **RES:** Univ of Med & Dent NJ Hosp, Newark, NJ 84-86; **HMO:** CIGNA QualCare NYLCare Oxford

🔲 🔲 🔲 🔲 🔲 2-4 Weeks

Siroty, Robert (MD)   IM **PCP**
Northwest Covenant Med Ctr

375 E Mcfarlan St; Dover, NJ 07801; (973) 361-6600; **BDCERT:** IM 68; **MS:** SUNY Syracuse 60; **RES:** IM, Kings County Hosp Ctr, Brooklyn, NY 60-62; IM, Montefiore Med Ctr, Bronx, NY 64-65; **FEL:** Hem, Montefiore Med Ctr, Bronx, NY 65-66; **FAP:** Asst Clin Prof UMDNJ New Jersey Sch Osteo Med; *SI: Blood Disorders; Coagulation Problems;* **HMO:** CIGNA Prucare US Hlthcre United Healthcare QualCare +

🔲 🔲 🔲 🔲 🔲 🔲 🔲 🔲 2-4 Weeks

Weine, Gary (MD)   IM **PCP**
Morristown Mem Hosp

95 Madison Ave 405; Morristown, NJ 07960; (973) 829-9998; **BDCERT:** IM 79; **MS:** Cornell U 76; **RES:** NY Hosp-Cornell Med Ctr, New York, NY 77-79; **FAP:** Asst Clin Prof Columbia P&S

🔲 🔲 🔲 🔲 🔲 🔲 A Few Days

MEDICAL ONCOLOGY

Adler, Kenneth (MD) Onc
Morristown Mem Hosp
100 Madison Ave; Morristown, NJ 07960; (973)
538-5210; **BDCERT:** Hem 78; IM 76; **MS:** Albany
Med Coll 73; **RES:** Albany Med Ctr, Albany, NY 73-
76; **FEL:** Albany Med Ctr, Albany, NY 76-78; **HMO:**
Aetna Hlth Plan US Hlthcre Oxford HIP Network
Sanus-NYLCare +

♿ 📺 💲 📠 🏥 2-4 Weeks **VISA** 💳

Casper, Ephraim (MD) Onc
Northwest Covenant Med Ctr
Memorial Sloan Kettering Cancer Center at
Northwest Covenant Medical Center, 23 Pocono
Rd; Denville, NJ 07834; (973) 983-7330; **BDCERT:**
IM 77; Onc 79; **MS:** Rush Med Coll 74; **RES:** Med,
Rush Presbyterian-St Lukes Med Ctr, Chicago, IL
75-77; **FEL:** Onc, Mem Sloan Kettering Cancer Ctr,
New York, NY 77-79; **HOSP:** Mem Med Ctr at
South Amboy; **SI:** *Gastrointestinal Cancer; Sarcoma;*
HMO: Prudential Empire Blue Cross & Shield

♿ 📷 🏥 📺 📠 🏥 A Few Days ▓▓ **VISA** 💳 💳

Papish, Steven (MD) Onc
Morristown Mem Hosp
261 James St; Morristown, NJ 07960; (973) 538-
5210; **BDCERT:** IM 77; Hem 80; **MS:** Univ Penn
74; **RES:** IM, Geo Wash U Med Ctr, Washington, DC
74-78; **FEL:** New England Med Ctr, Boston, MA 78-
79; Onc, Harvard Med Sch, Cambridge, MA 79-81;
HOSP: St Clare's Hosp & Health Ctr; **HMO:** CIGNA
US Hlthcre HMO Blue

♿ 📷 📺 💲 📠 🏥 1 Week **VISA** 💳

NEPHROLOGY

Fine, Paul (MD) Nep
Morristown Mem Hosp
Nephrology Hypertension Associates of Morris
County, 2 Franklin Pl; Morristown, NJ 07960;
(973) 267-7673; **BDCERT:** IM 82; Nep 84; **MS:**
Yale U Sch Med 79; **RES:** IM, NY Hosp-Cornell Med
Ctr, New York, NY 79-82; **FEL:** Nep, Columbia-
Presbyterian Med Ctr, New York, NY 82; **FAP:** Asst
Prof of Clin Med Columbia P&S; **HOSP:** Northwest
Covenant Med Ctr; **SI:** *Kidney Failure; Hypertension;*
HMO: Oxford CIGNA Blue Cross & Blue Shield
Prudential

♿ 📷 🏥 📺 💲 📠 🏥 🏥 2-4 Weeks **VISA** 💳

Goldstein, Carl (MD) Nep
Overlook Hosp
Medical Diagnostic Assoc, 417 W Broad St;
Westfield, NJ 07090; (908) 233-0895; **BDCERT:**
Nep 84; **MS:** Washington U, St Louis 78; **RES:** U
MN Med Ctr, Minneapolis, MN 78-81; **FEL:** Nep,
Hosp of U Penn, Philadelphia, PA 81-84; **FAP:**
Assoc Clin Prof Columbia P&S; **SI:** *High Blood
Pressure; Kidney Failure & Dialysis*

🅲 📷 📺 💲 📠 A Few Days **VISA** 💳

NEUROLOGICAL SURGERY

Beyerl, Brian (MD) NS
Morristown Mem Hosp
Neuro Surgical GroupChatham, 10 Parrott Mill Rd;
Chatham, NJ 07928; (973) 635-2597; **BDCERT:**
NS 90; **MS:** Johns Hopkins U 80; **RES:** S, Johns
Hopkins Hosp, Baltimore, MD 79-81; NS, Mass Gen
Hosp, Boston, MA 81-86; **FAP:** Asst Clin Prof
UMDNJ New Jersey Sch Osteo Med; **HOSP:** Overlook
Hosp; **SI:** *Brain Tumors; Stereotactic Neurosurgery*

♿ 📷 📺 💲 📠 🏥 1 Week ▓▓ **VISA** 💳 💳

Hodosh, Richard (MD)   NS
Overlook Hosp

Neurosurgical Group of Chatham, 10 Parrott Mill Rd Box 808; Chatham, NJ 07928; (973) 635-2597; **BDCERT:** NS 80; **MS:** U Cincinnati 72; **RES:** Parkland Mem Hosp, Dallas, TX 72-78; **FEL:** N, Kanto Hosp, Switzerland 75-76; Nat Hosp Neuro Diseases, Nat'l Hosp Neuro Diseases 75; **FAP:** Clin Prof NS UMDNJ New Jersey Sch Osteo Med; **HOSP:** Morristown Mem Hosp; *SI: Brain Tumors; Brain Aneurysms;* **HMO:** Aetna-US Healthcare CIGNA PHCS Oxford

⌖ 📷 🎬 💲 Mcr Mod Nfi 2-4 Weeks **VISA** 💳

Zampella, Edward (MD)   NS
Overlook Hosp

Neurosurgical Group of Chatham, 10 Parrott Mill Rd; Chatham, NJ 07928; (973) 635-2597; **BDCERT:** NS 91; **MS:** U Ala Sch Med 82; **RES:** NS, U of Alabama Hosp, Birmingham, AL 83-88; **FEL:** N, Queen Square/Maida Vale, 85; **FAP:** Assoc Prof UMDNJ New Jersey Sch Osteo Med; **HOSP:** Morristown Mem Hosp; *SI: Pediatric Neurosurgery; Pain Management*

LANG: Sp; ⌖ 📷 🎬 💲 Mcr Mod WC Nfi A Few Days **VISA** 💳

NEUROLOGY

Cerny, Kenneth (MD)   N
Morristown Mem Hosp

The Neuroscience Center of Northern NJ, 95 Madison Ave; Morristown, NJ 07960; (973) 285-1446; **BDCERT:** N 83; **MS:** Columbia P&S 76; **RES:** Barnes Hosp, St Louis, MO 76-78; Albert Einstein Med Ctr, Bronx, NY 78-81; *SI: Parkinson's Disease; Headache;* **HMO:** Oxford PHCS United Healthcare Blue Cross & Blue Shield First Option +

⌖ 📷 🎬 🎬 💲 Mcr WC Nfi 1 Week **VISA** 💳

Fox, Stuart (MD)   N
Morristown Mem Hosp

The Neuroscience Center of Northern NJ PA, 95 Madison Ave; Morristown, NJ 07960; (973) 285-1446; **BDCERT:** N 82; **IM** 78; **MS:** Cornell U 75; **RES:** IM, U Mich Med Ctr, Ann Arbor, MI 75-78; N, Albert Einstein Med Ctr, Bronx, NY 78-81; **FEL:** C/NPh, Long Island Jewish Med Ctr, New Hyde Park, NY 81-82; **FAP:** Asst Clin Prof Med Columbia P&S; **HOSP:** Overlook Hosp; *SI: Neuromuscular Disease; Headache;* **HMO:** Aetna Hlth Plan Prucare Blue Cross & Blue Shield CIGNA Oxford +

LANG: Sp; ⌖ 📷 🎬 💲 Mcr Mod WC Nfi 1 Week **VISA** 💳

OBSTETRICS & GYNECOLOGY

Christman, J Eric (MD)   ObG
Morristown Mem Hosp

Morristown Memorial Hospital, 100 Madison Ave Bx 1956; Morristown, NJ 07962; (973) 971-5900; **BDCERT:** ObG 79; **MS:** Ind U Sch Med 68; **RES:** USAF Med Ctr-Kessler AFB, , MS 71-75; **FEL:** GO, Stanford Med Ctr, Stanford, CA 84-86; **HOSP:** Overlook Hosp; *SI: Women's Cancer Problems;* **HMO:** PHCS CIGNA NYLCare HMO Blue

⌖ 📷 🎬 Mcr Mod 1 Week

Gluck, Ian (MD)   ObG
Morristown Mem Hosp

261 James St Ste 3C; Morristown, NJ 07960; (973) 538-1515; **BDCERT:** ObG 85; **MS:** NY Med Coll 79; **RES:** ObG, Grady Mem Hosp, Atlanta, GA 79-83; **HMO:** Blue Cross & Blue Shield CIGNA Oxford PHS Prucare +

⌖ 📷 🎬 🎬 💲 Mcr 4+ Weeks **VISA**

Iammatteo, Matthew (MD) ObG
Morristown Mem Hosp

Franklin Ob Gyn, 59 Franklin St; Morristown, NJ 07960; (973) 539-1024; **BDCERT:** ObG 91; **MS:** Dominica 85; **RES:** ObG, St Michael's Med Ctr, Newark, NJ 85-89; *SI: Hysteroscopy; High Risk OB;* **HMO:** Oxford Aetna Hlth Plan First Option Prucare PHCS +

€ 📷 🎬 💲 4+ Weeks **VISA** 💳

Jacobowitz, Walter (MD)   ObG
Morristown Mem Hosp

261 James St 3C; Morristown, NJ 07960; (973) 538-1515; **BDCERT:** ObG 89; **MS:** NYU Sch Med 58; **RES:** Bellevue Hosp Ctr, New York, NY 59-63; **SI:** *Menopause; Cervical Disease;* **HMO:** Guardian Oxford CIGNA Prudential PHS +

🅰 🔲 🔛 📅 🆂 M̅ A Few Days **VISA** 💳

Mohr, Robert (MD)   ObG
Morristown Mem Hosp

261 James St; Morristown, NJ 07960; (908) 719-2264; **BDCERT:** ObG 83; **MS:** Hahnemann U 77; **RES:** Northwest Mem Hosp, Chicago, IL 77-81

Steer, Robert (MD)   ObG
Morristown Mem Hosp

32 Maple Ave; Morristown, NJ 07960; (973) 993-1919; **BDCERT:** ObG 93; **MS:** Cornell U 86; **RES:** ObG, NY Hosp-Cornell Med Ctr, New York, NY 86-90; **HMO:** Aetna Hlth Plan Blue Choice Blue Cross & Blue Shield

🔲 📅 🆂 2-4 Weeks

Thornton, Yvonne S (MD)   ObG
Morristown Mem Hosp

100 Madison Ave; Morristown, NJ 07962; (973) 971-7900; **BDCERT:** ObG 79; MF 81; **MS:** Columbia P&S 73; **RES:** ObG, St Luke's Roosevelt Hosp Ctr, New York, NY 73-77; **FEL:** MF, Columbia-Presbyterian Med Ctr, New York, NY 77-79; **FAP:** Assoc Clin Prof Columbia P&S; **SI:** *Obstetrical Ultrasound; Chorionic Villus Sampling*

🅰 📅 🆂 1 Week 🅰🅴 **VISA** 💳 🔲

Wallis, Joseph (DO)   ObG   `PCP`
Northwest Covenant Med Ctr

600 Mt Pleasant Ave; Dover, NJ 07801; (973) 989-9000; **BDCERT:** ObG 77; **MS:** Philadelphia Coll Osteo Med 70; **RES:** ObG, St Michael's Med Ctr, Newark, NJ 72-75; **SI:** *Laparoscopic Surgery; Infertility;* **HMO:** CIGNA Blue Shield NYLCare QualCare US Hlthcre +

🅰 🄲 🔲 🔛 📅 🆂 M̅ 2-4 Weeks 🅰🅴 **VISA** 💳

OPHTHALMOLOGY

Pinke, Robert S (MD)   Oph
Northwest Covenant Med Ctr

66 Sunset Strip Ste 107; Succasunna, NJ 07876; (973) 584-4451; **BDCERT:** Oph 89; **MS:** Mt Sinai Sch Med 84; **RES:** Baylor Coll Med, Houston, TX 85-88

Silverman, Cary (MD)   Oph
NW Covenant Med Ctr-Riverside

Parsippany Eye Care Associates, 199 Baldwin Rd; Parsippany, NJ 07054; (973) 316-0387; **BDCERT:** Oph 87; **MS:** UMDNJ-NJ Med Sch, Newark 82; **RES:** Oph, Hahnemann U Hosp, Philadelphia, PA 83-86; **FAP:** Clin Prof UMDNJ New Jersey Sch Osteo Med; **HOSP:** St Barnabas Med Ctr-Livingston; **SI:** *Laser Refractive Surgery; Cataract Surgery;* **HMO:** Aetna Hlth Plan Blue Choice Blue Cross & Blue Shield CIGNA

LANG: Sp; 🅰 🆂🄳 🄲 🔲 🔛 📅 🆂 M̅ W̅C̅ N̅F̅I̅ 1 Week 🅰🅴 **VISA** 💳

ORTHOPAEDIC SURGERY

Hurley, John (MD)   OrS
Morristown Mem Hosp

TriCountry Orthopaedic, 160 E Hanover Ave PO Box 1446; Morristown, NJ 07962; (973) 538-2334; **BDCERT:** OrS 88; **MS:** NYU Sch Med 80; **RES:** OrS, Univ of Med & Dent NJ Hosp, Newark, NJ 81-85; **FEL:** SM, Cleveland Clinic Hosp, Cleveland, OH 85-86; **FAP:** Sr OrS; **SI:** *Sports Medicine; Knees & Shoulders;* **HMO:** Most

🅰 🔲 🔛 📅 🆂 M̅ A Few Days 🅰🅴 **VISA** 💳 🔲

Guide to symbols and abbreviations can be found on pages 110-113.

993

OTOLARYNGOLOGY

Rubin, Edward (MD)　　　Oto
St Clare's Hosp & Health Ctr
North Jersey Ear Nose & Throat, 16 Pocono Rd
112; Denville, NJ 07834; (973) 625-1818;
BDCERT: Oto 69; **MS:** NY Med Coll 63; **RES:** S, Beth
Israel Med Ctr, New York, NY 64-65; Oto, New
York Eye & Ear Infirmary, New York, NY; **HOSP:**
NW Covenant Med Ctr-Riverside; **HMO:** HMO Blue
Aetna-US Healthcare CIGNA QualCare NYLCare +

LANG: Ger, Sp, Itl; 🔲 🔲 🔲 🔲 🔲 🔲 🔲 🔲 🔲
A Few Days **VISA** 💳

Taylor, Howard (MD)　　　Oto
Chilton Mem Hosp
Ear Nose Throat & Facial Plstc surgery, 51 State
Highway 23 S; Riverdale, NJ 07457; (973) 831-
1220; **BDCERT:** Oto 80; **MS:** Columbia P&S 76;
RES: Oto, U Chicago Hosp, Chicago, IL 77-80; U
Chicago Hosp, Chicago, IL 77-80; **FEL:** Oto Facial
PlS, Hosp Med College of PA, Philadelphia, PA 80-
81; **FAP:** Asst Clin Prof UMDNJ New Jersey Sch
Osteo Med

🔲 🔲 🔲 🔲 🔲 🔲 🔲 🔲 A Few Days **VISA** 💳

PAIN MANAGEMENT

Rudman, Michael E (MD)　　PM
Morristown Mem Hosp
Morristown Memorial Hospital, Dept of Pain
Management, 100 Madison Ave; Morristown, NJ
07962; (973) 971-4444; **BDCERT:** Anes 93; PM
96; **MS:** Penn State U-Hershey Med Ctr 88; **RES:**
Anes, Hosp of U Penn, Philadelphia, PA 89-92;
HMO: +

🔲 🔲 🔲 🔲 🔲 🔲 🔲 1 Week

PEDIATRIC ALLERGY & IMMUNOLOGY

Chernack, William J (MD)　PA&I
Morristown Mem Hosp
28 Franklin Pl; Morristown, NJ 07960; (973) 538-
7271; **BDCERT:** Ped 75; A&I 75; **MS:** NY Med Coll
70; **RES:** Ped, Columbia-Presbyterian Med Ctr, New
York, NY 70-72; **FEL:** A&I, Columbia-Presbyterian
Med Ctr, New York, NY 72-74; **FAP:** Asst Clin Prof
Ped Columbia P&S; **SI:** *Bronchial Asthma; Sinusitis;*
HMO: Aetna-US Healthcare Blue Cross & Blue
Shield CIGNA Oxford Prudential +

🔲 🔲 🔲 🔲 A Few Days

Morrison, Susan (MD)　　PA&I
Clara Maass Med Ctr
36 Newark Ave; Belleville, NJ 07109; (973) 450-
0100; **BDCERT:** A&I 89; Ped Inf 94; **MS:** UMDNJ-NJ
Med Sch, Newark 81; **RES:** Ped, Univ of Med & Dent
NJ Hosp, Newark, NJ 81-85; **FEL:** Ped Inf, Univ of
Med & Dent NJ Hosp, Newark, NJ 85-88; **FAP:** Asst
Clin Prof UMDNJ-NJ Med Sch, Newark; **SI:** *Adult
A&I*

🔲 🔲 🔲 🔲 🔲 🔲 4+ Weeks

PEDIATRIC CARDIOLOGY

Donnelly, Christine (MD)　　PCd
Morristown Mem Hosp
100 Madison Ave; Morristown, NJ 07960; (973)
971-4340; **BDCERT:** PCd 85; Ped 85; **MS:**
Columbia P&S 78; **RES:** Ped, Columbia-
Presbyterian Med Ctr, New York, NY 78-81; **FEL:**
PCd, Columbia-Presbyterian Med Ctr, New York,
NY 81-84; **FAP:** Assoc Clin Prof Ped Columbia P&S;
HOSP: Columbia-Presbyterian Med Ctr; **SI:**
*Interventional Catheterization; Fetal
Echocardiography;* **HMO:** Aetna-US Healthcare
Oxford Prucare CIGNA/CoMed Blue Cross & Blue
Shield +

🔲 🔲 🔲 🔲 🔲 🔲 🔲 A Few Days 💳 **VISA** 💳

PEDIATRIC ENDOCRINOLOGY

Sills, Irene N (MD)　　　　PEn
Morristown Mem Hosp
Pediatric Endocrine Ctr, PO Box 1956; Morristown, NJ 07960; (973) 971-4340; **BDCERT:** Ped 80; PEn 83; **MS:** NYU Sch Med 76; **RES:** Univ Hosp SUNY Syracuse, Syracuse, NY 76-78; Children's Hosp of Buffalo, Buffalo, NY 78-79; **FEL:** PEn, Children's Hosp of Buffalo, Buffalo, NY 78-79; **FAP:** Assoc Prof of Clin Ped Columbia P&S; **HOSP:** Overlook Hosp; *SI: Growth and Development; Diabetes Mellitus;* **HMO:** CIGNA US Hlthcre First Option Oxford Prucare +
🦽 📷 🈵 🏧 $ Mcr　2-4 Weeks **VISA** 💳

Starkman, Harold (MD)　　　　PEn
Morristown Mem Hosp
100 Madison Ave; Morristown, NJ 07960; (973) 971-4340; **BDCERT:** PEn 83; **MS:** Albert Einstein Coll Med 76; **RES:** Mount Sinai Med Ctr, New York, NY 76-78; NY Hosp-Cornell Med Ctr, New York, NY 78-79; **FEL:** NY Hosp-Cornell Med Ctr, New York, NY 79-80; Joslin Diabetic Clinic, Boston, MA 80; **FAP:** Assoc Prof Columbia P&S; **HOSP:** Overlook Hosp; *SI: Diabetes; Growth Disorders;* **HMO:** US Hlthcre Prucare CIGNA United Healthcare Oxford +
🦽 🅲 📷 🈵 🏧 $ Mcr　2-4 Weeks ▦ **VISA** 💳 💳

PEDIATRIC NEPHROLOGY

Feld, Leonard (MD & PhD)　PNep
Morristown Mem Hosp
Atlantic Health Systems, 325 Columbia Tpke; Florham Park, NJ 07932; (973) 971-5649; **BDCERT:** PNep 85; Ped 84; **MS:** SUNY Buffalo 79; **RES:** Albert Einstein Med Ctr, Bronx, NY 79-81; **FEL:** PNep,; **FAP:** Prof Ped UMDNJ New Jersey Sch Osteo Med; **HOSP:** Overlook Hosp; *SI: Hypertension; Kidney Disease;* **HMO:** Most
🦽 🅲 📷 🈵 🏧 $ Mcr Mcd　A Few Days ▦ **VISA** 💳 💳

PEDIATRIC PULMONOLOGY

Atlas, Arthur (MD)　　　　PPul
Morristown Mem Hosp
Respiratory Center for Children, 100 Madison Ave; Morristown, NJ 07960; (973) 971-4142; **BDCERT:** Ped 89; PPul 92; **MS:** Mexico 82; **RES:** St Louis Children's Hosp, St Louis, MO 84-86; **FEL:** Pul A&I, St Louis Children's Hosp, St Louis, MO 87-89; Children's Hosp of Pittsburgh, Pittsburgh, PA 89-91; **HOSP:** Columbia-Presbyterian Med Ctr; **HMO:** Cost Care First Option HIP Network Oxford Prucare +
🦽 🅲 📷 🈵 🏧 $ Mcr Mcd　1 Week **VISA** 💳

PEDIATRICS

Cohen, Martin (MD)　　　Ped　[PCP]
Morristown Mem Hosp
Morristown Pediatrics Associates, 261 James St 1G; Morristown, NJ 07960; (973) 540-9393; **BDCERT:** Ped 72; **MS:** SUNY Hlth Sci Ctr 67; **RES:** Children's Hosp Med Ctr, Cincinnati, OH 67-70; **HMO:** Aetna Hlth Plan Blue Choice CIGNA Prucare Sanus-NYLCare +
LANG: Sp; 🦽 🈳 🅲 📷 🈵 🏧 $ Mcr　1 Week **VISA** 💳

Handler, Robert (MD)　　　Ped　[PCP]
Morristown Mem Hosp
1140 Parsippany Blvd; Parsippany, NJ 07054; (973) 263-0066; **BDCERT:** Ped 80; **MS:** UMDNJ-NJ Med Sch, Newark 75; **RES:** Children's Hosp Nat Med Ctr, Washington, DC 75-78; **FAP:** Asst Clin Prof Ped UMDNJ New Jersey Sch Osteo Med; **HOSP:** St Clare's Hosp & Health Ctr; **HMO:** CIGNA Blue Cross & Blue Shield Prucare US Hlthcre Oxford +
🦽 🈳 🅲 📷 🈵 $　2-4 Weeks **VISA** 💳

Lo Frumento, Mary Ann (MD)Ped
Morristown Mem Hosp
PO Box 1789; Morristown, NJ 07762; (973) 538-6116; **BDCERT:** Ped 86; **MS:** Univ Penn 81; **RES:** Columbia-Presbyterian Med Ctr, New York, NY 81-84; **HMO:** Oxford Prucare CIGNA Aetna-US Healthcare NYLCare +

🦽 🈂 📞 📷 🖼 🏨 💲 Med 2-4 Weeks **VISA** 💳 📧

Panza, Robert (MD) Ped
Morristown Mem Hosp
836 Mountain Ave; Westfield, NJ 07090; (908) 233-7171; **BDCERT:** Ped 89; **MS:** Italy 85

PHYSICAL MEDICINE & REHABILITATION

Mulford, Gregory (MD) PMR
Morristown Mem Hosp
Associates in Rehabilitation Medicine, 95 Mt Kemble Ave; Morristown, NJ 07960; (973) 267-2293; **BDCERT:** PMR 90; **MS:** UMDNJ-RW Johnson Med Sch 85; **RES:** S, Overlook Hosp, Summit, NJ 86; PMR, Columbia-Presbyterian Med Ctr, New York, NY 89; **FAP:** Asst Clin Prof Columbia P&S; **HOSP:** Overlook Hosp; **SI:** Sports Medicine; Electrodiagnosis; **HMO:** CapCare Aetna-US Healthcare Oxford Prudential Blue Cross & Blue Shield +

LANG: Sp, Itl, Kor; 🦽 📞 📷 🖼 🏨 💲 Mcr Mod WC NFl Immediately

PLASTIC SURGERY

Starker, Isaac (MD) PlS
Morristown Mem Hosp
124 Columbia Tpk; Florham Park, NJ 07932; (973) 822-3000; **BDCERT:** PlS 92; **MS:** NYU Sch Med 81; **RES:** S, St Luke's Roosevelt Hosp Ctr, New York, NY 81-86; PlS, Montefiore Med Ctr, Bronx, NY 86-88; **FEL:** HS, St Luke's Roosevelt Hosp Ctr, New York, NY 89; **HOSP:** St Barnabas Med Ctr-Livingston; **SI:** Cosmetic Surgery of Face; Body Contouring

LANG: Sp, Fr; 🦽 📷 🖼 🏨 💲 Mcr WC NFl 2-4 Weeks

PSYCHIATRY

Granet, Roger (MD) Psyc
Morristown Mem Hosp
261 James St 2E; Morristown, NJ 07960; (973) 540-9490; **BDCERT:** Psyc 78; **MS:** UMDNJ-NJ Med Sch, Newark 74; **RES:** NY Hosp-Cornell Med Ctr, New York, NY 74-77; **FAP:** Clin Prof Psyc Cornell U; **HOSP:** NY Hosp-Cornell Med Ctr; **SI:** Psychiatric Care of Cancer Patients; Anxiety and Depression

🦽 📷 🖼 🏨 💲 2-4 Weeks **VISA** 💳

Sofair, Jane (MD) Psyc
Morristown Mem Hosp
52 Maple Ave; Morristown, NJ 07960; (973) 292-0960; **BDCERT:** Psyc 86; **MS:** NYU Sch Med 80; **RES:** Psyc, New York University Med Ctr, New York, NY 81-84; **FAP:** Instr Columbia P&S; **SI:** Depression and Anxiety; Women's Health; **HMO:** Oxford Prucare

LANG: Fr; 📞 📷 💲 2-4 Weeks

Sundaram, Savitri (MD) Psyc
NW Covenant Med Ctr-Riverside
Atrium Bldg, 195 Rte 46 West; Mine Hill, NJ 07803; (973) 361-2550; **BDCERT:** Psyc 82; **MS:** India 68

PULMONARY DISEASE

Capone, Robert (MD) Pul
Morristown Mem Hosp
Pulmonary & Allergy Associates, PA, 101 Madison Ave Ste 205; Morristown, NJ 07966; (973) 267-9393; **BDCERT:** Pul 84; CCM 96; **MS:** Columbia P&S 78; **RES:** Med, Columbia-Presbyterian Med Ctr, New York, NY 79; Med, Columbia-Presbyterian Med Ctr, New York, NY 79-81; **FEL:** Pul, Bellevue Hosp Ctr, New York, NY 81-83; **FAP:** Clin Instr Med Columbia P&S; **HOSP:** Overlook Hosp; **SI:** Pulmonary Disease; Sleep Disorders

🦽 📷 🖼 🏨 💲 Mcr Mod WC **VISA** 💳

RADIATION ONCOLOGY

Cole, Robert (MD)　　RadRO
Morristown Mem Hosp
Radiation Oncology Associates of North Jersey, PA, 100 Madison Ave; Morristown, NJ 07962; (973) 971-5329; **BDCERT:** Rad 83; **MS:** Bowman Gray 79; **RES:** Rad, U of VA Health Sci Ctr, Charlottesville, VA 79-80; RadRO, U of VA Health Sci Ctr, Charlottesville, VA 80-83; **SI:** *Prostate Seed Implantation; Breast Conservation*; **HMO:** Blue Cross & Blue Shield Oxford HIP Network CIGNA First Option +

LANG: Sp, Pol, Chi, Rus, Ger; 🦽 📷 👤 🎚 Mcr Mcd WC Immediately **VISA** ⬤

Oren, Reva (MD)　　RadRO
Morristown Mem Hosp
Radiation Oncology Associates of North Jersey, 100 Madison Ave; Morristown, NJ 07960; (973) 971-5329; **BDCERT:** RadRO 77; **MS:** Italy 70; **RES:** Thomas Jefferson U Hosp, Philadelphia, PA 75-77; Onc, Thomas Jefferson U Hosp, Philadelphia, PA 71-72; **SI:** *Breast Cancer; Gynecological Oncology*; **HMO:** CIGNA Oxford Prudential Guardian +

🦽 📷 👤 🎚 Mcr Mcd A Few Days

Scher, Allan (MD)　　RadRO
Morristown Mem Hosp
Radiation Oncology Associates of North Jersey, 100 Madison Ave; Morristown, NJ 07960; (973) 971-5329; **BDCERT:** Rad 67; **MS:** Albert Einstein Coll Med 62; **RES:** Rad, Kings County Hosp Ctr, Brooklyn, NY 63-66; **SI:** *Head & Neck Cancers; Breast Cancer*; **HMO:** CIGNA Oxford Aetna-US Healthcare United Healthcare Blue Cross +

LANG: Sp, Ger, Pol, Yd; 🦽 📷 👤 🎚 Mcr Mcd WC A Few Days

RADIOLOGY

Palace, Fred (MD)　　Rad
Morristown Mem Hosp
Alliance Imaging, 65 Maple Ave; Morristown, NJ 07960; (973) 267-5700; **BDCERT:** Rad 65; NuM 76; **MS:** Yale U Sch Med 60; **RES:** Rad, Yale-New Haven Hosp, New Haven, CT 61-64; **SI:** *Mammography Ultrasound Open; MRI Cat Scans Fluoroscopy*; **HMO:** CIGNA Prucare Blue Cross & Blue Shield Amerihealth First Option +

🦽 SA/SD 🗝 📷 🎚 Mcr Mcd WC NFI Immediately **VISA**

REPRODUCTIVE ENDOCRINOLOGY

Dlugi, Alexander M (MD)　　RE
Morristown Mem Hosp
Center for Reproductive Endocrinology, Atlantic Health System, 95 Mt Kimble Ave; Morristown, NJ 07962; (973) 971-4600; **BDCERT:** ObG 85; RE 87; **MS:** Univ Penn 77; **RES:** ObG, Johns Hopkins Hosp, Baltimore, MD 78-81; **FEL:** RE, Yale-New Haven Hosp, New Haven, CT 82-83; **HOSP:** Overlook Hosp; **SI:** *Infertility; In Vitro Fertilization*

🦽 📷 👤 🎚 💲

RHEUMATOLOGY

Efros, Barry (MD)　　Rhu
Morristown Mem Hosp
95 Madison Ave Suite A04; Morristown, NJ 07960; (973) 540-8744; **BDCERT:** IM 77; Rhu 80; **MS:** UMDNJ-NJ Med Sch, Newark 74; **RES:** IM, Geo Wash U Med Ctr, Washington, DC 74-77; **FEL:** Rhu, Georgetown U Hosp, Washington, DC 77-79; **SI:** *Fibromyalgia*; **HMO:** Oxford US Hlthcre CIGNA PHS United Healthcare +

🦽 📷 👤 🎚 💲 Mcr 2-4 Weeks

Widman, David (MD)   Rhu
Morristown Mem Hosp

95 Madison Ave; Morristown, NJ 07960; (973) 540-9198; **BDCERT:** Rhu 80; IM 78; **MS:** Harvard Med Sch 75; **RES:** IM, Bellevue Hosp Ctr, New York, NY 75-78; **FEL:** Rhu, Yale-New Haven Hosp, New Haven, CT 78-80

[symbols] 2-4 Weeks

SURGERY

Carter, Mitchel (MD)   S
Morristown Mem Hosp

Associated Surgical Consultants, 261 James St; Morristown, NJ 07960; (973) 267-6400; **BDCERT:** S 94; **MS:** U Hlth Sci/Chicago Med Sch 79; **RES:** S, Albert Einstein Med Ctr, Bronx, NY 79-84; Montefiore Med Ctr, Bronx, NY 79-84; *SI: Laparoscopic Surgery; Breast Surgery*; **HMO:** Prucare Oxford United Healthcare Aetna-US Healthcare CIGNA +

[symbols] Immediately [symbols]
VISA [symbols] [symbols]

Chevinsky, Aaron (MD)   S
Morristown Mem Hosp

Morris County Surgical Associates, 182 South St Ste 3; Morristown, NJ 07960; (973) 539-5115; **BDCERT:** S 97; SCC 92; **MS:** SUNY Stony Brook 83; **RES:** S, Univ Hosp SUNY Stony Brook, Stony Brook, NY 83-88; **FEL:** S Onc, Ohio State U Hosp, Columbus, OH 89-90; **HOSP:** Northwest Covenant Med Ctr; *SI: Colon and Rectal Cancer; Breast Cancer*; **HMO:** Aetna-US Healthcare Oxford Prucare HMO Blue CIGNA/CoMed +

[symbols] Immediately

Diehl, William (MD)   S
Morristown Mem Hosp

Associated Surgical Consultants, 261 James St 2G; Morristown, NJ 07960; (973) 267-6400; **BDCERT:** S 87; **MS:** Mexico 81; **RES:** S, Morristown Mem Hosp, Morristown, NJ 81-86; **FEL:** S Onc, Mem Sloan Kettering Cancer Ctr, New York, NY 86-88; *SI: Breast Cancer; Liver Cancer*; **HMO:** Aetna-US Healthcare Prucare CIGNA Oxford Pinnacle +

LANG: Sp; [symbols] A Few Days
VISA [symbols]

Dougan, Hughes (MD)   S
Columbia-Presbyterian Med Ctr

Associated Surgical Consultants, 261 James St 2G; Morristown, NJ 07960; (973) 267-6400; **BDCERT:** S 81; **MS:** Dominica 72; **RES:** S, Morristown Mem Hosp, Morristown, NJ 75-80; *SI: Laparoscopic Surgery; Breast Cancer*; **HMO:** Prucare HMO Blue Aetna Hlth Plan CIGNA

LANG: Sp; [symbols]

Widmann, Warren (MD)   S
Morristown Mem Hosp

Morris County Surgical Associates, PC, 182 South St 3; Morristown, NJ 07960; (973) 539-5115; **BDCERT:** TS 69; **MS:** Yale U Sch Med 61; **RES:** S, Yale-New Haven Hosp, New Haven, CT 61-67; **FEL:** Cv, Yale-New Haven Hosp, New Haven, CT 62-63; **FAP:** Assoc Clin Prof Columbia P&S; *SI: Lung Cancer Surgery; Breast Cancer*; **HMO:** Aetna Hlth Plan CIGNA Blue Shield Anthem Health Prucare +

[symbols] A Few Days

THORACIC SURGERY

Luka, Norman L (MD)　　TS
Overlook Hosp
Thoracic Cardiovascular & Surgical Group, 220 St
Paul St; Westfield, NJ 07960; (908) 233-5859;
BDCERT: S 78; TS 82; **MS:** U Rochester 69; **RES:** S,
Strong Mem Hosp, Rochester, NY 70-72; TS,
Strong Mem Hosp, Rochester, NY 76-77; **FEL:** S,
Strong Mem Hosp, Rochester, NY 76-77; **HOSP:**
Rahway Hosp; *SI: Heart & Lungs; Circulation*; **HMO:**
HMO Blue US Hlthcre Prucare Oxford First Option
+

LANG: Sp; 🛇 🔂 🚹 🏨 🅂 Mcr Mcd WC NFl
Immediately **VISA** 💳

Parr, Grant (MD)　　TS
Morristown Mem Hosp
MidAtlantic Surgical Associates, 100 Madison Ave;
Morristown, NJ 07962; (973) 971-7300; **BDCERT:**
TS 79; **MS:** Cornell U 69; **RES:** S, U of Alabama
Hosp, Birmingham, AL 71-75; TS, U of Alabama
Hosp, Birmingham, AL 76-77; **FAP:** Asst Prof of
Clin S Columbia P&S; **HOSP:** Overlook Hosp; *SI:*
Minimally Invasive Heart Surgery; Heart Valve Repair;
HMO: Aetna-US Healthcare Empire Blue Shield
Blue Shield Oxford Prudential +

LANG: Sp; 🛇 🔂 🏨 🅂 Mcr Mcd　1 Week

UROLOGY

Atlas, Ian (MD)　　U
Morristown Mem Hosp
Adult & Pediatric Urology Grp, 261 James St 3A;
Morristown, NJ 07960; (973) 539-0333; **BDCERT:**
U 94; **MS:** Mt Sinai Sch Med 84; **RES:** U, Mount
Sinai Med Ctr, New York, NY 84-89; **FEL:** U, Mem
Sloan Kettering Cancer Ctr, New York, NY 89-92;
SI: Prostate Seed Implants; Bladder Cancer; **HMO:**
Blue Cross Oxford Aetna Hlth Plan US Hlthcre
Prucare +

🛇 🅲 🔂 🚹 🏨 🅂 Mcr Mcd WC NFl　1 Week 💳 **VISA**
💳

Schwartz, Malcolm (MD)　　U
Union Hosp-New Jersey
Consultants in Urology, 275 Orchard St; Westfield,
NJ 07090; (908) 654-5100; **BDCERT:** U 80; **MS:**
UMDNJ-NJ Med Sch, Newark 72; **RES:** U, New York
University Med Ctr, New York, NY 74-78; S, Mount
Sinai Med Ctr, New York, NY 72-74; **FAP:** Instr
Columbia P&S; **HOSP:** Overlook Hosp; *SI: Male*
Infertility; Urologic Oncology; **HMO:** Blue Choice
Blue Cross & Blue Shield CIGNA Prucare CIGNA +

LANG: Sp; 🛇 🅲 🔂 🚹 🏨 🅂 Mcr WC NFl
Immediately **VISA** 💳

Taylor, David (MD)　　U
Morristown Mem Hosp
261 James St 3A; Morristown, NJ 07960; (973)
539-0333; **BDCERT:** U 86; **MS:** U Mich Med Sch
79; **RES:** U, Barnes Hosp, St Louis, MO 75; **HMO:**
Aetna Hlth Plan Blue Cross & Blue Shield CIGNA
HIP Network

🛇 🔂 🚹 🏨 🅂 Mcr Mcd　A Few Days 💳 **VISA** 💳
💳

PASSAIC
COUNTY

PASSAIC COUNTY

Specialties in capital letters indicate Primary Care Specialties. However, many doctors will be certified in a subspecialty, but will practice predominantly primary care medicine. In our lists this will be indicated.

*Oncologists deal with Cancer

ALLERGY & IMMUNOLOGY

Klein, Robert (MD)   A&I
Gen Hosp Ctr At Passaic
1005 Clifton Ave; Clifton, NJ 07013; (973) 773-7400; **BDCERT:** Ped 81; **MS:** NY Med Coll 76; **RES:** Ped, Beth Israel Med Ctr, New York, NY 76-79; **FEL:** A&I, Columbia-Presbyterian Med Ctr, New York, NY 82-84; **FAP:** Asst Clin Prof Columbia P&S; **HOSP:** Beth Israel Med Ctr; *SI: Chronic Sinusitis; Bronchial Asthma;* **HMO:** Aetna-US Healthcare Oxford Blue Cross & Blue Shield CIGNA United Healthcare +

LANG: Sp; 🚻 🆘 🅰 👤 🎬 💲 Mcr A Few Days

CARDIOLOGY (CARDIOVASCULAR DISEASE)

Siepser, Stuart (MD)   Cv
Chilton Mem Hosp
Cardiology Assoc of North Jersey, 1777 Hamburg Tpke 302; Wayne, NJ 07470; (973) 831-9222; **BDCERT:** IM 72; Cv 75; **MS:** NYU Sch Med 68; **RES:** IM, New York University Med Ctr, New York, NY 69-70; Cv, New York University Med Ctr, New York, NY 70-72; **FAP:** Asst Clin Prof IM UMDNJ New Jersey Sch Osteo Med; **HOSP:** St Joseph's Hosp-Patterson; *SI: Hypertension—Heart Attack; High Cholesterol;* **HMO:** Oxford First Option CIGNA Aetna Hlth Plan Guardian +

🚻 🅰 👤 🎬 💲 Mcr Mcd WC NFI 1 Week **VISA** 💳

DERMATOLOGY

Maier, Herbert (MD)   D
Wayne Gen Hosp
220 Hamburg Tpke 22; Wayne, NJ 07470; (973) 595-6338; **BDCERT:** D 75; **MS:** Geo Wash U Sch Med 67; **RES:** D, Mount Sinai Med Ctr, New York, NY 75; *SI: Melanoma Evaluation; Atopic Eczema;* **HMO:** HIP Network Oxford First Option GHI QualCare +

🅰 👤 🎬 WC A Few Days

FAMILY PRACTICE

Ventimiglia, Anthony (MD)   FP   **PCP**
Wayne Gen Hosp
1500 Alps Rd Fl 1; Wayne, NJ 07470; (973) 628-8500; **BDCERT:** FP 80; **MS:** Italy 77; **RES:** Community Hosp, Glen Cove, NY 77-80

GASTROENTEROLOGY

Bleicher, Robert (MD)   Ge
Chilton Mem Hosp
330 Ratzer Rd B10; Wayne, NJ 07470; (973) 633-1484; **BDCERT:** IM 81; Ge 83; **MS:** Columbia P&S 78; **RES:** IM, Northwestern Mem Hosp, Chicago, IL 78-81; **FEL:** Ge, Northwestern Mem Hosp, Chicago, IL 81-83; **HOSP:** Wayne Gen Hosp; *SI: Hepatitis*
🚻 🅰 🎬 💲 Mcr Mcd WC Immediately 💳 **VISA** 💳 💳

Farkas, John (MD)   Ge
St Joseph's Hosp-Patterson
716 Broad St Fl 1; Clifton, NJ 07013; (973) 777-5717; **BDCERT:** IM 89; **MS:** West Indies 83; **RES:** IM, St Joseph's Hosp, Paterson, NJ 83-86; **FEL:** Ge, St Joseph's Hosp, Paterson, NJ 86-88; **HOSP:** Wayne Gen Hosp

Youner, Kenneth (MD)   Ge
Chilton Mem Hosp
Gastrointestinal Group, 1777 Hamburg Tpke 101;
Wayne, NJ 07470; (973) 839-7083; **BDCERT:** IM
74; Ge 93; **MS:** Med Coll Va 71; **RES:** Mount Sinai
Med Ctr, New York, NY 72-74; **FEL:** Ge, Mount
Sinai Med Ctr, New York, NY 74-76; **FAP:** Asst Mt
Sinai Sch Med; *SI: Inflammatory Bowel Disease;
Irritable Bowel Syndrome*

🔲 📷 👥 🎬 💲 Mcr Mcd   A Few Days **VISA** 💳

GYNECOLOGIC ONCOLOGY

Pineda, Albert (MD)   GO
St Joseph's Hosp-Patterson
1035 US Highway 46 202; Clifton, NJ 07013;
(973) 471-7272; **BDCERT:** ObG 70; **MS:** NYU Sch
Med 63; **RES:** ObG, Flower Fifth Ave Hosp, New
York, NY 68-69; **FEL:** GO, Metropolitan Hosp Ctr,
New York, NY 68-69; **FAP:** Clin Prof

LANG: Sp, Itl; 🔲 📷 🎬 💲   1 Week

INTERNAL MEDICINE

Brabston, Robert J (MD)   IM   **PCP**
Chilton Mem Hosp
525 Wanaque Ave; Pompton Lakes, NJ 07442;
(973) 839-3333; **BDCERT:** IM 74; Ger 90; **MS:**
UMDNJ-NJ Med Sch, Newark 64; **RES:** Jersey City
Med Ctr, Jersey City, NJ 64-66; Newark City Hosp,
Newark, NJ 66-68

🔲 📷 👥 🎬 💲 NFI   A Few Days **VISA** 💳

Gold, Jeffrey (MD)   IM
St Joseph's Hosp-Patterson
Pulmonary & Critical Care, 871 Allwood Rd;
Clifton, NJ 07014; (201) 471-2123; **BDCERT:** IM
83; **MS:** Mexico 77; **RES:** IM, St Joseph's Hosp-
Patterson, Paterson, NJ 78-81; **FAP:** Asst Clin Prof
UMDNJ New Jersey Sch Osteo Med; **HMO:** Aetna
Hlth Plan Blue Cross & Blue Shield CIGNA

Kreiger, Richard (MD)   IM
Chilton Mem Hosp
2035 Hamburg Tpke Suite F; Wayne, NJ 07470;
(973) 831-9228; **BDCERT:** IM 81; **MS:** UMDNJ-NJ
Med Sch, Newark 78; **RES:** IM, Hosp Med College of
PA, Philadelphia, PA 78-81; **FEL:** Inf, Hosp Med
College of PA, Philadelphia, PA; **HOSP:** Wayne Gen
Hosp

Loughlin, Bruce Timothy (DO) IM
Chilton Mem Hosp
705 Hamburg Tunpike; Wayne, NJ 07470; (201)
904-9898; **BDCERT:** IM 86; **MS:** Philadelphia Coll
Osteo Med 82; **RES:** Saddlebrook Gen Hosp,
Saddlebrook, NJ 82-83; Monmouth Med Ctr, Long
Branch, NJ 83-86

MEDICAL GENETICS

Hutcheon, R Gordon (MD)   MG
St Joseph's Hosp-Patterson
57 Willowbrook Blvd Fl 4; Wayne, NJ 07470;
(973) 754-2727; **BDCERT:** Ped 81; MG 87; **MS:**
Tulane U 77; **RES:** Columbia Presbyterian Med Ctr,
New York, NY 77-80; **FEL:** MG, Albert Einstein Med
Ctr, Bronx, NY 83-85

NEPHROLOGY

Vitting, Kevin (MD)   Nep
St Joseph's Hosp-Patterson
203 Hamburg Tpke; Wayne, NJ 07470; (973) 778-
4422; **BDCERT:** IM 85; Nep 88; **MS:** UMDNJ-RW
Johnson Med Sch 82; **RES:** Lenox Hill Hosp, New
York, NY 82-85; **FEL:** Lenox Hill Hosp, New York,
NY 85-87; **HOSP:** Wayne Gen Hosp

NEUROLOGY

Chodosh, Eliot (MD) N
Wayne Gen Hosp
North Jersey Neurologic Associates, 220 Hamburg
Tpke Ste 16; Wayne, NJ 07470; (201) 942-4778;
BDCERT: N 87; **MS:** Mexico 81; **RES:** N, Boston U
Med Ctr, Boston, MA 83-86; **FEL:** Cerebrovascular
Disease, Boston U Med Ctr, Boston, MA 86-87;
HOSP: Chilton Mem Hosp; **SI:** *Cerebrovascular
Disease*; **HMO:** Aetna Hlth Plan CIGNA Oxford
LANG: Sp, Itl; ♿ 🅰 🔲 💲 Mcr WC NFI   A Few Days
VISA 💳

OBSTETRICS & GYNECOLOGY

Burns, Les Alan (MD) ObG
Chilton Mem Hosp
Physicians For Women, 330 Ratzer Rd 7; Wayne,
NJ 07470; (201) 694-2222; **BDCERT:** ObG 88; **MS:**
Hahnemann U 81; **RES:** St Raphael's Hosp, New
Haven, CT 81-82; Danbury Hosp, Danbury, CT 82-
85

Seigal, Stuart (MD) ObG
Chilton Mem Hosp
1777 Hamburg Tpke; Wayne, NJ 07470; (973)
839-4242; **BDCERT:** ObG 69; **MS:** NY Med Coll 69;
RES: Metropolitan Hosp Ctr, New York, NY 67; **FEL:**
ObG, American Coll, Beirut, Lebanon 72

OPHTHALMOLOGY

Giliberti, Orazio (MD) Oph
Univ of Med & Dent NJ Hosp
415 Totowa Rd; Totowa, NJ 07512; (973) 595-
0011; **BDCERT:** Oph 89; **MS:** Grenada 82; **RES:**
Oph, Univ of Med & Dent NJ Hosp, Newark, NJ 84-
87; **FEL:** S, Hosp of U Penn, Philadelphia, PA 83-84;
FAP: Asst Prof Oph UMDNJ New Jersey Sch Osteo
Med; **SI:** *Laser Corrective Surgery; Laser Glaucoma
Cataract*; **HMO:** Blue Cross & Blue Shield Empire
Blue Cross & Shield Oxford CIGNA Prudential +
LANG: Itl, Prt, Sp; ♿ 🌙 🅰 🔲 💲 Mcr Mod WC
1 Week ▨ **VISA** 💳 💳

ORTHOPAEDIC SURGERY

Drillings, Gary (MD) OrS
Chilton Mem Hosp
1777 Hamburg Tpke; Wayne, NJ 07470; (201)
831-6666; **BDCERT:** OrS 93; **MS:** SUNY Syracuse
85; **RES:** Northwestern Mem Hosp, Chicago, IL 86-
90; **FEL:** SM, Lenox Hill Hosp, New York, NY 90-
91; **SI:** *Knee Injuries; Shoulder Injuries*; **HMO:** Oxford
PHCS CIGNA Blue Cross & Blue Shield Magnacare
+
♿ 🅰🅰 🌙 🅰 ✚ 🔲 💲 Mcr WC NFI   A Few Days **VISA**
💳

Reicher, Oscar (MD) OrS
Chilton Mem Hosp
Orthopaedic Surgery/ Sports Medicine Center,
2035 Hamburg Tpke Ste D; Wayne, NJ 07470;
(973) 616-0200; **BDCERT:** OrS 86; **MS:** Univ
Pittsburgh 79; **RES:** Vanderbilt U Med Ctr,
Nashville, TN 79-84; **HOSP:** Wayne Gen Hosp
♿ 🌙 🅰 ✚ 🔲 💲 Mcr WC NFI   Immediately **VISA** 💳

OTOLARYNGOLOGY

Cece, John (MD)   Oto
Passaic Beth Israel Hosp

Ear Nose Throat Facial Plastic Surgery and Sinus Group PA, 1001 Clifton Ave; Clifton, NJ 07013; (973) 835-8855; **BDCERT:** Oto 86; PlS 92; **MS:** UMDNJ-RW Johnson Med Sch 81; **RES:** Oto, Mount Sinai Med Ctr, New York, NY 81-86; **HOSP:** Clara Maass Med Ctr; *SI: Sinus Surgery; Facial Plastic Surgery;* **HMO:** Blue Cross & Blue Shield Prucare First Option PHCS

LANG: Itl, Sp; 🦽 📞 🅰 🏥 🆂 Mcr WC NFi 4+ Weeks **VISA** 💳

Kardos, Frank L (MD)   Oto
Wayne Gen Hosp

220 Hamburg Tpke; Wayne, NJ 07470; (913) 956-1200; **MS:** Italy 59; **RES:** Oto, Manhattan Eye, Ear & Throat Hosp, New York, NY 60-63; S, VA Med Ctr-East Orange, East Orange, NJ 63-64; **HOSP:** Barnert Hosp; *SI: Ear, Nose, Throat Diseases; Rhinoplasty;* **HMO:** Blue Cross & Blue Shield First Option QualCare Magnacare GHI +

LANG: Itl, Hun, Sp; 🦽 🅰 🦼 🏥 Mcr Mcd WC NFi A Few Days 📋 **VISA** 💳

Mattel, Stephen (MD)   Oto
Beth Israel Med Ctr

Norht Jersey Otolaryngology, PA, 1070 Clifton Ave; Clifton, NJ 07013; (973) 773-9880; **BDCERT:** Oto 81; **MS:** NYU Sch Med 77; **RES:** S, Mount Sinai Med Ctr, New York, NY 77-78; Oto, Bellevue Hosp Ctr, New York, NY 78-81; **FAP:** Clin Instr NYU Sch Med; **HOSP:** Gen Hosp Ctr At Passaic; *SI: Endoscopic Sinus Surgery; Laser Assisted Surgery;* **HMO:** Aetna Hlth Plan Prudential Oxford CIGNA HMO Blue +

🦽 📞 🅰 🦼 🏥 🆂 Mcr WC NFi Immediately **VISA** 💳 📋

Meyer, Robert Peter (MD)   Oto
Wayne Gen Hosp

246 French Hill Road; Wayne, NJ 07470; (201) 694-3599; **BDCERT:** Oto 75; **MS:** Germany 68; **RES:** Oto, Mtsde Hosp, Mountclair, NJ 70-72; Oto, Bellevue Hosp, New York, NY 72-75

Respler, Don (MD)   Oto
Hackensack Univ Med Ctr

Pediatric Otolaryngologic Associates of NJ, 777 Terrace Ave; Hasbrook Heights, NJ 07604; (201) 288-2700; **BDCERT:** Oto 86; **MS:** Mt Sinai Sch Med 81; **RES:** S, Beth Israel Med Ctr, New York, NY 81-83; Oto, Univ of Med & Dent NJ Hosp, Newark, NJ 83-86; **FEL:** Ped Oto, Children's Hosp of Pittsburgh, Pittsburgh, PA 86-87; Ped Oto, Children's Hosp Nat Med Ctr, Washington, DC 87-88; **FAP:** Asst Prof S UMDNJ New Jersey Sch Osteo Med; **HOSP:** Univ of Med & Dent NJ Hosp; *SI: Airways—Sinus, Ear; Tonsil, Head & Neck Tumors;* **HMO:** Oxford HIP Network Mastercare

🦽 📞 🅰 🦼 🏥 🆂 WC NFi 1 Week **VISA** 💳

PEDIATRIC PULMONOLOGY

Kanengiser, Steven (MD)   PPul
St Joseph's Hosp-Patterson

703 Main St; Paterson, NJ 07503; (973) 754-2550; **BDCERT:** Ped 88; **MS:** UC San Francisco 84; **RES:** The Children's Hosp,, Boston, MA 84-87; **FEL:** CCM, West Cnty Med Ctr, Valhalla, NY; NY Hosp-Cornell Med Ctr,, New York, NY; **HOSP:** Valley Hosp

PEDIATRICS

Eisenstein, Elliot (MD)   Ped   PCP
Chilton Mem Hosp

1055 Hamburg Tpke; Wayne, NJ 07470; (201) 696-4145; **BDCERT:** Ped 65; **MS:** Geo Wash U Sch Med 60; **RES:** Fitzsimons Gen Hosp, Denver, CO 60-61; Ped, Letterman Gen Hosp, San Francisco, CA 61-63; **HOSP:** St Joseph's Hosp-Patterson; **HMO:** United Healthcare CIGNA Blue Cross & Blue Shield PHS PHCS +

SA/SU 📞 🅰 🦼 🏥 🆂 Mcd WC NFi A Few Days

Scofield, Lisa (MD) Ped `PCP`
St Joseph's Hosp-Patterson
57 Willowbrook Blvd Fl 4; Wayne, NJ 07470;
(201) 754-4000; **BDCERT:** Ped 94; **MS:** UMDNJ-
RW Johnson Med Sch 90; **RES:** Ped, NY Hosp-
Cornell Med Ctr, New York, NY 90-94; **HMO:**
Prucare Oxford HMO Blue CIGNA US Hlthcre +

♿ 🏧 ➕ 📷 🐴 🛏️ 🆂 A Few Days 💳 *VISA* 💳

PSYCHIATRY

El-Rafei, Nabil (MD) Psyc
Valley Hosp
683 Lafayette Ave; Hawthorne, NJ 07506; (973)
427-1999; **BDCERT:** Psyc 71; ChAP 75; **MS:** Egypt
57; **RES:** CHIP, Montreal Children's Hosp,
Montreal, Canada 68-69; Psyc, Winnipeg Gen
Hosp, Winnipeg, Canada 66-67; **FEL:** ChAP,
Nassau County Med Ctr, East Meadow, NY 69-70;
FAP: Asst Clin Prof UMDNJ-NJ Med Sch, Newark;
HMO: Aetna Hlth Plan CIGNA Metlife

REPRODUCTIVE
ENDOCRINOLOGY

Ransom, Mark (MD) RE
St Joseph's Hosp-Patterson
North Jersey Ctr For Reprdctve, 1035 US Highway
46; Clifton, NJ 07013; (973) 470-0303; **BDCERT:**
RE 94; **MS:** UMDNJ-RW Johnson Med Sch 87;
HMO: Aetna Hlth Plan Blue Cross & Blue Shield
CIGNA

SURGERY

Buckley, Michael Kevin (MD) S
Gen Hosp Ctr At Passaic
Surgery Associates Of N Jersey, 1100 Clifton Ave
100; Clifton, NJ 07013; (201) 778-0100; **BDCERT:**
S 88; CRS 89; **MS:** Ireland 79; **RES:** S, RWJ Univ
Hosp-New Brunswick, New Brunswick, NJ 82-87;
FEL: CRS, Cook Cty Hosp, Chicago, IL 87-88; **HOSP:**
Passaic Beth Israel Hosp; *SI: Anal Diseases; Colon and
Rectal Cancer;* **HMO:** US Hlthcre Oxford Blue Shield
Prudential CIGNA +

♿ 📷 🐴 🛏️ 🆂 Mcr Mcd WC NFI A Few Days

Budd, Daniel (MD) S
Barnert Hosp
Vascular Diagnostic Svc, 525 Wanaque Ave;
Pompton Lakes, NJ 07442; (973) 742-3371;
BDCERT: S 75; **MS:** Duke U 69; **RES:** S, Columbia-
Presbyterian Med Ctr, New York, NY 69-74; **FAP:**
Assoc Prof S UMDNJ New Jersey Sch Osteo Med;
HOSP: Chilton Mem Hosp; *SI: Thyroid Surgery;
Endocrine Surgery;* **HMO:** Aetna-US Healthcare
Prucare Oxford CIGNA Blue Cross +

LANG: Sp, Ger; 📷 🛏️ 🆂 Mcr Mcd WC NFI A Few Days
VISA 💳

Feigenbaum, Howard (MD) S
Chilton Mem Hosp
227 Hamburg Tpke; Pompton Lakes, NJ 07442;
(973) 839-7999; **BDCERT:** S 79; CRS 88; **MS:** NYU
Sch Med 71; **RES:** S, Bellevue Hosp Ctr, New York,
NY 71-72; *SI: Gallbladder Biliary Tract; Colon
Surgery;* **HMO:** Oxford CIGNA US Hlthcre HMO
Blue Magnacare +

📷 🐴 🛏️ Mcr WC NFI A Few Days

Saperstein, Lewis (MD) S
Passaic Beth Israel Hosp
Surgery Associates of North Jersey, PA, 1100
Clifton Ave; Clifton, NJ 07013; (973) 778-0100;
BDCERT: S 96; **MS:** Albert Einstein Coll Med 70;
RES: Beth Israel Med Ctr, New York, NY 70-75;
HOSP: Gen Hosp Ctr At Passaic; **HMO:** Aetna-US
Healthcare Oxford United Healthcare Prucare Blue
Shield +

♿ 📷 🐴 🛏️ 🆂 Mcr Mcd WC NFI A Few Days

Warden, Mary Jane (MD)   S
Chilton Mem Hosp

2035 Hamburg Tpke F; Wayne, NJ 07470; (973) 694-4155; **BDCERT:** S 84; **MS:** UMDNJ-NJ Med Sch, Newark 78; **RES:** S, Univ of Med & Dent NJ Hosp, Newark, NJ; **FEL:** S Onc, Roswell Park Cancer Inst, Buffalo, NY 84-86; **HOSP:** Hackensack Univ Med Ctr; *SI: Breast Disease; Melanoma;* **HMO:** CIGNA Oxford QualCare First Option

♿ ✆ 📷 👤 🏠 Mcr NFl   A Few Days

THORACIC SURGERY

Ciocon, Hermogenes (MD)   TS
Children's Hosp of New Jersey

871 Oldwood Rd 2nd FL; Clifton, NJ 07013; (973) 779-2270; **BDCERT:** TS 74; **MS:** Philippines 61; **RES:** TS, Flower Fifth Ave Hosp, New York, NY 67-69; **HOSP:** St Mary's Hosp; *SI: Cardiovascular Surgery*

LANG: Fil, Sp; ♿ 📷 🏠 Mcr Mcd WC   2-4 Weeks

UROLOGY

Levine, Seth (MD)   U
Chilton Mem Hosp

Associates In Urology, 1777 Hamburg Tpke 301; Wayne, NJ 07470; (973) 616-8400; **BDCERT:** U 80; **MS:** Tufts U 71; **RES:** U, Mount Sinai Med Ctr, New York, NY 75-78; *SI: Impotence; Prostate Cancer;* **HMO:** Aetna Hlth Plan Blue Cross & Blue Shield CIGNA Oxford NYLCare +

📷 👤 🏠 S Mcr WC NFl   1 Week *VISA* 💳 💳

SOMERSET COUNTY

SOMERSET COUNTY

SPECIALTY & SUBSPECIALTY	ABBREVIATION	PAGE(S)
Cardiology (Cardiovascular Disease)	Cv	1011
Colon & Rectal Surgery	CRS	1011
FAMILY PRACTICE	FP	1011
Gastroenterology	Ge	1011
Geriatric Medicine	Ger	1011
Hematology	Hem	1011-1012
Infectious Disease	Inf	1012
INTERNAL MEDICINE	IM	1012
Medical Oncology*	Onc	1012
Neonatal-Perinatal Medicine	NP	1012
OBSTETRICS & GYNECOLOGY	ObG	1012
Ophthalmology	Oph	1013
Orthopaedic Surgery	OrS	1013
Otolaryngology	Oto	1013
Plastic Surgery	PlS	1013
Rheumatology	Rhu	1014
Surgery	S	1014

Specialties in capital letters indicate Primary Care Specialties. However, many doctors will be certified in a subspecialty, but will practice predominantly primary care medicine. In our lists this will be indicated.

*Oncologists deal with Cancer

CARDIOLOGY (CARDIOVASCULAR DISEASE)

Leeds, Richard (MD)   Cv
Somerset Med Ctr
Medicor Cardiology, 225 Jackson St; Bridgewater, NJ 08807; (908) 526-8668; **BDCERT:** IM 84; Cv 87; **MS:** NY Med Coll 81; **RES:** IM, Beth Israel Med Ctr, New York, NY 81-84; IM, Beth Israel Med Ctr, New York, NY 84-85; **FEL:** Cv, St Vincents Hosp & Med Ctr NY, New York, NY 85-87; **HOSP:** RWJ Univ Hosp-New Brnsw; **HMO:** Aetna-US Healthcare CIGNA Blue Cross & Blue Shield Prudential United Healthcare +

LANG: Sp, Chi, Grk, Rom, Hin; ♿ 🌙 📷 ⚕ 🏨 💲 🅜 🅜 1 Week **VISA** 💳

COLON & RECTAL SURGERY

Lott, James V (MD)   CRS
Somerset Med Ctr
Central Jersey Colon & Rectal, 704 US Highway 202 So; Bridgewater, NJ 08807; (908) 526-5600; **BDCERT:** CRS 76; **MS:** France 70; **RES:** S, Univ of Med & Dent NJ Hosp, Newark, NJ 71-75; CRS, Muhlenberg Regional Med Ctr, Plainfield, NJ 75-76; **FAP:** Asst Clin Prof S UMDNJ-NJ Med Sch, Newark; **HMO:** Most

♿ 🆚 🌙 📷 🏨 🅜 1 Week **VISA** 💳

FAMILY PRACTICE

Ziering, Thomas (MD)   FP   **PCP**
Morristown Mem Hosp
39 Olcott Sq; Bernardsville, NJ 07924; (908) 221-1919; **BDCERT:** FP 90; **MS:** UMDNJ-NJ Med Sch, Newark 87; **RES:** Somerset Med Ctr, Somerville, NJ 87-90; **SI:** *HIV Related Illness; Office Dermatology;* **HMO:** NYLCare CoMed US Hlthcre CIGNA

LANG: Sp; ♿ 🌙 📷 ⚕ 🏨 💲 🅜 🆆 A Few Days 💳 **VISA** 💳

GASTROENTEROLOGY

Accurso, Charles (MD)   Ge
Somerset Med Ctr
Digestive Health Care Center, PA, 56 Union Ave; Somerville, NJ 08876; (908) 218-9222; **BDCERT:** IM 87; Ge 89; **MS:** UMDNJ-NJ Med Sch, Newark 84; **RES:** IM, Univ of Med & Dent NJ Hosp, Newark, NJ 85-87; **FEL:** Ge, Univ of Med & Dent NJ Hosp, Newark, NJ 87-89; **FAP:** Asst Clin Prof UMDNJ-NJ Med Sch, Newark; **HOSP:** RWJ Univ Hosp-New Brnsw; **SI:** *Irritable Bowel Syndrome;* **HMO:** Aetna-US Healthcare CIGNA/CoMed Blue Cross & Blue Shield HMO Blue United Healthcare +

LANG: Itl, Kor; ♿ 🌙 📷 ⚕ 🏨 💲 🅜 🅜 🆆 🅽 Immediately **VISA** 💳

GERIATRIC MEDICINE

Ryan, Joseph (MD)   Ger
Morristown Mem Hosp
14 Church St Box 118; Liberty Corner, NJ 07938; (908) 580-0980; **BDCERT:** IM 74; Ge 81; **MS:** SUNY Downstate 70; **RES:** IM, Univ Hosp SUNY Buffalo, Buffalo, NY 70-73; **FEL:** Ge, St Vincents Hosp & Med Ctr NY, New York, NY 73-75; **FAP:** Asst Prof Columbia P&S

♿ 📷 ⚕ 🏨 💲 🅜 2-4 Weeks

HEMATOLOGY

Frimmer, Daniel (MD)   Hem
Muhlenberg Regional Med Ctr
Hematology Oncology Assoc, 7 Cedar Grove Ln 36; Somerset, NJ 08873; (732) 469-6501; **BDCERT:** IM 71; **MS:** SUNY Downstate 65; **RES:** Stanford Med Ctr, Stanford, CA 67-69; Univ Hosp SUNY Bklyn, Brooklyn, NY 66-67; **FEL:** Hem, U UT Hosp, Salt Lake City, UT 72-73; **FAP:** Asst Prof Rutgers U

Toomey, Kathleen (MD)   Hem
RWJ Univ Hosp-New Brnsw

107 Cedar Grove Ln; Somerset, NJ 08873; (732) 356-8300; **BDCERT:** Hem 90; IM 82; **MS:** Italy 79; **RES:** IM, St Peter's Med Ctr, New Brunswick, NJ 79-80; IM, RWJ Univ Hosp-Hamilton, Hamilton, NJ 80-82; **FEL:** Hem Onc, RWJ Univ Hosp-Hamilton, Hamilton, NJ 82-85; **HOSP:** Somerset Med Ctr; **SI:** *Breast Cancer; Hospice Care;* **HMO:** US Hlthcre CIGNA Oxford HMO Blue CoMed +

LANG: Itl, Chi; 🚪 🔒 ⛑ 🏥 $ ⚕ ⚕   Immediately
VISA

INFECTIOUS DISEASE

Herman, David (MD)   Inf
Somerset Med Ctr

Infectious Diseases Assoc NJ, 411 Courtyard Dr; Somerville, NJ 08876; (908) 725-2522; **BDCERT:** IM 88; Inf 90; **MS:** Univ Mo-Columbia Sch Med 85; **RES:** IM, Northwestern Mem Hosp, Chicago, IL 85-88; **FEL:** Inf, U MN Med Ctr, Minneapolis, MN 88

INTERNAL MEDICINE

Lipschutz, Herbert (MD)   IM   **PCP**
Overlook Hosp

31 Mountain Blvd # J; Warren, NJ 07059; (908) 756-8021; **BDCERT:** IM 74; **MS:** NYU Sch Med 63; **RES:** IM, Beth Israel Med Ctr, New York, NY 63-64; IM, Beth Israel Med Ctr, New York, NY 64-65; **FEL:** IM, VA Med Ctr-Manh, New York, NY 65-66; Cv, VA Med Ctr-Manh, New York, NY 66-67; **FAP:** Assoc Clin Prof Med UMDNJ-RW Johnson Med Sch; **HOSP:** Muhlenberg Regional Med Ctr; **SI:** *Coronary Artery Disease; Hypertension;* **HMO:** Aetna-US Healthcare Oxford CIGNA HMO Blue Sanus +

🚪 🏧 🔌 🔒 ⛑ 🏥 $ ⚕   A Few Days

MEDICAL ONCOLOGY

Wu, Hen-vai (MD)   Onc
Somerset Med Ctr

Somerset Hematology Oncology, 107 Cedar Grove Ln 101; Somerset, NJ 08873; (908) 356-8300; **BDCERT:** IM 77; Onc 81; **MS:** Taiwan 72; **RES:** IM, Mount Vernon Hosp, Mt Vernon, NY 72-74; IM, Helene Fuld Med Ctr, Trenton, NJ 74-75; **FEL:** RWJ Univ Hosp-New Brunswick, New Brunswick, NJ; **FAP:** Asst Clin Prof UMDNJ-NJ Med Sch, Newark; **HOSP:** St Peter's Med Ctr; **SI:** *Cancer Diagnosis; Blood Disorders;* **HMO:** US Hlthcre Oxford Blue Cross & Blue Choice Empire First Option +

LANG: Chi; 🚪 🔒 🏥 $ ⚕ ⚕   1 Week **VISA**

NEONATAL-PERINATAL MEDICINE

Chavez, Alberto (MD)   NP
Somerset Med Ctr

PO Box 356, 190 Fairfield Lane; Belle Mead, NJ 08502; (908) 685-2868; **BDCERT:** Ped 85; NP 97; **MS:** Peru 72; **RES:** Ped, U San Marcos, Peru 74-76; Ped, Univ of Med & Dent NJ Hosp, Newark, NJ 80-82; **FEL:** NP, Univ of Med & Dent NJ Hosp, Newark, NJ 82-85; **HMO:** US Hlthcre HIP Network Blue Cross & Blue Choice Heritage

LANG: Sp; 🚪 🔒 ⛑ 🏥 ⚕ ⚕   A Few Days

OBSTETRICS & GYNECOLOGY

Soffer, Jeffrey (MD)   ObG
Overlook Hosp

8 Mountain Blvd; Warren, NJ 07059; (908) 561-8444; **BDCERT:** ObG 83; **MS:** Howard U 75; **RES:** ObG, Hosp of U Penn, Philadelphia, PA 76-78; **HMO:** HMO Blue Blue Choice CIGNA Sanus-NYLCare Metlife +

LANG: Sp; 🚪 🔌 🔒 ⛑ 🏥 $ ⚕   2-4 Weeks ▨
VISA

OPHTHALMOLOGY

Ocken, Paul (MD)   Oph
Muhlenberg Regional Med Ctr
The Eye Center, 65 Mountain Blvd Ext; Warren, NJ 07059; (732) 356-6200; **BDCERT:** Oph 77; **MS:** UMDNJ-NJ Med Sch, Newark 73; **RES:** Eye, Assoc-UMDNJ, Piscataway, NJ 73-76; New York University Med Ctr, New York, NY 61-66; **FAP:** Prof UMDNJ-RW Johnson Med Sch; **SI:** *Glaucoma; Geriatric Ophthalmology*; **HMO:** Aetna-US Healthcare CIGNA First Option PHCS Amerihealth +

🔳 🔳 🔳 🔳 🔳 🔳 🔳 A Few Days **VISA** 🔳

ORTHOPAEDIC SURGERY

D'Agostini, Robert (MD)   OrS
Morristown Mem Hosp
2345 Lamington Rd 110; Bedminster, NJ 07921; (908) 234-2002; **BDCERT:** OrS 98; **MS:** UMDNJ-RW Johnson Med Sch 80; **RES:** OrS, Georgetown U Hosp, Washington, DC 81-85; **SI:** *Joint Surgery*; **HMO:** Oxford Blue Cross & Blue Shield CIGNA US Hlthcre

🔳 🔳 🔳 🔳 🔳 🔳 🔳 🔳 A Few Days **VISA** 🔳

Johnson, Albert (MD)   OrS
Somerset Med Ctr
Somerset Orthopedic Associates, 1081 Route 22 W; Bridgewater, NJ 08807; (908) 722-0822; **BDCERT:** OrS 77; **MS:** India 67; **RES:** S, New England Med Ctr, Boston, MA 71; OrS, New England Med Ctr, Boston, MA 72-75; **FEL:** HS, St Luke's Roosevelt Hosp Ctr, New York, NY; **SI:** *Hand Surgery; Total Hip & Knee Replacement*; **HMO:** CIGNA CoMed Blue Cross & Blue Shield Oxford

🔳 🔳 🔳 🔳 🔳 🔳 🔳 A Few Days 🔳 **VISA** 🔳

Sarokhan, Alan (MD)   OrS
Overlook Hosp
Orthopaedic Assoc also 33 Ovrlook Dr, Summit NJ, 8 Mountain Blvd; Warren, NJ 07059; (908) 757-4444; **BDCERT:** OrS 86; OrS 94; **MS:** Harvard Med Sch 77; **RES:** Peter Bent Brigham Hosp, Boston, MA 77-79; Harvard Comb Ortho Surg, Boston, MA 79-82; **FEL:** HS, Harvard Med Sch, Cambridge, MA 82; St Luke's Roosevelt Hosp Ctr, New York, NY 83; **HOSP:** St Barnabas Med Ctr-Livingston; **SI:** *Joint Replacement; Adult Reconstructive Surgery*

🔳 🔳 🔳 🔳 🔳 🔳 🔳 🔳 Immediately **VISA**

OTOLARYNGOLOGY

Bortniker, David (MD)   Oto
Somerset Med Ctr
242 E Main St; Somerville, NJ 08876; (908) 704-9696; **BDCERT:** Oto 85; **MS:** Albert Einstein Coll Med 80; **RES:** Montefiore Med Ctr, Bronx, NY 80-81; Albert Einstein Med Ctr, Bronx, NY 81-84; **FEL:** Head & Neck S, Beth Israel Med Ctr, New York, NY 94-95; **FAP:** Asst Prof UMDNJ-RW Johnson Med Sch; **HOSP:** Overlook Hosp; **SI:** *Nasal and Sinus Surgery; Facial Cosmetic Surgery*; **HMO:** US Hlthcre Oxford Prucare CIGNA United Healthcare +

🔳 🔳 🔳 🔳 🔳 🔳 🔳 🔳 Immediately **VISA** 🔳

PLASTIC SURGERY

Perry, Arthur (MD)   PlS
RWJ Univ Hosp-New Brnsw
3055 Route 27; Franklin Park, NJ 08823; (732) 422-9600; **BDCERT:** PlS 89; **MS:** Albany Med Coll 81; **RES:** S, Beth Israel Med Ctr, Boston, MA 81-84; PlS, U Chicago Hosp, Chicago, IL 85-87; **FEL:** Burns, New York University Med Ctr, New York, NY 84-85; Cosmetic S, Baker-Gordon Associates, Miami, FL 87; **FAP:** Assoc Clin Prof UMDNJ-RW Johnson Med Sch; **HOSP:** Somerset Med Ctr; **SI:** *Facial Cosmetics; Liposuction*; **HMO:** None

🔳 🔳 🔳 🔳 🔳 🔳 🔳 🔳 2-4 Weeks **VISA** 🔳

RHEUMATOLOGY

Brodman, Richard Rory (MD)Rhu
Muhlenberg Regional Med Ctr
345 Somerset St; North Plainfield, NJ 07060; (908) 561-7440; **BDCERT:** IM 76; Rhu 82; **MS:** SUNY Downstate 73; **RES:** IM, Rhode Island Hosp, Providence, RI 74-76; **FEL:** Rhu, Robert Brigham Hosp, Providence, RI 76-78; **FAP:** Assoc Clin Prof Med UMDNJ-RW Johnson Med Sch; **SI:** *Lupus; Rheumatoid Arthritis;* **HMO:** PHS PHCS Oxford First Option United Healthcare +

 🔲 📷 👥 🏠 **VISA** 💳

McWhorter, John (MD)   **Rhu**
Somerset Med Ctr
201 Union Ave 2D; Bridgewater, NJ 08807; (908) 722-5380; **BDCERT:** IM 73; **MS:** UMDNJ-NJ Med Sch, Newark 68; **RES:** IM, Thomas Jefferson U Hosp, Philadelphia, PA 68-71; IM, Harlem Hosp Ctr, New York, NY 71-72; **FEL:** Rhu, Columbia-Presbyterian Med Ctr, New York, NY 73-75; **FAP:** Asst UMDNJ-NJ Med Sch, Newark; **SI:** *Arthritis; Osteoporosis;* **HMO:** Aetna Hlth Plan CIGNA First Option Oxford Blue Cross & Blue Shield +

 🔲 📷 👥 🏠 💲 Mcr Mcd WC   1 Week

SURGERY

Drascher, Gary (MD)   **S**
Somerset Med Ctr
Surgical AssociatesCentral NJ, 515 Church St 1; Bound Brook, NJ 08805; (732) 356-0770; **BDCERT:** S 88; **MS:** Mt Sinai Sch Med 81; **RES:** S, St Luke's Roosevelt Hosp Ctr, New York, NY 82-87; **FEL:** GVS, Englewood Hosp, Englewood, NJ 87-89; **FAP:** Clin Instr S UMDNJ-RW Johnson Med Sch; **HOSP:** RWJ Univ Hosp-New Brnsw; **SI:** *Vascular Surgery; Laparoscopic Surgery;* **HMO:** Blue Cross & Blue Shield Aetna-US Healthcare Oxford CIGNA PHCS +

 🔲 📷 👥 🏠 💲 Mcr WC NFI   A Few Days **VISA** 💳

Goldson, Howard (MD)   **S**
Somerset Med Ctr
Surgical AssociatesCentral NJ, 515 Church St; Boundbrook, NJ 08807; (732) 356-0770; **BDCERT:** S 78; **MS:** SUNY Downstate 71; **RES:** S, U MN-Duluth Sch Med, Duluth, MN 72-74; S, Univ Hosp SUNY Bklyn, Brooklyn, NY 74-77; **HOSP:** RWJ Univ Hosp-New Brnsw; **SI:** *Laparoscopic Surgery; Vascular Surgery;* **HMO:** CIGNA Prucare NYLCare US Hlthcre Oxford +

 🔲 🔳 📷 🏠 💲 Mcr   A Few Days

Iacuzzo, John (MD)   **S**
Somerset Med Ctr
Raritan Valley Surgical Assoc, 201 Union Ave E; Bridgewater, NJ 08807; (908) 722-0030; **BDCERT:** S 77; Rad 87; **MS:** Jefferson Med Coll 71; **RES:** S, Columbia-Presbyterian Med Ctr, New York, NY 71-76; **HOSP:** St Peter's Med Ctr; **SI:** *Breast Surgery; Endoscopic Hernia Surgery;* **HMO:** US Hlthcre CIGNA Prucare Blue Cross & Blue Shield NYLCare +

LANG: Itl, Sp; 🔲 📷 🏠 💲 Mcr WC NFI   Immediately **VISA** 💳

UNION
COUNTY

SPECIALTY & SUBSPECIALTY	ABBREVIATION	PAGE(S)
Allergy & Immunology	A&I	1017
Anesthesiology	Anes	1017
Cardiology (Cardiovascular Disease)	Cv	1018
Child & Adolescent Psychiatry	ChAP	1018
Colon & Rectal Surgery	CRS	1019
Dermatology	D	1019
Diagnostic Radiology	DR	1019
Endocrinology, Diabetes & Metabolism	EDM	1020
FAMILY PRACTICE	FP	1020
Gastroenterology	Ge	1020-1021
Geriatric Medicine	Ger	1021
Hematology	Hem	1021-1022
Infectious Disease	Inf	1022
INTERNAL MEDICINE	IM	1022-1023
Medical Oncology*	Onc	1023-1024
Nephrology	Nep	1024
Neurological Surgery	NS	1024
Neurology	N	1024
OBSTETRICS & GYNECOLOGY	ObG	1024
Ophthalmology	Oph	1025
Orthopaedic Surgery	OrS	1025-1026
Otolaryngology	Oto	1026
Pain Management	PM	1026
Pediatric Cardiology	PCd	1027
Pediatric Pulmonology	PPul	1027
PEDIATRICS (GENERAL)	Ped	1027-1028
Physical Medicine & Rehabilitation	PMR	1028
Plastic Surgery	PlS	1028
Psychiatry	Psyc	1028-1029
Pulmonary Disease	Pul	1029
Radiation Oncology*	RadRO	1029
Rheumatology	Rhu	1029
Sports Medicine	SM	1029
Surgery	S	1030
Thoracic Surgery (includes open heart surgery)	TS	1030-1031
Urology	U	1031
Vascular Surgery (General)	GVS	1031

Specialties in capital letters indicate Primary Care Specialties. However, many doctors will be certified in a subspecialty, but will practice predominantly primary care medicine. In our lists this will be indicated.

*Oncologists deal with Cancer

ALLERGY & IMMUNOLOGY

Brown, David (MD) A&I
Overlook Hosp
Allergy , Asthma & Sinus Center of New Jersey, 33 Overlook Rd suite 307; Summit, NJ 07901; (908) 522-9696; **BDCERT:** A&I 87; IM 84; **MS:** MC Ohio, Toledo 81; **RES:** IM, Overlook Hosp, Summit, NJ 81-84; **FEL:** A&I, St Luke's Roosevelt Hosp Ctr, New York, NY 84-86; **HMO:** Blue Choice Blue Cross & Blue Shield CIGNA

♿ 🏠 📞 🏧 💲 Mcr A Few Days *VISA* 💳

Bukosky, Richard (MD) A&I
St Elizabeth Hosp
Allergy & Immunology, 926 N Wood Ave; Linden, NJ 07036; (908) 925-3318; **BDCERT:** A&I 77; **MS:** Med Coll Wisc 60; **RES:** IM, VA Hosp, Wood, WI 63-66; **FEL:** A&I, Milwaukee Cty Gen Hosp, Milwaukee, WI 66-68; **FAP:** Asst Clin Prof Med UMDNJ New Jersey Sch Osteo Med; **HOSP:** Union Hosp-New Jersey; **HMO:** Blue Choice Blue Cross & Blue Shield CIGNA Prudential

LANG: Pol, Sp; 📞 🔒 🅿 🏧 💲 Mcr Mcd WC NFl
1 Week

Goodman, Alan (MD) A&I
St Barnabas Med Ctr-Livingston
Allergy Asthma & Immunology, 381 Chestnut St; Union, NJ 07083; (908) 688-6200; **BDCERT:** IM 85; A&I 89; **MS:** SUNY Syracuse 82; **RES:** IM, Univ Hosp SUNY Syracuse, Syracuse, NY 82-83; IM, Washington Hosp Ctr, Washington, DC 83-85; **FEL:** A&I, St Luke's Roosevelt Hosp Ctr, New York, NY 86-88; **HOSP:** Union Hosp-New Jersey; *SI: Allergic Rhinitis; Sinus Problems;* **HMO:** Prudential Blue Cross & Blue Shield Oxford PHCS Guardian +

♿ 🏧 📞 🔒 🅿 🏧 💲 Immediately

Le Benger, Kerry (MD) A&I
Overlook Hosp
120 Summit Ave; Summit, NJ 07901; (908) 273-4300; **BDCERT:** A&I 85; IM 83; **MS:** NY Med Coll 80; **RES:** IM, Lenox Hill Hosp, New York, NY 80-83; **FEL:** A&I, NY Hosp-Cornell Med Ctr, New York, NY 83-85; **FAP:** Clin Instr Columbia P&S; **HOSP:** St Barnabas Med Ctr-Livingston; *SI: Asthma; Allergic Rhinitis;* **HMO:** Oxford Blue Cross Prucare CIGNA Guardian +

♿ 🏧 🔒 🅿 🏧 💲 Mcr A Few Days 🔶 *VISA* 💳

Maccia, Clement (MD) A&I
Muhlenberg Regional Med Ctr
Asthma Allergy Care, 19 Holly St; Cranford, NJ 07016; (908) 276-0666; **BDCERT:** A&I 85; **MS:** Italy 71; **RES:** Muhlenberg Regional Med Ctr, Plainfield, NJ 73-74; **FEL:** U Hosp, Cincinnati, OH 74-76; **FAP:** Clin Prof A&I UMDNJ-RW Johnson Med Sch; *SI: Allergic Rhinitis; Asthma;* **HMO:** CIGNA Blue Cross & Blue Shield US Hlthcre Oxford NYLCare +

LANG: Itl; ♿ 🏧 📞 🔒 🏧 💲 Mcd WC NFl A Few Days

Mendelson, Joel (MD) A&I
Newark Beth Israel Med Ctr
346 South Ave; Fanwood, NJ 07023; (908) 889-7454; **BDCERT:** A&I 89; **MS:** Dominican Republic 82; **RES:** St Lukes Rsvlt Ctr, New York, NY 82-85; **FEL:** UMDNJ-NJ Med Sch, 85-87; **HOSP:** Overlook Hosp; **HMO:** Oxford CIGNA Aetna Hlth Plan

ANESTHESIOLOGY

Novik, Edward (MD) Anes
Union Hosp-New Jersey
Union Anesthesia Associates, PA, 1000 Galloping Hill Rd; Union, NJ 07083; (908) 851-7161; **BDCERT:** PM 97; **MS:** Russia 88; **RES:** IM, St John's Epis Hosp-S Shore, Far Rockaway, NY 92-93; PM, Univ Hosp SUNY Bklyn, Brooklyn, NY 93-96; **FEL:** PM, Univ Hosp SUNY Bklyn, Brooklyn, NY 96-97

♿ 📞 🔒 🏧 💲 Mcr Mcd WC NFl A Few Days *VISA* 💳

Guide to symbols and abbreviations can be found on pages 110-113.

1017

CARDIOLOGY (CARDIOVASCULAR DISEASE)

Brodyn, Nicholas (DO)   Cv
Union Hosp-New Jersey
Suburban Heart Group, PA, 2333 Morris Ave D1;
Union, NJ 07083; (908) 964-7333; **BDCERT:** IM
87; Cv 91; **MS:** Univ Osteo Med & Hlth Sci 83; **RES:**
IM, St Michael's Med Ctr, Newark, NJ 83-87; **FEL:**
Cv, St Michael's Med Ctr, Newark, NJ 87-89; **FAP:**
Assoc Clin Prof Med Seton Hall Coll of Med; **HOSP:**
St Michael's Med Ctr; **SI:** *Transesophageal
Echocardiography*; **HMO:** CIGNA US Hlthcre Oxford
First Option

🅲 🅖 🅗 🏥 Mcr WC   A Few Days **VISA**

Inglesby, Thomas V (MD)   Cv
Overlook Hosp
Summit Medical Group, 120 Summit Ave; Summit,
NJ 07901; (908) 273-4300; **BDCERT:** IM 73; Cv
75; **MS:** U Md Sch Med 63; **RES:** IM, St Vincents
Hosp & Med Ctr NY, New York, NY 66-68; **FEL:** Cv,
Emory U Hosp, Atlanta, GA 68-71; **HMO:** Aetna
Hlth Plan Blue Cross & Blue Shield CIGNA

Kalischer, Alan (MD)   Cv
Muhlenberg Regional Med Ctr
2253 South Ave; Westfield, NJ 07090; (908) 654-
3080; **BDCERT:** IM 82; Cv 85; **MS:** NY Med Coll 77;
RES: IM, Kings County Hosp Ctr, Brooklyn, NY 78-
80; **FEL:** Cv, Columbia-Presbyterian Med Ctr, New
York, NY 80-84; **FAP:** Asst Prof of Clin Med
UMDNJ-RW Johnson Med Sch; **SI:** *General
Cardiology*; **HMO:** 1199 Aetna Hlth Plan Aetna-US
Healthcare Allied Health 21st Century +

LANG: Heb, Yd; 🅖 🅖 🅗 🏥 Mcr Mcd WC NFI
Immediately

Sachs, R Gregory (MD)   Cv
Overlook Hosp
Summit Medical Group, 120 Summit Ave; Summit,
NJ 07901; (908) 273-4300; **BDCERT:** IM 72; Cv
76; **MS:** Georgetown U 66; **RES:** IM, Georgetown U
Hosp, Washington, DC 67-68; Cv,; **HOSP:**
Morristown Mem Hosp; **SI:** *Internal Medicine*; **HMO:**
Aetna Hlth Plan Oxford Blue Choice Blue Cross
1199 +

LANG: Sp; 🅖 🏥 Mcr Mcd WC NFI   4+ Weeks ▓ **VISA**
💳 💳

Slama, Robert (MD)   Cv
Overlook Hosp
Summit Medical GroupCardiology, 120 Summit
Ave; Summit, NJ 07901; (908) 273-4300;
BDCERT: IM 74; Cv 77; **MS:** Temple U 71; **RES:**
Boston Med Ctr, Boston, MA; IM, Georgetown
University Hosp, Washington, DC; **FEL:** Cv, Boston
U Med Ctr, Boston, MA

Stein, Elliott (MD)   Cv
Union Hosp-New Jersey
Mid Atlantic Cardiology, 211 Mountain Ave;
Springfield, NJ 07081; (973) 467-0005; **BDCERT:**
IM 74; Cv 74; **MS:** Jefferson Med Coll 64; **RES:** IM,
Mount Sinai Med Ctr, New York, NY 68-69; Cv,
Mount Sinai Med Ctr, New York, NY 69-71; **FEL:**
Stockholm, Sweden; **HOSP:** Overlook Hosp

LANG: Rus, Sp; 🅖 🅖 🅗 🏥 🆂 Mcr Mcd WC   2-
4 Weeks **VISA** 💳

CHILD & ADOLESCENT PSYCHIATRY

Greenberg, Rosalie (MD)   ChAP
Columbia-Presbyterian Med Ctr
Medical Arts Phsychotherapy, 33 Overlook Rd Ste
406; Summit, NJ 07901; (908) 598-0200;
BDCERT: Psyc 82; ChAP 83; **MS:** Columbia P&S
76; **RES:** Psyc, Columbia-Presbyterian Med Ctr,
New York, NY 77-80; **FEL:** ChAP, Columbia-
Presbyterian Med Ctr, New York, NY 79-81; **FAP:**
Clin Instr Psyc Columbia P&S; **HOSP:** Overlook
Hosp; **HMO:** None

🅖 🅲 🅖 🅗 🏥 🆂   2-4 Weeks

COLON & RECTAL SURGERY

Eisenstat, Theodore (MD)   CRS
Muhlenberg Regional Med Ctr
1010 Park Ave; Plainfield, NJ 07060; (908) 756-6640; **BDCERT:** S 74; CRS 80; **MS:** NY Med Coll 68; **RES:** Thomas Jefferson U Hosp, Philadelphia, PA 69-71; Pennsylvania Hosp, Philadelphia, PA 71-73; **FEL:** CRS, RWJ Univ Hosp-New Brunswick, New Brunswick, NJ 78-79; **FAP:** Clin Prof UMDNJ-RW Johnson Med Sch; **HOSP:** JFK Med Ctr; **SI:** *Colon Cancer; Inflammatory Bowel Disease;* **HMO:** CIGNA Magnacare Metlife

🚶 💳 🔧 🏧 Mcr Mcd   Immediately *VISA* 💳

Groff, Walter (MD)   CRS
Overlook Hosp
37 Overlook Rd Ste 412; Summit, NJ 07901; (908) 578-0220; **BDCERT:** CRS 80; S 80; **MS:** Albany Med Coll 70; **RES:** S, St Vincents Hosp & Med Ctr NY, New York, NY 70-72; **FEL:** CRS, Muhlenberg Regional Med Ctr, Plainfield, NJ 79-80; **FAP:** Assoc Clinical Columbia P&S; **SI:** *Rectal Cancer; Colonoscopy;* **HMO:** HMO Blue US Hlthcre Prucare CIGNA Magnacare +

🚶 💳 📷 🔧 🏧 💲 Mcr Mcd   Immediately

Oliver, Gregory (MD)   CRS
JFK Med Ctr
Assoc Colon & Rectal Surgeons, 1010 Park Ave; Plainfield, NJ 07060; (908) 756-6640; **BDCERT:** CRS 86; **MS:** Geo Wash U Sch Med 76; **RES:** S, Geo Wash U Med Ctr, Washington, DC 76-83; S, UMDNJ-RW Johnson, Plainfield, NJ 84-85; **FAP:** Assoc Clin Prof UMDNJ-RW Johnson Med Sch; **HOSP:** Muhlenberg Regional Med Ctr; **SI:** *Anal Incontinence; Inflammatory Bowel Disease;* **HMO:** Oxford Prucare CIGNA HMO Blue

LANG: Sp; 🚶 📷 🔧 🏧 Mcr Mcd   Immediately *VISA* 💳

Rubin, Robert (MD)   CRS
JFK Med Ctr
Associated Colon & Rectal Surgeons,PA, 1010 Park Ave; Plainfield, NJ 07060; (908) 756-6640; **BDCERT:** CRS 73; S 62; **MS:** Jefferson Med Coll 53; **RES:** S, Mount Sinai Med Ctr, New York, NY 54-55; S, Philadelphia Gen Hosp, Philadelphia, PA 57-59; **FAP:** Clin Prof UMDNJ-RW Johnson Med Sch; **HOSP:** Muhlenberg Regional Med Ctr; **SI:** *Rectal Cancer;* **HMO:** First Option Blue Cross & Blue Shield Oxford CIGNA Prucare +

🚶 📷 🔧 🏧 Mcr Mcd NFI   Immediately *VISA* 💳

DERMATOLOGY

Gruber, Gabriel (MD)   D
Overlook Hosp
Summit Medical Group,PA, 120 Summit Ave; Summit, NJ 07901; (908) 273-4300; **BDCERT:** D 77; IM 77; **MS:** Harvard Med Sch 72; **RES:** IM, Boston Med Ctr, Boston, MA 72-74; D, Mass Gen Hosp, Boston, MA 74-77; **HOSP:** St Barnabas Med Ctr-Livingston; **SI:** *Psoriasis; Phototherapy;* **HMO:** US Hlthcre Oxford Aetna Hlth Plan CIGNA Metlife +

🚶 🅂🄳 💳 📷 🔧 🏧 💲 Mcr   2-4 Weeks 💳 *VISA* 💳

DIAGNOSTIC RADIOLOGY

Perl, Louis (MD)   DR
Overlook Hosp
Summit Radiological Associates PA, 151 Summit Ave; Summit, NJ 07901; (908) 277-3314; **BDCERT:** DR 76; **MS:** Tufts U 72; **RES:** DR, Columbia-Presbyterian Med Ctr, New York, NY 73-76; **HMO:** Oxford NYLCare CIGNA

🚶 🅂🄳 💳 🏧 💲 Mcr Mcd WC NFI   Immediately *VISA* 💳

Guide to symbols and abbreviations can be found on pages 110-113.

1019

ENDOCRINOLOGY, DIABETES & METABOLISM

Chen, James (MD) EDM
Muhlenberg Regional Med Ctr
Park Assoc Thyroid Center, 445 Chestnut St A;
Union, NJ 07083; (908) 668-2787; **BDCERT:** NuM
87; EDM 85; **MS:** Taiwan 80; **RES:** IM, Muhlenberg
Regional Med Ctr, Plainfield, NJ 80-83; **FEL:** EDM,
Johns Hopkins Hosp, Baltimore, MD 83-85; NuM,
Johns Hopkins Hosp, Baltimore, MD 86-88; **FAP:**
Asst Clin Prof Med UMDNJ-RW Johnson Med Sch;
HOSP: Union Hosp-New Jersey; *SI: Thyroid Nodule;
Hypothyroid & Hyperthyroid;* **HMO:** CIGNA Prucare
Oxford First Option US Hlthcre +

LANG: Chi; ⬙ 🆂🅾 🄶 🎬 🆂 ﾒ⊂ 2-4 Weeks

Silverman, Mitchell (MD) EDM
Newark Beth Israel Med Ctr
FACE, 2333 Morris Ave Ste B9; Union, NJ 07082;
(908) 964-5511; **BDCERT:** IM 83; EDM 88; **MS:**
Duke U 80; **RES:** IM, Emory U Hosp, Atlanta, GA
80-83; **FEL:** EDM, NY Hosp-Cornell Med Ctr, New
York, NY 84-88; **HOSP:** St Barnabas Med Ctr-
Livingston; *SI: Diabetes; Thyroid Diseases;* **HMO:** First
Option Magnacare Multiplan QualCare

⬙ ⓒ 🄶 🎬 🆂 ﾒ⊂ 🆆🅲 🅽🅵🅸 1 Week **VISA** 💳

FAMILY PRACTICE

Eisenstat, Steven (DO) FP 🄿🄲🄿
Union Hosp-New Jersey
440 Chestnut St; Union, NJ 07083; (908) 688-
4845; **MS:** Switzerland 84; **HOSP:** Overlook Hosp

Kaye, Susan (MD) FP 🄿🄲🄿
Overlook Hosp
Overlook Hosp-Dept Med Ed, PO Box 220, 99
Beauvoir at Sylvad Rd; Summit, NJ 07902;
BDCERT: FP 82; FP 94; **MS:** NY Med Coll 79; **RES:**
Overlook Hosp, Summit, NJ 79-82; **FEL:** FP, Fac
Develop Ctr, Waco, TX 82-83; **FAP:** Assoc Clin Prof
Med Columbia P&S

Tabachnick, John F (MD) FP 🄿🄲🄿
Overlook Hosp
563 Westfield Ave; Westfield, NJ 07090; (908)
232-5858; **BDCERT:** FP 82; **MS:** Mt Sinai Sch Med
79; **RES:** FP, Overlook Hosp, Summit, NJ 79-82;
FAP: Asst Clin Prof UMDNJ New Jersey Sch Osteo
Med; **HOSP:** St Barnabas Med Ctr-Livingston; **HMO:**
CIGNA CoMed US Hlthcre HMO Blue United
Healthcare +

⬙ 🆂🅾 ⓒ 🄶 🆂 ﾒ⊂ ﾒ⊂⊂ 2-4 Weeks

GASTROENTEROLOGY

Belladonna, Joseph (MD) Ge
Overlook Hosp
Summit Medical Group, 120 Summit Ave; Summit,
NJ 07901; (908) 273-4300; **BDCERT:** IM 73; Ge
75; **MS:** Cornell U 69; **RES:** IM, NY Hosp-Cornell
Med Ctr, New York, NY 69-71; **FEL:** Ge, Mem Sloan
Kettering Cancer Ctr, New York, NY 73-75; **FAP:**
Asst Clin Prof Columbia P&S; *SI: Gastroesophageal
Reflux; Colitis;* **HMO:** Aetna Hlth Plan CIGNA Blue
Cross & Blue Shield Prucare Oxford +

⬙ 🎬 🆂 ﾒ⊂ 🅰🅼🅴🆇 **VISA** 💳

Goldenberg, David (MD) Ge
Muhlenberg Regional Med Ctr
1165 Park Ave; Plainfield, NJ 07060; (908) 754-
2992; **BDCERT:** IM 77; Ge 81; **MS:** NY Med Coll 74;
RES: IM, Metropolitan Hosp Ctr, New York, NY 74-
77; **FEL:** Ge, Emory U Hosp, Atlanta, GA 80; **FAP:**
Asst Clin Prof UMDNJ New Jersey Sch Osteo Med;
SI: Inflammatory Bowel Disease; Biliary Disorders;
HMO: Blue Cross & Blue Shield Aetna-US
Healthcare PHCS CIGNA +

LANG: Sp, Ger; ⓒ 🄶 🎬 🎬 🆂 ﾒ⊂ A Few Days

Kerner, Michael (MD)   Ge
Overlook Hosp

25 Morris Ave; Springfield, NJ 07081; (973) 467-1313; **BDCERT:** IM 75; **MS:** Bowman Gray 71; **RES:** New York University Med Ctr, New York, NY; **FEL:** VA Med Ctr-Manh, New York, NY; **FAP:** Asst Clin Prof Med Columbia P&S; **HOSP:** St Barnabas Med Ctr-Livingston; **SI:** *Colonoscopy*; **HMO:** CIGNA Prucare Aetna Hlth Plan HMO Blue United Healthcare +

LANG: Sp, Heb; 🚫 🌙 🔲 👤 🔟 $ Mcr Mcd
Immediately *VISA* 💳

Levinson, Joel (MD)   Ge
Overlook Hosp

25 Morris Ave; Springfield, NJ 07081; (973) 467-1313; **BDCERT:** IM 70; Ge 72; **MS:** Georgetown U 63; **RES:** Georgetown U Hosp, Washington, DC 63-65; Vanderbilt U Med Ctr, Nashville, TN 67-68; **FEL:** Ge, U Chicago Hosp, Chicago, IL 68-70; **FAP:** Asst Clin Prof Columbia P&S; **HOSP:** St Barnabas Hosp-Bronx; **SI:** *Gastrointestinal Disorders; Liver Disease*; **HMO:** CIGNA Oxford Blue Cross & Blue Shield United Healthcare Aetna-US Healthcare +

LANG: Sp; 🚫 🌙 🔲 👤 🔟 $ Mcr Mcd   Immediately
VISA 💳

Mahal, Pradeep (MD)   Ge
Union Hosp-New Jersey

Millennium Medical Group PC, 1308 Morris Ave 2; Union, NJ 07083; (908) 851-6767; **BDCERT:** Ge 81; Onc 83; **MS:** India 74; **RES:** Univ of Med & Dent NJ Hosp, Newark, NJ 75-78; **FEL:** Onc, MD Anderson Cancer Ctr, Houston, TX 78-80; Ge, MD Anderson Cancer Ctr, Houston, TX 78-80; **HOSP:** St Elizabeth Hosp; **SI:** *Gastrointestinal Cancer*; **HMO:** Prucare US Hlthcre Oxford CIGNA First Option +

LANG: Sp, Hin, Pun; 🚫 🌙 🔲 👤 🔟 $ Mcr WC NFI
A Few Days

Tempera, Patrick (MD)   Ge
Union Hosp-New Jersey

Mellennium Gastroenterology Associates, 1308 Morris Ave 2; Union, NJ 07083; (908) 851-7799; **BDCERT:** IM 90; Ge 93; **MS:** Grenada 86; **RES:** IM, St Michaels Med Ctr, Newark, NJ; IM, Seton Hall Med Sch, Newark, NY; **FEL:** Ge, Seton Hall Coll Med, Newark, NJ

LANG: Sp, Prt; 🚫 🌙 👤 🔟 $ Mcr WC   Immediately

GERIATRIC MEDICINE

Solomon, Robert (MD)   Ger   **PCP**
Overlook Hosp

744 Galloping Hill Rd; Roselle Park, NJ 07204; (908) 241-0044; **BDCERT:** IM 80; Ger 80; **MS:** SUNY Hlth Sci Ctr 77; **RES:** Westchester County Med Ctr, Valhalla, NY 77-80; **FEL:** Ger, NY Hosp-Cornell Med Ctr, New York, NY 80-81; **HOSP:** Union Hosp-New Jersey; **SI:** *Alzheimer's Disease*; **HMO:** Aetna Hlth Plan Oxford HMO Blue First Option CIGNA +

🚫 🌙 🔲 👤 🔟 $ Mcr   1 Week

HEMATOLOGY

Arkel, Yale S (DO)   Hem
Overlook Hosp

Overlook Blood Disorder Center, 99 Beauvoir Ave; Summit, NJ 07901; (908) 522-4989; **BDCERT:** IM 69; Hem 72; **MS:** Chicago Coll Osteo Med 61; **RES:** Med, Montefiore Med Ctr, Bronx, NY 65; Med, VA Med Ctr-Manh, New York, NY 63; **FEL:** Montefiore Med Ctr, Bronx, NY 66; **SI:** *Hemostasis; Thrombosis*

🚫 🔲 👤 🔟 Mcr   2-4 Weeks

Rifkin, Paul (MD)   Hem
St Elizabeth Hosp

230 W Jersey St 301; Elizabeth, NJ 07202; (908) 355-5300; **BDCERT:** IM 72; **MS:** Georgetown U 67; **RES:** U of Pittsburgh Med Ctr, Pittsburgh, PA 68-70; **FEL:** Hem, New York University Med Ctr, New York, NY 70-72; **SI:** *Medical Oncology; Blood Diseases*; **HMO:** Blue Shield First Option CIGNA PHS

🚫 🔲 👤 🔟 Mcr   Immediately

Wax, Michael (MD)   Hem
Overlook Hosp

Summit Medical Group, 120 Summit Ave; Summit, NJ 07901; (908) 273-4300; **BDCERT:** IM 80; Onc 83; **MS:** Med Coll PA 77; **RES:** IM, Hosp Med College of PA, Philadelphia, PA 78-80; Hahnemann U Hosp, Philadelphia, PA 77-78; **FEL:** Onc, U WA Med Ctr, Seattle, WA 80; **FAP:** Instr Columbia P&S; **HOSP:** St Barnabas Med Ctr-Livingston; **HMO:** Blue Cross CIGNA Aetna Hlth Plan Oxford Prucare +

♿ 🆒 📷 🎦 🏧 Mcr Mod WC 2-4 Weeks ▦ **VISA** 💳 💳

INFECTIOUS DISEASE

Roland, Robert (DO)   Inf   PCP
Elizabeth Gen Med Ctr

Infectious Disease Specialists/Millennium Medical Group, 1308 Morris Ave 204; Union, NJ 07083; (908) 810-9200; **BDCERT:** IM 90; Inf 92; **MS:** Kirksville Coll Osteo Med 85; **RES:** IM, Union Hosp, Union, NJ 85-86; **FEL:** Inf, Kennedy Mem Hosp, Stratford, NJ 89-91; **FAP:** Asst Clin Prof Med NY Coll Osteo Med; **HOSP:** Union Hosp-New Jersey; *SI: HIV/AIDS; Travel Medicine;* **HMO:** First Option Blue Cross & Blue Shield Chubb CIGNA

LANG: Sp; ♿ 🌙 🎦 🏧 S Mcr Mod Immediately **VISA** 💳

INTERNAL MEDICINE

Bell, Kevin (MD)   IM   PCP
St Barnabas Med Ctr-Livingston

Warren Watchung Internal Medicine, 8 Mountain Blvd; Warren, NJ 07059; (908) 561-8600; **BDCERT:** IM 78; **MS:** Columbia P&S 75; **RES:** U WI Sch Med, Milwaukee, WI 75-79; **HOSP:** Overlook Hosp; **HMO:** Metlife Oxford

♿ 🆒 🌙 📷 S Mcr Immediately **VISA** 💳

Burstin, Stuart J (MD & PhD) IM
Overlook Hosp

Summit Medical Group, 120 Summit Ave; Summit, NJ 07901; (908) 273-4300; **BDCERT:** IM 78; Inf 80; **MS:** NYU Sch Med 75; **RES:** Montefiore Med Ctr, Bronx, NY 76-78; **FEL:** Inf, Peter Bent Brigham Hosp, Boston, MA 78; **FAP:** Asst Clin Prof Med Columbia P&S; **HOSP:** St Barnabas Hosp-Bronx; *SI: Viral Infections; Endocarditis;* **HMO:** CIGNA Oxford US Hlthcre Aetna Hlth Plan Blue Cross +

LANG: Sp, Prt; ♿ 🆒 🌙 📷 🎦 🏧 S Mcr WC NFI 1 Week ▦ **VISA** 💳 💳

Cassidy, Brian (MD)   IM   PCP
Muhlenberg Regional Med Ctr

1314 Park Ave; Plainfield, NJ 07060; (908) 755-4232; **BDCERT:** IM 88; **MS:** West Indies 85; **RES:** Muhlenberg Regional Med Ctr, Plainfield, NJ 85-88

♿ 📷 🎦 🏧 S Mcr 1 Week ▦ **VISA** 💳 💳

Feldman, Jeffrey (MD)   IM   PCP
Union Hosp-New Jersey

440 Chestnut St 2; Union, NJ 07083; (908) 686-9330; **BDCERT:** IM 79; Nep 81; **MS:** Hahnemann U 76; **RES:** IM, Bronx Muncipal Hosp Ctr, Bronx, NY 76; Albert Einstein Med Ctr, Bronx, NY 79; **FEL:** Nep, Univ Hosp SUNY Bklyn, Brooklyn, NY 79-81; **HOSP:** Overlook Hosp; *SI: Hypertension; Cholesterol;* **HMO:** Prucare US Hlthcre CIGNA Oxford HMO Blue +

♿ 🆒 🌙 📷 🎦 🏧 S Mcr NFI A Few Days

Fuhrman, Robert (MD)   IM   PCP
Overlook Hosp

552 Westfield Ave; Westfield, NJ 07090; (908) 654-3377; **BDCERT:** IM 71; EDM 72; **MS:** U Hlth Sci/Chicago Med Sch 66; **RES:** IM, Mount Sinai Med Ctr, New York, NY 67-70; **FEL:** EDM, Mount Sinai Med Ctr, New York, NY 69-70; NuM, VA Med Ctr-Bronx, Bronx, NY 69-70; **FAP:** Assoc Clin Prof Med Columbia P&S; *SI: Diabetes, Thyroid Disease; Osteoporosis;* **HMO:** PHS Oxford CIGNA United Healthcare Blue Cross +

LANG: Sp; ♿ 🆒 📷 🎦 🏧 S Mcr Mod NFI 2-4 Weeks **VISA**

Gray, Samuel (DO)   IM   PCP
Overlook Hosp
Westfield Associates, 512 E Broad St; Westfield, NJ 07090; (908) 232-6151; **BDCERT:** IM 74; Ge 75; **MS:** Chicago Coll Osteo Med 67; **RES:** IM, Montefiore Med Ctr, Bronx, NY 70-72; **FEL:** Ge, Montefiore Med Ctr, Bronx, NY 72-74; **FAP:** Assoc Clin Prof Columbia P&S; **HOSP:** St Barnabas Med Ctr-Livingston; *SI: Swallowing Problems/Heartburn; Cancer Surveillance*; **HMO:** Prudential CIGNA Oxford Blue Cross United Healthcare +

▨ ⬚ ▨ ▥ ▦ S ▣   A Few Days *VISA* ●

Hwang, Cheng-hong (DO)   IM   PCP
Union Hosp-New Jersey
1457 Raritan Rd 201; Clark, NJ 07066; (908) 272-2270; **BDCERT:** IM 83; **MS:** Coll Of Osteo Med-Pacific 78; **RES:** USPHS Hosp, Baltimore, MD 78-79; IM, USPHS Hosp, Baltimore, MD 79-81; **FEL:** Pul, Univ of Med & Dent NJ Hosp, Newark, NJ 81-83; **HOSP:** Rahway Hosp; *SI: Pulmonary Disease*; **HMO:** Aetna Hlth Plan Blue Cross & Blue Shield

€ ⬚ ▥ ▦ ▣ ▣ ▣ ▣   1 Week

Khimani, Karim (MD)   IM   PCP
St Elizabeth Hosp
815 Salem Ave; Elizabeth, NJ 07208; (908) 352-5071; **BDCERT:** IM 86; **MS:** Dominican Republic 82; **RES:** IM, St Elizabeth Hosp, Elizabeth, NJ 82-85; *SI: Geriatrics*

LANG: Hin; ▨ ▨ € ⬚ ▥ S ▣ ▣   1 Week

Rosenbaum, Robert (MD)   IM
Overlook Hosp
Summit Medical Group, 120 Summit Ave; Summit, NJ 07901; (908) 273-4300; **BDCERT:** IM 78; EDM 81; **MS:** Columbia P&S 75; **RES:** IM, Montefiore Med Ctr, Bronx, NY; **FEL:** EDM, Montefiore Med Ctr, Bronx, NY; **FAP:** Asst Clin Prof Columbia P&S; *SI: Thyroid Diseases, Diabetes; Osteoporosis*; **HMO:** Aetna Hlth Plan CIGNA US Hlthcre Oxford Blue Cross & Blue Shield +

▨ ▨ € ⬚ ▥ ▦ S ▣ ▣   2-4 Weeks *VISA* ●

Toth, William (MD)   IM
Overlook Hosp
Summit Medical Group, 120 Summit Ave; Summit, NJ 07901; (908) 273-4300; **BDCERT:** IM 67; **MS:** Hahnemann U 60; **RES:** IM, Brooke Army Med Ctr, San Antonio, TX 61-64; **FAP:** Asst Clin Prof Med Columbia P&S; **HMO:** Aetna Hlth Plan CIGNA Oxford United Healthcare HMO Blue +

▨ ▨ ⬚ ▥ ▦ S ▣   2-4 Weeks ▨ *VISA* ●

Whitman III, Hendricks (MD) IM
Overlook Hosp
Summit Medical Group, 40 Stirling Rd; Watchung, NJ 07060; (908) 769-0100; **BDCERT:** IM 78; Rhu 80; **MS:** U NC Sch Med 75; **RES:** IM, U Chicago Hosp, Chicago, IL 75-76; IM, NY Hosp-Cornell Med Ctr, New York, NY 76-78; **FEL:** Rhu, Hosp For Special Surgery, New York, NY 78-80; **FAP:** Asst Clin Prof Cornell U; **HOSP:** St Barnabas Med Ctr-Livingston; *SI: Rheumatoid Arthritis; Scleroderma*; **HMO:** Aetna-US Healthcare CIGNA Oxford

▨ ⬚ ▥ ▦ S ▣   2-4 Weeks ▨ *VISA* ●

Worth, David (MD)   IM
Overlook Hosp
1990 Hillside Ave; Union, NJ 07083; (908) 686-6616; **BDCERT:** IM 74; Rhu 78; **MS:** U Rochester 71; **RES:** IM, Montefiore Med Ctr, Bronx, NY 71-74; **FEL:** Rhu, Montefiore Med Ctr, Bronx, NY 77-78; **FAP:** Instr Columbia P&S; **HOSP:** Union Hosp-New Jersey; *SI: Rheumatoid Arthritis; Osteoporosis*

▨ € ⬚ ▥ ▦ S ▣   A Few Days

MEDICAL ONCOLOGY

Moriarty, Daniel (MD)   Onc
Overlook Hosp
Medical Diagnostic Associates, 150 Morris Ave; Springfield, NJ 07081; (973) 376-5777; **BDCERT:** IM 82; Onc 87; **MS:** Univ Vt Coll Med 92; **RES:** Cambridge Hosp, Cambridge, MA 80-82; **FEL:** Hem Onc, St Elizabeth's Med Ctr, Boston, MA 82-84; **FAP:** Instr Columbia P&S; **HMO:** Blue Cross & Blue Shield US Hlthcre CIGNA Aetna Hlth Plan

▨ ⬚ ▥ ▦ S ▣   Immediately ▨ *VISA* ●

Pliner, Lillian (MD)　　　Onc
Union Hosp-New Jersey

Med Onc Assocs of St Barnabas, 1050 Galloping
Hill Rd; Union, NJ 07083; (908) 810-6470;
BDCERT: Onc 89; IM 84; MS: SUNY Hlth Sci Ctr
80; RES: IM, Boston U Med Ctr, Boston, MA 80-83;
FEL: Hem Onc, Mem Sloan Kettering Cancer Ctr,
New York, NY 83-86; FAP: Clin Prof UMDNJ-NJ
Med Sch, Newark; HOSP: St Barnabas Med Ctr-
Livingston; SI: *Breast Cancer; Sarcoma*; HMO: Aetna
Hlth Plan Prucare US Hlthcre Oxford HMO Blue +

⟦symbols⟧ A Few Days

NEPHROLOGY

Alterman, Lloyd (MD)　　　Nep
Overlook Hosp

Summit Medical Group, 120 Summit Ave; Summit,
NJ 07901; (908) 273-4300; BDCERT: IM 80; MS:
Wayne State U Sch Med 77; RES: IM, Overlook
Hosp, Summit, NJ 77-80; FEL: Nep, Montefiore Med
Ctr, Bronx, NY 80-82; FAP: Asst Clin Prof
Columbia P&S; HOSP: St Barnabas Hosp-Bronx; SI:
Hypertension; Kidney Disease; HMO: Oxford Aetna-
US Healthcare CIGNA Prudential Blue Cross +

⟦symbols⟧ 4+ Weeks VISA ⬤

NEUROLOGICAL SURGERY

Fineman, Sanford (MD)　　　NS
Union Hosp-New Jersey

Union County Neurosurgery, 2333 Morris Ave Ste
A12; Union, NJ 07083; (908) 688-8800; BDCERT:
NS 85; MS: Temple U 76; RES: Thomas Jefferson U
Hosp, Philadelphia, PA 77-81; U of Pittsburgh Med
Ctr, Pittsburgh, PA 81-82; HOSP: Elizabeth Gen
Med Ctr; SI: *Brain Tumors; Pain Management*; HMO:
HIP Network QualCare Blue Cross & Blue Choice
First Option CompSource +

⟦symbols⟧ A Few Days

NEUROLOGY

Pollock, Jeffrey (MD)　　　N
Overlook Hosp

47 Maple St 104; Summit, NJ 07901; (908) 277-
2722; BDCERT: N 87; MS: Med Coll Ga 82; RES:
IM, Rutgers U Med Ctr, New Brunswick, NJ 82-83;
N, Univ of Med & Dent NJ Hosp, Newark, NJ 83-86;
FEL: VA Med Ctr-East Orange, East Orange, NJ 83-
86; HMO: Most

⟦symbols⟧ 1 Week VISA ⬤

Sachs, Stephen (MD)　　　N
Union Hosp of the Bronx

Neurological Associates, 700 N Broad St 201;
Elizabeth, NJ 07208; (908) 354-3994; BDCERT: N
77; MS: Univ Penn 71; RES: N, Columbia-
Presbyterian Med Ctr, New York, NY 73-76; IM,
Bellevue Hosp Ctr, New York, NY 72-73; FAP: Asst
Clin Prof N UMDNJ New Jersey Sch Osteo Med

Sananman, Michael (MD)　　　N
Elizabeth Gen Med Ctr

Neurological Associates, 700 N Broad St 201;
Elizabeth, NJ 07208; (908) 354-3994; BDCERT: N
71; MS: Columbia P&S 64; RES: Med, UC San
Francisco Med Ctr, San Francisco, CA 65-66; N,
Columbia-Presbyterian Med Ctr, New York, NY 66-
69; FEL: EEG, Columbia-Presbyterian Med Ctr, New
York, NY; FAP: Assoc Clin Prof N UMDNJ New
Jersey Sch Osteo Med; HOSP: Union Hosp-New
Jersey; SI: *Headache; Seizures*; HMO: CIGNA Prucare
First Option HMO Blue Oxford +

LANG: Sp, Itl, Ger, Rus, Fr; ⟦symbols⟧
1 Week VISA

OBSTETRICS & GYNECOLOGY

Frattarola, Michael (MD)　　　ObG
Union Hosp-New Jersey

975 Leehigh Ave; Union, NJ 07083; (908) 688-
8545; BDCERT: ObG 84; MS: UMDNJ-NJ Med Sch,
Newark 73; RES: ObG, UMDNJ, 73-76

LANG: Sp; ⟦symbols⟧ 1 Week VISA ⬤

OPHTHALMOLOGY

Burke, Jordan D (MD)   Oph
Overlook Hosp

Summit Eye Group, 369 Springfield Ave; Berkeley Heights, NJ 07922; (908) 464-4600; **BDCERT:** Oph 68; **MS:** U Mich Med Sch 62; **RES:** Oph, Kings County Hosp Ctr, Brooklyn, NY 63-66; **FAP:** Asst Clin Prof S UMDNJ New Jersey Sch Osteo Med; *SI: Cataracts;* **HMO:** Aetna Hlth Plan Blue Choice Blue Cross & Blue Shield

[SA/SU] [C] [⊞] [Mcr]   2-4 Weeks

Natale, Benjamin (DO)   Oph
Union Hosp-New Jersey

Associated Eye Physicians & Surgeons of NJ, 1020 Galloping Hill Rd; Union, NJ 07083; (908) 964-7878; **BDCERT:** Oph 91; **MS:** Coll Of Osteo Med-Pacific 80; **RES:** FP, Union Hosp, Union, NJ 80-82; Oph, Univ of Med & Dent NJ Hosp, Newark, NJ 83-85; **FEL:** Newark Eye & Ear Infirmary, Newark, NJ 85-86; **FAP:** Adjct Clin Prof NY Coll Osteo Med; **HOSP:** St Francis Hosp-Jersey City; *SI: Laser Refractive Surgery; Cataract Surgery-Stitchless;* **HMO:** Blue Cross & Blue Shield Prudential United Healthcare Aetna-US Healthcare Oxford +

LANG: Itl, Sp, Fr, Arm; [⅄] [C] [⌂] [⅊] [⊞] [$] [Mcr] [WC] 1 Week [▦] **VISA** [●]

Tchorbajian, Kirk (MD)   Oph
Union Hosp-New Jersey

Associated Eye Physicians, 1020 Galloping Hill Rd; Union, NJ 07083; (908) 964-7878; **BDCERT:** Oph 91; **MS:** France 81; **RES:** France Hosp, Paris, France 80; St Clare Hospital, New York, NY 81-82; **FEL:** Oph, UMDNJ- Newark, Newark, NJ 82-85; *SI: Cataract Surgery; Glaucoma*

LANG: Sp; [⅄] [⌂] [⊞] [$] [Mcr] [WC] 1 Week [▦] **VISA** [●]

ORTHOPAEDIC SURGERY

Barmakian, Joseph (MD)   OrS
Overlook Hosp

Orthopedics,Hand & Upper Extremeties Center,PA, 555 Westfield Ave; Westfield, NJ 07090; (908) 654-1100; **BDCERT:** OrS 92; HS 93; **MS:** UMDNJ-RW Johnson Med Sch 84; **RES:** Columbia-Presbyterian Med Ctr, New York, NY 89; **FEL:** HS, Hosp For Joint Diseases, New York, NY 89-90; **HOSP:** JFK Med Ctr; *SI: Hand Surgery*

[⅄] [C] [⌂] [⅊] [⊞] [$] [Mcr] [WC] [NFI] 2-4 Weeks **VISA** [●]

Botwin, Clifford (DO)   OrS
Union Hosp-New Jersey

900 Stuyvesant Ave; Union, NJ 07083; (908) 964-6600; **BDCERT:** SM 85; OrS 82; **MS:** Univ Hlth Sci Coll -Osteo Med 71; **RES:** OrS, Delaware Valley Hospital, Bristol, PA 72-76; Union Hospital, Union, NJ 71-72; **HOSP:** Bayonne Hosp; *SI: Arthroscopic Surgery; Total Knee & Hip Surgery;* **HMO:** Aetna Hlth Plan Blue Cross & Blue Choice First Option GHI

[⅄] [C] [⌂] [⅊] [⊞] [$] [Mcr] [WC] [NFI] 2-4 Weeks **VISA** [●]

Gallick, Gregory (MD)   OrS
Overlook Hosp

2780 Morris Ave; Union, NJ 07083; (908) 686-6665; **BDCERT:** OrS 88; **MS:** UMDNJ-NJ Med Sch, Newark 80; **RES:** S, Univ of Med & Dent NJ Hosp, Newark, NJ 81; OrS, Univ of Med & Dent NJ Hosp, Newark, NJ 82-85; **FEL:** SM, Van Nuys Hosp, Van Nuys, CA 86; **HOSP:** St Barnabas Med Ctr-Livingston; *SI: Sports Medicine*

LANG: Sp; [⅄] [C] [⅊] [⊞] [$] [Mcr] [WC] [NFI] 1 Week **VISA** [●]

Innella, Robin (DO)   OrS
Union Hosp-New Jersey
Associated Orthopaedics, 900 Stuyvesant Ave;
Union, NJ 07083; (908) 964-6600; **BDCERT:** OrS
89; **MS:** Philadelphia Coll Osteo Med 82; **RES:** OrS,
Somerset Med Ctr, Somerville, NJ 82-87; **FAP:** Asst
Clin Instr S UMDNJ New Jersey Sch Osteo Med;
HOSP: Bayonne Hosp; **SI:** *Sports Medicine; Joint
Surgery;* **HMO:** Aetna Hlth Plan Blue Cross Prucare
Oxford US Hlthcre +

[符号] Immediately **VISA** [符号]

OTOLARYNGOLOGY

Drake, William (MD)   Oto
Overlook Hosp
Westfield Ear Nose & Throat, 789 Elm St; Westfield,
NJ 07090; (908) 233-5500; **BDCERT:** Oto 95; **MS:**
UMDNJ-NJ Med Sch, Newark 89; **RES:** Mount Sinai
Med Ctr, New York, NY 89-94; **HOSP:** VA Med Ctr-
Bronx; **SI:** *Nasal & Sinus Surgery; Head & Neck
Surgery;* **HMO:** QualCare Blue Cross CIGNA United
Healthcare Oxford +

[符号] 2-4 Weeks

Kwartler, Jed (MD)   Oto
Overlook Hosp
Ear Specialty Group, 55 Morris Ave 304;
Springfield, NJ 07081; (973) 379-3330; **BDCERT:**
Oto 88; **MS:** UMDNJ-NJ Med Sch, Newark 83; **RES:**
S, Univ of Med & Dent NJ Hosp, Newark, NJ 83-85;
Oto, Univ of Med & Dent NJ Hosp, Newark, NJ 85-
88; **FEL:** St Vincent Med Ctr, Los Angeles, CA 89-
90; **FAP:** Assoc Clin Prof UMDNJ New Jersey Sch
Osteo Med; **HOSP:** St Barnabas Med Ctr-Livingston;
SI: *Ear Diseases Hearing Loss; Balance Disorders;*
HMO: HIP Network HMO Blue Magnacare CIGNA
Oxford +

[符号] 1 Week [符号] **VISA**
[符号]

Saporta, Diego (MD)   Oto
Elizabeth Gen Med Ctr
315 Elmora Ave Ste 104; Elizabeth, NJ 07083;
(908) 851-9777; **BDCERT:** Oto 90; **MS:** Uruguay
79; **RES:** Oto, Colum Presb Hosp, New York, NY 86-
90

Scharf, Richard (DO)   Oto
Union Hosp-New Jersey
Associated Ear Nose & Throat, 505 Chestnut St;
Roselle Park, NJ 07204; (908) 241-0200;
BDCERT: Oto 93; PlS 93; **MS:** U of Hlth Sci, Coll
Osteo Med 82; **RES:** Oto, Flint Hosp, Flint, MI 87-
90; S, Flint Hosp, Flint, MI 87-90; **HOSP:** Bayonne
Hosp; **SI:** *Sinus Surgery; Facial Cosmetic Surgery;*
HMO: Aetna Hlth Plan Prucare Oxford US Hlthcre
CIGNA +

[符号] A Few Days [符号]
VISA [符号]

PAIN MANAGEMENT

Weinberger, Michael (MD)   PM
Overlook Hosp
Summit Pain Management, 33 Overlook Rd Ste 3R;
Summit, NJ; (908) 598-0196; **BDCERT:** Anes 90;
PM 91; **MS:** Columbia P&S 83; **RES:** IM, St Vincents
Hosp & Med Ctr NY, New York, NY 83-86; Anes,
Columbia-Presbyterian Med Ctr, New York, NY 86-
89; **FEL:** PM, Mem Sloan Kettering Cancer Ctr, New
York, NY 90; **SI:** *Cancer Pain Management; Back
Pain;* **HMO:** Magnacare

[符号] Immediately [符号]
VISA [符号]

PEDIATRIC CARDIOLOGY

Leichter, Donald (MD)   PCd
Overlook Hosp
Medical Art Center, 33 Overlook Rd SUITE103;
Summit, NJ 07901; (908) 522-5340; **BDCERT:** Ped
88; PCd 96; **MS:** Cornell U 80; **FEL:** PCd, Children's
Hosp Nat Med Ctr, Washington, DC 81-83; **FAP:**
Dir PCd; **HOSP:** Morristown Mem Hosp

PEDIATRIC PULMONOLOGY

Nutman, Jacob (MD)   PPul
Overlook Hosp
33 Overlook Rd 207; Summit, NJ 07901; (908)
273-2300; **BDCERT:** Ped 89; PPul 89; **MS:** Israel
77; **RES:** Ped, Beilinson Hosp, Tel Aviv, Israel 81-
84; **FEL:** Pul, Rainbow Babies & Children's Hosp,
Cleveland, OH 84-87; **FAP:** Asst Prof Ped Columbia
P&S; **HOSP:** Clara Maass Med Ctr; **HMO:** Blue
Choice Blue Cross & Blue Shield Metlife US Hlthcre
♿ 🚻 📷 🍼 🏨 Mcd   Immediately

PEDIATRICS

Corbo, Emanuel (MD)   Ped   **PCP**
Elizabeth Gen Med Ctr
Park Pediatrics, 443 E Westfield Ave; Roselle Park,
NJ 07204; (908) 245-2442; **BDCERT:** Ped 92; **MS:**
Grenada 85; **RES:** Ped, Newark Beth Israel Med Ctr,
Newark, NJ 87-90; **FEL:** Ped, Newark Beth Israel
Med Ctr, Newark, NJ 90-91; **HOSP:** Overlook Hosp;
HMO: Blue Choice Oxford CIGNA HMO Blue First
Option +
LANG: Itl, Sp; 🚻 ☺ 📷 🍼 🏨 $ Mcr Mcd
A Few Days **VISA** ●

Davis, Kenneth J (MD)   Ped   **PCP**
Elizabeth Gen Med Ctr
815 Salem Ave; Elizabeth, NJ 07208; (908) 354-
9500; **BDCERT:** Ped 85; **MS:** Albert Einstein Coll
Med 80; **RES:** Bellevue Hosp Ctr, New York, NY 80-
83; **HOSP:** Overlook Hosp; **HMO:** First Option
Oxford QualCare PHCS HIP Network +
LANG: Sp; ♿ 🚻 ☺ 📷 🏨 $ Mcd   Immediately
VISA ●

Panzner, Elizabeth (MD)   Ped   **PCP**
St Barnabas Med Ctr-Livingston
Pediatric Medical Group, 1050 Galloping Hill Rd
Ste 200; Union, NJ 07083; (908) 810-6440;
BDCERT: Ped 89; **MS:** Mexico 84; **RES:** Ped, Univ of
Med & Dent NJ Hosp, Newark, NJ 85-88; **HOSP:**
Union Hosp-New Jersey; **HMO:** Prucare Blue Cross
& Blue Shield Aetna Hlth Plan Prucare Oxford +
LANG: Sp, Fr; ♿ ☺ 🚻 📷 🍼 🏨 $ Mcd
A Few Days ▦ **VISA** ● ▦

Sank, Lewis (MD)   Ped   **PCP**
Overlook Hosp
SummitWarren Pediatric Assoc, 33 Overlook Rd
403; Summit, NJ 07901; (908) 277-0050;
BDCERT: Ped 72; **MS:** Johns Hopkins U 61; **RES:**
Ped, Jacobi Med Ctr, Bronx, NY 61-64; **FEL:** ChAP,
Jacobi Med Ctr, Bronx, NY 63-64; **FAP:** Asst Clin
Prof Columbia P&S; **SI:** *Hyperactivity; Attention
Deficit Disorder;* **HMO:** Aetna-US Healthcare HMO
Blue CIGNA United Healthcare +
♿ ☺ 📷 🍼 🏨 $ Mcd   A Few Days **VISA** ●

Vigorita, John (MD)   Ped   **PCP**
Overlook Hosp
Summit Pediatric Assoc, 33 Overlook Rd 101;
Summit, NJ 07901; (908) 273-1112; **BDCERT:** Ped
89; **MS:** Mexico 74; **RES:** Ped, Overlook Hospital,
Summit, NJ 74-78; **FAP:** Assoc Clin Prof Ped
Columbia P&S; **SI:** *Learning Disabilities; Sports
Medicine;* **HMO:** CIGNA Aetna Hlth Plan Empire
Blue Cross & Shield Oxford US Hlthcre +
LANG: Sp; ♿ ☺ 📷 🍼 🏨 $ Mcd   A Few Days

Zanger, Norman (MD)   Ped   **PCP**
St Barnabas Med Ctr-Livingston

Pediatric Medical Group, 1050 Galloping Hill Rd; Union, NJ 07083; (908) 810-6440; **BDCERT:** Ped 72; **MS:** Belgium 66; **RES:** Ped, Newark Beth Israel Med Ctr, Newark, NJ 70-72; **FAP:** Asst Clin Prof UMDNJ New Jersey Sch Osteo Med; **HOSP:** Overlook Hosp; **SI:** *General Pediatrics;* **HMO:** Aetna Hlth Plan Prudential First Option CIGNA Oxford +

LANG: Fr, Sp; 🅰 🆘 📞 👪 🛏 💲 🅼   Immediately

PHYSICAL MEDICINE & REHABILITATION

Bucksbaum, Mark J (MD)   PMR
St Barnabas Med Ctr-Livingston

440 Chestnut St; Union, NJ 07083; (908) 686-5800; **BDCERT:** PMR 89; **PM** 90; **MS:** West Indies 84; **RES:** IM, Montefiore Med Ctr, Bronx, NY 84-85; PMR, Montefiore Med Ctr, Bronx, NY 85-88; **HOSP:** Union Hosp-New Jersey; **SI:** *Pain Management; Electrodiagnosis;* **HMO:** Blue Cross & Blue Shield CIGNA US Hlthcre United Healthcare

🅰 🆘 🅲 📞 👪 🛏 💲 🅼 🅼 🆆 🅽   1 Week

PLASTIC SURGERY

Hyans, Peter (MD)   PlS
Overlook Hosp

Summit Medical Group, 120 Summit Ave; Summit, NJ 07901; (908) 273-4300; **BDCERT:** PlS 95; **S** 92; **MS:** UMDNJ-RW Johnson Med Sch 86; **RES:** S, Thomas Jefferson U Hosp, Philadelphia, PA 86-91; **FEL:** PlS, U Hosp, Cincinnati, OH 91-93; **HOSP:** St Barnabas Med Ctr-Livingston; **SI:** *Cosmetic Surgery; Breast Reconstruction;* **HMO:** CIGNA Aetna Hlth Plan HMO Blue Prudential Oxford +

🅰 🅲 📞 👪 🛏 🅼 🆆 🅽   1 Week ▦ **VISA** 💳

Tepper, Howard (MD)   PlS
Overlook Hosp

522 E Broad St; Westfield, NJ 07090; (908) 654-6540; **BDCERT:** PlS 83; **MS:** Albert Einstein Coll Med 75; **RES:** Montefiore Med Ctr, Bronx, NY 75-78; **FEL:** PlS, St Luke's Roosevelt Hosp Ctr, New York, NY 78; Montefiore Med Ctr, Bronx, NY 79-81; **HOSP:** Union Hosp-New Jersey; **SI:** *Facial Rejuvenation; Breast Surgery;* **HMO:** Aetna Hlth Plan Blue Choice Blue Cross & Blue Shield CIGNA Sanus +

LANG: Heb, Fr, Sp, Yd; 🅰 📞 👪 🛏 💲 🅼 🆆 🅽   2-4 Weeks **VISA** 💳

West, Gerald (DO)   PlS
Union Hosp-New Jersey

505 Chestnut St; Roselle Park, NJ 07204; (908) 241-0200; **BDCERT:** Oto 74; PlS 74; **MS:** Univ Hlth Sci Coll -Osteo Med 67; **RES:** Metropolitan Hosp, Philadelphia, PA 68-71; **HOSP:** Bayonne Hosp; **SI:** *Rhinoplasty; Collagen;* **HMO:** Oxford Blue Cross & Blue Shield US Hlthcre CIGNA Guardian +

LANG: Sp; 🅰 🅲 📞 👪 🛏 💲 🅼 🅼 🆆 🅽   Immediately **VISA** 💳

PSYCHIATRY

Herridge, Peter L (MD)   Psyc
Overlook Hosp

1 Seward Pl; Chester, NJ 07930; (908) 522-2226; **BDCERT:** Psyc 87; **MS:** Albert Einstein Coll Med 80; **RES:** Psyc, McLean Hosp-Harvard U Belmont, Boston, MA 81-84; Med, St Vincents Hosp & Med Ctr NY, New York, NY 80-81; **FEL:** Rutgers School of Law, Newark, NJ 94-97; **SI:** *Mood Disorders; Neuropsychiatry*

🅰 📞 👪 🅼   A Few Days

Miller, David (MD)   Psyc
St Barnabas Hosp-Bronx

Summit Psychiatric Assoc, 47 Maple St 401; Summit, NJ 07901; (908) 277-1550; **BDCERT:** Psyc 86; **MS:** UMDNJ-RW Johnson Med Sch 80

🅲 📞 🛏 💲 🅼 🆆   A Few Days **VISA** 💳

Villafranca, Manuel (MD)   Psyc
Union Hosp-New Jersey
220 Lenox Ave; Westfield, NJ 07090; (908) 232-9369; **BDCERT:** Psyc 82; **MS:** Philippines 71; **RES:** St Vincents Hosp & Med Ctr NY, New York, NY 78-80; Psyc, St Vincents Hosp & Med Ctr NY, New York, NY 76-78; **HMO:** Blue Cross & Blue Shield

🧑 📷 👨 🏥 💲 Mcr   2-4 Weeks

PULMONARY DISEASE

Sussman, Robert (MD)   Pul
Overlook Hosp
Pulmonary & Allergy Associates, 530 Morris Ave; Springfield, NJ 07081; (973) 467-3334; **BDCERT:** IM 84; Pul 87; **MS:** Albert Einstein Coll Med 81; **RES:** IM, Montefiore Med Ctr, Bronx, NY 81-84; Pul, New York University Med Ctr, New York, NY 85-87; **FAP:** Asst Clin Instr Med Columbia P&S; **HMO:** Aetna Hlth Plan Blue Choice Blue Cross & Blue Shield CIGNA HIP Network +

🧑 📷 👨 🏥 Mcr Mcl NFl   2-4 Weeks **VISA** 💳

Zimmerman, Mark (MD)   Pul
Overlook Hosp
Summit Medical Group, 120 Summit Ave; Summit, NJ 07901; (908) 273-4300; **BDCERT:** Pul 92; CCM 93; **MS:** NYU Sch Med 85; **RES:** New York University Med Ctr, New York, NY 86-88; **FEL:** CCM, Mount Sinai Med Ctr, New York, NY 89-92; **FAP:** Asst Clin Prof Med Columbia P&S; **HMO:** Aetna Hlth Plan Blue Cross & Blue Shield CIGNA

🧑 📷 👨 🏥 Mcr WC NFl   2-4 Weeks 💳 **VISA** 💳

RADIATION ONCOLOGY

Schwartz, Louis (MD)   RadRO
Overlook Hosp
33 Overlook Rd Ste L05; Summit, NJ 07901; (908) 522-2871; **BDCERT:** RadRO 75; Ped 75; **MS:** SUNY Hlth Sci Ctr 74; **RES:** RadRO, Columbia-Presbyterian Med Ctr, New York, NY 77-79; Ped, New York Methodist Hosp, Brooklyn, NY 75-76; *SI: Radiosurgery; Conformal Radiation*; **HMO:** CIGNA Oxford Blue Choice HMO Blue First Option +

🧑 📷 👨 🏥 Mcr Mcl   Immediately

RHEUMATOLOGY

Wilmot, Richard (MD)   Rhu
Overlook Hosp
8 Magnolia; Boonton Township, NJ 07005; (908) 273-4300; **BDCERT:** IM 96; **MS:** Albert Einstein Coll Med 88; **RES:** IM, Albany Med Ctr, Albany, NY 89-91; **FEL:** Rhu, Columbia-Presbyterian Med Ctr, New York, NY 91-93; **FAP:** Asst Prof Med Columbia P&S; **HOSP:** St Barnabas Med Ctr-Livingston; *SI: Fibromyalgia- Soft Tissue; SLE—Arthritis*; **HMO:** Oxford CIGNA US Hlthcre Blue Cross & Blue Shield

🧑 SA 🌙 📷 👨 🏥 💲 Mcr WC   4+ Weeks

SPORTS MEDICINE

Levy, Andrew (MD)   SM
Univ of Med & Dent NJ Hosp
N J Orthopaedic Institute - Overlook Hospital, 33 Overlook Rd MAC103; Summit, NJ 07001; (908) 522-5895; **BDCERT:** SM 95; **MS:** Temple U 87; **RES:** Albert Einstein Med Ctr, Philadelphia, PA 90-94; **FEL:** SM, Duke U Med Ctr, Durham, NC 94-95; **FAP:** Asst Prof OrS UMDNJ-NJ Med Sch, Newark; **HOSP:** Overlook Hosp; *SI: Shoulder & Knee Injuries*; **HMO:** Most

LANG: Pol, Sp; 🧑 🌙 📷 👨 🏥 💲 Mcr Mcl WC NFl
1 Week 💳 **VISA** 💳

SURGERY

Befeler, David (MD)   S
Overlook Hosp
General Surgical Assoc, 709 Springfield Ave;
Summit, NJ 07901; (908) 277-3232; **BDCERT:** S
66; **MS:** Columbia P&S 59; **RES:** S, St Vincents Hosp
& Med Ctr NY, New York, NY 59-60; *SI: Breast
Disease; Gallbladder Disease;* **HMO:** Most

⬛ ⬛ ⬛ ⬛ ⬛ ⬛ ⬛ A Few Days ⬛ *VISA* ⬛
⬛

Frost, James (MD)   S
Union Hosp-New Jersey
Elizabeth Surgical Group, 700 N Broad St 301;
Elizabeth, NJ 07208; (908) 354-3779; **BDCERT:** S
89; RE 97; **MS:** Mexico 82; **RES:** S, U IL Med Ctr,
Chicago, IL 83-88; *SI: Breast and Colon Cancer;*
HMO: Oxford Blue Cross US Hlthcre Prudential First
Option +

LANG: Sp; ⬛ ⬛ ⬛ ⬛ ⬛ ⬛ ⬛ ⬛ ⬛ 1 Week ⬛
VISA ⬛ ⬛

Matkiwsksy, Zenon (DO)   S
Union Hosp-New Jersey
1020 Galloping Hill Rd; Union, NJ 07083; (908)
687-6688; **BDCERT:** S 78; **MS:** Philadelphia Coll
Osteo Med 62; **RES:** S, Cherry Hill Med Ctr, Cherry
Hill, NJ 66-69; **HOSP:** Overlook Hosp; *SI:
Laparoscopic Surgery;* **HMO:** Aetna Hlth Plan CIGNA
US Hlthcre Oxford First Option +

⬛ ⬛ ⬛ ⬛ ⬛ ⬛ ⬛ ⬛ ⬛ Immediately

Nitzberg, Richard (MD)   S
Overlook Hosp
Summit Medical Group, 120 Summit Ave; Summit,
NJ 07901; (908) 273-4300; **BDCERT:** S 89; GVS
92; **MS:** Harvard Med Sch 83; **RES:** S, Columbia-
Presbyterian Med Ctr, New York, NY 83-88; **FEL:**
GVS, New England Med Ctr, Boston, MA 88-90; *SI:
Laporoscopic Surgery; Melanoma/Sentinel Nodes;*
HMO: Oxford CIGNA US Hlthcre Blue Cross
Travelers +

LANG: Sp; ⬛ ⬛ ⬛ ⬛ ⬛ ⬛ ⬛ Immediately ⬛
VISA

Simpson, Thomas (MD)   S
New York University Med Ctr
33 Overlook Rd; Summit, NJ 07901; (908) 522-
3100; **BDCERT:** S 84; **MS:** NYU Sch Med 76; **RES:** U
Louisville Hosp, Louisville, KY 78-83; New York
University Med Ctr, New York, NY 76-78

Starker, Paul (MD)   S
Overlook Hosp
General Surgical Associates, PA, 507 Westfield
Ave; Westfield, NJ 07090; (908) 277-3232;
BDCERT: S 87; SCC 89; **MS:** Columbia P&S 80;
RES: S, Columbia-Presbyterian Med Ctr, New York,
NY 82-86; **FEL:** Columbia-Presbyterian Med Ctr,
New York, NY 81-82; **FAP:** Asst Clin Prof S
Columbia P&S; *SI: Laparoscopic Surgery;* **HMO:**
Aetna-US Healthcare Blue Cross & Blue Shield
CIGNA Oxford

⬛ ⬛ ⬛ ⬛ ⬛ ⬛ ⬛ ⬛ ⬛ A Few Days ⬛ *VISA*
⬛

THORACIC SURGERY

Bolanowski, Paul J P (MD)   TS
Univ of Med & Dent NJ Hosp
Bolanwoski Surgical Group, 623 Union Ave;
Elizabeth, NJ 07208; (908) 352-8110; **BDCERT:** TS
74; S 73; **MS:** UMDNJ-NJ Med Sch, Newark 65;
RES: S, Yale-New Haven Hosp, New Haven, CT 65-
68; S, Univ of Med & Dent NJ Hosp, Newark, NJ 69-
70; **FEL:** Cv, Univ of Med & Dent NJ Hosp, Newark,
NJ 71-72; **FAP:** Asst Prof S UMDNJ-NJ Med Sch,
Newark; **HOSP:** St Elizabeth Hosp; *SI: Tracheal
Stenosis; Thymectomy of Myastenics;* **HMO:** Aetna-
US Healthcare CIGNA Oxford Blue Cross & Blue
Shield CHA +

⬛ ⬛ ⬛ ⬛ ⬛ ⬛ ⬛ ⬛ 1 Week

Brenner, Richard (MD)   TS
Overlook Hosp
120 Summit Ave; Summit, NJ 07901; (908) 273-
4300; **BDCERT:** S 67; TS 67; **MS:** Columbia P&S
58; **RES:** TS, St Luke's Roosevelt Hosp Ctr, New
York, NY 58-63; Childrens Mem Med Ctr, Chicago,
IL 65-67; **HOSP:** Morristown Mem Hosp

⬛ ⬛ ⬛ ⬛ ⬛ ⬛ ⬛ ⬛ Immediately *VISA* ⬛

Lozner, Jerrold (MD)   TS
Overlook Hosp

Summit Medical Group, 120 Summit Ave; Summit, NJ 07901; (908) 273-4300; **BDCERT:** TS 81; S 79; **MS:** KY Med Sch, Louisville 71; **RES:** S, U Hosp, Cincinnati, OH 71-76; **FEL:** TS, U Hosp, Cincinnati, OH 76-78; **FAP:** Assoc Clin Instr S Columbia P&S; *SI: Lung Cancer; Cancer of the Breast;* **HMO:** Aetna Hlth Plan Blue Cross & Blue Shield CIGNA Oxford Prudential +

LANG: Sp; 🔲 🔲 🔲 🔲 🔲 🔲 🔲 🔲 Immediately **VISA** 💳

UROLOGY

Lehrhoff, Bernard (MD)   U
Overlook Hosp

Consultants In Urology, 275 Orchard St; Westfield, NJ 07090; (908) 654-5100; **BDCERT:** U 84; **MS:** UMDNJ-NJ Med Sch, Newark 76; **RES:** New York University Med Ctr, New York, NY; Mem Sloan Kettering Cancer Ctr, New York, NY 78-82; **FAP:** Clin Instr Columbia P&S; **HOSP:** St Barnabas Med Ctr-Livingston; *SI: Prostate Cancer; Impotence;* **HMO:** Aetna Hlth Plan HMO Blue Oxford Guardian

LANG: Sp, Prt; 🔲 🔲 🔲 🔲 🔲 🔲 🔲 🔲 🔲 A Few Days **VISA** 💳

Ring, Kenneth (MD)   U
Overlook Hosp

Consultants in Urology, 275 Orchard St; Westfield, NJ 07090; (908) 654-5100; **BDCERT:** U 93; **MS:** Mt Sinai Sch Med 85; **RES:** S, Mount Sinai Med Ctr, New York, NY 85-87; U, Columbia-Presbyterian Med Ctr, New York, NY 87-91; **HOSP:** Union Hosp-New Jersey; *SI: Pediatric Urology; Urologic Oncology;* **HMO:** Oxford HMO Blue United Healthcare US Hlthcre Blue Cross & Blue Shield +

LANG: Sp; 🔲 🔲 🔲 🔲 🔲 🔲 🔲 🔲 🔲 Immediately **VISA** 💳

Ritter, Joseph (MD)   U
Overlook Hosp

Summit Medical Group, 120 Summit Ave; Summit, NJ 07901; (908) 273-4300; **BDCERT:** U 71; **MS:** UMDNJ-NJ Med Sch, Newark 63; **RES:** U, Albert Einstein Med Ctr, Bronx, NY 65-68; **FAP:** Asst Clin Prof U Columbia P&S; **HOSP:** Union Hosp-New Jersey; **HMO:** Most

🔲 🔲 🔲 🔲 🔲 🔲 🔲 1 Week 🔲 **VISA** 💳 🔲

VASCULAR SURGERY (GENERAL)

Sales, Clifford (MD)   GVS
St Barnabas Med Ctr-Livingston

220 Saint Paul St; Westfield, NJ 07090; (908) 233-5859; **BDCERT:** GVS 95; **MS:** Mt Sinai Sch Med 86; **RES:** S, Montefiore Med Ctr, Bronx, NY 86-91; **FEL:** GVS, Montefiore Med Ctr, Bronx, NY 91-93; **HOSP:** Overlook Hosp; *SI: Varicose Veins; Artery Surgery*

🔲 🔲 🔲 🔲 🔲 🔲 🔲 Immediately **VISA** 💳

THE STATE OF CONNECTICUT

PHYSICIAN'S LISTING

FAIRFIELD COUNTY

THE STAMFORD HOSPITAL

Stamford Health System

SHELBURNE RD. AT WEST BROAD ST.
STAMFORD, CT 06904
PHONE (203) 325-7000
FAX (203) 325-7699

Sponsorship	Voluntary Not-for-Profit
Beds	305 acute
Accreditation	Joint Commission on Accreditation of Healthcare Organizations (JCAHO)

STAMFORD HEALTH SYSTEM

Stamford Health System is a health care delivery system that offers the community quality care in all stages of its citizens' lives. Health care providers within the system offer acute care, long-term care, sub-acute care, home care, rehabilitation, as well as hospice services and off-site diagnostic and ambulatory surgery services.

THE STAMFORD HOSPITAL

The Stamford Hospital is a major teaching hospital in Fairfield County that provides acute care, emergency and outpatient services to medical/surgical, obstetric, pediatric and psychiatric patients. The hospital offers the latest in diagnostic technology and treatment protocols.

RESIDENCY PROGRAMS

The Stamford Hospital offers residency programs in medicine, OB/GYN, surgery and psychiatry. These excellent teaching programs allow the hospital to provide a level of advanced care typically only available at university-based hospitals.

SPECIAL SERVICES

Cancer Care	The hospital offers comprehensive cancer services, including a free-standing cancer center, cancer genetic counseling and Autologous Bone Marrow Transplants. The hospital is the only community hospital in the state to offer ABMT.
Trauma Center	The Stamford Hospital is designated as a Level II Trauma Center by the American College of Surgeons Committee on Trauma.
Maternity Services	The Family Birthing Center offers home-like labor/delivery rooms, a Level II+ Neonatal unit and pediatricians in-house 24 hours a day. The hospital also offers fertility services, and perinatal services, including genetics counseling, fetal monitoring and in-utero procedures.

AFFILIATED SERVICES

Rehab Services	Stamford Health System offers all levels of rehab care through the William and Sally Tandet Center for Continuing Care, The Rehab Center and the Van Munching Center for Rehabilitation at St. Joseph Medical Center.
Home Care Services	Stamford Health System provides all levels of home care services–from skilled nursing to homemaker services–through VNA Care, Inc. Hospice services are also provided.
Community Education	Stamford Health System offers a range of community education and outreach programs, including lectures with local and national speakers; health screenings; yoga and tai chi classes; smoking cessation and weight control programs; support groups; diabetes and asthma education; and a membership program for adults 50 or older.
Physician Referral	MedMatch is a free, computer-based physician referral service offered by Stamford Health System. The coordinator is an experienced registered nurse who assists in finding family physicians, specialists or second opinions. To reach our physician referral service, please call (203) 325-7900.

SPECIALTY & SUBSPECIALTY	ABBREVIATION	PAGE(S)
Addiction Psychiatry	AdP	1039
Allergy & Immunology	A&I	1039-1040
Anesthesiology	Anes	1040
Cardiac Electrophysiology	CE	1040
Cardiology (Cardiovascular Disease)	Cv	1040-1042
Child & Adolescent Psychiatry	ChAP	1042
Colon & Rectal Surgery	CRS	1042
Dermatology	D	1043
Diagnostic Radiology	DR	1044
Emergency Medicine	EM	1044
Endocrinology, Diabetes & Metabolism	EDM	1045
FAMILY PRACTICE	FP	1045-1046
Gastroenterology	Ge	1046-1047
Geriatric Medicine	Ger	1047
Geriatric Psychiatry	GerPsy	1047
Gynecologic Oncology*	GO	1047-1048
Hand Surgery	HS	1048
Hematology	Hem	1048-1049
Infectious Disease	Inf	1049-1050
INTERNAL MEDICINE	IM	1050-1053
Maternal & Fetal Medicine	MF	1054
Medical Genetics	MG	1054
Medical Oncology*	Onc	1054-1056
Neonatal-Perinatal Medicine	NP	1056
Nephrology	Nep	1056-1057
Neurological Surgery	NS	1057-1058
Neurology	N	1058-1059
Nuclear Medicine	NuM	1059
OBSTETRICS & GYNECOLOGY	ObG	1059-1060
Occupational Medicine	**OM**	**1060**
Ophthalmology	Oph	1060-1061
Orthopaedic Surgery	OrS	1061-1062
Otolaryngology	Oto	1062-1064
Pain Management	PM	1064
Pediatric Cardiology	PCd	1064
Pediatric Hematology–Oncology*	PHO	1065
Pediatric Pulmonology	PPul	1065
Pediatric Surgery	PS	1065
PEDIATRICS (GENERAL)	Ped	1065-1067
Physical Medicine & Rehabilitation	PMR	1067-1068
Plastic Hand Surgery	**HS (PIS)**	**1068**
Plastic Surgery	PlS	1068-1069
Psychiatry	Psyc	1069-1070
Pulmonary Disease	Pul	1070-1071
Radiation Oncology*	RadRO	1072
Radiology	Rad	1072-1073
Reproductive Endocrinology	RE	1073
Rheumatology	Rhu	1073-1074
Sports Medicine	SM	1074
Surgery	S	1074-1076
Thoracic Surgery (includes open heart surgery)	TS	1076
Urology	U	1077-1078
Vascular Surgery (General)	GVS	1078

Specialties in capital letters indicate Primary Care Specialties. However, many doctors will be certified in a subspecialty, but will practice predominantly primary care medicine. In our lists this will be indicated.

*Oncologists deal with Cancer

ADDICTION PSYCHIATRY

Frances, Richard (MD) AdP
Hackensack Univ Med Ctr
208 Valley Rd; New Canaan, CT 06840; (203) 966-3561; **BDCERT:** Psyc 76; **MS:** NYU Sch Med 71; **RES:** Albert Einstein Med Ctr, Bronx, NY 71-74; **FAP:** Clin Prof Psyc NYU Sch Med; **SI:** *Psychiatry; Dual Diagnosis;* **HMO:** PHS Blue Cross VBH Medco

LANG: Sp, Fr, Rus, Ar, Itl; 🔯 📷 👪 🏥 💲 Mcr
Immediately ▨ *VISA* 💳

ALLERGY & IMMUNOLOGY

Askenase, Philip (MD) A&I
Yale-New Haven Hosp
333 Cedar St LCI904; New Haven, CT 06520; (203) 785-4242; **BDCERT:** A&I 74; **MS:** Yale U Sch Med 65; **RES:** IM, Boston Med Ctr, Boston, MA 65-67; Rhu, Nat Inst Health, Bethesda, MD 67-69; **FEL:** A&I, British American Heart Fellow London Hosp Med Coll, London, England 69-70; Inf, Yale-New Haven Hosp, New Haven, CT 70-71; **FAP:** Prof Yale U Sch Med; **SI:** *Asthma; Urticaria & Angioedema;* **HMO:** Aetna Hlth Plan US Hlthcre Oxford PHS

LANG: Sp, Fr; 🔯 📷 👪 🏥 💲 Mcr Mod NFI 2-4 Weeks
VISA 💳

Bell, Jonathan (MD) A&I
Danbury Hosp
107 Newtown Rd # 1B; Danbury, CT 06810; (203) 748-7433; **BDCERT:** Ped 87; **MS:** Georgetown U 80; **RES:** Ped, St Christopher's Hosp For Children, Philadelphia, PA; **FEL:** A&I/Pul, Children's Hosp of Philadelphia, Philadelphia, PA; **HMO:** Aetna Hlth Plan Blue Cross & Blue Shield CIGNA Oxford

🔯 📞 📷 👪 🏥 💲 Mcr Immediately *VISA* 💳

Coleman, Monroe (MD) A&I
Stamford Hosp
144 Morgan St; Stamford, CT 06905; (203) 324-9525; **BDCERT:** A&I 72; **MS:** SUNY Downstate 42; **RES:** Kings County Hosp Ctr, Brooklyn, NY 46-48; **FEL:** Kingsbrook Jewish Med Ctr, Brooklyn, NY 53-54; **FAP:** Clin Instr Med NY Med Coll; **SI:** *Asthma; Insect Bites;* **HMO:** Most

LANG: Sp; 🔯 📞 📷 👪 🏥 Mcr Mod WC NFI
Immediately

Linder, Paul (MD) A&I
Stamford Hosp
22 5th St; Stamford, CT 06905; (203) 978-0072; **BDCERT:** A&I 91; IM 89; **MS:** SUNY Buffalo 85; **RES:** IM, Univ Hosp SUNY Buffalo, Buffalo, NY 85-86; IM, Stamford Hosp, Stamford, CT 87-89; **FEL:** A&I, Nassau County Med Ctr, East Meadow, NY 89-91; **FAP:** Clin Instr NY Med Coll; **HOSP:** St Joseph's Med Ctr-Stamford; **SI:** *Asthma; Hayfever;* **HMO:** Aetna Hlth Plan United Healthcare Blue Cross Oxford Prudential +

LANG: Itl, Dan; 🔯 📞 📷 👪 🏥 Mcr Mod A Few Days

Litchman, Mark (MD) A&I
Greenwich Hosp
2 1/2 Dearfield Dr; Greenwich, CT 06831; (203) 869-2080; **BDCERT:** Rhu 88; A&I 91; **MS:** Rush Med Coll 84; **RES:** Greenwich Hosp, Greenwich, CT 84-87; **FEL:** Rhu/A&I, Yale-New Haven Hosp, New Haven, CT 86-89; Yale-New Haven Hosp, New Haven, CT; **FAP:** Asst Clin Prof Yale U Sch Med; **HOSP:** Yale-New Haven Hosp; **SI:** *Asthma; Clinical Immunology;* **HMO:** Oxford Health Source Health Choice Connecticut Health Blue Cross & Blue Shield +

🔯 📷 👪 🏥 💲 Mcr 1 Week *VISA* 💳

Rockwell, William (MD) A&I
Bridgeport Hosp
Allergy Assoc Of Fairfield, 4675 Main St; Bridgeport, CT 06606; (203) 374-6103; **BDCERT:** A&I 81; Ped 79; **MS:** Albany Med Coll 73; **RES:** Ped, Bridgeport Hosp, Bridgeport, CT 73-76; **FEL:** A&I, Long Island Coll Hosp, Brooklyn, NY 79-81; **HOSP:** St Vincent's Med Ctr-Bridgeport; **HMO:** MD Health Plan CIGNA Aetna Hlth Plan Yale Preferred Oxford +

🔯 📷 👪 🏥 💲 Mcr Mod 1 Week

Santilli, John (MD)   A&I
Bridgeport Hosp
Allergy Assoc of Fairfield, 4675 Main St;
Bridgeport, CT 06606; (203) 374-6103; **BDCERT:**
A&I 83; **MS:** Georgetown U 68; **RES:** Ped,
Georgetown U Hosp, Washington, DC 68-71; **FEL:**
A&I, Georgetown U Hosp, Washington, DC 71-73;
HOSP: St Vincent's Med Ctr-Bridgeport; **SI:** *Mold
Allergy; Sinusitis;* **HMO:** Aetna Hlth Plan CIGNA
Oxford Blue Cross MD Health Plan +

⬧ 🅲 🗗 🖾 🎟 🆂 Mcr Mcd   2-4 Weeks **VISA** 💳

Sweeney, Margaret (MD)   A&I   **PCP**
Norwalk Hosp
148 East Ave 1G1; Norwalk, CT 06851; (203)
838-1588; **BDCERT:** A&I 93; IM 90; **MS:** Austria
80; **RES:** Norwalk Hosp, Norwalk, CT 83; **FEL:** A&I,
U of WI Hosp, Madison, WI 85; **HMO:** PHS CIGNA
Oxford MD Health Plan Aetna Hlth Plan +

LANG: Ger; ⬧ 🆂🅳 🅲 🗗 🖾 🎟 🆂 Mcr WC NFl
A Few Days

ANESTHESIOLOGY

Gacso, William (MD)   Anes
St Vincent's Med Ctr-Bridgeport
Medical Anesthesiology Associates, PC, 2800 Main
St; Bridgeport, CT 06606; (203) 576-5152;
BDCERT: Anes 72; **MS:** Tufts U 62; **RES:** Milwaukee
City Hosp, Milwaukee, WI 65-67; Thomas Jefferson
U Hosp, Philadelphia, PA 66-67; **HMO:** PHS MD
Health Plan Bluecare

⬧ 🆂🅳 🅲 🗗 🖾 🎟 Mcr Mcd WC NFl   Immediately **VISA**
💳

Tribble, Cassandra (MD)   Anes
Greenwich Hosp
Greenwich Anesthesiology Assiciates, PC, PO Box
772; Greenwich, CT 06830; (203) 661-5330;
BDCERT: Anes 96; **MS:** U Mich Med Sch 90; **RES:**
Anes, New York University Med Ctr, New York, NY
91-94; **FEL:** Anes, Mass Gen Hosp, Boston, MA 91-
94; **SI:** *Pain Management;* **HMO:** Aetna Hlth Plan
PHS Oxford PHCS United Healthcare +

⬧ 🗗 🖾 🎟 Mcr WC   A Few Days 🎟 **VISA** 💳 💳

CARDIAC ELECTROPHYSIOLOGY

Turetsky, Arthur (MD)   CE   **PCP**
Bridgeport Hosp
15 Corporate Dr; Trumbull, CT 06601; (203) 259-
5153; **BDCERT:** CE 77; **MS:** Albert Einstein Coll
Med 74; **RES:** CE, Jacobi Med Ctr, Bronx, NY 77-79;
HMO: Aetna Hlth Plan Blue Choice Blue Cross &
Blue Shield CIGNA +

⬧ 🗗 🖾 🎟 🆂 Mcr Mcd WC   2-4 Weeks **VISA** 💳 💳

CARDIOLOGY (CARDIOVASCULAR DISEASE)

Brodsky, Samuel (MD)   Cv
Stamford Hosp
Cardiology Associates of Fairfield County, PC, 1275
Summer St; Stamford, CT 06905; (203) 353-1133;
BDCERT: IM 79; Cv 81; **MS:** SUNY Syracuse 76;
RES: IM, Boston U Med Ctr, Boston, MA 76-79; **FEL:**
Cv, Boston U Med Ctr, Boston, MA 79-81; **FAP:** Asst
Clin Prof Med NY Med Coll; **HOSP:** St Joseph's Med
Ctr-Stamford; **HMO:** US Hlthcre Oxford PHS Aetna
Hlth Plan CIGNA +

⬧ 🗗 🖾 🎟 🆂 Mcr Mcd WC NFl   1 Week 🎟 **VISA** 💳

Bull, Marcia (MD)   Cv
Stamford Hosp
PO Box 9317; Stamford, CT 06904; (203) 325-
7480; **BDCERT:** Cv 69; **MS:** Columbia P&S 62; **RES:**
IM, Columbia-Presbyterian Med Ctr, New York, NY
62-63; IM, Columbia-Presbyterian Med Ctr, New
York, NY 63-64; **FEL:** Cv, Columbia-Presbyterian
Med Ctr, New York, NY 64-69; **FAP:** Assoc Clin
Prof Med NY Med Coll; **SI:** *Hypertension; Women's
Cardiovascular Health;* **HMO:** Aetna Hlth Plan
Connecticare Medspan

⬧ 🗗 🎟 Mcr   A Few Days

Casale, Linda (MD)　　　　　Cv
Bridgeport Hosp
Cardiac Specialist of Fairfield, PC, 1305 Post Rd;
Fairfield, CT 06432; (203) 255-3441; **BDCERT:** Cv
90; IM 90; **MS:** NY Med Coll 86; **RES:** IM,
Montefiore Med Ctr, Bronx, NY 86-89; **FEL:** Cv, UC
San Diego Med Ctr, San Diego, CA 89-92; *SI:*
Women's Cardiac Health

🚹 A Few Days

Cleman, Michael (MD)　　　　Cv
Yale-New Haven Hosp
Yale Cardiology, 15 Homewood Rd; Woodbridge,
CT 06525; (203) 785-4129; **BDCERT:** IM 80; **MS:**
Johns Hopkins U 77; **RES:** IM, U FL Shands Hosp,
Gainesville, FL 77-80; **FEL:** Cv, Yale-New Haven
Hosp, New Haven, CT 80-81; **FAP:** Lecturer Med
Yale U Sch Med; **HOSP:** Hosp of St Raphael; *SI:*
Angioplasty; Cardiac Catheterization; **HMO:** CIGNA
Oxford Aetna Hlth Plan MD Health Plan Blue Cross
+

🚹 📷 🚼 🛏 💲 Mcr Mcd WC NFl Immediately 📧
VISA 💳 💳 💳

Cohen, Lawrence (MD)　　　　Cv
Yale-New Haven Hosp
333 Cedar St PO Box 208017; New Haven, CT
06520; (203) 785-4128; **BDCERT:** IM 66; Cv 67;
MS: NYU Sch Med 58; **RES:** Yale-New Haven Hosp,
New Haven, CT 58-60; Yale-New Haven Hosp,
New Haven, CT 64-65; **FEL:** Cv, Harvard Med Sch,
Cambridge, MA 62-64; *SI: Coronary Artery Disease*

🚹 📷 🚼 🛏 Mcr Mcd 1 Week 📧 *VISA* 💳 💳

Fisher, Lawrence (MD)　　　　Cv
Danbury Hosp
Danbury Internal Med Assoc, 92 Locust Ave;
Danbury, CT 06810; (203) 794-0090; **BDCERT:**
IM 88; Cv 91; **MS:** SUNY Buffalo 85; **RES:** IM,
Bronx Muncipal Hosp Ctr, Bronx, NY 86-88; **FEL:**
Albert Einstein Med Ctr, Bronx, NY 88-90; **HMO:**
Most

🚹 📷 🚼 🛏 💲 Mcr Mcd WC 1 Week *VISA* 💳

Hankin, Edwin (MD)　　　　Cv
Bridgeport Hosp
Cardiac SpecialistsFairfield, 1305 Post Rd; Fairfield,
CT 06430; (203) 255-3441; **BDCERT:** IM 69; Cv
75; **MS:** Columbia P&S 62; **RES:** IM, Bronx
Muncipal Hosp Ctr, Bronx, NY 62-66; **FEL:** Cv,
Montefiore Med Ctr, Bronx, NY 67; **FAP:** Assoc Clin
Prof Yale U Sch Med; *SI: Hypertension; Cholesterol
Lowering;* **HMO:** CIGNA United Healthcare PHS MD
Health Plan Blue Cross & Blue Shield +

🚹 📷 🚼 🛏 💲 Mcr Immediately 📧 *VISA* 💳

Herman, Michael (MD)　　　　Cv
St Vincent's Med Ctr-Bridgeport
2800 Main St; Bridgeport, CT 06606; (203) 576-
5440; **BDCERT:** Cv 71; **MS:** Northwestern U 62;
RES: IM, Peter Bent Brigham Hosp, Boston, MA 62-
64; **FEL:** Cv, Peter Bent Brigham Hosp, Boston, MA
64-66; **FAP:** Prof NY Med Coll; **HMO:** Blue Cross &
Blue Shield Connecticut Health CIGNA Empire Blue
Cross Med Span +

🚹 📷 🛏 Mcr Mcd 1 Week

Kosinski, Edward (MD)　　　　Cv
St Vincent's Med Ctr-Bridgeport
Cardiology Phycisians, 1275 Post Rd 208; Fairfield,
CT 06430; (203) 255-5514; **BDCERT:** Cv 89; **MS:**
Bowman Gray 73; **RES:** Columbia-Presbyterian
Med Ctr, New York, NY 73-76; **FEL:** Peter Bent
Brigham Hosp, Boston, MA 76-78

🚹 📷 🛏 Mcr Immediately

Neeson, Francis (MD)　　　　Cv
Greenwich Hosp
Greenwich Medical Group, 8 Greenwich Office
Park; Greenwich, CT 06831; (203) 869-6960;
BDCERT: IM 88; Cv 91; **MS:** NYU Sch Med 85; **RES:**
IM, Bronx Muncipal Hosp Ctr, Bronx, NY 85-88;
FEL: Cv, Albert Einstein Med Ctr, Bronx, NY 88-91;
FAP: Clin Instr Yale U Sch Med; **HMO:** Aetna Hlth
Plan PHS CIGNA Health Choice United Healthcare
+

LANG: Itl, Sp; 🚹 📷 🚼 🛏 💲 Mcr Mcd A Few Days
VISA 💳

Zaret, Barry (MD) Cv
Yale-New Haven Hosp

PO Box 208017, 333 Cedar St; New Haven, CT
06520; (203) 785-4127; **BDCERT:** Cv 73; IM 73;
MS: NYU Sch Med 66; **RES:** Bellevue Hosp Ctr, New
York, NY 67-69; **FEL:** Cv, Johns Hopkins Hosp,
Baltimore, MD 69-71; **FAP:** Chf Cv Yale U Sch Med;
SI: Cardiology Diagnostic Test; Cardiac Care/General;
HMO: Aetna Hlth Plan US Hlthcre MD Health Plan
CIGNA

[symbols] **VISA** [symbols]

CHILD & ADOLESCENT PSYCHIATRY

Cohen, Donald (MD) ChAP
Yale-New Haven Hosp

230 S Frontage Rd; New Haven, CT 06520; (203)
785-5759; **BDCERT:** Psyc 72; ChAP 76; **MS:** Yale
U Sch Med 66; **RES:** Psyc, Mass Mental Hlth Ctr,
Boston, MA 68-69; **FEL:** ChAP, Children's Hosp,
Boston, MA 69-70; **FAP:** Prof Yale U Sch Med; *SI:
Autism/Attention Deficit Disorders; Tourette's
Syndrome*

LANG: Fr, Ger, Sp, Yd; [symbols]
A Few Days [symbols] **VISA** [symbol]

Schowalter, John (MD) ChAP
Yale-New Haven Hosp

230 S Frontage Rd; New Haven, CT 06520; (203)
785-2516; **BDCERT:** ChAP 69; Psyc 68; **MS:** U
Wisc Med Sch 60; **RES:** Psyc, Cincinnati Gen Hosp,
Cincinnati, OH 61-63; **FEL:** ChAP, Yale-New Haven
Hosp, New Haven, CT 63-65; **FAP:** Prof Yale U Sch
Med; **HMO:** Health Choice PHS Bluecare Consumer
Hlth Network Connecticare +

[symbols] A Few Days

COLON & RECTAL SURGERY

Caushaj, Philip (MD) CRS
Bridgeport Hosp

Bridgeport Hospital, Dept of Colon & Rectal Surgery,
267 Grant St; Bridgeport, CT 06610; (203) 384-
3273; **BDCERT:** CRS 86; S 96; **MS:** Johns Hopkins
U 79; **RES:** S, Columbia-Presbyterian Med Ctr, New
York, NY 79-84; **FEL:** CRS, Lahey Clinic,
Burlington, MA 84-85; **FAP:** Prof S Yale U Sch Med;
HOSP: VA Ct Healthcare Sys; *SI: Ostomy
Alternatives; Colorectal Cancer*; **HMO:** PHS CIGNA
Connecticut Health Oxford

LANG: Alb, Fr; [symbols]
A Few Days

Guthrie, James (MD) CRS
Norwalk Hosp

148 East Ave 3B; Norwalk, CT 06851; (203) 853-
1705; **BDCERT:** CRS 75; **MS:** NYU Sch Med 61;
RES: S, Bellevue Hosp Ctr, New York, NY 61-66;
FEL: St Mark's Hosp, London, England 74; **FAP:**
Asst Prof S Yale U Sch Med; *SI: Proctology*; **HMO:**
United Healthcare CIGNA Aetna Hlth Plan Oxford
Connecticare +

[symbols] Immediately [symbol]

Littlejohn, Charles (MD) CRS
Stamford Hosp

70 Mill River St; Stamford, CT 06902; (203) 323-
8989; **BDCERT:** CRS 85; **MS:** Dartmouth Med Sch
78; **RES:** S, Rochester Gen Hosp, Rochester, NY 78-
80; S, UMDNJ Mental Health Ctr, Piscataway, NJ
80-83; **FEL:** CRS, UMDNJ Mental Health Ctr,
Piscataway, NJ 83-84; **HOSP:** St Joseph's Med Ctr-
Stamford; **HMO:** Oxford CIGNA Aetna Hlth Plan
PHCS

[symbols] 2-4 Weeks **VISA** [symbol]

DERMATOLOGY

Bolognia, Jean (MD) D
Yale-New Haven Hosp
Yale Dermatolgy Associates, 140 Patten Rd; North
Haven, CT 06473; (203) 785-4632; **BDCERT:** D
85; **MS:** Yale U Sch Med 80; **RES:** IM, Yale-New
Haven Hosp, New Haven, CT 80-82; D, Yale-New
Haven Hosp, New Haven, CT 82-85; **FAP:** Prof Yale
U Sch Med; **SI:** *Melanoma; Moles;* **HMO:** Blue Cross
PHS Aetna Hlth Plan MDNY

LANG: Sp; ♿ 🚗 📶 🏥 💲 Mcr Mcd WC 4+ Weeks **VISA**
💳

Branom Jr, Wayne (MD) D
Greenwich Hosp
Wayne Branom Jr MD, PC, 49 Lake Ave;
Greenwich, CT 06830; (203) 869-4242; **BDCERT:**
D 65; **MS:** NYU Sch Med 60; **RES:** D, New York
University Med Ctr, New York, NY 61-64

🚗 🏥 💲 Mcr 2-4 Weeks

Braverman, Irwin (MD) D
Yale-New Haven Hosp
PO Box 208059; New Haven, CT 06520; (203)
785-4632; **BDCERT:** D 63; **MS:** Yale U Sch Med 55;
RES: IM, Yale-New Haven Hosp, New Haven, CT
55-56; IM, Yale-New Haven Hosp, New Haven, CT
58-59; **FEL:** D, Yale-New Haven Hosp, New Haven,
CT 59-62; **FAP:** Prof D Yale U Sch Med; **SI:**
Cutaneous T-Cell Lymphoma; Lupus; **HMO:** Blue
Cross & Blue Shield CIGNA Aetna Hlth Plan PHS
MD Health Plan +

LANG: Sp; ♿ 🚗 🚗 🏥 💲 Mcr Mcd WC 1 Week 📷 **VISA**
💳 💳

Edelson, Richard (MD) D
Yale-New Haven Hosp
800 Howard Ave; New Haven, CT 06520; (203)
785-3466; **BDCERT:** D 77; **MS:** Yale U Sch Med 70;
RES: U Chicago Hosp, Chicago, IL 70-71; D, Mass
Gen Hosp, Boston, MA 71-72; **FAP:** Chrmn Yale U
Sch Med; **SI:** *Cutaneous T Cell Lymphoma; Mycosis
Fungioides*

♿ 🚗 🚗 🏥 💲 Mcr Mcd WC 4+ Weeks **VISA**

Friedman, Michael (MD) D
Stamford Hosp
144 Morgan St; Stamford, CT 06905; (203) 325-
3576; **BDCERT:** D 70; **MS:** U Mich Med Sch 63;
RES: D, New York University Med Ctr, New York,
NY 67-70; **FAP:** Asst Clin Prof Albert Einstein Coll
Med; **HMO:** Aetna Hlth Plan Blue Cross & Blue
Shield United Healthcare Oxford PHS +

♿ 🚗 🚗 🏥 💲 Mcr 2-4 Weeks 📷 **VISA** 💳 💳

Heald, Peter (MD) D
Yale-New Haven Hosp
Yale-New Haven Hosp—Derm, PO Box 208059;
New Haven, CT 06520; (203) 785-7057; **BDCERT:**
IM 79; **MS:** Duke U 79; **RES:** Duke U Med Ctr,
Durham, NC 19; **FEL:** Hosp of U Penn, Philadelphia,
PA 84; **HMO:** Most

♿ 🚗 🏥 💲 Mcr Mcd WC NFI 2-4 Weeks 📷 **VISA** 💳
💳

Leffell, David (MD) D
Yale-New Haven Hosp
800 Howard Ave; New Haven, CT 06520; (203)
785-3466; **BDCERT:** IM 84; N 87; **MS:** Canada 81;
RES: IM, NY Hosp-Cornell Med Ctr, New York, NY
81-84; D, Yale-New Haven Hosp, New Haven, CT
84-87; **FEL:** Dermatologic S, U Mich Med Ctr, Ann
Arbor, MI 87-88; **SI:** *Skin Cancer—Melanoma; Laser
Surgery; Moh's Surgery;* **HMO:** Aetna Hlth Plan
CIGNA PHS Oxford MD Health Plan +

LANG: Fr; ♿ 🚗 🚗 🏥 💲 Mcr Mcd WC NFI 📷 **VISA**
💳

Sibrack, Laurence (MD) D
Danbury Hosp
Dermatology Associates of Western Connecticut,
73 Sand Pit Rd 207; Danbury, CT 06810; (203)
792-4151; **BDCERT:** D 78; **MS:** U Mich Med Sch
74; **RES:** IM, Hosp of U Penn, Philadelphia, PA; **FEL:**
D, Yale-New Haven Hosp, New Haven, CT; **HOSP:**
Yale-New Haven Hosp; **HMO:** Most

LANG: Sp; ♿ 🏥 🅲 🚗 🏥 💲 Mcr Mcd WC 2-4 Weeks
VISA 💳

DIAGNOSTIC RADIOLOGY

Cohen, Steven (MD) DR
Stamford Hosp

Stamford Radiological Assocs PC, PO Box 1092; Stamford, CT 06904; (203) 359-0130; **BDCERT:** DR 87; **MS:** NY Med Coll 83; **RES:** IM, Stamford Hosp, Stamford, CT 83-84; DR, Montefiore Med Ctr, Bronx, NY 84-87; **FEL:** Diagnostic Imaging, Thomas Jefferson U Hosp, Philadelphia, PA 88-89; **FAP:** Asst Clin Prof Rad NY Med Coll; *SI: Ultrasound; Body Imaging;* **HMO:** Aetna Hlth Plan Blue Cross & Blue Shield CIGNA

🦽 Immediately *VISA* 💳

Lee, Ronald (MD) DR
Norwalk Hosp

Norwalk Radiology Consultants, PC, Ave; Norwalk, CT 06851; (203) 852-2720; **BDCERT:** Rad 91; **MS:** NYU Sch Med 86; **RES:** IM, Albert Einstein Med Ctr, Bronx, NY 86-87; Rad, New York University Med Ctr, New York, NY 87-91; **FEL:** MRI, Johns Hopkins Hosp, Baltimore, MD 91-92; *SI: MRI; CT Scan;* **HMO:** Aetna Hlth Plan PHS Connecticare CIGNA Oxford +

🦽 🅢🅞 🌙 ⏰ 🚹 🏧 💲 Mcr Mcd WC A Few Days *VISA* 💳

McCarthy, Shirley (MD & PhD)DR
Yale-New Haven Hosp

333 Cedar St; New Haven, CT 06520; (203) 785-6144; **BDCERT:** DR 83; **MS:** Yale U Sch Med 79; **RES:** Rad, Yale-New Haven Hosp, New Haven, CT 83; **FEL:** UC San Francisco Med Ctr, San Francisco, CA; *SI: Gynecologic Imaging*

🦽 ⏰ 🚹 🏧 Mcr Mcd WC NFI A Few Days

EMERGENCY MEDICINE

Dell'Aria, Joseph (MD) EM
St Vincent's Med Ctr-Bridgeport

St Vincent's Med Ctr Emergency Medicine, 2800 Main St; Bridgeport, CT 06606; (203) 576-5438; **BDCERT:** EM 97; **MS:** SUNY Buffalo 84; **RES:** EM, NC Baptist Hosp, Winston-Salem, NC 84-87; *SI: Emergency Care; Trauma Care;* **HMO:** Blue Cross & Blue Shield PHS MD Health Plan CIGNA

LANG: Sp; 🦽 🅢🅞 🌙 ⏰ 🚹 🏧 Mcr Mcd WC NFI Immediately

Maisel, Jonathan (MD) EM
Bridgeport Hosp

Bridgeport Hospital, 267 Grant St; Bridgeport, CT 06610; (203) 384-3319; **BDCERT:** EM 88; IM 85; **MS:** SUNY Downstate 82; **RES:** IM, Bronx Muncipal Hosp Ctr, Bronx, NY 82-85; EM, Bronx Muncipal Hosp Ctr, Bronx, NY 85-87; **FAP:** Asst Clin Prof Yale U Sch Med; *SI: Acute Stroke Treatments; Rabies Immunization;* **HMO:** Blue Cross & Blue Shield CIGNA Metlife

🦽 🅢🅞 🌙 ⏰ 🚹 🏧 Mcr Mcd WC NFI 1 Week ▦ *VISA* 💳 ▦

Smothers, Kevin (MD) EM
Greenwich Hosp

Greenwich Hosp-Dept of Emerg Medicine, Five Perryridge Rd; Greenwich, CT 06830; (203) 863-3632; **BDCERT:** EM 90; IM 84; **MS:** SUNY Stony Brook 81; **RES:** EM, Mt Zion Hosp, San Francisco, CA 81-84

🦽 🅢🅞 🌙 ⏰ 🚹 🏧 💲 Mcr Mcd WC NFI Immediately ▦ *VISA* 💳 ▦

Turnbull, Dorothy (MD) EM
Stamford Hosp

The Stamford Hospital Emergency Department, 41 Maywood Rd; Stamford, CT 06902; (203) 325-7595; **BDCERT:** EM 96; IM 79; **MS:** Med Coll PA 76; **RES:** IM, Stamford Hosp, Stamford, CT 76-77; IM, Stamford Hosp, Stamford, CT 77-79; **FAP:** Clin Instr NY Med Coll

🦽 🅢🅞 🌙 ⏰ 🚹 🏧 💲 Mcr Mcd WC NFI Immediately ▦ *VISA* 💳 ▦

ENDOCRINOLOGY, DIABETES & METABOLISM

Arden-Cordone, Mary (MD)EDM
Greenwich Hosp
4 Dearfield Dr 107; Greenwich, CT 06831; (203) 622-9160; **BDCERT:** IM 92; EDM 95; **MS:** NYU Sch Med 89; **RES:** IM, Columbia-Presbyterian Med Ctr, New York, NY 89-92; **FEL:** EDM, Columbia-Presbyterian Med Ctr, New York, NY 92-95; **FAP:** Clin Instr EDM Columbia P&S; *SI: Osteoporosis/Thyroid Disease*
⬧ 🔊 ▣ ▦ $ ☒ 2-4 Weeks

Burrow, Gerard (MD)   EDM
Yale-New Haven Hosp
PO Box 208055; New Haven, CT 06520; (203) 733-7932; **BDCERT:** IM 65; **MS:** Yale U Sch Med 58; **RES:** Yale-New Haven Hosp, New Haven, CT 58-59; **FEL:** EDM, Yale-New Haven Hosp, New Haven, CT 63-65; *SI: Thyroid; Thyroid & Pregnancy;* **HMO:** Aetna Hlth Plan Anthem Health CIGNA Connecticare Kaiser Permanente +
⬧ 🔊 ▦ ☒ ☒ ☒ ☒ 2-4 Weeks ▦ **VISA** ●

Engel, Samuel (MD)   EDM
Norwalk Hosp
83 East Ave 213; Norwalk, CT 06851; (203) 853-2746; **BDCERT:** IM 81; EDM 83; **MS:** NYU Sch Med 78; **RES:** IM, Bronx Muncipal Hosp Ctr, Bronx, NY 78-81; **FEL:** EDM, Albert Einstein Med Ctr, Bronx, NY 81-83; **FAP:** Assoc Clin Prof Med Albert Einstein Coll Med
⬧ 🔊 ▦ $ 1 Week

Padilla, Alfred (MD)   EDM
Greenwich Hosp
4 Dearfield Dr 102; Greenwich, CT 06831; (203) 622-9160; **BDCERT:** IM 75; **MS:** Northwestern U 72; **RES:** IM, Rush Presbyterian-St Lukes Med Ctr, Chicago, IL 72-73; IM, U Chicago Hosp, Chicago, IL 73-75; **FEL:** EDM, Columbia-Presbyterian Med Ctr, New York, NY 75-77; **FAP:** Asst Clin Prof Yale U Sch Med; **HOSP:** Montefiore Med Ctr
LANG: Sp, Ger, Fr; ⬧ 🔊 ▣ ▦ $ 1 Week

Robin, Noel (MD)   EDM
Stamford Hosp
PO Box 9317; Stamford, CT 06904; (203) 325-7485; **BDCERT:** IM 70; **MS:** SUNY Hlth Sci Ctr 65; **RES:** Long Island Jewish Med Ctr, New Hyde Park, NY 65-68; **FEL:** EDM, Peter Bent Brigham Hosp, Boston, MA; **FAP:** Prof Med NY Med Coll
LANG: Sp, Itl; ⬧ 🔊 ▣ ▦ ☒ ☒ 1 Week

Rosen, Stephen (MD)   EDM
Stamford Hosp
Stamford Endocrinology, PC, 166 W Broad Rd 303; Stamford, CT 06902; (203) 359-2444; **BDCERT:** EDM 85; IM 82; **MS:** NYU Sch Med 78; **RES:** Med, Barnes Hosp, St Louis, MO 78-81; **FEL:** Metabolism, Barnes Hosp, St Louis, MO 81-83; **FAP:** Assoc Clin Prof Med Cornell U; **HOSP:** Greenwich Hosp; *SI: Diabetes Mellitus; Thyroid Diseases;* **HMO:** Aetna Hlth Plan Oxford United Healthcare Blue Cross PHS +
⬧ 🔊 ▦ $ ☒ 1 Week **VISA** ●

FAMILY PRACTICE

Acosta, Rod (MD)   FP   PCP
Stamford Hosp
Stamford Family Practice, 2009 Summer St; Stamford, CT 06905; (203) 977-2566; **BDCERT:** FP 87; Ger 92; **MS:** U Tex SW, Dallas 84; **RES:** St Joseph's Med Ctr-Stamford, Stamford, CT 84-87; **HOSP:** St Joseph's Med Ctr-Stamford; *SI: Preventive Care;* **HMO:** Aetna Hlth Plan Oxford PHS CIGNA Prudential +
LANG: Itl, Sp; ⬧ ▦ ☒ 🔊 ▣ ▦ $ ☒ ☒ ☒ A Few Days **VISA** ●

Filiberto, Cosmo (MD)   FP   PCP
St Vincent's Med Ctr-Bridgeport
Family Practice Assoc, 3715 Main St; Bridgeport, CT 06606; (203) 372-4065; **BDCERT:** FP 80; Ger 90; **MS:** Italy 76; **RES:** Lutheran Med Ctr, Brooklyn, NY 76-80; **HOSP:** Bridgeport Hosp; *SI: Geriatric Medicine*
⬧ ▦ ☒ 🔊 ▣ $ ☒ ☒ ☒ ☒ 2-4 Weeks **VISA** ●

Zalichin, Henry (MD)   FP   PCP
Stamford Hosp

New England Primary Care, 555 Newfield Ave; Stamford, CT 06905; (203) 359-4444; **BDCERT:** FP 70; **MS:** SUNY Hlth Sci Ctr 53; **RES:** Stamford Hosp, Stamford, CT 54; **HOSP:** St Joseph's Med Ctr-Stamford; **SI:** *Cardiology*

LANG: Rus, Yd, Ger, Fr; ♿ 🅿 🚹 🏨 $ Mcr Mcd WC NFI A Few Days **VISA** ●

GASTROENTEROLOGY

Gardner, Peter (MD)   Ge
Stamford Hosp

Gastroenterology Consultants, 166 W Broad St 303; Stamford, CT 06905; (203) 967-2100; **BDCERT:** IM 82; Ge 87; **MS:** Georgetown U 79; **RES:** IM, St Vincent's Med Ctr-Bridgeport, Bridgeport, CT 79-82; **FEL:** Ge, U Conn Hlth Ctr, Farmington, CT 82-84; **FAP:** Assoc Prof NY Med Coll; **HOSP:** St Joseph's Med Ctr-Stamford; **HMO:** Aetna Hlth Plan Oxford US Hlthcre PHS CIGNA +

♿ 🚹 🏨 $ A Few Days **VISA** ●

Gordon, Donald G (MD)   Ge
Danbury Hosp

16 Hospital Ave 303; Danbury, CT 06810; (203) 731-3173; **BDCERT:** Ge 87; **MS:** Emory U Sch Med 81; **RES:** Emory U Hosp, Atlanta, GA 81-82; **FEL:** Med Coll of GA Hosp, Augusta, GA 84-86; **HMO:** Blue Cross Bluecare PHS Aetna Hlth Plan

LANG: Sp; ♿ SA/SU 🅿 🚹 🏨 $ Mcr Mcd NFI A Few Days **VISA** ●

Grossman, Edward (MD)   Ge
St Vincent's Med Ctr-Bridgeport

Gastroenterology Assoc of Fairfield Cty PC, 1305 Post Rd; Fairfield, CT 06430; (203) 255-3441; **BDCERT:** Ge 73; IM 70; **MS:** Albert Einstein Coll Med 63; **RES:** Albert Einstein Med Ctr, Bronx, NY 63-64; **FEL:** NY Hosp-Cornell Med Ctr, New York, NY 68-70; **FAP:** Assoc Clin Prof Yale U Sch Med; **HMO:** PHS CIGNA Aetna Hlth Plan Prucare

♿ SA/SU 🅿 🚹 🏨 $ Mcr Mcd 2-4 Weeks ●

Gruss, Claudia (MD)   Ge
Norwalk Hosp

73 Redding Rd; Georgetown, CT 06829; (203) 544-9517; **BDCERT:** IM 80; Ge 83; **MS:** Brown U 77; **RES:** Rhode Island Hosp, Providence, RI 77-80; **FEL:** Ge, Rhode Island Hosp, Providence, RI 80-82; **HOSP:** Danbury Hosp

Mauer, Kenneth (MD)   Ge
St Vincent's Med Ctr-Bridgeport

1305 Post Rd; Fairfield, CT 06430; (203) 255-3441; **BDCERT:** IM 86; Ge 89; **MS:** NYU Sch Med 83; **RES:** Bronx Muni Hosp Ctr, Bronx, NY 83-87; **FEL:** Ge, Mount Sinai Med Ctr, New York, NY 87-89

Scheinbaum, Richard (MD)   Ge
Stamford Hosp

1275 Summer St; Stamford, CT 06905; (203) 348-5355; **BDCERT:** Ge 87; **MS:** Temple U 79; **RES:** S, Mount Siani Hosp, New York, NY 80-81; Stamford Hosp, Stamford, CT 81-83; **FEL:** Ge, Cedars-Sinai Med Ctr, Los Angeles, CA 83-87

Taubin, Howard L (MD)   Ge
Bridgeport Hosp

Gastroenterology Associates, 2590 Main St; Stratford, CT 06497; (203) 375-1200; **BDCERT:** IM 72; Ge 72; **MS:** U Va Sch Med 65; **RES:** IM, Montefiore Med Ctr, Bronx, NY 65-67; IM, Yale-New Haven Hosp, New Haven, CT 69-70; **FEL:** Ge, Yale-New Haven Hosp, New Haven, CT 70-73; **FAP:** Assoc Clin Prof Yale U Sch Med; **HMO:** Aetna Hlth Plan Blue Cross & Blue Shield CIGNA MD Health Plan PHS +

♿ 🅿 🚹 🏨 $ Mcr Mcd A Few Days

Traube, Morris (MD)   Ge
Yale-New Haven Hosp
Yale Faculty PraticeSection of Digestive Diseases,
333 Cedar; New Haven, CT 06520; (203) 785-
4395; **BDCERT:** IM 81; Ge 83; **MS:** SUNY Hlth Sci
Ctr 78; **RES:** IM, Maimonides Med Ctr, Brooklyn,
NY 78-81; **FEL:** Ge, Yale-New Haven Hosp, New
Haven, CT 81-84; **FAP:** Prof Med Yale U Sch Med;
SI: Swallowing Disorders; Esophageal Diseases

🚻 📠 🅿 🎬 Mcr Mcd

Waldstreicher, Stuart (MD)   Ge
Stamford Hosp
Gastroenterology Consultants, 166 W Broad St
#303; Stamford, CT 06902; (203) 967-2100;
BDCERT: IM 85; **MS:** NY Med Coll 82; **RES:**
Overlook Hosp, Summit, NJ 83-85; **FEL:** NY Med
Coll, Valhalla, NY 85-87; *SI: Endoscopic Laser
Therapy; Inflammatory Bowel Disease*; **HMO:** PHS
Oxford Aetna Hlth Plan US Hlthcre CIGNA +

LANG: Heb; 🚻 📠 🅿 🎬 💲 Mcr Mcd   Immediately
VISA 💳

GERIATRIC MEDICINE

Spivack, Barney (MD)   Ger
Stamford Hosp
Stamford Hospital, Dept of Geriatric Medicine, 26
Palmer's Hill Rd; Stamford, CT 06904; (203) 967-
6120; **BDCERT:** Ger 90; Rhu 84; **MS:** Mt Sinai Sch
Med 78; **RES:** IM, Bellevue Hosp Ctr, New York, NY
78-81; **FEL:** Rhu, Rhode Island Hosp, Providence,
RI 81-83; **FAP:** Assoc Prof Columbia P&S; *SI:
Mobility Problems; Dementia*; **HMO:** Oxford Blue
Cross PHS

🚻 📠 🅿 🎬 Mcr Mcd   A Few Days

Tinetti, Mary (MD)   Ger
Yale-New Haven Hosp
20 York St; New Haven, CT 06504; (203) 785-
5238; **BDCERT:** Ger 88; **MS:** U Mich Med Sch 78;
FEL: Ger, Strong Mem Hosp, Rochester, NY 81-84;
SI: Mobility and Falls; Geriatric Assessment

🚻 🅿 🎬 Mcr Mcd   2-4 Weeks

GERIATRIC PSYCHIATRY

van Dyck, Christopher H (MD) GerPsy
Yale-New Haven Hosp
333 Cedar St Rm CB2041; New Haven, CT 06520;
(203) 785-5286; **BDCERT:** 94; **MS:** Northwestern
U 84; **RES:** Psyc, Yale-New Haven Hosp, New
Haven, CT 84-88; **FAP:** Prof Psyc Yale U Sch Med

GYNECOLOGIC ONCOLOGY

Chambers, Joseph (MD)   GO
Yale-New Haven Hosp
PO Box 208063; New Haven, CT 06520; (203)
785-5778; **BDCERT:** ObG 85; GO 87; **MS:**
Georgetown U 77; **RES:** U of VA Health Sci Ctr,
Charlottesville, VA 77-81; **FEL:** GO, Yale-New
Haven Hosp, New Haven, CT 82-84; **FAP:** Assoc
Prof Yale U Sch Med

Kohorn, Ernest (MD)   GO
Yale-New Haven Hosp
Yale University Dept Gynecology, PO Box 208063;
New Haven, CT 06520; (203) 785-4013; **BDCERT:**
GO 74; **MS:** England 52; **RES:** S, Hosp For Sick
Children, London, England 57-58; ObG, Charlotte
Chelsea Hosp, England 61-62; **FEL:** GO, Middlesex
Hosp, London, England 62-64; **FAP:** Prof Yale U
Sch Med; **HOSP:** Greenwich Hosp; *SI: Stress Urinary
Incontinence; Prolapse Pelvic Organs*

LANG: Ger; 🚻 📠 🎬 Mcr Mcd WC   Immediately

Koulos, John (MD)   GO
St Vincents Hosp & Med Ctr NY

U Conn Health Center, 153 W 11th St GynOnc Rm
L2092; Farmington, CT 06032; (860) 674-2570;
BDCERT: ObG 86; GO 92; **MS:** Northwestern U 78;
RES: ObG, Northwestern Mem Hosp, Chicago, IL
79-82; **FEL:** GO, Mem Sloan Kettering Cancer Ctr,
New York, NY 82-84; **FAP:** Asst Prof GO U Conn
Sch Med; *SI: Gynecologic Oncology;* **HMO:** Empire
Blue Cross & Shield Oxford US Hlthcre GHI Prucare
+

♿ 📷 🚗 🏨 **S** Mcr Mcd

Schwartz, Peter (MD)   GO
Yale-New Haven Hosp

333 Cedar St Suite FM13316; New Haven, CT
06520; (203) 785-4135; **BDCERT:** GO 78; ObG 73;
MS: Albert Einstein Coll Med 66; **RES:** S, U KY Hosp,
Lexington, KY 66-67; ObG, Yale-New Haven Hosp,
New Haven, CT 67-71; **FEL:** GO, MD Anderson
Cancer Ctr, Houston, TX 71-73; **FAP:** Prof Yale U
Sch Med; **HOSP:** Greenwich Hosp; *SI: Ovarian
Cancer; Gynecological Surgery*

♿ 📷 🏨 **S** Mcr Mcd   A Few Days

HAND SURGERY

Ariyan, Stephan (MD)   HS
Yale-New Haven Hosp

60 Temple St; New Haven, CT 06511; (203) 773-
8000; **BDCERT:** PlS 77; S 78; **MS:** NY Med Coll 66;
RES: S, UC San Diego Med Ctr, San Diego, CA 67-
68; Yale-New Haven Hosp, New Haven, CT 71-73;
FEL: Yale-New Haven Hosp, New Haven, CT 70-71;
PlS, Yale-New Haven Hosp, New Haven, CT 73-76;
FAP: Prof S Yale U Sch Med; **HOSP:** Hosp of St
Raphael; *SI: Cosmetic Surgery; Melanoma*

♿ 🚗 🏨 **S** Mcr   A Few Days   *VISA* 💳

Rago, Thomas (MD)   HS
Bridgeport Hosp

Hand Surgery of CT, 3101 Main St; Bridgeport, CT
06606; (203) 374-5892; **BDCERT:** OrS 86; HS 97;
MS: Columbia P&S 77; **RES:** S, Roosevelt Hosp, New
York, NY 78-79; OrS, Presby Hosp-Upittsburgh,
Pittsburgh, PA 79-82; **FEL:** HS, Columbia-
Presbyterian Med Ctr, New York, NY 82-83; **FAP:**
Instr OrS Columbia P&S; **HOSP:** St Vincent's Med
Ctr-Bridgeport; **HMO:** PHS Prucare Aetna Hlth
Plan CIGNA

♿ 🚗 🏨 **S** Mcr Mcd WC   Immediately *VISA* 💳

Sprague, Bruce (MD)   HS
Norwalk Hosp

Surgery of the Hand and Upper Extremity, PC, 148
East Ave 2E; Norwalk, CT 06851; (203) 853-2967;
BDCERT: OrS 73; HS 89; **MS:** Univ Penn 64; **RES:** S,
U IA Hosp, Iowa City, IA 67-69; OrS, U Tenn Hosp,
Memphis, TN 69-72; **FEL:** HS, U IA Hosp, Iowa City,
IA 68; **FAP:** Asst Clin Prof Columbia P&S; **HOSP:**
Stamford Hosp; **HMO:** Blue Cross & Blue Shield
Travelers Oxford Aetna Hlth Plan

♿ 🚗 🏨 **S** WC   Immediately

HEMATOLOGY

Bar, Michael (MD)   Hem
Stamford Hosp

Hematology Oncology, 34 Shelburne Rd; Stamford,
CT 06902; (203) 325-7199; **BDCERT:** Onc 89;
Hem 90; **MS:** Columbia P&S 83; **RES:** Columbia-
Presbyterian Med Ctr, New York, NY 83-86; **FEL:**
Hem, UC San Francisco Med Ctr, San Francisco, CA
86; **HOSP:** St Joseph's Med Ctr-Stamford; *SI: Bone
Marrow Transplantation; Hematologic Disorders;*
HMO: Oxford Aetna Hlth Plan Blue Cross & Blue
Shield CIGNA Prudential +

LANG: Sp; ♿ 📷 🚗 🏨 **S** Mcr Mcd   A Few Days

Beardsley, Diana (MD & PhD) Hem
Yale-New Haven Hosp

333 Cedar St; New Haven, CT 06520; (203) 785-4640; **BDCERT:** Ped 87; **MS:** Duke U 87; **RES:** Children's Hosp, Boston, MA 76-77; **FEL:** Hem, Children's Hosp, Boston, MA; *SI: Hemophilia; Vascular Anomalies/Hemangioma*

 ⌖ ▣ ▣ ▦ Mcr Mcd WC NFl Immediately

Duffy, Thomas (MD)   Hem
Yale-New Haven Hosp

333 Cedar St; New Haven, CT 06520; (203) 785-4144; **BDCERT:** IM 72; Hem 74; **MS:** Johns Hopkins U 62; **RES:** Johns Hopkins Hosp, Baltimore, MD 62-66; **FEL:** Hem, Johns Hopkins Hosp, Baltimore, MD 68-70; **FAP:** Prof Yale U Sch Med; *SI: Mast Cell Disease; Diagnostic Hematology Problems*

 ⌖ ▣ ▦ Mcr Mcd 2-4 Weeks

Forget, Bernard (MD)   Hem
Yale-New Haven Hosp

Yale University School of Medicine Faculty Practice Plan, 333 Cedar St; New Haven, CT 06510; (203) 785-4144; **BDCERT:** IM 71; Hem 73; **MS:** Canada 63; **RES:** IM, Mass Gen Hosp, Boston, MA 63-65; **FEL:** Hem, Peter Bent Brigham Hosp, Boston, MA 69-71; **FAP:** Prof Hem Yale U Sch Med; *SI: Hemolytic Anemias; Thalassemia*; **HMO:** Blue Cross & Blue Shield Aetna Hlth Plan PHS

LANG: Fr; ⌖ ▣ ▣ ▦ Mcr Mcd NFl 2-4 Weeks ▦
VISA ● ▣

Kloss, Robert (MD)   Hem
Danbury Hosp

Danbury Office Of Physicians, 95 Locust Ave FL2; Danbury, CT 06810; (203) 797-7029; **BDCERT:** IM 79; Onc 81; **MS:** Jefferson Med Coll 76; **RES:** IM, Univ Hosp SUNY Buffalo, Buffalo, NY 76-79; **FEL:** Hem Onc, Columbia-Presbyterian Med Ctr, New York, NY 79-81; *SI: Breast Cancer; Leukemia*; **HMO:** Aetna Hlth Plan Blue Cross & Blue Shield CIGNA Oxford Prucare +

 ⌖ ▣ ▦ S Mcr Mcd A Few Days ▦ ***VISA*** ● ▣

INFECTIOUS DISEASE

Hindes, Robert G (MD)   Inf
Danbury Hosp

Danbury Hosp, 24 Hospital Ave; Danbury, CT 06810; (203) 797-7413; **BDCERT:** Inf 86; IM 83; **MS:** UMDNJ-NJ Med Sch, Newark 80; **RES:** Hosp Med College of PA, Philadelphia, PA 80-83; **FEL:** Inf, New England Deaconess Hosp, Boston, MA; Harvard Med Sch, Boston, MA

Kim, Grace (MD)   Inf
St Vincent's Med Ctr-Bridgeport

2800 Main St; Bridgeport, CT 06606; (203) 576-5330; **BDCERT:** IM 90; Inf 97; **MS:** Northwestern U 86; **RES:** IM, St Vincent's Med Ctr-Bridgeport, Bridgeport, CT 87-90; **FEL:** Inf, Yale-New Haven Hosp, New Haven, CT 90-92; *SI: Traveler's Pre & Post Evaluation*

LANG: Kor; ⌖ ▣ ▣ ▦ Mcr Mcd WC NFl 1 Week

Kunkel, Mark (MD)   Inf
Danbury Hosp

24 Hospital Ave; Danbury, CT 06810; (203) 797-7413; **BDCERT:** IM 78; Inf 80; **MS:** Tufts U 75; **RES:** Boston U Med Ctr, Boston, MA 75-77; **FEL:** Inf, Albert Einstein Med Ctr, Bronx, NY 77-80; **FAP:** Asst Clin Prof Med Yale U Sch Med; *SI: Lyme Disease; Travel Medicine*; **HMO:** Most

LANG: Sp; ⌖ ▣ ▦ S Mcr Mcd WC 1 Week ▦ ***VISA***
● ▣

McLeod, Gavin (MD)   Inf
Stamford Hosp

Infectious Disease Associates, 190 W Broad St; Stamford, CT 06902; (203) 325-0146; **BDCERT:** Inf 92; IM 88; **MS:** U Conn Sch Med 85; **RES:** NY Hosp-Cornell Med Ctr, New York, NY 85-88; **FEL:** Boston Med Ctr, Boston, MA 89-92; **HOSP:** St Joseph's Med Ctr-Stamford; *SI: General Infections; HIV*; **HMO:** Oxford PHS Aetna Hlth Plan Blue Cross

 ⌖ ▣ ▣ ▦ S Mcr Mcd WC NFl A Few Days

Guide to symbols and abbreviations can be found on pages 110-113.

1049

Parry, Michael (MD)　　　Inf
Stamford Hosp

Infectious Disease Assoc, PO Box 9317; Stamford, CT 06904; (203) 325-0146; **BDCERT:** IM 74; Inf 78; **MS:** Columbia P&S 70; **RES:** Med, Columbia-Presbyterian Med Ctr, New York, NY 73-74; **FEL:** Inf, Columbia-Presbyterian Med Ctr, New York, NY 74-76; **FAP:** Prof of Clin Med Columbia P&S; *SI: HIV Infection; Hospital Acquired Infections*; **HMO:** Aetna Hlth Plan PHCS Med Span Oxford

LANG: Sp; ☒ 2-4 Weeks

Quagriarello, Vincent (MD)　Inf
Yale-New Haven Hosp

28 Justine Dr; North Haven, CT 06473; (203) 785-7570; **BDCERT:** Inf 89; IM 85; **MS:** Washington U, St Louis 80; **RES:** IM, Yale-New Haven Hosp, New Haven, CT 80-84; **FEL:** Inf, U of VA Health Sci Ctr, Charlottesville, VA 84-87; **FAP:** Assoc Prof Yale U Sch Med; *SI: Meningitis; Pneumonia*

☒ ▦ ⓢ Mcr Mod 2-4 Weeks ▦ **VISA** ⬤

Sabetta, James (MD)　　　Inf
Greenwich Hosp

5 Perryridge Rd; Greenwich, CT 06830; (203) 869-8838; **BDCERT:** Inf 84; IM 81; **MS:** Brown U 78; **RES:** IM, U NC Hosp, Chapel Hill, NC 78-79; IM, RI Hosp/Brown U, Providence, RI 79-81; **FEL:** Inf, Yale-New Haven Hosp, New Haven, CT 81-84; **HMO:** Aetna Hlth Plan PHCS

☒ ⓞ ▦ ▦ ⓢ Mcr WC A Few Days

Saul, Zane (MD)　　　　　Inf
Bridgeport Hosp

2600 Post Rd; Southport, CT 06490; (203) 259-8087; **BDCERT:** IM 90; Inf 84; **MS:** Grenada 85; **RES:** IM, Brooklyn Hosp Ctr, Brooklyn, NY 86-88; Hackensack U Med Ctr, Hackensack, NJ 88-90; **HOSP:** Norwalk Hosp; *SI: Lyme Disease; HIV*; **HMO:** Most

☒ ⓞ ▦ ▦ ⓢ Mcr Mod WC NFI A Few Days

Yee, Arthur (MD)　　　Inf　PCP
Norwalk Hosp

40 Cross St; Norwalk, CT 06851; (203) 845-2136; **BDCERT:** IM 86; Inf 88; **MS:** U Conn Sch Med 82; **RES:** IM, Columbia-Presbyterian Med Ctr, New York, NY 82-85; **FEL:** Inf, Hosp of U Penn, Philadelphia, PA 85-88; **FAP:** Asst Clin Prof Med Yale U Sch Med; *SI: Lyme Disease; Respiratory Infections*; **HMO:** Oxford Aetna Hlth Plan Blue Cross & Blue Choice US Hlthcre +

☒ ▦ ⓒ ⓞ ▦ ▦ ⓢ Mcr Mod WC A Few Days **VISA** ⬤

INTERNAL MEDICINE

Barry, Michele (MD)　　　IM
Yale-New Haven Hosp

PO Box 208025, 333 Cedar St; New Haven, CT 06520; (203) 688-2476; **BDCERT:** IM 80; **MS:** Albert Einstein Coll Med 77; **RES:** Med, Yale-New Haven Hosp, New Haven, CT 77-81; **FEL:** Rhu, Yale-New Haven Hosp, New Haven, CT 80-81; Walter Reed Army Med Ctr, Washington, DC 81; **FAP:** Prof Med Yale U Sch Med; *SI: Tropical Diseases; Travelers Health*; **HMO:** Blue Cross & Blue Shield Aetna Hlth Plan CIGNA

☒ ▦ ▦ Mcr Mod 2-4 Weeks

Benjamin, Burton (MD)　　IM　PCP
Stamford Hosp

Internal Medicine Associates of Stamford, PC, 51 Schuyler Ave; Stamford, CT 06902; (203) 327-1187; **BDCERT:** IM 87; **MS:** Columbia P&S 61; **RES:** IM, U of VA Health Sci Ctr, Charlottesville, VA 61-65; **FAP:** Assoc Clin Prof Med Columbia P&S; **HMO:** Aetna-US Healthcare CIGNA Oxford PHS Anthem Health +

LANG: Sp; ☒ ▦ ⓞ ▦ ▦ ⓢ Mcr NFI 1 Week **VISA** ⬤

Blumberg, Joel (MD)   IM   PCP
Greenwich Hosp

2 1/2 Dearfield Dr; Greenwich, CT 06831; (203) 661-4242; **BDCERT:** IM 72; Cv 74; **MS:** NYU Sch Med 66; **RES:** IM, Bellevue Hosp Ctr, New York, NY 69-71; **FEL:** Cv, NY Hosp-Cornell Med Ctr, New York, NY 71-73; **FAP:** Asst Clin Prof Yale U Sch Med; *SI: Preventive Cardiology; Hypertension*; **HMO:** Aetna-US Healthcare Health Choice Health Source PHCS Connecticut Health +

  2-4 Weeks

Boyd, D Barry (MD)   IM
Greenwich Hosp

Greenwich Medical Group, 8 Greenwich Office Park; Greenwich, CT 06831; (203) 869-6960; **BDCERT:** IM 82; Onc 87; **MS:** Cornell U 79; **RES:** IM, NY Hosp-Cornell Med Ctr, New York, NY 79-82; **FEL:** Hem Onc, NY Hosp-Cornell Med Ctr, New York, NY 83-86; **FAP:** Asst Clin Prof Yale U Sch Med; *SI: Nutrition in Cancer Treatment; Prevention of Cancer*; **HMO:** Oxford PHS CIGNA United Healthcare

LANG: Itl, Sp;   A Few Days **VISA**

Brenner, Stephen D (MD)   IM   PCP
Yale-New Haven Hosp

129 York St; New Haven, CT 06511; (203) 789-8888; **BDCERT:** IM 75; **MS:** SUNY Syracuse 70; **RES:** IM, Philadelphia Gen Hosp, Philadelphia, PA 70-72; IM, Roger Williams Med Ctr, Providence, RI 74-75; **FAP:** Assoc Clin Prof Med Yale U Sch Med; **HOSP:** Hosp of St Raphael; *SI: Preventive Health Care-Risk Reduction; Health Maintenance*; **HMO:** Oxford CIGNA CIGNA Connecticare Medspan +

  2-4 Weeks

Cooper, Milton (MD)   IM   PCP
St Vincent's Med Ctr-Bridgeport

Medical Specialists of Fairfield, 425 Post Rd; Fairfield, CT 06430; (203) 255-4545; **BDCERT:** IM 58; **MS:** Cornell U 48; **RES:** Mary Hitchcock Mem Hosp, Hanover, NH 48-49; **FEL:** Mayo Clinic, Rochester, MN 53-56; **HMO:** Blue Choice Blue Cross & Blue Shield CIGNA Travelers US Hlthcre +

  A Few Days

Cooper, Robert (MD)   IM
Danbury Hosp

Danbury Internal Med Assoc, 92 Locust Ave; Danbury, CT 06810; (203) 792-5303; **BDCERT:** Onc 74; IM 74; **MS:** Univ Pittsburgh 71; **RES:** Pennsylvania Hosp, Philadelphia, PA 71-74; **FEL:** U CO Hosp, Denver, CO 74-76; **FAP:** Asst Clin Prof Med Yale U Sch Med; *SI: Innovative Treatments*; **HMO:** Blue Cross Oxford Aetna Hlth Plan PHS

  1 Week **VISA**

Covey, William (MD)   IM   PCP
Bridgeport Hosp

Pri Med, LLC, 2590 Main St; Stratford, CT 06497; (203) 377-2626; **BDCERT:** IM 68; Hem 74; **MS:** Columbia P&S 62; **RES:** Kings County Hosp Ctr, Brooklyn, NY 63-67; **FEL:** Hem, Yale-New Haven Hosp, New Haven, CT 67-69; **FAP:** Assoc Prof Yale U Sch Med; *SI: Diseases of Blood*; **HMO:** PHS CIGNA Aetna Hlth Plan Oxford

  1 Week **VISA**

Dreyer, Neil (MD)   IM   PCP
Stamford Hosp

Internal Medicine Assoc of Stamford, PC, 51 Schuyler Ave; Stamford, CT 06902; (203) 327-1187; **BDCERT:** IM 72; Nep 74; **MS:** NYU Sch Med 67; **RES:** IM, Bellevue Hosp Ctr, New York, NY 67-68; IM, Bronx Muncipal Hosp Ctr, Bronx, NY 70-72; **FEL:** Nep, Albert Einstein Med Ctr, Bronx, NY 72-73; *SI: Hypertension; Preventive Medicine*; **HMO:** Aetna Hlth Plan Oxford PHS CIGNA Connecticare +

LANG: Sp;   1 Week **VISA**

Garrell, Marvin (MD)   IM
St Vincent's Med Ctr-Bridgeport

Primed, 2228 Black Rock Tpke 211; Fairfield, CT 06432; (203) 366-3869; **BDCERT:** IM 63; **MS:** Univ Vt Coll Med 52; **RES:** VA Med Ctr-Brooklyn, Brooklyn, NY 53; **FAP:** Assoc Clin Prof IM Yale U Sch Med; **HMO:** Blue Cross & Blue Shield CIGNA

  1 Week **VISA**

Herbin, Joseph (MD)   IM   PCP
St Vincent's Med Ctr-Bridgeport

2228 Black Rock Tpke 211; Fairfield, CT 06432; (203) 366-3869; **BDCERT:** IM 72; **MS:** Switzerland 65; **RES:** IM, St Vincent's Med Ctr-Bridgeport, Bridgeport, CT 67-70; **FEL:** Inf, Med Ctr Hosp of VT, Burlington, VT 70-71; **FAP:** Asst Clin Prof Yale U Sch Med; **SI:** *Lyme Disease*; **HMO:** US Hlthcre PHS Oxford United Healthcare CIGNA +

LANG: Ger; ♿ 📷 🅿 🏨 $ Mcr Mcd   Immediately **VISA**

Horwitz, Ralph (MD)   IM   PCP
Yale-New Haven Hosp

Yale Faculty Practice, 333 Cedar St; New Haven, CT 06520; (203) 785-4119; **BDCERT:** IM 78; **MS:** Penn State U-Hershey Med Ctr 73; **RES:** IM, Royal Victoria Hosp, Montreal, Canada 74-75; IM, Mass Gen Hosp, Boston, MA 77-78; **FEL:** Yale-New Haven Hosp, New Haven, CT 75-77; **FAP:** Chrmn IM Yale U Sch Med; **HMO:** Aetna Hlth Plan PHS CIGNA

♿ 📷 🅿 🏨 Mcr Mcd   A Few Days ▦ **VISA** 💳 💳

Johns, William (MD)   IM   PCP
Danbury Hosp

24 Hospital Ave; Danbury, CT 06810; (203) 797-9797; **BDCERT:** NuM 92; IM 92; **MS:** U Conn Sch Med 83; **RES:** IM, Danbury Hosp, Danbury, CT 83-86; NuM, Brigham & Women's Hosp, Boston, MA 86-88; **HMO:** PHS Blue Choice Blue Cross & Blue Shield CIGNA Travelers +

♿ SA/SU 🌙 📷 🅿 🏨 $ Mcr WC   A Few Days **VISA** 💳

Kernan, Walter (MD)   IM   PCP
Yale-New Haven Hosp

PO Box 208025, 333 Cedar St; New Haven, CT 06520; (203) 688-2984; **BDCERT:** IM 87; **MS:** Dartmouth Med Sch 84; **RES:** Johns Hopkins Hosp, Baltimore, MD 84-87; **FEL:** EDM, Yale-New Haven Hosp, New Haven, CT 87-89; **FAP:** Assoc Prof Yale U Sch Med; **SI:** *Stroke*

LANG: Sp; ♿ 🌙 📷 🅿 🏨 $ Mcr Mcd WC NFI   2-4 Weeks ▦ **VISA** 💳 💳

Klein, Neil (MD)   IM   PCP
Stamford Hosp

1450 Washington Blvd; Stamford, CT 06902; (203) 327-9321; **BDCERT:** IM 67; Ge 75; **MS:** Cornell U 60; **RES:** NY Hosp-Cornell Med Ctr, New York, NY 60-61; NY Hosp-Cornell Med Ctr, New York, NY 64-65; **FEL:** Ge, NY Hosp-Cornell Med Ctr, New York, NY 65-67; **FAP:** Clin Prof Med NY Med Coll; **HMO:** Oxford PHS Aetna Hlth Plan PHS Aetna Hlth Plan +

♿ SA/SU 📷 🅿 🏨 $ Mcr

Molloy, Edward Michael (MD) IM   PCP
St Vincent's Med Ctr-Bridgeport

134 Round Hill Rd FL2; Fairfield, CT 06430; (203) 255-0695; **BDCERT:** IM 74; **MS:** UMDNJ-NJ Med Sch, Newark 66; **RES:** IM, St Vincent's Med Ctr-Bridgeport, Bridgeport, CT 69-72; **SI:** *Diabetes; Arthritis*; **HMO:** PHS MD Health Plan Oxford CIGNA PHCS +

LANG: Sp; ♿ SA/SU 📷 🅿 🏨 $ Mcr Mcd WC NFI   Immediately

Mushlin, Stuart (MD)   IM   PCP
Stamford Hosp

1290 Summer St; Stamford, CT 06901; (203) 324-8900; **BDCERT:** IM 76; **MS:** Cornell U 73; **RES:** IM, Peter Bent Brigham Hosp, Boston, MA 73-75; Peter Bent Brigham Hosp, Boston, MA 76; **FEL:** Rhu, Robert B Bringham Hosp, Boston, MA 77; **FAP:** Asst Cornell U; **HOSP:** St Joseph's Med Ctr-Stamford; **SI:** *Complicated Diagnoses*; **HMO:** PHS Aetna Hlth Plan CIGNA Prucare

♿ SA/SU 📷 🅿 🏨 $ A Few Days ▦ **VISA** 💳

O'Connor, Patrick (MD)   IM   PCP
Yale-New Haven Hosp

Yale-New Haven Hosp—Int Med, 333 Cedar St; New Haven, CT 06520; (203) 688-6532; **BDCERT:** IM 86; **MS:** Albany Med Coll 82; **RES:** IM, U Rochester-Strong Mem Hosp, Rochester, NY 82-86; **FEL:** IM, Yale-New Haven Hosp, New Haven, CT 86-88; **HMO:** Health Choice Aetna Hlth Plan MD Health Plan Yale Preferred

LANG: Sp; ♿ 🌙 📷 🅿 🏨 Mcr Mcd WC NFI   A Few Days

Pinto, Edward (MD)   IM   **PCP**
Bridgeport Hosp
Cardiology Assoc, 52 Beach Rd 107; Fairfield, CT
06430; (203) 254-1663; **BDCERT:** IM 74; Cv 77;
MS: India 70; **RES:** Bridgeport Hosp, Bridgeport, CT
71-75; **FEL:** Hosp of U Penn, Philadelphia, PA 75-
76; MS Hershey Med Ctr, Hershey, PA 76-77

🚹 🈯 📷 💉 🏥 💲 📠 2-4 Weeks

Quartararo, Paul (MD)   IM   **PCP**
Stamford Hosp
Stamford Medical Group, 1450 Washington Blvd;
Stamford, CT 06902; (203) 327-9321; **BDCERT:**
IM 92; **MS:** Albert Einstein Coll Med 86; **RES:** IM, U
Hosp, Cincinnati, OH 86-89; **FEL:** Pul, Rhode Island
Hosp, Providence, RI 89-92; *SI: Lung Diseases*;
HMO: Oxford Aetna Hlth Plan PHS Blue Cross &
Blue Shield United Healthcare +

🚹 🈯 📷 💉 🏥 💲 📠 Immediately 💳 **VISA** 💳
📠

Sennett, Margaret (MD)   IM   **PCP**
Greenwich Hosp
Greenwich Medical Group, 8 Greenwich Office
Park; Greenwich, CT 06831; (203) 869-6960;
BDCERT: IM 79; Ge 94; **MS:** SUNY Syracuse 76;
RES: IM, Greenwich Hosp-Yale, Greenwich, CT 77-
79; **FAP:** Clin Instr Yale U Sch Med; **HMO:** Aetna-
US Healthcare Oxford Physician's Health Plan MD
Health Plan United Healthcare +

LANG: Sp; 🚹 🈯 📷 💉 💲 📠 📠 ♿ A Few Days
VISA 💳

Simkovitz, Philip (MD)   IM
St Vincent's Med Ctr-Bridgeport
1275 Post Rd 211; Fairfield, CT 06430; (203) 254-
3433; **BDCERT:** IM 85; Pul 88; **MS:** Boston U 82;
RES: IM, U Conn Hlth Ctr, Farmington, CT 82-85; U
Conn Hlth Ctr, Farmington, CT 85-86; **FEL:** Pul,
McGill Teaching Hosp, Montreal, Canada 86-88;
CCM, McGill Teaching Hosp, Montreal, Canada 88-
89; **FAP:** Clin Instr NY Med Coll; **HOSP:** Bridgeport
Hosp; *SI: Shortness of Breath; Asthma*; **HMO:** PHS
MD Health Plan Bluecare

🚹 📷 💉 🏥 💲 📠 📠 ♿ 📠 A Few Days

Spano, Frank (MD)   IM   **PCP**
Bridgeport Hosp
Fairfield County Medical Group, 4695 Main St;
Bridgeport, CT 06606; (203) 373-0899; **BDCERT:**
IM 87; **MS:** Albert Einstein Coll Med 84; **RES:** Albert
Einstein Med Ctr, Bronx, NY 84-87; **HMO:** PHS
Aetna Hlth Plan Oxford Blue Cross & Blue Shield
Metlife +

🚹 📷 💉 💲 📠 A Few Days **VISA** 💳

Thomas, Byron (MD)   IM   **PCP**
Danbury Hosp
Medical Associates of Danbury Hosp, 72 Wolfpits
Rd; Bethel, CT 06801; (203) 797-7173; **BDCERT:**
IM 78; Ger 92; **MS:** Univ Pittsburgh 75; **RES:** IM,
Mount Sinai Hosp, Cleveland, OH 75-78; **FAP:** Asst
Clin Prof Yale U Sch Med; *SI: Geriatrics*

🚹 📞 📷 💉 🏥 💲 📠 📠 📠 A Few Days 💳 💳 **VISA**
💳 📠

Weiner, Jay (MD)   IM   **PCP**
Danbury Hosp
Danbury Internal Medicine Associates, 92 Locust
Ave; Danbury, CT 06810; (203) 744-4511;
BDCERT: IM 67; Ger 94; **MS:** Univ Penn 59; **RES:**
IM, Montefiore Med Ctr, Bronx, NY 59-63; **HMO:**
Aetna Hlth Plan CIGNA Anthem Health Kaiser
Permanente Suburban +

🚹 📷 💉 🏥 💲 📠 📠 A Few Days **VISA** 💳

Wenick, Diane (MD)   IM
Danbury Hosp
30 Gertown Rd; Danbury, CT 06810; (203) 794-
1979; **BDCERT:** IM 88; **MS:** NYU Sch Med 85; **RES:**
IM, Danbury Hosp, Danbury, CT 85-88

Whitcomb, Michael (MD)   IM   **PCP**
Greenwich Hosp
Glenville Med Assocs, 7 Riversville Rd; Greenwich,
CT 06831; (203) 531-1808; **BDCERT:** IM 84; **MS:**
Northwestern U 81; **RES:** Greenwich Hosp,
Greenwich, CT 82-84

🚹 📷 🏥 💲 ♿ Immediately 💳 **VISA** 💳

MATERNAL & FETAL MEDICINE

Foye, Gerard (MD) MF
Danbury Hosp
Candlewood ObGyn, 300 Federal Rd; Brookfield, CT 06804; (203) 775-1217; **BDCERT:** ObG 72; MF 79; **MS:** Ireland 65; **RES:** ObG, Univ Hosp SUNY Bklyn, Brooklyn, NY 65-70; **FAP:** Asst Clin Prof ObG Yale U Sch Med; ***SI:*** *High Risk Ob-Gyn; Pre-Natal Diagnosis*; **HMO:** CIGNA PHS Blue Cross & Blue Shield MD Health Plan
LANG: Sp; ♿ ☾ ☎ 📅 $ [Mcr] [Mcd] [WC] 1 Week

MEDICAL GENETICS

Mahoney, Maurice (MD) MG
Yale-New Haven Hosp
Yale Genetics Consultation Serv, 333 Cedar St PO Bx 208005; New Haven, CT 06520; (203) 785-2661; **BDCERT:** Ped 67; MG 82; **MS:** Univ Pittsburgh 62; **RES:** Ped, Johns Hopkins Hosp, Baltimore, MD 63-65; **FEL:** MG, Yale-New Haven Hosp, New Haven, CT 68-70; **FAP:** Prof MG Yale U Sch Med; ***SI:*** *Prenatal Diagnosis; Inborn Errors of Metabolism*; **HMO:** Aetna Hlth Plan Blue Cross & Blue Shield MD Health Plan United Healthcare PHS +
♿ ☎ 👤 📅 [Mcr] [Mcd] A Few Days AMERICAN EXPRESS VISA MasterCard DISCOVER

Pober, Barbara (MD) MG
Yale-New Haven Hosp
Department of GeneticsYale University School of Medicine, PO Box 208005; New Haven, CT 06437; (203) 785-2660; **BDCERT:** Ped 83; MG 90; **MS:** Yale U Sch Med 78; **RES:** Ped, New England Med Ctr, Boston, MA 78-81; **FEL:** Ge, Mass Gen Hosp, Boston, MA 83-87; **FAP:** Assoc Prof Yale U Sch Med; ***SI:*** *Williams Syndrome; Dysmorphology*; **HMO:** Blue Cross & Blue Shield PHS
♿ ☎ 📅 [Mcr] [Mcd] 2-4 Weeks

Seashore, Margaretta (MD) MG
Yale-New Haven Hosp
333 Cedar St Rm WWW 305; New Haven, CT 06520; (203) 785-2660; **BDCERT:** MG 82; Ped 70; **MS:** Yale U Sch Med 65; **RES:** Yale-New Haven Hosp, New Haven, CT 65-68; **FEL:** Yale-New Haven Hosp, New Haven, CT 68-70; **FAP:** Prof Yale U Sch Med; ***SI:*** *Clinical Genetics; Inborn Errors of Metabolism*; **HMO:** Aetna Hlth Plan Connecticare MD Health Plan CIGNA Bluecare +
♿ ☎ 👤 📅 [Mcr] [Mcd] 1 Week

MEDICAL ONCOLOGY

Burd, Robert (MD) Onc
St Vincent's Med Ctr-Bridgeport
Medical Specialists of Fairfield, LLC, 425 Post Rd; Fairfield, CT 06430; (203) 255-4545; **BDCERT:** Hem 72; Onc 75; **MS:** Columbia P&S 63; **RES:** IM, Albert Einstein Med Ctr, Bronx, NY 63-66; **FEL:** Hem, Montefiore Med Ctr, Bronx, NY 66-67; **FAP:** Assoc Prof of Clin Med Yale U Sch Med; **HOSP:** Bridgeport Hosp; ***SI:*** *Breast Cancer; Lymphoma*; **HMO:** Blue Choice Blue Cross CIGNA PHS Travelers +
♿ ☾ ☎ 👤 📅 $ [Mcr] [Mcd] 1 Week VISA MasterCard

Cooper, Dennis (MD) Onc
Yale-New Haven Hosp
Yale Oncology, 333 Cedar St; New Haven, CT 06520; (203) 785-6007; **BDCERT:** IM 83; **MS:** Rush Med Coll 79; **RES:** Yale-New Haven Hosp, New Haven, CT 79-82; U of Pittsburgh Med Ctr, Pittsburgh, PA 82-83; **FEL:** Yale-New Haven Hosp, New Haven, CT 83-86; **FAP:** Assoc Prof Yale U Sch Med; ***SI:*** *Lymphoma; Stem Cell Transplants*; **HMO:** Aetna Hlth Plan Oxford Connecticare Blue Cross MD Health Plan +
LANG: Sp; ♿ 👤 📅 $ [Mcr] [Mcd] [WC] AMERICAN EXPRESS VISA MasterCard

Guide to symbols and abbreviations can be found on pages 110-113.

Coscia, Anthony (MD) Onc
Norwalk Hosp
Norwalk Medical Group, Whittingham Cancer Ctr; Norwalk, CT 06856; (203) 845-2121; **BDCERT:** Onc 75; IM 72; **MS:** Cornell U 68; **RES:** NY Mem Hosp, New York, NY 69-71; **FEL:** Onc, Mem Sloan Kettering Cancer Ctr, New York, NY 73-74

🦽 🔟 🛏 🟥 Mcr Mcd A Few Days **VISA** 🌀

Erichson, Robert (MD) Onc
Stamford Hosp
Hematology Oncology, 34 Shelburne Rd; Stamford, CT 06902; (203) 325-2695; **BDCERT:** IM 68; Onc 73; **MS:** Cornell U 60; **RES:** Univ Hosp SUNY Syracuse, Syracuse, NY 60-62; Montefiore Med Ctr, Bronx, NY 62-64; **FEL:** Hem, Montefiore Med Ctr, Bronx, NY 64-65; **FAP:** Clin Prof Med NY Med Coll; **HOSP:** St Joseph's Med Ctr-Stamford; **HMO:** Most

🦽 🆂🆂 🔟 🛏 Mcr Mcd A Few Days

Folman, Robert (MD) Onc
Bridgeport Hosp
Oncology Associates Of Bpt, 15 Corporate Dr 210; Trumbull, CT 06611; (203) 459-0262; **BDCERT:** IM 75; Onc 77; **MS:** SUNY Buffalo 72; **RES:** IM, Univ Hosp SUNY Buffalo, Buffalo, NY 72-75; **FEL:** Onc, Mem Sloan Kettering Cancer Ctr, New York, NY 75-77; **HOSP:** St Vincents Hosp & Med Ctr NY; **SI:** *Breast Cancer Treatment; Lung Cancer Chemotherapy;* **HMO:** PHS Anthem Health MD Health Plan Oxford

LANG: Sp; 🦽 🔟 🔟 🛏 Mcr Mcd A Few Days

Hollister Jr, Dickerman (MD) Onc
Greenwich Hosp
Greenwich Hospital, Dept of Hematology, 77 Lafayette Place Pl; Greenwich, CT 06830; (203) 863-3737; **BDCERT:** Onc 83; Hem 81; **MS:** U Va Sch Med 75; **RES:** IM, NY Hosp-Cornell Med Ctr, New York, NY 75-78; **FEL:** Onc, Mem Sloan Kettering Cancer Ctr, New York, NY 78-81; Hem, Mem Sloan Kettering Cancer Ctr, New York, NY 78-81; **FAP:** Asst Prof Yale U Sch Med; **SI:** *Breast Cancer; Lung & Colon Cancer;* **HMO:** Aetna Hlth Plan Oxford PHS Health Source Health Direct +

🦽 🔟 🔟 🛏 🟥 A Few Days **VISA** 🌀

Lo, K M Steve (MD) Onc
Stamford Hosp
Bennett Cancer Center Hematology Oncology, 34 Shelburne Rd; Stamford, CT 06902; (203) 325-7199; **BDCERT:** Onc 91; Hem 92; **MS:** Harvard Med Sch 85; **RES:** IM, Brigham & Women's Hosp, Boston, MA 85-88; **FEL:** Hem Onc, Dana-Farber Cancer Inst, Boston, MA 89-91; Hem, Dana-Farber Cancer Inst, Boston, MA 92; **HOSP:** St Joseph's Med Ctr-Stamford; **SI:** *Breast Cancer; Bone Marrow Transplant;* **HMO:** PHS Aetna Hlth Plan Blue Cross & Blue Shield Oxford

🦽 🔟 🔟 🛏 🟥 Mcr Mcd A Few Days

Poo, Wen Jen (MD) Onc
Yale-New Haven Hosp
333 Cedar St 224 WW; New Haven, CT 06520; (203) 785-4113; **BDCERT:** IM 85; **MS:** UC Irvine 82; **RES:** Onc, Yale-New Haven Hosp, New Haven, CT; **FAP:** Assoc Prof Yale U Sch Med; **SI:** *Melanoma; Genitourinary Cancer;* **HMO:** Aetna Hlth Plan CIGNA

LANG: Chi; 🦽 🔟 🔟 🛏 Mcr Mcd WC NFl 1 Week

Rosenberg, Arthur (MD) Onc **PCP**
Greenwich Hosp
77 Lafayette Pl; Greenwich, CT 06830; (203) 863-3777; **BDCERT:** Hem 72; Onc 73; **MS:** Columbia P&S 59; **RES:** U IL Med Ctr, Chicago, IL 62-63; Mount Sinai Med Ctr, New York, NY 63-64; **FEL:** Hem, Mount Sinai Med Ctr, New York, NY 64-65; **FAP:** Asst Prof Yale U Sch Med; **SI:** *Breast Cancer; Lymphoma;* **HMO:** Aetna Hlth Plan PHS Oxford CIGNA US Hlthcre +

🦽 🔟 🔟 🛏 🟥 Mcr Mcd WC A Few Days **VISA** 🌀

Sacks, Kenneth (MD) Onc
St Vincent's Med Ctr-Bridgeport
Medical Specialists of Fairfield LLC, 425 Post Rd; Fairfield, CT 06430; (203) 255-4545; **BDCERT:** IM 73; Onc 75; **MS:** Univ Pittsburgh 69; **RES:** IM, UCLA Med Ctr, Los Angeles, CA 69-71; IM, Geo Wash U Med Ctr, Washington, DC 71-72; **FEL:** Onc, Nat Inst Health, Bethesda, MD 72-74; Hem Onc, UCLA Med Ctr, Los Angeles, CA 74-75; **FAP:** Assoc Clin Prof Yale U Sch Med

🦽 🔟 🔟 🛏 🟥 Mcr Mcd A Few Days **VISA** 🌀

Guide to symbols and abbreviations can be found on pages 110-113.

1055

Weinstein, Paul (MD)   Onc
Stamford Hosp

Bennett Cancer Center - HemOncology, 34
Shelburne Rd; Stamford, CT 06902; (203) 325-
7199; **BDCERT:** Onc 77; Hem 78; **MS:** Univ IL Coll
Med 70; **RES:** IM, Montefiore Med Ctr, Bronx, NY
70-73; Hem, Montefiore Med Ctr, Bronx, NY 73-
74; **FEL:** Onc, Montefiore Med Ctr, Bronx, NY 74-
75; **FAP:** Asst Clin Prof NY Med Coll; **HOSP:** St
Joseph's Med Ctr-Stamford; *SI: Breast Cancer; Cancer
Genetics & High Risk*; **HMO:** Oxford PHS Aetna-US
Healthcare CIGNA Blue Cross +

🔲 🔲 🔲 🔲 🔲 🔲 🔲 🔲 🔲 A Few Days

NEONATAL-PERINATAL MEDICINE

Herzlinger, Robert (MD)   NP
Bridgeport Hosp

215 Curtis Ter; Fairfield, CT 06432; (203) 384-
3486; **BDCERT:** Ped 73; NP 76; **MS:** NY Med Coll
69; **RES:** Ped, NY Med Coll, New York, NY 69-71;
Ped, Columbia-Presbyterian Med Ctr, New York,
NY 71-72; **FEL:** NP, Columbia-Presbyterian Med
Ctr, New York, NY 72-73; NP, Albert Einstein Med
Ctr, Bronx, NY 75-76

🔲 🔲 🔲 🔲 🔲 🔲 🔲 🔲

Menzies, Cheryl (MD)   NP
Bridgeport Hosp

215 Old Post Rd; Fairfield, CT 06430; (203) 384-
3486; **BDCERT:** Ped 89 89; NP 91; **MS:** Vanderbilt
U Sch Med 84

Theofandis, Stylianos (MD)   NP
Greenwich Hosp

5 Perryridge Rd; Greenwich, CT 06830; (203) 863-
3515; **BDCERT:** Ped 89; **MS:** Greece 80; **RES:** Ped,
St Luke's Roosevelt Hosp Ctr, New York, NY 82-85;
FEL: NP, NY Hosp-Cornell Med Ctr, New York, NY
85-87; **FAP:** Asst Clin Prof Yale U Sch Med; **HOSP:**
Yale-New Haven Hosp; **HMO:** Oxford Aetna Hlth
Plan CIGNA Prucare Health Choice +

LANG: Grk; 🔲 🔲 🔲 🔲 🔲 🔲 🔲 Immediately

NEPHROLOGY

Brown, Eric (MD)   Nep
Stamford Hosp

Dialysis Associates, 166 W Broad St T3; Stamford,
CT 06896; (203) 324-7666; **BDCERT:** IM 88; Nep
90; **MS:** Emory U Sch Med 85; **RES:** Johns Hopkins
Hosp, Baltimore, MD 85-88; **FEL:** Nep, Yale-New
Haven Hosp, New Haven, CT 88-90; **FAP:** Asst Clin
Prof Yale U Sch Med; **HOSP:** St Joseph's Med Ctr-
Stamford; **HMO:** Aetna Hlth Plan Oxford PHS
NYLCare US Hlthcre +

🔲 🔲 🔲 🔲 🔲 🔲 Immediately

Fogel, Mitchell (MD)   Nep
St Vincent's Med Ctr-Bridgeport

900 Madison Ave 209; Bridgeport, CT 06606;
(203) 335-0195; **BDCERT:** IM 86; Nep 88; **MS:**
Univ Penn 82; **RES:** IM, Boston U Med Ctr, Boston,
MA 82-85; **FEL:** Nep, Boston U Med Ctr, Boston,
MA 85-88; **FAP:** Asst Clin Prof NY Med Coll; **HOSP:**
Bridgeport Hosp; *SI: Renal Vascular Disease; Lupus;
Lupus & Glomerulonephritis*; **HMO:** PHS Blue Cross &
Blue Shield CIGNA

🔲 🔲 🔲 🔲 🔲 🔲 🔲 2-4 Weeks

Garfinkel, Howard (MD)   Nep
Danbury Hosp

24 Hospital Ave; Danbury, CT 06810; (203) 797-
7104; **BDCERT:** IM 72; **MS:** Tufts U 65; **RES:** Med,
Cleveland Metro Gen Hosp, Cleveland, OH 68-70;
FEL: New England Med Ctr, Boston, MA 70-72;
FAP: Assoc Clin Prof Med Yale U Sch Med; *SI:
Hypertension*; **HMO:** Aetna Hlth Plan Blue Choice
CIGNA

🔲 🔲 🔲 🔲 🔲 1 Week 🔲 *VISA* 🔲 🔲

Hines, William (MD)   Nep
Stamford Hosp

166 W Broad St T3; Stamford, CT 06902; (203)
324-7666; **BDCERT:** Nep 86; IM 84; **MS:** Cornell U
81; **RES:** IM, Hosp of U Penn, Philadelphia, PA 81-
84; **FEL:** Nep, Hosp U of PA, Philadelphia, PA 84;
FAP: Assoc Clin Prof NY Med Coll; **HOSP:** St
Joseph's Med Ctr-Stamford; *SI: Kidney Disease;
Hypertension*; **HMO:** Aetna Hlth Plan Oxford Blue
Cross PHS

LANG: Fr; 🔲 🔲 🔲 🔲 🔲 🔲 A Few Days

Kennedy, Thomas (MD)   Nep
Bridgeport Hosp

Mill Hill Med Consultants Bridgeport Hosp, 267
Grant St; Bridgeport, CT 06610; (203) 384-4031;
BDCERT: Ped 77; PNep 79; **MS:** Cornell U 72; **RES:**
Ped, Children's Hosp of Philadelphia, Philadelphia,
PA 73-75; **FEL:** Nep, Children's Hosp of
Philadelphia, Philadelphia, PA 77-79; **FAP:** Clin
Prof Ped Yale U Sch Med; **HMO:** Oxford PHS Aetna
Hlth Plan Blue Cross & Blue Shield Yale Preferred +

🦽 📷 👱 🛏 Med   A Few Days

Mahnensmith, Rex (MD)   Nep
Yale-New Haven Hosp

Yale Nephrology Group, 789 Howard Ave; New
Haven, CT 06520; (203) 785-4184; **BDCERT:** IM
82; **MS:** Yale U Sch Med 77; **RES:** IM, Yale-New
Haven Hosp, New Haven, CT 77-81; **FEL:** Nep,
Yale-New Haven Hosp, New Haven, CT 82-84;
FAP: Assoc Prof Yale U Sch Med; **HMO:** Aetna Hlth
Plan PHS Oxford CIGNA MD Health Plan +

🦽 📷 👱 🛏 S Mcr Med WC   A Few Days 🖼 **VISA**
💳 💳

Walsh, Francis X (MD)   Nep   PCP
Greenwich Hosp

42 Sherwood Pl; Greenwich, CT 06830; (203)
661-9433; **BDCERT:** Nep 74; **MS:** NY Med Coll 67;
RES: IM, Greenwich Hosp, Greenwich, CT 67-70;
FEL: Nep, Duke U Med Ctr, Durham, NC 70-72;
FAP: Asst Clin Prof Yale U Sch Med; *SI: End Stage
Renal Disease; Chronic & Acute Dialysis*; **HMO:** Aetna
Hlth Plan Oxford

🦽 📷 👱 🛏 S Mcr Med WC NFI   A Few Days 🖼 **VISA**
💳 💳

NEUROLOGICAL SURGERY

Camel, Mark (MD)   NS
Greenwich Hosp

27 Bridge St; Stamford, CT 06805; (203) 324-
6620; **BDCERT:** NS 90; **MS:** Washington U, St
Louis 81; **RES:** NS, Barnes Hosp, St Louis, MO 81-
86; **FEL:** NS, Barnes Hosp, St Louis, MO 81-87;
HOSP: Stamford Hosp; *SI: Brain Tumor; Spinal
Disease*

🦽 📷 🛏 S Mcr WC   A Few Days **VISA** 💳

Dila, Carl (MD)   NS
Stamford Hosp

1290 Summer St; Stamford, CT 06905; (203) 324-
3504; **BDCERT:** NS 73; **MS:** Wayne State U Sch
Med 62; **RES:** Georgetown U Hosp, Washington, DC
62-63; NS, Montreal Neur Inst, Montreal, Canada
67-71; **FEL:** Neuropathology, Montreal Neur Inst,
Montreal, Canada 70; *SI: Spine Surgery; Brain
Tumors*; **HMO:** Aetna Hlth Plan Connecticare PHS
CIGNA Blue Cross +

LANG: Fr; 🦽 📷 🛏 S Mcr Med WC NFI

Duncan, Charles C (MD)   NS
Yale-New Haven Hosp

Yale Neurosurgical Group, 333 Cedar St TMP 416;
New Haven, CT 06520; (203) 785-2809; **BDCERT:**
NS 79; **MS:** Duke U 71; **RES:** NS, Duke U Med Ctr,
Durham, NC 72-77; **FAP:** Prof Yale U Sch Med;
HOSP: VA Med Ctr-Northport; *SI: Pediatric
Neurosurgery*; **HMO:** Yale Preferred PHS MD Health
Plan Blue Cross & Blue Shield Bluecare +

🦽 📷 🛏 S Mcr Med WC   1 Week

Mintz, Abraham (MD)   NS
St Vincent's Med Ctr-Bridgeport

340 Capitol Ave; Bridgeport, CT 06606; (203) 336-
3303; **BDCERT:** NS 92; **MS:** Mexico 82; **RES:** NS,
Jackson Mem Hosp, Miami, FL 82-89; **HOSP:**
Bridgeport Hosp; *SI: Spinal Diseases*; **HMO:** PHS
CIGNA Aetna Hlth Plan Blue Cross Oxford +

LANG: Sp; 🦽 📷 👱 🛏 S Mcr Med WC NFI
Immediately 💳

Rosenstein, C Cory (MD)   NS
Stamford Hosp

Neurological Surgeons of Stamford, 1290 Summer St 5000; Stamford, CT 06905; (203) 324-3504; **BDCERT:** NS 94; **MS:** Case West Res U 85; **RES:** NS, U Hosp of Cleveland, Cleveland, OH 85-90; **FEL:** U Hosp of Najoya, Japan 89; **SI:** *Diseases of the Spine; Intra-Cranial Vascular Surgery;* **HMO:** Aetna Hlth Plan PHS Oxford CIGNA Blue Cross & Blue Shield +

LANG: Sp, Fr; ⬛ ⬛ ⬛ ⬛ ⬛ ⬛ ⬛ ⬛ 1 Week

Shahid, S Javed (MD)   NS
Danbury Hosp

148 East Ave 3D; Norwalk, CT 06851; (203) 853-0003; **BDCERT:** NS 83; **MS:** Pakistan 72; **RES:** S, Kings County Hosp Ctr, Brooklyn, NY 73-74; NS, Kings County Hosp Ctr, Brooklyn, NY 74-75; **HOSP:** Norwalk Hosp; **SI:** *Brain Tumors; Neck and Back Surgery;* **HMO:** CIGNA Aetna Hlth Plan Blue Cross & Blue Shield

⬛ ⬛ ⬛ ⬛ ⬛ ⬛ ⬛ 1 Week **VISA** ⬛

Spencer, Dennis (MD)   NS
Yale-New Haven Hosp

Yale Neurosurgery Group, 333 Cedar St TMP4; New Haven, CT 06520; (203) 785-2811; **BDCERT:** NS 80; **MS:** Washington U, St Louis 71; **RES:** S, Barnes Hosp, St Louis, MO 71-72; NS, Yale-New Haven Hosp, New Haven, CT 72-76; **FAP:** Prof Yale U Sch Med; **HOSP:** Hosp of St Raphael; **SI:** *Epilepsy Surgery; Brain Tumors;* **HMO:** Aetna Hlth Plan Anthem Health CIGNA PHS MD Health Plan +

⬛ ⬛ ⬛ ⬛ ⬛ ⬛ ⬛ ⬛ A Few Days ⬛ **VISA** ⬛

NEUROLOGY

Engel, Murray (MD)   N
Greenwich Hosp

1290 Summer St 3300; Stamford, CT 06905; (203) 359-1790; **BDCERT:** N 80; Ped 79; **MS:** U Chicago-Pritzker Sch Med 72; **RES:** N, Yale - New Haven Hospial, New Haven, CT 72-76; N, Columbia Presbyterian Hospital, New York, NY 76-77

Goldstein, Jonathan (MD)   N
Yale-New Haven Hosp

Yale U, Dept of Neurology, LVI 702, PO Box 208018; New Haven, CT 06520; (203) 785-4867; **BDCERT:** N 91; **MS:** Brown U 86; **RES:** New England Deaconess Hosp, Boston, MA 86-87; N, Yale-New Haven Hosp, New Haven, CT 87-90; **FEL:** Yale-New Haven Hosp, New Haven, CT 90-92; **FAP:** Asst Prof N Yale U Sch Med; **SI:** *Neuropathy; Muscular Dystrophy;* **HMO:** Aetna Hlth Plan CIGNA Oxford PHS MD Health Plan +

LANG: Itl, Sp; ⬛ ⬛ ⬛ ⬛ ⬛ ⬛ ⬛ 4+ Weeks ⬛ **VISA** ⬛ ⬛

Murphy, John (MD)   N
Danbury Hosp

Associated Neurologists, PC, 69 Sand Pit Rd 300; Danbury, CT 06810; (203) 748-2551; **BDCERT:** N 91; **MS:** UMDNJ-RW Johnson Med Sch 85; **RES:** Univ of Med & Dent NJ Hosp, Newark, NJ 86-89; **FAP:** Asst Clin Prof N NY Med Coll; **SI:** *Parkinson's Disease;* **HMO:** Aetna Hlth Plan MD Health Plan PHS CIGNA

⬛ ⬛ ⬛ ⬛ ⬛ ⬛ ⬛ ⬛ 2-4 Weeks **VISA** ⬛

Resor, Louise (MD)   N
St Joseph's Med Ctr-Stamford

1290 Summer St Ste 3200; Stamford, CT 06905; (203) 978-0283; **BDCERT:** Psyc 80; N 80; **MS:** Washington U, St Louis 74; **RES:** Columbia-Presbyterian Med Ctr, New York, NY 75-78; **FEL:** Babies Hosp, New York, NY 78-79; **HMO:** PHS Aetna Hlth Plan Connecticare

⬛ ⬛ ⬛ ⬛ ⬛ 4+ Weeks

Seigel, Sheryl (MD)   N
Greenwich Hosp

The Greenwich Ctr for Traditional & Holistic Medicine, 239 Glenville Rd; Greenwich, CT 06831; (203) 531-1932; **BDCERT:** N 92; **MS:** Albert Einstein Coll Med 82; **RES:** N, Albert Einstein, Bronx, NY 85-88; **FAP:** Asst Prof NY Med Coll; **HOSP:** St Agnes Hosp; **SI:** *Headache; Pain;* **HMO:** Blue Cross & Blue Choice CIGNA Champus Prudential +

LANG: Sp; ⬛ ⬛ ⬛ ⬛ ⬛ ⬛ ⬛ ⬛ ⬛
A Few Days

1058

Sena, K N (MD)　　　　　　N
Bridgeport Hosp
Neurological Specialist, 325 Reef Rd; Fairfield, CT 06430; (203) 377-5988; **BDCERT:** N 79; **MS:** Sri Lanka 68; **RES:** N, Yale-New Haven Med, New Haven, CT 73-76; IM, Bridgeport Hosp, Bridgeport, CT 72-73; **FAP:** Assoc Clin Prof N Yale U Sch Med; **HMO:** Aetna Hlth Plan Blue Cross & Blue Shield CIGNA

🚻 🎔 🔓 🔏 📅 🅂 Mcr WC NFI　Immediately

Siegel, Kenneth C (MD)　　　N
St Vincent's Med Ctr-Bridgeport
Associated Neurolgists of Southern Conneticut, 4699 Main St; Bridgeport, CT 06606; (203) 372-8111; **BDCERT:** N 75; **MS:** Meharry Med Coll 69; **RES:** N, New York University Med Ctr, New York, NY 70; New York University Med Ctr, New York, NY 73; **SI:** *Parkinson's Disease; Headache;* **HMO:** CIGNA PHS Anthem Health Oxford +

🚻 🔓 🔏 📅 🅂 Mcr Mcd WC NFI　2-4 Weeks **VISA** ⬤

Waxman, Stephen (MD & PhD)N
Yale-New Haven Hosp
Dept of Neurology, Yale University School of Medicine Box208018; New Haven, CT 06520; (203) 785-5947; **BDCERT:** N 77; Psyc 77; **MS:** Albert Einstein Coll Med 72; **RES:** N, Boston Med Ctr, Boston, MA 72-75; **FAP:** Chrmn N Yale U Sch Med; **HOSP:** VA Ct Healthcare Sys; **SI:** *Multiple Sclerosis; Spinal Cord Injury*

🚻 📅 Mcr Mcd WC NFI　4+ Weeks 🔲 **VISA** ⬤

NUCLEAR MEDICINE

Gupta, Shiv (MD)　　　　NuM
Danbury Hosp
24 Hospital Ave; Danbury, CT 06810; (203) 397-7222; **BDCERT:** NuM 81; **MS:** India 69; **RES:** U Conn Hlth Ctr, Farmington, CT; Danbury Hosp, Danbury, CT; **FEL:** IM/NuM, Auckland Hosp, New Zealand; **FAP:** Clin Prof NuM U Conn Sch Med; **SI:** *Osteoporosis*

LANG: Sp, Hin, Ur, Pun, Guj; 🚻 🔓 📅 Mcr Mcd WC
Immediately

OBSTETRICS & GYNECOLOGY

Ayoub, Thomas (MD)　　　ObG
Norwalk Hosp
Women's Health Care, PO Box 2108; Norwalk, CT 06852; (203) 966-3777; **BDCERT:** ObG 86; **MS:** NYU Sch Med 80; **RES:** Bellevue Hosp Ctr, New York, NY 80-84; **HMO:** PHS Oxford MD Health Plan Aetna-US Healthcare Blue Cross +

LANG: Sp; 🚻 🅂🅄 🎔 🔓 🔏 📅 🅂 Mcr Mcd WC NFI　2-4 Weeks

Besser, Gary (MD)　　　　ObG
Stamford Hosp
OB/GYN Associates, 166 W Broad St 203; Stamford, CT 06902; (203) 325-4321; **BDCERT:** ObG 98; **MS:** SUNY Hlth Sci Ctr 82; **RES:** Stamford Hosp, Stamford, CT 82-86; **FAP:** Asst Prof NY Med Coll; **SI:** *Laparoscopic Surgery; High Risk Obstetrics;* **HMO:** PHS Oxford Prucare Medspan Blue Cross & Blue Shield +

LANG: Sp; 🚻 🔓 🔏 📅 🅂 Mcr　2-4 Weeks 🔲 **VISA** ⬤

Blair, Emily (DO)　　　　　ObG
Bridgeport Hosp
ObGyn of Fairfield County, 4920 Post Rd; Fairfield, CT 06430; (203) 256-3990; **BDCERT:** ObG 92; **MS:** Univ Osteo Med & Hlth Sci 86; **RES:** ObG, Bridgeport Hosp, Bridgeport, CT; **HOSP:** St Vincent's Med Ctr-Bridgeport; **SI:** *High Risk Obstetrics; High Risk Gynecology;* **HMO:** Aetna Hlth Plan Blue Cross & Blue Shield Aetna-US Healthcare PHS Connecticare +

LANG: Fr, Sp; 🚻 🔓 🔏 📅 🅂 Mcr WC　A Few Days **VISA** ⬤

Fine, Emily (MD)　　　　　ObG
Yale-New Haven Hosp
60 Washington Ave Ste 201; Hamden, CT 063518; (203) 230-2939; **BDCERT:** ObG 84; **MS:** Yale U Sch Med 78; **RES:** ObG, Yale-New Haven Hosp, New Haven, CT 79-82; **FAP:** Asst Clin Instr Yale U Sch Med; **HMO:** Most

🚻 🅂🅄 🔓 🔏 📅 🅂 Mcr Mcd　4+ Weeks **VISA** ⬤

Nelson, James (MD)   ObG
Stamford Hosp
Stamford Hosp Dept ObGyn, PO Box 9317;
Stamford, CT 06904; (203) 325-7853; **BDCERT:**
ObG 62; GO 82; **MS:** NYU Sch Med 54; **RES:** ObG,
US Naval Hosp, Brooklyn, NY 54-58; **FEL:** GO, Univ
Hosp SUNY Bklyn, Brooklyn, NY 61-64; **SI:** *Ovarian
& Uterine Cancer; Laparoscopic Surgery;* **HMO:** PHS
Oxford Aetna-US Healthcare Blue Shield Kaiser
Permanente +

♿ ☐ S Mcr Mcd

Nelson, Noreen (MD)   ObG
Westchester Med Ctr
PO Box 9317; Stamford, CT 06904; (203) 325-
7853; **BDCERT:** ObG 87; **MS:** Boston U 80; **RES:**
Mass Gen Hosp, Boston, MA 80-84

Rosenman, Stephen (MD)   ObG
Bridgeport Hosp
ObGyn Of Fairfield County, 2499 Main St;
Stratford, CT 06497; (203) 380-4666; **BDCERT:**
ObG 98; **MS:** Belgium 72; **RES:** ObG, Bridgeport
Hosp, Bridgeport, CT 71-75; **SI:** *Major Gynecologic
Surgery; Pelvic Reconstruction Surgery;* **HMO:** Aetna
Hlth Plan Blue Cross CIGNA PHS MD Health Plan +

♿ ☇ ⚑ ☐ S Mcr Mcd   2-4 Weeks ▦

Santomauro, Anthony (MD)ObG
Bridgeport Hosp
Infertility Institute, 4675 Main St 1; Bridgeport, CT
06606; (203) 372-9998; **BDCERT:** ObG 76; **MS:**
Columbia P&S 69; **RES:** ObG, Columbia-
Presbyterian Med Ctr, New York, NY 70-74; **HOSP:**
Yale-New Haven Hosp; **SI:** *Endometriosis; Advanced
Laparoscopy;* **HMO:** Blue Cross & Blue Shield Kaiser
Permanente MD Health Plan PHS Oxford +

LANG: Sp, Fr, Itl; ♿ ☇ ⚑ ☐ S Mcr   2-4 Weeks
VISA 💳 ▨

Weinstein, David (MD)   ObG
Stamford Hosp
OBS/GYN Associates, 166 W Broad St 203;
Stamford, CT 06902; (203) 325-4321; **BDCERT:**
ObG 76; **MS:** U Chicago-Pritzker Sch Med 69; **RES:**
NY Hosp-Cornell Med Ctr, New York, NY 70-74;
FAP: Assoc Prof ObG Cornell U; **SI:** *High Risk
Obstetrics;* **HMO:** Aetna-US Healthcare Oxford
CIGNA Prudential

LANG: Fr; ♿ ☇ ⚑ ☐ S Mcr Mcd

OCCUPATIONAL MEDICINE

Cullen, Mark R (MD)   OM
Yale-New Haven Hosp
Yale Occupational and Environmental Medicine
Program, 135 College St Rm392; New Haven, CT
06510; (203) 785-4197; **BDCERT:** OM 86; IM 79;
MS: Yale U Sch Med 76; **RES:** IM, Yale-New Haven
Hosp, New Haven, CT 76-80; **FAP:** Prof Med Yale U
Sch Med; **SI:** *Occupational Diseases; Environmental
Health;* **HMO:** Health Choice Anthem Health Yale
Preferred Oxford Aetna Hlth Plan +

LANG: Sp; ♿ ☇ ⚑ ☐ Mcr Mcd WC NFI   1 Week

OPHTHALMOLOGY

Eisner, Leslie (MD)   Oph
Stamford Hosp
70 Mill River St; Stamford, CT 06902; (203) 359-
2020; **BDCERT:** Oph 73; **MS:** Canada 78; **RES:**
Georgetown U, Washington, DC 80-83; **HOSP:** St
Joseph's Med Ctr-Stamford

Musto, Anthony (MD)   Oph
Bridgeport Hosp

Opticare, PC, 3060 Main St; Stratford, CT 06497;
(203) 375-5819; **BDCERT:** Oph 75; **MS:**
Georgetown U 68; **RES:** IM/Oph, USPHS, New
York, NY 69-71; Oph, Manhattan Eye, Ear &
Throat Hosp, New York, NY 71-73; **HOSP:** St
Vincents Hosp & Med Ctr NY; **SI:** *Cataract Surgery;*
Oculoplastic Surgery; **HMO:** PHS MD Health Plan
Blue Cross & Blue Shield Connecticare CIGNA +

🔳 🔳 🔳 🔳 🔳 Mcr Mcd WC NFI   1 Week **VISA** 💳

Siderides, Elizabeth (MD)   Oph
Stamford Hosp

Stamford Ophthalmology, 70 Mill River St;
Stamford, CT 06902; (203) 327-5808; **BDCERT:**
Oph 91; **MS:** Columbia P&S 85; **RES:** Oph, New
York University Med Ctr, New York, NY 86-89;
FEL: Retina, New York University Med Ctr, New
York, NY 89-90; **SI:** *Diabetes;* **HMO:** Aetna-US
Healthcare Oxford PHS CIGNA Connecticare +

LANG: Sp, Grk, Ger, Sgn; 🔳 🔳 🔳 🔳 🔳 Mcr Mcd WC
A Few Days **VISA** 💳

Wasserman, Eric (MD)   Oph
Stamford Hosp

1275 Summer St; Stamford, CT 06905; (203) 978-
0800; **BDCERT:** Oph 88; **MS:** NY Med Coll 79; **RES:**
IM, Danbury Hosp, Danbury, CT 79-80; Oph, NY
Med Coll, Valhalla, NY 80-83; **FEL:** John N Sheets
Eye Foundation, Odessa, TX 83-84; **HOSP:** St
Joseph's Med Ctr-Stamford; **SI:** *Cataract; Anterior*
Segment; **HMO:** Aetna-US Healthcare CIGNA PHS
Blue Cross & Blue Shield Oxford +

LANG: Itl; 🔳 🔳 🔳 🔳 🔳 🔳 Mcr WC   2-4 Weeks
VISA 💳 💳

ORTHOPAEDIC SURGERY

Bindelglass, David (MD)   OrS
Bridgeport Hosp

Orthopaedic Specialty Group, 325 Reef Rd 203;
Fairfield, CT 06430; (203) 255-2839; **BDCERT:**
OrS 94; **MS:** Columbia P&S 85; **RES:** S, Beth Israel
Med Ctr, New York, NY 85-87; OrS, Columbia-
Presbyterian Med Ctr, New York, NY 87-90; **FEL:**
Joint Replacement S, Kerlan-Jobe Ortho Clinic,
Inglewood, CA 90-91; **FAP:** Clin Instr Yale U Sch
Med; **SI:** *Arthritis; Joint Replacement;* **HMO:** PHCS
MD Health Plan Aetna Hlth Plan CIGNA Blue
Shield +

LANG: Sp; 🔳 🔳 🔳 🔳 🔳 Mcr Mcd WC NFI
A Few Days 🔳 **VISA** 💳 💳

Carolan, Patrick (MD)   OrS
St Vincent's Med Ctr-Bridgeport

Merritt Orthopaedic Assoc, 3909 Main St;
Bridgeport, CT 06606; (203) 372-4565; **BDCERT:**
OrS 72; **MS:** UMDNJ-NJ Med Sch, Newark 63; **RES:**
Letterman Gen Hosp, San Francisco, CA 66-70; **SI:**
Total Joint Replacement; Arthroscopic Surgery; **HMO:**
CIGNA Oxford PHS Aetna Hlth Plan MD Health
Plan +

🔳 🔳 🔳 🔳 🔳 Mcr Mcd WC NFI   A Few Days **VISA** 💳

Crowe, John (MD)   OrS
Greenwich Hosp

Orthopaedic Associates, 500 W Putnam Ave;
Greenwich, CT 06830; (203) 869-3131; **BDCERT:**
OrS 77; **MS:** Cornell U 71; **RES:** St Luke's Roosevelt
Hosp Ctr, New York, NY 71-73; Hosp For Special
Surgery, New York, NY 73-76; **FEL:** St Luke's
Roosevelt Hosp Ctr, New York, NY; **HOSP:** Hosp For
Special Surgery; **SI:** *Joint Replacement; Upper*
Extremity/Sports; **HMO:** Aetna Hlth Plan Oxford
PHCS Health Source

🔳 🔳 🔳 🔳 WC NFI   A Few Days **VISA** 💳 💳

Guide to symbols and abbreviations can be found on pages 110-113.

1061

Hughes, Peter (MD)   OrS
Stamford Hosp

90 Morgan St; Stamford, CT 06905; (203) 325-4087; **BDCERT:** OrS 78; **MS:** NY Med Coll 72; **RES:** NY Med Coll, Valhalla, NY 73-76; **FEL:** Hips, Hosp For Special Surg, New York, NY 76-77; **HOSP:** St Joseph's Med Ctr-Stamford; **HMO:** Aetna Hlth Plan Blue Cross & Blue Shield CIGNA United Healthcare PHS

LANG: Grk; 🔲 🔲 🔲 🔲 🔲 🔲 🔲 1 Week **VISA** 🔲 🔲

Jokl, Peter (MD)   OrS
Yale-New Haven Hosp

1 Longwhorf; New Haven, CT 06511; (203) 785-2579; **BDCERT:** OrS 74; **MS:** Yale U Sch Med 68; **RES:** Vanderbilt U Med Ctr, Nashville, TN 68-69; Yale-New Haven Hosp, New Haven, CT 69-72; **FAP:** Prof Yale U Sch Med; **HOSP:** Hosp of St Raphael; **SI:** *Sports Medicine; Knee Surgery*

LANG: Ger; 🔲 🔲 🔲 🔲 🔲 🔲 🔲 A Few Days 🔲 **VISA** 🔲 🔲

Rubinstein, Henry (MD)   OrS
Stamford Hosp

61 4th St; Stamford, CT 06905; (203) 324-0307; **BDCERT:** OrS 77; **MS:** Canada 70; **RES:** S, Mount Sinai Hosp, Cleveland, OH 71-72; OrS, Bellevue Hosp Ctr, New York, NY 72-75; **SI:** *Athletic Injuries; Joint Replacement;* **HMO:** CIGNA Oxford Aetna Hlth Plan PHS Blue Cross & Blue Shield +

🔲 🔲 🔲 🔲 🔲 🔲 🔲 🔲 🔲 A Few Days 🔲 **VISA** 🔲

Stovell, Peter (MD)   OrS
Norwalk Hosp

148 East Ave; Norwalk, CT 06851; (203) 853-1811; **BDCERT:** OrS 76; **MS:** Columbia P&S 68; **RES:** S, St Luke's Roosevelt Hosp Ctr, New York, NY 68-70; OrS, Hosp For Special Surgery, New York, NY 72-75; **FAP:** Clin Instr OrS Yale U Sch Med; **SI:** *Joint Reconstruction; Sports Medicine;* **HMO:** Oxford Blue Choice Blue Cross & Blue Shield CIGNA

🔲 🔲 🔲 🔲 🔲 🔲 🔲 🔲 🔲 1 Week **VISA** 🔲

Troy, Allen (MD)   OrS
Stamford Hosp

61 4th St; Stamford, CT 06905; (203) 324-0307; **BDCERT:** OrS 89; **MS:** SUNY Downstate 79; **RES:** S, New York University Med Ctr, New York, NY 79-80; OrS, New York University Med Ctr, New York, NY 80-84; **FEL:** Foot & Ankle, Hosp For Special Surgery, New York, NY 84-85; **HOSP:** St Joseph's Med Ctr-Stamford; **SI:** *Ankle Adult; Foot Adult;* **HMO:** Aetna Hlth Plan CIGNA Oxford PHS MD Health Plan +

🔲 🔲 🔲 🔲 🔲 🔲 🔲 🔲 🔲 A Few Days 🔲 **VISA** 🔲

Wilchinsky, Mark (MD)   OrS
St Vincent's Med Ctr-Bridgeport

Merritt Orthopaedic Assoc, 3909 Main St; Bridgeport, CT 06606; (203) 372-4565; **BDCERT:** OrS 86; **MS:** Tulane U 79; **RES:** S, U Mass Med Ctr, Worcester, MA 79; OrS, U Mass Med Ctr, Worcester, MA 80-84; **FAP:** Asst Clin Prof; **SI:** *Knee Shoulder-Arthroscopy; Joint Replacement;* **HMO:** PHS MD Health Plan Oxford Blue Cross Anthem Health +

LANG: Itl; 🔲 🔲 🔲 🔲 🔲 🔲 🔲 🔲 🔲 A Few Days **VISA** 🔲

OTOLARYNGOLOGY

Beres, Milan (MD)   Oto
Bridgeport Hosp

1681 Barnum Ave; Stratford, CT 06497; (203) 378-1267; **BDCERT:** Oto 74; **MS:** Czechoslovakia 59; **RES:** Oto, U Conn Hlth Ctr, Farmington, CT 71-73; Oto, U Conn Hlth Ctr, Farmington, CT 73-74; **FEL:** Oto, Cleveland Clinic Hosp, Cleveland, OH 70-71; **FAP:** Asst Clin Prof U Conn Sch Med; **SI:** *Head and Neck Surgery; Sleep Apnea, Snoring & Cancer;* **HMO:** Anthem Health Multiplan PHS MD Health Plan

LANG: Slv, Sp, Pol; 🔲 🔲 🔲 🔲 🔲 🔲 🔲 🔲 Immediately **VISA** 🔲

Coffey, Tom (MD)   Oto
St Vincent's Med Ctr-Bridgeport

CT Ear Nose Throat Specialists, 15 Corporate Rd; Trumble, CT 06611; (203) 452-7081; **BDCERT:** Oto 92; **MS:** Columbia P&S 86; **RES:** S, Yale-New Haven Hosp, New Haven, CT 87-88; Oto, Yale-New Haven Hosp, New Haven, CT 88-91; **FAP:** Clin Instr Yale U Sch Med; **HMO:** Aetna Hlth Plan Blue Cross MD Health Plan Oxford PHS +

♿ ☽ 📷 📅 Mcr WC Immediately **VISA** 💳

Gaynor, Edward (MD)   Oto
Norwalk Hosp

40 Cross St 230; Norwalk, CT 06851; (203) 226-0095; **BDCERT:** Oto 71; **MS:** SUNY Downstate 66; **RES:** Temple U Hosp, Philadelphia, PA 68-71; **FAP:** Asst Prof S Yale U Sch Med; **SI:** *Pediatric Otolaryngology*

♿ 📷 📅 📅 $ Mcr WC NFI Immediately **VISA** 💳

Klarsfeld, Jay (MD)   Oto
Danbury Hosp

107 Newtown Rd 2A; Danbury, CT 06810; (203) 830-4700; **BDCERT:** Oto 86; **MS:** Mt Sinai Sch Med 81; **RES:** S, Mount Sinai Med Ctr, New York, NY 81-83; Oto, Mount Sinai Med Ctr, New York, NY 83-86; **FAP:** Clin Instr Mt Sinai Sch Med; **SI:** *Sinus Disease Treatment; Thyroid and Parathyroid*; **HMO:** Aetna Hlth Plan CIGNA PHS US Hlthcre Oxford +

LANG: Prt, Sp, Fr; ♿ 📷 📅 📅 $ Mcr Mod WC NFI Immediately **VISA** 💳 💳

Klenoff, Bruce (MD)   Oto
Stamford Hosp

188 North St; Stamford, CT 06901; (203) 324-4123; **BDCERT:** Oto 76; **MS:** Tufts U 69; **RES:** S, St Elizabeth's Med Ctr, Boston, MA 72-73; Oto, Mass Eye & Ear Infirmary, Boston, MA 73-76; **FAP:** Instr NY Med Coll; **HOSP:** St Joseph's Med Ctr-Stamford; **SI:** *Ear Surgery; Sinus Surgery*; **HMO:** Aetna Hlth Plan Oxford Anthem Health PHS Medspan +

📷 📅 📅 $ Mcr Mod WC NFI 1 Week

Kveton, John (MD)   Oto
Yale-New Haven Hosp

333 Cedar St; New Haven, CT 06519; (203) 785-2593; **BDCERT:** Oto 82; **MS:** St Louis U 78; **RES:** Yale-New Haven Hosp, New Haven, CT 78-82; **FEL:** OntNeu Group, Nashville, TN 82-83; **FAP:** Prof Oto Yale U Sch Med; **SI:** *Acoustic Neuromas; Hearing Loss*; **HMO:** Aetna Hlth Plan PHS Oxford

♿ 📷 📅 📅 $ Mcr Mod WC NFI 1 Week 💳 **VISA** 💳 💳

Levin, Richard (MD)   Oto
St Vincent's Med Ctr-Bridgeport

1305 Post Rd; Fairfield, CT 06430; (203) 259-4700; **MS:** Tufts U 87; **RES:** Oto, Mount Sinai Hosp, Cleveland, OH

♿ ☽ 📷 📅 $ Mcr Mod NFI 2-4 Weeks

Lipton, Richard Jeffrey (MD) Oto
Danbury Hosp

107 Newton Rd Suite 2A; Danbury, CT 06810; **BDCERT:** Oto 90; **MS:** Mayo Med Sch 85; **RES:** S, Mayo Clinic, Rochester, MN 85-86; Oto, Mayo Clinic, Rochester, MN 86-90; **SI:** *Head & Neck Surgery*; **HMO:** Blue Cross & Blue Choice PHS US Hlthcre CIGNA

LANG: Sp, Fr; ♿ 📷 📅 📅 $ Mcr Mod WC NFI

McKee, David (MD)   Oto
Stamford Hosp

166 W Broad St Ste 304; Stamford, CT 06902; (203) 324-9297; **BDCERT:** Oto 71; **MS:** NYU Sch Med 59; **RES:** Oto, New York Eye & Ear Infirmary, New York, NY 64-67; **HOSP:** St Joseph's Med Ctr-Stamford; **HMO:** Most

♿ 📷 📅 📅 $ Mcr WC A Few Days **VISA** 💳

Miles, Richard (MD)   Oto
Stamford Hosp

125 Strawberry Hill Ave Ste 302; Stamford, CT 06902; (203) 327-5500; **BDCERT:** Oto 94; **MS:** Med Coll Va 87; **RES:** Oto, New York University Med Ctr, New York, NY 87-93; **FEL:** PlS, Deaconess, St Louis, MO 94; **FAP:** Clin Instr Yale U Sch Med; **SI:** *Sinus Disorders; Snoring and Sleep Disorders*; **HMO:** Aetna-US Healthcare CIGNA PHS United Healthcare Oxford +

♿ 📷 📅 📅 $ Mcr A Few Days

Guide to symbols and abbreviations can be found on pages 110-113.

1063

Salzer, Stephen (MD)   Oto
Greenwich Hosp
49 Lake Ave 5; Greenwich, CT 06830; (203) 869-
2030; **BDCERT:** Oto 95; **MS:** Johns Hopkins U 89;
RES: Yale-New Haven Hosp, New Haven, CT 89-
94; **FEL:** Head & Neck S, Laennel Hosp, Paris,
France; *SI: Sinus Surgery; Head and Neck Cancer;*
HMO: Aetna Hlth Plan Oxford United Healthcare
Blue Cross & Blue Shield

LANG: Itl, Sp; 🚹 🏧 🌙 📠 🚼 🏥 Mcr Mod WC NFI
Immediately

Sasaki, ClarenceT (MD)   Oto
Yale-New Haven Hosp
Yale ENT Group, 800 Howard Ave FL4; New
Haven, CT 06520; (203) 785-2592; **BDCERT:** Oto
73; **MS:** Yale U Sch Med 66; **RES:** S, Dartmouth,
Hanover, CT 67-68; Oto, Yale-New Haven Hospital,
New Haven, CT 70-73; **FAP:** Prof Yale U Sch Med;
HOSP: Hosp of St Raphael; *SI: Head and Neck
Surgery; Voice and Swallowing;* **HMO:** Aetna Hlth
Plan CIGNA Bluecare PHS Connecticare +

LANG: Sp; 🚹 📠 🏥 💲 Mcr Mod WC NFI 2-4 Weeks▨
VISA 💳

Townsend, Gary (MD)   Oto
Danbury Hosp
13 Hosp Ave; Danbury, CT 06810; (203) 830-
2015; **BDCERT:** Oto 71; **MS:** Yale U Sch Med 66;
RES: Oto, Mayo Clinic, Rochester, MN 68-71

Watts, Joe (MD)   Oto
Greenwich Hosp
Associates Of Otolaryngology, 49 Lake Ave;
Greenwich, CT 06830; (203) 869-0178; **BDCERT:**
Oto 78; **MS:** U Mich Med Sch 71; **RES:** S, NY Hosp-
Cornell Med Ctr, New York, NY 71-73; Oto, New
York University Med Ctr, New York, NY 73-76;
FAP: Asst Clin Instr NYU Sch Med; *SI: Pediatric
ENT; Sinus Disease;* **HMO:** Aetna Hlth Plan Oxford
Pomco Health Choice United Healthcare +

🚹 🏧 📠 🚼 🏥 💲 Mcr WC A Few Days▨ **VISA**
💳

PAIN MANAGEMENT

Gudin, Jeffrey A (MD)   PM
Hosp of St Raphael
Comprehensive Pain & Headache Treatment Ctrs,;
New Haven, CT 06510; (203) 732-1570; **BDCERT:**
Anes 97; **MS:** Albany Med Coll 92; **RES:** Anes, Yale-
New Haven Hosp, New Haven, CT 93-96; **FEL:**
Yale-New Haven Hosp, New Haven, CT 96-97; *SI:
Detoxification Services;* **HMO:** Most

🚹 📠 🏥 💲 Mcr Mod WC NFI 1 Week

PEDIATRIC
CARDIOLOGY

Berkwits, Kieve (MD)   PCd
Bridgeport Hosp
50 Ridgefield Ave 203; Bridgeport, CT 06610;
(203) 384-3783; **BDCERT:** Ped 86; **MS:** Mexico 79;
RES: Ped, Beth Israel Med Ctr, Boston, MA 81-83;
FEL: PCd, NY Hosp-Cornell Med Ctr, New York, NY
83-85; **FAP:** Asst Clin Prof Ped Yale U Sch Med
LANG: Sp; 🚹 📠 🚼 🏥 💲 Mod 2-4 Weeks

Hellenbrand, William E (MD) PCd
Yale-New Haven Hosp
333 Cedar St; New Haven, CT 06520; (203) 785-
2022; **MS:** SUNY Downstate 70; **RES:** Ped A&I,
Yale-New Haven Hosp, New Haven, CT 71-72; **FEL:**
PCd, Yale-New Haven Hosp, New Haven, CT 72-
73; PCd, Yale-New Haven Hosp, New Haven, CT
75-76; **FAP:** Prof Ped Yale U Sch Med; *SI: Cardiac
Catheterization-pediatric; Interventional
Catheterization;* **HMO:** Aetna Hlth Plan PHS CIGNA
Blue Choice Oxford +

LANG: Sp; 🚹 🌙 📠 🚼 🏥 Mcr Mod 1 Week

PEDIATRIC HEMATOLOGY-ONCOLOGY

Beardsley, G Peter (MD & PhD)PHO
Yale-New Haven Hosp
Yale Univ Sch Med - Dept of Pediatrics, 333 Cedar St; New Haven, CT 06520; (203) 785-4640; **BDCERT:** Ped 92; **MS:** Duke U 74; **RES:** Ped, Yale-New Haven Hosp, New Haven, CT 74-76; **FEL:** PHO, Children's Hosp, Boston, MA 76-79; PHO, Harvard Med Sch, Cambridge, MA 76-79; **FAP:** Prof Yale U Sch Med; **SI:** *Leukemia; Bone Tumors;* **HMO:** Blue Cross & Blue Shield United Payors PHS

LANG: Sp; ♿ 🅂🄰 📷 📋 🎬 Mcd Immediately ▦
VISA 💳 💳

McIntosh, Sue (MD) PHO
Yale-New Haven Hosp
405 Church St; Guilford, CT 06437; (203) 453-2013; **BDCERT:** Ped 74; 74; **MS:** U Tenn Ctr Hlth Sci, Memphis 69; **RES:** Yale-New Haven Hosp, New Haven, CT 70-71; **FEL:** Yale-New Haven Hosp, New Haven, CT 71-73

LANG: Sp; ♿ 🎬 🆂 Mcr Mcd WC 2-4 Weeks

PEDIATRIC PULMONOLOGY

Dworkin, Gregory (MD) PPul
Danbury Hosp
Danbury Office of Physician Services, 24 Hospital Ave; Danbury, CT 06810; (203) 797-7027; **BDCERT:** Ped 87; PPul 98; **MS:** Albany Med Coll 82; **RES:** Ped, Mount Sinai Med Ctr, New York, NY 82-85; Ped, Mount Sinai Med Ctr, New York, NY 85-86; **FEL:** PPul, Mount Sinai Med Ctr, New York, NY 86-89; **FAP:** Asst Clin Prof NY Med Coll; **SI:** *Asthma; Habit Cough*

♿ 🄲 📷 🎬 🆂 Mcr Mcd WC A Few Days ▦ **VISA**
💳

Hen Jr, Jacob (MD) PPul
Bridgeport Hosp
Mill Hill Med Consultants, 267 Grant St Box 5000; Bridgeport, CT 06610; (203) 384-3711; **BDCERT:** Ped 80; PCCM 87; **MS:** UMDNJ-NJ Med Sch, Newark 75; **RES:** Ped, Univ of Med & Dent NJ Hosp, Newark, NJ 76-77; **FEL:** PPul, Yale-New Haven Hosp, New Haven, CT 78-81; **FAP:** Assoc Clin Prof Yale U Sch Med; **HOSP:** Yale-New Haven Hosp; **SI:** *Asthma; Critical Care;* **HMO:** PHS Aetna-US Healthcare MD Health Plan Oxford Blue Cross & Blue Choice +

♿ 📷 🅙 🎬 🆂 Mcd NFI 1 Week

PEDIATRIC SURGERY

Touloukian, Robert (MD) PS
Yale-New Haven Hosp
Yale Pediatric Surgery, 333 Cedar St; New Haven, CT 06520; (203) 785-2701; **BDCERT:** PS 93; **MS:** Columbia P&S 60; **RES:** S, Columbia-Presbyterian Med Ctr, New York, NY 62-64; S, Bellevue Hosp Ctr, New York, NY 64-65; **FEL:** Ped S, Babies Hosp, New York, NY 66; **FAP:** Prof Yale U Sch Med; **SI:** *Hirschsprung's Disease; Solid Tumors;* **HMO:** Aetna Hlth Plan Oxford PHS MD Health Plan CIGNA +

♿ 🄲 📷 🎬 🆂 Mcr Mcd WC NFI Immediately ▦
VISA 💳 💳

PEDIATRICS

Cass, Alison (MD) Ped
Greenwich Hosp
Greenwich Pediatric Assoc, 8 W End Ave; Old Greenwich, CT 06870; (203) 637-3212; **BDCERT:** Ped 87; **MS:** U Conn Sch Med 83; **RES:** Ped, Bridgeport Hosp, Bridgeport, CT 83-86; **HOSP:** Stamford Hosp; **HMO:** Aetna Hlth Plan Oxford PHS United Healthcare Health Source +

🅂🄰 📷 🅙 🎬 🆂 A Few Days **VISA** 💳

Guide to symbols and abbreviations can be found on pages 110-113.

1065

Chessin, Robert (MD)   Ped   **PCP**
St Vincent's Med Ctr-Bridgeport
Pediatric Healthcare Assoc, PC, 4699 Main St 215;
Bridgeport, CT 06606; (203) 372-1000; **BDCERT:**
Ped 78; **MS:** Johns Hopkins U 73; **RES:** Ped, Duke U
Med Ctr, Durham, NC 73-76; **FAP:** Assoc Clin Prof
Yale U Sch Med; **HOSP:** Bridgeport Hosp; **HMO:**
PHS Aetna-US Healthcare Bluecare CIGNA Oxford
+

♿ ♻ ⚇ ⚇ ⚇ ⚇ ⚇ ⚇ 1 Week

Ertl, John (MD)   Ped
Danbury Hosp
Pediatric Associates of Western CT, 41
Germantown Rd 201; Danbury, CT 06810; (203)
744-1680; **BDCERT:** Ped 77; **PHO** 78; **MS:** SUNY
Downstate 70; **RES:** Ped, Rhode Island Hosp,
Providence, RI 71-73; **FEL:** PHO, UC Davis Med Ctr,
Sacramento, CA 75-77; *SI: Hematology*

♿ ⚇ ⚇

Hofreuter, Nancy (MD)   Ped   **PCP**
Stamford Hosp
New England Pediatrics, 166 W Broad St 103;
Stamford, CT 06902; (203) 323-1770; **BDCERT:**
Ped 92; **MS:** Univ Penn 88; **RES:** Children's Hosp of
Pittsburgh, Pittsburgh, PA 88-92; *SI: Eating
Disorders*; **HMO:** Aetna Hlth Plan Oxford PHS
United Healthcare
LANG: Sp; ♿ ♻ ⚇ ⚇ ⚇ ⚇ ⚇ ⚇ 1 Week
VISA ⚇

Juan, Paul (MD)   Ped
Greenwich Hosp
42 Sherwood Pl; Greenwich, CT 06830; (203)
661-2440; **BDCERT:** Ped 94; **MS:** NY Med Coll 90;
RES: VA Commonwealth Sch Med, , VA 90-93; *SI:
Development; Asthma*

Keller, Barry (MD)   Ped   **PCP**
Danbury Hosp
16 Hospital Ave 304; Danbury, CT 06810; (203)
743-1201; **BDCERT:** Ped 71; **MS:** SUNY Hlth Sci
Ctr 65; **RES:** Kingsbrook Jewish Med Ctr, Brooklyn,
NY 66; Montefiore Med Ctr, Bronx, NY 68; **FEL:**
EDM, Jacobi Med Ctr, Bronx, NY; *SI: Growth
Disorders*; **HMO:** PHS Aetna Hlth Plan CIGNA Blue
Cross & Blue Shield PHCS +

LANG: Fr; ♿ ♻ ⚇ ⚇ ⚇ ⚇ A Few Days

Klenk, Rosemary (MD)   Ped   **PCP**
Stamford Hosp
New England Pediatrics, 166 W Broad St 103;
Stamford, CT 06902; (203) 323-1770; **BDCERT:**
Ped 87; **MS:** Cornell U 80; **RES:** Ped, Columbia-
Presbyterian Med Ctr, New York, NY 80-83; **FAP:**
Instr Ped Columbia P&S; **HMO:** Aetna Hlth Plan
Oxford PHCS Sanus-NYLCare Connecticare +

LANG: Sp; ♿ ♻ ⚇ ⚇ ⚇ ⚇ ⚇ ⚇ A Few Days
⚇ ⚇

Korval, Arnold (MD)   Ped   **PCP**
Greenwich Hosp
Greenwich Pediatrics Assoc, 8 W End Ave; Old
Greenwich, CT 06870; (203) 637-0186; **BDCERT:**
Ped 79; **MS:** St Louis U 74; **RES:** Ped, Children's
Hosp of Philadelphia, Philadelphia, PA 74-77;
HOSP: Stamford Hosp; *SI: General Pediatrics;
Adolescents*; **HMO:** Aetna Hlth Plan Oxford PHS
CIGNA PHCS +

♻ ⚇ ⚇ ⚇ ⚇ ⚇ Immediately **VISA** ⚇

Levine, Dorothy (MD)   Ped   **PCP**
Stamford Hosp
New England Pediatrics, 166 W Broad St 103;
Stamford, CT 06902; (203) 323-1770; **BDCERT:**
Ped 85; **MS:** Albert Einstein Coll Med 80; **RES:** Ped,
Columbia-Presbyterian Med Ctr, New York, NY 80-
83; **FAP:** Asst Ped Columbia P&S; **HMO:** PHS
Oxford Connecticare Medspan Aetna Hlth Plan +
LANG: Sp; ♿ ♻ ⚇ ⚇ ⚇ ⚇ ⚇ A Few Days

Mongillo, Nicholas (MD) Ped PCP
Bridgeport Hosp
Pedicare PC, 7365 Main St; Stratford, CT 06497;
(203) 381-9990; **BDCERT:** Ped 95; **MS:** Grenada
87; **RES:** Ped, Bridgeport Hosp, Bridgeport, CT 87-
90; **HOSP:** Stamford Hosp; **SI:** *Pediatric HIV Disease;
Sports Medicine;* **HMO:** PHS MD Health Plan Oxford
Anthem Health CIGNA +

LANG: Sp, Itl; ♿ 🈂 🌙 📷 📅 💲 A Few Days ⬤

Morelli, Alan (MD) Ped PCP
Stamford Hosp
New England Pediatrics LLP, 166 W Broad St 103;
Stamford, CT 06902; (203) 323-1770; **BDCERT:**
Ped 87; **MS:** NY Med Coll 82; **RES:** Yale-New Haven
Hosp, New Haven, CT 82-85; **FAP:** Clin Instr Ped
Yale U Sch Med; **SI:** *Public Health Issues;
Immunizations;* **HMO:** PHS Oxford Aetna Hlth Plan
United Healthcare Medspan +

LANG: Sp, Fr, Ger; ♿ 🈂 🌙 📷 📹 📅 💲 Med
Immediately ▨ **VISA** ⬤

Romanowitz, Harry (MD) Ped PCP
Stamford Hosp
Stamford Hospital Department of Pediatrics, 190 W
Broad St; Stamford, CT 06904; (203) 325-7082;
BDCERT: Ped 89; **MS:** Yale U Sch Med 73; **RES:**
Ped, Strong Mem Hosp, Rochester, NY 73-76; **FAP:**
Asst Prof Ped Yale U Sch Med; **HOSP:** Yale-New
Haven Hosp; **HMO:** Aetna Hlth Plan PHS Oxford

LANG: Rus, Yd, Heb; ♿ 📷 📹 📅 💲 Med NFI 1 Week

Schutzengel, Roy (MD) Ped PCP
St Vincent's Med Ctr-Bridgeport
Main Street Pediatrics, 3543 Main St FL2;
Bridgeport, CT 06606; (203) 371-7111; **BDCERT:**
Ped 96; **MS:** Univ Penn 84; **RES:** Ped, UC Davis Med
Ctr, Sacramento, CA 84-88; **FEL:** PEn, Nat Inst
Health, Bethesda, MD 85-86; **PHO:** Yale-New
Haven Hosp, New Haven, CT 88-89; **HOSP:** Yale-
New Haven Hosp; **SI:** *Growth Disorders;
Developmental Disorders;* **HMO:** Aetna-US
Healthcare PHS Connecticare Blue Cross

♿ 🈂 🌙 📷 📹 📅 💲 Med 1 Week **VISA** ⬤

Smith, Marilyn (MD) Ped
St Vincent's Med Ctr-Bridgeport
St Vincent's Med Center Bridgeport-Dept of Ped,
3543 Main St; Bridgeport, CT 06606; (203) 371-
7111; **BDCERT:** Ped 98; **MS:** U Cincinnati 87; **RES:**
Ped, Yale-New Haven Hosp, New Haven, CT 87-90;
HOSP: Bridgeport Hosp

♿ 🈂 🌙 📷 📅 Mcr Med

Swidler, Sanford (MD) Ped PCP
Stamford Hosp
Pediatric Center, 126 Morgan St; Stamford, CT
06902; (203) 327-1055; **BDCERT:** Ped 87; **MS:**
NYU Sch Med 80; **RES:** Bellevue Hosp Ctr, New
York, NY 80-84; **HMO:** Aetna Hlth Plan CIGNA
Oxford PHS Anthem Health +

LANG: Fr, Sp; ♿ 🈂 🌙 📷 📹 📅 💲 Med **VISA** ⬤

PHYSICAL MEDICINE & REHABILITATION

Brennan, Michael (MD) PMR
Bridgeport Hosp
Rehabilitation Center, 226 Mill Hill; Bridgeport, CT
06610; (203) 336-7349; **BDCERT:** PMR 90; **MS:**
SUNY Downstate 85; **RES:** PMR, NY Hosp-Cornell
Med Ctr, New York, NY 86-89; **SI:** *Chronic Pain;
Back Pain;* **HMO:** PHS CIGNA US Hlthcre MD
Health Plan Blue Cross & Blue Shield +

LANG: Fr, Sp; ♿ 🌙 📷 📹 📅 💲 Mcr Med WC NFI
A Few Days ▨ **VISA** ⬤ ▨

Grant, Linda (MD) PMR
Greenwich Hosp
Greenwich HospDept PM&R, 5 Perryridge Rd;
Greenwich, CT 06830; (203) 863-3290; **BDCERT:**
PMR 90; **MS:** Rutgers U 85; **RES:** PMR, New York
University Med Ctr, New York, NY 86-89; **FAP:**
Instr NYU Sch Med; **SI:** *Musculoskeletal Injuries;
Neurological Disabilities;* **HMO:** Oxford PHS Aetna
Hlth Plan CIGNA Prucare +

LANG: Sp, Itl, Jpn; ♿ 📹 📅 Mcr Med WC NFI 1 Week
▨ **VISA** ⬤

Mashman, Jan (MD)   PMR
Danbury Hosp

Datahr Rehabilitation Inst, 135 Old State Rd; Brookfield, CT 06804; (203) 775-4700; **BDCERT:** N 71; **MS:** Univ Vt Coll Med 65; **RES:** N, Albert Einstein Med Ctr, Bronx, NY 65-69; **FAP:** Asst Clin Prof Yale U Sch Med; *SI: Acquired Brain Injury; Multiple Sclerosis;* **HMO:** Aetna Hlth Plan Oxford CIGNA Anthem Health PHS +

[♿] [▣] [♠] [⊞] [$] [Mcr] [WC] 1 Week **VISA** [●]

PLASTIC HAND SURGERY

Flagg, Stephen (MD)   HS (PlS)
Yale-New Haven Hosp

2 Church South 201; New Haven, CT 06519; (203) 789-2288; **MS:** Columbia P&S 62; **RES:** HS, St Luke's Roosevelt Hosp Ctr, New York, NY 70-71; New York University Med Ctr, New York, NY 66-70; **FEL:** HS, St Luke's Roosevelt Hosp Ctr, New York, NY 66-63; **FAP:** Asst Clin Prof PlS Yale U Sch Med

[♿] [▣] [♠] [⊞] [$] [Mcr] [WC] 2-4 Weeks

PLASTIC SURGERY

Calabrese, Carmine (MD)   PlS
Bridgeport Hosp

148 Riverview East St; Norwalk, CT 06851; (203) 853-9331; **BDCERT:** PlS 77; S 73; **MS:** Johns Hopkins U 65; **RES:** Albert Einstein Med Ctr, Bronx, NY 69-72; U NC Hosp, Chapel Hill, NC 73-75; **FEL:** S, Yale-New Haven Hosp, New Haven, CT 65-66; **HOSP:** Norwalk Hosp; *SI: Cosmetic Surgery; Skin Cancer Surgery;* **HMO:** PHS Aetna Hlth Plan Blue Cross & Blue Shield United Healthcare Oxford +

LANG: Itl; [♿] [▣] [♠] [⊞] [$] [Mcr] [Mcd] [WC] [NFI] A Few Days **VISA** [●]

Gewirtz, Harold (MD)   PlS
Stamford Hosp

70 Mill River St; Stamford, CT 06902; (203) 325-1381; **BDCERT:** PlS 84; HS 90; **MS:** Johns Hopkins U 75; **RES:** UCLA Med Ctr, Los Angeles, CA 75-80; **FEL:** PlS, New York University Med Ctr, New York, NY; **HOSP:** St Joseph's Med Ctr-Stamford; *SI: Cosmetic Surgery; Microsurgery;* **HMO:** Aetna Hlth Plan PHCS United Healthcare

[♿] [▣] [⊞] [$] [Mcr] [WC] 1 Week [▤] **VISA**

Goldenberg, David (MD)   PlS
Danbury Hosp

27 Hosp Ave 101; Danbury, CT 06810; (203) 791-9661; **BDCERT:** PlS 90; **MS:** NY Med Coll 82; **RES:** Montefiore Med Ctr, Bronx, NY 82-86; Albert Einstein Med Ctr, Bronx, NY; **FEL:** PlS, Montefiore Med Ctr, Bronx, NY 86-88; **HMO:** CIGNA Aetna Hlth Plan PHS Blue Cross & Blue Shield Oxford +

[♿] [SA/SD] [☾] [▣] [♠] [⊞] [Mcr] [Mcd] [WC] [NFI] Immediately **VISA** [●]

Rein, Joel (MD)   PlS
Greenwich Hosp

2 1/2 Dearfield Dr; Greenwich, CT 06831; (203) 869-9850; **BDCERT:** PlS 73; S 71; **MS:** Columbia P&S 63; **RES:** S, Columbia-Presbyterian Med Ctr, New York, NY 68-70; PlS, Columbia-Presbyterian Med Ctr, New York, NY 70-72; **FEL:** HS, St Luke's Roosevelt Hosp Ctr, New York, NY 72; *SI: Breast Surgery; Facial Cosmetic Surgery;* **HMO:** Aetna Hlth Plan CIGNA Oxford Blue Cross & Blue Shield PHS +

[♿] [▣] [♠] [⊞] [$] [Mcr] [NFI] A Few Days **VISA** [●]

Rosen, Rick (MD)   PlS
Norwalk Hosp

2600 Post Rd; Southport, CT 06490; (203) 254-3733; **BDCERT:** PlS 89; **MS:** Mexico 79; **RES:** S, St Vincent's Med Ctr-Bridgeport, Bridgeport, CT 83-85; S, N Shore Univ Hosp-Manhasset, Manhasset, NY 80-82; **FEL:** PlS, Nassau County Med Ctr, East Meadow, NY; **HOSP:** St Vincent's Med Ctr-Bridgeport; *SI: Breast Surgery; Facial Surgery;* **HMO:** MD Health Plan Aetna Hlth Plan Oxford Connecticare +

[♿] [☾] [▣] [♠] [⊞] [$] [Mcr] [WC] [NFI] Immediately **VISA** [●]

Rosenstock, Arthur (MD) PlS
Stamford Hosp
1290 Summer St 3100; Stamford, CT 06905;
(203) 359-1959; **BDCERT**: PlS 85; **MS**: Belgium
76; **RES**: S, NY Med Coll, Valhalla, NY 76-81; **FEL**:
PlS, Med Coll VA Hosp, Richmond, VA 81-83;
HOSP: Greenwich Hosp; *SI: Cosmetic Surgery; Breast
Reconstruction*; **HMO**: Aetna Hlth Plan United
Healthcare
LANG: Fr; 🦽 🔲 🎦 🏥 💲 ⓌⒸ ⓃⒻ 2-4 Weeks

PSYCHIATRY

Caraccio, Babette (MD) Psyc
Greenwich Hosp
23 Mianus View Ter; Cos Cob, CT 06807; (203)
622-7428; **BDCERT**: Psyc 88; ChAP 89; **MS**: NYU
Sch Med 82; **RES**: New York University Med Ctr,
New York, NY; **FEL**: NY Hosp-Cornell-Westchester,
White Plains, NY; *SI: Depression and Anxiety;
Parenting; Psychopharmacology*
🔲 🔲 🎦 🏥 💲 1 Week

Dolan, John (MD) Psyc
St Vincent's Med Ctr-Bridgeport
Saint Vincent's Medical Ctr, 2800 Main St;
Bridgeport, CT 06606; (203) 576-6000; **BDCERT**:
Psyc 75; **MS**: UMDNJ-NJ Med Sch, Newark 62; **RES**:
Psyc, St Louis U Hosp, St Louis, MO 70-72; N,
Barnes Hosp, St Louis, MO 66-69; **FAP**: Assoc Clin
Prof NY Med Coll; *SI: Depression; Anxiety*
🦽 🔲 🎦 🏥 💲 Ⓜⓡ Ⓜⓓ ⓌⒸ ⓃⒻ A Few Days

Hart, Sidney (MD) Psyc
Greenwich Hosp
2 1/2 Dearfield Dr; Greenwich, CT 06831; (203)
622-1722; **BDCERT**: Psyc 73; **MS**: Albert Einstein
Coll Med 64; **RES**: Psyc, Bronx Muncipal Hosp Ctr,
Bronx, NY 68-71; **FEL**: Montefiore Med Ctr, Bronx,
NY 71-73; *SI: Anxiety Disorders; Depressive
Disorders*; **HMO**: None
🦽 🔲 🔲 🎦 🏥 1 Week

Lamba, Ameet (MD) Psyc
Stamford Hosp
32 Imperial Ave; Westport, CT 06880; (203) 454-
3457; **BDCERT**: Psyc 85; **MS**: India 74; **RES**: Psyc,
Nassau County Med Ctr, East Meadow, NY 77-79;
Fairfield Hills Hosp, Newton, CT 79-81; **FAP**: Asst
Clin Prof Yale U Sch Med; *SI: Psychopharmacology;
Psychotherapy*
LANG: Hin, Pun; 🦽 🔲 🔲 🎦 🏥 💲 ⓌⒸ ⓃⒻ
Immediately

Lorefice, Laurence (MD) Psyc
Greenwich Hosp
404 Sound Beach Ave; Old Greenwich, CT 06870;
(203) 637-4006; **BDCERT**: Psyc 79; **MS**: Univ
Penn 75; **RES**: Psyc, Mass Gen Hosp, Boston, MA
75-79; **FAP**: Asst Clin Prof NY Med Coll; **HOSP**:
Stamford Hosp; *SI: Depression and Manic Depression;
Anxiety Panic Disorder*
🔲 🔲 🎦 🏥 💲 A Few Days

Mueller, F Carl (MD) Psyc
Stamford Hosp
1275 Summer St 203; Stamford, CT 06905; (203)
357-7773; **BDCERT**: Psyc 87; Ger 91; **MS**: U Conn
Sch Med 82; **RES**: Psyc, Yale-New Haven Hosp,
New Haven, CT 82-83; **FEL**: Psyc, Yale-New Haven
Hosp, New Haven, CT 83-86; **FAP**: Asst Prof Yale U
Sch Med; **HOSP**: St Joseph's Med Ctr-Stamford; *SI:
Psychopharmacology; Neuropsychiatry*; **HMO**:
CIGNA MD Health Plan Connecticare PHCS
🦽 🔲 🔲 🏥 💲 Ⓜⓡ ⓌⒸ 2-4 Weeks **VISA** 💳

Nelson, J Craig (MD) Psyc
Yale-New Haven Hosp
20 York St; New Haven, CT 06504; (203) 688-
2157; **BDCERT**: Psyc 92; **MS**: U Wisc Med Sch 68;
RES: Herrick Mem Hosp, Berkeley, CA 68-69; Psyc,
Yale-New Haven Hosp, New Haven, CT 69-70; *SI:
Psychopharmacology; Geriatric Psychiatry*
🦽 🏥 Ⓜⓡ Ⓜⓓ

Rifkin, Boris (MD)   Psyc
Hosp of St Raphael

100 York St 2B; New Haven, CT 06511; (203) 776-1213; **BDCERT:** Psyc 68; **MS:** South Africa 54; **RES:** Psyc, Yale-New Haven Hosp, New Haven, CT 62-65; Psyc, Fairfield Hills Hosp, Newton, CT 62-65; **FAP:** Assoc Clin Prof Yale U Sch Med; *SI: Anxiety Disorders; Major Depression;* **HMO:** Blue Cross MD Health Plan PHS Medspan

♿ ☐ ☐ ☐ **S** Mcr   A Few Days

Rousell, Charles (MD)   Psyc
Greenwich Hosp

Northeast Center For Trauma Recovery, 38 Lake Ave; Greenwich, CT 06830; (203) 661-9393; **BDCERT:** Psyc 77; **MS:** Columbia P&S 72; **RES:** Psyc, Bronx Muncipal Hosp Ctr, Bronx, NY 73-76; Psyc, Bronx Muncipal Hosp Ctr, Bronx, NY 75-76; **FEL:** Psyc, Bronx Muncipal Hosp Ctr, Bronx, NY 76-77; **FAP:** Asst Prof Psyc Albert Einstein Coll Med; *SI: Hypnosis; Post Traumatic Stress Disorder;* **HMO:** None

☸ ☐ ☐ ☐ **S**   2-4 Weeks **VISA**

Schechter, Justin (MD)   Psyc
Stamford Hosp

22 5th St Fl 3; Stamford, CT 06905; (203) 323-7760; **BDCERT:** Psyc 86; **MS:** SUNY Hlth Sci Ctr 81; **RES:** Med, Greenwich Hosp, Greenwich, CT 81-82; Psyc, Yale-New Haven Hosp, New Haven, CT 82-85; **FAP:** Asst Clin Prof Yale U Sch Med; **HOSP:** St Joseph's Med Ctr-Stamford; *SI: Mood Disorders; Anxiety Disorders;* **HMO:** Aetna Hlth Plan Oxford PHS CIGNA Bluecare +

LANG: Fr; ♿ ☸ ☐ ☐ ☐ **S** Mcr Mod WC   1 Week **VISA** ●

Shapiro, Bruce (MD)   Psyc
Stamford Hosp

190 W Broad St PO Box 9317; Stamford, CT 06900; (203) 325-7439; **BDCERT:** Psyc 76; **MS:** NY Med Coll 72; **RES:** Metropolitan Hosp Ctr, New York, NY 72-75

♿ WC

Sheftell, Fred (MD)   Psyc
Greenwich Hosp

77 Long Ridge Rd; Stamford, CT 06902; (203) 968-1799; **BDCERT:** Psyc 72; **MS:** NY Med Coll 66; **RES:** Metropolitan Hosp, New York, NY 67-70

Smith, Jo Ann (MD)   Psyc
St Vincent's Med Ctr-Bridgeport

160 Hawley Lane; Trumbull, CT 06611; (203) 377-0111; **BDCERT:** Psyc 80; **MS:** SUNY Hlth Sci Ctr 74; **RES:** Georgetown U Hosp, Washington, DC 76-79; **FAP:** Asst Clin Prof Psyc NY Med Coll; *SI: Mood Disorders; Menopause;* **HMO:** PHS Blue Cross & Blue Shield

LANG: Fr; ♿ ☐ ☐ ☐ **S**   A Few Days

Solnit, Albert (MD)   Psyc
Yale-New Haven Hosp

Yale Child Study Center, 230 S Frontage Rd; New Haven, CT 06520; (203) 785-2518; **BDCERT:** Psyc 51; **ChAP** 60; **MS:** UC San Francisco 43; **RES:** San Francisco Gen Hosp, San Francisco, CA 47-48; **FEL:** Yale-New Haven Hosp, New Haven, CT; *SI: Child Psychoanalysis*

♿ ☸ ☐ Mcr Mod   4+ Weeks

PULMONARY DISEASE

Elias, Jack (MD)   Pul
Yale-New Haven Hosp

Yale Univ School of Med, 333 Cedar St 105LCI; New Haven, CT 06525; (203) 785-4163; **BDCERT:** IM 79; Pul 82; **MS:** Univ Penn 76; **RES:** New England Med Ctr, Boston, MA 76-78; Hosp of U Penn, Philadelphia, PA 78-79; **FEL:** A&I/Pul, Hosp of U Penn, Philadelphia, PA 79-80; Pul, Hosp of U Penn, Philadelphia, PA 80-82; **FAP:** Prof Med Yale U Sch Med; *SI: Asthma; Sarcoidosis*

♿

Gentry, Eric (MD)   Pul
St Vincent's Med Ctr-Bridgeport

Associates In Pulmonary & Internal Medicine,
4699 Main St Ste 203; Bridgeport, CT 06606;
(203) 372-7715; **BDCERT:** IM 90; Pul 94; **MS:**
SUNY Hlth Sci Ctr 87; **RES:** Montefiore Med Ctr,
Bronx, NY 88-90; **FEL:** Pul/CCM, Boston U Med Ctr,
Boston, MA 91-94; **SI:** *Sleep Apnea; Critical Care;*
HMO: CIGNA PHS United Healthcare Blue Cross &
Blue Shield

LANG: Sp, Itl, Prt, Rus; ♿ ⬚ ⬚ $ ⬚   A Few Days

Krasnogor, Lester (MD)   Pul
Stamford Hosp

Pulmonary Associates of Stamford, PC, 190 W
Broad St; Stamford, CT 06902; (203) 348-2437;
BDCERT: CCM 92; Pul 72; **MS:** NYU Sch Med 63;
RES: IM, Duke U Med Ctr, Durham, NC 63-65; IM,
U of Pittsburgh Med Ctr, Pittsburgh, PA 68-69; **FEL:**
Pul, Yale-New Haven Hosp, New Haven, CT 67-68;
FAP: Assoc Clin Prof Med NY Med Coll; **HOSP:** St
Joseph's Med Ctr-Stamford; **SI:** *Shortness of Breath
Asthma; Emphysema Cough Lung Cancer*

♿ ⬚ ⬚ ⬚ $ ⬚ ⬚ ⬚ ⬚   A Few Days

Krinsley, James (MD)   Pul
Stamford Hosp

190 W Broad St; Stamford, CT 06902; (203) 348-
2437; **BDCERT:** Pul 86; CCM 89; **MS:** Cornell U 80;
RES: IM, VA Med Ctr-Manh, New York, NY 80-83;
FEL: Pul, Yale-New Haven Hosp, New Haven, CT
84-86; **HOSP:** St Joseph's Med Ctr-Stamford; **SI:**
Asthma; Sleep Apnea; **HMO:** Aetna Hlth Plan PHS
Oxford

♿ ⬚ ⬚ ⬚ $ ⬚ ⬚ ⬚   Immediately

Kurtz, Caroline (MD)   Pul   **PCP**
Norwalk Hosp

Norwalk Pulmonary Consultants PC, 30 Stevens St
Ste C; Norwalk, CT 06850; (203) 855-3888;
BDCERT: IM 88; Pul 90; **MS:** NYU Sch Med 84;
RES: Mount Sinai Med Ctr, New York, NY 84-87;
FEL: Pul/CCM, Mount Sinai Med Ctr, New York, NY
89-90; **SI:** *Asthma; Emphysema;* **HMO:** Oxford
Aetna-US Healthcare Connecticare MD Health Plan
Empire Blue Cross & Shield +

Immediately ▨ *VISA* ⬤

Marino, A Michael (MD)   Pul
Greenwich Hosp

5 Perryridge Rd; Greenwich, CT 06830; (203) 661-
5379; **BDCERT:** IM 70; Pul 72; **MS:** Georgetown U
64; **RES:** IM, VA Med Ctr, Washington, DC 65-67;
FEL: Pul, VA Med Ctr, Washington, DC 67-69; **FAP:**
Assoc Prof Yale U Sch Med; **SI:** *Chronic Obstructive
Lung Disease; Asthma;* **HMO:** Oxford Aetna Hlth
Plan PHS Prucare MD Health Plan +

LANG: Itl, Sp, Chi; ♿ ⬚ ⬚ $ ⬚ ⬚ ⬚   1 Week

McCalley, Stuart (MD)   Pul
Greenwich Hosp

Greenwich Medical Group, 8 Greenwich Office
Park; Greenwich, CT 06831; (203) 869-6960;
BDCERT: IM 72; Pul 74; **MS:** Case West Res U 69;
RES: Med, Med Ctr Hosp of VT, Burlington, VT 71-
72; Med Ctr Hosp of VT, Burlington, VT; **FEL:** Chest
Med, Albert Einstein Med Ctr, Bronx, NY 72-74;
Chest Med, Bronx Muncipal Hosp Ctr, Bronx, NY
73-74; **FAP:** Asst Clin Prof Med Yale U Sch Med

Sachs, Paul (MD)   Pul
Stamford Hosp

Pulmonary Associates, 190 W Broad St; Stamford,
CT 06902; (203) 348-2437; **BDCERT:** IM 85; CCM
89; **MS:** NYU Sch Med 82; **RES:** IM, NY Hosp-
Cornell Med Ctr, New York, NY 82-85; **FEL:** PM,
Albert Einstein Med Ctr, Bronx, NY 85-87; **FAP:**
Asst Clin Prof Med NY Med Coll; **HOSP:** St Joseph's
Med Ctr-Stamford; **SI:** *Chronic Obstructive Lung;
Asthma—Sleep Disorders;* **HMO:** Aetna Hlth Plan
Blue Choice GHI Oxford +

♿ ⬚ ⬚ ⬚ $ ⬚ ⬚ ⬚   2-4 Weeks

Tanoue, Lynn (MD)   Pul
Yale-New Haven Hosp

Yale Univeristy School of Medicine, 333 Cedar St;
New Haven, CT 06510; (203) 785-6359; **BDCERT:**
Pul 88; CCM 91; **MS:** Yale U Sch Med 82; **RES:** IM,
Yale-New Haven Hosp, New Haven, CT 83-85;
Yale-New Haven Hosp, New Haven, CT 85-86; **FEL:**
Pul/CCM, Yale-New Haven Hosp, New Haven, CT
86-88; **FAP:** Asst Prof Med Yale U Sch Med; **SI:**
Pulmonary Medicine; Critical Care Medicine

♿ ⬚ ⬚ ⬚ ⬚ ⬚ ⬚   2-4 Weeks

RADIATION ONCOLOGY

Dakofsky, LaDonna J (MD)RadRO
Norwalk Hosp

Norwalk Hospital Cancer Center, 24 Stevens St; Norwalk, CT 06856; (203) 855-3625; **BDCERT:** RadRO 93; **MS:** NYU Sch Med 87; **RES:** IM, NY Hosp-Cornell Med Ctr, New York, NY 87-88; RadRO, Hosp of U Penn, Philadelphia, PA 88-91; **FAP:** Asst Clin Prof Yale U Sch Med; *SI: Prostate Cancer; Breast Cancer;* **HMO:** Aetna Hlth Plan Oxford CIGNA Blue Cross & Blue Shield Prudential +

  🚹 🆘 📷 🚼 🏨 Mcr Mcd NFl Immediately 🏦 *VISA* 💳 📇

Dowling, Sean (MD)   RadRO
Stamford Hosp

Radiation Oncology Associates, Stamford Hosp Bennett Cancer Center; Stamford, CT 06902; (203) 325-7886; **BDCERT:** IM 90; RadRO 90; **MS:** Yale U Sch Med 83; **RES:** IM, Yale-New Haven Hosp, New Haven, CT 83-86; RadRO, Yale-New Haven Hosp, New Haven, CT 86-89; *SI: Breast Cancer; Gynecologic Oncology;* **HMO:** Oxford CIGNA Aetna Hlth Plan PHS

LANG: Sp, Fr, Itl; 🚹 📷 🚼 🏨 🆂 Mcr Mcd A Few Days

Fass, Daniel (MD)   RadRO
Greenwich Hosp

77 Lafayette Pl; Greenwich, CT 06830; (203) 863-3773; **BDCERT:** RadRO 87; **MS:** Howard U 83; **RES:** RadRO, New York University Med Ctr, New York, NY 83-86; **FEL:** Brachytherapy, Mem Sloan Kettering Cancer Ctr, New York, NY 86-87; **FAP:** Asst Prof Cornell U; *SI: Breast Cancer; Prostate Cancer;* **HMO:** Oxford PHS Aetna Hlth Plan SWCHP Health Choice +

  🚹 🅲 📷 🚼 🏨 Mcr WC NFl Immediately *VISA* 💳

Masino, Frank A (MD)   RadRO
Stamford Hosp

Radiation Oncology Associates, PC, 34 Shelburne Rd; Stamford, CT 06902; (203) 325-7886; **BDCERT:** Rad 82; **MS:** Albert Einstein Coll Med 78; **RES:** Rad, Yale-New Haven Hosp, New Haven, CT 79-82; **FAP:** Clin Instr Yale U Sch Med; *SI: Breast Cancer; Prostate Cancer;* **HMO:** PHS Kaiser Permanente Oxford Blue Cross & Blue Shield Aetna Hlth Plan +

LANG: Fr, Sp, Itl; 🚹 📷 🏨 🆂 Mcr Mcd 1 Week

Spera, John (MD)   RadRO
Danbury Hosp

24 Hospital Ave; Danbury, CT 06810; (203) 797-7190; **BDCERT:** RadRO 87; **MS:** Georgetown U 79; **RES:** S, Hosp of U Penn, Philadelphia, PA 79-81; U, Hosp of U Penn, Philadelphia, PA 81-83; **FEL:** RadRO, Hosp of U Penn, Philadelphia, PA 84-87; **FAP:** Clin Instr Yale U Sch Med; *SI: Breast Cancer; Prostate Cancer*

LANG: Sp; 🚹 📷 🚼 🏨 Mcr Mcd A Few Days *VISA* 💳

RADIOLOGY

Mullen, David (MD)   Rad
Greenwich Hosp

Greenwich Radiological Group, 49 Lake Ave; Greenwich, CT 06830; (203) 869-6220; **BDCERT:** Rad 87; **MS:** Albert Einstein Coll Med 83; **HMO:** Most

  🚹 🏨 Mcr Mcd WC Immediately 🏦 *VISA* 💳 📇

Russo, Robert (MD)   Rad
St Vincent's Med Ctr-Bridgeport

4699 Main St 108; Bridgeport, CT 06606; (203) 331-4555; **BDCERT:** Rad 77; **MS:** Georgetown U 43; **RES:** Rad, Georgetown U Hosp, Washington, DC 44-46; **HMO:** Blue Choice Blue Cross & Blue Shield CIGNA Metlife Prucare +

  🚹 🆘 🅲 📷 🏨 Mcr Mcd WC A Few Days 🏦 *VISA* 💳 📇

Strauss, Edward (MD)   Rad
Norwalk Hosp
Norwalk Radiology Consultants, 148 East Ave 1H;
Norwalk, CT 06851; (203) 852-2715; **BDCERT:**
Rad 83; **MS:** Yale U Sch Med 79; **RES:** Rad, Yale-
New Haven Hosp, New Haven, CT 80-83; **FEL:**
NuM, Yale-New Haven Hosp, New Haven, CT 83-
84; Yale-New Haven Hosp, New Haven, CT 84-85;
SI: Vascular/Interventional; Nuclear Medicine

🚫 ⏳ 🔵 🔲 🔳 🎬 Mcr Mcd WC NFI   Immediately 🔲
VISA 🔵 🔲

REPRODUCTIVE
ENDOCRINOLOGY

Ginsburg, Frances (MD)   RE
Stamford Hosp
Center For Fertility, The Stamford Hospital, PO Box
9317; Stamford, CT 06904; (203) 325-7559;
BDCERT: ObG 96; RE 96; **MS:** NYU Sch Med 80;
RES: ObG, Bellevue Hosp Ctr, New York, NY 80-84;
FEL: RE, Bellevue Hosp Ctr, New York, NY 84-86;
SI: Infertility; Menopause; **HMO:** Aetna Hlth Plan
PHS Oxford United Healthcare Aetna Hlth Plan +

🚫 🔲 🔳 🎬 🔵 Mcr Mcd   2-4 Weeks

RHEUMATOLOGY

Cooney, Leo (MD)   Rhu
Yale-New Haven Hosp
20 York St TMP17; New Haven, CT 06504; (203)
785-2204; **BDCERT:** IM 74; **MS:** Yale U Sch Med
69; **RES:** Boston Med Ctr, Boston, MA; **FEL:**
Rheumatology, Boston, MA; **FAP:** Prof Rhu Yale U
Sch Med; *SI: Back Pain in Elderly;* **HMO:** CIGNA PHS
Blue Cross & Blue Shield Oxford

🚫 🔲 🔳 🎬 🔵 Mcr Mcd WC NFI   A Few Days 🔲 **VISA**
🔵 🔲

Craft, Joseph (MD)   Rhu
Yale-New Haven Hosp
PO Box 208005, 333 Cedar St LCI 609; New
Haven, CT 06520; (203) 785-7063; **BDCERT:** IM
80; **MS:** U NC Sch Med 77; **RES:** Yale-New Haven
Hosp, New Haven, CT 77-78; **FEL:** Yale-New Haven
Hosp, New Haven, CT 82-85

🚫 🔵 Mcr Mcd   4+ Weeks 🔲 **VISA** 🔵

Dalgin, Paul (MD)   Rhu   PCP
Stamford Hosp
Medical AssociatesStamford, 1100 Bedford St;
Stamford, CT 06905; (203) 239-8032; **BDCERT:**
IM 73; **MS:** SUNY Buffalo 68; **RES:** IM, Univ Hosp
SUNY Bklyn, Brooklyn, NY 68-70; IM, Bellevue
Hosp Ctr, New York, NY 72-73; **FEL:** Rhu,
Columbia-Presbyterian Med Ctr, New York, NY 73-
75; Rhu, Columbia-Presbyterian Med Ctr, New
York, NY; **FAP:** Asst Clin Prof Yale U Sch Med;
HOSP: St Joseph's Med Ctr-Stamford; *SI:
Investigational Drugs for; Rheumatoid &
Osteoarthritis;* **HMO:** Aetna Hlth Plan Blue Cross
NYLCare Oxford PHS +

🚫 🔲 🔳 🎬 🔵 Mcr   A Few Days **VISA** 🔵 🔲

Danehower, Richard L (MD) Rhu
Greenwich Hosp
49 Lake Ave 2; Greenwich, CT 06830; (203) 869-
5715; **BDCERT:** IM 71; Rhu 74; **MS:** Univ Penn 65;
RES: IM, U Mich Med Ctr, Ann Arbor, MI 66-69;
FEL: Rhu, U Mich Med Ctr, Ann Arbor, MI 69-70;
FAP: Asst Clin Prof Yale U Sch Med

Miller, Kenneth (MD)   Rhu
Danbury Hosp
Arthritis Associates, 27 Hospital Ave 205;
Danbury, CT 06810; (203) 794-0599; **BDCERT:**
IM 78; Rhu 80; **MS:** Rush Med Coll 75; **RES:** IM,
Geo Wash U Med Ctr, Washington, DC 75-78; **FEL:**
Rhu, St Vincent Hosp, Worcester, MA 78-80; *SI:
Arthritis; Osteoporosis;* **HMO:** Aetna-US Healthcare
CIGNA Blue Cross & Blue Shield MD Health Plan
Kaiser Permanente +

🚫 🔵 🔲 🔳 🎬 🔵 Mcr WC NFI   2-4 Weeks **VISA** 🔵

Novack, Stuart N (MD)   **Rhu**
Norwalk Hosp

Norwalk Medical Group, 40 Cross St; Norwalk, CT 06851; (203) 845-2129; **BDCERT:** IM 71; Rhu 72; **MS:** SUNY Hlth Sci Ctr 66; **RES:** Maimonides Med Ctr, Brooklyn, NY 66-68; UCLA Med Ctr, Los Angeles, CA 68-69; **FEL:** UCLA Med Ctr, Los Angeles, CA 69-70; **FAP:** Assoc Clin Prof Med Yale U Sch Med; **SI:** *Lupus Rheumatoid Arthritis-Systemic Lupus; Osteoporosis;* **HMO:** Blue Cross & Blue Shield Oxford PHS Aetna Hlth Plan United Healthcare +

LANG: Sp; ♿ 🏧 📷 📄 🎬 $ Mcr 1 Week **VISA** 💳

SPORTS MEDICINE

Hermele, Herbert (MD)   **SM**
Bridgeport Hosp

Orthopaedic Specialty Group, 2900 Main St; Stratford, CT 06497; (203) 377-5108; **BDCERT:** OrS 75; **MS:** Albert Einstein Coll Med 69; **RES:** OrS, Albert Einstein Med Ctr, Bronx, NY 70-74; **FAP:** Asst Clin Prof Yale U Sch Med; **SI:** *Sports Medicine;* **HMO:** PHS Independent Health Plan CIGNA Blue Cross & Blue Shield Aetna Hlth Plan +

LANG: Sp; ♿ 📷 📄 🎬 Mcr Mcd WC NFI **VISA** 💳

Plancher, Kevin (MD)   **SM**
Stamford Hosp

Plancher Hand & Sports Medicine, 1275 Summer St 102; Stamford, CT 06905; (203) 325-8888; **BDCERT:** HS 97; SM 96; **MS:** Georgetown U 86; **RES:** S, Brigham & Women's Hosp, Boston, MA 91; OrS, Massachusets GH, Boston, MA 87-91; **FEL:** HS, Indianapolis Hand Ctr, Indianapolis, IN 92-93; SM, Steadman-Hawkins Clinic, Vail, CO 93-94; **FAP:** Asst Prof Med Albert Einstein Coll Med; **HOSP:** United Hosp Med Ctr; **SI:** *Arthroscopy—Shoulder, Wrist; Knee & Hand Surgery;* **HMO:** Oxford United Healthcare Aetna Hlth Plan PHS Empire +

LANG: Ger, Sp, Fr; ♿ 🏧 🌙 📷 📄 🎬 $ Mcr WC NFI Immediately 💳 **VISA** 💳 💳

Weiner, Avi (MD)   **SM**
St Joseph's Med Ctr-Stamford

47 Oak St; Stamford, CT 06905; (203) 356-1450; **BDCERT:** OrS 88; **MS:** Israel 81; **RES:** OrS, Bronx Lebanon Hosp Ctr, Bronx, NY 81-82; OrS, Bronx Lebanon Hosp Ctr, Bronx, NY 82-86; **HOSP:** Stamford Hosp; **SI:** *General Orthopaedic; Sport Medicine;* **HMO:** Oxford PHS Connecticare Aetna-US Healthcare CIGNA +

LANG: Heb; ♿ 📷 📄 🎬 $ Mcr WC NFI Immediately

SURGERY

Andersen, Dana (MD)   **S**
Yale-New Haven Hosp

PO Box 208062; New Haven, CT 06520; (203) 785-5231; **BDCERT:** S 80; **MS:** Duke U 72; **RES:** Duke U Med Ctr, Durham, NC 72-74; S, Duke U Med Ctr, Durham, NC 76-79; **FEL:** Ge, Nat Inst Health, Bethesda, MD 74-76; Duke U Med Ctr, Durham, NC 79-80; **FAP:** Prof S Yale U Sch Med; **SI:** *Pancreatic Disease; Pancreatic-Endocrine Tumors;* **HMO:** Most

♿ 📷 📄 🎬 $ Mcr Mcd WC NFI 2-4 Weeks **VISA** 💳

Barone, James (MD)   **S**
Stamford Hosp

190 W Broad St; Stamford, CT 06902; (203) 325-7470; **BDCERT:** S 77; SCC 87; **MS:** Jefferson Med Coll 71; **RES:** S, St Vincents Hosp & Med Ctr NY, New York, NY 71-76; **FAP:** Assoc Prof NY Med Coll

♿ 📷 📄 🎬 $ Mcr Mcd WC NFI Immediately

Blackwood, M Michele (MD)   **S**
Stamford Hosp

1250 Summer St 303; Stamford, CT 06905; (203) 406-9774; **BDCERT:** S 94; **MS:** Med U SC, Charleston 88; **RES:** Stamford Hosp, Stamford, CT 88-93; **FEL:** Mem Sloan Kettering Cancer Ctr, New York, NY 93-94; **HOSP:** St Joseph's Med Ctr-Stamford; **HMO:** Most

♿ 📷 📄 🎬 $ Mcr Mcd WC Immediately 💳 **VISA** 💳

Brown, Lionel (MD) S
Danbury Hosp
55 Federal Rd; Danbury, CT 06810; (203) 792-4263; **BDCERT:** S 78; HS 89; **MS:** Univ SD Sch Med 64; **RES:** S, UC San Francisco, San Francisco, CA; **FEL:** HS, UC San Francisco, San Francisco, CA

Bull, Sherman (MD) S
Stamford Hosp
22 Long Ridge Rd 2; Stamford, CT 06905; (203) 327-2777; **BDCERT:** S 69; **MS:** Columbia P&S 62; **RES:** S, Francis Delafield Hosp, New York, NY 65-68; S, Columbia-Presbyterian Med Ctr, New York, NY 64-67; **FEL:** S, Columbia-Bellevue Hospital, New York, NY 63-64; **PdS**, Babies Hospital, New York, NY 68-69; **FAP:** Instr S Columbia P&S; **HOSP:** St Joseph's Med Ctr-Stamford; *SI: Breast Surgery; Surgical Oncology*; **HMO:** Oxford PHS Aetna Hlth Plan CIGNA

♿ 🔊 🖊 🛏 S WC NFI Immediately

Garvey, Richard (MD) S
Bridgeport Hosp
General Surgeons Of Bridgeport, 310 Mill Hill Ave; Bridgeport, CT 06610; (203) 366-3211; **BDCERT:** S 80; **MS:** Georgetown U 74; **RES:** S, Boston U Sch of Med, Boston, MA 75-79

♿ 🕐 🔊 🛏 Mcr Mcd WC NFI Immediately

Kovacs, Karen (MD) S
Danbury Hosp
69 Sand Pit Rd; Danbury, CT 06818; (203) 748-5622; **BDCERT:** S 87; **MS:** Geo Wash U Sch Med 76; **RES:** Yale-New Haven Hosp, New Haven, CT 77-82; **FEL:** PS, Children's Hosp, Columbus, OH

♿ 🔊 🖊 🛏 S Mcr Mcd Immediately *VISA* 💳 💳

McWhorter, Philip (MD) S
Greenwich Hosp
4 Dearfield Dr 104; Greenwich, CT 06831; (203) 869-0338; **MS:** Cornell U 73; **RES:** S, New York Hospital, New York, NY 72-77; **FEL:** Breast Surgery, Memorial Sloan Kettering Cancer Center, New York, NY 77; *SI: Laparascopic Surgery*; **HMO:** PHS Oxford Aetna Hlth Plan NYLCare United Healthcare +

♿ 🔊 🖊 🛏 S Mcd WC NFI Immediately

Napp, Marc (MD) S
Danbury Hosp
Surgical Associates of Western Connecticut, 69 Sand Pit Rd 202; Danbury, CT 06810; (203) 748-5622; **BDCERT:** S 91; **MS:** Albert Einstein Coll Med 85; **RES:** S, Mount Sinai Med Ctr, New York, NY 85-90; *SI: Laparoscopy; Gastrointestinal Surgery*; **HMO:** Aetna Hlth Plan PHS CIGNA Kaiser Permanente Oxford +

LANG: Prt, Sp; ♿ 🔊 🖊 🛏 Mcr Mcd WC A Few Days
VISA 💳 💳

Passarelli, Nicholas (MD) S
Yale-New Haven Hosp
General Surgery, PC, 2 Church St South; New Haven, CT 06519; (203) 776-2500; **BDCERT:** S 66; **MS:** Yale U Sch Med 59; **RES:** Grace New Haven Hosp, New Haven, CT 60-65; **FAP:** Asst Clin Prof Yale U Sch Med; **HOSP:** Hosp of St Raphael; *SI: Gall-Bladder & Liver; Pancreas—Stomach—Colon*

LANG: Itl; ♿ 🔊 🖊 🛏 S Mcr Mcd WC A Few Days

Passeri, Daniel (MD) S
St Vincent's Med Ctr-Bridgeport
888 White Plains Rd Fl 2; Trumbull, CT 06611; (203) 459-2666; **BDCERT:** S 91; **MS:** Yale U Sch Med 75; **RES:** Yale-New Haven Hosp, New Haven, CT 75-80; **HOSP:** Bridgeport Hosp; *SI: Cancer; Breast Surgery*; **HMO:** PHS MD Health Plan Oxford Suburban Aetna Hlth Plan +

LANG: Itl; ♿ 🕐 🔊 🖊 🛏 Mcr Mcd WC NFI 1 Week

Reed, David (MD) S
Stamford Hosp
166 W Broad St; Stamford, CT; (203) 324-2381; **BDCERT:** S 94; **MS:** Jefferson Med Coll 78; **RES:** S, Episcopal Hosp, Philadelphia, PA 78-82; GVS, Albert Einstein Med Ctr, Philadelphia, PA 82-83; **FEL:** S Onc, Roswell Park Cancer Inst, Buffalo, NY 83-85; *SI: Laparoscopic Surgery*; **HMO:** Most

♿ 🕐 🔊 🛏 Mcr Mcd WC NFI A Few Days

Guide to symbols and abbreviations can be found on pages 110-113.

1075

Smego, Douglas (MD)   **S**
Stamford Hosp

1250 Summer St 303; Stamford, CT 06905; (203)
327-6755; **BDCERT:** S 83; **MS:** UMDNJ-NJ Med
Sch, Newark 77; **RES:** NY Hosp-Cornell Med Ctr,
New York, NY 77-82; **FEL:** Trauma, U Louisville
Hosp, Louisville, KY; **FAP:** Asst Clin Prof S NY Med
Coll; **HOSP:** St Joseph's Med Ctr-Stamford; **SI:**
Vascular Surgery; Image Directed Breast Surgery
🦽 📷 👥 🏨 💲 Mcr Mcd WC 2-4 Weeks **VISA** 💳

Ward, Barbara (MD)   **S**
Yale-New Haven Hosp

800 Howard Ave; New Haven, CT 06510; (203)
785-6214; **BDCERT:** S 91; **MS:** Temple U 83; **RES:**
Yale-New Haven Hosp, New Haven, CT 83-85;
Yale-New Haven Hosp, New Haven, CT 87-90; **FEL:**
S Onc, Nat Cancer Inst, Bethesda, MD 85-87; **FAP:**
Assoc Prof S Yale U Sch Med; **SI:** *Breast Disease;*
HMO: Anthem Health Aetna Hlth Plan PHS MD
Health Plan

LANG: Sp; 🦽 📷 👥 🏨 💲 Mcr Mcd WC NFI 1 Week 💳
VISA 💳

Wasson, Dennis (MD)   **S**
Bridgeport Hosp

2900 Main St 2B; Stratford, CT 06497; (203) 378-
4500; **BDCERT:** S 68; **MS:** Ireland 57; **RES:** Boston
U Med Ctr, Boston, MA 64-66; Royal Victoria Hosp,
Ireland 59-63; **FEL:** Havard Surgical Service,
Boston, MA 63-64

🏨

Wilbanks, Tyr (MD)   **S**
Stamford Hosp

22 Long Ridge Rd; Stamford, CT 06905; (203)
327-2777; **BDCERT:** S 91; **MS:** Cornell U 83; **RES:**
Columbia-Presbyterian Med Ctr, New York, NY 83-
85; **FEL:** Columbia-Presbyterian Med Ctr, New
York, NY 85-87; **HOSP:** St Joseph's Med Ctr-
Stamford; **HMO:** Aetna Hlth Plan
🦽 📷 👥 🏨 💲 WC NFI Immediately

THORACIC SURGERY

De France, John (MD)   **TS**
Danbury Hosp

27 Hospital Ave Ste 405; Danbury, CT 06810;
(203) 797-1811; **BDCERT:** TS 96; S 75; **MS:**
Jefferson Med Coll 69; **RES:** S, Polyclinic Hosp,
Harrisburg, PA 70-74; Cv, VA Med Ctr, Asheville,
NC 74-76; **SI:** *Lung Cancer; Aortic Aneurysms;* **HMO:**
PHS Medspan Oxford United Healthcare Anthem
Health +

🦽 📷 👥 🏨 💲 Mcr Mcd WC NFI A Few Days

Elefteriades, John (MD)   **TS**
Yale-New Haven Hosp

Yale University School of Medicine, 333 Cedar St
121FMB; New Haven, CT 06510; (203) 785-2705;
BDCERT: S 82; TS 85; **MS:** Yale U Sch Med 76; **RES:**
S, Yale-New Haven Hosp, New Haven, CT 76-77;
FEL: TS, Yale-New Haven Hosp, New Haven, CT
81-83; **FAP:** Chf TS Yale U Sch Med; **HOSP:** Hosp of
St Raphael; **SI:** *Coronary Artery Disease; Aortic
Aneurysm;* **HMO:** MD Health Plan PHS Blue Cross &
Blue Shield CIGNA Aetna Hlth Plan +

LANG: Fr, Sp, Grk, Rus, Ger; 🦽 📷 👥 🏨 Mcr Mcd WC
NFI Immediately

Newton, Charles (MD)   **TS**
Bridgeport Hosp

Cardiac & Thoracic Surgery, 52 Beach Rd; Fairfield,
CT 06430; (203) 254-2022; **BDCERT:** TS 92; S 83;
MS: Washington U, St Louis 75; **RES:** S, Johns
Hopkins Hosp, Baltimore, MD 76-80; TS, Brigham
& Women's Hosp, Boston, MA 80-82; **FEL:** Cancer
S, Cleveland Clinic Hosp, Cleveland, OH 82-83
🦽 💲 Mcr Mcd WC NFI 1 Week

Rose, Daniel (MD)   **TS**
St Vincent's Med Ctr-Bridgeport

2800 Main St; Bridgeport, CT 06606; (203) 576-
5708; **BDCERT:** TS 83; **MS:** U Colo Sch Med 74;
RES: Bellevue Hosp Ctr, New York, NY 74-79; **FEL:**
TS, Bellevue Hosp Ctr, New York, NY 80-82; TS,
Nat Heart Inst, Bethesda, MD 79-80; **SI:** *Minimally
Invasive Surgery;* **HMO:** PHS US Hlthcre CIGNA
Oxford

LANG: Sp; 🦽 📷 👥 🏨 Mcr Mcd WC NFI A Few Days
💳 **VISA** 💳 💳

UROLOGY

Anderson, Kevin (MD)   U
Yale-New Haven Hosp
PO Box 208041; New Haven, CT 06520; (203) 783-8215; **BDCERT:** U 95; **MS:** UC San Diego 86; **RES:** UC Davis Med Ctr, Sacramento, CA 87-92

Andriani, Rudy (MD)   U
Stamford Hosp
166 W Broad St 404; Stamford, CT 06902; (203) 356-9692; **BDCERT:** U 89; **MS:** NY Med Coll 81; **RES:** St Vincents Hosp & Med Ctr NY, New York, NY 81-83; Duke U Med Ctr, Durham, NC 83-87; **FAP:** Clin Instr NY Med Coll; **HOSP:** Greenwich Hosp; *SI: Urologic Cancer; Urologic Stone Management*

🦽 📞 👥 🏧 $ Mcr Wc   1 Week **VISA** 💳

Burbige, Kevin (MD)   U
Greenwich Hosp
Greenwich Hospital, Dept of Pediatric Urology, 49 Lake Ave; Greenwich, CT 06830; (203) 869-1285; **BDCERT:** U 84; **MS:** Wayne State U Sch Med 72; **RES:** U, Boston U Med Ctr, Boston, MA 77-81; **FEL:** Ped U, Children's Hosp, Boston, MA 81-82; **FAP:** Asst Prof U Columbia P&S; **HOSP:** Columbia-Presbyterian Med Ctr; *SI: Hypospadias; Hernia*; **HMO:** Oxford PHS Aetna Hlth Plan CIGNA

🦽 📞 🏧 $ Mcr Mcd   A Few Days **VISA** 💳

Gorelick, Jeffrey (MD)   U
Danbury Hosp
Urology Associates of Danbury, PC, 73 Sand Pit Rd 204; Danbury, CT 06810; (203) 748-0330; **BDCERT:** U 91; **MS:** Northwestern U 83; **RES:** S, NY Hosp-Cornell Med Ctr, New York, NY 83-89; U, NY Hosp-Cornell Med Ctr, New York, NY 88; **FAP:** Clin Instr U Conn Sch Med; *SI: Prostate Cancer; Urinary Incontinence*; **HMO:** Aetna-US Healthcare CIGNA PHS Oxford Prucare +

LANG: Sp; 🦽 📞 👥 🏧 $ Mcr Mcd Wc   A Few Days **VISA** 💳

Ranta, Jeffrey (MD)   U
Greenwich Hosp
Greenwich Urological Assoc, 49 Lake Ave 21; Greenwich, CT 06830; (203) 869-1285; **BDCERT:** U 86; **MS:** Georgetown U 79; **RES:** S, Georgetown U Hosp, Washington, DC 79-81; **FEL:** Lahey Clinic, Burlington, MA 81-84; *SI: Prostate Cancer; Kidney Stones*; **HMO:** Aetna Hlth Plan Oxford PHS PHCS Empire +

🦽 📞 👥 🏧 $ Mcr Mcd Wc NFI   A Few Days **VISA** 💳

Roach, James (MD)   U
St Vincent's Med Ctr-Bridgeport
3715 Main St 403; Bridgeport, CT 06606; (203) 372-8550; **BDCERT:** U 68; **MS:** NY Med Coll 58; **RES:** Albany Med Ctr, Albany, NY 62-65; **HOSP:** Yale-New Haven Hosp; **HMO:** PHS MD Health Plan Blue Shield Oxford

🦽 📞 🏧 $ Mcr Mcd Wc   Immediately

Viner, Nicholas (MD)   U
Bridgeport Hosp
Urological Assoc Of Bridgeport, 1305 Post Rd 212; Fairfield, CT 06430; (203) 255-6825; **BDCERT:** U 77; **MS:** Vanderbilt U Sch Med 68; **RES:** S, Greenwich Hosp, Greenwich, CT 68-70; U, Vanderbilt U Med Ctr, Nashville, TN 70-74; *SI: Prostate Cancer; Urinary Tract Stones*

🦽 📞 👥 🏧 $ Mcr Mcd Wc   A Few Days 💳 **VISA** 💳

Waxberg, Jonathan (MD)   U
Stamford Hosp
Urology Associates, 35 Hoyt St; Stamford, CT 06905; (203) 324-2268; **BDCERT:** U 89; **MS:** U Cincinnati 80; **RES:** St Francis Hosp Med Ctr, Hartford, CT 80-82; Maimonides Med Ctr, Brooklyn, NY 82-86; **HOSP:** St Joseph's Med Ctr-Stamford; *SI: Prostate Cancer; Incontinence*; **HMO:** Aetna Hlth Plan PHS Blue Cross US Hlthcre Oxford +

🦽 🌙 📞 👥 🏧 $ Mcr Mcd   2-4 Weeks 💳 **VISA** 💳

Zuckerman, Howard (MD)   U
Bridgeport Hosp

Urological Assoc Of Bridgeport, 160 Hawley Ln 2;
Trumbull, CT 06611; (203) 375-3456; **BDCERT:** U
77; **MS:** St Louis U 67; **RES:** Albert Einstein Med Ctr,
Bronx, NY 72-75; Med Coll VA Hosp, Richmond,
VA 68-69; **FEL:** Med Coll VA Hosp, Richmond, VA
67-68; **HOSP:** St Vincent's Med Ctr-Bridgeport; *SI:
Urinary Incontinence; Sexual Dysfunction*; **HMO:** PHS
MD Health Plan Oxford Aetna Hlth Plan Health
Choice +

LANG: Sp, Ger; ⬛ ⬛ ⬛ ⬛ ⬛ ⬛ ⬛ ⬛
A Few Days ⬛ *VISA* ⬛

Sumpio, Bauer (MD)   GVS
Yale-New Haven Hosp

Yale U Sch MedSurg, 333 Cedar-137FMB St; New
Haven, CT 06520; (203) 785-2561; **BDCERT:** S
88; GVS 90; **MS:** Cornell U 80; **RES:** S, Yale-New
Haven Hosp, New Haven, CT 82-86; **FEL:** GVS, U
NC Hosp, Chapel Hill, NC 86-87; **FAP:** Assoc Prof S
Yale U Sch Med

LANG: Sp; ⬛ ⬛ ⬛ ⬛ ⬛ ⬛ ⬛ ⬛ ⬛ 2-4 Weeks
⬛ *VISA* ⬛ ⬛

VASCULAR SURGERY (GENERAL)

Blabey, Robert (MD)   GVS
Stamford Hosp

166 W Broad St 305; Stamford, CT 06902; (203)
357-1010; **BDCERT:** GVS 75; **MS:** Columbia P&S
67; **RES:** Columbia-Presbyterian Med Ctr, New
York, NY 67-72; **FEL:** Babies Hosp, New York, NY
72-73; Columbia-Presbyterian Med Ctr, New York,
NY 73-74; **HOSP:** Stamford Hosp; *SI: Breast
Diseases; Parathyroid Thyroid Disease*; **HMO:** Aetna-
US Healthcare Oxford Magnacare United
Healthcare PHCS +

⬛ ⬛ ⬛ ⬛ ⬛ ⬛ ⬛ ⬛ ⬛ A Few Days

Pasternak, Bart M (MD)   GVS
Norwalk Hosp

Vascular Surgery PC, 162 Kings Hwy North;
Westport, CT 06880; (203) 454-4416; **BDCERT:**
GVS 81; S 71; **MS:** Poland 63; **RES:** England 63-67;
Mayo Med Sch, Minneapolis, MN 67-70; **FEL:** GVS,
Baylor Med Ctr, Dallas, TX 70-71; **FAP:** Assoc Prof
Yale U Sch Med; **HOSP:** Stamford Hosp; **HMO:** Most

LANG: Pol; ⬛ ⬛ ⬛ ⬛ ⬛ ⬛ ⬛ A Few Days

SECTION THREE

CENTERS OF EXCELLENCE

CENTERS OF EXCELLENCE

Health care consumers are not only interested in information on hospitals; they also want to know in which specialties hospitals are leaders or have special programs dealing with a specific disease or health issue. Many hospitals in the region have devoted significant resources to developing superior programs of patient care in these areas. We have invited those institutions selected for inclusion in the Castle Connolly Guide to present information on programs they believe would be of interest to and meet the special needs of our readers.

CENTERS OF EXCELLENCE

Obstetrics and Gynecology

Orthopaedics

Parkinson's Disease

Psychiatry

Women's Health

Wound Care

AIDS/HIV

Saint Vincents Comprehensive HIV Center

203 WEST 12TH STREET,
NEW YORK, NY 10011
212-604-1700

People with HIV and AIDS have been turning to Saint Vincent's for help, support and hope since the onset of the epidemic. From 1981 onward, our doctors and nurse practitioners have provided treatment and services recognized as "leading edge" by our peers. Most important, patients who face many turning points in their battle with the virus trust us with their lives.

HIV complicates everyday life. Our center, newly expanded in 1997, is designed to address complex needs with more resources than ever. Quality of care is our hallmark. In national surveys by *U.S. News and World Report* and *American Health,* in fact, our HIV program was recognized as one of the top 50 in the nation.

*"Your nurses made sure my brother
kept his dignity at all times. Their caring
and concern were truly remarkable."*

– Family Member of a Patient with AIDS

Saint Vincent's is the city's premier one-stop source for HIV care and the latest-breaking therapies. Testing, counseling, support groups, and early intervention services are all available in our convenient and compassionate setting. So is access to our innovative HIV-fighting drugs. Today, our patients can participate in over 50 clinical drug trials.

What truly distinguishes our program, however, is the continuity and outstanding quality of care seldom seen in large city hospitals. As reported in *New York Magazine* our patients and their families often describe our nursing care as second to none. And, whether an individual comes to our outpatient center or our dedicated inpatient unit they're treated by the same professional team, which is a source of reassurance to everyone.

Bringing hope and healing to HIV patients and families means playing a critical role in their lives. Our comprehensive case management services are designed to fit around their very personal, individual needs. Our unique offerings include an Early Intervention Program; a Family-Centered AIDS Program for children, adolescents and women; a Peer Education Counseling Program to reduce the spread of HIV; home care; special programs for immigrants and the elderly; and a research and educational program to share our knowledge with the larger medical community.

CANCER

Cabrini Medical Center
Cancer Care Center

227 EAST 19TH STREET • NEW YORK, NY 10003
PHONE 212-CABRINI (212-222-7464)

Effective Cancer Care With A Compassionate Touch

Cabrini Medical Center offers one of the most comprehensive and effective cancer care programs in New York City, using the most sophisticated technology available to screen for and treat all types of benign and malignant tumors. A team of expertly skilled cancer specialists, from oncologists and radiologists to physicists and surgeons, provide high quality care in a patient-friendly, compassion-driven environment. CMC's Oncology and Radiation Oncology Departments successfully treat a broad spectrum of cancer, including breast, prostate, lung, colon and gastrointestinal. Treatment is tailored to individual needs with the goal of curing patients, who are walked through the process and comforted by everyone involved in their care. CMC even meets special patient needs, like transportation. One of the few institutions to offer permanent implants for prostate cancer, CMC provides services that include cutting-edge early diagnosis procedures (especially for breast, prostate and colon cancer), surgery, aggressive chemotherapy and radiation treatment, follow-up care and education outreach. In addition, CMC offers hospice care for those with advanced illness.

Breakthrough Technology

CMC uses breakthrough technology to simulate treatment before it is actually administered, enabling radiation oncologists to map out treatment areas with utmost precision. Custom-blocking tumor regions allows radiation to reach the cancer while shielding healthy tissue. High-tech X-ray-producing equipment treats tumors at all depths and is capable of surface treatment without deep body penetration. CMC performs the latest techniques in bone marrow transplantation curatives, in which a cancer patient's bone marrow is frozen-stored allowing massive chemotherapy treatment. The Mammography Center uses highly advanced technology for the screening for and early detection of breast cancer. CMC's Tumor Board meets weekly to evaluate patient progress, while a Cancer Committee oversees everything from diagnosis and surgery to patient care and follow-up.

ABBI TREATMENT

When breast cancer is detected accurately and treated early, survival is above 90%. Cabrini was the first Manhattan hospital to acquire ABBI, a minimally invasive, breast cancer detection biopsy procedure using imaging technology, allowing surgeons to accurately identify and completely remove a lesion in one step. Patients resume normal activity the same day. Call the Breast Diagnostic & Treatment Center at 212•995•6656.

INDIGO TREATMENT

Half the American male population over age 50 suffers from prostate enlargement— most resorting to invasive surgery or drug therapy. For moderate-to-severe symptoms of benign prostate enlargement, Cabrini offers Indigo Laser Treatment— a minimally invasive, successful alternative that shrinks the prostate with laser energy. There's no incision or hospitalization, less anesthesia and fewer side effects. Call the Urology Department at 212•995•6769.

Calvary Hospital Cancer

1740 EASTCHESTER ROAD • BRONX, NY 10461
PHONE (718) 518-2300   FAX (718) 518-2670

Palliative Care

Calvary Hospital Palliative Care--addressing the symptoms of the disease, not its cure--is the active, total care of patients whose disease is unresponsive to curative treatment. The relief of pain and other physical symptoms, and of the psychological, social, and spiritual problems, are paramount. It is intended to assist patients and their families in living as fully as possible, thus, our claim that "Life Continues at Calvary Hospital."

It is generally conceded that palliative care's most important contribution to the care of patients has been the bringing back of humanity into medicine. The qualities that define it: kindness, compassion, privacy, patient autonomy, beneficence, justice, and non-abandonment, have always been the hallmarks of ideal care of the sick. Calvary has been proud to provide that brand of care for nearly a century.

The Palliative Care Institute at Calvary Hospital was established with the vision of becoming a recognized source for research into the whole spectrum of palliative care and the development of innovative educational models. Within its mission is the intent to educate not only the health care community but the community-at-large. It continues to articulate and publicize Calvary Hospital's commitment to kindness, non-abandonment, and the importance of "caring" people who care for the patient.

In order to achieve our goal of making patients as comfortable as possible, Calvary Hospital offers care programs that address the full range of end-of-life needs. These programs include inpatient care, discharge planning, outpatient care, home care, hospice (to begin third quarter, 1998) and support programs for families and friends. If you would like additional information about Calvary Hospital's programs and services or about palliative care, please call us. Our staff would be happy to answer your questions.

Continuum Health Partners, Inc.

The Cancer Center

OF BETH ISRAEL AND ST. LUKE'S-ROOSEVELT
PHONE (800) 420-4004

A major cancer care provider in New York City, The Cancer Center provides a complete range of services for cancer patients and their families at every stage of the diagnostic, treatment and follow-up process. The Cancer Center features world renowned cancer specialists—including top-rated surgeons, medical oncologists, physicians, radiation oncologists, radiologists, oncology nurses and more.

Comprehensive diagnostic and treatment services are available for breast cancer, prostate cancers, head and neck cancers, skin cancer, lung cancer, colorectal and other gastrointestinal cancers, Lymphoma/Hodgkin's Disease, gynecological cancers, and cancers of the brain and central nervous system. Delivered efficiently in a friendly and supportive environment, services include prevention programs—such as community education, screenings and early detection—expert diagnosis, outpatient treatment, inpatient services, home care, and when necessary, hospice care. In addition, the Cancer Center Research Program offers patients access to investigational protocols through a wide number of clinical trials.

Support services play an important role at The Cancer Center. Nurses, social workers, psychiatrists, chaplains, pharmacists, rehabilitation therapists and nutritionists—each with specialized knowledge and expertise in the field of oncology—work closely together to ensure that patients' medical, emotional and family needs are addressed appropriately and in a timely manner.

The Comprehensive Breast Center at St. Luke's-Roosevelt combines state-of-the-art diagnosis and treatment of breast cancer with a supportive approach to health care that addresses emotional as well as physical needs. With radiology, pathology and consultation services available on site, a suspected malignancy can be confirmed or ruled out quickly and treatment options—including plastic surgery—can be outlined in a single visit. Services also include genetic testing, gynecologic cancer screening, referral to alternative therapies, psychiatric care and support groups.

THE SAINT VINCENTS
COMPREHENSIVE CANCER CENTER

A SALICK HEALTH CARE AFFILIATE

SMITH PAVILION
170 WEST 12TH STREET, 7TH FLOOR
NEW YORK, NY 10011
1-888-44-CANCER (1-888-442-2623)

Helping our patients and their families meet the very special challenges they face is the central focus of our cancer center. Largely because of this supportive philosophy that strengthens our excellent medical care, we've attracted some of the best cancer doctors in the world. In fact, our oncologists and other cancer experts have spearheaded leading research that has resulted in many of the newest breakthroughs in the diagnosis and treatment of cancer.

We understand that our patients are juggling everyday responsibilities while meeting the extraordinary demands caused by their illness. They want to work, carry on household duties, and simply enjoy home life. Overall, they want to remain in control of their lives, unrestrained by cancer. We help by offering care on a 24-hour basis to work with their busy schedules. And providing them with a convenient, truly one-stop outpatient experience.

"With such a team on my side, I can rest easy and just focus on getting better."

– Pauline Kalahele

Our collective expertise covers the entire range of specific cancers: from the most common to the rarest conditions, from the most basic to the most complex treatments. Even diseases like multiple myeloma – typically hard to manage – are treated here with advanced techniques like bone marrow and blood stem cell transplants.

All of our patients receive state-of-the-art care within the highest standard of practice. They may also have the option of receiving the latest-breaking therapies through our participation in clinical trials.

Recovery hinges on emotional well-being as much as physical strength. For that reason, we help our patients and their families with every need: medical, emotional, spiritual, nutritional, informational, and psychosocial. All of our current services will soon be available in a new 70,000 square-foot facility. Like our existing center, it will be open 24 hours a day, 365 days a year for screening, diagnosis, treatment, follow-up and emergency care.

The Valley Hospital Oncology Services

223 NORTH VAN DIEN AVENUE
RIDGEWOOD, NEW JERSEY 07450
(201) 447-8000
1-800-VALLEY 1 FOR PHYSICIAN REFERRAL

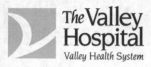

The Valley Hospital
Valley Health System

Oncology Services centered on "Total Care Approach"

Designated a **Comprehensive Community Hospital Cancer Program** by the American College of Surgeons, The Valley Hospital's Oncology Services are guided by a multidisciplinary Cancer Committee that emphasizes a **"Total Care Approach."** Placing a priority on early detection as well as supporting the emotional needs of patients and their families, the hospital supplements its state of the art technology and physician expertise with extensive screenings and a wide variety of support groups and social services.

Innovative treatments, affiliations, and services are hallmarks of Valley's Oncology Program

Through its affiliation with Columbia-Presbyterian Medical Center in New York, patients are offered participation in the latest clinical trials for new treatment protocols. Operating the busiest Radiation Oncology service in the state, Valley is known for its prostate seed implant therapy program. Plans to add Intensity Modulated Radiation Therapy in 1998 are underway. Breast cancer cases are reviewed at **Prospective Breast Cancer Review Conferences**, a multidisciplinary team review of cases to determine optimal diagnosis and treatment. Home care nursing is also offered.

New services include a **cancer genetics** program — **the first of its kind in New Jersey** — which evaluates a participant's risk for cancer, and **pediatric oncology**, led by the Director of Pediatric Oncology for Babies and Children's Hospital, Columbia-Presbyterian Medical Center. Future plans include an off site, full-service Cancer Center, designed to combine clinical and social services for patients and their families in one easily-accessible location.

CARDIAC SURGERY

Continuum Health Partners, Inc.

Cardiology Services

555 W. 57TH STREET • NEW YORK, NY 10019
PHONE (800) 420-4004

The partnership between Beth Israel and St. Luke's-Roosevelt brings together the expertise and excellence of two of Manhattan's best cardiac care teams. The skill and caliber of its cardiologists, cardiovascular surgeons, primary care physicians and other physician specialists is matched only by its state-of-the-art facilities—including the most technologically advanced cardiac care units, catheterization and electrophysiology labs, cardiac surgery suites, open heart recovery units, and cardiopulmonary stepdown telemetry units.

Together, Beth Israel and St. Luke's-Roosevelt offer every heart care service needed to prevent, diagnose, and treat heart disease, including leading-edge cardiac surgery, catheter-based diagnosis and treatment, hypertension diagnosis and treatment, heart failure diagnosis and treatment, and a hypertrophic cardiomyopathy program. Strong believers in prevention and early detection, the professionals at Beth Israel and St. Luke's-Roosevelt also provide complete medical evaluations, echocardiography, nuclear cardiology services, Coronary Artery Disease Prevention that assesses risk factors and recommends lifestyle changes, treatment centers for obesity and diabetes, smoking cessation programs, and complementary techniques for relaxation and stress reduction such as massage therapy and therapeutic touch.

Some of the unique features available at either Beth Israel or St. Luke's-Roosevelt include the Ross Procedure—a pulmonary autograft replacement of the aortic valve; the only PET scanner in Manhattan designated solely for cardiac evaluations; and a nationally recognized arrhythmia service.

THE HEART INSTITUTE

In an effort to bridge its many cardiac care programs and provide patients with more streamlined access to its full range of services, Beth Israel established The Heart Institute in 1998. This interdisciplinary cardiology, cardiac surgery and cardiac rehabilitation team consists of clinicians, surgeons, nurses and nurse practitioners, physician assistants, social workers, complementary care experts and rehabilitation specialists—all working together to give patients a full range of individualized treatment choices and services.

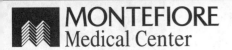

MONTEFIORE
Medical Center

**The University Hospital for the
Albert Einstein College of Medicine**

The Montefiore-Einstein Heart Center

111 EAST 210 STREET
BRONX, NY 10467-2490

1825 EASTCHESTER ROAD
BRONX, NEW YORK 10461-2373

Call 1-800-MD-MONTE (1-800-636-6683)
to find a Montefiore-Einstein Heart Center Physician

Web Site www.montefiore.org

National Leader in Cardiac Care

The Montefiore-Einstein Heart Center offers adult and pediatric patients in Greater New York and around the world a model approach to state-of-the-art cardiac care.

Cardiothoracic surgeons perform over 1,400 heart surgeries each year, including coronary artery bypasses and valve repairs. Interventional cardiologists perform more than 4,000 catheterizations. The Center includes active arrhythmia and pacemaker centers and one of the region's top pediatric cardiology programs. Diagnostic technology includes PET scanners & nuclear cameras.

Montefiore researchers are pushing the next frontiers of cardiac care with stimulation of diseased blood vessels to perform a "natural bypass" through a process called angiogenesis; beta-blockers to defer congestive heart failure and programs to improve post-surgical "quality of life."

Specialty programs, with large volumes of patients, include: Emergency Chest Pain, Congestive Heart Failure, Non-invasive Cardiology (Stress Testing, Echocardiography — including special fetal echocardiography service), Interventional Cardiology (Catheterization, Electrophysiology and Arrhythmia), Thoracic Surgery, Pediatric Cardiology, and Rehabilitation.

Emphasis on preventive care and early detection is exemplified in the Healthy Heart Program, a screening program available to the families of all heart patients. The "conditioning" program for congestive heart failure patients is a national model .

There is easy access to The Heart Center programs through a network of community-based cardiologists in the Bronx, Westchester and surrounding areas, 34 Montefiore Medical Group primary care offices in the Bronx and lower Westchester, and a large faculty of subspecialists at the medical center's two campus specialty hubs.

NYU Medical Center Cardiac Surgery

550 FIRST AVENUE ● NEW YORK, NY 10016

PHONE (800) 557-7000   FAX (212) 263-0745
http://cvsurg.med.nyu.edu/cvsurg.html

On the Leading Edge of Care

NYU Medical Center surgeons perform open heart surgery for many patients using the latest in minimally invasive techniques. Instrumental in the development of new minimally invasive surgery, NYU surgeons have already helped hundreds of patients recover and return to productive lives more quickly and painlessly than ever before. With this experience, NYU Medical Center has been the international leader in port-access minimally invasive valve reconstruction and multi-vessel bypass.

A History of Excellence

With more than 30 years of experience in all forms of heart surgery, NYU Medical Center has set new national standards for quality treatment and research. Throughout its history, NYU Medical Center has been a leader and innovator in the diagnosis and treatment of heart disease, including the most advanced surgical techniques for adults and children.

Call 800-557-7000 to schedule an appointment or get more information from our team.

Stephen B. Colvin, M.D.

Aubrey C. Galloway, M.D.

Alfred T. Culliford, M.D.

Rick A. Esposito, M.D.

Greg H. Ribakove, M.D.

Eugene A. Grossi, M.D.

Lawrence R. Glassman, M.D.

Frank C. Spencer, M.D.

Patients' quality of life is a priority at NYU Medical Center, where we are dedicated to achieving the highest quality results through a comprehensive line of services, an advanced practice nursing staff and a world-class team of experienced cardiac surgeons.

Saint Vincents Comprehensive Cardiovascular Center

12TH STREET AND 7TH AVENUE,
NEW YORK, NY 10011
212-604-2220

At Saint Vincent's, heart care does not begin and end in a surgical suite. As we tell our patients, the most hardworking organ in your body requires the insights of many experts when something goes wrong. As a New York State designated Comprehensive Cardiac Care Center, Cardiac experts throughout our hospital – from the ER to the Intensive Care Unit – work together as one cohesive team. Our cardiologists and cardiac surgeons are equally involved in every case, offering procedures that are minimally invasive whenever possible. When bypass surgery is the only option, we offer the assurance of internationally renowned experts in cardiac surgery. And some of the highest survival rate statistics of any hospital in the State of New York.

> *"I thought he was the best doc*
> *a man with cardiac failure could have.*
> *Little did I know the whole*
> *medical world thought so, too."*
>
> *– Anthony Trezza, Staten Island*

Since Saint Vincent's operates one of the few Level I Trauma Centers in the city, we're obviously well-equipped to take on any cardiac emergency or critical care case. Valve replacements, angioplasty and cardiac catheterization are the daily work of our program. Thanks to our overall emphasis on preventive care, we're just as equipped to be a citywide resource for heart health information. Recently, we received a grant from the New York State Department of Health to promote heart-healthy nutrition and exercise within our community – as the best hospital in the city for the job.

Preventive care has been at the heart of our program since we opened the nation's first coronary care unit in 1964. Each year, we continue to perform free community based blood pressure screenings and low-cost cholesterol tests. And we get the message out on issues like women's risk of heart attack through free lectures. How many lives have been lengthened as a result? Make sure yours is one of them. Call 212-604-7572 to schedule a free blood pressure screening or low-cost cholesterol test.

The Valley Hospital
Cardiac Services

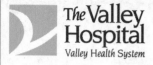

The Valley
Hospital
Valley Health System

223 NORTH VAN DIEN AVENUE
RIDGEWOOD, NEW JERSEY 07450
(201) 447-8000
1-800-VALLEY 1 FOR PHYSICIAN AND
PROGRAM REFERRAL

The Valley Hospital — A Full Service Center for Cardiac Care

The Valley Hospital offers a full range of diagnostic and interventional treatment options including open heart surgery for bypass and valve replacement and repair, as well as cardiac catheterization and diagnostic services, such as echocardiography, electrocardiography, and exercise stress testing. Interventional cardiology procedures conducted in the hospital's high-risk cardiac catheterization laboratory include coronary angioplasty, coronary atherectomy, coronary stents, and intra-vascular ultrasound. New cardiac services include the addition of an **electrophysiology studies** (EP) program to assist in the diagnosis of cardiac problems when detailed measurements are needed to understand irregular heartbeats. Patients who have undergone procedures at Valley may also receive cardiac nursing and education in their home.

First in the area to offer minimally invasive technique for bypass surgery

Recent innovations in treatment include the development of the modified Minimally Invasive Direct Coronary Artery Bypass (MIDCAB) procedure. Pioneered to wide acclaim by Valley's Director of Cardiac Surgery Bruce P. Mindich, M.D., the modification allows a greater number of cardiac patients with heart disease to have bypass surgery. The technique is performed through a three-inch incision in the chest and conducted while the heart continues to beat on its own. Because trauma to the body is reduced, patients experience a shorter recovery period.

DIAGNOSTIC

IMAGING

LONG BEACH MEDICAL CENTER IMAGING SERVICES

445 EAST BAY DRIVE, LONG BEACH, NY 11561
PHONE (516) 897-1360   FAX (516) 897-1363

First in the New York area with E-Cam

Long Beach Medical Center points with pride to a new era in diagnostic imaging.

First in the New York area with E-Cam dual digital, variable angle, single photo emission computerized tomography, this center of excellence provides more accurate and sensitive information in a fraction of the time used by previous technology.

Open MRI, Spiral CT, and a full complement of sophisticated nuclear equipment empower physicians with extensive diagnostic capabilities.

Dedicated cardiovascular diagnosis

"The Heart Station" is part of this complex, with noninvasive cardiovascular diagnosis in a comfortable setting. Directed by a team of board certified cardiologists, studies are performed by licensed and certified technologists.

Osteoporosis Center

State of the art technology measures bone density and mineral components. Each report is evaluated by a board certified Endocrinologist. Nutritional recommendations accompany the report to the primary physician.

A healing environment

Waterfront views are comforting and therapeutic.

Our commitment to excellence also extends to prompt appointments and prompt results.

From small beginnings in 1922, Long Beach Medical Center has become a major center of quality health care serving the south shore of Long Island.

Inpatient and outpatient services are marked by "the caring factor." Here, state of the art services are enhanced by continuing quality improvement and sincere interest in our patients. We care about you, as we care for you.

GERIATRICS

The Mount Sinai Medical Center

The Henry L. Schwartz Departmentof Geriatrics and Adult Development

ONE GUSTAVE L. LEVY PLACE
BOX 1070, NEW YORK, NY 10029
PHONE: (212) 241-7922   1-800-MD-SINAI

In recognition of the care we offer older patients, our specialists are cited time and time again as the finest in the nation. US News and World Report has ranked The Mount Sinai Hospital number one in New York for geriatric care many times.

A Heritage of Excellence:

The Mount Sinai Medical Center has long been a pioneer in geriatric medicine. A Mount Sinai physician coined the term "geriatrics" in 1909 and wrote the first textbook on medical care for older adults in 1914. In 1968, Mount Sinai established America's first approved residency and fellowship training programs in geriatrics. Today, every student at our Medical School is required to study geriatric medicine, and every physician, nurse and social worker in our Department is an expert in the special needs of older adults.

A Full Continuum of Care:

We offer comprehensive care, disease prevention and health maintenance, with a focus on healthy and productive aging. Our researchers continue to break ground in the understanding, prevention and treatment of age-related disorders. Our clinical services include The Phyllis and Lee Coffey Geriatrics Associates, offering comprehensive out-patient care; The Acute Care for the Elderly (ACE) Unit, especially designed to meet the needs of older adults who require hospitalization and to minimize the complications sometimes associated with an older person's hospital stay; the Consultation and Liaison Service, linking Geriatrics with other physicians at The Mount Sinai Hospital, to provide comprehensive care for patients on units other than ACE; the Orthopaedic-Geriatric Service, dedicated to the prevention and treatment of the bone fractures often associated with aging; the Geriatrics Home Medical Care Program, which provides optimal care for homebound older adults; and a Palliative Care team dedicated to assuring quality end-of-life care.

HOME
CARE

Valley Home Care

15 ESSEX ROAD
PARAMUS, NEW JERSEY 07652
(201) 291-6000

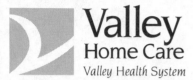

Valley
Home Care
Valley Health System

Quality Care...At Your Doorstep

Valley Home Care offers residents of northern and northwestern New Jersey comprehensive diagnostic and therapeutic health services. Affiliated with The Valley Hospital in Ridgewood, and Accredited with Commendation from the Joint Commission on Accreditation of Healthcare Organizations. Valley Home Care leads in providing skilled nursing and support services outside traditional healthcare settings.

A Variety of Service Offerings for Those Who Need Home Care

Specialty Nurse Clinician Program

Specially trained nurse clinicians are available for the following specialties: cardiology, oncology, IV therapy, enterostomal therapy, rehabilitation and psychiatry.

Maternal & Child Health

Prenatal and postnatal guidance as well as infant care instruction, pediatric nursing, pediatric asthma and rehabilitation therapy are available and provided by a specially trained staff of nurses, social workers, rehabilitation therapists, home health aides, volunteers and a nutritionist. Conditions treated include: complications from premature birth, nutrition deficiency, cardio-respiratory dysfunction, cerebral palsy and diabetes.

Rehabilitation Therapy

Physical, speech and occupational therapy is provided by a highly-trained staff. Patients benefiting from rehabilitation therapy include those who have experienced stroke, brain injury, orthopedic injury and many types of surgery.

Project Outreach

A program of medical, social, and spiritual support designed to improve an AIDS or HIV patient's comfort and quality of life through the relief of symptoms and provision of emotional support.

HOSPICE

Cabrini Medical Center
Cabrini Hospice

227 EAST 19TH STREET • NEW YORK, NY 10003
PHONE (212) 995-6480   FAX (212) 995-7015

Compassionate Care At Home

Caring for patients with advanced illness is at the core of CMC's century-old mission of providing compassionate, quality health care. At the heart of this mission is Cabrini Hospice — New York City's oldest and largest hospital-based hospice care program. Renowned nationally as a model program, Cabrini Hospice is noted for its dedicated team of care-givers committed to effectively and compassionately meeting the medical, emotional and spiritual needs of patients with advanced illness and their families. Under the program, patients remain in the familiar environment of their home, surrounded by family and friends. With the focus on quality of life, and not quantity of time, Cabrini Hospice care is designed to help patients deal with their illness and live their remaining days with meaning, dignity and comfort. Individualized home care is developed based upon thorough evaluation of patient needs. Physician specialists and registered nurses help with pain management and symptom-control, while social workers offer supportive counseling. Home health aides assist with personal care and daily living activities, while visits from music and art therapists promote self-expression and relaxation. Clergy members of all faiths are available for spiritual counseling, while trained volunteers offer companionship and perform errands. Patients and their families can take comfort in knowing that Cabrini Hospice care-givers are with them during their special time of need.

Inpatient Unit

Although the focus of hospice is care and support in the comfort of the home environment, the Cabrini Hospice Inpatient Unit is available to patients whose medical condition or pain-management requires hospitalization. The Cabrini Hospice Inpatient Unit has 45 inpatient beds set in an intimate environment with the comforts of home. It provides short-term acute care — usually one week — until the patient can return home. The Inpatient Unit offers overnight accommodations for family members and care partners of hospice patients. Daily around-the-clock visiting is permitted. There is a spacious lounge for patients and their visitors, a play room for children, and quiet rooms for private meditation and reflection.

PEDIATRIC HOSPICE

Children under age 16 with advanced illness receive compassionate, comforting, specialized care in the nurturing environment of their homes through Sister Loretta's Sunshine Kids Program. They are visited by Cabrini Hospice pediatric nurses who help keep their symptoms in check with therapeutic pain and symptom management. Music, art and play therapists work with the children to help them express their feelings and make their remaining days comfortable and fulfilling. Social workers and spiritual counselors offer emotional support, and a network of volunteers provides companionship and other services to the entire family. If a child requires inpatient short-term care, the hospice center has overnight accommodations for family members and a play room. Contact 212•995•6655.

Continuum Health Partners, Inc.

Department of Pain Medicine and Palliative Care

555 WEST 57TH STREET • NEW YORK, NY 10019
PHONE (800) 420-4004

In 1997, Beth Israel formed the first clinical department for pain medicine and palliative care at a major teaching hospital in the United States. The Department of Pain Medicine and Palliative Care provides services by a team of multidisciplinary specialists who work with patients to assess and treat pain, symptoms other than pain, or other problems related to progressive incurable diseases, including the need for end-of-life care.

Headed by Russell K. Portenoy, M.D., a world renowned pain medicine and palliative care expert, the department uses the expertise of board certified, multidisciplinary physicians, nurse clinicians, psychologists and social workers. In addition, it works closely with other health care professionals, including rehabilitation specialists, oncologists and physical therapists. Some of the services include an inpatient consultation service, an inpatient pain and palliative care unit, and outpatient services that include programs for chronic pain, headache pain due to nerve injury, and palliative care.

The department uses a comprehensive approach to diagnose and treat a broad range of problems, including back and neck pain, pain from cancer and AIDS, post-surgical pain, arthritis pain, headaches and more. Following a patient evaluation, the team prepares an individualized treatment plan, which may involve a singular technique or a combination of methods to achieve optimal results. In addition, the department features the Institute for Education and Research in Pain and Palliative Care to coordinate education and research programs in the rapidly growing fields of pain management and palliative care.

NEUROLOGY
NEUROSURGERY

Continuum Health Partners, Inc.

Hyman-Newman Institute for Neurology and Neurosurgery (INN)

170 EAST END AVENUE • NEW YORK, NY 10128
PHONE (800) 420-4004

The Hyman-Newman Institute for Neurology and Neurosurgery (INN) at Beth Israel Medical Center is one of the first multidisciplinary centers of its kind dedicated exclusively to the diagnosis and treatment of neurological disorders from infancy through adulthood. A "dream" of internationally renowned pediatric neurosurgeon, Fred J. Epstein, M.D., the INN was conceived and designed to deliver humanistic health care in one of the most technologically sophisticated of fields. It was a dream shared by his two co-directors, Alex Berenstein, M.D., interventional neuroradiologist and Matthew Fink, M.D., neurologist and president of Beth Israel.

Attracting patients from all over the world, the INN offers state-of-the-art facilities with the most advanced technology available today to treat brain and spinal cord tumors, strokes, aneurysms, epilepsy, ALS (Lou Gehrig's Disease), Parkinson's Disease, neuromuscular and neurobehavior disorders and more. Featuring world renowned physicians who are pioneers in their fields, the INN is committed to integrating the knowledge and experience of its full array of medical and surgical specialists, as well as professionals in allied health fields.

In addition to the most advanced technology and experienced health professionals, the INN also offers a unique, patient-centered environment that was designed specifically to ease the trauma of hospital stays, especially for pediatric patients. Also unique to the INN's approach to neurologic care is its complementary modalities, including music therapy, stress reduction and alternative approaches to pain management.

CENTER FOR ENDOVASCULAR SURGERY

The Center for Endovascular Surgery at the INN provides the latest technologic advances in the field of angiography (imaging of the vascular system to identify blockages), including the first machine that combines rotational CT scanner with angiography. The INN uses the most sophisticated diagnostic studies and surgical techniques available worldwide to treat patients suffering from stroke and cerebrovascular disorders. Interventional neuroradiology is used for the treatment of aneurysms, vascular malfunctions and vascular tumors as an adjunct or alternative to surgical treatment.

Hospital for Joint Diseases

301 East 17th Street (at Second Avenue)
New York, NY 10003
212-598-6000 FAX 212-260-1206
Physician Referral: 1-888-HJD-DOCS (1-888-453-3627)

The HJD Neurosciences Program Offers the Following Services and Treatments:

Orthopaedic Neurology

Multiple Sclerosis Comprehensive Care Center

Epilepsy Comprehensive Care Center

Initiative for Women with Disabilities (Gynecologic and Primary Care for Women with Physical Disabilities)

Clinical Neurophysiology

Neuroimmunology

Comprehensive Center for Adults with Cerebral Palsy

Attention Deficit Disorder Clinic

Functional Neurosurgery and Neurostimulation for Parkinson's disease and Movement Disorders

Neurorehabilitation and Traumatic Brain Injury

Neurorheumatology

The faculty of the Neurosciences Program are all board-certified neurologists with advanced training in their subspecialties. They are actively involved in research initiatives to enhance further patient care and treatment.

The Neurosciences Program at the Hospital for Joint Diseases — Orthopaedic Institute offers a full array of diagnostic and specialized treatment services for neurological disorders.

The clinical expertise of the faculty includes orthopaedic neurology, multiple sclerosis, neuroimmunology, epilepsy, neurophysiology, women's neurological disorders, neurorehabilitation, cerebral palsy, Parkinson's disease, attention deficit disorders, movement disorders, chronic pain management, and functional neurosurgery-neurostimulation.

OBSTETRICS
AND
GYNECOLOGY

The Brooklyn Hospital Center
Obstetrics/Gynecology

121 DEKALB AVENUE, BROOKLYN, NY 11201
PHONE (718) 4-CHOICE (424-6423)

Pioneering treatments in infertility . . . treating cardiology disorders in the womb. . a highly qualified staff . . These are some of the qualities and advantages our patients are continually discovering at The Brooklyn Hospital Center. Our 100 percent board certified staff has a total commitment to you, the patient, to render supportive, high-quality care.

Women's Health

More than 4,000 women a year choose The Brooklyn Hospital Center as the best place to deliver their babies, making the Obstetrics/Gynecology Service a leader in obstetric care throughout the region. The Obstetrics/Gynecology Service offers all the elements that ensure the best of care: state-of-the-art diagnosis and treatment, a warm and modern environment, and a caring medical staff who are 100 percent board certified. Among the first in Brooklyn to offer the latest treatments for infertility, the Service offers gynecologic oncology and perinatology.

The Fertility Institute

The Fertility Institute has pioneered the most sophisticated fertility treatments in Brooklyn while providing emotional support, privacy, and a relaxed atmosphere for men and women. Advanced treatments include laparoscopy, hysteroscopy, microsurgery, in vitro fertilization, GIFT, ICSI and assisted hatching, and egg donation. All sophisticated diagnostic services, treatment, and outpatient surgery are provided in-house for greater convenience. Highly qualified reproductive endocrinologists, led by George D. Kofinas, MD, founder of The Fertility Institute, render compassionate, high-quality, cost-effective care.

Perinatal Diagnostic Center

The Perinatal Diagnostic Center diagnoses and treats problems affecting the unborn baby and the management of complicated pregnancies. Offering personal attention and quality care, the Perinatal Diagnostic Center can help to protect the health of babies before they are born and enhance the pregnancy experience. Advanced diagnostic technology allows diagnosis and treatment of many disorders in the womb. Its services include cardiac treatment, transfusions, complete genetic services, and ultrasound examinations. The Perinatal Diagnostic Center is led by Drs. Alexander D. Kofinas and Michael F. Cabbad, who are board certified in Obstetrics/Gynecology and Maternal-Fetal Medicine.

The Valley Hospital Obstetric Services

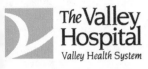

The Valley Hospital
Valley Health System

223 NORTH VAN DIEN AVENUE
RIDGEWOOD, NEW JERSEY 07450
(201) 447-8000
1-800-VALLEY 1 FOR PHYSICIAN
AND PROGRAM REFERRAL

Obstetric Services that Focus on Continuing Care for Mother and Baby

Located in the Family Wellness Care Center, The Valley Hospital offers more than 3,000 expectant families each year a comprehensive program of obstetric care and services that address not only the new mother and infant, but the needs of every family member. Focusing on a continuum of care that begins before birth and often ends with home care training and education, Valley's obstetrics program combines the skills of a highly-qualified medical staff with the compassion of a skilled nursing staff to make a family's experience meaningful.

Clinical and Support Services Offer Assistance Every Step of the Way

The service includes a Mother/Baby Unit with a series of specialized nurseries, birthing rooms, delivery rooms, and a recovery room; a newly renovated and enhanced Neonatal Intensive Care Unit (NICU) directed by two full-time neonatologists; perinatology services led by Charles Lockwood, M.D., who also serves as the Chairman of Obstetrics at New York University Medical Center; a comprehensive Maternal and Child Health home care program; and a Center for Child Development and Wellness where babies born with special needs can be followed and provided ongoing care. The completion of Labor/Delivery/Recovery/Post-Partum suites is scheduled for mid-1998.

Clinical services are complemented with a wide variety of support services including 18 parent education programs and a support group for parents of children born with special needs.

ORTHOPAEDICS

Cabrini Medical Center
Joint Replacement Center

227 EAST 19TH STREET • NEW YORK, NY 10003
PHONE 212-CABRINI (212-222-7464)

Total Joint Replacement

Cabrini's Total Joint Replacement Program is designed to provide prospective patients with the ability to make an informed decision on total joint replacement surgery. The program encourages them to view actual surgery, conduct hands-on examination of prosthetic equipment, and meet with orthopedic specialists before deciding on total joint replacement— primarily for patients with osteoarthritis, rheumatoid arthritis and other conditions. Hip and knee replacement surgery is performed in laminar flow surgical suites, providing a self-contained ultraclean air system designed to maximize sterile conditions and minimize risk of infection. Cabrini utilizes the latest surgical techniques, including breakthrough technology that minimizes the need for blood transfusions. Patients are usually moved to Cabrini's new 15-bed inpatient Physical Medicine and Rehabilitation Unit, which offers comprehensive rehabilitation services.

Rehabilitation Unit

When total joint replacement post-operative patients are brought to Cabrini's Rehabilitation Unit, their daily regimen is intensified and accelerated to a three-hour program of combined physical and occupational therapy designed to achieve safe and independent patient functioning. Bedside therapy begins with range of motion exercises, bed mobility and transfer, gait training, and room care management. A convenient on-site physical therapy gym offers traditional exercise and strengthening equipment (bicycles, treadmills, weights) to assist patients in achieving maximum physical performance within their capabilities. Patients are also taught how to safely use walking aides. Occupational therapy is provided in bathroom, kitchen and office-simulated rooms to retrain patients in self-care, homemaking and work skills. A dedicated interdisciplinary health care team of a physiatrist, physical, occupational and speech therapists, audiologists, nurses, social workers, nutritionists and other professionals assess patient progress after establishing goals and designing an individualized program that includes patient and care-partner education for at-home care. The Rehabilitation Unit also provides rehabilitative care for patients recovering from other surgeries, illness, trauma, stroke, amputation and long hospital stay. Patients requiring long-term therapy and sub-acute care are referred to Cabrini Center for Nursing and Rehabilitation.

GERIATRIC CARE UNIT

New York City has proportionately more elderly than the entire U.S., and with that distinction comes the responsibility of addressing health care needs of the aged. Cabrini's innovative 26-bed Geriatric Inpatient Unit for medical patients aged 75 and older meets the unique health care needs of the elderly. Specializing in the prevention, diagnosis, treatment and rehabilitation of disorders common to the elderly, the Geriatric Unit provides patient-friendly, compassionate care designed to maintain the dignity and functional abilities of patients during hospitalization, including a convenient on-site physical therapy program. Led by a geriatrician, a team of nurses, dietitians, audiologists, and physical, speech and occupational therapists provides comprehensive care tailored to individual patient needs. Contact 212•995•7028.

Continuum Health Partners, Inc.
Orthopaedics

555 W. 57TH STREET • NEW YORK, NY 10019
PHONE (800) 420-4004

From sports injuries to knee replacements to arthritis, the departments of orthopaedic surgery and physical medicine and rehabilitation at Beth Israel and St. Luke's-Roosevelt work in conjunction to provide diagnosis and treatment for all disorders of the musculoskeletal system. Its team of world-recognized orthopaedic surgeons is dedicated to serving the unique needs of the orthopaedic patients.

Featuring one of the largest programs in New York State for total replacement of knees, hips and other joints, Beth Israel and St. Luke's-Roosevelt offer a complete range of general and specialized procedures, including hand and upper extremity surgery, arthroscopy, pediatric orthopaedic surgery and spine surgery. Other key components in orthopaedics/sports medicine include special programs for the treatment of musculoskeletal disorders such as arthritis; comprehensive, multi-site rehabilitation care for non-surgical treatment of disorders and for post-surgical rehabilitation; and special programs for the prevention, diagnosis and treatment of sports-related injuries.

Beth Israel also features the Insall Scott Kelly Institute for Orthopaedics and Sports Medicine—a full-service, specialized center which focuses on the treatment of orthopaedic and sports-related ailments. Both Beth Israel and St. Luke's-Roosevelt feature comprehensive programs for the surgical treatment of all hand and many upper extremity problems. At St. Luke's-Roosevelt, the C.V. Starr Hand Surgery Center performs specialized work such as joint and shoulder reconstruction and surgery for compressive neuropathy and congenital deformities.

THE SPINE INSTITUTE

Featuring a multidisciplinary health care team, The Spine Institute offers patients an array of outpatient and inpatient services for congenital, chronic or acute spinal disorders as well as back problems of any kind or degree—from herniated discs to spinal stenosis to scoliosis to spinal deformities. Noninvasive treatment options include pain management, rehabilitation, and physical and occupational therapy. When surgical intervention is needed, The Spine Institute uses the latest in technology and innovation to perform the least invasive surgery possible with the most effective and safest results.

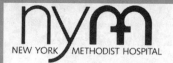

NEW YORK METHODIST HOSPITAL

New York Methodist Hospital
The Brooklyn Spine and Arthritis Center

519 SIXTH STREET BROOKLYN, N.Y. 11215
PHONE (718) 780-3104   FAX:(718) 780-5373

Physician Services

The Center's focus is on conservative treatment. At the time of the initial visit, each patient is matched with a physician whose area of expertise appears best suited to treat that patient's specific problems. After the initial diagnosis, patients may be referred for physical therapy or to another physician specialist if further medical consultation is necessary. Our interdisciplinary physician team includes specialists in spinal care/spinal surgery, rheumatology, upper extremity surgery, physiatry (rehabilitation medicine), pain management and joint replacement.

Joint Replacement Surgery

The Center uses the Joint Endeavor patient management program for all patients who undergo joint replacement of the hip or knee. This program, which is managed by a certified orthopedic nurse, includes formal patient education and aggressive post-operative rehabilitation.

Therapeutic Programs

Physical therapy is the basis of conservative treatment. It is prescribed to strengthen back, joint and limb muscles, improve range of motion and provide aerobic conditioning. In addition to active exercise and stretching, procedures such as ultrasound, heat and cold applications, electrical stimulation, massage, mobilization and manipulation can help reduce pain, discomfort or inflammation. All of these modalities are offered at the Center's physical therapy facility to provide patients with a wide variety of treatment options.

The Brooklyn Spine and Arthritis Center at New York Methodist Hospital is dedicated solely to the diagnosis and treatment of spinal and rheumatological disorders. This unique facility is located on the Hospital campus, thereby providing patients with easy access to the MRI/CT Center, x-ray, laboratory and other resources needed to diagnose and treat all types of arthritis and back problems.

NYU Medical Center / Hospital for Joint Diseases

1-888-HJD-2-NYU (1-888-453-2698)
FAX 212-598-6581

Leaders in adult and children's bone and joint disorders for more than a century.

The NYU/HJD Department of Orthopaedic Surgery Offers the Following Services and Treatments:

General Orthopaedics
Hip and Knee Replacement Center
Arthroscopic Surgery
Bone Tumor Service
Foot and Ankle Surgery
Hand Surgery
Limb Lengthening and Bone Growth
Occupational and Industrial Orthopaedic Care
Sports Medicine
Pediatric Orthopaedics
Shoulder Institute
Center for Neuromuscular and Developmental Disorders
The Geriatric Hip Fracture Program
The Scoliosis Program
The Spine Center
The Harkness Center for Dance Injuries
24-hour Urgent Orthopaedic Care

NYU/HJD Orthopaedics provides care at NYU Tisch Hospital, Hospital for Joint Diseases, Manhattan VA, Jamaica Hospital, and Bellevue Hospital Center where more than 12,000 surgical procedures are performed each year. The orthopaedic faculty maintains offices in all five boroughs as well as in Rockland County and New Jersey.

The NYU/HJD Department of Orthopaedic Surgery is the largest and most accomplished in the region for the diagnosis and treatment of musculoskeletal disorders as well as in research and education. The clinical expertise of the faculty represents all subspecialty areas of orthopaedic surgery, including spine, total joint replacement, sports medicine and arthroscopy, pediatric orthopaedics, shoulder, hand, and foot-and-ankle.

PARKINSON'S DISEASE

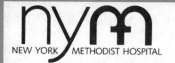

NEW YORK / METHODIST HOSPITAL

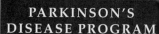

New York Methodist Hospital
The Parkinson's Disease Program

506 SIXTH STREET BROOKLYN, N.Y. 11215
PHONE (718) 780-5820   FAX (718) 780-3632

The Parkinson's Disease Program at New York Methodist Hospital offers the only comprehensive diagnostic and treatment program for Parkinson's and other tremor disorders in Brooklyn. The Center is staffed by neurologists and neurosurgeons who have special expertise in the treatment of Parkinson's disease and other tremor disorders.

Diagnosis and Medical Treatment

Patients who exhibit symptoms of Parkinson's disease or other tremor disorders receive a diagnostic examination, performed by a neurologist. Those who have already been diagnosed with Parkinson's or a related tremor disorder may also use this service to get a second opinion.

Once a diagnosis is substantiated, treatment can begin. Ordinarily, Parkinson's disease is initially controlled through medical (prescription drug) treatment. At some point in the course of the disease, medicine may become less effective and surgery may be indicated to relieve certain symptoms.

Surgical Treatment

All of the major surgical procedures performed to relieve symptoms of Parkinson's disease and other tremor disorders are performed at New York Methodist Hospital by an internationally renowned neurosurgeon, trained in this type of stereotactic surgery. Procedures performed to alleviate Parkinson's disease symptoms include pallidotomy (ablation or lesion in the internal globus pallidus), thalamotomy (ablation or lesion in the thalamus) and implantation of a deep brain stimulator. This region's first two stereotactic implantations of a deep brain stimulator to treat tremor caused by Parkinson's disease were successfully performed at New York Methodist Hospital in 1998.

PSYCHIATRY

Four Winds Hospital Psychiatric

800 CROSS RIVER ROAD • KATONAH, NY 10536
PHONE (914) 763-8151   FAX (914) 763-9597

Description

Four Winds Hospital provides a broad range of psychiatric treatment services, both inpatient and outpatient, for children ages 5 - 12, adolescents, adults and older adults. Located on 55 acres in Northern Westchester, near Connecticut, and Putnam and Dutchess counties, Four Winds is just an hour's drive from New York City, northern New Jersey, and western Long Island. Medically driven, multidisciplinary teams incorporate therapeutic milieu into the comprehensive treatment approach. Individual, group and family therapy is integrated with educational, and recreational therapies, psychodrama, and a range of other treatment modalities.

Admission & Referral Information

Four Winds accepts patients 24 hours a day, 7 days a week. Specialized programs are available for children, adolescents, adults, and older adults.

It is Four Winds' philosophy that quality treatment, delivered at the appropriate level, is not only clinically effective, but cost effective as well. Our goal is to ensure that every individual receives the exact services that are required during the course of their treatment.

Our referring community includes: clinicians, managed care organizations, schools, employers, EAP's, clergy, family members, community agencies, and self-referrals. Four Winds maintains regular contact with the referring professional during the admission process and throughout the treatment experience.

Most major medical policies cover treatment at Four Winds Hospital. Four Winds is a provider member of major managed care networks, Blue Cross, GHI, Medicare and Medicaid (NYS).

Four Winds is the largest specialized provider of child and adolescent mental health services in the Northeast.

Comprehensive inpatient and outpatient mental health treatment services are provided for children, as young as age 5 adolescents, adults and older adults.

Triage (evaluation and referral) services are provided 24 hours a day, 7 days a week.

WOMEN'S
HEALTH

Hospital for Joint Diseases

301 East 17th Street, New York, NY 10003
Main Number: 212-598-6000
Physician Referral 1-888-HJD-DOCS (1-888-453-3627)

Center for Arthritis and Autoimmunity

Most of the conditions treated at the Center for Arthritis and Autoimmunity affect women in ratios ranging from 2:1 to 10:1.

Fibromyalgia
Lupus
Lyme Disease
Osteoarthritis
Osteoporosis
Psoriatic Arthritis
Rheumatoid Arthritis
Scleroderma
Sjogren's Syndrome

Orthopaedic Surgery

Foot and Ankle
Neck, Back and Shoulder
Sports Medicine
The Spine Center
Blount's Disease
Developmental Disorders
Early Intervention and PreSchool for Children with Disabilities
  (birth through age 5)
Limb-lengthening
Neuromuscular Disorders
Pediatric Orthopaedics
Scoliosis

Neurosciences Program

Orthopaedic Neurology
Initiative for Women with Disabilities
Multiple Sclerosis
Epilepsy
Neuroimmunology
Neurohematology
Cerebral Palsy
Attention Deficit Disorder

Pain Program

Diagnosis and Treatment of Chronic Pain
Acupuncture
Biofeedback
Massage Therapy

Harkness Center for Dance Injuries

A range of services to the dance community including preventative screenings and care of acute injuries. Services are provided to dancers on a sliding scale according to income.

The Hospital for Joint Diseases is internationally known for expertise in treating orthopaedic, rheumatologic, and neuro-logic disorders. The hospital offers comprehensive clinical programs, many of which are particularly important to women as individuals, and as parents seeking the best medical care for their children. In addition, for immediate treatment after a fall or injury, the hospital offers walk-in 24-hour Orthopaedic care.

WOUND
CARE

Cabrini Medical Center
Wound Care Center

247 THIRD AVENUE • NEW YORK, NY 10003
PHONE (212) 995-6600   FAX (212) 979-3404

82% Healing Rate

Cabrini Wound Care Center®, part of a 160-member network of wound centers nationwide, has emerged as one of New York City's most comprehensive treatment facilities dedicated to caring for people with chronic wounds that resist healing because of complications of diabetes, poor circulation, swelling and extended immobility. Cabrini Wound Care Center®'s commitment to effectively preserving limbs and extremities and avoiding amputation is dramatized by its more than 82% healing rate. Its multidisciplinary wound management program effectively combines aggressive medical treatment, follow-up care, nutrition counseling and overall education. The Wound Care team consists of caring and experienced specialists in diabetes, podiatry, internal medicine, infectious disease, nursing, nutrition, and general, plastic, vascular, orthopedic and reconstructive surgeries. By administering the most advanced medical technology and wound care techniques and establishing individualized treatment programs based on patient needs, they have healed wounds that others deemed hopeless, and which might have resulted in amputation. A major element of treatment is patient education: at-home wound care, exercise, infection control and other measures that aid in the healing and prevention of wounds. Sometimes it's as simple as teaching a patient special walking techniques that help to reduce the potential of recurring sores. Cabrini Wound Care Center® provides comprehensive history and physical evaluation of patients, noninvasive vascular laboratory tests, radiology examination, surgical intervention and review of infection control practices.

Diabetes Foot Care Prevents Amputation

Foot ulcerations and other chronic wounds that arise from diabetes-related complications often lead to amputation. But the Diabetes Foot Care Program at Cabrini Wound Care Center® is a prevention initiative designed to avoid amputation — first by healing wounds, then by implementing thorough follow-up care and patient education. The centerpiece of the program is a noninvasive vascular laboratory, where patients are assessed, and a special unit which treats chronic leg swelling. Upon healing a wound, the program administers aggressive follow-up care and on-going education — including nutrition evaluation — to prevent recurrence. Something as routine as patients inspecting their own feet prevents chronic wounds and ensuing complications.

SECTION FOUR

APPENDICES

APPENDIX A

AMERICAN BOARD OF MEDICAL SPECIALTIES

PURPOSE OF THE AMERICAN BOARD OF MEDICAL SPECIALTIES

THE STATEMENT OF PURPOSE INCLUDED IN THE ARTICLES OF INCORPORATION IS:

- *To improve the standards of medical care.*

- *To act as spokesman for all approved specialty boards, as a group.*

- *To resolve problems encountered among and between specialty boards.*

- *To deal with the applications for approval of proposed new specialty boards, new types of certification, modification of existing types of certification, and related matters.*

- *To endeavor to avoid duplication of effort by specialty boards.*

- *To establish and maintain standards of organization and operation of specialty boards.*

Following is a list of the addresses of the various medical specialty boards approved by the ABMS. Note that there are 24 board organizations for 25 medical specialties. Psychiatry and Neurology share the same board.

To find out if a physician (M.D.) is certified, consumers can call the individual boards which will provide information for a fee, or they can call the ABMS at (800) 776-2378. (No fee)

BOARD SPECIALTIES

■ **American Board of Allergy and Immunology**
510 Walnut Street, Suite 1701
Philadelphia, PA 19106-3694
(215) 592-9466
General Certification in Allergy and Immunology; with Added Qualification in Diagnostic Laboratory Immunology. Certifications awarded since 1989 are valid for 10 years. For those certified prior to 1989 there is no recertification requirement.

■ **American Board of Anesthesiology**
4101 Lake Boone Trail
The Summit Suite 510
Raleigh, NC 27607-7506
(919) 881-2570
General Certification in Anesthesiology; with Special and Added Qualifications in Critical Care Medicine and Pain Management. In the subspecialty of Pain Management certifications awarded as of 1993 are valid for 10 years.

■ **American Board of Colon and Rectal Surgery**
20600 Eureka Road, Suite 713
Taylor, MI 48108
(313) 282-9400
General Certification is in Colon and Rectal Surgery. Certifications awarded since 1991 are valid for 8 years.

■ **American Board of Dermatology**
Henry Ford Hospital
One Ford Place
Detroit, MI 48202
(313) 874-1088
General Certification in Dermatology; with Special Qualifications in Dermatopathology, Dermatological Immunology/Diagnostic and Laboratory Immunology. Certifications awarded since 1991 are valid for 10 years. For those certified prior to 1991, there is no recertification requirement.

■ **American Board of Emergency Medicine**
3000 Coolidge Road
East Lansing, MI 48823
(517) 332-4800
General Certification in Emergency Medicine; with Special and Added Qualifications in Pediatric Emergency Medicine and Sports Medicine. Certifications are valid for a 10-year period.

■ **American Board of Family Practice**
2228 Young Drive
Lexington, KY 40505
(606) 269-5626
General Certification in Family Practice; with Added Qualifications in Geriatric Medicine and Sports Medicine. Certifications are valid for a 7-year period.

■ **American Board of Internal Medicine**
510 Walnut Street, Suite 1701
Philadelphia, PA 19106-3694
(215) 446-3500, (800) 441-ABIM
General Certification in Internal Medicine; with Special Qualifications in Cardiovascular Disease, Critical Care Medicine, Endocrinology, Diabetes and Metabolism, Gastroenterology, Hematology, Infectious Disease, Medical Oncology, Nephrology, Pulmonary Disease, and Rheumatology; and Added Qualifications in Adolescent Medicine, Cardiac Electrophysiology, Diagnostic Laboratory Immunology, Geriatric Medicine, and Sports Medicine. Certifications awarded since 1990 are valid for 10 years. For those certified prior to 1990 there is no recertification requirement.

■ **American Board of Medical Genetics**
9650 Rockville Pike
Bethesda, MD 20814
(301) 571-1825
General Certification in Clinical Genetics, Medical Genetics, Clinical Biochemical Genetics, Clinical Cytogenetics, Clinical Biochemical/Molecular Genetics and Clinical Molecular Genetics. Certifications are valid for a 10-year period.

■ **American Board of Neurological Surgery**
Smith Tower, Suite 2139
6550 Fannin Street
Houston, TX 77030-2701
(713) 790-6015
General Certification in Neurological Surgery. Presently, there is no recertification requirement.

■ **American Board of Nuclear Medicine**
900 Veteran Avenue, Room 12-200
Los Angeles, CA 90024-1786
(310) 825-6787
General Certification in Nuclear Medicine. Certifications awarded since 1992 are valid for 10 years. For those certified prior to 1992, there is no recertification requirement.

APPENDIX A

■ **American Board of Obstetrics and Gynecology**
2915 Vine Street
Dallas, TX 75204
(214) 871-1619
General Certification in Obstetrics and Gynecology; with Special Qualifications in Gynecologic Oncology, Maternal and Fetal Medicine, Reproductive Endocrinology and Added Qualification in Critical Care. Certifications awarded since 1986 are valid for 10 years. For those certified prior to 1986, there is no recertification requirement.

■ **American Board of Ophthalmology**
111 Presidential Boulevard, Suite 241
Bala Cynwyd, PA 19004
(610) 664-1175
Certifications awarded since 1992 are valid for 10 years. For those certified prior to 1992, there is no recertification requirement.

■ **American Board of Orthopaedic Surgery**
400 Silver Cedar Court
Chapel Hill, NC 27514
(919) 929-7103
General Certification in Orthopaedic Surgery; with Added Qualification in Hand Surgery. Certifications awarded since 1986 are valid for 10 years. For those certified prior to 1986, there is no recertification requirement.

■ **American Board of Otolaryngology**
2211 Norfolk, Suite 800
Houston, TX 77098-4044
(713) 528-6200
General Certification in Otolaryngology; with Added Qualification in Otology/Neurotology and Pediatric Otolaryngology. Presently, there is no recertification requirement.

■ **American Board of Pathology**
P.O. Box 25915
Tampa, FL 33622-5915
(813) 286-2444
General Certification in Anatomic and Clinical Pathology, Anatomic Pathology and Clinical Pathology; with Special Qualifications in Blood Banking/Transfusion Medicine, Chemical Pathology, Dermatopathology, Forensic Pathology, Hematology, Immunopathology, Medical Microbiology, Neuropathology and Pediatric Pathology and Added Qualification in Cytopathology. Presently, there is no recertification requirement.

■ **American Board of Pediatrics**
111 Silver Cedar Court
Chapel Hill, NC 27514-1651
(919) 929-0461
General Certification in Pediatrics; with Special Qualifications in Adolescent Medicine, Allergy & Immunology, Pediatric Cardiology, Pediatric Critical Care Medicine, Pediatric Emergency Medicine, Pediatric Endocrinology, Pediatric Gastroenterology, Pediatric Hematology-Oncology, Pediatric Infectious Diseases, Pediatric Nephrology, Pediatric Pulmonology, Neonatal-Perinatal Medicine and Pediatric Rheumatology. Added Qualifications in Diagnostic Laboratory Immunology, Medical Toxicology and Sports Medicine. Certifications valid for 7 years.

■ **American Board of Physical Medicine and Rehabilitation**
Norwest Center, Suite 674
21 First Street, S.W.
Rochester, MN 55902
(507) 282-1776
General Certification in Physical Medicine and Rehabilitation; with Special Qualifications in Spinal Cord Injury Medicine. Certifications awarded since 1993 are valid for 10 years.

■ **American Board of Plastic Surgery**
Seven Penn Center, Suite 400
1635 Market Street
Philadelphia, PA 19103-2204
(215) 587-9322
General Certification in Plastic Surgery; with Added Qualification in Hand Surgery. Certifications are valid for a 10-year period.

■ **American Board of Preventive Medicine**
9950 W. Lawrence Avenue, Suite 106
Schiller Park, IL 60176
(847) 671-1750
General Certification in Aerospace Medicine, Occupational Medicine and Public Health and General Preventive Medicine; with Added Qualification in Underseas Medicine and Medical Toxicology. In the subspecialty of Underseas Medicine and Medical Toxicology certifications are valid for a 10-year period.

■ **American Board of Psychiatry & Neurology**
500 Lake Cook Road, Suite 335
Deerfield, IL 60015
(847) 945-7900
General Certification in Psychiatry, Neurology and Neurology with Special Qualification in Child Neurology; with Special Qualification in Child and Adolescent Psychiatry and Added Qualification in Addiction Psychiatry, Clinical Neurophysiology, Forensic Psychiatry and Geriatric Psychiatry. Certifications are valid for a 10-year period.

APPENDIX A

■ **American Board of Radiology**
5255 E. Williams Circle, Suite 3200
Tucson, AZ 85711
(520) 790-2900
General Certification in Radiology, Diagnostic Radiology, Radiation Oncology and Radiological Physics; with Special Qualification in Nuclear Radiology and Added Qualifications in Neuroradiology, Pediatric Radiology and Vascular & Interventional Radiology. Certifications are valid for a 10-year period.

■ **American Board of Surgery**
1617 John F. Kennedy Boulevard, Suite 860
Philadelphia, PA 19103-1847
(215) 568-4000
General Certification in Surgery; with Special Qualifications in Pediatric Surgery and General Vascular Surgery and Added Qualifications in Surgery of the Hand, Surgical Critical Care and General Vascular Surgery. Certifications are valid for a 10-year period.

■ **American Board of Thoracic Surgery**
One Rotary Center, Suite 805
1560 Sherman Avenue
Evanston, IL 60201
(847) 475-1520
General Certification in Thoracic Surgery. Certifications awarded since 1976 are valid for 10 years. For those certified prior to 1976, there is no recertification requirement.

■ **American Board of Urology**
2216 Ivy Road, Suite 210
Charlottesville, VA 22903
(248) 646-9720
General Certification in Urology. Certifications awarded as of 1985 are valid for 10 years. For those certified prior to 1985, there is no recertification requirement.

APPENDIX B

OSTEOPATHIC BOARDS

American Osteopathic Association
142 E Ontario Street
Chicago, IL 60611
(800) 621-1773

GENERAL CERTIFICATION

■ **American Osteopathic Board of Anesthesiology**
Anesthesiology
- No time-limited certificates

■ **American Osteopathic Board of Dermatology**
Dermatology
- No time-limited certificates

■ **American Osteopathic Board of Emergency Medicine**
Emergency Medicine
- Beginning 1/1/94, 10-year certificates

■ **American Osteopathic Board of Family Physicians**
Family Practice
- No time-limited certificates

■ **American Osteopathic Board of Internal Medicine**
Internal Medicine
- Beginning 1/1/93, 10-year certificates

APPENDIX B

■ **American Osteopathic Board of Neurology and Psychiatry**
Neurology
Psychiatry
• Beginning 1/1/96, 10-year certificates

■ **American Osteopathic Board of Obstetrics and Gynecology**
Obstetrics and Gynecology
• No time-limited certificates

■ **American Osteopathic Board of Ophthalmology and Otorhinolaryngology**
Ophthalmology
• No time-limited certificates
Otorhinolaryngology
Facial Plastic Surgery
Otorhinolaryngology and Facial Plastic Surgery
• No time-limited certificates

■ **American Osteopathic Board of Orthopaedic Surgery**
Orthopaedic Surgery
• Beginning 1/1/94, 10-year certificates

■ **American Osteopathic Board of Pathology**
Laboratory Medicine
Anatomic Pathology
Anatomic Pathology and Laboratory Medicine
• Beginning 1/1/95, 10-year certificates

■ **American Osteopathic Board of Pediatrics**
Pediatrics
• Beginning 1/1/95, 7-year certificates

■ **American Osteopathic Board of Preventive Medicine**
Preventive Medicine/Aerospace Medicine
Preventive Medicine/Occupational-Environmental Medicine
Preventive Medicine/Public Health
• Beginning 1/1/94, 10-year certificates

■ **American Osteopathic Board of Proctology**
Proctology
• No time-limited certificates

■ **American Osteopathic Board of Radiology**
   Diagnostic Radiology
   Radiation Oncology
   • No time-limited certificates

■ **American Osteopathic Board of Rehabilitation Medicine**
   Rehabilitation Medicine
   • Beginning 6/1/95, 7-year certificates

■ **American Osteopathic Board of Special Proficiency in Osteopathic Manipulative Medicine**
   Special Proficiency in Osteopathic Manipulative Medicine
   • Beginning 1/1/95, 10-year certificates

■ **American Osteopathic Board of Surgery**
   Surgery (general)
   Plastic and Reconstructive Surgery
   Thoracic Cardiovascular Surgery
   Urological Surgery
   General Vascular Surgery
   • No time-limited certificates

Consumers may call the American Osteopathic Association at (800) 621-1773 for general certification information.

NOTES:

_____

_____

_____

_____

_____

_____

_____

_____

_____

_____

_____

_____

APPENDIX C

DESCRIPTIONS OF SPECIALTIES AND SUBSPECIALTIES

Addiction Psychiatry
A subspecialty certified by the American Board of Psychiatry and Neurology, Addiction Psychiatry deals with habitual psychological and physiological dependence on a substance or practice which is beyond voluntary control.

Adolescent Medicine
A subspecialty certified by both the American Board of Internal Medicine and the American Board of Pediatrics, Adolescent Medicine involves the primary care treatment of adolescents and young adults.

Allergy & Immunology
A specialty certified by the American Board of Allergy and Immunology, an allergist/immunologist diagnoses and treats allergies, asthma, and skin problems such as hives and contact dermatitis.

Cardiac Electrophysiology (Clinical)
A subspecialty certified by the American Board of Internal Medicine, Clinical Cardiac Electrophysiology involves complicated technical procedures to evaluate heart rhythms and determine appropriate treatment for them.

Cardiovascular Medicine
A subspecialty certified by the American Board of Internal Medicine, Cardiovascular Medicine involves the diagnosis and treatment of disorders of the heart, lungs, and blood vessels.

Child & Adolescent Psychiatry
A subspecialty certified by the American Board of Psychiatry and Neurology, Child & Adolescent Psychiatry deals with the diagnosis and treatment of mental diseases in children and adolescents.

Child Neurology
A specialty certification of Neurology. (See Neurology)

Colon and Rectal Surgery
A specialty certified by the American Board of Colon and Rectal Surgery, a colon and rectal surgeon surgically treats diseases of the intestinal tract, colon, and rectum, anal canal, and perianal area.

Critical Care Medicine
A subspecialty certified by the American Boards of Anesthesiology, Internal Medicine, Neurological Surgery, and Obstetrics & Gynecology, Critical Care Medicine involves diagnosing and taking immediate action to prevent death or further injury of a patient. Examples of critical injuries include shock, heart attack, drug overdose, and massive bleeding.

Dermatology
A specialty certified by the American Board of Dermatology, a dermatologist diagnoses and treats benign and malignant disorders of the skin, mouth, external genitalia, hair and nails, as well as a number of sexually transmitted diseases.

Diagnostic Radiology
A subspecialty certified by the American Board of Radiology, Diagnostic Radiology involves the study of all modalities of radiant energy in medical diagnoses and therapeutic procedures utilizing radiologic guidance.

Emergency Medicine
A specialty certified by the American Board of Emergency Medicine, an emergency physician deals with acute-care problems such as those seen in emergency room situations.

Endocrinology, Diabetes & Metabolism
A subspecialty certified by the American Board of Internal Medicine, Endocrinology, Diabetes & Metabolism involves the study and treatment of patients suffering from hormonal and chemical disorders.

Family Practice
A specialty certified by the American Board of Family Practice, a family practitioner deals with and oversees the total health care of individual patients and their family members. Family practitioners are more common in rural areas and may perform procedures more commonly performed by specialists (e.g., minor surgery).

DESCRIPTIONS OF SPECIALTIES AND SUBSPECIALTIES

Forensic Psychiatry
A subspecialty certified by the American Board of Psychiatry, Forensic Psychiatry concerns the evaluation of certain diagnostic groups of patients that include those with sexual disorders, antisocial personality disorders, paranoid disorders, and addictive disorders.

Gastroenterology
A subspecialty certified by the American Board of Internal Medicine, Gastroenterology is the study, diagnosis and treatment of diseases of the digestive organs including the stomachs, bowels, liver, and gallbladder.

Geriatric Medicine
A subspecialty certified by the American Boards of Family Practice and Internal Medicine, Geriatric Medicine deals with diseases of the elderly and the problems associated with aging.

Geriatric Psychiatry
A subspecialty certified by the American Board of Psychiatry and Neurology, Geriatric Psychiatry involves the diagnosis, prevention, and treatment of mental illness in the elderly.

Gynecologic Oncology
A subspecialty certified by the American Board of Obstetrics and Gynecology, Gynecologic Oncology deals with cancers of the female genital tract and reproductive systems.

Hand Surgery
A subspecialty certified by the American Boards of Orthopaedic Surgery, Plastic Surgery, and Surgery, Hand Surgery involves the treatment of injury to the hand through surgical techniques.

Hematology
A subspecialty certified by the American Boards of Internal Medicine and Pathology, Hematology involves the diagnosis and treatment of diseases and disorders of the blood, bone marrow, spleen, and lymph glands.

Infectious Disease

A subspecialty certified by the American Board of Internal Medicine, Infectious Disease is the study and treatment of diseases caused by a bacterium, virus, fungus, or animal parasite. AIDS is an infectious disease.

Internal Medicine

A specialty certified by the American Board of Internal Medicine, an internist diagnoses and nonsurgically treats diseases, especially those of adults. Internists may act as primary care specialists, highly trained family doctors, or they may subspecialize in specialties such as cardiology or nephrology.

Maternal & Fetal Medicine

A subspecialty certified by the American Board of Obstetrics and Gynecology, Maternal & Fetal Medicine involves the care of women with high-risk pregnancies and their unborn infants.

Medical Genetics

A specialty certified by the American Board of Medical Genetics, a medical geneticist is a physician or scientist who identifies the genetic causes of inherited diseases and ailments and prevents, when possible, their occurrence.

Medical Oncology

A subspecialty certified by the American Board of Internal Medicine, Medical Oncology refers to the study and treatment of tumors and other cancers.

Neonatal-Perinatal Medicine

A subspecialty certified by the American Board of Pediatrics, Neonatal-Perinatal Medicine involves the diagnosis and treatments of infants prior to, during, and one month beyond birth.

Nephrology

A subspecialty certified by the American Board of Internal Medicine, Nephrology is concerned with disorders of the kidneys, high blood pressure, fluid and mineral balance, dialysis of body wastes when the kidneys do not function, and consultation with surgeons about kidney transplantation.

Neurological Surgery

A specialty certified by the American Board of Neurological Surgery, a neurosurgeon performs surgery on the brain, spinal cord, and nervous system.

DESCRIPTIONS OF SPECIALTIES AND SUBSPECIALTIES

Neurology
A specialty certified by the American Board of Psychiatry and Neurology, a neurologist diagnoses and medically treats disorders of the brain, spinal cord, and nervous system.

Neurophysiology (Clinical)
A subspecialty certified by the American Board of Psychiatry and Neurology, Clinical Neurophysiology is the study of the makeup and functioning of the nervous system in patients as opposed to in a laboratory.

Neuroradiology
A subspecialty certified by the American Board of Radiology, Neuroradiology involves the utilization of imaging procedures during diagnosis as they relate to the brain, spine and spinal cord, head, neck, and organs of special sense in adults and children.

Nuclear Medicine
A specialty certified by the American Board of Nuclear Medicine, a nuclear medicine specialist, working in either a laboratory or with patients, evaluates the functions of all the organs in the body and treats thyroid disease, benign and malignant tumors, and radiation exposure through the use of radioactive substances.

Nuclear Radiology
A subspecialty certified by the American Boards of Nuclear Medicine and Radiology, Nuclear Radiology involves the use of radioactive substances to diagnose and treat certain functions and diseases of the body.

Obstetrics & Gynecology
A specialty certified by the American Board of Obstetrics & Gynecology, an obstetrician deals with the medical aspects of and intervention in pregnancy and labor.

Occupational Medicine
A subspecialty certified by the American Board of Preventive Medicine, Occupational Medicine concentrates on the effects of the work environment on the health of employees.

Ophthalmology
A specialty certified by the American Board of Ophthalmology, an ophthalmologist diagnoses and treats diseases of and injuries to the eye.

1145

APPENDIX C

Orthopaedic Surgery
A specialty certified by the American Board of Orthopaedic Surgery, an orthopaedic surgeon operates to correct injuries which interfere with the form and function of the extremities, spine, and associated structures.

Otolaryngology
A specialty certified by the American Board of Otolaryngology, an otolaryngologist (also known as ENT specialist) explores and treats diseases in the interrelated areas of the ears, nose and throat.

Otology/Neurotology
A subspecialty certified by the American Board of Otolaryngology, Otology/Neurotology concentrates on the management, prevention, cure and care of patients with diseases of the ear and temporal bone, including disorders of hearing and balance.

Pain Management
A subspecialty certified by the American Board of Anesthesiology, Pain Management involves providing a high level of care for patients experiencing problems with acute or chronic pain in both hospital and ambulatory settings.

Pediatric Allergy & Immunology
A subspecialty certified by the American Board of Pediatrics, Pediatric Allergy & Immunology involves the diagnosis and treatment of allergies, asthma and skin problems in children.

Pediatric Cardiology
A subspecialty certified by the American Board of Pediatrics, Pediatric Cardiology involves the diagnosis and treatment of heart disease in children.

Pediatric Critical Care Medicine
A subspecialty certified by the American Board of Pediatrics, Pediatric Critical Care Medicine involves the care of children who are victims of life threatening disorders such as severe accidents, shock, and diabetes acidosis.

Pediatric Emergency Medicine
A subspecialty certified by both the American Boards of Emergency Medicine and Pediatrics, Pediatric Emergency Medicine refers to the treatment of children in an acute-care situation.

DESCRIPTIONS OF SPECIALTIES AND SUBSPECIALTIES

Pediatric Endocrinology
A subspecialty certified by the American Board of Pediatrics, Pediatric Endocrinology involves the study and treatment of children with hormonal and chemical disorders.

Pediatric Gastroenterology
A subspecialty certified by the American Board of Pediatrics, Pediatric Gastroenterology is the study, diagnosis, and treatment of diseases of the digestive tract in children.

Pediatric Hematology-Oncology
A subspecialty certified by the American Board of Pediatrics, Pediatric Hematology-Oncology is the study and treatment of cancers of the blood and blood-forming parts of the body in children.

Pediatric Infectious Disease
A subspecialty certified by the American Board of Pediatrics, Pediatric Infectious Disease is the study and treatment of diseases caused by a virus, bacterium, fungus, or animal parasite in children.

Pediatric Nephrology
A subspecialty certified by the American Board of Pediatrics, Pediatric Nephrology deals with the diagnosis and treatment of disorders of the kidneys in children.

Pediatric Otolaryngology
A subspecialty certified by the American Board of Otolaryngology, Pediatric Otolaryngology involves the diagnosis and treatment of disorders of the ear, nose, and throat which affect children.

Pediatric Pulmonology
A subspecialty certified by the American Board of Pediatrics, Pediatric Pulmonology involves the diagnosis and treatment of diseases of the chest, lungs, and chest tissue in children.

Pediatric Radiology
A subspecialty certified by the American Board of Radiology, Pediatric Radiology involves diagnostic imaging as it pertains to the newborn, infant, child, and adolescent.

Pediatric Rheumatology
A subspecialty certified by the American Board of Pediatrics, Pediatric Rheumatology involves the treatment of diseases of the joints and connective tissues in children.

Pediatric Sports Medicine
A subspecialty certified by the American Board of Pediatrics, Pediatric Sports Medicine involves the diagnosis and treatment of injuries to the bone or soft tissue (muscles, tendons, ligaments) in children as a result of participation in athletic activity.

Pediatric Surgery
A subspecialty certified by the American Board of Surgery, Pediatric Surgery treats disease, injury, or deformity in children through surgical techniques.

Pediatrics
A specialty certified by the American Board of Pediatrics, a pediatrician diagnoses and treats diseases of childhood and monitors the growth, development, and well-being of preadolescents.

Physical Medicine & Rehabilitation
A specialty certified by the American Board of Physical Medicine & Rehabilitation, a physiatrist uses physical therapy and physical agents such as water, heat, light electricity, and mechanical manipulations in the diagnosis, treatment, and prevention of disease and body disorders.

Plastic Surgery
A specialty certified by the American Board of Plastic Surgery, a plastic surgeon specializes in reconstructive and cosmetic surgery of the face and other body parts.

Preventive Medicine
A specialty certified by the American Board of Preventive Medicine, a physician who specializes in preventive medicine focuses on health prevention and on the health of groups rather than individuals.

Psychiatry
A specialty certified by the American Board of Psychiatry and Neurology, a psychiatrist examines, treats, and prevents mental illness through the use of psychoanalysis and/or drugs.

DESCRIPTIONS OF SPECIALTIES AND SUBSPECIALTIES

Public Health & General Preventive Medicine
A subspecialty certified by the American Board of Preventive Medicine, Public Health and General Preventive Medicine involves the investigation of the causes of epidemic disease and the prevention of a wide variety of acute and chronic illness.

Pulmonary Disease
A subspecialty certified by the American Board of Internal Medicine, Pulmonary Disease involves the diagnosis and treatment of diseases of the chest, lungs, and airways.

Radiation Oncology
A subspecialty certified by the American Board of Radiology, Radiation Oncology involves the use of radiant energy and isotopes in the study and treatment of disease, especially malignant cancer.

Radiology
A specialty certified by the American Board of Radiology, a radiologist studies and uses various types of radiation, including X-rays, in the diagnosis and treatment of disease. Some imaging techniques no longer use radiation equipment (e.g., MRI and ultrasound).

Reproductive Endocrinology
A subspecialty certified by the American Board of Obstetrics and Gynecology, Reproductive Endocrinology deals with the endocrine system (including the pituitary, thyroid, parathyroid, adrenal glands, placenta, ovaries, and testes) and how its failure relates to infertility.

Rheumatology
A subspecialty certified by the American Board of Internal Medicine, Rheumatology involves the treatment of diseases of the joint, muscles, bones and associated structures.

Spinal Cord Injury Medicine
A subspecialty certified by the American Board of Physical Medicine & Rehabilitation, Spinal Cord Injury Medicine involves the prevention, diagnosis, treatment and management of traumatic spinal cord injuries.

Sports Medicine
A subspecialty certified by the American Boards of Emergency Medicine, Family

Practice, and Internal Medicine, Sports Medicine refers to the practice of an orthopaedist or other physician who specializes in injuries to bone or soft tissue (muscles, tendons, ligaments) caused by participation in athletic activity.

Surgery
A specialty certified by the American Board of Surgery, a surgeon treats disease, injury, and deformity by surgical procedures.

Surgery of the Hand
A subspecialty certified by the American Board of Surgery, Surgery of the Hand involves providing appropriate care for all structures in the upper extremity directly affecting the hand and wrist function.

Surgical Critical Care
A subspecialty certified by the American Board of Surgery, Surgical Critical Care involves the specialized care in the management of the critically ill patient, particularly the trauma victim and postoperative patient in the emergency department, intensive care unit, trauma unit, burn unit, and other similar settings.

Thoracic Surgery
A specialty certified by the American Board of Thoracic Surgery, a thoracic surgeon performs surgery on the heart, lungs, and chest area.

Urology
A specialty certified by the American Board of Urology, a urologist diagnoses and treats diseases of the genitals in men and disorders of the urinary tract and bladder in both men and women.

Vascular & Interventional Radiology
A subspecialty certified by the American Board of Radiology, Vascular & Interventional Radiology involves diagnosing and treating diseases by percutaneous methods guided by various radiologic imaging modalities.

Vascular Surgery (General)
A subspecialty certified by the American Board of Surgery, General Vascular Surgery involves the operative treatment of disorders of the blood vessels excluding those to the heart, lungs, or brain.

APPENDIX D
SELF-DESIGNATED MEDICAL SPECIALTIES

This list of self-designated medical specialty groups was obtained from the American Board of Medical Specialties. However, it is important to point out that these groups are not recognized by the ABMS, the governing board for the recognized twenty-four medical specialty boards (listed in Appendix A).

The organizations listed below range from highly organized groups that are attempting to formalize training and certification in their field to informal groups interested in a particular aspect of medicine.

If you wish to obtain information from any of these groups you will have to do some detective work. Because so many are informal, the location, phone and mailing addresses change frequently, depending upon the person who is functioning as secretary or administrator.

The best way to track down one of these groups is to consult this book's doctor listings to find a doctor who has expressed a special interest in that field, and call his or her office. You might also call a nearby academic health center in the area to see if they have a faculty or staff member known to be involved in that particular medical interest. If that fails, take the same approach with your community hospital.

A

Abdominal Surgeons
Acupuncture Medicine
Addiction Medicine
Addictionology
Adolescent Psychiatry
Aesthetic Plastic Surgery
Alcoholism and Other Drug
    Dependencies (AMSAODD)
Algology (Chronic Pain)
Alternative Medicine
Ambulatory Anesthesia
Ambulatory Foot Surgery
Anesthesia
Arthroscopic Surgery
Arthroscopy (Board of North America)

B

Bariatric Medicine
Bionic Psychology
Bloodless Medicine & Surgery

C

Chelation Therapy
Chemical Dependence
Clinical Chemistry
Clinical Ecology
Clinical Medicine and Surgery
Clinical Neurology
Clinical Neurophysiology
Clinical Neurosurgery
Clinical Nutrition
Clinical Orthopaedic Surgery
Clinical Pharmacology
Clinical Polysomnography
Clinical Psychiatry
Clinical Psychology
Clinical Toxicology
Cosmetic Plastic Surgery
Cosmetic Surgery
Council of Non-Board Certified Physicians
Critical Care in Medicine & Surgery

D

Dermalogy
Disability Analysis
Disability Evaluating Physicians

E

Electrodiagnostic Medicine
Electroencephalography
Electromyography & Electrodiagnosis
Environmental Medicine
Epidemiology (College)
Eye Surgery

F

Facial Cosmetic Surgery
Facial Plastic & Reconstructive Surgery
Family Practice, Certification
Forensic Examiners
Forensic Psychiatry
Forensic Toxicology

H

Hand Surgery
Head, Facial & Neck Pain & TMJ Orthopaedics
Health Physics
Homeopathic Physicians
Homeotherapeutics
Hypnotic Anesthesiology, National Board for

I

Independent Medical Examiners
Industrial Medicine & Surgery
Insurance Medicine
International Cosmetic & Plastic
    Facial Reconstructive Standards
Interventional Radiology

L

Laser Surgery
Law in Medicine
Longevity Medicine/Surgery

M

Malpractice Physicians
Maxillofacial Surgeons
Medical Accreditation (American Federation for)
Medical Hypnosis
Medical Laboratory Immunology
Medical-Legal Analysis of Medicine & Surgery
Medical Legal & Workers
    Comp. Medicine & Surgery
Medical-Legal Consultants
Medical Management
Medical Microbiology
Medical Preventics (Academy)
Medical Psychotherapists
Medical Toxicology
Microbiology (Medical Microbiology)
Military Medicine
Mohs Micrographic Surgery &
    Cutaneous Oncology

N

Neuroimaging
Neurologic & Orthopaedic Dental
    Medicine and Surgery
Neurological & Orthopaedic Medicine
Neurological & Orthopaedic Surgery
Neurological Microsurgery
Neurology
Neuromuscular Thermography
Neuro-Orthopaedic Dental Medicine & Surgery
Neuro-Orthopaedic Electrodiagnosis
Neuro-Orthopaedic Laser Surgery
Neuro-Orthopaedic Psychiatry
Neuro-Orthopaedic Thoracic Medicine/Surgery
Neurorehabilitation
Nutrition

O

Orthopaedic Medicine
Orthopaedic Microneurosurgery
Otorhinolaryngology

P

Pain Management (American Academy of)

Pain Management Specialties
Pain Medicine
Palliative Medicine
Percutaneous Diskectomy
Plastic Esthetic Surgeons
Prison Medicine
Professional Disability Consultants
Psychiatric Medicine
Psychiatry (American National Board of)
Psychoanalysis (American Examining
    Board in)
Psychological Medicine (International)

Q

Quality Assurance & Utilization Review

R

Radiology & Medical Imaging
Rheumatologic Surgery
Rheumatological & Reconstructive Medicine
Ringside Medicine & Surgery

S

Skin Specialists
Sleep Medicine (Polysomnography)
Spinal Cord Injury
Spinal Surgery
Sports Medicine
Sports Medicine/Surgery

T

Toxicology
Trauma Surgery
Traumatologic Medicine & Surgery
Tropical Medicine

U

Ultrasound Technology
Urologic Allied Health Professionals
Urological Surgery

W

Weight Reduction Medicine

NOTES:

_____

_____

_____

_____

_____

_____

_____

_____

_____

_____

_____

APPENDIX E
HIPPOCRATIC OATH

The Hippocratic Oath is administered to all medical students when they graduate from their respective medical schools. Today, some Deans of Medicine administer it to their students as they enter medical school in order to instill in them a sense of ethics, because even as students they will have contact with patients.

The oath is attributed to Hippocrates, a Greek physician who is often referred to as the Father of Medicine because of the degree to which he advanced medical practice and ethics. He died circa 377 B.C.

The oath has been modified by various medical schools and professional bodies and will be found in a variety of forms that typically embody the same principles.

Dorland's Illustrated Medical Dictionary. 27th ed. (Philadelphia) W.B. Saunders Co., 1988. Hippocratic Oath. [Hippocrates. Greek physician, 460-377 B.C.] An oath setting forward the duties of a physician to his patients as follows:

I swear by Apollo the physician, and Asklepios, and health, and All-Heal and all the gods and goddesses, that, according to my ability and judgement, I will keep this Oath and this stipulation — to reckon him who taught me this Art equally dear to me as my parents, to share my substance with him, and relieve his necessities if required; to look upon his offspring in the same footing as my own brothers, and to teach them this Art, if they should wish to learn it, without fee or stipulation; and that by precept, lecture and every other mode of instruction,

I will impart a knowledge of the Art to my own sons, and those of my teachers, and to disciples bound by a stipulation and oath according to the law of medicine, but to none others.

I will follow that system of regimen which, according to my ability and judgement, I consider for the benefit of my patients, and abstain from whatever is deleterious and mischievous. I will give no deadly medicine to anyone if asked nor suggest any such counsel; and in like manner I will not give to a woman a pessary to produce abortion. With purity and wholeness I will pass my life and practice my Art.

I will not cut persons labouring under the stone, but will leave this to be done by men who are practitioners of this work. Into whatever houses I enter, I will go into them for the benefit of the sick, and will abstain from every voluntary act of mischief and corruption; and, further, from the seduction of females or males, of freemen and slaves. Whatever, in connection with my professional practice, or not in connection with it, I see or hear, in the life of men, which ought not to be spoken of abroad, I will not divulge, as reckoning that all such should be kept secret. While I continue to keep this Oath unviolated, may it be granted to me to enjoy life and the practice of the art, respected by all men, in all times! But should I trespass and violate this Oath, may the reverse be my lot!

APPENDIX F
PATIENT RIGHTS

YOUR RIGHTS IN THE HOSPITAL

Most hospitals in New York State are required to adopt a bill of rights and many in New Jersey and Connecticut have as well. The following bill of rights is one that has been adopted by the American Hospital Association (AHA) and is in use in many hospitals throughout the nation.

The patient has the right to:

- *Considerate and respectful care.*
- *Complete information about his/her treatment and condition in terms the patient can reasonably understand.*
- *Know the identity of physicians, nurses, and others involved in their care, as well as when those involved are students, residents, or other trainees.*
- *Information necessary to give informed consent prior to the start of any procedure or treatment.*
- *Refuse treatment and be informed of the consequences.*
- *Have an advance directive (such as a living will, health care proxy, or durable power of attorney) for health care.*
- *Privacy concerning his/her treatment.*
- *Have all records and communications regarding medical treatment kept confidential.*

■ *Expect the hospital, within the limits of its capabilities, to respond to a request for services.*

■ *Obtain information regarding the relationship of the hospital to any other health care institutions.*

■ *Be advised if the hospital proposes human experimentation which affects his/her care.*

■ *Reasonable continuity of care.*

■ *An explanation of the bill, regardless of payment source.*

■ *Know what hospital rules and regulations apply to patient contact.*

(Source: American Hospital Association, Chicago, IL)

According to the American Hospital Association, this was last edited in 1992, so this version should be up to date. However, the AHA now has a "Fax on Demand" service at (312) 422-2020 through which consumers can obtain an up-to-date copy, free of charge, by sending their name, fax# and specifying document # 471124.

APPENDIX G
STATE AGENCIES

While there is a wealth of information available through these state agencies, much of it is not user-friendly. Complicated contractual agreements and other legal documents contain information that might prove to be valuable providing a consumer can locate it and then review it with some understanding. Often a department will suggest that a consumer visit the office for guidance in reviewing the documents. However, some of these agencies provide useful information on doctors, hospitals, and HMOs. They may also offer statistical reports and consumer-oriented studies.

CONNECTICUT

Doctors

    Department of Public Health
    Licensure and Registration
    410 Capitol Avenue, MS# 12MQA
    P.O. Box 340308
    Hartford, CT 06134-0308
    (860) 509-8000
    Attn: Physician renewal of verification

    Department of Health Service Legal Office
    410 Capitol Avenue
    MS#12LEG
    Hartford, CT 06134-0308
    (860) 509-7600

APPENDIX G

Hospitals
Connecticut State Department of Public Health
Division of Health Systems Regulation
410 Capitol Avenue, MS# 12HSR
P.O. Box 340308
Hartford, CT 06134-0308
(860) 509-7400

HMOs
Department of Insurance
P.O. Box 816
153 Market Street, 11th Floor
Hartford, CT 06103-0816
(860) 297-3800

Office of Health Care Access
410 Capitol Avenue
P.O. Box 340308
Hartford, CT 06134-0308
(860) 418-7001

NEW JERSEY

Doctors
New Jersey State Board of Medical Examiners
140 East Front Street, 2nd floor
Trenton, NJ 08608
(609) 826-7100

Hospitals
Department of Health
Division of Health Facilities Evaluation and Licensing
CN-367
Trenton, NJ 08625
(609) 588-7725

HMOs
Department of Health
Division of Health Facilities Evaluation and Licensing
CN-367
Trenton, NJ 08625
(609) 588-7725

1160

Department of Health
Alternative Health Systems
CN-367
Trenton, NJ 08625
(609) 588-2510 or (609) 588-7794

Department of Insurance
Division of Actuarial Services, Life and Health
Managed Healthcare Bureau
20 West State Street
CN-325, 11th floor
Trenton, NJ 08625
(609) 292-5436

NEW YORK

Doctors
New York State Department of Health
Office of Professional Medical Conduct
Corning Tower, Room 438
Empire State Plaza
Albany, NY 12237
(518) 474-8357

New York State Department of Education
Cultural Education Center
Division of Professional Licensing
Albany, NY 12230
(518) 486-5205

Hospitals
Office of Health Systems Management
Tower Building
Empire State Plaza
Albany, NY 12237-0701
(518) 474-7028

New York State Department of Health
Bureau of Biometrics
Concourse Room C-144
Empire State Plaza
Albany, NY 12237
(518) 474-3189

APPENDIX G

HMOs

> **Department of Insurance**
> **Health and Life Policy Bureau**
> Agency Building 1
> Empire State Plaza
> Albany, NY 12257
> (518) 474-4098
>
> **New York State Department of Health**
> **Office of Managed Care**
> Corning Tower, Room 1911
> Albany, NY 12237
> (518) 473-8944
>
> **New York State Department of Health**
> **Bureau of Management Analysis**
> **Records Access Office**
> Empire State Plaza Concourse, Room # C144
> Albany, NY 12237-0044
> (518) 474-8734

APPENDIX H
STATE & COUNTY
MEDICAL SOCIETIES

Although formed as professional associations of physicians, county medical societies also may be of importance to consumers through their referral services and to assist if a consumer has a complaint against a doctor.

Each county in New York State, New Jersey, and Connecticut has a medical society. Membership is open to licensed physicians and most have medical student chapters. (They also have active auxiliaries that raise money for medical student scholarships.) The county chapters relate to the state society which, in turn, relates to the American Medical Association. The relationship is conducted in a number of ways, but especially through elected officers serving on councils or boards at other levels (i.e. county to state, state to national).

County medical societies have a number of functions including education, advocacy for medicine and social camaraderie for doctors. (The membership in county medical societies ranges from about 50 percent to about 70 percent of doctors in a county.)

The educational function is usually carried out through an arm of the society, an Academy of Medicine, which offers continuing medical education (CME) programs for doctors in the region.

The county societies are organized by committee and usually include standing committees on legislation, public relations, ethics and peer review among others.

It is in the latter two areas that the public may be directly served and interact with the medical society.

County medical societies will review complaints by patients about doctors. Their review may be through an Ethics Committee in matters related to finance, legal, ethical or social issues; or through the Peer Review Committee in cases involving the quality or appropriateness of medical care.

If a doctor is found deficient in some respect, a medical society may censure the individual or, in more extreme cases, remove them from membership. Patients may contact the local medical society for further information if they have a problem and desire assistance.

Many county medical societies also sponsor physician referral lines for the public. All members of the medical society are eligible to participate in the referral service. Referrals are generally made on the basis of specialty, geographic proximity, languages spoken, house calls, evening hours, etc. Information such as medical school, board certification and status of medical license may also be provided.

The following is a listing of the county medical societies in the New York metropolitan area. They may be helpful if an individual needs information on a physician or has a problem with a physician.

CONNECTICUT STATE MEDICAL SOCIETY

160 Saint Ronan Street
New Haven, CT 06511
(203) 865-0587

COUNTY MEDICAL SOCIETY — CONNECTICUT

Fairfield County Medical Association
2285 Reservoir Avenue
Trumbull, CT 06611
(203) 372-4543

NEW JERSEY STATE MEDICAL SOCIETY

2 Princess Road
Lawrenceville, NJ 08648
(609) 896-1766

COUNTY MEDICAL SOCIETIES — NEW JERSEY

Bergen County Medical Society
1060 Main Street, Suite 2c
Riveredge, NJ 07661
(201) 489-3140

Essex County Medical Society
80 Pompton Avenue
Verona, NJ 07044
(973) 239-9392

Hudson County Medical Society
2 Jefferson Avenue
Jersey City, NJ 07306
(201) 798-0600

Mercer County Medical Society
199 Scotch Road
Trenton, NJ 08628
(609) 882-1048

Middlesex County Medical Society
575 Cranbury Road
East Brunswick, NJ 08816
(732) 257-6800

Monmouth County Medical Society
766 Shrewsbury Avenue
Tinton Falls, NJ 07724
(732) 530-3213

Morris County Medical Society
51 Elm Street
Morristown, NJ 07960
(973) 539-8888

Passaic County Medical Society
999 McBride Avenue, Suite B202
West Patterson, NJ 07424
(973) 890-0700

Somerset County Medical Society
c/o Somerset Medical Center
110 Rehill Avenue
Sommerville, NJ 08876
(908) 685-2910

Union County Medical Society
1164 Springfield Avenue
Mountainside, NJ 07092
(908) 789-8603

1165

NEW YORK STATE MEDICAL SOCIETY

420 Lakeville Road
Lake Success, NY 11042
(516) 488-6100

COUNTY MEDICAL SOCIETIES — NEW YORK

Bronx County Medical Society
2600 Netherlands Avenue, Suite # 118
Bronx, NY 10463
(718) 548-4401

Medical Society of the County of Kings
(Brooklyn)
1313 Bedford Avenue
Brooklyn, NY 11216
(718) 467-9000

Nassau County Medical Society
1200 Stewart Avenue
Garden City, NY 11530
(516) 832-2300

New York County Medical Society
(Manhattan)
15 East 26th Street, Suite 1101
New York, NY 10010
(212) 684-4670

Richmond County Medical Society
(Staten Island)
75 Vanderbilt Avenue
Bldg. #7
Staten Island, NY 10304
(718) 442-7267

Suffolk County Medical Society
1767-14 Veterans Memorial Highway
Islandia, NY 11722-1536
(516) 851-1400

Queens County Medical Society
112-25 Queens Boulevard
Forest Hills, NY 11375
(718) 268-7300

Rockland County Medical Society
33 West Nyack Road
Nanuet, NY 10954
(914) 623-3408

Westchester County Medical Society
3801 Purchase Street
Purchase, NY 10577
(914) 948-4100

APPENDIX I
HOW TO FILE
A COMPLAINT

Filing a complaint against a physician, other health-care practitioner or hospital is a serious matter. It should be undertaken with great thought and consideration, and is justified only if a patient feels seriously aggrieved and believes a law, regulation or professional ethic has been violated.

Before a complaint is filed, it may be helpful to contact the hospital administration if the problem is with a hospital. If it is a problem with a doctor at a hospital, the chief of the service, medical director or vice-president of medical affairs should be notified.

If these efforts fail, one may consider a formal complaint. If you wish to file a formal complaint against a medical practitioner, hospital, health-care facility or insurance company, you must file it with the State, which is the licensing authority. Contact the appropriate state agency and request a complaint form and any special forms that must be filed with your particular case. Include information such as name of offending party and date, place and nature of incident. Save all records and/or receipts relating to the incident (i.e., billing statements and medical and hospital records including lab reports).

CONNECTICUT

Doctors
> Department of Health Service
> Legal Office
> 410 Capitol Avenue, MS #12LEG
> P.O. Box 340308
> Hartford, CT 06134-0308
> (860) 509-7600

Hospitals
> Connecticut State Department of Public Health
> Division of Health Systems Regulation
> 410 Capitol Street
> MS#12HSR
> P.O. Box 340308
> Hartford, CT 06134-0308
> (860) 509-7400

HMOs
> Commission of Hospitals and Health Care
> Office of Health Care Access
> 410 Capitol Avenue
> P.O. Box 340308
> Hartford, CT 06134-0308
> (860) 418-7001

NEW JERSEY

Doctors
> New Jersey State Board of Medical Examiners
> 140 East Front Street, second floor
> Trenton, NJ 08608
> (609) 826-7100

Hospitals
> Department of Health
> Division of Health Facilities Evaluation and Licensing
> CN-367
> Trenton, NJ 08625
> (609) 633-6800
> (800) 792-9770 (NJ Only)

HMOs
> Department of Health and Senior Services
> Office of Managed Care
> P.O. Box 360
> Trenton, NJ 08625
> (609) 633-0660

NEW YORK

Doctors
> New York State Department of Health
> OPMC 433
> River Street, Suite 303
> Troy, NY 12180
> (518) 402-0836

Hospitals
> New York State Department of Health
> Bureau of Hospital Services
> Hedley Park Place
> 433 River Street, 6th Floor
> Troy, NY 12180-2299
> (518) 402-1003
> *(Will refer consumers to regional offices)*

HMOs
> New York State Department of Health
> Office of Managed Care
> 2001 Empire State Plaza
> Troy, NY 12237-0094
> (518) 474-5737

NOTES:

_____

_____

_____

_____

_____

_____

_____

_____

_____

_____

APPENDIX J

MEDICARE AND MEDICAID
STATE AGENCIES

The following phone numbers are those consumers may call to obtain information on Medicare and Medicaid.

CONNECTICUT

Medicaid	(800) 842-8440
Medicare	(800) 982-6819
(Hartford)	(203) 237-8592
(Meriden)	(800) 982-6819

NEW JERSEY

Medicaid	(609) 588-2600
Medicare	(717) 975-7333
or	(800) 462-9306

NEW YORK

Medicaid Consumers must contact the Department of Social Services at
(518) 473-3170
Medicare for counties of Bronx, Columbia, Delaware, Dutchess, Greene, Kings, Nassau, New York, Orange, Putnam, Richmond, Rockland, Suffolk, Sullivan, Ulster, Westchester:
(516) 244-5100
or (800) 442-8430
for county of Queens:
(212) 721-1770
for rest of state:
(800) 252-6550

NOTES:

APPENDIX K
SELECTED RESOURCES

American Ambulance Association
3800 Auburn Boulevard, Suite C
Sacramento, CA 95821
(800) 523-4447 phone
(916) 482-5473 fax
The American Ambulance Association can provide general information on EMS services.

Centers for Disease Control and Prevention (CDC)
Fax Information Service for International Travelers
(404) 639-2573 (information)
(404) 332-4565 (to order a document)
The CDC provides free, immediate faxed reports on disease risk and prevention and disease outbreaks in various parts of the world.

Commission on Accreditation of Ambulance Services
PO Box 619911
Dallas, TX 75261-9911
(214) 580-2829
The Commission on Accreditation of Ambulance Services is the accreditation body for all ambulance services. They provide information on accreditation status of all/any ambulance services.

Emergency Medical History & Assistance (EMX)
520 Madison Avenue —38th Floor
New York, New York 10022
(800)-325-5940
EMX is a company that supplies medical records, provided to it by a member of the service, to medical personnel at times of emergency. The medical information is accessed by a card which the member carries, as well as a pin number for identification and confidentiality.

Emergency Medical Systems, Inc.
2160 North Central Road, Suite 104
Ft. Lee, NJ 07024
(800) 317-5977 phone
(201) 461-8574 fax
Medi Vault is a series of products sponsored by Emergency Medical Systems Inc. that provide emergency and other medical records that are accessible through telephone, fax, beeper, area networks and the internet.

Health Care Rescue Network
Post Office Box 1326
Wheaton, Illinois 60189-1326
(800) 627-0552 voice mail
(708) 510-0256 fax
The Health Care Rescue Network is an alliance that educates the public on the benefits of medical savings accounts and the dangers of managed care. They will refer consumers to local organizations.

International Association for Medical Assistance To Travellers (IAMAT)
417 Center Street
Lewiston, New York 14092
(716) 754-4883 phone
IAMAT is a non-profit organization that disseminates information on health and sanitary conditions worldwide. Membership is free but donations are appreciated. Members will receive a membership card making them eligible to access English speaking physicians all over the world. The organization also provides information on immunization requirements, malaria, and other tropical diseases, and sanitary and climactic conditions around the world. For information, send request in writing.

Medic Alert Foundation
2323 Colorado Avenue
Turlock, CA 95382
(800) 432-5378 phone
The Medic Alert Foundation (a non-profit organization) provides an "ID tag" engraved with personal medical facts, as well as a 24-hour emergency response center which can release additional personal medical details. Membership is $15/year (waived for the first year) and members need to purchase the "ID tag" which sells for as low as $35.

The National Consumers League (NCL)
1701 K Street, NW, Suite 1200
Washington, DC 20006
(202) 835-3323 phone
NCL is a private, nonprofit consumer advocacy organization. NCL strives to investigate, educate, and advocate on a variety of issues including healthcare. Membership is $20 annually, but individuals can also write to the organization for a list of publications that non-members can purchase.

1174

National Insurance Consumer Helpline (800) 942-4242
The National Insurance Consumer Helpline advises consumers on how to choose an insurance company or broker. It also offers an analysis of life insurance and assists in insurance complaints.

Office of Alternative Medicine (OAM)
P.O. Box 8218
Silverspring, MD 20907
(888) 644-6226 phone
(301) 495-4957 fax
The OAM facilitates the evaluation of alternative medical treatment modalities to help determine their effectiveness and bring alternative medicine into mainstream medicine. This agency does not provide referrals but is in the process of setting up a clearinghouse of information.

People's Medical Society
462 Walnut Street
Allentown, PA 18102
(800) 624-8773 phone
The People's Medical Society is a nonprofit organization that educates and informs consumers about the confusing healthcare market. For a $20 fee, members will receive a newsletter as well as discounts on all publications. Non-members may still order publications from the organization directly. The Society publishes a number of excellent books on health care issues.

Physicians Who Care
10615 Perrin Beitel, Suite 201
San Antonio, Texas 78217
(800) 545-9305 phone
(210) 656-1545 fax
Physicians Who Care is an organization which serves as an advocate for quality health care. It offers brochures and newsletters for consumers with questions and concerns regarding managed care. Consumers may contact this organization with complaints concerning HMOs and other managed care organizations.

Public Citizen's Health Research Group
1600 20th Street, NW
Washington, DC 20009
(202) 588-1000 phone
The Health Research Group petitions and testifies before Congress and federal agencies on such issues as banning or relabeling of drugs, improved safety standards at work sites and safer medical devices. Their publications provide information on various health topics including quality of care, insurance, questionable doctors and hospitals, managed care and how to obtain medical records.

NOTES:

APPENDIX L
MEDICAL SCHOOLS

The following is a list of U.S. medical schools and the abbreviations used for each in the doctor listings. The abbreviations as they appear in the listings are in italics below.

ALABAMA

University of Alabama School of Medicine University of Alabama at Birmingham
U Ala Sch Med

University of South Alabama College of Medicine
U South Ala Coll Med

ARIZONA

University of Arizona College of Medicine
Arizona Health Sciences Center
U Ariz Coll Med

ARKANSAS

University of Arkansas College of Medicine
U Ark Sch Med

CALIFORNIA

University of California Davis School of Medicine
UC Davis
University of California Irvine College of Medicine
UC Irvine

University of California San Diego School of Medicine
UC San Diego

Loma Linda University School of Medicine
Loma Linda U

University of California Los Angeles UCLA School of Medicine
UCLA

University of Southern California School of Medicine
USC Sch Med

College of Osteopathic Medicine of the Pacific
Coll of Osteo Med-Pacific

University of California San Francisco School of Medicine
UC San Francisco

Stanford University School of Medicine
Stanford U

COLORADO

University of Colorado School of Medicine
U Colo Sch Med

CONNECTICUT

University of Connecticut School of Medicine
U Conn Sch Med

Yale University School of Medicine
Yale U Sch Med

DISTRICT OF COLUMBIA

George Washington University
School of Medicine and Health Science
Geo Wash U Sch Med

Georgetown University School of Medicine
Georgetown U

Howard University College of Medicine
Howard U

FLORIDA

University of Florida College of Medicine
U Fla Coll Med

University of Miami School of Medicine
U Miami Sch Med

Nova Southeastern University,
College of Osteopathic Medicine
Nova SE Univ, Coll of Osteo Med

University of South Florida
College of Medicine
U South Fla Coll Med

Florida College of Osteopathic Medicine
FL Coll of Osteo Med

GEORGIA

Emory University School of Medicine
Emory U Sch Med

Morehouse School of Medicine
Morehouse Sch Med

Medical College of Georgia
School of Medicine
Med Coll Ga

Mercer University School of Medicine
Mercer U Sch Med, Macon, GA

HAWAII

University of Hawaii John A. Burns
School of Medicine
U Hawaii JA Burns Sch Med

ILLINOIS

Arizona College of Osteopathic Medicine,
Midwestern University
Ariz Coll of Osteo Med

Chicago College of Osteopathic Medicine,
Midwestern University
Chicago Coll of Osteo Med

Northwestern University Medical School
Northwestern U

Rush Medical College of Rush University
Rush Med Coll

University of Chicago (Div Bio Sci)
Pritzker School of Medicine
U Chicago-Pritzker Sch Med

University of Illinois College of Medicine
U Ill Coll Med

Loyola University of Chicago - Stritch
School of Medicine
Loyola U-Stritch Sch Med, Maywood

University of Health Sciences Chicago
Medical School
U Hlth Sci/Chicago Med Sch

Southern Illinois University
School of Medicine

Southern Ill U

INDIANA

Indiana University School of Medicine
Ind U Sch Med

IOWA

University of Osteopathic Medicine
U of Osteo Med-IA

University of Iowa College of Medicine
U Iowa Coll Med

KANSAS

University of Kansas Medical Center School of Medicine
U Kans Sch Med

KENTUCKY

University of Kentucky College of Medicine
U Ky Coll Med

University of Louisville School of Medicine
KY Sch Med, Louisville

LOUISIANA

Louisiana State University School of Medicine New Orleans
LSU Sch Med, New Orleans

Tulane University School of Medicine
Tulane U

Louisiana State University School Of Medicine Shreveport
LSU Med Ctr, Shreveport

MARYLAND

Johns Hopkins University School of Medicine
Johns Hopkins U

University of Maryland School of Medicine
U Md Sch Med

F. Edward A. Hebert School of Medicine Uniformed Services University of Health Sciences
Uniformed Srvs U, Betheseda

MASSACHUSETTS

Boston University School of Medicine
Boston U

Harvard Medical School
Harvard Med Sch

Tufts University School of Medicine
Tufts U

University of Massachusetts Medical School
U Mass Sch Med

MICHIGAN

University of Michigan Medical School
U Mich Med Sch

Wayne State University School of Medicine
Wayne State U

Michigan State University College of Human Medicine
Mich St U

Michigan State University College of Osteopathic Medicine
Mich St Coll of Osteo Med

MINNESOTA

University of Minnesota Duluth School of Medicine
U Minn-Duluth Sch Med

University of Minnesota Medical School
U Minn

Mayo Medical School
Mayo Med Sch

MISSISSIPPI

University of Mississippi School of Medicine
U Miss Sch Med

MISSOURI

University of Missouri Columbia
School of Medicine
U Mo-Columbia Sch Med

Kirksville College of Osteopathic
Medicine
Kirksville Coll of Osteo Med

University of Health Sciences/College of
Osteopathic Medicine
U of Hlth Sci, Coll of Osteo Med

University of Missouri Kansas City
School of Medicine
U Mo-Kansas City Sch Med

Saint Louis University
School of Medicine
St Louis U

Washington University
School of Medicine
Wash U, St. Louis

NEBRASKA

Creighton University School of Medicine
Creighton U

University of Nebraska
College of Medicine
U Nebr Coll Med

NEVADA

University of Nevada School of Medicine
U Nevada

NEW HAMPSHIRE

Dartmouth Medical School
Dartmouth Med Sch

NEW JERSEY

University of Medicine and Dentistry
of New Jersey
UMDNJ-NJ Med Sch, Newark

University of Medicine and
Dentistry of New Jersey
UMDNJ-RW Johnson Med Sch

University of Medicine and Dentistry
of New Jersey/School of Osteopathic
Medicine
UMD-NJ Sch of Osteo Med

NEW MEXICO

University of New Mexico
School of Medicine
U New Mexico

NEW YORK

Albany Medical College
Albany Med Coll

Albert Einstein College of
Medicine of Yeshiva University
Albert Einstein Coll Med

State University of New York Health
Science Center at Brooklyn
SUNY Health Sci Ctr, Bklyn

State University of New York at Buffalo
School of Medicine & Biomedical
Sciences
SUNY Buffalo

New York College of Osteopathic
Medicine
NY Coll of Osteo Med

Columbia University College
of Physicians and Surgeons
Columbia P&S

Cornell University Medical College
Cornell U

Mt. Sinai School of Medicine of
the City University of New York
Mt Sinai Sch Med

New York University School
of Medicine
NYU Sch Med

University of Rochester
School of Medicine and Dentistry
U Rochester

State University of New York at Stony
Brook Health Sciences Center
SUNY Hlth Sci Ctr, Stony Brook

State University of New York Health
Science Center at Syracuse
SUNY Hlth Sci Ctr, Syracuse

New York Medical College
NY Med Coll

NORTH CAROLINA

University of North Carolina at Chapel
Hill School of Medicine
U NC Sch Med

Duke University School of Medicine
Duke U

East Carolina University School
of Medicine
E Carolina U

Bowman Gray School of Medicine
Bowman Gray

NORTH DAKOTA

University of North Dakota
School of Medicine
U ND Sch Med

OHIO

University of Cincinnati
College of Medicine
U Cincinnati

Case Western Reserve University
School of Medicine
Case West Res U

Ohio University, College
of Osteopathic Medicine
OH Coll of Osteo Med

Ohio State University
College of Medicine
Ohio State U

Wright State University
School of Medicine
Wright State U Sch Med

Northeastern Ohio University
College of Medicine
NE Ohio U

Medical College of Ohio
MC Ohio, Toledo

OKLAHOMA

University of Oklahoma
College of Medicine
U Okla Coll Med

Oklahoma State University
College of Osteopathic Medicine
OSU Coll of Osteo Med

OREGON

Oregon Health Science
University School of Medicine
U Oreg/Hlth Sci U, Portland

PENNSYLVANIA

Lake Erie College
of Osteopathic Medicine
Lake Erie Coll of Osteo Med

Pennsylvania State University
College of Medicine
Penn St U-Hershey Med Ctr

Hahnemann University
School of Medicine
Hahnemann U

Jefferson Medical College
of Thomas Jefferson University
Jefferson Med Coll

Medical College of Pennsylvania
Med Coll Penn

Philadelphia College
of Osteopathic Medicine
Philadelphia Coll of Osteo Med

Temple University
School of Medicine
Temple U

University of Pennsylvania
School of Medicine
U Penn

University of Pittsburgh
School of Medicine
U Pittsbrgh

PUERTO RICO

Universidad Central del Caribe School of Medicine
U del Caribe Escuela Med Cayey

Ponce School of Medicine
Ponce Med Sch

University of Puerto Rico School of Medicine
U Puerto Rico

RHODE ISLAND

Brown University Program in Medicine
Brown U

SOUTH CAROLINA

Medical University of South Carolina College of Medicine
Med U SC, Charleston

University of South Carolina School of Medicine
U SC Sch Med, Columbia

SOUTH DAKOTA

University of South Dakota School of Medicine
U SD Sch Med

TENNESSEE

East Tennessee State University James H. Quillen College of Medicine
E Tenn State U

University of Tennessee Memphis College of Medicine
U Tenn Memphis Coll Med

Meharry Medical College School of Medicine
Meharry Med Coll

Vanderbilt University School of Medicine
Vanderbilt U

TEXAS

Texas A&M University Health Science Center College of Medicine
Texas A&M U

University of Texas
U Texas, Dallas

University of North Texas Health Science Center/College of Osteopathic Medicine
U of North TX Coll of Osteo Med

University of Texas Medical School at Galveston
U Texas Med Br, Galveston

Baylor College of Medicine
Baylor

University of Texas Medical School at Houston
U Texas, Houston

Texas Tech University Health Science Center School of Medicine
Tex Tech U Sch Med

University of Texas Medical School at San Antonio
U Tex San Antonio

UTAH

University of Utah School of Medicine
U Utah

VERMONT

University of Vermont College of Medicine
U Vt Coll Med

VIRGINIA

University of Virginia School of Medicine
U Va Sch Med

Eastern Virginia Medical School of the Medical College of Hampton Roads
Eastern VA Med Sch, Norfolk

Virginia Commonwealth University Medical College of Virginia School of Medicine
Med Coll Va

WASHINGTON

University of Washington School of Medicine
U Wash, Seattle

WEST VIRGINIA

Marshall University School of Medicine
Marshall U

West Virginia School of Osteopathic Medicine
WV Sch Osteo Med

Robert C. Byrd Health Sciences Center of West Virginia University School of Medicine
W Va U Sch Med

WISCONSIN

University of Wisconsin School of Medicine
U Wisc Med Sch

Medical College of Wisconsin
Med Coll Wisc

CANADA

The University of Calgary Faculty of Medicine
U Calgary

Faculty of Medicine University of Alberta
U Alberta

University of British Columbia Faculty of Medicine
U British Columbia Fac Med

University of Manitoba Faculty of Medicine
U Manitoba

Memorial University of Newfoundland Faculty of Medicine
Meml U-St Johns, Newfoundland

Dalhousie University Faculty of Medicine
Dalhousie U

McMaster University Faculty of Health Sciences
McMaster U

Queen's University Faculty of Medicine
Queens U

University of Western Ontario Faculty of Medicine
U Western Ontario

University of Ottawa Faculty of Medicine
U Ottawa

University of Toronto Faculty of Medicine
U Toronto

McGill University Faculty of Medicine
McGill U

Laval University Faculty of Medicine
Laval U, Quebec

NOTES:

APPENDIX M
HOSPITAL LISTING

Following is an alphabetical listing of hospitals noted in doctors' entries. The abbreviations as they appear in the listings are in italics below. Due to the many mergers taking place in the hospital industry these days, the names on this list periodically may change.

Barnert Hospital
Barnert Hosp
680 Broadway
Paterson, NJ 07514
Passaic
(973) 977-6600

Bayley Seton Hospital
Bayley Seton Hosp
75 Vanderbilt Avenue
Staten Island, NY 10304
Richmond
(718) 354-6000

Bayonne Hospital
Bayonne Hosp
29 E. 29th Street
Bayonne, NJ 07002
Hudson
(201) 858-5000

Bayshore Community Hospital
Bayshore Community Hosp
727 N. Beers Street
Holmdel, NJ 07733
Monmouth
(732) 739-5900

Bellevue Hospital Center
Bellevue Hosp Ctr
462 1st Avenue
New York, NY 10016
New York (Manhattan)
(212) 562-4141

Bergen Pines County Hospital
Bergen Pines Cty Hosp
230 E. Ridgewood Avenue
Paramus, NJ 07652
Bergen
(201) 967-4000

Beth Israel Hospital
(See Passaic Beth Israel Hospital)

Institutions in bold are profiled in this edition of the Castle Connolly Guide.

APPENDIX M

Beth Israel Medical Center
Beth Israel Med Ctr
Part of Continuum Health Partners, Inc.
16th Street and First Avenue
New York, NY 10003
New York (Manhattan)
(212) 420-2000

Beth Israel Medical Center
Kings Highway Division
Beth Israel Med Ctr - Kings Hwy
Part of Continuum Health Partners, Inc.
3201 Kings Highway
Brooklyn, NY 11234
Kings
(718) 252-3000

Beth Israel Medical Center, North
Division
Beth Israel North
Part of Continuum Health Partners, Inc.
170 East End Avenue at 87th Street
New York, NY 10128
New York (Manhattan)
(212) 870-9000

Blythedale Children's Hospital
Blythedale Children's Hosp
Bradhurst Avenue
Valhalla, NY 10595
Westchester
(914) 592-7555

Bronx Children's Psychiatric Center
Bronx Children's Psych Ctr
1000 Waters Place
Bronx, NY 10461-2799
Bronx
(718) 892-0808

Bridgeport Hospital
Bridgeport Hosp
267 Grant Street
P.O. Box 5000
Bridgeport, CT 06610
Fairfield
(203) 384-3000

Bronx Lebanon Hospital Center
Concourse Division
Bronx Lebanon Hosp Ctr
1650 Grand Concourse
Bronx, NY 10457
Bronx
(718) 590-1800

Bronx Municipal Hospital Center
(See Jacobi Medical Center)

Brookdale University Hospital
and Medical Center
Brookdale Univ Hosp Med Ctr
One Brookdale Plaza
Brooklyn, NY 11212
Kings
(718) 240-5000

Bronx Psychiatric Center
Bronx Psychiatric Ctr
1500 Waters Place
Bronx, NY 10461
Bronx
(718) 931-0600

Brookhaven Memorial Hospital
Medical Center
Brookhaven Mem Hosp
Medical Center
101 Hospital Road
Patchogue, NY 11772
Suffolk
(516) 654-7100

The Brooklyn Hospital Center -
Caledonian Campus
Brooklyn Hosp Ctr - Caledonian
100 Parkside Avenue
Brooklyn, NY 11226
Kings
(718) 250-8000

Institutions in bold are profiled in this edition of the Castle Connolly Guide.

**The Brooklyn Hospital Center -
Downtown Campus**
Brooklyn Hosp Ctr - Downtown
121 DeKalb Avenue
Brooklyn, NY 11201
Kings
(718) 855-8242

Brunswick Hall
Brunswick Hall
80 Louden Avenue
Amityville, NY 11701
Suffolk
(516) 789-7100

Brunswick General Hospital
Brunswick Gen Hosp
366 Broadway
Amityville, NY 11701
Suffolk
(516) 789-7000

Burke Rehabilitation Hospital
Burke Rehabilitation Hosp
785 Mamaroneck Avenue
White Plains, NY 10605
Westchester
(914) 948-0050

Cabrini Medical Center
Cabrini Med Ctr
227 E. 19th Street
New York, NY 10003
New York (Manhattan)
(212) 995-6000

Calvary Hospital
Calvary Hosp
1740 Eastchester Road
Bronx, NY 10461
Bronx
(718) 518-2300

Capital Health System at Fuld
Capital Health Sys at Fuld
(formerly Helene Fuld Medical Center)
750 Brunswick Avenue
Trenton, NJ 08638
Mercer
(609) 394-6000

Capital Health System at Mercer
Capital Health Sys at Mercer
446 Bellevue Avenue
Trenton, NJ 08607
Mercer
(609) 394-4000

**Catholic Medical Center
of Brooklyn & Queens**
Catholic Med Ctr Bklyn & Qns
88-25 153rd Street
Jamaica, NY 11432
Queens
(718) 558-6900

Central Suffolk Hospital
Central Suffolk Hosp
1300 Roanoke Avenue
Riverhead, NY 11901
Suffolk
(516) 548-6000

Centrastate Medical Center
Centrastate Med Ctr
901 W. Main Street
Freehold, NJ 07728
Monmouth
(732) 431-2000

Charter Behavorial Health System
of New Jersey
Charter Behavorial Hlth Sys - NJ
19 Prospect Street
Summit, NJ 07901
Union
(908) 522-7000

**Children's Hospital of New Jersey at
Newark Beth Israel Medical Center**
Children's Hosp of NJ
Part of St. Barnabas Health Care System
201 Lyons Avenue at Osborne Terrace
Newark, NJ 07112
Essex
(973) 926-4000

Institutions in bold are profiled in this edition of the Castle Connolly Guide.

Chilton Memorial Hospital
Chilton Mem Hosp
97 W. Parkway
Pompton Plains, NJ 07444
Morris
(973) 831-5000

Christ Hospital
Christ Hosp
176 Palisade Avenue
Jersey City, NJ 07306
Hudson
(201) 795-8200

City Hospital Center at Elmhurst
(See Elmhurst Hospital Center)

Clara Maass Medical Center
Clara Maass Med Ctr
Part of St. Barnabas Health Care System
One Clara Maass Drive
Belleville, NJ 07109
Essex
(973) 450-2000

Columbia-Presbyterian Medical Center
Columbia-Presbyterian Med Ctr
Part of The New York
and Presbyterian Hospital
622 West 168th Street
New York, NY 10032
New York (Manhattan)
(212) 305-2500

Columbus Hospital
Columbus Hosp
495 N. 13th Street
Newark, NJ 07107
Essex
(973) 268-1400

Community Hospital at Dobbs Ferry
Community Hosp at Dobbs Ferry
128 Ashford Avenue
Dobbs Ferry, NY 10522
Westchester
(914) 693-0700

Community Hospital of Smithtown
Community Hosp of Smithtown
498 Smithtown By-Pass
Smithtown, NY 11787
Suffolk
(516) 979-9800

Coney Island Hospital
Coney Island Hosp
2601 Ocean Parkway
Brooklyn, NY 11235
Kings
(718) 616-3000

Danbury Hospital
Danbury Hosp
24 Hospital Avenue
Danbury, CT 06810
Fairfield
(203) 797-7000

Doctors Hospital of Staten Island
Doctors Hosp of Staten Island
1050 Targee Street
Staten Island, NY 10304
Richmond County
(718) 390-1400

East Orange General Hospital
East Orange Gen Hosp
300 Central Avenue
East Orange, NJ 07019
Essex
(973) 672-8400

Eastern Long Island Hospital
Eastern Long Island Hosp
201 Manor Place
Greenport, NY 11944
Suffolk
(516) 477-1000

Einstein Hospital
Einstein Hospital (See Jack D.
Weiler Hospital of the Einstein
College of Medicine)

Elizabeth General Medical Center
Elizabeth General Med Ctr
925 E. Jersey Street
Elizabeth, NJ 07201
Union
(908) 289-8600

Institutions in bold are profiled in this edition of the Castle Connolly Guide.

Elmhurst Hospital Center
Elmhrst Hosp Ctr
(Formerly City Hospital Center at Elmhurst)
79-01 Broadway
Elmhurst, NY 11373
Queens
(718) 334-4000

Englewood Hospital and Medical Center
Englewood Hosp & Med Ctr
350 Engle Street
Englewood, NJ 07631
Bergen
(201) 894-3000

Flushing Hospital Medical Center
Flushing Hosp Med Ctr
4500 Parsons Boulevard
Flushing, NY 11355
Queens
(718) 670-5000

Four Winds Hospital
Four Winds Hosp
800 Cross River Road
Katonah, NY 10536
Westchester
(914) 763-8151

Franklin Hospital Medical Center
Franklin Hosp Med Ctr
900 Franklin Avenue
Valley Stream, NY 11580
Nassau
(516) 256-6000

The General Hospital Center - Passaic
Gen Hosp Ctr Passaic
350 Boulevard
Passaic, NJ 07055
Passaic
(973) 365-4300

Good Samaritan Hospital
Good Samaritan Hosp
255 Lafayette Avenue
Suffern, NY 10901
Rockland
(914) 368-5000

Good Samaritan Hospital Medical Center
Good Samaritan Med Ctr
1000 Montauk Highway
West Islip, NY 11795
Suffolk
(516) 376-3000

Gracie Square Hospital
Gracie Square Hosp
421 E. 75th Street
New York, NY 10021
Manhattan
(212) 988-4400

Greenville Hospital
Greenville Hosp
1825 Kennedy Boulevard
Jersey City, NJ 07305
Hudson
(201) 547-6100

Greenwich Hospital
Greenwich Hosp
Five Perryridge Road
Greenwich, CT 06830
Fairfield
(203) 863-3000

Greystone Park Psychiatric Hospital
Greystone Park Psych Hosp
Greystone Park, NJ 07950
Morris
(973) 538-1800

Hackensack University Medical Center
Hackensack Univ Med Ctr
30 Prospect Avenue
Hackensack, NJ 07601
Bergen
(201) 996-2000

Hamilton Hospital
(See Robert Wood Johnson University Hospital
at Hamilton)

Institutions in bold are profiled in this edition of the Castle Connolly Guide.

1189

Harlem Hospital Center
Harlem Hosp Ctr
506 Lenox Avenue, Rm 2146
New York, NY 10037
New York (Manhattan)
(212) 939-1000

Hempstead General Hospital
Medical Center
Hempstead Gen Hosp Med Ctr
800 Front Street
Hempstead, NY 11550
Nassau
(516) 560-1200

Holliswood Hospital
Holliswood Hosp
87-37 Palermo Street
Queens, NY 11423
Queens
(718) 776-8181

Holy Name Hospital
Holy Name Hosp
718 Teaneck Road
Teaneck, NJ 07666
Bergen
(201) 833-3000

Hospital Center at Orange
Hosp Center at Orange
188 S. Essex Avenue
Orange, NJ 07050
Essex
(973) 266-2000

Hospital for Joint Diseases
Hosp for Joint Diseases
Orthopaedic Institute
301 E. 17 Street (at 2nd Avenue)
New York, NY 10003
New York (Manhattan)
(212) 598-6000

Hospital for Special Surgery
Hosp for Special Surgery
535 E. 70th Street
New York, NY 10021
New York (Manhattan)
(212) 606-1000

Hospital of St. Raphael
Hosp of St Raphael
1450 Chapel Street
New Haven, CT 06511
New Haven
(203) 789-3000

Hudson Valley Hospital Center at
Peekskill - Cortlandt
Hudson Valley Hosp
(Formerly Peekskill Community Hospital)
1980 Crompond Road
Peekskill, NY 10566
Westchester
(914) 737-9000

Huntington Hospital
Huntngtn Hosp
270 Park Avenue
Huntington, NY 11743
Suffolk
(516) 351-2000

Hurtado Health Center
Hurtado Health Ctr
11 Bishop Place
New Brunswick, NJ 08903
Middlesex
(732) 932-7401

Interfaith Medical Center - Brooklyn
Jewish Division
Interfaith Med Ctr-Bklyn Jewish Div
555 Prospect Place
Brooklyn, NY 11238
Kings
(718) 935-7000

Institutions in bold are profiled in this edition of the Castle Connolly Guide.

Interfaith Medical Center - St. John's
Episcopal Division
Interfaith Med Ctr - St John's Epis Div
1545 Atlantic Avenue
Brooklyn, NY 11238
Kings
(718) 604-6000

Irvington General Hospital
Irvngtn Gen Hosp
Part of St. Barnabas Health Care System
832 Chancellor Avenue
Irvington, NJ 07111
Essex
(973) 399-6000

Jacobi Medical Center
Jacobi Med Ctr
(Formerly Bronx Municipal Hospital Center)
1400 Pelham Pkwy. South
Bronx, NY 10461
Bronx
(718) 918-5000

Jamaica Medical Center
Jamaica Med Ctr
8900 Van Wyck Expressway
Jamaica, NY 11418
Queens
(718) 206-6000

Jersey City Medical Center
Jersey City Med Ctr
50 Baldwin Avenue
Jersey City, NJ 07304
Hudson
(201) 915-2000

Jersey Shore Medical Center
Jersey Shore Med Ctr
1945 Rte. 33
Neptune, NJ 07754
Monmouth
(732) 775-5500

JFK Medical Center
JFK Med Ctr
65 James Street
Edison, NJ 08818
Middlesex
(732) 321-7000

John T. Mather Memorial Hospital
of Port Jefferson
JT Mather Mem Hosp Pt Jfrson
North Country Road
Port Jefferson, NY 11777
Suffolk
(516) 473-1320

Kessler Institute for Rehabilitation
Kessler Inst for Rehab
East Orange Facility
240 Central Avenue
East Orange, NJ 07018-3460
Essex
(973) 414-4700

Kings County Hospital Center
Kings County Hosp Ctr
451 Clarkson Avenue
Brooklyn, NY 11203
Kings
(718) 245-3131

Kingsbrook Jewish Medical Center
Kingsbrook Jewish Med Ctr
585 Schenectady Avenue
Brooklyn, NY 11203
Kings
(718) 604-5000

Institutions in bold are profiled in this edition of the Castle Connolly Guide.

Lawrence Hospital
Lawrence Hosp
55 Palmer Avenue
Bronxville, NY 10708
Westchester
(914) 787-1000

Lenox Hill Hospital
Lenox Hill Hosp
100 E. 77th Street
New York, NY 10021
New York (Manhattan)
(212) 434-2000

Lincoln Medical & Mental Health Center
Lincoln Med & Mental Health Ctr
234 E. 149th Street
Bronx, NY 10451
Bronx
(718) 579-5000

Long Beach Medical Center
Long Beach Med Ctr
(Formerly Long Beach Memorial Hospital)
455 E. Bay Drive
Long Beach, NY 11561
Nassau
(516) 897-1000

The Long Island College Hospital
Long Island Coll Hosp
Part of Continuum Health Partners, Inc.
399 Hicks Street
Brooklyn, NY 11201
Kings
(718) 780-1000

Long Island Jewish Medical Center
Long Island Jewish Med Ctr
270-05 76th Avenue
New Hyde Park, NY 11040
Queens
(718) 470-7000

Lutheran Medical Center
Lutheran Med Ctr
150 55th Street
Brooklyn, NY 11220
Kings
(718) 630-7000

Maimonides Medical Center
Maimonides Med Ctr
4802 Tenth Avenue
Brooklyn, NY 11219
Kings
(718) 283-6000

Manhattan Eye, Ear & Throat Hospital
Manh Eye, Ear & Throat Hosp
210 E. 64th Street
New York, NY 10021
New York (Manhattan)
(212) 838-9200

Manhattan Psychiatric Center -
Ward's Island
Manh Psych Ctr - Ward's Is
600 E. 125th Street
New York, NY 10035
Manhattan
(212) 369-0500

Mary Immaculate Hospital
Mary Immaculate Hosp
152-11 89th Avenue
Jamaica, NY 11432
Queens
(718) 558-2000

Massapequa General Hospital
Massapequa Gen Hosp
750 Hicksville Road
Seaford, NY 11783
Nassau
(516) 520-6000

Institutions in bold are profiled in this edition of the Castle Connolly Guide.

Meadowlands Hospital Medical Center
Meadowlands Hosp Med Ctr
Meadowland Parkway
Secaucus, NJ 07096
Hudson
(201) 392-3100

Medical Center at Princeton
Med Ctr at Princeton
253 Witherspoon Street
Princeton, NJ 08540
Mercer
(609) 497-4000

Medical Center at Willowbrook
Med Ctr at Willowbrook
57 Willowbrook Boulevard
Wayne, NJ 07470
(973) 754-4000

Memorial Medical Center
at South Amboy
Mem Med Ctr at South Amboy
(Formerly South Amboy Memorial Hospital)
540 Bordentown Avenue
South Amboy, NJ 08879
Middlesex
(732) 721-1000

Memorial Sloan Kettering Cancer Center
Mem Sloan Kettering Cancer Ctr
1275 York Avenue
New York, NY 10021
New York (Manhattan)
(212) 639-2000

Mercy Medical Center
(Formerly Mercy Hospital)
Mercy Med Ctr
1000 North Village Avenue
Rockville Centre, NY 11570
Nassau
(516) 255-0111

Metropolitan Hospital Center
Metropolitan Hosp Ctr
1901 First Avenue
New York, NY 10029
New York (Manhattan)
(212) 423-6262

Mid-Island Hospital
Mid-Island Hosp
4295 Hempstead Turnpike
Bethpage, NY 11714
Nassau
(516) 579-6000

Middlesex Hospital
Middlesex Hosp
28 Cresent Street
Middletown, NJ 06457
Middlesex
(860) 344-6000

Monmouth Medical Center
Monmouth Med Ctr
Part of St. Barnabas Health Care System
300 Second Avenue
Long Branch, NJ 07740
Monmouth
(732) 222-5200

Montclair Community Hospital
Montclair Comm Hosp
120 Harrison Avenue
Montclair, NJ 07042
Essex
(973) 744-7300

Montefiore Medical Center
Montefiore Med Ctr
111 E. 210th Street
Bronx, NY 10467
Bronx
(718) 920-4321

Montefiore Medical Center-
Weiler/Einstein Division
1825 Eastchester Road
Bronx, NY 10461
(718) 904-2000

Morristown Memorial Hospital
Morristown Mem Hosp
100 Madison Avenue
Morristown, NJ 07960
Morris
(973) 971-5000

Institutions in bold are profiled in this edition of the Castle Connolly Guide.

The Mount Sinai Medical Center
Mount Sinai Med Ctr
One Gustave L. Levy Place
New York, NY 10029
New York (Manhattan)
(212) 241-6500

Mount Vernon Hospital
Mt. Vernon Hosp
12 N. Seventh Avenue
Mount Vernon, NY 10550
Westchester
(914) 664-8000

Mountainside Hospital
Mountainside Hosp
Bay and Highland Avenues
Montclair, NJ 07042
Essex
(973) 429-6000

Muhlenberg Regional Medical Center
Muhlenberg Regional Med Ctr
Park Avenue and Randolph Road
Plainfield, NJ 07061
Union
(908) 668-2000

Nassau County Medical Center
Nassau County Med Ctr
2201 Hempstead Turnpike
East Meadow, NY 11554
Nassau
(516) 572-0123

The New York Community Hospital
of Brooklyn
New York Comm Hosp of Bklyn
2525 Kings Highway
Brooklyn, NY 11229
Kings
(718) 692-5300

NYU Downtown Hospital
NYU Downtown Hosp
170 William Street
New York, NY 10038
New York (Manhattan)
(212) 312-5000

The New York Eye & Ear Infirmary
New York Eye & Ear Infirmary
2nd Avenue at 14th Street
New York, NY 10003
New York (Manhattan)
(212) 979-4000

**The New York Hospital -
Cornell Medical Center**
NY Hosp - Cornell Med Ctr
*Part of The New York and
Presbyterian Hospital*
525 East 68th Street
New York, NY 10021
New York (Manhattan)
(212) 746-5454

The New York Hospital - Cornell Medical
Center Westchester Division
NY Hosp - Cornell Med Westch
21 Bloomingdale Road
White Plains, NY 10605
Westchester
(914) 682-9100

New York Medical Center of Queens
NY Hosp Med Ctr of Queens
56-45 Main Street
Flushing, N.Y. 11355
Queens
(718) 670-1231

New York Methodist Hospital
New York Methodist Hosp
506 6th Street
Brooklyn, NY 11215
Kings
(718) 780-3000

New York State Psychiatric Institute
NYS Psychiatric Institute
722 W. 168th Street
New York, NY 10032
Manhattan
(212) 960-2200

Institutions in bold are profiled in this edition of the Castle Connolly Guide.

Newark Beth Israel Medical Center
Newark Beth Israel Med Ctr
Part of St. Barnabas Health Care System
201 Lyons Avenue at Osborne Terrace
Newark, NJ 07112
Essex
(973) 926-7000

North Central Bronx Hospital
North Central Bronx Hosp
3424 Kossuth Avenue
Bronx, NY 10467
Bronx
(718) 519-5000

North General Hospital
North General Hosp
1879 Madison Avenue
New York, NY 10035
New York (Manhattan)
(212) 423-4000

North Shore University Hospital,
Forest Hills
N Shore Univ Hosp - Forest Hills
102-01 66th Road
Forest Hills, NY 11375
Queens
(718) 830-4000

North Shore University Hospital,
Glen Cove
N Shore Univ Hosp - Glen Cove
101 St. Andrew's Lane
Glen Cove, NY 11542
Nassau
(516) 674-7300

North Shore University Hospital,
Manhasset
N Shore Univ Hosp - Manhasset
300 Community Drive
Manhasset, NY 11030
Nassau
(516) 562-0100

North Shore University Hospital-
Plainview
N Shore Univ Hosp - Plainview
888 Old Country Road
Plainview, NY 11803
Nassau
(516) 719-3000

North Shore University Hospital - Syosset
N Shore Univ Hosp - Syosset
221 Jericho Turnpike
Syosset, NY 11791
Nassau
(516) 496-6500

Northern Westchester Hospital Center
Northern Westchester Hosp Ctr
400 East Main Street
Mount Kisco, NY 10549
Westchester
(914) 666-1200

Northwest Covenant Medical Center -
Dover General Campus
NW Covenant Med Ctr - Dover
24 Jardine Street
Dover, NJ 07801
Morris
(973) 989-3000

Northwest Covenant Medical Center -
Denville Campus
NW Covenant Med Ctr - Riverside
(Formerly St. Clares - Riverside, Denville
Campus)
25 Pocono Road
Denville, NJ 07834
Morris
(973) 625-6000

Norwalk Hospital
Norwalk Hosp
Maple Street
Norwalk, CT 06856
Fairfield
(203) 852-2000

Institutions in bold are profiled in this edition of the Castle Connolly Guide.

Nyack Hospital
Nyack Hosp
160 N. Midland Avenue
Nyack, NY 10960
Rockland
(914) 348-2000

NYU Medical Center
NYU *Medical Ctr*
550 First Avenue
New York, N.Y. 10016
New York (Manhattan)
(212) 263-7300

Our Lady of Mercy Medical Center
Our Lady of Mercy Med Ctr
600 E. 233rd Street
Bronx, NY 10466
Bronx
(718) 920-9000

and
1870 Pelham Parkway South
Bronx, NY 10461
(718) 430-6000

Overlook Hospital
Overlook Hosp
99 Beauvoir Avenue
Summit, NJ 07902
Union
(908) 522-2000

Palisades Medical Center
Palisades Med Ctr
7600 River Road
North Bergen, NJ 07047
Hudson
(201) 854-5000

The Parkway Hospital
Parkway Hosp
70-35 113th Street
Forest Hills, NY 11375
Queens
(718) 990-4100

Pascack Valley Hospital
Pascack Valley Hosp
Old Hook Road
Westwood, NJ 07675
Bergen
(201) 358-3000

Passaic Beth Israel Hospital
Passaic Beth Israel Hosp
(Formerly Beth Israel Hospital)
70 Parker Avenue
Passaic, NJ 07055
Passaic
(973) 365-5000

Peekskill Community Hospital
(See Hudson Valley Hospital Center at
Peekskill)

Peninsula Hospital Center
Peninsula Hosp
51-15 Beach Channel Drive
Far Rockaway, NY 11691
Queens
(718) 945-7100

Phelps Memorial Hospital Center
Phelps Memorial Hosp
701 North Broadway
North Tarrytown, NY 10591
Westchester
(914) 366-3000

Queens Hospital Center
Queens Hosp Ctr
82-68 164th Street
Jamaica, NY 11432
Queens
(718) 883-3000

Rahway Hospital
Rahway Hosp
865 Stone Street
Rahway, NJ 07065
Union
(732) 381-4200

Raritan Bay Medical Center
Raritan Bay Med Ctr - P Amboy
Perth Amboy Division
530 New Brunswick Avenue
Perth Amboy, NJ 08861
Middlesex
(732) 442-3700

Raritan Bay Medical Center -
Old Bridge Division
Rritn Bay Med Ctr Old Brdg Div
One Hospital Plaza
Old Bridge, NJ 08857
Middlesex
(732) 360-1000

Riverview Medical Center
Riverview Med Ctr
One Riverview Plaza
Red Bank, NJ 07701
Monmouth
(732) 741-2700

Institutions in bold are profiled in this edition of the Castle Connolly Guide.

Robert Wood Johnson University
Hospital at Hamilton
RWJ Univ Hosp - Hamilton
(Formerly Hamilton Hospital)
One Hamilton Health Place
Hamilton, NJ 08690
Mercer
(609) 586-7900

Robert Wood Johnson University
Hospital at New Brunswick
RWJ Univ Hosp - New Brunswick
One Robert Wood Johnson Place
New Brunswick, NJ 08903
Middlesex
(732) 828-3000

Rockefeller University Hospital
Rockefeller Univ Hosp
1230 York Avenue
New York, NY 10021
New York (Manhattan)
(212) 327-8000

Roosevelt Hospital
Roosevelt Hosp
One Roosevelt Drive
Edison, NJ 08837
Middlesex
(732) 321-6800

Rye Hospital Center
Rye Hosp Ctr
754 Boston Post Road
Rye, NY 10580-2724
Westchester
(914) 967-4567

Saint Agnes Hospital
St Agnes Hosp
305 North Street
White Plains, NY 10605
Westchester
(914) 681-4500

Saint Barnabas Medical Center
St Barnabas Med Ctr - Livingston
Part of St. Barnabas Health Care System
94 Old Short Hills Road
Livingston, N.J. 07039
Essex
(973) 533-5000

Saint Vincents Hospital and
Medical Center Westchester Branch
St Vincents Med Ctr-Westchester
275 North Street
Harrison, NY 10528
Westchester
(914) 967-6500

Saint Vincents Hospital and Medical Center
Saint Vincents Hosp & Med Ctr
153 W. 11th Street
New York, NY 10011
New York (Manhattan)
(212) 604-7000

Schneider Children's Hospital
Schneider Children's Hosp
26901 76th Avenue
New Hyde Park, NY 11040
Queens
(718) 470-3000

Somerset Medical Center
Somerset Med Ctr
110 Rehill Avenue
Somerville, NJ 08876
Somerset
(908) 685-2200

Sound Shore Medical Center-Westchester
Sound Shore Med Ctr-Westchester
16 Guion Place
New Rochelle, NY 10802
Westchester
(914) 632-5000

South Amboy Memorial Hospital
(See Memorial Medical Center at South
Amboy)

South Beach Psychiatric Center
South Beach Psychiatric Ctr
777 Seaview Avenue
Staten Island, NY 10305-3436
Richmond
(718) 667-2300

Institutions in bold are profiled in this edition of the Castle Connolly Guide.

South Oaks Hospital
South Oaks Hosp
400 Sunrise Highway
Amityville, NY 11701
Suffolk
(516) 264-4000

South Nassau Communities Hospital
South Nassau Comm Hosp
2445 Oceanside Road
Oceanside, NY 11572
Nassau
(516) 763-2030

Southampton Hospital
Southhampton Hosp
240 Meeting House Lane
Southampton, NY 11968
Suffolk
(516) 726-8200

Southside Hospital
Southside Hosp
301 East Main Street
Bay Shore, NY 11706
Suffolk
(516) 968-3000

St. Barnabas Hospital
St Barnabas Hosp - Bronx
4422 Third Avenue
Bronx, NY 10457
Bronx
(718) 960-9000

St. Charles Hospital &
Rehabilitation Center
St Charles Hosp & Rehab Ctr
200 Belle Terre Road
Port Jefferson, NY 11777
Suffolk
(516) 474-6000

St. Clare's Hospital & Health Center
St Clare's Hosp & Health Ctr
415 W. 51st Street
New York, NY 10019
New York (Manhattan)
(212) 586-1500

St. Clares - Riverside, Denville Campus
(See Northwest Covenant Medical Center -
Riverside Campus)

St. Elizabeth Hospital
St Elizabeth Hosp
225 Williamson Street
Elizabeth, NJ 07207
Union
(908) 527-5000

St. Francis Medical Center
St Francis Med Ctr
601 Hamilton Avenue
Trenton, NJ 08629
Mercer
(609) 599-5000

St. Francis Hospital
St Francis Hosp - Jersey City
25 McWilliams Place
Jersey City, NJ 07302
Hudson
(201) 418-1000

St. Francis Hospital
St Francis Hosp - Roslyn
The Heart Center
100 Port Washington Boulevard
Roslyn, NY 11576
Nassau
(516) 562-6000

St. James Hospital of Newark
St James Hosp
155 Jefferson Street
Newark, NJ 07105
Essex
(973) 589-1300

St. John's Riverside Hospital
St John's Riverside Hosp
967 North Broadway
Yonkers, NY 10701
Westchester
(914) 964-4444

Institutions in bold are profiled in this edition of the Castle Connolly Guide.

St. John's Episcopal Hospital - Smithtown
St John's Epis Hosp - Smithtown
Route 25-A
Smithtown, NY 11787
Suffolk
(516) 862-3000

St. John's Episcopal Hospital -
South Shore
St John's Epis Hosp - S Shore
327 Beach 19th Street
Far Rockaway, NY 11691
Queens
(718) 869-7000

St. John's Queens Hospital
St John's Queens Hosp
9002 Queens Boulevard
Queens, NY 11373
Queens
(718) 558-1000

St. Joseph's Medical Center
St Joseph's Med Ctr - Stamford
128 Strawberry Hill Avenue
Stamford, CT 06904
Fairfield
(203) 353-2000

St. Joseph's Medical Center
St Joseph's Med Ctr - Yonkers
127 South Broadway
Yonkers, NY 10701
Westchester
(914) 378-7535

St. Joseph's Hospital and Medical Center,
Patterson
St Joseph's Hosp - Patterson
703 Main Street
Paterson, NJ 07503
Passaic
(973) 754-2000

St. Joseph's Hospital, Queens
St Joseph's Hosp Queens
15840 79th Avenue
Flushing, NY 11366
Queens
(718) 558-6200

St. Luke's - Roosevelt Hospital Center
St Luke's Roosevelt Hosp Ctr
Part of Continuum Health Partners Inc.
1111 Amsterdam Avenue
New York, NY 10025
New York (Manhattan)
(212) 523-4000

St. Mary's Hospital
St Mary's Hosp - Passaic
211 Pennington Avenue
Passaic, NJ 07055
Passaic
(973) 470-3000

St. Mary's Hospital of Brooklyn
St Mary's Hosp of Bklyn
170 Buffalo Avenue
Brooklyn, NY 11213
Kings
(718) 221-3000

St. Michael's Medical Center
St Michael's Med Ctr
268 Dr. Martin Luther King, Jr. Boulevard
Newark, NJ 07102
Essex
(973) 877-5000

St. Peter's Medical Center
St Peter's Med Ctr
254 Easton Avenue
New Brunswick, NJ 08901
Middlesex
(732) 745-8600

Institutions in bold are profiled in this edition of the Castle Connolly Guide.

St. Vincent's Medical Center of
Richmond
St Vincent's Med Ctr - Richmond
355 Bard Avenue
Staten Island, NY 10310
Richmond
(718) 876-1234

St. Vincent's Medical Center
St Vincent's Med Ctr - Bridgeport
2800 Main Street
Bridgeport, CT 06606
Fairfield
(203) 576-6000

The Stamford Hospital
The Stamford Hosp
Shelburn Road
at West Broad Street
Stamford, CT 06904
Stamford
(203) 325-7000

Staten Island University Hospital - North
Staten Island Univ Hosp - North
475 Seaview Avenue
Staten Island, NY 10305
Richmond
(718) 226-9000

Staten Island University Hospital - South
Staten Island Univ Hosp - South
375 Seguine Avenue
Staten Island, NY 10309
Richmond
(718) 226-2000

Stony Lodge Hospital
Stony Lodge Hosp
40 Croton Dam Road
Ossning, NY 10562
Westchester
(914) 941-7400

Union Hospital
Union Hospital - New Jersey
Part of St. Barnabas Health Care System
1000 Galloping Hill Road
Union, NJ 07083
Union
(908) 687-1900

Union Hospital of the Bronx
Union Hosp of the Bronx
260 E. 188th Street
Bronx, NY 10458
Bronx
(718) 220-2020

United Hospital Medical Center
United Hosp Med Ctr
406 Boston Post Road
Port Chester, NY 10573
Westchester
(914) 934-3000

University of Medicine and Dentistry
of New Jersey
Univ of Med & Dent of NJ Hosp
150 Bergen Street
Newark, NJ 07103
Essex
(973) 982-4300

University Hospital of Brooklyn
Univ Hosp SUNY Bklyn
SUNY Health Science Center of Brooklyn
450 Clarkson Avenue
Brooklyn, NY 11203
Kings
(718) 270-1000

University Hospital and Medical Center
Univ Hosp SUNY Stony Brook
SUNY at Stony Brook
Nicholls Road
Stony Brook, NY 11794
Suffolk
(516) 689-8333

Institutions in bold are profiled in this edition of the Castle Connolly Guide.

VA Connecticut Healthcare System
VA Ct Healthcare Sys
950 Campbell Avenue
West Haven, CT 06516
New Haven
(203) 932-5711

The Valley Hospital
Valley Hosp
223 North Van Dien Avenue
Ridgewood, NJ 07450
Bergen
(201) 447-8000

VA Medical Center - Bronx
VA Med Ctr - Bronx
130 W. Kingsbridge Road
Bronx, NY 10468-3904
Bronx
(718) 584-9000

VA Medical Center - Brooklyn
VA Med Ctr - Bklyn
800 Poly Place
Brooklyn, NY 11209-7104
Kings
(718) 836-6600

VA Medical Center
VA Med Ctr - E Orange
385 Tremont Avenue
East Orange, NJ 07018
Essex
(973) 676-1000

VA Medical Center - Manhattan
VA Med Ctr - Manh
423 E. 23rd Street
New York, NY 10010
Manhattan
(212) 686-7500

VA Medical Center-Northport
VA Med Ctr - Northport
79 Middleville Road
Northport, NY 11768
Suffolk
(516) 261-4400

Victory Memorial Hospital
Victory Memorial Hosp
699 92nd Street
Brooklyn, NY 11228
Kings
(718) 567-1234

Wayne General Hospital
Wayne General Hosp
Part of St. Barnabas Health Care System
224 Hamburg Turnpike
Wayne, NJ 07470
Passaic
(973) 942-6900

Jack D. Weiler Hospital of the
Albert Einstein College of Medicine
A Division of Montefiore
Medical Center
1825 Eastchester Road
Bronx, N.Y. 10461
Bronx
(718) 904-2000

Welkind Rehabilitation Hospital
Welkind Rehabilitation Hosp
201 Pleasant Hill Road
Chester, NJ 07930
Morris
(973) 584-7500

West Hudson Hospital
West Hudson Hosp
Part of St. Barnabas Health Care System
206 Bergen Avenue
Kearny, NJ 07032
Hudson
(201) 955-7000

Westchester Medical Center
Westchester Med Ctr
Route 100
Valhalla, NY 10595
Westchester
(914) 493-7000

Institutions in bold are profiled in this edition of the Castle Connolly Guide.

1201

Westchester Square Medical Center
Westchester Square Med Ctr
2475 St. Raymond Avenue
Bronx, NY 10461
Bronx
(718) 430-7300

Western Queens Community Hospital
Western Queens Comm Hosp
25-10 30th Avenue
Long Island City, NY 11102
Queens
(718) 932-1000

White Plains Hospital Center
White Plains Hosp Ctr
Davis Avenue at East Post Road
White Plains, NY 10601
Westchester
(914) 681-0600

Winthrop University Hospital
Winthrop Univ Hosp
259 First Street
Mineola, NY 11501
Nassau
(516) 663-0333

Woodhull Medical &
Mental Health Center
Woodhull Med Ctr
760 Broadway
Brooklyn, NY 11206
Kings
(718) 963-8000

Wyckoff Heights Medical Center
Wycoff Heights Med Ctr
374 Stockholm Street
Brooklyn, NY 11237
Kings
(718) 963-7272

Yale-New Haven Hospital
Yale-New Haven Hosp
20 York Street
New Haven, CT 06504
New Haven
(203) 785-4242

Yonkers General Hospital
Yonkers Gen Hosp
Two Park Avenue
Yonkers, NY 10703
Westchester
(914) 964-7300

Institutions in bold are profiled in this edition of the Castle Connolly Guide.

APPENDIX N
HMO/PPO AFFILIATIONS

Listed below are the HMOs and PPOs the doctors in the Castle Connolly Guide listed among their affiliations. We could not list all of those indicated by some doctors. They may belong to 20 or more! We included the first five they listed. It is wise to call and check with a doctor because these affiliations change frequently and many doctors belong to more plans than we had room to include.

A single HMO may offer a variety of plans. A doctor may be affiliated with some plans and not others. Also, the number of different plans of all HMOs and PPOs in the region would be in the hundreds so we could not list them all.

Again, because the multiple offerings are constantly changing, check with the doctor's office or plan affiliation.

Below is a list of the HMOs and PPOs doctors listed and abbreviations if they were used. We have presented them as the doctors described them even if the official corporate name might be different.

HMO/PPOS	ABBREVIATION IF USED	HMO/PPOS	ABBREVIATION IF USED
Aetna Health Plan		Amerihealth	
Aetna Managed Choice	Aetna Mng Choice	Atlanticare Health Plan	
		Better Health Plan	Btr Hlth Plan
Affordable Medical Networks	Aff Hlth Net	Blue Choice	
America's Health Plan	Am Hlth Plan	Blue Cross and Blue Shield	
American Medical Security	Am Med Sec	Blue Cross HealthEase	B C Hlthease
American Preferred Provider Plan	Am Pref Prov Plan	Blue Cross HealthNet	B C Hlthnet

APPENDIX N

HMO/PPOS	ABBREVIATION IF USED	HMO/PPOS	ABBREVIATION IF USED
Blue Cross Wraparound	B C Wrap	Harmony Health Plan	Harmony Hlth Plan
Bluecare Plus		Health Care Compare	Hlth Care Comp
The Bronx Health Plan		Health Care Payors Coalition of New Jersey	Hlth Care PC/NJ
Capital District Physicians Health Plan	Cap Dist Phys Hlth Plan	Health Care Plan	
Center Care		Health Network of America	Hlth Net Am
Champus		Health Services Medical Corporation	Hlth Serv Med Corp
Choice One			
Choicecare		Healthfirst PHSP	
ChubbHealth		Healthnet/Healthease B.C.	Hlthnet/ Hlthease BC
CIGNA			
CIGNA PPO		Healthplus	
CoMed		Healthsource	
Community Choice Health Plan	Comm Choice Hlth Plan	HIP Network	
		HIP Health Plan of New Jersey	HIP-NJ
Community Health Care & Development Corp.	Comm Hlth Care & Devl Corp	HMO Blue	
		Independent Health/MSSNY	Ind Hlth/MSSNY
ConnectiCare		Independent Practice Association-Metropolitan NY (MSSNY)	IPA Met NY/MSSNY
Consumer Health Network	Cons Hlth Net		
Constitution Health Care, Inc.	Const Hlth Care Inc		
Cost Care		Independent Health	Ind Hlth
Diocesan Plan		Independent Prepaid Health Plan	IPHP
District 47 Carpenters			
Elderplan		Intergroup	
Empire Blue Cross and Blue Shield	Emp Blue Cross & Shield	International Union of Operating Engineers	IUOE
		J J Newman	
Empire Metropolitan	Emp Met	John Hancock/Hancock Preferred/Sign. Hancock/ Sign. Health	John Han Pref /Sign Han/Sign Hlth
Empire PPO			
Ethix			
Fidelis Care		Kaiser Foundation Health Plan	Kaiser Found Hlth Plan
Fidelity Supplementary	Fidel Sup		
First Option		Lawrence HealthCare	Law Hlth Care
Foundation Health Plan	FHP	Liberty Health Plan	
Garden State Health Plan	Gdn St Hlth Plan	Magnacare	
Genesis Healthplan	Gen Hlth Plan	MagnaHealth	
GHI/Mass Mutual	GHI/MM	Mail Handlers Benefit Plan	Mail Hndlr Benef
GHI		Managed Health Care Systems	Mng Hlth Care Sys
GHI-CBP Plan only		Mastercare	
Global Medical Management	Global Med	Mayan	
Greater Atlantic Health Services	Greater Atlantic Hlth Serv	M.D. Health Plan	
Guardian		MDLI	

HMO/PPOS	ABBREVIATION IF USED	HMO/PPOS	ABBREVIATION IF USED
Med Source		PHS/Guardian	
Medicare		Physicians Health Services	PHS
Medichoice		Preferred Care	
Medigroup		Premier Health	
Metrahealth	Met Hlth Plan	Private Healthcare Systems	PHCS
Metroplus Health Plan		Prucare	
Metropolitan Empire	Met Emp	Qualcare	
Mohawk Valley Physicians Health Plan	Mohawk Valley Phys Hlth Plan	St. Barnabas Community Health Plan	St. Barn Comm Hlth Plan
Multiplan (ILGWU)		Sanus Health Plan	
N.J. Carpenters.		Sanus-NYLCare	
National Health Plan (1199)		Select Pro/Heathcare Compare	Sel Pro/Hlth Comp
National Preferred Provider Network	Nat PPN	Suffolk County Department of Health Services	Suffolk Health Plan
Neighborhood Health Providers	Neigh Hlth Prov	Total Care	
New England		Total Care Choice	
New York Health Plan		Travelers Health Network	Trav Hlth Net
North Medical Community Health Plan	N Med Comm Hlth Plan	Travelers/Metra Health	Trav/Met Hlth
Northcare		Universal Health Plan	
Northwestern National Life Ins. Co.	NW Nat Life Ins	University Health Plans	
		US Healthcare	US Hlthcre
Oxford		USA Healthnet	
Oxford Freedom		U.S. Life	
Pacific Mutual		Value Behavioral Health	VBH
Patient's Choice		Well Care	Well Care
		Vytra	

ACKNOWLEDGMENTS

We would like to thank the following people for their hard work in the production of this book:

Director of Publications:	*Adrienne Bonaparte*
Publications Assistant:	*Deborah Tropp*
Director of Information Services:	*Fred Ramen*
Director of Research:	*Jean Morgan, M.D.*
Research Associates:	*William Liss-Levinson, Ph.D.*
	Michael Wolf, Ph.D.
Research Staff:	*Maxine Atkins, Alicia Buckley,*
	Anita Holder, Connie Johnson,
	Paige Lewis, Ryder Syvertsen
Editorial Staff:	*Michael Wolf, Ph.D.*
	Cathy Granata
Director Provider Relations:	*Denise Walling*
Cover, Interior Design and Production:	*Lissa Milea, Harper & Case, Ltd., NYC*

SPECIAL
PRACTICE
INTEREST INDEX

DIRECTORY OF DOCTORS

Note: When reviewing this index, please recognize that the physicians may describe a given condition in different ways (ex: AIDS, HIV) so be sure to look under a number of key words, not just one (ex: Cosmetic Surgery, Aesthetic Surgery).

DIRECTORY OF DOCTORS

DIRECTORY OF DOCTORS

DIRECTORY OF DOCTORS

SPECIAL PRACTICE INTEREST INDEX

DIRECTORY OF DOCTORS

DIRECTORY OF DOCTORS

1222

SPECIAL PRACTICE INTEREST INDEX

DIRECTORY OF DOCTORS

SPECIAL PRACTICE INTEREST INDEX

SPECIAL PRACTICE INTEREST INDEX

DIRECTORY OF DOCTORS

DIRECTORY OF DOCTORS

1231

DIRECTORY OF DOCTORS

SPECIAL PRACTICE INTEREST INDEX

DIRECTORY OF DOCTORS

Bronx County

DIRECTORY OF DOCTORS

DIRECTORY OF DOCTORS

DIRECTORY OF DOCTORS

SPECIAL INTEREST	NAME	PAGE	SPECIAL INTEREST	NAME	PAGE
Fracture Treatment	Teicher, Joel (MD)	525	Heart Disease Prevention	Moskowitz, George (MD)	492
Gall Bladder Surgery	Adler, Harry (MD)	545	Heart Disease/Lung Disease	Husney, Joseph (MD)	503
Gallstone-Nonsurgical Removal	Iswara, Kadirawel (MD)	495	Heart Failure	Lichstein, Edgar (MD)	483
Gastric & Colonic Diseases	Cerulli, Maurice (MD)	494	Heart Failure	Lyon, Alan (MD)	484
Gastric Ulcer	Arya, Yashpal (MD)	494	Heart Failure	Ong, Kenneth (MD)	506
Gastroenterology	Piccione, Paul (MD)	496	Heart Illnesses	Turovsky, Leon (MD)	507
Gastroesophageal Reflux	Schwarz, Steven M (MD)	530	Heart Murmur	Kaplovitz, Harry (MD)	528
Gastrointestinal Cancer	Erber, William (MD)	494	Hematology	Friscia, Philip (MD)	508
Gastrointestinal Diseases	Leb, Alvin (MD)	495	Hemodialysis	Stam, Lawrence (MD)	513
Gastrointestinal Diseases	Richter, Robert (MD)	548	Hepatitis	Levendoglu, Hulya (MD)	495
Gastrointestinal Endoscopy	Gettenberg, Gary (MD)	495	Hepatitis	Lutwick, Larry Irwin (MD)	501
Gastrointestinal Endoscopy	Zimbalist, Eliot (MD)	497	Hepatitis	Rabinowitz, Simon (MD)	529
Gastrointestinal Malignancy	Youssef, Ezzat (MD)	543	Hepatology Specialist	Geders, Jane (MD & PhD)	495
Gastrointestinal Motility	Levendoglu, Hulya (MD)	495	Hernia	Siegman, Felix (MD)	549
Gastrointestinal Surgery	Brevetti, Gregorio (MD)	546	Hernia Repair	Borriello, Raffaele (MD)	546
General Endocrinology	Mann, David (MD)	490	Hernia Surgery	Choe, Dai-sun (MD)	546
General Medicine	Kurz, Larry (MD)	504	High Blood Pressure	Cohen, Barry (MD)	502
Genetics	Dosik, Harvey (MD)	499	High Blood Pressure	Kelter, Robert (MD)	504
Genital Abnormalities	Friedman, Steven (MD)	551	High Blood Pressure	Porush, Jerome (MD)	512
Geriatric Medicine	Bharathan, Thayyulla (MD)	501	High Pressure Diabetes	Husney, Joseph (MD)	503
Geriatric Neurology	Sobol, Norman (MD)	516	High Risk Obstetrics	Dor, Nathan (MD)	518
Geriatric Problems	Lipkowitz, Marvin (MD)	539	High Risk Obstetrics	Kofinas, Alexander (MD)	518
Geriatric Psychiatry	Goldberg, Jeffrey (DO)	538	High Risk Obstetrics	Lamarque, Madeleine (MD)	519
Geriatric Psychiatry	Licht, Arnold (MD)	539	High Risk Pregnancy	Shiffman, Rebecca (MD)	520
Geriatric Psychiatry	Samuelly, Israel (MD)	497	Hip and Knee Replacement	Mani, John (MD)	524
Geriatric Psychiatry, Anxiety	Berkowitz, Howard (MD)	538	Hip and Knee Surgery	Tischler, Henry (MD)	525
Geriatrics	Ellis, Earl A (MD)	502	Hip Dysplasia	Strongwater, Allan (MD)	525
Geriatrics	Falkow, Seymour (MD)	492	HIV	Berkowitz, Leonard B (MD)	500
Geriatrics	Goldberg, Richard (MD)	503	HIV	Brown, Lawrence S (MD)	502
Geriatrics	Levey, Robert (MD)	504	HIV AIDS	Viera, Jeffery (MD)	507
Geriatrics	Rosen, Evelyn (MD)	539	HIV/AIDS	Chapnick, Edward (MD)	500
Geriatrics	Schlecker, Austin (MD)	506	HIV-AIDS Pediatric	Mendez, Hermann (MD)	530
GI Cancer, Stomach & Colon-Cancer	Kodsi, Baroukh (MD)	495	Home Hemodialysis	Delano, Barbara (MD)	511
Glandular Disorders	Lamaute, Henry (MD)	547	Hyperlipidemia	Ginsberg, Donald (MD)	503
Glaucoma	Ackerman, Jacob (MD)	520	Hypertension	Chou, Shyan-yih (MD)	511
Glaucoma	Freedman, Jeffrey (MD & PhD)	521	Hypertension	Cohn, Steven (MD)	502
Glaucoma	Greenidge, Kevin (MD)	521	Hypertension	Del Monte, Mary (MD)	511
Glaucoma	Jaffe, Herbert (MD)	521	Hypertension	Friedman, Eli A (MD)	511
Glaucoma	Lazzaro, E Clifford (MD)	521	Hypertension	Kaiser, Stephen (MD)	504
Glaucoma	Sherman, Steven (DO)	523	Hypertension	Lipner, Henry (MD)	511
Glaucoma	Zellner, James (MD)	524	Hypertension	Louis, Bertin Magloi (MD)	505
Growth	Fennoy, Ilene (MD)	529	Hypertension	Parnes, Eliezer (MD)	512
Growth Disorders	Avruskin, Theodore W (MD)	529	Hypertension	Reiser, Ira (MD)	512
GYN Oncology-Cervix	Rotman, Marvin (MD)	542	Hypertension	Rosen, Herman (MD)	512
Hair Removal - Laser	Westfried, Morris (MD)	489	Hypertension	Shein, Leon (MD)	513
Hand Reconstruction	Woloszyn, Thomas T (MD)	549	Hypertension	Spitalewitz, Samuel (MD)	513
Hand Surgery	Gordon, Stanley (MD)	524	Hypertension	Tal, Avraham (MD)	507
Hand Surgery	Roth, Malcolm (MD)	537	Hypertension & Lupus	Shapiro, Warren (MD)	512
Head & Neck Malignancy	Youssef, Ezzat (MD)	543	Hypertension Prevention	Clark, Luther T (MD)	482
Head & Neck Pain	Consiglio, Michael (MD)	514	Hypertension/Dialysis	Sari Markell, Marian (MD)	512
Head & Neck Surgery	Habib, Mohsen (MD)	526	Impotence	Grunberger, Ivan (MD)	551
Head & Neck Surgery	Weiss, Michael H (MD)	527	Impotence	Wainstein, Sasha (MD)	553
Head & Neck Surgery-Thyroid	Khafif, Rene (MD)	547	In Vitro Fertilization	Lobell, Susan M (MD)	544
Head and Neck Cancer	Har-El, Gady (MD)	526	Incontinence	Mandel, Edmund (MD)	552
Headache	Drexler, Ellen (MD)	514	Infections in Children	Mendez, Hermann (MD)	530
Headache	Pincas, Martin (MD)	516	Infectious Disease	Sergiou, Harry (MD)	535
Headaches	Yellin, Joseph (DO)	516	Infectious Diseases	Bloom, Jerry (MD)	502
Hear Disease in Pediatrics	Nudel, Dov (MD)	534	Infectious Diseases	De Caprariis, Pascal (MD)	492
Hearing Loss	Shulman, Abraham (MD)	527	Infectious Diseases	Viera, Jeffery (MD)	507
Hearing Loss	Sperling, Neil Michael (MD)	527	Infertility	Bray, Mary (MD)	543
Heart Artery & Valve Disease	Kleeman, Harris J (MD)	483	Infertility	Kofinas, George (MD)	518
Heart Catheterization	Reddy, Chatla (MD)	484	Infertility	Lobell, Susan M (MD)	544
Heart Disease	Clark, Luther T (MD)	482	Infertility	Reyes, Francisco I (MD)	519

DIRECTORY OF DOCTORS

1242

SPECIAL PRACTICE INTEREST INDEX

DIRECTORY OF DOCTORS

SPECIAL PRACTICE INTEREST INDEX

Richmond (Staten Island) County

DIRECTORY OF DOCTORS

DIRECTORY OF DOCTORS

DIRECTORY OF DOCTORS

SPECIAL PRACTICE INTEREST INDEX

1251

DIRECTORY OF DOCTORS

SPECIAL INTEREST	NAME	PAGE	SPECIAL INTEREST	NAME	PAGE
Reconstructive Surgery	Garber, Perry (MD)	666	Stones, Urinary	Leventhal, Arnold (MD)	704
Reconstructive Surgery	Grant, Robert (MD)	685	Stones, Urinary	Shepard, Barry (MD)	704
Reconstructive Surgery	Hanna, Moneer (MD)	703	Strabismus	Rubin, Steven (MD)	668
Reconstructive Surgery	Kessler, Martin E (MD)	686	Stress Testing	Kuslansky, Phillip (MD)	633
Reconstructive, Cosmetic	Dubuoys, Elliot (MD)	684	Stroke Dementia Neuropathy	Mallin, Jeffrey (MD)	660
Rectal Cancer	Kalafatic, Alfredo (MD)	636	Sudden Death Prevention	Levine, Joseph H (MD)	629
Rectal Carcinoma	Lanter, Bernard (MD)	698	Systemic Erythematosus	Chiorazzi, Nicholas (MD)	627
Rectal Prolapse	Lanter, Bernard (MD)	698	Teenage Acne	Aprile, Georgette (MD)	636
Refractive Surgery	Hatsis, Alexander (MD)	666	Thallium Stress Testing	Rutkovsky, Edward (MD)	634
Relationship of Feelings to			Thoracic & Vascular Surgery	Damus, Paul S (MD)	700
Medical Illness	Hotchkiss, Edward (MD)	651	Thoracic & Vascular Surgery	Robinson, Newell B (MD)	701
Reproductive Endo-Infertility	Spector, Ira (MD)	664	Thoracic Surgery	Scott, William C (MD)	702
Respiratory Disease	Cohen, David (MD)	690	Thoracoscopy	Fox, Stewart (MD)	701
Rheumatic Fever	Kryle, Lawrence S (MD)	651	Thumb and Wrist Problems	Lane, Lewis B (MD)	646
Rheumatic Fever, Sports Med	Cooper, Rubin (MD)	675	Thyroid	Bhatt, Anjani (MD)	640
Rheumatoid Arthritis	Blau, Sheldon P (MD)	694	Thyroid Cancer	Margouleff, Donald (MD)	661
Rheumatoid Arthritis	Carsons, Steven (MD)	694	Thyroid Disease	Friedman, Seth (MD)	640
Rheumatoid Arthritis	Chiorazzi, Nicholas (MD)	627	Thyroid Disease	Klein, Irwin (MD)	651
Rheumatoid Arthritis	Furie, Richard (MD)	650	Thyroid Disease	Kolodny, Howard (MD)	641
Rheumatoid Arthritis	Tiger, Louis H (MD)	695	Thyroid Disease	Margouleff, Donald (MD)	661
Rheumatology	Porges, Andrew (MD)	694	Thyroid Disease	Margulies, Paul (MD)	641
Rhinitis	Spina, Christopher (MD)	628	Thyroid Disease	Rosenthal, David S (MD)	641
Sarcoidosis	Marcus, Philip (MD)	690	Thyroid Diseases	Katzeff, Harvey (MD)	640
School and Learning Problems	Heitler, Michael (MD)	682	Thyroid Diseases	Klass, Evan (MD)	640
Sciatica	Bluth, Mordecai (MD)	674	Thyroid Disorders	Greenfield, Martin (MD)	640
Sciatica/Back Pain	Hanania, Michael (MD)	674	Thyroid Surgery	Tawfik, Bernard (MD)	673
Second Opinion Pediatric Surgery	Bronsther, Burton (MD)	678	Thyroid/Parathyroid Surgery	Auguste, Louis T (MD)	696
Seizure Disorders	Haimovic, Itzhak (MD)	659	Total Joint Reconstruction	Orlin, Harvey (MD)	695
Seizures	Newman, Stephen (MD)	660	Total Joints	Ross, Bruce (MD)	671
Sexual Development	Castro-Magana, Mariano (MD)	676	Tourette's Syndrome	Budman, Cathy L (MD)	688
Sexual Dysfunction-Males	Bruno, Anthony (MD)	703	Tourette's Syndrome	Levy, Lewis (MD)	660
Short Stature	St Louis, Yolaine (MD)	683	Toxicology	Packy, Theodore (MD)	639
Short Stature in Children	Agdere, Levon (MD)	675	Toxicology Poison Prevention	Greensher, Joseph (MD)	681
Shoulder Surgery	Dines, David (MD)	669	Transesophageal Echocardiography	Schiff, Russell (MD)	675
Sinusitis	Corriel, Robert (MD)	627	Trauma	Gross, Lillian (MD)	688
Sjogren's Syndrome	Carsons, Steven (MD)	694	Trauma/Sports Medicine	Coryllos, Elizabeth (MD)	679
Skin Allergies	Fonacier, Luz (MD)	627	Treatment of Heart Disease	Chesner, Michael (MD)	630
Skin Cancer	Bruckstein, Robert (MD)	637	Tumors Pediatric	Kessler, Edmund (MD)	679
Skin Cancer	Falcon, Ronald (MD)	637	Ulcer Disease	Berger, David (MD)	649
Skin Cancer	Krivo, James (MD)	638	Ulcer Disease	Goldblum, Lester (DO)	643
Skin Cancer	Paltzik, Robert (MD)	638	Ulcerative Colitis	Talansky, Arthur (MD)	645
Skin Cancer Surgery	Spinowitz, Alan (MD)	638	Ulcers	Toffler, Allan (MD)	654
Skin Cancers	Feinstein, Robert (MD)	637	Ultrasonic Liposuction	Kaufman, Seth (MD)	686
Skin Surgery	Moynihan, Brian (DO)	642	Ultrasonography	Goodman, Ken J (MD)	692
Sleep/Insomnia	Martin, Robert (MD)	689	Ultrasound	Sherman, Scott J (MD)	693
Smoking Cessation	Wyner, Perry A (MD)	691	Urinary Tract Problems	Bruno, Anthony (MD)	703
Snoring	Rosner, Louis (MD)	673	Urogynecology	Rabin, Jill (MD)	664
Solid Tumors Breast/Lung	Vinciguerra, Vincent (MD)	647	Urological Cancer	Shepard, Barry (MD)	704
Spinal Cord Tumors	Overby, M Chris (MD)	658	Urological Cancers	Lieberman, Elliott (MD)	704
Spinal Procedures	Carras, Robert (MD)	658	Uterine Bleeding	Haselkorn, Joan (MD)	663
Spinal Reconstruction	Overby, M Chris (MD)	658	Uterine Cancer	Lovecchio, John (MD)	645
Spine	Biddle, David (MD)	659	Valvular Heart Disease	Gindea, Aaron (MD)	631
Spine Surgery	Cataletto, Mauro (MD)	669	Vascular Surgery	Mohtashemi, Manucher (MD)	701
Spine Surgery	Dimancescu, Mihai (MD)	658	Vein Disease of legs	Smirnov, Viktor (MD)	706
Sports Injuries	Putterman, Eric A (MD)	695	Vision Problems Pediatric	Rubin, Steven (MD)	668
Sports Injury	Ross, Bruce (MD)	671	Vulvovaginal Disorders	Krumholz, Burton (MD)	663
Sports Medicine	Dines, David (MD)	669	Women & Heart Disease	Spadaro, Louise A (MD)	634
Sports Medicine	Illman, Arnold (MD)	669	Women's Health	Lipstein-Kresch, Esther (MD)	651
Sports Medicine	Pellman, Elliot (MD)	694	Women's Health	Seltzer, Vicki (MD)	646
Sports Medicine	Simonson, Barry G (MD)	671	Women's Health Issues	Gorski, Lydia E (MD)	650
Sports Medicine	Watnik, Neil (MD)	671			
Stem Cell Transplantation	Kessler, Leonard (MD)	647			
Stereotactic Radiosurgery	Decker, Robert (MD)	658			

DIRECTORY OF DOCTORS

Westchester County

DIRECTORY OF DOCTORS

1256

DIRECTORY OF DOCTORS

SPECIAL PRACTICE INTEREST INDEX

1259

DIRECTORY OF DOCTORS

Rockland County

Bergen County

DIRECTORY OF DOCTORS

SPECIAL PRACTICE INTEREST INDEX

DIRECTORY OF DOCTORS

Essex County

Hudson County

DIRECTORY OF DOCTORS

Mercer County

DIRECTORY OF DOCTORS

SPECIAL INTEREST	NAME	PAGE
Sickle Cell Disease	Drachtman, Richard (MD)	965
Sports Medicine	Zawadsky, Joseph (MD)	963
Stroke	Friedlander, Marvin (MD)	961
Stroke	Gainey, Patrick (MD)	961
Stroke Prevention	Simpson, Alec (MD)	969
Surgical Oncology	Greco, Ralph S (MD)	968
Thyroid Disorders	Bucholtz, Harvey K (MD)	956
Thyroid Growths	Salas, Max (MD)	956
Treatment of Diabetes Mellitus	Amorosa, Louis (MD)	956
Ulcer Disease	Lenger, Ellis Steven (MD)	959
Upper Extremity	Leddy, Joseph (MD)	963
Women's Health	Lansing, Martha (MD)	957

Monmouth County

Abnormal Pap Smears	Goldstein, Steven (MD)	977
Anterior Cruciate Ligament	Sclafani, Michael (MD)	981
Anxiety	Rubin, Kenneth (MD)	980
Arthritis	Absatz, Michael (MD)	978
Arthroscopic Surgery	Berkowitz, Steven (MD)	978
Asthma	Davis, George (MD)	976
Asthma	Gross, Gary L (MD)	973
Asthma	Picone, Frank (MD)	973
Back and Neck Pain	Handlin, David (MD)	973
Biliary Disease	Schwartz, Mitchell (MD)	976
Blood Sugar Problems	Luria, Martin (MD)	974
Breast Cancer	Fitzgerald, Denis (MD)	976
Breast Cancer	Greenberg, Susan (MD)	976
Breast Cancer	Sharon, David (MD)	976
Breast Reconstruction	Hetzler, Peter (MD)	979
Breast Surgery	Averbach, David (MD)	981
Breast Surgery	Goldfarb, Michael (MD)	981
Breast Surgery	Samra, Said (MD)	979
Breast Surgery	Schwartz, Mark (MD)	982
Cancer	Arvanitis, Michael (MD)	973
Carpal Tunnel Syndrome	Chekofsky, Kenneth (MD)	975
Cataracts	Talansky, Marvin (MD)	978
Cervical Cancer	Hackett, Thomas (DO)	975
Chronic Neck and Lower Back Pain	Bram, Harris (MD)	979
Chronic Pain	Handlin, David (MD)	973
Colitis	Fiest, Thomas (DO)	975
Corneal Transplants	Goldberg, Daniel (MD)	978
Cough	Gross, Gary L (MD)	973
Depression	Rubin, Kenneth (MD)	980
Diabetes	Nassberg, B (MD)	974
Diabetes Mellitus	Burkett, Eric (MD)	975
Diabetic Eye Disease	Talansky, Marvin (MD)	978
Emphysema	Davis, George (MD)	976
Epilepsy	Gilson, Noah (MD)	977
Epilepsy	Herman, Martin (MD)	977
Facial Rejuvenation	Samra, Said (MD)	979
General Medical Oncology	Sharon, David (MD)	976
Gynecologic Surgery	Rothenberg, Eugene (MD)	977
Hypertension	Arbes, Spiros (MD)	977
Hypertension	Burkett, Eric (MD)	975
Hypertension	Flis, Raymond S (DO)	977
Incontinence	Ebani, Jack (MD)	982
Incontinence	Geltzeiler, Jules (MD)	982
Inflammatory Bowel Disease	Arvanitis, Michael (MD)	973
Inflammatory Bowel Disease	Turtel, Penny (MD)	975
Internal Radiation for GYN	Kornmehl, Carol (MD)	980
Kidney Disease	Arbes, Spiros (MD)	977
Kidney Disease	Flis, Raymond S (DO)	977
Lapapascopic Surgery	Rothenberg, Eugene (MD)	977

SPECIAL INTEREST	NAME	PAGE
Laparoscopic Surgery	Averbach, David (MD)	981
Laparoscopic Surgery	Schwartz, Mark (MD)	982
Laparoscopy	Goldfarb, Michael (MD)	981
Laser Vision Correction	Goldberg, Daniel (MD)	978
Liver Diseases	Turtel, Penny (MD)	975
Liver Disorders	Fiest, Thomas (DO)	975
Lung Cancer	Fitzgerald, Denis (MD)	976
Lung Cancer	Heleotis, Thomas (MD)	982
Lung Cancer	Sills, Charles (MD)	982
Lyme Disease	Schwartzberg, Mori (MD)	980
Lymphoma	Greenberg, Susan (MD)	976
Male Infertility	Litvin, Y Samuel (MD)	983
Mastectomy/Reconstructive	Dudick, Stephen T (MD)	979
Medical Genetics	Lefrak, Steven (MD)	979
Melanoma	Hetzler, Peter (MD)	979
Migraines	Herman, Martin (MD)	977
Multiple Sclerosis	Gilson, Noah (MD)	977
Nasal & Sinus Disease	Winarsky, Eric (MD)	979
Pacemakers	Sills, Charles (MD)	982
Pacemakers Defibrillators	Heleotis, Thomas (MD)	982
Pediatric Urology	Linn, Gary (MD)	983
Pediatrics	Rossos, Paul (MD)	978
Post Menopausal Health	Courtney, Barbara (MD)	976
Pre and Post Surgical Pain	Bram, Harris (MD)	979
Preventive Medicine	Glowacki, Jan S (MD)	976
Prostate Cancer	Ebani, Jack (MD)	982
Prostate Cancer	Geltzeiler, Jules (MD)	982
Prostate Cancer	Litvin, Y Samuel (MD)	983
Psoriasis	Grossman, Kenneth (MD)	974
Rheumatoid Arthritis	Schwartzberg, Mori (MD)	980
Shoulder Instability	Sclafani, Michael (MD)	981
Shoulder Surgery	Berkowitz, Steven (MD)	978
Sinus	Picone, Frank (MD)	973
Sinus Disease	Rossos, Paul (MD)	978
Skin Cancer	Grossman, Kenneth (MD)	974
Sleep & Snoring Disorders	Winarsky, Eric (MD)	979
Sleep Apnea	Kosinski, Robert (MD)	980
Stone Disease	Grebler, Arnold (MD)	982
Thyroid Disease	Nassberg, B (MD)	974
Thyroid Diseases	Luria, Martin (MD)	974
Total Joint Replacement	Absatz, Michael (MD)	978
Trauma	Dudick, Stephen T (MD)	979
Tumors as an outpatient	Kornmehl, Carol (MD)	980
Ultrasound	Goldstein, Steven (MD)	977
Urologic Cancer Surgery	Grebler, Arnold (MD)	982
Urologic Oncology	Linn, Gary (MD)	983
Uterine Cancer	Hackett, Thomas (DO)	975
Vascular Surgery	Arbour, Robert (MD)	981

Morris County

Adult A&I	Morrison, Susan (MD)	994
Anxiety and Depression	Granet, Roger (MD)	996
Arthritis	Ende, Leigh (MD)	989
Asthma	Applebaum, Eric (MD)	987
Bladder Cancer	Atlas, Ian (MD)	999
Blood Disorders	Siroty, Robert (MD)	990
Body Contouring	Starker, Isaac (MD)	996
Brain Aneurysms	Hodosh, Richard (MD)	992
Brain Tumors	Beyerl, Brian (MD)	991
Brain Tumors	Hodosh, Richard (MD)	992
Breast Cancer	Chevinsky, Aaron (MD)	998
Breast Cancer	Diehl, William (MD)	998
Breast Cancer	Dougan, Hughes (MD)	998

Passaic County

DIRECTORY OF DOCTORS

SPECIAL INTEREST	NAME	PAGE
Shoulder Injuries	Drillings, Gary (MD)	1005
Sinus Surgery	Cece, John (MD)	1006
Thyroid Surgery	Budd, Daniel (MD)	1007
Tonsil, Head & Neck Tumors	Respler, Don (MD)	1006

Somerset County

SPECIAL INTEREST	NAME	PAGE
Adult Reconstructive Surgery	Sarokhan, Alan (MD)	1013
Arthritis	McWhorter, John (MD)	1014
Blood Disorders	Wu, Hen-vai (MD)	1012
Breast Cancer	Toomey, Kathleen (MD)	1012
Breast Surgery	Iacuzzo, John (MD)	1014
Cancer Diagnosis	Wu, Hen-vai (MD)	1012
Coronary Artery Disease	Lipschutz, Herbert (MD)	1012
Endoscopic Hernia Surgery	Iacuzzo, John (MD)	1014
Facial Cosmetic Surgery	Bortniker, David (MD)	1013
Facial Cosmetics	Perry, Arthur (MD)	1013
Geriatric Ophthalmology	Ocken, Paul (MD)	1013
Glaucoma	Ocken, Paul (MD)	1013
Hand Surgery	Johnson, Albert (MD)	1013
HIV Related Illness	Ziering, Thomas (MD)	1011
Hospice Care	Toomey, Kathleen (MD)	1012
Hypertension	Lipschutz, Herbert (MD)	1012
Irritable Bowel Syndrome	Accurso, Charles (MD)	1011
Joint Replacement	Sarokhan, Alan (MD)	1013
Joint Surgery	D'Agostini, Robert (MD)	1013
Laparoscopic Surgery	Drascher, Gary (MD)	1014
Laparoscopic Surgery	Goldson, Howard (MD)	1014
Liposuction	Perry, Arthur (MD)	1013
Lupus	Brodman, Richard Rory (MD)	1014
Nasal and Sinus Surgery	Bortniker, David (MD)	1013
Office Dermatology	Ziering, Thomas (MD)	1011
Osteoporosis	McWhorter, John (MD)	1014
Rheumatoid Arthritis	Brodman, Richard Rory (MD)	1014
Total Hip & Knee Replacement	Johnson, Albert (MD)	1013
Vascular Surgery	Drascher, Gary (MD)	1014
Vascular Surgery	Goldson, Howard (MD)	1014

Union County

SPECIAL INTEREST	NAME	PAGE
Allergic Rhinitis	Goodman, Alan (MD)	1017
Allergic Rhinitis	Le Benger, Kerry (MD)	1017
Allergic Rhinitis	Maccia, Clement (MD)	1017
Alzheimer's Disease	Solomon, Robert (MD)	1021
Anal Incontinence	Oliver, Gregory (MD)	1019
Artery Surgery	Sales, Clifford (MD)	1031
Arthroscopic Surgery	Botwin, Clifford (DO)	1025
Asthma	Le Benger, Kerry (MD)	1017
Asthma	Maccia, Clement (MD)	1017
Attention Deficit Disorder	Sank, Lewis (MD)	1027
Back Pain	Weinberger, Michael (MD)	1026
Balance Disorders	Kwartler, Jed (MD)	1026
Biliary Disorders	Goldenberg, David (MD)	1020
Blood Diseases	Rifkin, Paul (MD)	1021
Brain Tumors	Fineman, Sanford (MD)	1024
Breast and Colon Cancer	Frost, James (MD)	1030
Breast Cancer	Pliner, Lillian (MD)	1024
Breast Disease	Befeler, David (MD)	1030
Breast Reconstruction	Hyans, Peter (MD)	1028
Breast Surgery	Tepper, Howard (MD)	1028
Cancer of the Breast	Lozner, Jerrold (MD)	1031
Cancer Pain Management	Weinberger, Michael (MD)	1026
Cancer Surveillance	Gray, Samuel (DO)	1023
Cataract Surgery	Tchorbajian, Kirk (MD)	1025

SPECIAL INTEREST	NAME	PAGE
Cataract Surgery-Stitchless	Natale, Benjamin (DO)	1025
Cataracts	Burke, Jordan D (MD)	1025
Cholesterol	Feldman, Jeffrey (MD)	1022
Colitis	Belladonna, Joseph (MD)	1020
Collagen	West, Gerald (DO)	1028
Colon Cancer	Eisenstat, Theodore (MD)	1019
Colonoscopy	Groff, Walter (MD)	1019
Colonoscopy	Kerner, Michael (MD)	1021
Conformal Radiation	Schwartz, Louis (MD)	1029
Cosmetic Surgery	Hyans, Peter (MD)	1028
Diabetes	Silverman, Mitchell (MD)	1020
Diabetes, Thyroid Disease	Fuhrman, Robert (MD)	1022
Ear Diseases Hearing Loss	Kwartler, Jed (MD)	1026
Electrodiagnosis	Bucksbaum, Mark J (MD)	1028
Endocarditis	Burstin, Stuart J (MD & PhD)	1022
Facial Cosmetic Surgery	Scharf, Richard (DO)	1026
Facial Rejuvenation	Tepper, Howard (MD)	1028
Fibromyalgia- Soft Tissue	Wilmot, Richard (MD)	1029
Gallbladder Disease	Befeler, David (MD)	1030
Gastroesophageal Reflux	Belladonna, Joseph (MD)	1020
Gastrointestinal Cancer	Mahal, Pradeep (MD)	1021
Gastrointestinal Disorders	Levinson, Joel (MD)	1021
General Cardiology	Kalischer, Alan (MD)	1018
General Pediatrics	Zanger, Norman (MD)	1028
Geriatrics	Khimani, Karim (MD)	1023
Glaucoma	Tchorbajian, Kirk (MD)	1025
Hand Surgery	Barmakian, Joseph (MD)	1025
Head & Neck Surgery	Drake, William (MD)	1026
Headache	Sananman, Michael (MD)	1024
Hemostasis	Arkel, Yale S (DO)	1021
HIV/AIDS	Roland, Robert (DO)	1022
Hyperactivity	Sank, Lewis (MD)	1027
Hypertension	Alterman, Lloyd (MD)	1024
Hypertension	Feldman, Jeffrey (MD)	1022
Hypothyroid & Hyperthyroid	Chen, James (MD)	1020
Impotence	Lehrhoff, Bernard (MD)	1031
Inflammatory Bowel Disease	Eisenstat, Theodore (MD)	1019
Inflammatory Bowel Disease	Goldenberg, David (MD)	1020
Inflammatory Bowel Disease	Oliver, Gregory (MD)	1019
Internal Medicine	Sachs, R Gregory (MD)	1018
Joint Surgery	Innella, Robin (DO)	1026
Kidney Disease	Alterman, Lloyd (MD)	1024
Laparoscopic Surgery	Matkiwsksy, Zenon (DO)	1030
Laparoscopic Surgery	Starker, Paul (MD)	1030
Laporoscopic Surgery	Nitzberg, Richard (MD)	1030
Laser Refractive Surgery	Natale, Benjamin (DO)	1025
Learning Disabilities	Vigorita, John (MD)	1027
Liver Disease	Levinson, Joel (MD)	1021
Lung Cancer	Lozner, Jerrold (MD)	1031
Medical Oncology	Rifkin, Paul (MD)	1021
Melanoma/Sentinel Nodes	Nitzberg, Richard (MD)	1030
Mood Disorders	Herridge, Peter L (MD)	1028
Nasal & Sinus Surgery	Drake, William (MD)	1026
Neuropsychiatry	Herridge, Peter L (MD)	1028
Osteoporosis	Fuhrman, Robert (MD)	1022
Osteoporosis	Rosenbaum, Robert (MD)	1023
Osteoporosis	Worth, David (MD)	1023
Pain Management	Bucksbaum, Mark J (MD)	1028
Pain Management	Fineman, Sanford (MD)	1024
Pediatric Urology	Ring, Kenneth (MD)	1031
Phototherapy	Gruber, Gabriel (MD)	1019
Prostate Cancer	Lehrhoff, Bernard (MD)	1031
Psoriasis	Gruber, Gabriel (MD)	1019

SPECIAL INTEREST	NAME	PAGE
Pulmonary Disease	Hwang, Cheng-hong (DO)	1023
Radiosurgery	Schwartz, Louis (MD)	1029
Rectal Cancer	Groff, Walter (MD)	1019
Rectal Cancer	Rubin, Robert (MD)	1019
Rheumatoid Arthritis	Whitman III, Hendricks (MD)	1023
Rheumatoid Arthritis	Worth, David (MD)	1023
Rhinoplasty	West, Gerald (DO)	1028
Sarcoma	Pliner, Lillian (MD)	1024
Scleroderma	Whitman III, Hendricks (MD)	1023
Seizures	Sananman, Michael (MD)	1024
Shoulder & Knee Injuries	Levy, Andrew (MD)	1029
Sinus Problems	Goodman, Alan (MD)	1017
Sinus Surgery	Scharf, Richard (DO)	1026
SLE-Arthritis	Wilmot, Richard (MD)	1029
Sports Medicine	Gallick, Gregory (MD)	1025
Sports Medicine	Innella, Robin (DO)	1026
Sports Medicine	Vigorita, John (MD)	1027
Swallowing Problems/Heartburn	Gray, Samuel (DO)	1023
Thrombosis	Arkel, Yale S (DO)	1021
Thymectomy of Myastenics	Bolanowski, Paul J P (MD)	1030
Thyroid Diseases	Silverman, Mitchell (MD)	1020
Thyroid Diseases, Diabetes	Rosenbaum, Robert (MD)	1023
Thyroid Nodule	Chen, James (MD)	1020
Total Knee & Hip Surgery	Botwin, Clifford (DO)	1025
Tracheal Stenosis	Bolanowski, Paul J P (MD)	1030
Transesophageal Echocardiography	Brodyn, Nicholas (DO)	1018
Travel Medicine	Roland, Robert (DO)	1022
Urologic Oncology	Ring, Kenneth (MD)	1031
Varicose Veins	Sales, Clifford (MD)	1031
Viral Infections	Burstin, Stuart J (MD & PhD)	1022

Fairfield County

Acoustic Neuromas	Kveton, John (MD)	1063
Acquired Brain Injury	Mashman, Jan (MD)	1068
Acute Stroke Treatments	Maisel, Jonathan (MD)	1044
Adolescents	Korval, Arnold (MD)	1066
Advanced Laparoscopy	Santomauro, Anthony (MD)	1060
Angioplasty	Cleman, Michael (MD)	1041
Ankle Adult	Troy, Allen (MD)	1062
Anterior Segment	Wasserman, Eric (MD)	1061
Anxiety	Dolan, John (MD)	1069
Anxiety Disorders	Hart, Sidney (MD)	1069
Anxiety Disorders	Rifkin, Boris (MD)	1070
Anxiety Disorders	Schechter, Justin (MD)	1070
Anxiety Panic Disorder	Lorefice, Laurence (MD)	1069
Aortic Aneurysm	Elefteriades, John (MD)	1076
Aortic Aneurysms	De France, John (MD)	1076
Arthritis	Bindelglass, David (MD)	1061
Arthritis	Miller, Kenneth (MD)	1073
Arthritis	Molloy, Edward Michael (MD)	1052
Arthroscopic Surgery	Carolan, Patrick (MD)	1061
Arthroscopy-Shoulder, Wrist	Plancher, Kevin (MD)	1074
Asthma	Askenase, Philip (MD)	1039
Asthma	Coleman, Monroe (MD)	1039
Asthma	Dworkin, Gregory (MD)	1065
Asthma	Elias, Jack (MD)	1070
Asthma	Hen Jr, Jacob (MD)	1065
Asthma	Krinsley, James (MD)	1071
Asthma	Kurtz, Caroline (MD)	1071
Asthma	Linder, Paul (MD)	1039
Asthma	Litchman, Mark (MD)	1039
Asthma	Marino, A Michael (MD)	1071
Asthma	Simkovitz, Philip (MD)	1053

SPECIAL INTEREST	NAME	PAGE
Asthma-Sleep Disorders	Sachs, Paul (MD)	1071
Athletic Injuries	Rubinstein, Henry (MD)	1062
Autism/Attention Deficit Disorders	Cohen, Donald (MD)	1042
Back Pain	Brennan, Michael (MD)	1067
Back Pain in Elderly	Cooney, Leo (MD)	1073
Body Imaging	Cohen, Steven (MD)	1044
Bone Marrow Transplant	Lo, K M Steve (MD)	1055
Bone Marrow Transplantation	Bar, Michael (MD)	1048
Bone Tumors	Beardsley, G Peter (MD & PhD)	1065
Brain Tumor	Camel, Mark (MD)	1057
Brain Tumors	Dila, Carl (MD)	1057
Brain Tumors	Shahid, S Javed (MD)	1058
Brain Tumors	Spencer, Dennis (MD)	1058
Breast Cancer	Burd, Robert (MD)	1054
Breast Cancer	Dakofsky, LaDonna J (MD)	1072
Breast Cancer	Dowling, Sean (MD)	1072
Breast Cancer	Fass, Daniel (MD)	1072
Breast Cancer	Hollister Jr, Dickerman (MD)	1055
Breast Cancer	Kloss, Robert (MD)	1049
Breast Cancer	Lo, K M Steve (MD)	1055
Breast Cancer	Masino, Frank A (MD)	1072
Breast Cancer	Rosenberg, Arthur (MD)	1055
Breast Cancer	Spera, John (MD)	1072
Breast Cancer	Weinstein, Paul (MD)	1056
Breast Cancer Treatment	Folman, Robert (MD)	1055
Breast Disease	Ward, Barbara (MD)	1076
Breast Diseases	Blabey, Robert (MD)	1078
Breast Reconstruction	Rosenstock, Arthur (MD)	1069
Breast Surgery	Bull, Sherman (MD)	1075
Breast Surgery	Passeri, Daniel (MD)	1075
Breast Surgery	Rein, Joel (MD)	1068
Breast Surgery	Rosen, Rick (MD)	1068
Cancer	Passeri, Daniel (MD)	1075
Cancer Genetics & High Risk	Weinstein, Paul (MD)	1056
Cardiac Care/General	Zaret, Barry (MD)	1042
Cardiac Catheterization	Cleman, Michael (MD)	1041
Cardiac Catheterization-pediatric	Hellenbrand, William E (MD)	1064
Cardiology	Zalichin, Henry (MD)	1046
Cardiology Diagnostic Test	Zaret, Barry (MD)	1042
Cataract	Wasserman, Eric (MD)	1061
Cataract Surgery	Musto, Anthony (MD)	1061
Child Psychoanalysis	Solnit, Albert (MD)	1070
Cholesterol Lowering	Hankin, Edwin (MD)	1041
Chronic & Acute Dialysis	Walsh, Francis X (MD)	1057
Chronic Obstructive Lung	Sachs, Paul (MD)	1071
Chronic Obstructive Lung Disease	Marino, A Michael (MD)	1071
Chronic Pain	Brennan, Michael (MD)	1067
Clinical Genetics	Seashore, Margaretta (MD)	1054
Clinical Immunology	Litchman, Mark (MD)	1039
Colorectal Cancer	Caushaj, Philip (MD)	1042
Complicated Diagnoses	Mushlin, Stuart (MD)	1052
Coronary Artery Disease	Cohen, Lawrence (MD)	1041
Coronary Artery Disease	Elefteriades, John (MD)	1076
Cosmetic Surgery	Ariyan, Stephan (MD)	1048
Cosmetic Surgery	Calabrese, Carmine (MD)	1068
Cosmetic Surgery	Gewirtz, Harold (MD)	1068
Cosmetic Surgery	Rosenstock, Arthur (MD)	1069
Critical Care	Gentry, Eric (MD)	1071
Critical Care	Hen Jr, Jacob (MD)	1065
Critical Care Medicine	Tanoue, Lynn (MD)	1071
CT Scan	Lee, Ronald (MD)	1044
Cutaneous T Cell Lymphoma	Edelson, Richard (MD)	1043
Cutaneous T-Cell Lymphoma	Braverman, Irwin (MD)	1043

DIRECTORY OF DOCTORS

SPECIAL INTEREST	NAME	PAGE	SPECIAL INTEREST	NAME	PAGE
Dementia	Spivack, Barney (MD)	1047	High Risk Obstetrics	Besser, Gary (MD)	1059
Depression	Dolan, John (MD)	1069	High Risk Obstetrics	Blair, Emily (DO)	1059
Depression and Anxiety	Caraccio, Babette (MD)	1069	High Risk Obstetrics	Weinstein, David (MD)	1060
Depression and Manic Depression	Lorefice, Laurence (MD)	1069	Hirschsprung's Disease	Touloukian, Robert (MD)	1065
Depressive Disorders	Hart, Sidney (MD)	1069	HIV	McLeod, Gavin (MD)	1049
Detoxification Services	Gudin, Jeffrey A (MD)	1064	HIV	Saul, Zane (MD)	1050
Development; Asthma	Juan, Paul (MD)	1066	HIV Infection	Parry, Michael (MD)	1050
Developmental Disorders	Schutzengel, Roy (MD)	1067	Hospital Acquired Infections	Parry, Michael (MD)	1050
Diabetes	Molloy, Edward Michael (MD)	1052	Hypertension	Blumberg, Joel (MD)	1051
Diabetes	Siderides, Elizabeth (MD)	1061	Hypertension	Bull, Marcia (MD)	1040
Diabetes Mellitus	Rosen, Stephen (MD)	1045	Hypertension	Dreyer, Neil (MD)	1051
Diagnostic Hematology Problems	Duffy, Thomas (MD)	1049	Hypertension	Garfinkel, Howard (MD)	1056
Diseases of Blood	Covey, William (MD)	1051	Hypertension	Hankin, Edwin (MD)	1041
Diseases of the Spine	Rosenstein, C Cory (MD)	1058	Hypertension	Hines, William (MD)	1056
Dual Diagnosis	Frances, Richard (MD)	1039	Hypnosis	Rousell, Charles (MD)	1070
Dysmorphology	Pober, Barbara (MD)	1054	Hypospadias	Burbige, Kevin (MD)	1077
Ear Surgery	Klenoff, Bruce (MD)	1063	Image Directed Breast Surgery	Smego, Douglas (MD)	1076
Eating Disorders	Hofreuter, Nancy (MD)	1066	Immunizations	Morelli, Alan (MD)	1067
Emergency Care	Dell'Aria, Joseph (MD)	1044	Inborn Errors of Metabolism	Mahoney, Maurice (MD)	1054
Emphysema	Kurtz, Caroline (MD)	1071	Inborn Errors of Metabolism	Seashore, Margaretta (MD)	1054
Emphysema Cough Lung Cancer	Krasnogor, Lester (MD)	1071	Incontinence	Waxberg, Jonathan (MD)	1077
End Stage Renal Disease	Walsh, Francis X (MD)	1057	Infertility	Ginsburg, Frances (MD)	1073
Endometriosis	Santomauro, Anthony (MD)	1060	Inflammatory Bowel Disease	Waldstreicher, Stuart (MD)	1047
Endoscopic Laser Therapy	Waldstreicher, Stuart (MD)	1047	Innovative Treatments	Cooper, Robert (MD)	1051
Environmental Health	Cullen, Mark R (MD)	1060	Insect Bites	Coleman, Monroe (MD)	1039
Epilepsy Surgery	Spencer, Dennis (MD)	1058	Interventional Catheterization	Hellenbrand, William E (MD)	1064
Esophageal Diseases	Traube, Morris (MD)	1047	Intra-Cranial Vascular Surgery	Rosenstein, C Cory (MD)	1058
Facial Cosmetic Surgery	Rein, Joel (MD)	1068	Investigational Drugs for	Dalgin, Paul (MD)	1073
Facial Surgery	Rosen, Rick (MD)	1068	Joint Reconstruction	Stovell, Peter (MD)	1062
Foot Adult	Troy, Allen (MD)	1062	Joint Replacement	Bindelglass, David (MD)	1061
Gall-Bladder & Liver	Passarelli, Nicholas (MD)	1075	Joint Replacement	Crowe, John (MD)	1061
Gastrointestinal Surgery	Napp, Marc (MD)	1075	Joint Replacement	Rubinstein, Henry (MD)	1062
General Infections	McLeod, Gavin (MD)	1049	Joint Replacement	Wilchinsky, Mark (MD)	1062
General Orthopaedic	Weiner, Avi (MD)	1074	Kidney Disease	Hines, William (MD)	1056
General Pediatrics	Korval, Arnold (MD)	1066	Kidney Stones	Ranta, Jeffrey (MD)	1077
Genitourinary Cancer	Poo, Wen Jen (MD)	1055	Knee & Hand Surgery	Plancher, Kevin (MD)	1074
Geriatric Assessment	Tinetti, Mary (MD)	1047	Knee Shoulder-Arthroscopy	Wilchinsky, Mark (MD)	1062
Geriatric Medicine	Filiberto, Cosmo (MD)	1045	Knee Surgery	Jokl, Peter (MD)	1062
Geriatric Psychiatry	Nelson, J Craig (MD)	1069	Laparascopic Surgery	McWhorter, Philip (MD)	1075
Geriatrics	Thomas, Byron (MD)	1053	Laparoscopic Surgery	Besser, Gary (MD)	1059
Growth Disorders	Keller, Barry (MD)	1066	Laparoscopic Surgery	Nelson, James (MD)	1060
Growth Disorders	Schutzengel, Roy (MD)	1067	Laparoscopic Surgery	Reed, David (MD)	1075
Gynecologic Imaging	McCarthy, Shirley (MD & PhD)	1044	Laparoscopy	Napp, Marc (MD)	1075
Gynecologic Oncology	Dowling, Sean (MD)	1072	Laser Surgery; Moh's Surgery	Leffell, David (MD)	1043
Gynecologic Oncology	Koulos, John (MD)	1048	Leukemia	Beardsley, G Peter (MD & PhD)	1065
Gynecological Surgery	Schwartz, Peter (MD)	1048	Leukemia	Kloss, Robert (MD)	1049
Habit Cough	Dworkin, Gregory (MD)	1065	Lung & Colon Cancer	Hollister Jr, Dickerman (MD)	1055
Hayfever	Linder, Paul (MD)	1039	Lung Cancer	De France, John (MD)	1076
Head & Neck Surgery	Lipton, Richard Jeffrey (MD)	1063	Lung Cancer Chemotherapy	Folman, Robert (MD)	1055
Head and Neck Cancer	Salzer, Stephen (MD)	1064	Lung Diseases	Quartararo, Paul (MD)	1053
Head and Neck Surgery	Beres, Milan (MD)	1062	Lupus	Braverman, Irwin (MD)	1043
Head and Neck Surgery	Sasaki, ClarenceT (MD)	1064	Lupus & Glomerulonephritis	Fogel, Mitchell (MD)	1056
Headache	Seigel, Sheryl (MD)	1058	Lupus Rheumatoid Arthritis-		
Headache	Siegel, Kenneth C (MD)	1059	Systemic Lupus	Novack, Stuart N (MD)	1074
Health Maintenance	Brenner, Stephen D (MD)	1051	Lyme Disease	Herbin, Joseph (MD)	1052
Hearing Loss	Kveton, John (MD)	1063	Lyme Disease	Kunkel, Mark (MD)	1049
Hematologic Disorders	Bar, Michael (MD)	1048	Lyme Disease	Saul, Zane (MD)	1050
Hematology	Ertl, John (MD)	1066	Lyme Disease	Yee, Arthur (MD)	1050
Hemolytic Anemias	Forget, Bernard (MD)	1049	Lymphoma	Burd, Robert (MD)	1054
Hemophilia	Beardsley, Diana (MD & PhD)	1049	Lymphoma	Cooper, Dennis (MD)	1054
Hernia	Burbige, Kevin (MD)	1077	Lymphoma	Rosenberg, Arthur (MD)	1055
High Risk Gynecology	Blair, Emily (DO)	1059	Major Depression	Rifkin, Boris (MD)	1070
High Risk Ob-Gyn	Foye, Gerard (MD)	1054	Major Gynecologic Surgery	Rosenman, Stephen (MD)	1060

DIRECTORY OF DOCTORS

ALPHABETICAL DOCTOR LISTING

DIRECTORY OF DOCTORS

NAME	SPECIALTY	PAGE	NAME	SPECIALTY	PAGE
A			Ahmed, Nafis (MD)	TS	550
			Ahmed, Tauseef (MD)	Onc	787
Abbate, Anthony (MD)	U	551	Ahn, Jung (MD)	PMR	329
Abbey, Albert (MD)	D	901	Ahronheim, Judith (MD)	Ger	197
Abdel-Dayem, Hussein M (MD)	NuM	255	Aiges, Harvey (MD)	PGe	676
Abell, Penny (MD)	Oph	268	Aisen, Paul (MD)	Rhu	376
Abemayor, Elie (MD)	Ge	773	Aisenberg, James (MD)	Ge	187
Abenavoli, T J (MD)	IM	779	Akhavan, Iraj (MD)	IM	209
Abiri, Michael (MD)	DR	177	Alaghabend, Mehran (MD)	D	418
Abittan, Meyer H (MD)	Cv	629	Albert, Joel (MD)	Ge	494
Abott, Michael (MD)	IM	501	Albertini, Francis (MD)	IM	568
Abouchedid, Claude (MD)	S	949	Albin, Joan (MD)	EDM	769
Abouzahr, Kamel (MD)	PlS	332	Albom, Michael (MD)	D	169
Abrahams, Irving (MD)	D	169	Alderman, Elizabeth (MD)	Ped	453
Abramowicz, Helen (MD)	Psyc	340	Alderson, Philip (MD)	Rad	370
Abrams, Jeffrey (MD)	OrS	943	Aldrich, Thomas (MD)	Pul	460
Abrams, Martin (MD)	PS	678	Aledo, Alexander (MD)	PHO	315
Abrams, Samuel (MD)	Psyc	341	Aledort, Louis (MD)	Hem	202
Abramson, Allan (MD)	Oto	672	Alexander, Martin (MD)	U	836
Abramson, Steven B (MD)	Rhu	376	Alexiades, Michael (MD)	OrS	285
Abright, Arthur Reese (MD)	ChAP	163	Alexopoulos, George (MD)	Psyc	821
Absatz, Michael (MD)	OrS	978	Alfonso, Antonio (MD)	S	545
Abud, Alfredo (MD)	GVS	951	Alger, Ian (MD)	Psyc	341
Abud, Ariel (MD)	NS	942	Alhasan, Harith (MD)	Anes	601
Abularrage, Joseph (MD)	Ped	583	Allegra, Donald (MD)	Inf	990
Accardi, Frank (MD)	Oph	268	Allen, Carol (MD)	EDM	420
Accettola, Albert (MD)	OrS	612	Allen, Jeffrey (MD)	N	245
Accurso, Charles (MD)	Ge	1011	Allen, Machelle (MD)	ObG	256
Acker, Gerald (MD)	PlS	684	Allen, Steven (MD)	Hem	646
Ackerman, Jacob (MD)	Oph	520	Allendorf, Dennis (MD)	Ped	320
Ackert, John (MD)	Ge	187	Almeida, Laila (MD)	D	987
Ackley Jr, Alexander (MD)	IM	940	Almeida, Victor (DO)	EM	901
Acosta, Rod (MD)	FP	1045	Almeyda, Elizabeth (MD)	PlS	332
Adachi, Akinori (MD)	ObG	794	Almond, Gregory (MD)	EM	179
Adams, Francis (MD)	Pul	363	Aloia, John (MD)	EDM	639
Adams, Marc (MD)	RadRO	619	Alpert, Barbara (MD)	IM	779
Addonizio, Gerard (MD)	Psyc	821	Alpert, Bertram (MD)	Nep	609
Adelman, Mark (MD)	GVS	407	Al-Salihi, Farouk (MD)	Ped	931
Adelman, Ronald (MD)	Ger	196	Altchek, David (MD)	OrS	285
Adesman, Andrew (MD)	Ped	679	Altchek, Edgar (MD)	PlS	332
Adler, Albert (MD)	Ped	738	Alter, Sheldon (MD)	IM	779
Adler, Edward (MD)	OrS	285	Alterman, Lloyd (MD)	Nep	1024
Adler, Harry (MD)	S	545	Altholz, Jeffrey (MD)	IM	779
Adler, Hilton C (MD)	PlS	740	Altman, Jill (MD)	Anes	758
Adler, Jack (MD)	Pul	363	Altman, Kenneth (MD)	IM	209
Adler, Jonathan (MD)	DR	865	Altman, R Peter (MD)	PS	318
Adler, Kenneth (MD)	Onc	991	Altman, Wayne (MD)	OrS	880
Adler, Melvin (MD)	OrS	446	Altorki, Nasser (MD)	TS	395
Adler, Mitchell (MD)	IM	209	Altschul, Larry (MD)	Cv	712
Adlersberg, Jay (MD)	Rhu	376	Altus, Jonathan (MD)	IM	648
Afif, Juan Simon (MD)	ObG	443	Alvarez, Manuel (MD)	ObG	877
Agarwal, Nanakram (MD)	S	464	Alweiss, Gary (MD)	N	876
Agdere, Levon (MD)	PEn	675	Aly, Sayed (MD)	NP	929
Agin, Carole (MD)	PM	449	Ambrose, John (MD)	Cv	153
Agre, Fred (MD)	Ped	320	Ames, Richard (MD)	Nep	238
Aguila, Helen (MD)	PPul	914	Amin, Jashvantkumar S (MD)	IM	904
Agulnek, Milton (MD)	Ped	679	Amin, Mahendra (MD)	IM	568
Agus, Bertrand (MD)	Rhu	376	Amiruddin, Qamar (MD)	S	545
Aharon, Raphael (MD)	Oph	577	Amis Jr, E Stephen (MD)	Rad	461
Ahlborn, Thomas (MD)	S	892	Amler, David (MD)	Ped	814
Ahluwalia, Brij Mohan Singh (MD)	N	791	Ammazzalorso, Michael (MD)	IM	648
Ahmad, Imtiaz (MD)	TS	950	Amorosa, Louis (MD)	EDM	956
Ahmed, Fakhiuddin (MD)	Onc	508	Amorosi, Edward (MD)	Hem	202
Ahmed, Maher (MD)	GVS	407	Amoruso, Robert (MD)	Pul	889

NAME	SPECIALTY	PAGE	NAME	SPECIALTY	PAGE
Anand, Vijay (MD)	Oto	299	Aruna, Pasalai N (MD)	Oto	963
Anant, Ashok (MD)	NS	513	Arvanitis, Michael (MD)	CRS	973
Ancona, Richard (MD)	Ped	738	Arya, Yashpal (MD)	Ge	494
Andersen, Bruce J (MD)	NS	513	Asad, Syed (MD)	Nep	725
Andersen, Dana (MD)	S	1074	Ascheim, Robert (MD)	IM	209
Anderson, Kevin (MD)	U	1077	Ascher, Enrico (MD)	GVS	553
Andrade, Joseph (MD)	Ped	453	Ascherman, Jeffrey (MD)	PlS	332
Andrews, David (MD)	OrS	285	Asheld, John (MD)	IM	648
Andriani, Rudy (MD)	U	1077	Ashikari, Roy (MD)	S	831
Andriola, Mary (MD)	ChiN	713	Ashinoff, Robin (MD)	D	169
Andron, Richard (MD)	IM	871	Askanas, Alexander (MD)	Cv	153
Andronaco, John (MD)	OrS	880	Askenase, Philip (MD)	A&I	1039
Anfang, David (MD)	S	933	Asnes, Russell (MD)	Ped	885
Angeli, Stephen (MD)	IM	871	Asnis, Gregory (MD)	Psyc	458
Angioletti, Louis (MD)	Oph	268	Asnis, Stanley (MD)	OrS	669
Angrist, Burton (MD)	Psyc	341	Aston, Sherrell (MD)	PlS	332
Angulo, Moris (MD)	MG	654	Astrow, Alan (MD)	Hem	202
Angus, L D George (MD)	S	545	Atakent, Pinar (MD)	PMR	536
Anhalt, Henry (DO)	PEn	528	Athanail, Steven (MD)	FP	491
Anker, Eli (MD)	GVS	749	Athanasian, Edward (MD)	HS	200
Ankobiah, William (MD)	IM	568	Atlas, Arthur (MD)	PPul	995
Annavajjhala, Durga (MD)	Ped	532	Atlas, Ian (MD)	U	999
Ansanelli, Vincent (MD)	S	382	Atlas, Scott (MD)	DR	177
Anselmi, Gregory (MD)	N	929	Attai, Lari (MD)	TS	468
Antell, Darrick (MD)	PlS	332	Attas, Lewis (MD)	Onc	874
Antman, Karen (MD)	Onc	230	Attia, Albert (MD)	Ge	187
Anto, Cecily (MD)	N	726	Attia, Evelyn (MD)	Psyc	341
Anto, Maliakal J (MD)	Cv	629	Attiyeh, Fadi (MD)	S	382
Antoine, Clarel (MD)	ObG	256	Auchincloss, Elizabeth (MD)	Psyc	341
Anton, John (MD)	PlS	740	Auerbach, Mitchell E (MD)	Ge	774
Antonacci, Anthony (MD)	S	382	Auerbach, Robert (MD)	D	169
Antonelle, Michael (MD)	Ge	773	Aufiero, Patrick (MD)	Inf	940
Antonelle, Robert (MD)	Ge	774	Aufses, Arthur (MD)	S	382
Antony, Michael (MD)	Ge	424	August, David (MD)	S	968
Apatoff, Brian R (MD & PhD)	N	245	August, Phyllis (MD)	Nep	238
Apisson, John (MD)	Oph	730	Auguste, Louis T (MD)	S	696
Appel, Gerald (MD)	Nep	238	Augustine, V M (MD)	Ped	738
Applebaum, Eric (MD)	A&I	987	Austin, John (MD)	DR	177
Applebaum, Seymour (MD)	Psyc	586	Ausubel, Herbert (MD)	IM	649
April, Max (MD)	Oto	299	Averbach, David (MD)	S	981
Aprile, Georgette (MD)	D	636	Aviv, Jonathan (MD)	Oto	300
Apuzzio, Joseph (MD)	ObG	909	Avram, Marc R (MD)	D	169
Apuzzo, Thomas (MD)	FP	771	Avram, Morrell M (MD)	Nep	510
Aranoff, Gaya S (MD)	PEn	312	Avruskin, Theodore W (MD)	PEn	529
Arbes, Spiros (MD)	Nep	977	Avvento, Louis (MD)	Hem	720
Arbour, Robert (MD)	S	981	Axelrod, Deborah (MD)	S	382
Arden, Martha (MD)	AM	627	Axelrod, Randi (MD)	NP	941
Arden-Cordone, Mary (MD)	EDM	1045	Ayoub, Thomas (MD)	ObG	1059
Arevalo, Carlos (MD)	EDM	563	Aziz, Hassan (MD)	Rad	542
Argyros, Thomas (MD)	Rhu	376	Azizirad, Hassan (MD)	Ped	583
Aries, Philip (MD)	Oph	730			
Ariyan, Stephan (MD)	HS	1048	**B**		
Arkel, Yale S (DO)	Hem	1021	Babu, Sateesh (MD)	GVS	839
Arkow, Stan (MD)	Psyc	341	Baccash, Emil (MD)	IM	501
Armbruster, Robert (MD)	ObG	794	Bachmann, Gloria (MD)	ObG	962
Armstrong, Donald (MD)	Inf	205	Baddoura, Rashid (MD)	EM	866
Arnold, Thomas E (MD)	GVS	750	Bade III, Harry A (MD)	SM	981
Arnon, Rica (MD)	PCd	310	Bader, Paul (MD)	IM	569
Arnstein, Ellis (MD)	Ped	453	Badikian, Arthur (MD)	Psyc	821
Aro, Dominic (DO)	ObG	443	Badlani, Gopal (MD)	U	593
Aron, Alan (MD)	ChiN	165	Baer, Jeanne (MD)	Rad	371
Aronoff, Michael (MD)	Psyc	341	Bailey, Michelle (MD)	Ped	453
Arpadi, Stephen M (MD)	Ped	320	Bailine, Samuel (MD)	Psyc	687
Artman, Michael (MD)	PCd	310	Bains, Manjit (MD)	TS	395

DIRECTORY OF DOCTORS

NAME	SPECIALTY	PAGE	NAME	SPECIALTY	PAGE
Bains, Yatinder (MD)	IM	928	Baumann, John (MD)	RadRÓ	948
Baiser, Dennis (MD)	Ped	946	Baurdy, Francis (MD)	Psyc	342
Bajorin, Dean (MD)	Onc	230	Baxi, Laxmi (MD)	ObG	256
Bakal, Curtis (MD)	VIR	406	Baxt, Saida (MD)	D	864
Baker, Barry (MD)	IM	430	Beardsley, Diana (MD & PhD)	Hem	1049
Baker, Daniel (MD)	PlS	332	Beardsley, G Peter (MD & PhD)	PHO	1065
Baker, David (MD)	ObG	728	Bearnot, H Robert (MD)	Ge	187
Baldassare, Jack L (MD)	DR	865	Beasley, Robert (MD)	HS	200
Baldwin, David (MD)	IM	209	Beaton, Howard L (MD)	S	383
Baldwin, Hilary (MD)	D	487	Beatty, Edward (MD)	ObG	256
Balk, Sophie (MD)	Ped	453	Bebawi, Magdi (MD)	S	383
Ball, Charles (MD)	Oph	910	Beccia, David (MD)	U	749
Balmaceda, Casilda (MD)	N	246	Beck, A Robert (MD)	PS	318
Balot, Barry (DO)	IM	721	Becker, Alfred (MD)	Rhu	849
Balsano, Nicholas (MD)	S	464	Becker, Carolyn (MD)	EDM	769
Balthazar, Emil J (MD)	Rad	371	Becker, David V (MD)	NuM	255
Bander, Neil (MD)	Onc	231	Becker, Jerrold (MD)	PS	678
Banerji, Mary (MD)	EDM	490	Becker, Joshua (MD)	Rad	542
Bangaru, Babu (MD)	PGe	314	Becker, Kenneth (MD)	FP	716
Bank, David (MD)	D	765	Becker, Richard (MD)	Cv	758
Bank, Simmy (MD)	Ge	565	Becker, Ted (MD)	Psyc	342
Banzon, Manuel (MD)	ObG	878	Beckerman, Barry (MD)	Oph	799
Bar, Michael (MD)	Hem	1048	Bederson, Joshua (MD)	NS	241
Barad, David (MD)	ObG	794	Bednarek, Karl (MD)	Ge	187
Barakat, Richard (MD)	GO	198	Bednoff, Stuart (MD)	ObG	661
Barandes, Martin (MD)	EDM	180	Beer, Maurice (MD)	IM	210
Barasch, Kenneth (MD)	Oph	268	Befeler, David (MD)	S	1030
Barbaccia, Ann (MD)	ObG	661	Behm, Dutsi (MD)	IM	501
Barbaris, Harry (MD)	U	702	Behr, Raymond (MD)	Psyc	687
Barbasch, Avi (MD)	Onc	231	Behrens, Fred (MD)	OrS	911
Barber, Hugh (MD)	GO	199	Behrens, Myles (MD)	Oph	269
Barbera, Jude (MD)	U	551	Beil, Arthur (MD)	TS	700
Barbuto, Joseph (MD)	Psyc	341	Beitler, Jonathan (MD)	RadRO	461
Bardeguez, Arlene (MD)	ObG	909	Bekirov, Huseyin (MD)	U	469
Bardes, Charles L (MD)	IM	209	Bell, Jonathan (MD)	A&I	1039
Baredes, Soly (MD)	Oto	912	Bell, Kevin (MD)	IM	1022
Barest, Herman (MD)	Oph	799	Belladonna, Joseph (MD)	Ge	1020
Barie, Philip (MD)	S	382	Bello, Jacqueline A (MD)	Rad	462
Barker, Barbara (MD)	Oph	268	Bello, Mary (MD)	FP	867
Barland, Peter (MD)	Rhu	464	Bellomo, Spartaco (MD)	Inf	927
Barmakian, Joseph (MD)	OrS	1025	Bellucci, Alessandro (MD)	Nep	657
Barnes, Edward (MD)	IM	210	Belmont, H Michael (MD)	Rhu	376
Barone, Clement (MD)	DR	178	Belok, Lennart (MD)	N	246
Barone, James (MD)	S	1074	Bender-Cracco, Joan (MD)	ChiN	486
Barone, Richard (MD)	Rhu	829	Benedicto, Ramon (MD)	S	591
Barry, Michele (MD)	IM	1050	Benisovich, Vladimir I (MD)	Onc	571
Barst, Robyn (MD)	PCd	310	Benjamin, Bry (MD)	IM	210
Bartlett, Jacqueline (MD)	ChAP	900	Benjamin, Burton (MD)	IM	1050
Bartolomeo, Robert (MD)	Ge	642	Benjamin, Ernest (MD)	CCM	168
Baruchin, Mitchell (MD)	Cv	925	Benjamin, Fred (MD)	ObG	661
Barzegar, Hooshang (MD)	ObG	517	Benjamin, John (MD)	Psyc	687
Basch, Samuel (MD)	Psyc	341	Benjamin, Vallo (MD)	NS	241
Bashevkin, Michael (MD)	Hem	498	Benkov, Keith (MD)	PGe	812
Baskin, David (MD)	IM	210	Bennett, Harvey S (MD)	ChiN	486
Baskin, Martin (MD)	Pul	363	Bennett, Ronald (MD)	Rhu	745
Baskind, Larry (MD)	Ped	814	Benninghoff, David (MD)	RadRO	744
Bastawros, Mary (MD)	Ped	614	Benovitz, Harvey (MD)	IM	210
Basuk, Pamela (MD)	D	713	Benson, Douglas (MD)	S	893
Basuk, Paul M (MD)	Ge	187	Benson, Mitchell C (MD)	U	399
Bauer, Joel (MD)	S	383	Bentivegna, Saverio (MD)	S	831
Bauer, Robert (MD)	Oph	799	Benvenia, Joseph (MD)	OrS	911
Baum, Carol (MD)	A&I	757	Benvenisty, Alan (MD)	GVS	407
Baum, Stephen (MD)	Inf	205	Benzil, Deborah (MD)	NS	791
Bauman, Phillip (MD)	OrS	285			

NAME	SPECIALTY	PAGE	NAME	SPECIALTY	PAGE
Ben-Zvi, Jeffrey (MD)	Ge	188	Berson, Anthony (MD)	RadRO	368
Bercow, Neil R (MD)	TS	700	Berson, Barry (MD)	Rad	371
Berdini, Jeffrey (MD)	U	895	Bertagnolli, Monica (MD)	S	383
Berdoff, Russell (MD)	Cv	153	Besser, Gary (MD)	ObG	1059
Berdon, Walter (MD)	PR	318	Besser, Louis (MD)	Cv	601
Berenson, Murray (MD)	Ge	188	Besser, Walter (MD)	OrS	285
Berenstein, Alejando (MD)	NRad	254	Best, Milton (MD)	Oph	269
Beres, Milan (MD)	Oto	1062	Bestak, Marc (MD)	PHO	451
Berger, Bernard (MD)	D	713	Bethal, Colin (MD)	PS	915
Berger, David (MD)	IM	649	Better, Donna (MD)	Cv	629
Berger, E Roy (MD)	Onc	724	Bevelaqua, Frederick (MD)	IM	210
Berger, Jack (MD)	Rhu	829	Beyda, Allan (MD)	IM	569
Berger, Joshua (MD)	D	419	Beyda, Bernadette (MD)	D	562
Berger, Judith (MD)	Inf	429	Beyerl, Brian (MD)	NS	991
Berger, Leonard (MD)	Ped	814	Beyrer, Charles R (MD)	Oph	730
Berger, Marvin (MD)	Cv	153	Bezahler, Harvey (MD)	Psyc	342
Berger, Matthew (MD)	IM	430	Bhalodkar, Narendra (MD)	Cv	416
Bergh, Paul A (MD)	RE	919	Bharathan, Thayyulla (MD)	IM	501
Bergman, Donald (MD)	EDM	180	Bhatt, Anjani (MD)	EDM	640
Bergman, Marion (MD)	Pul	743	Bhatt, Ashok (MD)	Psyc	688
Bergman, Michael I (MD)	Pul	539	Biagiotti, Emilio (MD)	IM	430
Bergstein, Michael (MD)	Oto	808	Biagiotti, Wendy (MD)	FP	422
Berk, Paul D (MD)	IM	780	Bialer, Martin G (MD)	MG	654
Berke, Andrew D (MD)	Cv	629	Bialkin, Robert (MD)	ObG	662
Berkeley, Alan S (MD)	RE	374	Biancaniello, Thomas (MD)	PCd	737
Berkey, Peter (MD)	Inf	778	Biasetti, John (MD)	IM	721
Berkman, Steven (MD)	ObG	878	Bickers, David (MD)	D	169
Berkower, Alan (MD & PhD)	Oto	448	Biddle, David (MD)	N	659
Berkowitz, Howard (MD)	Psyc	538	Bielory, Leonard (MD)	A&I	899
Berkowitz, Leonard B (MD)	Inf	500	Bienenstock, Harry (MD)	Rhu	544
Berkowitz, Norman (MD)	Ped	814	Bierman, Fredrick Z (MD)	PCd	580
Berkowitz, Rhonda (MD)	D	765	Biers, Martin (MD)	Hem	777
Berkowitz, Richard (MD)	ObG	257	Bigajer, Charles (MD)	Ge	494
Berkowitz, Robert (MD)	Cv	862	Bigliani, Louis (MD)	OrS	285
Berkowitz, Steven (MD)	OrS	978	Bilezikian, John Paul (MD)	EDM	180
Berkwits, Kieve (MD)	PCd	1064	Bilfinger, Thomas (MD)	TS	748
Berlin, Arnold (MD)	S	464	Biller, Hugh (MD)	Oto	300
Berliner, Stewart R (MD)	DR	768	Billett, Henny (MD)	Hem	428
Berman, Alvin (MD)	ObG	257	Bilmes, Ernest (MD)	FP	716
Berman, Ellin (MD)	Onc	231	Bindelglass, David (MD)	OrS	1061
Berman, Mark (MD)	OrS	881	Binder, Alan (MD)	Cv	629
Berman, Morton (MD)	Ped	815	Birch, Thomas (MD)	Inf	871
Berman, Sheldon (MD)	Psyc	538	Bird, Hector (MD)	ChAP	163
Berman, Steven (MD)	U	399	Birger, Daniel (MD)	Psyc	342
Bernanke, Harold (MD)	IM	430	Birkhoff, John (MD)	U	399
Bernard, Peter (MD)	Oto	300	Birnbaum, Jay (MD)	PlS	332
Bernard, Robert (MD)	IM	721	Birnbaum, Stanley (MD)	GO	199
Bernard, Robert (MD)	PlS	819	Birns, Douglas (MD)	U	399
Bernardini, Dennis (MD)	Pul	743	Birns, Robert (MD)	Pul	890
Bernaski, Edward (MD)	Cv	153	Biro, Laszlo (MD)	D	487
Bernhardt, Bernard (MD)	Onc	788	Birrer, Richard (MD)	FP	564
Bernot, Robert (MD)	IM	210	Bisaccia, Emil (MD)	D	988
Bernstein, Chaim (MD)	Pul	540	Bisberg, Dorothy Stein (MD)	PPul	914
Bernstein, Charles (MD)	D	603	Bizzoco, Sabina (MD)	Ped	320
Bernstein, Gerald (MD)	EDM	180	Blabey, Robert (MD)	GVS	1078
Bernstein, Larry (MD)	A&I	559	Blackinton, Charles (MD)	Psyc	888
Bernstein, Lawrence J (MD)	PMR	536	Blackwood, M Michele (MD)	S	1074
Bernstein, Leslie (MD)	IM	430	Blair, Emily (DO)	ObG	1059
Bernstein, Martin (MD)	Pul	540	Blair, Lester (MD)	Pul	364
Bernstein, Michael (MD)	S	546	Blaivas, Jerry G (MD)	U	399
Bernstein, Robert (MD)	ObG	661	Blake, James (MD)	Cv	153
Bernstein, Robert (MD)	Rad	462	Blanco, Jody (MD)	ObG	257
Berroya, Renato (MD)	GVS	705	Blank, Ellen (MD)	D	925
Berry, Richard (MD)	D	487			

DIRECTORY OF DOCTORS

NAME	SPECIALTY	PAGE	NAME	SPECIALTY	PAGE
Blank, Ellen (MD)	D	925	Bonforte, Richard (MD)	Ped	320
Blau, Sheldon P (MD)	Rhu	694	Bonilla, Mary Ann (MD)	PHO	812
Blaufox, M Donald (MD & PhD)	IM	431	Boniuk, Vivien (MD)	Oph	577
Blaugrund, Stanley (MD)	Oto	300	Boodish, Wesley (MD)	Ped	915
Bleiberg, Melvyn (MD)	Cv	758	Boozan, William (MD)	Oph	612
Bleicher, Robert (MD)	Ge	1003	Bopaiah, Vinod (MD)	CRS	486
Bleifeld, Charles (MD)	OrS	733	Borah, Gregory (MD)	PlS	965
Blitzer, Andrew (MD)	Oto	300	Borbely, Antal (MD)	Psyc	342
Bloch, Claude (MD)	Rad	371	Borek, Mark (MD)	Cv	712
Blood, David (MD)	Cv	862	Borer, Jeffrey (MD)	Cv	154
Bloom, Alan (MD)	Ge	424	Borg, Morton (MD)	PCd	310
Bloom, Jerry (MD)	IM	502	Borgen, Patrick (MD)	S	383
Bloom, Norman (MD)	S	383	Borkowsky, William (MD)	Ped	320
Bloom, Patricia (MD)	Ger	197	Borriello, Raffaele (MD)	S	546
Bloomenstein, Richard (MD)	PlS	887	Bortniker, David (MD)	Oto	1013
Bloomfield, Dennis A (MD)	Cv	601	Boscamp, Jeffrey (MD)	Ped Inf	884
Bloomgarden, David (MD)	EDM	770	Bosl, George (MD)	Onc	231
Bloomgarden, Zachary (MD)	EDM	180	Bosniak, Morton (MD)	Rad	371
Bluestone, Harvey (MD)	Psyc	458	Bossart, Peter (MD)	S	383
Blum, Alan (MD)	Pul	689	Bosso, John (MD)	A&I	845
Blum, Conrad (MD)	EDM	180	Bosworth, Jay (MD)	RadRO	692
Blum, David (MD)	EDM	770	Botet, Jose (MD)	Rad	829
Blum, Manfred (MD)	EDM	180	Botwin, Clifford (DO)	OrS	1025
Blum, Ronald (MD)	Onc	231	Botwinick, Nelson (MD)	HS	200
Blumberg, Denise (MD)	PEn	675	Boufford, Timothy (MD)	IM	780
Blumberg, Joel (MD)	IM	1051	Bourla, Steven (MD)	Nep	657
Blume, Ralph (MD)	Rhu	376	Bove, Joseph (MD)	EM	489
Blume, Sheila (MD)	AdP	711	Bowe, Edward (MD)	ObG	257
Blumencranz, Harriet (MD)	Ped	815	Bowen, Shawn (MD)	Ped	320
Blumenfield, Michael (MD)	Psyc	822	Boxer, Mitchell (MD)	A&I	627
Blumenthal, David S (MD)	Cv	153	Boxer, Robert A (MD)	PCd	674
Blumenthal, Jesse (MD)	GVS	407	Boyarsky, Andrew (MD)	S	968
Blumgart, Leslie H (MD)	S	383	Boyce, John G (MD)	GO	497
Blumstein, Meyer (MD)	Ge	565	Boyd, Arthur D (MD)	TS	395
Bluth, Mordecai (MD)	PM	674	Boyd, D Barry (MD)	IM	1051
Blyskal, Stanley (MD)	FP	717	Brabston, Robert J (MD)	IM	1004
Boal, Bernard (MD)	Cv	560	Bracero, Louis (MD)	ObG	575
Bobroff, Lewis (MD)	Rad	848	Brademas, Mary Ellen (MD)	D	169
Boccio, Richard (MD)	OrS	733	Bradley, Thomas (MD)	Hem	498
Bocian, Franklin (MD)	Oph	799	Brady, James (MD)	Rad	371
Bockman, Richard (MD & PhD)	EDM	181	Brady, Terence (MD)	CCM	562
Boczko, Stanley (MD)	U	400	Braff, Robert (MD)	Cv	154
Bodack, Mark (MD)	PMR	329	Bram, Harris (MD)	PM	979
Bodenheimer, Monty (MD)	Cv	560	Brancaccio, Ronald R (MD)	D	487
Bodenheimer Jr, Henry (MD)	Ge	188	Brancaccio, William (MD)	DR	715
Bodian, Eugene L (MD)	D	637	Brancucci, Marion (MD)	Psyc	822
Bodis-Wollner, Ivan (MD)	N	514	Brand, Howard (MD)	EDM	715
Bodner, William (MD)	RadRO	461	Brandeis, Steven (MD)	CRS	166
Bogaty, Stanley (MD)	Oph	731	Brandt, Lawrence (MD)	Ge	424
Bogin, Marc (MD)	Cv	602	Branom Jr, Wayne (MD)	D	1043
Bohrer, Stuart (MD)	PS	678	Braun, Carl (MD)	N	246
Boim, Marilynn (MD)	PEn	946	Braun, Norma (MD)	Pul	364
Bolanowski, Paul J P (MD)	TS	1030	Brauntuch, Glenn (MD)	Pul	890
Boley, Scott (MD)	PS	452	Brause, Barry (MD)	Inf	205
Bolognia, Jean (MD)	D	1043	Braverman, Irwin (MD)	D	1043
Boltin, Harry (MD)	Rad	848	Bray, Mary (MD)	RE	543
Bomback, Fredric (MD)	Ped	815	Brecher, Rubin (MD)	Oph	520
Bonagura, Vincent R (MD)	A&I	559	Breen, Charles (MD)	Psyc	538
Bonamo, Joel (MD)	OrS	613	Breen, James (MD)	ObG	909
Bonamo, John (MD)	OrS	285	Breen, William (MD)	Cv	629
Bonanno, Philip C (MD)	PlS	820	Bregman, Zachary (MD)	Pul	364
Bondi, Elliott (MD)	Pul	540	Breidbart, Scott (MD)	PEn	811
Bone, Stanley (MD)	Psyc	342	Breitbart, William (MD)	Psyc	342
Bonfils-Roberts, Enrique (MD)	TS	395	Breitstein, Robert (MD)	ObG	257

NAME	SPECIALTY	PAGE	NAME	SPECIALTY	PAGE
Brener, Bruce (MD)	GVS	922	Bruck, Harold (MD)	S	893
Brenholz, Pauline (MD)	MG	787	Bruckstein, Robert (MD)	D	637
Brennan, John P (MD)	ObG	517	Brunnquell, Stephen (MD)	IM	871
Brennan, Lawrence (MD)	Nep	657	Bruno, Anthony (MD)	U	703
Brennan, Michael (MD)	PMR	1067	Bruno, Michael (MD)	IM	211
Brennan, Murray (MD)	S	384	Bruno, Peter (MD)	IM	211
Brenner, Richard (MD)	TS	1030	Brusco, Louis (MD)	CCM	168
Brenner, Ronald (MD)	Psyc	888	Brust, John (MD)	N	246
Brenner, Stephen (MD)	OrS	881	Brustein, Harris (MD)	Oph	799
Brenner, Stephen D (MD)	IM	1051	Brustman, Lois (MD)	MF	787
Brenner, Steven (MD)	ObG	662	Bryk, David (MD)	Rad	542
Brescia, Michael J (MD)	Onc	436	Bryk, Eli (MD)	OrS	286
Brescia, Robert (MD)	Psyc	822	Buatti, Elizabeth (MD)	IM	431
Bressman, Susan (MD)	N	246	Buchalter, Maury (MD)	Ped	885
Brevetti, Gregorio (MD)	S	546	Buchbinder, Ellen (MD)	A&I	150
Brewer, Marlon (MD)	IM	569	Buchbinder, Mitchell (MD)	U	703
Brickman, Alan (MD)	EDM	490	Buchbinder, Shalom (MD)	Rad	462
Brickner, Gary (MD)	ObG	943	Bucholtz, Harvey K (MD)	EDM	956
Brief, Donald (MD)	S	919	Buckley, Michael Kevin (MD)	S	1007
Brill, Joseph (MD)	Pul	826	Bucksbaum, Mark J (MD)	PMR	1028
Brimberg, Arthur (MD)	RadRO	828	Buda, Joseph A (MD)	S	384
Brion, Luc (MD)	NP	438	Budd, Daniel (MD)	S	1007
Brisson, Paul (MD)	OrS	286	Budin, Joel A (MD)	DR	866
Brittis, Robert (MD)	Ped	815	Budman, Cathy L (MD)	Psyc	688
Brock, William (MD)	U	703	Budow, Jack (MD)	Cv	630
Brodey, Marvin (MD)	D	170	Bufalini, Bruno (MD)	S	893
Brodherson, Michael (MD)	U	400	Buiumsohn, Arno (MD)	Ge	424
Brodie, Jonathan (MD)	Psyc	342	Bukberg, Judith (MD)	Psyc	343
Brodkin, Roger (MD)	D	901	Bukberg, Phillip (MD)	EDM	181
Brodman, Michael (MD)	ObG	257	Bukosky, Richard (MD)	A&I	1017
Brodman, Richard (MD)	TS	468	Bulanowski, Michael (MD)	Rhu	745
Brodman, Richard Rory (MD)	Rhu	1014	Bull, Marcia (MD)	Cv	1040
Brodsky, Samuel (MD)	Cv	1040	Bull, Sherman (MD)	S	1075
Brodyn, Nicholas (DO)	Cv	1018	Bullock, Richard (MD)	IM	958
Brolin, Robert E (MD)	S	968	Bulmash, Max (MD)	Ped	533
Bromberg, Assia (MD)	IM	871	Burack, Bernard (MD)	Cv	154
Bromberg, Kenneth (MD)	Ped	532	Burack, Joshua H (MD)	TS	550
Bromberg, Warren (MD)	U	836	Burak, George (MD)	OrS	804
Bronheim, Harold (MD)	Psyc	343	Burbige, Kevin (MD)	U	1077
Bronin, Andrew (MD)	D	765	Burchell, Albert (MD)	S	384
Bronson, Michael (MD)	OrS	286	Burd, Robert (MD)	Onc	1054
Bronster, David (MD)	N	246	Burde, Ronald (MD)	Oph	445
Bronsther, Burton (MD)	PS	678	Burg, Richard (MD)	CRS	765
Brook, David W (MD)	Psyc	343	Burger, Steven (MD)	S	465
Brookler, Kenneth (MD)	Oto	300	Burk, Peter (MD)	D	419
Brower, Mark (MD)	Onc	231	Burke, Gary R (MD)	IM	211
Brower, Steven (MD)	S	384	Burke, Jordan D (MD)	Oph	1025
Brown, Alan (MD)	Oph	269	Burke, Patricia (MD)	Oph	879
Brown, Alan Joseph (MD)	N	792	Burke, Stanley J (MD)	Oph	665
Brown, Andrew (MD)	PMR	329	Burke, Stephen W (MD)	OrS	286
Brown, Arthur E (MD)	Inf	205	Burkett, Eric (MD)	IM	975
Brown, Charles (MD)	OrS	804	Burns, Elisa (MD)	ObG	794
Brown, David (MD)	A&I	1017	Burns, Godfrey (MD)	Nep	238
Brown, Eric (MD)	Nep	1056	Burns, John J (MD)	Cv	955
Brown, Jeffrey (MD)	Ped	815	Burns, Les Alan (MD)	ObG	1005
Brown, John C (MD)	Onc	231	Burns, Mark (MD)	Rhu	830
Brown, Jordan (MD)	U	400	Burns, Paul (MD)	PM	847
Brown, Lawrence S (MD)	IM	502	Burris, James (MD)	Oph	800
Brown, Lionel (MD)	S	1075	Burroughs, Valentine (MD)	IM	211
Brown, Mitchell Lee (MD)	Ger	927	Burrow, Gerard (MD)	EDM	1045
Brown, Richard (MD)	Psyc	343	Burrows, Lewis (MD)	S	384
Brownstein, Howard (MD)	Oto	526	Burstin, Harris E (MD)	Ped	320
Brown-Wagner, Marie (MD)	Oto	808	Burstin, Stuart J (MD & PhD)	IM	1022
Bruce, Jeffrey (MD)	NS	876	Buscaino, Giacomo (MD)	Cv	482

NAME	SPECIALTY	PAGE	NAME	SPECIALTY	PAGE
Bush, Michael (MD)	IM	211	Carone, Patrick F (MD)	Psyc	688
Bush Jr, Harry (MD)	GVS	407	Caronna, John J (MD)	N	247
Busillo, Christopher (MD)	Inf	205	Carpenter, Duncan (MD)	NS	876
Bussel, James (MD)	Ped	321	Carr, Elizabeth (MD)	D	487
Butler, David (MD)	ObG	878	Carr, Ronald (MD)	Oph	269
Butler, Robert (MD)	GerPsy	198	Carras, Robert (MD)	NS	658
Butt, Khalid (MD)	GVS	839	Carroll, Michael (MD)	OrS	669
Buxton, Douglas (MD)	Oph	269	Carson, Jeffrey (MD)	IM	959
Buxton, Jorge (MD)	Oph	269	Carsons, Steven (MD)	Rhu	694
Buyon, Jill P (MD)	Rhu	377	Carter, Mitchel (MD)	S	998
Buzzeo, Louis (MD)	Nep	789	Carty, Elyse (MD)	FP	939
Bye, Michael R (MD)	Ped	321	Carty, Robert (MD)	FP	939
Byrd, Lawrence H (MD)	Nep	907	Caruana, Joseph (DO)	FP	491
Bystryn, Jean Claude (MD)	D	170	Caruso, Anthony (MD)	Oto	735
			Caruso, Rocco (MD)	Onc	724
C			Carvajal, Simeon (MD)	Ge	424
			Carver, David (MD)	Ped	964
Cabbad, Michael (MD)	ObG	517	Casale, Linda (MD)	Cv	1041
Caccese, William (MD)	Ge	643	Casale Jr, Alfred Stanley (MD)	Cv	987
Cafferty, Maureen (MD)	N	246	Casden, Andrew (MD)	OrS	286
Cahan, Anthony (MD)	S	384	Case, David B (MD)	IM	211
Cahan, William George (MD)	S	384	Casey, Joan (MD)	IM	431
Cahill, John (MD)	FP	422	Casino, Joseph (MD)	Pul	826
Cahill, Kevin Michael (MD)	PrM	340	Casper, Daniel (MD)	Oph	800
Calabrese, Carmine (MD)	PlS	1068	Casper, Ephraim (MD)	Onc	991
Calamia, Vincent (MD)	EDM	604	Casper, Theodore (MD)	Pul	460
Calio, Anthony (MD)	IM	649	Cass, Alison (MD)	Ped	1065
Call, Pamela (MD)	Psyc	343	Cassel, Christine (MD)	Ger	197
Calman, Neil (MD)	FP	186	Cassell, Lauren (MD)	S	385
Cam, Jenny (MD)	EDM	926	Cassidy, Brian (MD)	IM	1022
Camacho, Fernando (MD)	Hem	428	Casson, Ira (MD)	N	573
Camel, Mark (MD)	NS	1057	Casson, Phillip (MD)	PlS	333
Camilien, Louis (MD)	ObG	517	Cassvan, Arminius (MD)	PMR	683
Camins, Martin B (MD)	NS	242	Castellano, Bartolomeo (MD)	Oto	614
Cammarata, Angelo (MD)	S	384	Castellano, Michael A (MD)	Pul	618
Campbell, Deborah (MD)	NP	438	Castellino, Ronald A (MD)	Rad	371
Campion, Robert E (MD)	Psyc	343	Castro, Zoila Yolanda (MD)	FP	926
Camunas, Jorge (MD)	TS	395	Castroll, Robert (MD)	Psyc	741
Cancellieri, Russell (MD)	A&I	711	Castro-Magana, Mariano (MD)	PEn	676
Cancro, Robert (MD)	Psyc	343	Catalano, Peter (MD)	Oto	300
Candelaria, Luis (MD)	FP	491	Cataletto, Mauro (MD)	OrS	669
Canino, Ian (MD)	Psyc	343	Caucino, Julie (DO)	A&I	937
Canter, Robert (MD)	EM	639	Caushaj, Philip (MD)	CRS	1042
Cantor, Michael C (MD)	Ge	188	Cavaliere, Gregg (MD)	SM	830
Capizzi, Anthony (MD)	S	746	Cavaliere, Ludovico (MD)	Rhu	464
Caplan, Ronald (MD)	ObG	257	Cayten, C Gene (MD)	S	465
Capobianco, Luigi (MD)	FP	641	Cea, Philip (MD)	U	469
Capone, Robert (MD)	Pul	996	Cece, John (MD)	Oto	1006
Capozzi, James (MD)	OrS	286	Cehelsky, John Ihor (MD)	S	831
Caputo, Anthony (MD)	Oph	910	Cemaletin, Nevber (MD)	Cv	154
Caputo, Thomas A (MD)	GO	199	Cenedese, Luis (MD)	PlS	333
Carabelli, Robert (MD)	PMR	946	Cerabona, Thomas D (MD)	SCC	835
Caracci, Giovanni (MD)	Psyc	343	Cerny, Kenneth (MD)	N	992
Caraccio, Babette (MD)	Psyc	1069	Ceron-Canas, L Carolina (MD)	Ped	680
Cardiello, Gary P (MD)	IM	928	Cerulli, Maurice (MD)	Ge	494
Cardoso, Erico R (MD)	NS	513	Cervia, Joseph (MD)	IM	211
Carey, Dennis (MD)	PEn	581	Chabot, John A (MD)	S	385
Carlon, Graziano (MD)	CCM	168	Chafizadeh, Mohsen (MD)	S	831
Carlson, Gabrielle A (MD)	Psyc	741	Chahrouri, Joseph (MD)	Rhu	544
Carmel, Peter (MD)	NS	907	Chaiken, Barry (MD)	Oph	269
Carmichael, David (MD)	IM	211	Chaiken, Rochelle (MD)	EDM	490
Carnevale, Nino (MD)	S	465	Chalas, Eva (MD)	ObG	728
Carney, Alexander (MD)	Rhu	949	Chambers, Joseph (MD)	GO	1047
Carolan, Patrick (MD)	OrS	1061	Chandler, James (MD)	S	949
Carolan, Stephen (MD)	ObG	794			

NAME	SPECIALTY	PAGE	NAME	SPECIALTY	PAGE
Chandler, Michael (MD)	A&I	150	Chou, Shyan-yih (MD)	Nep	511
Chandra, Pradeep (MD)	Onc	508	Choudhury, Muhammad (MD)	U	836
Chandra, Prasanta C (MD)	ObG	517	Chowdhury, Fazlur R (MD)	EDM	716
Chandrasekhar, Sujana (MD)	Oto	912	Chown, Judith (MD)	EDM	716
Chang, Edwin (MD)	NS	610	Chrisanderson, Donna (MD)	IM	904
Chang, James (MD)	DR	178	Christman, J Eric (MD)	ObG	992
Chang, John (MD)	GVS	705	Chu, Wing (MD)	Oph	270
Chang, Patrick (MD)	S	920	Chuang, Linus (MD)	GO	777
Chang, Stanley (MD)	Oph	269	Chun, Jin (MD)	PlS	333
Chanin, Irving (MD)	S	696	Chung, Henry (MD)	Psyc	344
Chapman, Mark (MD)	Ge	188	Chung-Loy, Harold (MD)	S	968
Chapnick, Edward (MD)	Inf	500	Chutorian, Abe (MD)	ChiN	165
Charap, Peter (MD)	IM	212	Ciccone, John (MD)	Cv	899
Charles, Norman (MD)	Oph	270	Ciccone, Patrick (MD)	U	921
Charney, Jonathan (MD)	N	247	Ciccone, Ralph (MD)	Pul	618
Charnoff, Judah (MD)	Cv	482	Cimino, Ernest (MD)	PlS	947
Charytan, Chaim (MD)	Nep	438	Cimino, James (MD)	IM	212
Chase, Norman (MD)	NRad	254	Cimino, James E (MD)	IM	431
Chaudhry, Rashid M (MD)	Oto	526	Cimino, Joseph (MD)	PrM	821
Chaudhry, Saqib S (MD)	GVS	594	Ciocon, Hermogenes (MD)	TS	1008
Chavez, Alberto (MD)	NP	1012	Cioroiu, Michael (MD)	S	385
Chazotte, Cynthia (MD)	MF	436	Cipollaro, Vincent (MD)	D	170
Checton, John (MD)	Cv	973	Citron, Charles (MD)	DR	715
Cheigh, Jhoong (MD)	Nep	239	Citron, Marc L (MD)	Onc	655
Chekofsky, Kenneth (MD)	HS	975	Ciuffo, Joseph (MD)	FP	564
Chen, Chia-maou (MD)	IM	607	Clain, David (MD)	IM	212
Chen, Hua Chin (MD)	Ped	533	Claps, Richard (MD)	DR	988
Chen, James (MD)	EDM	1020	Clark, Luther T (MD)	Cv	482
Chengot, Mathew (MD)	Cv	712	Clark, Richard (MD)	D	714
Chern, Relly (MD)	Oph	270	Clark, Sheryl (MD)	D	170
Chernack, William J (MD)	PA&I	994	Clarke, James (MD)	S	385
Chernaik, Richard (MD)	IM	431	Clay, Lucius (MD)	S	949
Chernaik, Robert (MD)	IM	721	Cleary, Joseph (MD)	S	385
Chernik, Norman (MD)	N	726	Cleman, Michael (MD)	Cv	1041
Cherofsky, Alan (MD)	PlS	617	Clemente, Jack (MD)	ChAP	900
Cherry, Sheldon (MD)	ObG	257	Clements, Jerry (MD)	FP	186
Chertoff, Harvey (MD)	Psyc	888	Close, Lanny Garth (MD)	Oto	301
Chervenak, Frank (MD)	ObG	258	Coco, Maria (MD)	IM	431
Chesner, Michael (MD)	Cv	630	Coddon, David R (MD)	N	247
Chess, Jeremy (MD)	Oph	800	Cody, Hiram (MD)	S	385
Chessin, Robert (MD)	Ped	1066	Coffey, Robert (MD)	Ped	321
Chevinsky, Aaron (MD)	S	998	Coffey, Tom (MD)	Oto	1063
Chia, Gloria (MD)	IM	780	Cofsky, Richard (MD)	Inf	500
Chianese, Maurice (MD)	Ped	680	Cohall, Alwyn (MD)	AM	149
Chiaramida, Salvatore (MD)	Cv	416	Cohen, Alfred M (MD)	CRS	166
Chiaramonte, Joseph (MD)	A&I	711	Cohen, Arnold (MD)	Psyc	344
Chideckel, Norman (MD)	GVS	407	Cohen, Barry (MD)	IM	502
Chin, Jean (MD)	ObG	258	Cohen, Ben (MD)	Oph	270
Chinitz, Marvin (MD)	Ge	774	Cohen, Bertram (MD)	PS	532
Chiorazzi, Nicholas (MD)	A&I	627	Cohen, Bradley (MD)	S	746
Chisolm, Alvin (MD)	Rad	829	Cohen, Burton A (MD)	DR	178
Chitkara, Dev (MD)	Oto	735	Cohen, Carl (MD)	GerPsy	497
Chiu, David T W (MD)	PlS	333	Cohen, Carmel (MD)	GO	199
Cho, Hyun (MD)	Oto	300	Cohen, Charmian (MD)	EDM	420
Cho, John (MD)	Hem	202	Cohen, Daniel (MD)	N	726
Chodock, Allen (MD)	Rhu	830	Cohen, Daniel H (MD)	Rhu	694
Chodosh, Eliot (MD)	N	1005	Cohen, David (MD)	Nep	239
Chodosh, Ronald (MD)	Pul	826	Cohen, David (MD)	Pul	690
Choe, Dai-sun (MD)	S	546	Cohen, Donald (MD)	ChAP	1042
Choi, Mihye (MD)	PlS	965	Cohen, Elliot L (MD)	U	400
Choi, Young (MD)	PM	963	Cohen, Harris L (MD)	DR	489
Chokroverty, Sudhans (MD)	N	247	Cohen, Herbert J (MD)	Ped	453
Chorney, Gail (MD)	OrS	286	Cohen, Joel (MD)	N	440
Chou, James (MD)	Psyc	344	Cohen, Jon (MD)	GVS	594

DIRECTORY OF DOCTORS

NAME	SPECIALTY	PAGE	NAME	SPECIALTY	PAGE
Cohen, Larry (MD)	Ge	188	Conte, Charles (MD)	S	696
Cohen, Lawrence (MD)	Cv	1041	Conway Jr, Edward E (MD)	Ped	815
Cohen, Lawrence (MD)	ObG	517	Cook, Jack (MD)	Oph	665
Cohen, Lee (MD)	ChAP	763	Cook, Perry (MD)	Onc	508
Cohen, Leeber (MD)	Oph	270	Cook, Stuart (MD)	N	908
Cohen, Martin (MD)	CRS	765	Cooke, Joseph T (MD)	Pul	364
Cohen, Martin (MD)	Cv	759	Cooney, Leo (MD)	Rhu	1073
Cohen, Martin (MD)	Ped	995	Cooper, Arnold (MD)	Psyc	344
Cohen, Maurice (MD)	Oto	526	Cooper, Dennis (MD)	Onc	1054
Cohen, Michael (MD)	IM	212	Cooper, Jay (MD)	RadRO	368
Cohen, Michael (MD)	Pul	690	Cooper, Jerome (MD)	Cv	759
Cohen, Michel (MD)	Ped	321	Cooper, Louis Z (MD)	Ped	321
Cohen, Neil (MD)	EDM	604	Cooper, Milton (MD)	IM	1051
Cohen, Noel (MD)	Oto	301	Cooper, Paul (MD)	NS	242
Cohen, Paul (MD)	Ge	494	Cooper, Robert (MD)	Ge	189
Cohen, Richard (MD)	Ped	964	Cooper, Robert (MD)	IM	1051
Cohen, Richard P (MD)	IM	212	Cooper, Rubin (MD)	PCd	675
Cohen, Sally (MD)	IM	872	Cooperman, Alan (MD)	ObG	909
Cohen, Seth (MD)	Ge	188	Cooperman, Avram M (MD)	S	831
Cohen, Seymour (MD)	Onc	231	Coplan, Jeremy (MD)	Psyc	344
Cohen, Stephen (MD)	U	895	Copland, Richard (MD)	Oph	270
Cohen, Steven (DO)	D	170	Copperman, Stuart (MD)	Ped	680
Cohen, Steven (MD)	DR	1044	Coppola, John (MD)	Cv	154
Cohen-Addad, Nicole (MD)	NP	237	Corapi, Mark (MD)	IM	649
Cohn, Steven (MD)	IM	502	Corbo, Emanuel (MD)	Ped	1027
Cohn, William (MD)	Ge	718	Cordero, Evelyn (MD)	FP	422
Coit, Daniel (MD)	S	385	Coren, Charles (MD)	PS	678
Colangelo, Daniel (MD)	IM	780	Corio, Laura (MD)	ObG	258
Colantonio, Anthony (MD)	S	696	Cornell, Charles (MD)	OrS	287
Colby, Steven (MD)	Inf	500	Cornell, James (MD & PhD)	CCM	864
Cole, Jeffrey L (MD)	PMR	585	Corpus, Marina (MD)	Ped	615
Cole, Robert (MD)	RadRO	997	Corpuz, Marilou (MD)	Inf	429
Cole, Steven A (MD)	Psyc	586	Correia, Joaquim (MD)	CE	899
Cole, William Joseph (MD)	Cv	154	Correoso, Lyla J (MD)	PM	449
Colella, Frank (MD)	Onc	508	Corriel, Robert (MD)	A&I	627
Coleman, D J (MD)	Oph	270	Corso, Salvatore (MD)	OrS	669
Coleman, John (MD)	U	400	Cortes, Engracio P (MD)	Onc	571
Coleman, Monroe (MD)	A&I	1039	Cortes, Hiram (MD)	Inf	500
Coleman, Morton (MD)	Onc	232	Cortese, Armand (MD)	S	385
Colen, Helen S (MD)	PlS	333	Coryllos, Elizabeth (MD)	PS	679
Colen, Stephen (MD)	PlS	333	Coscia, Anthony (MD)	Onc	1055
Colenda, Maryann (MD)	PA&I	883	Cossari, Alfred (MD)	Oph	731
Coll, Raymond (MD)	N	247	Costa, John (MD)	Ped	815
Collens, Richard (MD)	IM	212	Costa, Leon (MD)	OrS	944
Coller, Barry (MD)	IM	212	Costantino, Thomas (MD)	Cv	602
Collins, Adriane (DO)	Inf	720	Costin, Andrew (MD)	Cv	937
Collins, Allen H (MD)	Psyc	344	Coupey, Susan (MD)	AM	415
Coloka-Kump, Rodika (DO)	FP	771	Cournos, Francine (MD)	Psyc	344
Colombo, Antonio (MD)	Cv	154	Courtney, Barbara (MD)	IM	976
Colvin, Stephen (MD)	Cv	154	Coven, Barbara (MD)	Ped	816
Comes, Bina (MD)	Ped	533	Coven, Roger (MD)	ObG	878
Comfort, Christopher P (MD)	IM	431	Covey, William (MD)	IM	1051
Comrie, Millicent (MD)	ObG	518	Covit, Andrew (MD)	Nep	960
Concannon, Patrick (MD)	ObG	575	Cox, D Sayer (MD)	IM	213
Condo, Dominick (MD)	IM	928	Cox, Kathryn (MD)	ObG	258
Condon, Edward (MD)	IM	649	Coyle, Michael (MD)	HS	958
Connery, Cliff (MD)	TS	396	Craft, Joseph (MD)	Rhu	1073
Connolly, Adrian L (MD)	D	901	Craig, Edward V (MD)	OrS	287
Connolly, Mark (MD)	TS	550	Craig, Nicholas (MD)	S	746
Connor, Bradley A (MD)	Ge	188	Craig-Scott, Susan (MD)	PlS	334
Connor, Thomas (MD)	Ped	885	Cramer, Marvin (MD)	Cv	630
Consiglio, Michael (MD)	N	514	Crane, Richard (MD)	Rhu	377
Constad, William H (MD)	Oph	930	Crasta, Jovita (MD)	Psyc	741
Constantiner, Arturo (MD)	IM	212	Crawford, Bernard (MD)	TS	396

NAME	SPECIALTY	PAGE	NAME	SPECIALTY	PAGE
Cristofaro, Robert (MD)	OrS	805	Davies, Edward (MD)	Ped	321
Croen, Kenneth (MD)	IM	780	Davies, Terry (MD)	EDM	181
Croll, James (MD)	Nep	439	Davis, Anne (MD)	IM	213
Crovello, James (MD)	Psyc	741	Davis, George (MD)	IM	976
Crowe, John (MD)	OrS	1061	Davis, Jessica (MD)	MG	230
Cruickshank, David (MD)	U	749	Davis, Jonathan (MD)	NP	656
Cruz, Merle Correa (MD)	Cv	925	Davis, Joseph (MD)	U	400
Crystal, Howard (MD)	N	440	Davis, Joyce (MD)	D	170
Cullen, Mark R (MD)	OM	1060	Davis, Kenneth (MD)	Psyc	345
Cunha, Burke A (MD)	Inf	647	Davis, Kenneth J (MD)	Ped	1027
Cunningham, John (MD)	S	385	Davis, Raphael (MD)	NS	726
Cunningham, Joseph (MD)	TS	550	Davis, William J (MD)	A&I	150
Cunningham, Ward (MD)	IM	213	Davison, Edward (MD)	Cv	630
Cunningham-Rundles,			Daya, Rami (MD)	Hem	498
Charlotte (MD & PhD)	A&I	150	DeAlleaume, Lauren (MD)	FP	771
Cuomo, Frances (MD)	OrS	287	Deane, Leland M (MD)	PlS	684
Curras, Ernesto (MD)	S	465	De Angelis, Arthur (MD)	IM	780
Curtin, John P (MD)	GO	199	De Angelis, Lisa (MD)	N	247
Curtis, James (MD)	Psyc	344	De Angelis, Roger (MD)	S	831
Cusumano, Barbara (MD)	Ped	738	De Angelis, Vincent (MD)	S	746
Cusumano, Stephen (MD)	IM	649	De Antonio, Joseph (MD)	Ge	939
Cutler, Lawrence (MD)	ObG	258	De Araujo, Maria (MD)	PMR	457
Cutolo Jr, Louis C (MD)	PlS	617	De Bellis, Joseph L (MD)	PlS	740
Cutting, Court (MD)	PlS	334	DeBellis, Robert H (MD)	IM	213
Cuttner, Janet (MD)	Hem	202	DeBlasi, Henry (MD)	Oto	735
Cykiert, Robert (MD)	Oph	270	Deblasio, Maria (MD)	FP	422
			Debrovner, Charles (MD)	ObG	258
D			De Caprariis, Pascal (MD)	FP	492
			De Caprio, Vincent (MD)	S	832
D'Agostini, Robert (MD)	OrS	1013	De Carlo, Alan (MD)	Cv	712
D'Agostino, Ronald (MD)	Cv	630	Deck, Michael (MD)	Rad	372
Dakofsky, LaDonna J (MD)	RadRO	1072	Decker, Robert (MD)	NS	658
Dalena, John (MD)	Ge	989	Decorato, John (MD)	PlS	617
Dalgin, Paul (MD)	Rhu	1073	Decosimo, Diana R (MD)	IM	904
Daliana, Maurizion (MD)	S	386	Decosse, Jerome (MD)	S	386
Dalton, Jack F (MD)	RadRO	589	De Cristofaro, Joseph D (MD)	NP	725
Daly, John M (MD)	S	386	Decter, Edward (MD)	OrS	911
D'Amico, Richard (MD)	PlS	888	Decter, Julian A (MD)	Onc	906
D'Amico, Robert (MD)	Oph	271	Dedousis, John T (MD)	IM	928
D'Amico, Vincent M (MD)	ObG	794	De Fabritus, Albert (MD)	Nep	239
Damus, Paul S (MD)	TS	700	De France, John (MD)	TS	1076
Danehower, Richard L (MD)	Rhu	1073	Degann, Sona (MD)	ObG	258
D'Angelo, Enrico (MD)	FP	422	De Groote, Robert (MD)	GVS	896
Daniello, Nicholas (MD)	Oto	448	Deitch, Edwin (MD)	S	920
Daniels, Jeff (MD)	Cv	973	Deitz, Joel (MD)	IM	940
Danilowicz, Delores (MD)	PCd	310	Deitz, Marcia (MD)	D	488
D'Anna, John (MD)	S	620	Delaney, Brian (MD)	FP	422
Dantuono, Louise (MD)	ObG	258	Delano, Barbara (MD)	Nep	511
Dantzker, David (MD)	Pul	587	Delany, Harry (MD)	S	465
Daras, Michael (MD)	N	247	de Larosa, Maritza (MD)	FP	492
Dardik, Herbert (MD)	GVS	895	de Leo, Vincent A (MD)	D	170
D'Arienzo, Nicholas (MD)	Ped	583	DelGuercio, Louis (MD)	TS	835
Das, Seshadri (MD)	EDM	604	Delisa, Joel (MD)	PMR	916
Dasgupta, Indira (MD)	PHO	451	Dell'Aria, Joseph (MD)	EM	1044
Das Gupta, Manash K (MD)	Nep	789	Della Rocca, Robert (MD)	Oph	271
Dash, Greg (MD)	Oto	735	Delman, Michael (MD)	IM	722
Dasmahapatra, Kumar (MD)	S	968	Del Monte, Mary (MD)	Nep	511
Daum, Fredric (MD)	PGe	676	Delorenzo, Lawrence (MD)	Pul	827
Dave, Mahendraray (MD)	Nep	439	De Los Reyes, Raul (MD)	NS	242
Davenport, Deborah M (MD)	ObG	728	Del Rowe, John (MD)	RadRO	461
David, Raphael (MD)	PEn	312	DeLuca, Albert (MD)	Cv	759
David, Sami (MD)	RE	374	Deluca, Frank Ross (MD)	S	465
Davidson, Morton (MD)	IM	213	Demar, Leon (MD)	D	170
Davidson, Steven (MD)	EM	489	De Maria, Frank (MD)	Ped	886
Davidson, William (MD)	Oto	945			

DIRECTORY OF DOCTORS

NAME	SPECIALTY	PAGE	NAME	SPECIALTY	PAGE
De Matteo, Robert (MD)	IM	780	Di Scala, Reno (MD)	FP	564
Demento, Frank (MD)	D	637	Distenfeld, Ariel (MD)	IM	213
Demetis, Spiro (MD)	CCM	487	Dittmar, Klaus (MD)	Hem	646
Demos, Nicholas (MD)	TS	933	Diuguid, David L (MD)	Hem	202
Denehy, Thad (MD)	GO	903	Divack, Daniel (MD)	ObG	662
Dennett, Ronald (MD)	IM	780	Dlugi, Alexander M (MD)	RE	997
Dennis, Robert (MD)	OrS	978	Dobbs, Joan (MD)	Onc	724
Denton, John (MD)	OrS	578	Dobson, Chauncey (MD)	OrS	805
De Pasquale, Joseph (MD)	Ge	902	Docherty, John P (MD)	Psyc	822
De Pietro, William (MD)	D	637	Doctor, Naishad (MD)	PlS	684
De Puey, Ernest (MD)	NuM	255	Dodick, Jack M (MD)	Oph	271
Derespinis, Patrick (MD)	Oph	612	Doidge, Robert (DO)	OrS	881
De Risi, Dwight (MD)	S	696	Dolan, Anna (MD)	Psyc	822
Derman, Robert (MD)	Psyc	741	Dolan, John (MD)	Psyc	1069
Dermksian, George (MD)	IM	213	Dolgin, Stephen (MD)	PS	319
De Rose, Joseph J (MD)	IM	502	Dolich, Barry (MD)	PlS	458
Dershaw, D David (MD)	DR	178	Dolitsky, Charisse (MD)	D	637
Dervan, John (MD)	Cv	712	Dolitsky, Jay (MD)	Oto	301
DeSilva Jr, Derrick M (MD)	IM	959	Don, Philip (MD & PhD)	D	419
Desnick, Robert (MD)	MG	230	Donath, Joseph (MD)	Pul	587
Desposito, Franklin (MD)	MG	906	Donnelly, Christine (MD)	PCd	994
D'Esposito, Michael (MD)	FP	717	Donnelly, Harrison (MD)	Inf	568
Deutsch, James A (MD)	Oph	520	Donnenfeld, Eric D (MD)	Oph	665
Devereux, Corinne (MD)	Rad	919	Donovan, Denis (MD)	FP	772
Devereux, Richard (MD)	IM	213	Dooley, Evelyn (MD)	IM	502
Devinsky, Orrin (MD)	N	247	Dor, Nathan (MD)	ObG	518
DeVivo, Darryl C (MD)	ChiN	165	Doshi, Leena (MD)	Rad	589
Dhar, Santi (MD)	Pul	540	Dosik, Harvey (MD)	Hem	499
Dharmarajin, T S (MD)	Nep	439	Dosik, Michael (MD)	Onc	724
Diamond, Betty A (MD)	Rhu	464	Dossa, Christos (MD)	GVS	622
Diamond, Ezriel (MD)	RadRO	692	Dottino, Joseph (MD)	ObG	662
Diamond, Sharon (MD)	ObG	258	Dottino, Peter (MD)	GO	199
Diamond, Steven (MD)	PHO	884	Dotto, Myles (MD)	ObG	878
Diamond, William (MD)	Ped	680	Douedi, Hani Ramses (MD)	IM	928
Diaz, Maria (MD)	IM	431	Dougan, Hughes (MD)	S	998
Diaz, Michael (MD)	Hem	202	Douglas, Carolyn (MD)	Psyc	345
Di Buono, Mark (MD)	Psyc	618	Douglas, Montgomery (MD)	FP	564
Di Cesare, Paul (MD)	OrS	287	Dower, Samuel (MD)	IM	905
Dick, Harold (MD)	OrS	287	Dowling, Sean (MD)	RadRO	1072
Dickoff, David (MD)	N	792	Dowling, Thomas (MD)	OrS	733
DiCosmo, Bruno F (MD)	Pul	827	Downey, John (MD)	PMR	329
Dieck, Eileen (MD)	IM	781	Dozor, Allen (MD)	PPul	813
Dieck, William (MD)	Oph	800	Drachtman, Richard (MD)	Ped	965
Diehl, William (MD)	S	998	Drake, William (MD)	Oto	1026
Dieterich, Douglas (MD)	Ge	189	Dranitzke, Richard (MD)	TS	748
Dietrich, Marianne (DO)	FP	422	Drapkin, Arnold (MD)	IM	214
Digiacinto, George (MD)	NS	242	Drascher, Gary (MD)	S	1014
Di Giacomo, William (MD)	IM	904	Drayer, Burton P (MD)	DR	178
Di Gregorio, Vincent (MD)	PlS	684	Dresdale, Robert (MD)	Cv	630
Diktaban, Theodore (MD)	PlS	334	Drew, Michael (MD)	S	591
Dila, Carl (MD)	NS	1057	Drexler, Andrew (MD)	EDM	181
Dilello Sr, Edmund (MD)	Ped	583	Drexler, Ellen (MD)	N	514
Di Leo, Frank (MD)	Oph	731	Dreyer, Neil (MD)	IM	1051
Dillon, Robert (MD)	U	400	Dreyfus, Norma (MD)	Ped	816
Dilorenzo, Randolph (MD)	IM	649	Drillings, Gary (MD)	OrS	1005
Dimaio, Mary (MD)	PPul	317	Drimmer, Marc Alan (MD)	PlS	947
Dimancescu, Mihai (MD)	NS	658	Driscoll, John (MD)	NP	237
Di Maso, Gerald (MD)	IM	607	Droller, Michael J (MD)	U	400
Dines, David (MD)	OrS	669	Dropkin, Lloyd (MD)	Oto	301
Dinnerstein, Stephen (MD)	Oph	271	Drucker, David (MD)	OrS	613
Di Pasquale, Laurene (MD)	IM	872	Drusin, Ronald (MD)	Cv	155
Di Pietro, Joseph (MD)	D	765	Druss, Richard (MD)	Psyc	345
Dipillo, Frank (MD)	Hem	498	Dubin, David (MD)	RadRO	891
DiPirro, Earl (MD)	PlS	888			

NAME	SPECIALTY	PAGE	NAME	SPECIALTY	PAGE
Dubois, Michel (MD)	PM	308	Eisenstein, Elliot (MD)	Ped	1006
Duboys, Elliot (MD)	PlS	684	Eisert, Jack (MD)	D	766
Dubrow, Eric N (MD)	OrS	733	Eisner, Leslie (MD)	Oph	1060
Dubuoys, Elliot (MD)	PlS	684	Elamir, Mazhar (MD)	Pul	932
Duchnowska, Alicja (MD)	Ped	615	Elbirt-Bender, Paula (MD)	Ped	321
Dudick, Stephen T (MD)	PlS	979	El-Dakkak, Mohammed (MD)	OrS	287
Duffy, Kent (MD)	NS	791	Elefteriades, John (MD)	TS	1076
Duffy, Thomas (MD)	Hem	1049	Elfenbein, Joseph (MD)	OrS	805
Dulit, Everett P (MD)	Psyc	822	Elias, Jack (MD)	Pul	1070
Duncan, Albert (MD)	S	546	Elias, Steven (MD)	S	893
Duncan, Charles C (MD)	NS	1057	Elkin, Rene (MD)	N	441
Dunst, Maurice (MD)	IM	502	Elkind, Barry M (MD)	Cv	925
Durante, Anthony (MD)	Oto	672	Ellis, Earl A (MD)	IM	502
Durban, Lawrence (MD)	TS	700	Ells, Peter F (MD)	IM	722
Dutcher, Janice P (MD)	Onc	437	Ellstein, Jerry (MD)	OrS	734
Duva, Joseph (MD)	Ge	718	El-Rafei, Nabil (MD)	Psyc	1007
Du Vigneaud, Vincent (MD)	ObG	794	El-Sadr, Wafaa (MD)	IM	214
Dworetzky, Murray (MD)	A&I	150	Eltan, Noam (MD)	Psyc	741
Dworkin, Brad (MD)	Ge	774	Elwyn, Katherine (MD)	S	832
Dworkin, Gregory (MD)	PPul	1065	Emre, Umit Berk (MD)	PPul	531
Dwyer, Edward (MD)	Cv	899	Ende, Leigh (MD)	HS	989
Dyal, Cherise M (MD)	OrS	446	Enden, Jay B (MD)	Pul	743
Dyson, Robert (MD)	ObG	443	Eng, Kenneth (MD)	S	386
			Engber, Peter (MD)	D	603
			Engel, Milton (MD)	IM	214
E			Engel, Murray (MD)	N	1058
			Engel, Samuel (MD)	EDM	1045
Easton, Lon (MD)	Ped	454	Engler, Alan (MD)	PlS	334
Eaton, Richard (MD)	OrS	287	Engler, Mitchell (MD)	IM	872
Ebani, Jack (MD)	U	982	English, Joseph T (MD)	Psyc	345
Ebarb, Raymond (MD)	FP	717	Enker, Warren (MD)	S	386
Eberle, Mark Allen (MD)	Rhu	377	Ente, Gerald (MD)	Ped	680
Eberle, Robert (MD)	Oto	301	Epstein, Carol (MD)	IM	781
Economos, Katherine (MD)	GO	199	Epstein, Edward (MD)	Nep	572
Edelson, Charles (MD)	OrS	805	Epstein, Fred (MD)	PS	319
Edelson, Henry (MD)	IM	214	Epstein, Stanley (MD)	Cv	759
Edelson, Richard (MD)	D	1043	Erber, William (MD)	Ge	494
Edelstein, David (MD)	Oto	301	Ergin, M Arisan (MD & PhD)	TS	396
Edelstein, Martin (MD)	FP	641	Erichson, Robert (MD)	Onc	1055
Eden, Alvin N (MD)	Ped	583	Ernst, Jerome (MD)	Pul	460
Eden, Avrim (MD)	Oto	301	Errico, Thomas (MD)	OrS	288
Eden, Edward (MD)	Pul	364	Ertl, John (MD)	Ped	1066
Edersheim, Terri (MD)	ObG	258	Escobar, Javier I (MD)	Psyc	966
Edis, Gloria (MD)	Ped	816	Eshghi, Majid (MD)	U	836
Edsall, John (MD)	IM	214	Esman, Aaron H (MD)	Psyc	345
Edwards, Bruce (MD)	A&I	627	Esser, Aristide (MD)	Psyc	848
Efferen, Linda S (MD)	Pul	540	Essig, Mitchell (MD)	ObG	259
Effron, Charles (MD)	N	248	Estabrook, Alison (MD)	S	386
Efros, Barry (MD)	Rhu	997	Esteban, Nora (MD)	Ped	454
Eftekhar, Nas (MD)	OrS	287	Eswar, Sounder (MD)	HS	567
Eggers, Howard M (MD)	Oph	271	Etingin, Orli (MD)	IM	214
Eghrari, Massoud (MD)	S	747	Etra, William (MD)	U	401
Ehrlich, Elyse (MD)	IM	431	Ettinger, Lawrence (MD)	Ped	965
Ehrlich, Martin (MD)	IM	432	Eufemio, Michael (MD)	EDM	770
Ehrlich, Paul (MD)	PA&I	309	Eviatar, Abraham (MD)	Oto	448
Eichenbaum, Joseph (MD)	Oph	271	Eviatar, Lydia (MD)	N	573
Eichenfield, Andrew (MD)	Ped Rhu	318	Ezratty, Ari M (MD)	Cv	630
Eid, Francois (MD)	U	401			
Eilen, Bonnie (MD)	ObG	795	**F**		
Eingorn, David (MD)	OrS	944			
Eisenberg, Lee (MD)	Oto	882	Faber, Andrew (MD)	IM	781
Eisenberg, Robert (MD)	PCd	450	Fabian, Christopher (MD)	Psyc	345
Eisenberg, Sheldon (MD)	Cv	862	Fabian, Dennis (DO)	OrS	288
Eisenstat, Barrett (MD)	D	766	Facelle, Thomas (MD)	S	849
Eisenstat, Steven (DO)	FP	1020	Fagin, Bernard (MD)	U	837
Eisenstat, Theodore (MD)	CRS	1019			

DIRECTORY OF DOCTORS

NAME	SPECIALTY	PAGE	NAME	SPECIALTY	PAGE
Fagin, James (MD)	PA&I	674	Ferzli, George (MD)	S	620
Fahn, Stanley (MD)	N	248	Festa, Robert (MD)	Ped	739
Fahoum, Bashar (MD)	S	546	Fetell, Michael R (MD)	N	248
Fakharzadeh, Frederick (MD)	HS	869	Feuer, Martin (MD)	IM	214
Falco, Thomas (MD)	Cv	712	Fiedler, Robert (MD)	IM	215
Falcon, Ronald (MD)	D	637	Field, Barry (MD)	Ge	774
Falencki, John J (MD)	FP	186	Field, Steven (MD)	Ge	189
Falk, Theodore (MD)	A&I	861	Fieldman, Robert (MD)	Oto	912
Falkow, Seymour (MD)	FP	492	Fields, Abbie (MD)	GO	427
Faller, Jason (MD)	Rhu	377	Fields, Sheila (MD)	IM	872
Faltz, Lawrence L (MD)	Rhu	830	Fields, Theodore (MD)	Rhu	377
Fantini, Gary (MD)	GVS	407	Fiest, Thomas (DO)	Ge	975
Faraci, Nick (MD)	Ped	615	Figgie, Mark (MD)	OrS	288
Farber, Bruce (MD)	Inf	647	Fikrig, Senih (MD)	Ped	533
Farber, Charles (MD)	Ge	643	Filiberto, Cosmo (MD)	FP	1045
Fares II, Louis G (MD)	S	950	Filippone, Dennis (MD)	S	920
Farkas, Edward (MD)	Psyc	889	Fine, Emily (MD)	ObG	1059
Farkas, John (MD)	Ge	1003	Fine, Eugene M (MD)	U	401
Farmer, H Stephen (MD)	Oto	945	Fine, Herbert (MD)	D	864
Farrell, Robert (MD)	U	593	Fine, James (MD)	Psyc	538
Farris, R Linsy (MD)	Oph	271	Fine, Paul (MD)	Nep	991
Fasano, Carl (MD)	Oph	930	Fine, Richard (MD)	PNep	737
Fass, Arthur (MD)	Cv	759	Fine, Stanley (MD)	A&I	559
Fass, Daniel (MD)	RadRO	1072	Fineman, Sanford (MD)	NS	1024
Fass, Richard (MD)	Hem	778	Finger, Paul (MD)	Oph	271
Faust, Glenn (MD)	GVS	705	Fink, Matthew Earl (MD)	N	248
Faust, Michael (MD)	IM	214	Fink, Max (MD)	Psyc	688
Faust, Michael (MD)	ObG	878	Finkel, Jay (MD)	Psyc	345
Fazekas, John T (MD)	RadRO	589	Finkelman, Martin (MD)	Ped	533
Fazio, Nelson M (MD)	IM	781	Finkelstein, Jacob (MD)	S	832
Fazio, Richard (MD)	IM	607	Finkelstein, Martin Samuel (MD)	Ger	197
Fazzari, Patrick (MD)	PMR	329	Finkelstein, Michael (MD)	IM	781
Federbush, Richard (MD)	IM	649	Finlay, Jonathan (MD)	PHO	315
Federman, Harold (MD)	IM	781	Finley, David (MD)	S	832
Feghali, Joseph (MD)	Oto	448	Finley, Maria (MD)	ObG	575
Feigelson, Eugene (MD)	Psyc	538	Fiore, Americo S (MD)	RadRO	744
Feigenbaum, Howard (MD)	S	1007	Fiore, John J (MD)	Onc	724
Fein, Alan (MD)	Pul	690	Fisch, Arthur (MD)	Cv	987
Feinberg, Arthur W (MD)	IM	650	Fisch, Harry (MD)	U	401
Feinberg, Joseph (MD)	PlS	684	Fisch, Morton (MD)	IM	215
Feinstein, Neil (MD)	Oph	521	Fisch, Robert (MD)	Oph	577
Feinstein, Robert (MD)	D	637	Fischberg, Juan (MD)	PMR	931
Feit, David (MD)	Ge	868	Fischer, Harry (MD)	Rhu	377
Feld, Leonard (MD & PhD)	PNep	995	Fischer, Murry (MD)	S	386
Feld, Michael (MD)	Cv	759	Fischer, Rita (MD)	NP	237
Feldman, Alan (MD)	Onc	509	Fish, Bernard (MD)	PCd	810
Feldman, B Robert (MD)	A&I	150	Fish, Irving (MD)	ChiN	165
Feldman, David (MD)	PlS	537	Fishbach, Mitchell (MD)	Cv	760
Feldman, Frieda (MD)	Rad	372	Fisher, George (MD)	FP	564
Feldman, Jeffrey (MD)	IM	1022	Fisher, John D (MD)	Cv	416
Feldman, Philip (MD)	D	488	Fisher, Laura (MD)	IM	215
Feldman, Richard (MD)	Cv	759	Fisher, Lawrence (MD)	Cv	1041
Feldman, Robert (MD)	OrS	288	Fisher, Michael (MD)	D	419
Feldman, Stuart (MD)	Onc	788	Fisher, Stanley (MD)	PGe	529
Felig, Philip (MD)	EDM	181	Fisher, Yale (MD)	Oph	272
Felman, Yehudi (MD)	D	488	Fishkin, Michael (DO)	FP	717
Felsenstein, Jerome M (MD)	D	766	Fishman, Allen (MD)	Oph	577
Feltheimer, Seth (MD)	IM	214	Fishman, Donald (MD)	IM	215
Fennoy, Ilene (MD)	PEn	529	Fishman, Loren (MD)	PMR	585
Fernandes, David R (MD)	Ped	533	Fishman, Miriam (MD)	D	865
Fernbach, Barry (MD)	Hem	870	Fitzgerald, Denis (MD)	Onc	976
Ferran, Ernesto (MD)	Psyc	345	Flagg, Stephen (MD)	HS (PlS)	1068
Ferrier, Genevieve (MD)	Ped	321	Flanagan, Steven Robert (MD)	PMR	916
Ferriter, Pierce (MD)	OrS	288	Flatow, Evan (MD)	OrS	288

NAME	SPECIALTY	PAGE	NAME	SPECIALTY	PAGE
Flax, Herschel (MD)	S	465	Frager, Joseph (MD)	Ge	424
Fleischer, Adiel (MD)	ObG	662	Fram, Daniel K (MD)	RadRO	948
Fleischer, Arie (MD)	PlS	537	Frances, Richard (MD)	AdP	1039
Fleischer, Marian (MD)	CRS	486	Francfort, John (MD)	GVS	750
Fleischer, Norman (MD)	EDM	421	Franco, John (MD)	FP	717
Fleischman, Jay (MD)	Oph	445	Frank, Graeme (MD)	PEn	581
Fleischner, Gerald (MD)	Ge	424	Frank, Martin (MD)	Hem	870
Fleishman, Philip (MD)	IM	722	Frank, Michael (MD)	Ge	424
Fleishman, Stewart (MD)	Psyc	688	Frank, William (MD)	IM	722
Fleiss, David (MD)	SM	381	Frankel, Jeffrey (MD)	N	908
Fletcher, Stephen H (MD)	S	920	Frankel, Victor H (MD)	OrS	288
Flink, Elisheva (MD)	OrS	446	Franklin, Bonita (MD)	Ped	322
Flis, Raymond S (DO)	Nep	977	Franks Jr, Andrew G (MD)	D	171
Flogaites, Theodore (MD)	S	386	Franzetti, Carl (DO)	FP	422
Flores, Lucio (MD)	GVS	594	Fraser, Richard (MD)	NS	242
Florio, Francis (MD)	U	551	Frater, Robert (MD)	TS	468
Florio, Philip (MD)	ObG	795	Frattarola, Michael (MD)	ObG	1024
Flynn, Maryirene (MD)	OrS	613	Freddo, Lorenza (MD)	N	441
Flynn, William (MD)	Oto	808	Freed, Jeffrey (MD)	CRS	166
Focseneanu, Marius (MD)	PMR	329	Freedberg, Irwin M (MD)	D	171
Fodstad, Harald (MD)	NS	242	Freedman, Alan (MD)	PlS	685
Fogel, Mitchell (MD)	Nep	1056	Freedman, Jeffrey (MD & PhD)	Oph	521
Fogler, Richard (MD)	S	546	Freedman, Michael L (MD)	Ger	197
Fojas, Antonio (MD)	IM	432	Freedman, Pamela (MD)	Ge	989
Foley, Carmel (MD)	ChAP	561	Freeman, Harold (MD)	S	387
Foley, Conn J (MD)	IM	569	Freeman, Leonard M (MD)	NuM	443
Foley, Kathleen M (MD)	PM	308	Freeman, Ruth (MD)	EDM	421
Folkert, Vaughn W (MD)	Nep	439	Freeman, Susan (MD)	DR	769
Folman, Robert (MD)	Onc	1055	Freiman, Hal (MD)	Ge	189
Fomberstein, Barry (MD)	Rhu	464	Frenkel, Renata (MD)	A&I	150
Fonacier, Luz (MD)	A&I	627	Freuman, Henry (MD)	ObG	259
Fondacaro, Paul (MD)	S	387	Frey, Howard (MD)	U	895
Fong, Raymond (MD)	Oph	272	Fried, Kenneth (MD)	S	893
Foo, Sun-hoo (MD)	N	248	Fried, Richard (MD)	IM	215
Foong, Anthony (MD)	Ge	189	Fried, Sharon (MD)	D	865
Forbes, Max (MD)	Oph	272	Friedberg, Dorothy (MD)	Oph	272
Ford, Edward (MD)	OrS	944	Friedberg, Neal (MD)	Hem	499
Forde, Kenneth (MD)	S	387	Frieden, Faith (MD)	MF	874
Forget, Bernard (MD)	Hem	1049	Friedlander, Charles (MD)	Ge	189
Forlenza, Ronald (MD)	S	696	Friedlander, Marvin (MD)	N	961
Forlenza, Thomas (MD)	IM	607	Friedling, Steven (MD)	IM	722
Forman, Mark (MD)	TS	921	Friedman, Alan (MD)	Oph	272
Forman, Scott (MD)	Oph	800	Friedman, David (MD)	PS	885
Fornari, Victor (MD)	ChAP	635	Friedman, David (MD)	Psyc	346
Forster, George (MD)	N	248	Friedman, Deborah (MD)	PCd	310
Fort, Pavel (MD)	PEn	676	Friedman, Eli A (MD)	Nep	511
Forte, Francis (MD)	Hem	870	Friedman, Eliot (MD)	Onc	788
Forte, Frank (MD)	Hem	606	Friedman, Eugene (MD)	Ped	680
Fortunoff, Stephen (MD)	U	703	Friedman, Eugene W (MD)	S	387
Fost, Arthur (MD)	PA&I	912	Friedman, Frederick (MD)	ObG	259
Foster, Craig Allen (MD)	PlS	334	Friedman, Gerald (MD)	Ge	189
Foster, Jeffrey (MD)	Psyc	345	Friedman, Harvey Y (MD)	ObG	878
Fox, Arthur Charles (MD)	Cv	155	Friedman, Ira (MD)	S	387
Fox, Elaine E (MD)	Ger	719	Friedman, Jeffrey (MD)	IM	215
Fox, Herbert (MD)	Psyc	345	Friedman, Lawrence (MD)	Psyc	346
Fox, Joyce (MD)	MG	655	Friedman, Lorna (MD)	Ped	583
Fox, Mark (MD)	Oto	808	Friedman, Lynn (MD)	ObG	259
Fox, Martin (MD)	Oph	272	Friedman, Michael (MD)	D	1043
Fox, Sarah J (MD)	ChAP	163	Friedman, Norman (MD)	ObG	795
Fox, Stewart (MD)	TS	701	Friedman, Richard Alan (MD)	Psyc	346
Fox, Stuart (MD)	N	992	Friedman, Robert (MD)	Oph	272
Foxx, Martin (MD)	CRS	418	Friedman, Sam (MD)	IM	845
Foye, Gerard (MD)	MF	1054	Friedman, Sanford (MD)	Cv	155
Fracchia, John (MD)	U	401	Friedman, Seth (MD)	EDM	640

DIRECTORY OF DOCTORS

NAME	SPECIALTY	PAGE	NAME	SPECIALTY	PAGE
Friedman, Stanley (MD & PhD)	Psyc	346	Gannon, Fredric (MD)	Psyc	538
Friedman, Steven (MD)	U	551	Garay, Stuart (MD)	Pul	364
Friedman, Steven I (MD)	S	696	Garber, Perry (MD)	Oph	666
Friedman-Kien, Alvin (MD)	D	171	Garbitelli, Vincent (MD)	IM	650
Friedrich, Ivan (MD)	Ge	868	Garcia, Ariel (MD)	PlS	741
Frieri, Marianne (MD)	A&I	628	Garcia Jr, Jose G (MD)	S	832
Frimer, Richard (MD)	Pul	827	Gardner, Bernard (MD)	S	920
Frimmer, Daniel (MD)	Hem	1011	Gardner, Peter (MD)	Ge	1046
Frischer, Zelik (MD)	U	749	Gardner, Richard A (MD)	Psyc	889
Friscia, Philip (MD)	Onc	508	Garfein, Oscar (MD)	Cv	155
Frishman, William (MD)	Cv	760	Garfinkel, Burton (MD)	ObG	662
Frogel, Michael (MD)	Ped	680	Garfinkel, Howard (MD)	Nep	1056
Frohman, Larry (MD)	Oph	910	Garfinkel, Matthew (MD)	OrS	962
Frosch, William (MD)	Psyc	346	Gargiulo, Juan (MD)	PM	736
Frost, Elizabeth (MD)	Anes	758	Garjian, Peggy Ann (MD)	Rhu	619
Frost, James (MD)	S	1030	Garner, Bruce (MD)	Rhu	544
Fruchtman, Steven (MD)	Hem	202	Garner, Steven (MD)	Rad	542
Fuchs, Richard (MD)	Cv	155	Garrell, Marvin (MD)	IM	1051
Fuchs, Wayne (MD)	Oph	272	Garrick, Renee (MD)	Nep	789
Fuchs, Yael (DO)	ObG	518	Garrow, Eugene (MD)	PS	931
Fuhrman, Robert (MD)	IM	1022	Garroway, Robert (MD)	OrS	669
Fuks, Joachim (MD)	Onc	437	Gartenberg, Gary (MD)	Inf	958
Fuks, Zvi (MD)	RadRO	368	Gartenhaus, Willa (MD)	Hem	647
Fullilove, Mindy (MD)	Psyc	346	Garvey, Glenda Josephine (MD)	Inf	206
Fulop, Robert (MD)	IM	607	Garvey, Julius W (MD)	GVS	705
Funt, David (MD)	PlS	685	Garvey, Richard (MD)	S	1075
Funt, Tina (MD)	D	637	Garvin, James (MD)	PHO	315
Furey, Robert J (MD)	U	401	Gasalberti, Richard (MD)	PMR	585
Furie, Richard (MD)	IM	650	Gately, Adrian (MD)	Ped	533
Furman, Seymour (MD)	TS	468	Gattereau-Edwards, M (MD)	Ped	583
Fusillo, Christine (MD)	A&I	757	Gauthier, Bernard (MD)	PNep	582
Fuster, Valentin (MD & PhD)	Cv	155	Gayle, Lloyd (MD)	PlS	334
Futran-Sheinberg, Jacobo (MD)	Rhu	830	Gaylin, Willard (MD)	Psyc	346
Futterweit, Walter (MD)	EDM	181	Gaynor, Edward (MD)	Oto	1063
Fyer, Minna R (MD)	Psyc	346	Gaynor, Mitchell (MD)	Onc	232
			Gayola, George (MD)	TS	835
G			Gazzara, Paul (MD)	IM	607
			Gecelter, Gary (MD)	Ge	718
Gabbay, Mona (MD)	IM	432	Geders, Jane (MD & PhD)	Ge	495
Gabel, Richard (MD)	Psyc	822	Gee, Timothy S (MD)	Onc	232
Gabelman, Gary (MD)	Cv	760	Geffen, Merwin (MD)	Rad	462
Gabriel, James (MD)	IM	215	Geisler, Edward (MD)	U	469
Gabriel, Michael (MD)	Ped	533	Geiss, Alan (MD)	S	696
Gabrilove, J Lester (MD)	EDM	181	Gelberg, Burt (MD)	IM	650
Gacso, William (MD)	Anes	1040	Gelbfish, Joseph (MD)	Cv	483
Gaerlan, Pureza (MD)	Ped	322	Gelfand, Janice (MD)	Psyc	459
Gaffney, Joseph (MD)	PCd	964	Gelfand, Mathew (MD)	IM	650
Gafori, Iraj (MD)	GO	869	Geller, Mark (MD)	Rad	848
Gagliardi, Anthony (MD)	Pul	364	Geller, Peter (MD)	S	387
Gainey, Patrick (MD)	N	961	Geltzeiler, Jules (MD)	U	982
Gal, David (MD)	GO	645	Genato, Romulo (MD)	S	546
Galanter, Marc (MD)	Psyc	346	Gendelman, Seymour (MD)	N	248
Galdieri, Ralph (MD)	TS	621	Gendler, Ellen (MD)	D	171
Galeno, John (MD)	OrS	805	Genn, David (MD)	Ge	774
Gallagher, John F (MD)	S	747	Gennace, Ronald (MD)	OrS	911
Gallagher, Pamela (MD)	PlS	685	Genovese, Matthew L (MD)	S	832
Galler, Marilyn (MD)	Nep	572	Gentile, Ralph (MD)	U	469
Gallick, Gregory (MD)	OrS	1025	Gentilesco, Michael (MD)	ObG	728
Gallin, Pamela (MD)	Oph	273	Gentry, Eric (MD)	Pul	1071
Gallo, Victor A (MD)	CRS	636	George, Abraham (MD)	Cv	937
Gallousis, Spiro (MD)	ObG	518	George, Louis (MD)	Rad	967
Galloway, Aubrey (MD)	TS	396	Georgis, Michael (MD)	ObG	575
Gamache, Francis (MD)	NS	243	Georgsson, Maria (MD)	Ge	868
Gambert, Steven R (MD)	Ger	903	Georgsson, Sverrir (MD)	U	401
Gandhi, Rajinder (MD)	PS	885			

NAME	SPECIALTY	PAGE	NAME	SPECIALTY	PAGE
Geraci, Kira (MD)	A&I	757	Gitlow, Stanley (MD)	IM	215
Geraghty, Michael (MD)	Onc	509	Gittler, Robert (MD)	EDM	182
Gerard, Perry (MD)	DR	489	Giuffrida, Regina (MD)	ObG	795
Gerardi, Anthony (MD)	A&I	757	Giuliano, Michael (DO)	FP	902
Gerardi, Michael (MD)	EM	988	Giusti, Robert (MD)	PPul	531
Gerberg, Lynda Frances (MD)	SM	591	Gizzi, Martin (MD & PhD)	N	961
Gerbino-Rosen, Ginny (MD)	Psyc	459	Glabman, Sheldon (MD)	Nep	239
Gereme, Sebahat (MD)	D	488	Gladstein, Michael (MD)	D	638
Geronemus, Roy (MD)	D	171	Gladstone, Lenore (MD)	PMR	457
Gershberg, Herbert (MD)	EDM	181	Glaser, Amy (MD)	Ped	533
Gershell, William J (MD)	Psyc	347	Glaser, Morton (MD)	Pul	743
Gershengorn, Marvin (MD)	EDM	182	Glaser, Stephen (MD)	Ped	322
Gershon, Anne (MD)	Ped	322	Glass, Leonard (MD)	Ped	534
Gershowitz, Judith (MD)	ObG	259	Glass, Richard (MD)	Psyc	347
Gerson, Charles (MD)	Ge	189	Glass, Walter (MD)	Oto	672
Gersony, Welton (MD)	PCd	311	Glassberg, Kenneth (MD)	U	551
Gerst, Paul (MD)	TS	468	Glassman, Alexander (MD)	Psyc	347
Gertler, Menard (MD)	Cv	155	Glassman, Charles (MD)	U	837
Gettenberg, Gary (MD)	Ge	495	Glassman, Mark (MD)	PGe	812
Geuder, James (MD)	S	893	Glassman, Morris (MD)	Oph	800
Gevirtz, Clifford (MD & PhD)	PM	308	Glatt, Hershel (MD)	Ped	681
Gewirtz, George (MD)	IM	905	Glazer, Jordan (MD)	Inf	606
Gewirtz, Harold (MD)	PlS	1068	Gleckel, Louis Wade (MD)	Cv	631
Gewitz, Michael (MD)	PCd	811	Glenn, Jules (MD)	Psyc	688
Gewolb, Eric B (MD)	Psyc	932	Glick, Robert A (MD)	Psyc	347
Ghajar, Jamshid (MD)	NS	243	Glick, Ronald (MD)	OrS	944
Ghosh, Snehanshu (MD)	ObG	575	Glickel, Steven (MD)	OrS	289
Ghossein, Nemetallah A (MD)	Rad	372	Gliedman, Marvin L (MD)	S	465
Giammarino, Anthony (MD)	ObG	728	Gliklich, Jerry (MD)	Cv	156
Giamo, Thomas (MD)	DR	604	Globus, David (MD)	IM	216
Giangola, Gary (MD)	GVS	408	Glowacki, Jan S (MD)	IM	976
Giannaris, Theodore (MD)	OrS	288	Gluck, Ian (MD)	ObG	992
Giannattasio, Thomas (MD)	Ped	681	Godec, Ciril (MD)	U	551
Gianvito, Louis (MD)	FP	605	Godfrey, Norman (MD)	PlS	334
Giardina, Elsa-Grace (MD)	Cv	155	Godfrey, Philip (MD)	PlS	335
Giardina, Patricia (MD)	PHO	315	Goland, Robin (MD)	EDM	182
Gidwani, Sonia (MD)	Ped	322	Golbe, Lawrence (MD)	N	961
Giegerich, Edmund (MD)	EDM	490	Gold, Alan (MD)	PlS	685
Gifford, Irina (MD)	PMR	537	Gold, Arnold (MD)	ChiN	165
Gil, Constante (MD)	IM	959	Gold, Arthur (MD)	Oph	666
Gilbert, Fred (MD)	MG	230	Gold, Burton (MD)	Rad	692
Gilbert, Marvin (MD)	OrS	289	Gold, David (MD)	PGe	676
Gilbert, Richard (MD)	IM	215	Gold, Ellen (MD)	Onc	232
Gilcrist, Brien (MD)	PS	532	Gold, Jay (MD)	IM	432
Gildengers, Jaime (MD)	S	933	Gold, Jeffrey (MD)	IM	1004
Giliberti, Orazio (MD)	Oph	1005	Gold, Jeffrey P (MD)	TS	469
Gilson, Noah (MD)	N	977	Gold, Kenneth (MD)	Hem	720
Gindea, Aaron (MD)	Cv	631	Gold, Scott (MD)	Oto	301
Gingold, Bruce (MD)	CRS	166	Goldberg, Arthur (MD)	Onc	232
Ginsberg, Donald (MD)	IM	503	Goldberg, Daniel (MD)	Oph	978
Ginsberg, Gerald (MD)	PlS	334	Goldberg, Eugene L (MD & PhD)	Psyc	347
Ginsberg, Robert (MD)	TS	396	Goldberg, Gary L (MD)	GO	427
Ginsberg, Stanley (MD)	U	593	Goldberg, Harvey (MD)	Cv	156
Ginsburg, Eugene (MD)	ObG	878	Goldberg, Itzhak D (MD)	Rad	589
Ginsburg, Frances (MD)	RE	1073	Goldberg, Jack (MD)	Cv	416
Ginsburg, Howard (MD)	PS	319	Goldberg, Jeffrey (DO)	Psyc	538
Ginsburg, Mark (MD)	TS	396	Goldberg, Joel (MD)	Cv	631
Ginzler, Ellen (MD)	Rhu	544	Goldberg, Jory (MD)	Pul	966
Gioia, Leonard (MD)	EDM	716	Goldberg, Leslie (MD)	Oph	666
Giordano, Michael F (MD)	Inf	206	Goldberg, Max (MD)	S	697
Giorgini Jr, Gino (MD)	Ge	719	Goldberg, Michael (MD)	GO	958
Girardi, Anthony (MD)	Oph	666	Goldberg, Myron (MD)	Ge	190
Giron, Fabio (MD)	GVS	750	Goldberg, Neil (MD)	D	766
Gitler, Bernard (MD)	Cv	760	Goldberg, Richard (MD)	IM	503

DIRECTORY OF DOCTORS

NAME	SPECIALTY	PAGE	NAME	SPECIALTY	PAGE
Goldberg, Robert (DO)	PMR	330	Golinko, Richard J (MD)	PCd	311
Goldberg, Robert T (MD)	Oph	577	Golomb, Frederick (MD)	S	387
Goldberg, Roy J (MD)	IM	781	Golub, James (MD)	A&I	757
Goldberg, Steven (MD)	Cv	631	Golub, Richard (MD)	CRS	486
Goldberg, Theodore H (MD)	Cv	862	Golub, Robert (MD)	CRS	562
Goldberger, Marianne (MD)	Psyc	347	Gombert, Myles (MD)	Inf	647
Goldblatt, Kenneth (MD)	Pul	948	Gomez, Rolando (MD)	S	832
Goldblatt, Robert (MD)	Ge	774	Gomez, William (MD)	OrS	944
Goldblum, Lester (DO)	Ge	643	Gonzalez, Orlando (MD)	ObG	611
Golde, David (MD)	Onc	232	Good, Leonard (MD)	Ped	681
Golden, Brian (MD)	Rhu	377	Goodgold, Albert (MD)	N	248
Goldenberg, David (MD)	Ge	1020	Goodman, Alan (MD)	A&I	1017
Goldenberg, David (MD)	PlS	1068	Goodman, Alvin (MD)	Nep	790
Goldfarb, Alisan B (MD)	S	387	Goodman, Berney (MD)	Psyc	348
Goldfarb, Joel (MD)	Ge	868	Goodman, Ken J (MD)	Rad	692
Goldfarb, Michael (MD)	S	981	Goodman, Mark (MD)	Cv	631
Goldfarb, Richard (MD)	NuM	255	Goodman, Robert R (MD)	NS	243
Goldfarb, Steven (MD)	IM	722	Goodman, Susan (MD)	Rhu	377
Goldfischer, Jerome D (MD)	Cv	862	Goodrich, Charles (MD)	IM	216
Goldfrank, Lewis (MD)	EM	179	Goodrich, James (MD)	NS	440
Goldin, Gurston (MD)	Psyc	347	Goodstein, Carolyn E (MD)	A&I	861
Goldin, Howard (MD)	Ge	190	Goodwin, Charles (MD)	OrS	289
Goldman, Arnold (MD)	OrS	578	Gopinathan, Govindan (MD)	N	249
Goldman, Arnold (MD)	Ped	681	Gordon, Donald G (MD)	Ge	1046
Goldman, David S (MD)	Psyc	347	Gordon, Garet M (MD)	Cv	416
Goldman, Gary (MD)	ObG	259	Gordon, Jeffrey (MD)	EDM	640
Goldman, George J (MD)	Cv	631	Gordon, Lawrence A (MD)	S	697
Goldman, Ira (MD)	Ge	643	Gordon, Marc L (MD)	N	574
Goldman, Jack S (MD)	IM	781	Gordon, Mark (MD)	S	832
Goldman, Joel (MD)	EDM	490	Gordon, Marsha (MD)	D	171
Goldman, Kenneth Alan (MD)	S	950	Gordon, Michael A (MD)	Oto	673
Goldman, Martin (MD)	Cv	156	Gordon, Richard (MD)	Rhu	949
Goldman, Michael (MD)	EDM	866	Gordon, Stanley (MD)	OrS	524
Goldman, Mitchell (MD)	ObG	728	Gorelick, Jeffrey (MD)	U	1077
Goldman, Neil C (MD)	A&I	757	Gorenstein, Lyall (MD)	S	849
Goldman, Neil S (MD)	Psyc	348	Gorfine, Stephen (MD)	CRS	167
Goldofsky, Elliot (MD)	Oto	672	Gorkin, Janet (MD)	IM	432
Goldsmith, Ari (MD)	Oto	526	Gorman, Jack (MD)	Psyc	348
Goldsmith, Michael (MD)	Onc	232	Gorman, Lauren (MD)	Psyc	459
Goldsmith, Stanley J (MD)	NuM	255	Gorski, Lydia E (MD)	IM	650
Goldson, Howard (MD)	S	1014	Gotkin, Robert (MD)	PlS	685
Goldstein, Barry (MD)	Nep	790	Gotlin, Robert S (DO)	PMR	330
Goldstein, Carl (MD)	Nep	991	Gottesfeld, Peter (MD)	FP	772
Goldstein, Dov (MD)	ObG	259	Gottesman, Lester (MD)	CRS	167
Goldstein, Irwin (MD)	ObG	662	Gottlieb, Alice (MD)	D	901
Goldstein, Jonathan (MD)	N	1058	Gottlieb, Robert (MD)	Ped	739
Goldstein, Jonathon (MD)	S	697	Gottridge, Joanne (MD)	IM	650
Goldstein, Judith (MD)	Ped	322	Gouge, Thomas (MD)	S	388
Goldstein, Lawrence (MD)	FP	772	Goulart, Hamilton (MD)	NS	876
Goldstein, Marc (MD)	U	401	Gould, Eric (MD)	Ped	681
Goldstein, Mark (MD)	Oto	672	Gould, Perry (MD)	Ge	643
Goldstein, Mark (MD)	Rhu	619	Goussis, Onoufrios (MD)	EDM	640
Goldstein, Martin (MD)	ObG	259	Grace, William (MD)	Onc	233
Goldstein, Marvin (MD)	IM	216	Grad, Joel (MD)	HS	201
Goldstein, Paul (MD)	IM	216	Gradler, Thomas (MD)	FP	492
Goldstein, Robert (MD)	PlS	458	Graham, Alan (MD)	GVS	970
Goldstein, Stanley (MD)	A&I	628	Grajower, Martin (MD)	IM	432
Goldstein, Steven (MD)	ObG	977	Granadir, Charles (MD)	OrS	931
Goldstein, Steven (MD)	PlS	820	Granet, Roger (MD)	Psyc	996
Goldstein, Steven J (MD)	Ped	584	Grano, Vanessa (MD)	ObG	795
Goldstone, Jonas (MD)	IM	216	Granstein, Richard (MD)	D	171
Golfinos, John (MD)	NS	243	Grant, Alfred (MD)	OrS	289
Golier, Francis (MD)	Cv	760	Grant, Linda (MD)	PMR	1067
Golimbu, Mircea (MD)	U	402	Grant, Robert (MD)	PlS	685

NAME	SPECIALTY	PAGE	NAME	SPECIALTY	PAGE
Grant, Susan (MD)	ObG	260	Grenell, Steven (MD)	N	441
Grapa, Octavian (MD)	FP	926	Grenis, Michael (MD)	OrS	944
Grasso, Cono M (MD)	Oph	577	Gribbin, Dorota (MD)	PMR	946
Grasso, Michael (MD)	Nep	907	Gribetz, Allen (MD)	Pul	364
Graver, L Michael (MD)	TS	593	Gribetz, Donald (MD)	Ped	322
Gray, Samuel (DO)	IM	1023	Gribetz, Irwin (MD)	Ped	322
Grayson, Martha (MD)	IM	216	Gribetz, Michael (MD)	U	402
Grazi, Richard (MD)	RE	543	Grieco, Anthony (MD)	IM	216
Grebler, Arnold (MD)	U	982	Grieco, Michael (MD)	A&I	151
Grecco, Michael (MD)	ObG	611	Grieco, Michael B (MD)	S	697
Greco, Helen (MD)	ObG	662	Grieg, Adolfo (DO)	NP	510
Greco, Ralph S (MD)	S	968	Griepp, Randall (MD)	TS	396
Gredysa, Leslaw (MD)	GVS	750	Griffith, Barbara (MD)	FP	772
Greeley, Norman (MD)	A&I	481	Grifo, James (MD)	RE	375
Green, Abraham (MD)	Ped	681	Grijnsztein, Jacob (MD)	Ped	584
Green, Arthur (MD)	ChAP	163	Gristina, Jerome (MD)	PMR	819
Green, Mark (MD)	N	792	Grizzanti, Joseph (DO)	Pul	890
Green, Peter (MD)	Ge	190	Grob, David (MD)	IM	503
Green, Robert (MD)	Oto	302	Grodman, Richard (MD)	Cv	602
Green, Stephen (MD)	Cv	632	Grodstein, Gerald (MD)	Nep	875
Green, Steven (MD)	OrS	289	Groeger, William (MD)	PlS	686
Green, Stuart (MD)	Rhu	544	Groff, Walter (MD)	CRS	1019
Green, Wayne Hugo (MD)	ChAP	163	Groopman, Jacob (MD)	Pul	540
Greenbaum, Allen (MD)	Oph	800	Gropen, Toby Ira (MD)	N	514
Greenbaum, Dennis (MD)	CCM	168	Grosman, Irwin (MD)	Ge	495
Greenbaum, Mark (MD)	PMR	457	Gross, Arthur H (MD)	ObG	879
Greenberg, Andrew (MD)	Rad	948	Gross, Elliott (MD)	N	792
Greenberg, Harly (MD)	Pul	587	Gross, Gary L (MD)	A&I	973
Greenberg, Mark (MD)	PCd	450	Gross, Harvey (MD)	FP	867
Greenberg, Maury (MD)	FP	717	Gross, Lillian (MD)	Psyc	688
Greenberg, Michael L (MD)	Hem	203	Gross, Peter (MD)	Inf	871
Greenberg, Robert (MD)	D	171	Gross, Susan (MD)	MG	436
Greenberg, Ronald (MD)	Ge	565	Grossbard, Lionel (MD)	Onc	233
Greenberg, Rosalie (MD)	ChAP	1018	Grossi, Robert (MD)	S	388
Greenberg, Steven (MD)	Oph	800	Grossman, Bernard (MD)	Onc	941
Greenberg, Steven M (MD)	Cv	632	Grossman, Edward (MD)	Ge	1046
Greenberg, Susan (MD)	Onc	976	Grossman, Elliot (MD)	ChiN	987
Greenblatt, David (MD)	RadRO	891	Grossman, Kenneth (MD)	D	974
Greenblatt, Louis (DO)	FP	717	Grossman, Marc (MD)	D	766
Greenblatt, Michael (MD)	IM	650	Grossman, Susan (MD)	Nep	609
Greene, Jeffrey (MD)	IM	216	Grossman, Will (MD)	Cv	156
Greene, Loren (MD)	EDM	182	Grosso, John (MD)	Oto	673
Greenfield, Martin (MD)	EDM	640	Gruber, Gabriel (MD)	D	1019
Greenhill, Laurence (MD)	ChAP	763	Grubman, Jerold (MD)	U	970
Greenidge, Kevin (MD)	Oph	521	Grubman, Samuel (MD)	A&I	151
Greenlee, Robert (MD)	ObG	795	Gruen, Peter (MD)	Psyc	348
Greensher, Joseph (MD)	Ped	681	Gruenstein, Steven (MD)	Onc	233
Greenspan, Alan (MD)	D	172	Gruenwald, Laurence D (MD)	Ped	915
Greenspan, Joel (MD)	Inf	720	Grunberger, Ivan (MD)	U	551
Greenstein, Adrian (MD)	S	388	Grunebaum, Amos (MD)	ObG	260
Greenstein, Stuart (MD)	S	466	Grunfeld, Lawrence (MD)	ObG	260
Greenwald, Blaine (MD)	GerPsy	567	Grunfeld, Paul (MD)	Ped	323
Greenwald, Bruce M (MD)	PCCM	312	Grunther, Howard (MD)	Rad	372
Greenwald, Edward (MD)	Onc	437	Grunzweig, Milton (MD)	IM	503
Greenwald, Marc (MD)	CRS	636	Gruss, Claudia (MD)	Ge	1046
Greenwald, Robert (MD)	Rhu	590	Gruss, Leslie (MD)	ObG	260
Gregoire, Clyde (MD)	DR	489	Grynbaum, Bruce (MD)	PMR	330
Gregori, Caterina (MD)	GO	904	Guarini, Ludovico (MD)	PHO	530
Greif, Richard H (MD)	Cv	760	Guarnaccia, Gary (MD)	ObG	575
Greifer, Ira (MD)	PNep	452	Gudavalli, Madhu R (MD)	NP	510
Greig, Fenella (MD)	PEn	313	Gudesblatt, Mark (MD)	N	727
Greisman, Stewart (MD)	Rhu	378	Gudin, Jeffrey A (MD)	PM	1064
Grello, Fred W (MD)	Ped	739	Gugliucci, Camillo (MD)	MF	229
Grendell, James H (MD)	Ge	190	Guida, Anthony (MD)	FP	717

DIRECTORY OF DOCTORS

NAME	SPECIALTY	PAGE	NAME	SPECIALTY	PAGE
Guida, Robert (MD)	Oto	302	Halpern, Neil (MD)	CCM	418
Guilbe, Rose (MD)	FP	422	Halpern, Steven (MD)	PHO	884
Guillory, Samuel (MD)	Oph	273	Hamburger, Max (MD)	Rhu	746
Guirguis, Fayez (MD)	ObG	518	Hamby, Robert I (MD)	Cv	632
Gulati, Subhash C (MD & PhD)	Hem	203	Hametz, Irwin (MD)	D	974
Gulotta, Stephen J (MD)	Cv	632	Hamilton, Audrey (MD)	Onc	609
Gulrajani, Ramesh (MD)	Pul	540	Hamilton, Richard H (MD)	Rad	372
Gumbs, Milton (MD)	S	466	Hamilton, William (MD)	OrS	290
Gumprecht, Jeffrey Paul (MD)	Inf	206	Hammel, Jay (MD)	Rad	693
Gundy, Edward (MD)	OrS	805	Hammer, Glenn (MD)	Inf	206
Gupta, Prem (MD)	Cv	483	Hammerman, Hillel (MD)	Ge	190
Gupta, Sanjeev (MD)	Ge	425	Hammerschlag, Paul E (MD)	Oto	302
Gupta, Saroj (MD)	PMR	585	Hanania, Michael (MD)	PM	674
Gupta, Shiv (MD)	NuM	1059	Handelsman, Dan (MD)	PEn	811
Gurland, Frances (MD)	Psyc	889	Handelsman, John (MD)	OrS	578
Gurland, Judith (MD)	Oph	445	Handler, Robert (MD)	Ped	995
Gurland, Mark (MD)	OrS	881	Handlin, David (MD)	Anes	973
Gursel, Erol (MD)	U	837	Handszer, Bernardo (MD)	ObG	260
Gusmorino, Paul (MD)	Psyc	348	Hankin, Dorie (MD)	Ped	584
Gusset, George (MD)	Ge	495	Hankin, Edwin (MD)	Cv	1041
Guthrie, James (MD)	CRS	1042	Hanley, Gerard (MD)	Cv	483
Gutin, Philip (MD)	NS	243	Hanna, Moneer (MD)	U	703
Gutman, David (MD)	Ge	643	Hannafin, Jo (MD & PhD)	OrS	290
Gutstein, Sidney (MD)	IM	782	Haramati, Linda (MD)	Rad	462
Gutwein, Isadore (MD)	Ge	425	Haramati, Nogah (MD)	Rad	462
Guy, Roscoe Bruce (MD)	Hem	428	Harary, Albert (MD)	Ge	190
Guzick, Howard (MD)	Ger	645	Hardy, Mark (MD)	S	388
Guzman, Rodolpho (MD)	EDM	421	Hardy III, Howard (MD)	CRS	938
			Har-El, Gady (MD)	Oto	526
			Harin, Anantham (MD)	Ped	615

H

NAME	SPECIALTY	PAGE	NAME	SPECIALTY	PAGE
Haas, Alexander (MD)	RadRO	967	Harish, Ziv (MD)	A&I	861
Haber, Patricia (MD)	Ped	454	Harlow, Paul (MD)	Ped	886
Haber, Stuart (MD)	Inf	778	Harman, John (MD)	Pul	948
Habermann, Edward (MD)	OrS	447	Harmon, Gregory K (MD)	Oph	273
Habib, Mohsen (MD)	Oto	526	Harooni, Robert (MD)	Ge	566
Hackett, Thomas (DO)	GO	975	Harper, Harry (MD)	Hem	870
Haddad, A John (MD)	FP	974	Harper, Rita (MD)	NP	656
Haddad, Heskel (MD)	Oph	273	Harrington, Elizabeth (MD)	GVS	408
Haddad, Joseph (MD)	Oto	302	Harrington, Martin (MD)	GVS	408
Hages, Harry (MD)	Ped	886	Harris, Alan I (MD)	Ge	719
Haggerty, Mary (MD)	IM	905	Harris, Alvin H (MD)	PlS	686
Haher, Jane (MD)	PlS	335	Harris, Harriet (MD)	D	603
Haher, Thomas R (MD)	OrS	289	Harris, Matthew N (MD)	S	388
Hahn, John Charles (MD)	Ge	926	Harris, Michael (MD)	PHO	884
Haight, David (MD)	Oph	273	Harris, Steven (MD)	U	703
Hailoo, Wajdy (MD)	OM	730	Harrison, Aaron R (MD)	Ge	719
Haimov, Moshe (MD)	GVS	408	Harrison, Louis (MD)	RadRO	368
Haimovic, Itzhak (MD)	N	659	Harrison, Raymond (MD)	Oph	273
Haines, Kathleen (MD)	PA&I	309	Harrison, Theodore J (MD)	Oto	302
Hainline, Brian (MD)	N	659	Harrison-Ross, Phyllis (MD)	ChAP	163
Hait, William (MD & PhD)	Onc	960	Hart, Catherine (MD)	IM	217
Hakim-Elahi, Enayat (MD)	ObG	575	Hart, Sidney (MD)	Psyc	1069
Halata, Michael (MD)	Ge	774	Hartman, Alan (MD)	TS	701
Halbach, Joseph (MD)	FP	772	Hartman, Barry Jay (MD)	Inf	206
Hall, Craig (MD)	PlS	888	Hartz, Cindi (MD)	Ped	816
Hallal, Edward (MD)	IM	722	Hartzband, Mark (MD)	OrS	881
Haller, Jack (MD)	PR	531	Harwin, Steven F (MD)	OrS	290
Halmi, Katherine (MD)	Psyc	822	Haselkorn, Joan (MD)	ObG	663
Halperin, Alan (MD)	D	766	Hashmat, Aizid (MD)	U	551
Halperin, Ira (MD)	IM	217	Hatcher, Virgil (MD)	D	172
Halperin, John (MD)	N	659	Hatsis, Alexander (MD)	Oph	666
Halperin, Jonathan (MD)	Cv	156	Hauben, Robert (MD)	Psyc	742
Halpern, Abraham L (MD)	Psyc	822	Hauptman, Martin (MD)	Ped	739

NAME	SPECIALTY	PAGE	NAME	SPECIALTY	PAGE
Hausman, Michael (MD)	OrS	290	Hertz, Howard M (MD)	IM	722
Haveson, Stephen (MD)	GVS	408	Hertz, Stanley (MD)	ChAP	635
Haydock, Timothy (MD)	EM	420	Hertzig, Margaret (MD)	ChAP	164
Hayes, Mary (MD)	Rad	372	Herzig, Geoffrey P (MD)	Hem	203
Hayes-McKenzie, Leslie (MD)	AM	481	Herzlich, Barry (MD)	A&I	481
Hayworth, Nan (MD)	Oph	801	Herzlinger, Robert (MD)	NP	1056
Hayworth, Robin (MD)	Oph	445	Herzog, David (MD)	IM	782
Hayworth, Scott (MD)	ObG	795	Herzog, David (MD)	ObG	611
Heagarty, Margaret (MD)	Ped	323	Hetzler, Peter (MD)	PlS	979
Heald, Peter (MD)	D	1043	Hetzler, Theresa (MD)	Ped	816
Healey, John (MD)	OrS	290	Hewlett, Dial (MD)	Inf	778
Healy, Elaine (MD)	IM	782	Heymann, A Douglas (MD)	S	388
Healy Jr, William (MD)	OrS	734	Hicks, Patricia (MD)	PA&I	883
Hecht, Alan (MD)	Cv	156	Hidalgo, David (MD)	PlS	335
Hecht, Pauline (MD)	S	388	Hiesiger, Emile (MD)	N	249
Heckman, Bruce (MD)	IM	782	Higgins, William (MD)	IM	782
Hedayati, Hossein (MD)	S	547	Hilaris, Basil (MD)	RadRO	461
Hefter, Harold (MD)	D	638	Hilton, Eileen (MD)	Inf	648
Heidenberg, William (MD)	Cv	761	Hindes, Robert G (MD)	Inf	1049
Heier, Stephen (MD)	Ge	775	Hines, George L (MD)	TS	701
Heiman, Peter (MD)	Psyc	348	Hines, William (MD)	Nep	1056
Heimann, Tomas (MD)	S	388	Hinterbuchner, Catherine (MD)	PMR	819
Heinegg, Philip (MD)	FP	772	Hipps, Linda (MD)	ObG	663
Heinemann, Murk-Hein (MD)	Oph	273	Hirsch, Glenn S (MD)	ChAP	164
Heitler, Michael (MD)	Ped	682	Hirsch, Lissa (MD)	GO	199
Helbraun, Mark (MD)	CRS	863	Hirschenstein, Eva (MD)	N	514
Held, Barry (MD)	Rad	372	Hirschman, Alan (MD)	Ped	454
Held, Douglas (MD)	S	697	Hirschman, Richard J (MD)	Hem	203
Heldman, Jay (MD)	D	865	Hirschowitz, Jack (MD)	Psyc	459
Heleotis, Thomas (MD)	TS	982	Hirsh, David M (MD)	OrS	447
Helfet, David L (MD)	OrS	290	Hirshaut, Yashar (MD)	Onc	233
Helfgott, David (MD)	Inf	206	Hirt, Paula (MD)	ObG	728
Hellenbrand, William E (MD)	PCd	1064	Hisler, Barbara (MD)	D	562
Heller, Keith (MD)	S	697	Ho, Alison G (MD)	ObG	260
Heller, Stanley (MD)	Psyc	348	Ho, Victor (MD)	NS	610
Hellerman, James (MD)	EDM	770	Hobson, Robert W, II (MD)	GVS	922
Hembree, Wylie (MD)	IM	217	Hochman, Herbert (MD)	D	172
Henderson, Cassandra (MD)	ObG	795	Hochster, Howard (MD)	Onc	233
Hendin, Herbert (MD)	Psyc	348	Hodes, David (MD)	Pul	848
Hendricks, Judith (MD)	IM	608	Hodes, Steven (MD)	Ge	957
Hen Jr, Jacob (MD)	PPul	1065	Hodgson, W John B (MD)	S	466
Henry, Jack (MD)	SM	381	Hodosh, Richard (MD)	NS	992
Hensle, Terry (MD)	U	402	Hoexter, Barton (MD)	CRS	636
Herbin, Joseph (MD)	IM	1052	Hoffman, Anthony (MD)	Onc	437
Herbstein, Diego (MD)	N	249	Hoffman, Ira (MD)	IM	217
Herman, David (MD)	Inf	1012	Hoffman, Janet C (MD)	Rad	589
Herman, Martin (MD)	N	977	Hoffman, Joel (MD)	Psyc	349
Herman, Michael (MD)	Cv	1041	Hoffman, Lloyd (MD)	PlS	335
Herman, Peter (MD)	DR	563	Hoffman, Mark Andrew (MD)	IM	928
Herman, Peter (MD)	N	249	Hoffman, Michael L (MD)	Rhu	590
Herman, Steven (MD)	PlS	335	Hoffman, Richard (MD)	EDM	604
Hermance, William (MD)	A&I	757	Hoffman, Ronald (MD)	Oto	302
Hermele, Herbert (MD)	SM	1074	Hoffman, Saul (MD)	PlS	335
Herr, Harry W (MD)	U	402	Hofreuter, Nancy (MD)	Ped	1066
Herridge, Peter L (MD)	Psyc	1028	Hofstetter, Stephen (MD)	S	389
Hersh, Peter (MD)	Oph	910	Holden, David (MD)	FP	492
Hershman, Elliott (MD)	OrS	290	Holden, Melvin (MD)	IM	651
Hershman, Jack (MD)	U	837	Holder, Jonathan (MD)	OrS	805
Hershman, Ronnie (MD)	Cv	632	Holgersen, Leif (MD)	PS	813
Hershon, Kenneth (MD)	IM	651	Holland, Claudia (MD)	ObG	260
Hershon, Stuart (MD)	SM	695	Holland, James F (MD)	Onc	233
Herskovitz, Steven (MD)	N	441	Holland, Jimmie (MD)	Psyc	349
Hertan, Hilary (MD)	Ge	425	Hollander, Eric (MD)	Psyc	349
			Hollander, Gerald (MD)	IM	503

DIRECTORY OF DOCTORS

NAME	SPECIALTY	PAGE
Holland Jr, Elbridge (MD)	FP	988
Hollier, Larry (MD)	GVS	408
Hollis, Peter (MD)	N	659
Hollister Jr, Dickerman (MD)	Onc	1055
Holt, Peter (MD)	Ge	190
Holzer, Barry D (MD)	ChAP	485
Holzman, Ian (MD)	NP	237
Homayuni, Ali (MD)	Cv	602
Hong, Andrew (MD)	PS	679
Hong, Joon (MD)	S	547
Honig, Stephen (MD)	Rhu	378
Hopkins, Arthur (MD)	IM	782
Hoppenfeld, Stanley (MD)	OrS	447
Horbar, Gary (MD)	IM	217
Hordof, Allan (MD)	PCd	311
Hornblass, Albert (MD)	Oph	273
Hornyak, Stephen (MD)	S	620
Horovitz, Joel (MD)	S	547
Horowitz, Harold (MD)	Inf	778
Horowitz, Lawrence (MD)	Ge	190
Horowitz, Marc (MD)	Oph	801
Horowitz, Mark D (MD)	Rhu	378
Horowitz, Roy (MD)	Ped	682
Horowitz, Steven (MD)	Cv	156
Horwich, Mark (MD)	N	249
Horwitz, Ralph (MD)	IM	1052
Hoskins, Iffath (MD)	ObG	260
Hoskins, William (MD)	GO	199
Hotchkiss, Edward (MD)	IM	651
Hotchkiss, Robert (MD)	OrS	291
Houghton, Alan (MD)	IM	217
Housman, Arno (MD)	U	837
Howard, George (MD)	Oph	274
Howard, James (MD)	ObG	795
Hryhorowych, Arthur N (MD)	PMR	330
Hsueh, John Tzu-Lang (MD)	Cv	560
Huberman, Harris (MD)	Ped	454
Huberman, Roberta (MD)	Psyc	947
Hubschmann, Otakar (MD)	NS	908
Hughes, Peter (MD)	OrS	1062
Huh, Chung-ho (MD)	Oto	526
Huh, Sun (MD)	RadRO	541
Hunter, John G (MD)	PlS	335
Hupart, Kenneth (MD)	EDM	421
Hurley, James (MD)	EDM	182
Hurley, John (MD)	OrS	993
Hurst, Lawrence (MD)	HS	720
Hurst, Wendy (MD)	ObG	879
Hurwitz, Harvey (MD)	IM	782
Husami, Nabil (MD)	ObG	261
Husk, Gregg (MD)	EM	179
Husney, Joseph (MD)	IM	503
Huston, Jan A (MD)	S	920
Hutcheon, R Gordon (MD)	MG	1004
Hutchinson, John (MD)	TS	894
Hutson, J Milton (MD)	ObG	261
Hwang, Cheng-hong (DO)	IM	1023
Hyans, Peter (MD)	PlS	1028
Hyatt, Alexander (MD)	Ped	886
Hyde, Phyllis (MD)	Hem	499
Hyler, Irene (MD)	ChAP	764
Hyman, David (MD)	MG	724
Hyman, George (MD)	Oph	521
Hymes, Kenneth (MD)	Hem	203

NAME	SPECIALTY	PAGE
I		
Iacuzzo, John (MD)	S	1014
Iammatteo, Matthew (MD)	ObG	992
Ibrahim, Ibrahim (MD)	S	893
Idupuganti, Sudharam (MD)	Psyc	539
Igel, Gerard (MD)	Ped	454
Ilamathi, Ekambaram M (MD)	Nep	726
Ilkhani, Rahman (MD)	GVS	553
Illman, Arnold (MD)	OrS	669
Illueca, Marta (MD)	PGe	314
Ilowite, Norman Todd (MD)	Ped Rhu	678
Imber, Gerald (MD)	PlS	335
Imperato, Pascal James (MD)	IM	503
Imperato-Mcginley, Julianne (MD)	EDM	182
Inamdar, Sarla (MD)	Ped	323
Inch, Eugene (MD)	Ped	816
Infantino, Michael (MD)	Cv	156
Inglesby, Thomas V (MD)	Cv	1018
Inglis, Allan (MD)	OrS	291
Innella, Robin (DO)	OrS	1026
Inra, Lawrence A (MD)	Cv	157
Insall, John (MD)	OrS	291
Insler, Harvey (MD)	OrS	447
Inwald, Gary (DO)	PMR	330
Irving III, Henry C (MD)	OrS	931
Irwin, Mark (MD)	U	552
Irwin, Michael (MD)	IM	432
Irwin, Robert (MD)	U	921
Isaacs, Ellen (MD)	IM	782
Isaacson, Steven (MD)	RadRO	368
Isay, Richard A (MD)	Psyc	349
Isom, O Wayne (MD)	TS	396
Israel, Alan (MD)	Hem	870
Israel, Michael (MD)	IM	723
Issenberg, Henry (MD)	PCd	450
Istrico, Richard A (DO)	FP	564
Iswara, Kadirawel (MD)	Ge	495
Iyengar, Devarajan P (MD)	Onc	929
J		
Jacob, Harold (MD)	Ge	643
Jacob, Jessica (MD)	ObG	663
Jacobowitz, Israel (MD)	Cv	483
Jacobowitz, Walter (MD)	ObG	993
Jacobs, Allan J (MD)	ObG	261
Jacobs, David R (MD)	EDM	182
Jacobs, Elliot (MD)	PlS	336
Jacobs, Jonathan (MD)	Inf	206
Jacobs, Joseph (MD)	Oto	302
Jacobs, Laurie (MD)	Ger	426
Jacobs, Michael (MD)	D	172
Jacobs, Theodore (MD)	Psyc	349
Jacobs, Thomas (MD)	EDM	182
Jacobson, Ira (MD)	Ge	191
Jacobson, Marc S (MD)	AM	559
Jacobson, Ronald (MD)	ChiN	764
Jacoby, Jacob (MD)	Psyc	932
Jafar, Jafar (MD)	NS	243
Jaffe, Fredrick (MD)	OrS	291
Jaffe, Herbert (MD)	Oph	521
Jaffe, Israeli A (MD)	Rhu	378
Jaffe, Kenneth (MD)	FP	492
Jaffe, William (MD)	OrS	291

NAME	SPECIALTY	PAGE	NAME	SPECIALTY	PAGE
Jagannath, Sundar (MD)	Onc	233	Kahn, Max (MD)	Ped	323
Jahn, Anthony (MD)	Oto	912	Kahn, Steven (MD)	S	950
Jain, Subhash (MD)	PM	308	Kaiden, Jeffrey (MD)	Oph	879
Jaitly, Sharad (MD)	Cv	560	Kaiden, Richard (MD)	Oph	880
Jamal, Habib (MD)	Oto	808	Kairam, Indira (MD)	IM	218
James, David F (MD)	ObG	261	Kaiser, Stephen (MD)	IM	504
Janniger, Camila (MD)	D	865	Kaitz, Ronald (MD)	Psyc	822
Janowitz, Henry (MD)	Ge	191	Kalafatic, Alfredo (MD)	CRS	636
Januzzi, James (MD)	IM	217	Kalanadhabhatta, Vivekannad (MD)	A&I	481
Jarowski, Charles (MD)	Onc	233	Kalchthaler, Thomas (DO)	IM	783
Jarrett, Adam (MD)	IM	872	Kaleya, Ronald (MD)	S	466
Jarrett, Mark (MD)	Rhu	620	Kalin, Marcia (MD)	EDM	183
Jay, Judith (MD)	Oto	808	Kalinich, Lila J (MD)	Psyc	349
Jayabose, Somasundaram (MD)	PHO	812	Kalinsky, Jay (MD)	ObG	796
Jayaram, Nadubetthi (MD)	OrS	613	Kalischer, Alan (MD)	Cv	1018
Jelin, Abraham (MD)	PGe	529	Kalman, Jeffery (MD)	Ge	605
Jelks, Glenn (MD)	PlS	336	Kamalakar, Peri (MD)	PHO	913
Jelveh, Mansoor (MD)	Cv	632	Kamelhar, David (MD)	Pul	365
Johanson, Waldemar (MD)	Pul	918	Kamen, Mazen (MD)	Cv	157
John, Joseph (MD)	Inf	958	Kamholz, Stephan (MD)	Pul	541
Johns, William (MD)	IM	1052	Kaminetsky, Jed (MD)	U	402
Johnson, Albert (MD)	OrS	1013	Kaminsky, Donald (MD)	IM	218
Johnson, Edward (MD)	Inf	904	Kaminsky, Sari J (MD)	ObG	261
Johnson, Mark (MD)	FP	902	Kamler, Kenneth (MD)	HS	646
Johnson, Robert (MD)	Ped	915	Kandalaft, Souheil (MD)	S	389
Johnson, Valerie (MD)	PNep	317	Kandall, Stephen (MD)	NP	237
Johnson, Warren (MD)	IM	217	Kane, John M (MD)	Psyc	586
Jokl, Peter (MD)	OrS	1062	Kane, Michael J (MD)	Onc	941
Jonas, Darrell (DO)	IM	783	Kanengiser, Steven (MD)	PPul	1006
Jonas, Murray (MD)	IM	503	Kang, Harriet (MD)	ChiN	418
Jonas, Saran (MD)	N	249	Kann, Ferdinand (MD)	FP	642
Jones, Harold (MD)	RadRO	891	Kanner, Ronald (MD)	N	574
Jones, Jacqueline (MD)	Oto	302	Kanter, Alan (MD)	Ped	886
Jones, James (MD)	ObG	261	Kantor, Alan (MD)	EDM	770
Jones, Vann (MD)	IM	504	Kantor, Irwin (MD)	D	172
Jones Jr, Frank (MD)	Psyc	966	Kantounis, Stratos (MD)	S	697
Jordan, Lawrence (MD)	S	950	Kaphan, Mitchell (MD)	OrS	447
Josef, Minna (MD)	EDM	845	Kapila, Rajendra (MD)	Inf	904
Joseph, John (MD)	IM	569	Kaplan, Barry (MD)	Onc	572
Joseph, Patricia (MD)	S	893	Kaplan, Bruce (MD)	PM	580
Josephson, Alan S (MD)	A&I	481	Kaplan, Deborah (MD)	IM	432
Josephson, Barry (MD)	A&I	757	Kaplan, Jerry (MD)	N	441
Josephson, Jordan S (MD)	Oto	303	Kaplan, Kenneth (MD)	IM	783
Josephson, Lynn (MD)	S	832	Kaplan, Mark (MD)	Inf	648
Jotkowitz, Seymour (MD)	N	877	Kaplan, Martin (MD)	Ped	739
Juan, Paul (MD)	Ped	1066	Kaplan, Robert (MD)	ObG	729
Juan, Paul L (MD)	ObG	261	Kaplan, Sherri (MD)	D	766
Judge, Peter (MD)	ObG	729	Kaplan, Sidney (MD)	S	832
Juechter, Kenneth (MD)	Oph	445	Kaplan, William (MD)	ChAP	603
Justman, Jessica (MD)	Inf	429	Kaplovitz, Harry (MD)	PCd	528
Juthani, Virendra (MD)	Ger	777	Kapoor, Deepak A (MD)	U	703
Jutkowitz, Robert (MD)	N	610	Kapoor, Satish (MD)	IM	783
			Kappel, Bruce (MD)	Onc	655
K			Karanfilian, Richard (MD)	GVS	839
Kabakow, Bernard (MD)	Onc	234	Karasu, T Byram (MD)	Psyc	350
Kadar, Avraham (MD)	A&I	151	Karatoprak, Ohan (MD)	FP	867
Kaell, Alan (MD)	Rhu	746	Karayalcin, Gungor (MD)	PHO	582
Kafka, Ernest (MD)	Psyc	349	Karbowitz, Stephen (MD)	Pul	588
Kagan, Andrew (MD)	S	894	Kardos, Frank L (MD)	Oto	1006
Kagen, Lawrence (MD)	Rhu	378	Karen, Joel (MD)	PlS	686
Kahan, Norman (MD)	U	470	Karetzky, Monroe (MD)	Pul	918
Kahn, Alvin (MD)	Oto	579	Karp, Adam (MD)	IM	218
Kahn, David Allen (MD)	Psyc	349	Karp, Jason (MD)	Pul	690
Kahn, Martin (MD)	IM	217	Karpatkin, Margaret (MD)	PHO	315

NAME	SPECIALTY	PAGE	NAME	SPECIALTY	PAGE
Karpinski, Richard (MD)	PlS	336	Kelly, Patrick (MD)	NS	243
Kasabian, Armen (MD)	PlS	336	Kelly, Stephen E (MD)	Oph	274
Kase, Steven (MD)	Oto	808	Kelly, Stephen P (MD)	FP	772
Kaskel, Frederick (MD)	Ped	454	Kelman, Charles D (MD)	Oph	274
Kasoff, Samuel (MD)	NS	791	Kelsen, David (MD)	Onc	234
Kasper, William (MD)	Oph	666	Kelter, Robert (MD)	IM	504
Kassel, Barry (MD)	S	833	Keltz, Theodore (MD)	Cv	761
Kassner, E George (MD)	Rad	543	Kemeny, Margaret Mary (MD)	S	389
Kates, Matthew (MD)	Oto	809	Kemeny, Nancy (MD)	Onc	234
Kattan, Meyer (MD)	PPul	317	Kemmann, Ekkehard (MD)	RE	967
Katus, Eli (MD)	Psyc	688	Kenan, Samuel (MD)	OrS	291
Katz, Arnold (MD)	Oto	736	Kenet, Barney (MD)	D	172
Katz, Bruce (MD)	D	172	Kenigsberg, Daniel (MD)	RE	745
Katz, Harry (MD)	Oto	882	Kennedy, Gary (MD)	Psyc	459
Katz, Henry (MD)	Ge	775	Kennedy, James (MD)	IM	218
Katz, Herbert I (MD)	U	933	Kennedy, Thomas (MD)	Nep	1057
Katz, Jack (MD)	Psyc	689	Kennish, Arthur (MD)	IM	218
Katz, Jeffrey (MD)	U	922	Kent, Joan (MD)	ObG	261
Katz, Kenneth (MD)	Ped	816	Kent, K Craig (MD)	S	389
Katz, L Brian (MD)	S	389	Keolamphu, Narong (MD)	S	466
Katz, Michael (MD)	OrS	579	Kerenyi, Thomas (MD)	ObG	261
Katz, Nadine (MD)	ObG	444	Kern, Jeffrey H (MD)	PCd	580
Katz, Paul (MD)	S	697	Kernan, Nancy A (MD)	PHO	315
Katz, Seymour (MD)	Ge	643	Kernan, Walter (MD)	IM	1052
Katz, Stanley (MD)	Cv	632	Kernberg, Otto (MD)	Psyc	823
Katz, Steven (MD)	U	895	Kernberg, Paulina (MD)	ChAP	764
Katz, Susan (MD)	D	419	Kerner, Michael (MD)	Ge	1021
Katzeff, Harvey (MD)	EDM	640	Kerpen, Howard Owen (MD)	Nep	657
Katzenelenbogen, Moshe (MD)	IM	504	Kerr, Angela (MD)	ObG	518
Kaufman, Alan (MD)	A&I	415	Kershaw, Paul (MD)	N	727
Kaufman, Allen M (MD)	Nep	239	Kessel, Daniel (MD)	D	938
Kaufman, Brian (MD)	CCM (Anes)	167	Kessler, Alan (MD)	ObG	262
Kaufman, Cindy (MD)	IM	218	Kessler, Brad (MD)	PGe	582
Kaufman, David (MD)	N	441	Kessler, Edmund (MD)	PS	679
Kaufman, David Lyons (MD)	IM	218	Kessler, Jeffrey (MD)	N	659
Kaufman, David M (MD)	Ped	323	Kessler, Joseph (MD)	Ger	426
Kaufman, Seth (MD)	PlS	686	Kessler, Leonard (MD)	Hem	647
Kaufman, Stephen (MD)	Rad	891	Kessler, Martin E (MD)	PlS	686
Kaufmann, Charles (MD)	Psyc	350	Kessler, Stuart (MD)	EM	974
Kaufmann, Cheryl (MD)	Oph	577	Kestenbaum, Alan (MD)	PM	308
Kay, Arthur (MD)	N	515	Kestenbaum, Clarice (MD)	ChAP	164
Kay, Richard (MD)	Cv	761	Keuskamp, P Arjen (MD)	NS	726
Kay, Scott (MD)	Oto	945	Khafif, Rene (MD)	S	547
Kaye, Jeremy J (MD)	Rad	372	Khalife, Michael (MD)	S	698
Kaye, Susan (MD)	FP	1020	Khan, Arfa (MD)	Rad	693
Kaynan, Arieh (MD)	GVS	595	Khan, Farida (MD)	EDM	490
Kazam, Elias (MD)	Rad	372	Khanna, Yash (MD)	Ped	915
Kazdin, Hal (MD)	IM	504	Khatib, Reza (MD)	NS	573
Kazenoff, Steven (MD)	D	938	Khimani, Karim (MD)	IM	1023
Kazim, Michael (MD)	Oph	274	Khouri, Phillippe John (MD)	Psyc	947
Kazmi, Mahmood Mehdi (MD)	N	441	Khoury, F Frederic (MD)	PlS	820
Keen, Monte (MD)	PlS	336	Khoury, Paul (MD)	Rad	829
Keilson, Marshall (MD)	N	515	Khulpateea, Taru (MD)	ObG	663
Keiser, Harold (MD)	Rhu	464	Kiernan, Howard (MD)	OrS	291
Kelemen, John (MD)	N	659	Kierszenbaum, Hugo (MD)	AdP	415
Keller, Alex (MD)	PlS	686	Killackey, Maureen (MD)	GO	200
Keller, Barry (MD)	Ped	1066	Killip, Thomas (MD)	Cv	157
Keller, Peter Karl (MD)	Cv	416	Kim, Dong (MD)	S	698
Keller, Steven M (MD)	TS	397	Kim, Grace (MD)	Inf	1049
Kellogg, F Russell (MD)	Ger	197	Kim, Hong (MD)	U	552
Kelly, Amalia (MD)	RE	375	Kim, Joyce M (MD)	ObG	262
Kelly, Carol (MD)	IM	433	Kim, Shihan (MD)	TS	835
Kelly, Michael (MD)	OrS	291	Kim, Zung Wan (MD)	S	833
Kelly, Nancy (MD)	Oph	801	Kimball, Annetta (MD)	IM	218

NAME	SPECIALTY	PAGE	NAME	SPECIALTY	PAGE
Kimmelman, Charles P (MD)	Oto	303	Knapp, Albert B (MD)	Ge	191
Kimmelstiel, Fred (MD)	S	389	Knuppel, Robert A (MD)	ObG	962
Kimura, Yukiko (MD)	Ped Rhu	885	Kocher, Jeffrey (MD)	Inf	871
King, Thomas (MD)	IM	846	Kocsis, James (MD)	Psyc	350
King, William (MD)	HS	201	Kodsi, Baroukh (MD)	Ge	495
Kinn, Mark (MD)	IM	219	Koenig, Eli (MD)	Ped	534
Kinne, David W (MD)	S	389	Koenigsberg, Mordecai (MD)	Rad	462
Kipen, Howard (MD)	OM	962	Koenigsberger, M Richard (MD)	N	908
Kirsch, Mitchell (MD)	Nep	726	Kofinas, Alexander (MD)	ObG	518
Kirschenbaum, Alexander (MD)	U	402	Kofinas, George (MD)	ObG	518
Kirschner, Paul A (MD)	TS	397	Kogan, Stanley J (MD)	U	837
Kirschner-Levy, Stacy (MD)	EDM	866	Kohan, Darius (MD)	Oto	303
Kirshblum, Steven C (MD)	PMR	917	Kohn, Brenda (MD)	PEn	313
Kirtane, Sanjay (MD)	Cv	632	Kohorn, Ernest (MD)	GO	1047
Kislak, Jay Ward (MD)	Inf	206	Kolker, Harvey (MD)	Ped	739
Klagsbrun, Samuel C (MD)	Psyc	823	Kolodny, Edwin H (MD)	N	249
Klapholz, Ari (MD)	Pul	365	Kolodny, Erwin (MD)	Pul	365
Klapholz, Marc (MD)	Cv	900	Kolodny, Howard (MD)	EDM	641
Klapper, Daniel (MD)	Oph	274	Kolsky, Neil (MD)	Ped	886
Klapper, Philip (MD)	Pul	460	Komisar, Arnold (MD)	Oto	303
Klar, Tobi (MD)	D	766	Konecky, Elizabeth (MD)	D	173
Klarsfeld, Jay (MD)	Oto	1063	Konigsberg, Stephen (MD)	S	969
Klass, Evan (MD)	EDM	640	Konka, Sudarsanam (MD)	IM	504
Kleber, Herbert (MD)	Psyc	350	Kopec, Anna V (MD)	D	926
Klecatsky, Lawrence (MD)	IM	783	Kopel, Samuel (MD)	Hem	499
Kleeman, Harris J (MD)	Cv	483	Kopelman, Rima (MD)	Rhu	892
Klein, Arthur (DO)	Inf	721	Kopf, Alfred (MD)	D	173
Klein, Donald (MD)	Psyc	350	Koplewicz, Harold (MD)	ChAP	164
Klein, George (MD)	U	402	Koplin, Richard (MD)	Oph	274
Klein, Gerald (MD)	S	981	Koppel, Barbara (MD)	N	792
Klein, Irwin (MD)	IM	651	Korelitz, Burton I (MD)	Ge	191
Klein, Israel (MD)	Psyc	350	Koren, Zeev (MD)	RE	463
Klein, Lester (MD)	D	767	Korin, Daniel (MD)	Ped	454
Klein, Neil (MD)	IM	1052	Korman, Elise (MD)	FP	718
Klein, Noah (MD)	Oph	274	Kornbluth, Arthur Asher (MD)	Ge	191
Klein, Norman (MD)	N	877	Kornfeld, Donald S (MD)	Psyc	350
Klein, Patricia (MD)	N	877	Kornmehl, Carol (MD)	RadRO	980
Klein, Robert (MD)	A&I	1003	Korval, Arnold (MD)	Ped	1066
Klein, Robert (MD)	Oph	666	Kosinski, Edward (MD)	Cv	1041
Klein, Robert M (MD)	Rad	829	Kosinski, Robert (MD)	Pul	980
Klein, Steven (MD)	FP	717	Koss, Jerome (MD)	Cv	560
Klein, Victor (MD)	MF	654	Kostadaras, Ari (MD)	Nep	572
Kleinbaum, Jerry (MD)	EDM	770	Kostis, John B (MD)	Cv	955
Kleinberg, David (MD)	EDM	183	Kostroff, Karen (MD)	S	698
Kleiner, Morton (MD)	Nep	609	Kostrzewa, Raymond (MD)	D	938
Kleinhaus, Sylvain (MD)	PS	452	Kotin, Neal (MD)	Ped	323
Kleinman, Andrew (MD)	PlS	820	Kotler, Donald P (MD)	Ge	191
Kleinman, Paul (MD)	OrS	447	Kottler, William (MD)	PPul	914
Klenk, Rosemary (MD)	Ped	1066	Koulos, John (MD)	GO	1048
Klenoff, Bruce (MD)	Oto	1063	Kovacs, Karen (MD)	S	1075
Kleyman, Felix (MD)	Psyc	350	Koval, Kenneth (MD)	OrS	292
Kligfield, Paul (MD)	Cv	157	Kowallis, George (MD)	Psyc	350
Klindt, Joyce (MD)	PlS	741	Koz, Gabriel (MD)	Psyc	350
Kline, Gary (MD)	TS	701	Kozel, Joseph Martin (MD)	IM	928
Kline, Mitchell (MD)	D	172	Kozicky, Orest (MD)	Ge	775
Klinger, Ronald (MD)	N	660	Kozin, Arthur (MD)	Nep	846
Klion, Franklin (MD)	Ge	191	Kozlowski, Jeffrey (MD)	Nep	875
Kliot, David (MD)	ObG	518	Kraft, Robert (MD)	PlS	585
Kloss, Robert (MD)	Hem	1049	Krakovitz, Evan (MD)	CRS	765
Kloth, Howard (MD)	Cv	157	Kramer, Elissa (MD)	NuM	255
Klotz, Donald (MD)	PS	532	Kramer, Neil (MD)	IM	905
Klugman, Susan (MD)	ObG	796	Kramer, Philip (MD)	Oph	612
Klyde, Barry J (MD)	EDM	183	Kramer, Robert (DO)	ObG	729
Knackmuhs, Gary (MD)	IM	872	Kramer, Sara (MD)	Rhu	378

DIRECTORY OF DOCTORS

NAME	SPECIALTY	PAGE
Kranzler, Elliot (MD)	Psyc	351
Kranzler, L Stephan (MD)	N	792
Krasinski, Keith M (MD)	Ped Inf	316
Krasna, Irwin (MD)	PS	964
Krasnogor, Lester (MD)	Pul	1071
Krause, Cynthia (MD)	ObG	262
Krauss, Alfred N (MD)	NP	238
Krauss, Denis (MD)	Oto	303
Kreel, Isadore (MD)	S	389
Kreiger, Richard (MD)	IM	1004
Kreitzer, Joel (MD)	PM	308
Kreitzer, Paula (MD)	PEn	581
Krellenstein, Daniel (MD)	TS	397
Kremberg, M Roy (MD)	Psyc	351
Krespi, Yosef (MD)	Oto	303
Kressner, Michael (MD)	Ge	775
Krieger, Ben-Zion (MD)	Ped	534
Krieger, Karl (MD)	S	390
Krilov, Leonard (MD)	Ped	682
Krim, Eileen (MD)	ObG	663
Krinick, Ronald M (MD)	OrS	292
Krinsley, James (MD)	Pul	1071
Kris, Mark (MD)	Onc	234
Krishnamurthy, Shanker (MD)	OrS	805
Krivo, James (MD)	D	638
Krol, Kristine (MD)	A&I	601
Kroll, Richard (MD)	U	850
Kron, Leo (MD)	ChAP	164
Krongrad, Ehud (MD)	PCd	311
Kronzon, Itzhak (MD)	Cv	157
Kropinicki, William (MD)	IM	940
Krown, Susan (MD)	Onc	234
Krumholz, Burton (MD)	ObG	663
Krumholz, Michael (MD)	Ge	191
Kryle, Lawrence S (MD)	IM	651
Kudowitz, Paul (MD)	PM	580
Kuflik, Paul (MD)	OrS	292
Kugaczewski, Jane T (MD)	PS	738
Kugler, David (DO)	EDM	716
Kuhel, William (MD)	Oto	303
Kuhn, Leslie (MD)	Cv	157
Kukar, Narinder (MD)	EDM	563
Kula, Roger W (MD)	N	515
Kulick, Roy (MD)	HS	427
Kulick, Stephen (MD)	N	610
Kulpa, Jolanta (MD)	PHO	530
Kumar, Dharamjit (MD)	IM	569
Kumar, Sampath (MD)	S	547
Kummer, Bart (MD)	Ge	192
Kuncham, Sudha (MD)	ObG	663
Kunkel, Mark (MD)	Inf	1049
Kupersmith, Mark J (MD)	N	249
Kurani, Devendra (MD)	Psyc	932
Kuriloff, Daniel (MD)	Oto	304
Kurtin, Stephen (MD)	D	173
Kurtz, Caroline (MD)	Pul	1071
Kurtz, Lewis (MD)	S	698
Kurtz, Neil J (MD)	OrS	734
Kurtz, Robert C (MD)	IM	219
Kurz, Larry (MD)	IM	504
Kuslansky, Phillip (MD)	Cv	633
Kutcher, Rosalyn (MD)	Rad	829
Kutin, Neil (MD)	PS	679
Kutnick, Richard (MD)	Cv	157

NAME	SPECIALTY	PAGE
Kutnick, Robert (MD)	Pul	365
Kutscher, Martin (MD)	ChiN	764
Kveton, John (MD)	Oto	1063
Kwartler, Jed (MD)	Oto	1026
Kwon, Tae (MD)	GO	777
Kyi, Michael (MD)	EM	769
Kyriakides, Christopher (DO)	PMR	585

L

NAME	SPECIALTY	PAGE
La Barbera, Marianne (MD)	FP	605
LaBarbera, Philip (MD)	IM	723
Labissiere, Jean-Claude (MD)	IM	905
Lachmann, Elisabeth A (MD)	PMR	330
Lachs, Mark (MD)	Ger	197
La Corte, Michael (MD)	PCd	528
Lacqua, Frank (MD)	S	547
Lafferty, James (MD)	Cv	602
Lafontant, Jennifer (MD)	ObG	262
Lagoda, Boleslaw (MD)	Oph	930
Lahita, Robert (MD)	Rhu	378
Laitman, Robert (MD)	IM	433
Lajam, Fouad E (MD)	TS	397
Lajam, Frank E (MD)	TS	593
Lalli, Corradino (MD)	IM	723
La Marca, Charles (MD)	Oto	579
Lamarque, Madeleine (MD)	ObG	519
Lamaute, Henry (MD)	S	547
Lamba, Ameet (MD)	Psyc	1069
Lambroza, Arnon (MD)	Ge	192
La Mendola, Christopher (MD)	Cv	633
Lamm, Carin (MD)	PPul	317
Lamm, Steven (MD)	IM	219
Lamparello, Patrick (MD)	GVS	408
Lan, Sam (MD)	S	466
Lancefield, Margaret (MD)	IM	940
Landau, Leon (MD)	Hem	428
Landau, Steven (MD)	Ge	775
Landers, David (MD)	Cv	862
Landreth, Barbara (MD)	Ped	323
Landrigan, Philip (MD)	PrM	340
Lane, Fredrick M (MD)	Psyc	351
Lane, Lewis B (MD)	HS	646
Lang, Enid (MD)	Psyc	351
Lang, Jeffrey (MD)	DR	420
Lange, Dale J (MD)	N	250
Langelier, Carolyn (MD)	IM	219
Langman, Ronald (DO)	FP	565
Langone, Daniel (MD)	Oph	521
Langsner, Alan (MD)	PCd	913
Lanman, Geraldine (MD)	Ger	645
Lans, David (DO)	IM	783
Lansen, Thomas (MD)	NS	791
Lansigan, Nicholas (MD)	S	620
Lansing, Martha (MD)	FP	957
Lansman, Steven (MD)	TS	397
Lanter, Bernard (MD)	S	698
Lanyi, Valery (MD)	PMR	330
Lanzkowsky, Philip (MD)	PHO	677
Laor, Eliahu (MD)	U	470
La Quaglia, Michael (MD)	PS	319
Laragh, John (MD)	Cv	158
Laraja, Raymond (MD)	S	390
Larkin, Aimee (MD)	A&I	758
Larsen, John (MD)	Ped	323

NAME	SPECIALTY	PAGE	NAME	SPECIALTY	PAGE
Larson, Signe S (MD)	Ped	324	Lefkovits, Albert M (MD)	D	173
Larson, Steven (MD)	NuM	255	Lefkovitz, Zvi (MD)	Rad	373
Lasala, Patrick (MD)	NS	440	Lefkowitz, Harvey (MD)	Rad	693
Laskey, Richard S (MD)	Oto	931	Lefkowitz, Matthew (MD)	PM	528
Laskin, Richard (MD)	OrS	292	Lefrak, Steven (MD)	Ped	979
Lateiner, Lloyd (MD)	Oph	801	Legato, Marianne J (MD)	IM	220
Latov, Norman (MD)	N	250	Lehach, Joan (MD)	A&I	415
La Trenta, Gregory (MD)	PlS	336	Lehman, Thomas (MD)	Ped Rhu	318
Lau, Henry (MD)	IM	872	Lehman, Wallace B (MD)	OrS	292
Laub, Edward (MD)	IM	940	Lehrer, Joel (MD)	Oto	882
Laude, Teresita A (MD)	D	488	Lehrfeld, Jerome (MD)	FP	642
Laufer, Ira (MD)	EDM	183	Lehrhoff, Bernard (MD)	U	1031
Lauricella, Joseph (MD)	Cv	862	Lehrman, David B (MD)	RadRO	828
Lavyne, Michael H (MD)	NS	243	Lehrman, Gary (MD)	Pul	827
Lawrence, David (MD)	Oto	809	Lehrman, Stuart (MD)	Pul	827
Lawson, William (MD)	Oto	304	Leib, Martin L (MD)	Oph	275
Lax, James (MD)	IM	219	Leibel, Steven A (MD)	RadRO	368
Layne, Jeffrey (MD)	U	704	Leibowitz, Michael D (MD)	Psyc	351
Lazar, Eliot (MD)	Cv	483	Leichter, Donald (MD)	PCd	1027
Lazar, Emanuel (MD)	Ped	615	Leichter, Jair (MD)	DR	866
Lazarus, George (MD)	Ped	324	Leifer, Bennett (MD)	IM	872
Lazarus, Herbert (MD)	Ped	324	Leifer, Edgar (MD & PhD)	IM	220
Lazzaro, E Clifford (MD)	Oph	521	Leifer, Marvin W (MD)	Psyc	947
Leahy, Mary (MD)	IM	846	Leipzig, Rosanne (MD)	Ger	197
Leb, Alvin (MD)	Ge	495	Leipziger, Lyle S (MD)	PlS	687
Le Benger, Kerry (MD)	A&I	1017	Le Leiko, Neal S (MD)	PGe	314
Lebinger, Martin (MD)	Psyc	459	Lell, Mary-Elizabeth (MD)	ChiN	166
Lebinger, Tessa (MD)	PEn	811	Lempel, Herbert (MD)	IM	569
Lebofsky, Martin (MD)	IM	783	Lenger, Ellis Steven (MD)	IM	959
Lebovics, Edward (MD)	Ge	775	Lense, Lloyd (MD)	Cv	712
Lebovitz, Harold (MD)	EDM	490	Lenzo, Salvatore (MD)	OrS	292
Lebowicz, Joseph (MD)	Onc	509	Leong, Pauline (MD)	IM	651
Lebowitz, Arthur (MD)	IM	219	Leonidas, John (MD)	PR	582
Lebowitz, Mark (MD)	Oph	521	Lepor, Herbert (MD)	U	402
Lebwohl, Mark (MD)	D	173	Lepore, Frederick (MD)	N	961
Lebwohl, Oscar (MD)	Ge	192	Leppard, John (MD)	OrS	670
Lechner, Michael (MD)	IM	783	Lerman, Jay (MD)	D	767
Leddy, Joseph (MD)	OrS	963	Lerner, Chester (MD)	Inf	207
Lederberg, Marguerite (MD)	Psyc	351	Lerner, Harvey (MD)	IM	723
Lederman, Gil (MD)	RadRO	619	Lerner, Robert (MD)	Hem	203
Lederman, Josiane (MD)	D	603	Lesesne, Cap (MD)	PlS	336
Lederman, Martin (MD)	Oph	801	Lesniewski, Peter (MD)	OrS	670
Lederman, Sanford (MD)	ObG	519	L'Esperance, Francis A (MD)	Oph	275
Ledger, William (MD)	ObG	262	Lesser, Robert (MD)	Rhu	545
Lee, April (MD)	AM	601	Lessing, Jeffrey (MD)	U	621
Lee, Chol (MD)	Psyc	618	Lester, Richard (MD)	Oph	275
Lee, Chong Sung (MD)	S	833	Lester, Thomas (MD)	IM	784
Lee, Kwang Soo (MD)	Psyc	742	Levchuck, Sean G (MD)	PCd	675
Lee, Marjorie (MD)	IM	219	Levendoglu, Hulya (MD)	Ge	495
Lee, Mathew H (MD)	PMR	330	Levenson, Mark (MD)	Oto	304
Lee, Norris K (MD)	Oto	304	Leventhal, Arnold (MD)	U	704
Lee, Ronald (MD)	DR	1044	Leventhal, Elaine (MD & PhD)	IM	959
Lee, Sicy H (MD)	Rhu	378	Levere, Richard (MD)	IM	220
Lee, Stanley (MD)	Hem	499	Levey, Mark (MD)	Oto	912
Lee, Won Jay (MD)	Rad	589	Levey, Robert (MD)	IM	504
Lee, Youngick (MD)	TS	894	Levie, Mark (MD)	ObG	444
Leeds, Gary (MD)	FP	186	Levin, Aaron (MD)	PCd	811
Leeds, Richard (MD)	Cv	1011	Levin, Andrew Paul (MD)	Psyc	823
Leeman, Cavin P (MD)	Psyc	351	Levin, David (MD)	Nep	875
Leevy, C M (MD)	Ge	902	Levin, Henry (MD)	Oph	801
Lefer, Jay (MD)	Psyc	351	Levin, Howard (MD)	OrS	806
Leff, Alan (MD)	Anes	152	Levin, Leroy (MD)	S	698
Leff, Sanford (MD)	Cv	483	Levin, Linda (MD)	Ped	324
Leffell, David (MD)	D	1043	Levin, Mark (MD)	Hem	500

DIRECTORY OF DOCTORS

NAME	SPECIALTY	PAGE	NAME	SPECIALTY	PAGE
Levin, Nathan (MD)	IM	504	Lichtiger, Simon (MD)	Ge	192
Levin, Paul Edward (MD)	OrS	734	Lieber, Ernest (MD)	MG	508
Levin, Richard (MD)	Oto	1063	Lieberman, Beth (MD)	ObG	262
Levin, Sheryl (MD)	PMR	457	Lieberman, David M (MD)	Oph	522
Levine, Allwyn (MD)	ChAP	863	Lieberman, Elliott (MD)	U	704
Levine, David (MD)	N	250	Lieberman, James (MD)	PMR	331
Levine, Dorothy (MD)	Ped	1066	Lieberman, Kenneth (MD)	PNep	317
Levine, Evan (MD)	Cv	761	Lieberman, Theodore (MD)	Oph	275
Levine, Harold (MD)	Ped	682	Liebert, Peter (MD)	PS	813
Levine, Jeremiah (MD)	Ped	682	Liebeskind, Arie (MD)	NuM	255
Levine, Jerome (MD)	Inf	871	Liebling, Anne (MD)	Ped Rhu	531
Levine, Joseph H (MD)	CE	629	Liebowitz, Michael R (MD)	Psyc	352
Levine, Laurie J (MD)	D	638	Liebowitz, Solomon (MD)	Oph	275
Levine, Lenore (MD)	PEn	313	Lief, Philip (MD)	IM	433
Levine, Marc Joel (MD)	Oto	847	Lifshitz, Benjamin (MD)	IM	505
Levine, Martin S (DO)	FP	926	Lifshitz, Fima (MD)	PEn	529
Levine, Milton (MD)	IM	651	Lifshitz, Miriam (MD)	Ped	739
Levine, Mitchell E (MD)	N	660	Lightdale, Charles (MD)	Ge	192
Levine, Randy (MD)	IM	220	Ligouri, Lorene (MD)	ObG	519
Levine, Richard U (MD)	ObG	262	Liguori, Michael (MD)	IM	220
Levine, Seth (MD)	U	1008	Lim, Aquillina (MD)	ObG	444
Levine, Shirley (MD)	Hem	428	Lindenmayer, Jean-Pierre (MD)	Psyc	352
Levine, Steven (MD)	Ped	816	Linder, Paul (MD)	A&I	1039
Levinson, Joel (MD)	Ge	1021	Lindner, Arthur (MD)	Ge	192
Levitan, Stephan (MD)	Psyc	352	Lindsay, Gaius K (MD)	U	552
Levites, Kenneth (MD)	FP	718	Linn, Gary (MD)	U	983
Levitt, Miriam (MD)	Ped	817	Linstrom, Christopher (MD)	Oto	304
Levitt, Selwyn (MD)	U	837	Lipinsky, Edward John (MD)	Oto	736
Levitzky, Munro (MD)	Oph	275	Lipkowitz, Marvin (MD)	Psyc	539
Levitzky, Susan (MD)	Ped	324	Lipman, Marvin (MD)	IM	784
Levowitz, Bernard (MD)	GVS	553	Lipner, Henry (MD)	Nep	511
Levy, Albert (MD)	FP	186	Lipper, Evelyn (MD)	Ped	324
Levy, Andrew (MD)	SM	1029	Lipschitz, Robin (MD)	Rhu	379
Levy, Brian (MD)	EDM	183	Lipschutz, Herbert (MD)	IM	1012
Levy, Howard (MD)	OrS	292	Lipset, Richard (MD)	DR	178
Levy, James (MD)	Cv	761	Lipshutz, Mark (MD)	Onc	725
Levy, Joseph (MD)	PGe	314	Lipsitz, Philip (MD)	NP	572
Levy, Judith (MD)	ObG	444	Lipsky, William M (MD)	Inf	648
Levy, Lewis (MD)	N	660	Lipstein-Kresch, Esther (MD)	IM	651
Levy, Morton (MD)	Ped	682	Lipsztein, Roberto (MD)	RadRO	589
Levy, Roger (MD)	OrS	292	Lipton, Brian (MD)	Psyc	352
Levy, Ross (MD)	D	767	Lipton, Jeffrey F (MD)	PHO	315
Lew, Arthur (MD)	Psyc	823	Lipton, Mark (MD)	IM	221
Lew, Mark (MD)	Ped	534	Lipton, Richard Jeffrey (MD)	Oto	1063
Lewin, Margaret (MD)	IM	220	Lisman, Richard (MD)	Oph	275
Lewin, Sharon (MD)	IM	220	Liss, Donald (MD)	PMR	887
Lewis, Benjamin (MD)	Cv	158	Liss, Mark (MD)	Ge	775
Lewis, Blair (MD)	Ge	192	Lissak, Louis (MD)	ObG	262
Lewis, Dorothy Otnow (MD)	ChAP	164	Litchman, Mark (MD)	A&I	1039
Lewis, Lawrence (MD)	Oto	809	Liteplo, Ronald (MD)	D	419
Lewis, Owen (MD)	ChAP	164	Litman, Nathan (MD)	Ped	454
Lewis, Ralph (MD)	S	969	Litman, Richard (MD)	Oto	736
Lewis-Mantell, Laura (MD)	PM	308	Littlejohn, Charles (MD)	CRS	1042
Li, Ronald (MD)	Oto	945	Lituchy, Stanley (MD)	Psyc	823
Liang, Howard (MD)	S	390	Litvin, Yair (MD)	EDM	867
Libby, Daniel (MD)	Pul	365	Litvin, Y Samuel (MD)	U	983
Libman, Richard (MD)	N	574	Liu, Kang (MD)	FP	492
Libow, Leslie (MD)	Ger	198	Liu, Lena (MD)	PCd	311
Li Calzi, Luke (MD)	GVS	705	Liu, Paul (MD)	GO	200
Lichstein, Edgar (MD)	Cv	483	Livelli, Frank (MD)	Cv	863
Licht, Arnold (MD)	Psyc	539	Livingston, David (MD)	S	920
Lichtblau, Sheldon (MD)	OrS	293	Livingston, Lawrence (MD)	OrS	881
Lichtenstein, David (MD)	IM	569	Livingstone, Ian (MD)	N	942
Lichter, Stephen M (MD)	Onc	509	Lloyd, J Mervyn (MD)	OrS	881

NAME	SPECIALTY	PAGE	NAME	SPECIALTY	PAGE
Lo, K M Steve (MD)	Onc	1055	Luks, Howard J (MD)	SM	831
Lobell, Susan M (MD)	RE	544	Luntz, Maurice (MD)	Oph	275
Lobo, Rogerio (MD)	RE	375	Lupiano, John (MD)	IM	221
Lockshin, Michael Dan (MD)	Rhu	379	Luria, Martin (MD)	EDM	974
Lockwood, Charles (MD)	MF	229	Lurio, Joseph (MD)	FP	423
Loeb, Laurence (MD)	Psyc	823	Lusman, Paul (MD)	A&I	711
Loeb, Thomas (MD)	PlS	586	Lustbader, Ian (MD)	Ge	193
Lo Frumento, Mary Ann (MD)	Ped	996	Lustig, Ilana (MD)	ObG	263
Lo Galbo, Peter (MD)	A&I	559	Lutwick, Larry Irwin (MD)	Inf	501
Logan, Bruce (MD)	IM	221	Lutz, Gregory (MD)	PMR	946
Lo Gerfo, Paul L (MD)	S	390	Lyman, Neil (MD)	Nep	907
Loiacono, Anthony F (MD)	ObG	796	Lynn, Robert (MD)	Nep	439
Lois, William (MD)	S	547	Lynn, Stephan (MD)	EM	179
Lomasky, Steven (MD)	EDM	641	Lyon, Alan (MD)	Cv	484
Lombard, Jay (MD)	N	441	Lyon, Ross (MD)	GVS	470
Lombardi, Joseph (MD)	OrS	963			
Lombardo, Gerard (MD)	Pul	541	**M**		
Lombardo, James (MD)	Oph	522	Ma, Dong M (MD)	PMR	331
Lombardo, John (MD)	Oph	522	Macatangay, Angelo (MD)	Oto	614
Lombardo, Peter C (MD)	D	173	Maccabee, Paul J (MD)	N	515
Lombardo, Robert (MD)	Ge	192	Macchia, Richard (MD)	U	552
London, Ronald (MD)	Ped	455	Maccia, Clement (MD)	A&I	1017
Longobardi, Raphael (MD)	OrS	881	Macher, Mark (MD)	RadRO	967
Loo, Marcus (MD)	U	403	Mack, Walter J (MD)	Rad	745
Lopez, Clark (MD)	FP	492	Mackay, Cynthia J (MD)	Oph	276
Lopez, Deborah (MD)	PCCM	450	Mackenzie, C Ronald (MD)	IM	221
Lopez, Ralph (MD)	AM	149	Mackenzie, James (MD)	TS	969
Lopez, Robert (MD)	Oph	666	Mackler, Karen (MD)	D	767
Lorber, Daniel (MD)	EDM	563	Mackool, Richard (MD)	Oph	578
Lorefice, Laurence (MD)	Psyc	1069	Macris, Nicholas T (MD)	A&I	151
Loren, Gary Mark (MD)	PM	945	Maddalo, Anthony (MD)	OrS	806
Lotongkhum, Vichai (MD)	Cv	484	Magaro, Joseph (MD)	Oph	801
Lott, James V (MD)	CRS	1011	Maggio, John (DO)	ObG	263
Loughlin, Bruce Timothy (DO)	IM	1004	Magid, Steven K (MD)	Rhu	379
Louie, Eddie (MD)	Inf	207	Maguire, George (MD)	Pul	827
Louis, Bertin Magloi (MD)	IM	505	Magun, Arthur (MD)	Ge	193
Lovecchio, John (MD)	GO	645	Mahal, Pradeep (MD)	Ge	1021
Lovelace, Robert Edward (MD)	N	250	Mahler, Richard J (MD)	EDM	183
Lovelle-Allen, Susan (MD)	PlS	617	Mahnensmith, Rex (MD)	Nep	1057
Low, Ronald (MD)	Oto	883	Mahon, Eugene (MD)	Psyc	352
Lowe, Franklin (MD)	U	403	Mahoney, Maurice (MD)	MG	1054
Lowenheim, Mark Saul (MD)	PGe	737	Maidman, Jack (MD)	ObG	263
Lowenstein, Jerome (MD)	Nep	239	Maier, Herbert (MD)	D	1003
Lowenthal, Dennis (MD)	Onc	906	Maiman, Mitchell (MD)	GO	606
Lowinson, Joyce (MD)	Psyc	352	Maisel, James (MD)	Oph	667
Lowy, Joseph (MD)	Pul	365	Maisel, Jonathan (MD)	EM	1044
Lowy, Robert (MD)	Ge	566	Maizel, Barry (MD)	Ge	496
Lozner, Jerrold (MD)	TS	1031	Majlessi, Heshmat (MD)	GVS	839
Lu, Gabriel (MD)	PM	810	Maklansky, Daniel (MD)	DR	178
Lubat, Edward (MD)	Rad	891	Malach, Barbara (MD)	IM	608
Lubell, David (MD)	Ped	817	Malamud, Stephen (MD)	Onc	234
Lubell, Harry R (MD)	Ped	817	Malik, Asim (MD)	IM	505
Lubin, Martin (MD)	Psyc	586	Malik, Rubina (MD)	Ger	426
Lubliner, Jerry (MD)	OrS	293	Mallin, Jeffrey (MD)	N	660
Lucak, Basil K (MD)	Ge	193	Mallouh, Camille (MD)	U	837
Lucariello, Ralph (MD)	IM	433	Malone, Charlie (MD)	HS	201
Lucariello, Richard (MD)	Cv	417	Malovany, Robert (MD)	Pul	890
Lucente, Frank (MD)	Oto	527	Malpeso, James (MD)	Cv	602
Luciani, R L (MD)	ObG	909	Mamelok, Alfred E (MD)	Oph	276
Luciano, Anthony (MD)	IM	652	Mamtani, Ravinder (MD)	PrM	821
Lugo, Raul (MD)	S	390	Mandel, Edmund (MD)	U	552
Luka, Norman L (MD)	TS	999	Mandelbaum, Sid (MD)	Oph	276
Lukash, Barbara (MD)	D	767	Mandell, Lynda (MD & PhD)	RadRO	368
Lukash, Frederick (MD)	PlS	687	Mandeville, Edgar (MD)	ObG	575

DIRECTORY OF DOCTORS

NAME	SPECIALTY	PAGE	NAME	SPECIALTY	PAGE
Manevitz, Alan (MD)	Psyc	352	Martin, Eric C (MD)	VIR	406
Manfredi, Orlando (MD)	Rad	619	Martin, George (MD)	Ge	566
Manginello, Frank (MD)	NP	875	Martin, Robert (MD)	Psyc	689
Mango, Enrico S (MD)	OrS	734	Martin, Sidney A (MD)	Oph	731
Mani, John (MD)	OrS	524	Martinez, Alfred (MD)	S	747
Maniatis, Theodore (MD)	Pul	618	Martins, Publius (MD)	Pul	618
Maniscalco, Albert (MD)	Nep	610	Marush, Arthur (MD)	IM	505
Maniscalco, Anthony (MD)	N	515	Masciello, Michael (MD)	Cv	713
Mann, Charles (MD)	ObG	729	Maseda, Nelly (MD)	Ped	455
Mann, David (MD)	EDM	490	Masella, Peter A (MD)	Ped	455
Mann, Ronald (MD)	OrS	806	Maselli, Frank (MD)	FP	423
Manners, Richard (MD)	Ped	739	Mashman, Jan (MD)	PMR	1068
Manning, Frank (MD)	ObG	263	Masino, Frank A (MD)	RadRO	1072
Manning, Reginald (MD)	SM	545	Massad, Susan (MD)	IM	505
Manno, Joseph (MD)	S	894	Masson, Lalitha (MD)	ObG	930
Manolas, Panos (MD)	S	591	Mastrantonio, John (MD)	ObG	796
Manson, Aaron (MD)	IM	221	Matalon, Martin (MD)	ObG	729
Mansouri, Hormoz (MD)	S	698	Matalon, Robert (MD)	Nep	239
Mansouri, Mehran (MD)	S	698	Matarasso, Alan (MD)	PlS	336
Manzione, Nancy (MD)	Ge	425	Match, Ronald M (MD)	OrS	670
Marano, Anthony (MD)	Cv	761	Matera-Abouzahr, Cristina (MD)	ObG	263
Marans, Hillel (MD)	U	403	Mathur, Ambrish P (MD)	TS	550
Marans, Zvi (MD)	PCd	883	Matilsky, Michael (MD)	Cv	713
Marchetta, Paula (MD)	Rhu	379	Matkiwsksy, Zenon (DO)	S	1030
Marcus, Eric R (MD)	Psyc	352	Matkovic, Christopher (MD)	IM	723
Marcus, Judith (MD)	Ped	817	Matos, Jeffrey (MD)	Cv	158
Marcus, Michael (MD)	PPul	614	Matos, Marshall (MD)	Cv	761
Marcus, Norman (MD)	PM	308	Matossian, Cynthia (MD)	Oph	943
Marcus, Philip (MD)	Pul	690	Matta, Raymond (MD)	IM	221
Marcus, Ralph (MD)	Rhu	892	Mattana, Joseph (MD)	IM	652
Marcus, Richard (MD)	Ped	915	Mattel, Stephen (MD)	Oto	1006
Marcus, Stephen (MD)	OrS	670	Mattes, Leonard (MD)	Cv	158
Mardirossian, Jonathan (MD)	Oph	801	Matthews, Gerald J (MD)	U	838
Margouleff, Donald (MD)	NuM	661	Mattison, Timothy (MD)	D	767
Margulies, Paul (MD)	EDM	641	Mattoo, Nirmal (MD)	Nep	572
Margulis, Stephen (MD)	Ge	868	Mattucci, Kenneth (MD)	Oto	673
Marin, Deborah B (MD)	Psyc	353	Matz, Robert (MD)	IM	784
Marin, Lorraine A (MD)	RadRO	692	Mauer, Kenneth (MD)	Ge	1046
Marino, A Michael (MD)	Pul	1071	Maulik, Dev (MD)	ObG	663
Marino, John (MD)	Onc	655	Maurer, Virginia (MD)	S	699
Marino, Ronald (DO)	Ped	683	Mauser, Donald (MD)	N	660
Marino, William (MD)	Pul	460	Mauskop, Alexander (MD)	N	250
Marion, Robert (MD)	MG	436	Maxfield, Roger (MD)	Pul	365
Markell, Mariana (MD)	Nep	511	Mayer, Daniel (MD)	A&I	711
Markenson, Joseph (MD)	IM	221	Mayer, Ira (MD)	Ge	496
Markowitz, Allan (MD)	Oph	802	Mayer, Lloyd (MD)	IM	221
Markowitz, Arlene (MD)	Oto	304	Mayers, Marguerite (MD)	Ped	455
Markowitz, David (MD)	Ge	193	Mayers, Martin (MD)	Oph	445
Markowitz, James (MD)	Ped	683	Maytal, Joseph (MD)	ChiN	635
Markowitz, John (MD)	Psyc	353	Mazella, John S (MD)	OrS	806
Markowitz, Morri (MD)	PEn	451	Mazza, David Stephen (MD)	A&I	151
Marks, Alan (MD)	Oph	667	Mazzara, James (MD)	Cv	158
Marks, Andrea (MD)	AM	149	Mazzarino, Aldo (MD)	U	552
Marks, David A (MD)	N	908	McCaffrey, Raymond (MD)	ObG	263
Marks, Jon (MD)	U	403	McCalley, Stuart (MD)	Pul	1071
Marks, Richard (MD)	S	390	McCampbell, Edwin (MD)	FP	902
Marks, Stephen (MD)	N	792	McCann, Peter (MD)	OrS	293
Marks Jr, Clement E (MD)	Pul	365	McCarthy, Joseph (MD)	Rad	829
Marrero, Vito A (MD)	S	833	McCarthy, Shirley (MD & PhD)	DR	1044
Marrone, Vincent (MD)	IM	505	McCarton, Cecelia (MD)	Ped	324
Marsh, Jonathan (MD)	Hem	647	McClung, John A (MD)	Cv	761
Marshall, Merville (MD)	EDM	770	McConnell, John (MD)	CRS	864
Marsh Jr, Franklin (MD)	IM	221	McConnell, Robert (MD)	EDM	183
Martens Jr, Frederick W (MD)	ObG	263	McCormack, Barbara (MD)	ObG	879

NAME	SPECIALTY	PAGE	NAME	SPECIALTY	PAGE
McCormack, Patricia (MD)	D	603	Melone Jr, Charles P (MD)	OrS	293
McCormack, William M (MD)	Inf	501	Melton, R Christine (MD)	Oph	276
McCormack Jr, Richard R (MD)	HS	201	Meltzer, Jay I (MD)	Nep	239
McCormick, Beryl (MD)	RadRO	369	Meltzer, Marc (MD)	IM	652
McCormick, John R (MD)	TS	921	Menche, David (MD)	OrS	293
McCormick, Paul C (MD)	NS	244	Menchell, David (MD)	A&I	559
McDonough, Michael (MD)	Pul	918	Mendelowitz, Alan (MD)	Psyc	586
McElhinney, A James (MD)	S	466	Mendelowitz, Lawrence (MD)	ObG	796
McEvoy, Robert (MD)	EDM	183	Mendelowitz, Mark (MD)	ObG	796
McGill, Frances (MD)	ObG	263	Mendelsohn, Frederic (MD)	N	727
McGinn, Regina (MD)	IM	608	Mendelsohn, Irwin (MD)	Psyc	689
McGinn, Thomas (MD)	IM	433	Mendelsohn, Lois (MD)	A&I	758
McGinn Jr, Joseph (MD)	TS	621	Mendelsohn, Sara L (MD)	OM	730
McGovern, Thomas P (MD)	U	403	Mendelsohn, Steven (MD)	DR	639
McGovern Jr, Patrick Joseph (MD)	S	933	Mendelson, Harold (MD)	Psyc	823
McGowan, James M (MD)	Psyc	353	Mendelson, Joel (MD)	A&I	1017
McGrath, Patrick (MD)	Psyc	353	Mendes, Donna (MD)	GVS	408
Mc Groarty, James (MD)	Oph	522	Mendez, Hermann (MD)	Ped Inf	530
McHugh, Margaret (MD)	Ped	324	Mendoza, Francis (MD)	OrS	293
McIntosh, Sue (MD)	PHO	1065	Mendoza, Glenn (MD)	NP	846
McIvor, John (MD)	Rad	745	Menegus, Mark (MD)	Cv	417
McKee, David (MD)	Oto	1063	Menezes, Placido (MD)	OrS	524
McKee, Heather (MD)	Oph	802	Mennin, Gerald (MD)	Oph	802
McKee, Melissa Diane (MD)	FP	423	Menon, Latha (MD)	IM	433
McKinley, Matthew (MD)	Ge	644	Mensch, Alan (MD)	IM	652
McLeod, Gavin (MD)	Inf	1049	Menzies, Cheryl (MD)	NP	1056
McManus, Edward (MD)	Inf	990	Merav, Avraham (MD)	TS	469
McMullen, Robert (MD)	Psyc	353	Mercado, Myra (MD)	NP	238
McMurtry, James (MD)	NS	244	Mercando, Anthony (MD)	Cv	762
McSherry, Charles K (MD)	S	390	Mercurio, Peter (MD)	Cv	762
McVeigh, Anne Marie (MD)	Oph	276	Mercuro, T John (MD)	Cv	937
McWhorter, John (MD)	Rhu	1014	Meredith, Gary (MD)	Rhu	694
McWhorter, Philip (MD)	S	1075	Merhige, Kenneth (MD)	Oph	276
Meacham, Kevin (MD)	ObG	796	Merkatz, Irwin R (MD)	ObG	444
Mears, John Gregory (MD)	Hem	203	Merker, Edward (MD)	EDM	184
Mechanic, Alan (MD)	NS	658	Merker, Edward (MD)	FP	772
Mechanick, Jeffrey (MD)	EDM	184	Mermelstein, Erwin (MD)	Cv	955
Medina, Emma (MD)	Cv	762	Mermelstein, Harold (MD)	D	419
Medow, Norman (MD)	Oph	276	Mermelstein, Steve (MD)	Pul	690
Meed, Steven D (MD)	Rhu	379	Mernick, Mitchel (MD)	IM	222
Meek, Allen (MD)	RadRO	744	Merriam, John C (MD)	Oph	276
Megalli, Maguid (MD)	U	838	Merrill, Joan T (MD)	Rhu	379
Meggs, Leonard (MD)	Nep	790	Messana, Ida (MD)	IM	570
Megibow, Alec Jeffrey (MD)	DR	178	Messina, John (MD)	PCd	884
Megna, Daniel (MD)	Ge	605	Messo, Ralph K (DO)	IM	608
Mehra, Sunil (MD)	Pul	588	Mettu, Sudhaker (MD)	IM	784
Mehta, Dinesh (MD)	Oto	449	Mevs, Clifford (MD)	Ped	615
Mehta, Rajeev (MD)	NP	510	Meyer, Richard (MD)	IM	222
Mehta, Rekha (MD)	Ge	775	Meyer, Robert Peter (MD)	Oto	1006
Meier, Diane (MD)	Ger	198	Meyers, Barnett (MD)	Psyc	823
Meiland, Hanne (MD)	ObG	264	Meyers, Donald (MD)	Psyc	459
Meinhard, Bruce (MD)	OrS	670	Meyers, Helen (MD)	Psyc	459
Meisenberg, Eugene (MD)	U	552	Meyers, John H (MD)	D	638
Meislin, Aaron G (MD)	Ped	325	Meyers, Paul (MD)	Ped	325
Meiteles, Lawrence (MD)	Oto	809	Meyers, Samuel (MD)	Ge	193
Meixler, Steven (MD)	Pul	827	Mezey, Andrew (MD)	Ped	455
Melamed, Marc (MD)	IM	872	Miarrostami, M Rameen (MD)	Pul	541
Melillo, Nicholas (MD)	Pul	966	Michaelson, Richard (MD)	Onc	907
Mellinger, Brett (MD)	U	704	Michalos, Peter (MD)	Oph	731
Mellins, Robert (MD)	PPul	317	Michelis, Mary Ann (MD)	A&I	861
Mellman, Lisa (MD)	Psyc	353	Michelis, Michael (MD)	Nep	240
Melman, Arnold (MD)	U	403	Michels, Robert (MD)	Psyc	353
Melman, Martin (MD)	IM	784	Michelsen, W Jost (MD)	NS	440
Melnick, Hugh (MD)	ObG	264	Michler, Robert (MD)	TS	397

DIRECTORY OF DOCTORS

NAME	SPECIALTY	PAGE	NAME	SPECIALTY	PAGE
Mickatavage, Robert (MD)	Oph	802	Mohr, Jay Preston (MD)	N	250
Miclat Jr, Marciano (MD)	PlS	820	Mohr, Robert (MD)	ObG	993
Middleton, John (DO)	IM	959	Mohrer, Jonathan (MD)	IM	570
Midoneck, Shari (MD)	IM	222	Mohtashemi, Manucher (MD)	TS	701
Mignone, Biagio (MD)	Oph	802	Moideen, Ahamed (MD)	TS	593
Miguel, Eduardo (MD)	IM	873	Mojtabai, Shaparak (MD)	IM	433
Milano, Andrew (MD)	IM	222	Moldover, Jonathan (MD)	PMR	331
Milburn, Peter (MD)	D	488	Moldwin, Robert (MD)	U	594
Mildener, Barry (MD)	Psyc	586	Mollin, Joel (MD)	DR	563
Mildvan, Donna (MD)	Inf	207	Molloy, Edward Michael (MD)	IM	1052
Miles, Richard (MD)	Oto	1063	Molnar, Thomas (MD)	FP	565
Milhorat, Thomas H (MD)	NS	514	Molofsky, Walter (MD)	ChiN	166
Miller, Aaron (MD)	N	515	Molson, Robert (MD)	ObG	519
Miller, Albert (MD)	Pul	588	Molt, Patrick (MD)	S	833
Miller, Ann (MD)	N	442	Mondestin, Harry (MD)	Ped	946
Miller, Anne (MD)	HS	869	Mondrow, Stanley (MD)	Pul	588
Miller, Brian (MD)	Oph	802	Mones, Richard (MD)	PGe	314
Miller, Charles (MD)	S	390	Mongillo, Nicholas (MD)	Ped	1067
Miller, Daniel (MD)	FP	772	Monrad, E Scott (MD)	Cv	417
Miller, David (MD)	Psyc	1028	Monsanto, Enrique (MD)	HS	498
Miller, Dennis (MD)	Inf	207	Monteferrante, Judith (MD)	Cv	762
Miller, Ellen G (MD)	FP	773	Monteleone, Bernard B (MD)	Cv	633
Miller, Hyman (MD)	TS	835	Monteleone, Frank (MD)	S	699
Miller, James R (MD)	N	250	Montero, Carlos (MD)	OrS	670
Miller, Jeffrey (MD)	HS	990	Monti, Louis G (MD)	Ped	325
Miller, John I (MD)	NS	573	Mooney, Robert (MD)	Oph	802
Miller, Karen (MD)	DR	769	Moore, Anne (MD)	Onc	234
Miller, Kenneth (MD)	Rhu	1073	Moore, Eric (MD)	GVS	409
Miller, Lawrence (MD)	Psyc	618	Moore, Frank (MD)	NS	244
Miller, Richard L (MD)	D	714	Moore, Joanne (MD)	Psyc	353
Miller, Seth (MD)	Ge	644	Moorjani, Harish (MD)	Inf	778
Millman, Arthur (MD)	Oph	277	Moorthy, Chitti (MD)	RadRO	828
Millman, Robert B (MD)	Psyc	353	Mootabar, Hamid (MD)	ObG	796
Mills, Christopher B (MD)	S	391	Moqtaderi, Farideh (MD)	PM	309
Mills, Nancy Ellyn (MD)	Onc	788	Morabito, Carmine D (MD)	Oph	731
Milman, Perry (MD)	Ge	644	Moraille, Pascale (MD)	Psyc	932
Milone, Richard (MD)	Psyc	824	Moreau, Donna (MD)	ChAP	164
Milstein, David (MD)	NuM	443	Morehouse, Helen (MD)	DR	420
Mindel, Joel (MD)	Oph	277	Morelli, Alan (MD)	Ped	1067
Minkoff, Jeffrey (MD)	OrS	293	Morelli, Michael (MD)	IM	784
Minkowitz, Susan (MD)	IM	222	Morello, Robert (MD)	Oph	802
Minnefor, Anthony (MD)	Ped Inf	914	Moreno, Fernando (MD)	ObG	264
Minsky, Bruce (MD)	RadRO	369	Moreta, Henry (MD)	N	727
Mintz, Abraham (MD)	NS	1057	Moretti, Michael (MD)	ObG	611
Mintz, Fredric (MD)	IM	652	Moriarty, Daniel (MD)	Onc	1023
Miranda, Luis (MD)	U	621	Morris, Robert (MD)	Oph	731
Mirsky, Stanley (MD)	IM	222	Morrison, Susan (MD)	PA&I	994
Mirza, M Ather (MD)	HS	720	Morrissey, Kevin (MD)	S	391
Miskoff, A R (DO)	Onc	960	Morrow, Robert (MD)	FP	423
Miskovitz, Paul (MD)	Ge	193	Morrow, Todd (MD)	PlS	917
Mitchell, Janet L (MD)	ObG	519	Mortiz, Michael (MD)	PNep	452
Mitchell, John P (MD)	Oph	277	Moscatello, Augustine (MD)	Oto	809
Mitchell, Michael (MD)	Ped	325	Moscoso, Juan (MD)	Oto	579
Mitnick, Hal J (MD)	Rhu	379	Moser, Stuart (MD)	Cv	762
Mitnick, Julie (MD)	DR	179	Moses, Jeffrey W (MD)	Cv	158
Mittelman, Abraham (MD)	Onc	788	Moshe, Solomon (MD)	N	442
Mittman, Neal (MD)	Nep	512	Moskovich, Ronald (MD)	OrS	294
Mitty, Harold (MD)	Rad	373	Moskovits, Tibor (MD)	Hem	203
Mizrachy, Benjamin (MD)	S	391	Moskowitz, George (MD)	FP	492
Modlin, Saul (MD)	Oto	673	Moskowitz, Richard (MD)	CRS	987
Mogan, Glen (MD)	Ge	903	Moskowitz, Robert (MD)	IM	505
Moggio, Richard (MD)	TS	835	Moskowitz, Sam (MD)	Ge	496
Mogilner, Leonard (MD)	Ped	534	Moss, Richard (MD)	ObG	264
Mohaideen, A Hassan (MD)	S	547	Mossey, Robert (MD)	Nep	657

1306

NAME	SPECIALTY	PAGE	NAME	SPECIALTY	PAGE
Most, Richard W (MD)	Oph	803	Nassberg, B (MD)	EDM	974
Motahedeh, Faraj (MD)	ObG	519	Natale, Benjamin (DO)	Oph	1025
Motola, Jay Alan (MD)	U	838	Natarajan, Sam (MD)	Nep	790
Moulin, Nicole (MD)	Oto	449	Nath, Sunil (MD)	Pul	588
Moussa, Ghias (MD)	Cv	925	Nattis, Richard (MD)	Oph	731
Moynihan, Brian (DO)	FP	642	Navot, Daniel (MD)	RE	891
Moynihan, Gavan (MD)	D	714	Nawabi, Ismat (MD)	Hem	500
Muchnick, Richard (MD)	Oph	277	Nayak, Devdutt (MD)	Psyc	539
Muecke, Edward (MD)	U	403	Nealon, Nancy (MD)	N	251
Mueller, F Carl (MD)	Psyc	1069	Nedunchezian, Deeptha (MD)	Inf	607
Mueller, Richard (MD)	Cv	158	Needle, Mark (MD)	Nep	876
Muhlbauer, Helen (MD)	Psyc	459	Neelakantappa, Kotresha (MD)	Nep	512
Muhlfelder, Thomas (MD)	Hem	428	Neeson, Francis (MD)	Cv	1041
Muldoon, Thomas (MD)	Oph	277	Neff, Martin (MD)	Nep	573
Mulford, Gregory (MD)	PMR	996	Neibart, Eric (MD)	Inf	207
Mullen, David (MD)	Rad	1072	Nejat, Moosa (MD)	Cv	633
Mullen, Edward (MD)	RadRO	744	Nelson, David (MD)	Oph	667
Mullen, Michael (MD)	IM	222	Nelson, Deena (MD)	IM	223
Multz, Alan (MD)	Pul	588	Nelson, James (MD)	ObG	1060
Mundheim, Marshall (MD)	Rhu	379	Nelson, J Craig (MD)	Psyc	1069
Munoz, Eric (MD)	S	920	Nelson, Jeffrey (MD)	N	251
Munoz, Jose (MD)	IM	570	Nelson, John C (MD)	Onc	788
Muraca, Glenn (DO)	FP	565	Nelson, Noreen (MD)	ObG	1060
Murali, Raj (MD)	NS	244	Nelson, Peter (MD)	DR	179
Murphy, John (MD)	N	1058	Nelson, William (MD)	ObG	797
Murphy, Ramon J C (MD)	Ped	325	Nelson Jr, John M (MD)	OrS	806
Murray, Joseph P (MD)	Oto	809	Neophytices, Andreas (MD)	N	251
Murray, Simon (MD)	IM	941	Nerenberg, Alan (MD)	ObG	576
Muscillo, George (MD)	ObG	444	Nersessian, Edward (MD)	Psyc	354
Mushlin, Stuart (MD)	IM	1052	Nerwen, Clifford (MD)	Ped	584
Musiker, Seymour (MD)	Ped	739	Neschis, Martin (MD)	Ge	776
Muskin, Philip (MD)	Psyc	354	Neschis, Ronald (MD)	Psyc	824
Musto, Anthony (MD)	Oph	1061	Nessel, Mark (MD)	Psyc	354
Mutterperl, Mitchell (MD)	IM	928	Neubardt, Selig (MD)	ObG	797
Myers, Dale (MD)	Rad	891	Neubauer, Peter B (MD)	Psyc	354
Myers, Stanley (MD)	PMR	331	Neuwirth, Michael (MD)	OrS	294
Myers, Wayne A (MD)	Psyc	354	Nevins, Michael (MD)	IM	873
Myssiorek, David (MD)	Oto	579	Nevins, Stuart (MD)	Oto	809
			New, Maria (MD)	PEn	313
			Newhouse, Jeffrey (MD)	Rad	373
N			Newhouse, Robert P (MD)	Oph	278
Nachman, Ralph L (MD)	Onc	234	Newhouse, Stanley (MD)	IM	505
Nacier, Paul (MD)	IM	505	Newman, George (MD & PhD)	N	727
Nadel, Alfred (MD)	Oph	277	Newman, Lawrence C (MD)	N	442
Nadelman, Robert (MD)	Inf	779	Newman, Leonard (MD)	PGe	812
Nadler, Scott (DO)	PMR	917	Newman, Stephen (MD)	N	660
Nagel, Ronald (MD)	Hem	428	Newman-Cedar, Meryl (MD)	Ped	325
Nagler, Harris M (MD)	U	403	Newmark, Ian (MD)	Pul	690
Nagler, Jerry (MD)	Ge	193	Newton, Charles (MD)	TS	1076
Nagler, Willibald (MD)	PMR	331	Newton, Michael (MD)	Oph	278
Nahass, Ronald (MD)	Inf	940	Ngeow, Jeffrey (MD)	PM	309
Naidich, David P (MD)	Rad	373	Nicholas, James (MD)	OrS	294
Namerow, David (MD)	Ped	886	Nicholas, Stephen (MD)	OrS	294
Namm, Joel (MD)	DR	938	Nicholas, William (MD)	A&I	628
Napp, Marc (MD)	S	1075	Nichols, Francis (MD)	TS	894
Narins, Rhoda (MD)	D	767	Nichols, Jeffrey (MD)	Ger	426
Narula, Amarjot (MD)	Psyc	889	Nickerson, Katherine (MD)	Rhu	380
Narula, Pramod (MD)	PPul	677	Nickles, Steven (DO)	FP	867
Nash, Bernard (MD)	IM	723	Nicolas, Fred (MD)	S	548
Nash, Martin (MD)	Ped	325	Nicosia, Thomas A (MD)	Cv	633
Nash, Thomas (MD)	IM	222	Niederman, Michael (MD)	Pul	691
Nash, Warner (MD)	ObG	264	Nieporent, Hans (MD)	Psyc	539
Naso, Kristin (DO)	Ge	719	Nightingale, Jeffrey (MD)	Oph	278
Nass, Jack (MD)	Psyc	742	Nigro, Antoinette (MD)	ObG	797
Nass, Ruth (MD)	N	250			

DIRECTORY OF DOCTORS

NAME	SPECIALTY	PAGE	NAME	SPECIALTY	PAGE
Nigro, Emil (MD)	EM	769	Offit, Kenneth (MD)	Onc	235
Nimaroff, Michael (MD)	ObG	664	Ofodile, Ferdinand (MD)	PlS	337
Nini, Kevin (MD)	PlS	965	Oghia, Hady (MD)	Ped	534
Nininger, James (MD)	Psyc	354	O'Hea, Brian (MD)	S	747
Nir, Yehuda (MD)	Psyc	354	Okadigwe, Chukuma (MD)	TS	550
Nirenberg, Jason (MD)	Oph	445	Oktay, Kutluk (MD)	RE	544
Nisce, Lourdes (MD)	RadRO	369	Okun, Alex (MD)	Ped	455
Nisi, Rudolph (MD)	Cv	417	Olanow, C Warren (MD)	N	251
Nisonson, Barton (MD)	OrS	294	Olarte, Marcelo (MD)	N	251
Nissenblatt, Michael (MD)	Onc	960	Oldham, John (MD)	Psyc	355
Nitowsky, Harold (MD)	MG	436	Olds, David (MD)	Psyc	355
Nitzberg, Richard (MD)	S	1030	O'Leary, John (MD)	Anes	758
Nizin, Joel (MD)	CRS	864	O'Leary, Patrick (MD)	OrS	294
Noble, Kenneth (MD)	Oph	278	Oleske, James (MD)	Ped	915
Nochimson, David (MD)	MF	960	Oliver, Gregory (MD)	CRS	1019
Noel, Gary (MD)	Ped Inf	316	Oloumi, Mohammad (MD)	S	548
Nordli, Douglas (MD)	ChiN	166	Olsson, Carl (MD)	U	404
Nori, Dattatreyudu (MD)	RadRO	369	O'Malley, Grace M (MD)	Oph	732
Norris, John (MD)	Oph	910	Ong, Kenneth (MD)	IM	506
Norton, Karen (MD)	DR	179	Opler, Lewis (MD)	Psyc	355
Norton, Larry (MD)	Onc	235	Oppedisano, Carlyn (MD)	Ped	455
Nosko, Michael (MD & PhD)	NS	961	Oppenheim, Jeffery (MD)	NS	846
Notaro, Antoinette (MD)	D	714	Oratz, Ruth (MD)	Onc	235
Noto, Richard (MD)	Ped	817	Orbuch, Philip (MD)	D	173
Noto, Rocco (MD)	IM	784	Ordorica, Steven (MD)	ObG	264
Notterman, Daniel A (MD)	PCCM	312	O'Reilly, Richard (MD)	PHO	316
Novack, Stuart N (MD)	Rhu	1074	Oren, Reva (MD)	RadRO	997
Novak, Gerald P (MD)	ChiN	562	Orentreich, David (MD)	D	173
Novendstern, Joel (MD)	ObG	797	Orentreich, Norman (MD)	D	174
Novetsky, Allan (MD)	Onc	509	Orland, Steven (MD)	U	950
Novick, Brian (MD)	A&I	559	Orlin, Harvey (MD)	SM	695
Novik, Edward (MD)	Anes	1017	Orlow, Seth (MD)	D	174
Novogroder, Michael (MD)	Ped	886	Orofino, Michael (MD)	ObG	797
Nowak, Eugene (MD)	S	391	O'Rourke, James (MD)	Oph	803
Nowygrod, Roman (MD)	GVS	409	Orsher, Stuart (MD)	IM	223
Nozad, Steve (MD)	Cv	484	Orsini, William (MD)	D	974
Nucci, Annamaria (MD)	Psyc	917	Osborn, Harold (MD)	EM	420
Nudel, Dov (MD)	Ped	534	Osborne, Michael (MD)	S	391
Nudelman, Jeffrey Stuart (MD)	Oph	732	Osei, Clement (MD)	Pul	848
Nunberg, Henry (MD)	Psyc	354	Osei-Tutu, John (MD)	Psyc	459
Nunes, Edward (MD)	Psyc	354	O'Shaughnessy, Jane (MD)	EM	604
Nunez, Domingo (MD)	S	391	Ossias, A Lawrence (MD)	Hem	204
Nussbaum, Arnold (MD)	Ped	534	Oster, Martin (MD)	Onc	235
Nussbaum, Michel (MD)	Ge	566	Ostrovsky, Paul (MD)	Rad	373
Nussbaum, Moses (MD)	S	391	Ostrow, Stanley (MD)	Onc	725
Nutman, Jacob (MD)	PPul	1027	Ott, Allen (MD)	ObG	729
Nydick, Martin (MD)	IM	223	Ottaviano, Lawrence (MD)	Ge	193
Nyer, Kenneth (MD)	IM	433	Overby, M Chris (MD)	NS	658
			Owens, George (MD)	U	838
			Oxenhorn, Sanford (MD)	Psyc	742

O

Oberfield, Richard (MD)	Psyc	355	Oz, Mehmet (MD)	Cv	158
Oberfield, Sharon (MD)	PEn	313	Ozick, Hershel (MD)	Cv	762
Oberlander, Samuel (MD)	ObG	797	Ozuah, Philip (MD)	Ped	455
O'Brien, John D (MD)	Oph	732			
O'Brien, Stephen J (MD)	OrS	294			

P

Obstbaum, Stephen (MD)	Oph	278	Pace, Benjamin (MD)	S	591
Ocken, Paul (MD)	Oph	1013	Pacernick, Lawrence (MD)	D	638
O'Connell, Barbara E (MD)	Psyc	824	Pachter, H Leon (MD)	S	391
O'Connell, Daniel (MD)	FP	423	Pacienza, Vincent (MD)	Cv	633
O'Connell, Ralph (MD)	Psyc	824	Packard, William (MD)	Psyc	742
O'Connor, Kathleen (MD)	D	419	Packer, Milton (MD)	Cv	159
O'Connor, Patrick (MD)	IM	1052	Packer, Paul (MD)	ObG	444
Odell, Peter (MD)	Oph	278	Packer, Samuel (MD)	Oph	667
Oestreich, Herbert (MD)	NS	791	Packy, Theodore (MD)	EM	639

NAME	SPECIALTY	PAGE	NAME	SPECIALTY	PAGE
Padberg, Frank (MD)	S	921	Patel, Pankaj (MD)	AdP	899
Padilla, Alfred (MD)	EDM	1045	Patel, Sunil (MD)	IM	570
Padilla, Crisologo (MD)	S	548	Patrick, Albert (MD)	Ped	615
Padilla, Maria (MD)	IM	223	Patterson, Andrew (MD)	OrS	295
Paget, Stephen (MD)	Rhu	380	Patton-Greenidge, Loretta (MD)	FP	565
Paglia, Michael (MD)	S	391	Paul, Edward (MD)	AdP	149
Pagliaro, Salvatore (MD)	Psyc	824	Paul, Seth (MD)	OrS	670
Pagnani, Daniel J (MD)	ObG	664	Pawel, Michael (MD)	Psyc	355
Pahuja, Murlidhar (MD)	S	620	Pawl, Nancy (MD)	ObG	797
Pahwa, Savita (MD)	PA&I	674	Pearl, Richard (MD)	OrS	295
Pai, Narayan (MD)	S	466	Pearlman, Hubert (MD)	OrS	524
Pak, Jayoung (MD)	Ped	916	Pearlman, Steven (MD)	PlS	337
Palace, Fred (MD)	Rad	997	Pearlstein, Eric (MD)	Oph	522
Palatt, Terry (MD)	TS	748	Peck, Harvey (MD)	Rad	848
Palestro, Christopher (MD)	NuM	574	Pedley, Timothy (MD)	N	251
Paley, Carole (MD)	PHO	677	Pegler, Cynthia (MD)	AM	149
Pallotta, John (MD)	ObG	729	Pelavin, Martin (MD)	IM	873
Palmieri, Thomas J (MD)	HS	646	Pellettieri, John (MD)	ObG	576
Paltzik, Robert (MD)	D	638	Pellicci, Paul (MD)	OrS	295
Palumbo, John (MD)	Oph	803	Pellicci, Virginia (MD)	D	865
Pane, Carmella (MD)	NP	875	Pellman, Elliot (MD)	Rhu	694
Panella, Vincent (MD)	Ge	868	Pelosi, Marco A (MD)	ObG	930
Panetta, Thomas F (MD)	S	548	Pelosi, Richard (MD)	NS	876
Pang, Kenneth (MD)	Ped	615	Pena, Alberto (MD)	PS	583
Panicek, David (MD)	Rad	373	Penchaszadeh, Victor (MD)	MG	230
Panter, Gideon (MD)	ObG	264	Peng, Benjamin (MD)	U	404
Panza, Robert (MD)	Ped	996	Pennisi, Joseph (MD)	ObG	576
Panzner, Elizabeth (MD)	Ped	1027	Pepe, John (MD)	Nep	610
Paolino, James (MD)	Rhu	919	Pepper, Gary (MD)	EDM	491
Papish, Steven (MD)	Onc	991	Pereira, Frederick (MD)	D	563
Pappas, Steven (MD)	IM	784	Perel, Allan (MD)	N	610
Pappas, Thomas W (MD)	Cv	633	Peress, Richard (MD)	OrS	806
Pareja, N John (MD)	Psyc	355	Perez, Iris (MD)	PPul	452
Parikh, Divyang (MD)	Ge	605	Perez, Louis A (MD)	NR	793
Paris Cammer, Barbara (MD)	Ger	198	Perez, Maritza (MD)	D	174
Parisien, J Serge (MD)	OrS	294	Perkel, David (DO)	FP	867
Parisier, Simon (MD)	Oto	304	Perl, Harold (MD)	NP	875
Park, Constance (MD & PhD)	EDM	184	Perl, Louis (MD)	DR	1019
Park, Tai (MD)	IM	785	Perla, Elliott (MD)	IM	223
Parker, Albert (MD)	ObG	797	Perlman, Barry Bruce (MD)	Psyc	824
Parker, Margaret (DO)	Ped	740	Perlman, David (MD)	Inf	207
Parker, Robert (MD)	PHO	737	Perlmutter, Barbara (MD)	IM	928
Parnell, Vincent (MD)	TS	701	Perron, Reed (MD)	N	877
Parnes, Eliezer (MD)	Nep	512	Perry, Arthur (MD)	PlS	1013
Parness, Ira (MD)	PCd	311	Perry, Bradford (MD)	Psyc	824
Parr, Grant (MD)	TS	999	Perry, Henry (MD)	Oph	667
Parrish, Edward (MD)	Rhu	380	Perry, Kathleen (MD)	ObG	611
Parry, Michael (MD)	Inf	1050	Perry, Richard (MD)	Psyc	355
Pascal, Mark (MD)	Onc	874	Perskin, Michael (MD)	IM	223
Pascario, Ben (MD)	ObG	264	Persky, Mark (MD)	Oto	305
Pasmantier, Mark (MD)	Onc	235	Person, Ethel (MD)	Psyc	355
Passarelli, Nicholas (MD)	S	1075	Pertsemlidis, Demetrius (MD)	S	392
Passeri, Daniel (MD)	S	1075	Pervil, Paul (MD)	Ge	644
Pasternak, Bart M (MD)	GVS	1078	Pesiri, Vincent (MD)	S	699
Pastewski, Andrew (MD)	S	747	Peterson, Stephen J (MD)	IM	785
Pastore, Louis (MD)	U	749	Petito, Frank (MD)	N	251
Pastorek, Norman (MD)	Oto	305	Petratos, Marinos (MD)	D	174
Pastrich, Howard Jay (MD)	Ge	719	Petrek, Jeanne (MD)	S	392
Patel, Jitendra K (MD)	Rhu	545	Petrillo, Anthony (MD)	S	747
Patel, Kamalesh (MD)	Ge	957	Petro, Jane (MD)	PlS	820
Patel, Kamini (MD)	NuM	793	Petrossian, George A (MD)	Cv	633
Patel, Mahendra (MD)	NRad	574	Pettei, Michael (MD)	PGe	582
Patel, Mahendrakumar (MD)	PlS	458	Peyser, Donald (MD)	IM	905
Patel, Mukund (MD)	HS	498	Peyser, Ellen (MD)	Psyc	355

NAME	SPECIALTY	PAGE	NAME	SPECIALTY	PAGE
Peyser, Herbert (MD)	Psyc	355	Ponterio, Jane M (MD)	ObG	611
Pfeffer, Cynthia (MD)	Psyc	356	Poo, Wen Jen (MD)	Onc	1055
Phillips, Donna (MD)	OrS	295	Poole, Thomas (MD)	Oph	279
Phillips, Elizabeth (MD)	Onc	788	Pooley, Richard (MD)	TS	835
Phillips, Howard (MD)	Oph	803	Poon, Eric (MD)	Ped	326
Phillips, Malcolm (MD)	Cv	417	Popovich, Joseph F (MD)	S	933
Phillips, Reed (MD)	Onc	655	Popper, Laura (MD)	Ped	326
Pica, Vincent (MD)	Oph	943	Porder, Joseph (MD)	Cv	159
Piccione, Paul (MD)	Ge	496	Porder, Michael (MD)	Psyc	356
Piccirilli, Dora (MD)	FP	773	Poretsky, Leonid (MD)	EDM	184
Picone, Frank (MD)	A&I	973	Porges, Andrew (MD)	Rhu	694
Pierson, Richard (MD)	NuM	256	Porges, Robert (MD)	ObG	264
Pile-Spellman, John (MD)	Rad	373	Porreca, Francis (MD)	S	467
Pillari, Vincent (MD)	ObG	611	Portenoy, Russell (MD)	PM	309
Pilnik, Samuel (MD)	S	392	Portlock, Carol S (MD)	Onc	235
Pinals, Robert (MD)	Rhu	949	Porush, Jerome (MD)	Nep	512
Pincas, Martin (MD)	N	516	Porwancher, Richard (MD)	Inf	940
Pincus, Robert (MD)	Oto	305	Posner, David (MD)	Pul	366
Pineda, Albert (MD)	GO	1004	Posner, Jerome (MD)	N	252
Pines, Jeffrey (MD)	Psyc	356	Posner, Martin (MD)	HS	201
Pinke, Robert S (MD)	Oph	993	Post, Kalmon (MD)	NS	244
Pinkernell, Bruce (MD)	Cv	159	Post, Martin (MD)	Cv	159
Pinsker, Kenneth (MD)	Pul	460	Post, Robert (MD)	ObG	576
Pintauro, Frank (MD)	IM	434	Postley, John E (MD)	IM	223
Pintauro, Robert (MD)	IM	434	Potaznik, Daniel (MD)	Ped	616
Pinto, Edward (MD)	IM	1053	Pott, Nicholas (DO)	Psyc	742
Piomelli, Sergio (MD)	PHO	316	Pousada, Lidia (MD)	Ger	777
Pipala, Joseph (MD)	Onc	655	Prager, Kenneth (MD)	Pul	366
Piper, James (MD)	S	833	Prakash, Anaka (MD)	Ge	927
Pitchumoni, Capecomo (MD)	Ge	425	Preis, Oded (MD)	Ped	535
Pitem, Michael (DO)	N	516	Present, Daniel (MD)	Ge	194
Pitman, Gerald (MD)	PlS	337	Press, Joseph H (MD)	IM	506
Pitman, Mark (MD)	OrS	295	Press, Robert (MD)	Inf	207
Pitt, Jane (MD)	Ped	325	Pressman, Peter (MD)	S	392
Pizzarello, Louis (MD)	Oph	732	Presti, Salvatore (MD)	PCd	528
Pizzi, Francis (MD)	NS	942	Prestia, Alan (MD)	D	714
Pizzurro, Joe (MD)	OrS	882	Preven, David (MD)	Psyc	356
Plancher, Kevin (MD)	SM	1074	Prezant, David (MD)	Pul	460
Plantilla, Eduardo (MD)	TS	550	Prezioso, Paula (MD)	Ped	326
Pleasset, Maxwell (MD)	IM	785	Price, Andrew (MD)	OrS	295
Pliner, Lillian (MD)	Onc	1024	Price, Mitchell (MD)	PS	964
Plotkin, Roger (MD)	Oto	847	Priebe, Cedric J (MD)	PS	738
Plottel, Claudia (MD)	Pul	366	Primack, Marshall (MD)	IM	223
Plum, Fred (MD)	N	251	Prince, Andrew (MD)	Oph	279
Plummer, Robert (MD)	S	467	Pringle, Sheryl (MD)	FP	423
Pober, Barbara (MD)	MG	1054	Prioleau, Philip G (MD)	D	174
Pochapin, Mark (MD)	Ge	194	Prisco, Douglas L (MD)	IM	652
Podell, David (MD)	Oph	278	Pritzker, Henry (MD)	Rad	462
Podos, Steven (MD)	Oph	278	Procaccino, Angelo (MD)	S	699
Podwal, Mark (MD)	D	174	Procaccino, John (MD)	CRS	636
Poh, Maureen (MD)	D	174	Proshan, Steven Gerald (MD)	CRS	938
Policastro, Anthony (MD)	S	833	Provet, John (MD)	U	404
Polkow, Melvin (MD)	Pul	890	Pruzansky, Mark E (MD)	OrS	295
Pollack, Geoffrey (MD)	Oto	305	Prystowsky, Barry (MD)	Ped	916
Pollack, Jed (MD)	RadRO	692	Prystowsky, Janet (MD)	D	174
Pollak, Harvey (MD)	IM	652	Prystowsky, Milton (MD)	Ped	916
Pollina, Robert M (MD)	GVS	750	Prywes, Arnold (MD)	Oph	667
Pollock, Jeffrey (MD)	N	1024	Puccio, Carmelo (MD)	Onc	788
Polsky, Bruce (MD)	Inf	207	Pucillo, Anthony (MD)	Cv	762
Pomerantz, Barry (MD)	IM	846	Puder, Douglas (MD)	Ped	847
Pomeranz, Lee (MD)	S	699	Pugkhem, Tretorn (MD)	TS	593
Pomeroy, John (MD)	ChAP	713	Pulle, Dunstan (MD)	IM	434
Pomper, Stuart (MD)	S	620	Purcell, Ralph (MD)	HS	777
Pond, William (MD)	IM	990	Puritz, Elliot (MD)	D	714

NAME	SPECIALTY	PAGE	NAME	SPECIALTY	PAGE
Purow, Henry (MD)	Ped	616	Rao, Addagada (MD)	S	548
Purpura, Anthony (MD)	FP	493	Rao, Madu (MD)	PPul	531
Putignano, Joseph (MD)	U	838	Raphael, Bruce (MD)	Hem	204
Putterman, Eric A (MD)	SM	695	Rapin, Isabelle (MD)	ChiN	418
			Rapoport, Samuel (MD)	N	252
Q			Rapp, Lynn (MD)	ObG	611
			Rappaport, Irwin (MD)	PA&I	310
Qadir, Shuja (MD)	IM	570	Raps, Mitchell S (MD)	N	252
Quagliarello, John (MD)	EDM	184	Raskin, Jonathan (MD)	Pul	366
Quagriarello, Vincent (MD)	Inf	1050	Raskin, Keith (MD)	OrS	296
Quartararo, Paul (MD)	IM	1053	Raskin, Noel (MD)	TS	397
Quest, Donald (MD)	NS	876	Raskin, Raymond (MD)	Psyc	356
Quinn, Joseph (MD)	Ped	740	Ratner, Lynn (MD)	Onc	235
Quitkin, Frederic (MD)	Psyc	356	Ratzan, Sanford (MD)	OrS	734
Quittell, Lynne (MD)	Ped	326	Raucher, Harold (MD)	Ped	326
			Rauscher, Gregory (MD)	PlS	888
R			Rausen, Aaron (MD)	PHO	316
			Ravetz, Valerie (MD)	FP	186
Raab, Edward (MD)	Oph	279	Ravikumar, Sunita (MD)	IM	785
Rabhan, Nathan B (MD)	D	175	Ray, Audell (MD)	Oph	803
Rabin, Aaron (MD & PhD)	N	877	Rayner, Martha (MD)	IM	506
Rabin, Jill (MD)	ObG	664	Raynor, Richard B (MD)	NS	244
Rabinowicz, Morris (MD)	Ped	683	Razaboni, Rosa (MD)	PlS	337
Rabinowitz, Jack G (MD)	Rad	373	Razmzan, Shahram (MD)	ObG	797
Rabinowitz, Simon (MD)	PGe	529	Reader, Robert (MD)	S	392
Rabinowitz, Stanley (MD)	Pul	691	Reale, Mario (MD)	NP	789
Raboy, Adley (MD)	U	621	Reape, Donald (MD)	IM	224
Racanelli, Joseph (MD)	IM	224	Rebold, Bruce (MD)	ObG	664
Rackoff, Paula (MD)	Rhu	380	Reckler, Jon Michael (MD)	U	404
Rackow, Eric (MD)	IM	224	Reda, Dominick (MD)	IM	785
Radel, Eva (MD)	PHO	451	Reddy, Chatla (MD)	Cv	484
Radin, Allen (MD)	Rhu	380	Reddy, Gaddam D (MD)	Ped	584
Radparvar, Dariush (MD)	Rad	463	Reddy, Malikar Juna (MD)	FP	565
Rafia, Sameer (MD)	RadRO	542	Reddy, Munagala (MD)	Ger	645
Rafii, Shahrokh (MD)	Cv	484	Reddy, Stanley (MD)	Psyc	689
Rafla, Sameer Demetrious (MD)	RadRO	542	Rednor, Jeffrey (DO)	FP	939
Raggi, Robert (MD)	Anes	861	Reduto, Lawrence (MD)	Cv	634
Ragnarsson, Kristjan (MD)	PMR	331	Reed, David (MD)	S	1075
Ragno, Philip David (MD)	Cv	634	Reed, George (MD)	TS	836
Rago, Thomas (MD)	HS	1048	Reed, Lawrence S (MD)	PlS	337
Ragone, Philip (MD)	N	660	Reed, Louis Juden (MD)	IM	434
Rahal, James (MD)	Inf	568	Reed, Mary K (MD)	Onc	437
Rai, Kanti (MD)	Hem	568	Rehman, Hafiz (MD)	Ped	740
Rajdeo, Heena (MD)	S	833	Rehnstrom, Jaana (MD)	ObG	265
Rajput, Ashok (MD)	Psyc	586	Rehrer, Lisa (MD)	ObG	265
Raju, Raghava (MD)	PlS	617	Reich, Edward (MD)	N	252
Raju, Ramanathan (MD)	S	548	Reich, J Douglas (MD)	FP	493
Raju, Samanthi (MD)	U	552	Reich, Raymond (MD)	Oph	522
Rakowitz, Frederic (MD)	IM	652	Reichel, Joseph (MD)	Pul	461
Ramanathan, Kumudha (MD)	Rad	543	Reicher, Oscar (MD)	OrS	1005
Rambler, Louis (MD)	DR	866	Reichman, Lee (MD)	IM	905
Ramenofsky, Max (MD)	PS	532	Reichstein, Robert (MD)	Cv	159
Ramgopal, Mekala (MD)	Ge	566	Reid, Roberto (MD)	U	470
Ramirez, Mark A (MD)	Onc	437	Reidenberg, Marcus (MD)	IM	224
Ramsay, David L (MD)	D	175	Reiffel, James (MD)	Cv	159
Ramsey Jr, Walter S (MD)	S	699	Reiffel, Robert (MD)	PlS	820
Ranawat, Chitranjan (MD)	OrS	296	Reilly, John (MD)	OrS	613
Rand, Jacob (MD)	Hem	204	Reilly, John Patrick (MD)	Onc	437
Rand, James (MD)	Ge	566	Reilly, Kevin B (MD)	ObG	798
Randolph, Audrey (MD)	PMR	819	Reilly, Kevin D (MD)	ObG	444
Randolph, Paula (MD)	ObG	264	Reilly, Thomas (MD)	IM	570
Rangraj, Madhu S (MD)	S	834	Rein, Joel (MD)	PlS	1068
Raniolo, Robert (MD)	S	834	Reiner, Mark (MD)	S	392
Ransom, Mark (MD)	RE	1007	Reinersman, Gerold (MD)	NP	438
Ranta, Jeffrey (MD)	U	1077			

DIRECTORY OF DOCTORS

NAME	SPECIALTY	PAGE	NAME	SPECIALTY	PAGE
Reinhardt, Henry (MD)	ObG	664	Roach, James (MD)	U	1077
Reinitz, Elizabeth (MD)	Rhu	830	Robbins, John (MD)	N	792
Reisberg, Barry (MD)	GerPsy	198	Robbins, Michael (MD)	Cv	560
Reisch, Milton (MD)	D	175	Robbins, Noah (MD)	Inf	429
Reiser, Ira (MD)	Nep	512	Roberts, Calvin (MD)	Oph	280
Reiss, Joseph (MD)	A&I	628	Roberts, Larry P (MD)	U	838
Reiss, Ronald (MD)	ObG	265	Robilotti, James (MD)	Ge	194
Reitman, Milton (MD)	PCd	737	Robin, Noel (MD)	EDM	1045
Reizis, Igal (MD)	ObG	519	Robins, Perry (MD)	D	175
Rella, Anthony (MD)	S	849	Robinson, John (MD)	S	747
Relland, Maureen (MD)	Oph	279	Robinson, Newell B (MD)	TS	701
Remy, Prospere (MD)	Ge	425	Rocchio, Joseph (MD)	Ped	326
Rentrop, K Peter (MD)	Cv	159	Rochelson, Burton (MD)	ObG	729
Repice, Michael (MD)	Rhu	746	Rochman, Andrew (MD)	S	699
Reppucci, Vincent (MD)	Oph	279	Rock, Erwin (MD)	Oto	809
Resmovits, Marvin (MD)	Ped	584	Rockwell, William (MD)	A&I	1039
Resnick, David (MD)	A&I	415	Rodke, Gae (MD)	ObG	265
Resnick, Richard (MD)	Psyc	356	Rodman, John (MD)	IM	224
Resor, Louise (MD)	N	1058	Rodriguez-Sains, Rene (MD)	Oph	280
Respler, Don (MD)	Oto	1006	Roeder, Werner (MD)	S	834
Reyes, Francisco I (MD)	ObG	519	Roff, George (MD)	Psyc	824
Reyniak, Victor (MD)	RE	375	Rogal, Gary J (MD)	Cv	900
Reynolds, Benedict (MD)	S	467	Roger, Ignatius Daniel (MD)	HS	567
Rezk, George (MD)	Ge	496	Rogers, Brad (MD)	U	950
Rhee, Jung (MD)	Ped	931	Rogers, Murray (MD)	IM	224
Rhoads, Frances (MD)	Ped	965	Rogg, Gary (MD)	IM	434
Ricca, Richard (MD)	S	747	Rohman, Michael (MD)	TS	469
Ricci, Mario (MD)	IM	434	Rokito, Andrew (MD)	SM	382
Ricciardelli, Charles (MD)	OrS	806	Roland, Robert (DO)	Inf	1022
Ricciardi, Daniel (MD)	Rhu	545	Rom, William N (MD)	Pul	366
Rice, Emanuel (MD)	Psyc	356	Romagnoli, Mario (MD)	Inf	208
Rich, Andrea (MD)	Ped	916	Romanelli, John (MD)	Oph	732
Rich, Daniel (MD)	OrS	670	Romanello, Paul (MD)	Cv	160
Richard, Jack (MD)	EDM	184	Romano, Alicia (MD)	PEn	812
Richards, Arnold (MD)	Psyc	357	Romano, John (MD)	D	175
Richards, Ernest (MD)	IM	785	Romano, Rosario (MD)	IM	723
Richards, Renee (MD)	Oph	279	Romanowitz, Harry (MD)	Ped	1067
Richel, Peter (MD)	Ped	817	Romas, Nicholas A (MD)	U	404
Richter, Robert (MD)	S	548	Romero, Carlos (MD)	S	699
Ricketti, Anthony (MD)	A&I	937	Romeu, Jose (MD)	Ge	194
Ricotta, John (MD)	GVS	750	Romita, Mauro C (MD)	PlS	337
Ridge, Gerald (MD)	IM	785	Romo III, Thomas (MD)	PlS	337
Rie, Jonathan (MD)	Nep	790	Roose, Steven (MD)	Psyc	357
Riechers, Roger (MD)	U	838	Root, Barry (MD)	PMR	683
Rieder, Ronald (MD)	Hem	500	Root, Leon (MD)	OrS	296
Riegelhaupt, Elliot (MD)	Cv	159	Rosch, Elliott (MD)	IM	785
Rifkin, Arthur (MD)	Psyc	587	Rose, Arthur L (MD)	ChiN	486
Rifkin, Boris (MD)	Psyc	1070	Rose, Daniel (MD)	TS	1076
Rifkin, Paul (MD)	Hem	1021	Rose, David (MD)	IM	570
Rifkin, Terry (MD)	ObG	664	Rose, Donald J (MD)	OrS	296
Rifkind, Kenneth (MD)	S	592	Rose, Eric A (MD)	Cv	160
Rifkinson-Mann, Stephanie (MD)	Ped	817	Rose, Henry (MD)	Pul	890
Rigel, Darrell (MD)	D	175	Rose, Howard Anthony (MD)	OrS	296
Riles, Thomas (MD)	GVS	409	Rose, Louis (MD)	OrS	447
Riley, David (MD)	Pul	966	Rosello, Lori (MD)	Ped	326
Ring, Kenneth (MD)	U	1031	Rosemarin, Jack (MD)	Ge	776
Ritch, Robert (MD)	Oph	279	Rosen, Arnold M (MD)	Psyc	357
Ritter, Joseph (MD)	U	1031	Rosen, Bruce (MD)	Psyc	742
Ritter, Sam (MD)	PCd	614	Rosen, Evelyn (MD)	Psyc	539
Rivenson, Melanie (MD)	A&I	758	Rosen, Herman (MD)	Nep	512
Rivers, Steven P (MD)	GVS	470	Rosen, Mark J (MD)	Pul	366
Rivlin, Richard (MD)	IM	224	Rosen, Norman (MD)	Onc	789
Rizzo, Frank (MD)	N	252	Rosen, Richard (MD)	Oph	280
Rizzo, Thomas (MD)	OrS	806	Rosen, Rick (MD)	PlS	1068

DIRECTORY OF DOCTORS

NAME	SPECIALTY	PAGE	NAME	SPECIALTY	PAGE
Rudin, Leonard (MD)	U	850	Saleh, Anthony (MD)	Pul	541
Rudman, Michael E (MD)	PM	994	Salem, Noel (MD)	Rhu	892
Rudolph, Steven (MD)	N	252	Salemi, Mozafar (MD)	Ped	584
Rudorfer, Alvin (DO)	FP	493	Sales, Clifford (MD)	GVS	1031
Ruggiero, Joseph (MD)	Hem	204	Salik, James (MD)	Ge	195
Rummo, Nicholas (MD)	IM	786	Salkin, Paul (MD)	Psyc	358
Runowicz, Carolyn (MD)	ObG	444	Salky, Barry (MD)	S	393
Ruoff, Michael (MD)	Ge	194	Salmon, Jane (MD)	Rhu	380
Rusch, Valerie (MD)	TS	398	Saltzman, Martin (MD)	Nep	790
Rush, Stephen (MD)	RadRO	692	Saltzman, Simone (MD)	Inf	429
Rush, Thomas (MD)	Inf	779	Salvati, Eduardo (MD)	OrS	297
Russakoff, L Mark (MD)	Psyc	825	Salvati, Eugene (MD)	CRS	956
Russell, Robin (MD)	Ger	427	Salzano, Anthony (MD)	PMR	819
Russo, Paul (MD)	U	404	Salzberg, C Andrew (MD)	PlS	820
Russo, Robert (MD)	Rad	1072	Salzer, Peter (MD)	S	700
Rutkovsky, Edward (MD)	Cv	634	Salzer, Richard (MD)	OrS	882
Rutkovsky, Lisa Rosner (MD)	PCd	580	Salzer, Stephen (MD)	Oto	1064
Ryan, Joseph (MD)	Ger	1011	Salzman, Jacqueline (MD)	Oph	803
Ryan, Samuel (MD)	ObG	265	Sama, Andrew (MD)	EM	639
Ryback, Hyman (MD)	Oto	810	Sama, Jahir (MD)	ObG	909
Rydzinski, Mayer (MD)	Cv	561	Samach, Michael (MD)	Ge	989
			Samberg, Eslee (MD)	Psyc	358
S			Sami, Sherif (MD)	Psyc	689
			Sampogna, Dominick (MD)	Oto	736
Saada, Simon (MD)	U	553	Samra, Said (MD)	PlS	979
Saal, Stuart (MD)	Nep	240	Samuel, Edward (MD)	Onc	725
Sabba, Stephen (MD)	IM	786	Samuelly, Israel (MD)	GerPsy	497
Sabetta, James (MD)	Inf	1050	Samuels, Steven (MD)	Inf	721
Sable, Robert (MD)	Ge	425	Samuels, Steven (MD)	Psyc	358
Sabot, Lawrence M (MD)	Psyc	689	Sananman, Michael (MD)	N	1024
Sacchi, Terrence J (MD)	Cv	484	Sand, Jay P (MD)	FP	926
Sacco, Ralph L (MD)	N	253	Sander, Norbert (MD)	IM	434
Sachar, David (MD)	Ge	194	Sanders, Abraham (MD)	Pul	366
Sachdev, Ved (MD)	NS	244	Sandhaus, Jeffrey (MD)	U	594
Sachs, Jonathan (MD)	Ge	939	Sandhu, M Y (MD)	Cv	925
Sachs, Paul (MD)	Pul	1071	Sandler, Benjamin (MD)	ObG	266
Sachs, R Gregory (MD)	Cv	1018	Sands, Andrew (MD)	OrS	297
Sachs, Stephen (MD)	N	1024	San Filippo, J Anthony (MD)	PS	814
Sacker, Ira (MD)	AM	481	Sanford, Marie (MD)	Ped	327
Sacks, Kenneth (MD)	Onc	1055	Sanger, Joseph J (MD)	NuM	256
Sacks, Michael (MD)	Psyc	357	Sanjana, Veeraf (MD & PhD)	Inf	208
Sacks, Steven (MD)	Oto	305	Sank, Lewis (MD)	Ped	1027
Sacks-Berg, Anne (MD)	Inf	721	San Roman, Gerardo (MD)	ObG	729
Sadan, Sara (MD)	Onc	789	Santamaria II, Jaime (MD)	Oph	962
Sadanandan, Swayam (MD)	PHO	530	Santiamo, Joseph (MD)	IM	608
Sadarangani, Gurmukh J (MD)	RadRO	369	Santilli, John (MD)	A&I	1040
Sadeghi, H (MD)	N	929	Santilli, Veronica (MD)	Ped	535
Sadick, Neil (MD)	D	175	Santomauro, Anthony (MD)	ObG	1060
Sadiq, Saud (MD)	N	253	Santorineou, Maria (MD)	Ped	456
Sadler, Arthur (MD)	OrS	448	Santoro, Elissa (MD)	S	921
Sadock, Benjamin (MD)	Psyc	358	Santoro, Michael (MD)	U	704
Sadock, Virginia (MD)	Psyc	358	Santoro, Nanette (MD)	ObG	445
Sadovsky, Richard (MD)	FP	493	Saperstein, Lewis (MD)	S	1007
Saenger, Paul (MD)	PEn	451	Saphir, Richard L (MD)	Ped	327
Safai, Bijan (MD)	D	768	Saponara, Eduardo (MD)	Onc	789
Saffra, Norman (MD)	Oph	523	Saporta, Diego (MD)	Oto	1026
Safier, Henry L (MD)	Ge	566	Sara, Gabriel (MD)	Onc	235
Safirstein, Benjamin (MD)	Pul	918	Sarabu, Mohan (MD)	TS	836
Sage, Jacob (MD)	N	961	Saraf, Varsha (MD)	RE	590
Sagy, Meyer (MD)	PCCM	581	Saraiya, Narendra (MD)	Ped	535
Saha, Chanchal (MD)	TS	701	Sari Markell, Marian (MD)	Nep	512
Sailon, Peter (MD)	ObG	265	Sarokhan, Alan (MD)	OrS	1013
Salama, Meir (MD)	Ge	776	Sarokhan, John (MD)	S	981
Salas, Max (MD)	EDM	956	Sarosi, Peter (MD)	ObG	266
Salcedo, Jose (MD)	PNep	914			

NAME	SPECIALTY	PAGE	NAME	SPECIALTY	PAGE
Sas, Norman (MD)	S	467	Schiller, Robert (MD)	FP	186
Sasaki, ClarenceT (MD)	Oto	1064	Schiowitz, Emanuel (DO)	FP	493
Sasso, Louis (MD)	Pul	619	Schlaeger, Ralph (MD)	Rad	374
Sassoon, Robert (MD)	ObG	266	Schlecker, Austin (MD)	IM	506
Satnick, Steven (MD)	A&I	711	Schlegel, Peter (MD)	U	405
Saubermann, Albert J (MD)	Anes	416	Schleider, Michael (MD)	Onc	874
Sauer, Mark (MD)	RE	375	Schleifer, Steven (MD)	Psyc	917
Saul, Zane (MD)	Inf	1050	Schlesinger, Irwin (MD)	N	660
Savasatit, Panas (MD)	S	592	Schley, W Shain (MD)	Oto	305
Savatsky, Gary (MD)	SM	892	Schliftman, Alan (MD)	D	768
Savetsky, Lawrence (MD)	Oto	305	Schmelkin, Ira (MD)	Ge	644
Savino, John (MD)	S	834	Schmer, Veronica (MD)	PCd	528
Savino, Michael (MD)	U	621	Schmerin, Michael (MD)	Ge	195
Sawczuk, Ihor S (MD)	U	404	Schmidt, Philip (MD)	IM	506
Sawyer, David (MD)	Psyc	358	Schmidt-Sarosi, Cecilia (MD)	RE	375
Saxe, Bruce (MD)	RadRO	692	Schnabel, Freya (MD)	S	393
Saxena, Anil (MD)	IM	506	Schneck, Gideon (MD)	Oph	732
Sayad, Karim (MD)	IM	225	Schneebaum, Cary (MD)	IM	225
Sayegh, Naseem E (MD)	S	834	Schneider, Arlene (MD)	A&I	482
Sayegh, Neil (MD)	U	838	Schneider, George (MD)	EDM	902
Scaduto, Phillip (MD)	IM	990	Schneider, Howard (MD)	Oph	280
Scarpa, Nicholas P (DO)	Rhu	932	Schneider, Karen (MD)	Oph	446
Scerbo, Joseph (MD)	Pul	932	Schneider, Kenneth L (MD)	Oto	306
Schaefer, John A (MD)	N	253	Schneider, Lewis (MD)	Ge	195
Schaefer, Steven (MD)	Oto	305	Schneider, Robert (MD)	Onc	789
Schaeffer, Henry (MD)	Ped	535	Schneider, Ronald (MD)	ObG	798
Schaeffer, Janis (MD)	PPul	678	Schneider, Samuel (MD)	Psyc	947
Schaffer, Dean (MD)	Oto	810	Schneider, Steven (MD)	IM	225
Schanzer, Harry (MD)	GVS	409	Schneider, Steven Jack (MD)	NS	658
Scharf, Richard (DO)	Oto	1026	Schneyer, Barton (MD)	Pul	743
Scharf, Robert (MD)	Psyc	358	Schob, Clifford (MD)	OrS	911
Scharf, Stephen (MD)	NuM	256	Schoen, Roy M (MD)	ObG	266
Scharfman, Edward (MD)	Psyc	825	Schoeneman, Morris J (MD)	PNep	531
Schaul, Neil (MD)	N	574	Schoenwald, Robert (MD)	S	747
Schaumburg, Herbert (MD)	N	442	Schonberg, Samuel Kenneth (MD)	Ped	456
Schechner, Richard (MD)	S	467	Schore, Arthur (MD & PhD)	Psyc	358
Schechter, Justin (MD)	Psyc	1070	Schorn, Karen (MD)	Rhu	694
Schechter, Miriam (MD)	Ped	456	Schowalter, John (MD)	ChAP	1042
Schechter, Ronald (MD)	Oph	523	Schrader, Zalman (MD)	Ge	903
Scheer, Max (MD)	IM	653	Schrager, Alan (MD)	U	839
Scheidt, Stephen (MD)	Cv	160	Schreiber, Carl (MD)	Cv	634
Schein, Jonah (MD)	Psyc	358	Schreiber, Michael (MD)	Pul	827
Scheinbaum, Richard (MD)	Ge	1046	Schreiber, Zwi (MD)	Hem	429
Schell, Harold S (MD)	S	950	Schreibman, Barbara (MD)	EM	866
Scher, Allan (MD)	RadRO	997	Schubert, Herman N (MD)	Oph	281
Scher, Howard (MD)	Onc	236	Schulder, Michael (MD)	NS	908
Scher, Jonathan (MD)	ObG	266	Schullinger, John (MD)	PS	319
Scher, Richard K (MD)	D	175	Schulman, David (MD)	Psyc	359
Scherl, Michael (MD)	Oto	883	Schulman, Ira (MD)	Cv	160
Scherl, Newton (MD)	Ge	869	Schulman, Lawrence (MD)	OrS	807
Scherl, Sharon (MD)	D	865	Schulman, Nathan (MD)	IM	653
Scheuch, Robert (MD)	Pul	743	Schulman, Norman (MD)	PlS	338
Scheuer, James (MD)	Cv	417	Schulman, Susan (MD)	Ped	535
Schianodicola, Joseph (MD)	Anes	482	Schulster, Rita B (MD)	Pul	691
Schiavello, Henry (MD)	ObG	576	Schultz, Barbara (MD)	Pul	366
Schiavone, Frederick M (MD)	EM	715	Schultz, Neal (MD)	D	176
Schick, David (MD)	Cv	417	Schultz, Sidney (MD)	Rad	980
Schiff, Carl (MD)	IM	506	Schulze, Ruth (MD)	ObG	879
Schiff, Howard (MD)	U	404	Schuss, Steven (MD)	Ped	887
Schiff, Peter B (MD & PhD)	RadRO	369	Schussler, George (MD)	EDM	491
Schiff, Russell (MD)	PCd	675	Schuster, Joseph (MD)	IM	873
Schiffer, Mark (MD)	Cv	160	Schuster, Stephen (MD)	ObG	576
Schiller, Carl (MD)	PlS	538	Schuster, Victor L (MD)	Nep	439
Schiller, Myles (MD)	Cv	160	Schutz, James (MD)	Oph	281

DIRECTORY OF DOCTORS

NAME	SPECIALTY	PAGE	NAME	SPECIALTY	PAGE
Schutzengel, Roy (MD)	Ped	1067	Seidenfeld, Andrew (MD)	Oph	578
Schvey, Malcolm H (MD)	Oto	306	Seigal, Stuart (MD)	ObG	1005
Schwab, Richard (MD)	EM	866	Seigel, Sheryl (MD)	N	1058
Schwager, Robert (MD)	PlS	338	Seigle, Robert (MD)	PNep	317
Schwartz, Aaron (MD)	S	467	Seiler, Jerome (MD)	ObG	576
Schwartz, Arthur (MD)	Psyc	966	Seinfeld, David (MD)	Cv	161
Schwartz, Charles (MD)	Cv	602	Seitzman, Peter (MD)	IM	225
Schwartz, Ernest (MD)	EDM	421	Sekons, David (MD)	S	393
Schwartz, Evan (MD)	OrS	579	Selesnick, Samuel H (MD)	Oto	306
Schwartz, Gary (MD)	Ge	644	Self, Edward (MD)	OrS	882
Schwartz, Joel (MD)	Rad	849	Selman, Jay E (MD)	N	793
Schwartz, Judith (MD)	ObG	266	Seltzer, Murray (MD)	S	921
Schwartz, Kenneth (MD)	GVS	840	Seltzer, Terry (MD)	IM	225
Schwartz, Louis (MD)	RadRO	1029	Seltzer, Vicki (MD)	GO	646
Schwartz, Malcolm (MD)	U	999	Selzer, Jeffrey A (MD)	Psyc	587
Schwartz, Mark (MD)	S	982	Semple, Sandra (MD)	ObG	798
Schwartz, Marlene (MD)	Pul	541	Sen, Dilip (MD)	PNep	531
Schwartz, Michael (MD)	Psyc	742	Sena, K N (MD)	N	1059
Schwartz, Miles (MD)	Cv	161	Sender, Joel (MD)	Pul	461
Schwartz, Mitchell (MD)	IM	976	Sennett, Margaret (MD)	IM	1053
Schwartz, Paula R (MD)	Onc	655	Sensakovic, John (MD)	Inf	958
Schwartz, Peter (MD)	GO	1048	Senz, Ronald (MD)	FP	974
Schwartz, Peter (MD)	Oph	668	Sepkowitz, Douglas (MD)	Inf	501
Schwartz, Robert A (MD)	D	901	Seplowitz, Alan (MD)	EDM	184
Schwartz, Simeon (MD)	Hem	778	Serby, Michael J (MD)	GerPsy	198
Schwartz, Stephen (MD)	Ped	327	Seremetis, Stephanie (MD)	IM	225
Schwartz, William (MD)	Cv	161	Sergiou, Harry (MD)	Ped	535
Schwartzberg, Mori (MD)	Rhu	980	Seriff, Nathan (MD)	IM	225
Schwartzman, Alexander (MD)	S	548	Serle, Janet (MD)	Oph	281
Schwartzman, Sergio (MD)	Rhu	380	Serur, Eli (MD)	GO	567
Schwarz, Richard (MD)	ObG	730	Setzen, Michael (MD)	Oto	673
Schwarz, Steven M (MD)	PGe	530	Shabry, Fryderyka (MD)	ChAP	485
Schwechter, Leon (DO)	IM	653	Shabsigh, Ridwan (MD)	U	405
Schweitzer, Philip (MD)	Ge	426	Shabto, Uri (MD)	Oph	281
Schwimmer, Richard (MD)	Ped	535	Shachner, Arthur (MD)	FP	493
Schwinn, Hans Diete (MD)	FP	718	Shaffer, David (MD)	ChAP	165
Sciales, John (MD)	IM	571	Shah, Jatin (MD)	S	393
Sciallis, Gabriel F (MD)	D	938	Shah, Jitendra (MD)	IM	506
Sciarra, Daniel (MD)	N	253	Shah, Mahendra (MD)	IM	435
Scibetta, Maria (MD)	IM	873	Shah, Pravin (MD)	GVS	840
Scigliano, Eileen (MD)	Hem	204	Shah, Vijay (MD)	Inf	721
Sciortino, Patrick (MD)	Oph	523	Shahid, S Javed (MD)	NS	1058
Sclafani, Michael (MD)	SM	981	Shahrivar, Farrokh (MD)	NP	238
Sclafani, Salvatore (MD)	OrS	524	Shalit, Shimon (MD)	U	839
Scofield, Lisa (MD)	Ped	1007	Shalita, Alan (MD)	D	488
Sconzo, Frank (MD)	S	748	Shamoon, Harry (MD)	EDM	421
Scott, Norman (MD)	FP	493	Shane, Elizabeth (MD)	EDM	184
Scott, Rachelle (MD)	D	176	Shani, Jacob (MD)	Cv	484
Scott, William C (MD)	TS	702	Shanies, Harvey (MD)	IM	571
Scott, W Norman (MD)	OrS	297	Shank, Brenda (MD)	RadRO	370
Sculco, Thomas (MD)	OrS	297	Shapir, Yehuda (MD)	PCd	581
Sculerati, Nancy (MD)	Oto	306	Shapiro, Barry (MD)	Oto	810
Seaman, Cheryl (MD)	Psyc	825	Shapiro, Bruce (MD)	Psyc	1070
Seashore, Margaretta (MD)	MG	1054	Shapiro, Kenneth (MD)	Nep	846
Seaver, Robert (MD)	ChAP	764	Shapiro, Lawrence (MD)	IM	435
Seebacher, J Robert (MD)	OrS	807	Shapiro, Lawrence R (MD)	MG	787
Seed, William T (MD)	Ped	327	Shapiro, Neil (MD)	Ge	776
Seedor, John (MD)	Oph	281	Shapiro, Nella (MD)	S	467
Seelagy, Marc (MD)	Pul	948	Shapiro, Peter (MD)	Psyc	359
Segal, Nancy (MD)	EDM	771	Shapiro, Theodore (MD)	Psyc	359
Segura-Bustamante, Alina (MD)	Psyc	359	Shapiro, Warren (MD)	Nep	512
Seibold, James R (MD)	Rhu	967	Shaps, Jeffrey (MD)	Ge	605
Seibt, R Stephen (MD)	D	901	Sharon, David (MD)	Onc	976
Seicol, Noel (MD)	IM	786	Sharon, Ezra (MD)	Rhu	591

NAME	SPECIALTY	PAGE	NAME	SPECIALTY	PAGE
Shaw, Jennifer (MD)	Ped	916	Siegel, Jerome H (MD)	Ge	195
Shaw, Ronda R (MD)	Psyc	359	Siegel, Kenneth C (MD)	N	1059
Shebairo, Raymond (MD)	OrS	671	Siegel, Randall (MD)	DR	956
Sheehy, Albert (MD)	IM	786	Siegel, Wayne (MD)	Ge	927
Sheftell, Fred (MD)	Psyc	1070	Siegler, Eugenia (MD)	Ger	497
Shein, Leon (MD)	Nep	513	Siegman, Felix (MD)	S	549
Shelley, Gabriella (MD)	GerPsy	567	Siepser, Stuart (MD)	Cv	1003
Shelov, Steven (MD)	Ped	535	Siever, Larry J (MD)	Psyc	359
Shelton, Ronald M (MD)	D	176	Siffert, Robert (MD)	OrS	297
Shemen, Larry (MD)	Oto	306	Sigal, Leonard (MD)	Rhu	968
Shepard, Barry (MD)	U	704	Siglock, Timothy (MD)	Oto	810
Shepherd, Gillian M (MD)	A&I	152	Silane, Michael F (MD)	GVS	409
Sherbell, Stanley (MD)	IM	507	Silber, Austin (MD)	Psyc	359
Sherling, Bruce E (MD)	Pul	828	Silberman, Deborah (MD)	Oph	523
Sherman, Frederic (MD)	IM	507	Silberman, Mark (MD)	PlS	687
Sherman, Fredrick (MD)	Ger	198	Silbert, Glenn (MD)	Oph	880
Sherman, Howard (MD)	Ge	426	Silich, Robert (MD)	S	620
Sherman, Mark (MD)	OrS	613	Sills, Charles (MD)	TS	982
Sherman, Raymond (MD)	Nep	240	Sills, Irene N (MD)	PEn	995
Sherman, Richard (MD)	IM	959	Silva, Jose (MD)	U	405
Sherman, Scott J (MD)	Rad	693	Silver, Bennett (MD)	Psyc	917
Sherman, Spencer (MD)	Oph	281	Silver, Carl (MD)	S	467
Sherman, Steven (DO)	Oph	523	Silver, Jonathan M (MD)	Psyc	359
Sherman, Warren (MD)	Cv	161	Silver, Lester (MD)	PlS	338
Sherman, William H (MD)	Onc	236	Silver, Richard (MD)	Onc	236
Shevde, Ketan (MD)	Anes	482	Silverberg, Arnold (MD)	EDM	491
Shiffman, Rebecca (MD)	ObG	520	Silverberg, Shonni J (MD)	EDM	185
Shike, Moshe (MD)	Ge	195	Silverman, Barney (MD)	ObG	798
Shikowitz, Mark (MD)	Oto	579	Silverman, Cary (MD)	Oph	993
Shimony, Rony (MD)	IM	225	Silverman, David (MD)	IM	226
Shin, Choon (MD)	GVS	554	Silverman, Jason (MD)	Ped	818
Shinbach, Kent (MD)	Psyc	359	Silverman, Joel (MD)	Pul	588
Shinnar, Shlomo (MD)	ChiN	418	Silverman, Joseph (MD)	Ped	327
Shinya, Hiromi (MD)	Ge	195	Silverman, Marc (MD)	SM	591
Ship, Arthur G (MD)	PlS	338	Silverman, Mitchell (MD)	EDM	1020
Shlofmitz, Richard A (MD)	Cv	634	Silverman, Rubin (MD)	Cv	417
Shojai, E Mohajer (MD)	ObG	798	Silvers, David (MD)	D	176
Shookoff, Charlene (MD)	Ped	456	Simberkoff, Michael S (MD)	Inf	208
Shoreibah, Ahmed (MD)	IM	435	Simkovitz, Philip (MD)	IM	1053
Shorofsky, Morris (MD)	IM	226	Simon, Clifford J (MD)	Pul	890
Short, Joan (MD)	Ped	616	Simon, John (MD)	S	748
Shugar, Joel (MD)	Oto	306	Simon, Lawrence (MD)	S	849
Shulman, Abraham (MD)	Oto	527	Simon, Lloyd (MD)	IM	723
Shulman, Joanna (MD)	ObG	445	Simon, Steven (MD)	D	488
Shulman, Julius (MD)	Oph	281	Simone, Don (MD)	IM	929
Shulman, Susan (MD)	Ped	536	Simonson, Barry G (MD)	OrS	671
Shulman, Yale (MD)	U	934	Simpson, Alec (MD)	S	969
Shum, Kee (MD)	Onc	572	Simpson, Roger (MD)	PlS	687
Shupack, Jerome (MD)	D	176	Simpson, Thomas (MD)	S	1030
Shypula, Gregory (MD)	Onc	960	Sincero, Domenico (MD)	FP	773
Sibony, Patrick (MD)	Oph	732	Singer, Carol (MD)	Inf	568
Sibrack, Laurence (MD)	D	1043	Singer, Elliot (MD)	Psyc	825
Sibulkin, David (MD)	D	176	Singer, Lewis (MD)	PCCM	451
Sicklick, Marc (MD)	A&I	628	Singer, Paul (MD)	Psyc	360
Siddiqi, Ahmed Mutee (MD)	S	592	Singh, Ajay (MD)	Nep	941
Siderides, Elizabeth (MD)	Oph	1061	Singh, Avtar (MD)	N	793
Sidoti, Eugene (MD)	Ped	817	Singhal, Pravin (MD)	Nep	573
Siebel, Wayne D (MD)	Ge	927	Sinha, Gopal Krishna (MD)	FP	957
Siebert, John (MD)	PlS	338	Sinha, K (MD)	PM	674
Siegal, Elliot (MD)	Ped	847	Sinnreich, Abraham (MD)	Oto	614
Siegal, Frederick P (MD)	A&I	560	Siracuse, Jeffrey F (MD)	NP	609
Siegal, Michael S (MD)	Cv	161	Siris, Ethel (MD)	EDM	185
Siegel, Beth (MD)	S	592	Siris, Samuel G (MD)	Psyc	587
Siegel, George (MD)	IM	226	Sirota, David King (MD)	IM	226

DIRECTORY OF DOCTORS

NAME	SPECIALTY	PAGE	NAME	SPECIALTY	PAGE
Siroty, Robert (MD)	IM	990	Smotrich, Gary (MD)	PlS	947
Siskind, Steven Jay (MD)	Cv	561	Smouha, Eric (MD)	Oto	736
Sisler, Glenn (MD)	TS	969	Snow, Robert (MD)	NS	245
Sison, Joseph (MD)	NP	875	Snyder, Arthur (MD)	IM	226
Sisti, Michael (MD)	NS	244	Snyder, David (MD)	N	253
Sisto, Donato (MD)	TS	469	Snyder, Gary (MD)	Oto	580
Sitarz, Anneliese (MD)	PHO	316	Snyder, Jon (MD)	ObG	266
Sithian, Nedunchezia (MD)	GVS	622	Snyder, Michael (MD)	PCd	811
Sitron, Alan (MD)	DR	639	Snyder, Richard (MD)	A&I	482
Sivak, Mark (MD)	N	253	Snyder, Stephen (MD)	Psyc	360
Sivak, Steven L (MD)	IM	226	Soave, Rosemary (MD)	Inf	208
Sixsmith, Diane (MD)	EM	563	Sobel, Howard (MD)	D	176
Skeist, Loren (MD)	Psyc	360	Sobol, Norman (MD)	N	516
Skilbred, Arne (MD)	OrS	735	Sockolow, Robbyn (MD)	PGe	677
Skinner, David B (MD)	TS	398	Socolow, Edward (MD)	EDM	771
Skirtkus, Aldonna (MD)	Ped	931	Soeiro, Ruy (MD)	Inf	429
Sklansky, B Donald (MD)	PlS	687	Sofair, Jane (MD)	Psyc	996
Sklar, Barrett (MD)	FP	642	Soffen, Edward (MD)	RadRO	948
Sklar, Charles A (MD)	PEn	313	Soffer, Jeffrey (MD)	ObG	1012
Sklarek, Howard (MD)	Pul	743	Softness, Barney (MD)	Ped	328
Sklaroff, Herschel (MD)	IM	226	Sogani, Pramod (MD)	U	405
Sklower, Jay A (DO)	FP	926	Sohn, Norman (MD)	CRS	167
Sklower Brooks, Susan (MD)	MG	609	Sokal, Myron (MD)	NP	510
Skog, Donald (MD)	Ped	327	Soley, Robert (MD)	PlS	821
Skolnik, Richard A (MD)	PlS	338	Solnit, Albert (MD)	Psyc	1070
Skrokov, Robert (MD)	D	714	Solomon, Edward (MD)	Oph	880
Skuza, Kathryn (MD)	PEn	913	Solomon, Gary (MD)	Rhu	381
Sladowski, Catherine (MD)	ObG	910	Solomon, Gregory (MD)	IM	435
Slama, Robert (MD)	Cv	1018	Solomon, Ira (MD)	Oph	803
Slamovits, Thomas (MD)	Oph	446	Solomon, Joel (MD)	Oph	282
Slankard, Marjorie (MD)	A&I	152	Solomon, Michael (MD)	U	970
Slater, Gary (MD)	S	393	Solomon, Randall (MD)	Psyc	742
Slater, Jonathan (MD)	ChAP	764	Solomon, Robert (MD)	Ger	1021
Slatkin, Richard (MD)	ObG	520	Solomon, Robert (MD)	NS	245
Slavin, Michael (MD)	Oph	578	Solomon, Ronald (MD)	HS	498
Slavit, David H (MD)	Oto	306	Solomon, Seymour (MD)	N	442
Slim, Michel (MD)	PS	814	Solomon, Sherry (MD)	Oph	804
Sloan, Don (MD)	ObG	266	Soloway, Barrie D (MD)	Oph	282
Sloan, William (MD)	Ge	903	Soloway, Bruce (MD)	FP	423
Sloane, Lori (MD)	Rhu	830	Soltren, Rafael (MD)	IM	786
Slotwiner, Paul (MD)	N	516	Som, Peter (MD)	DR	179
Slovin, Alvin (MD)	TS	702	Somasundaram, Mahend (MD)	N	516
Small, Steven (MD)	OrS	807	Somerstein, Michael (MD)	Nep	942
Smallberg, Gerald (MD)	N	253	Sommer, Bruce (MD)	S	549
Smego, Douglas (MD)	S	1076	Sommers, Gara M (MD)	GO	927
Smiles, Stephen (MD)	Rhu	380	Sonnenblick, Edmund (MD)	IM	435
Smirnov, Viktor (MD)	GVS	706	Sonpal, Girish (MD)	Rhu	591
Smith, Alford (MD)	FP	493	Sood, Harish (MD)	IM	653
Smith, Aloysius G (MD)	S	393	Sood, Sunil (MD)	Ped Inf	677
Smith, Anthony (MD)	Pul	367	Sorabella, Philip (MD)	Rad	891
Smith, Arthur (MD)	U	704	Soriano, Dale (MD)	D	768
Smith, Charles (MD)	N	442	Soriano, John (MD)	Ge	989
Smith, Craig R (MD)	TS	398	Soroko, Theresa (MD)	IM	905
Smith, Daniel (MD)	GO	200	Sorra, Toomas (MD)	Ge	496
Smith, David (MD)	Ped	327	Sosa, R Ernest (MD)	U	405
Smith, Edward (MD)	Oph	523	Soskel, Neil (DO)	FP	642
Smith, James (MD)	Pul	367	Sossi, Anthony (MD)	IM	571
Smith, Jo Ann (MD)	Psyc	1070	Sostman, H Dirk (MD)	Rad	374
Smith, Leon G (MD)	IM	905	Soter, Nicholas A (MD)	D	176
Smith, Margaret D (MD)	Rhu	381	Soterakis, Jack (MD)	Ge	644
Smith, Marilyn (MD)	Ped	1067	Sotsky, Gerald (MD)	Cv	863
Smith, Michael O (MD)	Psyc	460	Sottile, Vincent M (MD)	Ge	606
Smith, Peter (MD)	Pul	541	Southern, D Loren (MD)	A&I	937
Smothers, Kevin (MD)	EM	1044	Southren, A Louis (MD)	EDM	771

NAME	SPECIALTY	PAGE	NAME	SPECIALTY	PAGE
Spadaro, Louise A (MD)	Cv	634	Starr, Michael (MD)	Oph	282
Spaide, Richard (MD)	Oph	282	Stassa, George (MD)	Rad	374
Spano, Frank (MD)	IM	1053	Stathopoulos, Peter (MD)	IM	608
Sparano, Joseph (MD)	IM	435	Statile, Lorna (MD)	Anes	152
Sparr, Steven (MD)	N	443	Steadman, E Thomas (MD)	ObG	266
Speaker, Mark (MD)	Oph	282	Steckowych, Jayde (MD)	Oto	883
Spector, Ira (MD)	ObG	664	Steeg, Carl (MD)	PCd	450
Speiser, Phyllis W (MD)	PEn	676	Steele, Andrew M (MD)	NP	656
Spencer, Dennis (MD)	NS	1058	Steele, Mark (MD)	Oph	282
Spencer, Elizabeth (MD)	ChAP	165	Steer, Robert (MD)	ObG	993
Spencer, Frank C (MD)	TS	398	Steigbigel, Neal H (MD)	Inf	429
Spera, John (MD)	RadRO	1072	Steiger, David (MD)	CCM	168
Sperber, Alan B (MD)	U	405	Steigman, Elliott G (MD)	U	934
Sperber, Kirk (MD)	IM	226	Stein, Alan (MD)	Inf	501
Spergel, Gabriel (MD)	EDM	491	Stein, Alvin (MD)	Onc	656
Sperling, Neil Michael (MD)	Oto	527	Stein, Arnold (MD)	Oph	523
Sperling, Richard (MD)	PlS	888	Stein, Barry B (MD)	Ped	328
Spero, Marc (MD)	IM	227	Stein, Elliott (MD)	Cv	1018
Speyer, James (MD)	Onc	236	Stein, Jeffrey Alan (MD)	Ge	195
Spielberg, Alan (MD)	Ge	719	Stein, Jeffrey S (MD)	GVS	409
Spielman, Gerald (MD)	Ped	328	Stein, Lawrence (MD)	Ge	989
Spielvogel, Arthur (MD)	Hem	870	Stein, Mark (MD)	U	470
Spiera, Harry (MD)	Rhu	381	Stein, Martin F (MD)	Nep	790
Spiera, Robert (MD)	Rhu	381	Stein, Mitchell (MD)	Oph	804
Spierer, Gary (MD)	ObG	612	Stein, Perry (MD)	PMR	537
Spiler, Ira (MD)	EDM	957	Stein, Richard (MD)	IM	227
Spina, Christopher (MD)	A&I	628	Stein, Richard A (MD)	Cv	161
Spindola-Franco, Hugo (MD)	Rad	463	Stein, Ruth (MD)	Ped	456
Spinelli, Henry M (MD)	PlS	338	Stein, Sidney (MD)	IM	227
Spinner, Morton (MD)	OrS	671	Stein, Stefan (MD)	Psyc	360
Spinowitz, Alan (MD)	D	638	Stein, William (MD)	IM	227
Spinowitz, Bruce (MD)	Nep	573	Steinberg, Alan (MD)	GerPsy	720
Spira, Robert S (MD)	Ge	927	Steinberg, Charles (MD)	IM	227
Spiro, Alfred (MD)	ChiN	418	Steinberg, Gregory (MD)	Cv	161
Spiro, Ronald H (MD)	S	393	Steinberg, Harry (MD)	Pul	588
Spitalewitz, Samuel (MD)	Nep	513	Steinberg, Herman (MD)	Ge	195
Spitz, Henry (MD)	Psyc	360	Steinberg, L Gary (MD)	PCd	581
Spitzer, Adrian (MD)	PNep	452	Steinberger, Alfred A (MD)	NS	245
Spitzer, Daniel (MD)	NS	847	Steinbruck, Richard (MD)	S	621
Spivack, Barney (MD)	Ger	1047	Steiner, Henry (MD)	S	549
Spivak, William (MD)	PGe	314	Steinfeld, Alan (MD)	RadRO	370
Splain, Shepard (DO)	OrS	525	Steinfeld, Leonard (MD)	PCd	311
Sporn, Aaron (MD)	OrS	944	Steinglass, Kenneth (MD)	TS	398
Spotnitz, Alan J (MD)	Cv	955	Steinglass, Peter (MD)	Psyc	360
Spotnitz, Henry (MD)	TS	398	Steinhagen, Randolph (MD)	CRS	167
Sprague, Bruce (MD)	HS	1048	Steinherz, Laurel (MD)	PCd	311
Spreecher, Stanley (MD)	Rad	590	Stelzer, Paul (MD)	TS	398
Spriggs, David (MD)	Onc	236	Stenzel, Kurt H (MD)	Nep	240
Springfield, Dempsey (MD)	OrS	298	Stern, Harvey (MD)	Rad	463
Squire, Anthony (MD)	Cv	161	Stern, Jack (MD)	NS	791
Squires, Sandra (MD)	Psyc	918	Stern, Jordan (MD)	Oto	306
Stabile, John (MD)	Oph	880	Stern, Leonard (MD)	Nep	240
Stacy, Charles B (MD)	N	253	Stern, Peter (MD)	PMR	819
Stahl, Jeffrey (MD)	Cv	634	Stern, Richard (MD)	Rhu	381
Stahl, Theodore (MD)	NuM	962	Stewart, Charles (MD)	PNep	737
Stam, Lawrence (MD)	Nep	513	Stickevers, Susan (MD)	PMR	617
Stamatos, John (MD)	PM	309	Stillman, Margaret (MD)	Ped	818
Stampfer, Morris (MD)	Cv	763	Stillman, Michael (MD)	D	768
Stangel, John (MD)	EDM	771	Stillwell, William (MD)	OrS	735
Starke, Charles (MD)	IM	786	Stilwell, Anne Marie (MD)	Anes	601
Starker, Isaac (MD)	PlS	996	Stingle, Walter (MD)	Oto	307
Starker, Paul (MD)	S	1030	St Louis, Yolaine (MD)	Ped	683
Starkman, Harold (MD)	PEn	995	Stock, Howard (MD)	Psyc	825
Staro, Frank (MD)	Oto	736	Stock, Richard (MD)	RadRO	370

DIRECTORY OF DOCTORS

NAME	SPECIALTY	PAGE	NAME	SPECIALTY	PAGE
Stolar, Charles (MD)	PS	319	Sussman, Robert (MD)	Psyc	825
Stoller, Gerald (MD)	Oph	733	Sussman, Robert (MD)	Pul	1029
Stone, Alex (MD)	S	700	Sutaria, Maganlal (MD)	TS	702
Stone, Michael (MD)	Psyc	360	Sutton, Ira (MD)	FP	773
Stone, Richard K (MD)	Ped	328	Suvannavejh, Chaisurat (MD)	ObG	798
Stoopler, Mark (MD)	Onc	236	Svitra, Paul (MD)	Oph	668
Storper, Ian (MD)	Oto	307	Swaminathan, A P (MD)	S	969
Stovell, Peter (MD)	OrS	1062	Swamy, Samala (MD)	Cv	602
Stover-Pepe, Diane E (MD)	Pul	367	Swee, David (MD)	FP	957
Strain, James (MD)	Psyc	360	Sweeney, Eugene (MD)	D	865
Strange, Theodore (MD)	Ger	606	Sweeney, Margaret (MD)	A&I	1040
Strashun, Arnold M (MD)	NuM	516	Sweeney, William (MD)	Rad	967
Strassberg, Barbara (MD)	Ped	456	Sweeting, Joseph (MD)	IM	227
Strauch, Berish (MD)	PlS	458	Swerdlow, Frederick H (MD)	IM	227
Straus, David (MD)	Hem	204	Swerdlow, Michael (MD)	N	443
Strauss, Barry (MD)	Onc	725	Swidler, Sanford (MD)	Ped	1067
Strauss, Bernard (MD)	U	922	Swiller, Hillel (MD)	Psyc	361
Strauss, Edward (MD)	Rad	1073	Swirsky, Michael (MD)	DR	769
Strauss, Michael (MD)	IM	227	Swistel, Alexander (MD)	S	394
Streisand, Robert (MD)	TS	836	Sy, Wilfrido M (MD)	NuM	517
Strider, William (MD)	ObG	267	Szabo, Andrew John (MD)	EDM	185
Striker, Paul (MD)	PlS	339			
Strobeck, John (MD)	Cv	863	**T**		
Stroh, Jack (MD)	Cv	955			
Strominger, Mitchell (MD)	Ped	536	Tabachnick, John F (MD)	FP	1020
Strong, Elliot (MD)	S	394	Tabaddor, Kamran (MD)	NS	440
Strong, Leslie (MD)	S	394	Tabbal, Nicolas (MD)	PlS	339
Strongin, Michael J (MD)	ObG	267	Tabershaw, Richard (MD)	OrS	735
Strongwater, Allan (MD)	OrS	525	Taddonio, Rudolph (MD)	OrS	807
Strongwater, Richard (MD)	FP	773	Taffet, Sanford (MD)	Ge	776
Stuchin, Steven (MD)	OrS	298	Taffet, Simeon (MD)	Oph	804
Sturm, Richard (MD)	Oph	668	Taintor, Zebulon C (MD)	Psyc	361
Sturza, Jeffrey (MD)	D	768	Taitsman, James (MD)	OrS	945
Stylianos, Steven (MD)	PS	319	Tal, Avraham (MD)	IM	507
Suarez, Joseph (MD)	OrS	613	Talansky, Arthur (MD)	Ge	645
Subramanian, Valavanur (MD)	TS	398	Talansky, Marvin (MD)	Oph	978
Sudarsky, R David (MD)	Oph	283	Talavera, Wilfredo (MD)	Pul	367
Sudhakar, Telechery (MD)	Nep	942	Talor, Zvi (MD)	IM	571
Suggs, William (MD)	GVS	470	Tamarin, Steven (MD)	FP	186
Sukumaran, Muthiah (MD)	Pul	367	Tan, Mark (MD)	Rhu	746
Sulkowicz, Kerry (MD)	Psyc	360	Tanchajja, Supoj (MD)	S	549
Sullivan, Ann Marie (MD)	Psyc	361	Tancredi, Laurence R (MD)	Psyc	361
Sullivan, Bessie (MD)	A&I	955	Tannenbaum, Gary (MD)	GVS	840
Sullivan, Brenda (MD)	IM	786	Tanoue, Lynn (MD)	Pul	1071
Sullivan, James (MD)	Rhu	695	Tanowitz, Herbert (MD)	Inf	430
Sullivan, Timothy (MD)	Psyc	825	Tanz, Alfred (MD)	ObG	267
Sullum, Stanford (MD)	ObG	267	Tapper, Michael (MD)	Inf	208
Sultan, Joseph (MD)	Psyc	539	Tarantola, Vincent (MD)	Pul	619
Sultan, Mark (MD)	PlS	339	Tarasuk, Albert (MD)	U	594
Sultan, Ronald H (MD)	S	933	Tardiff, Kenneth (MD)	Psyc	361
Sumpio, Bauer (MD)	GVS	1078	Tartaglia, Joseph J (MD)	Cv	763
Sunaryo, Francis (MD)	PGe	913	Tartell, Jay (MD)	Rad	590
Sundaram, Revathy (MD)	PHO	530	Tartter, Paul (MD)	S	394
Sundaram, Savitri (MD)	Psyc	996	Tash, Robert R (MD)	Rad	849
Sundaresan, Narayan (MD)	NS	245	Taub, Robert (MD & PhD)	Onc	236
Sunderwirth-Bailly, Ramona (MD)	EM	420	Taubin, Howard L (MD)	Ge	1046
Sung, Kap-jae (MD)	S	592	Taubman, Lowell (MD)	IM	653
Sunshine, Robert (MD)	U	704	Taubman, Richard (MD)	ObG	665
Surks, Martin (MD)	EDM	421	Tawfik, Bernard (MD)	Oto	673
Surow, Jason (MD)	Oto	883	Taylor, David (MD)	U	999
Sussman, Barry (MD)	GVS	896	Taylor, Howard (MD)	Oto	994
Sussman, Cindy (MD)	EM	939	Taylor, James R (MD)	TS	702
Sussman, John (MD)	Oph	804	Taylor, Noel (MD)	Psyc	361
Sussman, Norman (MD)	Psyc	361	Taylor, William (MD)	IM	227
			Tchorbajian, Kirk (MD)	Oph	1025

NAME	SPECIALTY	PAGE	NAME	SPECIALTY	PAGE
Tedesco, Salvatore (MD)	S	621	Tornambe, Robert (MD)	PlS	339
Teffera, Fassil (MD)	IM	435	Torre, Arthur (MD)	Ped	916
Teich, Steven (MD)	Oph	283	Torres Gluck, Jose (MD)	NS	440
Teicher, Joel (MD)	OrS	525	Tortolani, Anthony (MD)	TS	399
Teirstein, Alvin (MD)	Pul	367	Toth, William (MD)	IM	1023
Tejani, Nergesh (MD)	ObG	798	Toueg, Elia (MD)	Oph	283
Tellis, Vivian (MD)	S	468	Touloukian, Robert (MD)	PS	1065
Telzak, Edward E (MD)	Inf	430	Tow, Tony (MD)	Pul	743
Tempera, Patrick (MD)	Ge	1021	Townsend, Gary (MD)	Oto	1064
Templeton, Hilda (MD)	Psyc	918	Townsend, Janet (MD)	FP	423
Tenenbaum, Joseph (MD)	Cv	162	Tozzi, Robert (MD)	PCd	884
Tenenbaum, Marvin J (MD)	Inf	648	Tozzo, Pellegrino (MD)	U	839
Tenet, William (MD)	Cv	561	Tracer, Robert (MD)	Ge	496
Tenner, Michael (MD)	NRad	793	Trachtenberg, Albert (MD)	Rad	745
Tepler, Jeffrey (MD)	Onc	236	Trachtman, Howard (MD)	PNep	582
Tepler, Melvin (MD)	OrS	525	Trainin, Eugene (MD)	Ped	536
Tepper, Howard (MD)	PlS	1028	Traister, Michael (MD)	Ped	328
Tepperberg, Jerome (MD)	ChiN	486	Tranbaugh, Robert (MD)	TS	399
Terkelsen, Kenneth (MD)	Psyc	825	Traube, Charles (MD)	Cv	485
Termine, Charles (MD)	Cv	561	Traube, Morris (MD)	Ge	1047
Tesauro, William (MD)	ObG	730	Travin, Sheldon (MD)	Psyc	826
Tesher, Martin (MD)	FP	187	Treiber, Ruth Kaplan (MD)	D	768
Tesser, Mark (MD)	D	177	Tretter, Wolfgang (MD)	ObG	267
Tessler, Arthur (MD)	U	405	Tribble, Cassandra (MD)	Anes	1040
Tessler, Sidney (MD)	CCM	487	Trokel, Stephen (MD)	Oph	283
Testa, Noel (MD)	OrS	298	Trotman, Bruce W (MD)	Ge	903
Teusink, J Paul (MD)	Psyc	361	Troy, Allen (MD)	OrS	1062
Theofandis, Stylianos (MD)	NP	1056	Troy, Kevin (MD)	IM	228
Thies, Harold (MD)	Nep	657	Truchly, George (MD)	OrS	298
Thomas, Byron (MD)	IM	1053	Truman, John (MD)	PHO	316
Thomas, Rogelio (MD)	Ger	427	Tsin, Daniel (MD)	ObG	576
Thomashow, Byron (MD)	Pul	367	Tsoukas, Elias (MD)	S	894
Thomashow, Peter (MD)	Psyc	361	Tucci, Paul (MD)	U	839
Thomsen, Stephen (MD)	Nep	907	Tuchman, Alan (MD)	N	254
Thorne, Charles (MD)	PlS	339	Tugal, Oya (MD)	PHO	813
Thornhill, Herbert (MD)	PMR	331	Tuhrim, Stanley (MD)	N	254
Thornton, Yvonne S (MD)	ObG	993	Tumminello, Calogero (MD)	IM	571
Tibaldi, Joseph (MD)	EDM	564	Tunis, Leonard (MD)	U	553
Tierney, Peter (MD)	FP	957	Turato, Mariann (MD)	Psyc	826
Tiger, Louis H (MD)	Rhu	695	Turcios, Nelson (MD)	PPul	915
Tinetti, Mary (MD)	Ger	1047	Turetsky, Arthur (MD)	CE	1040
Tirschwell, Perry (MD)	TS	702	Turino, Gerard M (MD)	IM	228
Tischler, Gary L (MD)	Psyc	826	Turnbull, Alan (MD)	S	394
Tischler, Henry (MD)	OrS	525	Turnbull, Dorothy (MD)	EM	1044
Tiszenkel, Howard (MD)	CRS	562	Turner, Ira (MD)	N	661
Tiwari, Ram (MD)	Oph	446	Turner, James (MD)	S	592
Toback, Arnold C (MD)	D	177	Turovsky, Leon (MD)	IM	507
Tobias, Geoffrey (MD)	Oto	307	Tursi, William (MD)	IM	608
Tobias, Hillel (MD)	Ge	196	Turtel, Allen (MD)	FP	642
Tobias, Theodore (MD)	ObG	879	Turtel, Penny (MD)	Ge	975
Todd, George (MD)	S	394	Tutela, Rocco (MD)	PlS	917
Toffler, Allan (MD)	IM	654	Tutino, Jody (MD)	IM	507
Tohme, Jack (MD)	EDM	867	Tyberg, Theodore (MD)	Cv	162
Tolchin, Deborah (MD)	Ped	456	Tydings, Lawrence (MD)	ObG	665
Tolchin, Joan G (MD)	Psyc	361	Tyras, Denis (MD)	TS	702
Toles, Allen (MD)	ObG	576			
Tom, Jack (MD)	D	714	**U**		
Tomao, Frank (MD)	Onc	656	Uday, Kalpana (MD)	IM	435
Tomasula, John (MD)	S	834	Udell, Ira (MD)	Oph	668
Tonnesen, Marcia (MD)	D	715	Ulin, Richard (MD)	OrS	298
Toomey, Kathleen (MD)	Hem	1012	Ullman, Joel (MD)	ObG	798
Topilow, Harvey (MD)	Oph	283	Underberg, James (MD)	IM	228
Toriello, Edward (MD)	OrS	579	Unger, Allen (MD)	Cv	162
Torman, Julie (MD)	Ge	776	Unterricht, Sam (MD)	Oph	523

DIRECTORY OF DOCTORS

NAME	SPECIALTY	PAGE	NAME	SPECIALTY	PAGE
Urken, Mark (MD)	Oto	307	Vogel, Louis (MD)	D	177
Usas, Craig (MD)	RadRO	828	Voges, Peter (MD)	S	834
Usiskin, Keith (MD)	EDM	988	Vogl, Steven Edward (MD)	Onc	437
Uy, Rodolfo (MD)	Ped	456	Volcovici, Guido (MD)	Pul	828
Uy, Vena (MD)	ObG	930	Volpe, Anthony Peter (MD)	IM	873
			Volpe, Salvatore (MD)	Ped	616
V			Volpi, David (MD)	Oto	307
Vadde, Nirmala (MD)	Ped	616			
Vaillancourt, Phillippe (MD)	N	727	**W**		
Valacer, David J (MD)	PPul	318	Wachtel, Alan (MD)	Psyc	362
Valda, Victor (MD)	PS	885	Wadler, Scott (MD)	Onc	438
Vallarino, Ramon (MD)	PMR	537	Wager, Marc (MD)	Ped	818
Vallejo, Alvaro (MD)	RadRO	370	Wager, Steven (MD)	Psyc	362
Vallone, Ambrose (MD)	PCd	675	Wagle, Sharad (MD)	Psyc	889
Van Amerongen, Robert (MD)	EM	489	Wagner, Ira (MD)	CCM	168
van Dyck, Christopher H (MD)	GerPsy	1047	Wagner, John (MD)	Nep	657
Van Engel, Daniel (MD)	N	877	Wagner, Michael L (MD)	IM	929
van Gilder, Max (MD)	Ped	328	Wagner, Rudolph (MD)	Oph	911
Van Praagh, Ian (MD)	ObG	267	Wainstein, Sasha (MD)	U	553
Vapnek, Jonathon M (MD)	U	405	Waintraub, Stanley (MD)	Onc	875
Varada, Koteswar (MD)	NP	510	Wait, Richard B (MD)	S	549
Vardi, Joseph R (MD)	GO	497	Wajnberg, Alexander (MD)	Cv	955
Varriale, Philip (MD)	Cv	162	Waldbaum, Robert (MD)	U	705
Vas, George A (MD)	N	516	Waldorf, Donald (MD)	D	845
Vasavada, Balendu (MD)	Cv	485	Waldstreicher, Stuart (MD)	Ge	1047
Vastola, A Paul (MD)	Oto	527	Walerstein, Steven J (MD)	IM	654
Vasudeva, Kusum (MD)	ObG	665	Walfish, Jacob (MD)	IM	228
Vaswani, Ashok N (MD)	EDM	641	Walker, Yvette (MD)	IM	436
Vaughan, Edwin D (MD)	U	406	Wallace, Claudina (MD)	Ped	328
Vazzana, Thomas (MD)	Cv	603	Wallach, Robert C (MD)	ObG	267
Vecchiotti, Arthur (MD)	Oto	810	Wallach, Stanley (MD)	EDM	185
Vega-Rich, Carlos (MD)	NP	438	Wallack, Joel (MD)	Psyc	362
Veith, Frank (MD)	S	468	Wallack, Marc (MD)	S	394
Velcek, Francisca (MD)	PS	319	Waller, John F (MD)	OrS	298
Veloso, Manuel (MD)	ObG	665	Wallis, Joseph (DO)	ObG	993
Ventimiglia, Anthony (MD)	FP	1003	Walser, Lawrence (MD)	Pul	744
Verde, Robert (MD)	OrS	525	Walsh, Bruce (MD)	S	834
Verga, Michelle (MD)	PlS	339	Walsh, B Timothy (MD)	Psyc	362
Versfelt, Mary (MD)	Ped	818	Walsh, Christina (MD)	Hem	975
Vickery, Carlin (MD)	PlS	339	Walsh, Christine A (MD)	PCd	450
Videtti, Nicholas (MD)	Psyc	889	Walsh, Francis X (MD)	Nep	1057
Viederman, Milton (MD)	Psyc	362	Walsh, Joseph (MD)	Oph	283
Viera, Jeffery (MD)	IM	507	Walsh, William (MD)	OrS	807
Vigorita, John (MD)	Ped	1027	Walsky, Robert (MD)	S	894
Vikram, Bhadrasain (MD)	RadRO	461	Walther, Robert (MD)	D	177
Villafranca, Manuel (MD)	Psyc	1029	Waltz, Joseph (MD)	NS	440
Villamena, Patricia (MD)	IM	228	Waltzer, Wayne (MD)	U	749
Villegas, Emilio (MD)	Ped	585	Wan, Livia (MD)	ObG	267
Vinas, Sonia (MD)	Ped	536	Wang, Christopher (MD)	FP	187
Vincent, Miriam (MD)	FP	493	Wang, Frederick (MD)	Oph	283
Vinciguerra, Vincent (MD)	Hem	647	Wang, Jen Chin (MD)	Hem	647
Viner, Nicholas (MD)	U	1077	Wang, John (MD)	Nep	240
Viscardi, Anthony (MD)	ObG	879	Wangenheim, Paul (MD)	IM	906
Visco, Ferdinand (MD)	Cv	561	Wantz, George (MD)	S	394
Visconti, Ernest (MD)	Ped	616	Wapnir, Irene (MD)	S	969
Viswanathan, Kusum (MD)	Ped	536	Ward, Barbara (MD)	S	1076
Viswanathan, Ramasmy (MD)	Psyc	539	Ward, Robert (MD)	Oto	307
Vitale, Gerard (MD)	S	700	Ward, Robert J (MD)	S	700
Vitenson, Jack (MD)	U	895	Warden, Mary Jane (MD)	S	1008
Vitting, Kevin (MD)	Nep	1004	Wardlaw, Sharon (MD)	EDM	185
Vivek, Seeth (MD)	Psyc	587	Ware, J Anthony (MD)	Cv	417
Vladeck, Bob (MD)	S	849	Warm, Hillard (MD)	S	748
Vlay, Stephen C (MD)	Cv	713	Warner, Richard (MD)	Ge	196
Vogel, James M (MD)	Onc	237	Warner, Robert (MD)	D	177

NAME	SPECIALTY	PAGE	NAME	SPECIALTY	PAGE
Warren, Michelle (MD)	RE	375	Weinstein, Richard (MD)	OrS	448
Warren, Russell (MD)	OrS	298	Weinstein, Toba (MD)	PGe	677
Wasnick, Robert (MD)	U	749	Weinstock, Gary (MD)	A&I	628
Wasser, Kenneth (MD)	Rhu	980	Weinstock, Judith (MD)	ObG	520
Wasser, Walter (MD)	Nep	240	Weinstock, Murray (MD)	Cv	863
Wasserman, Eric (MD)	Oph	1061	Weintraub, Gerald (MD)	IM	228
Wasserman, Eugene (MD)	Ped	818	Weintraub, Michael (MD)	N	793
Wasserman, Gary (MD)	U	895	Weintraub, Neil (MD)	GVS	840
Wasserman, Kenneth (MD)	IM	873	Weisblatt, Steven (MD)	GerPsy	427
Wasserman, Robert L (MD)	Oph	733	Weiselberg, Lora (MD)	Onc	656
Wasson, Dennis (MD)	S	1076	Weisenseel, Arthur (MD)	Cv	162
Watnik, Neil (MD)	OrS	671	Weiser, Robert (MD)	GVS	554
Watts, Joe (MD)	Oto	1064	Weisfeldt, Myron L (MD)	Cv	162
Wax, Michael (MD)	Hem	1022	Weisholtz, Steven (MD)	IM	874
Waxberg, Jonathan (MD)	U	1077	Weiss, Arthur H (MD)	N	254
Waxenbaum, Steven (MD)	CRS	864	Weiss, Carl (MD)	OrS	671
Waxman, Samuel (MD)	Hem	204	Weiss, Carol J (MD)	AdP	149
Waxman, Stephen (MD & PhD)	N	1059	Weiss, Gary (MD)	U	594
Waye, Jerome (MD)	Ge	196	Weiss, Gerson (MD)	ObG	910
Wayne, Peter (MD)	Ge	776	Weiss, Harvey (MD)	Hem	204
Wazen, Jack (MD)	Oto	307	Weiss, Karen (MD)	ObG	665
Weber, Pamela (MD)	Oph	733	Weiss, Leonard (MD)	OrS	671
Wechsler, Michael (MD)	U	406	Weiss, Louis (MD)	Inf	430
Weck, Steven (MD)	Rad	693	Weiss, Lynne (MD)	PNep	964
Weg, Arnold (MD)	Ge	567	Weiss, Marshall (MD)	S	395
Weg, Ira (MD)	Cv	561	Weiss, Melvin (MD)	Cv	763
Wehmann, Robert (MD & PhD)	EDM	867	Weiss, Michael (MD & PhD)	Oph	283
Wei, Fong (MD)	Nep	942	Weiss, Michael H (MD)	Oto	527
Weiland, Andrew J (MD)	HS	201	Weiss, Rita (MD)	Onc	656
Weill, Terry (MD)	Psyc	362	Weiss, Robert (MD)	Ge	196
Wein, Paul (MD)	Cv	485	Weiss, Robert Allen (MD)	PNep	813
Weinberg, Gerard (MD)	PS	453	Weiss, Robert E (MD)	U	970
Weinberg, Harlan (MD)	IM	786	Weiss, Stanley (MD)	Nep	240
Weinberg, Harold (MD)	N	254	Weiss, Stanley H (MD)	Onc	907
Weinberg, Harvey (MD)	D	988	Weiss, Steven (MD)	A&I	899
Weinberg, Hubert (MD)	PlS	339	Weissberg, David (MD)	OrS	735
Weinberg, Jeffrey (MD)	PMR	617	Weissberg, Josef (MD)	Psyc	362
Weinberg, Martin (MD)	Oph	880	Weiss-Harrison, Adrienne (MD)	Ped	818
Weinberg, Samuel (MD)	D	639	Weissman, Allan Mark (MD)	PM	528
Weinberger, Jessie (MD)	N	254	Weissman, Michael H (MD)	Ped	818
Weinberger, Michael (MD)	PM	1026	Weissman, Ronald (MD)	Cv	763
Weinberger, Sylvain M (MD)	Ped	328	Weisstuch, Joseph (DO)	Nep	241
Weinblatt, Mark (MD)	PHO	677	Weisz, Daniel (MD)	TS	702
Weine, Gary (MD)	IM	990	Weitzman, Lee (MD)	Cv	635
Weiner, Avi (MD)	SM	1074	Weizman, Howard (MD)	IM	874
Weiner, Bernard M (MD)	Nep	439	Welch, John (MD)	ChAP	485
Weiner, Jay (MD)	IM	1053	Welch, Peter (MD)	Inf	779
Weiner, Jerome (MD)	Pul	744	Welsh, Howard (MD)	Psyc	362
Weiner, Lon S (MD)	OrS	299	Welt, H (MD)	Rad	949
Weiner, Michael (MD)	PHO	316	Wengerter, Kurt (MD)	GVS	896
Weiner, Richard (MD)	Ped	456	Wenick, Diane (MD)	IM	1053
Weinerman, Stuart (MD)	EDM	641	Wenick, Gary (MD)	Ped	818
Weingarten, Jacqueline (MD)	PCCM	312	Wernz, James (MD)	Onc	237
Weingarten, Marvin J (MD)	DR	845	Werres, Roland (MD)	Cv	900
Weinstein, Arthur (MD)	Rhu	830	Wert, Sanford (MD)	OrS	525
Weinstein, David (MD)	ObG	1060	Werther, J Lawrence (MD)	Ge	196
Weinstein, Jay (MD)	IM	228	Wertkin, Martin (MD)	S	835
Weinstein, Joel (MD)	OrS	882	Weseley, Alan (MD)	Oph	524
Weinstein, Joseph (MD)	Oph	668	Weseley, Martin (MD)	OrS	525
Weinstein, Joshua (MD)	FP	423	West, Gerald (DO)	PlS	1028
Weinstein, Mark (MD)	Inf	648	Westfried, Morris (MD)	D	489
Weinstein, Melvin (MD)	Inf	958	Wetherbee, Roger (MD)	Inf	208
Weinstein, Michael (MD)	CRS	167	Wexler, Craig Barry (DO)	EDM	716
Weinstein, Paul (MD)	Onc	1056	Wheeler, Mary (MD)	EDM	491

DIRECTORY OF DOCTORS

NAME	SPECIALTY	PAGE	NAME	SPECIALTY	PAGE
Whelan, Richard (MD)	CRS	167	Wolpin, Martin (MD)	OrS	526
Whitcomb, Michael (MD)	IM	1053	Wong, Martha (MD)	Ped	457
White, Dorothy (MD)	Pul	367	Wong, Michael (MD)	Oph	943
White, Ronald (MD)	CRS	864	Wong, Raymond (MD)	Oph	284
Whiteside, Timothy (MD)	IM	228	Wong, Richard (MD)	Oph	943
Whitman III, Hendricks (MD)	IM	1023	Wood-Smith, Donald (MD)	PlS	340
Whitmore, Wayne (MD)	Oph	284	Wooh, Kenneth (MD)	Oto	614
Whitsell, John (MD)	TS	399	Woolf, Paul (MD)	PCd	811
Wickiewicz, Thomas (MD)	OrS	299	Wormser, Gary (MD)	Inf	779
Wickremesinghe, Prasanna (MD)	Ge	606	Worth, David (MD)	IM	1023
Widman, David (MD)	Rhu	998	Wozniak, D (MD)	IM	929
Widmann, Warren (MD)	S	998	Wright, Albert (MD)	S	549
Wiernik, Peter H (MD)	Onc	438	Wu, Bernard (MD)	Ped	616
Wierum, Carl (MD)	IM	874	Wu, Chia (MD)	IM	906
Wiesen, Mark (MD)	EDM	867	Wu, Ching-hui (MD)	EDM	716
Wilbanks, Tyr (MD)	S	1076	Wu, Hen-vai (MD)	Onc	1012
Wilchinsky, Mark (MD)	OrS	1062	Wyner, Perry A (MD)	Pul	691
Wilentz, James (MD)	Cv	162			
Willard, David (MD)	EDM	939	**Y**		
Williams, Christine (MD)	PrM	821			
Williams, Daniel T (MD)	ChAP	635	Yadoo, Moshe (MD)	Ped	683
Williams, Gail S (MD)	Nep	241	Yaffe, Bruce (MD)	IM	229
Williams, John (MD)	U	406	Yaghoobian, Jahangui (MD)	Rad	543
Willner, Joseph (MD)	N	877	Yagoda, Arnold (MD)	Oph	284
Willner, Judith P (MD)	MG	230	Yahalom, Joachim (MD)	RadRO	370
Wilmot, Richard (MD)	Rhu	1029	Yale, Suzanne (MD)	ObG	268
Wilner, Philip (MD)	Psyc	363	Yancovitz, Stanley (MD)	Inf	208
Wilson, Roger (MD)	Anes	152	Yang, Chin-tsun (MD)	Pul	691
Wilson, Thomas (MD)	Ped	740	Yankelowitz, Stanley (MD)	Oto	449
Winant, John (MD)	PA&I	946	Yannuzzi, Lawrence (MD)	Oph	284
Winarsky, Eric (MD)	Oto	979	Yanoff, Allen (MD)	IM	229
Winawer, Sidney G (MD)	Ge	196	Yapalater, Greg (MD)	Ped	329
Windsor, Russell (MD)	OrS	299	Yatco, Ruben (MD)	S	592
Winick, Martin (MD)	PS	738	Yee, Arthur (MD)	Inf	1050
Winston, Jonathan (MD)	Nep	241	Yeh, Ming-neng (MD)	ObG	268
Winston, Marvin (MD)	D	715	Yellin, Joseph (DO)	N	516
Winter, Steven (MD)	IM	608	Yellin, Paul (MD)	NP	238
Winters, Richard (MD)	Psyc	363	Yen, Owen (MD)	Cv	713
Wisch, Nathaniel (MD)	Hem	205	Yerys, Paul (MD)	SM	695
Wise, Gilbert (MD)	U	553	Yhu, Hyung Harry (MD)	PMR	537
Wise, Leslie (MD)	S	549	Yi, Peter (MD)	Onc	941
Wiseman, Paul (MD)	IM	228	Yiengpruksawan, Anusak (MD)	S	894
Wishnick, Marcia M (MD & PhD)	Ped	328	Yip, Chun (MD)	Pul	368
Wisnicki, H Jay (MD)	Oph	284	Yoo, Jinil (MD)	Nep	439
Wisoff, Jeffrey H (MD)	NS	245	Youn, Hyung Joong (MD)	IM	507
Witt, Barry (MD)	ObG	799	Youner, Craig (MD)	Rad	590
Witte, Arnold (MD)	N	943	Youner, Kenneth (MD)	Ge	1004
Wohlberg, Gary (MD)	Pul	744	Young, Bruce (MD)	ObG	268
Wolf, Barry (MD)	Pul	966	Young, Charles (MD)	Oph	284
Wolf, David J (MD)	IM	229	Young, Constance (MD)	ObG	799
Wolf, Ellen L (MD)	Rad	463	Young, Iven (MD)	IM	229
Wolf, Kenneth (MD)	Oph	446	Young, Melvin (MD)	Cv	635
Wolf, Leonard (MD)	ObG	267	Young, Rosemarie (MD)	A&I	711
Wolfe, Mary (MD)	IM	786	Young, Stuart (MD)	A&I	152
Wolff, Edward (MD)	IM	654	Young, Zenaida (MD)	ObG	799
Wolf-Klein, Gisele (MD)	Ger	645	Younger, Joseph (MD)	Oph	668
Wolfman, Cyrus (MD)	Psyc	689	Youngerman, Jay (MD)	Oto	673
Wolfson, David (MD)	Ge	496	Youngerman, Joseph (MD)	ChAP	165
Wolintz, Arthur (MD)	Oph	524	Younus, Bazaga (MD)	ObG	577
Wolk, Joel (MD)	Ped	536	Youssef, Ezzat (MD)	Rad	543
Wolk, Michael (MD)	Cv	162	Yudin, Howard (MD)	FP	773
Wolmer, Donald (MD)	Ped	887	Yurt, Roger (MD)	S	395
Wolodiger, Fred (MD)	GVS	896			
Woloszyn, Thomas T (MD)	S	549			

NAME	SPECIALTY	PAGE	NAME	SPECIALTY	PAGE
			Zonszein, Joel (MD)	EDM	421
Z			Zucker, Arnold (MD)	Psyc	826
Zabetakis, Paul (MD)	Nep	241	Zucker, Howard A (MD)	PCCM	312
Zablow, Andrew (MD)	RadRO	918	Zucker, Ira (MD)	Ge	869
Zachary, Mary (MD)	FP	494	Zucker, Mark (MD)	IM	906
Zackson, David A (MD)	Nep	241	Zuckerman, Andrea (MD)	PNep	813
Zackson, Ephraim (MD)	FP	642	Zuckerman, Howard (MD)	U	1078
Zaffuto, Stephen (MD)	Oph	578	Zuckerman, Joseph (MD)	OrS	299
Zaharia, Veronica (MD)	Hem	205	Zullo, Joseph (MD)	S	969
Zahtz, Gerald (MD)	Oto	580	Zumoff, Barnett (MD)	EDM	185
Zaidman, Gerald (MD)	Oph	804	Zupnick, Henry (MD)	IM	508
Zakim, David (MD)	Ge	196	Zweibel, Lawrence (MD)	Oph	733
Zalichin, Henry (MD)	FP	1046	Zweibel, Stuart M (MD)	D	768
Zalkowitz, Alan (MD)	Rhu	892	Zweifach, Philip (MD)	Oph	284
Zaloom, Robert (MD)	Cv	485	Zweig, Julian (MD)	HS	568
Zalusky, Ralph (MD)	Hem	205			
Zambetti, George (MD)	OrS	299			
Zampella, Edward (MD)	NS	992			
Zanger, Norman (MD)	Ped	1028			
Zanzi, Italo (MD)	NuM	661			
Zarbin, Marco (MD)	Oph	911			
Zaremski, Benjamin (MD)	Cv	163			
Zaret, Barry (MD)	Cv	1042			
Zarlengo, Marco (MD)	IM	787			
Zarowitz, William (MD)	IM	787			
Zauber, N Peter (MD)	Hem	904			
Zawadsky, Joseph (MD)	OrS	963			
Zeale, Peter (MD)	IM	229			
Zeitlin, Alan (MD)	GVS	595			
Zelefsky, Melvin (MD)	Rad	463			
Zelefsky, Michael (MD)	RadRO	370			
Zelicof, Steven (MD & PhD)	OrS	807			
Zellner, James (MD)	Oph	524			
Zelman, Warren (MD)	Oto	674			
Zerykier, Abraham (MD)	Oph	612			
Zevon, Sanford (MD)	Cv	763			
Zevon, Scott (MD)	PlS	340			
Zide, Barry (MD)	PlS	340			
Ziegelbaum, Michael M (MD)	U	705			
Ziemba, David (MD)	IM	507			
Ziering, Thomas (MD)	FP	1011			
Zimbalist, Eliot (MD)	Ge	497			
Zimberg, Sheldon (MD)	Psyc	363			
Zimetbaum, Marcel (MD)	Ge	426			
Zimmerman, Alan (MD)	OrS	672			
Zimmerman, Franklin (MD)	Cv	763			
Zimmerman, Jerald (MD)	PMR	887			
Zimmerman, Lester (MD)	Ped	819			
Zimmerman, Mark (MD)	Pul	1029			
Zimmerman, Saul (MD)	FP	494			
Zimmerman, Sol (MD)	Ped	329			
Zimmerman, Zeva (MD)	Psyc	363			
Zingler, Barry (MD)	Ge	869			
Zinkin, Lewis (MD)	CRS	956			
Zinn, Keith (MD)	Oph	284			
Zippin, Allen (MD)	N	727			
Zitani Jr, Alfred M (MD)	GVS	934			
Zito, Joseph (MD)	Rad	693			
Zitsman, Jeffrey (MD)	PS	453			
Zitsman, Jeffrey (MD)	PS	814			
Zitzmann, Eric (MD)	OrS	807			
Ziviello, Alfred (MD)	S	748			
Zolkind, Neil (MD)	Psyc	826			
Zoltan, Irving (MD)	Ped	457			

OTHER CASTLE CONNOLLY GUIDES

The ABCs of HMOs: How to Get the Best from Managed Care
ISBN 1 883769 74-4
$12.95

The Buyer's Guide to the Best Health Care
ISBN 1 883769 61-2
$12.95

*How to Find the Best Doctors, Hospitals & HMOs for You
and Your Family-Pocket Guide*
ISBN 1 883769 70-1
$9.95

The Parent's Helper: Who to Call on Health and Family Issues
ISBN 1 883769 72-8
$15.95

To order call 1(800)399-DOCS (3627)

Visit our website at : www.bestdocs.com